Drugs and Nursing Implications

Drugs and Nursing Implications

Edition 5

LAURA E. GOVONI, Ph.D., R.N.

Lecturer and Consultant, Medical-Surgical Nursing and Pharmacology
Formerly, Professor of Nursing, Graduate Division
School of Nursing, University of Connecticut

JANICE E. HAYES, Ph.D., R.N.

Distinguished Visiting Scholar in Nursing
Worcester State College
Lecturer and Consultant, Pathophysiology and Pharmacology
Formerly, Professor of Nursing, Graduate Division
School of Nursing, University of Connecticut

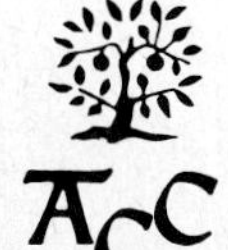

ACC APPLETON-CENTURY-CROFTS/Norwalk, Connecticut

Notice: Our knowledge in clinical sciences is constantly changing. As new information becomes available, changes in treatment and in the use of drugs become necessary. The author(s) and the publisher of this volume have taken care to make certain that the doses of drugs and schedules of treatment are correct and compatible with the standards generally accepted at the time of publication. The reader is advised to consult carefully the instruction and information material included in the package insert of each drug or therapeutic agent before administration. This advice is especially important when using new or infrequently used drugs.

85 86 87 88 89 / 10 9 8 7 6 5 4 3 2 1

Prentice-Hall of Australia, Pty. Ltd., Sydney
Prentice-Hall Canada, Inc.
Prentice-Hall Hispanoamericana, S.A., Mexico
Prentice-Hall of India Private Limited, New Delhi
Prentice-Hall International (UK) Limited, London
Prentice-Hall of Japan, Inc., Tokyo
Prentice-Hall of Southeast Asia (Pte.) Ltd., Singapore
Whitehall Books Ltd., Wellington, New Zealand
Editora Prentice-Hall do Brasil Ltda., Rio de Janeiro

Library of Congress Cataloging-in-Publication Data

Govoni, Laura E.
Drugs and nursing implications.

Bibliography: p.
Includes index.
1. Nursing. 2. Pharmacology. I. Hayes, Janice E.
II. Title. [DNLM: 1. Nursing Care. 2. Pharmacology.
QV 38 G721d]
RM300.G66 1985 617'.5'024613 85–13407
ISBN 0–8385–1788–9

Cover Design: Mary Chandler Martylewski
Text Design: Jean M. Sabato-Morley

PRINTED IN THE UNITED STATES OF AMERICA

CONTENTS

PREFACE

The Fifth Edition of *Drugs and Nursing Implications* continues to reflect our conviction that involvement in the total pharmacotherapeutic regimen is one of the most significant responsibilities of the professional health-care provider. Safe, effective drug therapy results from recognition, integration, and clinical application of two sets of characteristics:

1. The uniqueness of the patient/client (physiologic status, culture, age, and degree of ability to be medically independent)
2. Specific properties of the drug (i.e., pharmacokinetics and pharmacodynamics). Drug descriptions and suggested interventions in this volume are designed to make it possible for the practitioner to scientifically and rationally treat pharmacotherapeutics not as an adjunct but as an integral component of the total patient/client care plan.

The following features have been added or greatly augmented in this edition:

- Investigational and unlabeled drug uses
- FDA categories for drug use during pregnancy
- Canadian trade names
- Comprehensive drug classification (based on structure, effects, uses)
- Smoking–drug, food–drug, drug–drug interactions
- An expanded Index with cross-referenced generic–trade names, broad classification listings, drug-induced symptoms (as indicators for nursing action), pharmacotherapeutically-derived clinical interventions
- Age-related factors affecting drug therapy (particularly the newborn and the elderly age groups)

As in the past, the feature of each monograph is the section on Nursing Implications with its focus on drug-related issues and nursing interventions. This section is basically designed to reenforce the primary aim of health care plans, i.e., to move the patient/client from the dependency of illness to self-care in optimum health. The reader will note that nursing implications are derived primarily from clinical nursing specialties, and also from dental and other medical specialties and the sciences of nutrition and pharmacology. Drug-related implications include the following:

- Drug administration (e.g., with or without meals, flow rates of infusions, immediate precautions, etc.)
- Expected therapeutic responses
- Pertinent background information that may have relevance to the clinical condition being treated
- Recommended baseline and continuing clinical and physical assessment data
- Suggested measures for promoting and reenforcing clinical goals of drug therapy
- Adaptations to pharmacotherapy because of age or clinical status of patient

- Significant and reportable side effects and suggested practices to ameliorate drug induced clinical problems
- The consequences of interactions: smoking–drug, food–drug, drug–drug
- Withdrawal, toxicity, and overdosage symptoms and treatment
- Patient/family teaching plan
  - Relationship between prescribed drug therapy and clinical signs and symptoms (including what and when to report)
  - Drug therapy and activities of daily living
  - Measures to promote compliance with the prescribed drug regimen
  - Cautions about self-diagnosis and self-dosing with self-selected drugs
  - Prevention of potential drug related clinical problems
- Drug solution incompatibilities and stability information
- Storage of drug

Consistent with our interest in pharmacotherapeutics is our belief that the nurse is the health professional of choice to be making the necessary assessments of drug responses that indicate efficacy or untoward reactions. Unexpected responses and suspected or obvious adverse reactions should be documented and reported. To encourage such reporting we have included an example of the Department of Health and Human Services "Drug Experience Report" form in the Appendix.

Although *Drugs and Nursing Implications* was first conceived as a book for nursing students and nurse practitioners, we are pleased that our readership has expanded to include other health-care providers.

As in previous editions, we have found that the writing of the fifth edition has mandated constant study and analysis of reported clinical findings not only in nursing and pharmacotherapy but also in related disciplines in order to identify the nursing implications of drug therapy.

Comments, queries, and suggestions from our readers are not only welcomed but are solicited to help provide accuracy and relevance in future editions.

PREFACE TO THE FOURTH EDITION

Since the publication of the last edition, knowledge about pharmacology and the dynamics of drug use has undergone a quantum increase. Lay literature focusing on drug therapy has proliferated in response to an alerted and concerned public. During the same period, the scope of nursing functions and responsibilities has continued to expand, placing great demands on the practitioner to be well informed about current therapies and capable of translating this knowledge into safe, effective nursing action. The natural outgrowth of increased available information about drugs is the more comprehensive discussion of nursing implications in pharmacotherapy recorded in this edition.

The following areas of information (from which many nursing implications are derived) have also been expanded: 1) pharmacokinetics: drug half-life, protein binding, dynamics of absorption and excretion, drug-receptor relationships; 2) variations in drug response imposed by both immaturity and aging; 3) expected and potential drug–drug and drug–food interactions; and 4) drug interferences with diagnostic tests and procedures.

Additional features of this edition include: 1) expansion of the sections on absorption and fate which provide significant information to planners of the dose schedules; 2) increased numbers of trade names for each drug (in response to regional differences in drug availability); 3) arrangement of adverse reactions for most drugs by functional or systemic constellations to facilitate observation and interpretation; 4) the listing of fixed combination drugs that incorporate the agent under discussion; 5) an increased number of specifically designed nursing interventions (see Index) related to particular pharmacotherapeutic regimens, and 6) expanded data bases for informed observations, analysis, and prediction of drug response (e.g., RDA, clinical signs and symptoms, diagnostic tests, normal laboratory values).

The reader is reminded that clinical studies of patient response to drugs and new laboratory evidence often result in dose changes. The authors have made every effort to provide accurate information about dose regimens; however, we advise constant checking of product information supplied with the drug when dispensed and/or other up-to-date authoritative sources of drug information before administering a drug, particularly if it is infrequently used or is a new product.

Several points should be made about the use of this edition:

1. Referral to a prototype drug for more detailed discussion includes the assumption that listed drug–drug interactions and diagnostic test interferences apply to both prototype and referred drug(s), unless specified otherwise
2. Although alphabetical sequence prevents arrangement of drugs by class, the reader may locate the drugs within a given group or class by using the Index
3. The reader is reminded that the drug may be listed in the Index in four ways: by generic name, by trade name, by pharmacologic action, and by chemical classification

The user of this volume is provided with concise, scholarly, and professional suggestions meant to assist in the design and implementation of interventions in pharmacotherapy, reinforce the development of nurse-patient relationships based on mutual understanding about the drug regimen, and permit the adaptation of drug therapy to meet the particular needs of the patient.

In conclusion, we have found that the writing of the fourth edition has mandated not only constant study and analysis of reported clinical findings in nursing and pharmacotherapy but also the acquisition of new scientific background in pharmacology and related disciplines in order to identify the critical elements basic to nursing interventions in drug therapy.

ACKNOWLEDGMENTS

As with each new edition, many individuals, including students, professional colleagues, and friends from the lay public have influenced the preparation of this edition. Again, we are most grateful and professionally honored to have had the expert assistance of Paul G. Pierpaoli, Director, Department of Pharmacy, Rush-Presbyterian, St. Luke's Medical Center; Dr. Patricia Mullins, Pharm.D., Drug Information Center, Medical College of Virginia; and Sheldon S. Sones, R.Ph., Associate Administrator, World War II Veterans' Memorial Hospital, Meriden, Connecticut. Their critical reading of drug descriptions and resultant comments and suggestions were invaluable. We are also grateful to Alex Cardoni, M.S. (Pharm.), Director, Drug Information Center, University of Connecticut Health Center, Clinical Professor, University of Connecticut School of Pharmacy; Dr. Henry Palmer, Pharm.D., Clinical Professor, Assistant Dean, Clinical Affairs, University of Connecticut School of Pharmacy; Dr. Gilles L. Fraser, Pharm.D., Central Maine Medical Center Department of Pharmacy for their generous help and willingness to provide documented answers to our questions at a moment's notice. Much appreciation is also extended to Lisa Bellini, B.S., R.D., Consultant in Community Nutrition, N.Y.C., and Carol J. Lami-Keefe, Ph.D., Assistant Professor, Nutritional Sciences, University of Connecticut, for their valuable contributions with respect to drug-nutrition relationships.

We owe a special debt of gratitude to Charles Bollinger, Senior Editor, and to Joanne Jay, Director of Art/Editorial Production, of Appleton-Century-Crofts for their valuable production ideas and for their constant patience and unswerving support. Specifically, we could not have accomplished the demands required for publication without the competent assistance of Joanne Jay.

The book is dedicated to our parents Augusto Govoni and Marjorie Hayes for their love, endurance, and understanding throughout the preparation of this edition.

To ensure accuracy as well as adequacy of coverage this edition like the others required the assistance of many practitioners. We are especially indebted to the following contributors for their helpful comments and suggestions and for their willingness to be readily available as resources for clinical information:

Linn Belanger, R.N., Staff Nurse, Hartford Hospital

Barbara Bilodeau, R.N., Clinical Specialist, Oncology, New Britain General Hospital

Manon Bissonette, R.N., Staff Nurse, Hartford Hospital

Ann Burinskas, R.N., Head Nurse, Hartford Hospital

Shiela Burke, R.N., Staff Nurse, Hartford Hospital

H. David Crombie, Jr., M.D., General Surgery, Hartford, Connecticut

Laura Diskavich, R.N., Nurse Practitioner, Communicable Disease Clinic, City of Hartford

Marilyn Bellini Fall, B.S., R.N., Bayside Clinic Department of Public Health, Virginia Beach

Kathleen Getty, A.D., R.N., Respiratory Therapist, Medical Center Hospital of Vermont

Anita Gorman, R.N., M.S., Diabetes Nurse Clinician, Hartford Hospital, Connecticut

Ann Gunberg, R.N., Instructor of IV Therapy, Hartford Hospital

Debbie Hartman, R.N., Assistant Head Nurse, Hartford Hospital

Jean Ihli, R.N., IV Therapy, Hartford Hospital

Mary Sue Infante, Ed.D., R.N., Professor, School of Nursing, University of Connecticut

Mark W. Izard, M.D., Internal Medicine, Hartford, Connecticut

Alan W. James, D.M.D., Elmwood, Connecticut

Christine Johnson, R.N., M.S., Assistant Director, Medical and Rehabilitation Nursing, Hartford Hospital

Eric Johnson, Pharm.D., Drug Information Center, University of Connecticut Health Center

Kathleen Kelly, R.N., M.S., Clinical Specialist, North Adams, Massachusetts

Judy Koblect, R.N., Head Nurse, Hartford Hospital

Diane LaRochelle, R.N., Ph.D., Professor of Nursing, College of Nursing, University of Florida

Edmund Lowrie, M.D., Senior Vice President, National Medical Care, Inc.

Ernestine Lowrie, R.N., Vice President of Clinical Services, National Medical Care, Inc.

Elizabeth Luginbuhl, R.N., M.S.N., Pediatric Nurse Coordinator, Hartford Hospital

Steven Marcham, Registered Pharmacist, Vincent Pharmacy, Rockville, Connecticut

Diane Neri, Clinical Specialist, Oncology, New Britain General Hospital

Janice Noel, R.N., Staff Nurse, Hartford Hospital

Patricia O'Brien, R.N., M.S., C.P.N.P., Instructor, Worcester State College, Worcester, Massachusetts

William O'Brien, M.D., Obstetrics and Gynecology, Royal Society of Medicine ASGL

Bernard John Podurgiel, M.D., Norwich, Connecticut

Marie Roberto, R.N., M.S.N., Director, Division of Community Nursing and Home Health, Department of Health Services, Connecticut

Donald Rotenberg, M.D., Internal Medicine and Nephrology, Hartford, Connecticut

John R. Shepherd, D.D.S., Periodontist, West Hartford, Connecticut

William G. Wilcox, D.M.D., Elmwood, Connecticut

We wish to thank Christine Maynard and William Maynard for transcribing the manuscript onto microcomputer diskettes and for their expert and invaluable assistance in the many other activities related to preparing the manuscript.

We also wish to thank our many dear friends and relatives who greatly helped in various stages of the manuscript preparation. Grateful appreciation is due especially to Eva A. Bellini, Beth McGarity, Barbara Ransom, Cheryl Wentzel, and Jill Wentzel for their conscientious and reliable secretarial assistance.

LAURA E. GOVONI

JANICE E. HAYES

1985

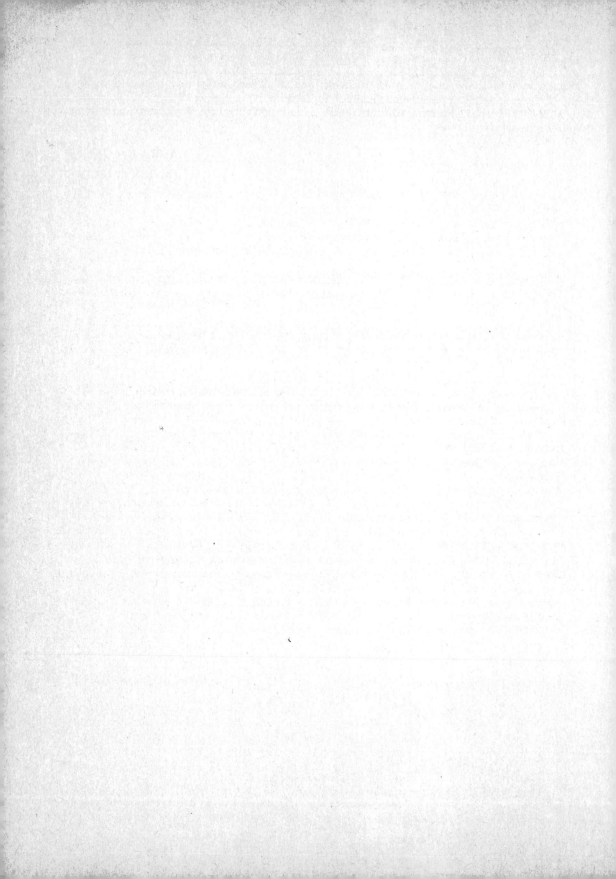

A

ABSORBABLE GELATIN SPONGE

(Gelfoam)

Hemostatic (topical)

ACTIONS AND USES. Sterile, water-insoluble, nonantigenic sponge prepared from purified gelatin solution. Capable of absorbing many times its weight in blood and provides an absorbable matrix into which clot forms and granulation tissue may grow. Since gelatin sponge must remain securely anchored to bleeding site, it is not as effective for brisk arterial bleeding. Entirely absorbed in 4 to 6 weeks when implanted in tissue. When applied to bleeding areas of skin, or nasal, rectal, or vaginal mucosa, completely liquefies in 2 to 5 days.

Used as adjunct to control bleeding and capillary oozing in highly vascular areas that are difficult to suture, and as an aid in healing of wounds and decubitus ulcers. Also available in powder form.

CONTRAINDICATIONS AND PRECAUTIONS. Frank infection, to control postpartum hemorrhage or menorrhagia, use as sole hemostatic agent in patients with blood dyscrasias, use in closure of skin edges.

ROUTE AND DOSAGE. *Hemostasis:* use sterile technique. Cut to desired size (minimal amount is applied to cover area). **When applied dry:** piece(s) are compressed before application to bleeding surface and held in place with moderate pressure for 10 to 15 seconds. **When applied moist:** piece(s) are immersed in either sterile isotonic saline injection or thrombin solution. Remove from solution, squeeze to remove air bubbles, and leave immersed in solution until needed. Sponge should swell to original size and shape. If it does not, remove from solution and knead vigorously until all air is expelled, and immerse again in solution. Wet piece may be blotted with gauze before applying it to bleeding point. Hold in place for 10 to 15 seconds with cotton pledget or gauze; remove carefully with a few drops of sterile water to prevent disturbing gelatin sponge. *Decubitus ulcer:* Following debridement, gelatin sponge is placed aseptically in ulcer and covered with DSD. Dressing may be changed daily, but gelatin sponge should not be disturbed: new sponges may be added as required. If infection develops, sponge should be removed and appropriate therapy given. *Dentistry:* **When applied dry:** roll between fingers, apply to cavity or socket, then hold in place with light pressure for 1 to 2 minutes. **When used moist:** immerse in sodium chloride solution, then remove, squeeze out all air bubbles, immerse again and allow it to swell to original size. Remove from solution, blot on sterile gauze and place in cavity.

Available as sponges, packs, dental packs, prostatectomy cones.

NURSING IMPLICATIONS

Since gelatin sponge absorbs fluid and expands, overpacking of cavity or closed tissue space can cause pressure on adjacent structures. Report to physician if patient complains of pain or discomfort.

Be alert to signs of infection: malaise, fever, tenderness, redness, swelling.

Use contents as soon as possible after opening package. Discard unused portions.

Manufacturer cautions not to resterilize product because absorption time may be affected.

Since gelatin sponge is completely absorbed, there is no need to remove it.

PROTOTYPE

ACETAMINOPHEN

(a-seat-a-mee′noe-fen)
Analgesic, antipyretic

(Acephen, APAP, Atasol, Campain, Datril Extra Strength, Dolanex, Liquiprin, Robigesic, Rounox, Tapar, Tempra, Tylenol, Valadol)

ACTIONS AND USES. Principal active metabolite of acetanilid and phenacetin. Analgesic and antipyretic actions, approximately equivalent to those of aspirin, appear to be related to inhibition of prostaglandin synthesis. Unlike aspirin, acetaminophen lacks antiplatelet action, generally produces no gastric bleeding and has weak antiinflammatory, uricosuric, and antirheumatic properties. Produces analgesia by unknown mechanism, perhaps by action on peripheral nervous system. Reduces fever by direct action on hypothalamus heat-regulating center with consequent peripheral vasodilation, sweating, and dissipation of heat. Reportedly has antidiuretic activity. Acetaminophen is available OTC in combination with aspirin and caffeine (e.g., Excedrin, Trigesic, Vanquish); with pamabrom and pyrilamine maleate (Pamprin, Premesyn PMS); and with sodium bicarbonate (Bromo Seltzer). Also available by prescription with butabarbital (Bancap); with chlorzoxazone (Parafon Forte); and with narcotic analgesics: codeine (Proval #3), hydrocodone (T-Gesic), oxycodone (Percocet, Tylox), and propoxyphene (Darvocet-N, Wygesic).

Used for temporary relief of mild to moderate pain, such as simple headache, minor joint and muscle pains, neuralgia, and dysmenorrhea, and for control of fever. Generally used as substitute for aspirin when the latter is not tolerated, or is contraindicated (as in antico agulated patients). Use of combined dosage of acetaminophen and aspirin (rather than 2 tablets of each) appears to minimize side/toxic effects without reduction of pharmacologic action.

ABSORPTION AND FATE. Rapidly and almost completely absorbed from GI tract and well distributed in body fluids. Peak blood levels in ½ to 2 hours; duration of action 3 to 4 hours. Variable bioavailability with rectal suppository. About 25% protein bound. Half-life: 1 to 3.5 hours. Metabolized in liver. 85% excreted in urine as conjugated acetaminophen and other (active and inactive) metabolites; 2 to 4% excreted unchanged. Crosses placenta. Excreted in breast milk.

CONTRAINDICATIONS AND PRECAUTIONS. Hypersensitivity to acetaminophen; children under 3 years of age unless directed by a physician; repeated administration to patients with anemia, or hepatic, renal, cardiac, or pulmonary disease; G6PD deficiency. *Cautious Use:* arthritic or rheumatoid conditions affecting children under 12 years of age; alcoholism, malnutrition, thrombocytopenia.

ADVERSE/SIDE EFFECTS. Negligible with recommended dosage. **Acute poisoning:** *2 to 24 hours postingestion:* anorexia, nausea, vomiting, dizziness, lethargy, generalized weakness, diaphoresis, chills, epigastric or abdominal pain, diarrhea; *24 to 48 hours postingestion* (often asymptomatic): onset of hepatotoxicity: elevation of serum transaminases (ALT, AST) and bilirubin; 3 to 5 days postingestion: vomiting, jaundice, RUQ tenderness, hepatic necrosis, abnormal liver function tests, hypoglycemia, metabolic acidosis, hypoprothrombinemia, hepatic coma, acute renal failure, CNS stimulation or depression, hypothermia, circulatory and acute renal failure. **Chronic ingestion:** hemoglobinemia, neutropenia, pancytopenia, leukopenia, hemolytic anemia (rare), thrombocytopenic purpura, agranulocytosis; rarely: methemoglobinemia (cyanosis of skin, nails, mucous membranes, CNS stimulation, then depression); sulfhemoglobinemia, hypoglycemia or hyperglycemia, splenomegaly, acute pancreatitis, psychologic changes, hepatic and renal damage. **Hypersensitivity (rare):** erythematous or urticarial skin rash, drug fever, mucosal lesions, laryngeal edema.

ROUTE AND DOSAGE. Adults, children (over 11 years): Oral, rectal: 325 to 650 mg at 4- to 6-hour intervals, as necessary; maximum dosage for 1 day: 4 Gm. Dosage for long-term therapy not to exceed 2.6 Gm daily. **Pediatric: Oral, rectal:** 1.5 Gm/m^2 a day in divided doses, or the following approximate doses every 4 to 6 hours; **Children (11 years):** 480 mg; **Children (9 to 10 years):** 400 mg; **Children (6 to 8 years):** 320 mg; **Children (4 to 5 years):** 240 mg; **Children (2 to 3 years):** 160 mg. Rectal doses for children up to 2 years must be individualized. **Oral: Children (1 to 2 years):** 120 mg; **Infants (4 to 11 months):** 80 mg; **Infants (up to 3 months):** 40 mg. Available forms: tablet, chewable tablet, capsule, drops, elixir, oral solution, oral suspension, syrup, rectal suppository.

NURSING IMPLICATIONS

Tablet may be crushed before administation and taken with fluid of patient's choice. Chewable tablets should be thoroughly chewed and wetted before swallowing.

Coadministration with a high carbohydrate meal may significantly retard absorption rate.

Caution patient not to exceed recommended dosage. Overdosing and chronic use can cause liver damage and other toxic effects.

Patients on prescribed high doses or long-term therapy are advised to have periodic tests of hepatic, renal, and hematopoietic function.

Individuals with poor nutrition or who have ingested alcohol over prolonged periods are prone to hepatotoxicity even from moderate acetaminophen doses.

Remind patients who self-medicate that reduction of fever by acetaminophen may mask serious illness.

Acetaminophen should not be used by adults and children for self-medication of pain beyond 3 to 5 days without consulting a physician. Additionally, it should not be used for fever persisting longer than 3 days, and never for fever over 39.5°C (103°F), or for recurrent fever without medical direction.

There is no basis for the claim that acetaminophen is safer than aspirin and there is little evidence that combination analgesic formulations have any therapeutic advantage over single component products.

High abuse potential; psychologic dependence can occur.

Self-administered acetaminophen is intended for temporary use only.

Withdrawal of acetaminophen following long-term use may be associated with restlessness and excitement.

Most poisonings result from suicide attempts or accidental ingestion by children. Caution patient to keep acetaminophen out of the reach of children.

Treatment of acute poisoning: Contact regional poison center or Rocky Mountain Poison Center (800–525–6115) for directions in use of acetylcysteine (antidote). Acetylcysteine may prevent hepatic necrosis if administered within 16 hours of acetaminophen overdose. Stomach contents are evacuated by emesis induced with ipecac syrup (qv) or gastric lavage. (Administration of activated charcoal is not recommended because it may interfere with absorption of acetylcysteine; however, if it has been used it should be thoroughly removed by lavage.) The commercially available acetylcysteine (Mucomyst) 20% solution is used orally: 140 mg/kg loading dose, diluted: 1 part acetylcysteine to 3 parts liquid (cola, grapefruit juice, or plain water). Treatment is continued with acetylcysteine 70 mg/kg every 4 hours for 17 additional doses. If patient vomits within 1 hour after a given dose, repeat dose and continue treatment protocol; duodenal tube may be necessary if emesis is a problem. Obtain serum acetaminophen concentration no sooner than 4 hours postingestion. Liver function tests: SGOT (AST), SGPT (ALT), bilirubin, prothrombin time should be obtained initially and every 24 hours for 96 hours.

Patient who has ingested a toxic dose should be hospitalized because the onset of hepatic damage is usually insidious and may not be apparent for several days after overdosage.
Preserved in tightly covered, light-resistant containers, at room temperature preferably between 15° and 30°C (59° and 86°F), unless otherwise directed by manufacturer.

Diagnostic Test Interferences. Acetaminophen may cause (1) false increases in **urinary 5-HIAA** (5-hydroxyindoleacetic acid) by-product of serotonin, (2) false decreases in **blood glucose** (by glucose oxidase-peroxidase procedure), and (3) false increases in **serum uric acid** (with phosphotungstate method).

Drug Interactions: Acetaminophen

Plus	Interactions
Alcohol (Ethanol) chronic or excessive ingestion	Increased risk of hepatotoxicity
Anticoagulants, oral	Possibility of increased anticoagulant (hypoprothrombinemic) effect
Chloramphenicol (Chloromycetin, Mychel)	Increased risk of chloramphenicol toxicity (by decreased drug metabolism). Monitor chloramphenicol serum levels
Contraceptives, oral	Decreased acetaminophen analgesic effect (drug metabolism increased)
Diazepam (Valium)	Increased diazepam effects (decreased diazepam renal excretion)
Phenothiazines	Possibility of severe hypokalemia

PROTOTYPE

ACETAZOLAMIDE

(Acetazolam, Ak-Zol, Apo-Acetazolamide, Cetazol, Dazamide, Diamox, Diamox Sequels, Hydrazol)

ACETAZOLAMIDE SODIUM

(Diamox Parenteral)

(a-set-a-zole'a-mide)
Anticonvulsant; carbonic anhydrase inhibitor diuretic
Alkalizer (systemic, urinary)
Sulfonamide derivative

ACTIONS AND USES. Nonbacteriostatic sulfonamide derivative. Diuretic effect is due to inhibition of carbonic anhydrase activity in proximal renal tubule thereby preventing formation of carbonic acid (H_2CO_3), source of hydrogen (H^+) and bicarbonate (HCO_3^-) ions. Absence or reduced availability of H^+ inhibits renal tubular reabsorption of Na thereby promoting its elimination with that of K, bicarbonate, and water. The net result is alkaline diuresis with conservation of chloride and ammonia. After 3 or 4 days of continuous inhibition, mild metabolic acidosis develops with concomitant reduction in diuresis. Inhibition of carbonic anhydrase in the eye reduces rate of aqueous humor formation with consequent lowering of intraocular pressure. This effect is apparently independent of systemic acid–base balance and diuretic action. Mechanism of anticonvulsant action unknown, but thought to involve inhibition of CNS carbonic anhydrase, which retards abnormal paroxysmal discharge from CNS neurons.

Used adjunctively in treatment of several forms of epilepsy, especially absence seizures (petit mal), generalized tonic–clonic (grand mal), and focal seizures; to reduce intraocular pressure in open- and closed-angle glaucoma, and secondary glaucoma; for preoperative treatment of acute closed-angle glaucoma prior to laser iridotomy; and in treatment of edema. Also used to correct metabolic alkalosis, to treat hypokalemic and hyperkalemic forms of familial periodic paralysis, and to relieve symptoms of acute mountain sickness.

ABSORPTION AND FATE. Rapidly absorbed from GI tract. Effects begin in 30 minutes to 1 hour; plasma levels peak within 2 to 4 hours and persist 8 to 12 hours. Sustained-release form: onset: 2 hours; peaks in 8 to 12 hours with duration: 18 to 24 hours. Acts within 2 minutes after IV administration; duration 4 to 5 hours. Wide distribution including CNS penetration; especially high concentrations in erythrocytes, pancreas, gastric mucosa, and renal cortex. Highly bound to plasma proteins. Half-life: 2.4 to 5.8 hours. Excreted unchanged in urine (90 to 100%) within 24 hours. Crosses placenta.

CONTRAINDICATIONS AND PRECAUTIONS. Hypersensitivity to sulfonamides; renal and hepatic dysfunction; Addison's disease or other types of adrenocortical insufficiency, hyponatremia, hypokalemia, hyperchloremic acidosis, prolonged administration to patients with hyphema, or chronic noncongestive angle closure glaucoma. Safe use in fertile women or during pregnancy not established. *Cautious Use:* history of hypercalciuria, diabetes mellitus, gout, digitalized patients, obstructive pulmonary disease.

ADVERSE/SIDE EFFECTS. CNS: paresthesias (especially of tongue, lips, anus, and extremities) and drowsiness are common; disorientation, depression, nervousness, excitement, fatigue, flaccid paralysis, headache, dizziness, convulsions. **EENT:** transient myopia, tinnitus. **GI:** anorexia, nausea, vomiting, weight loss, constipation, diarrhea, melena. **Hematologic/electrolyte imbalance (as for other sulfonamides):** bone marrow depression with agranulocytosis, thrombocytopenic purpura, hemolytic anemia, leukopenia, pancytopenia; increased serum bilirubin. Increased excretion of Ca, K, Mg, Na, thiamine, pyridoxine; hyperchloremic acidosis, hyperglycemia, hyperuricemia. **Hypersensitivity:** pruritus, rash, urticaria, fever. **Renal:** glycosuria, urinary frequency, polyuria, dysuria, alkaline urine, hematuria, crystalluria, ureteral colic, nephrolithiasis. **Other:** fatigue, weakness, hirsutism, loss of libido, impotence, exacerbation of gout, altered taste and smell; thirst, hepatic dysfunction, hyperpnea, cyanosis, pain at IM injection site.

ROUTE AND DOSAGE. Adults: *Glaucoma:* **Oral:** 250 mg every 6 hours (extended-release preparations may be prescribed every 12 to 24 hours); **Intravenous, intramuscular:** Initial: 500 mg repeated in 2 to 4 hours, if necessary. *Anticonvulsant, diuretic:* 250 mg to 1 Gm daily in divided doses. *Acute mountain sickness:* **Oral:** 250 mg twice daily or extended release form 500 mg once daily, beginning 3 or 4 days before ascent and continuing during descent. **Pediatric: Oral, intravenous, intramuscular:** *Anticonvulsant; glaucoma:* 5 to 10 mg/kg every 6 hours; *diuretic:* 5 mg/kg once daily. *Familial periodic paralysis:* 125 mg two or three times daily.

NURSING IMPLICATIONS

Not to be confused with acetohexamide.

Acetazolamide may be taken with food to minimize possibility of GI upset.

The long-acting preparation (Diamox Sequels) may be opened but contents should not be crushed, chewed, or swallowed dry. It may be spread on soft food.

Teach patient not to accept brand interchange unless approved by physician. Bioequivalence varies among different products.

If necessary, one regular tablet (not sustained release form) may be softened in 2 tsp of hot water and added to 2 tsp of honey or syrup (e.g., chocolate, raspberry, cherry) to disguise bitter taste. The drug does not dissolve in fruit juices. Alternatively, tablet(s) may be crushed and suspended in syrup (250 to 500 mg per 5 ml syrup).

High alkalinity (pH approximately 9.2) of the parenteral solution causes intense pain when injected IM; therefore, this route is not commonly employed.

Diuretic dose is generally administrated in the morning to avoid interrupted sleep from diuresis.

Monitor intake and output when drug used to reduce edema. Effectiveness as a diuretic diminishes in a few days; therefore, it is usually given on alternate days or for 2 days followed by a day or two without medication.

Adequate fluid intake (1.5 to 2.5 L/24 hr) should be maintained during acetazolamide therapy to reduce risk of kidney stone formation. Check with physician.

Patients should be weighed under standard conditions before drug therapy is initiated and daily thereafter: use same scale, with similar clothing, preferably in morning after voiding but before eating or defecating. Daily weight is a useful index of patient's response to diuretic action.

Transient nearsightedness (myopia) may occur following initiation of therapy. Report to physician. Symptom usually responds readily to dosage reduction or drug withdrawal.

Advise patient to report numbness, tingling, burning, and other paresthesias, and drowsiness (common side effects). Note implications for the ambulatory patient. Caution patient to avoid driving a car and other potentially hazardous activities if these symptoms are prominent.

Caution patient to report sore throat or mouth, unusual bleeding, fever, skin or renal problems (indications to discontinue acetazolamide).

Acetazolamide may cause substantial increases in blood glucose in diabetics and in prediabetics. Observe these patients closely. Changes in antidiabetic drug dose or diet may be indicated.

Hypokalemia and severe metabolic acidosis are direct extensions of the pharmacologic actions of acetazolamide. Note that concomitant use of steroids or ACTH may contribute to hypokalemia. Hypokalemia can sensitize the heart to toxic effects of digitalis.

Observe for and advise patient to report signs of hypokalemia (malaise, fatigue, depressed reflexes, muscle weakness and cramps, rapid, irregular pulse, vomiting, mental confusion, abdominal distention, polyuria), and signs of metabolic acidosis (lethargy, headache, weakness, abdominal pain, nausea, vomiting, dyspnea, hyperpnea progressing to Kussmaul breathing, dehydration).

When acetazolamide is given in high doses or for prolonged periods physician may prescribe potassium-rich diet and K supplement. *See Index: Food sources.*

Excessive salt intake should be avoided. *See Index: Food sources.*

Blood pH, blood gases, urinalysis, complete blood counts, and serum electrolyte determinations are recommended initially and at periodic intervals during prolonged drug therapy or during concomitant therapy with other diuretics or digitalis.

The sustained release drug form is not recommended for treatment of epilepsy.

When used as an anticonvulsant, drug withdrawal, if contemplated, should be gradual to prevent precipitating seizure activity.

Because the parenteral solution contains no antibacterial preservative, its use within 24 hours of reconstitution is strongly recommended by manufacturer. (Each 500-mg vial should be reconstituted with at least 5 ml sterile water for injection prior to use.)

Oral preparations are preserved in tightly covered, light-resistant containers. Store preferably between 15° and 30°C (59° and 86°F) unless otherwise directed by manufacturer.

Diagnostic Test Interferences. False-positive **urinary protein** determinations; falsely high values for **urine urobilinogen;** depressed **iodine uptake** values (exception: hypothyroidism).

Drug Interactions: Acetazolamide

Plus	Interactions
Amphetamines	Enhanced amphetamine effect. (Drug-induced alkaline urine decreases amphetamine excretion rate)
Amphotericin B (Fungizone) Corticosteroids Corticotropin	Concurrent use may cause severe hypokalemia
Anticonvulsants	Predisposes patient to anticonvulsant-induced osteomalacia (adult rickets) by increasing calcium excretion rate
Digitalis glycosides	Acetazolamide-induced hypokalemia may predispose patient to digitalis toxicity
Insulins and oral antidiabetic agents	Hypoglycemic effect may be reduced (possibly because of hypokalemia)
Lithium	Drug-induced alkaline urine increased lithium excretion and decreases plasma levels
Methenamine compounds	Drug-induced alkaline urine inhibits antibacterial effect of methenamine (requires acid urine to be effective)
Primidone (Mysoline)	Decreased anticonvulsant (reduced GI absorption of primidone). *See Anticonvulsants*
Procainamide (Procan, Pronestyl)	Enhanced procainamide effect (drug-induced alkaline urine delays procainamide excretion)
Pseudoephedrine (Sudafed)	Risk of pseudoephedrine toxicity (drug-induced alkaline urine delays pseudoephedrine excretion). Concurrent use generally avoided
Quinidine	Drug-induced alkaline urine decreases rate of quinidine excretion with possible toxicity
Salicylates	Increased risk of salicylate toxicity in patients receiving large salicylate doses. Concurrent use generally avoided

---

ACETOHEXAMIDE

(Dimelor, Dymelor)

(a-seat-oh-hex'a-mide)
Antidiabetic agent (oral)
Hypoglycemic
Sulfonylurea

ACTIONS AND USES. Intermediate-acting sulfonylurea that promotes increased effectiveness of endogenous insulin. Chemically related to sulfonamides, but has no antibacterial action. More potent and has longer action than tolbutamide (qv), but uses, precautions, and adverse reactions are similar. Also has moderate uricosuric effect, probably due to its primary metabolite, hydroxyhexamide.

Used in mild to moderately severe stable type II, NIDDM (noninsulin dependent diabetes mellitus). Also used to reduce insulin requirements in select patients with type I, IDDM (insulin dependent diabetes mellitus). Preferred by some clinicians for patients who also have gout.

ABSORPTION AND FATE. Rapidly absorbed from GI tract. Onset of action in 1 hour; peak activity in about 4 to 5 hours. Duration of action: 12 to 24 hours (prolonged in kidney dysfunction). Well distributed into extracellular fluids. Metabolized in liver; highly protein bound. Active metabolite, hydroxyhexamide about 2½ times more potent than parent drug. Half-life: 5 to 6 hours. (Parent compound has half-life of approximately 1.3 to 1.5 hours.) About 80 to 95% of dose excreted in urine within 24 hours (about 50% as the active metabolite). Approximately 15% eliminated in bile. Excreted in breast milk.

CONTRAINDICATIONS AND PRECAUTIONS. Hypersensitivity to sulfonylureas; severe impairment of hepatic, renal, thyroid or other endocrine function; as sole therapy for NIDDM, and in diabetes complicated by ketosis, acidosis, coma, infection, trauma; hyperglycemia and glycosuria associated with primary renal disease. Safe use in pregnancy, in women of childbearing age, and in children not established. *Cautious Use:* renal insufficiency, history of hepatic porphyria. *See also Tolbutamide.*

ADVERSE/SIDE EFFECTS. (Generally dose-related). **GI:** nausea, vomiting, heartburn, diarrhea, GI hemorrhage (rare). **Hematologic:** agranulocytosis, leukopenia, pancytopenia, thrombocytopenia, aplastic anemia, hemolytic anemia; increases in urinary protein, serum alkaline phosphatase, and blood ammonia; severe hypoglycemia. **Hypersensitivity:** erythema, urticaria, pruritus, skin rash, photosensitivity. **Other:** headache, cholestatic and mixed hepatic jaundice, hepatic porphyria. *See also Tolbutamide.*

ROUTE AND DOSAGE. **Oral** (highly individualized): 250 mg daily before breakfast. May be increased every 5 to 7 days by 250 to 500 mg as needed to maximum of 1.5 Gm daily. Patients on 1 Gm/day or less usually can be controlled on once daily dosage. Those receiving 1.5 Gm/day usually benefit from twice daily dosage given before morning and evening meals.

NURSING IMPLICATIONS

Patient must understand that the mainstays of diabetic care continue to be compliance with prescribed diet, maintenance of ideal body weight, meticulous personal hygiene, graded exercise program, and scheduled follow-up care.

Blood and urine glucose concentrations should be closely monitored during the first 24 hours after therapy is initiated.

The elderly, malnourished and debilitated patients, patients with impaired hepatic or renal function, or who have adrenal or pituitary insufficiency or who are taking beta-adrenergic blocking drugs (e.g., propranolol) require particularly close monitoring because they have a tendency to manifest an exaggerated hypoglycemic response, which may be difficult to recognize.

Patients first started on acetohexamide are usually given at least 7 days trial period to determine therapeutic response. Favorable response is indicated by reduction in diabetes symptoms (elevated blood sugar, glycosuria, ketonuria, polydipsia, polyuria, polyphagia, pruritus).

During the initial trial period, patient should communicate with physician daily. Patients are generally examined weekly during the first month of therapy, to determine adequacy of response to acetohexamide. Thereafter, evaluations should be scheduled at regular intervals as indicated.

Although patients with type II diabetes are not prone to ketosis, they should also test for ketones during times of severe stress (surgery, trauma, fever, acute infection, severe diarrhea, nausea or vomiting, and other acute illnesses). Loss of blood glucose control may require administration of insulin.

Instruct patient to ingest some form of sugar such as orange juice, sugar cube, table sugar (dissolved in water), corn syrup, or honey if symptoms of hypoglycemia develop. Review cause of hypoglycemia. Adjustment in dosage or diet may be needed.

To convert from insulin to acetohexamide: transition may be made abruptly for insulin dosages up to 20 units daily. For insulin dosages greater than 20 units daily, a 25 to 30% reduction in insulin, daily or every second day, is advisable.

In general, transfer from another oral antidiabetic agent to acetohexamide can be made without a transitional period.

During conversion from one antidiabetic agent to another, patient should check urine for glucose and ketones (acetone) at least three times a day and report to physician as directed. Blood glucose monitoring may also be prescribed.

Caution patient not to take any other medication unless approved or prescribed by physician.

Warn patient that alcoholic beverages may produce a disulfiram reaction: drop in blood sugar with flushing, sweating, pounding headache, slurred speech, upset stomach, palpitation.

Dermatologic reactions tend to be transient and frequently subside even with continuation of therapy. However, if they persist or are severe drug discontinuation may be necessary.

Caution patient to avoid prolonged direct exposure to sun to prevent photosensitivity reaction.

Because hepatotoxicity is a possible complication of therapy, periodic tests of liver function are recommended, i.e., bilirubin, cholesterol, SGOT (AST), SGPT (ALT).

Keep drug out of the reach of children.

Store between 15° and 30°C (59° and 86°F) in a well-closed container, unless otherwise directed by manufacturer.

See Tolbutamide (prototype sulfonylurea).

Diagnostic Test Interferences. **Serum uric acid** levels may be appreciably reduced. *See also Tolbutamide.*

Drug Interactions: Acetohexamide

Plus	Interactions
Alcohol (Ethanol)	Disulfiram reaction
Anticoagulants, oral; aspirin, and other salicylates; chloramphenicol (Chloromycetin, Mychel-S) Clofibrate (Atromid-S) Fenfluramine (Pondimin) Guanethidine (Ismelin) MAOIs Oxyphenbutazone (Oxalid, Tandearil) Oxytetracycline (Oxymycin, Terramycin) Phenylbutazone (Azolid, Butazolidin) Probenecid (Benemid, Probalan) Salicylates Sulfinpyrazone (Anturane) Sulfonamides	Concurrent use enhances hypoglycemic effect of acetohexamide

Plus (cont.)	Interactions (cont.)
Diazoxide (Hyperstat, Proglycem)	Mutual antagonism. Pharmacologic effects of both drugs reduced
Phenytoin (Dilantin) and other hydantoins	Pharmacologic effects of acetohexamide may be decreased
Propranolol (Inderal) and other β-adrenergic blockers	May decrease pharmacologic effects of acetohexamide and mask clinical manifestations of hypoglycemia
Thiazides	Decreased hypoglycemic response

ACETOHYDROXAMIC ACID

(AHA, Lithostat)

(a-set-oh-hye-drox-am′-ic)
Enzyme inhibitor; antilithic ammonia detoxicant

ACTIONS AND USES. Synthetic compound derived from hydroxylamine and ethyl acetate with structural similarity to urea and hydroxyurea. Irreversibly inhibits urease (bacterial enzyme) apparently by complexing with it. As a result, suppresses conversion of urea to ammonia in urine infected with urease producing (urea splitting) organisms, e.g., *Proteus* species. Indirectly acidifies urine by reducing ammonia formation and bicarbonate and carbonate production. This action leads to reduction in growth of existing crystals or stones, and prevention of new formation of struvite or carbonate-apatite crystals. Acetohydroxamic therapy is not considered a substitute for surgical treatment or antibiotic therapy. Has no direct antibacterial activity except in high concentrations, but appears to enhance the action of certain antimicrobial agents.

Used in carefully selected patients as adjunct in treatment of chronic urinary tract infection caused by urease producing bacteria and characterized by staghorn or branched-type (struvite) renal stones. *Investigational Use:* to reduce blood ammonia concentration in management of hepatic coma.

ABSORPTION AND FATE. Well absorbed (chiefly from upper GI tract). Peak blood levels in 15 to 60 minutes. Well distributed throughout body water. Plasma half-life: approximately 3.5 to 10 hours (longer in patients with impaired renal function). Metabolized in part to acetamide, which lacks ability to inhibit urease. About 35 to 65% of dose excreted unchanged in urine (site of desired action) within 24 to 48 hours.

CONTRAINDICATIONS AND PRECAUTIONS. Advanced renal insufficiency (serum creatinine > 2.5 mg/dl and/or creatinine clearance (Ccr) < 20 mg/minute); pregnancy (category X), fertile women, nursing mother. *Cautious Use:* Impaired renal or hepatic function; history of thrombophlebitis, phlebothrombosis; varicose veins.

ADVERSE/SIDE EFFECTS. CNS (usually mild and transient): headache, depression, anxiety, nervousness, tremulousness. **CV:** superficial phlebitis, deep vein phlebothromboses, pulmonary emboli, palpitation. **GI** (usually mild and transient): nausea, vomiting, anorexia, diarrhea, constipation. **Hematologic:** reticulocytosis, hypochromic anemia, Coombs' negative hemolytic anemia, transient thrombocytopenia, leukocytopenia. **Skin:** nonpruritic macular rash, scalp tenderness, alopecia. **Other:** general malaise, renal impairment.

ROUTE AND DOSAGE. Adult: Initial: 250 mg three or four times daily, at 6- to 8-hour intervals. Total recommended dose: 10 to 15 mg/kg/day (not to exceed 1.5 Gm/day). Impaired renal function: total dose should not exceed 1 Gm daily given in divided doses at 12-hour intervals. **Children:** 10 mg/kg/day in two or three divided doses.

NURSING IMPLICATIONS

Administered on an empty stomach (at least 1 hour before or 2 hours after a meal).

Headache commonly occurs during first 48 hours of therapy and usually disappears spontaneously in 30 to 60 minutes.

Review patient's drug history. Caution against taking any OTC preparations without medical advice. Alcoholic beverages should be avoided or at least limited. *See Drug Interactions.*

Acetohydroxamic acid may interfere with absorption of dietary iron by forming a chelate. If patient requires iron therapy, parenteral iron should be prescribed.

Advise patient or responsible family member to be aware of intake and output ratio and pattern. Report immediately any suspicion of deteriorating renal function.

Review with patient preventive measures for minimizing risk of thrombophlebitis:

- Do not cross legs
- Avoid tight garters and undergarments
- Avoid standing still or sitting for prolonged periods
- Avoid injury to legs
- Maintain prescribed physical exercise program
- Weight control plan for obese patients (obesity contributes to venous stasis)

Bear in mind that inactive patients are most likely to develop thrombi. Physicians may prescribe support hose for these patients and for patients with extensive varicosities.

Instruct patient to report immediately to physician the onset of phlebitis (hard, tender, reddened area on extremity), or any other unusual symptoms.

A *CBC,* including reticulocyte and platelet counts, renal and liver function tests, are advisable after 2 weeks of therapy and at 3-month intervals for duration of therapy. Dosage should be reduced if reticulocytes exceed 6%. (*Normal:* 0.5 to 1.5% of total RBC count.) These tests may be prescribed more frequently in patients with impaired renal functions.

Severe forms of hemolytic anemia are occasionally accompanied by anorexia and other GI symptoms, fatigue, lethargy, and generalized malaise. Report symptoms to physician. Be aware that hematologic complications occur most commonly in patients with renal function impairment.

Drug should not be started in a fertile woman until the possibility of pregnancy has been ruled out and effective contraception started. Warn patient to notify physician promptly should pregnancy occur.

When prescribed for children, close monitoring of chemical response and hematologic status is essential since dosage has not been firmly established for this age group.

Advise patient to remain under close medical supervision. Optimal length of therapy has not been defined.

Drug Interactions: Acetohydroxamic acid

Plus	Interactions
Alcohol	May cause rash 30 to 45 minutes after ingestion of alcohol
Iron (oral) and possibly other heavy metals	Chelate formation reduces absorption of both drugs

ACETOPHENAZINE MALEATE
(Tindal)

(a-set-oh-fen'a-zeen)
Psychotropic: antipsychotic (neuroleptic)
Antiemetic
Phenothiazine

ACTIONS AND USES. Phenothiazine of the piperazine group with similar actions, contraindications, and adverse reactions as chlorpromazine (qv). Produces moderate extrapyramidal and sedative effects and has weak to moderate anticholinergic activity. Has prominent antiemetic action.

Used in treatment of acute and chronic schizophrenia; manic phase of manic–depressive psychosis; involutional, senile, organic, and toxic psychoses, with exception of delirium tremens.

CONTRAINDICATIONS AND PRECAUTIONS. Hypersensitivity to phenothiazines. Safe use during pregnancy, in nursing mothers, and in the pediatric age group not established. *Cautious Use:* patients receiving atropine or related drugs. *See also Chlorpromazine.*

ADVERSE/SIDE EFFECTS. CNS: Extrapyramidal symptoms, drowsiness, delirium (high doses). **CV:** orthostatic hypotension, tachycardia, ECG abnormalities. **GI:** dry mouth, constipation, anorexia. **Ophthalmic:** mydriasis, cycloplegia, lenticular deposits and opacities (prolonged use of high doses). **Reproductive:** gynecomastia, galactorrhea, menstrual changes, decreased libido. **Skin:** photosensitivity, rash, decreased sweating. **Other:** nasal congestion, cholestatic jaundice, blood dyscrasias. *See also Chlorpromazine.*

ROUTE AND DOSAGE. Oral: 20 mg three or four times daily. (Elderly, debilitated patients, and adolescents usually respond to lower dosages.) Hospitalized patients: 80 to 120 mg daily (dosages as high as 600 mg daily have been used).

NURSING IMPLICATIONS

In patients with sleeping problems, the last dose is usually given 1 hour before retiring. The drug has mild sedative effects.

Explain to patient importance of reporting side effects. Extrapyramidal symptoms (tremor, parkinsonism, dystonia, akathisia) should be reported immediately. Drug regimen changes may be indicated. Anticholinergic side effects may decrease with time, but some indicate need for nursing intervention (e.g., dry mouth, constipation).

Dry mouth may be relieved by frequent sips of water or use of saliva substitute. *See Index: Nursing Interventions: dry mouth.*

Bedsides and supervision of ambulation may be advisable during period of adjustment to dosage or adverse drug response.

Allergic reactions (rare) usually occur in the first few months of treatment.

Warn patient not to self-medicate and not to drink alcoholic beverages without advise of physician. Alcohol, sedatives, and other CNS depressants have additive effects and may impair psychomotor skills and cause both hypotension and excessive drowsiness. Caution patient to avoid driving and other potentially hazardous activities until response to drug is known.

Inform patient that acetophenazine may color urine pink or red or red-brown.

Patients on long-term therapy should be seen periodically to evaluate maintenance dosage regimen.

Advise patient to avoid direct sunlight and to use a sunscreen lotion if necessary. Photosensitivity is a possible side effect.
See Chlorpromazine: Nursing Implications and *Diagnostic Test Interferences.*

Drug Interactions: Acetophenazine

Plus	Interactions
Alcohol (Ethanol)	Additive pharmacologic effects of both drugs
Barbiturates, atropine and other anticholinergics	Reduce acetophenazine effect (possibly by increasing drug metabolism). Concurrent use generally avoided or acetophenazine dose increased
Guanethidine (Ismelin)	Antihypertensive effect of guanethidine reduced; (neuronal uptake inhibited by acetophenazine). Concurrent use generally avoided

Also see Chlorpromazine (prototype phenothiazine).

ACETYLCHOLINE CHLORIDE
(Miochol)

(a-se-teel-koe′leen)
Cholinergic (direct acting)
(Parasympathomimetic)
Miotic

ACTIONS AND USES. Quaternary ammonium compound. Acts directly on postjunctional effector cells of eye to produce intense miosis by stimulating contraction of iris sphincter muscles when introduced into anterior chamber of eye.

Used to obtain rapid and complete miosis after delivery of lens in cataract surgery; also in penetrating keratoplasty, iridectomy, and other surgical procedures of anterior segment.

ABSORPTION AND FATE. Miosis occurs within 10 seconds and may be maintained for about 10 minutes. Rapidly hydrolyzed by acetylcholinesterase to choline and acetic acid.

ADVERSE/SIDE EFFECTS. Low toxicity. With systemic absorption: transient hypotension, bradycardia, bronchospasm, flushing, sweating. Also reported: temporary lens opacities and iris atrophy following use of hypertonic solutions.

ROUTE AND DOSAGE. Intraocular instillation by physician: 0.5 to 2 ml 1% solution instilled into anterior chamber.

NURSING IMPLICATIONS

Immediately before use, cap should be dusted, label should be peeled off, and whole vial immersed in 70% ethanol or other sterilizing solution for 30 minutes or more. Stream of gas (e.g., ethylene oxide) should not be used.

Using aseptic technique, rubber stopper is pressed down sufficiently to dislodge center rubber plug seal, thus releasing solvent (sterile water) from upper chamber.

Vial should be shaken gently to dissolve and mix drug in lower chamber. If center rubber plug seal does not go down or is down, do not use vial.

After plunger-stopper is cleansed with 70% alcohol or other suitable germicide, desired dose is drawn into dry sterile syringe with sterile new 18- to 20-gauge needle. Needle is replaced with suitable atraumatic cannula for intraocular instillation.

Because solution is unstable, it should be reconstituted immediately before use. Discard unused portion.

Pilocarpine 2% or physostigmine 0.25% (long-acting miotics) may be prescribed topically before dressing is applied to maintain miosis.

Systemic reactions are treated with intravenous atropine 0.6 to 0.8 mg.

ACETYLCYSTEINE

(Airbron, Mucomyst, *N*-Acetylcysteine, Parvolex)

(a-se-til-sis′tay-een)
Mucolytic
Antidote

ACTIONS AND USES. Derivative of naturally occurring amino acid L-cysteine. Probably acts by disrupting disulfide linkages of mucoproteins in purulent and nonpurulent secretions, thereby lowering viscosity and facilitating their removal. Acetylcysteine is a precursor of hepatic glutathione, which normally inactivates a hepatotoxic metabolite of acetaminophen.

Used as adjuvant therapy in patients with abnormal, viscid, or inspissated mucous secretions in acute and chronic bronchopulmonary diseases, and in pulmonary complications of cystic fibrosis and surgery, tracheostomy, and atelectasis. Also used in diagnostic bronchial studies. *Investigational Use:* As an antidote for acute acetaminophen poisoning. Commercially available in combination with isoproterenol (e.g., Mucomyst with Isoproterenol).

ABSORPTION AND FATE. Liquefaction of mucus occurs within 1 minute after inhalation or instillation; maximum effects in 5 to 10 minutes. Most drug appears to participate in sulfhydryl–disulfide reaction; remainder is absorbed from epithelium, deacetylated by liver to cysteine and subsequently metabolized.

CONTRAINDICATIONS AND PRECAUTIONS. Hypersensitivity to acetylcysteine. Safe use during pregnancy and in nursing mothers not established. *Cautious Use:* patients with asthma, the elderly, debilitated patients with severe respiratory insufficiency.

ADVERSE/SIDE EFFECTS. CNS: drowsiness. **GI:** nausea, vomiting, stomatitis. **Respiratory:** bronchospasm, rhinorrhea, bronchorrhea, burning sensation in upper respiratory passages, hemoptysis. **Other:** fever, chills, clamminess, sensitization (rarely), transient maculopapular rash (after frequent and extended use).

ROUTE AND DOSAGE. Inhalation: by nebulization into face mask, mouthpiece, or tracheostomy: 1 to 10 ml of 20% solution, or 2 to 20 ml of 10% solution every 2 to 6 hours. **Nebulization** into closed tent or croupette (10 or 20% solution): use volume that will maintain a heavy mist for desired treatment period. Highly individualized according to equipment used. **Direct instillation:** tracheostomy or via bronchoscope: 1 to 2 ml of 10 to 20% solution every 1 to 4 hours. The 20% solution may be diluted to lesser concentration with either sterile normal saline or sterile water for injection. **Oral:** acetaminophen poisoning: initial loading dose 140 mg/kg, followed by 17 additional doses of 70 mg/kg every 4 hours. *See Acetaminophen.*

NURSING IMPLICATIONS

Intermittent aerosol treatments are commonly administered when patient arises, before meals, and prior to retiring at night.

For maximum effect, patient should be instructed to clear his or her airway, if possible, by coughing productively prior to aerosol administration.

Have suction apparatus immediately available. Following drug administration, increased volume of respiratory tract fluid may be liberated. If patient cannot cough adequately, suction or endotracheal aspiration will be necessary to establish and maintain an open airway. Elderly and debilitated patients require close monitoring to prevent aspiration of excessive secretions.

Unpleasant odor of the drug (rotten egg odor of hydrogen sulfide) and excess volume of liquefied bronchial secretions may cause nausea and possibly vomiting, particularly when face mask is used. Assure patient that the odor becomes less noticeable with continued inhalation.

Bronchospasm is most likely to occur in patients with asthma, and it may happen unpredictably. If it occurs, drug should be discontinued immediately. Consult physician beforehand about emergency use of bronchodilator (by nebulization) such as isoproterenol.

Solutions of acetylcysteine release hydrogen sulfide and become discolored when autoclaved and upon contact with rubber and certain metals (particularly iron and copper). When administering by nebulization, it is recommended to use equipment made of plastic, glass, stainless steel, aluminum, chromed metal, sterling silver, tantalum, or other nonreactive metals. Silver may tarnish, but this does not affect drug potency.

When drug is administered by nebulization, compressed air should be used to provide pressure. Oxygen may be used if prescribed, but close monitoring of blood gases must be observed since it may aggravate CO_2 retention.

Prolonged nebulization causes solution to become more concentrated impeding drug delivery. Therefore, after three-quarters of initial volume has been nebulized, the remainder may be diluted with an approximately equal volume of sterile water for injection.

Cleanse nebulizing equipment immediately after use to prevent occluded openings and corrosion of metal parts. Wash face and mask and have patient rinse mouth with water. The drug leaves a sticky coating.

Acetylcysteine should not be placed into the chamber of a heated (hot pot) nebulizer.

As a rule, hand bulb nebulizers are not recommended because output may be too small and particle size is generally too large.

For treatment of acetaminophen poisoning, contact regional poison center or Rocky Mountain Poison Center (800–525–6115) for directions in use of acetylcysteine. *See Acetaminophen.*

Acetylcysteine is a reducing agent and therefore it is incompatible with oxidizing agents such as hydrogen perioxide. Solutions of acetylcysteine are incompatible with ampicillin, amphotericicin B (Fungizone), chymotrypain (Avazyme), tetracyclines, erythromycin lactobionate, iodinized oil, and trypsin.

Collaborate with physician and respiratory therapist in constructing a teaching plan for the patient with chronic pulmonary insufficiency. *See Index: Nursing Interventions: chronic pulmonary insufficiency.*

Once opened, vial should be stored in refrigerator to retard oxidation, and used within 96 hours. A light purple color apparently does not significantly impair its mucolytic effectiveness.

Unopened vial should be stored at room temperature, preferably between 15° and 30°C (59° and 86°F), unless otherwise directed by manufacturer.

ACRISORCIN
(Akrinol)

(ak-ri-sor′-sin)
Antiinfective (topical): antibiotic, antifungal

ACTIONS AND USES. Synthetic compound prepared from 9-aminoacridine and hexylresorcinal. Bactericidal, bacteriostatic, and fungicidal agent with activity against *Malassezia furfur,* causative organism of tinea versicolor. Also believed to be mildly keratolytic.

Used topically in treatment of tinea versicolor.

CONTRAINDICATIONS AND PRECAUTIONS. Safe use during pregnancy and in nursing mothers not established.

ADVERSE/SIDE EFFECTS. Low order of toxicity. Blisters, erythematous vesicular eruptions, pruritus, urticaria, irritation, burning sensation, worsening of tinea versicolor.

ROUTE AND DOSAGE. **Topical cream (0.2%):** small quantity rubbed gently into affected areas twice daily, morning and night.

NURSING IMPLICATIONS

Prior to application of cream, area should be thoroughly cleansed. Soap reduces drug effectiveness, therefore it must be completely rinsed off and skin thoroughly dried before applying the cream. Pay particular attention to friction areas.

Night applications should be preceded by a warm soapy bath, and use of a stiff bath brush on lesions.

Wash hands before and after treatment.

Do not use acrisorcin near the eyes.

To avoid reinfection, towels and all clothing worn next to skin must be laundered after each treatment.

Caution patient that exposure to sunlight and ultraviolet lamp may cause pruritus.

Treatment should be discontinued if signs of irritation or sensitization occur, or if condition worsens.

Acrisorcin therapy should be continued for at least 6 weeks, even if improvement or clearing of lesions occurs. Sometimes a second or third course of therapy is needed. Urge patient not to interrupt therapy until advised to do so by physician.

Since there are no reliable laboratory studies for determining causative organism of tinea versicolor *(M. furfur),* diagnosis and therapeutic response are determined by clinical appearance, lesion scrapings, and by Wood's light examination of lesions. (The lesions of tinea versicolor are macular, with fine scales and hyperpigmented to hypopigmented patches.)

See Index: Nursing Intervention: fungal infection for patient teaching points.

Store at controlled temperature 15° to 30°C (59° to 86°F) unless otherwise directed by manufacturer.

PROTOTYPE

ACYCLOVIR
(Acycloguanosine, Zovirax)

ACYCLOVIR SODIUM

(ay-sye′-kloe-ver)
Antiinfective, antiviral

ACTIONS AND USES. Synthetic acyclic purine nucleoside analogue, derived from guanine. Selectively absorbed by virus infected cells. Drug activity depends chiefly on its phosphorylation to acyclovir triphosphate by virus-coded enzymes in cells infected with herpes virus. Acyclovir's virostatic action interferes with DNA synthesis of herpes simplex virus types 1 and 2 (HSV-1 and HSV-2) and varicella-zoster virus, thereby inhibiting viral replication. Demonstrates antiviral activity against herpes virus simiae (B virus), Epstein-Barr (infectious mononucleosis) and cytomegalovirus. Does not eradicate the latent herpes virus.

Used systemically for treatment of initial and recurrent mucosal and cutaneous herpes simplex (HSV-1 and HSV-2) infections in immunocompromised adults and children and for severe initial episodes of herpes genitalis in immunocompetent (normal immune system) patients. Used topically for initial episodes of herpes genitalis and in limited nonlife-threatening mucocutaneous herpes simplex virus infections in immunocompromised patients. *Investigational Use:* In immunocompromised patients to treat herpes zoster (shingles), varicella (chickenpox), and other herpetic infections. Oral formulation is being studied for long-term use in prevention and treatment of recurrent herpes genitalis, and in treatment of initial genital herpes.

ABSORPTION AND FATE. Peak serum levels in about 1 hour following IV administration with maximal renal concentration within 2 hours. Minimal systemic absorption follows topical application. Widely distributed to most body tissues including brain, kidneys, lungs, liver, and to body fluids and secretions, including vesicular fluids, CSF, and saliva. About 9 to 30% protein-binding. Biphasic decline in plasma concentration: initial half-life: ≈0.34 hour; terminal half-life: ≈3 hours (in patients with renal impairment up to 20 hours). Probably metabolized by liver. More than 95% of IV dose excreted in urine as unchanged drug within 24 hours; less than 2% eliminated in feces. Crosses placenta; distribution into breast milk not known.

CONTRAINDICATIONS AND PRECAUTIONS. History of acyclovir hypersensitivity; rapid or bolus injection of acyclovir; pregnancy (category C); herpes zoster, labialis, or simplex in immunocompromised patient. *Cautious Use:* nursing mother, neurologic, renal, hepatic or electrolyte abnormalities; hypoxia, dehydration, history of neurologic reactions to cytotoxic drugs; concomitant administration of nephrotoxic drugs or intrathecal methotrexate or interferon.

ADVERSE/SIDE EFFECTS. (generally minimal and infrequent): **CNS:** lethargy, obtundation, tremors, confusion, hallucinations, agitation, seizures, light-headedness, dizziness, headache, jitteriness, delirium, coma. **CV:** hypotension. **GI:** nausea, vomiting, abdominal or epigastric pain. **Hematologic:** thrombocytosis, thrombocytopenia, transient elevations of: BUN, serum creatinine, AST (SGOT), ALT (SGPT), alkaline phosphatase; leukopenia, lymphopenia, megaloblastic hematopoiesis, bone marrow hypoplasia. **Renal:** hematuria, renal tubular damage, acute renal failure. **Skin:** rash, urticaria, pruritus, burning, stinging sensation, irritation, sensitization. **Other:** inflammation or phlebitis at IV injection site, sloughing (with extravasation); diaphoresis, unusual thirst, substernal burning sensation, vulvitis.

ROUTE AND DOSAGE. **Intravenous:** *Mucosal and cutaneous herpes simplex* (HSV-1 and HSV-2) *infections in immunocompromised patients:* **Adults and Children (12 years and over):** 5 mg/kg every 8 hours for 7 days. **Children (under 12 years):** 250 mg/m² every 8 hours for 7 days. *Severe initial episodes of herpes genitalis:* Same dose as above but administered for 5 days. Acyclovir should be infused at a prescribed rate. Dosages for patients with impaired renal function based on creatinine clearance values. **Topical:** 5% ointment: approximately 1.25 cm (one-half inch) ribbon of ointment per 2.5 cm² (4 square inches) surface area. Rub gently onto affected area every 3 hours, six times daily for 7 days. (Ointment contains propylene glycol base.)

NURSING IMPLICATIONS

Parenteral Administration:

Acyclovir sodium is reconstituted first by adding 10 ml sterile water for injection to 500 mg vial (provide concentration of 50 mg/ml). Shake well to assure complete dissolution of drug. This solution should be used within 12 hours.

For infusion, withdraw appropriate dose of reconstituted solution from vial and add to designated compatible IV infusion solution. To reduce risk of renal injury and phlebitis, final concentration should be 7 mg/ml or less. Once prepared for infusion, solution should be used within 24 hours.

Manufacturer approves use of standard commercially available electrolyte and glucose solutions for the infusion solution. Acyclovir sodium is reportedly incompatible with biologicals and colloidal solutions, e.g., blood products and protein containing solutions.

Acyclovir sodium is intended **for IV infusion only** and it must be administered over a period of at least 1 hour to prevent renal tubular damage. Rapid or bolus IV, and IM or SC administration must be avoided.

Monitor IV flow rate and observe infusion site during and for a few days following infusion.

Maximum drug concentration in urine occurs within the first 2 hours following infusion. Keep patient adequately hydrated during this time to maintain sufficient urinary flow and thus prevent precipitation of drug in renal tubules.

Consult physician about amount and length of time oral fluids need to be pushed after IV drug treatment.

Monitor intake and output ratio and pattern. *Note:* unusual tiredness and weakness are suggestive symptoms of early renal failure.

Baseline and periodic renal function studies (BUN, serum creatinine, creatinine clearance) should by done. Elevations indicate need for dosage adjustment, discontinuation of drug, or correction of fluid and electrolyte balance.

Refrigeration may cause precipitation; however, crystals will redissolve at room temperature.

Store acyclovir powder and reconstituted solutions at controlled room temperature preferably between 15° and 30°C (59° and 86°F) unless otherwise directed by manufacturer.

Topical Administration:

Advise use of liquid soap for hand washing to prevent cross-contamination. Recent evidence suggests "in use" bar soap may harbor viable microorganisms for as long as 48 hours after hand washing.

Teach patient to be thorough in hand washing before and after treatment of lesions and after cautious handling and disposition of secretions. Virus is killed by thorough washing with soap and water. Reportedly it cannot be spread by dry towels or sheets or by bathtubs and swimming pools.

Cleanse area with soap and water three or four times daily; dry well. Hair dryer may be helpful. Advise patient to wear loose fitting clothing and absorbent (e.g., cotton) underclothing.

Instruct patient to apply topical preparation with finger cot or surgical glove to prevent further self-infection as well as spread of virus to others. Use sufficient ointment to completely cover lesions.

Avoid drug contact in or around the eyes. Any unexplained eye symptoms (e.g., redness, pain) should be reported immediately. Untreated infection can lead to corneal keratitis and blindness.

Warn patient to avoid use of self-prescribed emollient creams or ointments unless specifically prescribed by physician. These agents tend to delay healing and may even spread the lesions.

Notify physician if local reactions are pronounced or annoying, and if no improvement is noted within 1 week.
Store topical preparation in dry place, preferably at 15° and 25°C (59° and 78°F) unless otherwise directed by manufacturer.

General:
The incidence of genital herpes has increased 10-fold from 1966 to 1980.
Acyclovir therapy is most effective when started as soon as possible after onset of signs and symptoms.
Diagnosis of HSV-1 and HSV-2 virus infection is based on presence of characteristic lesions and on finding multinucleated giant cells in exudate and scrapings of lesions, and by positive cultures. Possibility of other sexually-transmitted diseases should be ruled out.
Risk of virus transfer is negligible. If sheets, underclothing, toilet seats, etc., are dry, contact is safe. If moisture is present handle fomites with surgical gloves.
When virus is on plastic or other hard surfaces, life span is only several minutes.
Caution patient to refrain from sexual intercourse if either partner has signs and symptoms of herpes infection. It is generally true that asymptomatic persons cannot transmit the disease, however, transmission can occur although signs and symptoms are so mild that person is not aware of them. (Symptoms of initial genital herpes occur within 2 to 10 days after exposure through sexual contact.)
Pregnant patients should be followed closely to detect reinfection.
Women with genital herpes reportedly are at a high risk level for developing cervical cancer. Urge patient to have a Papanicolaou (Pap) smear at least annually to detect early cervical changes.
Acyclovir is not a cure for herpetic infections. HSV-1 virus (cold sore or fever blister) remains latent in the trigeminal ganglia for life and may emerge periodically to cause symptoms. In some instances it attacks new sites such as the brain or eyes. HSV-2 virus, responsible for most genital herpes, lodges in sacral ganglia and can cause repeated infections.
Be aware that symptoms of genital herpes caused by either HSV-1 or HSV-2 may appear to be similar but the rate and frequency of occurrence is much lower in HSV-1 infections.
Children are unlikely to contract genital herpes except by incest or sexual assault.
The patient should be aware that even after the HSV infection is controlled by acyclovir, the latent virus can be activated by such stimuli as: stress, exposure to sunlight, sexual intercourse, treatment with immunosuppressive drugs.
Before the patient is discharged from medical supervision he or she should understand how long acyclovir is to be used, and when a return visit is scheduled. Urge compliance with treatment and assessment schedules.
If patient is interested in confidential information resources about genital herpes, suggest contacting the local health department or Planned Parenthood Chapter, or call the American Social Health Association VD National Hotline, toll free (800–227–8922).

Drug Interactions: Acyclovir

Plus	Interactions
Agents that decrease renal function or compete for renal excretion (e.g., aminoglycocides, amphotericin B)	Increased risk of nephrotoxicity. Used with caution
Interferon Methotrexate (Mexate)	Possibility of neurologic abnormalities with concurrent use. Used with caution
Probenecid (Benemid, Probalan)	Decreases renal clearance of acyclovir

ADENOSINE PHOSPHATE

(a-den′oh-seen)
Antiinflammatory agent

(Adeno, Adenosine 5-Monophosphate, AMP, A5MP, Cobalasine, Muscle Adenylic Acid)

ACTIONS AND USES. Natural nucleotide constituent of muscle tissue (adenine riboside) essential for formation of coenzymes involved in energy transfer mechanisms, biologic oxidation, and metabolism of carbohydrates and fats. Therapeutic effect of the drug adenosine phosphate may result from its action in elevating blood concentrations of ATP (adenosine triphosphate) or to its vasodilating action and ability to reduce inflammation and edema.

Used as adjunct in treatment of complications associated with varicose veins (e.g., ulcers, chronic thrombophlebitis), and in symptomatic treatment of acute and chronic bursitis, tendonitis, tenosynovitis, intractable pruritus, and multiple sclerosis.

CONTRAINDICATIONS AND PRECAUTIONS. History of myocardial infarction; cerebral hemorrhage. Safe use during pregnancy, in fertile women, and in children not established. *Cautious Use:* patient with history of allergy.

ADVERSE/SIDE EFFECTS. CV: generalized flushing, dizziness, headache, palpitation, hypotension. **GI:** epigastric discomfort, nausea, diarrhea. **Hypersensitivity:** anaphylactoid reaction (following injection of sustained-action preparation): feeling of chest tightness, difficulty in breathing. **Other:** diuresis, rash, increase in symptoms of bursitis and tendonitis, local erythema at IM site.

ROUTE AND DOSAGE. Intramuscular: Initial: 25 to 50 mg daily or 50 mg three times weekly until symptoms subside. Highly individualized. Doses may be reduced and intervals lengthened as condition improves. Maintenance: 25 mg two or three times weekly.

NURSING IMPLICATIONS

Administered only by IM injection. Aspirate carefully to avoid inadvertent entry into blood vessel.

Drug should be discontinued if dyspnea or tightness in chest occurs.

Some patients experience transient flushing, palpitation, and dizziness with high doses. Advise these patients to avoid strenuous activities until dosage is stabilized.

Patients being treated for bursitis or tendonitis may experience exacerbation of symptoms after 5 to 10 days of therapy. Symptoms usually subside in 1 or 2 days.

Preparation of adenosine phosphate in gelatin vehicle is no longer commercially available.

ALBUMIN HUMAN

(al-byoo′min)
Blood derivative
Plasma volume expander

(Albuminar, Albutein, Buminate, Normal Human Serum Albumin, Normal Serum Albumin [Human], Plasbumin)

ACTIONS AND USES. Obtained by fractionating pooled venous and placental human plasma, which is then pasteurized to minimize possibility of transmitting hepatitis B virus. Risk of sensitization is reduced because it lacks cellular elements. Expands volume of circulating blood by exerting osmotic pull on tissue fluids. Exerts about 80% effective osmotic pressure of blood. Each volume of the 25% solution draws about 3.5 volumes of interstitial fluid into the circulation within 15 minutes. Supplied in two strengths: 5% (approximately isotonic and isosmotic with normal human plasma), and 25% (equivalent to 5 volumes of 5% albumin in producing hemodilution). Both strengths now contain sodium 130 to 160 mEq/L. (Formerly, the 25% solution was labeled "salt-poor.")

Used to restore plasma volume and colloidal osmotic pressure in hypovolemic shock (as in hemorrhage, burns, surgery, trauma), in prevention and treatment of cerebral edema, as adjunct in exchange transfusion for hyperbilirubinemia, and erythroblastosis fetalis; and in treatment of hypoproteinemia to increase plasma protein level, and to promote diuresis in refractory edema. Also used as pump primer for preoperative blood dilution before cardiopulmonary bypass procedures. Has been used for patients with varicella zoster infections.

CONTRAINDICATIONS AND PRECAUTIONS. Severe anemia, cardiac failure, patients with normal or increased intravascular volume. *Cautious Use:* low cardiac reserve, pulmonary disease, absence of albumin deficiency; hepatic or renal failure, dehydration, restricted sodium intake.

ADVERSE/SIDE EFFECTS. (Possibly due to allergy or protein overload): fever, chills, nausea, urticaria, rash, flushing, circulatory overload, pulmonary edema (with rapid infusion); hypotension, tachycardia, nausea, vomiting, increased salivation, headache, back pain, relative anemia (large doses).

ROUTE AND DOSAGE. Highly individualized according to patient's clinical response. **Adults and children (emergency): Intravenous:** Initial: 25 Gm repeated in 15 to 30 minutes, if necessary. Not to exceed 250 Gm of albumin (5 L of 5% solution or 1 L of 25% solution) in 48 hours. Whole blood or plasma usually prescribed if patient requires more. **Pediatric (nonemergency):** 25 to 50% of adult dose. Hyperbilirubinemia, erythroblastosis fetalis: 1 Gm/kg of 25% solution 1 or 2 hours before transfusion. **Premature:** hypoproteinemia (prophylaxis): 1.4 to 1.8 ml of 25% solution.

NURSING IMPLICATIONS

Albumin may be administered without regard to blood typing and crossmatching.

Albumin is a yellow or amber, clear, moderately viscous liquid. Solutions that show a sediment or appear turbid should not be used.

Note that albumin is supplied in two strengths: 5 and 25%.

In general the 5% solution is used for hypovolemic patients, whereas the more concentrated 25% solution is used when fluid (and sodium) intake must be restricted as in hypoproteinemia, cerebral edema, and in pediatric patients.

See manufacturer's instructions for proper use of provided administration set.

Once vial is opened, solution should be used within 4 hours since it contains no preservatives or antimicrobials. Discard unused portion.

As with any oncotically active solution, infusion rate should be relatively slow. Some patients may require monitoring of central venous pressure or pulmonary artery wedge pressure to evaluate vascular volume status.

Rate of infusion will depend on patient's age, diagnosis, clinical condition and response, and on concentration of solution. Specific flow rate should be ordered by physician.

Administration rate for hypovolemic shock: initially administered as rapidly as necessary to restore blood volume. When blood volume approaches normal, rate should be reduced to avoid circulatory overload and pulmonary edema. The 5% concentration is usually administered undiluted at rate of 2 to 4 ml/minute; the 25% concentration may be given diluted or undiluted no faster than 1 ml/minute.

Administration rate for patients with normal blood volume: 5% albumin human solution not to exceed 5 to 10 ml/minute; 25% solution not to exceed 2 or 3 ml/minute.

Reportedly, albumin may be administered in combination with or in conjunction with dextrose, sodium lactate, and sodium chloride injections, whole blood or plasma. Consult pharmacist for compatible IV infusion fluids.

Monitor blood pressure, pulse and respiration, and flow rate. Frequency of readings and dosage depend on patient's condition and clinical response. Flow rate adjustments may be required to avoid too rapid a rise in blood pressure.

Laboratory parameters used to monitor dosage of albumin include: *plasma albumin (normal:* 3.5 to 5 Gm/dl), *total protein (normal* 6 to 8.4 Gm/dl), Hgb, Hct, and serum electrolytes.

Observe patient closely during infusion for signs of circulatory overload (increased venous pressure, distended neck veins), and pulmonary edema: shortness of breath, cyanosis, persistent productive cough (frothy sputum may be blood-tinged), expiratory rales, restlessness, anxiety, increased heart rate, sense of chest pressure. If these signs and symptoms appear, slow the infusion rate just sufficiently to keep vein open, and report immediately to physician.

Make careful observations of patients with injuries or those who have had surgery in order to detect bleeding points that failed to bleed at lower blood pressure.

Monitor intake and output ratio and pattern. Report changes in urinary output. Increase in colloidal osmotic pressure by albumin usually causes mobilization of extracellular fluid and diuresis, which may persist 3 to 20 hours.

When albumin is given to patients with cerebral edema, fluids are generally withheld completely during succeeding 8 hours. Meticulous mouth care is indicated.

Intact containers may be stored at room temperature, but not exceeding 37°C (98.6°F).

Diagnostic Test Interferences. False rise in **alkaline phosphatase** when albumin is obtained partially from pooled placental plasma (levels reportedly decline over period of weeks).

ALBUTEROL

(Proventil, Salbutamol, Ventolin)

(al-byoo'-ter-ole)

Beta-adrenergic agonist (sympathomimetic)

Smooth muscle relaxant (respiratory)

Bronchodilator

ACTIONS AND USES. Moderately selective beta-2-adrenergic agonist with comparatively long action. Has more prominent effect on beta-2-receptors (particularly bronchial, uterine, and vascular smooth muscle, and mast cells) than on beta-1- (heart) and alpha-adrenergic receptors. Acts by stimulating the conversion of intracellular ATP (adenosine triphosphate) to cAMP (cyclic adenosine monophosphate), a mediator of cell responses including beta-adrenergic activity. Produces bronchodilation, regardless of administration route, by relaxing smooth muscles of bronchial tree. This decreases airway resistance, facilitates mucus drainage, and increases vital capacity. As effective as isoproterenol and metaproterenol, but produces more prolonged bronchodilation and causes little direct cardiac stimulation. Reportedly improved cardiac output due to lowered left ventricular afterload.

Used to relieve bronchospasm in patients with reversible obstructive airway disease (e.g., asthma). *Investigational Uses:* to prevent exercise-induced bronchospasm; as adjunct in treatment of refractory heart failure; to arrest preterm labor; and to stimulate intracellular transport of K in hyperkalemic familial periodic paralysis.

ABSORPTION AND FATE. Inhalation: Gradually absorbed from bronchi; (small swallowed portions absorbed from GI tract). Onset of bronchodilation in 5 to 15 minutes with physiologic effects related to topical action rather than to blood levels. Peak effect in ½ to 2 hours; duration: 3 to 6 hours; half-life: 3.8 hours. About 65 to 90% of dose excreted in urine within 24 hours, as unchanged drug (28%) and metabolite (44%). **Oral tablet:** Onset of bronchodilation within 30 minutes. Peak plasma levels in 2½ hours. Peak effect in 2 to 3 hours; duration: 4 to 6 or more hours; half-life: 2.7 to 5 hours; metabolized in liver. Approximately 76% of dose excreted in urine over 3 days (most is eliminated in first 24 hours). Apparently does not cross blood–brain barrier, but may cross placenta. Distribution to breast milk not known.

CONTRAINDICATIONS AND PRECAUTIONS. Safe use during pregnancy (category C), breast feeding, and in children below age 12 not established. *Cautious Use:* cardiovascular disease, hypertension, hyperthyroidism, diabetes mellitus, hypersensitivity to sympathomimetic amines or to fluorocarbon propellant used in inhalation aerosols.

ADVERSE/SIDE EFFECTS. CNS: tremor (most commonly with oral drug), dizziness, vertigo, stimulation, nervousness, restlessness, irritability, insomnia, weakness, headache, hallucinations, paranoia. **CV:** palpitation, increased or decreased blood pressure; reflex tachycardia, angina (with high doses). **GI:** nausea, vomiting, heartburn. **Other:** paradoxical bronchospasm, difficulty in voiding, unusual taste; hyperemia, drying and irritation of oropharynx; muscle cramps, aggravation of preexisting diabetes mellitus and ketoacidosis; inhibition of uterine contractions; hypokalemia (theoretically possible).

ROUTE AND DOSAGE. Adults and children (12 years and older): Metered spray: (albuterol): 2 inhalations repeated every 4 to 6 hours (each actuation delivers 90 mcg (0.09 mg) albuterol). **Oral tablet** (albuterol sulfate): initially, 2 mg three times daily, titrated to 2 to 4 mg three or four times daily, as necessary. **Elderly:** doses started at lower range and increased cautiously as needed.

NURSING IMPLICATIONS

Patient should receive explicit directions on use of medication and inhaler and follow them precisely. Review patient instruction sheet dispensed with medication. Caution patient to avoid contact of drug with eyes.

Summary of instructions for using metered dose inhalers:

- Shake container well before using.
- Place mouthpiece well into mouth and close lips firmly around it.
- Exhale (some clinicians advise exhaling normally; others direct patient to exhale a little more than normal). Clarify with physician.
- Take slow deep breath through mouth while actuating the inhaler.
- After holding breath as long as possible, remove mouthpiece and exhale slowly.
- Remove drug canister from inhaler assembly following treatment.
- Wash inhaler assembly with warm running water at least daily. Dry thoroughly.

If patient is to receive a second inhalation, check with physician about dose interval (may vary from 1 to 10 minutes). Spacing doses ensures maximum bronchial penetration by drug.

If patient is also receiving beclomethasone (Vanceril) inhalation treatments, albuterol should be administered 20 to 30 minutes before, to allow deeper penetration of beclomethasone into lungs, unless otherwise directed by physician.

Significant subjective improvement in pulmonary function should occur within 60 to 90 minutes after drug administration. Advise patient to notify physician if albuterol fails to provide relief. Reevaluation of patient's condition and therapy may be indicated.

All patients with asthma should have a thorough initial history and physical examination to help identify factors that provoke attacks.

Baseline and periodic evaluations of pulmonary function should be done to monitor patient's progress: forced expiratory volume in 1 second, (FEV_1), maximal midexpiratory flow (MMEF), peak flow rate, vital capacity (VC); and arterial blood gases to assess pH: Pco_2 and Po_2.

The most common adverse effect associated with the oral drug is fine tremor in fingers, which may interfere with precision handwork (believed to be caused by direct stimulation of skeletal muscles). Keep physician informed of any unusual symptoms.

Drug-induced dry mouth and throat may be relieved by rinsing mouth well with water immediately after each inhalation treatment.

If paradoxical bronchospasm (wheezing) occurs discontinue drug immediately, and notify physician.

Emphasize dangers of using self-prescribed OTC drugs without physician's approval. Many remedies (e.g., cold medicines) contain sympathomimetics that may intensify albuterol action.

The ideal approach in asthma management is to prevent relapses, to maintain good pulmonary function, and to provide prompt therapy when an emergency situation arises.

Advise patient to maintain optimal health in order to prevent an overlay of stress on respiratory tract: e.g., avoid crowds and individuals with known respiratory infections; adhere to immunization schedules for influenza and pneumonia.

Patient-Teaching Plan for COPD: Constructed in collaboration with physician, respiratory therapist, patient and responsible family member(s) should include the following guidelines and advice:

- ✓ Review of drug action and expected effects
- ✓ Importance of precise compliance with drug regimen
- ✓ Avoid environmental irritants (e.g., dust, smoke, animal dander, sprays, feathers)
- ✓ Maintain optimum environmental humidification, especially in winter
- ✓ Avoid temperature extremes
- ✓ Planned rest and physical reconditioning program; balanced diet
- ✓ Prevent respiratory tract infections
- ✓ No smoking
- ✓ Keep follow-up appointments
- ✓ Carry medical identification (e.g., Medic Alert)

Albuterol tablets should be stored between 2° and 30°C (36° and 86°F) in tight, light-resistant container, unless otherwise directed by manufacturer.

Store canisters between 15° and 30°C (59° and 86°F) away from heat and direct sunlight. Since contents of inhalers are under pressure, do not puncture and never throw container into incinerator or fire for disposal.

Diagnostic Test Interferences. Transient small increases in **plasma glucose** may occur.

Drug Interactions: Albuterol

Plus	Interactions
Epinephrine (Adrenalin) and other adrenergic aerosol bronchodilators	Possibility of additive effects. Concurrent use not recommended
MAO inhibitors, tricyclic antidepressants	Potentiate albuterol action on vascular system
Propranolol (Inderal) and other beta-adrenergic blocking agents	Mutual inhibitory effect

ALCOHOL IN DEXTROSE INFUSION

(5% or 10% Alcohol and 5% Dextrose in Water)

Caloric agent
Tocolytic

ACTIONS AND USES. Intravenous alcohol (Ethanol) lowers concentration of oxytocin in maternal blood. Precise mechanism of tocolytic action unknown. Appears to act by suppressing release of hypophyseal oxytocin and by altering myometrial membrane sensitivity, thus inhibiting myometrial contractions. Reportedly inferior to other tocolytics, e.g., ritodrine, terbutaline. Not effective in blocking labor after membranes have ruptured, or after full cervical effacement or dilatation of more than 3 cm has occurred. Alcohol may cause marked diuresis by suppressing antidiuretic hormone (ADH). Dextrose, a monosaccharide, provides 3.4 calories/Gm and alcohol provides 5.6 calories/ml. The commercially prepared 5% alcohol, 5% dextrose in water supplies 450 calories/L; the 10% alcohol and 5% dextrose in water supplies 750 calories/L. Metabolism rate for alcohol is 10 to 20 ml/hour. Sedative effects occur if infusion rate exceeds rate of alcohol metabolism. Dextrose can be infused up to 0.5 to 0.85 Gm/kg/hour without producing significant glycosuria.

Used to increase caloric intake. Also, widely used to prevent or delay premature labor.

ABSORPTION AND FATE. Alcohol is metabolized in liver to acetaldehyde or acetate. (Metabolism rate is increased by starvation and decreased by insulin.) Promptly crosses placenta and enters fetal circulation. Excreted in breast milk.

CONTRAINDICATIONS AND PRECAUTIONS. Epilepsy, urinary tract infection, alcohol addiction, diabetic coma. Safe use during pregnancy not established (category C). *Cautious Use:* renal or liver impairment, subclinical or overt diabetes mellitus; shock, postpartum hemorrhage, following cranial surgery; gout, porphyria.

ADVERSE/SIDE EFFECTS. **In large doses or if infused too rapidly:** sedation, inebriation (alcohol breath, nausea, vomiting, vertigo, ataxia, disorientation, restlessness, stupor, flushing, fever, maternal and fetal hypotension; acidosis, impaired gag reflex, hypoglycemia, hypervolemia, pulmonary edema, respiratory depression); marked diuresis, abnormal bone marrow morphology (prematures). **Local reactions:** pain, tissue irritation at injection site, venous thrombosis, phlebitis. **With prolonged therapy:** vitamin deficiencies, liver function alterations, increase in serum uric acid, precipitation of acute gout, and acute intermittent porphyria.

ROUTE AND DOSAGE. **Intravenous infusion only:** *Parenteral nutrient* (5% solution): **Adults:** 1 to 2 L; rarely exceeds 3 L/24 hours. **Children:** 40 ml/kg/24 hours or 350 to 1000 ml depend ing on size and clinical response. *To inhibit preterm labor* (10% solution): 7.5 ml/kg/hour for 2 hours, then maintenance: 1.5 ml/kg/hour until uterine contractions have stopped for several hours (up to 10 hours). Some clinicians limit treatment to maximum of three courses.

NURSING IMPLICATIONS

IV infusion is made into the largest available peripheral vein, using a small bore needle. Administered slowly.

Use solution only if it is clear and seal was intact. Discard unused portions.

Sedative effect (CNS depression) and glycosuria can be minimized by controlling rate of infusion *(see Actions and Uses).* Observe and report onset of restlessness, reduced responsiveness, or other changes in mental status.

Alcohol can cause increase in gastric secretions and impairment of gag reflex. Aspiration is a constant danger particularly in the elderly. If patient complains of nausea, foods and fluids should be withheld temporarily. Have suction equipment readily available.

Patients with diabetes require close monitoring to avoid loss of blood sugar control.
Observe injection site for signs of extravasation. IV infusion should be interrupted immediately if it occurs.
Fluid, electrolyte, and acid–base balance, and blood sugar should be monitored during therapy.

Drug Interactions: Alcohol in dextrose

Plus	Interactions
Antidiabetic agents	Potentiation of hypoglycemic action. Hyperglycemia also reported with sulfonylureas
Antihypertensive agents	May potentiate hypotensive effects
Barbiturates and other CNS depressants	Possibility of additive CNS depression
Cimetidine (Tagamet)	May cause increase in plasma alcohol levels
Cefamandole (Mandol) Cefoperazone (Cefobid) Disulfiram (Antabuse) Metronidazole (Flagyl) Moxalactam (Moxam) Sulfonylureas Tolazoline (Priscoline)	Disulfiram (antabuse)-like reaction is a possibility (flushing, headache, palpitation, nausea, confusion)

—PROTOTYPE

ALLOPURINOL

(al-oh-pure′i-nole)

(Alloprin, Apo-Allopurinol, Lopurin, Novopurol, Purinol, Roucol, Zyloprim)

Antigout agent; enzyme inhibitor; antilithic

ACTIONS AND USES. In contrast to uricosuric agents, which act by increasing renal excretion of uric acid, allopurinol reduces endogenous uric acid by selectively inhibiting action of xanthine oxidase, enzyme responsible for converting hypoxanthine to xanthine and xanthine to uric acid (end product of purine metabolism). Thus, urate pool is decreased by the lowering of both serum and urinary uric acid levels, resorption of tophaceous deposits begins, and hyperuricosuria is prevented. Has no analgesic, antiinflammatory, or uricosuric actions; therefore not useful for acute gouty attack and may actually aggravate and prolong it. May inhibit hepatic microsomal enzymes and thus affect metabolism of certain drugs. Unlike uricosuric agents, action is not antagonized by salicylates.

Used to control primary hyperuricemia that accompanies severe tophaceous gout complicated by advanced renal insufficiency or uric renal calculi. Has been used to prevent other types of recurrent renal calculi. Also used prophylactically for secondary hyperuricemia, a potential of antineoplastic and radiation therapies (both of which greatly increase plasma uric acid levels by promoting nucleic acid degradation), myeloproliferative neoplastic diseases (e.g., leukemia, lymphoma, sarcoma), Lesch-Nyhan syndrome, polycythemia vera, G6PD deficiency, and therapy with thiazides or ethambutol.

ABSORPTION AND FATE. Approximately 80% of oral dose is absorbed. Plasma level peaks in 2 to 4 hours. Widely distributed to all extracellular fluid; less concentration in brain. Not bound to plasma proteins. Rapidly cleared from plasma (probable half-life 2 to 3 hours). About 5 to 7% of dose excreted unchanged in urine within 6 hours; 20% eliminated unchanged in feces within 48 to 72 hours. Remainder rapidly metabolized to active metabolites, chiefly oxypurinol (half-life of 18 to 30 hours) thought to be primarily responsible for xanthine oxidase inhibition. Metabolite is excreted slowly; therefore, it may accumulate with chronic administration of allopurinol.

CONTRAINDICATIONS AND PRECAUTIONS. Hypersensitivity to allopurinol as initial treatment for acute gouty attacks, idiopathic hemochromatosis (or those with family history), children (except those with hyperuricemia secondary to neoplastic disease and chemotherapy). Safe use during pregnancy or in fertile women and nursing mothers not established. *Cautious Use:* impaired hepatic or renal function, history of peptic ulcer, lower GI tract disease, bone marrow depression.

ADVERSE/SIDE EFFECTS. **GI:** nausea, vomiting, metallic taste, diarrhea, abdominal discomfort, precipitation of peptic ulcer. **Hematologic:** agranulocytosis (fever, sore throat, unusual fatigue, malaise), anemia, aplastic anemia, transient leukopenia or leukocytosis, bone marrow depression, pancytopenia, thrombocytopenia. **Hypersensitivity or idiosyncracy (rare):** fever, chills, stomatitis, dysphagia, oliguria, pyelonephritis, dermatitis, vasculitis, polyarteritis, necrotizing angiitis (rare); arthralgia, permanent deafness, congestive heart failure, eosinophilia. **Neurologic:** drowsiness, headache, vertigo, peripheral neuritis (numbness, tingling, pain, weakness of hands and feet). **Ophthalmic:** retinopathy, macular degeneration, cataracts (may accompany severe dermatitis). **Skin (possibly indications of hypersensitivity):** pruritic maculopapular rash (common); exfoliative, urticarial, and purpural dermatitis; erythema multiforme including Stevens-Johnson syndrome; toxic epidermal necrolysis, alopecia (rare); severe furunculosis of nose, ichthyosis. **Other:** lymphadenopathy, lymphedema, tachycardia, xanthine renal calculi, especially in children with Lesch-Nyhan syndrome; pancreatitis, hepatotoxicity, hyperlipemia, adrenal insufficiency; precipitation of acute gout.

ROUTE AND DOSAGE. Highly individualized; dosage adjusted on basis of serum uric acid levels and renal function. Manufacturer recommends dividing doses greater than 300 mg. **Oral: Adults:** *Gout:* initially 100 mg for 3 or 4 days, increased by 100 mg increments at weekly intervals until serum urate falls to 6 mg/dl or less or until maximal dosage of 800 mg daily is reached. Maintenance: 300 mg as a single daily dose. *Secondary hyperuricemia:* 200 to 800 mg daily for 2 or 3 days or longer. **Pediatric (Children 6 to 10 years):** 100 mg three times daily or 300 mg as single daily dose; **(Children under 6 years):** 50 mg three times daily.

NURSING IMPLICATIONS

Generally the drug is best tolerated when taken following meals. If necessary, tablet may be crushed before administration and taken with fluid or mixed with food.

When used to prevent secondary hyperuricemia associated with antineoplastic therapy, allopurinol should be prescribed 1 or 2 days before chemotherapy begins.

Instruct patient to report promptly the onset of itching or rash especially if ampicillin is prescribed concurrently, or any other unusual sign or symptom *(See Adverse/Side Effects).*

A skin rash, which may appear after 1 to 5 weeks (and reportedly even after 2 years) of therapy, is the most common adverse reaction and is an indication to stop drug therapy.

Hypersensitivity reaction (sometimes fatal) has followed the onset of a skin rash. It commonly occurs in patients with impaired renal function and is generally accompanied by malaise, fever, and aching.

Patients with renal disorders should be closely monitored for any further deterioration of kidney function. These patients tend to have a higher than usual incidence of renal stones and dermatologic (hypersensitivity) problems.

Advise patient to minimize exposure and to shield eyes from ultraviolet or sunlight. Ultraviolet light may stimulate the development of cataracts. Patients should be examined periodically for lens changes.

Aim of therapy is to lower serum urate level gradually to about 6 mg/dl. Serum uric acid levels should be evaluated at least every 1 to 2 weeks to check adequacy of dosage. A sudden decrease in serum uric acid can precipitate an acute gouty attack.

Baseline complete blood counts and liver and kidney function tests should be performed before initiating therapy and monthly, particularly during first few months of therapy.

Acute gouty attacks are most likely to occur during first 6 weeks of allopurinol therapy, possibly because of mobilization of urates from tissue deposits. Concurrent maintenance therapy with colchicine may be prescribed, as prophylaxis, for the first 3 to 6 months of allopurinol therapy.

When allopurinol is prescribed for patient who has been taking a uricosuric, dose of the latter should be reduced slowly over several weeks while allopurinol is being increased gradually to desired dose.

Allopurinol may cause drowsiness and vertigo. Caution patient to avoid driving or performing other complex tasks until reaction to drug has been evaluated.

It is advisable to maintain fluid intake sufficient to produce urinary output of at least 2000 ml daily (fluid intake of at least 3000 ml daily) and to keep urine neutral or slightly alkaline by oral administration of sodium bicarbonate or potassium citrate. These measures are prescribed to reduce risk of xanthine stone formation.

Intake-output ratio and pattern should be monitored. Since allopurinol and metabolites are excreted chiefly by kidneys, decreased renal function causes drug accumulation. Instruct patient to report diminishing urinary output, cloudy urine, unusual color or odor to urine, pain or discomfort on urination.

A rigid low purine diet is not usually prescribed for patients with gout. However, physician may advise patient to omit or limit certain of these high purine foods: organ meats (e.g., kidney, liver, sweetbreads, brains), anchovies, sardines, salmon, meat soups, gravies, lentils, dried peas and beans.

Weight reduction may be prescribed and should be undertaken slowly and during quiescent phase of the disease to avoid precipitating a gouty attack *(see Colchicine).*

Food–Drug Interaction: Excessive alcohol or coffee consumption can cause secondary hyperuricemia and therefore should be avoided.

Allopurinol is generally continued indefinitely. Advise patient to remain under medical supervision. The drug can cause severe adverse reactions.

Therapeutic response to allopurinol is indicated by normal serum and urinary uric acid levels (usually by 1 to 3 weeks), gradual decrease in size of tophi, absence of new tophaceous deposits (after approximately 6 months), with consequent relief of joint pain and increased joint mobility.

Store at room temperature preferably between 15° and 30°C (59° and 86°F) in a well-closed container.

Teaching Plan for Patient with Chronic Gout: *See Colchicine*

Diagnostic Test Interferences. Possibility of elevated blood levels of **alkaline phosphatase** and **serum transaminases** (AST, ALT), and decreased blood **Hct, Hgb, leukocytes.**

Drug Interactions: Allopurinol

Plus	Interactions
Alcohol (Ethanol)	Excessive alcohol promotes formation of lactic acid and ketone bodies which inhibit renal excretion of uric acid
Ampicillin	Increased risk of skin rash
Anticoagulants, oral	Enhanced anticoagulant effects. (Allopurinol inhibits hepatic drug metabolizing enzymes.) May require lower anticoagulant dosage
Azathioprine (Imuran)	Increased toxicity (Azathioprine metabolism depends on xanthine oxidase). Generally prescribe lower initial azathioprine dosage
Chlorpropamide	Hypoglycemic effects increased (chlorpropamide excretion decreased). Monitor for excessive hypoglycemia
Cyclophosphamide	Potentiates cyclophosphamide. Monitor closely for bone marrow depression
Diuretics	May interfere with renal excretion of uric acid
Iron preparations	Increased hepatic deposition of iron (based on animal studies)
Mercaptopurine (Purinethol)	Increased risk of mercaptopurine toxicity (metabolism depends on xanthine oxidase)
Phenytoin (Dilantin), and other hydantoins	Possibility of increased phenytoin effects. (Allopurinol inhibits hepatic drug metabolism)
Probenecid (Benemid, Probalan)	Allopurinol inhibits probenecid metabolism. Probenecid reduces allopurinol effect by enhancing urinary excretion of its active metabolite
Pyrazinamide	May interfere with renal excretion of uric acid
Theophylline	Theophylline toxicity increases with high allopurinol dosages. (Allopurinol inhibits hepatic drug metabolism)
Thiazides (and possibly other diuretics)	Increased risk of allopurinol toxicity and hypersensitivity (especially with impaired renal function). Monitor renal and hepatic function
Tamoxifen (Nolvadex)	Possibility of hepatotoxicity
Vitamin C (Ascorbic acid) in large doses, and other urinary acidifiers	May increase possibility of renal calculi
Vidarabine (Vira-A)	Increased vidarabine toxicity (reduced drug metabolism). Concurrent use generally avoided

---

ALPHAPRODINE

(Nisentil)

(al-fa-proe′-deen)
Narcotic analgesic (opiate agonist)
C II

ACTION AND USES. Synthetic phenylpiperidine derivative chemically and pharmacologically similar to meperidine (qv), but produces more rapid onset of action, greater sedation and analgesia, and has shorter duration of effect. Acts principally on CNS. Like meperidine, also increases smooth muscle tone and spasm and demonstrates some anticholinergic and histamine-releasing properties.

Used for sedation and analgesia in minor surgery, urologic examinations and procedures, for obstetric analgesia, and preoperatively in major surgery. May be administered with atropine or scopolamine or as supplement with nerve block or inhalation anesthesia. Used in children via submucosal route only, for analgesia during dental procedures.

ABSORPTION AND FATE. Following SC injection, onset of action in 5 to 10 minutes; duration 1 to 2 or more hours (depending on dose). Onset of action following IV administration in 1 to 2 minutes; duration 30 to 90 minutes. Half-life: 2.2 hours. Metabolized chiefly in liver. Rapidly excreted, mainly in urine as free drug and metabolites. Crosses placenta. Distribution into breast milk not known.

CONTRAINDICATIONS AND PRECAUTIONS. Severe CNS or respiratory depression; pulmonary edema resulting from chemical respiratory irritants; for relief of chronic pain; pregnancy (category C). Safe use in children except for dental procedures not established. *Cautious Use:* increased intracranial pressure, head injury, bronchial asthma, alcoholism, COPD, cor pulmonale, cardiac arrhythmias, impaired renal or hepatic function, history of convulsions; gallstones, gallbladder disease, ureteral structure, prostatic hypertrophy, urinary tract surgery, Addison's disease, hypothyroidism; critically ill, debilitated patients; the very young or the elderly.

ADVERSE/SIDE EFFECTS. CNS: dizziness, light-headedness, unusual fatigue, drowsiness, sedation, headache, tremors, uncoordinated muscle movements, euphoria, dysphoria, confusion, mental depression, excitement, especially in children (paradoxical reaction); hallucinations, **CV:** flushing, hypotension, palpitation, tachycardia, bradycardia, syncope. **GI:** nausea, vomiting, constipation, dry mouth, anorexia, abdominal cramps, biliary tract spasm. **Hypersensitivity:** rash, hives, pruritus; wheal and flare at IV site; bronchoconstriction, laryngeal edema, anaphylactoid reaction (especially with rapid IV). **Ophthalmic:** blurred vision, diplopia, constricted pupils (overdosage). **Respiratory:** shortness of breath, slow or irregular respiratory rate, respiratory depression. **Other:** urinary retention, oliguria, diaphoresis, pain and tissue irritation at SC injection site, phlebitis. For other possible but not reported adverse reactions, *see Meperidine.*

ROUTE AND DOSAGE. Adults: Intravenous: 0.4 to 0.6 mg/kg administered slowly. Initial dose not to exceed 30 mg IV. If required, one-fourth of the initial dose given after 15 minutes. **Subcutaneous:** 0.4 to 1.2 mg/kg. Initial dose not to exceed 60 mg SC. If required one-fourth of the initial dose given after 30 minutes. During labor, repeated as necessary at 2-hour intervals. Total dose by either route not to exceed 240 mg/24 hours. **Pediatric dentistry: Submucosal:** 0.3 to 0.6 mg/kg. Lower dosage range in very old, very young, debilitated or very ill patients.

NURSING IMPLICATIONS

Whenever alphaprodine is to be administered, a narcotic antagonist such as naloxone (Narcan) and equipment and personnel necessary for assisted or controlled ventilation should be immediately available.

Submucosal injection (used in pediatric dentistry), has been associated with fatalities resulting from CNS or respiratory depression. If necessary, drug action can be reversed at any time by administration of naloxone (Narcan).

Patients receiving the drug IV should be lying down. Monitor respiratory and cardiac function. Advise patient to remain recumbent for at least 1½ hours, unless otherwise directed by physician, to reduce risk of hypotension, light-headedness, dizziness, nausea, and vomiting.

Close monitoring of respirations (ability to deep breathe and sigh), pulse, and blood pressure is particularly essential with IV administration or when given to elderly, very young, debilitated patients, or to patients with pulmonary disease.

A comparatively high incidence of hypotension, lightheadedness, and nausea occurring in ambulatory patients may be alleviated by having patient lie supine.

IM administration is not recommended because absorption from muscle is erratic and unpredictable.

When administered to provide analgesia during labor, alphaprodine is given after cervical dilation has begun. Neonates must be closely observed for signs of CNS or respiratory depression.

Monitor intake and output ratio and pattern in patients receiving repeated doses. Report oliguria or urinary retention. Palpate for full bladder.

Alphaprodine is contraindicated for chronic pain because of its short duration of action. Tolerance, physical and psychologic dependence (morphine type) can develop with repeated use.

Warn patient to avoid driving or other potentially hazardous activities, at least for duration of drug action.

Classified as Schedule II drug under the Federal Controlled Substances Act.

Stored at controlled room temperature, preferably between 15° and 30°C (59° and 86°F) unless otherwise directed by manufacturer. Do not use discolored solutions or solutions with particulate sediment.

Diagnostic Test Interferences. Alphaprodine can cause increased **CSF,** increased plasma **amylase** and plasma **lipase** for up to 24 hours after drug administration.

Drug Interactions: Alphaprodine

Plus	Interactions
Alcohol Anesthetics (general) Barbiturates and other sedative-hypnotics Cimetidine (Tagamet) MAO inhibitors Narcotic analgesics, other skeletal muscle relaxants Psychotropics	Potentiation of CNS depression; possibility of cerebral damage. Alphaprodine used with extreme caution (if at all) and in reduced dosage

---

ALPRAZOLAM

(Xanax)

(al-pray'-zoe-lam)
Psychotropic; anxiolytic
Benzodiazepine
C IV

ACTIONS AND USES. Shares CNS depressant actions of other benzodiazepines, but compared to most drugs of this group, duration of activity is relatively short and associated with significantly less drowsiness. Has antidepressant as well as anxiolytic actions.

Used in management of anxiety disorders or for short-term relief of anxiety symptoms. Also used as adjunct in management of anxiety associated with depression, and for panic disorders, such as agoraphobia.

ABSORPTION AND FATE. Rapidly and well absorbed following oral administration. Peak blood levels in 1 to 2 hours. Protein binding about 80%. Half-life: 12 to 15 hours (in elderly males may be 19 to 20 hours). Oxidative metabolism in liver results in few metabolites, therefore drug accumulation is minimal. Steady state plasma levels usually achieved within 2 or 3 days. Unchanged drug and metabolites excreted rapidly, principally in urine. Probably crosses placenta; enters breast milk.

CONTRAINDICATIONS AND PRECAUTIONS. Sensitivity to benzodiazepines; acute narrow angle glaucoma; use alone in primary depression or psychotic disorders; during pregnancy (category D), fertile women, nursing mothers, children below age 18. *Cautious Use:* impaired renal or hepatic function; history of alcoholism; geriatric and debilitated patients. Effectiveness of alprazolam for long-term treatment (beyond 4 months) not established.

ADVERSE/SIDE EFFECTS. **CNS:** drowsiness, light-headedness, dizziness, syncope, headache, confusion, fatigue, depression, nervousness, clumsiness, unsteadiness, rigidity, tremor, restlessness (akathisia), paradoxical excitement, insomnia, hallucinations, muscle spasticity. **CV:** tachycardia, palpitation, hypotension. **GI:** constipation, diarrhea, nausea, vomiting, increased salivation, dry mouth. **Skin:** dermatitis, itching (allergy). **Other:** nasal congestion, weight gain or loss, blurred vision. *See Chlordiazepoxide for additional adverse/side effects.*

ROUTE AND DOSAGE. **Oral:** Initial, 0.25 to 0.5 mg three times daily. Total dose not to exceed 4 mg/day in divided doses. Highly individualized. **Elderly and debilitated patients, patients with liver disease or low serum albumin:** Initial: 0.25 mg two or three times daily; gradually increased if necessary and tolerated.

NURSING IMPLICATIONS

Alprazolam is not intended for management of anxieties and minor distresses associated with everyday life. Ideally, diagnosis of underlying difficulties should be attempted before drug is prescribed.

Oversedation, drowsiness, unsteadiness, light-headedness, and other adverse reactions, which may occur during early high dose therapy, usually disappear with continuing therapy. Advise patient to keep physician informed; dosage adjustments may be indicated. Note implications especially for elderly and debilitated patients (bedsides; supervise ambulation).

Warn patient that alprazolam will potentiate effects of alcoholic beverages and other CNS depressants *(see Drug Interactions).* Caution patient not to use OTC medications containing antihistamines (sleep aids, cold, hayfever or allergy remedies) without consulting physician.

Advise patient to avoid driving and other potentially hazardous activities until reaction to drug is determined.

Patients receiving continuing therapy should have periodic blood counts, urinalyses, and blood chemistry studies.

Need for further therapy should be reassessed at least in 4 months. (Effectiveness of alprazolam and other benzodiazepines beyond this period has not been established.)

Following continuous use, dosage should be tapered off before drug is stopped. Abrupt discontinuation of drug may cause withdrawal symptoms (nausea, vomiting, abdominal and muscle cramps, sweating, confusion, tremors, convulsions).

Classified as Schedule IV drug under the Federal Controlled Substances Act.

Psychic and physical dependence may occur with large doses given over prolonged periods of time.

Store in tightly-covered, light-resistant containers preferably between 15° and 30°C (59° and 86°F), unless otherwise directed by manufacturer.

Drug Interactions: Alprazolam

Plus	Interactions
Alcohol (Ethanol) and other CNS depressants: anticonvulsants, antihistamines, barbiturates, narcotic analgesics, other psychotropics	Additive CNS depression: increased sedation, impaired psychomotor performance
Cimetidine (Tagamet) Disulfiram (Antabuse)	Increased alprazolam effects especially excessive sedation (decreased alprazolam metabolism). Lower alprazolam dose may be indicated
Oral contraceptives	Increased or decreased alprazolam effects (altered hepatic metabolism)
Rifampin (Rifadin, Rimactane) Valproic acid (Depakene)	Decreased alprazolam effect (increased metabolism). Higher alprazolam dose may be indicated

See also Chlordiazepoxide, prototype benzodiazepine, for additional possible interactions.

ALPROSTADIL

(al-pross'-ta-dil)

(PGE_1, Prostaglandin E, Prostin VR Pediatric)

Ductus arteriosus patency adjunct
Hormone
Prostaglandin

ACTIONS AND USES. Naturally occurring substance derived from fatty acids. Pharmacologic actions include vasodilation, inhibition of platelet aggregation, and stimulation of intestinal and uterine smooth muscles. Preserves ductal patency by relaxing smooth muscle of ductus arteriosus. This results in improved oxygenation of blood and perfusion of lower body of neonates with certain congenital cardiac anomalies, e.g., cyanotic heart disease (pulmonary atresia and stenosis, tricuspid atresia, tetralogy of Fallot, transposition of great arteries); and noncyanotic heart disease (interruption of the aortic arch, coarctation of aorta, aortic atresia). In high doses, lowers blood pressure by reducing peripheral resistance. Heart rate and cardiac output may rise reflexly.

Used as temporary measure to maintain patency of ductus arteriosus in infants with ductal dependent congenital heart defects, until corrective surgery can be performed.

ABSORPTION AND FATE. Onset of action in cyanotic congenital heart disease: 15 to 30 minutes; noncyanotic congenital heart disease: 1½ to 3 hours. Rapidly and completely metabolized. Approximately 68 to 80% metabolized (primarily by oxidation) in "one pass" through lungs. Metabolites excreted chiefly by kidneys within 24 hours.

CONTRAINDICATIONS AND PRECAUTIONS. Respiratory distress syndrome (hyaline membrane disease). *Cautious Use:* bleeding tendencies.

ADVERSE/SIDE EFFECTS. CNS: fever, apnea, seizures; (less frequent): cerebral bleeding, hyperextension of neck, hyperirritability, hypothermia, jitteriness, lethargy, stiffness. **CV:** flushing (most commonly with intraarterial administration), bradycardia, hypotension, tachycardia, cardiac arrest, edema; (less frequent): congestive heart failure, hyperemia, second degree heart block, spasm of right ventricle infundibulum, supraventricular tachycardia, ventricular fibrillation, shock. **GI:** diarrhea, gastric regurgitation. **Hematologic:** disseminated intravascular clotting (DIC); (infrequent): anemia, hyperbilirubinemia, thrombocytopenia. **Renal:** (infrequent): oliguria, anuria, hematuria. **Respiratory:** (infrequent): bradypnea, wheezing, hypercapnia, tachypnea, respiratory distress, respiratory depression. **Skeletal:** cortical proliferation of long bones, pain and swelling around bones (reversible following drug withdrawal). **Other:** sepsis, hypokalemia; (infrequent): peritonitis, bleeding, hypoglycemia. **Overdosage:** apnea, bradycardia, pyrexia, hypotension, flushing.

ROUTE AND DOSAGE. **Intravenous:** Continuous IV infusion (preferred route) into large vein; **Intraarterial** (through umbilical artery catheter placed in ductal opening). **Intraaortic:** Infusion rate: initial: 0.05 to 0.1 mcg/kg/minute. With therapeutic response, rate is reduced to lowest effective dosage level; with unsatisfactory response, rate is increased gradually to 0.2 mcg/kg/minute, up to 0.4 mcg/kg/minute.

NURSING IMPLICATIONS

Administered only by trained clinicians in facilities fully equipped to provide intensive care and immediate ventilatory assistance.

Arterial pressure is measured intermittently throughout infusion by umbilical cord catheter, auscultation, or with Doppler transducer. Also monitor respiratory status, temperature, and pulse throughout therapy.

Infusion rate should be reduced immediately if arterial pressure drops significantly or if fever occurs. If apnea or bradycardia occurs, infusion should be discontinued promptly.

Cardiovascular and CNS symptoms, including apnea, reportedly occur more frequently in neonates weighing less than 2 kg (4.4 lb) at birth, during first hour of drug infusion.

Flushing (peripheral arterial vasodilation) is usually controlled by repositioning catheter (by qualified personnel).

Prolonged infusion not recommended because it increases risk of ductal rupture by contributing to its fragility, and increases risk of damage to pulmonary artery and aorta.

Summary of monitoring that should be done intermittently throughout the infusion for all patients receiving alprostadil: (1) arterial pressure; (2) arterial blood gases Po_2 and Pco_2; (3) arterial blood pH; (4) ECG; (5) heart and respiratory rate, and rectal temperature.

Patients with aortic arch abnormalities should also be monitored for systemic blood pressure, pulmonary artery and descending aorta pressures, return of palpable femoral pulse, and urinary output.

Therapeutic response in infants with cyanotic heart disease (restricted pulmonary blood flow) is indicated by increase in blood oxygenation (Po_2) usually evident within 30 minutes. *(Normal Po_2 for neonates is 60 to 70 mm Hg.)*

Therapeutic response in infants with restricted systemic blood flow is indicated by increased pH in those with acidosis; increased systemic blood pressure and urinary output, return of palpable pulses, and decreased ratio of pulmonary artery to aortic pressure.

Infusion solution is prepared by diluting 500 mcg alprostadil with sodium chloride or dextrose injection to volume appropriate for pump delivery system being used. Prepare fresh solution every 24 hours. Discard unused portions.

Store alprostadil between 2° and 8°C (36° and 46°F) unless otherwise directed by manufacturer. Protect from freezing.

ALSEROXYLON
(Rauwiloid)

(al-ser-ox'i-lon)
Antihypertensive
Rauwolfia alkaloid

ACTIONS AND USES. Fat soluble mixture of alkaloids derived from *Rauwolfia serpentina.* Contains reserpine (1 mg is approximately equivalent to 0.1 mg reserpine). Similar to reserpine (qv) in actions, uses, contraindications, and adverse reactions. May lower convulsive threshold.

Used alone or with a diuretic in treatment of mild essential hypertension, or adjunctively with other antihypertensive agents for more severe forms.

ABSORPTION AND FATE. Slow onset of action; sustained duration of effects. Crosses placenta and appears in breast milk.

CONTRAINDICATIONS AND PRECAUTIONS. Patients with known hypersensitivity to rauwolfia alkaloids; mental depression, especially with suicidal tendencies; patients receiving electroshock therapy; glaucoma, active peptic ulcer, ulcerative colitis, gallstones, epilepsy. Safe use during pregnancy and lactation not established. *Cautious Use:* severe cardiac or cerebrovascular disease. *See also Reserpine.*

ADVERSE/SIDE EFFECTS. CNS: drowsiness, lethargy, fatigue, mental depression, insomnia, nightmares, increased headaches, nervousness, anxiety. **CV:** anginalike symptoms, bradycardia, skin flushing, dizziness, orthostatic hypotension (infrequent with recommended dosage). **EENT:** pinpoint pupils (overdose), nasal congestion, dry mouth. **GI:** nausea, vomiting, diarrhea, increased gastric secretion, peptic ulcer, weight gain (sodium and water retention if diuretic is not given concomitantly). **Other:** impotence. *See also Reserpine.*

ROUTE AND DOSAGE. Oral: Initial: 1 to 4 Gm daily, in single or divided doses. Maintenance: 2 mg or less daily.

NURSING IMPLICATIONS

Advise patient to take alseroxylon with meals or milk and at the same time each day.

Adjustments in dosage are made every 7 to 14 days, if necessary, because of long drug half-life *(see Reserpine: Absorption and Fate).*

Blood pressure and pulse should be monitored closely when alseroxylon is given with other antihypertensive drugs.

Caution patient to avoid potentially hazardous activities such as driving, until reaction of drug is known.

The drug should be discontinued at the first sign of mental depression (e.g., loss of appetite, self deprecation, dejection, early morning insomnia). Drug-induced depression may persist for several months after drug withdrawal and may be severe enough to result in suicidal tendencies.

Unusual headaches, fatigue, anxiety, nightmares, and impotence should be reported to physician. Dosage adjustment or drug withdrawal may be indicated.

Nasal stuffiness commonly occurs and should be reported to physician if it persists. Caution patient not to use OTC nasal decongestants without consulting the physician or pharmacist (may contain an adrenergic agent that can raise blood pressure).

Instruct patient to check ankles and legs daily for edema and to monitor weight. Report unusual weight gain to physician.

Advise patient to remain under medical care. Blood pressure and serum electrolytes should be checked at periodic intervals.

The commercial preparation Rauwiloid contains tartrazine, which can cause an allergic type reaction including asthma in susceptible individuals. It occurs frequently in persons with aspirin hypersensitivity.

See Reserpine (prototype Rauwolfia alkaloid) for: Nursing Implications, including teaching plan for patients with hypertension.

Diagnostic Test Interferences. *See Reserpine.*

Drug Interactions. *See Reserpine.*

ALUMINUM ACETATE SOLUTION

Antipruritic (topical)
Astringent

(Acid Mantle, Burow's Solution, Otic Domeboro)
(Modified Burow's Solution: Bluboro, Domeboro, Pedi-Boro)

ACTIONS AND USES. Prepared from aluminum subacetate and glacial acetic acid. Modified Burow's solution contains aluminum sulfate and calcium acetate. Has antiinflammatory, antipruritic, mild astringent, and antiseptic properties. Reportedly maintains protective acidity of skin.

Used in treatment of mildly irritated or inflamed skin and mucous membranes associated with, e.g., diaper rash, insect bites, poison ivy, athlete's foot, acne, allergy, eczema, otitis externa, bruises, anal pruritus. Also has been used as astringent gargle, as irrigating solution to remove tissue debris, and for soaks, douche, and sitz bath.

ROUTE AND DOSAGE. Topical (wet dressings): 1:10 to 1:40 solution. Applied for 15 to 30 minutes at 4- to 8-hour intervals. **Gargle:** 1:10 solution. **Otic preparation** (Otic Domeboro): 4 to 6 drops instilled slowly along wall of external ear. Repeat every 2 or 3 hours. Cream, lotion, and solution preparations available.

NURSING IMPLICATIONS

Buro-Sol powder: 1 packet (2.36 Gm) in 1 pint of water produces 1:15 clear Burow's solution. Domeboro or Bluboro: 1 packet or 1 tablet in 1 pint of water produces a *modified* 1:40 Burow's solution.

Following instillation of otic preparation (e.g., Otic Domeboro), have patient maintain position with affected ear uppermost for about 2 minutes. If physician prescribes an ear wick, solution may be added to wick as often as directed.

For wet dressings, warm or cold solution (as ordered) may be carefully poured on dressing at prescribed intervals. May be bandaged lightly and loosely, but do not cover with plastic or other occlusive material without consulting the physician.

Protect eyes from solution.

Use should be discontinued if irritation or extension of inflammatory condition occurs.

Burow's and modified Burow's solutions have limited compatibility with vitamin A, neomycin, and other water soluble antibiotics.

The activity of products containing benzalkonium chloride (qv) e.g., Buro-Sol, is antagonized by soap and soap substitutes such as pHisoHex, pHisoDerm. If these agents have been used, skin should be rinsed thoroughly prior to treatment.

Store drug below 30°C (86°F). Avoid freezing.

ALUMINUM CARBONATE GEL, BASIC

(Basaljel)

Antilithic
Antacid

ACTIONS AND USES. Nonsystemic antacid with similar actions, uses, contraindications, and adverse reactions as aluminum hydroxide gel. Neutralizing ability is greater than that of aluminum hydroxide gel and demonstrates greatest phosphate binding capacity of all aluminum-containing antacids. Lowers serum phosphate by binding dietary and gastrointestinal phosphates to form insoluble, nonabsorbable aluminum phosphate, which is excreted in feces. This prevents formation of phosphatic urinary calculi by decreasing excretion of phosphate in urine. Sodium content of available preparations: regular suspension: 2.3 mg/5 ml; extra strength suspension: 23.0 mg/5 ml; capsule: 2.8 mg; tablet: 2.1 mg.

Used primarily in conjunction with a low phosphate diet to reduce hyperphosphatemia in patients with renal insufficiency and for prophylaxis and treatment of phosphatic renal calculi. Also used as an antacid.

CONTRAINDICATIONS AND PRECAUTIONS. Hypersensitivity to aluminum, patients on fluid restriction or who are dehydrated, decreased bowel motility (e.g., patients receiving anticholinergics, antidiarrheals, antispasmodics), intestinal obstruction. *Cautious Use:* elderly patients, impaired renal function, patients on Na restriction.

ADVERSE/SIDE EFFECTS. Constipation, fecal impaction, intestinal concretions and obstruction, hypophosphatemia, transient hypercalciuria, dialysis dementia (thought to be due to aluminum intoxication).

ROUTE AND DOSAGE. Oral: *antacid:* 10 ml of regular suspension, or 5 ml of extra strength suspension, or 2 capsules or tablets every 2 hours, if necessary between meals and at bedtime. *For serum phosphate lowering or phosphatic renal calculi prevention:* 10 to 30 ml of regular suspension, or 5 to 15 ml of extra strength suspension, or 2 to 6 capsules, or tablets 1 hour after meals and at bedtime.

NURSING IMPLICATIONS

Shake liquid well before pouring.

Antacid dose may be followed by a little water or fruit juice to assure passage into stomach; it is generally given between meals and at bedtime.

For serum phosphate lowering or prevention of phosphate stones, mix dose in a full glass of water or fruit juice. Usually given 1 hour after meals and at bedtime.

If used to control urinary calculi, measure and record intake and output, and strain all urine through gauze. Since calculi may traumatize tissue, be on the alert for evidence of bleeding and infection: fever, chills, dysuria, and hematuria.

Physician will prescribe a high fluid intake for the patient with urinary calculi. The amount prescribed is variable. Some sources suggest 10 or more glasses of fluid daily; some recommend daily intake in excess of 3000 ml; others advise sufficient liquids to produce a daily urinary output at least 2000 to 3000 ml or more. Assist patient in developing a plan to accomplish this objective.

Food–Drug Interactions: Some physicians prescribe a moderate acid ash diet to acidify the urine thereby discouraging phosphate calculi formation. High acid ash foods include: cheese, corn, lentils, breads, pasta, bacon, cranberry juice, plums, prunes. Ascorbic acid also has been used to acidify urine. Phosphorus-rich foods (i.e., milk and selected milk products, eggs, fish, lean meat, carbonated beverages, fruits, instant beverages sold as powders) may be restricted. Often, control of phosphorus intake entails control of protein intake. Collaborate with dietitian.

Patients on Na restriction should be advised about Na content of the various forms of aluminum carbonate *(see Actions and Uses).* Mild sodium restriction generally means to reduce Na intake to 2000 mg (90 mEq) or less per day.

Since aluminum carbonate adsorbs phosphates, excessive doses for prolonged periods can lead to *hypophosphatemia,* manifested by muscle weakness, anorexia, malaise, absent deep tendon reflexes, bone pain, tremors, negative calcium balance, osteomalacia, osteoporosis. In general, hypophosphatemia is a problem only in patients who are also on a low phosphate diet or who have sustained diarrhea.

Periodic determinations should be made of urinary pH and serum calcium, phosphates, and other electrolytes in patients on long-term therapy.

Immobilization and voluntary suppression of voiding stimulus enhance urinary stasis and development of urinary calculi. If allowed, ambulation should be encouraged, as well as regularly scheduled passive and active exercises.

Note number and consistency of stools; intestinal obstruction from fecal concretions is a possibility. If constipation is a problem, physician may prescribe concurrent therapy with a magnesium antacid or may advise patient to take a laxative or stool softener.

Aluminum carbonate can cause premature absorption of enteric-coated tablets; it also has a high potential for interfering with the absorption of tetracycline and many other oral drugs. As a general rule, it is best not to administer other oral drugs within 1 to 2 hours of any antacid.

Patient-Teaching Plan to Prevent Renal Calculi: Should be constructed in cooperation with physician, dietitian, patient, and responsible family member(s). It should include:

- ✓ Fluid intake: at least 3000 ml/day (approximately 1 full glass every hour)
- ✓ Types of liquids to avoid or limit
- ✓ Dietary restrictions based on stone analysis
- ✓ Medication regimen, including OTC drugs to avoid or limit

Aluminum carbonate contains approximately 5% aluminum hydroxide and 2.4% carbon dioxide. On exposure to air, carbon dioxide is lost; therefore, keep container tightly covered.

Store preferably between 15° and 30°C (59° and 86°F) unless otherwise directed by manufacturer.

See Aluminum Hydroxide Gel for management of peptic ulcer, and Drug Interactions.

ALUMINUM CHLORIDE HEXAHYDRATE

Astringent

(Drysol)

ACTIONS AND USES. The antiperspirant (Drysol) contains 20% aluminum chloride hexahydrate in absolute alcohol. Controls sweating by astringent action which coagulates protein in sweat glands and causes temporary reduction in duct size or closure. Also has mild antibacterial action. An ingredient in several OTC preparations.

Used to control hyperhidrosis of palms, soles, and axillae. Also used in treatment of athlete's foot (dermatophytosis of foot or tinea pedis).

ROUTE AND DOSAGE. *Hyperhidrosis* (20%): Apply to affected area once daily, only at bedtime. When excessive sweating is controlled, applied once or twice weekly or as needed. *Athlete's foot* (2 to 20%): twice daily applications until symptoms such as odor, wetness, and whiteness subside, then once daily to complete healing.

NURSING IMPLICATIONS

Inform patient that medication may produce a burning, prickly sensation.

Avoid contact with eyes. Advise patient to wash hands thoroughly with soap and water after each application.

Treated areas should be washed and dried thoroughly each day.

Dry area completely before applying medication.

Preparation should not be applied to broken, irritated, or recently shaved skin.

Treatment of hyperhidrosis: for maximum effect, treated parts can be covered with a plastic wrap held in place by clothing. Do not use tape. Complete occlusion of axillary area with plastic wrap may promote development of boils or furuncles.

Excessive sweating is usually controlled after a few days of treatment.

Review with patient some predisposing factors that should be controlled to prevent athlete's foot: (1) Avoid ill-fitting footwear that does not allow ventilation (stockings made from synthetic materials, and rubber-soled shoes should be avoided). Wear cotton socks if possible. (2) Poor foot hygiene. Advise patient to wash feet daily and dry thoroughly; change stockings daily, and alternate shoes. (3) Going barefoot in infected areas (wear protective sandals). (4) Excessive perspiration of feet (lamb's wool between toes to evaporate perspiration; liberal dusting with corn starch may help to control wetness).

Instruct patient to discontinue drug if irritation or sensitization occurs, and to report to physician.

Inform patient that medication may damage certain fabrics.

Store in airtight container.

PROTOTYPE

ALUMINUM HYDROXIDE

($Al(OH)_3$ Gel, ALternaGEL, Alu-Cap, Alu-Tab, Amphojel, Dialume)

Antacid
Antilithic

ACTIONS AND USES. Nonsystemic antacid with limited neutralizing action. Reacts with gastric acid to form aluminum chloride, believed to be responsible for astringent and constipating effects. Chloride is reabsorbed in small intestines, thus preserving systemic acid–base balance. Neutralizing capacity of liquid suspension is reported to surpass that of dried gel because particle size is much smaller. Decreases rate of gastric emptying and has demulcent, adsorbent, and mild astringent properties. Lowers serum phosphate by binding dietary phosphorus to form insoluble aluminum phosphate, which is excreted in feces. This prevents formation of urinary phosphatic calculi by decreasing excretion of phosphates in urine. Phosphate-binding capacity not as great as that of aluminum carbonate. Each tablet, capsule, or 5 ml provides about 6.5 to 12 mEq acid-neutralizing capacity, and contains 0.06 to 0.30 mEq of Na (approximately 1.4 mg Na per 0.3 Gm tablet or capsule, and 6.9 mg Na per 5 ml) depending upon product. (23 mg of sodium equals 1 mEq.)

Used for symptomatic relief of gastric hyperacidity associated with gastritis, esophageal reflux, and hiatus hernia; used as adjunct in treatment of gastric and duodenal ulcer. Also has been used in management of hyperphosphatemia of renal failure and in treatment of phosphatic urinary calculi. More commonly used in combination with other antacids. Available in fixed-dose combination with magnesium hydroxide: Algenic Alka Improved, Aludrox, Creamalin, Delcid, Kolantyl, Maalox, Magmalin, Rulox, WinGel; Di-Gel, Gelusil, and Mylanta also contain simethicone. Also available with magnesium trisilicate: Alma-Mag, Gaviscon (also contains alginic acid and sodium bicarbonate), Neutracomp.

ABSORPTION AND FATE. Slow onset of action; duration about 20 to 40 minutes if drug is taken on empty stomach, and approximately 2 hours with food in stomach. Excreted in feces, primarily as insoluble phosphates. Minimal amounts of aluminum may be absorbed; traces excreted in urine.

CONTRAINDICATIONS AND PRECAUTIONS. Sensitivity to aluminum; prolonged use of high doses in presence of low serum phosphate, or in patients on sodium restriction. *Cautious Use:* renal impairment, gastric outlet obstruction, elderly patients, decreased bowel activity (e.g., patients receiving anticholinergic, antidiarrheal, or antispasmodic agents), patients who are dehydrated or on fluid restriction.

ADVERSE/SIDE EFFECTS. Constipation (common), nausea, vomiting, fecal impaction, intestinal concretions, and obstruction. **Phosphorus deficiency syndrome:** (malaise, anorexia, profound muscle weakness, tremors, absent deep tendon reflexes, mental depression, bone pain, negative Ca balance: hypercalciuria, urinary calculi, osteoporosis, osteomalacia); dialysis dementia (thought to be due to aluminum intoxication), hypomagnesemia.

ROUTE AND DOSAGE. Oral: OTC *(antacid)* use: 5 to 10 ml (1 or 2 tsp), or 1 or 2 tablets or capsules, four to six times a day if necessary, between meals and at bedtime. Not to exceed 18 tsp/24 hr nor taken longer than 2 weeks except under advice and supervision of a physician. *Ulcer therapy, esophageal reflux:* 5 to 10 ml, 1 and 3 hours after meals and at bedtime. May be ordered every hour for severe symptoms. **Intragastric drip:** One part diluted with two or three parts water or milk as prescribed (generally 1500 ml in 24 hours at 15 to 20 drops/minute). *Phosphate lowering:* 40 ml PO 1 hour after meals and at bedtime.

NURSING IMPLICATIONS

Shake liquid well before pouring.

If administered in tablet form, instruct patient to chew the tablet until thoroughly wetted before swallowing (swallowing undissolved particles increases risk of developing intestinal concretions). *For antacid use:* follow tablet with one-half glass of water or milk; follow liquid preparation (suspension) with sip of water to assure passage into stomach. *For phosphate lowering:* follow tablet, capsule, or suspension with full glass of water or fruit juice.

Drug is sometimes left at the bedside if it is to be given frequently, but only if the patient is able to assume responsibility for following a prescribed schedule.

During the 4- to 6-week period required for healing an active peptic ulcer, some physicians prescribe antacid 1 and 3 hours after meals, and at bedtime. Others alternate antacid and meals on a 2-hour schedule and advise patients to take an extra antacid dose when discomfort is felt.

The objective of therapy for an active ulcer is not to leave the stomach empty, i.e., without food or antacid, for more than 2 hours. Food itself has considerable buffering capacity. For example, if antacid is given 1 hour after a meal, buffering action will persist an additional 2 hours; administration 3 hours after a meal extends buffering action another hour.

The value of milk and cream ulcer diet is not supported by objective evidence; therefore this adjunct of therapy has largely been abandoned. The neutralizing effect of milk or cream is slight; large amounts may actually stimulate gastric acid secretion for at least 3 hours after ingestion.

Note: the traditional bedtime milk snack is particularly to be avoided to prevent an excess of unbuffered gastric acid during sleep.

Since frequency of meals may vary in the elderly particularly, explain specifically the best time to take an antacid.

Pain is used as a clinical guide for adjusting dosage. Advise patient to keep physician informed. Pain that persists beyond 72 hours may signify serious complications such as perforation or malignancy.

Food–Drug Interactions: Patients receiving large doses of antacids for prolonged periods and who eat a diet low in phosphorus (e.g., avoiding milk, milk products, poultry, whole grain cereals) and low in protein can develop phosphorus deficiency syndrome *(see Adverse/ Side Effects).* It has occurred within 2 weeks of continuous antacid use. The elderly patient in poor nutritional state is at high risk. Both vitamin A and thiamine deficiencies also can occur in some patients because of reduced absorption.

Note number and consistency of stools. Constipation occurs commonly and is dose-related. Intestinal obstruction from fecal concretions has been reported. If constipation is a problem, physician may prescribe alternate or combination therapy with an antacid with laxative action, such as magnesium hydroxide, magnesium oxide, or magnesium trisilicate.

Explain to patient that antacid may cause stools to appear speckled or whitish in color.

The American Dietetic Association advocates a liberal, nutritionally complete diet for the patient with peptic ulcer. Although strict dietary control is no longer considered a crucial aspect of therapy, the patient and responsible family members should be advised about dietary management such as: (1) to avoid known food intolerances; (2) avoid or at least minimize use of recognized stimulants of gastric secretion such as smoking, caffeine-containing beverages, alcohol, black pepper, harsh spices, extremely hot and cold foods, and ulcerogenic drugs such as aspirin; (3) chew food thoroughly; (4) avoid overeating; (5) create a relaxed atmosphere at mealtimes, control anxiety-provoking situations and environmental factors that are irritating.

Length of antacid therapy for patients with duodenal ulcer is usually 4 to 6 weeks, and for gastric ulcers until healing has taken place.

Serum calcium and phosphorus levels should be determined at periodic intervals in patients receiving prolonged high dose therapy or who have impaired renal function.

Patients with *gastroesophangeal reflux* associated with hiatus hernia are generally advised to (1) avoid possible causes of heartburn (a prominent symptom) such as overeating, fatty foods (which also delay gastric emptying), foods known to cause heartburn or gas (based on individual intolerance), concentrated fruit juices, chocolate, coffee, alcohol; (2) limit fluid intake during meals; (3) eat meals at regular intervals in a relaxed atmosphere. Eat and drink slowly to avoid gulping air; (4) avoid lying down sooner than 1 hour after a meal; (5) elevate head of bed 6 to 8 inches on bed blocks (use of pillows alone tends to "jackknife" abdomen); (6) avoid straining and heavy lifting; (7) avoid tight abdominal garments; (8) maintain ideal weight, if possible. (Discuss these teaching points with physician.)

Caution individuals who self-medicate with antacids to seek medical help if indigestion is accompanied by shortness of breath, sweating, or chest pain, if stools are very dark or tarry, or if symptoms are recurrent.

Self-prescribed antacid use should not exceed 2 weeks before seeking medical advice and supervision.

Store preferably between 15° and 30°C (59° and 86°F) in tightly closed container, unless otherwise directed by manufacturer.

See Aluminum Carbonate Gel, Basic for management of phosphatic urinary calculi.

Drug Interactions. An increase in pH (as with antacid therapy) delays gastric emptying time leading to variation and unpredictability in drug absorption. Therefore, in general, it is best to avoid taking an antacid any sooner than 1 hour before or until 2 to 3 hours after another oral medication, unless otherwise advised. **Digoxin, indomethacin, iron salts,** and **tetracycline** particularly should be spaced as far from an antacid as possible. Also note that antacid-induced elevations in gastric pH may increase rate of absorption of buffered or enteric coated preparations by causing premature dissolution.

Concurrent use of aluminum-hydroxide or other aluminum-containing antacids inhibits absorption of:

- Anticholinergic agents
- Chlordiazepoxide (Librium)
- Chloroquine (Aralen)
- Cimetidine (Tagamet)
- Corticosteroids
- Diazepam (Valium)
- Digoxin (Lanoxin)
- Indomethacin (Indocin)
- Iron salts
- Isoniazid (INH)
- Penicillamine (Cuprimine)
- Phenothiazines
- Phenytoin (Dilantin)
- Tetracyclines
- Vitamin A and possibly other fat soluble vitamins

Plus	**Interactions**
Dicumarol Pseudoephedrine (Sudafed)	Concurrent use of antacid may increase drug absorption (by decreasing drug excretion)
Sodium polystyrene sulfonate (Kayexalate)	Coadministration with nonsystemic antacid can cause significant rise in blood bicarbonate level, and may impair potassium lowering ability of sodium polystyrene sulfonate

---

ALUMINUM PHOSPHATE

Antacid

(Phosphaljel)

ACTIONS AND USES. Slow-acting nonsystemic antacid with properties similar to those of aluminum hydroxide (qv), but does not increase fecal excretion of phosphate. Reported to have one-fourth the neutralizing capacity of aluminum hydroxide. Phosphagel is sugar-free; it contains 0.54 mEq (12.5 mg) of Na per 5 ml.

Used as antacid in preference to aluminum hydroxide gel when a high phosphorus diet cannot be maintained or to reverse hypophosphatemia induced by aluminum hydroxide, or in patients with diarrhea or pancreatic insufficiency.

CONTRAINDICATIONS AND PRECAUTIONS. Sensitivity to aluminum; high dose therapy in patients with impaired renal function, or who are on sodium-restricted diets.

ADVERSE/SIDE EFFECTS. Constipation (common), hyperphosphatemia (patients with impaired renal function).

ROUTE AND DOSAGE. Oral: 15 to 30 ml, undiluted every 2 hours, between meals and at bedtime. For intragastric therapy, diluted 1:3 or 1:4.

NURSING IMPLICATIONS

Shake liquid well before pouring.

May be given undiluted and followed by sufficient liquid to assure passage into stomach.

Monitor input and output ratio and pattern and serum phosphate levels in patients receiving prolonged therapy.

If serum phosphate level is elevated (normal: 2.5 to 4.5 mg/dl), a low phosphate diet may be prescribed (e.g., decreased intake of milk and dairy products).

Note number and consistency of stools. If constipation is a problem, physician may prescribe concurrent therapy with a magnesium antacid, or administration of a laxative or stool softener as needed.

See Aluminum Hydroxide (prototype aluminum-containing antacid).

Drug Interactions. In common with other antacids, aluminum phosphate can cause premature dissolution of enteric-coated tablets and also has a high potential for interfering with the absorption of tetracycline and many other oral medications. As a general rule, it is best not to administer other oral drugs within 1 or 2 hours of an antacid. *See also Aluminum Hydroxide.*

AMANTADINE HYDROCHLORIDE

(Symmetrel)

(a-man′ta-deen)
Anticholinergic (antimuscarinic)
Parasympatholytic
Antiparkinson agent
Antiviral

ACTIONS AND USES. Synthetic tricyclic amine with virostatic action. Believed to act by inhibiting penetration of host cell by virus, or by preventing uncoating of viral nucleic acid. Because it does not suppress antibody formation it can be administered for interim protection in combination with influenza A virus vaccine until antibody titer is adequate, or to augment prophylaxis in a previously vaccinated individual. Active against several strains of influenza A virus; not effective against influenza B infections. Has mild anticholinergic activity. Mechanism of action in Parkinson's disease not understood, but may be related to release of dopamine and other catecholamines from neuronal storage sites. Reportedly less effective than levodopa, but produces more rapid clinical response and causes fewer adverse reactions.

Used in initial therapy or as adjunct with anticholinergic drugs or levodopa in treatment of all forms of parkinsonism (arteriosclerotic, idiopathic, postencephalitic) and for relief of drug-induced extrapyramidal reactions, and symptomatic parkinsonism caused by carbon monoxide poisoning. Also used for prophylaxis and symptomatic treatment of influenza A infections. *Investigational Use:* primary enuresis.

ABSORPTION AND FATE. Readily and almost completely absorbed from GI tract. Maximal blood concentrations after 1 to 4 hours. Onset of action within 48 hours. Half-life about 24 hours (range 9 to 37 hours), prolonged in patients with impaired renal function. Not metabolized. Distributed to saliva, nasal secretions, breast milk; crosses blood–brain barrier. Approximately 90% of dose excreted unchanged in urine. Acidification of urine increases rate of elimination. Crosses placenta. Excreted in breast milk.

CONTRAINDICATIONS AND PRECAUTIONS. Known hypersensitivity to amantadine; nursing mothers. Safe use during pregnancy (category C), in women of childbearing potential, and in children under 1 year not established. *Cautious Use:* history of epilepsy or other types of seizures; congestive heart failure, peripheral edema, orthostatic hypotension, recurrent eczematoid dermatitis, psychoses, severe psychoneuroses, hepatic disease, renal impairment; elderly patients with cerebral arteriosclerosis.

ADVERSE/SIDE EFFECTS. Usually dose related: **CNS:** dizziness, light-headedness, headache, ataxia, drowsiness, fatigue, weakness, irritability, anxiety, nervousness, difficulty in concentrating, depression, psychosis, confusion, slurred speech, visual and auditory hallucinations, insomnia, nightmares, tremor, convulsions. **CV:** orthostatic hypotension, peripheral edema, dyspnea, congestive heart failure. **Dermatologic:** dermatitis, livedo reticularis, photosensitization. **GI:** anorexia, nausea, vomiting, constipation, dry mouth. **GU:** urinary retention, frequency. **Hematologic:** leukopenia, neutropenia (rare). **Ophthalmic:** blurring or loss of vision, oculogyric episodes.

ROUTE AND DOSAGE. **Oral:** *Parkinsonism:* **Adults:** 100 mg twice daily. For patients with associated severe medical problems or who are taking other antiparkinson drugs: initial: 100 mg once daily for 1 to several weeks; then 100 mg twice daily, if necessary. *Drug-induced extrapyramidal symptoms:* 100 mg twice daily; up to 400 mg daily in divided doses, if necessary. *Influenza A prophylaxis and treatment:* **Adults and children (over 9 years):** 200 mg once daily or 100 mg every 12 hours. **Children (1 to 9 years):** 4.4 to 8.8 mg/kg in 2 or 3 equal doses, not to exceed 150 mg/day. Available in capsules and syrup.

NURSING IMPLICATIONS

Capsule may be emptied and contents swallowed with water or mixed with food.

To be effective for influenza prophylaxis, amantadine should be started in anticipation of exposure or as soon as possible after initial contact with infected individuals and continued for at least 10 days. When repeated exposure is a possibility prophylaxis is continued up to 90 days.

In influenza epidemics, amantadine should be continued throughout epidemic (usually 6 to 8 weeks). (Infectious period for influenza is shortly before onset of symptoms and up to 1 week after symptoms appear.)

Although use of influenza vaccine is the preferred prophylactic method, amantadine is used when the vaccine is either not available or contraindicated, or for unvaccinated patient at high risk: e.g., the elderly, individuals with chronic respiratory, cardiovascular, metabolic, neuromuscular, and renal disease, and immunosuppression.

Amantadine may be used in conjunction with influenza A vaccine (generally in high risk patients who have not been vaccinated previously), until protective antibodies develop (10 to 21 days) after vaccine administration.

To be effective in treatment of influenza, amantadine must be administered preferably within 24 hours but no later than 48 hours after onset of symptoms and should be continued for 24 to 48 hours after symptoms disappear.

Administration of last daily dose too close to retiring may produce insomnia. If insomnia is a problem, medication should be scheduled several hours before bedtime. Suggest that patient limit number of daytime naps.

CNS and psychic disturbances are most likely to appear within 1 day to a few days after initiation of drug therapy, or after dosage has been increased. Symptoms tend to subside when drug is given in two divided doses.

Solicit help of family members to establish a baseline profile of the patient's disabilities. This information is essential for accurate differentiation between disease symptoms (e.g., dementia) and drug-induced neuropsychiatric adverse reactions. A quantitative scoring system may be of help.

Patients receiving doses above 200 mg daily should be closely observed for amantadine toxicity. Monitor vital signs for at least 3 or 4 days following increases in dosage.

Elderly patients with cerebrovascular disease or impaired renal function are more prone to develop symptoms of toxicity.

Because orthostatic hypotension may be a problem, caution patient not to go to sleep in a sitting position, and advise elderly male patients particularly to sit down to urinate, especially at night.

Advise patient to make all position changes slowly, particularly from recumbent to upright position, and to dangle legs a few minutes before standing. Caution patient to lie down immediately if faint or dizzy.

Instruct patient and responsible family members to report to physician onset of shortness of breath, peripheral edema, significant weight gain, dizziness, inability to concentrate, and other changes in mental status, dysuria.

Activities requiring mental alertness such as driving a car should be avoided until patient's response to the drug has been evaluated.

Patients with parkinsonism may show reduction of salivation, akinesia, and rigidity within 4 to 48 hours after initiation of therapy. Generally, drug has little effect on tremors. If significant improvement is not noted within 1 or 2 weeks, drug is usually discontinued.

Patient should remain under close medical supervision while receiving amantadine therapy. Maximum therapeutic response generally occurs within 2 weeks to 3 months. Effectiveness sometimes wanes after 6 to 8 weeks of treatment. Report to physician. Decision may be made to increase dosage or to discontinue drug temporarily or to use another antiparkinsonian agent.

Livedo reticularis occurs most frequently in women receiving amantadine for 1 month or longer for parkinsonism. It is a diffuse, rose-colored mottling of skin, usually confined to lower extremities, but it may also appear on arms. Caused by local release of catecholamines, which results in vasoconstriction and abnormal capillary permeability. Sometimes preceded by or accompanied by ankle edema. More noticeable when patient stands or is exposed to cold; color fades when legs are elevated. Generally, this side effect appears within 1 month to 1 year following initiation of drug therapy and may subside with continued therapy, but disappears gradually in 2 to 12 weeks after drug is discontinued.

Abrupt discontinuation of amantadine therapy in patients with parkinsonism may precipitate *parkinsonian crisis* within 24 hours to 3 days (severe akinesia, rigidity, tremor). Warn patient to adhere to established dosage regimen.

Treatment of overdosage: immediate gastric lavage or induction of emesis. Have on hand physostigmine and chloropromazine for neurologic manifestations. General supportive measures: maintenance of airway, administration of oxygen, fluids, urinary acidifier. Monitor urinary output and pH, serum electrolytes, vital signs. Observe for seizures.

Plan of care should address problems that frequently accompany parkinsonism: (1) Mental depression. (2) Sleep disturbances. (3) Constipation. (4) Urinary retention especially in elderly males with enlarged prostate. (5) Complications related to inactivity (decubiti, contractures, postural deformities). Patients should have medical follow-up at regular intervals.

Store in tightly closed container preferably between 15° and 30°C (59° and 86°F) unless otherwise directed by manufacturer. Avoid freezing.

Drug Interactions: Amantadine

Plus	Interactions
Alcohol, and other CNS depressants	Additive CNS effects
Anticholinergics	Amantadine may potentiate CNS effects of large doses of anticholinergic drugs. Dosage of either should be reduced.
Hydrochlorothiazide plus triamterene (Dyazide)	Increase in amantadine toxicity

AMBENONIUM CHLORIDE
(Mytelase)

(am-be-noe'nee-um)
Cholinergic
Cholinesterase inhibitor

ACTIONS AND USES. Synthetic quaternary ammonium compound. Slowly reversible cholinesterase inhibitor approximately six times more potent than neostigmine (qv), but similar with respect to uses, contraindications, and adverse reactions. Principle action results in prolonged effects of ACh (neurotransmitter) at the postsynaptic receptor site. Produces fewer severe cholinergic (muscarinic) effects than neostigmine, but has more prolonged duration of action and possibly greater tendency to accumulate.

Used in symptomatic treatment of myasthenia gravis for patients who cannot tolerate neostigmine bromide or pyridostigmine bromide because of bromide sensitivity. Has been used in conjunction with corticosteroids, ephedrine sulfate, and/or potassium chloride to increase muscle strength.

ABSORPTION AND FATE. Poorly absorbed from GI tract. Onset of action: 20 to 30 minutes. Duration of action: 3 to 8 hours (variable).

CONTRAINDICATIONS AND PRECAUTIONS. Intestinal or urinary tract obstruction, patients receiving mecamylamine. Safe use during pregnancy not established. *Cautious Use:* epilepsy, bradycardia, cardiac arrhythmias, recent coronary occlusion, bronchial asthma, hyperthyroidism, vagotonia, peptic ulcer, megacolon.

ADVERSE/SIDE EFFECTS. *Exaggerated cholinergic (muscarinic) effects:* **CNS:** headache, confusion, dizziness, incoordination, fasciculations, muscle weakness, paralysis, respiratory depression. **CV:** bradycardia, hypotension, tachycardia. **GI:** nausea, vomiting, diarrhea, abdominal discomfort, excessive salivation. **GU:** urinary frequency, incontinence. **Ophthalmic:** miosis, blurred vision, lacrimation. **Respiratory:** bronchospasm, increased bronchial secretions. **Other:** muscle cramps. *See also Neostigmine.*

ROUTE AND DOSAGE. Oral: Adults: Initial: 2.5 to 5 mg three or four times a day. Highly individualized. Dosage adjustments made as needed every 1 to 2 or more days. Some patients require as much as 50 to 75 mg three or four times a day. **Children:** Initial: 0.3 mg/kg/24 hours in three or four divided doses. Maintenance: 1.5 mg/kg/24 hours divided into three or four doses.

NURSING IMPLICATIONS

Administration with food or milk may minimize muscarinic side effects.

Hazards of cumulative effects and overdosage are high.

Atropine sulfate should always be immediately available to treat severe cholinergic reactions.

During dosage adjustment periods, facilities for cardiopulmonary rescusitation, endotracheal intubation, suctioning, tracheostomy, respiratory ventilation and cardiac monitoring should be readily available.

Dosage requirements may vary according to disease exacerbations and remissions, and stress provoking factors. The effects of a given dosage change may not appear for several days because of cumulative action. If a dosage increase produces no effect, physician may reduce dose to previous level. Keep physician informed.

In general, medication schedule is planned so that larger doses are given when patient experiences the most fatigue or muscle weakness. Patients who have difficulty in eating may benefit by taking drug 30 to 45 minutes before meals.

Usually medication is not required throughout the night because action is prolonged.

It is important to record time that adverse symptoms appear. When muscle weakness occurs within 1 hour after drug administration, suspect overdosage. Other signs of overdosage include headache, weakness of muscles of neck and of chewing, and salivation. Weakness that begins 3 or more hours after drug administration is probably due to underdosage or drug resistance.

Patients and responsible family members should be taught to recognize adverse effects, how to modify the doses accordingly, and when and how atropine should be taken.

Patients on long-term therapy may become refractory to ambenonium. Responsiveness usually returns when dosage is reduced or drug is withdrawn for several days.

Store preferably between 15° and 30°C (59° and 86°F) unless otherwise directed by manufacturer.

See Neostigmine bromide (prototype cholinergic).

Drug Interactions: Ambenonium

Plus	Interactions
Aminoglycosides Anesthetics, general and local Antiarrhythmics Mecamylamine (Inversine) Polymyxin antibiotics Quinidine	May antagonize ambenonium actions
Succinylcholine (Anectine, Quelicin)	Increased neuromuscular blocking effects with possibility of respiratory depression

---

AMCINONIDE
(Cyclocort)

(am-sin'oh-nide)
Corticosteroid (topical)
Antiinflammatory agent

ACTIONS AND USES. Synthetic fluorinated topical agent. Has vasoconstrictor, antipruritic, and antiinflammatory actions equal to those produced by betamethasone and triamcinolone.

Used adjunctively in treatment and relief of inflammatory and pruritic manifestations of corticoid-responsive dermatoses, such as psoriasis, eczematous and contact dermatitis.

CONTRAINDICATIONS AND PRECAUTIONS. History of hypersensitivity to corticosteroids; ophthalmic use, markedly impaired circulation, systemic or local viral infection, fungal infection, tuberculosis of skin. Safe use during pregnancy (category C) or in nursing mothers, not established. *Cautious Use:* children. *See Hydrocortisone.*

ADVERSE/SIDE EFFECTS. (Most frequently with occlusive dressings): burning, itching, irritation, dryness, folliculitis, hypertrichosis, acneiform eruptions, perioral dermatitis, patchy hypopigmentation, allergic contact dermatitis, skin maceration, atrophy, striae, miliaria, secondary infection. *See Hydrocortisone for possible systemic effects.*

ROUTE AND DOSAGE. Topical: 0.1% (emulsified) cream, ointment: apply 2 or 3 times a day.

NURSING IMPLICATIONS

Cleanse area to be treated before applying cream to reduce risk of infection. Unless otherwise directed, use tepid water. Discuss specific procedure with prescribing physician.

Apply a thin film of medication to cleansed affected areas and rub in gently and thoroughly until it disappears. Do not use in or near the eyes. Note carefully evidence of limited response, irritation, or skin changes such as atrophy, telangiectasis, hypopigmentation, and report to physician.

Do not bandage or otherwise cover treated area or apply occlusive dressing unless prescribed by physician.

Application of occlusive dressing: Following application of medication, cover affected area with thin plastic film, seal edges with nonallergenic adhesive or hold in place with gauze, elastic bandage, stockinette, or stocking. Occlusive dressings are usually changed every 12 hours.

Occlusive dressings should not be used if lesions are exudative, weeping, or infected.

Be aware that greater drug absorption may occur when occlusive dressings are used, and when drug is applied to thin skin surfaces: e.g., axilla, groin, neck; or on child's skin (because of thin stratum corneum) or on skin of the elderly (atrophic skin).

Systemic absorption, which could lead to growth retardation (in children) and adrenal suppression, may occur with use of topical corticosteroid on large skin areas for prolonged periods and particularly if occlusive dressings are used.

Periodic evaluation of need to continue drug is essential, especially in children.

Advise patient to avoid exposure of treated areas to sunlight. Severe sun burn may occur, especially when occlusive dressings have been used.

Report evidence of intercurrent infection, which will require prompt control by adjunctive treatment. Question physician about continuation of amcinonide therapy during antifungal or antimicrobial treatment.

Warn patient to use medication only for disorder prescribed and only as directed (schedule, method of application, and length of treatment time).

Store preferably between 15° and 30°C (59° and 86°F) in well-closed container unless otherwise directed by manufacturer.

See Hydrocortisone (prototype corticosteroid) for further discussion of topical applications.

AMIKACIN SULFATE

(Amikin)

(am-i-kay'sin)
Antiinfective
Antibiotic
Aminoglycoside

ACTIONS AND USES. Semisynthetic derivative of kanamycin with broadest range of antimicrobial activity of the aminoglycosides. Pharmacologic properties essentially the same as those of gentamicin (qv). Unlike other aminoglycosides, resists destruction by bacterial enzymes, (except acetyltransferase and an adenylating enzyme). Like other aminoglycosides, inhibits protein synthesis in bacterial cell and is bactericidal. Effective against a wide variety of gram-negative bacilli including *Escherichia coli, Enterobacter, Klebsiella pneumoniae,* most strains of *Pseudomonas aeruginosa,* and many strains of *Proteus* species, *Serratia, Providencia stuartii, Citrobacter freundii, Acinetobacter.* Also effective against penicillinase and non-penicillinase-producing staphylococci. Active against *Mycobacterium tuberculosis* and atypical mycobacteria, but not against majority of other gram-positive anaerobic bacteria, or rickettsiae, fungi, and viruses.

Used primarily for treatment of serious nosocomial gram-negative bacillary infections resistant to gentamicin and tobramycin. Has been used in combination with carbenicillin or ticarcillin for severe pseudomonas infections.

ABSORPTION AND FATE. Serum levels peak in 45 minutes to 2 hours following IM administration and within 30 minutes following IV. Half-life: about 2 to 3 hours in adults and 4 to 8 hours in neonates; 28 to 86 hours in anephric patients. Small amounts (4 to 8%) protein bound. Primarily distributed to extracellular fluid; progressively accumulates in renal cortex and fluid of inner ear over course of therapy. Penetrates CSF particularly when meninges are inflamed. Excreted unchanged in urine; 94 to 98% of dose excreted within 24 hours. Crosses placenta. Excretion into breast milk not known.

CONTRAINDICATIONS AND PRECAUTIONS. History of hypersensitivity or toxic reaction with aminoglycosides. Safe use during pregnancy or breast feeding not determined. *Cautious Use:* impaired renal function, eighth cranial nerve impairment, dehydration, fever, the elderly, neonates and infants, myasthenia gravis, parkinsonism, hypocalcemia.

ADVERSE/SIDE EFFECTS. **CNS (neurotoxicity):** drowsiness, headache, unsteady gait, weakness, clumsiness, paresthesias, tremors, neuromuscular blockade with respiratory depression. **CV:** hypotension, tachycardia. **GI:** nausea, vomiting, stomatitis. **Hematologic:** (infrequent): anemia, leukopenia, granulocytopenia, thrombocytopenia. **Hypersensitivity:** skin rash, urticaria, pruritus, generalized burning sensation, drug fever, arthralgia, eosinophilia. **Ototoxicity:** *auditory:* high frequency hearing loss, complete hearing loss (occasionally permanent); tinnitus; fullness, ringing, or buzzing in ears; *vestibular:* dizziness, vertigo, ataxia, nausea, vomiting, nystagmus. **Renal (nephrotoxicity):** oliguria, urinary frequency, red and white blood cells in urine, frank hematuria, casts, albuminuria, azotemia, increase in BUN and serum creatinine, decrease in creatinine clearance, specific gravity; renal damage and failure. **Other:** unusual thirst, difficult breathing, superinfections, peripheral neuritis; rare: hypocalcemia with symptoms of tetany; weakness, lethargy, and associated with hypokalemia and hypomagnesemia. *See also Gentamicin.*

ROUTE AND DOSAGE. Dosage calculations should be based on estimate of ideal body weight (IBW). **Intramuscular, intravenous infusion: Adults, children, and older infants:** 5 mg/kg every 8 hours or 7.5 mg/kg every 12 hours. Not to exceed 15 mg/kg/day. Duration of therapy usually 7 to 10 days. *Uncomplicated urinary tract infection:* 250 mg every 12 hours. **Intrathecal, intraventricular** *(investigational):* 4 to 20 mg as single daily dose in conjunction with IM or IV dosage. **Neonates:** Initial: 10 mg/kg IM or IV infusion then 7.5 mg/kg every 12 hours.

NURSING IMPLICATIONS

Not to be confused with Amicar.

Culture and susceptibility tests should be performed before initial dose, but therapy may begin pending test results. Most infections respond to amikacin therapy in 24 to 48 hours. If therapeutic response does not occur in 3 to 5 days, susceptibility tests should be repeated and therapy reevaluated.

Baseline weight, vital signs, and tests of renal function and eighth cranial (vestibulocochlear) nerve function should be performed before therapy and at regular intervals during therapy.

Renal function and eighth cranial nerve function should be closely monitored in the elderly, in patients with history of ear problems, patients with renal impairment, or during high dose or prolonged therapy.

Ototoxicity is primarily cochlear (auditory); however, vestibular toxicity can also occur *(see Adverse/Side Effects).* High frequency deafness usually appears first and can be detected only by audiometer.

Patient should be questioned periodically about hearing, and symptoms related to vestibular disturbances.

Tinnitus is not a reliable index of ototoxicity in the very old who may already have hearing problems to begin with, or in the very young who cannot talk. In these patients blood drug levels must be monitored to follow therapy.

Monitor intake and output. Report any change in intake and output ratio or pattern, oliguria, hematuria, or cloudy urine. Keeping patient well hydrated reduces chemical irritation of renal tubules (nephrotoxicity). Consult physician regarding optimum fluid intake.

Be aware of renal function test results. Decreasing urine specific gravity and creatinine clearance, and increasing creatinine, BUN, and white and red blood cells in urine are significant indicators of declining renal function.

Usual duration of treatment is 7 to 10 days. If treatment is continued for more than 10 days, daily tests of renal function and weekly audiograms and vestibular tests are advised.

To reduce risk of nephrotoxicity and ototoxicity, periodic measurements of serum amikacin levels in addition to serum creatinine, and creatinine clearance (generally preferred) are recommended. These values are used as guidelines for determining dosage adjustments needed to maintain desired serum concentrations.

Blood for determining peak amikacin level is drawn 1 hour after IM administration and 1 hour after IV infusion begins.

Therapeutic peak serum amikacin concentrations range from 20 to 25 mcg/ml; therapeutic trough levels are 5 to 10 mcg/ml. High trough or peak levels are associated with toxicity.

Monitor vital signs. Amikacin serum levels are reportedly lower in patients with fever.

Be on the alert for symptoms of respiratory tract infections and other symptoms indicative of superinfections. Notify physician should they occur.

To prepare IV solution, dilute calculated dose in 100 or 200 ml sterile diluent recommended by manufacturer and administer over 30- to 60-minute period for adults. In pediatric patients, volume of diluent depends on patient need. Infants should be given a 1- to 2-hour infusion. Monitor drip rate prescribed by physician. A rapid rise in serum level can cause respiratory depression and other signs of toxicity.

Manufacturer recommends that no other drug be combined with amikacin; that is, it should be administered separately.

Color of solution may vary from colorless to light straw color or very pale yellow. Discard dark colored solutions.

Stored preferably between 15° and 30°C (59° and 86°F) unless otherwise directed by manufacturer. Protect from freezing. *See also Gentamicin.*

Drug Interactions: Amikacin

Plus	**Interactions**
Concurrent or sequential administration of drugs with potential for nephrotoxicity, ototoxicity, or neurotoxicity is generally avoided, e.g.:	

- Aminoglycosides, other amphotericin B (Fungizone)
- Bacitracin
- Capreomycin (Capastat)
- Cephalothin (Keflin)
- Cisplatin (Platinol)
- Colistimethate (Coly-Mycin M)
- Diuretics (potent): e.g., bumetanide (Bumex), ethacrynic acid (Edecrin), furosemide (Lasix)
- Methoxyflurane (Penthrane)
- Polymyxin B (Aerosporin)

Plus	Interactions
Anesthetics (general) skeletal muscle relaxants (nondepolarizing), e.g., succinyl choline	Additive neuromuscular blocking action; used with caution
Dimenhydrinate and other antiemetics	May mask symptoms of ototoxicity
Penicillins	Possibility of aminoglycoside inactivation. Also, administered separately, because of physical incompatibility

AMILORIDE HYDROCHLORIDE

(Midamor)

(a-mill'-oh-ride)

Diuretic (potassium-sparing)

ACTIONS AND USES. Potassium-sparing diuretic, structurally similar to triamterene, with mild diuretic and antihypertensive actions. Induces urinary excretion of sodium, e.g., bicarbonates, and calcium and reduces excretion of potassium and hydrogen ions by direct action on distal renal tubules. Potassium-sparing action results in rise of total body concentration of potassium; reduction in hydrogen ions causes moderate increase in urinary pH. Effect on serum uric acid is reportedly variable and requires further study. Like triamterene, diuretic action is independent of aldosterone and carbonic anhydrase.

Used for its potassium-sparing effect in prevention or treatment of diuretic-induced hypokalemia in patients with congestive heart failure, hepatic cirrhosis, or hypertension. Also used in management of primary hyperaldosteronism. Usually combined with a potassium-wasting (kaliuretic) diuretic such as a thiazide or loop diuretic. Commercially available in fixed-dose combination with hydrochlorothiazide (Moduretic). The combination is more effective than either drug alone, and risk of hyperkalemia is reduced.

ABSORPTION AND FATE. Approximately 50% absorbed from GI tract following oral administration. Onset of diuretic action within 2 hours, peaks at 6 to 10 hours, and is completed in 24 hours. Approximately 23% protein bound; half-life: 6 to 9 hours (longer in patients with impaired renal function). Excreted unchanged 20 to 50% via kidneys, 40% in feces. In animals, crosses placenta and enters breast milk. Human studies incomplete.

CONTRAINDICATIONS AND PRECAUTIONS. Elevated serum potassium (> 5.5 mEq/L), concomitant use of other potassium-sparing diuretics; anuria, acute or chronic renal insufficiency, evidence of diabetic nephropathy; type I (insulin-dependent) diabetes mellitus, metabolic or respiratory acidosis, hepatic function impairment. Safe use in pregnancy (category B), nursing mothers, and children not established. *Cautious Use:* debilitated patients, diet-controlled or uncontrolled diabetes mellitus, cardiopulmonary disease, elderly.

ADVERSE/SIDE EFFECTS. Generally well tolerated. **CNS:** headache, dizziness, tremors, nervousness, insomnia, somnolence, confusion, depression, paresthesias. **CV:** orthostatic hypotension, angina, palpitation, cardiac arrhythmias. **Electrolyte Imbalance/Hematologic:** hyperkalemia, hyponatremia, metabolic acidosis; rare (causal relationship not established): eosinophilia, leukopenia, neutropenia, aplastic anemia, elevated Hct, positive Coombs' test. **ENT:** tinnitus, nasal congestion. **GI:** diarrhea or constipation, anorexia, nausea, vomiting, abdominal cramps, abdominal bloating, flatulence, heartburn; dry mouth, alterations of taste, thirst, jaundice; reactivation of peptic ulcer (causal relationship not established). **GU:** polyuria, dysuria, bladder spasms, urinary frequency. **Ophthalmic:** visual disturbances, increased intraocular pressure. **Respiratory:** cough, dyspnea, shortness of breath. **Skin:** erythematous rash, pruritus, alopecia, photosensitivity reactions. **Other:** weakness, fatigue, muscle cramps and musculoskeletal discomfort, impotence, decreased libido, minor psychiatric symptoms. Transient rises in: BUN, serum creatinine, uric acid, AST (SGOT), and alkaline phosphatase; transient glycosuria, mild proteinuria (rare).

ROUTE AND DOSAGE. Oral: Initial: 5 mg/day. Increased to 10 mg/day, if necessary; up to 20 mg/day.

NURSING IMPLICATIONS

Administered preferably with food to reduce possibility of gastric distress.

Generally taken in the morning to avoid interrupting nighttime sleep. Advise patient to take amiloride at the same time each day.

Serum K levels (normal: 3.5 to 5 mEq/L) should be monitored for all patients particularly when therapy is initiated, whenever dosage adjustments are made, and during any illness that may affect kidney function.

Hyperkalemia occurs in about 10% of patients receiving amiloride. Even with concurrent thiazide therapy (a combination designed to decrease K retention) serum K can rise suddenly and without warning. *Symptoms of hyperkalemia* (serum K > 6.5 mEq/L): life-threatening cardiac arrhythmias, unusual fatigue, weakness or heaviness of limbs, general muscle weakness, muscle cramps, paresthesias, flaccid paralysis of extremities, shortness of breath, nervousness, confusion.

Hyperkalemia frequency is higher in the elderly, and in patients with diabetes or renal disease (fosters potassium retention).

In addition to periodic serum K concentrations, intermittent evaluations of BUN, creatinine, and ECG are advised for patients with renal or hepatic dysfunction, diabetes mellitus, or who are elderly or debilitated.

Potassium supplements, salt substitutes, high intake of dietary K *(see Index: Food sources)* are all contraindicated. Exception: these measures may be prescribed by physician for patients with severe or refractory hypokalemia, along with close monitoring of serum K levels.

Because amiloride can cause visual disturbances and dizziness particularly during early therapy, advise patient to be cautious when driving or performing other potentially hazardous tasks.

Instruct patient to consult physician before self-medicating with OTC products. Many preparations contain adrenergic agents that may aggravate high blood pressure (e.g., nasal decongestants, cough, cold or asthma remedies, and appetite suppressants).

For other teaching points for patients with hypertension, see Reserpine.

Store preferably between 15° and 30°C (59° and 86°F) in a well-closed container, unless otherwise directed by manufacturer.

Diagnostic Test Interferences. Manufacturer advises discontinuing amiloride in patients with diabetes mellitus at least 3 days prior to **glucose tolerance** tests.

Drug Interactions: Amiloride

Plus	Interactions
Antihypertensives	Potentiation of antihypertensive effects. Used concomitantly with caution
Blood from blood banks (plasma content: plasma may contain up to 30 mEq/L; whole blood may contain up to 65 mEq/L when stored over 10 days) Captopril (Capoten) Diuretics, potassium-sparing: spironolactone (Aldactone), triamterene (Dyrenium) Potassium-containing medications, e.g., parenteral penicillin G potassium, potassium supplements Salt substitutes (high in potassium chloride)	Possibility of hyperkalemia

Plus (cont.)	Interactions (cont.)
Digoxin (Lanoxin)	Possibility of altered digoxin response and reduced inotropic effect
Cation-exchange resins (e.g., sodium polystyrene sulfonate (Kayexalate)	Reduce serum K levels by replacing K with Na (also may increase fluid retention)
Glucose–insulin infusion Sodium bicarbonate	Reduces serum K levels by promoting shift of K ions into cells
Lithium	Amiloride reduces lithium renal excretion with possibility of toxicity. Concurrent use not recommended

---

AMINO ACID INJECTION

(Aminosyn, Crystalline amino acid solution, FreAmine III, Travasol, Veinamine)

(a-mee'noe)

Caloric agent

ACTIONS AND USES. Mixture of approximately 15 essential and nonessential amino acids (but no peptides). Supplied in a variety of concentrations both alone and with electrolytes. Solutions containing 3.5% amino acids may be administered by peripheral vein. The more concentrated formulations are intended for infusion into a large (central) vein, such as the jugular or subclavian, in *total parenteral nutrition* (TPN), also called intravenous hyperalimentation (IVH). TPN is the technique of providing total nutritional support by IV infusion of amino acids, a nonprotein source of calories (e.g., dextrose), electrolytes, vitamins, and trace elements. TPN solutions are usually administered together with a concentrated dextrose solution which, in addition to supplying calories essential for incorporation of amino acids into protein, also stimulates insulin production (important for amino acid transport). At least 100 to 150 nonprotein calories per gram of nitrogen is recommended.

Used as adjunct in TPN to prevent nitrogen loss or to correct negative nitrogen balance when there is interference with ingestion, digestion, or absorption of proteins, particularly over long periods. Also used for short-term, protein-sparing therapy to improve nitrogen balance, e.g., surgical patients, and patients with severe trauma or sepsis. Also commercially available in combination with a variety of electrolytes.

CONTRAINDICATIONS AND PRECAUTIONS. Hypersensitivity to any component; severe uncorrected electrolyte and acid–base imbalances; decreased circulating blood volume; anuria, oliguria, severe kidney or liver disease, hyperammonemia, bleeding abnormalities, inborn errors of amino acid metabolism. Safe use during pregnancy (category C) and children not established. *Cautious Use:* impaired renal or hepatic function, cardiac insufficiency, hypertension, diabetes mellitus.

ADVERSE/SIDE EFFECTS. (Dose-related): **CNS:** headache, dizziness, mental confusion, lassitude, unconsciousness. **CV:** flushing of skin and sensations of warmth (rapid infusion); pulmonary edema, exacerbation of hypertension. **GI:** nausea, vomiting, abdominal pain, fatty liver. **Hypersensitivity reactions:** skin rash, papular eruptions. **Infusion catheter site:** infection, including pyogenic arthritis, phlebitis, venous thrombosis, tissue sloughing. With extravasation (subclavian vein site): shoulder pain or burning, edema of neck and face. **Metabolic:** acidosis, alkalosis, hypophosphatemia, hypocalcemia, osteoporosis, electrolyte imbalance, glycosuria, hyperglycemia, rebound hypoglycemia, hypervolemia, hyperammonemia, and elevated liver enzymes (especially pediatric patients with liver disease); hypo- or hypervitaminosis. Following use of hyperosmolar preparations: osmotic diuresis, dehydration, coma. **Other:** flushing, fever, sensation of warmth, diaphoresis.

ROUTE AND DOSAGE. Dosage depends on patient's metabolic requirements and clinical response. **Intravenous: Adults:** 1 to 1.5 Gm/kg daily. **Pediatric:** 2 to 3 Gm/kg daily.

NURSING IMPLICATIONS

Effectiveness of TPN is largely dependent upon a team approach and a carefully prepared protocol.

TPN solutions should be prepared daily, preferably in hospital pharmacy, under a laminar flow filtered air hood, using strict aseptic technique.

Mixed solutions should be used immediately. If not used within an hour, refrigerate and use preferably in less than 24 hours, unless otherwise directed by manufacturer.

A volumetric infusion pump is recommended to maintain constant rate of infusion. An inline microfilter is used to remove particulate matter and microorganisms from the solution. Do not administer solution unless it is absolutely clear.

Scrupulous observation of aseptic technique is essential when inserting and changing catheter, when changing bottles, tubing or filters, and when giving care to catheter site.

All IV apparatus should be replaced every 24 hours (IV lines, filter, and bottle). Follow agency policy.

If infusion schedule falls behind, do not attempt to compensate by speeding up infusion rate since this may subject patient to glucose (dextrose) overload. However, do remedy cause of the incorrect flow rate.

Guidelines for monitoring patient receiving TPN:

Check vital signs at least every 4 hours.

Observe infusion catheter entry site for signs of infection, drainage, edema (extravasation).

Follow agency policy for care of skin puncture site. Usually, skin is first cleansed with a defatting substance such as acetone to remove oils. Site is then cleaned with povidone–iodine and an antimicrobial ointment is applied. Area is covered with an occlusive dressing and changed every 48 hours. Mask and gloves should be worn during procedure.

Sepsis is a constant threat and the most frequent serious complication of therapy. Fever or other possible signs of infection or hypersensitivity should be reported and investigated promptly. Solution and tubing are generally replaced and cultured. If source of fever still remains obscure, infusion catheter should be aseptically withdrawn and tip cultured.

Hyperalimentation line should not be used for collecting blood samples, giving blood, administration of medications, or for any other purpose but nutrition.

Urine should be tested for glucose, acetone, and specific gravity every 6 hours until infusion rate is stabilized, then two times daily. Blood glucose is usually obtained daily then twice weekly. In patients receiving high glucose loads or who are cardiacs, blood glucose may be done at same time urine is checked, until infusion rate is stable.

Use Clinistix, Keto-Diastix, or Tes-Tape to test for urine glucose. These specific tests for glucose are not affected by reducing substances that may be present in hyperalimentation solutions.

Patient may manifest high blood and urine glucose levels during first few days of therapy, depending on tolerance to the concentrated dextrose being administered concomitantly. If levels are sufficiently high, supplementary insulin may be necessary to prevent dehydration and coma.

Sudden fluctuations in urine glucose may indicate infection and should be reported.

If TPN therapy must be interrupted for whatever reason, 5% or 10% dextrose in water is usually given by peripheral vein to avoid rebound hypoglycemia.

Monitor intake and output and pattern, and caloric intake. Inform patient that he or she will have fewer bowel movements while receiving TPN. Report significant changes.

Patients receiving hyperalimentation frequently imagine they taste or smell food. Explain that these sensations occur commonly and suggest some distracting activity during mealtimes.

Administer meticulous mouth care at regular intervals to prevent parotitis. Encourage patient to use a soft toothbrush with a fluoride toothpaste, and to floss teeth daily.

Weigh patient daily under standard conditions: same time (preferably in the morning after voiding), same weight clothing, same scale. Once patient is stabilized, weights may be done two or three times weekly.

Be on the alert for and report signs of *circulatory overload:* edema, distended neck veins, dyspnea, cough, dizziness, pulmonary rales, elevated blood pressure, pulse, and CVP.

Observe pediatric patients and patients with impaired hepatic function for symptoms of *hyperammonemia:* lethargy, decreased appetite, vomiting, asterixis (flapping tremor), decreased responsiveness, seizures.

The following values are generally determined at start of TPN therapy and at regular intervals thereafter: CBC with differential and platelet count, serum electrolytes, blood glucose, urine glucose and ketones, prothrombin time, renal and hepatic function tests, trace elements (e.g., copper, zinc, manganese, iodine, cobalt, iron), plasma lipid levels.

A BUN to creatinine ratio in excess of 1:10 may mean that patient is receiving too much protein per unit of glucose. Reportedly, 100 to 150 Gm carbohydrate calories per gram of nitrogen are required to use amino acids effectively.

Patients should be mobilized as soon as feasible, beginning with passive exercises and progressing gradually into a muscle reconditioning program.

Patients receiving protein-sparing therapy should have daily BUN determinations. If BUN increases 10 to 15 mg% for more than 3 days, therapy is usually interrupted or a full protein caloric regimen started.

Recommended RDA dietary allowance of protein is approximately 0.9 Gm/kg/day for healthy adults and 1.4 to 2.2 Gm/kg/day for healthy infants and children. Protein and caloric requirements are substantially increased in traumatized and malnourished patients.

Drug Interactions. Antianabolic action of **tetracyclines** may reduce protein-sparing effects of amino acids.

AMINOCAPROIC ACID

(Amicar, Epsilon-Aminocaproic Acid [EACA])

(a-mee-noe-ka-proe'ik)
Hemostatic
Enzyme inhibitor
Antidote

ACTIONS AND USES. Synthetic monoaminocarboxylic acid with specific antifibrinolysis action. Acts principally by inhibiting plasminogen activator substance; to a lesser degree slightly inhibits activity of plasmin (fibrinolysin), which is concerned with destruction of clots. Does not control bleeding caused by loss of vascular integrity.

Used to control excessive bleeding resulting from systemic hyperfibrinolysis, a pathologic condition that may accompany heart surgery, portocaval shunt, abruptio placentae, aplastic anemia, and carcinoma of lung, prostate, cervix, and stomach. Also used in urinary fibrinolysis associated with severe trauma, anoxia, shock, urologic surgery, and neoplastic diseases of GU tract. Has been used to prevent hemorrhage in hemophiliacs undergoing dental extraction, as a specific antidote for streptokinase or urokinase toxicity, to prevent recurrence of subarachnoid hemorrhage especially when surgery is delayed, for management of amegakaryocytic thrombocytopenia, and to prevent or abort hereditary angioedema episodes.

ABSORPTION AND FATE. Rapidly absorbed from GI tract following oral administration; peak plasma levels achieved in about 2 hours. Widely distributed through both extravascular and intravascular compartments. Readily penetrates red blood cells and other body cells; does not appear to be bound to plasma proteins. Approximately 80% of single dose eliminated within 12 hours as unmetabolized drug.

CONTRAINDICATIONS AND PRECAUTIONS. Severe renal impairment, active disseminated intravascular clotting (DIC); upper urinary tract bleeding. Safe use during pregnancy not established. *Cautious Use:* cardiac, renal, or hepatic disease, history of thromboses.

ADVERSE/SIDE EFFECTS. CNS: dizziness, malaise, headache, unusual fatigue, weakness, tinnitus, hallucinations (auditory, visual, kinesthetic), acute delirium, psychotic reactions, seizures. **CV:** faintness, orthostatic hypotension; transient hypotension, bradycardia and other arrhythmias (with rapid IV); thrombophlebitis, generalized thromboses. **Dermatologic:** skin rash, pruritus, erythema. **EENT:** nasal stuffiness, conjunctival erythema. **GI:** nausea, vomiting, cramps, diarrhea, bloating, heartburn, anorexia. **GU:** diuresis, dysuria, urinary frequency, oliguria, reddish-brown urine (myoglobinuria), acute renal failure; inhibition of ejaculation, prolonged menstruation with cramping. **Other:** necrotic changes in heart and liver, liver failure (patients with cirrhosis), skeletal myopathy (rhabdomyolysis, myoglobinuria); increases in: CPK, serum aldose, SGOT, SGPT.

ROUTE AND DOSAGE. Oral; intravenous infusion (slowly): Adults: Initial priming dose: 4 to 5 Gm during the first hour, followed by 1 to 1.25 Gm at hourly intervals for about 8 hours until bleeding is controlled. Not to exceed 30 Gm/24 hours. **Children:** Initial priming dose: 100 mg/kg (3 Gm/m^2) during the first hour, followed by 33.3 mg/kg (1 Gm/m^2) per hour, by continuous infusion. Not to exceed 18 Gm/m^2 in 24 hours. Intravenous preparation must be diluted before use. Utilize compatible intravenous vehicles (sterile water for injection, physiologic saline, 5% dextrose, or Ringer's injection).

NURSING IMPLICATIONS

Before initiating aminocaproic acid therapy, a clinical diagnosis or laboratory findings indicative of hyperfibrinolysis (hyperplasminemia) should be obtained, i.e., normal platelet count, negative protamine paracoagulation test, and decreased euglobulin clot lysis.

If oral therapy is prescribed, note that patient may have to take as many as 10 tablets or 4 tsp for a 5 Gm dose during the first hour of treatment. (Each tablet contains 500 mg; syrup contains 250 mg/ml.)

Parenteral aminocaproic acid should always be diluted before use *(See Route and Dosage).*

Physician will order specific IV flow rate. Rapid administration should be avoided to prevent hypotension, faintness, and bradycardia or other arrhythmias.

Fresh whole blood, fibrinogen infusions, and other emergency measures may be required for some patients. (Plasma level of 0.13 mg/ml of drug is reportedly necessary to inhibit systemic fibrinolysis.) Patient's condition should be reevaluated after 8 hours of continuous therapy.

Check IV site at frequent intervals for extravasation. Observe for signs of thrombophlebitis (redness, heat, swelling, tenderness).

Inform patient that because drug may cause postural hypotension, he or she should change positions slowly and in stages, avoid standing still, and to lie down if feeling faint. Report symptoms to physician; they can be reversed by lowering dosage.

Monitor vital signs and intake and output. Record response to aminocaproic therapy and keep physician informed.

Report possible signs of myopathy: muscle weakness, myalgia, diaphoresis, fever, reddish-brown urine (myoglobinuria), oliguria. Drug should be discontinued promptly.
Patients receiving prolonged therapy should have routine laboratory measurements of creatine phosphokinase activity and urinalyses for early detection of myopathy.
Be alert to and report signs of thrombotic complications: arm or leg pain, tenderness, or swelling, Homan's sign, prominence of superficial veins, chest pain, breathlessness, dyspnea.
Store in tightly closed containers at room temperature, preferably between 15° and 30°C (59° and 86°F), unless otherwise directed by manufacturer. Protect from freezing.

Diagnostic Test Interferences. Serum **potassium** may be elevated (especially in patients with impaired renal function).

Drug Interactions. Possibility of hypercoagulation with concomitant administration of **oral contraceptives** or **estrogens.**

AMINOGLUTETHIMIDE

(Cytadren)

(a-mee-noe-gloo-teth′-i-mide)
Enzyme inhibitor
Adrenal suppressant

ACTIONS AND USES. Analogue of glutethimide. Blocks adrenal corticosteroid biosynthesis (i.e., mineralocorticoids, glucocorticoids, and other steroids) by inhibiting enzymatic conversion of cholesterol to pregnenolone precursors of cortisol and aldosterone. Also blocks aromatase thereby preventing conversion of androgens to estrogens in peripheral tissues. Because estrogens are supplied principally by the adrenals in postmenopausal and oophorectomized women, aminoglutethimide-induced lowering of plasma estrogen levels (by adrenal suppression) is reportedly as effective as that produced by surgical adrenalectomy. Goiter and mild hypothyroidism can develop with prolonged use because drug may block iodination of tyrosine. Aminoglutethimide has weak anticonvulsant properties.

Used for temporary treatment of selected patients with Cushing's syndrome associated with adrenal carcinoma, ectopic ACTH-producing tumors, or adrenal hyperplasia. *Investigational Use:* to produce medical adrenalectomy in postmenopausal women with positive estrogen receptor test, metastatic breast cancer, or who fail or relapse with tamoxifen (Nolvadex), and for patients with prostatic carcinoma. Former use as an anticonvulsant supplement has been abandoned, because of its adrenal suppressant activity.

ABSORPTION AND FATE. Onset of adrenal suppression: 3 to 5 days. Approximately 20 to 25% protein bound. Half-life: 13 hours (decreases to about 7 hours with prolonged use because aminoglutethimide accelerates its own metabolism by inducing hepatic enzymes). Recovery of adrenal responsiveness to stress usually occurs in 36 to 72 hours, following discontinuation of aminoglutethimide. Metabolized in liver. Excreted by kidneys: 50% of dose as unchanged drug and 20 to 50% as mildly active metabolites. Crosses placenta. Distribution into breast milk not known.

CONTRAINDICATIONS AND PRECAUTIONS. Hypersensitivity to aminoglutethimide or to glutethimide; hypothyroidism; infection. Safe use in pregnancy (category D), nursing mothers, and in children not established. Use with caution in the elderly.

ADVERSE/SIDE EFFECTS. CNS: lethargy, drowsiness, orthostatic dizziness or light-headedness, uncontrolled eye movements (dose related); clumsiness, ataxia, fever, headache, mental depression, confusion, respiratory depression, coma (overdosage). **CV:** orthostatic or persistent hypotension, tachycardia. **Endocrine:** masculinization including hirsutism, adrenal insufficiency. **GI:** nausea, vomiting, anorexia, elevation of liver enzymes (SGOT, alkaline phosphatase), cholestatic jaundice (possibly hypersensitivity). **Hematologic** (rare): neutropenia, leukopenia, thrombocytopenia, pancytopenia, agranulocytosis, decreased Hgb and Hct, anemia, Coombs' negative hemolytic anemia. **Skin:** measles-like (morbilliform) rash, pruritus, urticaria, darkening of skin. **Other:** myalgia, arthralgia, hypothyroidism, goiter (with prolonged use).

ROUTE AND DOSAGE. Oral: *metastatic breast cancer:* Initial: 250 mg two or three times daily for approximately 2 weeks (usually combined with hydrocortisone). Maintenance: 250 mg four times daily, preferably every 6 hours. *Cushing's syndrome:* Initial: 250 mg every 6 hours; increased in increments of 250 mg daily every 1 or 2 weeks, if necessary, up to 2 Gm daily.

NURSING IMPLICATIONS

Therapy is generally initiated in the hospital until dosage is stabilized. Certain carefully selected patients may be followed closely in the ambulatory care unit.

Baseline and periodic determinations should be made of: 8 AM fasting *plasma cortisol* levels (normal: 5 to 30 mcg/dl; excessively low levels indicate adrenal insufficiency); CBC; serum alkaline phosphatase (clue for early bone recurrence); AST (SGOT); bilirubin; thyroid function tests; *urinary aldosterone* (normal: 2 to 26 mcg/24 hours); serum electrolytes; CO_2.

Baseline and regularly scheduled blood pressure readings indicate the effect of reduced aldosterone levels on BP. Orthostatic and persistent hypotension (subjectively experienced as dizziness, light-headedness, weakness) results from reduced aldosterone production. Some patients require mineralocorticoid replacement, e.g., fludrocortisone.

Advise patient to make position changes gradually, pausing between each change. Also warn patient not to stand still for prolonged periods. Support hose may be helpful. Consult physician.

The elderly are particularly sensitive to the CNS effects of aminoglutethimide (e.g., lethargy, ataxia, orthostatic dizziness, lightheadedness). Note implications for ambulation.

Drowsiness, nausea, and anorexia often disappear spontaneously within 1 to 2 weeks of continuing therapy. Caution patient not to stop taking drug but to inform physician if symptoms persist or become pronounced.

Report skin rash that persists beyond 5 to 8 days. Physician may discontinue drug and possibly restart it after rash disappears.

Tolerance to lethargy and ataxia usually develops after 4 weeks of therapy (metabolism of aminoglutethimide accelerates with continuing use). If symptoms are severe, however, drug discontinuation may be necessary.

Emphasize importance of contacting physician immediately in times of stress such as surgery, dental work, acute illness, acute emotional situations. Steroid supplements, i.e., glucocorticoids (cortisone) and mineralocorticoids (fludrocortisone) may be indicated because normal body response to stress including infection and inflammation is impeded by adrenal suppression. Physician may temporarily stop aminoglutethimide.

Patients with Cushing's syndrome may show reduced effect (increasing cortisol levels) with continuing therapy possibly because ACTH rises reflexly in response to declining glucocorticoid levels. These patients are generally not treated beyond 3 months with aminoglutethimide.

Adrenal insufficiency (hypoadrenalism) symptoms include: anorexia, nausea, vomiting, weight loss, weakness, hypotension, dizziness, hypoglycemia, oliguria, low serum sodium, elevated K and BUN, arthralgia, myalgia, hyperpigmentation.

Because *hypothyroidism* may be induced, make appropriate observations. Report: cool, pale, dry skin; puffiness of hand and face (especially periorbital edema); constipation; sensitivity to cold; fatigue; slow relaxation phase in deep tendon reflexes, enlarged thyroid. Some patients require supplementary thyroid hormone therapy.

If patient becomes pregnant or must take aminoglutethimide during pregnancy she should be apprised of potential fetal deformities. Advise patient to notify physician immediately if pregnancy is suspected.

When aminoglutethimide is to be discontinued, dosage tapering is not necessary because the adrenal cortex returns to pretreatment level rather rapidly after drug is withdrawn.

Because of the possibility of drowsiness and dizziness, warn patient to avoid driving and other potentially hazardous activities until the reaction to drug is known.

Advise patient to carry card or jewelry (e.g., Medic Alert) indicating medical diagnosis, medication(s), physician's name, address, and telephone number.

Reinforce importance of continuous medical follow-up.

Store preferably between 15° and 30°C (59° and 86°F) in well-closed containers, unless otherwise directed by manufacturer.

Drug Interactions: Aminoglutethimide

Plus	Interactions
Dexamethasone	Acceleration of dexamethasone metabolism

AMINOPHYLLINE

(am-in-off'i-lin)

(Amoline, Corophyllin, Lixaminol, Mini-Lix, Palaron, Phyllocontin, Rectalad-Aminophylline, Somophyllin, Somophyllin-DF, Theophylline Ethylenediamine, Truphylline)

Smooth muscle relaxant: bronchodilator

Xanthine

ACTIONS AND USES. Ethylenediamide salt of theophylline with effects similar to those of other xanthines, e.g., caffeine and theobromine. Action is dependent on theophylline content (approximately 79%). Only xanthine derivative given IV for acute bronchial asthma attack. *See Theophylline.*

Used to prevent and relieve symptoms of acute bronchial asthma, and treatment of bronchospasm associated with chronic bronchitis and emphysema. Also used as a respiratory stimulant in Cheyne-Stokes respiration and for treatment of apnea and bradycardia in prematures. Use as cardiac stimulant and diuretic, in treatment of congestive heart failure, and as antispasmodic for acute biliary attack, has largely been replaced by more effective drugs.

ABSORPTION AND FATE. Time to peak serum concentrations: IV administration: within 30 minutes; oral solution: 1 hour; uncoated tablet: 2 hours; chewable tablet: 1 to 1.5 hours; enteric-coated tablet: 5 hours; extended release form: 4 to 7 hours (varies with product); retention enema: 1 to 2 hours. Retention enema: blood levels comparable to those for IV administration in contrast to suppository form, which is absorbed erratically. Metabolized in liver and excreted by kidneys, primarily as metabolites. Crosses placenta; excreted in breast milk.

CONTRAINDICATIONS AND PRECAUTIONS. Hypersensitivity to xanthine derivatives or to ethylenediamine component. *Cautious Use:* severe hypertension, cardiac disease, arrhythmias, impaired hepatic or renal function, diabetes mellitus, hyperthyroidism, glaucoma, prostatic hypertrophy, fibrocystic breast disease, history of peptic ulcer, neonates and young children, patients over 55, COPD, acute influenza or patients receiving influenza immunization. *See Theophylline.*

ADVERSE/SIDE EFFECTS. CNS: nervousness, restlessness, severe depression, insomnia, irritability, headache, dizziness, light-headedness, hyperactive reflexes, muscle twitching, convulsions. **CV:** flushing, palpitation, tachycardia, PVCs; with rapid IV: hyperventilation, precordial pain, severe hypotension, cardiac arrest. **GI:** nausea, vomiting, anorexia, bitter aftertaste, hematemesis, diarrhea, epigastric pain. **Hypersensitivity:** urticaria, contact dermatitis, exfoliative dermatitis, pruritus, angioedema. **Other:** rectal burning or irritation (suppository form), local pain and tissue sloughing (IM use), dehydration (from diuresis), hyperglycemia, tinnitus, flashes of light (toxicity).

ROUTE AND DOSAGE. *Individualized.* **Oral: Adults:** Initial: 500 mg; maintenance: 200 to 300 mg every 6 to 8 hours. **Pediatric:** Initial: 7.5 mg/kg; maintenance: 3 or 6 mg/kg every 6 to 8 hours. **Controlled release** (equivalent to 178 mg anhydrous theophylline tablet):Initial: 1 or 2 tablets. After 1 to 3 days (if desired response not achieved and if there are no adverse effects): **Adult:** 17 mg/kg/day; **Pediatric (9 to 16 years):** 23 to 25 mg/kg/day; **Children (6 to 9 years):** 30 mg/kg/day. **Intravenous:** Loading dose: 6 mg/kg administered over 30 minutes; not to exceed 25 mg/minute; maintenance: **Smoking adult (1 or 2 packs/day), and young adult (9 to 16 years):** 0.8 to 1.0 mg/kg/hour. **Nonsmoking adult:** 0.5 to 0.7 mg/kg/hour. **Pediatric (6 months to 9 years):** 1.0 to 1.2 mg/kg/hour. **Intramuscular** (not recommended): **Adult:** 500 mg. **Rectal solution: Adult:** 300 mg one to three times daily or 450 mg two times daily. **Pediatric:** 5 mg/kg every 6 to 8 hours. **Rectal suppository: Adult:** 500 mg one or two times daily. **Pediatric:** 7 mg/kg.

NURSING IMPLICATIONS

Some patients may require an around-the-clock dosage schedule.

Toxic effects are generally related to theophylline serum levels over 20 mcg/ml (therapeutic range 10 to 20 mcg/ml).

Dosages are based on ideal body weight because aminophylline (theophylline) is not distributed to fatty tissue.

Smoking–Drug Interaction. Smoking (tobacco or marijuana) tends to increase aminophylline elimination (prolongs half-life) and therefore dosage requirements may be higher and dosage intervals shorter than in nonsmokers. Reportedly, 3 months to 2 years of no smoking may be required to attain normal theophylline utilization.

Absorption may be delayed but is not reduced by presence of food in stomach.

Oral drug is absorbed faster if taken with a full glass of water on an empty stomach (½ to 1 hour before or 2 hours after meals).

GI symptoms may be minimized by administering oral drug with or immediately following a meal or food. It may be necessary to lower dosage or discontinue therapy if GI symptoms persist.

Extended (controlled) release preparations should not be chewed or crushed before swallowing; however, some tablets are scored and can be broken in half, then swallowed.

The contents of extended release capsules may be mixed with soft food and swallowed without chewing if patient desires.

To avoid overdosing, patient should be questioned whether he or she has received any aminophylline or theophylline preparation during previous 12 to 24 hours, before aminophylline regimen is started.

Rectally administered preparations are generally ordered when the patient must fast or cannot tolerate the drug orally. Drug absorption is enhanced if rectum is empty; therefore, if possible, schedule drug administration in relation to patient's evacuation time.

Because peristaltic activity is stimulated reflexly by presence of food in stomach, patient may experience less difficulty in retaining rectal medication if it can be given before a meal. Also advise patient to remain recumbent for 15 to 20 minutes or until defecation reflex subsides.

High incidence of toxicity is associated with rectal suppository use because of erratic rate of absorption. Children in contrast to adults absorb drug more quickly by rectum (use is generally avoided in children).

Administered IV aminophylline solution should be at room temperature.

Intramuscular route is generally avoided because injection causes prolonged intense pain. Note that IV and IM preparations are not interchangeable.

Patients receiving parenteral aminophylline should be closely observed for signs of hypotension, arrhythmias, and convulsions until serum theophylline stabilizes within the therapeutic range.

Monitor vital signs; measure and record intake and output. Improvements in quality and rate of pulse and respiration, as well as diuresis, are expected clinical effects. A sudden, sharp, unexplained rise in heart rate is a useful clinical indicator of toxicity.

The elderly, acutely ill, and patients with severe respiratory problems, liver dysfunction, or pulmonary edema are at greater risk of toxicity because of reduced drug clearance.

Dizziness is a relatively common side effect, particularly in the elderly. Take necessary safety precautions and forewarn patient of this possibility.

Children appear to be more susceptible than adults to the CNS stimulating effects of xanthines (nervousness, restlessness, insomnia, hyperactive reflexes, twitching, convulsions). Dosage reduction may be indicated.

When a change is made from one administration route to another observe patient closely until dosage is regulated. Changes in brands or dosage forms must be prescribed by physician.

Many popular OTC remedies for treatment of asthma or cough contain ephedrine in combination with various salts of theophylline. Caution patient to take only those medications approved by physician.

Aminophylline should not be mixed in a syringe with other drugs. Because aminophylline solutions are strongly alkaline, they are incompatible with alkali-labile drugs such as epinephrine (adrenalin), levarterenol (norepinephrine), isoproterenol, or penicillin G potassium. Aminophylline solutions are also incompatible with strong acid solutions, e.g., ascorbic acid. Consult pharmacist for specific compatibility information.

Do not use aminophylline solutions if discolored or if crystals are present.

Stored preferably between 15° and 30°C (59° and 86°F) in tightly closed containers unless otherwise directed by manufacturer.

Follow manufacturer's directions regarding storage of suppositories. Some are stored at room temperature, others must be refrigerated.

See Theophyline for Patient Teaching, Food–Drug Interactions, Diagnostic Test Interferences, and Drug Interactions.

AMINOSALICYLATE SODIUM

(a-mee-noe-sal-i′-si-late)

(Para-aminosalicylate Sodium, Parasal Sodium, PAS Sodium, Teebacin)

AMINOSALICYLIC ACID

(a-mee-noe-sal-i-sil-ik)

(Para-aminosalicylic Acid, PAS)

Antiinfective

Antituberculosis agent

ACTIONS AND USES. Structurally similar to para-aminobenzoic acid (PABA); mechanism of action resembles that of sulfonamides. Aminosalicylic acid and salts are highly specific bacteriostatic agents that suppress growth and multiplication of *Mycobacterium tuberculosis* by preventing folic acid synthesis. Despite close chemical relationship to salicylic acid, pharmacodynamics are not similar and apparently it does not produce syndrome of salicylism. Aminosalicylates reportedly have potent hypolipemic action and reduce serum cholesterol and triglycerides by lowering LDL and VLDL. Mechanism of this effect has not been established. Incidence of GI disturbances and crystalluria is reportedly greater with aminosalicylic acid than with its salts. Aminosalicylate sodium contains 73% aminosalicylic acid equivalent and 54.5 mg sodium per 500 mg tablet.

Used in combination with streptomycin or isoniazid or both in treatment of pulmonary and extrapulmonary tuberculosis to delay emergence of strains resistant to these drugs. Has been used for its lipid-lowering effect.

ABSORPTION AND FATE. Readily and almost completely absorbed from GI tract. Produces maximal blood concentrations within 1½ to 2 hours that persist about 4 hours. Aminosalicylate sodium is absorbed faster and more completely than the acid. Well-distributed to most tissues and body fluids, except CSF, unless meninges are inflamed. Rapidly penetrates pleural and caseous tissue. Half-life approximately 1 hour. About 50 to 73% protein bound. Metabolized in liver. Over 80% eliminated in urine within first 7 to 10 hours, in part as free drug and as acetylated compounds. Scant amounts excreted in bile and breast milk.

CONTRAINDICATIONS AND PRECAUTIONS. Hypersensitivity to aminosalicylates, salicylates, or to compounds containing para-aminophenyl groups (e.g., sulfonamides, certain hair dyes); G6PD deficiency, use of the sodium salt in patients on sodium restriction or congestive heart failure. Safe use during pregnancy not established. *Cautious Use:* impaired renal and hepatic function, blood dyscrasias, goiter, gastric ulcer.

ADVERSE/SIDE EFFECTS. CNS: headache, mental depression, confusion, psychotic reactions, encephalopathy. **GI:** anorexia, nausea, vomiting, abdominal distress, diarrhea, peptic ulceration, gastric hemorrhage. **Hematologic:** leukopenia, agranulocytosis, eosinophilia, lymphocytosis, thrombocytopenia, acute hemolytic anemia. **Hypersensitivity:** high temperature with intermittent spiking or low-grade fever, chills, generalized malaise, joint pain, sore throat, skin rash, fixed-drug eruptions, pruritus; vasculitis; syndrome resembling infectious mononucleosis; Loeffler's syndrome (lung tissue changes, fever, cough, breathlessness), neurologic manifestations. **Metabolic:** acidosis (especially in children), hypokalemia, pancreatitis (elevated serum amylase levels), glycosuria, jaundice, acute hepatitis, prothrombinemia. **Renal:** renal irritation, crystalluria. **Other:** impaired intestinal absorption of iron, lipids, folic acid, and vitamin B_{12}, development of megaloblastic anemia. With long-term administration: goiter with or without myxedema.

ROUTE AND DOSAGE. Oral: Adults: *Aminosalicylic acid:* 10 to 12 Gm daily in 2 or 3 divided doses. *Aminosalicylate sodium:* 12 to 15 Gm daily in 2 to 4 divided doses. **Children:** *Aminosalicylic acid:* 200 to 300 mg/kg daily in 3 or 4 divided doses. *Aminosalicylate sodium:* 240 to 360 mg/kg in 3 or 4 divided doses.

NURSING IMPLICATIONS

Administer with or immediately following meals to reduce irritative gastric effects. Physician may order an antacid to be given concomitantly. Generally, GI side effects disappear after a few days of therapy. If they persist, however, it may be necessary to reduce dosage or interrupt therapy for several days, then start with lower doses, or it may be necessary to terminate therapy.

Aminosalicylic acid is mildly sour to the taste, and it sometimes leaves a bitter aftertaste that may be relieved by rinsing mouth with clear water, or by chewing sugar-free gum or candy.

Appropriate bacteriologic studies, including sputum smears and cultures, blood cell counts should be performed initially and regularly throughout therapy.

Intake and output should be monitored and fluids encouraged. High concentrations of the drug are excreted in urine, and this can cause crystalluria and hematuria.

Food–Drug Interaction. Foods that promote alkaline urine include milk and dairy products, high intake of fruits and fruit juices (except prune and cranberry), and vegetables. Collaborate with physician and dietitian. Risk of crystalluria may be minimized by administering the sodium salt of aminosalicylic acid (prescribed) or by keeping urine neutral or alkaline with adjunctive drugs, such as antacids or with diet therapy.

Inform patient that urine may turn red on contact with hypochlorite bleach used in commercial toilet bowl cleaners.

Hypersensitivity reactions may occur after a few days, but most commonly in the fourth or fifth week.

Monitor temperature. Abrupt onset of fever, particularly during the early weeks of therapy, and a clinical picture resembling that of infectious mononucleosis (malaise, fatigue, generalized lymphadenopathy, splenomegaly, sore throat), as well as minor complaints of pruritus, joint pains, and headache, are strongly suggestive of hypersensitivity; these symptoms should be reported promptly. Continued administration of drug in the presence of hypersensitivity reactions can lead to hepatic damage, pancreatitis, and nephritis.

Instruct patient to notify physician if sore throat or mouth, malaise, unusual fatigue, bleeding or bruising occur (symptoms of blood dyscrasia).

Check weight semiweekly under standard conditions.

Therapeutic response to drug therapy is indicated by a feeling of well-being, improved appetite, weight gain, reduced fever, lessening of fatigue, decreased cough and sputum, improved chest x-rays, and negative sputum cultures.

Generally, chemotherapy is continued about 2 years. Patient and responsible family members must understand signs and symptoms of drug toxicity, the importance of maintaining an established drug regimen, and the need for remaining under close medical supervision to detect covert adverse drug effects. Point out that resistant strains develop more rapidly when drug regimen is interrupted or is sporadic.

Caution patient not to take aspirin or other OTC drugs without physician's approval.

A brownish or purplish discoloration of the drug signifies decomposition; should this occur, discard drug.

Aminosalicylic acid is an unstable drug that deteriorates rapidly on contact with heat, air, and moisture. Store in tight, light-resistant containers in a cool, dry place, preferably between 15° and 30°C (59° and 86°F), unless otherwise directed by manufacturer. Solutions of aminosalicylate generally should be used within 24 hours.

Diagnostic Test Interferences. Aminosalicylates (PAS) may interfere with urine **urobilinogen** determinations (using Ehrlich's reagent), and may cause false-positive **urinary protein** and

VMA determinations (with diazoreagent); false-positive **urine glucose** may result with cupric sulfate tests, e.g., Benedict's solution, but reportedly not with glucose oxidase reagents, e.g., Tes-Tape, Clinistix. Reduces **serum cholesterol,** and possibly **serum potassium, serum PBI,** and 24-hour **I-131 thyroidal uptake** (effect may last almost 14 days).

Drug Interactions: Aminosalicylic acid

Plus	Interactions
Alcohol, ethyl (Ethanol)	May diminish hypolipemic effect of PAS
Anticoagulants, oral	PAS enhances hypoprothrombinemic effect
Ammonium chloride Ascorbic acid (vitamin C)	Acidifying doses may increase possibility of PAS-induced crystalluria. Concurrent use generally avoided
Cyanocobalamin (vitamin B_{12}) Folic acid (Folacin)	PAS may decrease GI absorption of oral vitamins. Parenteral administration may be necessary
Digoxin	Possibility of reduced serum digoxin levels (PAS decreases GI absorption). Monitor serum digoxin concentration
Diphenhydramine (Benadryl) and other antihistamines	May impair GI absorption of PAS. Concurrent use generally avoided
Isoniazid (INH)	Increases isoniazid plasma levels (PAS decreases rate of isoniazid metabolism)
Para-aminobenzoic acid (PABA)	May inhibit activity of PAS. Concurrent use not recommended
Phenytoin (Dilantin)	PAS (in combination with isoniazid) may increase phenytoin blood levels
Probenecid (Benemid) Sulfinpyrazone (Anturane)	Increases PAS effect by inhibiting renal excretion. Used with caution
Rifampin	Certain PAS preparations (containing bentonite) may impair rifampin absorption. Separate by 8 to 12 hours
Salicylates	May enhance PAS toxicity

AMIODARONE

(Cordarone)

(a-mee'-oh-da-rone)

Antiarrhythmic (Class III)

ACTIONS AND USES. Iodinated benzofuran derivative structurally related to thyroxine. Exhibits antiarrhythmic, antianginal, and antiadrenergic properties (antagonizes both alpha and beta responses to catecholamines). Totally unrelated to other antiarrhythmics. By direct action on cardiac tissue, increases SA node conduction and recovery time, and thus depresses sinus, atrial, and AV nodal function. Other hemodynamic effects: increased cardiac output, decreased peripheral and coronary vascular resistance, and bradycardia. May induce refractoriness to cardioversion; prolongs QT interval. During early treatment period (first 3 months) thyroid hormone metabolism is altered as evidenced by elevated serum T_4 and lowered T_3 concentrations. Usually normal levels are restored (unknown reason) after this period even with continuation of therapy.

Used to treat refractory supraventricular and ventricular tachyarrhythmias, particularly in patients with atrial fibrillation complicated by Wolff–Parkinson–White (WPW) syndrome.

ABSORPTION AND FATE. Serum concentration peaks in 2 to 10 hours, but onset of clinical effect is slow *(see Nursing Implications).* Half-life: 13 to 107 days (with chronic therapy). Extensively metabolized in liver releasing 6 mg iodine/200 mg dose daily. Eliminated in urine.

CONTRAINDICATIONS AND PRECAUTIONS. Severe sinus bradycardia, advanced AV block, severe liver disease. *Cautious Use:* Hashimoto's thyroiditis, goiter.

ADVERSE/SIDE EFFECTS. CNS/Neurologic: tremor, abnormal gait, ataxia, peripheral neuropathy (proximal muscle weakness, numbness, tingling), headache, depression, insomnia, nightmares, hallucinations. **CV:** bradycardia, myocardial depression, hypotension, sinoatrial block, sinus arrest, cardiogenic shock. **GI:** anorexia, nausea, vomiting, abdominal pain, constipation. **Ophthalmic:** blurred vision, colored halos around lights, yellow-brown corneal microdeposits, photophobia. **Respiratory (pulmonary toxicity):** alveolitis, pulmonary fibrosis, hypersensitivity pneumonitis, necrotizing pneumonitis. **Skin:** slate-blue discoloration (slowly reversible), photosensitivity. **Other (with chronic use):** high frequency of drug-induced hyperthyroidism and hypothyroidism; hepatic toxicity, significant elevations in AST, ALT; bone marrow depression, transient ischemic attacks (TIAs).

ROUTE AND DOSAGE. Oral (dosages vary widely): *Dose range:* 200 to 800 mg/day; up to 1.4 Gm/day in divided doses. **Intravenous:** 5 to 10 mg/kg/day. Smallest effective dose is advised regardless of route. (Each 200 mg tablet contains 75 mg iodine.)

NURSING IMPLICATIONS

Onset of pharmacologic effects range from 5 to 30 days. Full clinical effects may not be apparent for 1½ to 3 months.

Neurologic symptoms may develop within a week after therapy with amiodarone begins.

Amiodarone-induced thyroid dysfunction depends on environmental factors: i.e., if patient is in a geographic area of iodine deficiency, hyperthyroidism is common; but if iodine intake in normal, hypothyroidism can occur.

During early treatment period, especially, watch for and report symptoms of drug-induced thyroid dysfunction: *hypothyroidism:* periorbital edema, lethargy, puffy hands and feet; cool, pale skin; vertigo, nocturnal cramps, decreased GI motility, enlarged thyroid gland. *Hyperthyroidism* (thyrotoxicosis): warm, flushed, moist skin; tachycardia, exophthalmos, infrequent lid blinking, lid edema, weight loss in spite of increased appetite, frequent urination, menstrual irregularity, breathlessness, hypoventilation, congestive heart failure.

Baseline and periodic assessments should be made of liver, lung, thyroid, and neurologic function.

Skin and corneal discoloration *(lipofuscinosis)* seen in most patients who receive drug for 2 months or more, is reportedly reversible but may take several months to fade completely.

Generally, corneal deposits do not interfere with vision.

After drug steady state is established, regular drug holidays may minimize or interrupt development of corneal deposits.

Photophobia may be eased by wearing dark glasses but some patients are unable to go outdoors at all in the daytime even with such protection.

Alert patient to the possibility of a photosensitivity reaction; advise use of sun screen lotion (SPF above 15) and protective clothing to reduce reaction in exposed skin areas.

Be alert to symptoms of pulmonary toxicity: progressive dyspnea, fatigue, cough, pleuritic pain, fever. Drug will be stopped pending diagnosis.

Monitor heart rate and rhythm until drug response has stabilized. Report promptly symptomatic bradycardia (light-headedness, syncope, fatigue) and onset of worsening arrhythmia.

After patient is stabilized, cardiac rhythm should be checked daily (as prescribed) by patient or primary caregiver.

Proximal muscle weakness, a common side effect, intensified by tremors present a great hazard to the ambulating patient. Assess severity of these drug-induced effects and protect patient from falling if he or she walks, or restrict ambulation if necessary.

Noncardiac side effects of this drug (especially lipofuscinosis, photophobia, insomnia) are major factors in noncompliance even though reversible. Check periodically to reinforce importance of adhering to the established drug regimen.

Report adverse reactions promptly. Bear in mind that long elimination half-life means that drug effects will persist long after regimen adjustment or discontinuation, and that it serves, too, as a camouflage for noncompliance.

Drug Interactions: Amiodarone

Plus	Interactions
β-blockers, e.g., propranolol (Inderal); Calcium channel blockers, e.g., verapamil (Calan, Isoptin)	Possibility of additive bradycardia; used with caution
Digoxin (Lanoxin)	Possibility of elevated serum digoxin levels; used with caution
Disopyramide (Norpace); Quinidine	Pharmacologic effects of disopyramide and quinidine may be increased with development of atypical ventricular tachycardia. Used with caution, if at all
Lidocaine	Severe bradycardia and sinoatrial arrest can occur. Monitor closely
Warfarin	Enhanced anticoagulant effect. Initial anticoagulant doses reduced by 32 to 50%

AMITRIPTYLINE HYDROCHLORIDE

(a-mee-trip′ti-leen)

(Amitid, Amitril, Apo-Amitriptyline, Elavil, Emitrip, Endep, Enovil, Levate, Meravil, Novotriptyn, SK-Amitriptyline)

Psychotropic: antidepressant
Tricyclic

ACTIONS AND USES. Dibenzocycloheptene tricyclic antidepressant with greater anticholinergic and sedative actions than imipramine. May suppress alpha rhythm in EEG; most active of the tricyclic antidepressants (TCAs) in inhibition of serotonin uptake from synaptic gap. Has H_2-receptor blocking activity (inhibits gastric acid secretion). Antimigraine effect appears to be independent of antidepressant action. Actions, uses, contraindications, precautions, adverse effects similar to those of other TCAs; *see Imipramine.*

Used to treat endogenous depression. *Investigational Use:* as prophylaxis for cluster, migraine, and chronic tension headaches, intractable pain, peptic ulcer disease, and to increase muscle strength in myotonic dystrophy. Available in fixed combination with chlordiazepoxide (Limbitrol) and with perphenazine (Triavil, Etrafon).

ABSORPTION AND FATE. Rapidly absorbed from GI tract and injection sites. Peak plasma concentrations (for oral and IM routes) occur within 2 to 12 hours. Steady state attained in 4 to 10 days. Half-life: 10 to 50 hours; 96% protein bound. Metabolized in liver; intermediate active metabolite is nortriptyline. About 25 to 50% of dose excreted in urine as inactive metabolites within 24 hours. Small amounts eliminated in feces via bile. Crosses placenta and enters breast milk.

CONTRAINDICATIONS AND PRECAUTIONS. Acute recovery period following myocardial infarction; pregnancy (category C), nursing mothers, children under 12. *Cautious Use:* prostatic hypertrophy, history of urinary retention or obstruction, angle-closure glaucoma, history of seizures, diabetes mellitus, hyperthyroidism, patient with cardiovascular, hepatic, or renal dysfunction; patient with suicidal tendency or on electroschock therapy; schizophrenia, respiratory disorders; elderly, adolescent age groups. *See also Imipramine.*

ADVERSE/SIDE EFFECTS. CNS: drowsiness, dizziness, nervousness, restlessness, fatigue, headache, disorientation, confusion, insomnia, nightmares, paresthesias, ataxia, tremors. **CV:** orthostatic hypotension, hypertension, palpitation, tachycardia, ECG changes. **ENT:** tinnitus, nasal congestion. **GI:** increased appetite, weight gain or loss, epigastric distress, dry mouth, sour or metallic taste, constipation, nausea, vomiting. **Hypersensitivity:** rash, pruritus, urticaria, photosensitivity. **Ophthalmic:** blurred vision, ophthalmoplegia. **Other:** urinary retention, SIADH (rare), leukopenia. *See also Imipramine.*

ROUTE AND DOSAGE. Highly individualized. **Oral: Adults** *(Hospitalized):* Initial: 100 mg/day; gradually increased to 200 to 300 mg/day, if necessary. *(Outpatient):* 75 mg/day in divided doses; may be increased to 150 mg/day. Alternate regimen: Initial: 50 to 100 mg at bedtime, increased gradually to 150 mg/day, if necessary. **Adolescents, elderly:** 10 mg three times daily with 20 mg at bedtime. Maintenance: 25 to 100 mg/day in single dose at bedtime. **Intramuscular:** 20 to 30 mg four times daily (until patient can or will take tablet form).

NURSING IMPLICATIONS

Oral drug may be taken with or immediately after food to reduce possibility of gastric irritation.

Tablet may be crushed if patient is unwilling to take it whole; administer with food or fluid.

Dose increases by 25 to 50 mg are preferably made in late afternoon and/or at bedtime because sedative action precedes antidepressant effect.

Because amitriptyline is long-acting, physician may prescribe entire oral dose at one time. A single dose at bedtime is useful for patients who complain of insomnia or dizziness or when daytime sedation interferes with work productivity. Drug effect on depression is not affected by time of day dose is taken.

Smoking–Drug Interaction. Smoking increases metabolism of tricyclics. A higher dose of amitriptyline may be required for heavy smokers than for non- or moderate smokers. Urge patient to stop or at least reduce cigarette smoking.

Monitor blood pressure and pulse rate in patients with cardiovascular disease. Withhold drug if there is a significant fall in systolic BP (10 to 20 mm Hg) or a sudden increase in pulse rate. Notify physician.

Desired therapeutic effects for depression may not be evident until after 3 to 4 weeks of therapy, because of long serum half-life. Dosage should then be reduced gradually to lowest effective level.

Maintenance regimen is usually continued for at least 3 months to prevent relapse. Typical length of therapy for depression is 6 months to 1 year. Patient should be evaluated at regular intervals to determine need for continued drug therapy.

Parenteral preparation is for IM use only.

Baseline and periodic leukocyte and differential counts, BP, cardiac and hepatic function tests are recommended in patients receiving high doses or prolonged therapy.

Plasma levels (therapeutic range: 125 to 250 ng/ml) do not always correlate with clinical effectiveness and therefore are not done routinely.

The actions of both alcohol and amitriptyline are potentiated when used concurrently during therapy and for up to 2 weeks after drug is discontinued. Consult physician about safe amount of alcohol, if any, that can be taken.

If a patient uses excessive amounts of alcohol it should be borne in mind that the potentiation of amitriptyline effects may increase the dangers of overdosage or suicide attempt.

Suicide is an inherent risk with any depressed patient and may remain until there is significant improvement. Supervise patient closely during early phase of therapy. The amount of amitriptyline dispensed to the patient should be strictly controlled.

Tolerance or adaptation to distressing anticholinergic actions (dry mouth, constipation, blurred vision, urinary retention) usually develops after patient goes on maintenance regimen.

During initial therapy be alert to orthostatic hypotensive and sedative effects, and confusional episodes, especially in the elderly. Institute measures to prevent falling. Instruct patient to change from recumbency to upright position slowly and in stages. Support hose may help. Consult physician.

Caution patient to avoid potentially hazardous activities such as driving until response to the drug is known.

Monitor weight. Amitriptyline may increase the appetite for carbohydrate foods.

Withdrawal symptoms (headache, nausea, malaise, musculoskeletal pain, weakness) can be avoided by tapering dosage over a 2-week period.

When used for migraine prophylaxis, therapeutic effect may occur in 1 to 6 weeks. Drug is usually discontinued after patient has been headache-free for 1 to 2 months. If headache recurs, physician may prescribe another course of treatment.

Amitriptyline may impart blue green color to urine.

Store drug at 15° to 30°C (59° to 86°F) unless otherwise instructed by manufacturer. Protect from light. *See Imipramine (prototype tricyclic antidepressant).*

Drug Interactions: Amitriptyline

Plus	Interactions
Anticoagulants, oral	Decreased hypoprothrombinemic effects. Monitor closely
Antihypertensives: clonidine (Catapres), guanethidine (Ismelin), methyldopa (Aldomet)	Antihypertensive action may be decreased. Combination avoided, when possible
CNS depressants, e.g., alcohol (Ethanol), barbiturates, sedatives, hypnotics	Potentiation of CNS depression. Also, barbiturates reduce TCA blood levels. Used with caution
Disulfiram (Antabuse)	Possibility of acute organic brain syndrome: confusion, psychosis. Described for amitriptyline only. Used with caution
Furazolidone (Furoxone), MAO inhibitors	Possibility of severe reactions (toxic psychosis, hyperpyrexia, tachycardia, seizures). Used with extreme caution
Levodopa (Dopar, Larodopa), Sympathomimetics	Possibility of sympathetic hyperactivity with hypertension and hyperpyrexia. Used with caution

See also Imipramine.

AMMONIA SPIRIT, AROMATIC

Central stimulant: respiratory

(Ammonia Aromatic)

ACTIONS AND USES. Aromatic solution of ammonia, alcohol, and a mixture of oils (lemon, lavender, nutmeg). Stimulates respiratory and vasomotor centers in medulla reflexly by peripheral irritation of sensory receptors in nasal membrane, mucosa of esophagus, and fundus of stomach. Also acts as an antacid and carminative.

Used as mild stimulant ("smelling salts") to prevent or treat fainting.

ROUTE AND DOSAGE. Inhalation: inhale vapors as required. **Oral:** 2 to 4 ml well diluted with water (at least 30 ml).

NURSING IMPLICATIONS

For inhalation, available in single dose glass vials (pearls) covered with woven fabric. Wrap in gauze or cloth and crush between fingers.

Although fainting is not generally an indication of a health problem, it can be. After patient recovers from faint, inquire about history of events that preceded it. Some possible causes of faintness include: head injury, combination of alcohol and drugs, prolonged standing, straining at stool or urination (Valsalva maneuver), slow or irregular heartbeat, heart failure, loss of blood volume, low blood sugar, sudden inactivity following vigorous exercise.

Medical referral is indicated if patient has had other recent episodes of fainting or if person is 40 years of age or over.

Preserved in tight, light-resistant containers in a cool place, at temperature not exceeding 30°C (86°F), unless otherwise directed by manufacturer.

AMMONIUM CHLORIDE

Acidifier, systemic and urinary
Diuretic

ACTIONS AND USES. Acidifying property is due to conversion of ammonium ion (NH_4^+) to urea in liver with liberation of H^+ and Cl^-. Chloride anions displace bicarbonate producing acidosis that causes temporary (1 to 3 days) increased excretion of Na^+ and hence diuresis. Potassium excretion also increases, but to a lesser extent. Tolerance to diuretic effect occurs by compensatory mechanisms, including renal excretion of H^+ and K^+ cations and formation of ammonia by renal cells, with recovery of corresponding amounts of sodium ions. Also has mild expectorant action. Contains 18.7 mEq each of ammonium and chloride ions per gram.

Used as systemic acidifier in patients with metabolic alkalosis (e.g., produced by excess alkalinizing medications, chloride loss from gastric suction, vomiting, gastric fistula drainage), to correct chloride depletion following diuretic therapy, as adjunct to lower urinary pH in treatment of urinary tract infections, and as an aid in excretion of certain alkalinizing drugs. Limited use as a primary diuretic. Has been used to increase solubility of calcium and phosphate ions in urinary phosphatic calculi, and in treatment of bromism and Meniere's syndrome. Common ingredient in OTC cough mixtures.

ABSORPTION AND FATE. Complete absorption occurs in 3 to 6 hours (enteric-coated tablet absorption is erratic). Metabolized in liver to form HCl and urea. Primarily excreted in urine; 1 to 3% excreted in feces.

CONTRAINDICATIONS AND PRECAUTIONS. Renal, hepatic, and pulmonary insufficiency, primary respiratory acidosis. Safe use during pregnancy and in children not established. *Cautious Use:* cardiac edema.

ADVERSE/SIDE EFFECTS. *(Most are secondary to ammonia toxicity):* **CNS:** headache, progressive drowsiness, confusion, twitching, convulsions, excitement alternating with coma. **CV:** bradycardia and other arrhythmias. **GI:** gastric irritation, nausea, vomiting, anorexia, diarrhea. **Metabolic:** *metabolic acidosis* (nausea, vomiting, increased rate and depth of respirations [Kussmaul breathing], thirst, weakness, flushed face, full bounding pulse, lethargy, progressive drowsiness, mental confusion, combativeness, excitement alternating with coma); hypercalcinuria, calcium deficiency, tetany, hyponatremia, hypokalemia, hypomagnesemia, hyperglycemia. **Other:** skin rash, glycosuria, hyperventilation, EEG abnormalities; pain and irritation at IV site. With rapid IV administration: *hyperammonemia:* vomiting, pallor, sweating, irregular breathing, bradycardia, asterixis (liver flap), hyperreflexia, tonic convulsions, coma.

ROUTE AND DOSAGE. Oral: *Urine acidifier; diuretic:* **Adults:** 4 to 12 Gm/day in divided doses at 4- to 6-hour intervals. For diuresis, administered in intermittent 3- or 4-day courses followed by rest period of a few days. **Intravenous:** *Metabolic alkalosis* (Dosages calculated on basis of CO_2 combining power, serum chloride deficit, and serum bicarbonate): **Adults and children:** approximately 10 ml/kg of 2.14% solution. Infusion rate: 0.9 to 1.3 ml/minute, not to exceed 2 ml/minute.

NURSING IMPLICATIONS

GI side effects may be minimized by giving drug immediately after meals or by use of enteric-coated tablets.

The concentrated ammonium chloride parenteral preparation (26.75%) must be diluted prior to infusion. See manufacturer's package insert or consult pharmacist.

Ammonium chloride should be administered slowly IV to avoid serious side effects (ammonia toxicity), and local irritation and pain.

Ammonium chloride preparations are not intended to be used subcutaneously, intraperitoneally, or rectally.

Baseline and periodic determinations of CO_2 combining power, serum electrolytes, and urinary and arterial pH should be made during therapy to avoid serious acidosis. For some patients, dosage may be monitored by repeated serum chloride and CO_2 content (bicarbonate), determinations and urinary pH.

Normal values: blood ammonia: 15 to 110 mcg/100 ml; *serum chloride:* 100 to 106 mEq/L; *CO_2 content* (as bicarbonate): 20 to 30 mEq/L; *arterial blood pH:* 7.35 to 7.45; *Pco_2:* 35 to 45 mm Hg; *serum potassium:* 3.5 to 5 mEq/L; *urinary pH:* normal range 4.8 to 7.8.

Food–Drug Interaction. Unless contraindicated, diet of patients on diuretic therapy should include foods high in potassium, e.g., bananas, oranges, cantaloupe, honeydew melon, milk (all types), yogurt, spinach, tomatoes, mushrooms, potatoes.

Note rate and depth of respirations. Shortness of breath and increased ventilation at rest are signs of acidosis *(see Adverse/Side Effects).* Intravenous sodium bicarbonate or sodium lactate may be used to treat severe acidosis.

Report change in intake and output ratio. Because of compensatory mechanisms the diuretic effect of ammonium chloride lasts only 1 or 2 days.

In the elderly, vigorous diuresis may precipitate renal insufficiency, urinary retention in males with prostatic hypertrophy, incontinence in both sexes, and acute Na^+ and K^+ depletion. Report signs of weakness and confusion and changes in voiding pattern and comfort.

Check urine specific gravity of the older person on diuretic therapy: elevation accompanying even mild diuresis is suggestive of renal insufficiency.

Hyperglycemia and glycosuria are potential side effects. Note implications for the diabetic patient.

Concentrated solutions of ammonium chloride tend to crystallize at low temperatures. Crystals will dissolve by placing intact container in a warm water bath and warming to room temperature.

Diagnostic Test Interferences. Ammonium chloride (NH_4Cl) may increase **blood ammonia** and **SGOT (AST)**, decrease **serum magnesium** (by increasing urinary magnesium excretion), decrease urine **urobilinogen.**

Drug Interactions: Ammonium chloride

Plus	Interactions
Aminosalicylic acid (PAS)	By increasing urine acidity NH_4Cl enhances possibility of crystalluria and PAS toxicity. Used with caution
Anorexigenics, e.g., amphetamines Antidepressants, tricyclics Ephedrine Methadone Pseudoephedrine (Sudafed) Sulfonylureas, e.g., chlorpropamide	Increase in urine acidity by NH_4Cl reduces renal tubular reabsorption and thus may decrease effects of these drugs
Salicylates	Acidification of urine increases renal tubular reabsorption and thus increases plasma salicylate concentrations
Spironolactone (Aldactone)	Possibility of severe systemic acidosis. Used with caution

AMOBARBITAL
(Amytal, Isobec, Novamobarb)
AMOBARBITAL SODIUM
(Amytal Sodium)

(am-oh-bar'bi-tal)
Sedative/hypnotic
Anticonvulsant
Barbiturate
C II

ACTIONS AND USES. Intermediate-acting barbiturate with actions, uses, contraindications, and precautions similar to those of phenobarbital (qv).

Used as sedative, to relieve anxiety, and as short-term hypnotic to treat insomnia. Also used parenterally to control status epilepticus or acute convulsive episodes, agitated behavior, and for narcoanalysis and narcotherapy. Amobarbital sodium is available in combination with secobarbital (Tuinal).

ABSORPTION AND FATE. Oral administration: onset of action within 1 hour; duration of action approximately 6 to 8 hours. IV administration: onset of effects within 5 minutes; duration about 3 to 6 hours. Protein binding: 61%. Half-life: 16 to 40 hours. Inactivated in liver by hydroxylation. About 40 to 50% of oral dose excreted in urine as inactive metabolites; less than 1% excreted unchanged.

CONTRAINDICATIONS AND PRECAUTIONS. Hypersensitivity to barbiturates; history of addiction; family or patient history of porphyria; severe respiratory disease. *Cautious Use:* impaired hepatic function, hypotension, hypertension, cardiac disease. *See Phenobarbital.*

ADVERSE/SIDE EFFECTS. Light-headedness, dizziness, nausea, vomiting, slurred speech; with rapid injection: hypotension, apnea, respiratory depression; with extravasation or intraarterial injection: thrombophlebitis, tissue necrosis. *See also Phenobarbital.*

ROUTE AND DOSAGE. Adults: Oral: *Sedative:* 30 to 50 mg two or three times daily (range 15 to 120 mg two to four times/day). *Hypnotic:* 65 to 200 mg. Preoperative: 200 mg 1 or 2 hours before surgery. *Labor:* Initial: 200 to 400 mg, may be repeated at 1- to 3-hour intervals; not to exceed 1 Gm daily. *Anticonvulsant:* 65 mg two to four times daily. **Intravenous, intramuscular:** Maximum IM dose: 500 mg. Maximum IV dose: 1 Gm. IV rate of injection not to exceed 100 mg/minute for adults. **Pediatric: Oral:** *Sedative:* 2 mg/kg (or 60 mg/m^2) three times a day; *Anticonvulsant: Hypnotic:* **Intramuscular, intravenous:** 3 to 5 mg/kg or (125 mg/m^2)/dose. IV rate of injection not to exceed 60 mg/m^2/minute for children. Available in tablets, elixir, capsules, powder (for injection).

NURSING IMPLICATIONS

Rate of absorption is increased if oral drug is taken on an empty stomach. Caution patient not to take alcoholic beverages or other CNS depressants.

For insomnia, dose is generally administered 30 to 60 minutes before bedtime.

Hypnotic use should be limited to 2 weeks. Amobarbital effectiveness appears to decrease by second week of continued use. Some clinicians recommend tapering dosage over 5 to 6 days to prevent any rebound effects.

Prolonged use may lead to tolerance and dependence.

Amobarbital sodium hydrolyzes in dry form or in solution when exposed to air. Drug should be injected within 30 minutes after opening ampule.

Parenteral solution is reconstituted with sterile water for injection. After adding diluent, rotate vial to facilitate solution. Do not shake vial. If solution does not clear within 5 minutes or contains a precipitate, do not use.

IM injection should be deep in a large muscle mass, e.g., gluteus maximus. Superficial injections are painful and can cause sterile abscess or sloughing.

No more than 5 ml should be injected IM into any one site.

IV amobarbital sodium is given only to hospitalized patients under close supervision. Vital signs should be monitored during injection and for several hours after drug administration. Caution patient not to get out of bed without assistance. Bedsides are indicated.

Personnel and equipment for management of respiratory depression and hypotension should be immediately available when drug is administered IV.

Barbiturates may produce paradoxical restlessness, excitement, confusion, and depression in the elderly and in some children. Dosage adjustments may be required.

Paradoxical excitement may occur in patients receiving barbiturates, with onset of pain. Barbiturates are not intended for pain relief.

Advise patient not to drive or engage in potentially hazardous activities until reaction to drug is known.

Classified as a Schedule II drug under Federal Controlled Substances Act.

Store oral and unopened parenteral forms preferably between 15° and 30°C (59° and 86°F) unless otherwise directed by manufacturer. Avoid freezing.

See Phenobarbital (prototype barbiturate).

Drug Interactions: Amobarbital

Plus	Interactions
Anorexiants, e.g., amphetamines	Antagonistic pharmacologic effects. Concurrent use generally avoided

Plus (cont.)	Interactions (cont.)
CNS depressants, e.g., alcohol, sedatives, hypnotics	Increased CNS depression. Used with extreme caution
MAO inhibitors, e.g., tranylcypromine (Parnate)	Prolongs amobarbital effects; excessive CNS depression (inhibits metabolism). Used with caution
Methoxyflurane anesthesia (Penthrane)	Risk of nephrotoxicity. Barbiturate should be discontinued 7 days in advance

See also Phenobarbital (prototype barbiturate).

AMOXAPINE

(Asendin)

(a-mox'a-peen)
Psychotropic: antidepressant
Tricyclic

ACTIONS AND USES. Dibenzoxazepine derivative tricyclic antidepressant (TCA). Action mechanism not clear. Appears to reduce reuptake of norepinephrine (particularly) and serotonin, and to block response to dopamine by dopaminergic receptors. Antidepressant activity is equivalent to that of imipramine, but amoxapine is more effective in relieving agitation and anxiety. Unlike other TCAs, not associated with severe cardiotoxicity. Has mild sedative and anticholinergic actions. Similar to imipramine (qv) in actions, uses, limitations and interactions.

Used to treat neurotic and endogenous depression accompanied by anxiety or agitation.

ABSORPTION AND FATE. Rapidly absorbed. Peak blood levels reached in 1 to 2 hours. About 90% protein bound. Metabolized in liver to active metabolites. Half-life of parent drug: 8 hours; major active metabolite has antidepressant activity and half-life of about 30 hours. About 60% dose excreted in urine, primarily as conjugated metabolites, within 6 days; approximately 7 to 18% eliminated in feces. Excreted in breast milk.

CONTRAINDICATIONS AND PRECAUTIONS. Hypersensitivity to other tricyclic antidepressants; children under 16 years of age; pregnancy (category C), nursing mothers, acute recovery period following MI. *Cautious Use:* history of convulsive disorders, schizophrenia, manic depression, alcohol abuse, urinary retention, angle closure glaucoma, cardiac abnormalities. *See also Imipramine.*

ADVERSE/SIDE EFFECTS. CNS: drowsiness, dizziness, headache, fatigue, akathisia (motor restlessness), acute dystonic reactions, panic attacks, parkinsonism, tardive dyskinesia, seizures (overdosage). **CV:** hypotension; irregular, unusually slow or rapid heart beat. **GI:** constipation, flatulence, dry mouth, peculiar taste, nausea, craving for sweets, weight gain. **GU:** loss of libido, ejaculatory disturbances, amenorrhea, oligomenorrhea, breast tenderness and swelling, galactorrhea. **Other:** blurred vision, elevated serum prolactin levels, nephrotoxicity (overdosage).

ROUTE AND DOSAGE. Oral: Adult: Initial: 50 mg two or three times daily. Depending upon tolerance, increased on third day of treatment to 100 mg three times daily. If no response in 2 weeks, dose is increased to 400 mg depending upon tolerance. When effective dose is established, administered as single dose (not to exceed 300 mg) at bedtime. If daily dose is more than 300 mg, give in divided doses. For hospitalized patients, may be increased cautiously to 600 mg/day in divided doses. **Elderly:** Initial: 25 mg three times daily; if tolerated by end of first week, increased to 50 mg two or three times daily. If necessary, increased gradually up to 300 mg/day. Maintenance: lowest effective dose. If depression reappears, dosage increased to earlier level until symptoms are controlled.

NURSING IMPLICATIONS

Tablet may be crushed before administration and taken with fluid of patient's choice.

Initial antidepressant effect (mild euphoria, increased energy) may occur within 4 to 7 days; however, most patients do not have minimal clinical response until after 2 or 3 weeks of drug therapy.

Patient may experience sedation during early therapy, mostly when dosage increases are made. Note implications for ambulation particularly in the elderly.

Maintenance dose is generally taken as a single dose at bedtime to minimize daytime sedation and other annoying drug side effects.

Monitor intake and output ratio and bowel elimination pattern. Report to physician if patient has continuing constipation. Teach patient importance of drinking at least 2000 ml fluid daily and eating foods with high fiber content (if allowed), to provide needed roughage.

If xerostomia (dry mouth) is a clinical problem, institute prophylactic and symptomatic treatment. *See Imipramine.* A saliva substitute may be helpful (e.g., Moi-stir).

Although sedation is usually mild, warn patient that alertness and skill in performing hazardous tasks, such as driving, may be impaired particularly during early therapy.

Urine and blood glucose levels should be checked periodically in patients on prolonged therapy.

The effects of alcohol and amoxapine are potentiated when used concurrently during therapy and for up to 2 weeks after the TCA is discontinued. Consult physician about alcohol use.

If a patient uses excessive amounts of alcohol it should be borne in mind that the potentiation of TCA effects increases the dangers of overdosage or suicide attempt.

Suicide is an inherent risk with any depressed patient and may remain even when there is significant improvement. Supervise patient closely during therapy.

Tolerance to amoxapine antidepressant effects develops in some patients after 1 to 3 months of drug therapy. Close medical follow-up is essential.

Impress on patient necessity to maintain established dosage regimen. Tell patient not to skip, reduce, or double doses or change dose intervals. Also caution not to "loan" or give any of TCA to another individual.

OTC drug use should be approved by the physician.

Stored at 15° to 30°C (59° to 86°F) in well-closed container, unless otherwise directed by manufacturer.

See Imipramine (prototype tricyclic antidepressant).

Drug Interactions: Amoxapine

Plus	Interactions
Anticoagulants, oral	Decreased hypoprothrombinemic effect. Monitor closely
Antihypertensives: clonidine (Catapres), guanethidine (Ismelin), methyldopa (Aldomet)	Antihypertensive action may be decreased. Combination avoided, when possible
CNS depressants, e.g., alcohol (Ethanol), barbiturates, ethchlorvynol (Placidyl), and other sedatives/hypnotics	Potentiation of CNS depression. Also, barbiturates reduce TCA blood levels. Used with caution

Plus (cont.)	Interactions (cont.)
Furazolidone (Furoxone) MAO inhibitors	Possibility of severe reactions (toxic psychosis, hyperpyrexia, tachycardia, seizures). Used with extreme caution
Levodopa (Dopar, Larodopa) Sympathomimetics	Possibility of sympathetic hyperactivity with hypertension and hyperprexia. Used with caution

See also Imipramine.

AMOXICILLIN

(Amoxil, Amoxycillin, Larotid, Moxilean, Novamoxin, Polymox, Sumox, Trimox, Utimox, Wymox)

(a-mox-i-sill'in)
Antiinfective; antibiotic (Beta lactam)
Penicillin

ACTIONS AND USES. Broad spectrum, acid-stable, semisynthetic aminopenicillin and analogue of ampicillin. Like ampicillin, it is bactericidal, has essentially the same antibacterial spectrum, and is inactivated by penicillinase. Reportedly, rash and diarrhea occur less frequently than with ampicillin, and at equal doses produces higher serum levels because it is more completely absorbed. Less effective in treatment of shigellosis than ampicillin and is more expensive.

Used in infections of ear, nose, and throat, GU tract, skin and soft tissue caused by susceptible strains of *E. coli, P. mirabilis, H. influenzae,* streptococci (including *S. faecalis* and *S. pneumoniae*), and nonpenicillinase-producing staphylococci. Also used in uncomplicated gonorrhea. Available in combination with potassium clavulanate (Augmentin), which extends antibacterial spectrum of amoxicillin.

ABSORPTION AND FATE. Absorption is rapid and nearly complete following oral administration. Resists inactivation by gastric acid. Serum levels peak in about 2 hours after administration of capsule and in 1 hour following oral suspension. Measurable serum levels still present after 8 hours. Diffuses into most tissues and body fluids except synovial fluid and CSF (unless meninges are inflamed). Approximately 20% bound to plasma proteins. Half-life: 1 to 1.3 hours. About 60% of dose excreted in urine in 6 to 8 hours, as intact amoxicillin and penicillinoic acid. Crosses placenta. Excreted in breast milk in very small amounts.

CONTRAINDICATIONS AND PRECAUTIONS. Hypersensitivity to penicillins or cephalosporins; infectious mononucleosis. Safe use during pregnancy not established. *Cautious Use:* history of or suspected atopy or allergy (hives, eczema, hay fever, asthma); history of GI disease; severely impaired renal function.

ADVERSE/SIDE EFFECTS. As with other penicillins: **GI:** abdominal cramps, diarrhea, nausea, vomiting. **Hypersensitivity:** pruritus, erythema, urticaria, or other skin eruptions, severe morbilliform rash (patients with infectious mononucleosis), fever, wheezing; anaphylaxis, serum sickness (rare); hemolytic anemia, thrombocytopenia, purpura, eosinophilia, leukopenia, agranulocytosis, pseudomembranous colitis (rare). **Other:** superinfections, conjunctival ecchymosis, numbness and tingling of extremities. *See Penicillin G.*

ROUTE AND DOSAGE. Oral: Adults and Children (weighing 20 kg or more): 250 to 500 mg every 8 hours. *For gonorrhea:* 3 Gm (with probenecid, 1 Gm) as a single dose. **Children (under 20 kg):** 20 to 40 mg/kg/day in equally divided doses every 8 hours. Available in capsules, chewable tablets, oral suspension, pediatric drops.

NURSING IMPLICATIONS

If necessary, capsule may be emptied and contents swallowed with water.

Chewable tablet should be chewed or crushed before swallowing with a liquid.

Serum levels are not significantly affected by food; therefore, amoxicillin may be given without regard to meals.

Oral suspension and pediatric drops are reconstituted when they are dispensed from pharmacy. Date and time of reconstitution, and discard date, should appear on container. Stable for 7 days at room temperature, i.e., around 25°C (77°F) or 14 days if refrigerated, depending on product. (Refrigeration is preferable, but not required.) Shake well before using.

For children, reconstituted pediatric drops may be placed directly on child's tongue for swallowing or added to formula, milk, fruit juice, water, ginger ale, or other soft drink. Have child drink all of the prepared dose promptly.

Pediatric drops should be dispensed with a calibrated liquid measure.

Instruct patient to take medication around the clock, not to miss a dose, and to continue therapy until all medication is taken, unless otherwise directed by physician.

Before therapy is initiated, careful history should be obtained of patient's previous exposure and sensitivity to penicillins and cephalosporins, and other allergic reactions of any kind.

Therapy may be instituted prior to obtaining results of bacteriologic and susceptibility tests.

Periodic assessments of renal, hepatic, and hematologic functions should be made during prolonged therapy.

When amoxicillin is used to treat urinary tract infections, frequent bacteriologic and clinical evaluations are recommended.

Patients being treated for gonorrhea and suspected of having syphilis should have dark-field examination before receiving amoxicillin as well as monthly serologic tests, for a minimum of 4 months.

For most infections, treatment is continued for a minimum of 48 to 72 hours beyond the time that patient is asymptomatic or cultures are negative.

Patients with hemolytic streptococcal infections should receive at least 10 days of treatment to prevent occurrence of acute rheumatic fever.

Advise patient to report to physician the onset of itching, skin rash or hives, wheezing, diarrhea, and symptoms of superinfection (sore mouth, malodorous vaginal discharge, rectal or vaginal itching, cough, return of fever).

Store tablets, capsules in tightly-covered containers preferably between 15° and 30°C (59° and 86°F), unless otherwise directed by manufacturer.

See Penicillin G (prototype for the penicillins).

Diagnostic Test Interferences. Elevations of **SGOT (AST)** and **SGPT (ALT)**.

Drug Interactions: Amoxicillin

Plus	Interactions
Chloramphenicol (Chloromycetin) Erythromycins Tetracyclines	May inhibit bactericidal activity of amoxicillin. Concurrent therapy generally avoided

PROTOTYPE

AMPHETAMINE SULFATE

(Racemic Amphetamine Sulfate)

(am-fet'a-meen)
Central stimulant
Anorexigenic
Amphetamine
C II

ACTIONS AND USES. Indirect-acting synthetic sympathomimetic amine (noncatecholamine) with alpha- and beta-adrenergic activity. Chemically and pharmacologically related to ephedrine. Marked stimulant effect on CNS thought to be due to action on cortex and possibly reticular activating system. Acts indirectly on adrenergic receptors by increasing synaptic release of norepinephrine and dopamine in brain and by blocking reuptake at presynaptic membranes. CNS stimulation results in marked analeptic effect, diminished sense of fatigue, alertness, wakefulness, and elevation of mood. In hyperkinetic children exerts a paradoxic sedative effect by unclear mechanism. Peripheral actions produce mydriasis without cycloplegia, nasal decongestion, weak bronchodilator and respiratory stimulation, vasoconstriction, increased systolic and diastolic blood pressures, and decreased urinary bladder tone coupled with sphincter constriction. Anorexigenic effect thought to result from direct inhibition of lateral hypothalamic appetite area and possibly from drug-induced loss of acuity of smell and taste, as well as mood elevation.

Used as adjunct in certain depressive reactions characterized by apathy and psychomotor retardation and to stimulate subjective feeling of improvement in postencephalitic parkinsonism. Also used in treatment of narcolepsy, attention deficit disorder in children (hyperkinetic behavioral syndrome, minimal brain dysfunction), and to counteract drug-induced respiratory depression. Use as short-term adjunct to control exogenous obesity not generally recommended because of its potential for abuse. Has been used as adjunct in treatment of persistent hiccups, urinary incontinence, and nocturnal enuresis.

ABSORPTION AND FATE. Rapid absorption and distribution to all tissues. Duration of effect: 4 to 24 hours depending on dose. High concentration in brain and CSF results from rapid passage across blood–brain barrier. Half-life: 10 to 30 hours, depending on urine pH. Some deamination and conjugation probably occurs in liver. Elimination accelerated in acidic urine and slowed in alkaline urine. Excreted in breast milk.

CONTRAINDICATIONS AND PRECAUTIONS. Hypersensitivity to sympathomimetic amines, history of drug abuse, hyperthyroidism, severe agitation, endogenous depression, renal disease, diabetes mellitus, moderate to severe hypertension, angina pectoris or other cardiovascular disorders, glaucoma, arteriosclerotic parkinsonism, Gilles de la Tourette disorder; use as anorexic in children under 12 years or for behavioral syndrome in children under 3 years; during pregnancy and in nursing mothers. *Cautious Use:* elderly, debilitated, or asthenic patients; anorexia, insomnia, psychopathic personality, history of suicidal tendencies.

ADVERSE/SIDE EFFECTS. Allergy: urticaria, fixed-drug reaction, periarteritis nodosa, Tourette's syndrome. **CNS:** overstimulation, restlessness, nervousness, agitation, talkativeness, dizziness, severe headache (high doses), insomnia, mental depression, euphoria, dysphoria, psychoses, tremors, hyperactive reflexes, dyskinesia, convulsions, respiratory failure. **CV:** palpitation, increased or decreased blood pressure; tachycardia or bradycardia, angina (high doses), pallor or flushing. **Endocrine (with high doses):** impotence, change in libido, gynecomastia. **GI:** dry mouth, metallic taste, anorexia, unusual weight loss, nausea, vomiting, diarrhea or constipation, abdominal cramps. **Hematologic:** aplastic anemia (high doses), pancytopenia (prolonged use). **Other:** excessive sweating, chills, fever, fatigue, mydriasis, difficult micturition.

ROUTE AND DOSAGE. Oral: *Narcolepsy:* **Adults (12 years and older):** Initial: 10 mg daily. **Children (6 to 12 years):** Initial: 5 mg daily. *Attention deficit disorder in children:* **Children (6 years and older):** Initial: 5 mg one or two times a day. Dosage rarely exceeds 40 mg/day; **Children**

(3 to 5 years): Initial: 2.5 mg a day. *Exogenous obesity:* 5 to 10 mg ½ to 1 hour before meals. Doses usually raised at weekly intervals in increments equal to initial dose until optimum response is achieved.

NURSING IMPLICATIONS

To avoid insomnia, last dose should be administered no later than 6 hours before retiring.

When used as an anorexigenic, drug is generally administered ½ to 1 hour before meals.

Since tolerance (tachyphylaxis) to the anorexigenic and mood-elevating effects commonly occurs within a few weeks, continuous weight reduction cannot be achieved without additional dietary restriction. A structured weight reduction program (which includes desirable caloric intake, increase in activity level, and behavior modification) should be planned in collaboration with physician, dietitian, patient, and responsible family members.

Keep physician informed of clinical response.

In a state of fatigue, amphetamine exerts a stimulating effect that masks the feeling of being tired. After the exhilaration has disappeared there is usually greater fatigue and depression than before, and a longer period of rest is needed. Therefore, inform patient that amphetamine does not obviate the need for planned rest.

Because of potential effect of amphetamine on appetite and weight, insulin dose may require adjustment. Monitor closely.

Alert patient to the possibility that the drug may impair ability to engage in hazardous activities such as operating a car or machinery.

The following measures may help to relieve mouth dryness: frequent rinses with clear water, especially after eating (avoid overuse of astringent or antiseptic mouth washes because they may change oral flora); increase fluid intake, if allowed; sugarless chewing gum. Advise patient to be meticulous about daily oral hygiene (flossing, use of soft, small toothbrush and fluoride toothpaste) since decreased or absence of saliva encourages demineralization of tooth surfaces and mucosal erosion. Use of a commercially available oral lubricant such as Moi-Stir or Xero-Lube can relieve soft tissue problems and reduce the potential of caries.

Following prolonged administration of high doses, amphetamine should gradually be withdrawn. Abrupt withdrawal may result in lethargy, profound depression, or other psychotic manifestations that may persist for several weeks.

Response to the drug is more variable in children than in adults. Acute toxicity has occurred over a wide range of dosage.

Effect of amphetamines on growth in children is not known. Close monitoring is advised.

Treatment of overdosage: Gastric lavage or emesis; barbiturate for sedative effect (used with caution); acidification of urine (e.g., with ammonium chloride) to enhance amphetamine excretion; chlorpromazine (Thorazine) to control CNS symptoms; antihypertensive for marked hypertension.

Amphetamines have a high abuse potential because of their excitatory and euphoric effects.

Addiction potential is controversial. Most authorities seem to agree that long-term therapy is unlikely to produce addiction and that habituation or psychic dependence is caused by psychologic factors rather than by pharmacologic action. Pronounced tolerance develops with repeated use.

Lay terms used for amphetamines include "pep pills," "wake-ups," "bennies," and "speed" (when injected IV), among others. Mixture of an opioid with amphetamine is called "speedball."

Classified as Schedule II drug under the Federal Controlled Substances Act.

Stored preferably between 15° and 30°C (59° and 86°F) unless otherwise directed by manufacturer.

Drug Interactions: Amphetamines

Plus	Interactions
Acetazolamide (Diamox), sodium bicarbonate	Alkalinization of urine by these drugs decreases amphetamine excretion thus prolonging its effects. Amphetamine dose reduction may be necessary
Ammonium chloride, ascorbic acid (vitamin C)	Increase in urine acidity by these drugs increases amphetamine excretion thus reducing its effects. Amphetamine dose increase may be necessary
Barbiturates	May antagonize pharmacologic effects of amphetamines
Furazolidone (Furoxone)	May increase pressor (BP) effects of amphetamines. Effects may even occur several weeks after furazolidone is discontinued. Combination avoided
Guanethidine (Ismelin)	Amphetamines may antagonize antihypertensive effect of guanethidine. Combination avoided
MAO inhibitors, e.g., phenelzine (Nardil), tranylcypromine (Parnate)	Potentiate pharmacologic effects of amphetamines and can cause hypertensive crisis. Fatalities reported. Amphetamine should not be administered during or within 14 days following MAO inhibitors
Phenothiazines	Phenothiazines inhibit mood elevating effects of amphetamines

---

AMPHOTERICIN B

(Fungizone)

(am-foe-ter′i-sin)

Antiinfective: antibiotic (macrolide)

Antifungal

ACTIONS AND USES. Polyene fungistatic antibiotic produced by *Streptomyces nodosus.* Fungicidal at higher concentrations, depending on sensitivity of fungus. Exerts antifungal action on both resting and growing cells. Binds sterols in fungus cell membrane, with resultant increase in membrane permeability, thus allowing leakage of K and other intracellular constituents. Because it may also interfere with function of human cell membrane, it can produce severe adverse effects. Not effective against bacteria, rickettsiae, or viruses.

Used intravenously for a wide spectrum of potentially fatal systemic fungal (mycotic) infections including aspergillosis, blastomycosis, coccidioidomycosis, cryptococcosis, disseminated candidiasis, histoplasmosis, sporotrichosis, and others. Has been used to potentiate antifungal effects of flucytosine (Ancobon), and to provide anticandidal prophylaxis in certain susceptible patients receiving rifampin or tetracycline therapy. Used topically for cutaneous and mucocutaneous infections caused by *Candida* (Monilia). *Investigational Use:* treatment of oral thrush, candidal cystitis or vaginitis, leishmaniasis, rhinocerebral phycomycosis, amebic meningoencephalitis, coccidioidal and cryptococcal meningitis. Available in fixed combination with tetracycline, e.g., Mysteclin-F.

ABSORPTION AND FATE. Topical applications poorly absorbed. Peak blood levels in 1 to 2 hours after IV injection. Approximately 90 to 95% bound to serum proteins; plasma half-life about 24 hours. Minimal amounts enter CSF, aqueous humor, pleural, pericardial, and synovial fluid. Serum and urine concentrations similar. Metabolic pathways and distribution unknown. Approximately 40% excreted by kidneys over 7-day period. Can be detected in blood and urine for at least 7 to 8 weeks after discontinuation of therapy. Excretion increased in alkaline urine. Crosses placenta.

CONTRAINDICATIONS AND PRECAUTIONS. Hypersensitivity to amphotericin; severe bone marrow depression or renal function impairment. Safe use during pregnancy and in nursing mothers not established.

ADVERSE/SIDE EFFECTS. CNS/Neuromuscular: headache, sedation, muscle or nerve pain, arthralgia, weakness, paresthesias; peripheral neuropathy, foot drop (rare), convulsions. **CV:** flushing, arrhythmias, hypertension, hypotension; ventricular fibrillation and cardiac arrest (rapid IV). **ENT (ototoxicity):** tinnitus, vertigo, loss of hearing. **GI:** nausea (especially during IV infusion): vomiting, diarrhea, epigastric cramps, hemorrhagic gastroenteritis, anorexia, weight loss. **Hematologic:** leukopenia, coagulation defects, thrombocytopenia, agranulocytosis, eosinophilia, anemia (normochromic, normocytic), Coombs' positive hemolytic anemia (rare), hypokalemia, hypomagnesemia, hyponatremia. **Hypersensitivity:** pruritus, urticaria, skin rashes, fever, shaking chills, anaphylaxis. **Ophthalmic:** blurred vision, diplopia. **Renal:** difficult micturition; nephrotoxicity, (oliguria, hematuria, granular and hyaline casts in urine, renal tubular acidosis, renal damage); nephrocalcinosis. **Topical use:** dry skin, erythema, pruritus, burning sensation; allergic contact dermatitis, exacerbation of lesions. **Other:** pain, tissue irritation (with extravasation); thrombi, thrombophlebitis (IV site); chemical meningitis, acute liver failure, superinfections, severe pulmonary reaction in patients receiving leukocyte transfusions.

ROUTE AND DOSAGE. Adult and pediatric: Intravenous infusion: Initial, 0.25 mg/kg daily infused over 6 hours; or 1 mg in 250 ml of 5% dextrose infused over 2 to 4 hours. Dosage increased gradually to 1 mg/kg/day as tolerance permits. Not to exceed 1.5 mg/kg/day. If therapy is interrupted for longer than 1 week, restarted at initial dosage and again increased gradually. **Intrathecal:** Initial: 0.025 to 0.1 mg diluted with 10 to 20 ml of CSF, two or three times per week. Dose increases made gradually; range: 0.5 to 1 mg (maximum). **Topical** (3% cream, lotion, ointment): apply enough to cover affected area and rub in gently two to four times a day.

NURSING IMPLICATIONS

Intravenous administration: Amphotericin B is administered IV only to hospitalized patients or to those under close clinical supervision who have a confirmed diagnosis of progressive, potentially fatal mycotic infection susceptible to the drug.

Prior to systemic therapy, diagnosis is confirmed by positive cultures or histologic studies.

Check with physician regarding IV flow rate. Generally the drug is administered slowly over a 6-hour period. If a reaction occurs, interrupt therapy and report promptly to physician.

During initial IV therapy, monitor vital signs every 30 minutes for at least 4 hours and observe patient closely for adverse effects. Febrile reactions (fever and chills) usually occur in 1 to 2 hours after onset of therapy and subside within 4 hours after drug is discontinued.

Severity of adverse reactions may be reduced by prophylactic use of aspirin or acetaminophen, antiemetics, antihistamines, and corticosteroids.

Renal and hematologic status should be determined before therapy. During dosage regulation period, hemograms, serum electrolytes (especially K, Mg, Na, Ca), renal function tests including urinalysis are performed twice weekly, then at least weekly during therapy. Liver function tests are also done periodically throughout therapy.

Nephrotoxicity is a predictable complication in patients receiving intensive therapy. Monitor intake and output. Report immediately oliguria, any change in intake and output ratio and pattern, or appearance of urine, e.g., sediment, pink or cloudy urine (hematuria), or abnormal renal function tests. Renal damage is usually reversible if drug is discontinued when first signs of renal dysfunction appear.

If BUN exceeds 40 mg/dl, or serum creatinine rises above 3 mg/dl, withhold drug and report to physician. Dosage should be reduced or drug discontinued until renal function improves.

Amphotericin B may cause local inflammatory reaction or thrombosis at injection site, particularly if extravasation occurs. Risk of thrombophlebitis associated with IV infusion may be reduced by using pediatric scalp vein needle in the most distal vein possible, by alternating veins, by addition of heparin to the infusion, and by alternate day dosage schedule.

Frequently check IV site for leakage. It is more apt to occur in the elderly patient because loss of tissue elasticity with aging may promote extravasation around the needle.

Hypokalemia occurs commonly and occasionally can be life-threatening. Report immediately the onset of these possible signs of hypokalemia: anorexia, drowsiness, profound muscle weakness, hypoactive reflexes, paresthesias, polyuria, polydypsia, dizziness.

The drug is potentially ototoxic. Report promptly any evidence of hearing loss or complaints of tinnitus, vertigo, or unsteady gait. Keep in mind that tinnitus may not be present in an elderly person who may have hearing problems to begin with, or in the very young. Other signs of ototoxicity (i.e., vertigo or hearing loss) are more reliable in these age groups.

Check weight at weekly intervals, or more frequently if patient has anorexia.

A flow chart may be useful for organizing significant observations.

Several weeks of therapy (approximately 6 to 12 weeks) are usually required to assure adequate response and to prevent relapse. Some infections require 9 to 12 months of therapy, e.g., sporotrichosis, aspergillosis.

Preparation and administration: Keep dry powder refrigerated and protected from exposure to light. Avoid freezing.

Amphotericin B is reconstituted with sterile water for injection without preservatives or bacteriostatic agent. Follow manufacturer's directions. Dilutents containing a preservative or bacteriostatic agent such as benzyl alcohol, or acidic solutions, sodium chloride or other electrolyte solutions should not be used because they may cause precipitation.

Following reconstitution with sterile water for injection, solution is stable for 24 hours at room temperature and for 1 week under refrigeration. Discard any solution before this time if it is cloudy or contains a precipitate.

For IV infusion, the reconstituted amphotericin B is added to dextrose 5% in water, with pH above 4.2. If pH is less, a sterile buffer must be added, using strict aseptic technique. See package insert. Solutions prepared for IV infusion must be used promptly.

An in-line membrane filter can be used during IV infusion. If used, the mean pore diameter should be no less than 1 micron, to avoid reducing concentration of amphotericin B delivered.

Although manufacturer recommends protecting aqueous solutions of amphotericin B from light during IV infusion, short-term exposure (e.g., less than 8 hours) does not appreciably affect potency. Follow agency policy.

Topical applications: Do not cover with plastic wrap or other occlusive dressings.

Request physician to specify when and how lesions are to be washed.

Cream or lotion is preferred for intertriginous areas such as creases of neck, groin, armpit. Some clinicians advise exposure of skin to air or the warmth of an electric bulb several times a day to enhance drying.

Topical treatment should be discontinued promptly if signs of hypersensitivity, irritation, or worsening of lesions occurs.

The appearance of mild erythema surrounding lesions may be an indication to reduce frequency of application. Consult physician about applying a protective circle of petroleum jelly on normal skin surrounding easily accessible lesions.

Advise patient to notify physician if improvement does not occur within 1 to 2 weeks, or if lesions appear to worsen.

Most skin lesions require about 1 to 3 weeks of drug therapy. Paronychia and interdigital lesions may not respond before 2 to 4 weeks of treatment. Nail infections (onychomycoses) usually require several months or longer.

Towels and clothing in contact with affected areas should be washed after each treatment.

Topical cream slightly discolors the skin. Generally, lotion and ointment do not stain skin when rubbed into lesion, but nail lesions may be stained.

To remove cream or lotion from fabric, wash with soap and water. Ointment may be removed from fabric with a standard cleaning fluid.

Patient-Teaching Points to Prevent Spread and Recurrence of Lesions (Relevance Depends on Location of Lesions):

- ✓ Careful handwashing technique before and after application of medication. Dry hands well.
- ✓ Avoid pulling hangnails.
- ✓ Avoid squeezing pimples or picking at scabs. In general, keep hands off skin.
- ✓ Wear nonconstricting, absorbent underclothing.
- ✓ Anything that contacts skin should be kept separate, e.g., washcloths, towels, bed linen.
- ✓ Use freshly laundered clothing and bedding every day.
- ✓ Keep affected areas dry and exposed to air, if possible.
- ✓ Follow prescribed treatment as directed.
- ✓ Keep follow-up appointments.

Store topical forms in well-closed containers at room temperature, preferably 15° to 30°C (59° to 86°F), unless otherwise directed by manufacturer.

Drug Interactions: Amphotericin

Plus	Interactions
Drugs with nephrotoxic potential, e.g., aminoglycosides, capreomy cin (Capastat), cisplatin (Plat inol), colistin (Coly-Mycin S), cyclosporine (Sandimmune), methoxyflurane (Penthrane), polymyxin B (Aerosporin), vancomycin (Vancocin)	Synergistic nephrotoxicity and ototoxicity. Concurrent and sequential use generally avoided, if possible
Corticosteroids	Potentiate amphotericin B-induced hypokalemia. Used only when necessary to counteract adverse reactions
Digitalis glycosides	Amphotericin B-induced hypokalemia may increase potential for digitalis toxicity. Used with caution
Flucytosine (Ancoban)	Effects of either may be increased. Used with caution
Miconazole	Antagonistic antifungal effects. Concurrent use generally avoided
Skeletal muscle relaxants (nondepolarizing)	Amphotericin B-induced hypokalemia may potentiate effects of curariform drugs. Used with caution
Urinary alkalizers, e.g., acetazolamide (Diamox)	May increase excretion of amphotericin B

PROTOTYPE

AMPICILLIN

(am-pi-sill'in)
Antiinfective
Antibiotic (beta lactam)
Penicillin

(Amcap, Amcill, Ampicin, Ampilean, D-Amp, Novo-Ampicillin, Omnipen, Pfizerpen-A, Polycillin, Principen, SK-Ampicillin, Supen, Totacillin)

AMPICILLIN SODIUM

(Omnipen-N, Polycillin-N, SK-Ampicillin-N, Totacillin-N)

ACTIONS AND USES. Broad spectrum semisynthetic aminopenicillin derived from 6-aminopenicillanic acid, the basic penicillin nucleus. Relatively stable in gastric acid. Highly bactericidal even at low concentrations, but is inactivated by penicillinase (beta-lactamase). Resembles penicillin G (qv) in its activity against gram-positive microorganisms such as alpha- and beta-hemolytic streptococci, *Diplococcus pneumoniae,* and non-penicillinase-producing staphylococci. Major advantage over penicillin G is enhanced action against most strains of enterococci, and several gram-negative strains including *Escherichia coli, Neisseria gonorrhoea, N. meningitidis, Haemophilus influenzae, Proteus mirabilis, Salmonella* (including typhosa), and shigella. Ampicillin sodium contains approximately 3 mEq (69 mg) of sodium per gram. (1 mEq of sodium = 23 mg).

Used in infections of urinary, respiratory, and gastrointestinal tracts, and skin and soft tissues. Also used in the treatment of gonococcal infections, bacterial meningitis, and otitis media, septicemia, and for prophylaxis of bacterial endocarditis. Used parenterally only for moderately severe to severe infections. Commercially available in combination with probenecid e.g., Ampicin-PRB, Polycillin-PRB, Principen w/Probenecid, Probampacin.

ABSORPTION AND FATE. Approximately 30 to 60% of oral dose absorbed from GI tract. Serum levels peak within 2 hours (oral route), within 1 hour (IM route), and within 5 minutes (IV route). Equivalent oral and parenteral doses produce higher blood concentrations by parenteral route. Diffuses into most body tissues and fluids; high concentrations in CSF only when meninges are inflamed. About 20 to 25% bound to plasma proteins. Half-life: 50 to 110 minutes; higher in infants and prematures (due to immature kidney function). Appears to be partially inactivated by liver; enters enterohepatic circulation. Excreted unchanged; high concentrations in urine and bile (through feces). Crosses placenta. Eliminated in breast milk.

CONTRAINDICATIONS AND PRECAUTIONS. Hypersensitivity to penicillin derivatives or cephalosporins. Safe use during pregnancy not established. *Cautious Use:* history of or suspected atopy or allergy (hay fever, asthma, hives, eczema); renal, liver, or GI disease; infectious mononucleosis, hyperuricemia, lymphatic leukemia, prematures and neonates.

ADVERSE/SIDE EFFECTS. (Similar to Penicillin G). **CNS (with high doses):** headache, convulsive seizures. **GI:** diarrhea, abdominal pain, nausea, vomiting, pseudomembranous colitis (rare). **Hypersensitivity:** drug fever, pruritus, urticaria, and other skin eruptions, eosinophilia, hemolytic anemia, thrombocytopenia, leukopenia, agranulocytosis, delayed respiratory distress syndrome, interstitial nephritis, anaphylactoid reaction, serum sickness. **Other:** severe pain (following IM); phlebitis (following IV); hypokalemia (large IV doses); morbilliform rash (ampicillin rash), superinfections. *See Penicillin G.*

ROUTE AND DOSAGE. **Oral:** **Adults:** 250 to 500 mg every 6 hours. **Children:** 25 to 50 mg/kg/day in equally divided doses at 6 to 8 hour intervals. **Intramuscular, intravenous:** (ampicillin sodium): **Adults:** 250 to 500 mg every 6 hours. **Children:** 25 to 50 mg/kg/day in equally divided doses at 6 to 8-hour intervals. *Septicemia and bacterial meningitis:* **Adults and children:** 150 to 200 mg/kg/day in equally divided doses every 3 or 4 hours. Treatment initiated with IV administration, then continued IM. *Gonorrheal urethritis:* **Adults: Intramuscular or intravenous** 500 mg at 8- to 12-hour intervals for two doses. **Oral:** 3.5 Gm simultaneously with probenecid 1 Gm as a single dose.

NURSING IMPLICATIONS

A careful history should be taken before therapy begins, to determine previous hypersensitivity reactions to penicillins, cephalosporins, and other allergens.

As a guide to therapy, culture and sensitivity tests should be done prior to and periodically during therapy. Therapy may be initiated before results are known.

Although ampicillin is comparatively acid-stable, food hampers its absorption. Maximum absorption is achieved if it is taken with a glass of water on an empty stomach (at least 1 hour before or 2 hours after meals).

If necessary, tablet may be crushed before administration and taken with fluid of patient's choice. Capsule may be emptied and contents swallowed with water or mixed with food.

Following reconstitution of oral suspension or pediatric drops (by pharmacist), solutions are stable for 14 days under refrigeration. Date and time of reconstitution, and discard date, should appear on container; medication should be dispensed with a calibrated measuring device. Shake well before using.

Ampicillin sodium (for parenteral use) may be reconstituted with sterile water for injection. Follow manufacturer's directions for amount of diluent to use. Solutions for IM or direct IV should be administered within 1 hour after preparation.

Administration of drug by direct IV should be done slowly, over at least 10 to 15 minutes. Rapid administration can result in seizures (neurotoxicity).

For administration by IV infusion, the reconstituted solution (see above) must be added to suitable IV fluid. Consult product information for list of acceptable diluents, concentration to use, and stability period.

Note that the sodium content must be taken into consideration in patients on sodium restriction.

Contact dermatitis occurs frequently in sensitized individuals. Those who must handle ampicillin repeatedly are advised to wear disposable gloves.

Inspect skin daily and instruct patient to do the same. The appearance of a rash should be carefully evaluated to differentiate an ampicillin rash (nonallergic) from a hypersensitivity reaction. Report promptly to physician if it appears.

Ampicillin rash is characteristically dull red, macular or maculopapular, and mildly pruritic. It generally begins on light-exposed or pressure areas such as knees, elbows, palms, soles, and may spread in a symmetric pattern over most of body. The rash usually develops after 5 to 14 days of treatment, but occasionally appears on first day of therapy or after therapy has stopped. It disappears within a week after discontinuation of drug therapy.

The incidence of ampicillin rash is higher in patients with infectious mononucleosis or other viral infections, Salmonella infections, lymphocytic leukemia, and in patients taking allopurinol or who have hyperuricemia.

Since ampicillin rash is believed to be nonallergic in origin, its appearance is not an absolute contraindication to future therapy with ampicillin or other penicillins.

Advise patient to report diarrhea and not to self-medicate. A detailed report should be given to the physician regarding onset, duration, character of stools, associated symptoms, and patient's temperature and weight to help rule out the possibility of drug-induced, potentially fatal pseudomembranous colitis.

Baseline and periodic assessments of renal, hepatic, and hematologic functions are advised particularly during prolonged or high-dose therapy.

Frequent bacteriologic and clinical evaluations are essential in the treatment of urinary tract and intestinal infections. Follow-up for several months after cessation of therapy may be indicated.

Female patients receiving ampicillin for treatment of gonorrhea should have cultures of endocervical and anal canal to determine cure.

Superinfections are more likely to occur with broad spectrum derivatives of penicillin, such as ampicillin. Instruct patient to report the onset of black, hairy tongue; oral lesions (stomatitis, glossitis); rectal or vaginal itching; vaginal discharge; loose, foul-smelling stools; unusual odor to urine.

Instruct patient to take medication around the clock, not to miss a dose, and to continue taking medication until it is all gone, unless otherwise directed by physician or pharmacist.

If no improvement is noted within a few days after therapy is started, physician should be notified.

Treatment for most infections is continued 48 to 72 hours beyond the time that patient becomes asymptomatic or negative cultures are obtained. A minimum of 10 days is recommended for group A beta-hemolytic streptococci to help prevent rheumatic fever.

Capsules and unopened vials are stored preferably between 15° and 30°C (59° and 86°F) unless otherwise directed by manufacturer.

See also Penicillin G.

Diagnostic Test Interferences. Elevated **CPK** levels may result from local skeletal muscle injury following IM injection. **Urine glucose:** high urine drug concentrations can result in false-positive test results with Clinitest, Benedict's, or Fehling's solution; (enzymatic glucose oxidose methods, e.g., Clinistix, Diastix, Tes-Tape not affected). SGOT(AST) may be elevated (significance not known). *See also Penicillin G.*

Drug Interactions: Ampicillin

Plus	Interactions
Allopurinol	Allopurinol may predispose patient to "ampicillin rash"
Bacteriostatic antibiotics e.g., chloramphenicol (Chloromycetin), erythromycins, tetracyclines	Bactericidal effects of ampicillin may be reduced. Concurrent administration generally avoided
Contraceptives, oral	Ampicillin may interfere with contraceptive action (by decreasing urinary excretion of endogenous estrogens). Female patients should be advised to consider use of a nonhormonal contraceptive
See also Penicillin G.	

AMRINONE

(Inocor)

(am′-ri-none)
Cardiac inotropic agent

ACTIONS AND USES. Bipyridine derivative, the first of a new chemical class of cardiac inotropic agents with vasodilator activity. Action mechanism uncertain, but thought to be related to increased calcium (Ca) concentration in myocardial cytoplasm. Mode of action appears to differ from that of the digitalis glycosides and beta-adrenergic stimulants. In patients with depressed myocardial function, amrinone enhances myocardial contractility, increases cardiac output and stroke volume, and reduces right and left ventricular filling pressure, pulmonary capillary wedge pressure, and systemic vascular resistance. Vasodilating action, produced by direct relaxant effect on vascular smooth muscle, reduces strain on failing heart. Improves hemodynamics at rest and during exercise, and increases exercise capacity without adverse effects on heart rate, rhythm, or blood pressure.

Used for short-term management of congestive heart failure in patients not adequately controlled by traditional therapy, such as digitalis, diuretics, and vasodilators, and may be used in conjunction with these agents. Administration with hydralazine (Apresoline) produces synergistic effects and allows reduction in dosage of both drugs.

ABSORPTION AND FATE. Following oral administration, onset of hemodynamic action within 30 to 120 minutes; peak effect: 1 to 4 hours; duration: 4 to 6 hours. Following IV administration, hemodynamic action begins in 2 to 5 minutes, peaks within 10 minutes. Duration depends upon dose: 0.75 mg/kg lasts about 30 minutes; 3 mg/kg lasts about 2 hours. Approximately 35 to 49% protein bound. Half-life: 3.6 to 7.5 hours. Metabolized in liver. Excreted principally via urine as unchanged drug (10 to 40%) and metabolites in 24 hours. Some excretion into feces. Distribution to placenta and into breast milk not known.

CONTRAINDICATIONS AND PRECAUTIONS. Hypersensitivity to amrinone or to bisulfites; severe aortic or pulmonic valvular disease in lieu of appropriate surgery, acute myocardial infarction, uncorrected hypokalemia or dehydration. Safe use during pregnancy (category C), in nursing women, and in children not established. *Cautious Use:* compromised renal or hepatic function.

ADVERSE/SIDE EFFECTS. CV: arrhythmias, hypotension. **Endocrine:** nephrogenic diabetes insipidus (dose related and reversible). **GI:** nausea, vomiting, anorexia, abdominal cramps, diarrhea, hepatotoxicity (particularly with long-term oral therapy). **Hematologic:** asymptomatic thrombocytopenia. **Hypersensitivity** (causal relationship uncertain): pericarditis, pleuritis; myositis with interstitial shadows on chest x-ray and elevated sedimentation rate; vasculitis with nodular pulmonary densities; hypoxemia, ascites, jaundice. **Other:** drug fever, headache, chest pain, reduced taste and smell perceptions, hiccoughs; burning and necrosis at injection site.

ROUTE AND DOSAGE. Oral: 1 to 3 mg/kg at 8 hour intervals. **Intravenous:** Initial: 0.75 mg/kg bolus given slowly over 2 to 3 minutes, continued with maintenance infusion 5 to 10 mcg/kg/minute. If necessary, additional 0.75 mg/kg bolus may be repeated 30 minutes after initiation of therapy. Recommended total daily dose, including bolus, not to exceed 10 mg/kg. For limited number of patients, up to 18 mg/kg/day has been given for short duration only. May be administered as supplied, or diluted with normal or half-normal (0.45%) saline to concentration of 1 to 3 mg/ml.

NURSING IMPLICATIONS

During IV administration, monitor blood pressure and heart rate and keep physician informed. Rate of administration and duration of therapy are prescribed according to clinical response or adverse effects. Consult physician for guidelines.

Monitor infusion site to prevent extravasation.

Monitor intake and output ratio and pattern, and daily weights. If patient is on diuretic therapy, dosage adjustments may be necessary. Improvement in cardiac output enhances diuresis with consequent danger of hypokalemia and arrhythmias, particularly in digitalized patients. Hypokalemia should be corrected before and during amrinone therapy.

Principal hemodynamic parameters indicating clinical improvement include: increased cardiac output, decreased pulmonary capillary wedge pressure (PCWP). Central venous pressure (CVP) may be used to assess hypotension and blood volume (hydration state).

Other measurements used to evaluate patient response are: lessening of dyspnea, orthopnea, paroxysmal nocturnal dyspnea (PND), fatigue, and edema; reduction or stabilization of weight, increase in exercise capacity.

The following laboratory values should be closely monitored throughout therapy to detect adverse effects of amrinone: platelet counts, liver enzymes, serum electrolytes, renal function studies.

Thrombocytopenia may occur during prolonged therapy. Close monitoring of platelet counts, appropriate dosage reduction or drug discontinuation should prevent symptoms and allow reversibility. If platelet count falls below 150,000/mm³ report immediately to physician.

Amrinone IV preparation contains sodium metabisulfite, a reducing agent to which certain susceptible individuals are allergic. Drug should be discontinued immediately if patient manifests clinical symptoms suggestive of hypersensitivity reactions.

Patient must be closely observed when drug is withdrawn following prolonged therapy because clinical deterioration may occur within hours.

Natural color of IV amrinone is clear yellow. Examine ampul before use. Discard solutions that are discolored or that contain a precipitate.

Do not dilute IV amrinone with dextrose or glucose solutions because a chemical interaction occurs slowly over a 24-hour period. However, manufacturer states that amrinone may be injected into a *running* dextrose (glucose) infusion, through Y-connector or into tubing.

All diluted solutions should be used within 24 hours. Discard unused portions.

Store at room temperature, preferably between 15° and 30°C (59° and 86°F) unless otherwise directed by manufacturer. Protect ampuls from light.

Drug Interactions: Amrinone

Plus	Interactions
Disopyramide (Norpace)	Possibility of excessive hypotension. Used with caution

AMYL NITRITE

(am′il)
Vasodilator (coronary)
Nitrite

ACTIONS AND USES. Short-acting vasodilator and smooth muscle relaxant with actions, contraindications, and adverse reactions similar to those of nitroglycerin (qv). Action in treatment of cyanide poisoning based on ability of amyl nitrite to convert hemoglobin to methemoglobin which forms a nontoxic complex with cyanide ion.

Used to relieve pain of renal and gallbladder colic and to change intensity of heart murmurs. Also used as an adjunct in the immediate treatment of cyanide poisoning. (Because of expense, adverse effects, and unpleasant odor, infrequently used to treat angina pectoris.)

ABSORPTION AND FATE. Rapidly absorbed from mucous membranes and lungs. Onset of action, 10 to 30 seconds; duration, 3 to 5 minutes. Excreted by kidneys.

CONTRAINDICATIONS AND PRECAUTIONS. Hypersensitivity to nitrites or nitrates; cerebral hemorrhage, head trauma, hypotension, glaucoma.

ADVERSE/SIDE EFFECTS. Headache, transient flushing, orthostatic hypotension, dizziness, weakness, syncope, palpitation, tachycardia, methemoglobinemia (large doses). *See Nitroglycerin.*

ROUTE AND DOSAGE. Inhalation: *Acute angina pectoris:* 0.18 ml or 0.3 ml as required. *Cyanide poisoning:* **Adults and children:** 0.3 ml ampul crushed every minute and vapor inhaled for 15 to 30 seconds until sodium nitrite infusion is prepared. *To change intensity of heart murmur:* vapor inhaled *only* until reflex tachycardia develops.

NURSING IMPLICATIONS

Amyl nitrite is available in 0.18-ml and 0.3-ml pearls (thin, friable glass ampuls enveloped with woven fabric cover). To prepare for administration, wrap ampul in gauze or cloth and crush between fingers.

Inform patient that drug has a strongly ethereal or fruity odor.

Syncope, due to a sudden drop in systolic blood pressure, sometimes follows amyl nitrite inhalation; therefore, patient should be sitting during and immediately after drug is administered. If syncope occurs place patient in recumbent position and instruct to breathe deeply and move legs and ankles to facilitate venous return and to increase cerebral blood flow.

After administration of drug, note length of time required for pain to subside; monitor vital signs until they are stable. Rapid pulse, which usually lasts for a brief period, is an expected baroreceptor response to the fall in blood pressure produced by the nitrite ion.

Patients taking amyl nitrite for angina pectoris should be advised to consult physician or go to the hospital emergency immediately if no relief is experienced after 3 doses 5 minutes apart.

When used to change the intensity of heart murmur, those resulting from stenotic valves become louder; those associated with aortic or mitral regurgitation become softer.

Amyl nitrite is volatile and highly flammable. When mixed with air or oxygen it forms a mixture that can explode if ignited.

Tolerance may develop with repeated use over prolonged periods.

Generally, if continued therapy is indicated, a less expensive vasodilator such as nitroglycerin is prescribed.

Amyl nitrite, called "amy," "poppers," "snappers," and "whiffenpoppers" in street language, has been used illicitly to increase intensity of sexual orgasm.

Store in a cool place, preferably between 8° and 15°C (46° and 59°F), unless otherwise directed by manufacturer. Protect from light.

See Nitroglycerin (prototype for nitrates–nitrites).

ANISINDIONE

(Miradon)

(an-iss-in-dye′one)
Anticoagulant
Indandione

ACTIONS AND USES. Indandione derivative with slow onset of effect and long action. Related chemically to phenindione. Similar to coumarin anticoagulants but with potentially greater spectrum of adverse effects. Reserved for use only in patients who cannot tolerate coumarin anticoagulants. *See Warfarin.*

ABSORPTION AND FATE. Readily absorbed from GI tract. Peak prothrombin time effect in 2 to 3 days; duration: 1 to 3 days. Half-life: 3 to 5 days. Considerable differences in individual absorption and metabolism rates. Almost completely bound to plasma proteins. Metabolized by liver; excreted primarily in urine as metabolites. Crosses placenta; enters breast milk.

ADVERSE/SIDE EFFECTS. Agranulocytosis, leukopenia or leukocytosis, hepatitis, jaundice, nephropathy, diarrhea, blurred vision, fever, oral ulcers, urticaria, exfoliative dermatitis. *See also Warfarin.*

ROUTE AND DOSAGE. Oral: Initial: 300 mg on first day, 200 mg on second day, 100 mg on third day. Maintenance: 25 to 250 mg daily. Dosages based on prothrombin time determinations and clinical findings.

NURSING IMPLICATIONS

During period of dosage adjustment, prothrombin time should be checked daily by physician and a dose order obtained.

When patient is controlled on maintenance dose, prothrombin times may be prescribed at 1- to 4-week intervals, depending on uniformity of patient's response.

Periodic blood studies and liver function tests advised for patients on prolonged therapy. Urine should be checked regularly for albumin and blood, and stools tested for occult blood.

Advise patient to withhold medication and to report immediately the onset of bleeding, fever, chills, sore throat or mouth, marked fatigue, jaundice, skin rash, pink or cloudy urine, diminished urination, peripheral edema, blurred vision, or any other unusual signs or symptoms.

Metabolites of anisindione may impart a harmless red orange color to alkaline urine. Alert patient to this possibility. Acidification of urine causes color to disappear (preliminary test for differentiating it from hematuria).

Caution patient not to start or stop taking any other medication (including OTC drugs) while receiving an anticoagulant without approval of physician.

Advise patient to inform all doctors and dentists who may administer care to him that he is taking anisindione.

Store in tightly closed container in temperature between 15° and 30°C (59° and 86°F).

See Warfarin (prototype for oral anticoagulant).

ANISOTROPINE METHYLBROMIDE

(Octatropine methylbromide, Valpin 50)

(an-iss-oh-troe'peen)

Anticholinergic, antimuscarinic, antispasmodic

ACTIONS AND USES. Synthetic quaternary ammonium compound similar to atropine (qv) in actions, contraindications, precautions, and adverse/side effects. Reportedly associated with fewer side effects such as mydriasis and dry mouth than either atropine or homatropine. Inhibits secretion of gastric acid and reduces GI motility by blocking action of acetylcholine at parasympathetic nerve endings.

Used as adjunct in treatment of peptic ulcer.

ABSORPTION AND FATE. Onset of action: 1 to 2 hours; duration: 4 to 6 hours. Data on distribution and fate incomplete. Less than 10% of dose absorbed from GI tract (because it is completely ionized); poor penetration into CNS and eye. Urine believed to be principal route of excretion; some excretion in feces.

CONTRAINDICATIONS AND PRECAUTIONS. Glaucoma, prostatic hypertrophy, intestinal atony, paralytic ileus, or other obstructive diseases of GU or GI tract, severe ulcerative colitis, myasthenia gravis, unstable cardiovascular status. Safe use in pregnancy and in women of childbearing age not established. *Cautious Use:* hepatic or renal disease, hyperthyroidism, hiatal hernia, autonomic neuropathy.

ADVERSE/SIDE EFFECTS. Allergic: urticaria, skin rashes, anaphylaxis. **CNS:** dizziness, drowsiness, headache, weakness; nervousness, confusion, hallucinations, excitement, insomnia, neuromuscular blockade (overdosage). **CV:** palpitation, tachycardia. **GI:** dry mouth, nausea, vomiting, loss of taste, constipation, paralytic ileus. **GU:** urinary hesitancy and retention, impotence. **Ophthalmic:** blurred vision, mydriasis, photophobia. **Other:** decreased sweating, fever, suppression of lactation. *See Atropine.*

ROUTE AND DOSAGE. Oral: 50 mg three times a day.

NURSING IMPLICATIONS

Administered 30 minutes to 1 hour before meals.

Elderly patients may be more susceptible to adverse drug reactions, such as mental confusion, excitement, dizziness, and unsteady gait. Small doses are advised initially to determine patient's response to drug.

Advise patient to report to physician any change in intake and output ratio, difficulty in urination, or constipation. Constipation should be treated promptly particularly in the elderly, to prevent fecal impaction.

Caution patient to avoid driving a car or other potentially hazardous activities until reaction to drug is known.

Warn patient that he or she will be more susceptible to effects of elevated environmental temperatures. Risk of heat stroke is high because drug may interfere with regulation of body temperature by impairing ability to perspire.

Mouth dryness may be relieved by fastidious oral hygiene: (1) floss teeth daily; (2) brush with soft toothbrush after eating; (3) increase fluid intake, if allowed; (4) frequent rinses with water (preferred to commercial rinses which may change oral flora with overuse); (5) sugarless gum or lemon drops; (6) saliva substitute, e.g., Moi-Stir, Salivart.

Stored in tightly closed container at room temperature unless otherwise directed by manufacturer. Protect from light and heat.

See Atropine sulfate (prototype anticholinergic).

ANTHRALIN

(an'thra-lin)

(Anthra-Derm, Anthraforte, Anthranol, Dithranol, Drithocreme, Dritho-Scalp, Lasan)

Cytostatic, antipsoriatic

ACTIONS AND USES. Inhibits nucleic protein synthesis, which results in decreased rate of mitosis and proliferation of epidermal cells in psoriasis. Carcinogenic-tumorigenic activity has been demonstrated in long-term studies with mice.

Used as topical treatment of chronic plaque psoriasis.

ABSORPTION AND FATE. Absorption appears to be low. That which is absorbed from skin is excreted in urine partly as chrysophanic acid and unchanged drug.

CONTRAINDICATIONS AND PRECAUTIONS. Hypersensitivity to anthralin or to any components in product; renal disease; applications to acute eruptions or where inflammation is present, pregnancy (category C), nursing mothers and in children. *Cautious Use:* erythema, or intertriginous and flexural areas, and face.

ADVERSE/SIDE EFFECTS. Sensitivity reactions, erythema of adjacent normal skin, possible renal irritation, folliculitis, temporary discoloration of gray or white hair, fingernails, and skin; fabric stains may be permanent.

ROUTE AND DOSAGE. Usually lowest concentration is first employed, then increased until irritation or the desired response occurs. **Topical:** cream, ointment (0.1 to 1%): once or twice daily.

NURSING IMPLICATIONS

Anthralin ointment is usually applied at bedtime and should remain on skin for length of time specified by physician (time varies from 10 to 20 minutes to 8 to 12 hours).

Apply ointment carefully to affected sites in thin coat. Neighboring uninvolved skin may need protection with petrolatum or plain zinc oxide. Ointment may be dusted with talc and covered with stockinette or gauze bandage. Consult physician.

If patient has a limited number of plaques, paper tape applied to anthralin covered sites has been shown to provide effective occlusion, and to largely eliminate staining of clothing and bedding. Tape should be applied well beyond the lesions in case tape loosens. Consult physician.

Care must be taken when applying medication to avoid uninvolved skin, acute eruptions, or inflamed skin. Wear a finger cot or plastic glove or use a tongue depressor and wash hands thoroughly after completing treatment.

Consult physician about procedure for cleansing skin before reapplying medication. Ointments and oils do not permit evaporation from skin surfaces. Continued applications without intermittent cleansing allow moisture and desquamated epidermis to become trapped and may cause maceration. Warmed mineral oil is a common agent for cleansing.

Avoid getting anthralin (a powerful ocular irritant) into the eyes or on mucous membranes. Do not apply to face, intertriginous areas, or to genitalia unless directed to do so by physician.

Scalp treatment (Lasan Unguent 0.4%): Manufacturer recommends application of a thin protective film of petrolatum (vaseline) to uninvolved skin surrounding scalp margin and on and behind ears, before doing treatment. Apply medication sparingly to affected areas of scalp only. Cover pillow with plastic to avoid staining. Scalp is shampooed at end of prescribed contact period.

Manufacturer advises rinsing bath, shower, or sink with hot water immediately after shampooing with Dritho-Scalp to prevent discoloration, and to use suitable cleanser to remove any surface deposits.

For excessive scalp scaliness, physician may prescribe warm olive oil massage and hot wet towel turban to head prior to shampoo. After shampoo, scale removal can be facilitated by use of fine tooth comb through hair.

Because some patients are hypersensitive to anthralin, it is advisable to make a preliminary test for sensitivity on a small area of skin. Red-haired individuals may be particularly sensitive to the drug.

The appearance of erythema on normal skin may indicate the need to reduce frequency or strength of medication.

Treatment should be discontinued if lesions appear to be spreading or with onset of skin irritation or pustular folliculitis. Folliculitis is most likely to appear in hairy areas.

Weekly urine tests are recommended to determine evidence of renal irritation. *Note:* alkaline urine may take on a brown stain.

Anthralin therapy is generally continued for 2 to 4 weeks.

Psychologic effects of psoriasis on the patient and family members can be especially severe. Direct relationship between stressful situations and flares of psoriasis has been emphasized by some investigators.

A purplish-brown discoloration may appear gradually on lesion margins, but will disappear after treatment is discontinued. Use of excess medication can cause unnecessary staining of skin and clothing as well as skin irritation.

Preserved in tightly covered containers preferably between 15° and 30°C (59° and 86°F) and protected from light unless otherwise directed by manufacturer.

ANTIHEMOPHILIC FACTOR

(an-tee-hee-moe-fill'ik)
Hemostatic
Factor VIII

(AHF, Antihemophilic Globulin [AHG], Antihemophilic Factor, Human; Factorate, Factorate Generation II, Factor VIII, Hemofil, Hemofil T, Koate, Profilate)

ACTIONS AND USES. Stable lyophilized concentrate of human antihemophilic factor (AHF) obtained from large pools of fresh normal human plasma; therefore, carries risk of transmitting viral hepatitis. Factor VIII is essential in the body for conversion of prothrombin to thrombin in blood clotting and for maintaining effective hemostasis. Administration of AHF corrects or prevents bleeding episodes by replacing the missing factor and obviates the need of administering large volumes of plasma, thus avoiding risk of hypervolemia and hyperproteinemia.

Used in treatment of hemophilia A (deficiency of Factor VIII) and in patients with acquired circulating Factor VIII inhibitors.

ABSORPTION AND FATE. Following IV administration, rapidly cleared from plasma. Half-life is biphasic ranging from 4 to 15 hours. Does not readily cross placenta.

CONTRAINDICATIONS AND PRECAUTIONS. Safe use during pregnancy (category C) not established. *Cautious Use:* hepatic disease, patients with blood types A, B, and AB.

ADVERSE/SIDE EFFECTS. (Generally related to rate of administration) **CNS:** headache, paresthesias, somnolence, lethargy, clouding or loss of consciousness. **CV:** hypotension, tachycardia, intravascular hemolysis (with administration of large doses in patients with type A, B, or AB blood). **Hypersensitivity:** chills, fever, backache, flushing, erythema, urticaria, bronchospasm, stinging of infusion site, acute hemolytic anemia (rare). **Other:** dizziness, nausea, vomiting, transient chest discomfort and cough; disturbed vision, jaundice, viral hepatitis.

ROUTE AND DOSAGE. Intravenous: 10 to 20 units/kg by slow IV injection or infusion every 8 to 12 hours. Dosages highly individualized according to weight of patient, severity of bleeding, and coagulation studies.

NURSING IMPLICATIONS

Reconstitute according to manufacturer's directions and with diluent supplied. Prior to reconstitution the dried concentrate and diluent should be warmed to room temperature 20° to 30°C (68° to 86°F). Temperature should not exceed 37°C (98.6°F).

Expiration date should be checked carefully.

Following the addition of diluent to the vial, rotate or agitate *gently* until concentrate is completely dissolved. Administer within 3 hours to avoid microbial contamination. Do not refrigerate or keep at less than room temperature after reconstitution, as precipitation may occur.

If syringe is necessary, use a plastic one (antihemophilic factor solutions tend to stick to surface of ground glass).

Physician will prescribe IV flow rate. Preparations containing 34 or more antihemophilic factor (AHF) units/ml should be administered at carefully controlled rate, not exceeding 2 ml/minute. Preparations containing less than 34 AHF units/ml are administered at rate of 10 to 20 ml over 3 minutes, as prescribed.

Vital signs should be monitored and patient closely observed for vasomotor and hypersensitivity reactions. Take vital signs before and during therapy. If there is a significant increase in pulse rate, IV flow rate should be reduced or administration stopped. Consult physician for permissible parameters.

Some patients manifest an acute, transient allergic reaction (erythema, urticaria, backache, fever) during or following administration of certain preparations. The reaction generally subsides within 20 minutes. Physician may prescribe diphenhydramine (Benadryl) before treatment to avert a reaction.

Factor VIII activity is determined before therapy and daily during therapy. Normal value is 100% (range 50 to 200%).

Tests for Factor VIII inhibitor also should be determined before initiation of therapy. Patients with inhibitor levels greater than 5 to 10 Bethesda units/ml may not respond to AHF.

Hematocrit (Hct) and direct Coombs' test should be monitored in patients with blood types A, B, or AB who are receiving large or frequently repeated doses, to detect intravascular hemolysis. (AHF preparations contain small amounts of group A and B isohemagglutinins.)

Bear in mind that the preparation may contain the causative agents of homologous serum hepatitis. Active immunization with hepatitis B virus may be given as a precautionary measure for patients receiving multiple doses of AHF.

Commercially prepared antihemophilic factor (AHF) is not to be confused with the cryoprecipitated form of Factor VIII. The latter is prepared in hospital blood banks by rapid freezing and slow thawing of fresh plasma. It is obtained from individual donors and therefore is less likely than commercial preparations to transmit hepatitis.

Cryoprecipitated Factor VIII must be kept frozen until ready to use. Then it should be thawed to room temperature by placing it in a warm water bath at no higher than 37°C (98.6°F). Higher temperatures may cause loss of Factor VIII activity. Bag should be gently agitated to assure dissolution. Once thawed it should be used within 3 hours. Administered through a filter.

Cryoprecipitated Factor VIII is especially appropriate for patients with Willebrand's disease because, in addition to Factor VIII, it also supplies about 250 mg fibrinogen (Factor I), which they lack.

The most common bleeding sites in patients with hemophilia are the knees, elbows, and ankles. Early therapy is essential to prevent severe swelling and pain, and possibly joint damage.

Patients with hemophilia and other blood disorders tend to bleed longer but no more rapidly than normal. Frequently, these patients sense early bleeding episodes even before objective confirmation is feasible.

Patients with hemophilia should be cautioned not to take aspirin, aspirin-containing analgesics, or other drugs that inhibit platelet aggregation.

Most large cities have hemophilia diagnostic and treatment centers that provide comprehensive care for patients with severe hemophilia.

Store dried concentrate preparations in refrigerator at 2° to 8°C (35° to 46°F), unless otherwise directed by manufacturer. Avoid freezing.

Unless otherwise directed by manufacturer, concentrate should be refrigerated preferably between 2° and 8°C (35° and 46°F) until ready for use. Do not freeze.

ANTIMONY POTASSIUM TARTRATE

(Tartar Emetic)

(an'ti-moe-nee)
Antiinfective
Anthelmintic

ACTIONS AND USES. Potent trivalent antimony compound chemically similar to arsenic. Parasiticidal action believed to be due to ability to block anaerobic glucose metabolism by inhibiting phosphofructokinase. Powerful emetic action results from irritation of gastric mucosa; in toxic doses emesis is also produced by stimulation of CTZ in medulla. Reflexly stimulates salivary and bronchial secretions.

Used primarily in treatment of *Schistosoma japonicum* (blood fluke) infection. Used also for granuloma inguinale and mycosis fungoides. Because of toxicity, use as an emetic and expectorant has been largely replaced by other drugs.

ABSORPTION AND FATE. Rapidly bound to erythrocytes following IV administration. Slow renal excretion. Following a single dose, 10% may be recovered in urine within 24 hours, and about 30% within 1 week. Still detectable in urine for about 100 days after drug is discontinued.

CONTRAINDICATIONS AND PRECAUTIONS. Renal, hepatic, or cardiac insufficiency; febrile conditions other than those caused by Schistosoma; concomitant administration of other heavy metals; antiemetics.

ADVERSE/SIDE EFFECTS. CV: ECG changes, marked bradycardia, hypotension, shock syndrome, syncope, cardiac arrest. **GI:** nausea, vomiting, diarrhea, abdominal colic. **Hematologic:** thrombocytopenic purpura, hemolytic anemia. **Hepatotoxicity:** depressed hepatic function, hepatitis, jaundice. **Hypersensitivity:** skin rash, pruritus, urticaria, anaphylactoid reaction. **Injection site reactions:** cellulitis, necrosis (with extravasation), phlebitis. **Nephrotoxicity:** depressed renal function, albuminuria, renal damage. **Respiratory:** cough (common), dyspnea, apnea, pneumonia. **Other:** headache, vertigo, weakness, severe dermatitis, facial edema, fever, chills, diaphoresis, joint and muscle pain, acute arthritis.

ROUTE AND DOSAGE. Intravenous: Initial: 40 mg (8 ml) repeated every 2 days, with dose increase of 20 mg (4 ml) until 140 mg (28 ml) is reached; then 140 mg every other day to a total of 2.5 Gm. Administer slowly. Usually given as 0.5% (5 mg/ml) solution freshly prepared in sterile water for injection or 5% dextrose injection.

NURSING IMPLICATIONS

Anemia and malnutrition should be treated before therapy is initiated.

Preparation is administered by a physician and is usually given 2 hours after a light meal.

Too rapid injection can result in hypotension, dizziness, tachycardia, and acute circulatory failure.

Paroxysms of coughing and vomiting occur in most patients during and following IV injection, but symptoms usually subside within a few minutes. In some patients, nausea and vomiting may persist even after drug administration. Position patient so that aspiration of secretions is prevented.

Patient must be closely observed while receiving this toxic drug. Margin between toxicity and therapeutic safety is narrow. Have the antidote dimercaprol (BAL) and suction equipment immediately available.

Following injection, patient should remain recumbent for 1 hour or longer if necessary. Monitor vital signs.

Drug is a powerful tissue irritant; extravasation into perivascular tissues can cause cellulitis and necrosis. Observe injection sites.

Instruct patient to refrain from vigorous exercise during drug therapy. Many patients show ECG changes which may persist for 2 months after treatment is completed. These changes are apparently not associated with permanent cardiac injury.

Antiemetics should not be used during therapy because they may mask nausea and vomiting, which are warning signs of hepatotoxicity.

Therapy should be discontinued if vomiting persists or is severe or if patient develops blood dyscrasia, evidence of renal function impairment, fever, or dermatitis.

Joint and muscle pain and bradycardia occur most commonly near end of a course of treatment. Vital signs should be monitored during entire course of therapy.

Depressed hepatic function is not uncommon during drug therapy and may persist for several months after cessation of treatment. Periodic hepatic function tests should be performed during follow-up care.

Compliance (i.e., returning for repeat treatments and for medical surveillance) tends to be low because of discomfort caused by drug side effects, and is reportedly the major reason for therapeutic failure.

The common name for infections caused by *Schistosoma japonicum* is bilharziasis or blood fluke. Source of infection is from freshwater snail adults and larvae that penetrate the skin in contaminated water.

APOMORPHINE HYDROCHLORIDE

(a-poe-mor'feen)
Emetic
C II

ACTIONS AND USES. Centrally acting emetic prepared by treating morphine with dilute hydrochloric acid results in marked reduction of analgesic activity but enhanced emetic action. Produces CNS excitation and depression; induces vomiting by direct stimulant action on chemoreceptor trigger zone (CTZ), and possibly by excitation of vestibular centers. Depresses medullary center that controls respiration and vasomotor tone, and stimulates salivation. Elevates plasma levels of human growth hormone and reduces serum prolactin levels by stimulating dopamine receptors. Reduces tremor and rigidity in parkinsonism as well as levopoda-induced tremor, choreiform movements, and dyskinesia. Has sedative and hypnotic action in small nonemetic doses.

Used to produce emesis, particularly in acute oral drug overdosage or after oral ingestion of certain poisons.

ABSORPTION AND FATE. Vomiting usually occurs within 10 to 15 minutes in adults and within 1 or 2 minutes in children, following SC injection. Metabolized in liver. Excreted in urine; small amounts excreted unchanged.

CONTRAINDICATIONS AND PRECAUTIONS. Hypersensitivity to morphine derivatives and related opiates; after ingestion of caustics or corrosives (e.g., lye, acids) or volatile oils. Use for petroleum distillates or liquid hydrocarbons (gasoline, kerosene, fuel oil, paint thinner, cleaning fluid, and the like) depends on amount ingested and relative toxicity of substance. Other contraindications: strychnine poisoning, unconsciousness, during seizures; absent gag reflex, inebriated patients, shock, narcosis due to alcohol, barbiturates, opiates, and other CNS depressants. Safe use during pregnancy and in nursing mothers not established. *Cautious Use:* children, elderly and debilitated patients, impaired cardiac function, epilepsy, predisposition to nausea and vomiting.

ADVERSE/SIDE EFFECTS. Salivation, nausea, lacrimation, perspiration, weakness, fatigue, dizziness, sedation, hypnosis, orthostatic hypotension, fainting; *CNS stimulation* (euphoria, restlessness, tremors, polypnea, tachycardia). **With large doses:** violent and persistent vomiting, retching, *CNS depression* (dyspnea, depressed respirations, hypnosis, coma, bradycardia, acute circulatory failure); in patients with parkinsonian syndrome: myoclonia, dyskinesia, reversible renal damage.

ROUTE AND DOSAGE. Subcutaneous: Adults: 5 to 6 mg (range 2 to 10 mg) as a single dose. Not to be repeated. **Pediatric:** 0.07 to 0.1 mg/kg as a single dose. Not to be repeated.

NURSING IMPLICATIONS

For the adult patient, administration of 200 to 300 ml of water or preferably evaporated milk immediately before injection induces more efficient emesis. Smaller amounts of liquid are recommended for the small child.

Emesis may be enhanced by gently bouncing the child. Emetic effect is potentiated by motion and reduced by recumbency.

Position patient on side to prevent aspiration of vomitus.

Vomiting occurs in about 5 minutes and may be preceded by salivation and nausea. When vomiting ceases, patient usually falls into a profound sleep. Sedative effects persist for about 2 hours. Bedsides are indicated. Caution patient not to get out of bed without assistance.

If apomorphine fails to induce vomiting, dose is not repeated because it not likely to work. Also, additional drug would increase the risk of CNS or respiratory depression.

If patient has ingested an adsorbable poison, activated charcoal may be given immediately after apomorphine-induced vomiting is completed. If delay in giving the emetic is anticipated, activated charcoal is administered before the injection, to reduce absorption of poisons in stomach.

Monitor vital signs closely for at least 2 hours after drug administration. Since apomorphine may not evacuate all of the toxic substance ingested, patient should be observed closely for signs of poisoning after vomiting is complete.

Have on hand equipment for gastric lavage, suction, seizure precautions, and respiratory assistance; naloxone (opiate antagonist) to combat respiratory depression; and atropine (for treatment of cardiac depression).

Apomorphine is reported to be incompatible with iodides, iron salts, tannins, and oxidizing agents.

Classified as Schedule II drug under Federal Controlled Substances Act.

Apomorphine is dispensed as soluble hypodermic tablets. Solution is prepared by pharmacist, under aseptic conditions, by dissolving 6 mg tablet in 1 to 2 ml 0.9% sodium chloride or sterile water for injection. Resulting solution must then be filtered prior to administration. Do not heat sterilize. Stable for 2 days when protected from light and air and stored in refrigerator at between 2° to 8°C (35° to 43°F).

Apomorphine deteriorates with age and on exposure to light and air. Solutions that are green or brown or otherwise discolored or that contain a precipitate should not be used. Note expiration date of prepared solutions of apomorphine.

Store tablets in tight, light-resistant container, preferably between 15° and 30°C (59° and 86°F), unless otherwise directed by manufacturer.

APROBARBITAL

(Alurate)

(a-proe-bar'-bi-tal)

Sedative, hypnotic, barbiturate

C III

ACTIONS AND USES. Intermediate-acting barbiturate with actions, uses, precautions, and adverse reactions similar to those of phenobarbital (qv).

ABSORPTION AND FATE. Onset of action occurs within 1 hour, peaks in about 3 hours, and lasts approximately 6 to 8 hours. Mean half-life: 27 hours. Partly metabolized in liver. Excreted in urine as inactive metabolite; about 25% of a single dose excreted as unchanged drug. Rate of drug excretion increased by alkalinization of urine and increase in urinary output.

ROUTE AND DOSAGE. Oral: *Sedative:* 20 to 40 mg three times a day; *hypnotic:* 40 to 160 mg before retiring. (Dosage should be reduced for the elderly and debilitated. Pediatric dosage not established.)

NURSING IMPLICATIONS

Available as elixir only; 5 ml contains 40 mg aproparbital. Contains 20% alcohol.

Not generally used beyond 2 weeks because barbiturates appear to lose sleep-inducing effect after this time.

May be habit forming.

Aprobarbital is classified as a Schedule III drug under the Federal Controlled Substances Act.

See Phenobarbital (prototype barbiturate).

ASCORBATE, CALCIUM
ASCORBATE, SODIUM
(Cenolate, Cevita)
ASCORBIC ACID
(Apo-C, Arco-Cee, Ascorbicap, Best-C, Cecon, Ceebate, C-Long, Cemill, Cevalin, Cevi-Bid, Cetane, Ce-Vi-Sol, Cevita, Cevitamic Acid, Dull-C, Flavorcee, Redoxon, Schiff Effervescent Vitamin C, Vita-C, Vitamin C)

(a-skor'bate)
Antiscorbutic, antioxidant
Vitamin C
Acidifier, urinary

ACTIONS AND USES. Water-soluble vitamin essential for synthesis and maintenance of collagen and intercellular ground substance of body tissue cells, blood vessels, cartilage, bones, teeth, skin, and tendons. Necessary for wound healing. Powerful antioxidant and reducing agent essential for many cellular enzymatic activities. Functions in carbohydrate metabolism, the conversion of folic acid (folacin) to folinic acid (leucovorin), metabolism of phenylalanine and tyrosine, reduction of plasma transferrin to liver ferritin, the formation of serotonin, and in maintenance of vascular tone and integrity. Ascorbate sodium contains approximately 5 mEq (115 mg) of sodium per Gm.

Used for prophylaxis and treatment of scurvy, to facilitate intestinal absorption of non-heme iron, for treatment of methemoglobinemia, to promote tissue healing, and in a wide variety of malnutrition, deficiency, and hemorrhagic states. Ascorbic acid (not the ascorbates) has been used with limited success with methenamine to acidify urine when ammonium chloride is contraindicated or not tolerated. Also has been used in megadoses to prevent and treat the common cold, to inhibit sperm agglutination in male infertility, and to treat type VI Ehlers-Danlos syndrome. Widely used as an antioxidant in formulations of parenteral tetracycline and other drugs, and to protect color and flavor of foods.

ABSORPTION AND FATE. Readily absorbed following oral or parenteral administration; widely distributed to body tissues, with highest concentrations in glandular tissue, leukocytes, platelets, and lens. Reportedly better utilized following IM rather than IV administration. Limited body storage. Rapidly excreted from body when plasma level exceeds renal threshold of 1.4 mg/dl. Metabolized in liver. Excess amounts excreted chiefly in urine as unchanged drug, oxalic acid, and other metabolites. Crosses placenta. Excreted in breast milk. Removed by hemodialysis.

CONTRAINDICATIONS AND PRECAUTIONS. Use of sodium ascorbate in patients on sodium restriction; use of calcium ascorbate in patients receiving digitalis. *Cautious Use:* excessive doses in patients with G6PD deficiency, iron overload associated with repeated blood transfusions, hemochromatosis, thalassemia, sideroblastic anemia; sickle cell anemia; patients prone to gout or renal calculi. Safe use during pregnancy (category C) and in nursing mothers not established.

ADVERSE/SIDE EFFECTS. Acute hemolytic anemia (patients with deficiency of G6PD); sickle cell crisis (patients with sickle cell anemia); decreased urine urobilinogen excretion. *With excessive doses:* nausea, vomiting, heartburn, diarrhea, abdominal cramps, fatigue, flushing, headache; insomnia or sleepiness, increase in urination, urine acidification, and possibly crystalluria, (oxalate, cystine, or urate stones); dental erosion with high doses and prolonged use of chewable tablets. **Parenteral administration:** mild soreness at IV injection site; dizziness and temporary faintness with rapid administration, deep venous thrombosis; tissue necrosis following IM calcium ascorbate in infants.

ROUTE AND DOSAGE. Oral, intramuscular, intravenous: *Antirachitic:* **Adults and children:** 300 mg to 1 Gm or more daily in divided doses; *prophylactic:* 45 to 60 mg daily. **Infants:** *therapeutic:* 100 to 300 mg daily in divided doses; *prophylactic:* 20 to 50 mg daily. *Urinary acidification:* 4 to 12 Gm/day in divided doses every 4 hours. Available as tablets, chewable tablets, capsules, timed-release capsules and tablets, and drops, syrup, liquid, solution for injection.

NURSING IMPLICATIONS

Ampuls containing ascorbic acid injection should be opened with caution. After prolonged storage, decomposition may occur with release of carbon dioxide and resulting increase in pressure within ampul.

Parenteral vitamin C is incompatible with many drugs. Consult pharmacist for compatibility information.

Large doses of vitamin C (i.e., 1000 mg/day) are given in divided amounts because the body utilizes only what is needed at a particular time and excretes the rest in urine. Megadoses may increase pH of the small intestine leading to interference with absorption of vitamin B_{12}.

Oral solutions of vitamin C may be dropped directly in mouth or mixed with food.

Effervescent tablet form should be dissolved in a glass of water immediately before ingestion.

Minimum daily requirement of vitamin C to prevent scurvy is 10 mg. Recommended daily dietary allowance for adults is 60 mg (equivalent to about 4 ounces of orange juice); during pregnancy, 80 mg; during lactation, 100 mg; for infants, 35 mg; and for children, 45 mg.

High doses of vitamin C are not recommended during pregnancy. Fetus can adapt to high levels by developing the capacity to inactivate vitamin C. Rebound scurvy can result when vitamin C intake in reduced to normal.

Infants fed on cow's milk alone require supplemental vitamin C. A daily dose of 35 mg has been recommended during first week of life if formula contains two to three times the amount of protein found in human milk.

Normal plasma concentration of ascorbic acid: approximately 0.4 to 1.5 mcg/dl.

Vitamin C requirements are significantly increased in conditions that elevate metabolic rate, e.g., hyperthyroidism, fever, infection, burns and other severe trauma, postoperative states, neoplastic disease, chronic alcoholism. Reportedly, patients taking oral contraceptives also require vitamin C supplements.

Subclinical vitamin C deficiency may exist in persons who subsist on diets low in fruits and vegetables. Particularly vulnerable are the indigent, the elderly, food faddists, drug addicts, alcoholics, patients on restricted therapeutic diets, and those receiving prolonged

IV fluids, parenteral hyperalimentation, or chronic hemodialysis without adequate supplementation.

Symptoms of vitamin C deficiency usually become objectively evident after 3 to 5 months of inadequate intake: irritability, emotional disturbances, general debility, pallor, anorexia, sensitivity to touch; limb and joint pain, follicular hyperkeratosis (particularly on thighs and buttocks), easy bruising, petechiae, bloody diarrhea, delayed wound healing, loosening of teeth, sensitive, swollen, bleeding gums, anemia.

Smoking–Drug Interaction. Smokers appear to have increased requirements for ascorbic acid because the vitamin is oxidized and excreted more rapidly than in nonsmokers. Advise patient with vitamin C deficiency to modify or stop smoking. Replacement dosages will be greater for the smoker.

Most fruits and vegetables contain vitamin C, with highest levels in citrus fruits, strawberries, rose hips, guava, cantaloupe, leafy vegetables, tomatoes, potatoes, cabbage, green peppers, and parsley. A 6-ounce glass of juice from the fruit of the acerola tree or Puerto Rican cherry yields about 8650 mg of vitamin C, approximately 85 times as much as an equal amount of orange juice. (Orange or grapefruit juice, fresh or concentrated, contains approximately 0.5 mg/dl.)

Further studies are needed to determine the value of ascorbic acid in the prevention of atherosclerosis and in the prophylaxis or treatment of the common cold.

Vitamin C is rapidly oxidized when exposed to air (deterioration is accelerated by light and heat). Slight darkening of tablets may occur without loss of potency.

Food–Drug Interaction. Vitamin C increases the absorption of iron when taken at the same time as iron-rich foods.

Large losses of vitamin C may result from: (1) Prolonged exposure to light and air (e.g., storage of foods and fruit juices in uncovered containers; early precutting). (2) Prolonged cooking. (3) Prolonged soaking. (4) Addition of sodium bicarbonate to foods. (5) Contact with copper and iron utensils.

Stored in airtight, light-resistant, nonmetallic containers, away from heat and sunlight, preferably between 15° and 30°C (59° and 86°F), unless otherwise directed by manufacturer.

Diagnostic Test Interferences. High doses of vitamin C can produce false-negative results for **urine glucose** with glucose oxidase methods (Clinitest, Tes-Tape, Diastix); false-positive results with copper reduction methods (Benedict's solution, Clinitest); and false increases in **serum uric acid** determination (by enzymatic methods). Interferes with **urinary steroid** (17-OHCS) determinations (by modified Reddy, Jenkins, Thorn procedure), and decreases in **serum bilirubin.** May cause false-negative tests for **occult blood** in stools.

Drug Interactions: Ascorbic acid in megadoses (high enough to increase urine acidity)

Plus	Interactions
Aminosalicylic acid (PAS)	Increases risk of crystalluria
Amphetamines Antidepressants, tricyclics	Effects of these drugs may be decreased
Contraceptives, oral	May enhance effect of oral contraceptive, but contraceptive failure may result with abrupt discontinuation of vitamin C
Disulfiram (Antabuse)	May reduce disulfiram reaction
Digitalis	Calcium ascorbate may precipitate arrhythmias in patients taking digitalis
Phenothiazines	Decreases phenothiazine blood levels

Plus (cont.)	Interactions (cont.)
Salicylates	Potentiates salicylate effects (vitamin C decreases salicylate excretion). Salicylates may inhibit uptake of vitamin C
Sulfonamides	Increases risk of crystalluria

ASPARAGINASE

(Elspar, L-Asparaginase)

(a-spar'a-gi-nase)
Antineoplastic
Enzyme

ACTIONS AND USES. A highly toxic drug with a low therapeutic index. This enzyme, isolated from *Escherichia coli* is active in solution at pH 6.5 to 8.0 and functions chiefly during postmitotic G_1 phase of cell division. Catalyzes hydrolysis (breakdown) of asparagine to ammonia and aspartic acid, thus depleting extracellular supply of an amino acid essential to synthesis of DNA and other nucleoproteins. Reduced availability of asparagine has little effect on most normal cells but tumor cells unable to synthesize their own supply are destroyed. Because some normal cells have high rates of protein synthesis, they also depend on an extracellular source of asparagine; thus drug-induced deficiency interferes with synthesis of important proteins by cells in, e.g., liver (clotting factors), pancreas (insulin), lymphocytes (antibodies). Bone marrow depression or cytotoxic effects on cells of GI tract, oral mucosa, hair follicles rarely occurs. Resistance to cytotoxic action develops rapidly; therefore asparaginase is not effective in treatment of solid tumors and is not recommended for maintenance therapy. No cross-resistance to other antineoplastic agents has been demonstrated.

Used primarily in combination regimens with other antineoplastic agents to treat acute lymphocyte leukemia (ALL). Has been used investigationally alone or in combination regimens in treatment of other leukemias, lymphosarcoma, and (intraarterially) in treatment of hypoglycemia due to pancreatic islet cell tumor.

ABSORPTION AND FATE. Distribution is primarily within the intravascular space (80%). About 3 hours after IV dose, remaining drug (20%) is distributed in lymph and (low levels) in CSF, pleural and peritoneal fluids. Plasma half-life, 8 to 30 hours, is unaffected by age, hepatic or renal function, or by diagnosis or extent of disease. Metabolic fate unknown; small amounts of the enzyme are found in urine; presence in milk has not been demonstrated.

CONTRAINDICATIONS AND PRECAUTIONS. History of previous hypersensitivity to asparaginase; history of or existing pancreatitis. Safe use during pregnancy (category C) and in nursing mothers not established. *Cautious Use:* liver impairment, diabetes mellitus, infections, history of urate calculi or of gout, patients who have had previous antineoplastic and/or radiation therapy.

ADVERSE/SIDE EFFECTS. CNS: depression, headache, irritability, personality disorders, fatigue, lethargy, confusion, agitation, hallucinations, coma, seizures (rare), organic brain syndrome, Parkinson-like syndrome with tremor and progressive increase in muscle tone. **GI:** severe vomiting, nausea, anorexia, abdominal cramps, diarrhea, oral and intestinal ulcerations, malabsorption syndrome (rare), acute pancreatitis. **GU:** uric acid nephropathy, azotemia, renal shutdown or insufficiency, proteinuria. **Hematologic:** hypofibrino ginemia, reduced clotting factors (especially V, VII, VIII, IX), decreased circulating platelets, marked leukopenia. **Hepatotoxicity:** liver function abnormalities: jaundice, fluctuations in total serum lipids, increases in: blood ammonia, alkaline phosphatase, SGOT (AST), SGPT (ALT), BUN, bilirubin, cholesterol. **Hypersensitivity:** skin rashes, urticaria, arthralgia; anaphylaxis. **Other:** chills, fever, perspiration, weight loss, fatal hyperthermia, hyperglycemia, glycosuria, polyuria, hypoalbuminemia associated with peripheral edema, hypocalcemia, hyperuricemia, infections.

ROUTE AND DOSAGE. (Highly individualized regimens): **Intravenous: Adults and children:** *Sole induction agent:* 200 IU/kg daily for 28 days. *Combination therapy* as with prednisone and vincristine (dosages vary widely): 1000 IU/kg/day for 10 successive days, injected slowly over 30 minutes. **Intramuscular:** 6000 IU/m^2 every third day until remission.

NURSING IMPLICATIONS

Administered preferably to hospitalized patients who can be under constant supervision of a clinician experienced in cancer chemotherapy.

Patient should be informed before treatment is initiated of the positive and negative effects of drug therapy. Some degree of toxicity generally occurs.

Caution is warranted in handling, administering, and disposing of antineoplastic drugs because of their carcinogenic, mutagenic, and teratogenic potential. Follow agency policy.

Have immediately available: personnel, drugs (epinephrine, antihistamine, diphenhydramine, IV corticosteroid), oxygen, and equipment for treating anaphylactic reaction, whenever drug is administered.

Because of the possibility of allergic reactions, an intradermal skin test is performed before the initial dose of asparaginase and when the drug is readministered after an interval of a week or more.

Observe test site for at least 1 hour for evidence of positive reaction (wheal, erythema). A negative skin test, however, does not preclude possibility of an allergic reaction.

Positive reactors can be desensitized with increasing IV doses at 10-minute intervals (provided no allergic reaction occurs) until patient's total dose for that day is reached. Be aware that desensitization itself can be hazardous because asparaginase is a large foreign protein and is antigenic.

Unlike many other desensitization regimens, asparaginase desensitization does not eliminate risk of subsequent allergic reactions with retreatments.

During asparaginase administration, monitor vital signs and be alert to evidence of hypersensitivity reactions or anaphylaxis: hypotension, irregular pulse, feeling of lump in throat or hoarseness (laryngeal edema), bronchospasm (wheezing), dyspnea, cyanosis, chest constriction. Anaphylaxis usually occurs within ½ to 1 hour after dose has been given. It is more apt to happen with intermittent administrations and when IM route is used.

When given concurrently with or immediately before a course of prednisone and vincristine, toxicity potential is increased.

Maintenance of adequate fluid intake, alkalinization of urine and/or administration of allopurinol may accompany treatment as prophylaxis against uric acid stones.

Tests for glycosuria should be done regularly. Report polyuria, polydipsia, or positive urine test to the physician.

Surveillance of body weight is important. Instruct patient to notify physician of continued loss of weight or onset of foot and ankle swelling.

Serum amylase, blood glucose, plasma coagulation factor determinations, ammonia and uric acid levels, hepatic and renal function tests, peripheral blood counts, and bone marrow function are monitored regularly during treatment. Liver function tests are done at least twice weekly during therapy.

Circulating lymphoblasts decrease markedly in the first several days of treatment and leukocyte counts may fall below normal. Protection from infection during this period is crucial. Dressings and treatments should be done with sterile technique and health personnel and visitors with respiratory or other infections should be restricted. Reverse precautions may be ordered. Signs of infection in the patient (chill, fever, aches, sore throat) should be reported promptly.

Report sudden severe abdominal pain with nausea and vomiting, particularly if these symptoms occur after medication is discontinued (may indicate pancreatitis).

Elevations of BUN and serum ammonia are expected findings because of enzymatic action. Blood ammonia levels are elevated in most patients as high as 700 to 900 mcg/dl (normal 80 to 110 mcg/dl). Watch for signs of *hyperammonemia:* anorexia, vomiting, lethargy, weak pulse, depressed temperature, irritability, asterixis, seizures, coma. The treatment is usually *low-protein diet* (i.e., low protein breads, most vegetables and fruits, avoidance of meat, sea food, legumes) with ample amounts of simple carbohydrate e.g., jellies, syrups, honey, sugar, candy, to increase colonic intake. Collaborate with dietitian and physician.

Because of potential serious hepatic dysfunction, enzymatic detoxification of other drugs may be reduced; therefore anticipate possibility of prolonged or exaggerated effects of concurrently given drugs and/or their toxicity; report incidence promptly.

Asparaginase toxicity is reportedly less in children than in adults. In general, because of the low therapeutic index characteristic of this agent, a therapeutic response will most likely be accompanied by some toxicity in all patients.

Nausea, vomiting, and anorexia can interrupt scheduled doses at first, but lessen with continued treatment. Instruct patient to try to continue all prescribed medications if at all possible but if not possible, the physician should be notified without delay.

Urge patient to report the onset of unusual bleeding, bruising, petechiae, melena, skin rash or itching, yellowed skin and sclera, joint pain, puffy face, or dyspnea.

CNS function (general behavior, emotional status, level of consciousness, thought content, motor function) should be evaluated before and during therapy.

Drowsiness, decreased alertness, and shakiness are symptoms that can accompany treatment with this drug. Driving or operating equipment that requires alertness and skill can be hazardous. Urge caution and inform patient that these effects can continue several weeks after last dose of the drug.

Reinforce necessity to keep scheduled appointments for evaluation of therapy.

The lyophilized powder is reconstituted with sterile water for injection for IV administration or with NaCl for injection for IV and IM administration. Shake vial well to promote dissolution of powder. Avoid vigorous shaking: ordinary shaking does not inactivate the enzyme or cause foaming of content.

For IV infusion, the reconstituted solution should be further diluted with NaCl or 5% dextrose injection and administered into tubing of an already running infusion, in not less than 30 minutes. If a filter is used it should be a 5-micron filter. Use of a 0.2-micron filter can reduce potency of asparaginase solution.

Limit the IM injection volume to 2 ml in one site. Select a second site if volume exceeds 2 ml.

Unless otherwise directed by manufacturer, store sealed vial of lyophilized powder below 8°C (46°F); reconstituted solutions can be stored at 2° to 8°C (36° to 46°F) for up to 8 hours, then discard. Do not use cloudy solution.

Diagnostic Test Interferences. Asparaginase may interfere with interpretation of **thyroid function** tests (pretreatment values return within 4 weeks after drug is discontinued).

Drug Interactions: Asparaginase

Plus	Interactions
Antigout agents	Since asparaginase raises blood uric acid levels adjustment of antigout drug dose may be necessary

Plus (cont.)	Interactions (cont.)
Corticosteroids (glucocosteroids) especially prednisone	Increase hyperglycemic effect of asparaginase and may increase risk of neuropathy and erythropoietic pathology
Hypoglycemics	Hypoglycemic effect reduced; dose adjustment required during and after asparaginase treatment
Immunosuppressives or radiation therapy	Effects enhanced by asparaginase
Methotrexate (Mexate)	Antineoplastic effect of methotrexate blocked when administered immediately before or with asparaginase
Vincristine (Oncovin)	*See corticosteroids (above)*

PROTOTYPE

ASPIRIN

(Acetylsalisylic Acid, Ancasal, A.S.A., Aspergum, Astrin, Bayer, Cosprin, Easprin, Ecotrin, Empirin, Entrophen, Hipirin, Measurin, Novasen, Supasa, Triaphen-10, Zorprin)

(as'pir-in)

NSAID, analgesic/antipyretic, antiplatelet, enzyme inhibitor, antirheumatic

Salicylate

ACTIONS AND USES. A salicylic ester of acetic acid; each gram contains about 760 mg salicylate. Major actions, i.e., analgesic, antiinflammatory, and antipyretic appear to be associated with inhibition of synthesis and release of prostaglandins. *Analgesic action:* principally peripheral with limited action in the CNS possibly on the hypothalamus, and results in relief of mild to moderate pain. *Antiinflammatory action:* aspirin and other salicylates inhibit cyclooxygenase, an enzyme required for prostaglandin synthesis. Prostaglandins directly mediate many of the signs of inflammation, e.g., release of lysosomal substance, increased lymphocyte activation, formation of autoantibodies. As an antiinflammatory agent, aspirin appears to be involved in increased antigen removal, reduction of spread of inflammation in ground substances, and depression of the total inflammatory process. These antiinflammatory effects also contribute to analgesic effects. As an *antipyretic,* aspirin lowers body temperature in fever by inhibiting prostaglandin synthesis and release, and by indirectly causing centrally mediated peripheral vasodilation and sweating. Aspirin (but not other salicylates) is a powerful inhibitor of platelet aggregation and prolongs bleeding time (measurable *antiplatelet effect* may persist 3 to 7 days). It may decrease leukocytosis and erythrocyte sedimentation rate in rheumatic fever (by an unknown mechanism) and reportedly increases fibrinolysis. Antithrombotic action may be limited to males but studies are continuing to evaluate the effect of low dosage of aspirin in preventing first or subsequent heart attacks and thromboembolic disorders in both sexes. Urate excretion *(uricosuric effect)* is enhanced by high doses of aspirin (over 5 Gm/day) and suppressed by usual analgesic doses (less than 2 Gm/day). Has hypocholesterolemic and hypoglycemic effects in large doses.

Used to relieve pain of low to moderate intensity, such as headache, dysmenorrhea, neuralgia, myalgia, arthalgia, discomforts of common cold, cancer pain, postoperative (after second or third day), and postpartum pain. Also used for various inflammatory conditions, such as acute rheumatic fever, systemic lupus erythematosus, rheumatoid arthritis, osteoarthritis, bursitis, calcific tendonitis, and to reduce fever in selected febrile conditions. *Investigational Use:* to reduce recurrence of TIA (transient ischemic attack) and risk of stroke, as prophylactic against thromboembolism, to prevent recurrence of myocardial infarction, and to prevent progression of diabetic retinopathy. Buffered aspirins generally contain aspirin with magnesium or aluminum hydroxide (e.g., Ascriptin, Buff-A, Cope) or with magnesium carbonate (e.g., Bufferin). Unbuffered products containing aspirin in combination with caffeine alone include Anacin, P-A-C, Excredin (also contains acetaminophen). Aspirin is combined with sodium bicarbonate and citric acid (e.g., Alka-Seltzer Effervescent Pain Reliever and Antacid) but is not an ingredient in Alka-Seltzer Antacid.

ABSORPTION AND FATE. Rapidly and completely absorbed from stomach and upper bowel. Administration with food retards absorption rate, but does not reduce total amount absorbed. Erratic absorption times reported for enteric-coated, rectal suppository, and extended release forms. Readily absorbed by most body fluids and all tissues. Peak plasma levels in 1 to 2 hours. Extensively bound to plasma proteins. Half-life is dose dependent (about 2 to 3 hours with low or single doses and 5 to 18 hours with moderate doses). Rapidly hydrolyzed in GI tract, plasma, and liver to salicylate. Additional metabolism by liver microsomal system. Individual differences in metabolism and excretion rates reported. At low doses, 50% of dose excreted in urine in 2 to 4 hours, and in 15 to 30 hours at high doses. Eliminated as salicyluric acid and conjugates; about 1% excreted unhydrolyzed. Urinary excretion rate is pH dependent. Alkaline salts increase absorption rate and renal clearance; urinary acidification promotes retention. Readily crosses placenta; excreted in breast milk.

CONTRAINDICATIONS AND PRECAUTIONS. Hypersensitivity to salicylates including methyl salicylate (oil of wintergreen), to other NSAIDs or to tartrazine; patients with **"aspirin triad"** (rhinitis, nasal polyps, asthma); chronic rhinitis, history of GI ulceration or bleeding; hemophilia or other bleeding disorders, carditis; use during pregnancy (category D), especially in third trimester, in nursing mothers, and in prematures, neonates, and children under 2 years, except under advice and supervision of physician. *Cautious Use:* otic diseases, allergies, gout, children with fever accompanied by dehydration; cardiac disease, renal or hepatic impairment, vitamin K deficiency, G6PD deficiency, anemia, preoperatively, Hodgkin's disease.

ADVERSE/SIDE EFFECTS. CV: with large doses: pulmonary edema (increase in plasma volume), rapid pulse. **GI:** gastric irritation (nausea, vomiting, heartburn, anorexia, stomach pain, GI ulceration and bleeding). **Hematologic:** easy bruising, ecchymoses, increased bleeding before and after delivery, hypoglycemia (especially in diabetics), iron-deficiency anemia, thrombocytopenia, purpura, leukopenia, agranulocytosis, hemolytic anemia (G6PD deficiency). **Hypersensitivity:** bronchospasm (wheezing), tightness in chest, severe rhinitis, skin eruptions, angioedema, urticaria, anaphylaxis. *Marked intoxication:* (symptoms as for mild intoxication, but more pronounced and occur more rapidly): hemorrhage, tachycardia, pulmonary edema, hypoglycemia or hyperglycemia, hyponatremia, hypokalemia, disturbances in acid–base balance, hyperpyrexia, nephropathy, hepatotoxicity, acute pancreatitis, dehydration, "*salicylic jag*" (CNS stimulation: restlessness, incoherent speech, hallucinations resembling alcoholic inebriation but without euphoria, convulsions); CNS depression, delirium, coma, respiratory failure. **Otic:** (dose related and usually reversible): tinnitus, decreased hearing, deafness. **Salicylism:** *mild intoxication:* rapid and deep breathing (hyperpnea), tinnitus, diminished hearing, dizziness, severe or continuing headache, dimmed vision, mental confusion, lassitude, drowsiness, fever, flushing, sweating, thirst, nausea, vomiting, diarrhea, anorexia, rapid pulse. **Other:** prolonged pregnancy, labor.

ROUTE AND DOSAGE. Oral, rectal suppository (rarely used): Adults: *Analgesic, antipyretic:* 325 to 650 mg (5 to 10 grains) every 4 to 6 hours, as necessary. *Arthritis and rheumatic conditions* (highly individualized): **Oral:** 2.6 to 5.2 Gm daily in divided doses. *Acute rheumatic fever* (highly individualized); up to 7.8 Gm daily in divided doses. *Thromboembolic disorders:* **Oral only** (numerous schedules): 80 to 650 mg once or twice daily or 325 mg four times daily. **Children (under 2 years):** *Analgesic, antipyretic:* dosage individualized by physician; **Children (2 to 4 years):** 160 mg; **Children (4 to 6 years):** 240 mg; **Children (6 to 9 years):** 320 mg; **Children (9 to 11 years):** 400 mg; **Children (11 to 12 years):** 480 mg. Doses given every 4 to 6 hours as necessary. For OTC use no more than 5 doses/24-hour period, unless otherwise directed by physician. Dosage by body surface area: **Children under 12 years:** 1.5 Gm/m² or 65 mg/kg/24 hours in four to six divided doses. Available as regular tablets, enteric-coated, chewable, and timed-released tablets, gum, capsules and rectal suppository.

NURSING IMPLICATIONS

GI side effects may be minimized by administering with a full glass of water (240 ml, preferably warm), milk, food, or an antacid. Exception: enteric-coated tablet; may dissolve too quickly if administered with milk. Also enteric coated tablet should not be crushed or chewed. The aim is to prevent direct contact of drug particles with gastric mucosa.

If patient has difficulty in swallowing tablets, plain aspirin can be crushed to a fine powder and mixed with applesauce or other food that patient likes.

Buffered aspirin or aspirin administered with an antacid may be better tolerated; however, large doses or repeated use can contribute to alkalinization of urine which enhances salicylate excretion.

Buffered aspirin preparations in an effervescent vehicle, e.g., Alka-Seltzer, are more rapidly absorbed than plain aspirin, and cause less GI irritation and bleeding. Alka-Seltzer, however, has a high sodium content, and therefore should not be used on a scheduled basis or in patients on sodium restriction. Additionally, repeated doses may raise urinary pH and increase excretion of certain drugs.

There is no convincing support to the claim that one brand of aspirin is more effective than another. Brands may differ in the binder used and moisture content per tablet, but all must pass the USP standard disintegration test.

Because aspirin lacks topical anesthetic action there is no logical basis for applying it locally for toothache or for using aspirin gargle or gum for sore throat. Any relief gained is due to systemic absorption, not local action.

When prescribed for dysmenorrhea, explain to patient that for best results aspirin should be taken 1 or 2 days before menses (to reduce prostaglandin-induced uterine contractions). Patients having heavy menstrual blood loss should be advised to take another analgesic, such as acetaminophen, instead of aspirin.

For treatment of rheumatic diseases, physician may prescribe daily dose increase of 1 or 2 tablets/day on basis of serum salicylate concentrations, or until therapeutic response occurs (usually within 3 to 5 days after beginning regular dosing), or symptoms of toxicity (salicylism) intervene. Symptoms of toxicity are often eliminated after dosage reduction of as little as 325 mg (5 grains).

Schedule aspirin administration at least 30 minutes before physical therapy or other planned exercise to keep discomfort at a minimum.

To reduce risk of bleeding, generally, aspirin therapy is discontinued about 1 week before surgery. Patients undergoing oral surgery should be advised not to take aspirin-containing gum or gargles and not to chew aspirin products for at least 1 week following surgery. Prolonged contact with aspirin can cause hemorrhage and injury to oral tissues.

Chronic administration of high-dose aspirin during the last 3 months of pregnancy may prolong pregnancy and labor, increase maternal bleeding before and after delivery, and cause weight increase and hemorrhage in the neonate.

Therapeutic range for rheumatic diseases: 20 to 30 mg/dl. Symptoms of toxicity generally occur when serum salicylate levels are over 30 mg/dl.

Previous nonreaction to salicylates does not guarantee future safety. Subsequent sensitivity especially to aspirin is not uncommon.

Patients with asthma, nasal polyps, perennial vasomotor rhinitis, or hay fever demonstrate a high frequency of salicylate hypersensitivity.

Advise patient to discontinue use with onset of ringing in the ears, impaired hearing, dizziness, GI discomfort or bleeding. Hearing impairment resulting from salicylate toxicity is generally reversible.

Tinnitus and decreased hearing are not always reliable indicators of toxicity because these changes may pass unnoticed in the hearing impaired, the elderly, and in children.

Potential for toxicity is high in the elderly who are chronic aspirin users because they have less serum proteins to bind salicylate and also are less able to excrete it.

Children tend to manifest salicylate toxicity by hyperventilation, agitation, mental confusion, lethargy, sweating, constipation.

Accidental ingestion of salicylates is one of the most common causes of poisoning and death in young children. Caution patients to keep drug out of the reach of children.

The following is a rough estimate for the appropriate dosage of aspirin for children: one grain (65 mg) daily per year up to age 10.

Children on high doses of aspirin are particularly prone to develop hypoglycemia. Monitor the diabetic child carefully for indicated need of insulin adjustment.

The American Academy of Pediatrics and the CDC warn not to give aspirin to children under 18 years with symptoms of varicella (chickenpox), influenza-like illnesses, or other viral infections because of the possible association of aspirin usage with Reye's syndrome. Children presenting symptoms of persistent vomiting, changes in level of consciousness, with or without lethargy, behavioral changes, severe headache, or fever should be evaluated immediately for Reye's syndrome.

Most low to moderate fevers do not require treatment beyond drinking liquids, wearing lighter clothing, and sponge baths. Additionally, the use of aspirin to reduce fever may mask serious illness. Nonprescribed use in children for this purpose should be discouraged. In adults, aspirin should not be used for self-medication of pain beyond 3 to 5 days without consulting a physician. Additionally, it should not be used longer than 2 or 3 days for fever and never for fever over 39.5°C (103°F), or for recurrent fever, without medical direction.

If aspirin has been prescribed, advise patient to check with clinician if fever continues more than 3 days or if it continues to rise or returns. In children, particularly, salicylate toxicity is enhanced by dehydration as might occur during fever. Monitor these patients closely.

Caution patient to avoid aspirin products if he or she has been drinking alcohol *(see Drug Interactions).*

Food–Drug Interaction: chronic ingestion of aspirin may be associated with depressed plasma ascorbic acid (vitamin C) and folate levels in some patients. Supplemental therapy may be indicated.

Prolonged use of high salicylate doses can lead to iron-deficiency anemia, especially in women. Average blood loss with daily use of several aspirin tablets is reportedly 2 to 6 ml; 10% of patients on chronic high doses may lose as much as 80 ml/day.

Instructions for patients receiving repeated or large doses of salicylates:

- Observe and report symptoms of salicylism *(see Adverse/Side Effects):* petechiae, ecchymoses, bleeding gums, bloody or black stools.
- Maintain adequate fluid intake (consult physician) to prevent salicylate crystalluria.
- Report for periodic hematocrit, prothrombin time, and blood and urine salicylate determinations as directed by physician. Hepatic and renal function tests are also recom-

mended at regular intervals, particularly for patients with systemic lupus erythematosus (SLE) and juvenile rheumatoid arthritis (JRA). Diabetic patients should be closely monitored *(see Drug Interactions).*

- Avoid other medications containing aspirin unless directed by physician, because of danger of overdosing. (There are more than 500 aspirin-containing compounds.)
- Supplemental ascorbic acid and folates, if prescribed.

Treatment of overdosage: Acute salicylate toxicity requires immediate emesis or gastric lavage and activated charcoal. Further treatment is designed to maintain hydration, electrolyte and acid–base balance, and to reduce hyperthermia (IV fluids); to reduce excitement or convulsions (diazepam or barbiturates); and to force diuresis by alkalinizing urine. Hemodialysis in adults, peritoneal dialysis in children, and exchange transfusion in infants may be required. Patients who have ingested sustained-release aspirin must be observed for at least 3 days after toxicity treatment.

Most aspirin tablets develop a hard shell with age, a change that lengthens disintegration time, increases risk of GI irritation, and delays onset of therapeutic action. Advise patient not to buy aspirin in large quantities.

Aspirin tablets rapidly hydrolyze on exposure to heat, moisture, and air. Instruct patient to smell tablet before taking it. If a vinegarlike (acetic acid) odor is detected discard all tablets.

Store preferably between 15° and 30°C (59° and 86°F) in airtight container, unless otherwise directed by manufacturer. Store suppositories in a cool place or refrigerate, but do not freeze.

Diagnostic Test Interferences. **Bleeding time** is prolonged 4 to 7 days (life of exposed platelets) following a single 325 mg (5 grains) dose of aspirin. Large doses of aspirin (5 Gm or more/day) may cause prolonged **prothrombin time,** interference with **pregnancy tests** (using mouse or rabbit), decrease in **serum cholesterol, potassium,** and **PBI. Serum uric acid** may increase when plasma salicylate levels are below 10 and decrease when above 15 mg/dl. **Urine 5-HIAA:** test interference by fluorescent methods. **Urine ketones:** interference with Gerhardt test (reaction with ferric chloride produces a reddish color that persists after boiling). **Urine glucose:** moderate to large doses of aspirin (2.4 Gm or more per day) may produce false-negative results with glucose oxidase methods (e.g., Clinistix, Tes-Tape), and false-positive results with copper reduction methods (Benedict's solution, Clinitest). Urinary **PSP excretion** may be reduced. **Urine VMA** falsely elevated (by most tests), or reduced (by Pisano method).

Drug Interactions: Aspirin (and other salicylates)

Plus	Interactions
Alcohol (Ethanol)	Potentiation of ulcerogenic effects. Concomitant ingestion not advised
Aminosalicylic acid (PAS)	Increased PAS toxicity (salicylates decrease renal excretion of PAS)
Ammonium chloride and other acidifying agents	Elevate serum salicylate levels (increases renal tubular reabsorption of salicylates by lowering urine pH)
Antacids, including sodium bicarbonate and other urinary alkalinizing agents	Reduce serum salicylate levels (alkalinization of urine, decreases renal tubular reabsorption of salicylate)
Anticoagulants	Additive hypoprothrombinemic effect (by decreasing plasma protein binding). Combination avoided, if possible

Plus (cont.)	Interactions (cont.)
Antidiabetic agents	Increased hypoglycemic activity with moderate to large salicylate doses, i.e., > 2 Gm/day (by decreased plasma protein binding). Concurrent use generally avoided. If used, dosage reduction of both drugs may be necessary
Carbonic anhydrase inhibitors, e.g., acetazolamide (Diamox)	May induce metabolic acidosis and thus enhance salicylate intoxication in patients receiving high salicylate doses
Corticosteroids	Decrease serum salicylate levels (possibly by increasing renal excretion); additive ulcerogenic effects. Concurrent use generally avoided
Indomethacin (Indocin) and other NSAIDs	Decreased serum indomethacin levels possibly by decreasing GI absorption; additive ulcerogenic effects. Concurrent use generally avoided
Methotrexate (Mexate)	Increased methotrexate levels (by decreasing renal clearance and decreasing plasma protein binding of methotrexate). Concurrent use generally avoided, if possible
Niacin	Aspirin blocks high dose niacin-induced flushing
Phenylbutazone (Butazolidin), Probenecid (Benemid), Sulfinpyrazone (Anturane)	Salicylates in small to moderate doses may antagonize uricosuric action of these drugs. Concurrent use generally avoided during uricosuric therapy
Sulfonamides	Salicylates reportedly increase serum sulfonamide levels, possibly by displacing them from serum protein binding sites
Tetracyclines	May form complex with aluminum- or magnesium-containing antacids in buffered aspirins. Salicylates should be administered at least 1 hour before or after tetracyclines

---

ATENOLOL
(Tenormin)

(a-ten′oh-lole)
Adrenergic blocking agent (beta$_1$-selective)
Antihypertensive

ACTIONS AND USES. In therapeutic doses this drug selectively blocks beta$_1$-adrenergic receptors located chiefly in cardiac muscle. With large doses preferential effect is lost and inhibition of beta$_2$-adrenergic receptors (especially in bronchial and vascular musculature) may lead to increased airway resistance, especially in patients with asthma or COPD. Unlike propranolol (a nonselective beta blocker), atenolol lacks membrane-stabilizing and intrinsic sympathomimetic (partial agonist) activities. Mechanisms for antihypertensive action include central effect leading to decreased sympathetic outflow to periphery, reduction in renin activity with consequent suppression of the renin–aldosterone–angiotensin system, and competitive inhibition of catecholamine binding at beta adrenergic receptor sites. Cardiac output is reduced, as is diastolic blood pressure. Atenolol increases peripheral vascular resistance both at rest and with exercise.

Used for the management of hypertension (step 1 drug) as a single agent or concomitantly with other antihypertensive agents, especially a diuretic. Also has been used in treatment of stable angina pectoris. Available in fixed combination with chlorthalidone (Tenoretic).

ABSORPTION AND FATE. About 50% oral dose rapidly absorbed from GI tract. Peak blood levels within 2 to 4 hours after ingestion. Minimal protein binding (6 to 16%); thus plasma blood levels are relatively consistent (with about a fourfold interpatient variation). Does not readily cross blood–brain barrier. Half-life: 6 to 7 hours; longer in patients with impaired renal function. Both beta blocking and resultant antihypertensive effects persist at least 24 hours. Little or no hepatic metabolism. Approximately 40 to 50% of dose eliminated unchanged in urine; remainder excreted unchanged in feces.

CONTRAINDICATIONS AND PRECAUTIONS. Sinus bradycardia, greater than first-degree heart block, overt cardiac failure, cardiogenic shock. Safe use during pregnancy (category C), in nursing women, and in children not established. *Cautious Use:* hypertensive patients with congestive heart failure controlled by digitalis and diuretics, asthma and chronic obstructive disease (COPD), diabetes mellitus, impaired renal function, hyperthyroidism.

ADVERSE/SIDE EFFECTS. (Usually well tolerated). **CNS:** dizziness, vertigo, light-headedness, fatigue, lethargy, drowsiness, headache, vivid dreams. **CV:** bradycardia, hypotension, congestive heart failure, cold extremities, leg pains. **GI:** nausea, vomiting, diarrhea. **Ophthalmic:** dry eyes, visual disturbances. **Respiratory:** wheezing, dyspnea, bronchospasm. **Other:** rash, increase in serum triglycerides. *See also Propranolol for potential adverse/side effects.*

ROUTE AND DOSAGE. Oral: Initial: 50 mg daily alone or added to diuretic therapy. If full effect is not achieved within 1 or 2 weeks, dose should be increased to 100 mg given as single daily dose. Higher dosages unlikely to produce further benefit. Dosage adjustment necessary in patients with creatinine clearance below 35 ml/min/1.73 m².

NURSING IMPLICATIONS

If necessary, tablet may be crushed before administration and taken with fluid of patient's choice.

Check apical pulse before administration of drug, especially in patients receiving digitalis (both drugs slow AV conduction). If below 60 bpm withhold dose and consult physician.

Monitor apical pulse, blood pressure, respirations, and peripheral circulation throughout dosage adjustment period. Consult physician for acceptable parameters.

Bradycardia and severe hypotension are treated with atropine. Isoproterenol or cardiac pacemaker may be required if AV block occurs.

If patient on atenolol therapy requires hemodialysis, patient should be hospitalized because marked drop in blood pressure can occur. Atenolol, 50 mg, is given after each dialysis.

Advise patient to adhere rigidly to dose regimen. Sudden discontinuation of drug can exacerbate angina and precipitate tachycardia or myocardial infarction in patients with coronary artery disease, and thyroid storm in patients with hyperthyroidism.

Caution patient to make position changes slowly and in stages, particularly from recumbent to upright posture.

Expected therapeutic effects in patients receiving atenolol for angina include the reduction in frequency of anginal attacks and in the amount of nitroglycerin required, and increase in exercise tolerance.

As with other beta-blockers, the decision to discontinue therapy before surgery remains controversial. If atenolol is to be withdrawn, it should be done 48 hours before surgery.

If treatment is to be continued, anesthetic agents that depress the myocardium (e.g., cyclopropane, ether, trichlorethylene) must be used with extreme caution.

Store in well-closed, light-resistant container between 15° and 30°C (59° and 86°F), unless otherwise directed by manufacturer.

See also Propranolol (prototype beta-blocker) for Nursing Implications, Diagnostic Test Interferences, Drug Interactions.

Drug Interactions: Atenolol

Plus	Interactions
Atropine and other anticholinergics	Atenolol effects may be increased (anticholinergics enhance GI absorption of atenolol)
Indomethacin (Indocin)	Indomethacin decreases hypotensive effect of beta-blockers. Combination generally avoided
Lidocaine	Possibility of increased lidocaine plasma levels and toxicity. Used concurrently with caution
Prazosin (Minipress)	Hypotensive effect of first prazosin dose may be more severe and of longer duration

See also Propranolol.

ATRACURIUM BESYLATE
(Tracrium)

(a-tra-kyoor′-ee-um)
Skeletal muscle relaxant: nondepolarizing
Neuromuscular blocking agent

ACTIONS AND USES. Synthetic nondepolarizing skeletal muscle relaxant with intermediate duration of action. Pharmacologically similar to tubocurarine (qv), but 2½ times more potent. Produces shorter duration of neuromuscular blockade, exhibits minimal direct effects on cardiovascular system, and has less histamine releasing action than tubocurarine. Has minimal cumulative tendency with subsequent doses provided recovery from the drug begins before dose is repeated. Similar to vecuronium in having unique pathways of metabolism and excretion independent of renal function, but unlike vecuronium it can be given without dosage reduction to patients with hepatic disease. Inhibits neuromuscular transmission by binding competitively with acetylcholine to motor endplate receptors. Lacks analgesic action and has no apparent effect on pain threshold, consciousness or cerebration. Given in general anesthesia only after unconsciousness has been induced by other drugs.

Used as adjunct for general anesthesia to produce skeletal muscle relaxation during surgery. Especially useful for patients with severe renal or hepatic disease or limited cardiac reserve. Also used to facilitate endotracheal intubation.

ABSORPTION AND FATE. Onset of action within 2 minutes after IV administration. Maximum neuromuscular blocking action in 3 to 5 minutes. Under balanced anesthesia, recovery begins in 20 to 35 minutes and usually is 95% complete in 60 to 70 minutes (children may recover more rapidly). Recovery time not influenced by plasma pseudocholinesterase concentrations. Biphasic decline in plasma concentration: initial half-life: approximately 2 minutes; terminal half-life: approximately 20 minutes. Well-distributed to tissues and extracellular fluids; 82% protein bound. Undergoes rapid spontaneous degradation in body at physiologic pH and normal body temperature. About 70 to 90% of dose excreted in urine within 5 to 7 hours chiefly as inactive metabolites; some excretion in feces via bile. Crosses placenta. Distribution into breast milk not known.

CONTRAINDICATIONS AND PRECAUTIONS. Safe use during pregnancy (category C), breast-feeding, in children younger than 2 years not established. *Cautious Use:* history of asthma or anaphylactoid reaction; significant cardiovascular disease, neuromuscular disease (e.g., myasthenia gravis, Eaton–Lambert syndrome), carcinomatosis, electrolyte or acid–base imbalances, dehydration, impaired pulmonary function.

ADVERSE/SIDE EFFECTS. (Generally mild and most likely due to histamine release): **CV:** transient changes in heart rate and blood pressure; cardiac arrest (rare). **Respiratory:** increased bronchial secretions, bronchospasm (wheezing), cyanosis, respiratory depression. **Skin:** erythema, transient flushing, pruritus, urticaria.

ROUTE AND DOSAGE. Intravenous: Adults and children (2 years old and over): Initial: 0.4 to 0.5 mg/kg. Maintenance: 0.08 to 0.1 mg/kg, 20 to 45 minutes after initial dose, if necessary. Dosages reduced in patients endangered by histamine release and in patients who have been anesthetized with isoflurane or other potent anesthetics (approximately 20 to 33% less).

NURSING IMPLICATIONS

Administered only by qualified clinicians.

Baseline determinations of serum electrolytes, acid–base balance, and renal function are generally done as part of preanesthetic assessment.

Peripheral nerve stimulator may be used by qualified individual, to avoid risk of overdosage and to identify residual paralysis during recovery period. It is especially indicated when cautious use of atracurium is specified *(see Contraindications and Precautions).*

Personnel and equipment required for endotracheal intubation, administration of oxygen under positive pressure, artificial respiration, assisted or controlled ventilation should be immediately available.

Patient may find oral communication difficult until head and neck muscles recover from blockade effects.

For treatment of overdosage, have on hand: cholinesterase inhibitors, such as edrophonium (Tensilon), neostigmine (Prostigmin), pyridostigmine (Mestinon), to reverse neuromuscular blockade. Also have available atropine or glycopyrolate (Robinul) to counteract muscarinic side effects of cholinesterase inhibitor drugs. Monitor vital signs at least every 15 minutes until stable, then every ½ hour for the next 2 hours. Also observe airway until assured that patient has fully recovered from drug effects. Note rate, depth, and pattern of respirations. Obese patients and patients with myasthenia gravis or other neuromuscular diseases may pose ventilation problems.

Evaluate patient for recovery from neuromuscular blocking (curare-like) effect as evidenced by ability to breathe naturally or to take deep breaths and cough, keep eyes open, lift head keeping mouth closed, adequacy of hand-grip strength. Notify physician if recovery is delayed. *(See Absorption and Fate.)*

Note that recovery time may be delayed in patients with cardiovascular disease, edematous states, and in the elderly.

Incompatible with alkaline solutions (e.g., barbiturates). Reportedly compatible with 5% dextrose, 0.9% sodium chloride, and lactated Ringer's injections. To preserve potency, store solution under refrigeration, preferably at 2° to 8°C (36° to 46°F), unless otherwise directed by manufacturer. Avoid freezing.

See Tubocurarine (prototype skeletal muscle relaxant (nondepolarizing).

Drug Interactions: Atracurium

Plus	Interactions
Aminoglycoside antibiotics, clindamycin (Cleocin), lincomycin (Lincocin)	Increased neuromuscular blocking effects (respiratory depression apnea)
Diuretics (loop): bumetanide (Bumex), ethacryic acid (Edecrin), furosemide (Lasix)	Possibility of increased or decreased neuromuscular blocking effects
Thiazides	Possibility of increased neuromuscular blocking effects
Quinidine, quinine Trimethaphan (Arfonad)	Increased neuromuscular blocking effects
Succinylcholine (Anectine, Quelicin)	Increases onset and depth of atracurium action. Not administered until patient has recovered from succinylcholine-induced neuromuscular blockade
Theophylline	May cause resistance to or reversal of neuromuscular action. Possibility of cardiac arrhythmias

PROTOTYPE

ATROPINE SULFATE

(Atropisol, Buf-Opto Atropine, Dey-Dose, Isopto Atropine, S.M.P. Atropine)

(a'troe-peen)
Anticholinergic (parasympatholytic)
Antimuscarinic; antispasmodic; mydriatic

ACTIONS AND USES. Naturally occurring alkaloid and tertiary amine derived from *Atropa belladonna* (deadly nightshade). Selectively blocks all muscarinic responses (antimuscarinic action) to acetylcholine (ACh) whether excitatory or inhibitory. Forms strong drug-receptor complex at postganglionic parasympathetic neuroeffector sites in smooth muscle, cardiac muscle, and exocrine glands, thereby blocking action of ACh and antagonizes action of 5-hydroxytryptamine (serotonin) and histamine. Blocks vagal impulses to heart with resulting increased heart rate and cardiac output, and shortened PR interval. Causes vasodilation of small blood vessels usually with little effect on blood pressure. Selective depression of CNS relieves rigidity and tremor of Parkinson's syndrome. Toxic doses cause CNS stimulation, still larger doses cause CNS depression. Reduces amplitude, tone, and frequency of smooth muscle contractions in stomach, intestinal tract, ureters, and urinary bladder; effect on gallbladder and bile ducts is not consistent. Antisecretory action causes suppression of sweating, lacrimation and salivation, as well as bronchial mucus and gastric secretions. Produces mydriasis and cycloplegia by blocking responses of iris sphincter muscle and ciliary muscle of lens to cholinergic stimulation; effects occur with both systemic and local administration.

Used as adjunct in symptomatic treatment of *GI disorders,* e.g., peptic ulcer, pylorospasm, hypermotility, irritable bowel syndrome. *Ophthalmic Use:* to produce mydriasis, and cycloplegia prior to refraction and for treatment of anterior uveitis and iritis. *Preoperative Use:* to suppress salivation, perspiration, and respiratory tract secretions and for its bronchodilating effect during surgery. *Cardiac and Other Uses:* to abolish vagal reflexes in cardiac arrest and to counteract bradycardia induced by propranolol and other drugs with cholinergic effects, organophosphorous insecticides, and *Amanita* mushroom poisoning, and in selected patients with early myocardial infarction for relief of sinus bradycardia associated with hypotension and increased ventricular irritability. Also used to diagnose sinus node dysfunction and to evaluate coronary artery disease during atrial pacing. *Investigational Use:* by inhalation for prophylactic treatment of bronchospasm. Available in fixed combination with meperidine, diphenoxylate (Lomotil), phenobarbital (Antrocol), and with belladonna products (atropine, hyocyamine, scopolamine), and phenobarbital, e.g., Donnatal.

ABSORPTION AND FATE. Well absorbed from all administration sites and widely distributed in body. Peak plasma concentrations within 1 hour following oral ingestion, 30 minutes following IM injection, and 1.5 to 4 hours after inhalation. Peak increase in heart rate following IV occurs in 2 to 4 minutes. Inhibition of salivation may last up to 4 hours. Mydriatic action following topical instillation peaks in 30 to 40 minutes, and may persist 7 to 12 days; effect on accommodation may last up to 14 days or longer. Crosses blood–brain barrier. About 18% bound to plasma proteins; plasma half-life: 2 to 3 hours. Metabolized in liver. Most (77 to 94% of dose) is excreted in urine within 24 hours as unchanged drug (30 to 50%) and metabolites. Crosses placenta. Traces appear in breast milk.

CONTRAINDICATIONS AND PRECAUTIONS. Hypersensitivity to belladonna alkaloids or to any ingredients in the formulaton; synechia, angle-closure glaucoma, parotitis, obstructive uropathy, e.g., bladder neck obstruction caused by prostatic hypertrophy; intestinal atony, paralytic ileus, obstructive diseases of GI tract, severe ulcerative colitis, toxic megacolon, tachycardia secondary to cardiac insufficiency or thyrotoxicosis; acute hemorrhage, myasthenia gravis. Safe use during pregnancy (category C) and in nursing women not established. *Cautious Use:* myocardial infarction, hypotension; coronary artery disease, congestive heart failure, tachyarrythmias, gastric ulcer, GI infections, hiatal hernia with reflux esophagitis, hyperthyroidism, chronic lung disease, hepatic or renal disease, the elderly, debilitated patients, children under 6 years of age, Down's syndrome, autonomic neuropathy, spastic paralysis, brain damage in children.

ADVERSE/SIDE EFFECTS. CNS: headache, drowsiness, ataxia, dizziness, restlessness, excitement, mental depression, confusion, disorientation, insomnia, hallucinations, delirium, toxic psychosis, hyperpyrexia, respiratory depression, coma. **CV:** hypertension or hypotension, tachycardia, palpitation, angina, ectopic ventricular beats, paradoxical bradycardia, AV dissociation, ventricular or atrial fibrillation. **Dermatologic and Allergic:** flushed, dry skin; anhidrosis, skin rash (face and upper trunk), uticaria, contact dermatitis, allergic conjunctivitis, fixed-drug eruption. **GI:** dry mouth (xerostomia) with thirst, dysphagia, loss of taste; nausea, vomiting, constipation, paralytic ileus, abdominal distention. **GU:** urinary hesitancy and retention, dysuria, impotence. **Ophthalmic:** mydriasis, blurred vision, photophobia, increased intraocular pressure, cycloplegia, eye pain, edema of eyelids, eye dryness, chronic conjunctivitis (with continued use). **Other:** leukocytosis, bronchial plugging, suppression of lactation, nasal dryness or congestion.

ROUTE AND DOSAGE. Oral, subcutaneous, intramuscular, intravenous: Adults: 0.4 to 0.6 mg may be repeated every 4 to 6 hours. **Children:** 0.01 mg/kg every 4 to 6 hours generally not to exceed 0.4 mg. **Adults: Inhalation:** 0.025 mg/kg diluted with 3 to 5 ml saline, administered through nebulizer three or four times daily. **Ophthalmic:** *Uveitis:* 1 or 2 drops of 0.5 to 1% solution or small amount (0.3 to 0.5 cm) of 1% ointment into eye(s) up to three times daily. *Refraction:* 1 drop of 1% solution or small amount (0.3 to 0.5 cm) of 1% ointment into eye(s) 1 hour before refraction. **Children: Inhalation:** 0.05 mg/kg diluted in saline and administered by nebulizer three or four times daily. **Ophthalmic:** *Uveitis:* 1 or 2 drops of 0.5% solution or 0.3 cm of 0.5% ointment into eye(s) up to three times daily. *Refraction:* 1 or 2 drops of 0.5% solution or small amount of (0.3 cm) of ointment in eye(s) two times daily for 1 to 3 days prior to exam and before refraction (solution instilled 1 hour before; usually longer for ointment, to avoid effect on corneal transparency).

NURSING IMPLICATIONS

Oral atropine is usually given 30 minutes before meals and at bedtime.

Smaller doses of atropine are indicated for the elderly because of the possibility of atropine-induced tachycardia, mydriasis, and increased intraocular pressure in this glaucoma-prone age group. Intraocular pressure should be determined before atropine is prescribed.

Monitor vital signs. Pulse is a sensitive indicator of patient's response to atropine. Be alert to changes in quality and rate of pulse and respiration and changes in blood pressure and temperature.

Initial paradoxic bradycardia following IV atropine usually lasts only 1 to 2 minutes. It is most likely to occur when IV is administered very slowly or when small doses (less than 0.5 mg) are used. Following parenteral administration, postural hypotension may occur if the patient ambulates too soon.

Atropine may contribute to the problem of urinary retention. On initiation of therapy, establish a baseline of 24-hour urinary output, and monitor daily output thereafter; especially important in older patients and in patients who have had surgery. Have patient void before giving atropine.

If constipation is a problem, check for abdominal distention and auscultate for bowel sounds. (Symptoms of *paralytic ileus* include abdominal distention, constipation, absent bowel sounds usually associated with nausea, vomiting, and epigastric pain.)

Increased fluid intake and increased bulk in the diet may help to overcome constipating effects of atropine.

The following measures may help to relieve dry mouth: small, frequent mouth rinses with tepid water; meticulous mouth and dental care; gum chewing or sucking hard, sour candy (sugarless); humidification of air; use of saliva substitute, e.g., Xero-Lube, Moi-stir, Orex (all available OTC). Avoid overuse of commercial mouthwashes because of the possibility of changing the normal oral flora. Additionally, most contain alcohol which enhances drying. Reduction of dosage may be necessary.

The elderly patient is especially prone to develop "atropine fever" (hyperpyrexia due to suppression of perspiration and heat loss) lending to the risk of heatstroke. Warn patient to avoid excessive heat. *Heatstroke* is a medical emergency. Initial symptoms may include dizziness, weakness, headache, sudden loss of consciousness, hot, red *dry* skin. Treatment consists of rapid cooling (temperatures sometimes rise above 41°C (106°F) by wetting skin with tap water and fanning (evaporative cooling), and ice packs to neck, axillae, groin, and abdomen.

Intraocular tension should be determined before and during therapy with ophthalmic preparations. Note that ophthalmic solutions and ointments are available in various strengths.

Suggested technique for administering eye drops: Wash hands. Have patient tilt head back and look up. Depress lower lid by applying pressure with index finger over bony prominence below lid. Apply gentle pressure to inner canthus (lacrimal duct) with middle finger. Instill medication into lower conjunctival sac. Once drug is introduced, direct patient to keep lids closed without squeezing, while gentle pressure is maintained on inner canthus, for 1 minute. This method obstructs drug flow to nasal mucosa and thus helps to prevent systemic absorption.

Instruct patient to prepare for impaired visual acuity of several days duration *(see Absorption and Fate)* and to protect eyes by wearing dark glasses during drug action period.

Caution patient that in addition to causing sensitivity to light and blurring of near vision, atropine will temporarily impair ability to judge distance. Advise patient to avoid driving and other activities requiring visual acuity while vision is affected.

Ophthalmic preparations should be discontinued if eye pain, conjunctivitis, palpitation, rapid pulse, or dizziness occurs. Report symptoms promply to physician.

Frequent and continued use of eye preparations, as well as overdosage, can produce systemic effects of atropine. Studies reveal that over one-half of atropine deaths have resulted from systemic absorption following ocular administration and have been in infants and children.

Ointment dosage form is preferred by some clinicians for use in children because it is less likely to be absorbed systemically than solution formulations.

Onset of mydriatic action may be slower and duration longer in persons with dark eyes.

Infants and children with spastic paralysis, brain damage, or Down's syndrome, and blonde, blue-eyed individuals appear to be highly sensitive to the effects of atropine.

Patients receiving atropine via inhalation sometimes manifest mild CNS stimulation with doses in excess of 5 mg and mental depression and other mental disturbances with larger doses.

Treatment of overdosage: If swallowed, remove drug from stomach by gastric lavage or emesis. Have available antidote physostigmine *(Antilirium)*, diazepam (Valium) to control CNS stimulation, oxygen, measures to treat respiratory depression and hyperpyrexia.

Protected in light-resistant containers at room temperature, preferably between 15° and 30°C (59° and 86°F) unless otherwise directed by manufacturer.

Diagnostic Test Interferences. **Upper GI series** findings may require qualification because of anticholinergic effects of atropine (reduced gastric motility).

Drug Interactions: Atropine (and other anticholinergic drugs)

Plus	Interactions
Amantadine (Symmetrel)	Enhanced anticholinergic effects (especially with high doses)
Antidepressants; tricyclics	Additive anticholinergic effects
Levodopa (Dopar, Larodopa)	Decreased levodopa effect; (delayed gastric emptying by anticholinergic drugs increases gastric degradation of levodopa). Used concurrently with caution
Methotrimeprazine (Levoprome)	Possibility of precipitating extrapyramidal symptoms. Used concurrently with caution
MAO inhibitors	Action of anticholinergic drugs may be potentiated
Nitrofurantoin (Furadantin)	Increased nitrofurantoin effect (decreased GI motility by anticholinergics results in increased nitrofurantoin absorption)
Phenothiazines	Decreased antipsychotic effect of phenothiazines. (Anticholinergics may reduce GI absorption of phenothiazines.) Used concurrently with caution

---

ATTAPULGITE, ACTIVATED

(Kaopectate tablets, Rheaban)

(a-ta pull'gyte)
Antidiarrheal

ACTIONS AND USES. Inert clay composed primarily of hydrous magnesium aluminum silicate. Claimed to be superior to kaolin as an absorbent and adsorbent.

Used for relief of acute diarrhea. Available in combination with pectin (Diar-Aid, Polymagma Plain), and with pectin and belladonna alkaloids (Diarkote).

ABSORPTION AND FATE. Not absorbed from GI tract.

CONTRAINDICATIONS AND PRECAUTIONS. Use for more than 2 days, or in presence of high fever; use of tablet form in children under 6 years; use of liquid form for children under 3 years, unless directed by a physician; use for diarrhea associated with pseudomembranous colitis or bacterial toxins.

ROUTE AND DOSAGE. Oral: *Liquid:* **Adults:** 2 Tbsp after initial bowel movement (BM) and 1 Tbsp after subsequent BMs. **Children (6 to 12 years):** 1 Tbsp after initial BM and ½ Tbsp after each subsequent BM; **Children (3 to 6 years):** ½ Tbsp after initial and after each subsequent BM. *Tablets:* **Adults:** 2 tablets after initial and after each subsequent BM. **Children (6 to 12 years):** 1 tablet after initial and after each subsequent BM.

NURSING IMPLICATIONS

Prolonged use may interfere with intestinal absorption of nutrients and may cause constipation.

Replacement of fluids and electrolytes is a part of diarrhea therapy.

Advise patient to report to physician if diarrhea persists for more than 2 days.

Attapulgite is a common ingredient of several commercially available antidiarrheal mixtures.

See Diphenoxylate for patient teaching.

PROTOTYPE

AUROTHIOGLUCOSE

(Gold thioglucose, Solganal)

(aur-oh-thye-oh-gloo'kose)
Gold compound
Antirheumatic, antiinflammatory

ACTIONS AND USES. Slow-acting preparation of approximately 50% gold. Available commercially as a suspension in anhydrous vegetable oils to delay absorption and prolong action. Major effect is suppression of joint inflammation in early arthritic disease; has no effect on separative process, but may significantly slow or arrest progression of the disease. Mechanism of antiinflammatory action not clearly understood. Gold uptake by macrophages with subsequent inhibition of phagocytosis and lysosomal enzyme activity may be a principle mechanism. Other proposed mechanisms include altered immune response and inhibition of prostaglandin synthesis.

Used in treatment of adult and juvenile active rheumatoid arthritis. Also has been used in psoriatic arthritis, and investigationally for pemphigus. Generally used as addition to basic conservative management with nonsteroidal antiinflammatory drugs (NSAIDs) such as aspirin. (Use of gold in treatment of disease is called aurotherapy or **chrysotherapy.**)

ABSORPTION AND FATE. Slowly and irregularly absorbed from IM injection site. Widely distributed in body, especially to synovial fluid, eyes, skin, bone marrow, reticuloendothelial system (liver, spleen), kidneys. Does not cross blood–brain barrier. Peak blood levels in 2 to 6 hours. About 95% bound to plasma proteins. Half-life: 3 to 27 days for 50 mg dose (varies with dose and duration of therapy). Metabolism unknown. Eliminated slowly; 85% of each dose is retained for at least 1 week. Almost 60 to 90% of dose ultimately excreted in urine and 10 to 40% in feces. (May be found in urine for more than 1 year following a course of therapy.) Crosses placenta; appears in breast milk.

CONTRAINDICATIONS AND PRECAUTIONS. Gold allergy or severe toxicity from previous therapy with gold or other heavy metals; severely debilitated patients, uncontrolled diabetes mellitus; renal or hepatic insufficiency, history of infectious hepatitis; congestive heart failure, tuberculosis, abnormalities of hematopoietic system, severe anemia, hemorrhagic conditions; disseminated lupus erythematosus, recent radiation therapy, colitis, urticaria, eczema, history of exfoliative dermatitis. Safe use during pregnancy (category C), in nursing women, and in children under 6 years not established. *Cautious Use:* elderly patients, history of drug allergies, history of blood dyscrasias, history of renal or hepatic disease, marked hypertension, compromised cerebral or cardiovascular circulation.

ADVERSE/SIDE EFFECTS. **Dermatologic:** (common): pruritus, erythema, "gold dermatitis," fixed-drug eruptions, exfoliative dermatitis with alopecia and shedding of nails; Stevens-Johnson syndrome, gray to blue pigmentation (chrysiasis), photosensitivity. *Mucous membranes:* ulcerative stomatitis, glossitis or gingivitis (may be preceded by metallic taste), pharyngitis, tracheitis, gastritis, colitis, vaginitis. **GI:** nausea, vomiting, abdominal cramps, anorexia, diarrhea, ulcerative enterocolitis, **Hematologic:** (rare): agranulocytosis, thrombocytopenia with or without purpura, leukopenia, eosinophilia, panmyelopathy, hemorrhagic diathesis, aplastic and hypoplastic anemia. **Hypersensitivity:** vasomotor (nitritoid) reaction: flushing, fainting, dizziness, sweating, malaise, weakness; anaphylactic shock, syncope, bradycardia, thickening of tongue, dysphagia, dyspnea, angioneurotic edema (face, lips, eyelids). **Ophthalmic:** conjunctivitis, iritis, corneal ulcer, gold deposits in eye. **Renal:** nephrotic syndrome with proteinuria, hematuria. **Respiratory:** dyspnea, gold bronchitis, interstitial pneumonitis, pulmonary fibrosis. **Other:** peripheral neuritis, headache, hepatitis, cholestatic jaundice, acute yellow atrophy of liver, EEG abnormalities, encephalitis, immunologic destruction of synovial fluid; arthralgia, myalgia (rare), fever.

ROUTE AND DOSAGE. **Intramuscular (only):** **Adults:** 10 mg first week; 25 mg second and third weeks; then 50 mg every week thereafter to cumulative dose of 800 mg to 1 Gm. If no improvement, therapy is discontinued. If patients shows improvement without adverse reactions, dosage is reduced to 50 mg every 2 weeks for four doses, then every 3 weeks for four doses, and finally 25 to 50 mg every 3 to 4 weeks for indefinite period. **Children (6 to 12 years):** One-fourth of adult dose. Alternatively, 1 mg/kg weekly for 20 weeks, then same dose at 2- to 4-week intervals as long as patient benefits from therapy. Single doses not to exceed 25 mg.

NURSING IMPLICATIONS

Before initiation of treatment, patient should be well-informed regarding dangers associated with gold therapy and requirements for compliance in receiving scheduled doses, for keeping laboratory appointments, and for prompt reporting of adverse effects. Minor or moderate transient toxicity occurs in 25 to 50% of patients, and serious toxicity in about 10% of patients.

Hold vial horizontally and shake thoroughly to assure uniform suspension. Heating vial to body temperature (by placing in a warm water bath) facilitates withdrawal. Aurothioglucose must not be injected intravenously. Needle and syringe must be dry.

Administer drug deep into upper outer quadrant of gluteal muscle. An 18- or 20-gauge, 1½-inch needle is recommended (for obese patients a 2-inch needle may be preferable). During early therapy some patients complain of arthralgia for 1 or 2 days postinjection.

Patient should remain recumbent for 10 minutes after injection to overcome possible nitritoid reaction (manufacturer's recommendation although reaction occurs infrequently). Observe patient for about 30 minutes after injection for anaphylactic shock, bradycardia, edema of tongue, face, eyelids, difficulty in breathing or swallowing.

Clinical observation and interview remain the most effective means for regulating dosage, and for predicting therapeutic effectiveness and gold toxicity. Provide patient with a list of possible adverse reactions that should be reported. If therapy is interrupted at the onset of gold toxicity, serious reactions can be avoided. Note that elderly patients are particularly sensitive to the effects of gold therapy.

Interview and examine patient before each injection to detect signs and symptoms suggestive of *gold toxicity.* Beginning toxicity generally involves skin and mucous membranes: pruritus, skin eruptions, erythema, metallic taste (frequently precedes mouth ulceration); sore mouth or tongue, cankers, sore throat, gray-blue discoloration of skin or mucous membranes, indigestion, abdominal cramps, diarrhea, jaundice. Use tongue blade and flashlight to examine mouth and throat. The onset of itching or any skin eruption, metallic taste or sore mouth should be looked upon with suspicion of gold reaction. A rapid improvement in joint pain and mobility also may indicate that patient is approaching toxic tissue levels.

Reactions are most likely to occur during second and third months of therapy, but they may appear at any time during therapy and for several weeks after treatment has been discontinued.

During first few months of therapy a urinalysis (for protein and blood), Hct, total and differential WBC, and platelet count should be done prior to each injection. Serum IgA (immunoglobulin) levels have been used also to predict gold toxicity. Thereafter these values are determined every 1 or 2 weeks throughout therapy.

Platelet counts below 100,000/mm^3 or leukocytes below 4000/mm^3, eosinophils over 5%, and presence of proteinuria or hematuria are all indications to discontinue therapy pending further studies.

Instruct patient to report any unusual color or odor to urine, or change in intake and output ratio and pattern.

Advise patient to report early signs of infection that may indicate onset of agranulocytosis (unusual fatigue or weakness, malaise, chills, fever, sore throat), and unusual bleeding (possible signs of thrombocytopenia): bleeding gums, nosebleeds, dark urine (hematuria), petechiae, easy bruising. Thrombocytopenia can occur abruptly or gradually and it can appear several months after gold therapy has been terminated.

Be alert to vulnerability of patient to secondary infection because of the possible immunosuppressive effect of gold. Caution patient to avoid contact with persons who have colds or other communicable diseases.

Therapeutic effectiveness may not be apparent before 6 to 8 weeks of gold therapy. There is little agreement regarding how long to continue therapy following a remission. Some rheumatologists prefer to continue patient indefinitely on gold treatment; others discontinue drug after a year of therapy.

Collaborate with physical therapist in providing adjunctive measures that may help to maintain or improve joint function and prevent deformities.

Record subjective and objective evidence of therapeutic effectiveness: reduction in pain, stiffness, and swelling of affected joints; improved mobility; improved grip strength; reduction of sedimentation rate.

Inform patient that the necessity to increase the amount of aspirin for analgesia is a significant indication of diminishing response to gold therapy, and therefore should be reported to physician.

Treatment of toxicity: antihistamines and systemic corticosteroids, e.g., prednisone, may be prescribed for rash and mucous membrane ulcerations. Gray-blue pigmentation (**chrysiasis**) of mucous membranes and light-exposed skin areas may be treated with Lugol's solution (strong iodine solution); advise patient to avoid sunlight. Severe toxic reactions are treated with dimercaprol (BAL), a chelating agent.

Gold therapy is contraindicated following a severe reaction, but may be attempted at reduced initial dosage schedule and careful monitoring after a mild reaction.

Symptomatic treatment of stomatitis: Use a soft tooth brush (may be softened with hot water) or finger covered with moistened cotton or moistened gauze (rub gently), to clean teeth after meals; floss gently with waxed dental floss once daily. Rinse mouth frequently with warm water, tea, or saline (if allowed). Some clinicians prefer occasional use of hydrogen peroxide (H_2O_2) diluted with normal saline or water 1:1 to 1:4; prepare solution immediately before use. Have patient rinse mouth with clear water or normal saline after using H_2O_2 and avoid overuse (can cause gum sponginess and decalcification of tooth surfaces). Other agents that might provide relief of discomfort include solutions of Mylanta or milk of magnesia. Avoid overuse of commercial mouth washes especially those that are bactericidal. Many contain alcohol which enhances drying and irritation and can change mouth flora. Advise patient to avoid concentrated fruit juices, hard or dry foods, smoking, and alcohol.

Stored in light-resistant containers at room temperature, preferably between 15° and 30°C (59° and 86°F) unless otherwise directed by manufacturer. Protect from freezing and light.

Diagnostic Test Interferences. Low **PBI** (by chloric acid method); test interference may persist for several weeks after gold therapy is discontinued.

Drug Interactions: Aurothioglucose

Plus	Interactions
Antimalarials Cytotoxic agents Immunosuppressants Oxyphenbutazone Phenylbutazone	Possibility of increased risk of blood dyscrasias. Concurrent use generally avoided

AZATADINE MALEATE
(Optimine)

(a-za'ta-deen)
Antihistamine
H_1-receptor antagonist

ACTIONS AND USES. Long-acting antihistamine acts by competitively antagonizing the effects of histamine at H_1-receptor sites on smooth muscle of blood vessels, bronchioles, and GI tract. This action blocks or reduces intensity of allergic responses and cell tissue injury associated with histamine release. In common with other antihistamines, has anticholinergic and sedative actions. Also reported to have antiserotonin activity.

Used for symptomatic relief of hay fever (seasonal allergic rhinitis), perennial (or nonseasonal) allergic rhinitis, and chronic urticaria. Available in fixed combination with pseudoephedrine (Trinalin).

ABSORPTION AND FATE. Readily absorbed from GI tract. Plasma levels peak in about 4 hours. Probably crosses blood–brain barrier since it causes CNS effects. Minimally bound to plasma proteins. Half-life: 9 to 12 hours. About 50% of dose excreted in urine within 5 days, 20% as unchanged drug. Appears to cross placenta. Distribution into breast milk not known.

CONTRAINDICATIONS AND PRECAUTIONS. Hypersensitivity to other H_1-receptor antagonists; MAO inhibitor therapy, lower respiratory tract disease including asthma. Safe use during pregnancy (category B), in nursing women, and in children under age 12 not established. *Cautious Use:* increased intraocular pressure, narrow-angle glaucoma, pyloroduodenal obstruction, stenosing peptic ulcer, prostatic hypertrophy, bladder neck obstruction; history of bronchial asthma, hyperthyroidism, hypertension, cardiovascular disease; patients with convulsive disorders.

ADVERSE/SIDE EFFECTS. CNS: drowsiness (common); dizziness, disturbed coordination, fatigue, confusion, paresthesias, neuritis; excitation, nervousness, euphoria. CNS stimulation: restlessness, hysteria, insomnia, tremor, irritability, convulsions. **CV:** hypotension, palpitation, tachycardia, extrasystoles. **ENT:** nasal stuffiness; dryness of nose, mouth and throat; tinnitus, labyrinthitis (vertigo). **GI:** epigastric distress, nausea, vomiting, anorexia, diarrhea or constipation. **GU:** urinary frequency, dysuria, urinary retention, early menses. **Hematologic** (rare): hemolytic anemia, thrombocytopenia, agranulocytosis. **Hypersensitivity:** urticaria, rash, photosensitivity, anaphylactic shock. **Ophthalmic:** blurred vision, diplopia, dilated pupils. **Respiratory:** thickening of bronchial secretions, chest tightness and wheezing. **Other:** excessive perspiration, chills, headache.

ROUTE AND DOSAGE. Oral: 1 or 2 mg twice a day, usually in the morning and evening.

NURSING IMPLICATIONS

GI side effects may be minimized by administering drug with food or milk.

Because drug commonly causes drowsiness, sedation, and dizziness, caution patient not to drive a car or engage in other potentially hazardous activities until reaction to drug is known.

Azatadine is most likely to cause sedation, dizziness, hypotension, and confusion in the elderly. Advise patient to report these effects. Reduction in dosage may be indicated.

Patient should be informed that azatadine may produce additive CNS depression with alcohol and other CNS depressants (e.g., sedatives, anxiolytics, sleep medications).

Dry mouth (xerostomia) may be relieved by the following measures: (1) frequent rinses with tepid water. Preferred to commercial mouth washes, overuse of which can change oral flora, also many contain alcohol which enhances drying; (2) increase fluid intake (if allowed) or at least maintain normal intake; (3) brush with soft tooth brush after every meal; (4) floss teeth daily with waxed floss or ribbon; (5) sugarless gum or sugarless lemon drops; (4) use of artificial saliva, e.g., Xero-Lube, Moi-Stir, Orex.

Treatment of overdosage is symptomatic and supportive. Vomiting is induced by ipecac syrup. Following emesis, activated charcoal slurry and if necessary gastric lavage is given. Have on hand vasopressors, short-acting barbiturates, diazepam (Valium) or paraldehyde, and equipment for respiratory assistance.

Stored in tightly closed container at room temperature, preferably between 2° and 30°C (36° and 86°F), unless otherwise directed by manufacturer.

Diagnostic Test Interferences. As a general rule, H_1-receptor antagonists are discontinued about 4 days before **skin testing** procedures are to be performed since they may produce false-negative results.

Drug Interactions: Azatadine

Plus	Interactions
Alcohol (Ethanol) and other CNS depressants	Possibility of additive CNS depression
Anticoagulants, oral	Action may be reduced by azatadine
MAO inhibitors	May prolong and intensify anticholinergic effects of azatadine
Tricyclic antidepressants	Possibility of additive CNS and anticholinergic effects

AZATHIOPRINE
(Imuran)

(ay-za-thye'oh-preen)
Immunosuppressant

ACTIONS AND USES. Imidazolyl derivative of mercaptopurine (6-mercaptopurine) to which it is metabolized in body. Precise mechanism of action not determined. Antagonizes purine metabolism and appears to inhibit DNA, RNA, and normal protein synthesis in rapidly growing cells. Suppresses T-cell effects before transplant rejection, i.e., during induction phase of antibody response.

Used as adjunctive agent to prevent rejection of kidney allografts, usually with other immunosuppressants. Also used in selective patients with severe, active rheumatoid arthritis (as specified by American Rheumatism Association); unresponsive to conventional therapy. *Investigational Use:* in patients with myasthenia gravis refractory to other therapy, and in treatment of systemic lupus erythematosus, Crohn's disease, polymyositis, idiopathic thrombocytopenia, and other systemic inflammatory and autoimmune diseases.

ABSORPTION AND FATE. Readily absorbed following oral or IV administration. Well distributed throughout body. Metabolized primarily by xanthine oxidase in liver to active metabolite mercaptopurine. About 30% bound to plasma proteins. Approximately 50% of dose eliminated in urine within 24 hours; small amount excreted as unchanged azathioprine and mercaptopurine. Half-life of active metabolite and azathioprine approximately 3 hours. Crosses placenta.

CONTRAINDICATIONS AND PRECAUTIONS. Hypersensitivity to drug; clinically active infection, anuria, pancreatitis, patients receiving alkylating agents (increased risk of neoplasms). Safe use during pregnancy and in women of childbearing potential not established. *Cautious Use:* impaired kidney and liver function, patients receiving cadaveric kidney.

ADVERSE/SIDE EFFECTS. GI: nausea, vomiting, anorexia, ulcerations of lips and mouth, esophagitis, diarrhea, steatorrhea. **Hematologic** (bone marrow depression): leukopenia, acute leukemia, macrocytic anemia, aplastic anemia, agranulocytosis, pancytopenia, thrombocytopenia. **Hepatotoxicity** with elevations in bilirubin, alkaline phosphatase, SGOT, SGPT; biliary stasis. **Hypersensitivity:** skin eruptions, formication (sensation of crawling ants), serum sickness, polyarthritis, polyneuritis, allergic hepatitis, interstitial pneumonitis. **Other:** secondary infection (immunosuppression); acute pancreatitis, dysphagia, dysarthria, alopecia, muscle wasting (negative nitrogen balance), drug fever, Raynaud's phenomenon, pulmonary edema, arthralgia retinopathy. Carcinogenic and teratogenic potential reported.

ROUTE AND DOSAGE. Highly individualized on basis of clinical response and hematopoietic toxicity. **Oral, intravenous** (azathioprine sodium): **Renal allotransplantation:** Initial: 3 to 5 mg/kg body weight daily; maintenance 1 to 2 mg/kg/day. *Rheumatoid arthritis:* **Oral:** Initial: 1 mg/kg/day. If response is not satisfactory after 6 to 8 weeks, dosage increased by 0.5 mg/kg/day, and again at 4-week intervals as necessary to maximum 2.5 mg/kg/day.

NURSING IMPLICATIONS

Gastric disturbances may be minimized by administering oral drug in divided doses (prescribed), or with or immediately after meals.

Azathioprine sodium for IV injection is reconstituted by adding 10 ml sterile water for injection into vial. Swirl vial until drug is dissolved. Stable for 24 hours at room temperature. For IV infusion, reconstituted solution may be further diluted with sodium chloride injection or 5% dextrose in sodium chloride injection.

Azathioprine therapy is usually instituted 1 to 5 days before kidney transplantation and restarted within 24 hours posttransplantation.

Azathioprine carries warning that chronic immunosuppression may increase risk of neoplasia and hematologic toxicity, and that it has mutagenic potential in both men and women.

Close medical supervision both in and out of hospital is necessary during therapy. The patient should understand toxicity potential, as well as expected benefits. Clinical effects of azathioprine appear within 2 to 4 days of administration.

Complete blood counts, including platelets, and liver and kidney function tests should be performed prior to and at least weekly during first month of therapy, twice monthly during second and third months, and monthly, or more frequently if indicated, thereafter.

Kidney function is monitored to prevent drug accumulation (urine protein, urine electrolytes, creatinine clearance, serum creatinine, BUN).

Surveillance of intake and output ratio is crucial. Up to a twofold increase in toxicity is possible in anephric or anuric patients. Note color, character, and specific gravity of urine. Report an abrupt decrease in urinary output or any change in intake and output ratio.

Azathioprine has a high toxic potential. Because it may have delayed action, dosage should be reduced or drug withdrawn at the first indication of a decreasing leukocyte or platelet count to avoid irreversible bone marrow depression.

Thrombocytopenia occurs less commonly than leukopenia; however, be alert to signs of abnormal bleeding (easy bruising, bleeding gums, petechiae, purpura, melena, epistaxis, hemoptysis, hematemesis).

If *hepatic dysfunction* develops (pruritus, abdominal pain, and distention, clay-colored stools, dark urine, yellow skin, and sclera) report promptly.

Intercurrent infection is a constant hazard of immunosuppressive therapy. Monitor vital signs. Warn patient to avoid contact with persons who have colds or other infections and to report signs of impending infection (coryza, fever, chills, sore throat, malaise) which are also possible symptoms of agranulocytosis. Personal hygiene should be scrupulous. Azathioprine dosage may be reduced until the infection is controlled by appropriate therapy.

Hospitalized patient may be on reverse isolation for protection. Explain significance to patient and family.

Therapeutic effectiveness in patients with rheumatoid arthritis usually occurs in 6 to 8 weeks of therapy (improvement in morning stiffness and grip strength). If no improvement has occurred after 12-week trial period, drug should be discontinued.

Monitoring should continue in patients who respond to the drug and gradual dosage reduction to lowest effective level attempted at some point during therapy.

Patients should be advised to practice birth control during azathioprine therapy and for 4 months after discontinuation.

Patient should be informed that vaccinations or other immunity conferring agents may cause unusually severe reactions because of the immunosuppressive effects of azathioprine.

Preserved in tightly closed, light-resistant containers at room temperature, preferably between 15° and 30°C (59° and 86°F), unless otherwise directed by manufacturer.

Diagnostic Test Interferences. Azathioprine may decrease plasma and urinary **uric acid** in patients with gout.

Drug Interactions: Azothioprine

Plus	Interactions
Allopurinol (Zyloprim)	Increased pharmacologic effect and toxicity of azothioprine (inhibition of xanthine oxidase by allopurinol interferes with degradation of active metabolite [mercaptopurine] to inactive products). Dosage of azothioprine should be reduced by one-third to one fourth
Anticoagulants, oral	Possibility of reduced anticoagulant effect
Tubocurarine, and other nondepolarizing skeletal relaxants	Neuromuscular blocking effect may be reversed or inhibited by azathioprine

AZLOCILLIN

(Azlin)

(az-loe-sill'in)

Antiinfective, antibiotic (beta lactam)

Penicillin

ACTIONS AND USES. Semisynthetic, extended spectrum, bactericidal acylureidopenicillin. Antibacterial spectrum similar to that of mezlocillin (Mezlin); but azlocillin is more active against *Pseudomonas aeruginosa* and less active against *Klebsiella.* Believed to act by interfering with bacterial cell wall synthesis. Effective against *Streptococcus faecalis* and most other gram-positive cocci (but not penicillinase-producing strains of *Staphylococci*), certain gram-negative bacilli, particularly *Pseudomonas aeruginosa,* and other species of *Pseudomonas, Escherichia coli, Hemophilus influenzae, Proteus mirabilis, Bacteroides fragilis,* and other anaerobes. Susceptible to inactivation by beta-lactamases produced by Enterobacteriaceae. Sodium content: 2.17 mEq/Gm (49.8 mg).

Used primarily for treatment of serious infections caused by *Pseudomonas aeruginosa* in lower respiratory tract, urinary tract, skin and skin structures, bone and joints, and for bacterial septicemia. Most often used concurrently with an aminoglycoside, e.g., amikacin (Amikin), gentamicin (Garamycin), tobramycin (Nebcin), for synergistic effects against *Pseudomonas* strains. Also used with cephalosporins, e.g., cefotaxime (Claform) to treat life-threatening infections.

ABSORPTION AND FATE. Following IV administration, distributed in active form to bile, serum, urine, bronchial and wound secretions, bone, and other tissues. Poor CSF penetration unless meninges are inflamed. Bile levels approximately 15 times higher than serum levels. Elimination half-life: 55 to 70 minutes (longer with impaired renal function); 25 to 45% protein bound. Less than 10% metabolized by liver. About 50 to 70% of dose eliminated unchanged in urine within 24 hours; 20 to 25% excreted unchanged in bile. Crosses placenta. Low concentrations in breast milk.

CONTRAINDICATIONS AND PRECAUTIONS. Hypersensitivity to any of the penicillins or cephalosporins; common bile duct obstruction. Safe use during pregnancy (category B) and in neonates not established. *Cautious Use:* impaired renal or hepatic function, history of drug allergy or hypersensitivity to multiple allergens; nursing mothers, history of bleeding disorders, GI disease; patients on restricted sodium intake, hypokalemia and other electrolyte imbalances, dehydration.

ADVERSE/SIDE EFFECTS. CNS: headache, dizziness; overdosage: neuromuscular hyperirritability, convulsive seizures. **GI:** disturbances of taste and smell, stomatitis, flatulence, nausea, vomiting, diarrhea, epigastric pain. **Hematologic:** eosinophilia, leukopenia, neutropenia, thrombocytopenia; decreased: Hgb and Hct, and serum uric acid; prolonged prothrombin and bleeding times, hypokalemia; increased: serum alkaline phosphatases, LDH, bilirubin, creatinine, BUN, SGPT (ALT), and SGOT (AST); hypernatremia. **Hypersensitivity:** rash, pruritus, urticaria, arthralgia, myalgia, drug fever, chills, chest discomfort, anaphylactic reactions. **Other:** superinfections, transient chest discomfort with rapid IV injection: pain and thrombophlebitis at IV site.

ROUTE AND DOSAGE. Intravenous (direct slow IV injection or intermittent IV infusion): **Adults:** 3 to 4 Gm every 4 to 6 hours; up to 24 Gm/day. Recommendations for patients with impaired renal function: (1) creatinine clearance (Ccr) less than 30 ml/min: usual recommended dosage; (2) Ccr of 10 to 30 ml/min: 2 Gm every 8 hours; (3) Ccr less than 10 ml/min: 3 Gm every 12 hours. **Children:** (acute pulmonary exacerbations of cystic fibrosis) 75 mg/kg infused over 30 minutes, every 4 hours. Not to exceed 24 Gm/daily.

NURSING IMPLICATIONS

Culture and susceptibility tests should be performed before initiation of drug therapy and periodically thereafter to detect possible emergence of bacterial resistance. Treatment may begin pending test results.

Azlocillin is administered either by direct slow IV injection over 5 minutes or longer, or by IV infusion over 30 minutes. Rapid IV injection can cause transient chest pains.

A careful drug history should be obtained before initiation of therapy to determine patient's previous exposure and sensitivity to penicillin, cephalosporin, and other allergens.

When other antibiotics are prescribed concomitantly with azlocillin, it is advisable to administer each drug separately because mutual inactivation may occur when mixed together.

Baseline and periodic evaluation of renal, hepatic, and hematopoietic functions, and serum electrolytes, especially K and Na, is advisable during prolonged therapy.

Monitor intake and output ratio and pattern, particularly in patients with impaired renal function. Serum drug and creatinine levels and creatinine clearance are recommended to determine appropriate dosages.

Although rare, azlocillin can cause abnormalities in coagulation tests (thrombocytopenia), particularly in patients with renal impairment. Check values of clotting time, platelet aggregation, prothrombin, and partial prothrombin times. Instruct patient to report any unexplained bleeding or bruising (hematomas, petechiae, ecchymoses).

Superinfections occur commonly during prolonged use of extended spectrum antibiotics. Be alert to symptoms and report their onset immediately to physician, e.g., fever, cough, sore mouth or throat (oral thrush), vaginitis, diarrhea.

For treatment of anaphylactoid reactions, have on hand epinephrine, IV steroids, oxygen, equipment for intubation and for maintaining airway.

Therapy is generally continued for at least 2 days after signs and symptoms have disappeared. Usual duration of therapy is 10 to 14 days, but may be longer in complicated infections.

For direct IV injection: Each gram of azlocillin should be reconstituted with at least 10 ml of sterile water, 5% dextrose or 0.9% sodium chloride injection. Shake vigorously until dissolved. To minimize venous irritations, drug concentration should not exceed 10%. Resulting solution may be administered by direct IV injection or into IV tubing over 5 minutes or more.

For intermittent IV infusion: Initial dilution (see above) should be diluted further with suitable diluent (sterile water, 0.9% sodium chloride, 5% dextrose in 0.225% sodium chloride, 5% dextrose in 0.45% sodium chloride for injection, lactated Ringer's injection) to desired volume (50 to 100 ml) and administered over 30-minute period.

If Y-type or "piggyback" method of administration is used, infusion of any other solution should be temporarily discontinued during administration of azlocillin.

Reconstituted solutions should be clear, colorless to pale yellow, and free of particulate matter. Solutions are stable at room temperature for 24 hours (potency loss less than 10%) in suitable diluents (see above). Concentrations up to 100 mg/ml are stable for 24 hours when refrigerated below 8°C (46.4°F).

Prior to reconstitution, store vial containing azlocillin below 30°C (86°F), unless otherwise directed by manufacturer.

Diagnostic Test Interferences. Transient lowering of **serum uric acid** levels. False-positive **urinary protein** reactions (pseudoproteinuria) with many methods; bromphenol blue (multi-stix) method reportedly reliable. **Platelet abnormalities** may persist for as long as 2 weeks following drug discontinuation.

Drug Interactions: Azlocillin

Plus	Interactions
Aminoglycosides	Synergistic effect; however, physiochemical inactivation can occur depending on contact time. Scheduling 1 hour apart may help
Anticoagulants, oral	Increased risk of bleeding (by platelet function impairment)
Chloramphenicol (Chloromycetin), Erythromycins, Sulfonamides, Tetracyclines	Possibility of azlocillin antagonism. Concurrent use generally avoided
Contraceptives, oral	Effectiveness of oral contraceptives may be reduced because of increased (unsubstantiated report) estrogen metabolism
Probenecid	Increased azlocillin serum levels and half-life (by decreasing renal tubular secretion of azlocillin)

B

BACAMPICILLIN HYDROCHLORIDE
(Spectrobid)

(ba-kam-pi-sill′in)
Antiinfective, antibiotic (beta lactam)
Penicillin

ACTIONS AND USES. Acid-stable, penicillinase-sensitive semisynthetic ester of ampicillin (qv) to which it is rapidly hydrolyzed in body. Has broad spectrum of antimicrobial activity and exerts antibacterial action by inhibiting bacterial cell wall biosynthesis. More rapidly and completely absorbed from GI tract than ampicillin, and incidence of diarrhea is claimed to be less. Significant disadvantage to its use is its high cost.

Used for treatment of infections caused by susceptible microorganisms of upper and lower respiratory tract, urinary tract, skin and skin structures.

ABSORPTION AND FATE. Rapidly absorbed from GI tract. Diffuses to most body tissues and fluids. About 20% protein bound. Approximately 75% eliminated in urine as active ampicillin within 8 hours of administration. Excreted in breast milk. Effective serum levels sustained when administered every 12 hours.

B

CONTRAINDICATIONS AND PRECAUTIONS. Hypersensitivity to penicillins, cephalosporins, and other allergens; history of asthma, hay fever, or urticaria; pregnancy (category B); mononucleosis, coadministration with disulfiram (Antabuse); children under 25 kg. *Cautious Use:* nursing mothers. *See also Ampicillin.*

ADVERSE/SIDE EFFECTS. Epigastric distress, diarrhea, hypersensitivity reactions, ampicillin rash, fixed drug eruption, superinfections. *See also Ampicillin.*

ROUTE AND DOSAGE. Oral: Adults and children weighing 25 kg or more: *mild to moderate infections:* 400 mg every 12 hours. *Severe infections:* 800 mg every 12 hours. *Acute gonorrhea:* 1.6 Gm and probenecid 1 Gm as single dose. Larger doses may be required for severe infections.

NURSING IMPLICATIONS

Because food does not retard absorption of bacampicillin, it may be administered without regard to food or meals.

Careful inquiry should be made before initiation of therapy concerning previous hypersensitivity reactions to penicillins, cephalosporins, and other allergens.

Prior to therapy, culture and susceptibility tests should be performed; however, therapy may be started pending results. Baseline and periodic checks of renal, hepatic, and hematopoietic systems are advised during prolonged therapy, particularly in patients with history of impaired function of these systems, and in prematures and neonates.

Instruct patient to report symptoms of an allergic reaction immediately (rash, fever, chills).

Emphasize need to take medication for the full course of therapy as prescribed.

For most infections, therapy should be continued for 48 to 72 hours beyond time that patient is asymptomatic or that bacteriologic eradication is achieved. Therapy for hemolytic streptococcal infections should be continued for at least 10 days to reduce risk of glomerulonephritis or acute rheumatic fever.

Stubborn infections may require several months of clinical and/or bacteriologic follow-up after therapy has stopped. Urge patient to keep follow-up appointments.

See also Ampicillin.

BACITRACIN

(Baciguent, Baciguent Ophthalmic, Bacitin, Bacitracin Ophthalmic)

(bass-i-tray′sin)
Antiinfective, antibiotic

ACTIONS AND USES. Antibiotic derived from cultures of *Bacillus subtilis.* Precise mechanism of action not known; appears to interfere with function of bacterial cell membrane by suppressing cell wall and protein synthesis. Spectrum of antibacterial activity similar to that of penicillin. Bactericidal against many gram-positive organisms including streptococci, staphylococci, pneumococci, corynebacteria, and clostridia. Also active against gonococci and meningococci; ineffective against most other gram-negative organisms. Has neuromuscular blocking action.

Used for treatment of infections due to susceptible organisms. Parenteral therapy restricted to infants with staphylococcal pneumonia and empyema due to susceptible organisms where adequate laboratory facilities and constant supervision are available. Used topically in treatment of superficial infections of skin and eye. Commercially available in fixed combination with neomycin and polymyxin B, e.g., Cortisporin, Mycitracin, Neosporin, Triple Antibiotic ointment.

ABSORPTION AND FATE. Poorly absorbed from intact or denuded skin or mucous membranes. Rapidly and completely absorbed following IM administration. Maximal bactericidal plasma concentrations in 1 to 2 hours, with duration of action 6 to 8 hours. Widely distributed in body and in ascitic and pleural fluids. Only traces in CSF unless meninges are inflamed. Minimally bound to plasma proteins. Slow renal excretion; 10 to 40% of single dose excreted within 24 hours.

CONTRAINDICATIONS AND PRECAUTIONS. Previous hypersensitivity to bacitracin or to any ingredient in the formulation; toxic reaction or renal dysfunction associated with bacitracin; impaired renal function; pregnancy. *Cautious Use:* myasthenia gravis or other neuromuscular disease. Patients sensitive to neomycin may be sensitive to bacitracin.

ADVERSE/SIDE EFFECTS. GI: anorexia, nausea, vomiting, diarrhea, rectal itching and burning, peculiar taste sensations. **Hypersensitivity:** urticaria, pruritus, burning sensation, erythema, skin rashes, anaphylaxis: tightness of chest, wheezing, dyspnea, swelling of lips and face hypotension cardiac arrest. **Nephrotoxicity** (dose related): frequent urination, oliguria, anuria, albuminuria, cylinduria, hematuria, increased blood urea nitrogen (BUN), uremia, renal tubular and glomerular necrosis. **Ophthalmic:** delayed corneal healing. **Other:** pain and inflammation at injection site, fever, superinfection, neuromuscular weakness with respiratory depression; tinnitus.

ROUTE AND DOSAGE. Intramuscular: Infants under 2.5 kg: not to exceed 900 U/kg/24 hours in two or three divided doses; **Infants over 2.5 kg:** not to exceed 1000 U/kg/24 hours in two or three divided doses. **Topical:** ointment (500 U/Gm) applied in thin layer to cleansed area two or three times a day, or as solution containing 250 to 1000 U/ml applied as wet dressing. **Ophthalmic:** ointment (500 U/Gm): Apply small amount in conjunctival sac several times a day.

NURSING IMPLICATIONS

Before systemic therapy is begun, determinations should be made of BUN and nonprotein nitrogen (NPN), and urine should be examined for albumin, casts, and cellular elements. Renal function should be monitored daily throughout therapy.

Culture and susceptibility tests should be performed initially and periodically during therapy, as indicated.

Bacitracin should not be reconstituted with diluents containing parabens because solution may precipitate or become cloudy.

Parenteral solution (for IM use only) should be dissolved in sodium chloride injection containing 2% procaine hydrochloride (prescribed). Alternate injection sites since injections are painful.

Administration of parenteral bacitracin for longer than 12 days not advised.

Monitor intake and output during parenteral therapy. Adequate urinary output should be maintained to reduce possibility of renal toxicity. If fluid intake is inadequate and/or urinary output decreases, report to physician.

To reduce renal irritation, urine should be kept at pH 6 or higher by systemic alkalinization with sodium bicarbonate or other alkali (prescribed).

Inspect urine for turbidity and hematuria, and be on the alert for other signs and symptoms of urinary tract dysfunction. Note and report any changes in urination pattern, e.g., oliguria, urinary frequency, nocturia.

As with other antibiotics, prolonged use of bacitracin may result in overgrowth of nonsusceptible organisms, especially *Candida albicans*. *See Index: Nursing Interventions: Superinfections.*

B

Instruct patient taking ophthalmic preparation to stop drug and notify physician if signs of hypersensitivity appear: itching, burning, swelling of eyelids.

Be alert to signs of local allergic manifestations (itching, burning, redness) in patients receiving topical applications. Local reactions have preceded life-threatening anaphylactic episodes.

Consult physician for guidelines for cleansing skin before reapplications of topical bacitracin.

Intramuscular bacitracin solution is stable for 1 week if refrigerated; inactivation occurs at room temperature. Dry bacitracin should be stored in refrigerator at 2° to 8°C (36° to 46°F); topical ointments should be stored in tightly closed containers at 15° to 30°C (59° to 86°F), unless otherwise directed by manufacturer.

Drug Interactions: Bacitracin (parenteral)

Plus	Interactions
Aminoglycoside antibiotics, Polymyxins	Possibility of additive nephrotoxic effects and neuromuscular blocking action. Concurrent use generally avoided
Tubocurarine and other nondepolaring skeletal muscle relaxants	Possibility of additive and prolonged neuromuscular blocking action with resulting respiratory depression. Used concurrently with caution, and only when necessary

BACLOFEN

(Lioresal, Lioresa DS)

(bak'loe-fen)
Skeletal muscle relaxant

ACTIONS AND USES. Centrally acting skeletal muscle relaxant. Depresses polysynaptic afferent reflex activity at spinal cord level thereby reducing skeletal muscle spasm caused by upper motor neuron lesions. Relaxes external sphincter of the hyperreflexic urinary bladder and appears to have an anticholinergic-like effect on involuntary bladder contractions.

Used to provide symptomatic relief of painful spasms in multiple sclerosis and in the management of detrusor sphincter dyssynergia in spinal cord injury or disease. *Investigational Use:* to reduce choreiform movements in patients with Huntington's chorea, to reduce rigidity in patients with parkinsonian syndrome, and to reduce spasticity in patients with cerebrovascular stroke, pneumatic disorders, or cerebral palsy.

ABSORPTION AND FATE. Rapidly absorbed from GI tract and widely distributed in body. Absorption thought to be dose-dependent; reduced absorption occurs at high dosage levels. Wide individual variations in extent of absorption and elimination. Peak serum levels appear in 2 to 3 hours; significant levels persist about 8 hours. Approximately 30% protein bound. Half-life: 3 to 4 hours. About 15% of dose metabolized in liver. Primarily eliminated in urine within 72 hours, mostly as unchanged drug (70 to 85%); remainder excreted in feces. Crosses placenta.

CONTRAINDICATIONS AND PRECAUTIONS. Hypersensitivity to baclofen. Safe use during pregnancy, in nursing mothers, and in children under 12 years not established. *Cautious Use:* impaired renal and hepatic function, epilepsy, diabetes mellitus, patients with psychiatric or brain disorders, peptic ulcer.

ADVERSE/SIDE EFFECTS. Allergic (uncommon): pruritus, skin eruptions. **CV:** hypotension (asymptomatic); rarely: dyspnea, palpitation, chest pain, fainting (syncope). **EENT:** tinnitus, nasal congestion, blurred vision, mydriasis, nystagmus, diplopia, strabismus, miosis. **GI:** nausea, vomiting, constipation or diarrhea, abdominal pain, dry mouth, taste disorders, anorexia, positive test for occult blood. **GU:** urinary frequency; rarely: enuresis; urinary retention, dysuria, nocturia, hematuria; inability to ejaculate, impotence. **Neuropsychiatric:** most common: transient drowsiness, vertigo, dizziness, weakness, fatigue; ataxia, headache, confusion, insomnia; rarely: paresthesias, tremors, dysarthria (slurred speech), muscle pain and rigidity, hypotonia, euphoria, excitement, depression, hallucinations, loss of seizure control in epileptic patients; respiratory depression, seizures, coma (overdosage). **Other:** ankle edema, weight gain, excessive perspiration.

ROUTE AND DOSAGE. Oral: 5 mg three times a day; increased by 5 mg per dose every 3 days until optimum response obtained. Total daily dosage not to exceed 80 mg.

NURSING IMPLICATIONS

If patient complains of GI distress, drug may be administered with food.

Supervise ambulation. In common with other skeletal muscle relaxants, initially, the loss of spasticity induced by baclofen may affect patient's ability to stand or walk. (In some patients, spasticity associated with multiple sclerosis and spinal cord disease helps patient to maintain upright posture and balance.)

Advise patient to report adverse reactions to physician. Most can be reduced by decreasing dosage. Incidence of CNS symptoms (drowsiness, dizziness, ataxia) reportedly high in patients over 40 years of age. Dose increases should be made with caution.

Caution patient that CNS depressant effects of baclofen will be additive to other CNS depressants, including alcohol.

Patients with epilepsy should be closely monitored by EEG, clinical observation and interview at regular intervals for possible loss of seizure control.

Inform diabetic patients that baclofen may raise blood glucose levels. Urge patient to report promptly changes in urine or blood tests to the physician. Dose adjustment of insulin may be indicated during and after baclofen treatment is stopped for a short period.

Warn patient to avoid driving and other potentially hazardous activities until the reaction to baclofen is determined.

Observe for and record patient's response to drug. Therapeutic effectiveness may be noted in a few hours to weeks by: decrease in frequency of spasms and in severity of knee and ankle clonus, increase in ease and range of joint motion and in performance of activities of daily living. If therapeutic effectiveness is not observed within a reasonable trial period (1 to 2 months), drug should be withdrawn.

Caution patient not to self-dose with OTC drugs without physician's approval.

The elderly are especially sensitive to this drug. Observe carefully for side effects: mental confusion, depression, hallucinations.

Inform patient that drug withdrawal should be accomplished gradually over a 1- to 2-week period. Abrupt withdrawal following prolonged administration may cause anxiety, agitated behavior, auditory and visual hallucinations, severe tachycardia, and acute exacerbation of spasticity.

Treatment of overdosage: If patient is alert, emesis is induced, followed by gastric lavage. If patient is obtunded: maintain adequate respiratory exchanges, without use of respiratory stimulants, and maintain high urinary output. Dialysis may be indicated in renal failure.

Store at room temperature, preferably between 15° and 30°C (59° and 86°F) in tightly closed container, unless otherwise directed by manufacturer.

Diagnostic Test Interferences. Possibility of increased **blood glucose,** serum **alkaline phosphatase,** and **SGOT** (AST) levels.

B

Drug Interactions: Baclofen

Plus	Interactions
CNS depressants, e.g., alcohol, antihistamines, general anesthetics, tricyclic antidepressants, barbiturates and other sedatives, and skeletal muscle relaxants	Additive CNS depression

BECLOMETHASONE DIPROPRIONATE

(Beclovent, Beconase, Vancenase, Vanceril)

(be-kloe-meth'a-sone)
Corticosteroid

ACTIONS AND USES. Synthetic corticosteroid with potent antiinflammatory activity. When applied topically (by oral and nasal inhalation) about 10 to 15% dose reaches mucous membranes of the bronchioles and bronchi; the remainder deposits in the oropharynx to be swallowed. Due to metabolic inactivation by first-pass metabolism, beclomethasone produces little or no glucocorticoid action usually associated with oral and parenteral corticosteroids. Action mechanism on lung tissue unknown, but its effect is to suppress signs and symptoms of bronchial asthma in patients not responding to bronchodilators or nonsteroid treatment. Unlike hydrocortisone (qv), this corticosteroid does not suppress the hypothalamus–pituitary–adrenal function.

Used to treat chronic steroid-dependent bronchial asthma adjunctively with other therapy (sympathomimetics, xanthines), and for treatment of seasonal and perennial rhinitis. Beclomethasone is prophylactic and fails to provide immediate benefit in acute asthma. Has been used for symptomatic treatment of nasal polyposis.

ABSORPTION AND FATE. Systemic absorption occurs promptly following inhalation. Rapidly metabolized in lung and GI tissues, and in liver; 87% bound to plasma protein. Half-life of inhaled dose: first phase, 3 hours; second phase, about 15 hours. Drug and its metabolites are excreted principally in feces (over 90%); remainder excreted in urine. Possibly crosses placenta, and secreted in breast milk.

CONTRAINDICATIONS AND PRECAUTIONS. Hypersensitivity to beclomethasone or to any ingredient in the formulation, e.g., oleic acid, fluorocarbons, asthma adequately controlled by bronchodilators or nonsteroidal medication; nonasthmatic bronchitis, primary treatment of status asthmaticus, acute attack of asthma, bronchopulmonary mycoses, or other untreated infections of mouth, throat or lungs. Safe use during pregnancy (category C), in the nursing mother, in women of childbearing potential and in children younger than 6 years not established. *Cautious Use:* patients receiving systemic corticosteroids; nasal septal ulcers, nasal trauma, or surgery. *See also Hydrocortisone.*

ADVERSE/SIDE EFFECTS. Candidal infection of oropharynx and occasionally larynx especially with oral inhalation (75% of patients, especially females); unmasking of previously suppressed allergic conditions; hoarseness, dry mouth, sore throat, sore mouth; rarely, bronchospasm; rash. With use of nasal inhaler: epistaxis, bloody mucus, nasopharyngeal itching, dryness, crusting, and ulceration; transient irritation, burning, sneezing. *See also Hydrocortisone.*

ROUTE AND DOSAGE. Oral inhalation: Adults: (approximately 42 mcg per metered spray): 2 inhalations three or four times daily. *Severe asthma:* start with 12 to 16 inhalations/day;

adjust dosage downward according to response. Not to exceed 20 inhalations daily. **Children (6 to 12 years):** 1 or 2 inhalations three or four times daily. *Transfer of patient from systemic corticosteroid to beclomethasone:* Initially given concurrently with usual maintenance dosage of systemic corticosteroid. After 1 week, begin gradual withdrawal: reduce daily or alternate daily dose by decrements not to exceed 2.5 mg prednisone or equivalent. **Intranasal: Adults and children (over 12 years):** (about 42 mcg per metered spray): 1 spray in each nostril two to four times daily, or two sprays in each nostril twice daily.

NURSING IMPLICATIONS

Instructions for inhaler use are included with package. Review information with patient to assure complete understanding.

If patient is also receiving bronchodilators by inhalation (isoproterenol, metaproterenol, epinephrine, etc.), bronchodilator should be used several minutes before beclomethasone aerosol to enhance penetration of the steroid into the bronchial tree and to reduce the potential toxicity of fluorocarbon propellants.

Improvement in pulmonary function may require as long as 3 weeks when beclomethasone is given to patient not receiving systemic steroids.

Rinsing mouth and gargling with warm water after each inhalation removes residual medication thereby preventing further drug absorption. Mouth care may also delay or prevent onset of oral dryness, hoarseness, and candidiasis.

Oral membranes should be inspected frequently for indications of candida infection (white patches, red, sore membranes) and patient should be questioned about symptoms, e.g., cough, sore mouth or throat. If present, antifungal therapy (e.g., Nystatin) will be instituted.

Warn patient not to use higher than recommended doses or regular doses at shorter intervals. If response is not adequate, notify physician.

Clean inhaler daily: remove cap and nosepiece from canister, rinse with warm water, and dry thoroughly.

When patient dependent on systemic steroids is transferred to beclomethasone, management may be troublesome because recovery from suppressed adrenal function may require as long as 12 months.

Monitor blood pressure and weight during withdrawal–transfer period. Hypotension and weight loss (signs of adrenal insufficiency) indicate need for temporary boost in systemic steroid and slower withdrawal schedule.

During period of steroid withdrawal, symptoms of adrenal insufficiency (joint and/or muscular pain, depression, lassitude, fatigue, weakness, dizziness, light-headedness [hypotension]) may occur in spite of maintenance and even improvement of respiratory function.

During transfer from systemic steroid therapy to aerosol administration, conditions previously suppressed (rhinitis, conjunctivitis, eczema) may be unmasked. Instruct patient to report to physician promptly.

Caution patient/significant other to report to the physician if stress (e.g., infection, trauma, surgery, gastroenteritis, emotional crisis) or a severe asthma attack occurs during transfer period. Supplemental treatment with large doses of systemic steroid will be required.

Patient should have a reserve supply of oral corticosteroid and be instructed to use it during time of extreme stress or a severe asthma attack.

Patient should carry a card indicating need for supplementary systemic steroid during a severe asthma attack or periods of stress.

Long-term effects of beclomethasone have not been determined. Specifically, local effects of drug deposits on oropharyngeal membranes and lung tissue as well as long-term systemic effects, are unknown.

B

When symptoms for which beclomethasone was prescribed are relieved, dosage should be reduced gradually to lowest effective level. Keep physician informed.
Urge patient to keep follow-up appointments. Periodic evaluation of therapy is essential.
Store inhaler and aerosol dispenser out of reach of children.
Keep inhaler away from open flame or heat above 120°F (may cause bursting). Do not puncture container and do not discard into fire or incinerator.
Store between 15° and 30°C (59° and 86°F), unless otherwise directed by manufacturer.
See Hydrocortisone, prototype corticosteroid.

BELLADONNA EXTRACT
BELLADONNA TINCTURE

(bell-a-don'a)
Anticholinergic (parasympatholytic), antispasmodic
Belladonna alkaloid

ACTIONS AND USES. Prepared from *Atropa belladonna* (deadly nightshade). Belladonna extract contains 12.5 mg of belladonna alkaloids per Gm, and the tincture contains 0.3 mg/ml. Shares same actions, precautions, and adverse reactions as other tertiary amine antimuscarinics; *see Atropine.*

Used as adjunct to suppress gastric secretions in gastric and duodenal ulcers, and to inhibit spasms and motility in spastic or irritable colon, mucous colitis, diarrhea, diverticulitis, and pancreatitis. Also has been used for dysmenorrhea, nocturnal enuresis, spasms of urinary tract, nausea and vomiting of pregnancy, vertigo, and for symptomatic relief of parkinsonism. Belladonna extract is available in fixed combination with phenobarbital, e.g., Belap, Chardonna-2, Pheno-Bella; with butabarbital (Butibel); and with amobarbital (Amobell). Bellafoline is a proprietary mixture of levorotatory belladonna alkaloids.

CONTRAINDICATIONS AND PRECAUTIONS. Obstructive uropathy, atony of urinary bladder, esophageal reflux, obstructive disease of GI tract, severe ulcerative colitis, toxic megacolon, myasthenia gravis, narrow-angle glaucoma, cardiovascular disease. *See also Atropine.*

ADVERSE/SIDE EFFECTS. Dry mouth, choking sensation, mydriasis, blurred vision, acute glaucoma, urinary hesitancy or retention (especially older males), constipation, headache, drowsiness, excitement/palpitation, mental confusion, tachycardia. *See also Atropine.*

ROUTE AND DOSAGE. Oral: *Belladonna Extract:* **Adult:** 15 mg three or four times a day. *Belladonna Tincture:* **Adult:** 0.6 to 1 ml three or four times a day. **Children:** 0.1 ml/kg/day (or 2.5 ml/m^2/day) in three or four divided doses. Not to exceed 3.5 ml daily.

NURSING IMPLICATIONS

When given for GI problems, usually administered 30 to 60 minutes before meals and at bedtime.
If patient is receiving antacid therapy, the antacid is given after meals. Space antacid at least 1 hour apart from belladonna preparations.
Dosage should be reduced if flushing or other signs of toxicity appear.
Because of the possibility of heat intolerance, caution patient to avoid hot baths, saunas, strenuous work or exercise during hot and humid weather.
Advise patient to refrain from driving and other potentially hazardous activities until reaction to drug is determined.

If mouth dryness is a problem instruct patient to practice meticulous oral hygiene. Sugarless gum or lemon drops may help. *See Atropine.*
Store preferably at 15° to 30°C (59° to 86°F) in tightly covered, light-resistant containers, unless otherwise directed by manufacturer.
See also Atropine.

BENDROFLUMETHIAZIDE

(Naturetin)

(ben-droe-floo-meth-eye'a-zide)
Diuretic
Thiazide

ACTIONS AND USES. Benzothiadazine (thiazide) derivative. Similar to chlorothiazide (qv) in pharmacologic actions, uses, contraindications, precautions, adverse effects, and interactions. Reportedly does not alter serum electrolyte concentrations appreciably at recommended doses. Bendroflumethiazide is available in fixed combination with nadolol (Corzide); with potassium chloride (Naturetin with K); with rauwolfia serpentina (Rautrax, Rauzide), and with potassium chloride and rauwolfia serpentina (Rautrax-N).

ABSORPTION AND FATE. Onset of diuretic effect in 1 to 2 hours; peaks between 6 to 12 hours and lasts 18 to 24 hours. Highly protein bound. Excreted unchanged in urine within 24 hours. *See Chlorothiazide.*

CONTRAINDICATIONS AND PRECAUTIONS. Anuria, hypersensitivity to thiazides, sulfonamides; pregnancy, lactation. *Cautious Use:* history of allergy, renal and hepatic disease, gout, diabetes mellitus, sympathectomy. *See also Chlorothiazide.*

ADVERSE/SIDE EFFECTS. Xerostomia, sialadenitis, anorexia, unusual fatigue, paresthesias, photosensitivity, vasculitis, orthostatic hypotension, agranulocytosis, electrolyte imbalance, hyperglycemia, impaired glucose tolerance, hyperuricemia, exacerbation of gout, SLE. *See also Chlorothiazide.*

ROUTE AND DOSAGE. **Oral: Adult:** *Antidiuretic* (in diabetes insipidus) *or diuretic:* Initial: 2.5 to 10 mg one to two times daily, once every other day, or once daily for 3 to 5 days/week; maintenance: 2.5 to 5 mg daily, once every other day or once daily for 3 to 5 days/week. *Antihypertensive:* Initial: 5 to 20 mg/day as single dose or in two divided doses; maintenance: 2.5 to 15 mg/day as single dose or in two divided doses. **Pediatric:** *Diuretic:* Initial: 0.1 to 0.4 mg/kg daily as single dose or in two divided doses; maintenance: 0.05 to 0.1 mg/kg in one or two doses. *Antihypertensive:* 0.05 to 0.4 mg/kg as single dose or in 2 divided doses.

NURSING IMPLICATIONS

Diuretic action lasts more than 18 hours permitting longer intervals between doses and therefore fewer problems with electrolyte balance.
Administer drug early in AM after eating (to reduce gastric irritation) to prevent possibility of interrupted sleep because of diuresis. If 2 doses are ordered, administer second dose no later than 3 PM.
Antihypertensive effects may be noted in 3 to 4 days; maximal effects may require 3 to 4 weeks.
Monitor blood pressure, intake and output ratio and pattern, and weight particularly during

B

first phase of antihypertensive therapy. Report a sudden fall in BP which may initiate severe postural hypotension and potentially dangerous perfusion problems of the extremities, especially in older patients.

Older patients may be sensitive to average doses. Orthostatic hypotension and hypokalemia may be the most distressing side effects.

Monitor patient for hypokalemia: dry mouth, anorexia, thirst, paresthesias, muscle cramps, cardiac arrhythmias. Report promptly. Physician may change dose and institute supplement therapy.

Hypokalemia is rarely severe in most patients even on long-term therapy with thiazides. To prevent onset, urge patient to eat a normal diet (usually includes K-rich foods such as fruit juices, potatoes, cereals, skim milk) and to include a banana (about 370 mg K) and at least 6 ounces orange juice (about 330 mg K) every day.

If hypokalemia develops, dietary K supplement of 1000 to 2000 mg (25 to 50 mEq) is usually an adequate treatment.

Dietary management is important in thiazide treatment for hypertension. The physician will specifically order the goal of diet, i.e., electrolyte, weight, or fluid control. Collaborate with dietitian and arrange for patient-dietitian planning for an individualized diet.

Asymptomatic hyperuricemia can be produced because of interference with uric acid excretion although thiazides rarely precipitate acute gout. Report onset of joint pain and limitation of motion. Patient with history of gout may be continued on a thiazide with adjusted dosage of uricosuric agent.

The prediabetic or diabetes mellitus patient should be watched carefully for loss of control of diabetes or early signs of hyperglycemia: drowsiness; flushed, dry skin; fruitlike breath odor, polyuria, anorexia, polydipsia. These symptoms are slow to develop and to recognize. Notify physician, and question need to adjust insulin dosage.

Counsel patient to avoid use of OTC drugs unless approved by physician. Many preparations contain both potassium and sodium and if misused, or if patient overdoses, could induce electrolyte side effects.

Notify the anesthetist that patient is on thiazide therapy.

Tablets contain tartrazine, which can cause an allergic reaction (including bronchial asthma) in susceptible persons. Frequently such individuals are also sensitive to aspirin.

Store tablets in tightly closed container, preferably at 15° to 30°C (59° to 86°F), unless otherwise specified by the manufacturer.

See Chlorothiazide (prototype thiazide diuretic).

Drug Interactions: Bendroflumethiazide

Plus	Interactions
Cholestyramine (Questran) Colestipol (Colestid)	Pharmacologic effects of thiazide may be reduced. Separate administration as far apart as possible
Diazoxide (Hyperstat)	Additive pharmacologic effects of both drugs. Monitor for hyperglycemia, hyperuricemia, hypotension
Digitalis glycosides	Thiazide induced hypokalemia can sensitize myocardium to digitalis toxicity. Monitor serum potassium
Lithium	Possibility of lithium toxicity (renal lithium excretion reduced). Monitor serum lithium levels
Tolbutamide and other sulfonylureas	Decreased hypoglycemic effects. Higher sulfonylurea doses may be necessary

See Chlorothiazide for other possible interactions.

BENOXINATE HYDROCHLORIDE WITH FLUORESCEIN SODIUM

(Fluress)

(ben-ox'i-nate)
Anesthetic (local)

ACTIONS AND USES. Benzoic acid ester chemically related to procaine combined with the disclosing agent fluorescein. Exerts surface anesthesia of short duration and has slight bacteriostatic properties. Instillation into eye does not change size of pupil, reaction to light, or accommodation. Reportedly, prolonged use does not produce local or systemic toxicity.

Used for its short-acting local anesthetic effect in minor ophthalmologic procedures such as tonometry, gonioscopy, or removal of foreign bodies from cornea or for short operative procedures on cornea or conjunctiva.

CONTRAINDICATIONS AND PRECAUTIONS. Hypersensitivity to local anesthetics or their components. *Cautious Use:* patients with known allergies, cardiac disease, hyperthyroidism, open lesions.

ADVERSE/SIDE EFFECTS. Occasionally: slight pain, temporary stinging, and burning immediately after instillation; conjunctival erythema. Rarely: allergic corneal reaction. Prolonged use: corneal opacity with vision loss, delayed corneal healing.

ROUTE AND DOSAGE. Topical instillation: 0.4% ophthalmic solution. *For tonometry and other minor procedures:* 1 or 2 drops in single instillations prior to procedure. *Deep ophthalmic anesthesia:* (benoxinate hydrochloride solution 0.4%) 2 drops into each eye at 90-second intervals for 3 instillations.

NURSING IMPLICATIONS

One drop instilled into conjuntival sac allows tonometry, gonioscopy or removal of foreign body within 60 seconds.

Three instillations of the benoxinate 0.4% solution at 90-second intervals produce sufficient anesthesia for short corneal and conjunctival procedures.

Protective eye patch is recommended following procedure to prevent drying and injury to corneal epithelium from loss of blink reflex.

Corneal reflex is fully restored in about 1 hour.

Caution patient to avoid touching eyes while protective reflexes are blocked.

BENTIROMIDE

(Chymex)

(ben-teer'-oh-mide)
Diagnostic agent

ACTIONS AND USES. Synthetic peptide containing PABA (para-aminobenzoic acid). Each 500 mg of bentiromide contains 170 mg of PABA. Use in evaluating exocrine pancreatic function is based on chymotrypin metabolism of bentiromide in small intestine and its ultimate absorption and elimination as PABA. Percentage of PABA metabolites (arylamines) recovered in urine reflects the enzymatic activity of chymotrypsin and thus provides an indirect measure of pancreatic function. Compared with other pancreatic tests, the bentiromide test is practical, noninvasive, and reportedly reliable.

Used as screening test in diagnosis of exocrine pancreatic insufficiency, and to monitor adequacy of pancreatic enzyme replacement therapy in patients with insufficiency. A modification of the bentiromide test utilizes a tracer dose of PABA labeled with radioactive carbon (^{14}C) concomitantly with bentiromide.

B

ABSORPTION AND FATE. Following oral administration, rapidly hydrolyzed in small intestine to free PABA. Peak plasma concentration in 2 to 3 hours. PABA is readily absorbed through intestinal mucosa and is partially metabolized in liver. About 40 to 45% of dose excreted in urine within 6 hours, principally as conjugated arylamines (PABA metabolites). Urinary excretion of PABA may be reduced in patients with impaired renal function. Distribution to brain, placenta, and breast milk not known.

CONTRAINDICATIONS AND PRECAUTIONS. History of hypersensitivity to bentiromide or PABA, or to ingredients in formulation, e.g., propylene glycol. Safe use during pregnancy (category B), in nursing mothers, and in children under 6 years not established.

ADVERSE/SIDE EFFECTS. (Low incidence and usually transient) **CNS:** headache, drowsiness, light-headedness. **GI:** diarrhea, flatulence, nausea, vomiting, abdominal pain, heartburn. **Hypersensitivity** (rare): acute respiratory distress, stridor. **Other:** elevations in liver function tests, weakness.

ROUTE AND DOSAGE. Oral: **Adults and children (12 years and older):** 500 mg in a single dose. **Children (under 12 years):** 14 mg/kg.

NURSING IMPLICATIONS

Bentiromide test (for exocrine pancreatic function) demands minute attention to detail for accuracy.

Careful instructions should be given to patient and responsible family member(s) regarding foods and drugs that should be omitted prior to the test *(see Food–Drug Interaction, following, and Drug Interactions).*

Food–Drug Interaction. Foods containing *arylamines* (e.g., apples, cranberries, plums, prunes) may interfere with bentiromide test results. These foods should be avoided for at least 3 days before drug is administered.

Diabetic patients may require insulin dosage adjustments while being tested because a period of fasting is required.

Following completion of test, patient should remain under observation to detect any evidence of hypersensitivity.

General directions for administering test (see package insert for details):

- Fast after midnight before test is performed.
- Urinate immediately before taking drug.
- Bentiromide is taken as a single dose, followed by 250 ml of water.
- To promote diuresis, take another 250 ml of water 2 hours later, and an additional 500 ml of water during the following 4 hours.
- All urine should be collected into a single container for exactly 6 hours after taking drug.
- Measure total urine volume after 6 hours and record. Retain 10 ml sample for analysis. Store urine specimen in cool place, preferably in refrigerator, to retard microbial growth.
- Patient may eat after 6 hours of urine collection.

Urine specimen is analyzed in laboratory for arylamines by modification of Bratton–Marshall test. A negative test suggests pancreatic exocrine insufficiency. Because test results are regarded as presumptive, confirmation by other pancreatic tests is essential.

If a second test is necessary, a 7-day interval should be allowed to avoid possibility of test interference.

False-positive test results may occur in patients with impaired renal or hepatic function, gastric stasis, impaired intestinal mucosa, malabsorption syndromes, and in patients re-

ceiving drugs metabolized to primary arylamines *(see Drug Interactions),* or arylamine-containing foods. *See Food–Drug Interaction.*
Store bentiromide at room temperature, preferably between 15° and 30°C (59° and 86°F), unless otherwise directed by manufacturer.

Diagnostic Test Interferences. Falsely elevated **bentiromide test** results can occur with PABA-containing drugs, or drugs that are metabolized to primary arylamines *(see Drug Interactions),* and foods containing arylamines *(see Food–Drug Interaction).*

Drug Interactions: Bentiromide

Plus	Interactions
Drugs that are metabolized to primary arylamines: Acetaminophen Benzocaine Lidocaine Procaine Procainamide PABA-containing drugs, e.g., selected multiple vitamins, sunscreens Sulfonamide diuretics (e.g., bumetanide (Bumex), furosemide (Lasix)) Thiazide diuretics	Falsely elevated bentiromide test results. These drugs should be discontinued 3 days prior to bentiromide administration
Pancreatic enzyme supplements, e.g., pancreatin, pancrelipase	Concurrent administration can cause false-negative bentiromide test results. In adults, these enzymes should be discontinued at least 5 days before administration of bentiromide, and 1 day in children with cystic fibrosis
Methotrexate (Mexate)	Possibility of increased methotrexate plasma levels (displacement of methotrexate from protein binding sites). Used with caution

---

BENZALKONIUM CHLORIDE

(Benza, Benzalchlor-50, Dermo-Sterol, Germicin, Mercurochrome II, Nonsul Jelly, Sabol, Zephiran)

(benz-al-koe'nee-um)
Antiinfective, topical

ACTIONS AND USES. Quaternary ammonium cationic surfactant with low surface tension and detergent, keratolytic, wetting, and emulsifying actions. Bactericidal or bacteriostatic action (depending on concentration), probably due to enzyme inactivation. Effective against bacteria, some fungi (including yeasts) and certain protozoa, e.g., *Trichomonas vaginalis.* Generally not effective against spore-forming organisms.

Used for antisepsis of intact skin, mucous membranes, superficial injuries, and infected wounds; also for irrigations of the eye and body cavities and for vaginal douching. A component of several contact lens wetting and cushioning solutions, and a preservative for ophthalmic solutions.

CONTRAINDICATIONS AND PRECAUTIONS. History of allergy to benzalkonium chloride in occlusive dressings, casts, and anal or vaginal packs. *Cautious Use:* irrigation of body cavities.

ADVERSE/SIDE EFFECTS. (Few or no toxic effects in recommended dilutions) Erythema, local burning, hypersensitivity (rarely). Systemic absorption: nausea, vomiting, muscle weakness, apprehension, confusion, dyspnea, respiratory paralysis, coma.

ROUTE AND DOSAGE. **Topical:** Minor wounds, preoperative skin preparation, cold sterilization: 1:750 aqueous solutions; deep infected wounds: 1:3000 to 1:20,000 aqueous solution; denuded skin and mucous membranes, eye irrigations: 1:5000 to 1:10,000 aqueous solution; vaginal douche, irrigation: 1:2000 to 1:5000 aqueous solution; bladder and urethral irrigation: 1:5000 to 1:20,000 aqueous solution; wet dressings: 1:5000 or less aqueous solution. **Vaginal instillation** (gel): Instill once daily at bedtime for 24 days. Resume treatment during last 3 days of the menstrual period and for 2 days following menses for three or more menstrual cycles.

NURSING IMPLICATIONS

Cationic detergent action is antagonized by pus and other organic matter, and by anionic compounds such as soaps and soap substitutes (e.g., pHisoHex, pHisoderm). If these agents have been used, rinse skin thoroughly with water, dry, and then apply benzalkonium.

Other potentially incompatible substances with benzalkonium chloride solutions: aluminum, caramel, citrates, fluorescein, iodine, kaolin, lanolin, nitrates, peroxide, pine oil, potassium permanganate, sulfonamide solutions, silver nitrate, zinc oxide, zinc sulfate, yellow oxide of mercury.

Patient-Teaching Points for Use of Vaginal Jelly: (1) Insert high in vagina with applicator provided. (2) Advise patient to avoid douches containing soap or soap substitutes; physician may prescribe a cleansing acidic douche (usually 1 tablespoon of white vinegar per quart of water). (3) Notify physician if burning or irritation develops.

For preoperative skin preparation, follow use of soap with thorough rinsing, first with water, then with 70% alcohol, before applying benzalkonium. Avoid pooling or prolonged contact of solution with skin.

Use sterile water for injection as diluent for aqueous solutions to be instilled in wounds or body cavities. For other uses, fresh sterile distilled water is used. Tap water (especially hard water) may contain metallic ions and organic matter that reduce antibacterial potency of benzalkonium chloride, and should not be used.

The tincture and spray preparations contain flammable solvents and should not be used near an open flame or cautery. Keep away from eyes and mucous membranes.

If solution stronger than 1:5000 enters the eyes, irrigate immediately and repeatedly with water; see a physician promptly.

Solutions used on denuded skin or inflamed or irritated tissues should be more dilute than those used on normal tissue.

Organic, inorganic, and synthetic materials, such as wool, rayon, gauze, cotton, plastic, rubber, cork, or other porous material, may adsorb benzalkonium chloride thus reducing its concentration and antibacterial potency.

Cationic detergents are unreliable substitutes for heat sterilization of surgical instruments; however, they may be used to preserve the established sterility of instruments.

Prolonged contact of metal with benzalkonium chloride will result in corrosion unless antirust tablets are added to the solution. A prepared solution for instrument sterilization is available from pharmacy.

Solutions used for cold sterilization should be checked for possible contamination and replenished at regular intervals (boil container and add fresh solution).

Recommended treatment for accidental ingestion: immediate administration of several glasses of mild soap solution, milk, or egg whites beaten in water, followed by gastric lavage with mild soap solution. Avoid alcohol, as it promotes gastric absorption. Have on hand oxygen, equipment for respiratory assistance.

Store at room temperature in airtight container, protected from light.

BENZOCAINE

(ben'zoe-caine)
Anesthetic, local
Antipruritic

(Aerocaine, Americaine, Americaine Anesthetic Lubricant, Americaine-Otic, Anbesol, Benzocol, Chigger-Tox, Col-Vi-Nol, Dermoplast, Ethyl Aminobenzoate, Foille, Hurricaine, Orabase with Benzocaine, Oracin, Rhulicream, Soft 'n Soothe, Solarcaine, Unguentine)

ACTIONS AND USES. Ethyl ester of para-aminobenzoic acid (PABA). Produces surface anesthesia by inhibiting conduction of nerve impulses from sensory nerves. Almost identical to procaine in chemical structure, but has lower solubility; therefore, it is slowly absorbed and has prolonged duration of anesthetic action.

Used for temporary relief of pain and discomfort in pruritic skin problems, minor burns and sunburn, minor wounds, and insect bites. Otic preparations used to relieve pain and itching in acute congestive and serous otitis media, swimmer's ear, and otitis externa. Preparations are also available for toothache, for application to mucous membranes, e.g., canker sores, hemorrhoids, rectal fissures, pruritus ani or vulvae, as male genital densitizer to slow onset of ejaculation, and for use as anesthetic–lubricant for passage of catheters and endoscopic tubes. An ingredient in certain OTC appetite suppressants, e.g., Ayds, Slim-Line (probable action is by dulling taste for food).

ABSORPTION AND FATE. Poorly absorbed through intact skin, but readily absorbed from mucous membranes and traumatized skin. Peak anesthetic effect in about 1 minute, duration 30 to 60 minutes. Hydrolyzed primarily by plasma cholinesterases and to lesser extent by hepatic cholinesterases. Metabolites excreted in urine.

CONTRAINDICATIONS AND PRECAUTIONS. Hypersensitivity to benzocaine or other PABA derivatives, (e.g., sun screen preparations), or to any of the components in the formulation; use of ear preparation in patients with perforated eardrum, applications to large areas; use in children under 1 year of age. Safe use in women of childbearing potential or during pregnancy not established. *Cautious Use:* history of drug sensitivity, denuded skin or severely traumatized mucosa, children under 6 years.

ADVERSE/SIDE EFFECTS. (Low toxicity) Sensitization in susceptible individuals; allergic reactions: contact urticaria, contact dermatitis, erythema; swelling, edema, or vesiculation of treated part; anaphylaxis. Methemoglobinemia reported in infants.

ROUTE AND DOSAGE. Topical: 0.5 to 20%. Available in ointment, cream, lotion, aerosol, spray, liquid, liquid gel, otic drops, lozenges. Lowest effective dose should be used. Lower strengths in elderly, debilitated or acutely ill patients, and children.

NURSING IMPLICATIONS

Follow directions on labels or as prescribed by physician.

Otic preparation should be warmed to body temperature (37°C or 98.6°F) by holding bottle in hands for a few minutes or by placing unopened container in a warm water bath.

Instillation of ear drops: Adult: have patient lying down with affected side up. Hold dropper

B

with hand resting on patient's head for support. Pull pinna up and back to straighten ear canal; instill drops along side of auditory canal to prevent air pocket. Advise patient to lie on unaffected side for 1 to 2 minutes. *Child younger than 3 years of age:* straighten external auditory canal by gently pulling pinna down and straight back; *child older than 3 years:* pull pinna up and back. Instill medication and hold child for 1 to 2 minutes after instillation. Instruct older patient or parent to avoid touching ear with dropper and not to rinse dropper.

Advise patient to use eardrops as prescribed and warn patient that haphazard use may mask symptoms of a fulminating middle ear infection. Also advise patient to report to physician if earache lasts longer than 48 hours or if ear itches or burns.

Avoid contact of all preparations with eyes and be careful not to inhale mist when spray form is used. Do not use spray near open flame or cautery and do not expose to high temperatures. Hold can at least 12 inches away from affected area when spraying.

Chemical burns should be washed and neutralized before applying benzocaine.

Before administration of hemorrhoidal preparation, thoroughly clean and dry rectal area. Usually administered morning and evening and after each bowel movement.

Bear in mind that when used on oral mucosa, benzocaine may interfere with second (pharyngeal) stage of swallowing. If possible, foods and liquids should be withheld for about 1 hour following administration to prevent possible aspiration and mouth injury.

Most local anesthetics are potentially sensitizing in susceptible individuals and when applied repeatedly or over extensive areas. Instruct patient to discontinue medication if the condition being treated persists, worsens, or if signs of sensitivity, irritation, or infection occur.

Patient should be given specific directions regarding administration procedure, how often to use medication, and how long to continue treatment.

Store preferably between 15° and 30°C (50° and 86°F) in tight, light resistant containers, unless otherwise specified by manufacturer.

Drug Interactions. Benzocaine may antagonize antibacterial activity of **sulfonamides.**

BENZOIN TINCTURE, COMPOUND

(ben'zoin)

Skin protectant, expectorant

ACTIONS AND USES. Mixture of benzoin, aloes, prepared storax, and tolu balsam in 90% alcohol. Reported to have local antiseptic, astringent, and protective properties; effectiveness as a stimulant expectorant unproven.

Used to protect skin under occlusive plasters and bandages; also has been used as an antiseptic and astringent in treatment of cracked nipples and skin fissures, and as steam inhalant in treatment of acute laryngitis, bronchitis, and croup. A common ingredient in OTC products for treatment of diaper rash and prickly heat.

CONTRAINDICATIONS AND PRECAUTIONS. Acutely inflamed skin.

ADVERSE/SIDE EFFECTS. Contact dermatitis.

ROUTE AND DOSAGE. Topical: Apply once or twice daily.

NURSING IMPLICATIONS

Skin should be clean and thoroughly dry before applying since it forms an occlusive coating and may foster retention of moisture and bacterial growth.

Examine skin daily for erythema, induration, discoloration, and blistering.

Care must be taken to allow tr. benzoin to dry thoroughly following application because it is tacky when moist and can strip skin if it sticks to bedclothing.

Decubitus ulcers (bed or pressure sores) cannot be prevented by the application of tr. benzoin or any other topical medication.

Measures for Preventing Decubitus Ulcers:

- Keep skin clean and free of moisture
- Turn patient at least every 2 hours
- Proper positioning and judicious use of pressure-relieving devices
- Keep underbedding dry and wrinkle free
- Stimulate circulation by active and passive exercises, gentle massage, and ambulation, as allowed
- Maintain nutritional status

Tr. of benzoin spray is prepared for use on skin only.

Tr. benzoin compound is frequently mixed with other topical medications such as zinc oxide, or aluminum and magnesium hydroxides (Maalox) for treatment of bedsores. Consult physician before applying such mixtures.

For steam inhalation add 1 tsp to 1 pint of hot water. Review procedure carefully with patient to prevent burning.

Store in a cool place.

PROTOTYPE

BENZONATATE

(Tessalon)

(ben-zoe'na-tate)
Antitussive

ACTIONS AND USES. Nonnarcotic antitussive chemically related to tetracaine. Antitussive activity reported to be somewhat less effective than that of codeine. Exerts selective topical anesthetic action on stretch receptors in respiratory passages, lungs, and pleura and thus suppresses initiation of cough reflex. Does not inhibit respiratory center at recommended doses. More effective in treatment of nonproductive cough than cough associated with copious sputum.

Used to decrease frequency and intensity of nonproductive cough in acute and chronic respiratory conditions. Also used in bronchoscopy, thoracentesis, and other procedures when coughing must be avoided.

ABSORPTION AND FATE. Action begins within 15 to 20 minutes and lasts 3 to 8 hours.

CONTRAINDICATIONS AND PRECAUTIONS. Hypersensitivity to benzonate or related compounds. Safe use during pregnancy and lactation not established.

ADVERSE/SIDE EFFECTS. (Low incidence) **CNS:** drowsiness, headache, mild vertigo. **Dermatologic:** skin rash, pruritus. **GI:** constipation, nausea. **Other:** transitory rise in blood pressure, hypersensitivity reactions (rare), nasal congestion, chilly sensation, burning sensation of eyes, numbness or tightness of chest. **Overdosage:** CNS stimulation (restlessness, tremors, convulsions).

ROUTE AND DOSAGE. Adults and children (over 10 years): Oral: 100 mg three times a day, as required; if necessary up to 600 mg daily. **Children (under 10 years):** 8 mg/kg in three to six divided doses.

NURSING IMPLICATIONS

Instruct patient to avoid chewing oral preparation (perle) or allowing it to dissolve in mouth; it should be swallowed whole. If it dissolves, local anesthesia of mouth, tongue and pharynx will result.

Antitussive agents are used selectively. Suppression of cough and gag reflex in the immediate postoperative period may lead to aspiration and development of atelectasis and pneumonitis.

A cough suppressant is justified when cough is excessive, not productive, and prevents rest and sleep.

Objective of treatment with an antitussive agent is to reduce overactive nonproductive coughing, not to suppress the cough completely.

Observe character and frequency of coughing and volume and quality of sputum. Keep physician informed.

Changing the patient's position at least every 2 hours helps to prevent pooling of lung secretions. Concomitant deep breathing exercises may stimulate productive coughing.

Teaching Points Related to Providing Relief of Nonproductive Cough:

✓ Limitation on talking
✓ No smoking
✓ Adequate fluid intake
✓ Cold mist or steam vaporizer or steam inhalations
✓ Maintenance of environmental humidity
✓ Use of sugarless hard candy, such as lemon drops, to increase flow of saliva (a normal protective demulcent to pharyngeal mucosa).

See Index: Nursing Interventions: breathing exercises; respiratory therapy.

Store in airtight containers, protected from light.

BENZOYL PEROXIDE

(ben'zoe-ill per-ox'ide)
Keratolytic

(Acetoxyl, Acne-Aid, Alquam-X, Ben-Aqua, Benoxyl, Benzac, Benzagel, Clearasil Lotion, Clear By Design, Cuticura Acne, Dermoxyl, Desquam-X, Dry and Clear, Fostex, Oxy-5, Oxy-10, PanOxyl, Persadox, Persadox HP, Persa-Gel, Topex, Xerac BP, Zeroxin)

ACTIONS AND USES. Slowly releases oxygen that exerts bactericidal action on *Propionibacterium (Corynebacterium) acnes,* anaerobic rods found in sebaceous follicles and comedones responsible for formation of irritating free fatty acids in sebum. In addition to being an oxidizing agent, it also has antiseborrheic (drying) and keratolytic (peeling) actions which help to keep pilosebaceous orifices open and draining properly. Reportedly not as effective as retinoic acid in comedolytic activity.

Used in adjunctive treatment of mild to moderate acne vulgaris and acne rosacea. Available in fixed-dose combination with hydrocortisone (Vanoxide-HC), and with sulfur (Sulfoxyl).

ABSORPTION AND FATE. Approximately 50% of dose may be absorbed through skin. Major metabolite is benzoic acid. Excreted in urine as benzoate.

CONTRAINDICATIONS AND PRECAUTIONS. Hypersensitivity to benzoyl peroxide and to benzoic acid derivatives. Use on inflamed, denuded, thin, or highly sensitive skin. Safe use during pregnancy (category C), in nursing mothers, and in children below age 12 not established.

ADVERSE/SIDE EFFECTS. Local skin irritation, feeling of warmth, stinging; excessive scaling, erythema, edema (especially with gel preparation), allergic contact dermatitis.

ROUTE AND DOSAGE. Topical: Apply one or two times a day. Fair-skinned individuals are advised to initiate treatment with one application of lower concentration at bedtime. Available as 5 to 10% bar, cream, liquid, lotion, sticks and pads, and 2.5 to 10% gel.

NURSING IMPLICATIONS

Avoid contact of medication with eyes, eyelids, lips, inside of nose, and sensitive skin areas of neck.

It is usually advisable to initiate acne therapy with a single application of a small amount of medication until patient's reaction to drug is known. Some clinicians recommend the following conservative approach which may be modified for individual patients: apply medication for 15 minutes the first evening then wash off with soap and water, and dry well. Increase length of exposure by 15 minutes every evening until tolerated for 2 hours, then leave on overnight and wash off in the morning. Morning applications may be started when indicated.

Inform patient that mild peeling and dryness are anticipated therapeutic actions. If these effects are not observed within 3 or 4 days, application should be increased to twice daily.

Because benzoyl peroxide is an oxidizing agent, it may bleach colored fabrics. Lotion and cleansing lotion formulations, particularly may also bleach hair.

Most benzoyl peroxide gels are available only by prescription. Other forms of benzoyl peroxide may be purchased OTC. The gels are reportedly more penetrating but also tend to be more drying and irritating.

Forewarn patient that medication may cause transitory redness and feeling of warmth or slight smarting. If symptoms are excessive, advise patient to remove medication with mild soap and water, dry skin well. Application may be attempted cautiously the following day using less medication at reduced frequency.

Advise patient that skin irritation caused by benzoyl peroxide may be further aggravated by harsh soap, vigorous scrubbing of skin, and by other acne medications.

Benzoyl peroxide may be worn under makeup, if desired.

Inform patient that if improvement does not occur within 2 weeks, consult a physician.

Some patients develop a delayed hypersensitivity reaction to benzoyl peroxide. If allergic sensitization is suspected, it may be confirmed by a patch test with 5% benzoyl peroxide in petrolatum.

Patient-Teaching Points for Acne:

- ✓ There is no single cause or treatment for acne. Therapy may control but does not cure it.
- ✓ Acne is not caused by inadequate washing. However, careful washing does help remove surface oil. If skin is oily, wash face several times a day with regular toilet soap; otherwise wash once or twice daily.
- ✓ Do not pick, squeeze, or finger lesions since infection and scarring may result.
- ✓ Use water base cosmetics.
- ✓ If skin is not irritated a *controlled* amount of sunlight may help to dry lesions.
- ✓ Shampoo frequently if hair is oily.
- ✓ Avoid greasy hair dressings and keep hair away from face.
- ✓ Based on present evidence, many clinicians are convinced that dietary restrictions are not warranted. However, if patient believes that certain foods cause flare-up of lesions he or she should be advised to omit these foods. Encourage patient to eat a well-balanced diet.

✓ Psychologic support is needed and should be provided. Patient should be encouraged to ask questions and to express concerns.
✓ Some physicians teach responsible family member to remove large comedones using a Schamberg loop extractor.

Preferably stored between 15° and 30°C (59° and 86°F), unless otherwise directed by manufacturer.

BENZPHETAMINE HYDROCHLORIDE

(Didrex)

(benz-fet'a-meen)
Central stimulant (sympathomimetic)
Anorexigenic
Amphetamine
C III

ACTIONS AND USES. Indirect acting sympathomimetic amine with amphetaminelike actions, but produces fewer side effects than amphetamine. Anorexiant effect thought to be secondary to central stimulation.

Used as short-term adjunct in management of exogenous obesity.

ABSORPTION AND FATE. Following oral administration, readily absorbed from GI tract; effects persist for about 4 hours.

CONTRAINDICATIONS AND PRECAUTIONS. Known hypersensitivity to sympathomimetic amines, angle-closure glaucoma, advanced arteriosclerosis, angina pectoris, severe cardiovascular disease, moderate to severe hypertension, hyperthyroidism, agitated states, history of drug abuse, children under 12 years of age. Safe use during pregnancy or in women of childbearing potential not established. *Cautious Use:* diabetes mellitus, the elderly.

ADVERSE/SIDE EFFECTS. CNS: euphoria, irritability, hyperactivity, tremor, nervousness, restlessness, insomnia, headache, light-headedness, dizziness. **CV:** palpitation, tachycardia, elevated blood pressure. **GI:** xerostomia, unpleasant taste, nausea, vomiting, diarrhea or constipation, abdominal cramps. **Other:** urticaria and other allergic skin reactions, sweating, changes in libido. *Chronic intoxication:* marked insomnia, irritability, hyperactivity, personality changes, psychosis, severe dermatoses. *See Amphetamine.*

ROUTE AND DOSAGE. Oral: 25 to 50 mg one to three times daily.

NURSING IMPLICATIONS

Administering drug before meals may serve as a reminder of the need for self-discipline during mealtime. A single daily dose is given preferably mid-morning or mid-afternoon, according to patient's eating habits.

To avoid insomnia, the last dose should be scheduled no later than 6 hours before patient retires.

Because dizziness and light-headedness are possible side effects, caution patient against driving a car or performing any other potentially hazardous activities until his reaction to drug is determined.

For maximal results, drug therapy should be used as part of a plan that includes reeducation and behavior modification with respect to eating habits and nutritional needs, resolution of underlying psychologic factors, and an appropriate exercise program.

Dosage of antidiabetic drug may require adjustment in diabetic patients because their food intake may change.
Note that commercially available tablet contains tartrazine, which can cause allergic reactions including bronchial asthma in susceptible individuals. Frequently such persons are also sensitive to aspirin.
Anorexiant effects are temporary, seldom lasting more than a few weeks; tolerance (tachyphylaxis) may occur. Therefore long-term use is not indicated.
Patients taking an anorexigenic agent should be seen at regular intervals to determine progress and to decide whether continuation of therapy is advisable.
Abrupt termination of therapy following prolonged high dosages can result in GI distress, stomach cramps, trembling, unusual tiredness, weakness, and mental depression.
The possibility of psychic dependence should be noted.
Classified as Schedule III drug under the Federal Controlled Substances Act.
Preserved in tight, light-resistant containers at room temperature preferably between 15° and 30°C (59° and 86°F), unless otherwise advised by manufacturer.

Drug Interactions: Benzphetamine

Plus	Interactions
Acetazolamide (Diamox) Sodium bicarbonate	Drugs that render urine alkaline increase renal tubular reabsorption of amphetamines. Monitor for enhanced effects
Barbiturates	May antagonize anorexigenic effects. Combination generally avoided
CNS stimulants, other	Additive CNS stimulation. Combination generally avoided
Guanethidine (Ismelin) and other antihypertensives	Decreased antihypertensive action. (Neuronal uptake of antihypertensive drug is inhibited.) Combination avoided
MAO inhibitors including drugs with significant MAO inhibitor activity, e.g., furazolidone (Furoxone)	Increased benzphetamine toxicity with possibility of severe hypertensive crisis. Combination avoided
Phenothiazines	May antagonize anorexigenic effects. Combination generally avoided
Tricyclic antidepressants	Effects of tricyclics may be enhanced. Used concurrently with caution

See Amphetamine (prototype for amphetamines) for other possible drug interactions.

BENZQUINAMIDE HYDROCHLORIDE
(Emete-Con)

(benz-kwin'a-mide)
Antiemetic

ACTIONS AND USES. Benzoquinolizine amide with antiemetic activity similar to that of phenothiazines and antihistamine antiemetics, but chemically unrelated to both. Mechanism of antiemetic action unknown, but believed to be by depression of CTZ. Also exhibits antihistaminic, antiserotonin, anticholinergic, and sedative properties.

Used for prevention and treatment of nausea and vomiting associated with anesthesia, surgery, and antineoplastic drugs.

B

ABSORPTION AND FATE. Rapidly and completely absorbed. Onset of antiemetic action within 15 minutes following IM or IV administration; duration 3 to 4 hours. Peak blood levels in about 30 minutes after IM and less than 15 minutes after IV injection. Distributed throughout body tissues, with highest concentrations in liver and kidneys. Approximately 58% protein-bound; half-life is about 40 minutes. Rapidly metabolized in liver. About 95% of dose excreted in urine and feces within 72 hours primarily as metabolites; less than 10% as unchanged drug. Distribution to placenta and to breast milk not known.

CONTRAINDICATIONS AND PRECAUTIONS. Hypersensitivity to the drug; IV administration to patients with cardiovascular disease, moderate to severe hypertension, or to those who have received preanesthetic and/or concomitant cardiovascular drugs. Safe use during pregnancy, in nursing women, and in children younger than 12 years not established. *Cautious Use:* elderly and debilitated patients.

ADVERSE/SIDE EFFECTS. CNS: drowsiness (common), insomnia, headache, excitement, restlessness, nervousness; extrapyramidal symptoms (in large doses): tremors, twitching, rigidity, hypersalivation, weakness, motor restlessness, fatigue. *Autonomic:* dry mouth or salivation, blurred vision, sweating, shivering, chills, flushing, hiccoughs. **CV:** (particularly following IV): sudden increase in blood pressure and respiration; hypotension, dizziness, tachycardia, atrial fibrillation, premature atrial and ventricular contractions. **GI:** anorexia, nausea, vomiting, abdominal cramps. **Other:** Allergic (rare): urticaria, skin rash, pyrexia.

ROUTE AND DOSAGE. Intramuscular (preferred route): 50 mg (0.5 to 1 mg/kg). First dose may be repeated in 1 hour; subsequent doses every 3 or 4 hours, if necessary. **Intravenous:** 25 mg (0.2 to 0.4 mg/kg) (Initially reconstituted with 2.2 ml sterile water for injection or bacteriostatic water for injection preserved with benzyl alcohol or parabens. Do not reconstitute with sodium chloride because precipitation may result. Subsequent doses given intramuscularly, if necessary.) Administered slowly IV at rate not exceeding 1 ml (25 mg) per ½ to 1 minute.

NURSING IMPLICATIONS

Benzquinamide should be administered at least 15 minutes prior to expected emergence from anesthesia or administration of antineoplastic drugs.

IM injection should be made well into mass of a large muscle. Aspirate carefully to avoid inadvertent intravascular injection.

Deltoid area may be used only if well developed. Expose entire upper arm for complete visualization. Do not inject into lower or mid-third of arm.

Monitor patient for cardiovascular effects such as hyper- or hypotension, and arrhythmias, particularly when drug is administered IV.

Drowsiness is a common side effect.

In common with other antiemetics, benzquinamide may mask signs and symptoms of overdosage from other drugs and obscure diagnosis of conditions associated with nausea and vomiting e.g., GI obstruction, brain pathology.

Do not use sodium chloride for reconstitution because precipitation may occur.

Reconstituted solutions maintain potency for 14 days at room temperature. Do not refrigerate.

Preserve in light-resistant containers. Unused vials and reconstituted solutions should be protected from light.

BENZTHIAZIDE

(Aquatag, Exna, Hydrex, Marazide, Proaqua)

(bens-thye'a-zide)
Diuretic, thiazide
Antihypertensive
Sulfonamide derivative

ACTIONS AND USES. Benzothiadiazine derivative chemically related to sulfonamides. Similar to chlorothiazide (qv) in actions, uses, contraindications, precautions, adverse reactions, interactions.

Used adjunctively (step 1) with other agents in stepped care approach for treatment of mild hypertension.

ABSORPTION AND FATE. Onset of diuretic effect in 2 hours, peaks in 4 to 6 hours; duration of action 12 to 18 hours. Distribution and fate assumed to be similar to those of other thiazides. Crosses placenta; appears in breast milk. *See Chlorothiazide.*

CONTRAINDICATIONS AND PRECAUTIONS. Anuria, hypersensitivity to thiazides or sulfonamides; pregnancy, lactation. *Cautious Use:* history of renal and hepatic disease, gout, diabetes mellitus, electrolyte imbalance. *See also Chlorothiazide.*

ADVERSE/SIDE EFFECTS. Xerostomia, anorexia, unusual fatigue, paresthesias, vasculitis, orthostatic hypotension, agranulocytosis, hyperglycemia, hypokalemia; hyperuricemia, photosensitivity. *See also Chlorothiazide.*

ROUTE AND DOSAGE. Oral: Adult: *Antidiuretic (diabetes insipidus) or diuretic:* 25 to 100 mg twice daily, once every other day, or once a day for 3 to 5 days/week. *Antihypertensive:* 25 to 100 mg two times daily. **Pediatric:** 1 to 4 mg/kg/day in divided doses.

NURSING IMPLICATIONS

Administer drug early in the morning to prevent interrupted sleep because of diuresis. If 2 doses are ordered give second dose no later than 3 PM.

Dosage regimens are highly individualized and based upon blood pressure response.

Antihypertensive effects may be noted in 3 to 4 days; maximal effects may require 3 to 4 weeks.

The elderly may be more sensitive to the average adult dose. Monitor carefully for signs of hypokalemia (dry mouth, anorexia, thirst, paresthesias, muscle cramps, hypoactive reflexes, weakness). Dose adjustment may be indicated.

Food–Drug Interactions:

- To prevent onset of hypokalemia, (rarely severe in most patients even on long-term therapy with thiazides): Urge patient to eat a normal diet (usually includes K-rich foods such as fruit juices, potatoes, cereals, skim milk). Also advise patient to include a banana (about 370 mg K) and at least 6 ounces orange juice (about 330 mg K) every day.
- If hypokalemia develops, dietary K supplement of 1000 to 2000 mg (25 to 50 mEq) is usually an adequate treatment.
- Dietary management is important in thiazide treatment of hypertension. The physician will specifically order goal of the diet: electrolyte, weight, fluid control. Collaborate with dietitian and arrange for patient–dietitian planning for an individualized diet.

Instruct patient to weigh self daily. Consult physician about acceptable range of weight change; report sudden weight gain.

Counsel patient to avoid use of OTC drugs unless approved by the physician. Many prepara-

B

tions contain K and sodium, and if misused, or if patient overdoses, electrolyte side effects could be induced.

Warn patient about the possibility of photosensitivity reaction and to notify the physician if it occurs (like an exaggerated sunburn). Thiazide-related photosensitivity is considered a photoallergy (ultraviolet radiation changes drug structure making it allergenic for some individuals) and occurs 1½ to 2 weeks after initial sun exposure.

Aquatag, 50 mg tablets, Exna, and Proaqua contain tartrazine, which may cause an allergic reaction (including bronchial asthma) in susceptible individuals. Frequently such persons are also sensitive to aspirin.

Store tablets in tightly closed container at temperature of 15° to 30°C (59° to 86°F), unless otherwise directed by manufacturer.

See Chlorothiazide (prototype thiazide).

Drug Interactions: Benzthiazide

Plus	Interactions
Cholestyramine (Questran) Colestipol (Colestid)	May decrease absorption of thiazines. Separate administration as far apart as possible
Diazoxide (Hyperstat)	Additive pharmacologic effects of both drugs. Monitor for hyperglycemia, hyperuricemia, hypotension
Digitalis glycosides	Thiazide-induced hypokalemia can sensitize myocardium to digitalis with possible toxicity. Monitor serum potassium
Lithium	Possibility of lithium toxicity (renal lithium excretion reduced), monitor serum lithium levels
Tolbutamide and other sulfonylureas	Decreased hypoglycemic effect. Higher sulfonylurea dosage may be needed

See Chlorothiazide (prototype thiazide) for other possible interactions.

BENZTROPINE MESYLATE

(Apo-Benzotropine, Bensylate, Cogentin)

(benz'troe-peen)
Anticholinergic (parasympatholytic)
Antiparkinsonian agent

ACTIONS AND USES. Synthetic centrally acting anticholinergic (antimuscarinic) agent, chemically similar to atropine and diphenhydramine. Also exhibits antihistaminic, and local anesthetic activity. Acts by diminishing excess cholinergic effect associated with dopamine deficiency. (Normal motor activity relies upon a balance between cholinergic and dopaminergic activity in corpus striatum.) Suppresses tremor and rigidity; does not alleviate tardive dyskinesia.

Used in symptomatic treatment of all forms of parkinsonism (arteriosclerotic, idiopathic, postencephalitic), and to relieve extrapyramidal symptoms associated with neuroleptic drugs e.g., haloperidol (Haldol), phenothiazines, thiothixene (Navane). Commonly used as supplement with trihexyphenidyl, carbidopa, or levodopa therapy.

ABSORPTION AND FATE. Onset of action following IM and IV injections occurs within 15 minutes; onset occurs about 1 hour following oral administration. Effects may persist 6 to 10 hours or more.

CONTRAINDICATIONS AND PRECAUTIONS. Hypersensitivity to benztropine or to any ingredients in the formulation; narrow angle glaucoma, myasthenia gravis, obstructive diseases of GU and GI tracts, tendency to tachycardia, patients with tardive dyskinesia, children under 3 years of age. Safe use during childbearing potential, pregnancy (category C), and in nursing women not established. *Cautious Use:* older children, elderly or debilitated patients, patients with poor mental outlook, mental disorders. *See also Atropine.*

ADVERSE/SIDE EFFECTS. CNS: sedation, dizziness, nervousness, paresthesias; in high doses: CNS depression, preceded or followed by stimulation, agitation, hallucinations, delirium, mental confusion, toxic psychosis, muscular weakness, ataxia. **CV:** palpitation, tachycardia. **GI:** nausea, vomiting, xerostomia, constipation, paralytic ileus. **GU:** dysuria, urinary retention. **Ophthalmic:** blurred vision, mydriasis, photophobia. **Other:** anhidrosis. *See Atropine for other possible adverse effects.*

ROUTE AND DOSAGE. *Parkinsonism:* **Oral:** Initial: 0.5 to 1 mg, gradually increased up to 6 mg/day if required and tolerated. (Generally low doses are given to patients with arteriosclerotic parkinsonism, the elderly, thin patients, and older children.) *Extrapyramidal reactions:* **Oral, intramuscular, intravenous:** 1 to 4 mg one or two times daily.

NURSING IMPLICATIONS

Administration of drug immediately after meals or with food may help to prevent gastric irritation. If patient cannot swallow tablet, it may be crushed prior to administration and sprinkled on or mixed with food.

Patients with arteriosclerotic or idiopathic parkinsonism generally experience greatest relief by taking benztropine at bedtime. Younger patients with postencephalitic parkinsonism usually require more frequent scheduling.

Physician will rely on accurate observations and reporting to establish patient's optimum dosage level and frequency of scheduling, and to determine appropriateness of therapy. For example, if extrapyramidal (acute dystonic) reactions are not relieved, causes other than drug-induced must be investigated, e.g., hypocalcemia.

Patients with mental illness should be closely observed for intensification of mental symptoms, particularly during early therapy.

When used as an adjunct to antipsychotic drugs, generally benztropine is not continued beyond 3 months because prolonged use may predispose patient to tardive dyskinesia.

Effects of benztropine are cumulative: therefore, clinical improvement may not be evident until 2 or 3 days after oral drug is started. Drug therapy is usually initiated at low doses, with subsequent increments of 0.5 mg made at 5- or 6-day intervals, if necessary.

Elderly patients should be kept under close surveillance especially at beginning of drug therapy or whenever dosage increases are made.

Monitor intake and output ratio and pattern. Advise patient to report difficulty in urination or infrequent voiding. Dosage reduction may be indicated.

Appearance of intermittent constipation, abdominal pain, and distention may herald onset of paralytic ileus. Patients receiving combination drugs with anticholinergic action should be closely monitored for these symptoms.

Therapeutic effect in the patient with parkinsonism is evidenced by lessening of rigidity, drooling (sialorrhea) and oculogyric crises, and by improvement in gait, balance, and posture. Usually, tremors are not appreciably relieved. Note that muscle weakness is an adverse side effect and requires dosage reduction.

Most of the atropinelike side effects of benztropine are controlled by adjustment of dosage. However, severe reactions, such as signs and symptoms of CNS depression or excitement, generally require interruption of drug therapy.

B

Caution patient about possibility of drowsiness and blurred vision, and advise against operating vehicles or machinery or other activities requiring alertness until reaction to the drug is known. Supervision of ambulation and bedsides may be indicated.

Inform patient that alcohol and other CNS depressants may cause additive drowsiness and therefore should be avoided. Also advise patient not to take OTC cold, cough, or hay fever remedies unless approved by physician because they commonly contain anticholinergic and antihistaminic agents.

Mouth dryness may be relieved by frequent rinsing of mouth with tepid water, or by sugarless gum or hard candy, diligent dental hygiene such as brushing with soft tooth brush after meals and at bedtime, use of fluoride toothpaste, and daily flossing. If symptom persists, and particularly if associated with difficulty in swallowing, anorexia, and weight loss, benztropine dosage should be reduced or drug should be discontinued temporarily.

Anhidrosis (diminished sweating) especially in hot weather, may require dose adjustments because of possibility of heat stroke. This condition is particularly apt to occur in the elderly patient. Check temperature daily in this age group. Caution patient to avoid doing manual labor or strenuous exercise in a hot environment.

Benztropine has drug abuse potential and has been misused by narcotic addicts for its hallucinogenic effects.

Preserved in tightly covered, light-resistant container at room temperature preferably between 15° and 30°C (59° and 86°F), unless otherwise directed by manufacturer.

Drug Interactions: Benztropine

Plus	Interactions
Alcohol (Ethanol) and other CNS depressants	Potentiation of sedative and other CNS depressant effects
Amantadine (Symmetrel) Antidepressants, tricyclic Antihistamines Haloperidol (Haldol) MAO inhibitors Phenothiazines Procainamide (Pronestyl) Quinidine (Cardioquin)	Additive anticholinergic (atropinelike) side effects: confusion, hallucinations, paralytic ileus. Used concomitantly with caution

---

BENZYL BENZOATE LOTION

(Scabanca)

(ben'zill ben'zoe-ate)
Antiinfective
Scabicide, pediculocide

ACTIONS AND USES. Produced synthetically by esterification of benzoic acid with benzyl alcohol. Widely used in other countries, but largely replaced by other agents in the U.S. Reportedly less toxic than lindane (gamma benzene hexachloride) and therefore preferred by many clinicians for use in the young. Destroys arthropod parasite that causes scabies *(Sarcoptes scabei).* Also active against head louse and crab louse.

Used for topical treatment of scabies, particularly in infants and young children, and for pediculosis pubis and capitis. Has been used as an insect repellent and to increase solubility and stability of dimercaprol.

CONTRAINDICATIONS AND PRECAUTIONS. History of hypersensitivity to benzyl benzoate and to benzoic acid derivatives; application to acutely inflamed, raw, or weeping surfaces, mucous membranes.

ADVERSE/SIDE EFFECTS. (Low toxicity) Irritation of skin, burning and stinging sensation (especially of scalp), pruritus, allergic skin sensitization, contact dermatitis.

ROUTE AND DOSAGE. Topical: *Scabies:* Patient should be instructed to bathe with soap and water to remove crusts and scales before initiation of therapy. Towel dry. While skin is still damp gently massage thin film of lotion (28%) onto all skin surfaces from neck to toes, including soles of feet. Apply second coat after first coat dries. Put on clean clothing and change bed clothes. Usual course of treatment consists of 3 consecutive applications as above, applied nightly or every other night. If necessary, course of therapy may be repeated after 7 to 10 days if live mites are seen or new lesions develop. *Pediculosis pubis and capitis:* Instruct patient to rub the lotion into hairy areas and to remove it with soap and water after 12 to 24 hours. If necessary, treatment may be repeated after 1 week. Use fine-toothed comb to remove nits.

NURSING IMPLICATIONS

Shake lotion well before using.

If 50% lotion is used, dilute with equal quantity of water before applying.

Wash hands thoroughly before and after treatments.

Avoid contact with face, eyes, genitalia, and other mucous membranes.

If irritation occurs, drug should be washed off and treatment discontinued.

Pruritus that persists for one to several weeks may occur from acquired sensitivity to mites. This symptom is not an indication of the need for further treatment with benzyl benzoate.

All clothing and bedding used by patient should be machine washed in hot water and detergent, or boiled, or dry cleaned following each application and completion of treatment to avoid reinfection.

Members of household and close contacts should be treated concurrently.

Store in well-covered container protected from light and excessive heat.

See Lindane (prototype scabicide); Malathim (prototype pediculocide).

BETA CAROTENE

(Solatene)

(bay-ta kare'oh-teen)
Antioxidant
Provitamin

ACTIONS AND USES. Carotenoid pigment and fat-soluble precursor of vitamin A found in green and yellow vegetables. Provides photoprotection by unclear mechanism but it may be a quelling effect on free radicals and singlet excited oxygen (antioxidant activity), through which photosensitizers appear to act. Bioavailability is dependent on bile in intestinal tract for its absorption, fat as a carrier, and adequate protein intake. 6 mcg dietary beta carotene is considered to be equivalent to 1 mcg vitamin A (retinol).

Used to protect against and to reduce severity of photosensitivity reactions in patients with erythropoietic protoporphyria.

ABSORPTION AND FATE. Before absorption, portions of dose are metabolized in intestinal tract to vitamin A in presence of fat and bile acids. Widely distributed and stored in various tissues, particularly in skin and fat depots. Small amounts metabolized to vitamin A and stored in liver. Release from storage is followed by conversion to retinal, then to retinol, which is further metabolized. Excreted in urine and feces as gluconurides.

CONTRAINDICATIONS AND PRECAUTIONS. Known sensitivity to beta carotene; pregnancy (category C); chronic diarrhea, steatorrhea. *Cautious Use:* impaired renal and hepatic function, nursing mothers.

ADVERSE/SIDE EFFECTS. Diarrhea (sporadic); arthralgia, ecchymoses (rare); hypercarotenemia, carotenodermia (yellow or orange skin pigmentation).

ROUTE AND DOSAGE. Adults: 30 to 300 mg (1 to 10 capsules) daily. **Children (under 14 years):** 30 to 150 mg (1 to 5 capsules) daily.

NURSING IMPLICATIONS

Although beta carotene is converted to vitamin A, chronic intake does not lead to elevated concentrations of blood vitamin A.

Administer capsules as single dose or in divided doses, preferably with meals.

Capsules may be opened and contents mixed with fruit juice to aid in administration. Do not swallow dry contents (powder). Always swallow with food or liquid.

Photosensitivity reactions caused by erythropoietic protoporphyria are severe: burning sensation, edema, erythema, pruritus, cutaneous lesions. Photoprotection, i.e., therapeutic effect of this drug, requires from 2 to 6 weeks to develop and is correlated with development of carotenodermia.

When palms, soles, and possibly face skin are yellowish, gradual exposure to sun or artificial (xenon arc) lights may begin.

Carotenodermia is differentiated from jaundice by the absence of yellow sclera and pruritus.

Drug-induced photoprotection is not complete nor is it a "sunscreen." Each individual will need to recognize personal limits with regard to amount and time of exposure to light and continue to protect his or her skin.

In the normal individual, beta carotene does not bestow sunscreen activity.

Reportedly, about 86% of patients treated with this drug quadrupled the time they can be out in the sun; 8% have doubled acceptable exposure time.

Intolerance to light returns in 1 to 2 weeks after drug is discontinued.

Food–Drug Interactions. Yellow (especially carrots and yellow corn) and green vegetables or their juices or extracts in large quantities contain beta carotene; however, large quantities may cause leukopenia or menstrual disorders. Warn patient not to substitute excess amounts of these vegetables for the prescribed medication. Inadequate protein intake reduces absorption, transportation and metabolism of carotene.

Warn patient against self-dosing with supplemental vitamin A because the usual dose of beta carotene provides the normal daily requirement.

Collaborate with dietitian in the design of an appropriate diet and in required patient teaching.

An oral preparation of beta carotene with canthoxanthin is available for cosmetic "tanning" (carotenodermia).

BETAMETHASONE

(bay-ta-meth'a-sone)
Corticosteroid

(Betinelan, Celestone)

BETAMETHASONE ACETATE AND BETAMETHASONE SODIUM PHOSPHATE

(Celestone Soluspan)

BETAMETHASONE BENZOATE

(Beben, Benisone, Uticort)

BETAMETHASONE DIPROPRIONATE

(Diprolene, Diprosone)

BETAMETHASONE SODIUM PHOSPHATE

(Celestone Phosphate, Cel-U-Jec, Selestoject)

BETAMETHASONE VALERATE

(Betacort, Betaderm, Beta-Val, Metaderm, Novobetamet, Valisone)

ACTIONS AND USES. Synthetic long-acting glucocorticoid with minor mineralocorticoid properties but strong immunosuppressive, antiinflammatory, and metabolic actions. Topical use provides relief of inflammatory manifestations of corticosteroid-responsive dermatoses. Has been administered parenterally to mothers to prevent hyaline membrane disease (respiratory distress syndrome) in neonates. With exception of use as replacement therapy in adrenocortical insufficiency and salt-losing forms of adrenogenital syndromes, betamethasone has the same indications for use, absorption and fate, limitations of use, and adverse/side effects as hydrocortisone (qv).

ROUTE AND DOSAGE. Doses highly individualized on basis of response of patient and disease being treated. **Oral:** (Betamethasone) 0.6 to 7.2 mg/day. **Intramuscular, intravenous** (Betamethasone phosphate): 0.5 to 9 mg/day (usually doses range from ⅓ to ½ oral dose given every 12 hours). **Intrabursal, intraarticular** (Bethamethasone acetate and sodium phosphate): (dose determined by joint size): *Respiratory distress syndrome (RDS):* 2 ml IM to mother once daily for 2 or 3 days before delivery. **Topical:** (Betamethasone benzoate, diproprionate, valerate) thin film applied to affected area 1 to 3 times daily. Available in aerosol, cream, gel, lotion, ointment.

NURSING IMPLICATIONS

Betamethasone acetate combined with betamethasone sodium phosphate (Celestone Soluspan) is used for intraarticular, intramuscular, and intralestional injection. Response following intraarticular, intralesional, or intrasynovial administration is within a few hours and persists for 1 to 4 weeks. Following IM administration response occurs in 2 to 3 hours and persists for 3 to 7 days. *Not intended for IV use.* Do not mix with diluents containing preservatives (e.g., parabens, phenol). If prescribed, 1 or 2% lidocaine hydrochloride may be used. (Withdraw betamethasone mixture first then lidocaine; shake syringe briefly).

With short-term use, mineralocorticoid (electrolyte) action is limited; therefore, dietary supplements of potassium or restriction of sodium are usually unnecessary. Betamethasone appears to cause weight gain, however.

Topical preparations: Lotions are generally better for use on weeping lesions or on areas subject to friction (e.g., axilla, groin), and also for hairy areas. *Aerosols and gels* are appropriate for use on hairy areas, especially scalp. Ointments are mostly suitable for dry scaly lesions. They are the most occlusive of all topical forms. *Creams* are good for general use.

Consult physician regarding cleansing skin before treatments. Some clinicians recommend thorough washing with mild soap and water before each application. Others prefer that area not be disturbed.

Absorption following use of aerosol preparation (Valisone) equals that of oral and parenteral administration. Avoid inhaling drug; do not spray mucous membranes or external ear canal. Protect eyes.

Aerosol administration: spray no more than 3 seconds and at a distance of no less than 6 inches. Do not apply to area that is to be covered by occlusive dressing.

The topically treated skin area should not be covered unless prescribed by physician. *See Hydrocortisone for special points about topical application.*

Percutaneous absorption is enhanced by occlusion of the medication by means of plastic wrap or occlusive drug vehicles. Adverse systemic steroid effects are most apt to occur if the skin is abraded or otherwise altered.

Advise patient to avoid exposing areas treated with topical corticosteroid to sunlight. Severe burns have been reported, especially when occlusive dressing are used.

Carefully and routinely note condition of skin to which topical betamethasone has been applied. Report evidence of limited response or intercurrent infection which may necessitate adjunctive treatment with an appropriate antifungal or antibacterial agent.

See manufacturer's directions for stability and storage.

See Hydrocortisone (prototype corticosteroid).

BETHANECHOL CHLORIDE

(Duvoid, Myotonachol, Urecholine)

(be-than'e-kole)

Cholinergic (parasympathomimetic)

ACTIONS AND USES. Synthetic choline ester with effects similar to those of acetylcholine (ACh); acts directly on postsynaptic receptors and, since it is not hydrolyzed by cholinesterase, its action is prolonged. Produces muscarinic effects primarily on GI tract and urinary bladder with minimal effects on CV system, autonomic ganglia, neuromuscular junction, sweat glands, salivary glands, and eyes. Increases tone and peristaltic activity of esophagus, stomach, and intestines; contracts detrusor muscle of urinary bladder, usually enough to initiate micturition.

Used in treatment of acute postoperative and postpartum nonobstructive (functional) urinary retention, and for neurogenic atony of urinary bladder with retention. Has been used in selected cases of adynamic ileus, gastric atony and retention, reflux esophagitis, congenital megacolon, familial dysautonomia. Also used for treatment of bladder and salivary gland inhibition induced by tricyclic antidepressants and for prophylaxis and treatment of phenothiazine-induced bladder dysfunction. *Investigative Use:* to increase ACh level in brain of patient with Alzheimer's disease.

ABSORPTION AND FATE. Onset of action occurs within 30 to 90 minutes following oral administration and in 5 to 15 minutes after SC injection. Effects persist about 1 hour after oral administration (reportedly up to 6 hours with large doses), and up to 2 hours after SC administration. Excreted via kidneys.

CONTRAINDICATIONS AND PRECAUTIONS. Hypersensitivity to bethanechol; obstructive pulmonary disease, history of or active bronchial asthma, hyperthyroidism, recent urinary bladder surgery, cystitis, bacteriuria, urinary bladder neck or intestinal obstruction, peptic ulcer, recent GI surgery, peritonitis, marked vagotonia, pronounced vasomotor instability, AV conduction defects, severe bradycardia, hypotension or hypertension, coronary artery disease, recent myocardial infarction, epilepsy, parkinsonism. Safe use during pregnancy (category C), in nursing women, and in children under 8 years not established.

ADVERSE/SIDE EFFECTS. CV: hypotension with dizziness, faintness; orthostatic hypotension (large doses); mild reflex tachycardia, atrial fibrillation (hyperthyroid patients), transient complete heart block, transient syncope with cardiac arrest. **GI:** nausea, vomiting, abdominal cramps, bloody diarrhea, borborygmi, belching, fecal incontinence (large doses), urge to defecate (or urinate). **Respiratory:** acute asthmatic attack, dyspnea (large doses). **Other:** flushing of skin, increased sweating, salivation and lacrimation, malaise, headache, blurred vision, miosis, substernal pain or pressure (possibly due to bronchoconstriction or esophageal spasm), hypothermia. *Cholinergic overstimulation:* may occur with overdosage, hypersensitivity, or when given inadvertently IV or IM: fall in blood pressure, bradycardia, reflex tachycardia, severe abdominal cramps, bloody diarrhea, shock, sudden cardiac arrest, circulatory collapse.

ROUTE AND DOSAGE. Oral: Adults: 10 to 50 mg two to four times daily to a maximum of 120 mg daily. **Pediatric:** 0.2 mg/kg or 6.7 mg/m² three times daily. **Subcutaneous: Adults:** 2.5 to 5 mg three or four times daily, as required. **Pediatric:** 0.15 to 0.2 mg/kg (or 5 to 6.7 mg/m²) three times a day. Highly individualized.

NURSING IMPLICATIONS

Bethanechol should be given on an empty stomach (1 hour before or at least 2 hours after meals) to lessen possibility of nausea and vomiting, unless otherwise advised by physician.

Bethanechol may be prescribed with meals following bilateral vagotomy in patients with gastric atony. The drug is given orally in incomplete gastric retention, and SC if retention is complete.

To determine minimum effective oral dose: physician may prescribe an initial test dose of 5 to 10 mg and a repeat of same dose at hourly intervals to a maximum of 30 mg, unless satisfactory response or disturbing side effects intervene. Alternatively, 10 mg followed at 6-hour intervals by 25 mg then 50 mg until desired response obtained.

To determine minimum effective subcutaneous dose: physician may prescribe an initial test dose of 2.5 mg and a repeat of the same dose at 15- to 30-minute intervals to a maximum of 4 doses, unless satisfactory response or disturbing side effects intervene.

Sterile solution of bethanechol is intended for subcutaneous use only. After inserting needle, aspirate carefully before injecting drug to avoid inadvertent entry into a blood vessel. Severe symptoms of cholinergic stimulation may occur if it is given IM or IV *(see Adverse/Side Effects).*

Adverse effects are most commonly associated with subcutaneous administration, and high oral doses. Monitor blood pressure and pulse in these patients. Observe patient for at least 1 hour following SC administration. Report early signs of overdosage: salivation, sweating, flushing, abdominal cramps, nausea.

Syringe containing atropine sulfate (specific antidote) should be ready for instantaneous use to abolish severe side effects, 0.6 to 1.2 mg for adults administered IM, slow IV, or SC; and 0.01 mg/kg for infants and children repeated every 2 hours, if necessary. Specific directions for administering antidote should be prescribed by physician.

Because orthostatic hypotension is a possible side effect, caution patient to make position changes slowly and in stages, particularly from recumbent to upright posture, not to stand still, to avoid hot baths or showers, and to lie down at first indication of faintness or light-headedness.

When bethanechol is administered to relieve urinary retention or abdominal distention, a bedpan or urinal should be readily available to the patient. It may be necessary to insert a rectal tube to facilitate passage of flatus.

Monitor intake and output. Observe and record patient's response to bethanechol, and report

B

any failure of the drug to relieve the particular condition for which it was prescribed.

Bear in mind that reflux infection can occur in patients with preexisting bacteriuria when urine is forced up into ureters and kidney by bethanechol-induced bladder contractions.

Store at room temperature, preferably between 15° and 30°C (59° and 86°F), unless otherwise directed by manufacturer.

Diagnostic Test Interferences. Bethanechol may cause increases in **serum amylase** and **serum lipase,** by stimulating pancreatic secretions, and may increase **SGOT, serum bilirubin,** and **BSP retention** by causing spasms in sphincter of Oddi.

Drug Interactions: Bethanechol

Plus	Interactions
Cholinergics, especially cholinesterase inhibitors, e.g., ambenonium (Mytelase), neostigmine (Prostigmin)	Additive cholinergic effects
Ganglionic blocking agents, e.g., mecamylamine (Inversine)	Concurrent use may cause severe abdominal symptoms and precipitous fall in blood pressure
Procainamide (Procan, Pronestyl) Quinidine	Antagonize cholinergic effects of bethanechol

BIPERIDEN HYDROCHLORIDE
(Akineton Hydrochloride)

BIPERIDEN LACTATE
(Akineton Lactate)

(bye-per'i-den)
Anticholinergic, (antimuscarinic)
Antiparkinsonian agent

ACTIONS AND USES. Analogue of trihexyphenidyl with similar actions, uses, contraindications, and adverse reactions. In common with other drugs of this group has atropinelike (anticholinergic) actions. Drying effects are reported to be relatively weak compared with atropine (qv).

Used in all forms of parkinsonism, but appears to be more effective in postencephalitic and idiopathic parkinsonism than in arteriosclerotic type. Also used to control extrapyramidal disorders associated with reserpine and phenothiazines.

CONTRAINDICATIONS AND PRECAUTIONS. Safe use during pregnancy (category C), in nursing women, and in children not established. *Cautious Use:* elderly or debilitated patients, prostatic hypertrophy, glaucoma, cardiac arrhythmias.

ADVERSE/SIDE EFFECTS. (Dose-related): dry mouth, blurred vision, constipation, drowsiness, dizziness, lack of coordination, disorientation, euphoria, agitation, confusion, urinary hesitancy or retention; hematuria, mild, transient postural hypotension (following parenteral administration). *See Atropine for other possible reactions.*

ROUTE AND DOSAGE. Oral (biperiden hydrochloride): 2 mg one to four times daily. **Intramuscular and intravenous** (biperiden lactate): 2 mg injected slowly; may be repeated every 30 minutes to maximum of 8 mg per 24-hour period.

NURSING IMPLICATIONS

GI disturbances may be alleviated by administering drug with or after meals.

Slight dryness of mouth and blurred vision are common dose-related side effects and may be relieved or eliminated by dosage reduction.

Patient should be recumbent when receiving parenteral biperiden. Postural hypotension, disturbances of coordination, and temporary euphoria may occur especially following IV injection. Monitor blood pressure and pulse. Advise patient to make position changes slowly and in stages, particularly from recumbent to upright position.

It is reported that certain susceptible patients may manifest mental confusion, drowsiness, dizziness, agitation, hematuria (rarely), and decrease in urinary flow. Report these symptoms immediately.

Biperiden usually reduces sweating, drooling, excessive oiliness of skin, and muscle rigidity. In patients with severe parkinsonism, tremors may increase as spasticity is relieved.

Caution patient to avoid driving and other potentially hazardous activities until reaction to drug is determined.

Patients on prolonged therapy can develop tolerance; an increase in dosage may be required.

Preserve in tightly closed, light-resistant containers at room temperature preferably between 15° and 30°C (59° and 86°F), unless otherwise directed by manufacturer.

See Atropine for Drug Interactions.

PROTOTYPE

BISACODYL

(bis-a-koe′dill)

(Apo-Bisacodyl, Bisacolax, Bisco-Lax, Cenalax, Deficol, Dulcolax, Fleet Bisacodyl, Nuyac, Theralax)

Laxative: stimulant

ACTIONS AND USES. Diphenylmethane laxative structurally related to phenolphthalein. On contact, sensory nerve endings in the colonic wall are stimulated and by reflex parasympathetic action, widespread colonic peristaltic contractions produce evacuation.

Used for temporary relief of constipation and for evacuation of colon before surgery, proctoscopic sigmoidoscopic, and radiologic examinations. Also used to cleanse colon prior to delivery and to relieve constipation in patients with spinal cord damage. Available as one component of bowel evacuant kits with a saline laxative (Tridrate Bowel Evacuant Kit; Fleet Prep Kit).

ABSORPTION AND FATE. Acts within 6 to 12 hours following oral administration; acts 15 to 60 minutes after insertion of rectal suppository. Approximately 5% may be absorbed from GI tract, metabolized in liver, and excreted in urine, bile, and milk in conjugated form.

CONTRAINDICATIONS AND PRECAUTIONS. Hypersensitivity to bisacodyl or to ingredients in formulation; acute surgical abdomen, nausea, vomiting, abdominal cramps, intestinal obstruction, fecal impaction: use of rectal suppository in presence of anal or rectal fissures, ulcerated hemorrhoids, proctitis.

ADVERSE/SIDE EFFECTS. Systemic effects not reported. Rarely: mild cramping, nausea, vertigo, diarrhea, fluid and electrolyte disturbances (especially potassium and calcium). Rectal burning, irritation, and proctitis following use of suppositories for several weeks.

ROUTE AND DOSAGE. **Oral:** **Adults:** 10 to 15 mg (up to 30 mg may be given in preparation for special procedures). **Children (6 years and over):** 5 to 10 mg. **Rectal suppository** (at the time a bowel movement is required): **Adults and children (over 2 years):** 10 mg; **Children (under 2 years):** 5 mg.

B

NURSING IMPLICATIONS

In view of action time, administer oral drug in the evening or before breakfast. Suppository may be inserted at time bowel movement is desired.

Tablets are enteric coated; therefore, to avoid gastric irritation, they should be swallowed whole and not cut, crushed, or chewed. Preferably taken with a full glass (240 ml) of water or other liquid.

Advise patient not to take tablets within 1 hour of antacids or milk. These substances may cause premature dissolution of enteric coating, with release of drug in stomach resulting in gastric irritation and loss of cathartic action.

Bisacodyl usually produces 1 or 2 soft formed stools. Periodically evaluate patient's need for continued use of bisacodyl.

Note that *Dulcolax* contains tartrazine, which can cause allergic reactions including bronchial asthma in susceptible individuals. Frequently such persons are also sensitive to aspirin.

Patients with hypertension and cardiovascular disease should be cautioned to avoid excessive straining *(Valsalva maneuver)* during defecation. Straining causes concurrent rises in intrathoracic and venous pressures, momentarily interfering with free flow of blood out of heart. When patient stops straining, blood is quickly rushed through heart; this may result in tachycardia and even cardiac arrest in the susceptible patient.

Because of OTC availability, laxative abuse, especially among the elderly, is widespread. Recognize that the elderly patient who is preoccupied with bowel function may erroneously believe that failure to have a daily bowel movement can lead to "autointoxication."

Inform the habitual laxative user that a normal pattern for elimination varies from three bowel movements a day to three a week, depending on a self-established functionally effective schedule.

Food–Drug Interactions:

- *High fiber* in the diet is frequently prescribed as a supplement and eventual substitute for laxative use. Examples of high fiber foods: fruits (don't peel), blackberries; vegetables; baked beans, beet greens, broccoli, lima beans; artichoke; bran, wheat cereals and breads; cornmeal, coconut, nuts, and seeds.
- Dietary fiber absorbs water, increases stool volume, decreases intracolonic pressure, and reduces fecal transit time.
- Indiscriminate use of laxatives or dietary fiber can lead to changes in intestinal bacterial flora; some high fiber cereals (containing phytates) bind and reduce absorption of calcium, iron, zinc, and other trace minerals.
- Both selection and amounts of high fiber foods to supplement diet should be part of the teaching aimed at reducing laxative dependence. Some physicians recommend a supplement of 6 to 12 teaspoons of unprocessed bran a day. Consult physician and dietitian.

Overuse or misuse of bisacodyl or other laxatives can lead to decreased absorption of vitamin K and oral anticoagulants because of decreased transit time in the intestine.

A teaching plan designed to interrupt an older person's dependency on laxatives should take into account several age-related phenomena which influence gut motility:

- Heavy reliance on processed foods
- Decreased salivary flow
- Decreased thirst and hunger perceptions
- Inadequate food and fluid intake
- Dental problems
- Inactivity

B

Teaching Points Regarding Prevention of Constipation:

- ✓ Adequate fluid intake (7 to 10 glasses if allowed)
- ✓ Regular meal times
- ✓ High fiber foods (increase gradually to reduce intestinal flatus)
- ✓ Daily exercise program, e.g., brisk walking (if allowed)
- ✓ Unhurried and regular defecation time (duodenocolic and defecation reflexes are most active after meals, especially breakfast)
- ✓ Control of emotional factors, such as anxiety and depression

Bisacodyl tablets and suppositories are preserved in tight containers at temperatures not exceeding 30°C (86°F).

Drug Interactions. In general it is best not to take a laxative within 2 hours of taking other medications.

BISACODYL TANNEX

(Clysodrast)

(bis-a-koe′dill)
Laxative: stimulant

ACTIONS AND USES. Water-soluble complex of bisacodyl (qv), and tannic acid, which decreases mucus secretions in the large intestine.

Used to prepare patient for radiographic examination of lower bowel and rectum.

CONTRAINDICATIONS AND PRECAUTIONS. Patients with extensive ulcerations of colon. Safe use in women of childbearing potential, during pregnancy, and in children under 10 years not established. *Cautious Use:* patients receiving multiple enemas, elderly, and debilitated patients.

ADVERSE/SIDE EFFECTS. Abdominal cramping, weakness, fainting, nausea; hepatotoxicity (due to tannic acid, if absorbed in sufficient quantity).

ROUTE AND DOSAGE. Rectal: *Cleansing enema:* 1 packet (equivalent to bisacodyl 1.5 mg and tannic acid 2.5 Gm) in a liter of warm water. *Preparation for barium enema:* total dosage for one colonic examination should not exceed 3 packets. No more than 6 mg bisacodyl and 10 Gm tannic acid (equivalent to 4 packets) should be administered within a 72-hour period.

NURSING IMPLICATIONS

Physician generally prescribes residue-free diet (clear fluids) the day before and castor oil 30 to 60 ml 16 hours before radiologic, sigmoidoscopic, or proctoscopic examination.

Reconstituted solutions should be used as soon as prepared.

The cleansing enema may be given on the day of examination and repeated, if necessary.

The tannic acid portion of this complex may cause constipation. Be sure normal bowel pattern is reestablished following the diagnostic procedure.

B

BISMUTH SUBSALICYLATE

(Pepto-Bismol)

Antidiarrheal
Salicylate

ACTIONS AND USES. Thought to be hydrolyzed with release of salicylic acid which inhibits synthesis of prostaglandins, responsible for GI hypermotility and inflammation. Effectiveness as a prophylactic against diarrhea believed to be due to direct antimicrobial action and neutralization of enterotoxins particularly of *Escherichia coli* and *Vibrio cholerae.* Also reported to have protective coating action. Converted in small intestine to bismuth carbonate and sodium salicylate.

Used for prophylaxis and treatment of traveler's diarrhea, and for temporary relief of indigestion.

CONTRAINDICATIONS AND PRECAUTIONS. Use for more than 2 days in presence of high fever or in children under 3 years of age, unless prescribed by physician. *Cautious Use:* patient taking salicylates.

ADVERSE/SIDE EFFECTS. Temporary darkening of stool and tongue. With high doses: fecal impaction, *bismuth toxicity* (disorientation, muscle twitching, metallic taste, bluish gum line); *salicylism:* tinnitus, hearing loss, bleeding tendencies.

ROUTE AND DOSAGE. Oral: *Diarrhea:* **Adults:** 30 ml or 2 tablets; **Children (3 to 6 years):** 5 ml or ½ tablet; **Children (6 to 10 years):** 10 ml or 1 tablet; **Children (10 to 14 years):** 20 ml. Doses are repeated every 30 to 60 minutes if needed, up to 8 doses for no longer than 2 days. *Prophylactic use for traveler's diarrhea:* **Adults:** 60 ml four times daily for 3 weeks. (Pepto-Bismol suspension contains 524 mg bismuth subsalicylate per 30 ml, and chewable tablets contain 300 mg/tablet.) Contains no sugar.

NURSING IMPLICATIONS

Instruct patient to chew (chewable tablet) or allow it to dissolve in mouth.

Inform patient that drug contains salicylate and therefore must be used with caution with aspirin and other salicylates.

Prolonged use in the elderly, particularly, has caused bismuth encephalopathy. Prophylactic use should be limited to 3 weeks or less.

Tell patient that temporary grayish, black discoloration of tongue and stool may occur. (Note that this side effect may mask GI bleeding.)

Protect drug from light.

See Diphenoxylate with Atropine for nursing implications of antidiarrheal therapy.

Diagnostic Test Interferences. Because bismuth subsalicylate is radiopaque, it may interfere with radiographic studies of GI tract.

Drug Interactions: *See Aspirin (prototype salicylate) for possible interactions.*

BLEOMYCIN SULFATE

(Blenoxane)

(blee-oh-mye'sin)
Antineoplastic
Antibiotic

ACTIONS AND USES. Mixture of cytotoxic glycopeptide antibiotics from a strain of *Streptomyces verticillus.* A toxic drug with low therapeutic index; intensely cytotoxic. By unclear mechanism, blocks DNA, RNA, and protein synthesis. A cell cycle-phase nonspecific. Causes minimal immunosuppression and has capacity to release intracellular pyrogens leading to profound hyperpyrexia. Weak antibiotic activity is overshadowed by potent cytotoxic effects. Has strong affinity for skin and lung tumor cells, in contrast to its low affinity for cells in hematopoietic tissue (perhaps due to the high levels of bleomycin degrading enzymes found in bone marrow).

Used as single agent or in combination with other chemotherapeutic agents as adjunct to surgery and radiation therapy. Used in treatment of squamous cell carcinomas of head, neck, penis, cervix, and vulva; also lymphomas (including reticular cell sarcoma, lymphosarcoma, Hodgkin's), and testicular carcinoma. Intrapleural administration: to prevent pleural fluid accumulation. *Investigational Use:* treatment of mycosis fungoides.

ABSORPTION AND FATE. Absorbed systemically following subcutaneous, IV, IM, intrapleural, intraperitoneal, or intraperiocardial administration. Concentrates mainly in skin, lungs, kidneys, lymphocytes, peritoneum. Metabolic fate poorly understood; protein binding about 1%. In patient with creatinine clearance of more than 35 ml/minute, half-life is about 2 hours; in patient with clearance less than 35 ml/minute, half-life increases exponentially as creatinine clearance decreases. 60 to 70% of dose recovered in urine as active bleomycin.

CONTRAINDICATIONS AND PRECAUTIONS. Hypersensitivity to bleomycin, pregnancy, women of childbearing age. *Cautious Use:* compromised hepatic, renal, or pulmonary function, patients who have had previous cytotoxic drug or radiation therapy.

ADVERSE/SIDE EFFECTS. Dermatologic (over 50% of patients): stomatitis, oral ulcerations, alopecia, hyperpigmentation, patchy hyperkeratosis, peeling of skin, rash, striae, pruritic erythema, vesiculation, peeling, bleeding, acne, pigmented banding of nails and thickening of nail bed, angioedema, radiation recall. **GI:** nausea, vomiting, anorexia, diarrhea, weight loss. **Hematologic (rare):** thrombocytopenia, leukopenia, mild anemia. **Respiratory:** (dose and age-related): interstitial pneumonitis, pneumonia, or fibrosis. **Other:** anaphylactoid reaction: fever, chills, severe hyperpyrexia, hypotension, mental confusion, wheezing; headache, cystitis, pain at tumor site, phlebitis; renal, hepatic, and CNS toxicity; Raynaud's phenomenon, necrosis at injection site.

ROUTE AND DOSAGE. Dosage regimen highly individualized based on published protocols. **Subcutaneous, intramuscular, intravenous:** *Reticular cell sarcoma, Hodgkin's disease, squamous cell carcinoma, lymphosarcoma, testicular carcinoma:* 0.25 to 0.5 units/kg once or twice weekly to a total of 300 to 400 units. *Hodgkin's disease:* maintenance (after 50% response) intravenous, intramuscular: 1 unit daily or 5 units weekly. **Intraarterial infusion:** *squamous cell carcinoma of head, neck, cervix:* 30 to 60 units/day over 1 hour to 24 hours.

NURSING IMPLICATIONS

Used only under constant supervision by medical personnel experienced in cancer chemotherapy.

Reconstituted solutions are stable at room temperature for 2 weeks or for 4 weeks if refrigerated. Discard unused solutions.

IV and intraarterial injections should be administered slowly over a 10-minute period, or the solution may be further diluted with 50- to 100-ml diluent for administration by regional infusion.

Inject IM bleomycin deeply into upper outer quadrant of buttock; change sites with each injection.

Favorable response, if any is to occur, is expected within 2 weeks for treatment of Hodgkin's or testicular tumor, and within 3 weeks for squamous cell cancers.

Profound hyperthermia (chills and fever) especially after a large single dose may occur 4 to 6 hours after administration and lasts 4 to 12 hours. This reaction can be fatal. It is most apt to appear in patients with lymphoma. Reactions become less frequent with continued use of the drug, but may recur sporadically. Tepid sponge baths may provide relief.

Anaphylactoid reactions, sometimes fatal, may occur several hours after first or second dose, especially in lymphoma patients (10%).

Usually a test dose of 2 units of bleomycin is given to these patients for the first 2 doses. Patient is closely observed for at least 24 hours. If there is no acute reaction (hypotension, fever, chills, confusion, wheezing), regular dosage schedule is resumed.

Treatment for anaphylaxis is symptomatic and includes pressor agents, antihistamine, corticosteroids, volume expansion. Have emergency equipment and drugs readily available at the time of each bleomycin injection.

Aspirin and diphenhydramine may be prescribed as premedication to reduce onset of drug fever and risk of anaphylaxis; however, these drugs are ineffective as treatment for drug-induced hyperpyrexia.

If the treatment regimen includes concomitant therapy with an oral antineoplastic (such as vinblastine), plan with the patient the most feasible schedule for taking medication. Stress complete adherence to the established regimen.

Counsel patient to avoid using OTC drugs during antineoplastic treatment period unless such drugs are approved by physician.

Although bone marrow toxicity is rare, unexplained bleeding or bruising should be promptly reported to the physician.

Monitor patient for evidence of deterioration of renal function, i.e., changed intake and output ratio and pattern, weight gain (edema), decreasing creatinine clearance. Bleomycin will be discontinued if kidney function diminishes, because of increased danger of toxicity. Reference limits for creatinine clearance: 90 to 120 ml/minute.

Pulmonary toxicity occurs in about 10% of all patients and most frequently in patients over 70 years of age or when the total of all doses approaches 400 units. It may also occur in young people, however, and with lower doses.

Subclinical pulmonary toxicity may be determined by changes in pulmonary diffusion capacity for carbon monoxide (DL_{CO}). If DL_{CO} decreases to 30 or 35% below pretreatment level, bleomycin will be discontinued. Sequential measurements of single breath DL_{CO} and determinations of vital capacity are monitored at regular intervals during therapy.

Monitor, by interrogation of patient, for nonproductive cough, chest pain, dyspnea; by auscultation for fine rales; and by serial chest x-rays for structural signs of pulmonary toxicity. If pulmonary fibrosis is present, drug will be discontinued.

Skin toxicity usually develops in second or third week of treatment and after 150 to 200 units of bleomycin have been administered. Report symptoms (hypoesthesias, urticaria, tender swollen hands) promptly; therapy may be discontinued.

Be alert to evidence of *radiation recall,* i.e., erythema that develops in a previously unradiated field. Most frequently occurs when chemotherapy is started during or shortly after radiation therapy, but it also may be observed several years after the treatment. Protect such an area or a pressure area by frequent observation, scheduled, gentle, soapless skin care, and programmed mobility.

Inform patient that hyperpigmentation may occur in areas subject to friction and pressure, skin folds, nail cuticles, scars, and intramuscular sites.

Stomatitis may be a dose-limiting factor because oral ulcerations can interfere with adequate nutrient intake leading to severe debilitation. Consult physician if an oral local anesthetic seems to be indicated. It may help patient to eat if agent is applied about 10 minutes before eating.

Check weight at regular intervals under standard conditions. Weight loss and anorexia may persist a long time after therapy has been discontinued. Arrange for a conference between the dietitian and patient to allow conjoint planning for strategies to maintain oral intake.

Although this drug causes nausea and vomiting, it is important that the established administration schedule for injections be maintained. Antiemetic drugs may be prescribed.

If patient is receiving bleomycin for testicular carcinoma, advise him to observe and report early signs of Raynaud's phenomenon: hands and feet constantly cold especially when exposed; intermittent blanching and cyanosis in finger and toe tips; swelling of fingers and toes. Signs can occur during or after therapy has been discontinued.

Store unopened ampuls between 15° and 30°C (59° and 86°F), unless otherwise specified by manufacturer.

Patient-Teaching Points for Mouth Care:

- ✓ Inspect oral membranes regularly for oral bleeding, pain, or ulceration. Report if present.
- ✓ Caries following radiation or chemotherapy must be controlled if teeth are to be retained. Mechanical removal of plaque is the best preventive measure.
- ✓ Initiate prophylactic and comfort measures: frequent rinses with warm water, saline, or diluted hydrogen peroxide solution; use a soft toothbrush or cotton-covered finger, flossing with waxed floss at least once daily, avoid overuse of commercial mouth rinses, avoid highly acid food and drink, and coarse physically "scratchy" foods.
- ✓ *See Mechlorethamine for additional points about mouth care*

Drug Interactions. **Antineoplastics,** other **radiation therapy** may lead to increased bleomycin toxicity including bone marrow depression. Pharmacologic effects of phenytoin (Dilantin) may be reduced. Monitor phenytoin plasma levels.

BORIC ACID

(Boracic Acid, Borofax)

(bor'ik)
Antiinfective (topical)

ACTIONS AND USES. Weak acid with fungistatic and feeble bacteriostatic properties.

Used externally for temporary relief of various minor conditions of eye, ear, skin, and mucous membranes. Commercially available in combination with sodium borate as sterile isotonic ophthalmic irrigation solutions, e.g., Blinx, Lauro, Trisol, for use following tonometry and gonioscopy procedures and to rinse eye free of foreign material. An ingredient with isopropyl alcohol in several ear preparations for infections of external ear canal, e.g., Auro-Dri, Dri-Ear, Ear-Dry, Swim Ear. Also available in combination with benzoic acid for treatment of athletes foot, e.g., Ting.

CONTRAINDICATIONS AND PRECAUTIONS. Application to abraded or denuded surfaces or to inflamed or granulating tissue; preparation of nipples for nursing; irrigation of closed wound cavities; use of otic preparations in perforated eardrum or excoriated ear canal.

ADVERSE/SIDE EFFECTS. *Following absorption or accidental ingestion:* nausea, vomiting, diarrhea, abdominal pain, muscular weakness, hypothermia, headache, restlessness, skin eruptions, hair loss, kidney damage, tachycardia, dyspnea, circulatory collapse, delirium, convulsions, coma.

ROUTE AND DOSAGE. Topical: aqueous solution, powder (1 to 4%), topical ointment (5%, 10%).

B

NURSING IMPLICATIONS

The Subcommittee on Accidental Poisoning of the American Academy of Pediatrics has recommended that boric acid be eliminated from newborn nurseries in all hospitals.

Boric acid should be applied only to intact skin. Application to abraded skin or open wounds has caused fatal poisoning in infants. Deaths from accidental ingestion have also been reported.

Applications of boric acid should not be made over large areas or for prolonged periods, in order to avoid possibility of absorption.

Use only sterile ophthalmic preparations for applications to the eyes. Apply as directed.

If irritation occurs, discontinue use and consult physician.

Because of danger of contamination, boric acid solution should be used as soon as reconstituted. Container should bear "poison" label as well as contents.

Boric acid is incompatible with polyvinyl alcohol and tannins.

Store at room temperature, preferably around 25°C (77°F), unless otherwise directed by manufacturer.

BRETYLIUM TOSYLATE

(Bretylate, Bretylol)

(bre-til'ee-um)
Adrenergic blocking agent (sympatholytic)
Antiarrhythmic (class III)

ACTIONS AND USES. Quaternary ammonium compound; mechanism of action is complex and not fully understood. Suppresses ventricular fibrillation by direct action on the myocardium and ventricular tachycardia by adrenergic blockade. Shortly after administration, norepinephrine is released from adrenergic postganglionic nerve terminals resulting in a moderate increase in blood pressure, heart rate, and ventricular irritability. Subsequently (1 to 2 hours) both release and reuptake of norepinephrine are blocked because of drug-induced depression of adrenergic nerve terminal excitability. Electrophysiologic events: initially bretylium causes hyperpolarization during diastole, increases conduction velocity, and shortens action potential (AP) and effective refractory period. After adrenergic blockade is established, Phase 3 (repolarization) is prolonged group III antiarrhythmic characteristic. Phase 4 (spontaneous depolarization of conducting system cells) is unaffected. These effects suppress arrhythmias with a reentry mechanism and decrease dispersion of ectopic foci. PR, QT, and QRS intervals are unchanged. Orthostatic hypotension occurs commonly as a result of peripheral adrenergic blockade; some degree of hypotension may occur even while patient is supine. Tolerance to this effect develops after several days in most patients as adrenergic receptors become more responsive to circulating catecholamines (as opposed to synaptic catecholamine). Has no apparent CNS or cholinergic blockade effects, and effect on GI motility is less than with other adrenergic blockers. Has weak local anesthetic properties. Because onset of desired action is delayed, bretylium is not a first-line antiarrhythmic agent.

Used for short-term treatment of life-threatening ventricular tachycardia in patients who have not responded to conventional therapy such as lidocaine, procainamide, direct current countershock (cardioversion). Formerly used orally for treatment of hypertension, but found to be unsuitable for long-term therapy because of tolerance and troublesome side effects (orthostatic hypotension, parotid pain).

ABSORPTION AND FATE. Antifibrillatory effect begins within minutes following IV administration. Suppression of ventricular tachycardia, PVCs, and other arrhythmias may require 20 minutes to 2 hours (delay is longer after IM than IV); maximal effect in 6 to 9 hours; duration up to 24 hours. Half-life: 4 to 17 hours (longer in patients with impaired renal function). Does not pass blood–brain barrier. Not metabolized. Eliminated unchanged by kidneys; 70 to 80% of dose excreted during first 24 hours, and an additional 10% over the following 3 days. Distribution to placenta and breast milk not known.

CONTRAINDICATIONS AND PRECAUTIONS. No contraindications for use in life-threatening ventricular fibrillation or arrhythmias. Contraindications for less serious arrhythmia: digitalis-induced arrythmias, patients with fixed cardiac output such as severe aortic stenosis, severe pulmonary hypertension (profound hypotension can result without compensatory increase in cardiac output). Safe use during pregnancy, in nursing mothers, and in children not established. *Cautious Use:* impaired renal function, sinus bradycardia, patients on digitalis maintenance.

ADVERSE/SIDE EFFECTS. CV: both supine and postural hypotension with dizziness, vertigo, light-headedness, faintness, syncope, transitory hypertension, bradycardia, increased frequency of PVCs, exacerbation of digitalis-induced arrhythmias, precipitation of angina, sensation of substernal pressure. **GI:** nausea, vomiting (particularly with rapid IV), loose stools, diarrhea, abdominal pain, anorexia. **Neuropsychiatric:** involuntary head movements, headache, muscle weakness, aching sensation in legs, generalized tenderness; confusion, paranoid psychosis, emotional lability, lethargy, anxiety. **Skin:** erythematous macular rash, flushing, sweating. **Other:** nasal stuffiness, mild conjunctivitis, hiccoughs, renal dysfunction, IM injection site reactions, shortness of breath, respiratory depression, hyperthermia.

ROUTE AND DOSAGE. *Life-threatening ventricular fibrillation:* **Intravenous:** *(undiluted solution):* 5 mg/kg by rapid IV injection; if fibrillation persists, dosage increased to 10 mg/kg and repeated every 15 to 30 minutes, as necessary to maximum of 30 mg/kg/day. Maintenance: *(diluted solution)* administered at 1 to 2 mg/minute by continuous IV infusion, or 5 to 10 mg/kg by *slow* intermittent infusion, over a period greater than 8 minutes every 6 hours. *Other ventricular arrhythmias:* **Intravenous use** (*diluted solution):* 5 to 10 mg/kg by IV infusion over period greater than 8 minutes; repeated at 1 to 2 hour intervals if arrhythmia persists. **Intramuscular use:** 5 to 10 mg/kg *(undiluted solution):* repeated in 1 to 2 hours if arrhythmia persists; thereafter, same dose every 6 to 8 hours for maintenance. **Directions for dilution:** dilute contents of ampul (500 mg) to minimum of 50 ml with dextrose 5% or sodium chloride injection.

NURSING IMPLICATIONS

Use of bretylium should be limited to patients in facilities adequately equipped and staffed for constant monitoring of ECG and blood pressure, and for cardiopulmonary resuscitation, and cardioversion, if necessary.

Administer no more than 5 ml in any one IM site. Avoid injecting into or near a major nerve. Keep a record of injection sites. Injection into same site can cause muscle atrophy, necrosis and fibrosis.

Monitor patient closely for initial transient rise in blood pressure, increased heart rate, PVCs and other arrhythmias, or worsening of existing arrhythmias which may occur within a few minutes to 1 hour after drug administration. Usually patients eventually stabilize to these effects.

Initial effect of hypertension is usually followed within 1 hour by a fall in supine blood pressure and by orthostatic hypotension.

The supine position is recommended until patient develops tolerance to the hypotensive effect of bretylium (generally in several days). Hypotension can occur in the supine position, particularly in patients with severely compromised cardiac function. It may not readily respond to therapy (e.g., vasopressors, fluids), therefore, early reporting is essential.

A systolic blood pressure greater than 75 mm Hg usually need not be treated unless associated

B

with symptoms of hypotension: faintness, light-headedness, dizziness. If systolic blood pressure drops to 75 mm Hg or below, it is cautiously treated with dopamine (Intropin) or low doses of diluted norepinephrine (Levarterenol, Levophed). Plasma or blood may be required for plasma volume expansion.

To prevent orthostatic hypotension, raise or lower head of bed slowly and advise patient to make position changes slowly. If patient is allowed to be out of bed caution to dangle legs for a few minutes before standing and not to stand still for prolonged periods. Advise male patient to sit on toilet to urinate.

IV administration is associated with a high incidence of nausea and vomiting. These side effects can be minimized by slow administration of drug (over 10 or more minutes).

Bretylium dosage should be reduced gradually and discontinued after 3 to 5 days under close ECG monitoring. Another antiarrhythmic agent may be substituted if indicated.

Unopened vials stored preferably between 15° and 30°C (59° and 86°F), unless otherwise directed by manufacturer.

Diagnostic Test Interferences. **Urinary VMA, epinephrine,** and **norepinephrine** levels may be decreased during bretylium therapy.

Drug Interactions: Bretylium

Plus	Interactions
Antiarrhythmics, other e.g., lidocaine, procainamide, propranolol (Inderal), quinidine	Cardiac effects may be antagonistic or additive; toxic effects may be additive when administered concomitantly with bretylium
Antihypertensive agents	Potentiation of hypotensive effect (during early bretylium therapy)
Digitalis glycosides	May worsen arrhythmias caused by digitalis toxicity. Bretylium and digitalis should not be given simultaneously as initial treatments

---

BROMOCRIPTINE MESYLATE
(Parlodel)

(broe-moe-krip'teen)
Dopamine receptor agonist
Antiparkinsonian agent

ACTIONS AND USES. Semisynthetic ergot alkaloid derivative, but devoid of oxytocic activity generally attributed to drugs of this class. Reduces elevated serum prolactin levels in men and women by activating postsynaptic dopaminergic receptors in hypothalamus to stimulate release of prolactin inhibiting factor and possibly luteinizing hormone release factor. Ovulation and ovarian function in amenorrheic women are restored (by direct action on ovary), thus correcting female infertility secondary to elevated prolactin levels. (Correction of male infertility has not been documented.) Growth hormone secretion is increased transiently in patient with normal concentrations but parodoxically is suppressed in some patients with acromegaly. Pretreatment levels are restored 2 to 4 weeks after bromocriptine is discontinued. Activates dopaminergic receptors in neostriatum of CNS, which may explain action in parkinsonian syndrome: improvement in symptoms 30 to 90 minutes after administration of the drug with maximum effects experienced in 2 hours. Bromocriptine also reduces blood pressure in the hypertensive and normotensive individual and may cause peripheral vasoconstriction (large doses) and increased sodium excretion.

Used for short-term management of amenorrhea/galactorrhea or female infertility associated with hyperprolactemia (when there is no indication of pituitary tumor) and to prevent physiologic lactation. Also used as adjunctive to levodopa or levodopa/carbidopa therapy to relieve symptoms of Parkinson's disease. *Investigational Use:* to relieve premenstrual symptoms, to treat hypogonadism and galactorrhea in hyperprolactinemic men, and to lower plasma growth hormone in patients with acromegaly.

ABSORPTION AND FATE. Approximately 28% of oral dose absorbed from GI tract. Plasma levels peak in about 1 to 2 hours; duration of action 4 to 8 hours. About 90 to 96% bound to serum albumin. Half-life: 3 to 8 hours. Completely metabolized in liver to inactive metabolites. Eighty-five percent of dose excreted within 5 days in feces via bile; about 3 to 6% eliminated in urine.

CONTRAINDICATIONS AND PRECAUTIONS. Sensitivity to ergot alkaloids; severe ischemic heart disease or peripheral vascular disease; patients with pituitary tumor; patients with normal prolactin levels, nursing women. Safe use during pregnancy and in children under 15 years not established. *Cautious Use:* hepatic and renal dysfunction, history of psychiatric disorder, history of myocardial infarction with residual arrhythmia.

ADVERSE/SIDE EFFECTS. (Mostly dose related.) **CV:** transient decrease in blood pressure, orthostatic hypotension, shock, palpitation, extrasystoles, digitospasm in response to cold (Raynaud's phenomenon), red, tender, hot, edematous extremities (erythromelalgia), exacerbation of angina, arrhythmias. **Dermatologic:** urticaria, rash, mottling, livedo reticularis. **GI:** nausea, vomiting, epigastric pain, abdominal cramps, constipation (long-term use) or diarrhea; metallic taste, dry mouth, dysphagia, anorexia, peptic ulcers, GI tract hemorrhage. **GU:** diuresis, urinary frequency, urinary incontinence, urinary retention. **Neuropsychiatric:** headache, dizziness, vertigo, light-headedness, fainting, sedation, nightmares, insomnia, dyskinesia, confusion, ataxia; visual and auditory hallucinations, paranoid delusions (particularly in patients with Parkinson's disease or those receiving high dosages); "on–off" phenomenon, mania, nervousness, anxiety, depression, seizures. **Ophthalmic:** blurred vision, burning sensation in eyes, blepharospasm, diplopia. **Other:** fatigue, asthenia, nasal congestion, ergotism (tingling and numbness of fingers, cramps in feet and legs, cold extremities), pulmonary infiltration, pleural effusion and thickening with long-term therapy (6 to 36 months), severe postpartum hypertension (causal relationship not established), hepatotoxicity (rare).

ROUTE AND DOSAGE. Oral: *Amenorrhea/galactorrhea; female infertility:* Initial: 1.25 to 2.5 mg daily; maintenance: 2.5 mg two or three times daily. Suppression of puerperal lactation: 2.5 mg one to three times daily with meals; for 14 up to 21 days, if necessary. *Parkinson's disease:* 2.5 to 100 mg daily in divided doses; maximum: 100 mg daily. *Acromegaly:* Initial: 1.25 to 2.5 mg daily; maintenance: 10 to 60 mg in divided doses.

NURSING IMPLICATIONS

General Information for All Patients:

Administer with meals, milk, or other food to reduce incidence of GI side effects.

Establish data regarding baseline vital signs. Therapy should not be initiated until vital signs are stable.

Since hypotension with dizziness and fainting may occur, particularly following first dose in sensitive patients, initial dose is usually prescribed for evening administration.

Blood pressure should be monitored closely during the first few days of therapy and periodically throughout therapy, for all patients. Compare readings with baseline data.

Instruct patient to make position changes slowly and in stages, especially from recumbent to upright posture, and to dangle legs over bed for a few minutes before ambulating. Caution patient to lie down immediately if lightheadedness or dizziness occurs.

Inform patient that a mild diuresis may occur due to vasodilating action of bromocriptine on renal arteries.

Side effects occur commonly but they are usually mild to moderate in degree and respond to dosage reduction or discontinuation of drug.

Since bromocriptine is associated with dose-related lightheadedness, dizziness, and syncope, caution patient to avoid driving and other potentially hazardous activities until reaction to drug has been determined.

Bromocriptine can cause digital vasospasm, particularly in patients with acromegaly and patients receiving high dosages. Advise patient to avoid exposure to cold and to report the onset of pallor of fingers or toes.

Patients should be advised that bromocriptine may make them more sensitive to the effects of alcohol.

Periodic evaluations should be made of hepatic, hematologic, cardiovascular, and renal function in patients on prolonged therapy.

Store in well-closed, light-resistant containers, preferably between 15° and 30°C (59° and 86°F), unless otherwise directed by manufacturer.

Parkinson's Disease:

Note that dosages for Parkinson's disease may be almost ten times larger than those for galactorrhea and amenorrhea. Close medical supervision is indicated in patients with Parkinson's disease. Psychotic symptoms occur most frequently in these patients.

In patients with Parkinson's disease, bromocriptine is administered with concomitant reduction of levodopa or levodopa/carbodopa dosages.

Patients should be evaluated at 2-week intervals during dosage titration to establish lowest effective dosage level.

Possible therapeutic effects in patients with Parkinson's disease include reduction in levodopa-induced dyskinesia (abnormal involuntary movements, tremor, rigidity), bradykinesia (slow movements), reduced frequency of "on–off" phenomenon (abrupt swings from immobility to mobility).

Suppression of Puerperal Lactation:

Because hypotension occurs most commonly in the postpartum patient, it is recommended that therapy not be started any sooner than 4 hours after delivery and then only if vital signs have stabilized.

Severe postpartum hypertension (including cerebrovascular accidents and seizures) have occurred 6 to 9 days after delivery. Causal relationship not established. Monitor blood pressure at regular intervals.

Patients receiving bromocriptine to suppress postpartum lactation may have temporary rebound breast enlargement and pain following drug withdrawal.

Amenorrhea/Galactorrhea; Infertility:

In patients with hyperprolactinemia, a complete evaluation of the sella turcica is recommended before initiation of therapy, including x-rays, posterior, anterior, and lateral tomography, to rule out pituitary tumor.

Patients being treated for amenorrhea/galactorrhea should be informed that restoration of regular menses occurs in 6 to 8 weeks (range: a few days to 24 weeks). (If patient has been amenorrheic more than 4 years, restoration of menses may require considerable time.) Galactorrhea suppression is usually seen after 7 to 12 weeks of therapy, but may not occur for more than 24 weeks. Maximum reduction of prolactin level generally occurs within the first 4 weeks of therapy. Normal plasma prolactin concentration is approximately 5 to 10 ng/ml.

Because long-term drug effects are not known, it is recommended that duration of therapy for amenorrhea and galactorrhea not exceed 6 months.

Recurrence rates of amenorrhea and galactorrhea are high (70 to 80%) following withdrawal of bromocriptine. Amenorrhea usually returns within 4 to 24 weeks; galactorrhea within 2 to 12 weeks; serum prolactin increases to pretreatment levels within 1 to 6 weeks.

Since restoration of fertility may result during therapy, patients being treated for amenorrhea and galactorrhea should be advised to use barrier type contraceptive measures until normal ovulating cycle is restored. Oral contraceptives are contraindicated because they may cause amenorrhea and galactorrhea.

Advise patient to inform physician immediately if pregnancy occurs during therapy. Bromocriptine should be discontinued without delay. These patients should be carefully observed throughout pregnancy. Because of the possible presence of a previously undetected prolactin-secreting pituitary tumor, which could cause optic nerve compression, visual fields should be checked monthly.

A pregnancy test is recommended at least every 4 months during the period of amenorrhea. Once menstruation is reestablished, a pregnancy test should be performed every time patient misses a menstrual period.

Diagnostic Test Interferences. Transient increases in **serum growth hormone (GH)** may occur in patients with normal levels, and paradoxical decreases in patients with acromegaly (GH returns to pretreatment levels within 2 weeks in acromegalic patients). **SGOT (AST), SGPT (ALT), alkaline phosphatase, GGPT, CPK, BUN, uric acid** may be transiently increased (generally not significant at therapeutic doses).

Drug Interactions: Bromocriptine

Plus	Interactions
Alcohol (ethanol)	Possibility of decreased tolerance to alcohol particularly patients with acromegaly
Antihypertensives	Additive hypotensive effects
Contraceptives, oral	May interfere with effect of bromocriptine by causing amenorrhea and galactorrhea
Amitriptyline Droperidol (Inapsine) Haloperidol (Haldol) Imipramine (Tofranil) Methyldopa (Aldomet) Phenothiazines Reserpine	Increases in serum prolactin levels induced by these drugs may interfere with bromocriptine action and require higher bromocriptine dosage
Levodopa	Possibility of additive effects allows reduction of levodopa dosage when given concomitantly with bromocriptine

BROMPHENIRAMINE MALEATE

(brome-fen-ir'a-meen)
Antihistamine
(H_1-receptor antagonist)

(Bromamine, Brombay, Bromphen, Codimal-A, Diamine T.D., Dimetane, Dimetane Extentabs, Veltane)

ACTIONS AND USES. Propylamine (alkylamine) antihistaminic similar to chlorpheniramine (qv) in actions, uses, pharmacokinetics, contraindications, and adverse effects. Produces less sedative effect than chlorpheniramine.

Used for symptomatic treatment of allergic manifestations. Also used in various cough mixtures and antihistamine-decongestant cold formulations.

ABSORPTION AND FATE. Serum levels peak in 2 to 5 hours following oral administration. Maximal antihistaminic effect with 3 to 9 hours; duration up to 48 hours. Half-life: 12 to 34 hours. About 40% of oral dose excreted in urine within 72 hours (5 to 10% as unchanged drug); 2% fecal elimination.

CONTRAINDICATIONS AND PRECAUTIONS. Hypersensitivity to antihistamines, use in newborns, nursing mothers, acute asthma, patients receiving MAO inhibitors. *Cautious Use:* prostatic hypertrophy, narrow angle glaucoma. *See also Chlorpheniramine.*

ADVERSE/SIDE EFFECTS. Sedation, drowsiness, dry mouth, dizziness, headache, disturbed coordination, urticaria, rash, agranulocytosis, thrombocytopenia. *See Chlorpheniramine.*

ROUTE AND DOSAGE. Oral: Adults: 4 mg every 4 to 6 hours as needed, or 8 to 12 mg of sustained action form every 8 to 12 hours as needed; not to exceed 24 mg/24 hours. **Children (over 6 years):** 2 mg every 4 to 6 hours as needed, or 8 to 12 mg of sustained release form every 12 hours as needed; not to exceed 12 mg/24 hours; **Children: (2 to 6 years)** 1 mg every 4 to 6 hours as needed; not to exceed 6 mg/24 hours. **Subcutaneous, intramuscular, intravenous: Adults:** 5 to 20 mg every 6 to 12 hours (not to exceed 40 mg in 24-hour period). **Children (under 12 years):** 0.5 mg/kg/24 hours divided into three or four doses.

NURSING IMPLICATIONS

If gastric distress occurs advise patient to take medication with meals or a snack.

Brompheniramine may be given IM or SC without dilution; IV administration may be undiluted or diluted with 5% dextrose or 0.9% sodium chloride, unless otherwise specified by manufacturer. IV should be administered slowly.

Drowsiness, sweating, transient hypotension, and syncope may follow IV administration. Patient should be recumbent while receiving injection, and reaction to drug should be evaluated. Keep physician informed.

Acute hypersensitivity reaction with sudden severe agranulocytosis reportedly can occur within minutes to hours after drug ingestion. The reaction is manifested by high fever, chills, and possible development of gangrenous ulcerations of mouth and throat, pneumonia, and prostration. Patient should seek medical attention immediately.

Elderly patients tend to be particularly susceptible to sedative effect, dizziness, and hypotension. Most symptoms respond to reduction in dosage.

Bear in mind that brompheniramine has an atropine-like effect (thickens bronchial secretions) that may make expectoration difficult.

Thickened bronchial secretions and dry mouth, nose, and throat may be relieved by increasing fluid intake (consult physician). Relief of dry mouth may be provided by sugarless gum or lemon drops, frequent rinses with warm water, diligent mouth care.

Blood counts should be performed in patients receiving long-term therapy, in order to preclude possibility of blood dyscrasias.

Caution patient to avoid driving a car or other potentially hazardous activities until reaction to drug is known.

Advise patient not to take alcoholic beverages and other CNS depressants, e.g., tranquilizers, sedatives, pain or sleeping medicines, without consulting physician.

In common with other antihistamines, brompheniramine may cause false-negative allergy skin tests. The drug should be discontinued about 4 days before such tests are done.

Store in tightly covered container, preferably between 15° and 30°C (59° and 86°F) unless otherwise directed by manufacturer. Elixir and parenteral form should be protected from

B

light. Crystals may form when parenteral solution is stored below 0°C. Redissolve by warming to 30°C (86°F). Avoid freezing.

See Chlorpheniramine (prototype propylamine antihistamine) for Nursing Implications and Drug Interactions.

BROMPTON'S COCKTAIL

(brom'tuns)
Narcotic analgesic
Opiate agonist
C II

ACTIONS AND USES. Brompton's Cocktail originated in Brompton Hospital in England. The term now includes a variety of analgesic mixtures containing the basic formula of a narcotic analgesic such as methadone, morphine, or diacetylmorphine (heroin), a CNS stimulant (e.g., cocaine or dextroamphetamine) to counteract narcotic-induced sedation and respiratory depression, up to 40% alcohol (as ethanol, gin, brandy, or sweet vermouth) to enhance sedation, and a flavoring agent such as syrup or honey to improve palatability. A phenothiazine (chlorpromazine, prochlorperazine, promethazine) may be given separately or combined in the mixture to alleviate nausea and to potentiate analgesic and sedative actions. Usually the principal ingredient is morphine in the U.S. and heroin in Great Britain. Advantage over use of a narcotic analgesic alone is that tolerance does not develop rapidly and patient can be maintained in a comparatively pain-free euphoric state without excessive sedation. Additionally, patient has a sense of control over pain.

Used to relieve chronic severe pain as in terminal cancer.

CONTRAINDICATIONS AND PRECAUTIONS. Increased intracranial pressure, respiratory depression. *See Morphine.*

ADVERSE/SIDE EFFECTS. Nausea, vomiting, constipation, sedation, drowsiness, insomnia, agitation, hypotension, respiratory depression, urinary retention, physical dependence. *See Morphine.*

ROUTE AND DOSAGE. The formula for Brompton's Cocktail varies from institution to institution. Dosage interval depends upon duration of action of component drugs. **Oral:** 10 to 20 ml (official formula). Formulations containing morphine are generally given every 3 or 4 hours; methadone containing mixtures are usually given every 6 to 8 hours. When necessary, dosage adjustments are made at 48- to 72-hour intervals.

NURSING IMPLICATIONS

Instruct patient and responsible family member to measure medication accurately by means of standard medicine cup.

Check expiration date before pouring. The officially recognized formula is stable for 4 weeks at room temperature (30°C) and for 6 months under refrigeration (4°C). Other mixtures should be discarded if unused after 2 weeks, following preparation.

Medication may be served over ice if desired, but do not mix with soft drinks or fruit juices if mixture contains cocaine. (Acidic pH enhances breakdown of cocaine in GI tract.)

If mixture contains cocaine, instruct patient to swish medication in mouth for about 15 seconds before swallowing, to facilitate absorption of cocaine through oral mucosa. Cocaine is degraded in GI tract and therefore is poorly absorbed otherwise.

Brompton's Cocktail is usually prescribed around the clock rather than PRN or on demand, and at sufficiently short intervals to keep pain under constant control.

B

Once dosage has been stabilized, changes in dosage requirements generally indicate alterations in the disease state rather than tolerance to analgesic action. Keep physician informed.
Successful management of pain requires control of factors that may increase pain awareness such as anxiety, fear, depression.
The risk of inducing tolerance and dependence is not usually considered of primary importance in patients with terminal illness.
The patient may require a stool softener to prevent constipation.
Respiratory function must be closely monitored whenever a dosage increase is made.
Brompton's Cocktail is classified as a Schedule II substance under the Federal Controlled Substances Act.

BUCLIZINE HYDROCHLORIDE

(Bucladin-S Softabs)

(byoo'kli-zeen)
Antihistamine
(H_1-receptor antagonist)
Antivertigo agent, antiemetic

ACTIONS AND USES. Piperazine antihistamine derivative of diphenylmethane structurally and pharmacologically related to other cyclizine compounds. In common with similar compounds, exhibits mild CNS depressant, central anticholinergic, antiemetic, and local anesthetic effects in addition to antihistaminic activity.

Used in management of mild anxiety states and to prevent and alleviate nausea, vomiting, and vertigo associated with motion sickness, labyrinthitis, and Meniere's syndrome.

ABSORPTION AND FATE. Duration of action 4 to 6 hours. Metabolic fate unknown. May be excreted in breast milk.

CONTRAINDICATIONS AND PRECAUTIONS. Hypersensitivity to cyclizines or to tartrazine. Safe use during pregnancy, in nursing mothers and in children not established. *Cautious Use:* narrow-angle glaucoma, prostatic hypertrophy, bladder neck obstruction, peptic ulcer.

ADVERSE/SIDE EFFECTS. Drowsiness, dizziness, headache, insomnia, nervousness, agitation; dry mouth, nose, and throat; anorexia, nausea, vomiting, blurred vision, mild hypotension.

ROUTE AND DOSAGE. Oral: 25 to 50 mg one to three times daily at 4- to 6-hour intervals. Maintenance: 50 mg twice daily.

NURSING IMPLICATIONS

Bucladin-S Softabs may be chewed, swallowed whole, or allowed to dissolve in the mouth.
When used to prevent motion sickness, buclizine should be taken at least 30 minutes before beginning travel. When travel time is extended, a second 50 mg tablet may be taken after 4 to 6 hours.
Warn patient of possibility of pronounced drowsiness and caution against driving a car or operating machinery or other activities requiring mental alertness.
Bucladin-S Softabs contains tartrazine, which may cause allergic type reaction including bronchial asthma in certain individuals, particularly those with aspirin sensitivity.
Bear in mind that concurrent use with ototoxic drug, e.g., aminoglycoside antibiotics, aspirin, may mask symptoms of ototoxicity.
Psychic dependence and addiction have not been reported, but they should be borne in

mind when drug is administered for tranquilizing effect, particularly in patients who may abuse its use. Watch to see that patient takes drug and does not hoard it.

Advise patient to avoid alcohol and not to take other CNS depressants, e.g., tranquilizers, pain or sleeping medicines without consulting physician.

Abrupt withdrawal of buclizine after extended use with large doses may cause sudden reversal of an improved state or may cause paradoxic reactions.

Store at room temperature preferably between 15° and 30°C (59° and 86°F), unless otherwise directed by manufacturer.

BUMETANIDE
(Bumex)

(byoo-met′a-nide)
Diuretic (loop)
Sulfonamide derivative

ACTIONS AND USES. Sulfonamide derivative structurally related to furosemide and with similar pharmacologic effects. Diuretic activity is 40 times greater, however, and duration of action is shorter than that of furosemide. Inhibits sodium and chloride reabsorption by direct action on ascending limit of the loop of Henle. Also appears to inhibit phosphate and bicarbonate reabsorption in proximal renal tubule. Produces only mild hypotensive effects at usual diuretic doses.

Used for edema associated with congestive heart failure, and hepatic or renal disease, including nephrotic syndrome. Has been used in management of postoperative and premenstrual edema and edema accompanying disseminated carcinoma, and for mild hypertension. May be used concomitantly with a potassium-sparing diuretic to prevent hypokalemia.

ABSORPTION AND FATE. Rapidly and almost completely absorbed following oral administration; completely absorbed following IM or IV injection. Onset of diuretic effect: 30 to 60 minutes after oral, about 40 minutes after IM, and within a few minutes following IV administration. With usual doses, diuresis is usually completed within 4 hours after oral or IM administration and 2 to 3 hours after IV. About 95% protein bound; half-life 60 to 90 minutes. Partially metabolized in liver. About 80% of dose excreted in urine within 48 hours (50% as unchanged drug); 10 to 20% eliminated in feces via bile. Excreted in breast milk.

CONTRAINDICATIONS AND PRECAUTIONS. Hypersensitivity to bumetanide or to other sulfonamides; anuria, markedly elevated BUN; hepatic coma, severe electrolyte deficiency. Safe use during pregnancy, in nursing mothers, and in children under 18 years not established. *Cautious Use:* hepatic cirrhosis, ascites.

ADVERSE/SIDE EFFECTS. CNS: dizziness, headache, weakness, fatigue. **CV:** hypotension, ECG changes, chest pain, hypovolemia, circulatory collapse with thromboses and emboli. **GI:** nausea, vomiting, abdominal or stomach pain, GI distress, diarrhea, dry mouth. **Hematologic/Electrolyte:** dehydration; increases or decreases Hgb, Hct, platelets, leukocytes; changes in differential count; hypokalemia, hyponatremia, hyperuricemia, hyperglycemia; decreases in blood magnesium, calcium, chloride, ammonium, bicarbonate, phosphorus; increased serum creatinine; azotemia. **Hepatic:** increased or decreased serum cholesterol, increased LDH, AST (SGOT), ALT (SGPT), alkaline phosphatase. **Musculoskeletal:** muscle cramps, muscle stiffness or tenderness, arthritic pain. **Ototoxicity:** ear discomfort, impaired hearing. **Reproductive:** breast or nipple tenderness, gynecomastia, premature ejaculation, difficulty maintaining erection. **Skin:** pruritus, urticaria, rash, purpura, Stevens-Johnson syndrome. **Other:** sweating, hyperventilation, renal failure (rare), glycosuria.

B

ROUTE AND DOSAGE. Oral: 0.5 to 2 mg once a day. Repeated doses at 4- to 5-hour intervals, if necessary. Not to exceed 10 mg/day. Intermittent dose schedule (may be used for maintenance): prescribed dose is administered on alternate days or for 3 or 4 consecutive days alternating with drug-free periods of 1 or 2 days. **Intramuscular, intravenous:** 0.5 to 1 mg. Administered slowly IV, over 1 to 2 minutes. Repeated doses at 2- to 3-hour intervals, if necessary. Not to exceed 10 mg/day.

NURSING IMPLICATIONS

Usually administered in the morning as a single dose, either daily or by intermittent schedule. For some patients, diuresis is reportedly more effective when administered in two divided doses, morning and evening. Optimum dosage schedule is still under study. Discuss with physician.

Monitor intake and output, BUN, and serum creatinine. Report promptly the onset of oliguria or other changes in intake and output ratio and pattern, and significant increases in BUN or serum creatinine.

Monitor weight, blood pressure, and pulse rate.

Large parenteral doses require breaking several ampules because bumetanide is presently available only in 0.5 mg. To prevent the possibility of glass particles entering the solution it has been suggested that solution be filtered through a sterile membrane filter. Discuss with pharmacist.

High doses or frequent administration, particularly in the elderly, can cause profound diuresis, hypovolemia, and resulting circulatory collapse with development of thrombi and emboli. Careful monitoring is essential.

Hypokalemia is a constant threat in all patients and particularly in those receiving digitalis, or who have congestive heart failure, hepatic cirrhosis, ascites, diarrhea, or potassium-losing nephropathy. Careful monitoring and hospitalization during initial therapy and dosage adjustment periods are advised in these patients.

Advise patient to report symptoms of electrolyte imbalance promptly to physician: weakness, dizziness, fatigue, faintness, confusion, muscle cramps, headache, paresthesias.

It is important for patient to maintain an adequate daily intake of potassium while taking bumetanide. *See Index: Food Sources.*

Patients with hepatic disease should be carefully observed. Alterations in fluid and electrolyte balance can precipitate encephalopathy (inappropriate behavior, altered mood, impaired judgment, confusion, drowsiness, coma).

Be alert to complaints about hearing difficulty or ear discomfort. Patients at risk of bumetanide-induced ototoxic effects include: patients receiving the drug IV, especially at high doses; rapid IV administration; patients with severely impaired renal function and those receiving other potentially ototoxic or nephrotoxic drugs.

Serum electrolytes, blood studies, liver and kidney function tests, and blood sugar (particularly diabetics) should be monitored at regular intervals especially in patients receiving prolonged treatment, high doses, or who are on Na restriction.

Note therapeutic effectiveness in patients being treated for edema: reductions in body weight, abdominal girth, ankle edema, blood pressure, and heart rate.

Instruct patient to keep scheduled appointments for medical evaluation.

For IV infusion, parenteral bumetanide is compatible with 5% dextrose, 0.9% sodium chloride, and lactated Ringer's. Infusion should be used within 24 hours after preparation.

Drug will discolor on exposure to light. Inspect parenteral bumetanide before administration. Discard if it contains particles or is discolored.

Stored in tight, light-resistant containers preferably at 15° to 30°C (59° to 86°F), unless otherwise directed by manufacturer.

Drug Interactions: Bumetanide

Plus	Interactions
Aminoglycosides, parenteral; Cisplatin (Platinol)	Increased risk of ototoxicity, particularly in patients with impaired renal function. Used together in low doses and with extreme caution, if at all
Digitalis glycosides	Bumetanide-induced hypokalemia predisposes patient to digitalis toxicity. Monitor serum potassium levels
Ibuprofen (Motrin); Indomethacin (Indocin), and possibly other inhibitors of prostaglandin synthesis	Pharmacologic effects of bumetanide may be reduced. Higher bumetanide doses may be required
Lithium (Eskalith)	Risk of lithium toxicity (possibly by reduced renal lithium excretion). Monitor lithium serum levels
Skeletal muscle relaxants (nondepolarizing), e.g., tubocurarine, gallamine	Possibility of prolonged neuromuscular blocking effects by bumetanide-induced hypokalemia
Probenecid	May reduce bumetanide diuretic activity. Concomitant use not recommended

---

BUSULFAN
(Myleran)

(byoo-sul'fan)
Antineoplastic, alkylating agent
Nitrosurea

ACTIONS AND USES. Potent cytotoxic alkylating agent that may be a carcinogen in itself. Cell cycle nonspecific. Acts predominantly on slowly proliferating stem cells by inducing cross linkage in DNA thus blocking replication and causing cell death. Reduces total granulocyte mass but has little effect on lymphocytes and platelets except in large doses. May cause widespread epithelial cellular dysplasia severe enough to make it difficult to interpret exfoliative cytologic examinations from lung, breast, bladder, and uterine cervix. May be mutagenic and carcinogenic. Acquired resistance may develop and is thought due to intracellular inactivation of busulfan before it reaches nuclear DNA.

Used in palliative treatment of chronic myelogenous (myeloid, granulocytic, myelocytic) leukemia for patients no longer responsive to radiation therapy or to previously tried antineoplastics. Does not appreciably extend survival time. Also used to treat polycythemia vera, severe thrombocytosis, and as adjunct in treatment of myelofibrosis.

ABSORPTION AND FATE. Within 5 minutes after IV administration and 4 hours after oral dose, a constant blood level of 1 to 3% of the dose is reached and maintained for about 4 hours. Metabolized in the liver. About 10 to 50% of dose excreted in urine as metabolites within 48 hours.

CONTRAINDICATIONS AND PRECAUTIONS. Prior irradiation or chemotherapy, therapy-resistant chronic myelocytic leukemia, neutrophilia, thrombocytopenia, infection, pregnancy (category D). Safe use during lactation not established. *Cautious Use:* men and women in childbearing years, history of gout or urate renal stones.

ADVERSE/SIDE EFFECTS. (Major toxic effects are related to bone marrow failure.) **Dermatologic:** alopecia, hyperpigmentation (especially if dark complexioned), cheilosis, urticaria, erythema multiforme and nodosum, porphyria cutanea tarda, excessive dryness and fragility

B

of skin with anhydrosis. **GI:** nausea, vomiting, diarrhea, glossitis, stomatitis, anorexia. **GU:** renal calculi, uric acid nephropathy, (hyperuricemia, hyperuricosuria), acute renal failure, gynecomastia, testicular atrophy, azoospermia, impotence, sterility in males, ovarian suppression, amenorrhea (potentially irreversible), menopausal symptoms. **Hematologic:** (usually dose-related): agranulocytosis (rare), pancytopenia, thrombocytopenia, leukopenia, anemia. **Respiratory:** irreversible pulmonary fibrosis ("busulfan lung"). **Other:** endocardial fibrosis, dizziness, cholestatic jaundice, cataracts, myasthenia gravis, Addisonlike syndrome: (weakness, severe fatigue, confusion, anorexia, nausea, vomiting, diarrhea, weight loss, melanoderma), cellular dysplasia, superinfections, hemorrhagic complications. Potentially mutagenic and carcinogenic.

ROUTE AND DOSAGE. Dosage highly individualized. **Oral: Adults:** 4 to 8 mg daily until maximal clinical and hematologic improvement is obtained. Maintenance (when remission is shorter than 3 months): 1 to 4 mg daily (individualized). Some clinicians prefer intermittent therapy rather than continuous maintenance. **Pediatric:** 0.06 to 0.12 mg/kg body weight/day or 1.8 to 4.6 mg/m²/day. Dosage titrated to maintain leukocyte count of 20,000/mm³.

NURSING IMPLICATIONS

Advise patient to take busulfan as directed, at the same time each day.

Establish data base with flow chart, recording initial vital signs and weight.

Hgb, Hct, total WBC, differential and quantitative platelet counts, liver and kidney function tests are obtained initially and at least weekly during therapy with busulfan.

Patients sensitive to busulfan may manifest abrupt onset of hematotoxicity. Recovery from busulfan-induced pancytopenia may take 1 month to 2 years. It may be irreversible in some patients.

Usually the leukocyte count does not start to decrease for about 10 to 15 days after therapy begins; it may actually increase during this period. Since the count continues to fall for more than a month after busulfan is withdrawn, usually therapy will be discontinued when the total leukocyte count reaches approximately 15,000/mm³; i.e., before the count reaches normal range.

During remission, patient is examined at monthly intervals at least. When total leukocyte count increases to approximately 50,000/mm³, induction dosage is resumed.

With recommended dosage of busulfan, the normal leukocyte count is usually achieved in about 2 months.

Remissions are characterized by increased appetite and sense of well-being within a few days after therapy begins. Leukocyte reduction in second or third week to below 10,000/mm³, regression of splenomegaly (to less than 3 cm below left costal margain), disappearance of sternal tenderness, increase in Hgb to more than 12 mg/dl, and platelet count between 100,000 and 350,000/mm³ are accepted criteria for "remission."

Monitor intake and output ratio and pattern. Urge patient to increase fluid intake to 10 to 12 glasses (8 ounces each) daily to assure adequate urinary output. Allopurinol and urine alkalinization are prescribed prophylactic measures with hydration to reduce incidence of hyperuricemia and/or hyperuricuria.

Weigh patient at least weekly. A slow but steady change in weight should be communicated to physician.

Make daily inspection of skin, oral membranes, and sites used for blood specimens for abnormal bleeding due to thrombocytopenia. Ecchymotic or petechial bleeding, epistaxis, or bleeding gums should be reported promptly.

If possible avoid IM administration of medication and other intrusive procedures (e.g., rectal temperature, enema, catheterization) during period of decreased platelet count.

Because of hyperpigmentation, signs of cholestatic jaundice may be overlooked. Caution patient to report yellow sclera, dark urine, or light-colored stools.

Advise patient to report immediately the onset of cough, low grade fever, dyspnea, possible symptoms of pulmonary fibrosis (busulfan lung), easy bruising or bleeding, sore mouth or throat, unusual fatigue (agranulocytosis), blurred vision (cataract), flank or joint pain, swelling of lower legs and feet (hyperuricemia).

Be alert to symptoms suggestive of superinfection: fever, white patches in mouth, black hairy tongue, foul smelling vaginal discharge or stools, anogenital itching, diarrhea.

Ovarian suppression and amenorrhea with menopausal symptoms commonly occur in premenopausal women. Effects are not apparent for 4 to 6 months. Amenorrhea may be irreversible.

Contraceptive measures should be used during busulfan therapy and for at least 3 months after drug is withdrawn.

Discuss possibility of alopecia with patient so that plans for temporary cosmetic substitution can be made, if desired. Advise patient to brush hair gently and not more than is necessary.

Busulfan is a highly toxic drug and additionally some patients eventually develop resistance to it. Therefore, urge patient to keep follow-up appointments.

Instruct patient that it is critically important to report promptly symptoms of bone marrow suppression: i.e., fever, sore throat, bleeding from any site, symptoms suggestive of anemia, signs of local infection. Any of these symptoms may indicate either busulfan toxicity or transformation of the disease to an acute "blastic" form.

See Mechlorethamine for nursing care of oral side effects.

Store drug in tightly capped, light-resistant container at temperature between 15° and 30°C (59° and 86°F), unless otherwise specified by the manufacturer.

Diagnostic Test Interferences. Busulfan may decrease **urinary 17-OHCS excretion,** and may increase **blood and urine uric acid** levels. Drug-induced cellular dysplasia may interfere with interpretation of **cytologic studies.**

Drug Interactions: Busulfan

Plus	Interactions
Antigout medication (e.g., probenecid)	Busulfan increases uric acid levels; dose of antigout agent may require adjustment

BUTABARBITAL SODIUM

(Butalan, Butatran, Buticaps, Butisol Sodium, Day-Barb, Neo-Barb, Sarisol No. 2, Secbutobarbitone Sodium)

(byoo-ta-bar′bi-tal)
Sedative, hypnotic
Barbiturate
C III

ACTIONS AND USES. Intermediate-acting barbiturate. Similar to phenobarbital (qv) in actions, contraindications, adverse reactions, and interactions.

Used as hypnotic in short-term treatment of simple insomnia, as sedative for relief of anxiety, and to provide sedation preoperatively. Available in fixed combination with belladonna, e.g., Butibel.

ABSORPTION AND FATE. Onset of action occurs in 40 to 60 minutes; duration of action is 6 to 8 hours. Half-life: 66 to 140 hours. Metabolized in liver. About 26% protein bound. Excreted in urine primarily as metabolites; 1 to 2% excreted as unchanged drug.

CONTRAINDICATIONS AND PRECAUTIONS. Hypersensitivity to barbiturates; porphyria, uncontrolled pain, severe respiratory disease, history of addiction. *Cautious Use:* renal or hepatic impairment. *See also Phenobarbital.*

ADVERSE/SIDE EFFECTS. Drowsiness, residual sedation ("hangover"), nausea, vomiting, skin rash. *See also Phenobarbital*

ROUTE AND DOSAGE. **Oral:** *Sedative:* **Adults:** 15 to 30 mg three or four times a day; *Hypnotic:* 50 to 100 mg at bedtime. **Children:** 7.5 to 30 mg three times a day. Alternatively, 6 mg/kg/day in three equally divided doses. Highly individualized. Low dosages advised for the elderly or debilitated, and patients with impaired renal function. Available in tablets, capsules, and elixir.

NURSING IMPLICATIONS

If patient has difficulty swallowing tablet, it may be crushed before administration and taken with fluid of patient's choice. Capsule may be emptied and contents swallowed with liquid or mixed with food.

Elderly and debilitated patients sometimes manifest morbid excitement, confusion, or depression. Some children also react with paradoxical excitement. Bedrails may be advisable. Report these reactions to physician.

Because butabarbital may cause drowsiness, caution patient not to drive, and to avoid other potentially hazardous activities until reaction to drug is known.

Advise patient not to drink alcoholic beverages while taking this drug. Also inform patient that other CNS depressants, e.g., sedatives, sleep or pain medications, tranquilizers, antihistamines, may produce additive CNS depression and should not be taken without approval of physician.

Butisol Sodium, Sarisol No. 2, and Buticaps contain tartrazine which may cause allergic-type reaction including asthma in susceptible individuals who frequently also have aspirin hypersensitivity.

Prolonged administration is not recommended because tolerance to butabarbital occurs in about 14 days.

Physical and psychologic dependence may develop with prolonged use. Following long-term use, drug should be withdrawn slowly to avoid precipitating withdrawal symptoms.

Subject to control under Federal Controlled Substances Act as Schedule III drug.

By inducing hepatic microsomal enzymes, the barbiturates tend to increase metabolism and thus may reduce response of many drugs, e.g., oral anticoagulants, beta blockers, corticosteroids, digitoxin, doxycycline, griseofulvin, oral contraceptives, phenytoin, quinidine.

Stored in tightly-covered containers, preferably between 15° and 30°C (59° and 86°F), unless otherwise directed by manufacturer.

See Phenobarbital (prototype barbiturate).

BUTORPHANOL TARTRATE

(byoo-tor'fa-nole)

(Stadol)

Analgesic (nonnarcotic)

ACTIONS AND USES. Synthetic, nonopiate, centrally acting analgesic with both narcotic agonist and antagonist capabilities. Pharmacologic properties closely resemble those of pentazocine. Site of analgesic action believed to be subcortical, possibly in the limbic system. On a weight basis, analgesic potency appears to be 5 times that of morphine, 40 times that of merperidine, and 20 times that of pentazocine. Narcotic antagonist potential is approximately 30 times that of pentazocine and $\frac{1}{40}$ that of naloxone. Two mg of butorphanol produces about the same degree of respiratory depression as 10 mg morphine. Respiratory depression does not increase appreciably with higher doses, as it does with morphine, but duration increases. Like pentazocine, analgesic doses may increase pulmonary arterial pressure and cardiac work load. Appears to have low potential for dependence. Tends to inhibit release of antidiuretic hormone (ADH) from hypothalamus.

Used for relief of moderate to severe pain, for preoperative or preanesthetic sedation and analgesia, and for obstetrical analgesia during labor. *Investigational Use:* for musculoskeletal and postepesiotomy pain.

ABSORPTION AND FATE. Rapidly absorbed. Analgesic effect occurs in 10 to 30 minutes following IM injection, peaks in 30 minutes to 1 hour with duration 3 to 4 hours. Following IV injection onset of analgesic activity in 1 minute, peaks in 4 to 5 minutes with duration of 2 to 4 hours. Plasma half-life: 2.5 to 3.5 hours following IV. Approximately 80% protein bound. Extensively metabolized in liver to inactive metabolites. Excreted primarily in urine; less than 5% of dose excreted unchanged. About 11 to 14% of dose eliminated in feces via bile. Readily crosses placenta. Excreted in breast milk.

CONTRAINDICATIONS AND PRECAUTIONS. Hypersensitivity to butorphanol; narcotic-dependent patients. Safe use during pregnancy (except labor) in nursing women, and in children under 18 years not established. *Cautious Use:* history of drug abuse or dependence, emotionally unstable individuals, head injury, increased intracranial pressure; acute myocardial infarction, ventricular dysfunction, coronary insufficiency, hypertension; patients undergoing biliary tract surgery; respiratory depression, bronchial asthma, and obstructive respiratory disease; renal or hepatic dysfunction.

ADVERSE/SIDE EFFECTS. CNS: drowsiness, sedation, headache, vertigo, dizziness, floating feeling, lethargy, confusion, light-headedness, nervousness, unusual dreams, agitation, euphoria, dysphoria, nervousness, unreality, hallucinations, depersonalization, respiratory depression. **CV:** increase or decrease in blood pressure, palpitation, bradycardia. **GI:** nausea, vomiting, dry mouth, abdominal cramps, constipation. **Ophthalmic:** diplopia, blurred vision, miosis (high doses). **Skin:** tingling sensation, flushing and warmth, cyanosis of extremities (acrocyanosis), diaphoresis, sensitivity to cold, skin rash, urticaria, pruritus. **Other:** transient increase in urinary output; dysuria; burning at IV site (rare), tinnitus.

ROUTE AND DOSAGE. Intramuscular: 2 mg (range 1 to 4 mg) every 3 to 4 hours, if necessary. **Intravenous:** 1 mg (range 0.5 to 2 mg) every 3 to 4 hours, if necessary.

NURSING IMPLICATIONS

When prescribed for emotionally unstable patients, butorphanol should be used only for relief of pain and never in anticipation of pain.

Drug-induced nausea may be controlled by lying down.

If butorphanol is used during labor or delivery, observe neonate for signs of respiratory depression.

Warn patient not to take alcohol or other CNS depressant without consulting physician because of possible additive effects.

Because butorphanol has agonist as well as antagonist actions, it can induce acute withdrawal symptoms in opiate-dependent patients.

Butorphanol causes sedation and dizziness; therefore, caution patient to avoid driving and other potentially hazardous activities until reaction to drug is known.

C

Although not currently classified as a controlled substance, bear in mind that butorphanol has habit-forming potential.

Abrupt withdrawal following chronic administration may produce vomiting, loss of appetite, restlessness, abdominal cramps, increase in blood pressure and temperature, mydriasis, "electric shock" feeling associated with faintness. (Patient does not manifest drug-seeking behavior.) Withdrawal symptoms peak in 48 hours after discontinuation of drug.

Treatment of overdosage: Naloxone (Narcan) IV is a specific antagonist of butorphanol; an IV dose of 0.2 to 0.8 mg reverses the respiratory depressant effects of 2 to 4 mg of IV butorphanol. It also reverses antitussive, GI inhibiting, and analgesic effects of butorphanol. Also have readily available: oxygen, IV fluids, and vasopressors and be prepared for assisted or controlled respiration, and continuous monitoring of cardiac and respiratory function.

Store preferably between 15° and 30°C (59° and 86°F), unless otherwise directed by manufacturer. Protect from light.

Diagnostic Test Interferences. Possibility of elevated **serum amylase** levels.

C

PROTOTYPE

CAFFEINE
(Caffedrine, Dexitac, NōDōz, S-250, Quick Pep, Tirend, Vivarin)
CAFFEINE AND SODIUM BENZOATE
CITRATED CAFFEINE

(kaf-een')
Central stimulant
Analeptic
Xanthine

ACTIONS AND USES. Methylxanthine with actions similar to those of other xanthines (e.g., theophylline qv). Releases epinephrine from adrenal medulla (and to a lesser extent, norepinephrine), producing CNS stimulation in descending fashion depending on dosage. Small doses improve psychic and sensory awareness and reduce drowsiness and fatigue by stimulating cerebral cortex. Higher doses stimulate medullary, respiratory, vasomotor, and vagal centers. Produces smooth muscle relaxation (especially bronchi) and dilatation of coronary, pulmonary, and systemic blood vessels by direct action on vascular musculature. Increases contractile force of heart and cardiac output by direct stimulation of myocardium. Also has diuretic action, but less than that produced by other xanthines (theobromine and theophylline). Relief of headache is perhaps due to mild cerebral vasoconstriction action and possibly to increased vascular tone.

Used parenterally as emergency respiratory stimulant in treatment of mild to moderate respiratory depression, particularly that due to alcohol, barbiturates, morphine, and electric shock. Also has been used to relieve headache caused by spinal puncture. Used orally as a mild CNS stimulant as an aid in staying awake and to restore mental alertness. Has been used parenterally and orally to control neonatal apnea. Use as an analeptic in treatment of respiratory depression associated with CNS depressants and electric shock largely replaced by more effective therapy. Used in combination with antihistamines to overcome sedative effects, and as a component of many OTC analgesic preparations due to its ability to enhance their actions (e.g., Anacin, APAP Fortified, Empirin, Excedrin, Vanquish). Used for its synergistic effect with ergotamine (e.g., Cafergot) in treatment of migraine.

ABSORPTION AND FATE. Readily absorbed following oral administration or injection. Peak plasma levels in 30 to 60 minutes. Rapidly demethylated and oxidized by liver. Crosses blood–brain barrier. Half-life: 3 to 10 hours (prolonged in pregnancy and with use of oral contraceptives); approximately 17% protein bound. Excreted in urine; 2 to 10% excreted as unchanged drug. Crosses placenta; appears in breast-milk in small amounts.

CONTRAINDICATIONS AND PRECAUTIONS. Hypersensitivity to caffeine, deep respiratory depression, acute myocardial infarction, gastric or duodenal ulcer. Safe use during pregnancy (category C), in nursing women, and use of oral form in children not established. *Cautious Use:* diabetes mellitus.

ADVERSE/SIDE EFFECTS. With large doses: **CNS:** restlessness, irritability, confusion, agitation, nervousness, fasciculations, hyperesthesia, insomnia, headache, anxiety neurosis, hyperexcitability, delirium, twitching, tremors, clonic convulsions, respiratory depression and arrest, psychosis. **CV:** tingling of face, flushing, palpitation, tachycardia or bradycardia, ventricular ectopic beats, hypotension. **GI:** nausea, vomiting, epigastric discomfort, gastric irritation (oral form), hematemesis, kernicterus (neonates). **Other:** scintillating scotomata, tinnitus, marked diuresis, hyperglycemia, tachypnea.

ROUTE AND DOSAGE. **Oral:** 100 to 250 mg every 4 hours as needed. **Intramuscular, intravenous:** *Caffeine and sodium benzoate:* 250 to 500 mg, repeated in 4 hours if necessary. (Single dose not to exceed 1 Gm.) **Infants and children:** 8 mg/kg; maximum 500 mg. Repeated every 4 hours if necessary.

NURSING IMPLICATIONS

Caffeine and sodium benzoate should be administered slowly.

Timed-release preparations should be administered not less than 6 hours before retiring.

Large doses may cause intensification rather than reversal of severe drug-induced depressions. Monitor vital signs closely.

Children are more susceptible than adults to the CNS effects of caffeine and other methylxanthines and therefore should be closely observed following administration. Neonates receiving caffeine and sodium benzoate have developed kernicterus (from the sodium benzoate component).

Food–Drug Interactions:

- Since tea and coffee contain tannins it has been suggested that they may interact with certain drugs (particularly pain relievers, tranquilizers, and antihistamines) and therefore should not be used to "wash down" medications. The addition of lemon or cream prevents the interaction since they combine with the tannins.
- Caffeine-containing beverages are contraindicated in patients with ulcers because caffeine stimulates gastric secretions. Patients who insist on drinking coffee should be advised to drink it with meals, well diluted with milk.
- Caffeine-containing beverages may decrease the effects of phenothiazines (e.g., chlorpromazine) and butyrophenone antipsychotics (e.g., haliperidol).

An average cup of coffee prepared by drip, percolation, or vacuum methods contains approximately 80 to 120 mg of caffeine. Instant coffee contains 66 to 100 mg/cup. Decaffeinated coffee contains 1 to 6 mg/cup. Tea (bag) may contain 42 to 100 mg/cup. Cola (8 oz) contains 30 to 35 mg. Chocolate bar contains about 25 mg; cocoa (5 oz) 50 mg.

According to recent evidence women with fibrocystic disease of the breast ("lumpy breasts") have responded favorably to elimination of all sources of caffeine and other methylxanthines, e.g., theophylline, theobromine (as in tea). Caffeine is a component of many prescription and nonprescription analgesic preparations.

C

Patients with diabetes should be advised that caffeine in large amounts may impair glucose tolerance.

Habituation to stimulating effects and tolerance to insomnia and diuretic action of caffeine are easily established. Psychological dependence can occur with ingestion of large amounts over prolonged periods.

Studies have shown that caffeine does not reverse the intoxicating effects of alcohol, nor does it overcome "hangover" effects.

Smoking–Drug Interaction: It is reported that smoking increases the metabolism and shortens the half-life of caffeine; therefore dose may be increased in the heavy smoker.

There is some evidence that headache, dizziness, anxiety, irritability, nervousness, and muscle tension may result from excessive use as well as from abrupt withdrawal of coffee (or oral caffeine) in heavy users. Withdrawal symptoms usually occur 12 to 18 hours following last coffee intake.

Treatment of overdosage: induce emesis or administer gastric lavage, follow with activated charcoal. Symptomatic and supportive therapy. Have on hand, diazepam (Valium), and phenobarbital to control seizures.

Diagnostic Test Interferences. Caffeine reportedly may interfere with diagnosis of pheochromocytoma or neuroblastoma by increasing urinary excretion of **catecholamines, VMA,** and **5-HIAA,** and may cause false positive increases in **serum urate** (by Bittner method).

Drug Interactions: Caffeine

Plus	Interactions
Cimetidine (Tagamet) Oral contraceptives	Possibility of increased pharmacologic effects of caffeine. (These drugs inhibit hepatic metabolism of caffeine)

CALCIFEDIOL

(Calderol, 25-OHD_3, 25-hydroxycholecalciferol)

(kal-si-fe-dye′ole)
(Serum) Calcium regulator
Vitamin D

ACTIONS AND USES. Vitamin D analog and major transport form of cholecalciferol (D_3); fat soluble. Because it is activated in the body and has regulatory effects it is sometimes called a hormone. Primary action leads to regulation of serum calcium, which is affected also by the activity of other vitamin D analogs (e.g., ergocalciferol, qv), parathyroid hormone, and calcitonin. Pharmacologic effects of calcifediol are related to intrinsic properties as well as to the properties of active metabolites (e.g., calcitriol) which result from renal metabolism.

Used in management of metabolic bone disease and hypocalcemia associated with chronic renal failure in patients undergoing renal dialysis. Has been used for treatment of osteopenia caused by prolonged glucocorticoid therapy and for osteomalacia secondary to hepatic disease.

ABSORPTION AND FATE. Rapidly absorbed from intestines. Peak serum concentrations reached after about 4 hours. Half-life: varies from 12 to 22 days, duration of action 15 to 20 days.

CONTRAINDICATIONS AND PRECAUTIONS. Hypersensitivity to vitamin D, vitamin D toxicity, hypercalcemia. Safe use of doses in excess of RDA during pregnancy (category C), in nursing women, and in children not established. *Cautious Use:* patients receiving digitalis glycosides.

C

ADVERSE/SIDE EFFECTS. *Vitamin D intoxication and hypercalcemia:* drowsiness, lethargy, headache, weakness, vertigo, anorexia, nausea, vomiting, dry mouth, thirst, constipation, abdominal cramps, metallic taste, muscle or bone pain, polyuria, hypercalciuria, hyperphosphatemia. Idiosyncratic reaction: headache, nausea, vomiting, diarrhea, fever. *See also Ergocalciferol.*

ROUTE AND DOSAGE. Oral: Initial: 300 to 350 mcg/week administered on daily or alternate day schedule. If necessary, dosage increases made at 4-week intervals. Patients with normal serum calcium may require only 20 mcg every other day. *Usual dosage range:* 50 to 100 mcg daily or 100 to 200 mcg on alternate days.

NURSING IMPLICATIONS

Baseline and periodic determinations should be made of serum calcium, phosphorus, magnesium, and alkaline phosphatase, and 24-hour urinary calcium and phosphorus levels.

In general, dosage is regulated to maintain serum calcium of 9 to 10 mg/dl. To guard against metastatic calcification, the product of serum calcium multiplied by phosphate ($Ca \times P$) should not be allowed to exceed 70. A fall in serum alkaline phosphatase usually signals the onset of hypercalcemia.

Serum calcium levels particularly should be monitored at least once weekly, or whenever dosage adjustments are made, and at periodic intervals thereafter. If hypercalcemia occurs, calcifediol should be discontinued until serum calcium returns to normal (9 to 10.6 mg/dl).

Effectiveness of therapy depends on an adequate daily intake of calcium. Since dietary calcium and phosphate are difficult to control, the physician may prescribe a calcium supplement as needed. *See Index for RDAs.*

Patients undergoing dialysis may require aluminum carbonate or hydroxide gels to bind intestinal phosphate and thus lower serum phosphate levels. Magnesium-containing antacids should not be used because of the possibility of hypermagnesemia.

Since calcitriol is a metabolite of vitamin D_3, all sources of vitamin D are usually withheld during therapy.

Patients receiving digitalis glycosides will require close monitoring. Elevated serum calcium in these patients may precipitate arrhythmias.

Instruct patient to withhold drug and report immediately signs and symptoms of hypercalcemia *(see Adverse/Side Effects).*

Advise patient to consult physician before taking an OTC medication. Magnesium-containing laxatives and antacids, mineral oil, and vitamin D preparations should be avoided.

Store preferably between 15° and 30°C (59° and 86°F) in tightly covered, light-resistant container unless otherwise directed by manufacturer.

See Ergocalciferol (prototype vitamin D).

Drug Interactions: Calcifediol

Plus	Interactions
Thiazide diuretics	Concurrent administration may result in hypercalcemia
Verapamil (Calan, Isoptin), and possibly other calcium channel blockers	Calcifediol-induced hypercalcemia may result in decreased verapamil effectiveness (antagonist action). Monitor closely
Digitalis glycosides	Calcifediol-induced hyperglycemia may precipitate arrhythmias

CALCITONIN (SALMON)

(Calcimar)

(kal-si-toe'nin)
Hormone
(Serum) Calcium regulator

C

ACTIONS AND USES. Synthetic polypeptide derived from salmon calcitonin. Inhibits bone resorption, lowers serum calcium concentration, and appears to accelerate bone formation and mineral deposition. (Opposes effects of parathyroid hormone on bone and kidneys.) Binds to specific receptor site on osteoclast cell membrane and alters transmembrane passage of calcium and phosphorus. Inhibition of bone resorption decreases both mineral release and collagen breakdown. Promotes renal excretion of calcium and phosphorus and causes transient sodium and water loss. Decreased volume and acidity of gastric juice and decreased volume of pancreatic trypsin and amylase are also transient effects. Increases small bowel secretion of potassium, chlorides, sodium, and water but not calcium. In Paget's disease, slows rate of bone turnover, with resultant decreases in serum alkaline phosphatase and urinary hydroxyproline, biochemical changes that seem to correspond with more normal bone formation. In some patients, long-term use initiates drug resistance due to formation of neutralizing antibodies. Transient hypocalcemia that follows therapeutic doses is asymptomatic and mild.

Used in treatment of symptomatic Paget's disease of bone (osteitis deformans), as short-term adjunctive treatment of severe hypercalcemia of cancer (with or without metastasis), immobilization, or hyperparathyroidism, particularly when renal, hepatic, or cardiac disease limits use of other forms of treatment. *Investigational Use:* diagnosis and management of medullary carcinoma of thyroid, treatment of postmenopausal osteoporosis, and osteogenesis imperfecta.

ABSORPTION AND FATE. Following IM or SC injection, action begins within 15 minutes, peaks in 4 hours, and persists 8 to 24 hours. Rapidly metabolized, primarily by kidneys. Excreted as inactive metabolites in urine. Does not cross placenta barrier; passage to CSF or to breast milk not established.

CONTRAINDICATIONS AND PRECAUTIONS. Hypersensitivity to fish and calcitonin; history of allergy; children, pregnancy, nursing mothers. *Cautious Use:* renal impairment, osteoporosis, pernicious anemia, Zollinger–Ellison syndrome.

ADVERSE/SIDE EFFECTS. Transient nausea, vomiting, local inflammatory reaction at injection site, swelling, tingling, and tenderness of hands, facial flushing, unusual taste sensation, headache, diarrhea, skin rash (rare), diuresis, calcitonin antibody formation, hypersensitivity (systemic) reaction, hypocalcemic tetany (rare).

ROUTE AND DOSAGE. **Subcutaneous, intramuscular:** *Hypercalcemia:* Initial: 4 IU (MRC)/kg every 12 hours. If inadequate response after 1 or 2 days dosage increased to 8 IU (MRC)/kg every 12 hours. If response still inadequate after 2 more days, administer 8 IU (MRC)/kg every 6 hours. *Paget's disease:* Initial: 100 IU (MRC) once a day: then 50 to 100 IU (MRC) daily or every other day. [Dosages expressed in IU (International Units) are equal to MRC (Medical Research Council) units.]

NURSING IMPLICATIONS

If patient is being taught to self-administer calcitonin, the SC route is preferred.

Teach patient to recognize and seek advice about local inflammatory reactions at site of injection. Careful avoidance of consecutive use of same area is as important as the required sterile technique.

When the volume of calcitonin to be injected exceeds 2 ml, the IM route is employed, and multiple sites should be used. Rotate injection sites.

Compliance with daily injections of calcitonin is based on complete understanding of rationale for treatment and a technique that is as free from discomfort as possible.

Since calcitonin is a protein, systemic allergic reaction is a possibility. Therefore, a skin test is usually done prior to initiation of therapy. The appearance of more than mild erythema or wheal 15 minutes after intracutaneous injection of calcitonin constitutes a positive response and indicates that the drug should not be given.

Have on hand epinephrine, antihistamines, oxygen in the event of a reaction. Also have readily available parenteral calcium, particularly during early therapy. Hypocalcemic tetany is a theoretical possibility.

Periodic laboratory examination of urine specimens for sediment is recommended when patient is on long-term therapy.

Paget's Disease:

- Diuresis that occurs during early therapy is thought to be related to improvement in circulation.
- Drug effect is monitored by evaluation of symptoms and periodic measurement of serum alkaline phosphatase (normal: 1.4 to 4.1 Bodansky units), 24-hour urinary hydroxyproline (15 to 20 mg), and serum calcium (9 to 10.6 mg/dl).
- Clinical response to calcitonin therapy in Paget's disease may not occur until after several months of therapy. It is evidenced by reduced bone pain, lowered skin temperature over involved bone, slight improvement or at least no further loss of hearing (hearing loss is due to compression of temporal bone on 8th cranial nerve), possible reversal of neurologic symptoms related to compression of spinal cord and nerves, measurable decreases in cardiac output, and decreases in serum alkaline phosphatase and urinary hydroxyproline values.
- Therapeutic effectiveness of long-term calcitonin treatment generally persists months after drug is withdrawn; pretreatment status usually returns after 1 to 2 years of therapy.
- If biochemical (hypercalcemia) or clinical relapse (return of painful symptoms of Paget's disease) occurs, calcitonin antibody titer and patient compliance should be evaluated.
- Test for high antibody titer: After overnight fasting, a sample of blood is drawn for determination of serum calcium prior to IM administration of calcitonin. Patient then eats usual breakfast. At 3 and 6 hours postinjection, additional blood samples are drawn. Findings: decrease from fasting serum calcium levels of 0.5 mg% or more is seen in the responsive patient. A decrease of 0.3 mg% or less constitutes inadequate hypocalcemic response. Further use of calcitonin will be ineffective.
- Circulating antibodies to salmon calcitonin may occur in 30 to 50% of patients after 2 to 18 months of treatment. A relapse after good initial response suggests probable treatment failure.

Hypercalcemia:

- Many patients have a return to the original elevated serum calcium after but a few days of emergency use of calcitonin. Hypercalcemia is suspected if the following symptoms are present: deep bone and flank pain, renal calculi, polyuria, anorexia, nausea, vomiting, thirst, constipation, muscle hypotonicity, pathologic fracture, bradycardia, lethargy, psychosis.
- Teach patient the importance of maintaining drug regimen even though symptoms have been ameliorated, to prevent early relapses.
- Theoretically, calcitonin can lead to hypocalcemic tetany (increased neuromuscular excitability). Latent tetany may be demonstrated by Chvostek's or Trousseau's signs *(see Index)* and by serum calcium values: (latent tetany) 7 to 8 mg/dl; (manifest tetany) below 7 mg/dl.

C

- If calcitonin is being used as an antihypercalcemic, the physician may prescribe reduced dietary calcium intake. High-calcium foods include greens, milk, and dairy products. Coordinate dietary planning with dietitian, patient, and family.

Advise patient to consult physician before using OTC preparations. Some supervitamins, hematinics, and antacids contain calcium.

Store calcitonin in refrigerator preferably at 2° to 8°C (36° to 46°F) unless otherwise directed by manufacturer.

CALCITRIOL

(kal-si-trye'ole)

(Rocaltrol)

(Serum) Calcium regulator

ACTIONS AND USES. Synthetic form of 1,25-dihydroxycholecalciferol, an active metabolite of ergocalciferol (qv). In the liver, cholecalciferol (vitamin D_3) and ergocalciferol (vitamin D_2) are enzymatically metabolized to calcifediol, an activated form of vitamin D_3. Calcifediol is biodegraded in the kidney to calcitriol, the most potent form of vitamin D_3. Patients with nonfunctioning kidneys are unable to synthesize sufficient calcitriol, and therefore must receive it pharmacologically. By increasing intestinal absorption of calcium, calcitriol elevates serum calcium levels, decreases elevated blood levels of phosphatase and parathyroid hormone, and decreases subperiosteal bone resorption and mineralization defects in some patients.

Used in management of hypocalcemia in patients undergoing chronic renal dialysis, and in patients with hypoparathyroidism or pseudohypoparathyroidism. *Investigational Use:* in selected patients with vitamin D–dependent rickets, familial hypophosphatemia (vitamin D–resistant rickets), and in management of hypocalcemia in premature infants.

ABSORPTION AND FATE. Rapidly and completely absorbed from the intestine. Onset of action in about 2 to 6 hours. Peak hypercalcemic effect in 10 to 12 hours; duration of action 3 to 5 days. Half-life: 3 to 6 hours. Metabolized in liver. Elimination is mainly fecal, being excreted with bile; about 4 to 6% excreted in urine. Approximately 65% of dose eliminated within 6 days.

CONTRAINDICATIONS AND PRECAUTIONS. Hypercalcemia or vitamin D toxicity. Safe use during pregnancy (category C), in nursing women, and in children not established. *Cautious Use:* hyperphosphatemia, patients receiving digitalis glycosides.

ADVERSE/SIDE EFFECTS. Vitamin D intoxication and **hypercalcemia** (drowsiness, headache, weakness, anorexia, nausea, vomiting, dry mouth, thirst, constipation, abdominal cramps, muscle or bone pain, metallic taste); hypercalciuria, hyperphosphatemia. *See also Ergocalciferol.*

ROUTE AND DOSAGE. Oral: Initial: 0.25 mcg/day. May be increased by 0.25 mcg/day at 4- to 8-week intervals for dialysis patients, and 2- to 4-week intervals for hypoparathyroid patients if necessary. Maintenance: 0.5 to 1 mcg daily.

NURSING IMPLICATIONS

Baseline and periodic determinations should be made of serum calcium, phosphorus, magnesium, alkaline phosphatase, creatinine, and 24-hour urinary calcium and phosphorus levels.

To guard against metastatic calcification, the product of serum calcium multiplied by phosphate (Ca × P) should not be allowed to exceed 70. A fall in serum alkaline phosphatase frequently signals the onset of hypercalcemia.

During early therapy, serum calcium levels particularly should be monitored twice weekly. Some clinicians prescribe weekly serum calcium levels for the first 12 weeks of therapy, and monthly after dosage is stabilized.

Effectiveness of therapy depends on an adequate daily intake of calcium and phosphate. Since dietary calcium and phosphate are difficult to control, the physician may prescribe a calcium supplement on an as needed basis. (RDA for calcium in children 1 to 10 years of age and in adults is 800 mg; for young people 11 to 18 years, it is 1200 mg.)

Excessive intake of calcium and phosphate can cause hypercalcemia, hypercalciuria, and hyperphosphatemia (also true of excessively high doses of calcitriol).

Review symptoms of hypercalcemia with patient and advise him or her to withhold drug and contact physician if they occur.

If hypercalcemia develops, calcitriol and calcium supplements (if being taken) should be discontinued until serum calcium returns to normal. Reduction of dietary calcium intake should also be considered. *(See Index: Food sources.)*

Since calcitriol is the most potent form of vitamin D_3 all sources of vitamin D should be withheld during therapy, to avoid possibility of hypercalcemia.

Patients undergoing dialysis may require aluminum carbonate or hydroxide gels to bind intestinal phosphate and thus lower serum phosphate levels. Magnesium-containing antacids are not to be used, to avoid possibility of hypermagnesemia.

Patients with normal renal function should maintain an adequate fluid intake. Consult physician for parameters.

Advise patient to consult physician before taking an OTC medication.

Treatment of overdosage: induction of emesis or gastric lavage. General supportive therapy. Monitor serial serum electrolytes (especially calcium), urinary calcium, and ECG. Discontinue supplemental calcium, and institute low calcium diet.

Capsules should be protected from heat, light, and moisture. Store in well-closed container preferably between 15° and 30°C (59° and 86°F), unless otherwise directed by manufacturer.

See also Ergocalciferol.

Drug Interactions: Calcitriol

Plus	Interactions
Digitalis glycosides	Calcitriol-induced hypercalcemia may precipitate arrhythmias. Close monitoring indicated
Thiazide diuretics	Pharmacologic effects of calcitriol may be increased with possibility of hypercalcemia. Monitor closely
Verapamil (Calan, Isoptin), and possibly other calcium channel blockers	Calcitriol-induced hypercalcemia may antagonize antiarrhythmic properties of verapamil. Monitor closely

C

CALCIUM CARBONATE, PRECIPITATED

Antacid
Replenisher: Calcium

(Alka-2, Amitone, BioCal, Calcilac, Calglycine, Cal-Sup, Caltrate, Chooz, Dicarbosil, Equilet, Mallamint, Os-Cal, Precipitated chalk, Titralac, Tums, Tums E-X)

ACTIONS AND USES. Reportedly regarded as antacid of choice by many physicians because of its rapid action, high neutralizing capacity, relatively prolonged duration of action, and low cost. Although classified as a nonsystemic antacid, a slight to moderate alkalosis usually develops with prolonged therapy. Acid rebound, which may follow as low a dose as 0.5 Gm, is thought to be caused by release of gastrin triggered by action of calcium in small intestines. Liberation of carbon dioxide in stomach causes belching in some patients. Contains 400 mg (20 mEq) of calcium per gram.

Used for symptomatic relief of hyperacidity associated with peptic ulcer and for relief of transient symptoms of acid indigestion, heartburn, sour stomach, peptic esophagitis, and hiatal hernia. Also used as calcium supplement when calcium intake may be inadequate (as in childhood and adolescence, during pregnancy, lactation, and postmenopause, in the aged), and in treatment of mild calcium deficiency states. Has been used for treatment of hyperphosphatemia in patients with chronic renal failure. Available in combination with aluminum and magnesium hydroxides, e.g., Camalox; in combination with magnesium carbonate, e.g., Marblen, Ratio, Spastosed; and in combination with magnesium oxide; e.g., Bisodol, Lo-Sal.

ABSORPTION AND FATE. Reacts within minutes with gastric acid to form calcium chloride, carbon dioxide, and water. Converted in part to soluble calcium salts that are absorbed from intestines; about 73 to 85% is reconverted to insoluble calcium chloride, phosphate, and calcium soaps and excreted in feces.

CONTRAINDICATIONS AND PRECAUTIONS. Hypercalcemia and hypercalciuria (e.g., hyperparathyroidism, vitamin D overdosage, decalcifying tumors, bone metastases), calcium loss due to immobilization, severe renal disease, renal calculi, GI hemorrhage or obstruction, dehydration, hypochloremic alkalosis, ventricular fibrillation, cardiac disease. *Cautious Use:* decreased bowel motility (patients receiving anticholinergics, antidiarrheals, antispasmodics), elderly patients.

ADVERSE/SIDE EFFECTS. Constipation or laxative effect, acid rebound, nausea, eructation, flatulence. *With prolonged use of high doses:* hypercalcemia with alkalosis and conjunctival and episcleral suffusion; metastatic calcinosis, hypercalciuria, hypomagnesemia, hypophosphatemia (when phosphate intake is low), renal calculi, renal dysfunction, vomiting, GI hemorrhage, fecal concretions, appendicolithiasis, milk-alkali syndrome.

ROUTE AND DOSAGE. **Oral:** *Antacid:* 0.5 to 2 Gm four to six times daily, if necessary. *Calcium supplement:* 1 to 1.5 Gm three times daily. Dosage should not exceed 8 Gm/day.

NURSING IMPLICATIONS

When used as antacid, taken between meals (e.g., 1 hour after meals) and at bedtime. When used as calcium supplement, taken with meals.

Available in tablet and powder form. For maximum effectiveness, tablet should be chewed well before swallowing, or allowed to dissolve completely in mouth; followed with water. Powder form is dispersed in water or may be sprinkled on food if taken as calcium supplement.

Because of acid rebound, which generally occurs after repeated use for 1 or 2 weeks, one can quickly become a chronic user of calcium carbonate. Explain to patient the potential dangers of self-medication.

C

Note number and consistency of stools. If constipation is a problem in patient on antacid therapy, physician may prescribe alternate or combination therapy with a magnesium antacid or advise patient to take a laxative or stool softener as necessary.

Weekly serum and urine calcium determinations *(see Index for Sulkowitch test)* are recommended in patients receiving prolonged therapy and in patients with renal dysfunction. (Normal serum calcium: 8.5 to 10.5 mg/dl; urinary calcium: 150 mg/day or less.) Note that a 24-hour urine specimen is collected for quantitative urinary calcium determinations and that a special bottle containing 10 ml of concentrated HCl is required. Follow agency policy.

Record amelioration of the following symptoms of *hypocalcemia:* depression, psychosis, neuromuscular hyperexcitability; cardiac arrhythmias, muscle spasms; paresthesias of feet, fingers, tongue; severe deficiency (tetany): carpopedal spasms, spasms of face muscle, laryngospasm, generalized convulsion.

Observe for signs and symptoms of *hypercalcemia* in patients receiving frequent or high doses: nausea, vomiting, anorexia, abdominal pain, constipation, nocturia, thirst, dry mouth, polyuria, cloudy memory, confusion, psychosis, lassitude, fatigue, loss of muscle tone, muscle weakness, joint pain, decreased renal function, renal calculi.

Food–Drug Interactions:

- When used as a supplement, avoid taking calcium carbonate with cereals or with foods high in oxylate. Phytic acid in the outer hulls of many cereal grains (especially in bran and wheat), and oxalates in leafy vegetables *(see Index: Food sources)* combine with calcium carbonate to form insoluble nonabsorbable compounds.
- Chronic usage of calcium carbonate taken together with foods high in vitamin D (such as milk) can cause *milk-alkali syndrome:* distaste for food, headache, confusion, nausea, vomiting, abdominal pain, hypercalcemia, hypercalciuria, soft tissue calcification (calcinosis), hyperphosphatemia, increased BUN and serum creatinine, renal insufficiency, metabolic alkalosis. Predisposing factors include renal dysfunction and electrolyte imlance.
- Principal sources of calcium are milk, milk products, meat, fish, eggs, cereal products, fruits, beans, and other vegetables. Certain foods interfere with absorption of calcium, e.g., oxalic acid (in spinach, rhubarb, chocolate, brewed tea), phytic acid (bran and whole grain cereals), and phosphorous (milk and dairy products). Collaborate with physician and dietitian regarding diet teaching plan.

Recommended dietary allowance (RDA) of calcium for infants ½ to 1 year is 540 mg; for children and adults 800 mg; during pregnancy and lactation + 400 mg; and during adolescence (ages 11 to 18) RDA is 1200 mg.

Store preferably between 15° and 30°C (59° and 86°F) in well-closed container, unless otherwise directed by manufacturer.

See Aluminum Hydroxide Gel for management of peptic ulcer; see Calcium gluconate, prototype calcium replenisher.

Drug Interactions: Calcium carbonate ($CaCO_3$)

Plus	Interactions
Quinidine	Alkalinization of urine induced by $CaCO_3$ may increase quinidine reabsorption. Monitor quinidine plasma levels
Salicylates	Alkalinization of urine induced by $CaCO_3$ increases renal excretion of salicylates. Dosage adjustments may be necessary in patients receiving chronic salicylate therapy

C

Plus (cont.)	**Interactions (cont.)**
Thiazides	Concurrent administration with high $CaCO_3$ doses can result in hypercalcemia
Verapamil (Calon, Isoptin), and possibly other calcium channel blockers	$CaCO_3$-induced hypercalcemia can antagonize antiarrhythmic properties of verapamil

In common with other antacids, calcium carbonate can cause premature dissolution and absorption of enteric-coated tablets and also may interfere with absorption of oral medications. As a general rule, it is best not to administer other oral drugs within 1 to 2 hours of an antacid.

CALCIUM CHLORIDE

Replenisher: Calcium

ACTIONS AND USES. Actions, uses, pharmacokinetics, contraindications, precautions, and adverse effects similar to those of calcium gluconate (qv). Ionizes more readily and thus is more potent than calcium gluconate and more irritating to tissues. Provides excess chloride ions that promote acidosis and temporary (1 to 2 days) diuresis secondary to excretion of sodium. Each gram (10 ml) supplies 272 mg (13.6 mEq) of calcium.

Used for treatment of cardiac resuscitation, to prevent hypocalcemia during transfusion with citrated blood, for treatment of hypermagnesemia, and for cardiac disturbances of hyperkalemia.

CONTRAINDICATIONS AND PRECAUTIONS. Ventricular fibrillation, hypercalcemia, digitalis toxicity, injection into myocardium or other tissue. Safe use during pregnancy (category C), in nursing women, and in children not established. *Cautious Use:* digitalized patients, renal insufficiency, sarcoidosis, history of renal stone formation, cor pulmonale, respiratory acidosis, respiratory failure.

ADVERSE/SIDE EFFECTS. Tingling sensation, chalky (calcium) taste. With rapid IV, sensations of heat, hypotension, bradycardia, cardiac arrhythmias, cardiac arrest, pain and burning at IV site, severe venous thrombosis, necrosis and sloughing (with extravasation).

ROUTE AND DOSAGE. **Intravenous:** **Adults:** 500 mg to 1 Gm repeated every 1 to 3 days if indicated. IV injection should be made slowly through small-bore needle into a large vein to minimize venous irritation and undesirable reactions. IV infusion rate not to exceed 1 ml/min. **Pediatric:** 25 mg/kg administered slowly. Rarely used because of small vasculature. Avoid use of scalp veins. **Intraventricular:** **Adults:** *cardiac resuscitation:* 200 to 800 mg (2 to 4 ml) directly into cardiac ventricle.

NURSING IMPLICATIONS

Monitor ECG, blood pressure, and flow rate and observe patient closely during administration.

IV injection may be accompanied by cutaneous burning sensation and peripheral vasodilation, with moderate fall in blood pressure. Following injection, advise ambulatory patient to remain in bed for ½ to 1 hour or more depending on response.

Extravasation must be avoided during IV injection, since cellulitis, necrosis, and sloughing can result. Local necrosis can occur with leakage from vein. If given IV to children, scalp veins should be avoided.

Calcium chloride should never be given subcutaneously or IM or by gavage, as it is a tissue irritant.
Severe thromboses of peripheral veins have been reported in patients receiving calcium chloride by IV push or for treatment of shock.
Digitalized patients must be closely observed since an increase in serum calcium increases risk of digitalis toxicity.
Frequent determinations of serum pH, calcium, and other electrolytes should be performed as guides to dosage adjustments.
The presence of alkalosis reduces ionization and thus absorption of calcium chloride. The presence of acidosis has the opposite effect.
Store preferably between 15° and 30°C (59° and 86°F), unless otherwise directed by manufacturer.
See Calcium gluconate (prototype calcium replenisher).

CALCIUM GLUCEPTATE

(gloo-sep'tate)
Replenisher: Calcium

ACTIONS AND USES. Contains approximately 23% calcium. Similar to calcium gluconate (qv) in actions, uses, pharmacokinetics, contraindications, and precautions, but reportedly less irritating. Preferred for use when IM administration is required as in neonatal tetany. Contains 82 mg (4.1 mEq) of calcium per gram.

ABSORPTION AND FATE. Duration of action following IV is 2 to 3 hours and after IM 1 to 4 hours.

ROUTE AND DOSAGE. Adults: Intravenous: 5 to 20 ml (1.1 Gm per 5 ml). **Intramuscular:** 2 to 5 ml. *Exchange transfusions in newborns:* 0.5 ml after each 100 ml of blood exchanged.

NURSING IMPLICATIONS

IM injection may produce mild local reactions. Generally, this route is used only in adults, when IV administration is not feasible.
Recommended IM site for adults is the upper outer quadrant of the buttock and in infants (if prescribed) the midlateral thigh.
Patient may complain of a transient tingling sensation and metallic taste following IV administration.
See Calcium gluconate (prototype calcium replenisher).

Drug Interactions: Calcium gluceptate

Plus	Interactions
Digitalis glycosides	Calcium chloride induced hypercalcemia may enhance digitalis toxicity and precipitate arrhythmias
Verapamil (Calan, Isoptin), and possibly other calcium channel blockers	Calcium-chloride-induced hypercalcemia may antagonize verapamil effectiveness. Monitor closely

PROTOTYPE

CALCIUM GLUCONATE

(Kalcinate)

(gloo'koe-nate)

Replenisher: Calcium

C

ACTIONS AND USES. Calcium is an essential element for regulating the excitation threshold of nerves and muscles, for blood clotting mechanisms, cardiac function (rhythm, tonicity, contractility), maintenance of renal function, for body skeleton and teeth. Also plays a role in regulating storage and release of neurotransmitters and hormones; regulating amino acid uptake and absorption of cyanocobalamin (vitamin B_{12}); gastrin secretion, and in maintaining structural and functional integrity of cell membranes and capillaries. Calcium gluconate acts like digitalis on heart, increasing cardiac muscle tone and force of systolic contractions (positive inotropic effect). Each gram (10 ml) contains 90 mg (4.5 mEq) of calcium.

Used to treat negative calcium balance (as in neonatal tetany, hypoparathyroidism, vitamin D deficiency, alkalosis, and intestinal malabsorption states). Also used to overcome cardiac toxicity of hyperkalemia, for cardiopulmonary resuscitation, to prevent hypocalcemia during transfusion of citrated blood, used as antidote for magnesium sulfate, for acute symptoms of lead colic, to decrease capillary permeability in sensitivity reactions, and to relieve muscle cramps in treatment of insect bites or stings, e.g., black widow spider. Oral calcium may be used to maintain normal calcium balance during pregnancy, lactation, and childhood growth period and to prevent primary osteoporosis. Also used in treatment of osteoporosis, osteomalacia, chronic hypoparathyroidism, rickets, and as adjunct in treatment of myasthenia gravis and Eaton-Lambert syndrome. *Investigational Use:* to antagonize aminoglycoside-induced neuromuscular blockade, and as "calcium challenge" to diagnose Zollinger-Ellison syndrome and medullary thyroid carcinoma.

ABSORPTION AND FATE. Cardiac response to IV injection is immediate and lasts ½ to 2 hours. Following oral administration, approximately one-third of dose is absorbed, primarily from proximal segments of small bowel. Vitamin D probably increases active transport of calcium from gut lumen. About 45% bound to plasma proteins. Largely excreted unchanged in feces; small amounts also excreted in urine, pancreatic juice, saliva, and breast milk. Crosses placenta.

CONTRAINDICATIONS AND PRECAUTIONS. Ventricular fibrillation, metastatic bone disease, injection into myocardium; administration by SC or IM routes; renal calculi, hypercalcemia. *Cautious Use:* digitalized patients, renal or cardiac insufficiency, sarcoidosis, history of lithiasis, immobilized patients.

ADVERSE/SIDE EFFECTS. Hypercalcemia: anorexia, nausea, thirst, vomiting, abdominal pain, constipation, ileus, somnolence, fatigue, headache, decreased excitability of muscles and nerves, pathologic fractures, muscle and joint pain, excessive thirst, nocturia, polyuria, azotemia, mental confusion, psychosis, renal calculi, acute pancreatitis, bradycardia and other arrhythmias. **IV injection:** tingling sensations, calcium (chalky) taste; **Rapid IV:** sense of oppression or "heat waves" (vasodilation), hypotension, bradycardia and other arrhythmias, syncope, cardiac arrest. **Local reactions:** tissue irritation, burning, cellulitis, soft tissue calcification, necrosis and sloughing (following IV extravasation). **Oral preparation:** constipation.

ROUTE AND DOSAGE. Adults: Oral: 1 to 2 Gm two to four times a day. *Supplement in osteoporosis:* 1 to 1.5 Gm daily. **Intravenous:** 0.5 to 2 Gm (5 to 20 ml) 10% solution given slowly at rate not exceeding 0.5 ml/minute. **Children:** 500 mg/kg/day in divided doses, orally or well diluted and given slowly by IV.

NURSING IMPLICATIONS

IV calcium should be administered slowly through a small bore needle into a large vein, to avoid possibility of extravasation and resultant necrosis. If administered to children, scalp veins should be avoided.

Physician will prescribe specific IV flow rate. High concentrations of calcium suddenly reaching the heart can cause fatal cardiac arrest.

During IV administration, ECG is monitored to detect evidence of hypercalcemia: decreased QT interval associated with inverted T wave.

Direct IV injection may be accompanied by cutaneous burning sensations and peripheral vasodilatation, with moderate fall in blood pressure. Injection should be stopped if patient complains of any discomfort. Patient should be advised to remain in bed for ½ to 1 hour or more following injection, depending on response.

Observe IV site closely. Extravasation may result in tissue irritation and necrosis.

Although sometimes prescribed for the adult, the IM route is not recommended. It is specifically contraindicated in children because it may result in abscess formation.

Oral calcium preparations are best utilized when administered 2 to 3 hours after meals. Calcium gluconate is reported to be nonirritating to GI mucosa.

Therapeutic effects in treatment of tetany (hypocalcemia) are evaluated by amelioration of neuromuscular hyperexcitability: paresthesias (numbness and tingling of fingers, toes, and lips), skeletal muscle spasms, twitching of facial muscles, intestinal hypermotility and colic, carpopedal spasm, laryngospasm, convulsions, and cardiac arrhythmias.

Latent tetany may be detected by Chvostek's and Trousseau's signs:

Chvostek's sign: Tap facial nerve (cranial nerve VII) just below temple where it emerges. Hyperirritability of nerve manifested by twitching of facial muscles is a positive sign of tetany.

Trousseau's sign: Apply sphygmomanometer cuff to upper arm and inflate until radial pulse is obliterated and keep inflated for about 3 minutes. The ischemia produced increases excitability of peripheral nerves and causes spasms of lower arm and hand muscles (carpal spasm) if tetany exists. Alternative method: Grasp patient's wrist firmly enough to constrict circulation for a few minutes.

If patient has hypocalcemia or if it is suspected, padded side rails are advisable. Also, have on hand mouth gag, airway, and suction apparatus in the event of laryngeal spasm. Control environmental stimuli, e.g., noise level.

Sulkowitch's test (may be prescribed for home patient or family member) is a simple test for urinary calcium, which gives an approximate index of serum calcium level. To rule out *hypercalcemia* (hypercalciuria), examine early morning specimen, since excretion is lowest at this time. For *hypocalcemia,* take urine sample after a meal, when Ca excretion is maximal. Results (qualitative): fine white cloud (normal), clear solution (decreased serum calcium), heavy precipitate (excessive serum calcium).

In sustained therapy, frequent determinations should be made of calcium and phosphorus (tend to vary inversely). Normal serum calcium is 8.5 to 10.5 mg/dl; normal serum inorganic phosphorus is 3 to 4.5 mg/dl.

RDA of calcium for infants younger than 6 months: 360 mg; for infants ½ to 1 year: 540 mg; for children 1 to 10 years and adults: 800 mg/day; for pregnant and lactating women and during adolescence (10 to 18 years): 1200 mg/day.

Food–Drug Interactions:

- Vitamin D is required for absorption of Ca; therefore it is used to fortify milk and calcium supplements.

C

- Milk products are best sources of calcium (and phosphorus); other sources include: green leafy vegetables (see below) as well as sardines, clams, and oysters.
- Avoid taking drug with cereals. Phytic acid (phytates) in outer hulls of many grains (especially wheat and bran) combine with Ca to form insoluble nonabsorable compounds.
- Ca absorption is blocked when its compounds are ingested with oxalate-rich foods: spinach, rhubarb, beets and beet greens, Swiss chard, collard greens, almonds, cashews, chocolate, cocoa.
- If diet is low in Ca and high in oxylate foods, calcium deficiency is enhanced.
- Ca absorption may be inhibited by zinc-rich foods: nuts, seeds, sprouts, legumes, soy products (tofu).
- Calcium should be taken 2 hours before or 3 hours after meals. This may be particularly important to the total vegetarian who often has marginal Ca intake.
- To facilitate intestinal absorption of calcium gluconate, physician may prescribe reduced phosphate intake (milk and other dairy products) or simultaneous administration of aluminum hydroxide, which forms insoluble phosphate salts.

Diagnostic Test Interferences. IV calcium may cause false decreases in **serum and urine magnesium** (by Titan yellow method) and transient elevations of **plasma 11-OHCS** levels by Glenn-Nelson technique. Values usually return to control levels after 60 minutes; **urinary steroid** values (17-OHCS) may be decreased.

Drug Interactions. Calcium gluconate and other Ca containing drugs enhance the inotropic and toxic effects of **digitalis glycosides** and may precipitate cardiac arrhythmias; may compete with **magnesium** for absorption with resulting magnesium deficiency (note that calcium can also produce false decrease in tests for serum Mg). Oral calcium forms a complex with **tetracyclines** and thus decreases their effect; do not administer within 3 hours of each other. (The two drugs are also incompatible in parenteral solutions.) Calcium gluconate-induced hypercalcemia may antagonize effectiveness of verapamil (Calan, Isoptin) and possibly other calcium channel blockers.

CALCIUM LACTATE

(lak'tate)
Replenisher: Calcium

ACTIONS AND USES. Oral calcium preparation reportedly well tolerated. Contains approximately 13% calcium. Similar to calcium gluconate (qv) in actions, uses, contraindications, and adverse reactions. Contains 130 mg (6.5 mEq) of calcium per gram.

Used to treat mild hypocalcemia and for maintenance calcium therapy.

ROUTE AND DOSAGE. Oral: Adults: 325 mg to 1.3 Gm three times a day with meals. **Children:** 500 mg/kg/24 hours in divided doses.

NURSING IMPLICATIONS

Tablets or powder can be dissolved in hot water; then add cool water to patient's taste.

May be administered with lactose (amount prescribed) to increase solubility.

Hospital pharmacy may prepare calcium lactate solution on request.

Blood calcium levels should be checked periodically. Hypercalcemia may occur during prolonged administration particularly if patient is also taking vitamin D.

Bear in mind that an increase in serum calcium in digitalized patients increases risk of digitalis toxicity.
Store in airtight containers.
See Calcium gluconate (prototype calcium replenisher).

C

CALCIUM PANTOTHENATE

(pan-toe-then′ate)

(Dextro Calcium Pantothenate, Pantholin, Vitamin B_5)

Vitamin B_5

ACTIONS AND USES. Calcium salt of pantothenic acid and member of the B-complex group; water-soluble. Precursor of coenzyme A, which functions in a variety of metabolic reactions involving transfer of acetyl groups. Is associated with release of energy from carbohydrates and the biosynthesis and degradation of fatty acids, sterols, and steroid hormones.

Used widely in conjunction with other B vitamins and multiple vitamin preparations and as nutritional supplement in enteral and parenteral alimentation. Its use for gray hair and in treatment of alopecia has not been successful. Available in combination with aluminum hydroxide and magnesium trisilicate, e.g., Durasil.

ABSORPTION AND FATE. Readily absorbed from GI tract and widely distributed in body tissues. About 70% excreted unchanged in urine and about 30% in feces. Appears in breast milk.

ROUTE AND DOSAGE. Oral: 10 mg daily, range 10 to 100 mg daily.

NURSING IMPLICATIONS

Well tolerated even in large doses.
Minimum daily requirement of pantothenic acid not established, but the following are estimates of adequate dietary intake: adults: 4 to 7 mg; adolescents and children: 3 to 4 mg; infants: 2 mg.
No human deficiency syndrome identified. Presumed signs of pantothenic acid deficiency include neurologic disturbances (burning feet and other paresthesias, steppage gait), muscle and abdominal cramps, flatulence, nausea, adrenocortical hypofunction (defective water excretion, sensitivity to insulin), dermatoses, weakness, fatigue, headache, insomnia, cardiovascular instability, mood changes, psychoses.
Pantothenic acid is widely distributed in animal and vegetable foods. Especially good sources: liver, kidney, muscle tissue, egg yolk, wheat bran, rice bran, dry milk, peanuts, legumes.
Incompatible with carbonates and phosphates.
Store preferably between 15° and 30°C (59° and 86°F) in well-closed container, unless otherwise directed by manufacturer.

CANTHARIDIN

(kan′thar-i-din)

(Canthacur, Cantharone)

Keratolytic

ACTIONS AND USES. Potent vesicant obtained from cantharides ("Spanish fly"). Preparation consists of cantharidin (0.7%) in a film-forming vehicle containing ether, alcohol, acetone, ethocel, and flexible collodion. Causes intraepidermal vesiculation without affecting basal

C

epidermal layer and with only minimal effect on corneum, and therefore does not result in scarring.

Used to remove benign epithelial growths such as warts (verrucae), including common wart, periungual, palpebral, and plantar warts. Also used to treat *Molluscum contagiosum.* Commercially available in fixed combination with salicylic acid and podophyllin (Canthacur-PS, and Cantharone Plus).

CONTRAINDICATIONS AND PRECAUTIONS. Diabetes mellitus, impaired peripheral circulation, use in presence of infection or inflammation, use on mucous membranes. Safe use during pregnancy, in nursing mothers, and in infants not established.

ADVERSE/SIDE EFFECTS. Blistering, tingling, burning sensation, extreme tenderness, annular warts; single report of chemical lymphangitis (following use of cantharidin with salicylic acid).

ROUTE AND DOSAGE. *Topical: Common and periungual warts:* Apply directly to wart with applicator stick; allow medication to dry. Cover with nonporous (occlusive) tape. Instruct patient to remove tape in 24 hours and replace with loose bandage. On next visit, necrotic tissue is removed and medication reapplied if necessary. *Plantar warts:* Pare away keratin covering wart. Using applicator stick, apply medication to wart and to 1 to 3 mm margin around wart. Allow a few minutes to dry. Secure with nonporous adhesive tape. After 3 days patient may bathe and replace dressing, as prescribed. Debridement is done 1 to 2 weeks after treatment. Small amount of medication may be reapplied to any viable wart remaining after debridement. Three or more treatments may be required. *Palpebral warts:* Apply small amount to wart surface with toothpick or fine probe. Leave uncovered. Repeat in 7 to 10 days, if required. *Molluscum contagiosum:* coat each lesion with thin film of medication. After 1 week treat remaining or new lesions; this time cover with small piece of occlusive tape. Remove tape in 4 to 6 hours.

NURSING IMPLICATIONS

Cantharidin must be applied by or under supervision of a physician and is not dispensed for patient use.

It is advisable to initiate therapy by treating only one or two lesions until patient's reaction to medication is determined. Note that fair-complexioned, blue-eyed individuals are prone to develop a reaction to cantharidin.

Avoid contact of drug with normal skin or mucous membranes as it may cause irritation and blistering.

If cantharidin contacts normal skin, remove immediately with acetone, alcohol, or tape remover, then wash vigorously with warm soapy water. Rinse well and dry.

For accidental contact of cantharidin with eye or mucous membranes, flush with water, remove precipitated collodion and flush with water for additional 15 minutes.

A small percentage of patients develop superficial annular warts following cantharidin therapy. Reassure patient that retreatment will control lesions.

If patient shows signs of sensitivity to cantharidin (tingling, burning, extreme tenderness) manufacturer recommends removing occlusive tape and soaking area in cool water for 10 to 15 minutes. Treatment may be repeated as necessary for relief of symptoms. If blisters form they may require puncturing under sterile conditions, following which they should be covered with an antiseptic, then bandaged. Cantharidin repeat treatment should be deferred if inflammatory reaction is intense.

Blenderm (3M Co.) tape is a commonly used nonporous tape. Some clinicians use old-fashioned fabric type adhesive as an occlusive tape.

Keep out of the reach of children. Cantharidin is highly toxic if taken internally and can cause severe renal damage.

Patient-Teaching Points

✓ *Molluscum contagiosum:* caused by a poxvirus. Diagnosis is confirmed by clinical examination and biopsy. Commonly transmitted by direct contact, often venereal. Indirect transmission through towels and washcloths is also possible. Although the disease is usually self-limiting, early treatment can control spread on self and to others. In addition to medication, lesions may require removal by cryosurgery or freezing, curettage, or light desiccation.

✓ *Warts (verrucae):* caused by a virus (papovavirus); mildly contagious and may be spread to other persons as well as to other parts of body. Plantar warts may be spread by swimming pools and common shower rooms. Folk remedies often appear to work because warts may disappear spontaneously, especially in young children. They are not precancerous.

CAPREOMYCIN SULFATE

(Capastat Sulfate)

(kap-ree-oh-mye'sin)
Antiinfective
Antibiotic (polypeptide)
Antituberculosis

ACTIONS AND USES. Polypeptide antibiotic derived from *Streptomyces capreolus.* Similar to viomycin in structure and action mechanism. Bacteriostatic in action; mechanism not clear. Active against human strains of *Mycobacterium tuberculosis* and other strains of *Mycobacterium.* Cross-resistance between capreomycin and both kanamycin and neomycin has been reported. Produces neuromuscular blockade in large doses.

Used in conjunction with other appropriate antitubercular drugs in treatment of pulmonary tuberculosis when bactericidal agents e.g., isoniazid and rifampin, cannot be tolerated or when causative organism has become resistant.

ABSORPTION AND FATE. Peak drug serum levels in 1 to 2 hours. Serum concentrations fall to low levels by 24 hours. Half-life: 4 to 6 hours. Approximately 52% is excreted in urine within 12 hours (if renal function is normal) essentially unchanged. Distribution to placenta and breast milk not known.

CONTRAINDICATIONS AND PRECAUTIONS. Hypersensitivity to capreomycin. Safe use during pregnancy, in nursing women and in infants and children not established. *Cautious Use:* extreme caution, if used at all in patients with renal insufficiency, auditory impairment, history of allergies (especially to drugs), preexisting liver disease, myasthenia gravis, parkinsonism.

ADVERSE/SIDE EFFECTS. Hematologic: leukocytosis, leukopenia, eosinophilia. **Hypersensitivity:** urticaria, maculopapular rash may be associated with febrile reaction, photosensitivity. **Nephrotoxicity** (long-term therapy): elevated BUN and NPN, abnormal urine sediment, hematuria, pyuria, albuminuria, depressed creatinine clearance and PSP excretion, tubular necrosis. **Ototoxicity:** eighth nerve (auditory and vestibular) damage: hearing loss, tinnitus, headache, vertigo. **Other:** hypokalemia, and other electrolyte imbalances (associated with disturbed renal function); impaired hepatic function (decreased BSP excretion); neuromuscular blockade (large doses): skeletal muscle weakness, respiratory depression or arrest; IM site reactions: pain, induration, excessive bleeding, sterile abscesses.

ROUTE AND DOSAGE. Intramuscular: 1 Gm daily (not to exceed 20 mg/kg body weight per day) given for 60 to 120 days, followed by 1 Gm two or three times weekly.

C

NURSING IMPLICATIONS

The following determinations are used as guidelines for therapy and should be performed before drug is started and at regular intervals during therapy: (1) appropriate bacterial susceptibility tests; (2) audiometric measurements (twice weekly or weekly) and tests of vestibular function (periodically); (3) complete blood counts; SMA-12 screening weekly: (4) weekly function studies (BUN, NPN, creatinine clearance, sediment); (5) liver function tests (periodically); (6) serum potassium levels (monthly).

IM injections should be made deep into large muscle mass. Superficial injections are more painful and are associated with sterile abscess. Aspirate carefully before injecting drug to avoid inadvertent entry into blood vessel (IV injection can cause neuromuscular blockade). Rotate injection sites.

Observe injection sites for signs of excessive bleeding and inflammation.

Monitor intake and output. Report immediately to physician any change in output or intake and output ratio, any unusual appearance of urine, or elevation of BUN above 30 mg/dl. (Normal BUN: 8 to 25 mg/dl.)

Instruct patient to report any change in hearing or disturbance of balance. Capreomycin can cause injury to both auditory and vestibular portions of cranial nerve VIII. These effects are sometimes reversible if drug is withdrawn promptly when first symptoms appear.

Hypokalemia is a significant side effect. Observe for and report muscle weakness, paresthesias, depressed reflexes, polyuria, polydipsia, gastric distention, unexplained anxiety.

Patient and responsible family members should be completely informed about adverse reactions. They should be urged to report immediately the appearance of any unusual symptom, regardless how vague it may seem.

Capreomycin is reconstituted by adding isotonic sodium chloride injection or sterile water for infection to vial; allow 2 to 3 minutes for drug to dissolve completely. See manufacturer's directions for volume of diluent.

Solution may become pale straw color and darken with time, but this does not indicate loss of potency or toxicity.

After reconstitution, solution may be stored 48 hours at room temperature and up to 14 days under refrigeration, unless otherwise directed by manufacturer.

Store preferably between 15° and 30°C (59° and 86°F), unless otherwise directed by manufacturer.

Drug Interactions: Capreomycin

Plus	Interactions
Drugs with high nephrotoxic or ototoxic potential, e.g., aminoglycoside antibiotics, colistin (Coly-Mycin S), polymyxin B (Aerosporin), vancomycin (Vancocin)	Increased risk of nephrotoxicity and ototoxicity. Concurrent or sequential use generally avoided
Aminoglycoside antibiotics Phenothiazines Tubocurarine and other nondepolarizing skeletal muscle relaxants	Possibility of additive neuromuscular blocking actions. Monitor for respiratory depression

CAPTOPRIL
(Capoten)

(kap'toe-pril)
Antihypertensive
Enzyme inhibitor

ACTIONS AND USES. Lowers blood pressure (renovascular and essential) by specific inhibition of the angiotensin-converting enzyme (ACE). This interrupts conversion sequences initiated by renin that ordinarily lead to formation of angiotensin II, a potent endogenous vasoconstrictor. ACE inhibition alters hemodynamics without compensatory reflex tachycardia or changes in cardiac output (except in patient with congestive heart failure). Peripheral vascular resistance is lowered by vasodilation but vascular bed perfusion in brain, heart, and peripheral circulation is maintained. Blockage of ACE also leads to decreased circulating aldosterone, a secretory response to angiotensin II stimulation. (Aldosterone, an adrenal cortex hormone promotes sodium and fluid retention.) Additionally, captopril is associated with interference with degradation of bradykinin (a potent vasodilator), increased plasma levels of a prostaglandin E_2 metabolite with vasodilator properties and a K-sparing effect (due to reduced aldosterone level). In heart failure, captopril administration is followed by a fall in CVP and pulmonary wedge pressure. Hypertensive action in essential hypertension appears to be unrelated to plasma renin levels. Available in fixed combination with hydrochlorothiazide (Capozide).

Used in treatment of mild to moderate hypertension; in severe hypertension resistant to conventional multidrug regimen (as step 4 agent in stepped care approach), and in conjunction with digitalis and diuretics in treatment of intractable edema or congestive heart failure. *Unlabeled Use:* treatment of arthritis.

ABSORPTION AND FATE. About 60 to 75% of dose absorbed rapidly following oral administration. Hypotensive effect of a single dose begins within 15 minutes, is maximal in 1 to 2 hours, and continues for 6 hours with small doses and up to 12 hours with larger doses. Rapid distribution to all tissues except CNS. Approximately 25 to 30% bound to plasma proteins. Half-life: less than 2 hours; increases to 20 to 40 hours when creatinine clearance is less than 20 ml/min. Over 95% of an absorbed dose excreted in urine as unchanged drug (40 to 50%) and metabolites. Removed by hemodialysis. It is not known if it crosses placenta, but it is distributed to breast milk.

CONTRAINDICATIONS AND PRECAUTIONS. Pregnancy (category C); safe use in nursing mothers and children not established. *Cautious Use:* impaired renal function; patient with solitary kidney; autoimmune diseases (particularly systemic lupus erythematosus), patients receiving immunosuppressants or other drugs that cause leukopenia or agranulocytosis; coronary or cerebrovascular disease; severe salt/volume depletion.

ADVERSE/SIDE EFFECTS. CV: slight increase in heart rate, hypotension, dizziness, fainting; rare: tachycardia, palpitation, angina pectoris, myocardial infarction, Raynaud's syndrome. **Dermatologic:** oncholysis, maculopapular rash (especially on upper extremities and trunk), urticaria, pruritus, angioedema, photosensitivity. **GI:** severe anorexia, GI distress. **Hematologic:** neutropenia, agranulocytosis, pancytopenia. **Renal:** proteinuria, urinary frequency, oliguria, impaired renal function, nephrotic syndrome, membranous glomerulonephritis. **Other:** reversible "scalded mouth sensation" (loss of taste perception, persistent salt or metallic taste); weight loss, cholestatic jaundice (rare), positive antinuclear antibody (ANA) titers, hyperkalemia.

ROUTE AND DOSAGE. Oral: Initial: 25 mg three times daily. Doses may be increased to 50 mg three times daily after 1 to 2 weeks, if necessary. If blood pressure control is still not satisfactory, a thiazide diuretic is added (e.g., hydrochlorothiazide 25 mg daily; increased to maximum antihypertensive level if necessary). If further control is indicated, captopril may be increased to 100 mg three times daily, then 150 mg three times daily, if required (diuretic therapy is continued). Maintenance: 25 to 150 mg three times daily. Maximum dose up to 450 mg daily.

NURSING IMPLICATIONS

If necessary, tablet may be crushed and taken with fluid. Best administered 1 hour before meals. Food reduces absorption by 30 to 40%.

Hyponatremia is a good predictor of potential first-dose phenomenon. Liberalized salt intake and termination of diuretic therapy are usual preparations 7 to 10 days before captopril treatment.

Bed rest and blood pressure monitoring are advised for the first 3 hours after the initial dose.

First dose phenomenon (hypotensive effect) (i.e., a precipitous drop in blood pressure) may occur within 1 to 3 hours of first dose, especially in the patient with very high blood pressure or one on a diuretic and controlled salt intake regimen. An IV infusion of normal saline for volume expansion will counteract the hypotensive response. (This initial response is not usually considered an indication to stop therapy with captopril.)

If patient is advised to restrict salt intake, emphasize that a salt substitute should be used only if prescribed. The abuse of a substitute (principal ingredient: K) can reinforce susceptibility to drug-induced hyperkalemia. *(See Index: Salt substitutes.)*

At least 2 weeks of therapy may be required before full therapeutic effects are achieved. If patient has impaired renal function, doses must be smaller and attainment of steady-state captopril levels will require more time.

Baseline urinary protein levels should be established prior to initiation of therapy and checked at monthly intervals for the first 8 months of treatment and then periodically thereafter.

Physician may request patient to test first voided morning urine at home using a dipstick (e.g., Chemstrip GP, Uristix), or collect a 24-hour specimen for laboratory quantification. Proteinuria occurs in 1 to 2% of patients receiving captopril and may reach levels as high as 1 Gm/day. (Normal value: <150 mg/24 hours.) If proteinuria persists (suggests renal disease), captopril therapy should be reevaluated.

WBC and differential counts are recommended before starting therapy and at approximately 2-week intervals for the first 3 months of therapy and then periodically thereafter. Differential counts are advised whenever leukocytes are 4000 mm^3 or less or half that of pretreatment level.

A patient with SLE is particularly prone to drug-induced neutropenia.

Urge patient to report to physician without delay the onset of unexplained fever, unusual fatigue, sore mouth or throat, easy bruising or bleeding (pathognomonic of agranulocytosis).

Since excessive vomiting, diarrhea, and perspiration can lead to depleted fluids with consequent drop in blood pressure, advise patient to consult physician if these symptoms occur.

Mild skin eruptions are most likely to appear during the first 4 weeks of therapy and may be accompanied by fever and eosinophilia. Advise patient to report to physician. Dosage reduction or discontinuation may be indicated.

Darkening, separating, or crumbling of nailbeds (onycholysis) has been reported. These changes usually disappear with dose reduction or termination.

Taste impairment (dysgeusia) occurs in 5 to 10% of patients and generally reverses in 2 to 3 months even with continued therapy. In some patients, it may be associated with anorexia and weight loss and may necessitate discontinuation of drug. If therapy is stopped, symptoms usually disappear within 3 to 4 weeks.

Treatment of overdosage involves correction of hypotension by blood volume expansion with IV infusions and possibly by hemodialysis.
See *Guanethidine* for teaching summary related to pharmacotherapy in hypertension.
Store in light-resistant containers at no more than 30°C (86°F) unless otherwise directed by manufacturer.

Diagnostic Test Interferences. In some patients elevated **urine protein levels** may persist even after captopril has been discontinued. Possibility of transient elevations of **BUN** and **serum creatinine,** slight increase in **serum potassium,** and **serum prolactin,** increases in **liver enzymes,** and false-positive **urine acetone.**

Drug Interactions: Captopril

Plus	Interactions
Antihypertensives that cause renin release [e.g., minoxidil (Loniten)]	Additive hypotensive action of captopril
Ganglionic blocking agents [e.g., mecamylamine (Inversine)]	Possible enhancement of hypotensive action of captopril (by reducing CNS support of blood pressure)
Nitroglycerin and other nitrates	Possibility of enhanced hypotensive effect (by vasodilation) of captopril
Indomethacin Salicylates	Antihypertensive effectiveness of captopril may be decreased. Dosage adjustments may be indicated
Potassium-sparing diuretics [e.g., amiloride (Midamor)] K supplements (e.g., potassium chloride)	Possibility of hyperkalemia
Probenecid	Pharmacologic effects of captopril may be increased

CARBACHOL

(Carbacel, Isopto Carbachol, Miostat Intraocular)

(kar'ba-kole)
Cholinergic, direct (parasympathomimetic)
Miotic

ACTIONS AND USES. Potent synthetic choline ester similar to acetylcholine in pharmacologic properties. Inactivation by cholinesterase is slow therefore its actions are more prolonged than those of acetylcholine; also more potent and longer-acting than pilocarpine. Acts directly on neuroeffectors of circular pupillary constrictor and ciliary muscles, producing miosis and spasms of accommodation, thus facilitating drainage from arterior chamber with consequent lowering of intraocular pressure. Usually prepared with wetting agent such as benzalkonium chloride to enhance corneal penetration.

Used intraocularly to produce pupillary miosis during ocular surgery. Used topically to reduce intraocular pressure in open-angle or narrow-angle glaucoma, particularly when patient has become intolerant of or resistant to pilocarpine.

ABSORPTION AND FATE. Poor penetration of intact cornea. Miotic action occurs in 10 to 20 minutes following topical application and lasts 4 to 8 hours. Miotic action occurs in 2 to 5 minutes following intraocular administration and persists about 24 hours.

CONTRAINDICATIONS AND PRECAUTIONS. Known hypersensitivity to any of the components; corneal abrasions, acute iritis. Safe use during pregnancy (category C) in nursing women, and in children not established. *Cautious Use:* acute cardiac failure, bronchial asthma, peptic ulcer, GI spasms, obstructive ileus, hyperthyroidism, urinary tract obstruction, Parkinson's disease; use following topical anesthetics or tonometry.

ADVERSE/SIDE EFFECTS. Headache, brow and eye pain, conjunctival hyperemia, ciliary spasm with temporary reduction in visual acuity, iritis. **Systemic absorption:** sweating, flushing, ciliary spasm, abdominal cramps, increased peristalsis, diarrhea, contractions of urinary bladder, transient fall in blood pressure with reflex tachycardia, asthma. Hypersensitivity reactions (infrequent).

ROUTE AND DOSAGE. Topical ophthalmic: 1 or 2 drops of 0.75 to 3% solution instilled into lower conjunctival sac two or four times daily. **Intraocular (administered by physician):** 0.5 ml of 0.01% intraocular solution instilled into anterior chamber before or after securing sutures.

NURSING IMPLICATIONS

Eye drops are sterile and therefore should be handled so as to avoid contamination.

Frequent administration of potent eye preparations presents the danger of systemic absorption if drug is allowed to drain into lacrimal system. Application of gentle pressure to nasolacrimal duct for 1 minute immediately after drop is instilled and before patient closes eyes prevents entry of drug into nasopharynx and general circulation. (For more complete description of administration technique, *See Index: Drug Administration: Eye drops.)*

Patient may blot lid with clean tissue, but advise patient not to rub or squeeze lids together.

Frequency and strength of drops are determined by patient's response and tolerance. Resistance may develop suddenly in some patients.

The patient with glaucoma should remain under medical supervision for periodic tonometer measurements, since patient usually will require miotics for the rest of his or her life. The patient must understand that even in the absence of symptoms progressive ocular damage can occur unless appropriate treatment is received.

Intraocular carbachol (e.g., Miostat) is intended for single-dose intraocular use only (administered by physician). Unused portions should be discarded.

Caution patient that drug may temporarily impair visual acuity particularly adaptation to dark and therefore to observe necessary safety precautions.

Store preferably between 15° and 30°C (59° and 86°F), unless otherwise directed by manufacturer.

CARBAMAZEPINE

(kar-ba-maz′e-peen)

(Tegretol)

Anticonvulsant

ACTIONS AND USES. Structurally related to tricyclic antidepressants but lacks antidepressant properties. Anticonvulsant actions appear qualitatively similar to those of phenytoin (Dilantin). Like phenytoin, provides relief in trigeminal neuralgia by reducing synaptic transmission within trigeminal nucleus. Also has sedative, anticholinergic, antidepressant, and muscle relaxant (by inhibition of neuromuscular transmission) and slight analgesic actions.

Used alone or concomitantly with other anticonvulsants in treatment of grand mal and psychomotor or temporal lobe epilepsy and mixed seizures in patients who have not responded satisfactorily to other agents. Also used for symptomatic treatment of trigeminal (tic douloureux) and glossopharyngeal neuralgias and for pain and paroxysmal symptoms associated with multiple sclerosis, and other neurologic disorders. *Investigational Use:* in prophylactic management of manic–depressive illness, for treatment of rage outbursts, restless legs syndrome, and for antidiuretic effect in diabetes insipidus.

C

ABSORPTION AND FATE. Slowly absorbed from GI tract; unpredictable absorption rate. Peak serum levels in 2 to 8 hours (variable). Widely distributed in body, especially in saliva, duodenal fluid, and bile; high concentrations in CSF. Half-life: 14 to 16 hours. Induces liver microsomal enzymes and thus may accelerate its own metabolism and that of drugs metabolized in liver. Highly bound (75 to 90%) to plasma proteins. Metabolites and less than 1% of unchanged drug excreted in urine and feces. Crosses placenta and appears in breast milk in high concentrations.

CONTRAINDICATIONS AND PRECAUTIONS. Hypersensitivity to carbamazepine and to tricyclic compounds; history of myelosuppression or hematologic reaction to other drugs; increased intraocular pressure; systemic lupus erythematosus (SLE); cardiac, hepatic, renal, or urinary tract disease; coronary artery disease; hypertension. Safe use in women of childbearing potential and during pregnancy, in nursing women, and in children younger than 6 years of age not established. *Cautious Use:* the elderly; history of cardiac disease.

ADVERSE/SIDE EFFECTS. CNS: dizziness, vertigo, drowsiness, disturbances of coordination, ataxia, confusion, headache, fatigue, tinnitus, abnormal hearing acuity, speech difficulty, development of minor motor seizures, hyperreflexia, involuntary movements, tremors, peripheral neuritis, paresthesias, visual hallucinations, activation of latent psychosis, mental depression with agitation and talkativeness. **CV:** edema, congestive heart failure, aggravation of coronary artery disease, hypertension, hypotension, syncope, arrhythmias, heart block, thrombophlebitis, circulatory collapse. **Dermatologic/Hypersensitivity:** skin rashes, urticaria, petechiae, Stevens-Johnson syndrome, photosensitivity reactions, altered skin pigmentation, exfoliative dermatitis, alopecia, aggravation of SLE; wheezing. **GI:** nausea, vomiting, anorexia, abdominal pain, diarrhea, constipation, dry mouth and pharynx, glossitis, stomatitis. **GU:** urinary frequency and retention, oliguria, impotence, albuminuria, glycosuria, elevated blood urea nitrogen (BUN), acute renal failure (rare). **Hematologic:** aplastic anemia, reticulocytosis, leukopenia, leukocytosis, agranulocytosis, eosinophilia, thrombocytopenia, purpura, hyponatremia. **Hepatotoxicity:** abnormal liver function tests, granulomatous hepatitis, cholestatic and hepatocellular jaundice. **Ophthalmic:** lens opacities, conjunctivitis, blurred vision, transient diplopia, oculomotor disturbances, nystagmus, mydriasis. **Other:** idiosyncratic virus-like infection (fever, chills, lymphadenopathy), diaphoresis, pneumonitis, myalgia, arthralgia, leg cramps, hypothyroidism.

ROUTE AND DOSAGE. Oral: *Epilepsy:* **Adults and children (over 12 years):** Initial: 200 mg two times a day, increased gradually by up to 200 mg/day. To minimize adverse effects, dosages in excess of 400 mg/day administered in three or four equally divided doses. Maintenance: 800 to 1200 mg daily in divided doses. Not to exceed 1000 mg/day in children 12 to 15 years or 1200 mg/day in patients over 15 years. **Children (6 to 12 years):** 100 mg twice daily increased gradually by 100 mg/day, using t.i.d. or q.i.d. regimen for doses in excess of 200 mg/day. Not to exceed 1000 mg day. Maintenance: 400 to 800 mg daily in divided doses. *Trigeminal neuralgia:* **Adults:** Initial: 100 mg twice a day; thereafter, dose is increased gradually by 100-mg increments every 12 hours until pain is relieved or side effects occur. Maintenance: 200 to 800 mg. Available in tablets and chewable tablets.

NURSING IMPLICATIONS

Absorption of drug is enhanced by administration with meals.

Prior to initiation of carbamazepine therapy, the following procedures for eliciting baseline data are recommended: (1) detailed health history; (2) physical examination, including

C

ophthalmoscopy (slit lamp, fundoscopy, tonometry) and ECG; (3) laboratory studies: complete blood counts including platelets, reticulocytes, and serum iron, liver function tests, BUN, and complete urinalysis.

Blood studies, as described above, should be repeated weekly during first 3 months of therapy, and monthly thereafter for at least 2 to 3 years (for early detection of bone marrow depression). Other tests (listed above) should be performed at regular intervals during drug treatment. Abnormal findings signal the need for dosage reduction or drug withdrawal.

Physician will rely on accurate observation and early reporting to determine lowest effective dosage level.

The following reactions occur commonly during early therapy: drowsiness, dizziness, lightheadedness, ataxia, gastric upset. If these symptoms do not subside within a few days, dosage adjustments may be indicated.

In general, therapy should be discontinued if any of the following signs of myelosuppression occur: erythrocyte count less than 4 million/mm^3, Hct less than 32%, Hgb less than 11 Gm/dl, leukocyte count less than 4000/mm^3, platelet count less than 100,000/mm^3, reticulocyte count less than 20,000/mm^3, serum iron greater than 150 mcg/dl.

Therapeutic serum levels reported to be 4 to 12 mcg/ml. Steady-state is generally reached in 2 to 4 days. Bear in mind that serum levels do not always reflect daily dosage requirements.

Home patients and responsible family members should be instructed to withhold drug and notify physician immediately if early signs of a possible hematologic problem appear, e.g., fever, sore throat or mouth, malaise, unusual fatigue, tendency to bruise or bleed, petechiae, ecchymoses, bleeding gums, nose bleeds.

Monitor intake and output ratio and vital signs during period of dosage adjustment. Report oliguria, signs of fluid retention (edema, night coughing, dyspnea), changes in intake and output ratio, and changes in blood pressure or pulse patterns.

Doses higher than 600 mg/day may precipitate arrhythmias in patients with heart disease.

The pain of tic douloureux is so excruciating that it has driven some patients to suicide. Learn from the patient what provokes attacks. Common triggering stimuli include drafts, shaving, washing face, talking, chewing, hot or cold fluids or foods, and jarring the bed.

Because dizziness, drowsiness, and ataxia are common side effects, warn patient to avoid hazardous tasks requiring mental alertness and physical coordination.

Impress on the patient and family the importance of remaining under close medical supervision throughout therapy.

Confusion and agitation may be aggravated in the elderly; therefore side rails and supervision of ambulation may be indicated.

Because photosensitivity reactions have been reported, caution patient to avoid excessive sunlight. Suggest application of a sunscreen (if allowed) with sun protection factor (SPF) of 12 or above to exposed skin areas when outdoors.

Patients taking oral contraceptives should be informed that carbamazepine may cause breakthrough bleeding and may also affect the reliability of oral contraceptives.

At least every 3 months throughout therapy it is recommended that physician attempt dosage reduction or termination of drug therapy, if possible, in patients with trigeminal neuralgia. Some patients develop tolerance to the effects of carbamazepine.

In patients with epilepsy, abrupt withdrawal of any anticonvulsant drug may precipitate seizures or even status epilepticus.

Store preferably between 15° and 30°C (59° and 86°F), unless otherwise directed by manufacturer.

Drug Interactions: Carbamazepine

Plus	Interactions
Anticoagulants, oral Doxycycline Oral contraceptives Phenytoin (Dilantin) Theophyllines	Carbamazepine appears to enhance metabolism of these drugs by inducing hepatic microsomal enzymes. Monitor closely for altered drug effectiveness when carbamazepine is initiated or discontinued
Erythromycins Isoniazid (INH) Niacinamide Propoxyphene (Darvon) Troleandomycin (TAO)	Carbamazepine actions may be increased (metabolism may be inhibited by these drugs). Monitor for carbamazepine toxicity
Lithium	Possibility of increased lithium effects and toxicity (may not be reflected in plasma lithium levels). Used concomitantly with caution
MAO inhibitors	Possibility of additive pharmacologic actions. Concomitant use avoided

---

CARBAMIDE PEROXIDE

(kar'ba-mide per-ox'ide)
Antiinfective, topical

(Cankaid, Debrox, Gly-Oxide, Murine Ear Drops, Orajel Brace-aid Rinse, Proxigel, Urea Peroxide)

ACTIONS AND USES. Urea compound combined with hydrogen peroxide 1:1 with foaming action and weak antibacterial properties due to release of nascent oxygen when exposed to moisture. Effervescence of liberated oxygen mechanically facilitates cleansing by loosening tissue debris or impacted or excessive ear wax. Commercial formulations contain anhydrous glycerin, which helps to penetrate and soften wax. Topical oral preparations contain 10 to 11% carbamide peroxide and otic preparations contain 6.5%.

Preparations intended for topical oral application are used for minor irritation, infection and inflammation of mouth and gums, such as aphthous ulcers (canker sores), gingivitis, stomatitis, Vincent's infection, and denture irritations. Also used as adjunct in oral hygiene. Otic formulations are used as aid in removal of excessive or hardened cerumen and to help prevent ceruminosis.

CONTRAINDICATIONS AND PRECAUTIONS. Use of otic preparations following otic surgery or in patients with perforated ear drum or with redness, tenderness, pain, dizziness, or ear drainage; use in children under 12 years. Use of topical mouth formulations in children under 3 years.

ADVERSE/SIDE EFFECTS. Redness, irritation, superinfections.

ROUTE AND DOSAGE. Topical: *Mouth lesions:* Apply several drops (undiluted) directly to affected area, four times daily. Expectorate after 1 to 3 minutes. If gel is used, apply undiluted (four times daily): gently massage medication on affected areas with finger or swab; do not drink or rinse for 5 minutes. Not to be used beyond 7 days. *For widespread inflammation or hard-to-reach surfaces:* place 10 drops on tongue; mix with saliva, swish for several minutes, then expectorate. *Ear wax:* instill 5 to 10 drops into affected ear twice daily for 3 or 4 days.

C

NURSING IMPLICATIONS

Topical oral preparation: used preferably after meals and at bedtime. Advise patient to rinse mouth of food debris before doing treatment.

Forewarn patient that medication will foam on contact with saliva.

Review essentials of good dental hygiene: use small soft-bristled toothbrush and a fluoride toothpaste. Floss teeth with dental floss once a day. At least rinse mouth thoroughly after each meal or after eating sweets.

Investigate cause of sore mouth. Dental referral may be indicated.

Advise patient to discontinue treatment and notify physician if redness, irritation, swelling, or pain increases or persists.

Instruct patient to examine mouth for signs of superinfection, e.g., black, hairy tongue.

Store medication in tightly covered container in a cool place. Protect from light.

Otic preparation:

- To administer ear drop to an adult: pull ear up and back. Support hand holding dropper on patient's head. Have patient tilt head so that affected ear is uppermost. Direct solution toward the canal, not the eardrum. Advise patient to keep head tilted for several minutes to assure contact of medication with ear wax.
- When instilling ear drops do not allow tip of bottle to enter ear canal.
- Gentle irrigation of ear with warm water or normal saline using a soft rubber ear washer placed on edge of ear canal may be necessary to facilitate removal of loosened wax. Ear canal should be dried after treatment. Many physicians prefer to use a chemical drying agent to dry ear canal instead of a swab: e.g., 70% isopropanol, Orlex Otic Solution, VōSol Otic Solution. Consult physician.
- Medication should be discontinued and physician notified promptly if patient develops dizziness, ear drainage, pain, tenderness, or redness.
- Ear wax in physiologic amounts is believed to be bacteriostatic, fungistatic, and to repel water.
- The most common causes of wax buildup are lack of humidity (causing wax to dry and harden), excessive hair growth in ears, attempts to remove wax with cotton swab which only jams the wax farther into ears.
- Protect medication from heat and direct sunlight.

PROTOTYPE

CARBARSONE

(kar-bar′sone)
Antiinfective
Amebicide

ACTIONS AND USES. Pentavalent organic arsenical containing 28.5% arsenic. Acts primarily in intestinal lumen against amebic intestinal trophozoites of *Entamoeba histolytica,* the source of cysts.

Used alone or in combination with other amebicides in treatment of acute and chronic intestinal amebiasis.

ABSORPTION AND FATE. Readily absorbed from GI tract. Presumed to be reduced in body to trivalent derivative, carbarsone oxide. Accumulates in tissues; slowly excreted by kidneys.

CONTRAINDICATIONS AND PRECAUTIONS. Hypersensitivity or intolerance to arsenic compounds, amebic hepatitis or other liver disease, kidney disease, contraction of visual or color fields or other visual disturbances. Safe use during pregnancy (category C), and in nursing women not established.

ADVERSE/SIDE EFFECTS. *Signs of arsenic toxicity:* **CNS:** hemorrhagic encephalitis, neuritis, convulsions, coma. **ENT:** sore throat, ulcerations of mucous membranes. **GI:** nausea, vomiting, gastritis, increased diarrhea, anorexia, epigastric pain and burning, increased GI motility, abdominal cramps, constipation, weight loss. **GU:** polyuria, albuminuria, kidney damage. **Hepatic:** hepatomegaly, hepatitis, jaundice, liver necrosis. **Hypersensitivity:** skin rash, pruritus, severe exfoliative dermatitis. **Ophthalmic:** retinal edema, papillitis, visual disturbances. **Other:** pulmonary congestion, fever, aplastic anemia, agranulocytosis, splenomegaly, edema of wrists, ankles, knees; shock.

ROUTE AND DOSAGE. Adults: Oral: 250 mg two or three times daily for 10 days. Course of therapy repeated if necessary after rest interval of 10 to 14 days. **Rectal** (as retention enema): 2 Gm dissolved in 200 ml warm 2% sodium bicarbonate solution, administered every other night for 5 doses. **Children:** average total dose over a 10 day period is about 75 mg/kg, administered in divided doses three times daily.

NURSING IMPLICATIONS

For children, it will be necessary to divide contents of a capsule and give in half a glass of milk or orange juice, in jelly or other food, or in a small volume of sodium bicarbonate solution 1%, if allowed.

Liver function tests are advised before initiation of carbarsone therapy and periodically during treatment.

Regular and careful inspection of skin, vision testing, and palpation of liver and spleen should be done during therapy.

Monitor intake and output. Amebiasis may produce liquid stools containing blood and mucus. Keep physician informed of number, frequency, and character of stools.

Low-residue diet may be prescribed, and patient is usually advised to limit physical activities during treatment period.

Because drug is excreted slowly, a rest period of 10 to 14 days must follow each 10-day course of therapy before starting another course, in order to prevent accumulation and toxicity. At the first appearance of adverse reaction, drug should be discontinued.

Instruct patient and responsible family members to report immediately GI upset, visual disturbances, sore throat, skin lesions, and urinary symptoms. Also report aggravation of symptoms already present or appearance of any other unusual signs or symptoms, even after therapy has been discontinued.

Carbarsone retention enema is generally ordered if patient has deep ulcers of lower colon.

The retention enema is instilled after a cleansing enema (following a delay sufficient that the urge to defecate has passed). Oral dose should be omitted when retention enema is given. A sedative may be prescribed to help patient retain medication.

Stools should be examined daily for amebic cysts. Presence of cysts indicates the need for an additional course of therapy.

Beginning 1 week after completion of therapy, stools should be examined for cysts on 3 alternate days and at monthly intervals for about 3 months to assure that amebae have been eliminated.

If enema is to be given to obtain stool specimen, normal saline or tap water should be used. Hypertonic solutions may alter appearance of amebae.

Stool specimen should be delivered promptly to laboratory for incubation. Characteristic movements of parasites are seen only when specimen is warm.

Microscopic examination should be made of feces of other household members, supplemented by search for source of infection and mode of transmission.

Amebic cysts are transmitted by water, vegetables (especially those served raw), and flies,

C

by hand-to-mouth transfer of fresh feces and by soiled hands of food handlers. In teaching the patient, emphasize personal hygiene, particularly sanitary disposal of feces, hand washing after defecation and before eating, and risks of eating raw foods.

Advise use of liquid soap (or patient's own bar of soap) for handwashing to prevent cross-contamination. Recent evidence suggests that "in use" bar soap may harbor viable microorganisms for as long as 48 hours after handwashing.

Isolation is not required, but patient must be excluded from preparing, processing, and serving foods until treatment is completed.

Treatment of arsenic toxicity: Have on hand the antidote dimercaprol (BAL), a chelating agent and specific antiarsenical. General symptomatic and supportive management: gastric lavage, oxygen, IV fluids, maintenance of body temperature.

CARBENICILLIN DISODIUM

(Geopen, Pyopen)

(kar-ben-i-sill'in)
Antiinfective
Antibiotic (beta lactam)
Penicillin

ACTIONS AND USES. Extended spectrum, penicillinase-sensitive, semisynthetic penicillin derived from penicillin G (benzylpenicillin). Similar to penicillin G (qv) in actions and adverse effects, but differs in having a broader range of antibacterial activity. Bactericidal against a variety of gram-negative and gram-positive microorganisms. Particularly effective against gram-negative infections caused by *Pseudomonas aeruginosa, Proteus* (especially indole-positive strains), susceptible strains of *Escherichia coli, Enterobacter* (Aerobacter), *Haemophilus influenzae,* and *Neisseria gonorrhoeae.* Effective also in severe infections caused by gram-positive *Streptococcus pneumoniae,* and enterocci *(Streptococcus faecalis).* Inhibits aggregation of newly formed and circulating platelets with resultant prolongation of bleeding and prothrombin times, particularly in high doses and in patients with impaired renal function. Contains 4.7 to 6.5 mEq (108 to 150 mg) of sodium per Gm of drug.

Used in the treatment of bacteremias, pneumonias, infections following burns, infections in patients with impaired immunologic defenses, and urinary tract infections caused by microorganisms resistant to penicillin G and ampicillin. May be used concurrently with gentamycin and tobramycin pending results of culture and susceptibility test and with probenicid to attain higher and more prolonged serum levels.

ABSORPTION AND FATE. Serum concentrations peak in 1 to 2 hours following IM injection, decline considerably by 3 hours, and are very low or absent by 6 hours. Blood levels are higher (in 15 to 30 minutes) following IV, but decrease more rapidly. Serum half-life about 67 minutes; prolonged to 10 to 15 hours in hepatic dysfunction and in renal impairment. Widely distributed in body tissues and fluids; low concentrations in CSF unless meninges are inflamed. Approximately 50% bound to plasma proteins. About 80 to 99% of single dose excreted unchanged in urine within 24 hours, most excreted in first 6 hours. Crosses placenta. Excreted in breast milk in small amounts.

CONTRAINDICATIONS AND PRECAUTIONS. Hypersensitivity to penicillins or cephalosporins. *Cautious Use:* history of or suspected atopy or allergies (asthma, hay fever, hives, eczema), renal or hepatic disease; coagulation disorders, patients on sodium restriction (cardiac patients; hypertensives). Safe use during pregnancy not established.

ADVERSE/SIDE EFFECTS. As for penicillin G (qv): **CNS:** with high doses: neurotoxicity (impaired sensorium, neuromuscular irritability, lethargy, hallucinations, asterixis, seizures). **GI:** nausea, vomiting, diarrhea, unpleasant taste. **Hematologic:** hemorrhagic manifestations (abnormal clotting and prothrombin times), hypernatremia and fluid overload, hypokalemia, hypokalemic alkalosis, anemia, neutropenia, leukopenia, thrombocytopenia, elevations of SGOT, SGPT (particularly in children); elevated CPK (from muscle injury following IM use). **Hypersensitivity:** pruritus, urticaria, skin rash, fever, chills, eosinophilia, anaphylactic reaction. **Renal:** hematuria, interstitial nephritis. **Other:** pain and induration (IM site), thrombophlebitis (IV site), superinfections.

ROUTE AND DOSAGE. Highly individualized according to severity of infection and status of renal function. **Intramuscular, intravenous:** *Urinary tract infections:* **Adults:** 200 mg/kg/day by IV drip or 1 to 2 Gm IM or IV every 6 hours. **Children:** 50 to 200 mg/kg/day in divided doses every 4 to 6 hours, IM or IV. *Soft tissue, respiratory infections, septicemia:* **Adults:** 15 to 40 Gm daily IV in divided doses or by continuous infusion. Not to exceed 40 Gm/day. **Children:** 250 to 500 mg/kg/day (not to exceed 40 Gm/day) IV by continuous infusion or in divided doses IV or IM. *Gonorrhea:* 4 Gm IM, divided between two injection sites. (Probenecid 1 Gm administered orally 30 minutes before injection.)

NURSING IMPLICATIONS

Culture and sensitivity tests are performed initially and at regular intervals throughout therapy in order to monitor drug effectiveness.

Careful inquiry should be made concerning hypersensitivity reactions to penicillin, cephalosporins, and other allergens.

Check expiration date.

IM injections should not exceed 2 Gm per individual injection site. Administer IM well into body of large muscle. Gluteus maximus and midlateral thigh are preferred sites for adults; midlateral thigh is the preferred site for children (follow agency policy). Rotate injection sites.

Pain and other local reactions associated with IM injections may be minimized by reconstituting drug with 0.5% lidocaine hydrochloride without epinephrine (prescribed by physician), or bacteriostatic water for injection containing 0.9% benzyl alcohol. The latter must *not* be used in neonates.

Follow manufacturer's directions explicitly regarding diluent and amount to use for initial reconstitution and for further dilution, to avoid tissue irritation and phlebitis.

After reconstitution, IM solutions retain their stability for 24 hours at room temperature, and for 72 hours if refrigerated. Indicate time and date of reconstitution on container. Follow manufacturer's recommendations for stability, storage, and compatibility information.

Monitor intake and output. Report any change in intake and output ratio, pattern, and unusual appearance of urine. Consult physician regarding advisable fluid intake.

Patients with impaired renal function are particularly susceptible to nephrotoxicity, neurotoxicity, and hemorrhagic manifestations and therefore must be closely monitored.

Bleeding tendency is most likely to occur 12 to 24 hours after initiation of therapy, in patients receiving high dose therapy and in those with impaired renal function. Observe patient for frank bleeding, nose bleed, bleeding gums, hematuria, purpura, petechiae, easy bruising or ecchymoses. If bleeding manifestations appear, drug should be stopped. Report promptly to physician.

C

Serum electrolytes, renal, hepatic, cardiac status and hematopoietic functions, and bleeding time assessments should be made prior to and at regular intervals during prolonged therapy, and in patients receiving high doses or who have impaired renal or hepatic function.

Serum electrolytes (particularly potassium and sodium) should be closely monitored in patients on sodium restriction.

Observe patients for symptoms of hypernatremia (confusion, neuromuscular excitability, muscle weakness, seizures); congestive heart failure (paroxysmal nocturnal dyspnea, cough, fatigue or dyspnea on exertion, tachycardia, edema, weight gain); and hypokalemia (paresthesias, muscle weakness, depressed reflexes, polyuria, disturbances in cardiac rhythm, gastric distention, ileus).

Report immediately signs and symptoms of hypersensitivity reaction. *(See Penicillin G, Adverse/Side Affects.)* Have on hand: epinephrine, IV corticosteroids, oxygen, suction, endotracheal tube, tracheostomy equipment.

Bear in mind that superinfections are particularly likely to occur in patients receiving extended spectrum penicillins. Report black, furry overgrowth on tongue, sore mouth, rectal or vaginal itching, vaginal discharge, loose foul-smelling stools, unusual odor to urine, cough, sudden fever.

Store preferably between 15° and 30°C (59° and 86°F), unless otherwise directed by manufacturer.

See Penicillin G (prototype penicillin).

Diagnostic Test Interferences. Elevated **serum sodium** levels with large carbenicillin doses due to high sodium content.

Drug Interactions: Carbenicillin

Plus	Interactions
Aminoglycoside antibiotics	Synergistic action when administered concurrently. However, carbenicillin activity may be impaired (1) if patient has severe renal impairment, (2) during aminoglycoside assay procedures, (3) if either is mixed in same infusion fluid. Combination generally avoided
Anticoagulants, oral; heparin	Possibility of increased risk of bleeding with high carbenicillin doses. Monitor prothrombin time closely
Tetracyclines	Bactericidal activity of carbenicillin may be reduced. Combination generally avoided

---

CARBENICILLIN INDANYL SODIUM

(Geocillin)

(kar-ben-i-sill'in)
Antiinfection
Antibiotic (beta lactam)
Penicillin

ACTIONS AND USES. Extended spectrum, semisynthetic penicillin and acid stable indanyl ester of carbenicillin, prepared for oral use. Rapidly hydrolyzed to carbenicillin in body. Like carbenicillin disodium (qv), it is penicillinase-sensitive and has similar antimicrobial activity, but achieves lower blood concentrations than parent compound.

Used mainly in the treatment of prostatitis and acute and chronic infections of upper and lower urinary tract caused by susceptible strains of *Escherichia coli, Enterobacter, Enterococci, Proteus,* and *Pseudomonas* species.

ABSORPTION AND FATE. Rapidly but incompletely absorbed from GI tract. Completely hydrolyzed to carbenicillin. Serum levels peak within ½ to 1 hour; usually not detectable in serum after 6 hours. Drug concentrations in urine higher than in serum. Excreted principally in urine as unchanged drug and metabolites.

CONTRAINDICATIONS AND PRECAUTIONS. Hypersensitivity to penicillins or cephalosporins. Safe use in children and during pregnancy not established. *Cautious Use:* history of or suspected atopy or allergies (asthma, hives, hay fever, eczema); impaired renal and hepatic function, patients on sodium restriction.

ADVERSE/SIDE EFFECTS. (Dose-related) **GI:** nausea, vomiting, diarrhea, abdominal cramps, flatulence, pseudomembranous enterocolitis (infrequent), dry mouth, unpleasant aftertaste. **Hematologic:** neutropenia, leukopenia, thrombocytopenia, hemolytic anemia, increased AST (SGOT). **Hypersensitivity:** rash, fever, urticaria, eosinophilia, pruritus, anaphylaxis. **Other:** superinfections, especially of vagina. *See Penicillin G.*

ROUTE AND DOSAGE. Oral: 1 to 2 tablets (equivalent to 382 to 764 mg) four times a day at 6-hour intervals. Given for 10 days or longer for *urinary tract infections* and for 2 to 4 days or longer for *prostatitis.*

NURSING IMPLICATIONS

Before treatment is initiated, a careful inquiry should be made concerning patient's previous exposure and sensitivity to penicillin and cephalosporins and other allergic reactions of any kind.

Best taken with a full glass (240 ml) of water on an empty stomach (either 1 hour before or 2 hours after meals) to attain maximum therapeutic drug levels in urine. Consult physician.

Explain to patient that tablets may be dispensed with a small pack of desiccant to keep tablets dry.

Culture and sensitivity test should be performed prior to and at regular intervals throughout therapy.

Drug-induced nausea, unpleasant aftertaste and smell, dry mouth, and furry tongue may be so objectionable as to necessitate drug withdrawal. Periodic mouth care may help to relieve mouth discomfort. Report to physician if symptoms persist.

Check with physician regarding optimum daily fluid intake. Instruct patient to report any change in quality or quantity of urine or in intake and output ratio.

During prolonged therapy, evaluations of renal, hepatic, and hematopoietic systems are advised at regular intervals. Patients with creatinine clearance of less than 10 ml/minute (normal: 105 to 130 ml/minute) will not attain therapeutic urine levels.

Observe patient for signs of electrolyte imbalance *(see Carbenicillin Disodium).* Each gram of drug contains approximately 1 mEq of sodium.

Instruct patient to take medication around the clock, not to miss any doses, and to continue taking medication until it is all gone, unless otherwise directed by physician.

Protect tablets from moisture. Unless otherwise specified by manufacturer, store at temperatures between 15° and 30°C (59° and 86°F).

See also Carbenicillin Disodium.

C

CARBIDOPA
(Lodosyn)
CARBIDOPA/LEVODOPA
(Sinemet)

(kar-bi-doe′pa)
Anticholinergic (parasympatholetic)
Antimuscarinic
Antiparkinsonian agent

ACTION AND USES. Carbidopa, a hydrazine derivative of methyldopa, is a peripheral dopa-decarboxylase inhibitor. When levodopa is given alone, large doses must be administered to compensate for peripheral decarboxylation in order to provide adequate amounts of dopamine at appropriate sites in the corpus striatum. Carbidopa prevents peripheral metabolism (decarboxylation) of levodopa and thereby makes more levodopa available for transport to the brain. Carbidopa does not cross blood–brain barrier and therefore does not affect metabolism of levodopa within the brain. Addition of carbidopa reduces amount of levodopa required by about 75%, because levodopa plasma levels and plasma half-life are increased. Carbidopa also prevents the inhibitory effect of pyridoxine (vitamin B_6) on levodopa. Although incidence of nausea and vomiting associated with levodopa is decreased, adverse CNS effects (e.g., dykinesias) may occur at lower dosages and sooner with carbidopa/levodopa combination than with levodopa alone and it does not affect "on–off" response to levodopa.

Indications for use are as for levodopa (qv). Available alone, from manufacturer on request by physician, for use with levodopa when separate titration of each agent is indicated, and for investigational use.

ABSORPTION AND FATE. For carbidopa: approximately 40 to 70% of dose absorbed following oral administration. Widely distributed in body with exception of CNS. About 36% protein bound. Plasma half-life: 1 to 2 hours. Excreted unchanged (30% in urine) within 24 hours.

CONTRAINDICATIONS AND PRECAUTIONS. Hypersensitivity to carbidopa or levodopa; narrow-angle glaucoma. Safe use in women of childbearing potential, during pregnancy and lactation, and in children under 18 years not established. *See also Levodopa.*

ADVERSE/SIDE EFFECTS. No reactions reported for carbidopa alone. Adverse reactions as for levodopa, e.g., involuntary movements (dyskinesia), ataxia, mental disturbances and depression, anorexia, nausea, orthostatic hypotension, palpitation, urinary retention, headache, dry mouth. *See also Levodopa.*

ROUTE AND DOSAGE. Highly individualized. **Oral:** *Patients not receiving levodopa:* Initial: 1 tablet containing 10 mg carbidopa and 100 mg levodopa or 25 mg carbidopa/100 mg levodopa three times daily, increased by 1 tablet every day or every other day up to 6 tablets daily. If further titration is necessary, 1 tablet of the 25/250 mixture three times a day is substituted; may be increased ½ to 1 tablet every day or every other day to a maximum of 8 tablets/day. *Patients receiving levodopa:* Initial: 1 tablet of the 25/250 mixture three or four times daily, or 1 tablet of the 10/100 mixture three or four times daily in patients who have required less than 1.5 Gm of levodopa; dosage adjustments made as necessary by adding or omitting ½ or 1 tablet per day.

NURSING IMPLICATIONS

Administer with meals or food as a precaution against GI disturbances.

Carbidopa/levodopa tablet may be crushed if patient cannot swallow it whole.

Carbidopa/levodopa is usually initiated with a morning dose after patient has been without levodopa for at least 8 hours.

Patients who have been taking levodopa must be carefully instructed regarding continuation or discontinuation of levodopa as prescribed by physician.

Monitor patient closely during dosage adjustment period. Both therapeutic and adverse effects appear more rapidly than with use of levodopa alone.

Observe for and report immediately the onset of CNS side effects such as choreiform, dystonic, and other involuntary movements. Dosage reduction may be required. Blepharospasm (involuntary winking) and muscle twitching are useful early signs of excessive dosage.

Orthostatic hypotension with weakness, dizziness, and faintness can occur. Observe necessary safety precautions. Advise patient to make position changes slowly and in stages.

Caution patient to avoid driving and other potentially hazardous activities until reaction to drug is known.

Stored in tightly covered, light-resistant container, preferably between 15° and 30°C (59° and 86°F) unless otherwise directed by manufacturer.

See Levodopa: Nursing Implications. Drug interactions are the same as those for levodopa, with exception of the statement regarding pyridoxine. Pyridoxine does not reverse the action of the carbidopa/levodopa combination.

Diagnostic Test Interferences. Carbidopa may cause significant increase in **serum prolactin** levels. **BUN, serum creatinine,** and **uric acid** levels may be lower than those attained with levodopa alone. *Also see Levodopa.*

CARBINOXAMINE MALEATE

(Clistin)

(kar-bi-nox'a-meen)
Antihistamine
H_1-receptor antagonist

ACTIONS AND USES. Ethanolamine derivative antihistamine similar to diphenhydramine (qv) in actions, contraindications, adverse effects, diagnostic test interferences, and interactions. Less pronounced sedative and antiemetic effects than diphenhydramine; anticholinergic activity is about equal.

Used in treatment of symptoms associated with allergic disorders. Commercially available in combination with pseudoephedrine (Rondec).

ABSORPTION AND FATE. Completely absorbed from GI tract. Onset of action in 30 to 60 minutes, with duration of 4 to 6 hours. Degraded in liver; excreted in urine in inactive form.

CONTRAINDICATIONS AND PRECAUTIONS. Hypersensitivity to antihistamines, patients receiving MAOI therapy; narrow-angle glaucoma, asthmatic attack, obstructive prostatic hypertrophy, prematures, neonates; nursing women. Safe use during pregnancy (category C) not established. *See also Diphenhydramine.*

ADVERSE/SIDE EFFECTS. Most frequent: drowsiness, thickening of bronchial secretions. Low incidence of other antihistamine-associated symptoms, e.g., blurred vision, difficult urination, anorexia, GI distress, dizziness, dry mouth.

ROUTE AND DOSAGE. **Oral: Adults:** 4 to 8 mg three or four times daily. Repeat-action tablet: 8 or 12 mg at 12-hour intervals. **Children (over 6 years):** 4 to 6 mg three or four times daily; **Children (3 to 6 years):** 2 to 4 mg three or four times/day; **Children (1 to 3 years):** 2 mg three or four times/day. Extended-release form is not recommended in children.

NURSING IMPLICATIONS

Administer with food as a precaution against GI disturbances.

Extended release tablet formulation should be swallowed whole.

C

Patient may develop tolerance to carbinoxamine sedative effect. If symptom persists notify physician.
Elderly patients are more likely to experience dizziness, sedation, confusion, and hypotension associated with antihistamines. Caution patient to make position changes slowly and in stages.
Thickening of bronchial secretions, a prominent side effect, may be relieved by increasing fluid intake (if allowed) and by humidification of environment.
Warn patient that alcohol and other CNS depressants, e.g., sleeping medications, sedatives, tranquilizers, may cause additive drowsiness and sedation. Advise patient to consult physician about the use of these agents.
Caution patient to avoid driving and other potentially hazardous activities until reaction to drug has been evaluated.
Advise patient to inform physician if large amounts of aspirin or other salicylates are being taken; for example for arthritis. Carbinoxamine may mask ototoxic effects of drugs.
Store in tightly closed light resistant containers preferably between 15° and 30°C (59° and 86°F), unless otherwise directed by manufacturer.
See Diphenhydramine hydrochloride (prototype ethanolamine antihistamine).

CARBOL-FUCHSIN TOPICAL SOLUTION
(Carfusin, Castaderm, Castellani's Paint)

(kar-bol-fook'sin)
Antiinfective
Antibiotic
Antifungal

ACTIONS AND USES. Dark purple dye containing a mixture of rosaniline and pararosaniline hydrochlorides. Appears red when applied to skin. Exhibits local anesthetic, bactericidal, and fungicidal actions, and is thought to stimulate granulation. Reported to be particularly effective for intertriginous areas and for oozing eczematous lesions. Original fuchsin formula known as Castellani's paint contained basic fuchsin 0.3%, boric acid 1%, phenol 4.5%, resorcinol 10%, acetone 5%, and ethyl alcohol 10%.

Used topically for treatment of subacute and chronic dermatophytoses, e.g., fungal infections such as tinea pedis (athlete's foot) and ringworm infections, e.g., tinea cruris ("jock itch").

CONTRAINDICATIONS AND PRECAUTIONS. Application to large denuded area.

ADVERSE/SIDE EFFECTS. Dermatologic: contact dermatitis. **Hematologic:** bone marrow hypoplasia (prolonged use).

ROUTE AND DOSAGE. Topical: apply to affected areas with applicator or swab one or two times daily.

NURSING IMPLICATIONS

An initial small test application of 1:2 or 1:3 dilution is recommended before applying full strength preparation, to determine possible sensitivity.
Areas to be treated should be cleaned with soap and water, and thoroughly dried before applying medication. Exposure of intertriginous areas to air, to controlled amount of sun, or to an ordinary lamp may help to clear lesions. Consult physician.

If sensitivity or irritation develops, advise patient to discontinue treatment and contact physician.
Instruct patient to stop medication if condition worsens or if there is no improvement after 1 week of therapy.
The drug is poisonous if ingested. Keep out of the reach of children.
Inform patient that fungal infections are transmitted by both direct and indirect contact. Fungi thrive best in warm, moist environments and tend to flare up during hot weather and after heavy sweating, prolonged wearing of wet bathing suit, wearing tight nylon undergarments, prolonged contact with wool, nylon or other synthetic fibers, sitting or driving for long periods of time.
Carbol-fuchsin will stain clothing, but stains may be removed by washing. The preparation is commercially available in a colorless solution (without basic fuchsin).
Carbol-fuchsin is incompatible with oxidizing and reducing agents.
Store in tightly covered, light-resistant containers preferably between 15° and 30°C (59° and 86°F), unless otherwise directed by manufacturer.

CARBOPROST TROMETHAMINE
(Prostin/15 M)

(kar'boe-prost)
Abortifacient, ocytocic
Prostaglandin
Hormone

ACTIONS AND USES. Synthetic analog of naturally occurring prostaglandin F_2 alpha with longer duration of biologic activity. Stimulates myometrial contractions of gravid uterus qualitatively similar to those occurring at term labor. Mean time to abortion 16 hours; mean dose required 2.6 ml. Length of time to abortion and total dose of carboprost required decreases with greater parity but increases with greater gestational age. Can be employed as abortifacient even if membranes are ruptured. Also stimulates smooth muscles in GI tract and bronchi, the cause of several troublesome adverse effects. *See Dinoprost.*

Used to induce abortion between 13th to 20th week of pregnancy, as calculated from first day of last menstrual period.

CONTRAINDICATIONS AND PRECAUTIONS. Hypersensitivity to carboprost; acute pelvic inflammatory disease, active cardiac, pulmonary, renal or hepatic disease. *Cautious Use:* history of asthma, adrenal disease, anemia, or hypotension; hypertension, diabetes mellitus, epilepsy, history of uterine surgery; cervical stenosis, fibroids.

ADVERSE/SIDE EFFECTS. (Generally transient and reversible with discontinuation of drug.) Nausea, diarrhea, vomiting, temperature increase greater than 2°F, flushing, chills, cough, headache, pain (muscles, joints, lower abdomen, eyes), hiccoughs, breast tenderness. *See also Dinoprost for other possible drug-related reactions.*

ROUTE AND DOSAGE. Intramuscular: Initial: 250 mcg (1 ml) repeated at 1½- to 3½-hour intervals if indicated by uterine response. Dosage may be increased to 500 mcg (2 ml) if uterine contractility is inadequate after several doses of 250 mcg (1 ml). Total dose should not exceed 12 mg.

NURSING IMPLICATIONS

Complete medical history and baseline physical examination should be performed before drug is administered. Patient should be completely informed of the potential risks associated with carboprost-induced abortions.

Carboprost is to be administered only by trained personnel in hospital settings with intensive care and operating room facilities.

An optional test dose of 100 mcg carboprost may be administered initially.

Because nausea and diarrhea occur in about 60% of patients, an antiemetic and an antidiarrheal agent may be prescribed before and during carboprost administration.

Administer carboprost deeply into muscle using tuberculin syringe. Aspirate carefully before injecting drug to avoid inadvertent entry into blood vessel which can result in bronchospasm, tetanic contractions, and shock. Do not use same site for subsequent doses.

Patient should not be left unattended during induced labor. Monitor uterine contractions (frequency, duration, intensity), and observe and report excessive vaginal bleeding and cramping pain. Save all clots and tissue for physician inspection and laboratory analysis.

Check vital signs at regular intervals. Carboprost-induced febrile reaction occurs in more than 10% of patients and must be differentiated from endometritis. Febrile reaction usually occurs from 1 to 16 hours following drug administration and is self-limiting. It defervesces after drug action is complete, and lochia is not foul smelling.

Because carboprost is not a feticide, it is possible that the expelled fetus may show signs of life. This may carry legal implications in certain states, particularly if gestational age is 20 weeks or over.

Carboprost (in common with other prostaglandin abortifacients), is potentially teratogenic. Therefore, if abortion failure or incomplete abortion occurs, pregnancy should be terminated by another method, after uterine effects of carboprost have stopped.

Because cervical injuries can be asymptomatic, cervix should be carefully examined postabortion for lacerations or other trauma.

In some women, ovulation may be reinstated as early as 2 weeks postabortion. Patient should be informed so that appropriate contraception may be started, if desired.

Advise patient to report promptly onset of bleeding, foul-smelling lochia, abdominal pain, or fever.

Store drug between 2° and 4°C (36° and 39°F), unless otherwise specified by manufacturer.

See Dinoprost (prototype prostaglandin abortifacient).

CARISOPRODOL

(kar-eye-soe-proe'dole)

(Rela, Soma, Soprodol)

Skeletal muscle relaxant (centrally acting)

ACTIONS AND USES. Propanediol derivative monocarbamate with central depressant action pharmacologically related to meprobamate and tybamate. Precise action mechanism is not clear. Skeletal muscle relaxant effect, unlike that of neuromuscular blocking agents, appears to be due to sedative (central depressant) action. Voluntary motor function is not lost, but there may be slight reduction in muscle tone leading to relief of pain and discomfort of muscle spasm.

Used for skeletal muscle spasm, stiffness, and pain in a variety of musculoskeletal disorders and to relieve spasticity and rigidity in cerebral palsy. Available in combination with aspirin (Carisoprodol Compound, Soma Compound), and also with aspirin and codeine (Soma Compound with Codeine).

ABSORPTION AND FATE. Rapidly absorbed from GI tract. Therapeutic effects usually appear within 30 minutes and persist 4 to 6 hours. Plasma half-life: about 8 hours. Metabolized by liver and excreted by kidney. Crosses placenta. Concentration in breast milk is two to four times that in plasma.

CONTRAINDICATIONS AND PRECAUTIONS. Hypersensitivity to carisoprodol and related compounds (e.g., meprobamate, tybamate); acute intermittent porphyria; children under 12 years of age; nursing mothers. Safe use in women of childbearing potential, during pregnancy, and in nursing women not established. *Cautious Use:* impaired liver or kidney function, addiction-prone individuals.

ADVERSE/SIDE EFFECTS. Low incidence of toxicity. **CNS:** drowsiness, dizziness, vertigo, ataxia, tremor, headache, irritability, depressive reactions, syncope, insomnia. **CV:** tachycardia, postural hypotension, facial flushing. **GI:** nausea, vomiting, hiccoughs. **Hypersensitivity:** skin rash, erythema multiforme, pruritus, eosinophilia, asthma, fever, anaphylactic shock. **Idiosyncratic reaction:** extreme weakness, transient quadriplegia, angioneurotic edema, smarting eyes, temporary loss of vision, diplopia, mydriasis, euphoria, confusion, agitation, disorientation, dysarthria.

ROUTE AND DOSAGE. Oral: 350 mg four times daily.

NURSING IMPLICATIONS

May be taken with food to reduce GI symptoms. Last dose should be taken at bedtime.

Drowsiness is a common side effect and may require reduction in dosage. Advise patient to avoid driving and other potentially hazardous activities until response to the drug has been evaluated.

Inform patient that carisoprodol may cause dizziness and faintness in some patients. Symptoms may be controlled by making position changes slowly and in stages. Report to physician if symptoms persist.

Allergic or idiosyncratic reactions generally occur within the period from the first to the fourth dose in patients taking the drug for the first time. Symptoms usually subside after several hours; they are treated by supportive and symptomatic measures.

Carisoprodol is used as an adjunct to rest, analgesics, and physical therapy modalities.

Caution patient not to take alcohol or other CNS depressants (effects may be additive) unless otherwise directed by physician.

Advise patient to discontinue drug and notify physician if skin rash, diplopia, dizziness, or other unusual signs or symptoms appear.

There are some indications that psychologic dependence may occur with long-term use.

Withdrawal symptoms may occur with abrupt termination of drug following prolonged use of doses higher than those recommended: abdominal cramps, insomnia, chilliness, headache, nausea.

The commercial preparation Rela contains tartrazine. This dye may cause allergic-type reaction, including bronchial asthma, in susceptible individuals, who also may be sensitive to aspirin.

Store in tightly closed container preferably between 15° and 30°C (59° and 86°F) unless otherwise directed by manufacturer.

C

CARMUSTINE
(BCNU, BiCNU)

(kar-mus'teen)
Antineoplastic
Alkylating agent
Nitrosurea

ACTIONS AND USES. Highly lipid-soluble nitrosurea derivative with cell cycle nonspecific activity against rapidly proliferating cell populations. Produces cross-linkage of DNA strands, thereby blocking DNA, RNA, and protein synthesis. Drug metabolites thought to be responsible for antineoplastic and toxic activities. Major toxic effect is bone marrow suppression.

Used as single agent or in combination with other antineoplastics in treatment of Hodgkin's disease and other lymphomas, melanoma, primary and metastatic tumors of brain, and GI tract malignancies. *Investigational Use:* treatment of carcinomas of breast, lungs; Ewing's sarcoma, Burkitt's tumor, and topically for mycosis fungoides.

ABSORPTION AND FATE. Rapid absorption and hepatic degradation. Intact drug leaves plasma within 15 minutes. Half-life: 5 to 15 minutes (active metabolites may persist in plasma for days). About 60 to 70% excreted in urine in 96 hours; 6 to 10% excreted as CO_2 by lungs, and about 1% via feces. Effectively crosses blood–brain barrier. Distributed into breast milk.

CONTRAINDICATIONS AND PRECAUTIONS. Previous sensitivity to carmustine; infection, decreased circulating platelets, leukocytes, or erythrocytes. Safe use during pregnancy and in nursing women not established. *Cautious Use:* hepatic and renal insufficiency; patient with previous cytotoxic medication, or radiation therapy.

ADVERSE/SIDE EFFECTS. CNS: dizziness, ataxia. **GI:** stomatitis, dysphagia, nausea, vomiting, diarrhea, anorexia. **Hematopoietic:** delayed myelosuppression (dose-related). **Hepatotoxic** (high doses): increases in transaminases, alkaline phosphatase, bilirubin, jaundice, encephalopathy. **Ophthalmic:** (with high doses): infarctions, retinal hemorrhage, suffusion of conjunctiva. **Pulmonary:** pulmonary infiltration and/or fibrosis. **Renal:** decrease in kidney size, progressive azotemia, renal failure. **Other:** skin flushing, burning pain at injection site, hyperpigmentation of skin (from contact), thrombosis (rare).

ROUTE AND DOSAGE. Intravenous: Adults: 200 mg/m^2 no more often than every 6 weeks as single dose, or divided doses such as 100 mg/m^2 on 2 successive days. Repeat course only if circulating blood elements have returned to accepted values: platelets, more than 100,000/mm^3; leukocytes, more than 4000/mm^3. Dose adjustments are made on basis of hematologic response.

NURSING IMPLICATIONS

Carmustine is to be used only when a physician experienced in cancer chemotherapy can provide constant supervision.

Wear disposable gloves when preparing carmustine. Contact of drug with skin can cause burning, dermatitis, and hyperpigmentation.

If possible avoid starting infusion into dorsum of hand, wrist, or the antecubital veins; extravasation in these areas can damage underlying tendons and nerves leading to loss of mobility of entire limb.

Slow infusion over a 1- to 2-hour period (by IV drip) and adequate dilution will reduce pain of administration. Frequently check rate of flow and blood return; palpate injection site for extravasation. If there is any question about patency, line should be restarted.

Carmustine is not a vesicant, but can cause burning discomfort even in the absence of extravasation. Instruct patient to report burning sensation immediately. Infusion will

C

be discontinued and restarted in another site. Ice application over the area may decrease the discomfort.

Inform patient that intense flushing of skin may occur during IV infusion. This side effect usually disappears in 2 to 4 hours.

Nausea and vomiting (dose related) may occur within 2 hours after drug administration and persist for up to 6 hours. Prior administration of an antiemetic may help to decrease or prevent these side effects.

Platelet nadir usually occurs within 4 to 5 weeks, and leukocyte nadir within 5 to 6 weeks after therapy is terminated. Thrombocytopenia may be more severe than leukopenia; anemia is less severe. Blood studies are continued following infusion, at weekly intervals, for at least 6 weeks.

Because carmustine causes myelosuppression, patient will be highly susceptible to infection and to hemorrhagic disorders. Be alert to hazardous periods of drug-induced lowered defense mechanisms that occur 4 to 6 weeks after a dose of carmustine. If possible, invasive procedures (e.g., IM injections, enemas, rectal temperatures) should be avoided during this period.

Check temperature daily. Avoid use of rectal thermometer to prevent injury to mucosa. An elevation of 0.6°F or more above usual temperature warrants reporting.

Infection prevention in all patient-related activities during period of leukopenia is imperative. Screen contacts to prevent exposure of patient to upper respiratory or other infections.

Antibiotics and red cell and platelet transfusions may be given to control infections during periods of drug-induced leukopenia and thrombocytopenia.

In addition to hematopoietic studies, baseline and periodic tests of hepatic, pulmonary, and renal function are recommended throughout therapy. Most patients receiving carmustine inevitably show some signs of toxicity.

Symptoms of lung toxicity (cough, shortness of breath, fever) should be reported to the physician immediately.

Be alert to signs of hepatic toxicity (jaundice, dark urine, pruritus, light colored stools) and renal insufficiency (dysuria, oliguria, hematuria, swelling of lower legs and feet).

Instruct patient to report promptly the onset of sore throat, weakness, fever, chills, infection of any kind, or abnormal bleeding (ecchymosis, petechiae, epistaxis, bleeding gums, hematemesis, melena).

Reconstituted solutions of carmustine are clear and colorless and may be stored at 2° to 8°C (36° to 46°F) for 24 hours protected from sunlight.

Reconstituted solutions, which are further diluted with NaCl for injection or 5% dextrose for injection, are stable for 48 hours when refrigerated and protected from light.

Note that carmustine powder contains no preservative, therefore storage requirements must be carefully observed. Signs of decomposition of carmustine in unopened vial: liquifaction and appearance of oil film at bottom of vial. Discard drug in this condition.

See Mechlorethamine (prototype antineoplastic agent).

Drug Interactions: Carmustine

Plus	Interactions
Cimetidine (Tagamet)	Carmustine-induced bone marrow toxicity may increase. Concurrent use generally avoided
Phentoin (Dilantin)	Possibility of reduced phenytoin absorption. Monitor phenytoin plasma levels

C

CASCARA SAGRADA

(kas-kar'a)

(Cascara Sagrada Aromatic Fluidextract, Cascara Sagrada Fluidextract)

Laxative
Anthraquinone

ACTIONS AND USES. Anthraquinone derivative obtained from bark of buckhorn tree *(Rhamnus purshiana).* Acts principally in large intestine. Causes propulsive movements of colon by direct chemical irritation. Fluid extract preparations contain about 18% alcohol. Casanthrol, which is present in a variety of OTC mixtures, is a derivative of cascara sagrada.

Used for temporary relief of constipation and to prevent straining at stool in various disease conditions. Available in combination with mineral oil (Kondremul with Cascara). Sometimes used with milk of magnesia ("black and white" mixture).

ABSORPTION AND FATE. Hydrolyzed in colon to active principles which are conveyed to colonic mucosa, bile, and saliva, and possibly other body tissues and fluids. Acts in 6 to 12 hours. Metabolized in liver. Excreted in feces and in urine. Also eliminated in breast milk. Following partial absorption, reaches large intestine indirectly via bloodstream and partly by direct passage through small intestine.

CONTRAINDICATIONS AND PRECAUTIONS. Nausea, vomiting, abdominal pain, fecal impaction; GI bleeding, ulcerations; appendicitis, gastroenteritis, intestinal obstruction, nursing mothers, congestive heart failure.

ADVERSE/SIDE EFFECTS. Large doses: anorexia, nausea, griping, abnormally loose stools, hypokalemia, impaired glucose tolerance, calcium deficiency, discoloration of urine. *Chronic Use:* constipation rebound, melanosis of colon.

ROUTE AND DOSAGE. Oral: Adult: *tablet:* 325 mg; *fluidextract:* 1 ml; *aromatic fluidextract:* 5 ml. **Children (2 to 12 years):** 50% of adult dose; **Children (under 2 years):** 25% of adult dose.

NURSING IMPLICATIONS

A single dose taken before retiring usually results in evacuation of soft stool 6 to 12 hours later.

For best results administer with a full glass of water on an empty stomach. Results may be delayed somewhat by food.

An increase in fluid intake will enhance laxative action. Unless contraindicated advise patient to drink a minimum of 6 to 8 full (8 oz) glasses a day.

Frequent or prolonged use of irritant cathartics disrupts normal reflex activity of colon and rectum and can lead to drug dependence for evacuation.

Constipation, which is especially common in the elderly, may be caused by poor eating habits, inadequate fluid intake, lack of exercise, or habitual use of cathartics based on the erroneous notion that autointoxication will result if bowels are not evacuated daily.

Evaluate patient's need for continued use of drug.

Prolonged ingestion of anthraquinone cathartics can cause benign melanotic pigmentation of rectal mucosa and may impart a reddish hue to alkaline urine and a yellowish brown color to acid urine.

Stored preferably between 15° and 30°C (59° and 86°F), in tightly covered, light-resistant containers, unless otherwise directed by manufacturer.

See Bisacodyl: prototype laxative for other patient teaching points.

Diagnostic Test Interferences. Possibility of interference with **PSP excretion test** because of urine discoloration.

Drug Interactions. Cathartics in large doses may result in decreased absorption of **vitamin K, oral anticoagulants,** and possibly other drugs by decreasing transit time in intestinal tract.

CASTOR OIL

Laxative (stimulant)

(Alphamul, Emulsoil, Fleet Castor Oil Stimulant Laxative, Kellogg's Castor Oil, Neoloid, Oleum Ricini, Purge, Unisoil)

ACTIONS AND USES. Obtained from the seeds of *Ricinus communis*. Hydrolyzed in small intestine to glycerol and ricinoleic acid, a local irritant. Stimulates motor activity in small intestine and inhibits antiperistalsis in colon, thus preventing normal fluid absorption from intestinal contents. Rapid evacuation of copious liquid or semiliquid stools follows, with little or no colic.

Used to prepare abdomen for radiographic examination of colon and kidneys and to evacuate irritants and poisons from intestinal tract. Rarely used to relieve constipation. Also applied locally to skin as emollient and protectant and to conjunctiva (sterile) to alleviate irritation caused by the presence of a foreign body.

ABSORPTION AND FATE. Poorly absorbed. Acts in 2 to 3 hours. Appears in breast milk.

CONTRAINDICATIONS AND PRECAUTIONS. Hypersensitivity to castor bean; dehydration, fecal impaction, abdominal pain, nausea, vomiting, appendicitis, GI bleeding, ulcerations, perforation, obstruction, use in conjunction with fat-soluble vermifuges; pregnancy, nursing women, menstruation.

ADVERSE/SIDE EFFECTS. Severe purgation, nausea, vomiting, abdominal cramps, flatus, rebound constipation, irritation of colon, pelvic congestion (rare); dehydration, electrolyte imbalance, elevation of blood glucose levels (extended use).

ROUTE AND DOSAGE. Oral: Adults: 15 to 60 ml. **Children (2 to 12 years):** 5 to 15 ml; **Children: (under 2 years):** 1 to 5 ml.

NURSING IMPLICATIONS

More active if taken on empty stomach. Because castor oil is a fat, it may retard gastric emptying time.

In general it is best not to schedule a laxative within 2 hours of taking other medications.

Action begins in 2 to 3 hours, depending on dose. Time the administration so as not to interfere with patient's sleep.

For visualization or surgical procedures, patient is generally given a residue free diet the day before and a cleansing enema on the day of the procedure. Some physicians prescribe standardized senna fluidextract to be taken 4 hours after castor oil.

Castor oil has objectionable odor, taste, and consistency. It may be made somewhat more palatable by chilling it and administering it with cold fruit juice or a carbonated beverage chaser.

Emulsified forms are reported to be less disagreeable to taste. Shake emulsion well before pouring. Mix with ½ to 1 glass (120 to 240 ml) of liquid (water, soft drink, fruit juice, milk).

Inform patient that castor oil causes complete emptying of intestinal contents, and therefore normal evacuation may be delayed for 2 days or more.

Long-term use may result in laxative dependence.

Preserved in tightly covered containers preferably between 15° and 30°C (59° and 86°F), unless otherwise directed by manufacturer. Avoid exposure to excessive light.

C

CEFACLOR

(Ceclor)

(sef'a-klor)
Antiinfective
Antibiotic (beta-lactam)
Cephalosporin

ACTIONS AND USES. Semisynthetic, second generation oral cephalosporin antibiotic similar to other drugs of this group. Possibly more active than other oral cephalosporins against gram-negative bacilli, especially beta-lactamase-producing *Haemophilus influenzae*, including ampicillin-resistant strains. Also active against *Escherichia coli, Proteus mirabilis, Klebsiella,* and certain gram-positive strains, e.g., *Streptococcus pneumoniae, S. pyogenes,* and *Staphylococcus aureus.*

Used in treatment of infections of upper and lower respiratory tract, urinary tract, skin and skin structures, and mainly for otitis media.

ABSORPTION AND FATE. Acid stable. Well absorbed following oral administration. Peak serum levels in 30 to 60 minutes when taken on an empty stomach. Half-life: 36 to 54 minutes (prolonged in impaired renal function). About 22 to 25% protein bound. Approximately 50 to 85% of dose eliminated within 8 hours unchanged in urine, with most of dose being excreted within first two hours. Crosses placenta; appears in breast milk.

CONTRAINDICATIONS AND PRECAUTIONS. Hypersensitivity to cephalosporins. Safe use during pregnancy, in nursing mothers, and infants younger than 1 month not established. *Cautious Use:* history of sensitivity to penicillins or other drug allergies; markedly impaired renal function.

ADVERSE/SIDE EFFECTS. GI: (common): diarrhea; nausea, vomiting, anorexia. **Hematologic:** transient leukopenia, transient leukocytosis, slight elevations of AST (SGOT), ALT (SGPT), alkaline phosphatase, BUN, serum creatinine; positive direct Coombs' test. **Hypersensitivity:** serum sickness-like reaction: urticaria, pruritus, morbilliform eruptions, eosinophilia, joint pain or swelling, fever. **Other:** superinfections. *See also Cephalothin.*

ROUTE AND DOSAGE. Oral: Adults: 250 to 500 mg every 8 hours. Not to exceed 4 Gm daily. **Children (1 month or older):** 20 to 40 mg/kg daily in divided doses every 8 hours. Not to exceed 1 Gm daily. Available in pulvules (capsules) and oral suspension.

NURSING IMPLICATIONS

Cefaclor may be administered without regard to meals. Although peak blood levels may be slightly lower and delayed when drug is administered with food, total amount absorbed is unchanged. Administration with food may help to reduce incidence of nausea and vomiting.

Before therapy is initiated, a careful inquiry should be made concerning previous hypersensitivity to cephalosporins, penicillins, and other drug allergies.

Culture and susceptibility tests recommended prior to and periodically during therapy.

Be on the alert for signs and symptoms of superinfections (black tongue, sore mouth, perianal irritation and itching, foul-smelling vaginal discharge, loose stools, sudden fever, cough).

Diarrhea, the most frequent adverse effect, may be due to a pharmacologic effect or to associated change in intestinal flora. If it persists interruption of therapy may be necessary.
Yogurt or buttermilk (if allowed) may serve as a prophylactic against intestinal superinfections by helping to maintain normal intestinal flora.
Instruct patient to take medication for the full course of therapy as directed by physician. Drug therapy for beta-hemolytic streptococcal infections should continue for at least 10 days to guard against risk of rheumatic fever.
After stock oral suspension is prepared, it should be kept refrigerated. Expiration date should appear on label. Discard unused portion after 14 days. Shake well before pouring. A calibrated liquid measuring device for home use should be included when dispensed by pharmacist.
Store pulvules preferably between 15° and 30°C (59° and 86°F) in tightly closed container, unless otherwise directed by manufacturer.
See Cephalothin Sodium (prototype cephalosporin).

Diagnostic Test Interferences. Cefaclor may produce positive direct Coombs' test, which can complicate **cross-matching procedures** and **hematologic studies.** False positive **urine glucose** determinations, using copper sulfate reduction methods, e.g., Clinitest, Benedict's reagent, or Fehling's solution, but not with glucose oxidase (enzymatic) tests such as Clinistix, Diastix, Tes-Tape.

Drug Interactions: Cefaclor

Plus	Interactions
Aminoglycosides, colistimethate and other potentially nephrotoxic drugs	Possibility of additive nephrotoxic effects. Monitor renal function
Probenecid	May result in higher and more prolonged serum cefaclor levels (probenecid inhibits cefaclor excretion). Used concomitantly with caution

CEFADROXIL

(Duricef, Ultracef)

(sef-a-drox'ill)
Antiinfective
Antibiotic (beta-lactam)
Cephalosporin

ACTIONS AND USES. Semisynthetic, first generation cephalosporin antibiotic with antibacterial spectrum similar to that of other members of this group. At equivalent doses, reportedly has longer duration in serum and urine than attained by other oral cephalosporins. Active against organisms that liberate cephalosporinase and penicillinase.

Used primarily in treatment of urinary tract infections caused by *Escherichia coli, Proteus mirabilis,* and *Klebsiella* species; infections of skin and skin structures caused by staphylococci and streptococci; and for treatment of Group A beta-hemolytic streptococcal pharyngitis.

ABSORPTION AND FATE. Acid stable. Rapidly and almost completely absorbed from GI tract. Peak serum levels in 1.2 to 1.5 hours. Measurable levels persist in serum 12 hours after administration. Approximately 20% protein bound. Half life: 1 to 2 hours. More than 90% of a single dose is excreted unchanged in urine within 8 hours; appreciable bacterial inhibitory levels persist for 20 to 22 hours. Crosses placenta; appears in breast milk.

C

CONTRAINDICATIONS AND PRECAUTIONS. Hypersensitivity to cephalosporins. Safe use during pregnancy (category B), in nursing mothers, and in children not established. *Cautious Use:* sensitivity to penicillins or other drug allergies; impaired renal function, history of GI disease, particularly colitis.

ADVERSE/SIDE EFFECTS. GI: nausea, vomiting, gastritis, bloating, cramps, diarrhea, pseudomembranous colitis (rare). **Hypersensitivity:** rash, swollen eyelids (angioedema), pruritus, chills. **Other:** dysuria, dizziness, headache, positive direct Coombs' test; increased SGOT, SGPT, alkaline phosphatase; transient neutropenia, superinfections.

ROUTE AND DOSAGE. Oral: 1 to 2 Gm in single dose or every 12 hours. For patients with renal function impairment, loading dose of 1 Gm; subsequent doses modified according to creatinine clearance. Available in capsules, tablets, and oral suspension.

NURSING IMPLICATIONS

The incidence of nausea (most frequent side effect) may be reduced by administration of drug with food. Rate of absorption and serum levels not affected by presence of food. If nausea persists, cessation of therapy may be necessary.

Before therapy is initiated a careful inquiry should be made concerning previous hypersensitivity to cephalosporins, penicillins, and other drug allergies.

Culture and susceptibility testing recommended prior to and periodically during therapy.

Baseline and periodic renal function studies should be performed in patients with renal function impairment, and intake and output ratio and pattern should be monitored.

Instruct patient to take medication for the full course of therapy as directed by the physician.

Drug therapy for beta-hemolytic streptococcal infections should continue for at least 10 days to guard against risk of rheumatic fever.

Be on the alert for signs and symptoms of superinfections (furry, black tongue; sore mouth; perianal itching or irritation; foul-smelling vaginal discharge; loose stools; and sudden fever; cough).

Store in tight container, preferably between 15° and 30°C (59° and 86°F), unless otherwise directed by manufacturer. Oral suspensions are stable for 14 days under refrigeration at 2° to 8°C (36° to 46°F). Avoid freezing. Note expiration date on label.

Diagnostic Test Interferences. False positive **urine glucose** determinations using copper sulfate reduction methods, such as Clinitest, Benedict's reagent, or Fehling's solution, but not with glucose oxidase (enzymatic) tests, e.g., Clinistix, Diastix, Tes-Tape. Cefadroxil-induced positive direct Coombs' test may interfere with **cross-matching procedures** and **hematologic studies.**

Drug Interactions: Cefadroxil

Plus	Interactions
Aminoglycosides, colistimethate and other potentially nephrotoxic drugs	Possibility of additive nephrotoxic effects. Monitor renal function
Probenecid	May result in higher and more prolonged serum cefadroxil levels (probenecid inhibits excretion). Used concomitantly with caution

CEFAMANDOLE NAFATE
(Mandol)

(sef-a-man′dole)
Antiinfective
Antibiotic (beta-lactam)
Cephalosporin

ACTIONS AND USES. Semisynthetic, second generation cephalosporin antibiotic similar to other drugs of this class. Reported to have a wider spectrum of antibacterial activity than other cephalosporins and to be effective against more strains of cephalosporinase- and penicillinase-producing gram-negative organisms (e.g., *E. coli, Enterobacter* species, indole-positive *Proteus,* and *H. influenzae*). In common with other cephalosporins, most strains of *Bacteroides fragilis, Serratia, Pseudomonas,* and *Acinetobacter calcoaceticus* are generally resistant to cefamandole. Formulated with sodium carbonate for pH adjustment; contains 3.3 mEq (76 mg) of sodium per gram of cefamandole.

Used in treatment of serious infections of respiratory, urinary, and biliary tracts, skin and soft tissue, bones and joints, and in septicemia and peritonitis.

ABSORPTION AND FATE. Peak serum levels in ½ to 2 hours after IM and in 10 minutes following IV administration. Serum half-life after IM: 60 to 120 minutes; after IV dose: 32 minutes. About 65 to 75% bound to serum proteins. Rapidly hydrolyzed in plasma to compound that is more active than parent drug. Poor penetration into CSF even when meninges are inflamed. Extensive enterohepatic circulation; high concentrations in bile. Excreted unchanged in urine; 60 to 95% eliminated within 6 to 8 hours.

CONTRAINDICATIONS AND PRECAUTIONS. Hypersensitivity to cephalosporins. Safe use during pregnancy (category B), in nursing mothers, and in children between 1 and 6 months not established. *Cautious Use:* history of sensitivity to penicillins, or other drug allergies; renal function impairment, history of GI disease, particularly colitis.

ADVERSE/SIDE EFFECTS. GI: nausea, vomiting, abdominal cramps, diarrhea, pseudomembranous colitis. **Hematologic** (rare): neutropenia, thrombocytopenia, hypoprothrombinemia (vitamin K deficiency), positive Coombs' test, transient elevations in SGOT, SGPT, alkaline phosphatase, BUN, decreased creatinine clearance. **Hypersensitivity:** rash, urticaria, drug fever, eosinophilia. **Other:** pain, redness and induration at IM site, thrombophlebitis (following IV), superinfections.

ROUTE AND DOSAGE. Intramuscular, intravenous: Adults: 500 mg to 1 Gm every 4 to 8 hours. Up to 2 Gm IV every 4 hours for life-threatening infections. **Pediatric (1 month and over):** 50 to 100 mg/kg/day in divided doses every 4 to 8 hours; up to 150 mg/kg/day, but not to exceed maximum adult dose.

NURSING IMPLICATIONS

Culture and susceptibility testing recommended prior to and periodically during therapy. Cefamandole therapy may be instituted pending test results.

Before therapy is initiated, careful inquiry should be made concerning previous hypersensitivity to cephalosporins, penicillins, and other drugs.

Administer IM deep into a large muscle mass such as gluteus maximus or lateral thigh. Reportedly, cefamandole IM produces less pain than cephalothin.

Baseline and periodic studies of renal function and prothrombin time determinations should be performed.

Monitor intake and output ratio and pattern particularly in patients with impaired renal function, patients over 50 years, or who are receiving high doses. Note number and consistency of stools.

C

Be on the alert for signs and symptoms of superinfection (ulceration or white patches in mouth, glossitis, black hairy tongue, anogenital itching, foul-smelling vaginal discharge, and diarrhea, sudden fever, cough).

Report the onset of diarrhea, which may or may not be dose-related and is seen especially in patients with history of drug-associated GI disturbances. Bear in mind that pseudomembranous colitis, a potentially life-threatening condition, starts with diarrhea. It is caused by overgrowth of resistant toxic-producing clostridia.

Cefamandole may inhibit production of vitamin K by normal bacterial flora. Although rare, hypoprothrombinemia with or without hemorrhage has been reported in patients with impaired renal function receiving high doses, patients who have had intestinal resection, the elderly or debilitated, and patients being maintained on IV fluids with no oral intake. Observe these patients for bleeding manifestation. Prophylactic administration of vitamin K may be necessary.

Drug therapy for beta-hemolytic streptococcal infections should continue for at least 10 days to guard against risk of rheumatic fever and glomerulonephritis.

For IM use: to each gram of cefamandole add 3 ml of sterile water for injection or bacteriostatic water for injection, 0.9% sodium chloride injection or 0.9% bacteriostatic sodium chloride injection. (Resulting solution will contain 285 mg cefamandole per ml.)

Prior to reconstitution store cefamandole powder preferably between 15° and 30°C (59° and 86°F), unless otherwise directed by manufacturer. The powder must be protected from prolonged exposure to light to prevent discoloration. Once reconstituted, cefamandole is no longer light sensitive. Solutions appear light yellow to amber in color. Do not use if otherwise colored or if a precipitate is present.

Clumping may be avoided by tapping powder to stopper end of vial, introducing diluent away from powder, and then quickly shaking vial vigorously for even dispersion. This prevents the insoluble lump that occurs when only the powder surface is wetted.

Following reconstitution, cefamandole is stable for 24 hours at room temperature (25°C or 77°F) and for 96 hours under refrigeration (5°C or 41°F).

After reconstitution, cefamandole may liberate carbon dioxide (CO_2) whether stored at room temperature or refrigerated. Pressure exerted by CO_2 allows medication to be withdrawn without injecting air. Manufacturer cautions not to store medication in syringes as pressure build-up from CO_2 may force plunger out of barrel. Gas production is apparently of little consequence when drug is stored in its original container or is added to IV solutions.

For direct IV administration, each gram of cefamandole should be reconstituted with 10 ml sterile water for injection, 5% dextrose injection, or 0.9% sodium chloride injection. Appropriate dose is administered slowly over 3 to 5 minutes.

Cefamandole may also be given by intermittent IV infusion via a Y-type administration set or volume control set, or by continuous IV in compatible IV infusion solutions. Consult package insert.

Because cefamandole is formulated with sodium carbonate, it is incompatible with fluids containing magnesium or calcium ions. Consult package insert for compatible IV infusion fluids and stability and storage times.

See Cephalothin Sodium (prototype cephalosporin).

Diagnostic Test Interferences. False-positive **urine glucose** determinations using copper sulfate reduction methods, e.g., Clinitest, Benedict's reagent, or Fehling's solution, but not with glucose oxidase (enzymatic) tests such as Clinistix, Diastix, Tes-tape. Cefamandole induced positive direct Coombs' test may interfere with **cross-matching procedures** and **hematologic studies.**

Drug Interactions: Cefamandole

Plus	Interactions
Alcohol	Ingestion of alcoholic beverages within 48 to 72 hours after cefamandole administation may produce a disulfiram reaction (flushing, throbbing headache, tachycardia). Concurrent use avoided
Aminoglycosides, colistimethate, and other potentially nephrotoxic drugs	Possibility of additive nephrotoxic effects. Monitor renal function
Probenecid	Higher and more prolonged serum cefamandole levels (cefamandole excretion inhibited by probenecid). Used concomitantly with caution

---

CEFAZOLIN SODIUM

(Ancef, Kefzol)

(sef-a'zoe-lin)
Antiinfective
Antibiotic (beta-lactam)
Cephalosporin

ACTIONS AND USES. Semisynthetic, first generation derivative of cephalosporin C. Broad-spectrum antibiotic similar to cephalothin (qv). Reported to be less irritating to tissue and less nephrotoxic than cephalothin, and to produce higher and more sustained serum levels at equivalent dosages. Appears to be less resistant to bacterial beta-lactamases (cephalosporinases and penicillinases) than other cephalosporins. Contains 2.1 mEq (48 mg) of sodium per Gm.

Used for treatment of severe infections of urinary and biliary tracts, skin, soft tissue, and bone, and for bacteremia and endocarditis caused by susceptible organisms. Also used for preoperative prophylaxis in patients undergoing procedures associated with high risk of infection such as open heart surgery.

ABSORPTION AND FATE. Peak serum concentrations in 1 to 2 hours following IM and in 5 minutes following IV injection. Average half-life: 69 to 130 minutes. Concentrations in gallbladder and bile may exceed those in serum; high concentrations in diseased bones also. Approximately 74 to 86% bound to plasma proteins. Excreted unchanged in urine, about 56 to 89% excreted within 6 hours, and 80 to 100% within 24 hours (slower excretion in patients with renal impairment). Readily crosses placenta. Excreted in small amounts in breast milk.

CONTRAINDICATIONS AND PRECAUTIONS. Hypersensitivity to any cephalosporin. Safe use during pregnancy (category B), in nursing mothers, and in infants under 1 month not established. *Cautious Use:* history of penicillin sensitivity, impaired renal function, patients on sodium restriction.

ADVERSE/SIDE EFFECTS. GI: nausea, vomiting, anorexia, abdominal cramps, diarrhea, pseudomembranous colitis (rare). **Hematologic:** neutropenia, leukopenia, thrombocytopenia, positive direct and indirect Coombs' test, transient rise in BUN, AST (SGOT), ALT (SGPT), alkaline phosphatase. **Hypersensitivity:** anaphylaxis, maculopapular rash, urticaria, fever, eosinophilia. **Other:** pain and induration at IM site, phlebitis (IV site), superinfections, seizure (high doses in patients with renal insufficiency).

ROUTE AND DOSAGE. Intramuscular, intravenous: Adults: *Infections:* 250 mg to 1 Gm every 6 to 8 hours, depending on severity of infection and susceptibility of causative organism. Up to 12 Gm/day has been used. *Acute uncomplicated urinary tract infections:* 500 mg to

C

1 Gm every 12 hours. *Perioperative prophylaxis:* (a) 1 Gm ½ to 1 hour before start of surgery. (b) For lengthy procedures 500 mg to 1 Gm during surgery. (c) 0.5 to 1 Gm every 6 to 8 hours for 24 hours or for 3 to 5 days after surgery. **Children and infants (over 1 month):** 25 to 50 mg/kg/day divided into three or four equal doses; total daily dose not to exceed 100 mg/kg even for severe infections. For patients with renal impairment, dosage and intervals are based on BUN and creatinine clearance.

NURSING IMPLICATIONS

Before therapy is initiated a careful inquiry should be made concerning history of hypersensitivity to cephalosporins, penicillins, and other drugs.

Culture and sensitivity testing is recommended prior to and during therapy. In serious infections, therapy may be initiated pending results.

IM injections should be made deep into large muscle mass. Pain on injection is usually minimal. Rotate injection sites.

Reconstituted with sterile water for injection, bacteriostatic water for injection, or 0.9% sodium chloride injection. Reconstituted solutions are stable for 24 hours at room temperature and for 96 hours if stored under refrigeration. (After reconstitution, shake well until drug is entirely dissolved.) Protect drug from light until used.

For IV infusion, solution is further diluted. Use only diluents recommended by manufacturer.

The risk of IV site reactions may be reduced by proper dilution of IV solution, use of small bore IV needle in a large vein, and rotating injection sites.

Be alert for signs and symptoms of superinfections: furry black tongue, sore mouth, perianal irritation or itching, foul-smelling vaginal discharge, loose stools, sudden fever, cough.

Report the onset of diarrhea, which may or may not be dose-related and is seen especially in patients with history of drug-related GI disturbances. Bear in mind that pseudomembranous colitis, a potentially life-threatening condition starts with diarrhea. It is caused by overgrowth of resistant toxic-producing clostridia.

Although clinical evidence of renal damage has not been reported, precautions outlined for cephalothin (qv) should be observed.

Store vials preferably between 15° and 30°C (59° and 86°F), unless otherwise directed by manufacturer.

See Cephalothin sodium (prototype cephalosporin).

Diagnostic Test Interferences. Because of cefazolin effect on the Combs' test, transfusion **cross-matching procedures** and **hematologic studies** may be complicated. False-positive **urine glucose** determinations with use of copper sulfate tests (e.g., Clinitest, Benedict's reagent, or Fehling's solution), but not with enzymatic tests such as Tes-Tape, Diastix, or Clinistix.

Drug Interactions: Cefazolin

Plus	Interactions
Alcohol	Ingestion of alcoholic beverages within 48 to 72 hours after cefazolin administration may produce a disulfiram reaction (flushing, throbbing headache, tachycardia). Concurrent use avoided
Aminoglycosides, colistimethate, and other potentially nephrotic drugs	Possibility of additive nephrotoxic effects. Monitor renal function
Probenecid	Higher and more prolonged serum cefazolin levels (probenecid inhibits cefazolin excretion). Used concomitantly with caution

CEFONICID SODIUM

(Monocid)

(se-fon′i-sid)
Antiinfective
Antibiotic (beta-lactam)
Cephalosporin

ACTIONS AND USES. Second generation, semisynthetic, broad-spectrum cephalosporin antibiotic structurally similar to cefamandole (Mandol), but with longer half-life that permits once daily dosage regimen. Reportedly less active than cefamandole against gram-positive cocci, including *Staphylococcus aureus, Streptococcus pyogenes,* and *S. pneumococci.* About twice as active against *Haemophilus influenza,* however, and slightly more active than cefamandole against gonococci. In common with cefamandole, it is also effective against many enteric gram-negative bacilli including *Citrobacter, Escherichia coli, Enterobacter, Klebsiella,* and *Proteus mirabilis.* Most strains of *Acinetobacter, Bacteroides fragilis, Enterococcus,* indole-positive *Proteus, Pseudomonas,* and *Serratia* are resistant. Highly resistant to beta-lactamases produced by *Staphylococcus, H. influenza,* and *Neisseria gonorrhea,* certain members of *Enterobacteriaceae,* and Richmond type I. Like other cephalosporins, acts by inhibiting bacterial cell wall synthesis. Has not been associated with disulfiram-like reaction with alcohol, prolonged bleeding time, overt bleeding or pseudomembranous colitis. Contains 3.7 mEq (85 mg) sodium per Gm.

Used in treatment of moderate to severe infections such as septicemia, infections of lower respiratory tract, bones and joints, skin and skin structure, and urinary tract. Also used for surgical prophylaxis.

ABSORPTION AND FATE. Peak serum concentrations within 5 minutes following IV, and in 1 hour after IM administration. Widely distributed in body tissues and fluid. Half-life: about 4.5 hours. Over 90% protein bound. Not metabolized. Approximately 90 to 99% of dose eliminated unchanged in urine within 24 hours. Small amounts excreted in breast milk.

CONTRAINDICATIONS AND PRECAUTIONS. Hypersensitivity to cephalosporins; severely impaired renal or hepatic function. Safe use during pregnancy (category B) and in children not established. *Cautious Use:* nursing mothers, penicillin-sensitive patients, allergy to other drugs.

ADVERSE/SIDE EFFECTS. GI: Nausea, vomiting, diarrhea. **Hematologic:** elevations of: BUN, serum creatinine, liver function tests: alkaline phosphatase, SGOT (AST), SGPT (ALT), LDH; elevated platelet counts, leukopenia, neutropenia, positive Coombs' test, eosinophilia, anemia. **Hypersensitivity:** fever, rash, pruritus, erythema, myalgia, anaphylactoid reaction. **Other:** pain with IM injection; burning sensation, phlebitis (IV administration), flu-like syndrome, superinfections.

ROUTE AND DOSAGE. Intramuscular, intravenous: direct (bolus) or infusion: 1 to 2 Gm once every 24 hours. Lower dosages for patients with renal insufficiency.

NURSING IMPLICATIONS

Culture and susceptibility tests should be performed prior to and periodically during therapy, if indicated. Therapy may be initiated before test results are available.

A careful inquiry should be made before therapy begins to determine history of hypersensitivity to cephalosporins, penicillins, or other drugs.

Although cephalosporins may be used in individuals with history of hypersensitivity to penicillin, they should not be used if individual has experienced an immediate reaction to penicillin, such as bronchospasm, urticaria, angioedema.

IM injections should be made deeply into large muscle mass. Pain and discomfort at IM site occurs commonly. Administer no more than 1 Gm into a single IM site. Rotate injection sites.

C

Bolus IV injections of reconstituted solution should be made slowly over 3 to 5 minutes. Injection may be made directly, or through IV tubing if patient is receiving a compatible parenteral fluid recommended by manufacturer. Examine IV site daily for evidence of inflammation.

When administered for surgical prophylaxis, cefonicid is usually given 1 hour before the surgical procedure. In cesarean section, administered only after umbilical cord has been clamped.

Monitor input and output ratio and pattern, particularly in patients with impaired renal function, patients over 50 years, or who are receiving high doses.

Monitor temperature. Report temperature alterations and the onset of flu-like symptoms (chills, malaise).

Report the onset of diarrhea. Although pseudomembranous colitis has not been reported with use of cefonicid, this life-threatening complication should be considered a possible cause of diarrhea.

Observe for superinfections (ulcerations of mouth, white patches in mouth, glossitis, black hairy tongue, anogenital itching, foul-smelling vaginal discharge or diarrhea, rectal or genital itching).

Because cefonicid is a comparatively new drug, inform pharmacist or physician of any unusual adverse reactions that may be associated with its use.

For IM injection or direct (bolus) IV injection, reconstitute with sterile water for injection and shake well to assure complete dissolution of drug (500 mg of drug to 2 ml of diluent or 1 Gm of drug to 2.5 ml diluent). Following reconstitution, inspect for particulate matter; if present, discard solution.

For IV infusion, the reconstituted solution (see above) is diluted in 50 to 100 ml of parenteral fluid recommended by manufacturer.

After reconstitution or dilution, solutions are stable for 24 hours at room temperature or 72 hours if refrigerated 5°C (41°F). Slight yellowing does not indicate loss of potency.

Diagnostic Test Interferences. A false-positive reaction for **urine glucose** may occur with copper sulfate reduction reagents, e.g., Benedict's or Fehling's solution, Clinitest; tests based on glucose oxidase reactions are apparently not affected, e.g., Tes-Tape, Clinistix, Diastix.

Drug Interactions: Cefonocid

Plus	Interactions
Probenecid	Slow renal excretion of cefonicid. Used therapeutically to achieve higher serum levels

---

CEFOPERAZONE SODIUM
(Cefobid)

(sef-oh-per′a-zone)
Antiinfective
Antibiotic (beta-lactam)
Cephalosporin

ACTIONS AND USES. Long-acting, semisynthetic, extra broad spectrum, third generation cephalosporin. Antimicrobial activity includes most clinically significant gram-positive and gram-negative aerobes, and anaerobic organisms. Particularly active against *Pseudomonas aeruginosa, Escherichia coli, Enterobacter, Haemophilus influenzae, Klebsiella,* and *Proteus mirabilis.* In common with other third generation members, not as active as first and second generation cephalosporins against gram-positive cocci, e.g., *Staphylococcus aureus, S. epidermides,* group A and B Streptococci, and *S. pneumoniae.* Highly resistant to beta-lactamases (cephalosporinases and penicillinases) produced by most gram-negative organisms. It may not be stable, however, against beta-lactamases produced by certain strains of *Enterobacter, Klebsiella,* and *Serratia.* Like other cephalosporins, acts by inhibiting mucopeptide synthesis in bacterial cell wall. Contains approximately 1.5 mEq (34 mg) of sodium per Gm.

Used in treatment of infections of skin and skin structures, bones and joints, urinary tract, respiratory tract, and in peritonitis and other intraabdominal infections, pelvic infections, and bacterial septicemia.

ABSORPTION AND FATE. Peak serum levels in 15 to 20 minutes after IV and in 1 to 2 hours following IM administration. IM serum concentrations are approximately ⅓ to ½ IV levels. Widely distributed in most body tissues and fluids. Highest concentrations in bile (100 times higher than serum). Low penetration in CSF except when meninges are inflamed. Half-life about 2 hours (higher in patients with hepatic disease or biliary obstruction); 82 to 93% protein bound (reduced in hepatic disease). Not appreciably metabolized. Dual excretion pattern: 70 to 75% eliminated unchanged in bile and 20 to 30% excreted unchanged in urine, within 6 to 12 hours. Compensatory increase in urinary excretion in patients with hepatic impairment or biliary obstruction. Crosses placenta. Small amounts eliminated in breast milk.

CONTRAINDICATIONS AND PRECAUTIONS. Hypersensitivity to cephalosporins. Safe use during pregnancy (category B) and in children younger than 12 years not established. *Cautious Use:* history of hypersensitivity to penicillins, history of allergy, particularly to drugs; hepatic disease, history of colitis or other GI disease, history of bleeding disorders; nursing mothers.

ADVERSE/SIDE EFFECTS. GI: abdominal cramps, bloating, loose stools or diarrhea, nausea, vomiting, pseudomembranous colitis with unusual weight loss (rare). **Hematologic:** reversible neutropenia (with prolonged use), reduction in: neutrophils, Hgb, Hct, positive direct Coomb's test, abnormal PT and partial thromboplastin time, hypoprothrombinemia, low platelet count. **Hepatic:** hepatitis (rare), elevated liver function tests: AST (SGOT), ALT (SGPT), alkaline phosphatase. **Hypersensitivity:** skin rash, urticaria, pruritus, drug fever, eosinophilia. **Renal:** transient increases in serum creatinine and BUN, oliguria. **Other:** hypertension, headache, dizziness, unusual fatigue or weakness, tremulousness, chills, unusual thirst, phlebitis (IV site), transient pain (IM site), superinfections, vitamin K deficiency.

ROUTE AND DOSAGE. Intramuscular, intravenous: 1 to 2 Gm every 12 hours. *Severe infections:* 6 to 12 Gm daily divided into two, three, or four doses, e.g., 1.5 to 3 Gm every 6 hours, 2 to 4 Gm every 8 hours, 3 to 6 Gm every 12 hours. Up to 16 Gm daily dose has been prescribed.

NURSING IMPLICATIONS

Culture and susceptibility studies should be performed prior to initiation of therapy and during therapy, as indicated. Therapy may begin pending test results.

Before therapy begins, a careful inquiry should be made concerning history of hypersensitivity to cephalosporins, penicillins, and other drug allergies.

Observe for and question patient about bleeding tendencies: wound bleeding (e.g., surgical patient), nose bleeds, bleeding gums, bloody sputum, hematuria. Hypoprothrombinemia and vitamin K deficiency are possible complications of therapy. Reversible with vitamin K and plasma, if necessary.

Vitamin K deficiency and hypoprothrombinemia can result in significant blood loss in some patients.

Vitamin K deficiency develops in conditions that reduce vitamin K-producing bacteria in GI tract. Patients at risk are those with poor nutritional states, malabsorption problems, patients on hyperalimentation regimens, and alcoholism. Vitamin K supplements may be prescribed for these patients, if indicated.

BT, partial thromboplastin time, and prothrombin time should be performed prior to and during therapy.

Report the onset of loose stools or diarrhea. Most patients respond to replacement of fluids, electrolytes, and proteins. *(See Index: Nursing Interventions: Rehydration).* Discontinuation of drug may be required for some patients. Although pseudomembranous colitis occurs rarely, this potentially life-threatening complication should be considered a possible cause of diarrhea during and after antibiotic therapy.

Cefoperazone serum levels (at steady state: 150 mcg/ml) should be monitored in patients with hepatic disease or biliary obstruction who are receiving over 4 Gm/daily, patients with both hepatic and renal disease receiving over 1 to 2 Gm daily, and patients with renal impairment on high dose therapy.

In general, cefoperazone therapy should be continued at least 48 to 72 hours after patient becomes afebrile or other signs of infection have subsided. Patients with group A beta hemolytic streptococcal infections should receive therapy for at least 10 days to reduce risk of glomerulonephritis or rheumatic fever.

Patient should be warned that ingestion of alcohol within 72 hours after drug administration will cause a disulfiram-like reaction: flushing, sweating, headache, tachycardia, hypotension, abdominal or stomach cramps, nausea, vomiting. Effects generally appear within 15 to 30 minutes after alcohol is taken and disappear spontaneously 1 to 2 hours later.

Observe for signs of superinfection: ulcerations of mouth; white patches in mouth or throat; black, hairy tongue; foul-smelling vaginal discharge or stools; anogenital itching.

If an aminoglycoside is prescribed to be given concomitantly with cefoperazone, the drugs should be administered into separate sites. Do not mix.

Rapid, direct (bolus) IV injections not recommended. Cefoperazone may be administered by intermittent IV over a 15- to 30-minute period or by continuous IV infusion, as prescribed. See manufacturer's directions for reconstitution and dilution and for compatible diluents.

To prepare IM injections appropriate diluents include sterile water for injection, bacteriostatic water for injection (containing benzyl alcohol or parabens), and 0.5% lidocaine. Manufacturer recommends using a lidocaine hydrochloride solution as a diluent when concentrations of 250 mg/ml or greater are administered. See package insert for reconstitution procedure.

Following reconstitution, solutions should be allowed to stand to allow foam to dissipate and solution to clarify. Vigorous and prolonged shaking may be necessary to assure complete dissolution of drug.

Prior to reconstitution, store preferably between 2° and 8°C (36° and 46°F), protected from light, unless otherwise directed by manufacturer.

After reconstitution, solutions retain potency for 24 hours at controlled room temperature 15° to 25°C (59° to 77°F) or for 5 days if refrigerated 2° to 8°C (36° to 46°F). After reconstitution, protection from light is unnecessary. See manufacturer's directions for details regarding stability.

Diagnostic Test Interferences. Cefoperazone can cause positive direct Coombs' test, which may result in interferences with **hematologic studies** and **cross-matching** procedures. False-positive results for **urine glucose** using copper sulfate tests (Benedict's, Fehling's, Clinitest), but not with glucose enzymatic tests, e.g., Clinistix, Tes-Tape, Diastix.

Drug Interactions: Cefoperazone

Plus	Interactions
Alcohol (Ethanol)	Disulfiram-like reaction *(see Nursing Implications)*
Aminoglycosides	Additive antibacterial activity. May be used therapeutically, but with close monitoring of renal function for possible nephrotoxicity
Anticoagulants	Increased risk of hypoprothrombinemia and bleeding. Dose lowering of one or both drugs may be necessary

---

CEFOTAXIME SODIUM

(Claforan)

(sef-oh-taks'eem)

Antiinfective, antibiotic (beta-lactam)

Cephalosporin

ACTIONS AND USES. Semisynthetic third generation cephalosporin antibiotic. First of the third generation drugs marketed in U.S. In common with other cephalosporins, acts by inhibiting bacterial cell wall synthesis. Less active against gram-positive bacteria, e.g., *Staphylococcus aureus,* group A and B Streptococci, and *Streptococcus pneumoniae* than first and second generation cephalosporins. Effective against a variety of gram-negative organisms resistant to first and second generation drugs, but not generally preferred over an aminoglycoside for this purpose. Reportedly, resistant strains of *Enterobacter, Pseudomonas aeruginosa,* and *Serratia* have developed during cefotaxime therapy. More resistant to inactivation of beta-lactamase (both penicillinases and cephalosporinases) than first and second generation cephalosporins except cefoxitin. Therefore, effective against many beta-lactamase-producing organisms including *Neisseria gonorrhoeae, Haemophilus influenzae,* and a wide variety of *enterobacteriaceae.* Contains 2.2 mEq (51 mg) of sodium/Gm.

Used for serious infections of lower respiratory tract, skin and skin structures, bones and joints, CNS including meningitis and ventriculitis, for gynecologic and genitorurinary tract infections, including uncomplicated and disseminated gonococcal infections caused by penicillinase-producing *Neisseria gonorrhoeae* (PPNG), bacteremia/septicemia, intraabdominal infections, and perioperative prophylaxis. Currently recommended by CDC for gonococcal ophthalmia caused by PPNG in adults, older children, and neonates.

ABSORPTION AND FATE. Peak serum levels within 30 minutes following IM, and in about 5 minutes after IV injection. Widely distributed to body tissues and fluids, particularly bile. Penetrates CSF when meninges are inflamed. Half-life about 1 hour; 35 to 64% protein bound. Partially metabolized in liver to active metabolites. About 40 to 62% of dose excreted unchanged in urine within 24 hours (most excreted within first 2 hours). Approximately 24% eliminated as active metabolites and about 10% excreted in feces via bile. Crosses placenta. Small amounts excreted in breast milk.

CONTRAINDICATIONS AND PRECAUTIONS. Hypersensitivity to cephalosporins. Safe use during pregnancy (category B) not established. *Cautious Use:* history of type I hypersensitivity to penicillins, history of allergy particularly to drugs, renal impairment, history of colitis or other GI disease, nursing mothers.

ADVERSE/SIDE EFFECTS. GI: diarrhea, abdominal pain, colitis, pseudomembranous colitis (rare); anorexia, nausea, vomiting. **Hematologic:** transient leukopenia, granulocytopenia, thrombocytopenia, neutropenia, eosinophilia, positive direct Coombs' test, transient increases in BUN and serum creatinine. **Hypersensitivity:** rash, pruritus, fever. **Other:** inflammatory reaction, phlebitis, thrombophlebitis (IV site); pain, induration, and tenderness (IM site), superinfections: moniliasis, vaginitis.

ROUTE AND DOSAGE. Intramuscular, intravenous: Adults: 1 Gm every 6 to 8 hours. Not to exceed 12 Gm daily. *Life-threatening infections:* 2 Gm IV every 4 hours. *Uncomplicated gonorrhea:* 1 Gm IM in single dose. *Disseminated gonorrhea:* 500 mg four times daily for at least 7 days. *Perioperative prophylaxis:* 1 Gm IM or IV ½ to 1½ hours before surgery; dose repeated intraoperatively, if necessary ½ to 2 hours after first dose. **Pediatric: Infants (0 to 1 week):** 25 to 50 mg/kg IV every 12 hours; **Infants (1 to 4 weeks):** 25 to 50 mg/kg IV every 8 hours; **Children (1 month to 12 years) (under 50 kg):** 50 to 180 mg/kg IM or IV divided into four to six doses.

NURSING IMPLICATIONS

Culture and sensitivity tests should be performed prior to initiation of therapy and periodically during therapy, if indicated. Therapy may be instituted pending test results.

Before therapy is initiated, a careful inquiry should be made to determine previous hypersensitivity reactions to cephalosporins, penicillins, and history of other allergies, particularly to drugs.

IM injections are prepared by adding 2, 3, or 5 ml of sterile water for injection or bacteriostatic water for injection to each 500 mg, 1 Gm, or 2 Gm vial, respectively.

Following reconstitution, shake well to dissolve drug, and inspect for particulate matter and discoloration. Solutions may range in color from light yellow to amber depending on drug concentration, diluent used, and storage conditions. Manufacturer states that this does not adversely affect product potency.

IM injections should be made deeply into large muscle mass such as upper outer quadrant of gluteus maximus. Aspirate carefully to avoid inadvertent entry of drug into blood vessel. Rotate injection sites.

Manufacturer recommends administration of no more than 1 Gm into a single IM site. Large doses may be extremely painful and can cause local tissue reactions.

For IV use, reconstitute all strengths with at least 10 ml of sterile water for injection. For infusion bottles add 50 or 100 ml of 0.9% sodium chloride injection, 5% dextrose injection or other diluents recommended by manufacturer.

Reconstituted solutions may be further diluted to 50 to 1000 ml with IV fluids recommended by manufacturer. These solutions maintain potency for 24 hours at room temperature and at least 5 days under refrigeration.

After reconstitution cefotaxime may be stored in disposable glass or plastic syringes for same time periods as for reconstituted solutions, i.e., 24 hours at room temperature, 5 days under refrigeration, and 13 weeks in frozen state.

For direct intermittent IV administration, injection is made over a 3- to 5-minute period. Drug may also be administered more slowly into tubing of a freshly flowing IV of compatible solution. See manufacturer's directions for details.

Report onset of loose stools or diarrhea. Most patients respond to replacement of fluids, electrolytes, and proteins *(see Index: Nursing Interventions: Rehydration).* Discontinuation of drug may be required for some patients. Although pseudomembranous colitis occurs rarely, this potentially life-threatening complication should be considered a possible cause of diarrhea during or after antibiotic therapy.

Monitor input and output ratio and pattern in patients with impaired renal function, or who are receiving high dosages, or an aminoglycoside concomitantly. Renal status (serum creatinine, creatinine clearance, BUN) should be evaluated at regular intervals.

C

Patients with impaired renal function do not usually need dosage adjustments until creatinine clearance falls below 20 ml/minute. Dosage is then usually halved.

Chronic urinary tract infections may require frequent clinical and bacteriologic follow-up for several months after drug has been discontinued.

Observe and report onset of superinfections: fever, sore mouth or throat, white patches in mouth, black hairy tongue, diarrhea, foul-smelling stools or vaginal discharge, vaginitis, anogenital itching, moniliasis (fungal infection of skin, vagina, bronchi, lungs).

Disulfiram-type reaction upon ingestion of alcohol not reported with cefotaxime, but since it has occurred with other cephalosporins, caution is warranted.

Cefotaxime therapy should continue for at least 48 to 72 hours after patient becomes afebrile or other signs of infection have disappeared.

Therapy for group A beta-hemolytic streptococci should be continued for a minimum of 10 days to reduce risk of glomerulonephritis and rheumatic fever.

If an aminoglycoside is prescribed, it must be administered separately and not mixed with cefotaxime. Also do not admix with sodium bicarbonate or any fluid with a pH above 7.5.

Store dry powder preferably between 15° and 30°C (59° and 86°F), unless otherwise directed by manufacturer. Protect from excessive light.

Diagnostic Test Interferences. False-positive reactions for **urine glucose** have not been reported using copper sulfate reduction methods, e.g., Benedict's, Fehling's, Clinitest. Because it has occurred with other cephalosporins, however, it may be advisable to use glucose oxidase tests (Clinistix, Tes-Tape, Diastix). Positive direct Coombs' test results may interfere with **hematologic studies** and **crossmatching** procedures.

Drug Interactions: Cefotaxime

Plus	Interactions
Aminoglycosides	Concomitant use may increase risk of nephrotoxicity and ototoxicity
Probenecid	May prolong cefotaxime plasma levels with possible toxicity

CEFOXITIN SODIUM

(Mefoxin)

(se-fox'i-tin)
Antiinfective
Antibiotic (beta-lactam)
Cephalosporin-like

ACTIONS AND USES. Semisynthetic broad-spectrum antibiotic, derivative of cephamycin C (produced by *Streptomyces lactamdurans*). Generally classified as second generation cephalosporin. Structurally and pharmacologically related to cephalosporins and penicillins, and like them exerts bactericidal action by inhibition of cell wall synthesis. Antimicrobial spectrum broader than that of cephalothin; more active against many gram-negative bacteria, e.g., strains of *Escherichia coli, Klebsiella, Proteus mirabilis,* and *Bacteroides fragilis.* Highly resistant to beta-lactamases (cephalosporinases and penicillinases) produced by gram-negative aerobic and anaerobic bacteria. Reportedly has only moderate activity against *Haemophilus influenzae.* Also less active against gram-positive cocci than first generation cephalosporins. Contains approximately 2.3 mEq (53 mg) of sodium per gram of cefoxitin.

Used in treatment of serious infections of lower respiratory tract, genitourinary tract, skin and soft tissue, bones and joints, and in gynecological infections, septicemia, peritonitis, and other intra-abdominal infections. Used as alternative to spectinomycin in treatment of penicillinase-producing *Neisseria gonorrhea* (PPNG) and gonococcal infections unresponsive to penicillin or tetracycline therapy. Also used for perioperative prophylaxis in patients undergoing surgery with high risk of infection.

ABSORPTION AND FATE. Peak serum levels within 20 to 30 minutes following IM and within 5 minutes or less after IV administration. Widely distributed to body tissues and fluids including pleural, synovial, ascitic fluid, and bile. About 50 to 60% bound to serum proteins. Half-life: 45 minutes to 1 hour, considerably longer with impaired renal function. Poor diffusion into CSF even when meninges are inflamed. Rapidly excreted in urine (approximately 85% of single dose excreted within 6 hours), mostly unchanged. Readily crosses placenta; small amounts appear in breast milk.

CONTRAINDICATIONS AND PRECAUTIONS. Hypersensitivity to cefoxitin or to cephalosporins. Safe use in women of childbearing potential, during pregnancy, in nursing mothers, and in children under 3 months not established. *Cautious Use:* history of sensitivity to penicillin or other allergies, particularly to drugs, impaired renal function.

ADVERSE/SIDE EFFECTS. GI (rare): nausea, vomiting, diarrhea. **Hematologic (rare):** transient leukopenia, neutropenia, pancytopenia, hemolytic anemia, positive direct Coombs' test, elevated serum creatinine, BUN, SGOT, SGPT, LDH (lactic dehydrogenase), alkaline phosphatase. **Hypersensitivity:** rash, exfoliative dermatitis, pruritus, urticaria, drug fever, eosinophilia. **Other:** superinfections, local reactions (common): pain, tenderness, and induration (with IM), thrombophlebitis (with IV); nephrotoxicity and oliguria (rare).

ROUTE AND DOSAGE. Intramuscular, intravenous: Adults: *Infections:* 1 to 2 Gm every 6 to 8 hours, depending on severity of infection. Up to 12 Gm daily in life-threatening infections. *Uncomplicated gonorrhea:* 2 Gm IM with 1 Gm oral probenecid at same time or approximately 30 minutes before cefoxitin. *Perioperative prophylaxis:* 2 Gm 30 to 60 minutes before surgery and 2 Gm every 6 hours thereafter for 24 hours (72 hours for prosthetic arthroplasty). *Impaired renal function:* initial loading dose of 1 to 2 Gm; dosage and frequency then modified according to creatinine clearance tests and severity of infection. **Children (3 months and older):** 80 to 160 mg/kg/day divided into 4 to 6 equal doses. Not to exceed 12 Gm daily. *Perioperative prophylaxis:* 30 to 40 mg/kg at same intervals as for adults.

NURSING IMPLICATIONS

Before therapy is initiated, careful inquiry should be made concerning previous hypersensitivity to cephalosporins, penicillins, and other drug allergies.

Culture and susceptibility testing is advised prior to and periodically during therapy.

Recommended diluents for IM use include sterile water for injection or 0.5 or 1% lidocaine hydrochloride (without epinephrine), used to reduce discomfort of IM injection. Consult physician before using lidocaine.

Lidocaine is used as diluent for IM administration only. If used, review package circular for precautions and adverse reactions.

After reconstitution for IM use, shake vial and allow solution to stand until it becomes clear. Solutions retain potency for 24 hours at room temperature, for 7 days if refrigerated, and for at least 26 weeks if frozen.

Administer IM injections deep into large muscle mass such as upper outer quadrant of gluteus maximus. Aspirate before injecting drug (particularly important when lidocaine is used). Rotate injection sites.

IV administration should be made over 3 to 5 minutes directly into vein, or slowly into tubing of compatible running IV infusion.
Incidence of thrombophlebitis following IV administration appears to be less with use of butterfly or scalp vein-type needle than with indwelling catheter.
Consult package circular for specific directions concerning reconstitution for IV administration, compatible IV infusion fluids, stability, and storage times.
Monitor intake and output ratio and pattern. Nephrotoxicity occurs most frequently in patients over 50 years of age, in patients with impaired renal function, the debilitated, and in patients receiving high doses or other nephrotoxic drugs.
Drug therapy for beta-hemolytic streptococcal infections should continue for at least 10 days to guard against risk of rheumatic fever.
Be alert to signs and symptoms of superinfections (furry, black tongue; sore mouth; perianal irritation or itching; foul-smelling vaginal discharge; loose stools).
Solutions range in color from colorless to light amber, but may darken on storage; reportedly this does not indicate change in potency.
Unused vials stored preferably between 15° and 30°C (59° and 86°F), unless otherwise directed by manufacturer.

C

Diagnostic Test Interferences. Positive direct Coombs' test may interfere with **cross-matching** procedures and **hematologic studies.** False positive **urine glucose** tests, using copper sulfate reduction methods, e.g., Clinitest, Benedict's reagent, or Fehling's solution, but not with glucose oxidase (enzymatic) tests such as Clinistix, Diastix, Tes-Tape. False elevations of serum or urine **creatinine** values (with Jaffe reaction if serum sample is drawn within 2 hours after cefoxitin is administered).

Drug Interactions. Like cephalosporins, possibility of increased risk of nephrotoxicity with nephrotoxic drugs such as **aminoglycoside antibiotics, colistin, polymixin B,** and **vancomycin.** Concomitant administration of **probenecid** produces higher and more prolonged cefoxitin levels (applied clinically primarily in treatment of gonorrhea).

CEFUROXIME SODIUM

(Zinacef)

(se-fyoor-ox'eem)
Antiinfective
Antibiotic (beta-lactam)
Cephalosporin

ACTIONS AND USES. Semi-synthetic second generation cephalosporin antibiotic. Resistance against beta-lactamase producing strains exceeds that of first generation cephalosporins. Has broader spectrum of activity against anaerobes and gram-negative microorganisms than most other second generation cephalosporins. Reported to be highly effective against *Streptococcus* (pneumococcus) *pneumoniae, Haemophilus influenza, Staphylococcus aureus, Neisseria gonorrhea, N. meningitides, Klebsiella, Escherichia coli,* and *Streptococcus pyogenes.* Like other cephalosporins, activity against *Streptococcus* (enterococcus) *faecalis* is generally limited. *Pseudomonas aeruginosa* and *Acinetobacter* are usually resistant to cefuroxime and it is inactivated by beta-lactamases of certain strains of *Enterobacter, Serratia, Bacteroides fragilis,* and *Providencia.* In common with other cephalosporins, acts by inhibiting bacterial cell wall synthesis. Contains 2.4 mEq (approximately 55 mg) of sodium/Gm.

Used in treatment of serious infections of lower respiratory tract, urinary tract, skin and skin structures, and for septicemia, meningitis, uncomplicated and disseminated gonococcal infections. Also used for preoperative prophylaxis.

ABSORPTION AND FATE. Peak serum levels in 15 to 60 minutes after IM injection and in about 3 minutes after IV administration. Widely distributed in body tissues and fluids. Crosses blood–brain barrier; therapeutic concentrations achieved in CSF even when meninges are not inflamed. Protein binding: 33 to 50%; half-life: 1 to 2 hours (prolonged in patients with impaired renal function). Very little if any is metabolized. About 90 to 100% eliminated unchanged in urine within 24 hours (most excreted within first 6 hours after drug administration). Excreted in breast milk.

CONTRAINDICATIONS AND PRECAUTIONS. Hypersensitivity to cephalosporins. Safe use during pregnancy (category B) and in children under 3 months not established. *Cautious Use:* history of allergy, particularly to drugs; penicillin sensitivity, renal insufficiency, history of colitis or other GI disease, nursing women.

ADVERSE/SIDE EFFECTS. GI: diarrhea, nausea, colitis, pseudomembranous colitis (rare). **Hematologic:** decreased Hgb and Hct, transient eosinophilia, neutropenia, leukopenia. **Hepatic:** transient increases in AST (SGOT), ALT (SGPT), alkaline phosphatase, LDH, and bilirubin. **Hypersensitivity:** rash, pruritus, urticaria, positive Coombs' test. **Renal:** increased serum creatinine and BUN, decreased creatinine clearance (causal relationship not established). **Other:** local reactions: thrombophlebitis (IV site); pain, burning, cellulitis (IM site).

ROUTE AND DOSAGE. Intramuscular, intravenous: Adults: 750 mg to 1.5 Gm every 8 hours for 5 to 10 days depending on severity of infection. *Life-threatening infections:* 1.5 Gm every 6 hours. *Bacterial meningitis:* not to exceed 3 Gm every 8 hours. *Uncomplicated gonococcal infections:* 1.5 Gm IM as single dose (but divided and given at two different sites), together with 1 Gm oral probenecid. *Preoperative prophylaxis:* 1.5 Gm IV ½ to 1 hour before surgery. Thereafter, 750 mg IV or IM every 8 hours during prolonged procedures for about 24 hours. **Children (over 3 months):** 50 to 100 mg/kg/day in equally divided doses every 6 to 8 hours. *Bacterial meningitis:* initially 200 to 240 mg/kg/day IV in divided doses every 6 to 8 hours. Reduced to 100 mg/kg/day upon clinical improvement. Patients with renal function impairment may require lengthening of time interval between doses or dosage reduction.

NURSING IMPLICATIONS

Culture and susceptibility tests should be performed prior to initiation of therapy and periodically during therapy, if indicated. Therapy may be instituted pending test results.

Before therapy is initiated, a careful inquiry should be made to determine previous hypersensitivity reactions to cephalosporins, penicillins, and history of allergies, particularly to drugs.

Shake IM suspension gently prior to administration. IM injections should be made deeply into large muscle mass such as upper outer quadrant of gluteus maximus or lateral part of thigh. Aspirate carefully before injecting drug to avoid inadvertent entry into blood vessel. Rotate injection sites.

Most patients complain of pain following IM administration, which lasts around 5 minutes. Reportedly, IM injections are less painful if IM concentrations recommended by manufacturer are used and if injections are made into gluteus maximus rather than lateral aspect of thigh.

Inspect IM and IV injection sites frequently for signs of phlebitis.

Monitor input and output ratio and pattern especially in severely ill patients receiving high doses. Report any significant changes. Also note serum creatinine, creatinine clearance and BUN values.

Report onset of loose stools or diarrhea. Most patients respond to replacement of fluids, electrolytes, and proteins *(see Index: Nursing Interventions: Rehydration).* Discontinuation of drug may be required in some patients. Although pseudomembranous colitis rarely occurs, this potentially life-threatening complication should be ruled out as the cause of diarrhea during and after antibiotic therapy.

Observe for signs of superinfections: fever, ulcerations and white patches in mouth or throat, black hairy tongue, foul-smelling vaginal discharge, diarrhea, fungal infection (moniliasis) of skin, nails, vagina, bronchi, lungs.

IV rather than IM administration is recommended especially for patients with septicemia and other life-threatening infections and in patients with low resistance particularly in the presence of shock.

For direct intermittent IV, solution is injected slowly into a vein over 3 to 5 minutes, or injection may be made slowly through tubing system of a freely running compatible IV solution.

If an aminoglycoside is to be given concomitantly with cefuroxime, administration should be into separate sites. Do not mix.

See manufacturer's directions for specifics regarding reconstitution, dilution, compatible solutions, and storage.

Inspect solutions for particulate matter and discoloration before administration. Cefuroxime powder and solutions of the drug may range in color from light yellow to amber without adversely affecting product potency.

When reconstituted as directed with sterile water for injection, solutions retain potency 24 hours at room temperature and 48 hours under refrigeration (5°C), then they should be discarded.

Store powder at controlled room temperature preferably 15° to 30°C (59° to 86°F) protected from light, unless otherwise directed by manufacturer.

Diagnostic Test Interferences. Cefuroxime can cause positive **direct Coombs' test** that can result in interferences with **hematologic studies** and **crossmatching** procedures. It also may cause false-positive results for **urine glucose** using copper reduction methods, e.g., Benedict's, Fehling's, Clinitest, but not with glucose oxidase tests, e.g., Clinistix, Tes-Tape, Diastix. Cefuroxime may induce false-negative **blood glucose** tests using ferricyanide methods.

Drug Interactions: Cefuroxime

Plus	Interactions
Aminoglycosides	Concomitant use increases potential for nephrotoxicity; monitor for nephrotoxicity and ototoxicity
Diuretics, potent	Increased potential for nephrotoxicity. Used with caution
Probenecid	Produces higher and more prolonged cefuroxime levels. May be used to therapeutic advantage

---

CELLULOSE SODIUM PHOSPHATE

(Calcibind, CSP, SCP, Sodium Cellulose Phosphate)

Antilithic
Resin exchange agent: cationic

ACTIONS AND USES. Synthetic sodium salt of the phosphate ester of cellulose; cation exchange resin. When taken with meals, releases sodium in exchange for divalent cations (e.g., dietary and secreted calcium and magnesium) in intestines to form a nonabsorbable complex. Binding

C

of these divalent ions renders them unavailable for complexing with oxalate (e.g., calcium oxalate or calcium phosphate in urine); thus formation of renal calculi is inhibited. Does not generally cause significant alterations in serum phosphate or calcium in most patients. Serum magnesium is predictably reduced, however, and therefore supplemention is necessary. Does not appear to affect serum concentrations of trace metals: copper, zinc, or iron. Contains about 25 to 50 mEq of exchangeable sodium per 15 Gm of CSP (1 mEq of sodium contains approximately 23 mg).

Used as adjunct to dietary restriction to reduce renal calculi formation in absorptive hypercalciuria type I with recurrent calcium oxalate and calcium phosphate nephrolithiasis. Has been used as adjunct in treatment of hypercalcemia (e.g., associated with parathyroid carcinoma or sarcoidosis) and in managment of calcinosis cutis.

ABSORPTION AND FATE. Not absorbed from GI tract. Partially hydrolyzed in intestines, causing release of phosphorus ions, which are absorbed by intestines. Nonabsorbable complex of calcium and cellulose phosphate excreted in feces along with unchanged resin.

CONTRAINDICATIONS AND PRECAUTIONS. Bone disease, hypocalcemia, hypomagnesemia, hyperoxaluria, primary and secondary hyperparathyroidism, including renal hypercalciuria, high fasting urinary calcium or hypophosphatemia, conditions associated with high skeletal mobilization of calcium. Safe use during pregnancy (category C), in nursing mothers, and in children under 16 years not established. *Cautious Use:* patients on sodium restriction—congestive heart failure, ascites, nephrotic syndrome.

ADVERSE/SIDE EFFECTS. GI: loose stools, diarrhea, GI discomfort, dyspepsia, anorexia, nausea, vomiting. With long-term use: hypomagnesemia, hypomagnesuria, hyperoxaluria, acute arthritis, arthralgia, hyperparathyroid bone disease, symptoms related to electrolyte imbalances, or depletion of trace metals (copper, zinc, iron).

ROUTE AND DOSAGE. Oral: *Patients with urinary calcium exceeding 300 mg/day:* Initial: 15 Gm/day (5 Gm three times a day, with each meal). Dosage decreased to 10 Gm/day (5 Gm with main meal, 2.5 Gm with each of two other meals) when urinary calcium declines to less than 150 mg/day.

NURSING IMPLICATIONS

Powder can be mixed with full glass (240 ml) of water, soft drink, or fruit juice and taken with meals. Cellulose sodium phosphate (CSP) is not very palatable.

Be sure that patient understands drug will not work unless taken with meals or at least within 30 minutes of a meal.

Oral magnesium supplements (e.g., magnesium gluconate) should be administered to prevent hypomagnesemia. They can be given at any time as long as it is at least 1 hour before or after CSP to avoid binding of magnesium.

Dose of oral magnesium supplements depends on dose of CSP. Patients receiving 15 Gm/day of CSP should take 1.5 Gm magnesium gluconate before breakfast and again at bedtime (separately from CSP). Patients taking 10 Gm/day of CSP should take 1 Gm magnesium gluconate twice a day.

Diagnosis of absorptive hypercalciuria type I must be substantiated at least by serum calcium and phosphorus determinations, fasting serum parathyroid hormone (PTH) levels obtained before breakfast, 24-hour urinary calcium excretion (while calcium and sodium are restricted), and fasting (12 hours) urinary calcium excretion.

A definitive diagnosis for absorptive hypercalciuria type I requires the following characteristic signs:

1. Recurrent calcium nephrolithiasis without clinical evidence of bone disease
2. Normal serum calcium and phosphorus
3. 24-hour urinary calcium exceeding 200 mg/day on a diet of 400 mg calcium and 100 mEq sodium/day
4. Normal parathyroid function
5. Normal fasting urinary calcium

Monitor intake and output ratio and pattern. Fluid intake should be encouraged to maintain a urinary output of at least 2 L/day (approximately 240 ml hourly while awake).

Serum parathyroid hormone (PTH) levels should be evaluated at least once between first 2 weeks to 3 months of therapy, and then every 3 to 6 months during therapy. Serum and urinary calcium and oxalate, and serum magnesium, copper, iron, and zinc, and CBC should also be monitored every 3 to 6 months throughout therapy.

Observe urinary calcium levels. A reduction of less than 30 mg per 5 Gm in urinary calcium in patients on moderate calcium and sodium restriction indicates treatment failure. Drug is usually discontinued.

Discontinuation of therapy is also indicated in patients on moderate oxalate restriction with urinary oxalate levels in excess of 55 mg/day. A rise in serum PTH above normal also points to the need to adjust dosage or stop the drug.

Food-Drug Interactions: To increase therapeutic effectiveness of CSP, dietary restriction of sodium, calcium, oxalate, and ascorbic acid is essential. Collaborate with physician and dietitian. The following dietary plan is generally prescribed as an adjunct to drug therapy:

- Limit sodium intake to less than 150 mEq/day (6.5 mg) by avoiding obviously salty foods and use of salt shaker
- Maintain moderate calcium intake by eliminating dairy foods
- Observe moderate restriction of oxalate-rich foods by avoiding spinach and similar dark greens, rhubarb, chocolate, brewed tea
- Do not self-dose with vitamin C supplements *(see Drug Interactions)*

Store in well-closed container, preferably between 15° and 30°C (59° and 86°F), protected from moisture, unless otherwise directed by manufacturer.

Drug Interactions: Cellulose sodium phosphate (CSP)

Plus	Interactions
Calcium supplements or calcium-containing medications	Counteract calcium lowering effect of CSP. Concurrent use generally avoided
Magnesium-containing medications	CSP binding of magnesium decreases its bioavailability. Separate administration by at least 1 hour from CSP
Thiazide diuretics	Additive action. Concurrent use generally avoided
Vitamin C (ascorbic acid)	Vitamin C is metabolized to oxalate, thereby counteracting CSP oxalate-lowering effect. Concurrent use generally avoided

C

CEPHALEXIN

(Keflex)

(sef-a-lex'in)
Antiinfective
Antibiotic (beta-lactam)
Cephalosporin

ACTIONS AND USES. Semisynthetic derivative of cephalosporin C. Broad-spectrum, first generation cephalosporin, antibiotic similar to cephalothin (qv), but reportedly less potent. In common with other cephalosporins, generally not effective against methicillin-resistant staphylococci.

Used as follow-up oral therapy in patients initially treated with parenteral cephalosporins. Has been used to treat infections caused by susceptible pathogens in respiratory and urinary tracts, middle ear, skin, soft tissue, and bone. Some clinicians recommend that it be reserved for treatment of urinary tract infections due to susceptible *Klebsiella* organisms resistant to other oral antibacterials.

ABSORPTION AND FATE. Stable in stomach acid; rapidly and almost completely absorbed from GI tract. (Absorption is delayed in young children and may be reduced in patients with pernicious anemia or obstructive jaundice.) Peak serum level in 1 hour. Measurable levels persist for 6 hours. Higher and more prolonged blood levels in patients with renal insufficiency and in neonates. Widely distributed in body fluids, with highest concentrations in kidney. About 6 to 15% bound to plasma proteins. Half-life: 0.6 to 1.2 hours. Over 90% of dose excreted in urine as unchanged drug within 8 hours. May cross placenta; appears in breast milk.

CONTRAINDICATIONS AND PRECAUTIONS. Hypersensitivity to cephalosporins. Safe use during pregnancy not established. *Cautious Use:* history of hypersensitivity to penicillin or other drug allergy; severely impaired renal function. *See Cephalothin.*

ADVERSE/SIDE EFFECTS. CNS: toxic paranoid reactions (high doses in patients with renal impairment); dizziness, headache, fatigue. **GI:** diarrhea (generally mild), nausea, vomiting, anorexia, abdominal pain. **Hematologic:** slightly elevated SGPT, SGOT, alkaline phosphatase; eosinophilia, positive direct Coombs' test. **Hypersensitivity:** angioedema, rash, urticaria, anaphylaxis. **Other:** superinfections.

ROUTE AND DOSAGE. Oral: Adults: 250 to 500 mg every 6 hours (usual dose range 1 to 4 Gm daily in divided doses). **Children:** 25 to 50 mg/kg/day in 4 equally divided doses. In severe infections, dosage may be doubled. Available in pulvules (capsules), tablets, oral suspension.

NURSING IMPLICATIONS

Cephalexin is not destroyed by gastric acid, but peak blood levels are slightly lower and delayed when administered with food. Total amount absorbed is unchanged however.

Before therapy is initiated, careful inquiry should be made concerning history of sensitivity to cephalosporins, penicillins, and other allergies particularly to drugs.

Culture and susceptibility testing is recommended prior to and periodically during therapy.

Physician should specify dosage interval. For example, four times a day may signify every 6 hours around the clock or it may mean to take the drug at evenly spaced intervals during waking hours, e.g., 7 AM, 12 noon, 5 PM, 10 PM.

Instruct patient to take medication for the full course of therapy as directed by physician.

Drug therapy for beta-hemolytic streptococcal infections should continue for at least 10 days to guard against risk of rheumatic fever.

Advise patient to keep physician informed if adverse reactions appear.

Periodic evaluations of renal and hepatic function should be made in patients receiving prolonged therapy.

Be alert to signs and symptoms of superinfections: furry, black tongue, sore mouth, anogenital irritation or itching, foul smelling vaginal discharge, loose stools, sudden fever, cough.

It has been reported that many IV drug abusers are taking cephalexin (Keflex) prophylactically to prevent cellulitis, phlebitis, and abscess formation. They procure it by manipulating prescriptions issued to friends or receive it from their drug supplier.

After reconstitution (by pharmacist), cephalexin oral suspension should be refrigerated; discard unused portions 14 days after preparation. Label should indicate expiration date. Keep tightly covered. Shake suspension well before pouring.

Store capsules and tablets preferably between 15° and 30°C (59° and 86°F) unless otherwise specified by manufacturer.

See Cephalothin sodium (prototype cephalosporin).

Diagnostic Test Interferences. False-positive **urine glucose** determinations using copper sulfate reduction tests such as Clinitest, Benedict's reagent, or Fehling's solution, but not with glucose oxidase (enzymatic) tests, e.g., Tes-Tape, Diastix, Clinistix. Positive Coombs' test may complicate transfusion **cross-matching procedures** and **hematologic studies.**

Drug Interactions: Cephalexin

Plus	Interactions
Aminoglycosides, colistimethate and other drugs with nephrotoxic potential	Possibility of additive nephrotoxic effects. Monitor renal function
Probenecid	Higher and more prolonged serum cephalexin levels (probenecid inhibits excretion of cephalexin). Use concomitantly with caution

PROTOTYPE

CEPHALOTHIN SODIUM

(Ceporacin, Keflin, Seffin)

(sef-a'loe-thin)
Antiinfective
Antibiotic (beta-lactam)
Cephalosporin

ACTIONS AND USES. Semisynthetic, broad spectrum, first generation cephalosporin derived from cephalosporin C, a substance produced by the fungus *Cephalosporium acremonium.* Structurally and pharmacologically related to penicillins. Inhibits synthesis of bacterial cell wall; has broad antibacterial spectrum. Primarily bactericidal but also bacteriostatic against most gram-positive organisms including nonpenicillinase and penicillinase-producing staphylococci, Group A beta-hemolytic Streptococci, *S. pneumoniae,* and *S. viridans;* and some gram-negative strains, particularly *Escherichia coli, Klebsiella, Haemophilus influenzae, P. mirabilis, Salmonella,* and *Shigella.* Most indole-positive *Proteus, Bacteroides, Serratia, Pseudomonas,* and motile *Enterobacter* species are resistant. Ineffective as prophylaxis against *Clostridium perfringens* (gas gangrene). Cephalothin is highly resistant to cephalosporinases (inactivating enzyme produced by certain bacteria). Formulated with sodium bicarbonate for pH adjustment and contains approximately 2.8 mEq (64 mg) of sodium per Gm.

Used in treatment of severe infections of respiratory, GI, and urinary tracts, bones, joints, soft tissue, and skin, and for septicemia, endocarditis, meningitis. Also used for perioperative prophylaxis in patients undergoing surgery with high risk of infection. Used intraperitoneally for bacterial peritonitis and has been used as systemic treatment for intraocular infections.

ABSORPTION AND FATE. Peak serum levels in 30 minutes after IM and 15 minutes after IV injection. Widely distributed in body tissues and fluids, including aqueous humor. Does not readily penetrate brain or CSF unless inflammation is present. Serum half-life is 30 to 60 minutes; 65 to 79% bound to plasma proteins. Partly deacetylated in liver and kidney. About 60 to 95% of dose excreted by kidneys within 6 hours, largely as unchanged drug and relatively active desacetyl metabolites. Readily crosses placenta; low concentrations in breast milk.

CONTRAINDICATIONS AND PRECAUTIONS. Hypersensitivity to cephalosporin antibiotics. Safe use during pregnancy not determined. *Cautious Use:* history of allergies, particularly to drugs, hypersensitivity to penicillins, impaired renal or hepatic function, patients on sodium restriction.

ADVERSE/SIDE EFFECTS. CNS: dizziness, vertigo, headache, fatigue, malaise, toxic paranoid reactions (patients with renal impairment). **GI:** nausea, vomiting, diarrhea, anorexia, abdominal cramps, pseudomembranous colitis (rare). **Hematologic:** neutropenia, leukopenia, pancytopenia (bone marrow toxicity), agranulocytosis, thrombocytopenia, hypoprothrombinemia, hemolytic anemia, direct positive Coombs' test (particularly patients with azotemia). **Hepatic:** transient rise in SGOT, SGPT, and alkaline phosphatase; increased plasma thymol turbidity and increased serum bilirubin. **Hypersensitivity:** maculopapular, morbilliform, or pruritic rash, urticaria, serum sickness-like reactions (arthralgia, myalgia, lymphadenopathy, fever), anaphylactic shock, eosinophilia, drug fever. **Renal:** nephrotoxicity (with high dose therapy): elevated BUN, decreased creatinine clearance, oliguria, renal failure. **Other:** superinfections; especially *Pseudomonas* or *Candida;* local reactions: pain, induration, slough, abscess (IM site); thrombophlebitis (IV site).

ROUTE AND DOSAGE. Intramuscular, intravenous: Adults: *Infections:* 500 mg to 1 Gm every 4 to 6 hours; up to 12 Gm/day for life-threatening infections. *Perioperative prophylaxis:* 1 to 2 Gm IV 30 to 60 minutes before surgery, repeated during prolonged surgery, then every 6 hours postoperatively for 24 hours. **Intraperitoneal:** up to 6 mg/100 ml added to dialysis fluid. **Pediatric:** *Infections:* 80 to 160 mg/kg/day in divided doses. *Perioperative prophylaxis:* 20 to 30 mg/kg at same intervals as for adults.

NURSING IMPLICATIONS

Culture and susceptibility studies should be performed prior to and during therapy. Therapy may be started pending test results.

A careful drug history should be elicited before therapy in order to determine previous hypersensitivity to cephalosporins, penicillins, and other allergies, particularly to drugs.

Physicians generally prefer other cephalosporins for IM injection because cephalothin causes intense pain and induration. If cephalothin IM is prescribed, administer injection deep into large muscle mass such as gluteus maximus or lateral aspect of thigh. Rotate injection sites.

IM injection is prepared by adding 4 ml of sterile water for injection to each gram of cephalothin (resultant solution: 500 mg per 2.2 ml). If vial contents do not completely dissolve add more diluent (0.2 to 0.4 ml), and warm vial slightly.

Observe IV sites for evidence of inflammatory reaction. IV infusions of doses larger than 6 Gm/day for more than 3 days can result in thrombophlebitis.

Reportedly, risk of phlebitis may be reduced by use of a small needle in a large vein. Some physicians add hydrocortisone to the infusion fluid as a prophylactic measure.

Report falling urinary output or change in intake and output ratio. Patients with renal dysfunction and those receiving high doses in the presence of dehydration are particularly susceptible to nephrotoxic reactions.

When renal function is reduced, as in the elderly or debilitated patient, dosage is based on creatinine clearance values and severity of infection.

Superinfections caused by emergence of nonsusceptible organisms may occur, particularly during prolonged use of cephalosporins. Mouth, vagina, anus, colon, and respiratory tract are susceptible areas; meticulous hygiene is indicated. White patches in mouth, black hairy tongue, mucosal erosions, itching, diarrhea, foul-smelling stools or vaginal discharge are early signs. Appropriate cultures should be taken if superinfection is suspected.

Report the onset of diarrhea. Bear in mind that pseudomembranous colitis may occur during or after cephalothin therapy. It is a superinfection life-threatening caused by clostridia.

Yogurt or buttermilk, 4 ounces of either (if allowed), may serve as a prophylactic against intestinal superinfection by helping to maintain normal intestinal flora.

Immediately report signs and symptoms of hypersensitivity reaction. If it occurs, drug should be discontinued.

Drug treatment for all infections should be continued for at least 48 to 72 hours after patient becomes asymptomatic or after evidence of bacterial eradication is obtained. For infections caused by beta-hemolytic streptococci, therapy should be continued at least 10 days in order to prevent the occurrence of rheumatic fever or glomerulonephritis.

Periodic hematologic studies and evaluations of renal and hepatic functions are recommended in patients receiving high doses and during prolonged therapy.

Kept at room temperature, solutions for IM injections and intermittent IV infusion should be administered within 12 hours after reconstitution. Solutions for continuous IV infusion should be started within 12 hours and completed within 24 hours of preparation.

Refrigeration protects potency for 96 hours after reconstitution with infusion fluids recommended by manufacturer. See manufacturer's literature for specific information regarding stability, storage, compatible fluids, and dilutions.

Slight discoloration of solution may occur especially when stored at room temperature, but this does not affect potency.

Storage at low temperature may cause precipitation. Redissolve crystals by warming vial to room temperature with constant agitation.

Do not store or freeze cephalothin in plastic syringes.

Solutions in sterile water for injection, 5% dextrose injection, or 0.9% sodium chloride injection that are frozen immediately after reconstitution in original container are stable up to 12 weeks at −20°C. Do not thaw until ready for use. Manufacturer warns to avoid heating after thawing and not to refreeze.

Store powder for injection preferably at 15° to 30°C (59° to 86°F), unless otherwise directed by manufacturer.

Diagnostic Test Interferences. Most cephalosporins cause confusing black-brown or green-brown color or false-positive **urine glucose** determinations with copper reduction reagents such as Benedict's, Fehling's, and Clinitest. Tests based on enzymatic glucose oxidase reactions, such as Clinistix, Tes-Tape, and Diastix, are not affected. With high doses, falsely elevated **serum and urine creatinine** (with Jaffe reaction) reported. Positive direct Coombs' test may interfere with **cross-matching procedures** and **hematologic studies.** False-positive **urinary protein** (sulfosalicylic acid method); falsely elevated **urinary 17-ketosteroids** (Zimmerman reaction); false-positive **direct Coombs'** test reported.

C

Drug Interactions: Cephalothin

Plus	Interactions
Aminoglycoside antibiotics, colistimethate, and other drugs with nephrotoxic potential	Possibility of additive nephrotoxic effect. Monitor renal function
Probenecid	Higher and more prolonged serum cephalosporin levels (probenecid inhibits their excretion). Used concomitantly with caution

---

CEPHAPIRIN SODIUM

(Cefadyl)

(sef-a-pye'rin)
Antiinfective
Antibiotic (beta-lactam)
Cephalosporin

ACTIONS AND USES. Semisynthetic, first generation, broad-spectrum cephalosporin antibiotic similar to cephalothin (qv). Reported to cause less tissue irritation and to be less nephrotoxic than either cephalothin. Each gram of cephapirin sodium contains 2.36 mEq (54 mg) of sodium.

Used in treatment of serious infections of respiratory and urinary tracts, skin and soft tissue and for osteomyelitis, septicemia, and endocarditis caused by susceptible pathogens, e.g., group A beta-hemolytic streptococci, penicillinase and nonpenicillinase producing *Staphylococcus aureus, Streptococcus pneumoniae, S. viridans, Haemophilus influenzae, Escherichia coli, Proteus mirabilis,* and *Klebsiella* species.

ABSORPTION AND FATE. Peak serum levels in 30 minutes following IM injection and in 5 minutes following IV administration. Half-life: 21 to 47 minutes; 44 to 50% bound to serum proteins. Partially metabolized in plasma, liver, and kidneys to metabolite with about 50% activity of parent compound. About 70 to 94% of dose excreted in urine within 6 hours as partially active desacetyl metabolite and unchanged drug. Crosses placenta; excreted in breast milk.

CONTRAINDICATIONS AND PRECAUTIONS. Hypersensitivity to cephalosporins. Safe use during pregnancy, in nursing mothers, and in children under 3 months of age not established. *Cautious Use:* history of sensitivity to penicillins, and other allergies particularly to drugs; patients on sodium restriction; impaired renal function.

ADVERSE/SIDE EFFECTS. GI: nausea, vomiting, diarrhea, abdominal cramps. **Hematologic** (rare): neutropenia, leukopenia, anemia, positive direct Coombs' test. **Hypersensitivity:** rash, urticaria, drug fever, eosinophilia, serum sickness-like reactions, anaphylaxis. **Other:** needle site reactions (infrequent); elevations in SGOT, SGPT, alkaline phosphatase, bilirubin, BUN. Same potential for adverse reactions as for other cephalosporins. *See Cephalothin Sodium.*

ROUTE AND DOSAGE. Intramuscular, intravenous: Adults: 500 mg to 1 Gm every 4 to 6 hours. Up to 12 Gm/day for life-threatening infections. Patients with moderate to severe impairment of renal function: 7.5 to 15 mg/kg every 12 hours. Dosage modified according to degree of impairment. **Children (over 3 months):** 40 to 80 mg/kg/24 hours in 4 equally divided doses.

NURSING IMPLICATIONS

Culture and susceptibility testing should be performed. Therapy may be initiated before results are obtained.

Before therapy begins, a careful inquiry should be made concerning previous hypersensitivity to cephalosporins, penicillins, and other allergies, particularly to drugs.

IM injections should be made deep into large muscle mass. Rotate injection sites.

Be on the alert for signs and symptoms of superinfections; most likely to be evident in mouth, vagina, anus, colon, wounds, respiratory tract.

Although clinical evidence of renal damage has not been reported, the precautions outlined for cephalothin should be observed.

For IM use, the 500-mg and 1-Gm vials are reconstituted with 1 or 2 ml sterile water for injection or bacteriostatic water for injection, respectively. Resulting solutions will contain 500 mg of cephapirin per 1.2 ml.

For direct IV the 1-Gm or 2-Gm vial is reconstituted with 10 ml or more 0.9% sodium chloride injection, bacteriostatic water for injection, or dextrose injection. Appropriate dose is then administered over a 4- to 5-minute period.

For intermittent IV infusion using Y-tube administration set, the contents of the 4-Gm vial should be diluted with 40 ml of bacteriostatic water for injection, dextrose injection, or sodium chloride injection. When this method is used, it is recommended that other solution be stopped while cephapirin is being administered.

Following reconstitution, depending on diluent and amount used, solutions retain potency for 12 to 48 hours at room temperature or for 10 days if refrigerated at 4°C. See package insert for specific information concerning compatible IV infusion solutions, dilutions, stability and storage times.

Solutions may become slightly yellow, but this does not affect potency.

See Cephalothin Sodium (prototype cephalosporin).

Diagnostic Test Interferences. False-positive **urine glucose** determinations, using copper sulfate reduction methods such as Clinitest, Benedict's reagent, or Fehling's solution, but not with glucose oxidase (enzymatic) tests, e.g., Clinistix, Diastix, Tes-Tape. Positive Coombs' test may complicate **cross-matching procedures** and **hematologic studies.**

Drug Interactions: Cephapirin Sodium

Plus	Interactions
Aminoglycosides, colistimethate, and other drugs with nephrotoxic potential	Possibility of additive nephrotoxic effects. Monitor renal function
Probenecid	Higher and more prolonged serum cephapirin levels (excretion inhibited by probenecid). Used concomitantly with caution

CEPHRADINE

(Anspor, Velosef)

(sef′ra-deen)
Antiinfective
Antibiotic (beta-lactam)
Cephalosporin

ACTIONS AND USES. Semisynthetic acid-stable, first generation, broad-spectrum cephalosporin similar to cephalothin (qv). Powder for parenteral use contains 3.5 mg anhydrous sodium carbonate (to increase solubility) per gram.

Used for serious infections of respiratory and urinary tracts, skin, and soft tissues, and for otitis media caused by susceptible pathogens. Has been used for perioperative prophylaxis in patients undergoing vaginal hysterectomy. Oral preparation is used primarily as follow-up to parenteral cephalosporin therapy and in treatment of urinary tract infections due to susceptible *Klebsiella* organisms resistant to other antibacterials.

ABSORPTION AND FATE. Well-absorbed from all routes. Peak serum levels obtained within 1 hour following oral administration, in 1 to 2 hours after IM, and in 5 minutes after IV administration. Half-life: 1 to 2 hours. Up to 20% bound to plasma proteins. Approximately 60 to 90% or more excreted unchanged in urine within 6 hours. Crosses placenta; excreted in breast milk.

CONTRAINDICATIONS AND PRECAUTIONS. Hypersensitivity to cephalosporins. Safe use during pregnancy, in nursing mothers, and children under 1 year not established. *Cautious Use:* history of penicillin or other allergies, particularly to drugs; renal function impairment, patients on sodium restriction (use of parenteral cephradine).

ADVERSE/SIDE EFFECTS. GI: nausea, vomiting, diarrhea or loose stools, abdominal pain, heartburn, pseudomembranous colitis (rare). **Hematologic:** neutropenia, leukopenia, positive direct Coombs' test, elevations of SGOT, SGPT, alkaline phosphatase, serum bilirubin, lactic dehydrogenase (following parenteral use), elevated BUN. **Hypersensitivity:** urticaria, rash, pruritus, joint pains, eosinophilia. **Other:** dizziness, tightness in chest, pain and induration at IM injection site; thrombophlebitis at IV injection site; paresthesias, superinfections, hepatomegaly (rare).

ROUTE AND DOSAGE. Adults: Oral: 250 to 500 mg every 6 hours or 500 mg to 1 Gm every 12 hours, depending on severity of infection. Not to exceed 4 Gm/day. **Intramuscular, intravenous:** 500 mg to 1 Gm every 6 to 12 hours; not to exceed 8 Gm/day. **Children (9 months or older): Oral:** 25 to 50 mg/kg daily in equally divided doses every 6 to 12 hours, up to 4 Gm daily. **Intramuscular, intravenous: Children (over 1 year):** 50 to 100 mg/kg/day in equally divided doses every 6 hours. Not to exceed 8 Gm daily. Dosages modified for patients with renal function impairment.

NURSING IMPLICATIONS

Before therapy is initiated, a careful inquiry should be made concerning previous hypersensitivity to cephalosporins, penicillins, and other drug allergies.

Culture and susceptibility tests and renal function studies should be performed prior to and periodically during drug therapy.

Recommended dosage schedule in patients with reduced renal function is lower than usual and is based on creatinine clearance determinations and severity of infection. Dosage recommendations vary widely.

Oral cephradine may be given without regard to meals, as it is not destroyed by gastric acid; however, the presence of food may delay absorption.

To minimize pain and induration of IM site, inject deep into large muscle mass such as gluteus maximus or lateral aspect of thigh. Sterile abscess has been reported with SC injection.

Following reconstitution, IM or direct IV solutions should be used within 2 hours at room temperature. With refrigeration (5°C), potency is retained 24 hours. Reconstituted solutions may vary in color from light straw to yellow; this does not affect potency.

Consult package insert for specific directions concerning types and amount of fluids used for reconstitution of cephradine for parenteral administration and for information on stability, storage, and compatible IV infusion fluids.

The risk of thrombophlebitis may be reduced by proper dilution of IV fluid, use of small IV needles and large veins, and by alternating injection sites.

C

Physician should specify dosage interval for patient taking cephradine at home. For example, four times a day may signify every 6 hours around the clock or it may indicate that drug should be taken at evenly spaced intervals during waking hours, e.g., 7 AM, 12 noon, 5 PM, 10 AM.

Instruct patient to take medication for the full course of therapy as directed by physician. Therapy is usually continued for at least 48 to 72 hours after patient becomes asymptomatic.

Drug therapy for beta-hemolytic streptococcal infections should continue for at least 10 days to guard against risk of rheumatic fever.

Be on the alert for symptoms of superinfections (furry, black tongue, sore mouth, anogenital irritation or itching, foul-smelling vaginal discharge, and loose stools, sudden fever, cough).

Report onset of diarrhea. Bear in mind that pseudomembranous colitis, a potentially life-threatening condition may occur during or after cephalosporin therapy. It is a superinfection caused by clostridia.

Following reconstitution, oral suspension may be stored at room temperature up to 7 days or in refrigerator for up to 14 days. Shake well before pouring. A calibrated liquid measuring device should be included when dispensed. Expiration date should be indicated on label.

All forms of cephradine, i.e., capsules, tablets, powder for oral suspension, and powder for injection are stored preferably between 15° and 30°C (59° and 86°F) unless otherwise directed by manufacturer. Protect drug from concentrated light or direct sunlight.

See Cephalothin Sodium (prototype cephalosporin).

Diagnostic Test Interferences. False-positive **urine glucose** determinations using copper sulfate reduction methods such as Clinitest, Benedict's reagent, or Fehling's solution, but not with glucose oxidase (enzymatic) tests such as Clinistix, Diastix, Tes-Tape. Note that cephradine may produce positive Coombs' test and therefore may complicate **cross-matching procedures** and **hematologic studies.**

Drug Interactions: Cephradine

Plus	Interactions
Aminoglycosides, colistimethate and other drugs with nephrotoxic potential	Possibility of additive nephrotoxic effects. Monitor renal function
Probenecid	Higher and more prolonged serum cephradine levels (probenecid inhibits renal excretion of cephradine). Used concomitantly with caution

CHARCOAL, ACTIVATED

(Activated Carbon, Adsorbent Charcoal, Charcocaps, CharcolantiDote, Liquid Antidose, Medicinal Charcoal)

Antidote
Adsorbent
Antiflatulent

ACTIONS AND USES. Residue from destructive distillation of various organic substances, treated to reduce particle size, which increases surface area and adsorptive power (referred to as activation). Activated charcoal is a chemically inert, odorless, tasteless, fine black powder with wide spectrum of adsorptive activity. Acts by binding (adsorbing) toxic substances thereby inhibiting their GI absorption, enterohepatic circulation, and thus bioavailability. Does not adsorb cyanide and is reportedly not very effective in poisonings due to ethanol, methanol, ferrous sulfate, caustic alkalis, and mineral acids.

Used as general purpose emergency antidote in treatment of certain common oral poisonings such as salicylates, acetaminophen, digitoxin, digoxin, phenobarbital, phenylpropanolamine, phenytoin propantheline, propoxyphene, tricyclic antidepressants, and others. Has been used to adsorb intestinal gases in treatment of dyspepsia, flatulence, and distention, but its value in these conditions is not established. Sometimes used topically as deodorant for foul-smelling wounds and ulcers. *Investigational Use:* via gastric dialysis to increase drug clearance, and also in uremia to adsorb various waste products from GI tract.

ABSORPTION AND FATE. Not absorbed from GI tract, and not metabolized. Excreted in feces.

ADVERSE/SIDE EFFECTS. Vomiting (rapid ingestion of high doses), constipation, diarrhea.

ROUTE AND DOSAGE. Oral: *Acute poisoning:* **Adults and children:** 30 to 100 Gm in 6 to 8 ounces of water. In general, dose should be approximately 5 to 10 times estimated weight of ingested poison. **Adults:** *GI disturbances:* 520 to 975 mg after meals, up to 4.16 Gm daily. *Gastric dialysis* (uremic patients): **Adults:** 20 to 50 Gm daily; (acute poisoning): **Adults:** multiple doses, e.g., 25 Gm at 6 hour intervals for 1 day.

NURSING IMPLICATIONS

Before using as an antidote, call a poison control center, or an emergency room, or physician immediately for advice.

Activated charcoal tablets or capsules are less adsorptive and thus less effective than powder or liquid form; therefore they are not recommended in treatment of acute poisoning.

Most effective when administered during early management of acute poisoning (preferably within 30 minutes after ingestion of poison), but even late administration may be of benefit.

Patient must be conscious, and emesis should be induced prior to administering activated charcoal.

Many physicians recommend that vomiting first be induced by ipecac syrup or apomorphine. Apomorphine may be given before or following activated charcoal, but ipecac must be administered before since it is adsorbed by activated charcoal.

In an emergency, dose may be approximated by stirring sufficient activated charcoal into tap water to make a slurry with consistency of thick soup.

Activated charcoal may be swallowed or used as the gastric lavage fluid. It is not a substitute for lavage. If administered too rapidly patient may vomit.

If necessary, palatability may be improved by adding small amount of concentrated fruit juice, cocoa, or chocolate powder. Reportedly, these agents do not appreciably alter adsorptive activity. Milk, ice cream, or sherbet, however, may significantly decrease efficacy of activated charcoal.

So-called universal antidote (e.g., Res-Q) contains 2 parts activated charcoal, 1 part antacid, such as magnesium oxide, and 1 part tannic acid. It is reportedly not as effective as activated charcoal used alone, and can cause hepatatoxicity.

Burnt toast is not a form of activated charcoal and is not a useful antidote in management of acute poisonings.

When used to relieve GI disorders, inform patient that tablet formulation may be chewed or allowed to dissolve in mouth, and followed by a small amount of water.

Prolonged use of activated charcoal may cause nutritional disturbances because the drug adsorbs digestive enzymes and valuable nutrients. It should not be taken for more than 3 days (72 hours).

Inform patient that activated charcoal will color feces black.

When administered via gastric dialysis, physician may prescribe a saline laxative, e.g., magnesium or sodium sulfate or magnesium citrate to reduce possibility of constipation or impaction.

Store in tightly-covered glass or metal container preferably between 15° and 30°C (59° and 86°F), unless otherwise directed by manufacturer.

C

Drug Interactions. When used as an antidote, charcoal should be administered as soon as possible. However, when used for relief of GI distress, other oral drugs should not be scheduled within 2 hours of activated charcoal, if possible (charcoal absorbs drugs, thereby limiting their bioavailability).

CHENODIOL

(kee-noe-dye′ole)

(CDCA, Chenic Acid, Chenix, Chenodeoxycholic Acid)

Antilithic

ACTIONS AND USES. One of the major naturally occuring human bile acids synthesized by liver. Following administration of chenodiol, total chenodiol in bile acid pool increases. Biliary cholesterol saturation decreases, perhaps due to drug-induced suppression of hepatic synthesis of cholesterol and decreased biliary cholesterol secretion. By decreasing cholesterol saturation in bile, chenodiol promotes dissolution of uncalcified cholesterol gallstones. (Pathogenesis of cholesterol gallstone formation: bile acids, e.g., chenodeoxycholic and cholic acids, form micellar aggregates with cholesterol and phospholipids, primarily lecithin. Cholesterol crystals form in excess; unsolubilized cholesterol and stones precipitate.) Chenodiol has no effect on calcified stones or on radiolucent bile pigment stones. Absorption of fluid in colon tends to be inhibited by chenodiol and therefore may cause loose stools or diarrhea. Increases in low-density lipoproteins (LDL) by about 10% may pose a potential risk to patients with atherosclerosis. Chenodiol does not affect serum or urinary bile acid levels with drug discontinuation cholesterol supersaturation of bile returns. Prophylactic use of low doses in preventing stone recurrence is ineffective.

Used to dissolve small or floating radiolucent cholesterol gallstones in carefully selected patients with radiographically well-visualized gallbladders and who are high surgical risks because of systemic disease or age.

ABSORPTION AND FATE. Rapidly absorbed from small intestine. Partially metabolized in intestines by anaerobic bacteria to form lithocholic acid (major metabolite). Distributed mainly into bile. Half-life following IV administration (biphasic): 3.1 minutes; 16.4 minutes. Approximately 96% protein bound; 60 to 80% of dose metabolized in liver on first pass; enters enterohepatic circulation. About 80% excreted in feces via bile, along with metabolite and unmetabolized chenodiol. Probably crosses placenta; distribution into breast milk not confirmed.

CONTRAINDICATIONS AND PRECAUTIONS. Hepatocellular dysfunction, bile duct abnormalities, nonvisualized gallbladder following two consecutive single doses, oral cholecystographic agent, patients with radiopaque stones, gallstone complications, compelling reasons for gallbladder surgery (e.g., unremitting acute cholecystitis, biliary obstruction, biliary GI fistula). Safe use during pregnancy (category X), or in fertile women, nursing mothers, children, and use beyond 6 months not established. *Cautious Use:* atherosclerosis.

ADVERSE/SIDE EFFECTS. GI: mild diarrhea (dose related), severe diarrhea (overdosage), fecal urgency, nausea, vomiting, dyspepsia, epigastric distress, anorexia, heartburn, flatulence, abdominal cramps, constipation (rare). **Hepatic:** elevated serum total cholesterol, transient elevations of SGPT (ALT), especially and/or SGOT (AST), elevated LDL, slight reduction of serum triglycerides, potential for hepatotoxicity. **Other:** leukopenia.

ROUTE AND DOSAGE. Oral: 250 mg two times daily, morning and evening, for first 2 weeks of therapy. Increased by 250-mg increments at weekly intervals to recommended dosage range: 13 to 16 mg/kg/day in two divided doses. Some clinicians prescribe total daily dose at bedtime.

C

NURSING IMPLICATIONS

Chenodiol should be taken with meals or milk. Food generally decreases rate but not extent of absorption.

Not recommended for fertile women unless effective contraception is practiced.

Women who become pregnant while taking chenodiol should be advised to notify physician as soon as possible. They should be informed of potential hazards to fetus.

Cholecystograms and/or ultrasonograms are recommended before initiation of therapy to determine presence of functioning gallbladder and radiolucent stones. Studies are repeated at 6- to 9-month intervals during therapy to monitor response to therapy, i.e., stone dissolution, and also to rule out recurrence. (Gallstones can be expected to recur in up to 50% of patients within 5 years.)

Diarrhea, usually mild and transient, occurs in about 30 to 40% of patients, more frequently at beginning of therapy, but may occur at any time during therapy. Treatment generally consists of temporary dosage reduction (by about ½) until diarrhea is controlled; dosage is then gradually increased to original level. Antidiarrheal agents may also be prescribed.

Patient should be informed that the crampy abdominal pain that sometimes accompanies bouts of diarrhea is to be distinguished from the pain of biliary colic. The latter pain occurs in right upper quadrant or epigastric region, is frequently associated with nausea and vomiting, and should be reported to physician immediately.

To reduce risk of stone recurrence, encourage patient to attain and maintain ideal body weight, to include high-fiber foods in diet, and to reduce cholesterol and carbohydrate intake. Collaborate with physician, dietitian, patient, and significant family members in design of a therapeutic diet plan.

Patient should be well informed about the requirements of the therapeutic regimen, and motivated to accept long-term therapy.

Safe use of chenodiol depends on careful monitoring of liver function:

1. Serum aminotransferases (transaminases), i.e., ALT (SGPT) and AST (SGOT), monthly for first 3 months, then every 3 months during therapy. If levels rise more than 3 times upper limit of normal, drug should be discontinued promptly. (*Normal SGPT:* 5 to 35 U/dl. *SGOT:* 8 to 40 U/dl.)
2. Alkaline phosphatase and bilirubin frequency as for serum aminotransferases. [*Normal alkaline phosphatase:* 1 to 4 U/dl (Bodansky); *bilirubin:* 0.2 to 1.5 mg/dl.]
3. Serum cholesterol and low-density lipoprotein (LDL) every 6 months during therapy. Chenodiol should be discontinued if values exceed patient's acceptable age-adjusted limits.

Dissolution of gallstones by chenodiol (confirmed by cholecystogram and/or ultrasonogram) may require 6 to 24 months. When complete dissolution has occurred, repeat studies should be performed after 1 to 3 months of continued chenodiol administration for verification.

If partial stone dissolution does not occur by 9 to 12 months, it is unlikely that further treatment will be effective. Therapy should be discontinued if no response has occurred by 18 months.

Store preferably between 15° and 30°C (59° and 86°F) in well-closed container, unless otherwise directed by manufacturer.

Drug Interactions: Chenodiol

Plus	Interactions
Cholestyramine (Questran), colestipol (Colestid), and other anion-exchange resins Aluminum-containing antacids	Cause binding of chenodiol, reducing its absorption. Simultaneous administration not advised
Estrogens, estrogen–progestin combinations, clofibrate (Atromid-S)	May counteract chenodiol effectiveness by increasing biliary cholesterol secretion

CHLORAL HYDRATE

(klor′al hye′drate)

(Aquachloral Supprettes, Noctec, Novochlorhydrate, SK-Chloral Hydrate)

Sedative, hypnotic

C IV

ACTIONS AND USES. Produces "physiologic sleep" by mild cerebral depression with little effect on respirations or blood pressure and little or no hangover. Principal action thought to be due in part to trichloroethanol, its reduction product. Does not affect sleep physiology (e.g., REM sleep) in low doses. The oldest chloral derivative and still regarded as a relatively safe, effective, and inexpensive sedative–hypnotic. Has little or no analgesic action. May cause enzyme induction and displace certain drugs from protein binding sites.

Used in short-term management of insomnia, for general sedation (especially in the young and the elderly), for sedation before and after surgery, to reduce anxiety associated with drug withdrawal, and alone or with paraldehyde to prevent or suppress alcohol withdrawal symptoms.

ABSORPTION AND FATE. Readily absorbed following oral or rectal administration. Hypnotic dose produces sleep within 30 minutes to 1 hour, lasting 4 to 8 hours. Rapidly reduced in body to active metabolite, trichloroethanol 70 to 80% of which is protein bound. Well distributed to body fluids and to all tissues. Plasma half-life: about 8 to 11 hours. Variable amount oxidized to inactive trichloroacetic acid metabolite in liver and kidney. Active and inactive metabolites excreted in urine in 24 to 48 hours. Small portion excreted in feces via bile. Crosses placenta; appears in breast milk in negligible amounts.

CONTRAINDICATIONS AND PRECAUTIONS. Known hypersensitivity to drug; severe hepatic, renal, or cardiac disease; rectal dosage form in patients with proctitis; oral use in patients with esophagitis, gastritis, gastric or duodenal ulcers. Safe use during pregnancy and in nursing women not established. *Cautious Use:* history of intermittent porphyria, asthma, history of or proneness to drug dependence, depression, suicidal tendencies.

ADVERSE/SIDE EFFECTS. (Generally well tolerated). **CNS:** light-headedness, dizziness, ataxia, drowsiness, headache, hangover (infrequent), nightmares; rarely: paradoxical excitement, somnambulistic reaction with disorientation and incoherence, paranoid behavior. **GI:** nausea, vomiting, diarrhea, flatulence, unpleasant taste. **Hypersensitivity:** fever, purpura, urticaria, erythematous rash, eczema, erythema multiforme, angioedema, eosinophilia. **Overdosage:** hypotension, hypothermia; respiratory depression, cardiac arrhythmias, miosis, are flexia, esophageal stricture, gastric necrosis. **Other:** breath odor, leukopenia, ketonuria, precipitation of acute intermittent porphyria. *Chronic Use:* fixed drug eruptions, severe gastritis, renal, and hepatic damage, sudden death.

ROUTE AND DOSAGE. Oral, rectal suppository, retention enema: Adults: *sedative:* 250 mg 3 times a day after meals; *hypnotic:* 500 mg to 1 Gm 15 to 30 minutes before bedtime.

Single dose should not exceed 2 Gm. **Children:** *sedative:* 8 to 25 mg/kg/24 hours divided into 3 or 4 doses; *hypnotic:* 50 mg/kg with maximum single dose of 1 Gm. Available as capsules, elixir, syrup, suppositories.

C

NURSING IMPLICATIONS

Chloral hydrate is not intended for relief of pain. When used in the presence of pain it may cause excitement and delirium.

Corrosive to skin and mucous membranes unless well diluted. Has an aromatic, pungent odor and bitter, pungent taste; these may be minimized by use of the capsule form or by dilution of liquid preparations in chilled fluids.

To minimize gastric irritation, administer drug after meals. Capsules should be swallowed whole and taken with a full glass of water, fruit juice, or ginger ale. Syrups or elixirs may be administered in half a glass of the same liquids.

Watch to see that drug is not cheeked and hoarded.

Suppository form: moisten suppository and the inserting finger with water only. When used rectally, observe skin area around anus for irritation.

When used as an hypnotic, prepare patient for sleep by providing maximum comfort measures and reducing environmental stimuli.

Because hypnotic doses may cause dizziness, caution patient not to ambulate without assistance and remove matches, cigarettes, etc., if patient is a smoker. Bed rails may be advisable for the elderly patient.

Prolonged use can lead to tolerance, physical dependence, and addiction. Sudden withdrawal from dependent patients may produce delirium, mania, or convulsions.

Allergic skin reactions may occur within several hours or as long as 10 days after drug administration.

Caution patient to avoid concomitant use of alcoholic beverages. The acute poisoning that occurs from the combination of chloral hydrate and alcohol (Mickey Finn or knockout drops) produces vasodilation, with flushing, headache, tachycardia, and hypotension.

Inform patient that driving and other potentially hazardous activities should be avoided while under the influence of chloral hydrate.

Evaluate patient's response to chloral hydrate and continued need for the drug.

Habituation may be minimized by evaluating and treating the underlying cause or causes of the symptom of insomnia.

Classified as Schedule IV drug under the Federal Controlled Substances Act.

Solutions are preserved in tightly covered, light-resistant containers. All forms preferably stored at between 15° and 30°C (59° and 86°F), unless otherwise directed by manufacturer.

Diagnostic Test Interferences. False-positive results for **urine glucose** with Fehling's and Benedict's solutions, and possibly with Clinitest, but not with glucose oxidase methods (e.g., Clinistix, Diastix, Tes-Tape). Possible interference with fluorometric test for **urine catecholamines** (if chloral hydrate is administered within 48 hours of test), and **urinary 17-OHCS** determinations (by modification of Reddy, Jenkins, Thorn procedure).

Drug Interactions: Chloral hydrate

Plus	Interactions
Alcohol, barbiturates, paraldehyde, tranquilizers, and other CNS depressants	Potentiation of CNS depression. Tachycardia, facial flushing may occur with alcohol. Combination generally avoided or used with great caution

Plus (cont.)	Interactions (cont.)
Anticoagulants, oral	Increased anticoagulant effects. Monitor prothrombin activity
Furosemide (Lasix) by IV route	Possibility of flushing, diaphoresis and blood pressure changes. Combination generally avoided

C

CHLORAMBUCIL

(Leukeran)

(klor-am'byoo-sil)
Antineoplastic
Alkylating agent
Nitrogen mustard

ACTIONS AND USES. Potent aromatic derivative of the alkylating agent, mechlorethamine (nitrogen mustard) and slowest acting and least toxic of the nitrogen mustards. A cell-cycle nonspecific (kills both resting and dividing cells), it causes cytotoxic cross linkage in DNA thus preventing synthesis of DNA, RNA, and proteins. Myelosuppression in therapeutic doses is moderate and rapidly reversible. Lymphocytic effect is marked. Has mutagenic and embryotoxic properties.

Used as single agent or in combination with other antineoplastics in treatment of chronic lymphocytic leukemia, malignant lymphomas including lymphosarcoma, Hodgkin's disease and giant follicular lymphoma, and in treatment of carcinoma of the ovary, breast, and testes. Also has been used in nonneoplastic conditions: vasculitis complicating rheumatoid arthritis, autoimmune hemolytic anemias associated with cold agglutinins, lupus glomerulonephritis, idiopathic nephrotic syndrome, and macroglobulinemia.

ABSORPTION AND FATE. Well-absorbed following oral administration. Plasma half-life: 90 minutes; fat storage may occur because of lipophilic properties. Believed to be highly bound to plasma and tissue proteins. Metabolized in liver. About 60% excreted in urine 24 hours after administration mostly as metabolites. Probably crosses placenta.

CONTRAINDICATIONS AND PRECAUTIONS. Hypersensitivity to chlorambucil or to other alkylating agents; administration within 4 weeks of a full course of radiation or chemotherapy; full dosage if bone marrow is infiltrated with lymphomatous tissue or is hypoplastic; small pox and other vaccines. Safe use during pregnancy and in nursing women not established. *Cautious Use:* excessive or prolonged dosage, pneumococcus vaccination.

ADVERSE/SIDE EFFECTS. Bone marrow depression: leukopenia, thrombocytopenia, anemia; sterility; hyperuricemia. Low incidence of gastric discomfort (high doses), drug fever, skin rashes, alopecia, peripheral neuropathy, sterile cystitis, pulmonary complications, hepatotoxicity, seizures (high doses). Suspect mutagenic, teratogenic, and carcinogenic potential.

ROUTE AND DOSAGE. Oral: Adults: Initial: 0.1 to 0.2 mg/kg/day for 3 to 6 weeks as required (reduced immediately on first indication of drop in WBC count). Maintenance: not to exceed 0.1 mg/kg/day; dosage may be as low as 0.03 mg/kg/day. **Children:** 0.1 to 0.2 mg/kg/day or 4.5 mg/m^2/day as single dose or in divided doses.

NURSING IMPLICATIONS

Nausea and vomiting may be controlled by giving entire daily dose at one time, 1 hour before breakfast or 2 hours after evening meal, or at bedtime. Consult physician.

If patient has difficulty swallowing tablet, ask pharmacist about the possibility of preparing an oral suspension.

C

CBC, hemoglobin, total and differential leukocyte counts, and serum uric acid should be checked initially and at least once weekly during treatment.

Body weight, size of spleen, and temperature charted before initiation of therapy and at the time of blood counts provide a useful profile for determining degree of bone marrow suppression.

Leukopenia usually develops after the third week of treatment; it may continue for up to 10 days after last dose then rapidly return to normal.

About one-fourth of the patients receiving a total dose of approximately 450 mg and one-half those receiving this dosage 8 weeks or less may develop severe neutropenia.

With confirmation of bone marrow depression (low platelet and neutrophil counts or peripheral lymphocytosis), it is recommended that dosage not exceed 0.1 mg/kg.

If possible, avoid or reduce to minimum injections and other invasive procedures (e.g., rectal temperatures, enemas) when platelet count is low because of danger of bleeding.

Clinical improvement is usually apparent by third week. Produces remission in a substantial number of patients.

During treatment with chlorambucil it is dangerous for the patient to go longer than 2 weeks without a clinical examination and blood studies. Reinforce importance of keeping appointments with the physician.

Advise patient to notify physician if the following symptoms occur: unusual bleeding or bruising, sores on lips or in mouth; flank, stomach or joint pain; fever, chills, or other signs of infection, sore throat, cough, dyspnea.

Skin reactions are rare, but all appear to show a consistent pattern: pustular eruption on mouth, chin, cheeks; urticarial erythema on trunk that spreads to legs. The rash occurs early in treatment period and lasts about 10 days after last dose. Responses become more and more severe with repeated challenges. Urge the patient to report immediately the onset of cutaneous reaction.

Urine alkalinization and allopurinol may be prescribed to prevent elevated serum uric acid levels (can lead to nephrotoxicity). If physician agrees, urge patient to drink at least 10 to 12 glasses (8 oz each) of fluid/day and to report to physician if urine output decreases below normal amounts.

Because of drug-impaired immune response, pneumococcus vaccine effectiveness is reduced and small pox vaccination can lead to progressive vaccinia; therefore neither is generally given during chlorambucil therapy.

Advise patient to report to physician immediately if she becomes pregnant. She should be informed of the potential hazard to the fetus.

Discuss possibility of gonadal suppression with patient (amenorrhea or azoospermia may be irreversible), which occurs especially with high doses.

During maintenance therapy, physician may occasionally interrupt drug schedule in order to determine if patient is in remission.

Store preferably at 15° to 30°C (59 to 86°F) in well-closed, light-resistant container.

See Mechlorethamine (prototype nitrogen mustard) for nursing implications of neoplastic therapy.

Drug Interactions: Chlorambucil

Plus	Interactions
Antigout agent	Dosage of antigout agent may have to be adjusted because chlorambucil causes hyperuricemia

C

CHLORAMPHENICOL

(Antibiopto, Chloromycetin, Chloroptic, Chloroptic S.O.P., Econochlor, Fenicol, Isopto Fenicol, Mychel, Novochlorocap, Ophthochlor, Pentamycetin, Sopamycetin)

CHLORAMPHENICOL PALMITATE

(Chloromycetin Palmitate)

CHLORAMPHENICOL SODIUM SUCCINATE

(Chloromycetin Sodium Succinate, Mychel-S)

(klor-am-fen′i-kole)
Antiinfective
Antibiotic
Antirickettsial

ACTIONS AND USES. Synthetic broad-spectrum antibiotic formerly derived from *Streptomyces venezuelae.* Principally bacteriostatic but may be bactericidal in certain species (e.g., *H. influenzae*) or when given in higher concentrations. Effective against a wide variety of gram-negative and gram-positive bacteria and most anaerobic microorganisms. Believed to act by interfering with synthesis of bacterial ribosomes.

Used only in severe infections when other antibiotics are ineffective or are contraindicated. Particularly effective against *Salmonella typhi* and other Salmonella species, *S. pneumoniae, Neisseria,* meningeal infections caused by *H. influenzae,* Rocky Mountain spotted fever and other *rickettsiae,* the lymphogranuloma-psittacosis group *(Chlamydia),* and *Mycoplasma.* Also used in cystic fibrosis antiinfective regimens and used topically for infections of skin, eyes, and external auditory canal. Commercially available for ophthalmic use in combination with polymycin B (Chloromyxin) and with prednisolone (Chloroptic-P S.O.P.).

ABSORPTION AND FATE. Readily and almost completely absorbed from GI tract. Peak plasma levels following oral and IV administration occur in 1 to 2 hours; therapeutic plasma levels still present after 8 hours. Half-life: 1.5 to 3.5 hours (longer in patients with impaired hepatic function). Approximately 50% bound to plasma proteins. Widely distributed in body, with highest concentrations in liver and kidney; therapeutic concentrations also in CSF and brain tissue. Measurable levels in pleural and ascitic fluid, bile, saliva, and aqueous and vitreous humor. Conjugates with glucuronic acid in liver, then is rapidly excreted in urine along with 5 to 15% free drug; 75 to 90% of dose is excreted within 24 hours. Small amounts excreted unchanged in bile and feces. Readily crosses placenta; appears in breast milk.

CONTRAINDICATIONS AND PRECAUTIONS. History of hypersensitivity or toxic reaction to chloramphenicol or to any component in the formulation; treatment of minor infections, prophylactic use; concomitant therapy with drugs that produce bone marrow depression. Safe use during pregnancy and in nursing mothers not established. *Cautious Use:* impaired hepatic or renal function, premenopausal women, premature and full-term infants, children; intermittent porphyria, patients with G6PD deficiency, patient or family history of drug-induced bone marrow depression.

ADVERSE/SIDE EFFECTS. CNS: (Neurotoxicity): headache, mental depression, confusion, delirium, digital paresthesias, peripheral neuritis. **GI:** nausea, vomiting, diarrhea, perianal irritation, enterocolitis, glossitis, stomatitis, unpleasant taste, xerostomia. **Gray syndrome:** abdominal distention, vomiting, pallid cyanosis, blotchy skin, vasomotor collapse, irregular respiration, hypothermia, death. **Hematologic:** Bone marrow depression (dose-related and reversible): reticulocytosis, leukopenia, vacuolation of erythroid cells, thrombocytopenia, increased plasma iron, reduced Hgb, anemia; non-dose-related and irreversible: pancytopenia, agranulocytosis, aplastic anemia (drug idiosyncrasy), hemolytic anemia (rare), paroxysmal nocturnal hemoglobinuria, leukemia. **Hypersensitivity:** topical itching, burning, stinging; angioedema, urticaria, contact dermatitis, maculopapular and vesicular rashes, fever, anaphylaxis; Herxheimer-like reaction (following therapy for typhoid fever, brucellosis, or syphilis). **Ophthalmic:** visual disturbances, optic neuritis, optic nerve atrophy, contact conjunctivitis. **Other:** jaundice, hypoprothrombinemia, fixed-drug eruptions, superinfections.

C

ROUTE AND DOSAGE. Oral, intravenous: Intravenous administration: may be injected directly as 10% (100 mg/ml) solution over period of at least 1 minute or by IV infusion. **Adults and children:** 50 mg/kg body weight daily in 4 equally divided doses, every 6 hours; up to 100 mg/kg/day for exceptionally severe infection. **Infants (up to 2 weeks) and children with immature metabolic function:** 25 mg/kg/day in 4 equally divided doses at 6 hour intervals. **Adults and children: Topical cream (1%):** gently rub into affected area 3 or 4 times daily after cleansing. **Ophthalmic ointment (1%):** apply small strip of ointment to lower conjunctival sac every 3 to 4 hours. **Ophthalmic solution (0.16, 0.25, 0.5%):** instill 1 or 2 drops every 1 to 6 hours. **Otic solution (0.5%):** Instill 2 or 3 drops into affected ear 3 times daily, at 6- to 8-hour intervals.

NURSING IMPLICATIONS

Oral drug is taken preferably with a full glass of water on an empty stomach, at least 1 hour before or 2 hours after a meal, to achieve optimum blood levels.

Generally patient is hospitalized during systemic chloramphenicol therapy to facilitate laboratory tests and close observation.

Bacterial culture and susceptibility tests are essential and may be performed concurrently with initiation of therapy and periodically thereafter.

Baseline CBC, platelets, serum iron, and reticulocyte cell counts are recommended prior to initiation of therapy, at 48-hour intervals during therapy, and periodically during follow-up period.

Inform patient that bitter taste may occur 15 to 20 seconds following IV injection and that it usually lasts only 2 to 3 minutes. Oral form is substituted as soon as feasible.

Chloramphenicol blood levels should be closely monitored (desired concentration between 5 and 20 mcg/ml).

Close observation of the patient is also crucial, because blood studies are not always reliable predictors of irreversible bone marrow depression.

Non-dose related irreversible bone marrow depression may appear weeks or months after drug therapy is terminated. The potential for this side effect is greatest in patients with impaired hepatic or renal function, infants, children, and premenopausal women.

Counsel patient to report immediately sore throat, fever, fatigue, petechiae, nose bleeds, bleeding gums, or other unusual bleeding or bruising, or any other suspicious sign or symptom. Drug therapy should be discontinued if abnormal bleeding occurs.

Check temperature at least every 4 hours. Usually chloramphenicol is discontinued if temperature remains normal for 48 hours. Some clinicians recommend that treatment for typhoid be continued 8 to 10 days after patient becomes afebrile to lessen the possibility of relapse.

Up to 10% of patients treated with chloramphenicol for typhoid reportedly become temporary or permanent carriers and therefore require further therapy with either ampicillin or amoxicillin. Chloramphenicol is not recommended for treatment of carriers.

Report any appreciable change in intake and output ratio or pattern.

Watch for signs and symptoms of superinfection by nonsusceptible organisms; stomatitis, glossitis with or without black tongue, anogenital irritation or itching, vaginal discharge, elevated temperature, diarrhea (enterocolitis), cough.

More frequent determinations of serum glucose are recommended in patients receiving oral antidiabetic agents *(see Drug Interactions).*

Gray syndrome has occurred 2 to 9 days after initiation of high dose chloramphenicol therapy in prematures and newborns, and in children up to 2 years of age. Report early signs: abdominal distention, failure to feed, pallor, changes in vital signs.

Chloramphenicol solution for injection may form crystals or a second layer when stored at low temperatures. Solution will clarify by shaking ampul. Do not use cloudy solutions.
Follow manufacturer's directions for dilution and storage of IV preparation.
Topical Use: Systemic absorption and toxicity can occur with prolonged or frequent intermittent use of topical preparations.
Topical preparations are *not* interchangeable. Use only as designated.
Advise patient to follow dosage and duration of therapy as prescribed by physician.
Instruct patient to stop medication immediately if signs of hypersensitivity, superinfection, or other adverse reactions appear.
Instillation of eye drops: apply light pressure to lacrimal duct for 1 minute to prevent drainage into nasopharynx and systemic absorption. *See Index: Drug administration: eye drops for more complete description.*
Applications to skin are generally preceded by a soap and water cleansing and thorough drying of part before reapplication of medication. Consult physician.
Avoid warming chloramphenicol solutions (e.g., otic solution) above body temperature, to prevent loss of potency.
Ophthalmic solution should be protected from light.
Store topical and oral forms, and unopened ampuls preferably between 15° and 30°C (59° and 86°F), unless otherwise directed by manufacturer. Note expiration date on label of oral suspension (generally stable for 30 days after reconstitution by pharmacist). Shake well before pouring.

Diagnostic Test Interferences. Possibility of false-positive results for **urine glucose** by copper reduction methods (e.g., Benedict's solution, Clinitest). Chloramphenicol may interfere with **17-OHCS** (urinary steroid) determinations (modification of Reddy, Jenkins, Thorn, procedure, not affected), with **urobilinogen excretion,** and with responses to **tetanus toxoid** and possibly other active immunizing agents.

Drug Interactions: Chloramphenicol

Plus	Interactions
Anticoagulants, oral; Chlorpropamide, tolbutamide, and possibly other sulfonylureas (oral antidiabetic agents); Cyclophosphamide (Cytoxan, Neosar); Phenytoin (Dilantin) and other hydantoins	By inhibiting hepatic microsomal enzyme activity, chloramphenicol may prolong half-life and potentiate action of drugs metabolized by this system. Used concurrently with caution
Phenobarbital and other barbiturates	Phenobarbital may reduce chloramphenicol plasma levels and phenobarbital effects may increase. Dosage adjustments may be indicated
Penicillins	Chloramphenicol may antagonize action of bactericidal antibiotics (theoretical possibility). Combination used with caution
Cyanocobalamin (vitamin B_{12}); Folic acid (Folvite); Iron preparations	By interfering with erythrocyte maturation, chloramphenicol may reduce response of these substances

PROTOTYPE

CHLORDIAZEPOXIDE HYDROCHLORIDE

(A-poxide, Libritabs, Librium, Lipoxide, Medilium, Murcil, Novopoxide, Reponans-10, Sereen, SK-Lygen, Solium)

(klor-dye-az-e-pox′ide)
Psychotropic anxiolytic
Benzodiazepine
C IV

C

ACTIONS AND USES. Benzodiazepine derivative, prototype of the anxiolytic agents. Exerts depressant effects on subcortical levels of CNS, and in high doses, on the cortex. Calming effect thought to be due to action on the limbic system. Produces mild sedative, anticonvulsant, and skeletal muscle relaxant effects. Has long-acting hypnotic properties. Causes mild suppression of REM sleep and of deeper phases, particularly stage 4, while increasing total sleep time. Usually does not result in withdrawal insomnia even with prolonged use.

Used for relief of various anxiety and tension states, preoperative apprehension and anxiety, and for management of withdrawal symptoms of acute alcoholism. Also used as an antidyskinetic. Available in fixed combination with amitriptyline (Limbitrol), with clidinium bromide (Librax), and with esterified estrogens (Menrium).

ABSORPTION AND FATE. Well-absorbed from GI tract. Peak plasma levels reached in 1 to 4 hours after oral administration, 15 to 30 minutes after IM, and 3 to 30 minutes after IV. Half-life: 5 to 30 hours. Metabolized in liver. Active and inactive metabolites slowly excreted, primarily in urine and small amount in feces. Urinary excretion continues for several days after last dose. Crosses placenta; excreted in breast milk.

CONTRAINDICATIONS AND PRECAUTIONS. Hypersensitivity to chlordiazepoxide and other benzodiazepines; narrow angle glaucoma, prostatic hypertrophy, shock, comatose states, primary depressive disorder or psychoses, pregnancy, lactation, oral use in children under 6 years of age, parenteral use in children under 12 years. *Cautious Use:* anxiety states associated with impending depression, history of impaired hepatic or renal function; addiction-prone individuals, allergic dermatoses, blood dyscrasias; in the elderly, debilitated patients, children; hyperkinesis, chronic obstructive pulmonary disease.

ADVERSE/SIDE EFFECTS. CNS: drowsiness, dizziness, lethargy (common), changes in EEG pattern (low-voltage fast activity); blurred vision, nystagmus, diplopia, vivid dreams, nightmares, headache, extrapyramidal symptoms, vertigo, syncope, tinnitus, confusion, hallucinations, parodoxic rage, depression, delirium, ataxia. **CV:** orthostatic hypotention, tachycardia, changes in ECG patterns. **GI:** xerostomia, nausea, constipation, increased appetite. **GU:** urinary frequency, menstrual irregularities, anovulation, increased or decreased libido. **Other:** edema, weight gain, pain in injection site, photosensitivity, skin rash, blood dyscrasias (including agranulocytosis), jaundice, acute intermittent porphyria, hiccoughs, elevation of LDH. **Overdosage:** somnolence, confusion, diminished reflexes, paradoxical excitation, depressed respirations, coma.

ROUTE AND DOSAGE. Highly individualized. Lower dosages for the elderly and debilitated. **Oral: Adults:** *Mild anxiety and tension; preoperative anxiety:* 5 to 10 mg, 3 or 4 times daily. *Severe anxiety and tension:* 20 to 25 mg, 3 or 4 times daily. *Withdrawal syndrome of acute alcoholism:* 50 to 100 mg followed by repeated doses as needed up to 300 mg/day; then reduced to maintenance levels. **Children (over 6 years):** *Mild anxiety and tension:* Initial: 5 mg, 2 to 4 times daily; may be increased to 10 mg, 2 or 3 times daily. **Parenteral: Adults:** *Preoperative anxiety:* IM: 50 to 100 mg one hour before surgery. *Acute* or *severe anxiety and tension:* IM or IV: Initial: 50 to 100 mg; then 25 to 50 mg, 3 to 4 times daily. *Withdrawal syndrome of acute alcoholism:* IM or IV: Initial: 50 to 100 mg; repeated in 2 to 3 hours if necessary. Available in capsule, tablets, powder for injection.

NURSING IMPLICATIONS

Patients who complain of gastric distress may obtain relief by taking the drug with or immediately after meals or with milk. If an antacid is prescribed, it should be taken at least 1 hour before or after chlordiazepoxide to prevent delay in drug absorption.

Tablet may be crushed before swallowing if patient cannot take it whole, or capsule may be emptied and contents swallowed with fluid or mixed with foods.

Supervise drug ingestion to prevent "cheeking" pills, a maneuver that leads to hoarding or omission of drug.

If patient is known to be addiction-prone, observe for signs of developing physical and/or psychologic dependency such as requests for change in drug regimen (dose and dose interval), diminishing favorable response (e.g., disturbed sleep pattern, increase in psychomotor activity), manipulative behavior, withdrawal symptoms. Investigate the symptoms of ataxia, vertigo, slurred speech; the patient may be taking more than the prescribed dose.

Advise patient to take drug specifically as prescribed: not to skip, increase, or decrease doses, change intervals, or terminate therapy without physician's advice. Emphasize that patient should not lend or offer any of drug to another person.

Benzodiazepines are not intended for management of episodic minor anxieties and tensions associated with every day living.

OTC drugs should not be taken unless prescribed. Check patient's self-medication habits. Sometimes a patient does not consider that a self-prescribed drug for minor pains and aches or for gastric distress or a cold is a "medication."

Prepare parenteral solution immediately before use; discard unused portion. Drug is unstable in light and when in solution.

Use special diluent provided by manufacturer to make the IM solution. Add diluent carefully to avoid bubble formation; gently agitate until solution is clear. Resulting solution: 50 mg/ml. Discard diluent if it is not clear.

For IV injection, sterile water for injection or sodium chloride 0.9% is added to the dry-filled ampul, agitated gently until dissolved. Do not use IM diluent for the IV solution because it may contain air bubbles.

Do not mix any other drug with chlordiazepoxide solution.

In early part of therapy, check blood pressure and pulse before giving benzodiazepine. If blood pressure falls 20 mm Hg or more or if pulse rate is above 120 beats/minute, delay medication and consult physician.

Orthostatic hypotension and tachycardia occur more frequently with parenteral administration. Patient should stay recumbent 2 to 3 hours after IM or IV injection; observe closely and monitor vital signs.

Instruct patient to change position from recumbency to standing slowly and in stages. Support hose may be helpful. Discuss with physician.

Until drug dosage is stabilized monitor intake and output. Report changes in intake and output ratio and dysuria to physician. Cumulative (overdosage) effects can result with renal dysfunction. The elderly are especially vulnerable (normal aging changes compromise kidney efficiency).

Observe intake of patient who is seriously agitated or depressed; willful reduction of fluids can be hazardous.

Paradoxic reactions (excitement, stimulation, disturbed sleep patterns, acute rage) may occur during first few weeks of therapy in psychiatric patients and in hyperactive and aggressive children receiving chlordiazepoxide. Withhold drug and report to physician.

Suicidal tendencies may be manifested in anxiety states accompanied by depression. Observe necessary protective precautions.

Long-term use of this drug may cause xerostomia. Good oral hygiene can alleviate the discomfort: frequent rinses with warm water, daily flossing with waxed floss, brushing

C

with small soft toothbrush and fluoride toothpaste, use of salivary substitute (e.g., Moi-stir), sugarfree gum, or lemon drops. For more complete description, *see Index: Nursing interventions: dry mouth.*

Observe patient's sleep pattern and quality. If dreams or nightmares (which usually occur during REM sleep) interfere with rest, notify physician. A change in the dosing schedule, dose, or an alternate drug may be prescribed.

If drug has been prescribed for anxiety-induced insomnia and is used every day, its effect begins in 2 or 3 nights; however, usefulness for this problem lasts only a few weeks.

Periodic blood cell counts and liver function tests are recommended during prolonged therapy.

Sore throat or mouth, upper respiratory infection, fever, and malaise should alert one to the possibility of agranulocytosis. Total and differential WBC counts should be ordered immediately, and protective isolation instituted.

Most signs and symptoms associated with chlordiazepoxide therapy are dose-related. Physicians will rely on accurate observations and reporting of patient's response to drug to determine lowest effective maintenance dose.

Adverse reactions, such as drowsiness, dizziness, lethargy, syncope, ataxia, confusion, constipation, and urinary retention, are dose-related but even at lower ranges may occur in elderly and debilitated patients. Supervision of ambulation is indicated, and possibly side rails.

Warn ambulatory patient that sedation may occur during early therapy. Activities requiring mental alertness and precision should be avoided until reaction to the drug has been evaluated.

Caution patient against drinking alcoholic beverages. When combined with chlordiazepoxide, effects of both are potentiated.

Smoking–Drug Interaction: Some studies suggest that smoking increases clearance rate of chlordiazepoxide. The heavy smoker may require higher dosage of the drug for therapeutic effectiveness than the nonsmoker.

If patient becomes pregnant during therapy or intends to become pregnant advise her to communicate with physician about continuing therapy.

Advise patient to avoid excessive sunlight. Photosensitivity has been reported. A sun screen lotion (SPF 12 or above) should be used (if allowed).

Effectiveness of chlordiazepoxide in long-term use for more than 6 months is not established. Periodic evaluations should be made of patient's response before continuing therapy.

Because drug is excreted slowly and is converted to active metabolites, habituation can occur. Incidence of physical dependency, however, is low.

Abrupt discontinuation of drug in patients receiving high doses for long periods has precipitated withdrawal symptoms, but not for at least 5 to 7 days because of slow elimination. Symptoms may include restlessness, unreal or distant feeling parethesias, abdominal and muscle cramps, tremors, insomnia, vomiting, anorexia, profuse sweating, psychomotor activity including convulsions and delirium. In most cases, after usual doses there is no withdrawal syndrome.

Chlordiazepoxide is classified as a Schedule IV drug under Federal Controlled Substances Act.

Management of overdosage: induce vomiting, monitor vital functions, provide general support measures (avoid use of barbiturates).

Store in tight, light-resistant containers at temperature between 15° and 30°C (50° and 86°F), unless otherwise specified by manufacturer. The special diluent supplied by manufacturer for IM preparation should be kept refrigerated, preferably between 2° and 8°C (36° and 46°F), until ready for use.

Diagnostic Test Interferences. Chlordiazepoxide increases **serum bilirubin, SGOT** and **SGPT;** decreases **radioactive iodine uptake;** and may falsely increase readings for urinary **17-OHCS** (modified Glenn-Nelson technique).

Drug Interactions: Chlordiazepoxide

Plus	Interactions
Alcohol (ethanol), and other CNS depressants	Potentiation of CNS depressant effects. (Reaction with alcohol may occur up to 10 hours after last dose of benzodiazepine)
Cimetidine (Tagamet)	Increased chlordiazepoxide plasma levels. (Cimetidine inhibits chlordiazepoxide metabolism.) Lower chlordiazepoxide doses may be indicated
Disulfiram (Antabuse)	Pharmacologic effects of chlordiazepoxide may be increased. Lower chlordiazepoxide doses may be necessary
Levodopa	Monitor for possibility of reduced antiparkinson effect (based on limited evidence)
MAO inhibitors	Enhanced benzodiazepine effects. Concurrent use generally avoided
Oral contraceptives	Pharmacologic effects of benzodiazepines may be increased or decreased. Dosage adjustments may be indicated
Phenytoin (Dilantin)	Serum levels of phenytoin may be increased with potentiation of pharmacologic effects. Monitor serum phenytoin levels

---

CHLORMEZANONE

(Trancopal)

(klor-mez'a-none)
Psychotropic
Anxiolytic

ACTIONS AND USES. A nonhypnotic anxiolytic with CNS depressant effects similar to those of meprobamate (qv). Believed to act on subcortical levels of CNS to produce mild sedation and skeletal muscle relaxant effects.

Used in symptomatic treatment of mild anxiety and tension states. Has been used as adjunct to rest, analgesics, and physical therapy for relief of painful musculoskeletal conditions.

ABSORPTION AND FATE. Rapidly absorbed from GI tract. Action begins in 15 to 30 minutes and may last up to 6 hours or longer. Plasma half-life: 24 hours. Widely distributed in most tissues, especially kidneys, heart, liver. Metabolized in liver. Excreted in urine as unchanged drug and metabolites. Passage across placenta or into breast milk unknown.

CONTRAINDICATIONS AND PRECAUTIONS. Hypersensitivity to chlormezanone; children less than 5 years of age. Safe use during pregnancy and in nursing women not established. *Cautious Use:* renal or hepatic disease, history of drug abuse.

ADVERSE/SIDE EFFECTS. CNS: drowsiness, dizziness, slurred speech, headache, weakness, ataxia, lethargy, mental depression, tremor, excitement, confusion, increased anxiety. **GI:** dry mouth, impaired sense of taste (ageusia), nausea, anorexia. **Hypersensitivity:** skin rash, fever, chills. **Other:** flushing, inability to void, cholestatic jaundice (rare), edema, tightness in throat.

ROUTE AND DOSAGE. Oral: Adults: 100 to 200 mg 3 or 4 times/day. **Children (5 to 12 years):** 50 to 100 mg 3 or 4 times/day. Reduced dosages in elderly and debilitated patients.

NURSING IMPLICATIONS

Effectiveness of drug should be periodically reassessed, particularly after 4 months of therapy.

Drowsiness is dose related. If it interferes with normal activity, dosage reduction is indicated. Report to physician.

Caution patient to avoid hazardous activities requiring mental alertness and physical coordination, such as driving, until reaction to the drug is known.

Long-term use of this drug may cause xerostomia. Good oral hygiene can alleviate the discomfort: frequent rinses with warm water, daily flossing with unwaxed floss, brushing with small, soft toothbrush and fluoride toothpaste, use of salivary substitute, e.g., Moistir, Orex, Xero-Lube (all available OTC), sugarless chewing gum or lemon drops.

Be alert to signs of overdosage and report to physician: slurred speech, lethargy, inattention to personal hygiene, lack of desire to undertake physical activity, heavy daytime sedation.

If patient has a history of drug abuse, supervise administration of chlormezanone to prevent patient from "cheeking" the drug, a maneuver to hoard or avoid medication.

When the drug is to be discontinued after long-term use, doses should be tapered gradually over a period of several days to avoid possibility of withdrawal symptoms.

Advise patient to consult physician before self-medicating with OTC drugs.

Patient should be advised that if she becomes pregnant during therapy or intends to become pregnant she should consult her physician about the desirability of discontinuing the drug.

Emphasize need to adhere to established drug regimen. Caution patient not to change dose or dose intervals, not to give any of the drug to another person, and not to use drug for a self-diagnosed problem.

If signs of hypersensitivity occur, withhold drug and inform physician.

Periodically check for evidence of jaundice, a reversible symptom with discontinuation of therapy.

Monitor intake and output ratio and pattern particularly in severely debilitated and elderly patients. Inability to void is a potential side effect of this drug.

Store in tightly closed container at temperature between 15° and 30°C (59° and 86°F), unless otherwise specified by the manufacturer.

Drug Interactions: Chlormezanone

Plus	Interactions
Alcohol (ethanol), and other CNS depressants	Additive CNS depression. Concomitant use generally avoided

PROTOTYPE

CHLOROQUINE HYDROCHLORIDE
(Aralen Hydrochloride)
CHLOROQUINE PHOSPHATE
(Aralen Phosphate)

(klor'oh-kwin)
Antiinfective
Antimalarial
4-Aminoquinoline

C

ACTIONS AND USES. Synthetic 4-aminoquinoline derivative. Antimalarial activity is believed to be based on ability to form complexes with DNA of parasite, thereby inhibiting replication and transcription to RNA and nucleic acid synthesis. Highly active against erythrocytic forms of plasmodia, providing suppressive prophylaxis and clinical cure. Not effective against exoerythrocytic tissue stages and therefore does not provide causal prophylaxis. Also has amebicidal activity, antiinflammatory action, quinidinelike effect on heart, antihistamine and antiserotonin properties, and inhibits prostaglandin effects on cells. Certain adverse effects are related to affinity of chloroquine for melanin-bearing cells particularly in ear and eyes.

Used for suppression and treatment of malaria caused by *P. malariae, P. ovale, P. vivax,* and susceptible forms of *P. falciparum* and in treatment of extraintestinal amebiasis. Concomitant therapy with primaquine (an 8-aminoquinoline) is necessary for radical cure of vivax and malariae malarias. Has been used in treatment of giardiasis, discoid and systemic lupus erythematosus, porphyria cutanea tarda, solar urticaria, polymorphous light eruptions, and in rheumatoid arthritis not controlled by other less toxic drugs. Commercially available in fixed-dose combination with primaquine (Aralen Phosphate with Primaquine Phosphate).

ABSORPTION AND FATE. Rapidly absorbed following oral administration. Maximum plasma concentration in 1 to 2 hours. Approximately 55% bound to plasma proteins. Plasma half-life about 3 to 5 days. High concentrations in liver, kidney, lung, brain, spinal cord, eyes, and erythrocytes. Partially metabolized in liver. Excreted slowly in urine as metabolites (25% of dose) and free drug (70% of dose); about 8% excreted unchanged in feces. Urinary excretion increased by acidification and decreased by alkalinization of urine. Small amounts of drug detectable in urine for months and sometimes for years following discontinuation of therapy. Crosses placenta. Excreted in breast milk.

CONTRAINDICATIONS AND PRECAUTIONS. Hypersensitivity to 4-aminoquinolines, psoriatic arthritis, porphyria, renal disease, 4-aminoquinoline-induced retinal or visual field changes; long-term therapy in children. Safe use during pregnancy, in nursing women, and women of childbearing potential not established. *Cautious Use:* impaired hepatic function, alcoholism, psoriasis, eczema, patients with G6PD deficiency, infants and children, hematologic, GI, and neurologic disorders.

ADVERSE/SIDE EFFECTS. CNS: mild transient headache, fatigue, irritability, confusion, psychic stimulation, psychoses, nightmares, skeletal muscle weakness, paresthesias, reduced reflexes. **CV:** quinidinelike effect (heart block, asystole with syncope, hypotension). **Dermatologic:** pruritus, lichen planuslike eruptions, eczema, exfoliative dermatitis, exacerbation of psoriasis, gray pigmentation of skin, nails, mucous membranes; bleaching of hair, patchy alopecia (reversible). **ENT:** tinnitus, vertigo, reduced hearing, auditory nerve damage. **GI:** diarrhea, abdominal cramps, nausea, vomiting, anorexia. **Hematologic:** anemia, leukopenia, thrombocytopenia, agranulocytosis, hemolytic anemia (patients with G6PD deficiency). **Ophthalmic:** visual disturbances, retinal artery constriction, extraocular muscle palsies, photophobia, night blindness, scotomata, visual field defects, optic atrophy, photophobia, corneal edema, opacity, or deposits; retinal changes. **Other:** slight weight loss, myalgia, lymphedema of hands and arms, acute intermittent porphyria. **Overdosage:** shock, cardiac arrhythmias, convulsions, respiratory and cardiac arrest, sudden death (infants and children).

ROUTE AND DOSAGE. Dosage is often expressed or calculated in terms of chloroquine base. Each 500 mg tablet (phosphate) = 300 mg (base). Each ml (50 mg) of the parenteral drug (hydrochloride) = 40 mg (base). *Acute malaria:* **Adults: Oral:** 600 mg (base) followed by 300 mg (base) at 6, 24, and 48 hours. **Intramuscular (chloroquine hydrochloride):** 160 to 200 mg (base) repeated in 6 hours if necessary. Not to exceed 800 mg base/24 hours. Oral therapy substituted as soon as possible. **Pediatric: Oral:** Initial: 10 mg (base)/kg, then 5 mg (base)/kg at 6, 24, and 48 hours. **Intramuscular:** 5 mg (base)/kg repeated in 6 hours. *Malarial suppression:* **Oral only: Adults and children:** 5 mg (base)/kg on exactly the same day each week, beginning 2 weeks before exposure. Not to exceed 300 mg (base)/week. *Extraintestinal amebiasis:* **Adults: Oral:** 600 mg (base) daily for 2 days followed by 300 mg (base) daily for at least 2 to 3 weeks. (Treatment usually combined with an intestinal amebicide.) **Intramuscular:** 160 to 200 mg (base) daily for 10 to 12 days. **Pediatric: Oral:** 10 mg/kg once daily for 2 to 3 weeks. Maximum 300 mg (base) daily. *Rheumatoid arthritis:* 200 mg (base) once daily with evening meal.

NURSING IMPLICATIONS

GI side effects may be minimized by administering oral drug immediately before or after meals.

Aspirate carefully before injecting drug IM to avoid inadvertent intravascular injection. IV injection may produce quinidinelike effects on heart (hypotension, depressed myocardial excitability, asystole with syncope). Rotate injection sites.

Children are susceptible to the effects of chloroquine (especially the parenteral drug) and other 4-aminoquinoline compounds. Oral administration should substitute parenteral drug as soon as possible. Long-term therapy is not recommended in children.

Complete blood cell counts and ECG are advised prior to initiation of therapy and periodically thereafter in patients on long-term therapy.

A test for G6PD deficiency is recommended for American blacks and individuals of Mediterranean ancestry, prior to therapy.

Baseline and regularly scheduled audiometric and ophthalmoscopic examinations, including slit lamp, fundus, and visual fields, should be performed.

Retinopathy (generally irreversible) can be progressive even after termination of therapy. Patient may be asymptomatic or complain of night blindness, scotomata, visual field changes, blurred vision, or difficulty in focusing. Chloroquine should be discontinued immediately.

Advise patient to report promptly visual or hearing disturbances, muscle weakness, or loss of balance, symptoms of blood dyscrasia (fever, sore mouth or throat, unexplained fatigue, easy bruising or bleeding).

Use of dark glasses in sunlight or bright light may reduce risk of ocular damage.

Patients on long-term therapy should be questioned regularly about skeletal muscle weakness, and periodic tests should be made of muscle strength and deep tendon reflexes. Positive signs are indications to terminate therapy.

If possible, suppressive therapy should begin 2 weeks before exposure and should be continued for 8 weeks after leaving endemic area.

Therapeutic effects in rheumatoid arthritis do not generally occur until after several weeks of therapy, and maximal benefit may not occur until 6 months to 1 year of therapy. Chloroquine is usually discontinued if no objective improvement occurs within 6 months.

Inform patient that chloroquine may cause rusty yellow or brown discoloration of urine.

Caution patient to keep chloroquine out of reach of children; a number of fatalities have been reported following accidental ingestion.

Treatment of overdosage is symptomatic and must be promptly administered. Stomach is immediately evacuated by emesis or gastric lavage; finely powdered activated charcoal in slurry is given after lavage. Have on hand ultra-short-acting barbiturate, vasopressors,

equipment for tracheal intubation, tracheostomy. Monitor patient closely for at least 6 hours. Follow-up therapy: force fluids, acidification of urine to pH 4.5 or lower with ammonium chloride (8 Gm daily in divided doses for a few days), monitor urine pH.
Store in well-closed container preferably between 15° and 30°C (59° and 86°F), unless otherwise directed by manufacturer.

C

Drug Interactions: Chloroquine

Plus	Interactions
Aluminum (e.g., Kaolin) or magnesium compounds (e.g., magnesium trisilicate)	Pharmacologic effects of chloroquine may be increased (aluminum and magnesium reduce GI absorption of chloroquine). Separate administration by at least 4 hours, if possible

PROTOTYPE

CHLOROTHIAZIDE

(klor-oh-thye'a-zide)

(Diachlor, Diuril, Ro-Chlorozide, SK-Chlorothiazide)

CHLOROTHIAZIDE SODIUM

(Sodium Diuril)

Diuretic
Antihypertensive
Thiazide

ACTIONS AND USES. Chemically related to sulfonamides. Primary action is production of diuresis by reducing sodium reabsorption and by increasing potassium secretion by the distal convoluted tubules. Promotes renal excretion of sodium, bicarbonate, and potassium; decreases renal calcium excretion and supports uric acid retention. Antihypertensive mechanism is unclear but correlates with contraction of extracellular and intravascular fluid volumes, and direct vasodilation effect on vascular wall. This initially reduces cardiac output with subsequent decrease in peripheral resistance through autoregulatory mechanisms. Thiazide-induced hypokalemia may promote hyperglycemia by suppressing release of endogenous insulin. Has paradoxic antidiuretic effect in diabetes insipidus, and increases total serum cholesterol and triglyceride levels. Cross-allergy reported among chemically related drugs, e.g., furosemide (Lasix), sulfonylureas, acetazolamide (Diamox), and other sulfonamides.

Used adjunctively to manage edema associated with congestive heart failure, hepatic cirrhosis, renal dysfunction, corticosteroid, or estrogen therapy. Used alone as step 1 agent in stepped care approach, or in combination with other agents for treatment of hypertension. Also used to reduce polyuria of central diabetes insipidus, and to prevent calcium-containing renal stones. Available in combination with methyldopa (Aldochlor), and with reserpine (Chloroserpine, Diupres).

ABSORPTION AND FATE. Diuretic response following oral administration: onset within 2 hours, peak effect, 4 hours; duration, 6 to 12 hours. Half-life: 1 to 3 hours. Following IV injection: onset of diuresis, in 15 minutes with maximal effect in 30 minutes that lasts 2 to 4 hours. Distributed throughout extracellular fluid; concentrates in renal tissues. Does not appear to be metabolized. About 95% of IV dose excreted in urine unchanged within 3 to 6 hours and 35 to 60% of oral dose within 24 hours. Readily crosses placenta and appears in breast milk.

CONTRAINDICATIONS AND PRECAUTIONS. Hypersensitivity to thiazides or sulfonamides; anuria, oliguria, renal decompensation; hypokalemia; IV use in infants and children. Hazardous potential in women of childbearing age, during pregnancy (category B), and in nursing mothers. *Cautious Use:* history of allergy, bronchial asthma, impaired renal or hepatic function, or gout; hypercalcemia, diabetes mellitus, lupus erythematosus, advanced arteriosclerosis; elderly or debilitated patients, pancreatitis, sympathectomy, jaundiced children.

ADVERSE/SIDE EFFECTS. CNS: unusual fatigue, dizziness, mental changes, vertigo, headache, paresthesias, yellow vision. **CV:** irregular heart beat, weak pulse, orthostatic hypotension. **GI:** nausea, xerostomia, sialadenitis, vomiting, anorexia, heartburn, acute pancreatitis, diarrhea, constipation, abdominal cramps. **Hematologic (rare):** leukopenia, agranulocytosis, thrombocytopenia, aplastic anemia, electrolyte imbalance (including hypochloremic alkalosis, hypokalemia, hypomagnesemia, hyponatremia); asymptomatic hyperuricemia, hyperglycemia, glycosuria, rise in blood ammonia level; parathyroid pathology with hypercalcemia and hypophosphatemia (rare), inappropriate antidiuretic hormone secretion (SIADH). **Hypersensitivity:** urticaria, purpura, photosensitivity, skin rash, fever, necrotizing vasculitis with hematuria (rare), respiratory distress, anaphylactic reaction. **Other:** dehydration, transient blurred vision, gout, jaundice, vascular thrombosis.

ROUTE AND DOSAGE. Oral, intravenous: Adults: *Edema:* 500 mg to 2 Gm once or twice daily. *Antihypertensive* (oral only): **Adults:** Initial: 500 mg to 2 Gm twice daily, with maintenance dosage determined by blood pressure response. **Pediatric: Oral:** *Edema:* **Children (under 6 months):** up to 33 mg/kg/day divided into 2 doses; **Children (up to 2 years of age):** 125 to 375 mg/day divided into 2 doses; **Children (2 to 12 years of age):** 375 mg to 1 Gm daily divided into 2 doses. **Geriatric:** usually less than average adult dose.

NURSING IMPLICATIONS

Tablets may be crushed, if necessary, to facilitate swallowing and taken with fluid of patient's choice.

Oral drug may be administered with or after food to prevent gastric irritation.

Schedule daily doses to avoid nocturia and interrupted sleep.

When used to promote diuresis, drug-free days (administration on alternate days or on 3 to 5 days each week) may reduce electrolyte imbalance or hyperuricemia.

Explain to patient that he or she will be urinating greater amounts and more frequently than usual, and that there will be an unusual sense of tiredness. With continued therapy, diuretic action decreases; hypotensive effects usually are maintained, and sense of tiredness diminishes.

Missed dose: If patient forgets to take AM dose, he or she should take it when remembered, so long as it is not later than 6 PM in order not to disturb sleep with diuresis. Warn patient not to double nor skip a dose of chlorothiazide.

To prepare IV solution: Reconstitute with no less than 18 ml sterile water for injection (500 mg/20 ml vial). Solution is further diluted for IV administration with dextrose or sodium chloride injection. Chlorothiazide is not compatible with whole blood or its derivatives. See manufacturer's directions regarding dilutions, stability, storage, and compatible fluids.

Do not administer chlorothiazide solution SC or IM. Thiazide preparations are extremely irritating to the tissues, and great care must be taken to avoid extravasation. Palpate entry site occasionally to confirm needle position. If infiltration occurs, stop medication, remove needle and apply ice, if area is small. Signs of infiltration: swelling (may or may not be painful), coolness, absence of back flow, sluggish flow rate. At first sign, discontinue infusion, immediately remove needle. Consult physician about treatment of infiltrated area if it is large.

Antihypertensive action of a thiazide diuretic requires several days before effects are observed, usually optimum therapeutic effect is not established for 3 to 4 weeks.

Stepped-care approach in treatment of hypertension starts with a thiazide diuretic. (If hypo-

C

kalemia develops, a K-sparing diuretic or K supplement is added.) Failure to produce desired clinical effects is an indication for the next steps: beta adrenergic blocker, vasodilator, another antihypertensive (added or substituted). As other antihypertensive agents are added to thiazide therapy, their dosage is reduced to prevent excessive hypotension.

Baseline and periodic determinations are indicated for blood count, serum electrolytes, CO_2, BUN, creatinine, uric acid, and blood sugar. For patients on maintenance doses, some physicians suggest repeat determinations every 6 to 8 weeks until stable and at least every 6 months therafter.

Thiazide therapy can cause hyperglycemia and glycosuria in diabetic and diabetic-prone individuals. Dosage adjustment of hypoglycemic drugs may be required. Correction of hypokalemia *(see Actions and Uses)* sometimes resolves problem of hyperglycemia.

Asymptomatic hyperuricemia can be produced because of interference with uric acid excretion, although thiazides rarely precipitate acute gout. Report onset of joint pain and limitation of motion. Patient with history of gout may be continued on a thiazide with adjusted doses of uricosuric agent.

Monitor intake and output ratio. Excessive diuresis (with consequent dehydration), or oliguria may cause electrolyte imbalance and necessitate prompt dosage adjustment. To prevent dehydration, urge patient to report GI illness accompanied by protracted vomiting or prolonged period of diarrhea.

Establish baseline weight prior to initiation of therapy. Weigh patient at the same time each morning under standard conditions. Consult physician about acceptable range of weight change. Usually a gain of more than 2 pounds within 2 or 3 days and a gradual weight gain over the week's period is reportable. Tell patient to check for signs of edema (hands, ankles, pretibial areas).

Blood pressure should be closely monitored during early drug therapy. Physician may want initial measurements for patients with hypertension taken in standing, sitting, and lying postitions to evaluate drug effects.

Consistency in technique and readings is essential. Some physicians advocate taking blood pressures in the arm with the higher reading (if one is higher), taking supine blood pressure after patient has been reclining for 10 minutes, and taking standing blood pressure after patient stands for 3 minutes. Discuss with physician.

If orthostatic hypotension is a troublesome symptom (and it may be, especially in the elderly), inform patient of measures that may help tolerate the effect, and to prevent falling: (1) change from sitting or lying down positions slowly and in stages; (2) suggest that men sit down to urinate, especially if they need to void at night; (3) use a commode or urinal; (4) avoid hot showers or baths, sun bathing, extremes of environmental heat, unaccustomed physical activity; (5) when on a long airplane flight, walk about when it is permissible to do so; (6) when traveling by automobile, stop every hour or so to stretch and walk about; (7) consult physician about wearing support panty hose and abdominal support; (8) lie down immediately if sensation of light-headedness, faintness, or dizziness occurs.

Skin and mucous membranes should be inspected daily for evidence of petechiae in patients receiving large doses and those on prolonged therapy.

Xerostomia and sialadenitis require fastidious oral hygiene because decreases in salivary lubrication of oral membranes and teeth promotes demineralization of tooth surfaces and membrane erosion. Urge patient to floss teeth daily and to use a soft tooth brush for frequent brushing especially after eating. Frequent rinses with clear water is preferred to use of commercial mouth rinses (overuse of which may change oral flora and cause irritation to tissues). Use of a saliva substitute, e.g., Moi-stir, Salivart, Xero-Lube (all available OTC) may benefit some patients.

In an attempt to relieve dry mouth, patient may significantly increase fluid intake. Consult physician about permissible intake volume. Because of the possibility of dehydration, caution patient against drinking large quantities of coffee or other caffeine drinks (sometimes the major type of self-selected fluid). Caffeine is a CNS stimulant with diuretic effects.

Patients on digitalis therapy should be observed closely for signs and symptoms of hypokalemia. Even moderate reduction in serum K can precipitate digitalis intoxication in these patients.

Hypokalemia is not clinically significant in many patients, but those most apt to develop electrolyte imbalance are the elderly or debilitated, or those with edema. Imbalance may occur after pathophysiologic loss of body fluids (e.g., vomiting) or after iatrogenic fluid loss (e.g., parencentesis, GI drainage).

Signs of hypokalemia include: dry mouth, anorexia, nausea, vomiting, thirst, paresthesias, mental confusion, irritability, drowsiness, muscle cramps and weakness, paralytic ileus, abdominal distention, hypoactive reflexes, dyspnea, hypotension, cardiac arrhythmias, polyuria.

Food–Drug Interactions:

- Hypokalemia may be prevented if the daily diet contains K-rich foods (e.g., banana, fruit juices, apricots, potatoes, beef, chicken, whole grain cereals, skim milk). Urge patient to eat a banana (about 370 mg K) and drink at least 6 ounces orange juice (about 330 mg K) every day. Collaborate with dietitian and physician.
- The patient should be aware that some K-rich foods are also high in Na, e.g., pressed cheese, canned spinach, tomato juice, carrots, sardines, raw clams, frozen peas, lima beans.
- Rigid sodium restriction is not usually prescribed; however, foods high in sodium content should be avoided when thiazides are in use (e.g., luncheon meats, instant or quick cooked foods, bouillon, beer, pretzels, snack foods, ham, bacon, Chinese foods).
- The physician may advise the patient not to add salt to food. Use of a salt substitute must be prescribed by the physician. Most substitutes are high in potassium, contain some sodium, and are contraindicated in renal pathology.
- If hypokalemia develops, dietary K supplement of 1000 to 2000 mg (25 to 50 mEq) is usually adequate treatment.

Weight control is an important adjunct to hypertension therapy. Some patients may require a diet tailored to correct lipid abnormalities and to prevent electrolyte imbalance problems.

Provide opportunity for the patient/family to work with the dietitian in planning an individualized diet based on patient's food preferences, life-style, customs, and habits.

The patient should be advised to avoid or at least to greatly reduce smoking. (Smoking raises blood pressure.)

Discuss self-medication habits with patient. Some frequently used OTC drugs contain liberal amounts of sodium (Alka-Seltzer, BiSoDol, Bromo-Seltzer, Rolaids, Soda Mints) and potassium (Alka-Seltzer, Gerutonic). Advise patient to consult physician before dosing with any nonprescribed medication.

Warn patient about the possibility of photosensitivity reaction and to notify physician if it occurs. Thiazide-related photosensitivity is considered a photoallergy (radiation changes drug structure and makes it allergenic for some individuals) and occurs 1½ to 2 weeks after initial sun exposure. Avoid use of PABA sunscreen products. *(See Drug Interactions.)*

Thiazide therapy need not be interrupted because of surgery, but the anesthesiologist should be made aware of such therapy.

Although the syndrome of inappropriate secretion of antidiuretic hormone (SIADH) is uncommon, it can occur in susceptible individuals even with a brief exposure to a thiazide. Be suspicious if the following clinical findings are present: low urine output (less than 500 ml/24 hours) and low specific gravity, weight gain, pitting edema in ankles and pretibial areas, elevated BP and pulse, nausea, vomiting, watery diarrhea, venous congestion, muscle cramps, twitching, and drowsiness, weakness, lethargy, confusion, disorientation, signs of pulmonary edema, low serum Na, K, Cl. Treatment is restoration of potassium and restricted water intake.

Patient Instructions Related to Antihypertensive Therapy Should Include the Following:

- ✓ Dosage regimen, drug action, reportable signs and symptoms
- ✓ Importance of compliance in preventing complications of hypertension
- ✓ Maintenance of weight
- ✓ Diet restrictions, if any; stop smoking
- ✓ Moderate exercise plan
- ✓ Dates for follow-up studies. Some physicians want the patient to be taught to take his or her own blood pressure at home and even at work

Overdosage is treated by evacuation of gastric contents, and supportive measures to maintain hydration, electrolyte balance, respiratory and cardiovascular–renal function.

Store tablets, oral solutions, and parenteral dosage forms at temperature between 15° and 30°C (59° and 86°F), unless otherwise directed by manufacturer. Unused reconstituted IV solutions may be stored at room temperature up to 24 hours. Use only clear solutions.

Diagnostic Test Interferences. Chlorothiazide (thiazides) cause marked increases in **serum amylase** values, decrease in **PBI** determinations, may increase excretion of **PSP,** and increase **BSP retention,** and possibly cause false-negative **phentolamine** and **tyramine** tests, and interfere with **urine steroid** determinations. Thiazides should be discontinued before **parathyroid function tests** because they alter (decrease) **calcium** excretion.

Drug Interactions: Chlorothiazide (thiazides)

Plus	Interactions
Amphotericin B, corticosteroids, and other drugs with hypokalemic effect	Intensification of hypokalemic effect. Monitor serum potassium
Antidiabetic agents (insulins, sulfonylureas)	Hypoglycemic effects antagonized by hyperglycemic action of thiazides. Monitor for decreased diabetic control
Cholestyramine (Questran), colestipol (Colestid)	Decreased thiazide effects (due to formation of complex). Administer thiazides at least 2 hours before these drugs
Diazoxide (Hyperstat, Proglycem)	Hyperglycemic, hypotensive, hyperuricemic effects of both drugs intensified. Used concomitantly with caution
Digitalis glycosides	Increased potassium and magnesium loss may lead to digitalis toxicity. Monitor serum potassium and magnesium levels
Lithium	Possibility of lithium toxicity (renal clearance suppressed by thiazides). Monitor serum lithium levels
Skeletal muscle relaxants (nondepolarizing), e.g., tubocurarine	Prolonged neuromuscular blocking effects. Used concomitantly with caution
PABA sunscreen products	Exaggerate thiazide-induced photosensitivity

C

CHLOROTRIANISENE

(Tace)

(klor-oh-trye-an'i-seen)
Antineoplastic
Estrogen

ACTIONS AND USES. Nonesteroidal synthetic estrogen derived from diethylstilbestrol. Properties similar to those of other estrogens *(see Estradiol).* Has weak estrogenic properties until metabolized.

Used to treat inoperable progressing prostatic cancer, and as short-term treatment of symptoms of estrogen deficiency, e.g., atrophic vaginitis, female hypogonadism, kraurosis vulvae, vasomotor symptoms of menopause. Use for prevention of postpartum breast engorgement no longer recommended because large doses required increase risk of thrombophlebitis.

ABSORPTION AND FATE. Stored in body fat from which it is slowly released, then converted in liver to active estrogen compound. *See Estradiol.*

CONTRAINDICATIONS AND PRECAUTIONS. Thromboembolic disorders, pregnancy (category X). Safe use during lactation not established. *Cautious Use:* history of jaundice, metabolic bone diseases, hypertension, impaired renal function, diabetes mellitus. *See also Estradiol.*

ADVERSE/SIDE EFFECTS. CNS: headache, dizziness, sudden loss of coordination, slurred speech, mental depression, irritability. **CV:** thromboembolism, thrombophlebitis, edema. **GI:** abdominal cramps, anorexia, nausea, vomiting, diarrhea. **Reproductive:** spotting, breakthrough bleeding, decrease in libido; testicular atrophy, gynecomastia (males); lumps in breast, breast tenderness, pigmentation of nipples and areola. **Other:** jaundice, loss of hair, shortness of breath, aggravation of migraine, photosensitivity, visual disturbances, intolerance to contact lenses.

ROUTE AND DOSAGE. Oral: *Prostatic cancer:* 12 to 25 mg daily. Highly individualized dosage. *Female hypogonadism* (cyclic therapy): 12 to 25 mg daily for 21 consecutive days followed immediately by IM progesterone; or oral progestin may be given during last 5 days of treatment. Next course may begin on day 5 of induced uterine bleeding. *Menopause:* 12 to 25 mg daily for 30 days; one or more courses may be prescribed. *Atrophic vaginitis, pruritus vulvae, kraurosis vulvae:* 12 to 25 mg daily for 30 to 60 days.

NURSING IMPLICATIONS

Instruct patient to swallow the capsule whole. It may be taken with or immediately after food to reduce nausea.

Tace contains tartrazine, which sometimes causes allergic reactions (including bronchial asthma) in susceptible persons. Frequently seen in patients who also have aspirin hypersensitivity.

Review package insert with patient to assure complete understanding about estrogen therapy.

Because of its long-acting effects, chlorotrianisene is less suitable for cyclic therapy than the shorter acting estrogens.

Patients with diabetes mellitus should be more closely monitored for loss of diabetes control.

If pregnancy occurs during therapy, stop medication and report promptly to physician.

Inform patient of the importance of keeping follow-up appointments.

Capsules should be stored in well-closed container in a dry place, preferably between 15° and 30°C (59° and 86°F). Protect from extremes of temperature and humidity above 50%.

See Estradiol (prototype estrogen).

CHLORPHENESIN CARBAMATE

(Maolate)

(klor-fen′e-sin)

Skeletal muscle relaxant (centrally active)

C

ACTIONS AND USES. Carbamate with centrally acting skeletal muscle relaxant action, pharmacologically and structurally related to methocarbamol. Muscle relaxant effects may be related to sedative properties. *See Cyclobenzaprine.*

Used as adjunct to rest, physical therapy, and other appropriate measures in the symptomatic treatment of skeletal muscle spasm and pain secondary to sprains, trauma, and other musculoskeletal conditions. *Investigational Use:* treatment of trigeminal neuralgia.

ABSORPTION AND FATE. Peak plasma levels in 1 to 3 hours following oral administrations; plasma half-life: 2.3 to 5.1 hours. Partly metabolized in liver. Excreted in urine primarily as glucuronide conjugates.

CONTRAINDICATIONS AND PRECAUTIONS. Hypersensitivity to chlorphenesin carbamate; severe hepatic disease. Safe use during pregnancy, in nursing mothers, and in children younger than 12 years not established. *Cautious Use:* impaired renal or hepatic function.

ADVERSE/SIDE EFFECTS. CNS: drowsiness, dizziness, confusion, headache, euphoria, paradoxical reactions (nervousness, hyperexcitement, insomnia, increased headache). **GI:** nausea, epigastric distress, constipation, GI bleeding (causal relationship not established). **Hematologic:** pancytopenia, leukopenia, thrombocytopenia, agranulocytosis. **Hypersensitivity:** rash, pruritus, drug fever, anaphylaxis.

ROUTE AND DOSAGE. Oral: Initial: 800 mg three times daily until desired response obtained; maintenance 400 mg four times daily. Duration of therapy not to exceed 8 weeks.

NURSING IMPLICATIONS

Best administered with meals or milk to reduce risk of GI problems.

Adverse reactions generally respond to dosage reduction.

Dizziness and drowsiness are the most common side effects. Caution patient to avoid driving a car or other potentially hazardous tasks requiring mental alertness or physical coordination until drug response has been determined.

Maolate tablets contain tartrazine. The dye has caused allergic reactions including bronchial asthma in susceptible individuals who frequently have history of aspirin sensitivity.

Safe use of chlorphenesin for periods exceeding 8 weeks has not been established.

Warn patient that alcohol and other CNS depressants may cause additive CNS depression.

Instruct patient to report signs and symptoms of blood dyscrasia; unusual fatigue, unexplained fever, easy bruising or bleeding, sore mouth or throat.

Baseline and periodic blood cell counts and liver function studies advised.

Store preferably between 15 and 30°C (59 and 86°F) unless otherwise directed by manufacturer.

See Cyclobenzaprine (prototype centrally-acting skeletal muscle relaxant).

PROTOTYPE

CHLORPHENIRAMINE MALEATE

(klor-fen-eer'a-meen)

(Alermine, Aller-Chlor, Allerid-O.D., Chlo-Amine, Chlorate, Chlor-Niramine, Chlor-Pro, Chlorspan, Chlortab, Chlor-Trimeton, Hal Chlor, Histrey, Phenetron, Telachlor S.R., Teldrin, Trymegan)

Antihistamine
H_2-receptor antagonist

C

ACTIONS AND USES. Propylamine (alkylamine) antihistamine, derivative of pheniramine. Generally produces less drowsiness than other antihistamines, but side effects involving CNS stimulation may be more common. Competes with histamine for H_1-receptor sites on effector cells, thus blocking the histamine action that promotes capillary permeability and edema formation and the constrictive action on respiratory, gastrointestinal, and vascular smooth muscles. Has antiemetic, antitussive, anticholinergic, and local anesthetic actions.

Used for symptomatic relief of various uncomplicated allergic conditions; to prevent transfusion and drug reactions in susceptible patients, and used as adjunct to epinephrine and other standard measures in anaphylactic reactions. Commercially available in combination with phenylpropanolamine (Allerest, Condrin, Contac), and with pseudephedrine (Chlor-Trimeton Decongestant, Sudafed Plus).

ABSORPTION AND FATE. Onset of action following oral administration occurs in 20 to 60 minutes; duration 8 to 12 hours. Half-life: 20 to 24 hours; 69 to 72% bound to plasma proteins. Detoxified in liver. Metabolites and some free drug excreted primarily in urine; 19% of dose excreted in 24 hours, and 34% in 48 hours.

CONTRAINDICATIONS AND PRECAUTIONS. Hypersensitivity to antihistamines of similar structure; lower respiratory tract symptoms (including asthma), narrow-angle glaucoma, obstructive prostatic hypertrophy or other bladder neck obstruction, GI obstruction or stenosis, pregnancy (category B), nursing mothers, premature and newborn infants, during or within 14 days of MAO inhibitor therapy. *Cautious Use:* convulsive disorders, increased intraocular pressure, hyperthyroidism, cardiovascular disease, hypertension, diabetes mellitus, history of bronchial asthma, elderly patients, patients with G6PD deficiency.

ADVERSE/SIDE EFFECTS. Low incidence of side effects. **CNS:** drowsiness, sedation, headache, dizziness, vertigo, tinnitus, fatigue, disturbed coordination, tingling, heaviness, weakness of hands, tremors, euphoria, nervousness, restlessness, insomnia. *Overdosage* (especially in children): hallucinations, excitement, agitation, feeling of terror, fever, ataxia, athetosis, convulsions, coma, cardiovascular collapse. **CV:** palpitation, tachycardia, mild hypotension or hypertension, cardiovascular collapse (overdosage). **ENT:** dryness of mouth, nose, and throat, tinnitus, vertigo, acute labyrinthitis, thickened bronchial secretions, wheezing, sensation of chest tightness. **GI:** epigastric distress, anorexia, nausea, vomiting, constipation or diarrhea. **GU:** urinary frequency or retention, dysuria. **Hematologic** (rare): leukopenia, agranulocytosis, thrombocytopenia, hemolytic anemia. **Hypersensitivity:** skin rash, urticaria, photosensitivity, anaphylactic shock. **Ophthalmic:** blurred vision, diplopia. **Other** (following parenteral administration): transitory stinging or burning at injection site, sweating, pallor, transient hypotension, early menses.

ROUTE AND DOSAGE. Adults: Oral: 2 to 4 mg three or four times daily; timed release form: 8 or 12 mg at bedtime or every 8 to 12 hours, not to exceed 24 mg/24 hours. **Subcutaneous, intramuscular, and intravenous:** 5 to 20 mg as single dose. Maximum 40 mg/daily. IV injection should be made over period of 1 minute. **Children (6 to 12 years): Oral:** 2 mg every 4 to 6 hours, not to exceed 12 mg/24 hours. **Children (2 to 6 years): Oral:** 1 mg 3 or 4 times daily. Sustained release form not recommended in children younger than 12 years. Available in tablet, chewable tablet, timed release tablet or capsule, syrup, injection.

NURSING IMPLICATIONS

Sustained release tablets should be swallowed whole and not crushed or chewed.

In patients receiving antihistamines for allergic manifestations, a careful history should be taken to discover the allergen involved, if possible. Some common precipitating factors of allergy include: changes in dietary habits, contact with animals, a new drug, changes in home environment (e.g., new rug, drapes, pillows), emotional upsets.

The 20 mg and 100 mg/ml preparations are intended for IM and SC use *only*. They should *not* be administered IV because they contain preservatives. The 10 mg/ml injection can be given by either IV, IM, or SC route. It contains no preservatives.

Solutions for injection should not be given intradermally.

If patient manifests any reaction following parenteral administration, drug should be discontinued. (Exception: patient may experience transitory stinging sensation that rarely lasts longer than a few minutes.)

Caution patient to avoid driving a car or other potentially hazardous activities until drug response has been determined.

Warn patient that antihistamines have additive effects with alcohol and other CNS depressants (e.g., hypnotics, sedatives, tranquilizers).

Patients on prolonged therapy should have periodic blood cell counts.

Antihistamines have no therapeutic effect on the common cold. Their continued popularity, despite having been debunked as cold cures, apparently stems from the comfort afforded by their drying effects. Patients with cough should be advised that this drying action may cause thickened bronchial secretions, thus making expectoration difficult.

Dry mouth may be relieved by sugarless gum or lemon drops, frequent rinses with water, increasing (noncaloric) fluid intake (if allowed), use of a saliva substitute, e.g., Moi-stir, Orex, Salivart, Xero-Lube. For a more complete description *see Index: Nursing Interventions: dry mouth.*

Chlorpheniramine maleate is a prescription drug and is also available OTC (e.g., Chlor-Trimeton).

Caution patient to store antihistamines out of reach of children. Fatalities have been reported.

Patients with allergies should be advised to carry at all times medical identification jewelry or card indicating specific allergy, name, and physician's name, address, and telephone number.

Store preferably between 15° and 30°C (59° and 86°F) unless otherwise directed by manufacturer. Syrup and injection forms should be protected from light to prevent discoloration.

Diagnostic Test Interferences. Antihistamines should be discontinued 4 days prior to **skin testing** procedures for allergy because they may obscure otherwise positive reactions.

Drug Interactions: Chlorpheniramine

Plus	Interactions
Alcohol (Ethanol) and other CNS depressants	Additive CNS depression (especially drowsiness and impaired psychomotor ability). Used with caution if at all
MAO inhibitors	Anticholinergic effects of antihistamines may be prolonged and intensified. Concomitant use avoided
Phenytoin (Dilantin) and possibly other hydantoins	Possibility of increased pharmacologic effects of phenytoin. Monitor phenytoin plasma levels

CHLORPHENTERMINE HYDROCHLORIDE

(Pre-Sate)

(klor-fen′ter-meen)
Anorexigenic
C III

C

ACTIONS AND USES. Amphetamine congener and sympathomimetic amine with actions, contraindications, precautions, adverse reactions, and interactions similar to those of amphetamine (qv). Reportedly produces fewer side effects attributable to CNS stimulation than amphetamine.

Used as temporary adjunct in treatment of exogenous obesity.

ABSORPTION AND FATE. Peak levels occur in 2 to 4 hours. Excreted primarily in urine.

CONTRAINDICATIONS AND PRECAUTIONS. Hypersensitivity to sympathomimetic amines, hyperthyroidism, glaucoma, agitated states, history of drug abuse, angina pectoris, cardiovascular disease, including arrhythmias; during or within 14 days of MAOI therapy, children under 12 years of age. Safe use during pregnancy and in women of childbearing potential not established. *Cautious Use:* mild hypertension.

ADVERSE/SIDE EFFECTS. CV: palpitation, tachycardia, rise in BP. **CNS:** overstimulation, restlessness, insomnia, paradoxical sedation, drowsiness, dizziness, headache, tremor. **GI:** unpleasant taste, dry mouth, constipation, diarrhea, nausea, vomiting. **Other:** urticaria, mydriasis, difficulty in initiating micturition. *See also Amphetamine.*

ROUTE AND DOSAGE. Oral: 65 mg (slow-release tablet) daily.

NURSING IMPLICATIONS

Administered after first meal of the day. CNS stimulant effect may interfere with sleep if extended release tablet is taken after 4 PM.

Blood pressure should be monitored in patients with drug-controlled hypertension.

Since caloric intake may be altered, patients with diabetes will require close monitoring. Dosage adjustment of antidiabetic drug may be necessary.

Inform patient of the possibility of paradoxical drowsiness and dizziness, and caution against potentially hazardous activities such as driving a motor vehicle or operating machinery until reaction to the drug is known.

Since tolerance to anorexigenic action often develops within a few weeks, therapy is usually discontinued at that time.

Habituation or addiction may result from long-term use, especially with large doses. Classified as Schedule III drug under Federal Controlled Substances Act.

Chlorphentermine is used as an adjunct in a regimen of weight reduction that includes reeducation with respect to eating habits, an appropriate exercise program, and psychologic support.

See Amphetamine Sulfate (prototype amphetamine).

PROTOTYPE

CHLORPROMAZINE
CHLORPROMAZINE HYDROCHLORIDE

(BayClor, Clorazine, Largactil, Novochlorpromazine, Ormazine, Promapar, Promaz, Thorazine, Thor-prom)

(klor-proe′ma-zeen)
Psychotropic
Antipsychotic (neuroleptic)
Antiemetic
Phenothiazine

ACTIONS AND USES. Aliphatic (propylamino) derivative of phenothiazine with actions at all levels of CNS. Mechanism that produce strong antipsychotic effects is unclear, but thought to be related to blockade of postsynaptic dopamine receptors in the brain. Actions on hypothalamus and reticular formation produce strong sedation, depressed vasomotor reflexes leading to centrally mediated hypotension, inhibition of hypothalamic and pituitary hormone release, and depressed temperature regulation. Has strong alpha-adrenergic blocking action and weak anticholinergic effects. Directly depresses the heart; may increase coronary blood flow. Either by local anesthetic or quinidinelike action exerts an antiarrhythmic effect. Other actions include centrally mediated skeletal muscle relaxation, weak anorexiant, antihistiminic, and antipruritic effects, lowered convulsive threshold, and depressed cough reflex. Recent reports suggest an inhibitory effect on dopamine reuptake, possibly the basis for moderate extrapyramidal symptoms.

Used to control manic phase of manic-depressive illness, in management of severe nausea and vomiting, to control excessive anxiety and agitation prior to surgery and for treatment of severe behavior problems in children, e.g., attention deficit disorder. Also used to relieve acute intermittent porphyria, hiccoughs and as adjunct in treatment of tetanus.

ABSORPTION AND FATE. Erratic absorption following oral administration: rapid absorption after IM injection. Widely distributed; accumulates in brain and other tissues with a rich blood supply. Wide intraindividual variation (perhaps genetic) in plasma concentrations. Average peak levels 2 to 4 hours after oral intake, 15 to 20 minutes after IM administration. Metabolized in liver. Approximately 95% bound to plasma proteins. Biphasic elimination half-lives: 2 hours, and 30 hours. Excreted in urine mostly as metabolites; less than 1% excreted unchanged within 72 hours. Crosses placenta and appears in breast milk.

CONTRAINDICATIONS AND PRECAUTIONS. Hypersensitivity to phenothiazine derivatives; withdrawal states from alcohol, barbiturates, and other nonbarbiturate sedatives; comatose states, brain damage, bone marrow depression, myasthenia gravis, Reye's syndrome; children younger than 6 months. Safe use during pregnancy and in nursing mothers not established. *Cautious Use:* agitated states accompanied by depression, seizure disorders, respiratory impairment due to infection or COPD; glaucoma, diabetes, hypertensive disease, peptic ulcer, prostatic hypertrophy; thyroid, cardiovascular, and hepatic disorders; patients exposed to extreme heat or organophosphate insecticides; previously detected breast cancer.

ADVERSE/SIDE EFFECTS. (Usually dose related.) **CNS:** sedation, drowsiness, dizziness, syncope, insomnia, reduced REM sleep, bizarre dreams, cerebral edema, convulsive seizures, hyperpyrexia, inability to sweat, depressed cough reflex, catatoniclike states, psychotic symptoms, adverse behavior effects, extrapyramidal symptoms *(see Nursing Implications),* EEG changes. **CV:** orthostatic hypotension, hypertension, palpitation, tachycardia, bradycardia, ECG changes (usually reversible): prolonged QT and PR intervals, blunting of T waves, ST depression. **Dermatologic:** fixed-drug eruption, urticaria, contact dermatitis, exfoliative dermatitis, photosensitivity reaction with cutaneous pigmentation producing blue-gray coloration of exposed skin surfaces; hirsutism (long-term therapy). **GI:** oral syndrome (xerostomia, loosened dentures, vesicular lesions on tongue and mucous membranes, cheilitis, white or black furry tongue, glossitis); constipation, adynamic ileus, cholestatic jaundice, aggravation of peptic ulcer, dyspepsia, increased appetite. **Hematologic:** agranulocytosis, thrombocytopenic purpura, pancytopenia (rare). **Ophthalmic:** blurred vision, increased intraocular pressure, lenticular opacities, mydriasis or miosis, photophobia. **Reproductive/GU:** anovulation, infertility, pseudopregnancy, menstrual irregularity, gynecomastia, galactorrhea, inhibition of ejaculation, reduced libido, urinary retention and frequency. **Respiratory:** nasal congestion, laryngospasm, bronchospasm, respiratory depression. **Other:** hypoglycemia, hyperglycemia, glycosuria (high doses), enlargement of parotid glands, peripheral edema, muscle necrosis (following IM), anaphylactoid reactions, SLE-like syndrome, sud den unexplained death.

ROUTE AND DOSAGE. Adults: Oral: 10 to 50 mg two to six times daily. **Elderly, emaciated, debilitated:** 25 mg three times daily. **Intramuscular, intravenous:** 25 to 50 mg one to four

C

times daily. **Rectal suppository:** 50 to 100 mg three or four times daily as needed. **Pediatric: Oral:** 0.55 mg/kg every 4 to 6 hours, as necessary. **Intramuscular, intravenous:** 0.55 mg/kg every 6 to 8 hours as needed. **Rectal suppository:** 1.1 mg/kg every 6 to 8 hours as needed. Available in tablet, timed release capsule, syrup, concentrate, suppository, injection.

NURSING IMPLICATIONS

Before initiating treatment with phenothiazine derivatives, establish baseline blood pressure in standing and recumbent positions, pulse, and respiratory capacity values.

Metabolic and elimination rates of antipsychotic medication decrease with advancing age. Smaller doses are used for the elderly; side effects (especially hypotensive neuromuscular) in this age group may be more pronounced.

Maintenance therapy is usually administered as a single dose at bedtime.

Hypotensive reactions, dizziness, and sedation are common during early therapy particularly in patients on high doses or in the elderly receiving parenteral doses. Patients usually develop tolerance to these side effects; however, lower doses or longer intervals between doses may be required.

Inform and reassure the patient that side effects are reversible with prompt dosage adjustment or discontinuation of drug; therefore urge patient to report unusual signs or symptoms without delay: dark-colored urine, pale stools, jaundice, impaired vision, unusual bleeding or bruising, skin rash, weakness, tremors, sore throat, fever.

Tablet may be crushed before administration and taken with fluid or mixed with food. Capsules should not be opened.

Watch to see that oral drug is swallowed and not hoarded. Suicide attempt is a constant possibility in the depressed patient, particularly when improving.

In some cases it may be advisable to put patient on the liquid preparation to permit more feasible control as well as improved compliance.

Chlorpromazine concentrate should be mixed just before administration in at least ½ glass juice, milk, water, coffee, tea, carbonated beverage, or with semisolid food.

Smoking–Drug Interaction: Smoking increases metabolism of phenothiazines resulting in shortened half-life, and more rapid clearance of drug. Higher dosage in smokers may be required. Advise patient to stop smoking, if possible.

Avoid drug contact with skin, eyes, and clothing because of its potential for causing contact dermatitis. Personnel who frequently handle injectable and liquid forms should use rubber gloves. Patient on maintenance doses of concentrate at home should be warned to flush spilled solution off skin promptly.

While titrating initial dosages, marked changes from established baseline data should be reported.

Inject IM preparations slowly and deep into upper outer quadrant of buttock; massage site well. Avoid SC injection; it may cause tissue irritation and nodule formation. If irritation is a problem consult physician about diluting medication with normal saline or 2% procaine. Rotate injection sites.

The patient should remain recumbent for at least ½ hour after parenteral administration. Observe closely. Hypotensive reactions may require head-low position and pressor drugs, e.g., phenylephrine Neosynephrine (Levarterenol, Levophed). Epinephrine and other pressor agents are contraindicated since they may cause sudden paradoxic drop in BP.

Phenothiazine derivatives form incompatible admixtures with many drugs; consult pharmacist before mixing with other drugs.

Avoid injecting undiluted chlorpromazine into a vein.

A specific flow rate should be ordered for the IV infusion. Usual rate: 1 to 2 mg/minute. Monitor blood pressure.

Lemon yellow color of parenteral preparation does not alter potency; if otherwise colored or markedly discolored, solution should be discarded.

Therapeutic effects of phenothiazine therapy include: emotional and psychomotor quieting in excited, hyperactive patients; reduction of paranoidal symptoms, hallucinations, delusions, fears, and hostility; stimulation of withdrawn patients and productive organization of thought and behavior.

Some patients fail to experience improvement for as long as 7 or 8 weeks of therapy; thus, they may not realize the importance of medication compliance. Stress necessity of keeping appointments for follow-up evaluation of dosage regimen.

Urge patient on home therapy not to alter dosing regimen; tell patient not to give the drug to another person.

Warn patient not to take any other drugs, especially OTC medications, without physician's approval.

Monitor dietary intake and bowel elimination pattern. Increased fluid intake and a gradual increase in high-fiber foods may help to prevent GI complications (fecal impaction, constipation).

Monitor intake and output ratio and pattern. Urinary retention due to depression and compromised renal function may occur. If serum creatinine becomes elevated, therapy should be discontinued.

Inform patient that phenothiazines may cause pink to red-brown discoloration of urine (due to a metabolite).

Note that chlorpromazine may suppress cough reflex. Be alert to danger of bronchopneumonia which may occur in the severely depressed patient, especially if elderly. Depressed thirst and lethargy can lead to dehydration, hemoconcentration, and reduced pulmonary ventilation.

Patients on home therapy should be advised which laxative to take, if needed. Many OTC drugs contain anticholinergic components that can precipitate adynamic ileus.

Support hose and elevation of legs when sitting may minimize drug induced hypotention (discuss with physician). Supervise ambulation. Instruct patient to make gradual position changes from recumbent to upright posture, and to dangle legs over bed a few minutes before ambulation. Caution against standing still for prolonged periods and advise against hot showers or baths, long exposure to environmental heat.

Since chlorpromazine may affect the temperature regulating mechanism, heed and report patient's complaint of feeling cold. Applying a blanket next to the body may help. Hot-water bottles and other heating devices are not recommended because phenothiazines tend to depress conditioned avoidance responses.

Chlorpromazine (phenothiazine) use is accompanied by loss of thermoregulation, and inability to sweat. Patient exposed to extremes in environmental temperature, or high fever due to illness, may develop heat stroke (red, dry hot skin; headache, dizziness, dilated pupils, dyspnea; full, bounding, strong pulse; temperature above 40.6°C (105°F), mental confusion, sudden loss of consciousness). Inform physician and prepare to institute measures to rapidly lower body temperature, e.g., move patient into shade; evaporative cooling (application of tap water with simultaneous fanning).

Antiemetic effect of chlorpromazine may obscure signs of overdosage of other drugs or other causes of nausea and vomiting.

Be alert to complaints of diminished visual acuity, reduced night vision, photophobia, and a perceived brownish discoloration of objects. Patient may be more comfortable with dark glasses. Facilitate periodic ophthalmic examination for patients on long-term therapy.

Photosensitivity associated with chlorpromazine therapy is a phototoxic reaction involving

C

photoactivated changes in cell structure. Severity of response depends on amount of ultra violet ray exposure and drug dose. Exposed skin areas have appearance of an exaggerated sunburn. If reaction occurs, patient should wear protective clothing and sun screen lotion (SPF above 12) when outdoors, even on dark days.

Xerostomia may be relieved by frequent sips of water, by rinsing mouth with warm water, or by increasing noncalorie fluid intake. Sugarfree candy or chewing gum may also help to stimulate salivary flow. Sucrose in regular gum or candy favors dental caries development and *Candida* growth. If these measures fail a saliva substitute may help, e.g., Moistir, Orex, Salivart, Xero-Lube (all available OTC).

Oral candidiasis occurs frequently in patients receiving chlorpromazine. Emphasize meticulous oral hygiene: daily flossing with waxed dental floss, brushing teeth with soft, small brush after eating, and use of a fluoride toothpaste. Overuse of antiseptic mouth rinses can change oral flora and should be discouraged. Inspect oral cavity of severely depressed patient; assist with oral hygiene if necessary.

Since chlorpromazine reduces REM sleep it is usually not used for nighttime sedation in patients with auditory or visual hallucinations.

Extrapyramidal symptoms occur most often in patients on high dosage, the pediatric patient with severe dehydration and acute infection, the elderly, and women. These symptoms are frightening to the uninformed. Be sure patient understands importance of prompt reporting to the physician the onset of symptoms. Usually symptoms disappear with dosage adjustment or over a period of time.

Extrapyramidal symptoms associated with antipsychotic drug use: *pseudoparkinsonism:* (slowing of volitional movement [akinesia], mask facies, rigidity and tremor at rest, especially upper extremities, pill rolling motion) occurs most frequently in women, the elderly of both sexes, and dehydrated patients; may be mistaken for depression. *Acute dystonia:* (abnormal posturing, grimacing, spastic torticollis and oculogyric crisis) occurs most frequently in men and patients under 25 years of age; may be misdiagnosed as hysteria or seizures. *Akathisia:* (compelling need to move without specific pattern; inability to sit still) occurs most frequently in women and is often misdiagnosed as agitation. *Tardive dyskinesia* (generally irreversible): involuntary rhythmic, bizarre movements of face, jaw, mouth, tongue, and sometimes extremities. Usual first sign of *tardive dyskinesia:* vermicular movements of the tongue. It is critical that this sign be noticed as soon as it appears and that the drug be withdrawn. Prompt action may prevent irreversibility.

Observe patient closely to recognize early indications of extrapyramidal symptoms. Maximal risk times following start of therapy for: pseudoparkinsonism and acute dystonia: 1 to 5 days; akathisia: 50 to 60 days; tardive dyskinesia: after months or years of treatment. (All patients on long-term phenothiazine treatment are at high risk for development of tardive dyskinesia.)

Some physicians prescribe an antiparkinson agent and instruct their patients to take it with the onset of symptoms such as restlessness, shakiness, or soreness.

Diabetics or prediabetics on long-term, high-dose therapy should be monitored for reduced glucose tolerance and loss of diabetes control. Urine and blood glucose should be checked regularly. Drug therapy may have to be discontinued or substituted by another agent.

If an antipsychotic must be used during pregnancy, drug treatment should be discontinued 1 to 2 weeks prior to delivery to avoid neonatal distress. The newborn may display hyperreflexia, jaundice, and prolonged extrapyramidal symptoms.

Close supervision of the infant is critical if the nursing mother must be on phenothiazine therapy.

Elevated temperature, sore mouth, gums, or throat, upper respiratory infection, fatigue and weakness (early manifestations of agranulocytosis) are most likely to occur within first 4 to 10 weeks of therapy, particularly in women and the elderly. Blood studies should be instituted promptly.

Cholestatic jaundice occurs more frequently in women, usually between second and fourth weeks, and is reversed by drug withdrawal. May begin with abrupt fever, flu-like symptoms, and abdominal discomfort, followed in about 1 week by jaundice. Pruritus, usually an early symptom of jaundice, may not be present because of the antipruritic effects of phenothiazines.

Complete blood counts, liver function tests, urinalysis, ocular examinations, EEG (in patients over 50 years of age) are recommended before and periodically during prolonged therapy.

Chlorpromazine may impair mental and physical abilities, especially during early therapy. Caution patient against driving a car or undertaking activities requiring precision and mental alertness until drug response is known.

Overdosage with chlorpromazine leads to CNS depression to the point of somnolence and coma. Treatment: early gastric lavage, close observation of patient, maintenance of open airway. Vomiting should not be induced because possible occurrence of dystonic reaction of head and neck coupled with drug-depressed cough reflex could lead to aspiration of vomitus. If overdosage involves spansules, a saline cathartic may hasten evacuation of medication pellets.

Abrupt withdrawal of drug or deliberate dose skipping, especially after prolonged therapy with large doses, can cause onset of extrapyramidal symptoms and severe GI disturbances. Urge patient to adhere to dosage regimen without changes. When treatment is to be discontinued, dosage must be reduced gradually over a period of several weeks.

Brand interchange of oral and suppository forms is not recommended.

Store preferably between 15° and 30°C (59° and 86°F) protected from light, unless otherwise specified by the manufacturer. Avoid freezing.

Diagnostic Test Interferences. Chlorpromazine may increase **cephalin flocculation,** and possibly other **liver function tests;** also may increase **PBI.** False-positive results may occur for **amylase, 5-hydroxyindole acetic acid, porphobilinogens, urobilinogen** (Ehrlich's reagent), **urine bilirubin** (Bili-Labstix) and **pregnancy tests** possibly caused by a metabolite of phenothiazines which discolors urine.

Drug Interactions: Chloropromazine (phenothiazines)

Plus	Interactions
Alcohol (Ethanol), and other CNS depressants	Enhanced CNS depression (hypotension, respiratory depression). Used concomitantly with caution if at all
Anorexigenic agents	Inhibition of anorexiant effect. Avoid combination, if possible
Antacids, antidiarrheals	Decreased absorption of oral phenothiazines. Space administration at least 2 hours apart
Amphetamines	Decreased amphetamine effects. Concurrent use generally avoided
Anticholinergics	Additive anticholinergic action, and reduced antipsychotic effect of phenothiazines. Used concomitantly with caution
Barbiturates	Possibility of increased metabolism of phenothiazines, (by induction of hepatic enzymes). Observe for reduced phenothiazine effects

C

Plus (cont.)	Interactions (cont.)
Barbiturate anesthetics	Increase in excitation (tremor, involuntary muscle movements), and hypotension. Combination generally avoided
Beta adrenergic blockers, e.g., propranolol	Additive hypotensive effects. Mutual inhibition of metabolism. Used concomitantly with caution. Dosage adjustment may be indicated
Guanethidine (Ismelin)	Phenothiazines may block antihypertensive action (inhibit neuronal uptake of guanethidine). Monitor patient closely
Lithium	Lowers plasma level of phenothiazines. Observe for reduced phenothiazine effects
Ototoxic medications	Phenothiazines may mask symptoms of ototoxicity
Phenytoin (Dilantin)	Inhibits phenytoin metabolism thus increased potential for its toxicity. Monitor phenytoin serum levels
Sympathomimetics, e.g., phenylpropanolamine	Possibility of sudden death. Mechanism not established. Used concurrently with caution
Tricyclic antidepressants	Mutual intensification of sedative and anticholinergic actions. Used concomitantly with caution

CHLORPROPAMIDE

(klor-proe′pa-mide)

(Apo-Chlorpropamide, Chloronase, Diabinese, Novopropamide, Stabinol)

Antidiabetic
Sulfonylurea
Sulfonamide derivative

ACTIONS AND USES. Longest-acting first generation sulfonylurea compound, structurally and pharmacologically related to tolbutamide (qv). Although a sulfonamide derivative, it has no antiinfective activity. Lowers blood glucose by stimulating beta cells in pancreas to release endogenous insulin. May potentiate available antidiuretic hormone (ADH), a property not shared by other sulfonylureas. Has longer duration of action and about six times the potency of tolbutamide, as well as a higher incidence of side effects. Reported to be associated with fewer primary and secondary failures. Not effective as sole therapy of diabetes.

Used in the management of mild to moderately severe, stable noninsulin-dependent diabetes mellitus (type II, NIDDM), in patients who cannot be controlled by diet alone, and who do not have complications of diabetes. *Unlabeled Use:* treatment of neurogenic diabetes insipidus, but use for this condition is debated by some clinicians.

ABSORPTION AND FATE. Promptly and completely absorbed from GI tract after oral ingestion. Wide distribution in extracellular fluid compartment. Action begins in 1 hour: peaks in 3 to 6 hours, with duration of 60 to 72 hours. Approximately 88 to 96% bound to plasma proteins. Half-life: 30 to 40 hours. Plasma levels become stabilized 5 to 7 days after initiation of therapy; therefore, undue accumulation in blood does not occur during prolonged therapy. As much as 80% may be metabolized in liver with formation of metabolites that may also have antidiabetic activity. Renal excretion is slow: 80 to 90% of a single dose excreted as unchanged drug and metabolites within 96 hours. Rate of excretion is accelerated in alkaline urine and is decreased in acidic urine. Excreted in milk.

CONTRAINDICATIONS AND PRECAUTIONS. Known hypersensitivity to sulfonylureas and to sulfonamides; type I (IDDM) diabetes, diabetes complicated by severe infection; acidosis; severe renal, hepatic, or thyroid insufficiency; pregnancy (category C); safe use in lactating women and in children not established. *Cautious Use:* elderly patients, Addison's disease, congestive heart failure. *See also Tolbutamide.*

ADVERSE/SIDE EFFECTS. Hypoglycemia; GI distress; skin reactions, drowsiness, muscle cramps, weakness, paresthesias, photosensitivity; cholestatic jaundice hypersensitivity reactions, leukopenia, thrombocytopenia, anemia (rare); agranulocytosis; disulfiram reaction; antidiuretic effect (SIADH): hyponatremia, hyposthenuria. *See also Tolbutamide.*

ROUTE AND DOSAGE. Oral: *Antidiabetic:* Initial: 250 mg daily (elderly patient: 100 to 125 mg daily). Dosage may be increased by 50 to 125 mg at 3- to 5-day intervals, as necessary. Maintenance: 100 to 500 mg daily; not to exceed 750 mg daily. *Antidiuretic:* 100 to 250 mg daily; dosage adjusted at 2- or 3-day intervals if necessary, up to 500 mg daily.

NURSING IMPLICATIONS

Chlorpropamide may be prescribed as a single morning dose with breakfast or divided into two or three doses and taken with meals to minimize GI side effects and to achieve maximum diabetes control.

Tablet may be crushed if patient is unable to swallow it whole. Be sure it is swallowed with an allowable liquid, not dry.

With long-acting hypoglycemic agents, mild CNS symptoms of hypoglycemia predominate, whereas other symptoms may go unnoticed or simply may be tolerated (e.g., abnormalities in sleep pattern, frequent nightmares, night sweats, morning headache). The patient and responsible family members should be alerted to the necessity of reporting all symptoms promptly to the physician.

Patient should be examined and evaluated during first 6 weeks of chlorpropamide therapy to determine drug effectiveness.

Ordinarily transfer from another antidiabetic medication to chlorpropamide does not require a conversion period.

If, prior to transfer to chlorpropamide, the patient required less than 40 units of insulin daily, the insulin may be withdrawn abruptly at the beginning of oral hypoglycemic therapy. If 40 U/day or more were needed, the insulin dose should be reduced by 50% for the first few transition days. Further adjustment is individualized. Some patients may need to be hospitalized 3 to 5 days for dose supervision and frequent feedings to prevent hypoglycemia which can occur during period of transition. IV glucose may be necessary.

Hypoglycemia can be severe in the type II diabetic patient although onset is not as fast or as dramatic as with use of insulin. If symptoms of impending hypoglycemia (feeling of hunger and weakness, lightheadedness, sweating, tachycardia, anxiety, numbness, tremor, headache) occur patient should take a soluble sugar (honey, orange juice, sugar cubes, corn syrup) and notify physician.

The controlled type II diabetic is usually advised to test urine for glucose at least 3 times daily, 2 hours after meals. If reagent strip tests are consistently high for 3 days, the patient should then also test for urine ketone and report the results to the physician.

Food–Drug Interactions: The individually planned diet for the type II patient is less rigid than for the type I insulin-dependent patient. In general it stresses: (1) 3 meals with or without a snack in the afternoon or evening; (2) avoiding excessive intake of carbohydrates at a single meal or large amounts between meals particularly as liquids and unaccompanied by other food types; (3) fiber rich diet. Modifications are not required for moderate exercise, missed meals, or mild intercurrent illness.

The elderly generally have decreased renal function, therefore close medical supervision

C

is essential because of the possibility of drug accumulation. Maintenance dosage of chlorpropamide is particularly hard to establish.

The more severe toxic effects, jaundice and agranulocytosis, are often preceded by skin eruptions, malaise, fever, or photosensitivity. Immediately report these symptoms to the physician. A change to another hypoglycemic agent may be indicated.

Periodic hematologic and hepatic studies are advisable particularly in patients receiving high doses. A CBC should be performed if symptoms of anemia appear: advise patient to report dizziness, shortness of breath, malaise, fatigue.

Caution patient not to self-dose with OTC drugs unless approved or prescribed by the physician.

Alcohol intolerance may occur in up to 30% of patients receiving normal doses of chlorpropamide. (Reaction occurs more frequently with chlorpropamide than with other oral antidiabetic agents.) Ingestion of alcohol causes chlorpropamide-alcohol flush (CPAI) a disulfiram reaction. Symptoms (facial flushing, pounding headache, sweating, slurred speech, abdominal cramps, nausea, vomiting, tachycardia) occur within 2 to 3 minutes, peak in 15 to 20 minutes, and may last 1 to 4 hours. Inform the patient about the possibility of this reaction.

Instruct the controlled diabetic patient to monitor weight and to be aware of intake and output ratio and pattern. Infrequently chlorpropamide produces an antidiuretic effect, with resulting severe hyponatremia, edema, and water intoxication. If fluid intake far exceeds output and edema develops (weight gain), the patient should report to the physician. The most noticeable early symptoms may include mental confusion, drowsiness, and lethargy. If not treated promptly, overt psychotic behavior, coma, grand mal convulsions, irreversible neurologic damage, and death may occur.

In the treatment of diabetes insipidus, the expected therapeutic effect of chlorpropamide is the promotion of a significant decrease in urinary output. Monitor intake and output ratio and check with physician regarding allowable parameters.

The patient on chlorpropamide needs to know: (1) how to administer insulin, because it is standard therapy if the diabetic is subjected to stress, e.g., severe trauma, infection, surgery; (2) how to recognize and counteract impending hypoglycemia, and (3) how to monitor diabetes control by blood and urine tests. *See Tolbutamide.*

Keep drug out of the reach of children. In accidental ingestion of this drug, complete elimination does not occur for 3 to 5 days. The patient should be hospitalized for close observation.

Store below 40°C (104°F), preferably between 15° and 30°C (59° and 86°F) in a well-closed container, unless otherwise directed by manufacturer.

See also Tolbutamide (prototype sulfonylurea antidiabetic agent).

Drug Interactions. Action of **barbiturates** may be prolonged by chlorpropamide. *See also Tolbutamide.*

CHLORPROTHIXENE

(klor-proe-thix'een)

(Taractan, Tarasan)

Psychotropic

Antipsychotic (neuroleptic)

ACTIONS AND USES. Thioxanthene derivative structurally and pharmacologically similar to the phenothiazines. Has strong antiemetic, sedative, and hypotensive actions but less anticholinergic and antihistaminic activity. Incidence of extrapyramidal symptoms is low. *See Chlorpromazine.*

Used for management of manifestations of psychotic disorders.

ABSORPTION AND FATE. Onset of effects occurs 10 to 30 minutes following IM administration. Presumably metabolized in liver and excreted in urine and feces as unchanged drug and sulfoxide metabolite.

CONTRAINDICATIONS AND PRECAUTIONS. Hypersensitivity to phenothiazine derivatives; epinephrine use, circulatory collapse, congestive heart failure, coronary artery disease, cerebral vascular disorders, comatose states. Safe use not established: during pregnancy, lactation, in women of childbearing potential, oral use in children under age 6 or parenteral use in those under age 12. *Cautious Use:* persons exposed to extreme heat or organophosphate insecticides, persons with suicide tendency; history of drug abuse, peptic ulcer, cardiovascular or respiratory disease, previously detected breast cancer, persons receiving ototoxic medications (especially aminoglycoside antibiotics).

ADVERSE/SIDE EFFECTS. Drowsiness, lethargy, dizziness, orthostatic hypotension, tachycardia, dry mouth, constipation, ocular disturbances, inability to sweat, contact dermatitis, photosensitivity, uricosuria, urinary retention, extrapyramidal symptoms, transient leukopenia, agranulocytosis pain and induration IM site (usually minimal). Shares toxic potential of phenothiazines. *See Chlorpromazine.*

ROUTE AND DOSAGE. Individually adjusted: **Oral: Adults:** 25 to 50 mg three or four times daily; increased as necessary and tolerated. Maximum dose usually no higher than 600 mg daily. **Elderly, debilitated, and children (over 6 years of age):** 10 to 25 mg three or four times daily. **Intramuscular:** 25 to 50 mg three or four times daily. Oral concentrate contains 100 mg/5 ml.

NURSING IMPLICATIONS

Oral concentrate may be given alone or diluted in water, milk, fruit juice, coffee, or carbonated beverage just before administration. Warn patient not to spill oral liquid on skin or clothing because drug can cause contact dermatitis.

If necessary, tablet may be crushed before administration and taken with fluid of patient's choice.

Administer IM in upper outer quadrant of buttock or midlateral thigh. Aspirate carefully to avoid inadvertent entry into blood vessel. Rotate injection sites.

Monitor intake and output ratio and bowel elimination pattern. Patient should know what laxative may be used if necessary. Consult physician about prescribing a high-fiber diet.

Since postural hypotension may occur in some patients, IM injection should be given with patient recumbent or seated. Observe patient until weakness or dizziness, if present, passes.

Observe patient closely when changeover from parenteral to oral doses is made. Oral dose is alternated with parenteral dose on same day, then oral dose only.

Be certain patient understands dosing regimen and that he or she should not change or omit doses. Also tell the patient not to give any of the drug to another person.

Antiemetic effect may mask toxicity of other drugs, or block recognition of such conditions as brain tumor or intestinal obstruction.

Geriatric and debilitated patients should be closely supervised particularly during ambulation. Lethargy and drowsiness are easily controlled by dosage adjustment.

Alcohol and other CNS depressants should be avoided during treatment with chlorprothixene.

Caution patient to avoid excessive exposure to sunlight. Use sunscreen lotion (SPF above 12) when outdoors, even if it is a cloudy day.

Therapy with chlorprothixene is accompanied by inability to sweat which can result in

C

increased body temperature. Patient exposed to extremes in environmental temperature (room, sun), or to high fever due to illness, may develop heat stroke (red, dry, hot skin; dilated pupils, dyspnea; full, bounding, pulse; temperature above 40.6°C (105°F), mental confusion). Inform physician and prepare to institute measures (evaporative cooling, and antipyretics) to rapidly lower body temperature.

Warn patient to avoid driving and other potentially hazardous activities until his reaction to drug is known.

Urge patient to keep follow-up appointments. Periodic evaluations should be made to determine possibility of dosage reduction or termination of drug therapy.

When therapy is to be discontinued, doses should be reduced gradually over a several-day period. Abrupt withdrawal may produce nausea, vomiting, gastritis, dizziness, and tremulousness.

Taractan tablets contain tartrazine which may cause an allergic reaction including bronchial asthma in susceptible individuals. These persons are frequently sensitive to aspirin also.

Chlorprothixene may discolor urine pink to red, or red brown.

Store in light-resistant, tightly covered container between 15° and 30°C (59° and 86°F) unless otherwise specified by manufacture.

See Chlorpromazine (prototype antipsychotic).

CHLORTETRACYCLINE HYDROCHLORIDE

(Aureomycin, Aureomycin Ophthalmic)

(klor-te-tra-sye′kleen)
Antiinfective
Antibiotic
Tetracycline

ACTIONS AND USES. Broad-spectrum antibiotic derived from *Streptomyces aureofaciens.* Closely related chemically and in actions to other tetracyclines. Primarily bacteriostatic in action. Effective against a variety of gram-negative and gram-positive pathogens.

Ophthalmic ointment is used as adjunct with oral therapy in the treatment of trachoma inclusion, conjunctivitis, chlamydial infections, and for superficial ocular infections caused by susceptible organisms. Skin ointment is used for treatment of superficial pyogenic skin infections.

CONTRAINDICATIONS AND PRECAUTIONS. Hypersensitivity to tetracyclines, or to any ingredients in the formulation. Safe use during pregnancy, in nursing women, and in children not established.

ADVERSE/SIDE EFFECTS. Hypersensitivity: itching, burning, urticaria, dermatitis, angioneurotic edema; superinfection.

ROUTE AND DOSAGE. Ophthalmic ointment (1%): apply small amount to infected eye every 2 hours, as condition and response indicate. **Skin ointment (3%):** apply directly to involved area, preferably on sterile gauze, one or more times daily.

NURSING IMPLICATIONS

The ophthalmic ointment and skin ointment are *not* interchangeable.

Use ophthalmic ointment only for eyes. Inform patient that vision will be temporarily blurred following administration. *See Index: Drug administration: eye ointment.*

Consult physician regarding procedure for cleansing infected skin area prior to reapplications of skin ointment.

Caution patient with skin problem to avoid prolonged exposure to sunlight unless otherwise advised by physician.

Advise patient to apply medication as directed by physician and not to exceed prescribed duration of therapy. Prolonged or frequent intermittent use of an antibiotic should be avoided because of danger of hypersensitization.

Instruct patient to discontinue medication and notify physician if an adverse reaction occurs.

Review personal hygiene practices.

Store in tightly closed container preferably between 15° and 30°C (59° and 86°F) unless otherwise directed by manufacturer.

CHLORTHALIDONE

(Hygroton, Hylidone, Novothalidone, Thalitone, Uridon)

(klor-thal'i-done)
Diuretic
Antihypertensive
Thiazide
Sulfonamide derivative

ACTIONS AND USES. Phthalimidine derivative of benzenesulfonamide. Structurally and pharmacologically related to thiazides, with similar actions, uses, contraindications, adverse reactions and interactions. Reportedly causes elevations in total cholesterol, LDL cholesterol, and triglycerides, in some patients. *See Chlorothiazide.*

Used to treat edema associated with congestive heart failure, renal decompensation, hepatic cirrhosis; as sole agent or with other antihypertensives to treat severe hypertension. Commercially available in combination with reserpine (e.g., Regroton), with clonidine (Combipres), and with atenolol (Tenoretic).

ABSORPTION AND FATE. Diuretic effect begins in 2 hours, peaks in 2 to 6 hours, and lasts 24 to 72 hours. About 90% bound primarily to carbonic anhydrase in red blood cells. Half-life: 35 to 54 hours if kidney function is normal. About 30 to 60% of dose excreted unchanged in urine. Crosses placenta and appears in breast milk.

CONTRAINDICATIONS AND PRECAUTIONS. Hypersensitivity to sulfonamide derivatives; anuria, hypokalemia, pregnancy (category B), lactation. *Cautious Use:* history of renal and hepatic disease, gout, systemic lupus erythematosus (SLE), diabetes mellitus. *See also Chlorothiazide.*

ADVERSE/SIDE EFFECTS. Orthostatic hypotension, hypercalcemia, hyperglycemia, hypokalemia, nausea and vomiting, unusual fatigue, paresthesias, vasculitis, acute pancreatitis, exacerbation of gout (rare), agranulocytosis, hemolytic anemia. *See also Chlorothiazide.*

ROUTE AND DOSAGE. Oral: Adults: *Edema:* 50 to 100 mg once daily, or 100 to 200 mg once every other day, or once daily for 3 days/week. *Antihypertensive:* Initial: 25 mg daily. If poor response, dosage may be increased to 100 mg once daily or a second antihypertensive may be added. **Pediatric:** 2 mg/kg body weight or 60 mg/m^2 body surface once daily three times a week. Maintenance dosage adjusted according to patient's needs; often lower than initial dosage.

NURSING IMPLICATIONS

If necessary, tablet may be crushed and administered with fluid of patient's choice.

When used as a diuretic, an intermittent dose schedule may reduce incidence of adverse reactions.

C

Divided doses are unnecessary. Administered as single dose in the morning to reduce potential for interrupted sleep because of diuresis.

Geriatric patients are more sensitive to adverse effects of drug-induced diuresis because of age-related changes in the cardiovascular and renal systems. Be alert to signs of hypokalemia (unusual fatigue, mental confusion, muscle cramps, irregular heart beat, GI disturbances). Report to physician; dose adjustment or termination of therapy may be indicated. K supplement (dietary or drug) or termination of chlorthalidone therapy may be indicated.

Advise patient to maintain adequate potassium intake, to monitor weight, and to make a daily estimate of intake and output ratio. *See Chlorothiazide.*

Controlled studies have shown that dosage increases above 25 mg/day are associated with a greater fall in serum potassium, rise in serum uric acid, and hyperglycemia in susceptible individuals, but little or no change in blood pressure.

The following laboratory values should be obtained initially and periodically throughout therapy: serum electrolytes (particularly K, Mg, Ca), serum uric acid, creatinine, BUN, and uric acid.

Store tablets in tightly closed container preferably between 15° and 30°C (59° and 86°F) unless otherwise advised by manufacturer.

See Chlorothiazide (prototype thiazide diuretic).

Drug Interactions: Chlorthalidone

Plus	Interactions
Cholestyramine (Questran) Colestipol (Colestid)	Pharmacologic effects of chlorthalidone may be reduced (decreased absorption). Separate administration as far apart as possible
Corticosteroids Digitalis glycosides	Increased risk of hypokalemia (with resultant predisposition of patient to digitalis toxicity). Monitor serum potassium
Diazoxide (Hyperstat)	Action of both drugs potentiated, with resultant hyperglycemia, hyperuricemia and hypotension. Used concomitantly with caution
Hypoglycemic agents, oral (sulfonylureas) and insulin	Chlorthalidone-induced elevation of blood sugar antagonizes hypoglycemic effect of antidiabetic drugs. Dosage adjustments may be required

CHLORZOXAZONE

(Paraflex)

(klor-zox'a-zone)

Skeletal muscle relaxant (centrally acting)

ACTIONS AND USES. Benzoxazole derivative, centrally acting muscle relaxant. Has no direct action on skeletal muscle. Produces skeletal muscle relaxation by depressing nerve transmission through polysynaptic pathways in spinal cord, subcortical centers, and brainstem, and possibly by sedative effect. Not effective for spastic or dyskinetic CNS disorders, e.g., cerebral palsy.

Used in symptomatic treatment of muscle spasm and pain associated with various musculoskeletal conditions. Commercially available in combination with acetaminophen (e.g., Chlorzoxazone with APAP, Chlorofon-F, Chlorzone Forte, Flexaphen, Flexin, Lobac, Paracet Forte, Parachlor, Parafon Forte, Polyflex, Zoxaphen).

ABSORPTION AND FATE. Readily absorbed. Onset of action usually within 1 hour; duration approximately 6 hours. Peak levels in about 3 to 4 hours. Half-life: approximately 66 minutes. Rapidly and extensively metabolized in liver; excreted in urine mainly as glucuronide conjugates. Distribution to placenta and into milk not established.

CONTRAINDICATIONS AND PRECAUTIONS. Impaired liver function. Safe use during pregnancy or in women of childbearing potential not established. *Cautious Use:* patients with known allergies or history of drug allergies; history of liver disease; elderly patients.

ADVERSE/SIDE EFFECTS. CNS: drowsiness, dizziness, lightheadedness, headache, malaise, overstimulation; amnesia, paresthesias (rare). **GI:** anorexia, heartburn, nausea, vomiting, constipation, diarrhea, abdominal pain, GI bleeding (rare). **Hematologic** (rare): granulocytopenia, anemia. **Hypersensitivity:** erythema, rash, pruritus, urticaria, petechiae, ecchymoses, angioneurotic edema, anaphylaxis. **Other:** hepatotoxicity: jaundice, liver damage (causal relationship not established).

ROUTE AND DOSAGE. Oral: Adults: 250 to 500 mg three or four times daily. If response is not adequate, dosage may be increased to 750 mg three or four times daily and reduced as improvement occurs. **Children:** 20 mg/kg/day in three or four divided doses or 125 to 500 mg three or four times a day, given according to age and weight.

NURSING IMPLICATIONS

May be taken with food or meals to prevent gastric distress. If necessary, tablet may be crushed and mixed with food or liquid, e.g., milk, fruit juice.

Since sedation, drowsiness, and dizziness may occur, advise patient not to undertake activities requiring mental alertness, judgment, and physical coordination until reaction to drug is known.

Some patients may require supervision of ambulation during early drug therapy.

Advise patient to check with physician before taking an OTC depressant (e.g., antihistamine, sedative, sleep medicine, alcohol) since effects may be additive.

Inform patient that drug metabolite may cause orange or purplish-red discoloration of urine and that it is of no clinical significance.

Drug should be discontinued if signs of hypersensitivity occur or if signs of liver dysfunction appear (dark urine, yellow sclerae or skin, pruritus).

Chlorzoxazone is used as an adjunct to rest and physical therapy.

Store in tight container preferably between 15° and 30°C (59° and 86°F) unless otherwise directed by manufacturer.

PROTOTYPE

CHOLESTYRAMINE RESIN

(Questran)

(koe-less-tir'a-meen)

Resin exchange agent (anion)
Bile acid sequestrant
Antilipemic

ACTIONS AND USES. Quaternary ammonium anion-exchange resin used for its cholesterol-lowering effect. Adsorbs and combines with intestinal bile acids in exchange for chloride ions to form an insoluble, nonabsorbable complex that is excreted in the feces. As a result, bile salts are continually (but not entirely) prevented from reentry to the enterohepatic circulation. Increased fecal loss of bile acids leads to lowered serum total cholesterol by decrease in low density lipoprotein (LDL) cholesterol and in reduction of bile acid deposit in dermal tissues. LDL is the main component of serum cholesterol and reportedly is involved in development of atherosclerosis. Serum triglyceride levels may increase or remain unchanged. Effectiveness of cholestyramine in patients with cholestatic pruritus is based on the assumption that it is the result of bile acid deposits in the skin. Sequestration of bile acids may interfere with absorption of calcium, dietary fat, and fat soluble vitamins A, D, and K. As an anion-exchange resin, cholestyramine may have a strong affinity for selected drugs given concomitantly.

Used primarily for relief of pruritus associated with partial biliary stasis, chronic renal failure, and polycythemia vera; as adjunct to diet therapy in management of primary hypercholesterolemia (type IIa and type IIb hyperlipoproteinemia) and to reduce the risk of atherosclerotic coronary artery disease and myocardial infarction. Also used in treatment of medication overdoses (particularly digitalis toxicity). *Unlabeled Uses:* to control diarrhea caused by excess bile acids in colon, as in hyperoxaluria, pseudomembranous colitis, erythroprotoporphyria; and for reducing half-life of the pesticide chlordecone in cases of poisoning and as adjunct in treatment of cardiac glycoside toxicity.

ABSORPTION AND FATE. Not absorbed from GI tract. Excreted in feces as insoluble complex.

CONTRAINDICATIONS AND PRECAUTIONS. Complete biliary obstruction, hypersensitivity to bile acid sequestrants. Safe use by pregnant women, nursing mothers, and children not established. *Cautious Use:* osteoporosis, impaired renal function, bleeding disorders, coronary artery disease, hemorrhoids, impaired GI function, peptic ulcer malabsorption states (e.g., steatorrhea), the elderly.

ADVERSE/SIDE EFFECTS. CNS: headache, anxiety, dizziness, fatigue, tinnitus, syncope, drowsiness, femoral nerve pain, paresthesia. **CV:** claudication, arteritis, thrombophlebitis, myocardial infarction, angina. **GI:** constipation (may be severe); fecal impaction, hemorrhoids, abdominal pain and distention, flatulence, bloating sensation, belching, nausea, vomiting, heartburn, anorexia, diarrhea, steatorrhea. The following have been reported but causal relationship not established: dysphagia, hiccoughs, sour taste, pancreatitis, diverticulitis, peptic ulcer, cholecystitis, cholelithiasis, black stools, rectal pain, hemorrhoidal bleeding. **Hypersensitivity:** urticaria, dermatitis, asthma, shortness of breath. **Musculoskeletal:** backache, muscle and joint pains, arthritis, osteoporosis. **Ophthalmic:** arcus juvenitis, uveitis. **Renal:** hematuria, dysuria, burnt odor to urine, diuresis. **Other:** xanthoma of hands and fingers, weight loss or gain, increased libido, swollen glands, edema, gingival bleeding, vitamin A, D, and K deficiencies, hypoprothrombinemia, hyperchloremic acidosis, decreased erythrocyte folate levels, rash, irritations of skin, tongue, and perianal areas.

ROUTE AND DOSAGE. Oral: Adult: Initial: 4 Gm three or four times daily before meals and at bedtime. Maintenance: 4 Gm daily in one dose or divided in three to four doses. *Pruritus:* up to 16 Gm/day. *Hyperlipoproteinemia:* up to 32 Gm/day. **Children (6 to 12 years):** 80 mg/kg 3 times/day; **(12 years and older):** adult dose. Each 9-Gm packet or scoopful contains 4 Gm of anhydrous cholestyramine.

NURSING IMPLICATIONS

A trial of diet therapy, exercise, and weight reduction is usually instituted before starting resin treatment.

Place contents of one packet or one level scoopful on surface of 2 to 6 ounces of the preferred liquid. Permit drug to hydrate by standing without stirring 1 to 2 minutes, twirling glass occasionally; then stir until suspension is uniform. A shaker may help. After ingestion of preparation, rinse glass with small amount liquid and have patient drink remainder to ensure taking entire dose. Administer before meals.

Water, highly flavored liquids, or other noncarbonated drinks, thin soups, pulpy fruits with high moisture content (applesauce, crushed pineapple) disguise the taste somewhat.

Always dissolve cholestyramine before administration; it is irritating to mucous membranes and may cause esophageal impaction if administered in dry form.

Cholestyramine color may vary with different batches but this does not affect drug action. Has a slight aminelike odor and a disagreeable taste; in solution its consistency is sandy or gritty.

Baseline serum cholesterol and triglyceride levels will be established at beginning of therapy and periodically evaluated to insure that desired levels are maintained. (Normal serum cholesterol: 120 to 220 mg/dl; triglyceride: 40 to 150 mg/dl.) Also, baseline and periodic determinations of serum electrolytes and hematologic studies should be made.

Serum cholesterol levels in hyperlipoproteinemia are reduced within 24 to 48 hours after treatment starts and may continue to decline for a year. After withdrawal of cholestyramine, cholesterol levels usually return to baseline level in about 2 to 4 weeks.

If response is unsatisfactory after 3 months of treatment drug is usually withdrawn. (Exception: treatment of xanthoma tuberosum which is continued as long as size and number of xanthomata decrease.)

Periodic erythrocyte folate levels are recommended, particularly in children.

Hyperchloremic acidosis (result of chloride liberation by cholestyramine) occurs most frequently in children and in adults receiving high doses. Serum levels should be monitored.

Supplemental water-miscible or parenteral vitamins A and D and folic acid may be required by patient on long-term therapy with cholestyramine.

Adjunctives to drug therapy for pruritus include: adequate fluid intake, use of mild soaps, and soft absorbent clothing, high ambient humidity, even room temperature. Relief of pruritus is an individual response, but therapy is usually continued at least 3 weeks before final evaluation. With improvement, dosage is lowered. Withdrawal of drug may result in return of pruritus within 1 to 2 weeks. (Cholestyramine effect on serum cholesterol of these patients varies considerably.)

With daily dosage higher than 24 Gm, side effects increase.

Preexisting constipation should be evaluated before starting treatment since it may be worsened by the drug, particularly in elderly patients, women, and when dose is high (more than 24 Gm/day). Instruct patient to report change in normal bowel elimination pattern promptly to physician.

If constipation becomes a problem, dosage may be lowered or temporarily interrupted. A stool softener is frequently ordered, especially if patient has heart disease or if hemorrhoids develop. Occasionally this side effect necessitates withdrawal of the drug.

High bulk diet (bran and other grains, fruit, raw vegetables) with adequate fluid intake is an essential adjunct to cholestyramine treatment and generally resolves the problems of constipation and bloating sensation. Collaborate with physician and dietitian.

Chronic use can cause increased bleeding tendency. Patient should be alert to early symptoms of hypoprothrombinemia (petechiae, ecchymoses, abnormal bleeding from mucous membranes, tarry stools) and report their occurrence promptly. Usually, parenteral vitamin K will reverse the symptoms. Oral vitamin K may be administered subsequently as a prophylactic.

The patient should completely understand the dose and drug schedule established for him or her when leaving direct medical supervision.

Warn patient not to omit doses. Sudden withdrawal of cholestyramine can promote uninhibited absorption of other drugs taken concomitantly leading to toxicity or overdosage.

Warn patient not to change dosage or dose intervals, or to stop taking medication even though it may be distasteful, without the physician's approval. Usually GI side effects subside after the first month of drug therapy. Distress following fat ingestion is apt to occur especially when the patient is on large cholestyramine doses.

Food–Drug Interactions:

- Diets for type IIa, IIb hyperlipoproteinemia usually low in cholesterol, high in polyunsaturated fat and low in saturated fat. Collaborate with dietitian in making out a dietary teaching plan.
- Foods with high cholesterol content include: egg yolk, turkey (dark meat and skin), gravies, organ meats, crab meat, shrimp, sardines, caviar, custard, cream, butter, cakes, pies, lady fingers, waffles. There is no cholesterol in plant foods such as fruits, vegetables, nuts, grains, cereals.
- Many foods high in cholesterol are also high in saturated fats: most animal products (including meats, dairy products, eggs, ice cream, cheese), solid and hydrogenated shortenings (lard, coconut oil, cocoa butter, palm oil, non-dairy cream substitutes).
- A controlled amount of polyunsaturated fats are usually allowed because they help to eliminate newly-formed cholesterol. Polyunsaturated fats are found in liquid vegetable oils e.g., safflower, sunflower, corn soybean, cottonseed, (olive oil and peanut oil are rich in monounsaturated fats. They neither raise nor lower serum cholesterol).

Patients with hypercholesterolemia should attempt to eliminate or at least alter risk factors such as smoking, obesity, faulty dietary habits, excessive alcohol intake, and sedentary lifestyle.

Warn patient to avoid self-medication with OTC drugs unless physician approves. Consult physician about use of alcohol; it may be restricted because it increases triglycerides.

The following symptoms may be drug-induced and should be reported promptly: severe gastric distress with nausea and vomiting (pancreatitis); unusual weight loss (steatorrhea, malabsorption); black stools, hemorrhoids; sudden back pain (osteoporosis—especially in postmenopausal women not on estrogens); sore throat, fever (agranulocytosis).

Questran contains tartrazine which can cause an allergic reaction (including bronchial asthma) in susceptible individuals. Frequently such persons are also sensitive to aspirin.

Store in tightly closed container at temperature between 15° and 30°C (59° and 86°F) unless otherwise specified by manufacturer.

Diagnostic Test Interferences. Cholestyramine therapy may be accompanied by increased serum **SGOT, phosphorus, chloride,** and **alkaline phosphatase** levels; decreased **serum calcium, sodium,** and **potassium** levels.

Drug Interactions. Cholestyramine may delay or decrease absorption of other oral drugs and thus reduce their effects. Therefore, as a general rule, **other medications should be administered at least 1 hour before or 4 to 6 hours after cholestyramine.** When cholestyramine is to be discontinued in patients taking potentially toxic drugs, monitor for toxicity. If possible concomitant administration with **warfarin** and other **oral anticoagulants** is avoided. If not, administer at least 6 hours apart and closely monitor anticoagulant response. Patients receiving **digitalis glycosides** should be monitored for underdigitalization; when cholestyramine is to be discontinued, monitor for digitalis toxicity.

CHOLINE SALICYLATE

(Arthropan)

(koe'leen)
Nonnarcotic analgesic
NSAID
Antirheumatic
Salicylate

ACTIONS AND USES. Choline salt of salicylic acid available commercially as a liquid salicylate preparation. Reported to be less potent than aspirin as an analgesic, antiinflammatory, and antipyretic, and produces less gastric irritation and bleeding. Clinical significance of the claim that it is absorbed more rapidly than aspirin is unclear. Unlike aspirin, believed to have no appreciable effect on platelet function.

Used as analgesic and antiinflammatory in rheumatoid arthritis, rheumatic fever, osteoarthritis, and other conditions for which oral salicylates are usually recommended. May be indicated for patients who have difficulty swallowing tablets or capsules or as an alternative preparation for patients who show gastric intolerance to aspirin or who should avoid sodium-containing salicylates. Available commercially in combination with magnesium salicylate, e.g., Trilisate.

ABSORPTION AND FATE. Rapidly absorbed from GI tract; peak blood levels occur in 10 to 30 minutes. Blood salicylate levels are higher and achieved more quickly than with comparable doses of aspirin in tablet form. Distribution and fate as for aspirin (qv).

CONTRAINDICATIONS AND PRECAUTIONS. Salicylate hypersensitivity. *See also Aspirin.*

ADVERSE/SIDE EFFECTS. Nausea, vomiting. *High doses:* tinnitus, deafness, dizziness, sweating, mental confusion, hyperventilation; hepatotoxicity. *See also Aspirin.*

ROUTE AND DOSAGE. Oral: Adults: 5 ml (870 mg) repeated every 3 to 4 hours as needed, but no more than six times/day. Each 5 ml (teaspoonful) contains 870 mg; equivalent to 650 mg (10 grains) of aspirin. *For arthritis:* 1 to 2 tsp up to four times a day. **Pediatric: (3 to 6 years):** 105 to 210 mg every 4 hours; **(6 to 12 years):** 210 to 420 mg every 4 hours.

NURSING IMPLICATIONS

Although the preparation is mint flavored, the taste is objectionable to some patients. May be mixed with or followed by fruit juice, a carbonated beverage, or water. Do not administer with an antacid.

If patient requires an antacid, administer choline salicylate prior to meals and the antacid 2 hours after meals.

Available OTC. Caution patient not to exceed recommended dosage and to keep medicine out of the reach of children.

Avoid concurrent use of other drugs containing aspirin or salicylates unless otherwise advised by physician.

Solutions of choline salicylate are stable at room temperature.

Store in tightly capped container at temperature between 15° and 30°C (59° and 86°F). Protect from freezing.

See Aspirin (prototype salicylate).

C

CHORIONIC GONADOTROPIN

(go-nad'oh-troe-pin)

(Android HCG, Antuitrin, A.P.L., Chorex, Corgonject-5, Follutein, Glukor, Gonic, Libigen, Pregnyl, Profasi HP)

Ovarian stimulant
Gonadotropin

ACTIONS AND USES. Human chorionic gonadotropin (HCG), a polypeptide hormone produced by the placenta and extracted from urine during first trimester of pregnancy with actions nearly identical to those of pituitary luteinizing hormone (LH). Promotes production of gonadal steroid hormones by stimulating interstitial cells of the testes (Leydig cells) to produce androgen, and the corpus luteum of the ovary to produce progesterone. Androgen stimulation in the male results in development of secondary sex characteristics and may cause testicular descent if there is no anatomic impediment; descent is usually reversible with termination of HCG therapy. Administration of HCG to women of child-bearing age with normal functioning ovaries causes maturation of the ovarian follicle and triggers ovulation. When given during normal pregnancy, it maintains corpus luteum after LH decreases, supports continuing secretion of estrogen and progesterone, and prevents ovulation. HCG has no known effect on fat metabolism, appetite, sense of hunger, or body fat distribution.

Used in treatment of prepubertal cryptorchidism not due to anatomic obstruction and male hypogonadism secondary to pituitary deficiency. Also used in conjunction with menotropins to induce ovulation and pregnancy in infertile women in whom the cause of anovulation is secondary.

ABSORPTION AND FATE. Peak blood levels within 6 hours following IM administration. Distributed mainly to sex organs and to kidney. Biphasic half-life: 11 hours to 23 hours. About 10 to 15% of dose excreted in urine in 24 hours; remainder eliminated within 3 to 4 days.

CONTRAINDICATIONS AND PRECAUTIONS. Known hypersensitivity to HCG, hypogonadism of testicular origin, hypertrophy or tumor of pituitary, prostatic carcinoma or other androgen-dependent neoplasms, precocious puberty. *Cautious Use:* epilepsy, migraine, asthma, cardiac or renal disease.

ADVERSE/SIDE EFFECTS. Headache, irritability, restlessness, depression, fatigue, gynecomastia, edema, precocious puberty, pain at injection site, increased urinary steroid excretion, ectopic pregnancy (incidence low). When used with menotropins (HMG): ovarian hyperstimulation: ascites with or without pain, pleural effusion, ruptured ovarian cysts with resultant hemoperitoneum, multiple births; arterial thromboembolism.

ROUTE AND DOSAGE. Highly individualized. Various regimens have been suggested e.g.: **Intramuscular:** *Prepubertal cryptorchidism:* 4000 USP units three times weekly for 3 weeks; or 5000 USP units every second day for 4 injections; or 15 injections of 500 to 1000 USP units over 6 weeks; or 500 to 1000 USP units three times weekly for 4 to 6 weeks. *Hypogonadotropic hypogonadism* in males: 500 to 1000 USP units three times/week for 3 weeks followed by same dose twice a week for 3 weeks; or 4000 USP units three times weekly for 6 to 9 months then 2000 USP units 3 times weekly for additional 3 months. *Induction of ovulation and pregnancy:* 5000 to 10,000 USP units one day following last dose of menotropins (qv).

NURSING IMPLICATIONS

HCG is given to the anovulatory patient only after failure to respond to therapy with clomiphene citrate.

Following reconstitution (diluent furnished by manufacturer), solution is stable 2 months when refrigerated; thereafter potency decreases.

When used for treatment of infertility, timing of coitus is important. Daily intercourse is encouraged from day before HCG is given until ovulation.

Be alert to signs of fluid retention; increase in weight, tight rings, shoes, or gloves, edema in dependent areas. A weight chart should be maintained for a bi-weekly record. Report to physician if weight gain is associated with edema to permit review of dosage regimen.

Treatment for prepubertal cryptorchidism is usually started between ages of 4 and 9. HCG can help predict whether or not orchidopexy will be needed in the future.

Induction of androgen secretion by HCG may induce precocious puberty in patient treated for cryptorchidism. Instruct parent to report to physician if the following appear: axillary, facial, pubic hair, penile growth, acne, deepening of voice.

Instruct patient to report promptly onset of abdominal pain and distention (ovarian hyperstimulation syndrome).

There is no substantial evidence that this drug is an effective adjunctive agent in the treatment of obesity.

Although the risk of ectopic pregnancy is low, be alert to symptoms that are usually clinically evident between 8 and 12 weeks of gestation: pain on affected side or referred to shoulder, irregular hemorrhage, shocklike signs, pallor, dizziness, weak pulse, tenderness on vaginal examination. Termination of ectopic pregnancy may be spontaneous by rupture into the peritoneal cavity or by abortion.

Vaginal bleeding during treatment of corpus luteum deficiency should be reported; drug will be discontinued.

CHYMOPAPAIN

(kye'moe-pa-pane)

(Chymodiactin, Discase)

Enzyme

ACTIONS AND USES. Proteolytic enzyme isolated from crude latex of papaya (Carica papaya) with molecular weight of approximately 27,000. When injected into the herniated nucleus palposus, causes solubilization of protein core of the chondromucoprotein. Net effect is reduction in intradiskal osmotic pressure, with resulting decrease in fluid absorption and accumulation and, ultimately, intradiskal pressure.

Used as chemonucleolytic agent as an alternative to surgery in patients with documented herniated lumbar intervertebral disks who have not responded to adequate trial(s) of conservative therapy.

ABSORPTION AND FATE. Detectable in plasma in low levels within 30 minutes following intradiskal administration. Rapidly inactivated in plasma. Small portions detected in urine.

CONTRAINDICATIONS AND PRECAUTIONS. Hypersensitivity to papaya, chymopapain, and other papaya derivatives; use in patients who had: previous injection of chymopapain or surgical treatment for the spinal disorder; use for spinal regions other than lumbar, severe spondylolisthesis, progressing paralysis or neurologic dysfunction; spinal cord or cauda equina lesion, intrathecal administration. Safe use during pregnancy (category C) and in children not established.

ADVERSE/SIDE EFFECTS. GI: nausea, paralytic ileus (rare). **Hypersensitivity:** erythema, piloerection, rash, pruritus, urticaria, vasomotor rhinitis, angioedema, conjunctivitis, GI disturbances; anaphylaxis: bronchospasm, laryngeal edema, arrhythmias, cardiac arrest, coma, death. **Neuromuscular:** back pain, stiffness, soreness, back spasms, sacral burning, paresthesias (tingling and numbness of legs and toes), lessened sensitivity to pain (hypalgesia), leg weakness, cramping in both calves, pain in opposite leg, foot drop (rare); acute transverse myelitis/myelopathy with paraplegia, and paraparesis (causal relationship not established); cerebral hemorrhage. **Other:** headache, dizziness, urinary retention, transient increases in urinary mucopolysaccharides.

C

ROUTE AND DOSAGE. Intradiskal: 2000 to 4000 U (preferably 3000 U) per disk. Maximum cumulative dose not to exceed 10,000 U. A single injection is made into each disk after needle is properly positioned as verified by image intensifier and diskography. At least 15 minutes must elapse between diskography and chymopapain administration to allow for dispersion and absorption of contrast medium. Manufacturer advises not to use automatic filling syringes since there is residual vacuum in vial as result of manufacturing process.

NURSING IMPLICATIONS

Only used in hospital settings by physicians with extensive training and experience in the diagnosis and management of spinal disorders, and who have had specialized training in the use of chymopapain.

Careful patient selection for the procedure and firm documentation of a herniated disk are mandatory.

Pretreatment laboratory work-up should include erythrocyte sedimentation rate (ESR), particularly in women.

Since chymopapain is a foreign protein, candidates for therapy should be carefully questioned about allergies, especially to papaya or its derivatives, and about history of any previous chymopapain injection. Also question patient about hypersensitivity to iodine or to contract media which must be used during myelography or diskography.

Papain is widely used as a meat tenderizer (Adolph's Meat Tenderizer) and in the processing of beer. It is also found in debriding ointments, digestive aids, and enzyme treatment for soft contact lenses. Therefore a large part of the U.S. population has probably developed sensitivity to papain.

In the period immediately following drug administration, patient must be monitored closely for anaphylactic reaction. The reaction may be immediate within 1 to 20 minutes lasting for minutes, or delayed (up to 1 hour, and lasting several hours or longer). Patients should be informed that delayed reactions have occurred as late as 15 days postinjection.

Anaphylaxis appears to occur ten times more frequently in female patients, particularly those with erythrocyte sedimentation rates greater than 20 mm/hour (normal: 0 to 20 mm/hour).

Monitor vital signs. Anticipate the possibility of anaphylaxis, e.g., signs of respiratory distress such as hoarseness, wheezing (bronchospasm), progressing to stridor (laryngeal edema). Also be alert to arrhythmias and signs of shock.

Have on hand epinephrine, antihistamine, equipment for intubation or tracheotomy, suction, oxygen, and have in place a free-flowing IV infusion. Some clinicians prefer to pretreat their patients with an antihistamine or with hydrocortisone and to use local rather than general anesthesia to reduce risk of anaphylaxis.

To allay anxiety, inform patient of the possibility of neuromuscular symptoms after drug administration. Back pain, stiffness, and soreness occur in 50% and back spasm in 30% of patients and may last for several days. Rarely, residual stiffness and soreness may persist for several weeks. Observe neuromuscular function and notify physician of any abnormalities.

Acute transverse myelitis/myelopathy with paraplegia or paraparesis has occurred 2 or 3 weeks after drug administration in 1 out of 18,000 patients. A causal relationship has not been established, but it appears to happen in patients receiving injections for two or more disks following diskography.

To reconstitute, cleanse top of vial stopper with alcohol. Allow alcohol to evaporate before inserting needle into vial. To produce solution containing 2000 U/ml, 5 ml of water for injection is added to vial containing 10,000 U of chymopapain.

Use care in selecting proper needle size and in introducing needle into vial, to reduce possibility of coring the stopper.

Following reconstitution with sterile water for injection, chymopapain solutions are enzymatically stable for 1 hour. Since solutions contain no preservative, they should be used within 1 hour. Discard unused portions.
Do not use bacteriostatic water for injection for reconstitution since it may inactivate chymopapain. Alcohol also inactivates chymopapain.
Solutions should be inspected for particulate matter and discoloration prior to administration.
Store in refrigerator at 2° to 8°C (36° to 46°F) until ready to be reconstituted, unless otherwise directed by manufacturer. Powder should not be exposed to temperatures above 54.4°C for longer than 48 hours.

C

Drug Interactions: Chymopapain

Plus	Interactions
Halothane	Risk of arrhythmias with epinephrine. Epinephrine may be necessary for treatment of chymopapain-induced anaphylaxis. Concomitant use of halothane and chymopapain generally avoided for this reason

---

CICLOPIROX OLAMINE

(Ciclopirox Ethanolamine, Loprox)

(sye-kloe-peer'ox)
Antiinfective
Antibiotic
Antifungal

ACTIONS AND USES. Synthetic broad spectrum antifungal agent with activity against pathogenic fungi including dermatophytes, yeasts, and *Malassezia furfur,* some species of *Mycoplasma* and *Trichomonas vaginalis,* and certain strains of gram-positive and gram-negative bacteria. Acts by inhibiting transport of essential elements within fungal cell, thereby interfering with synthesis of protein, RNA, and DNA.

Used topically for treatment of tinea cruris and tinea corporis (ringworm) due to *Trichophyton rubrum, T. mentagrophytes, Epidermophyton floccosum,* and *Microsporum canis,* and for tinea (pityriasis) versicolor due to *Malassezia furfur.* Also used for cutaneous candidiasis (moniliasis) caused by *Candida albicans.*

ABSORPTION AND FATE. Minimal amounts absorbed through intact skin. Following application, distributed to epidermis, corium, (dermis) including hair and hair follicles, and sebaceous glands. Half-life: 1.7 hours; 94 to 98% protein bound. Most of systemically absorbed drug is excreted, primarily by kidney, within 8 hours after drug application. Negligible amounts eliminated in feces. Distribution to placenta or to breast milk not known.

CONTRAINDICATIONS AND PRECAUTIONS. Hypersensitivity to ciclopirox olamine or to any excipients in the formulation. Safe use during pregnancy (category B) and in children younger than 10 years not established. *Cautious Use:* nursing women.

ADVERSE/SIDE EFFECTS. (Generally well tolerated) Pruritus, burning, worsening of clinical condition. Contact sensitization not reported.

ROUTE AND DOSAGE. Topical (1% cream in water-miscible base): Gently massage cream into affected area and surrounding skin twice daily, morning and evening.

C

NURSING IMPLICATIONS

Instruct patient to use medication for the prescribed time even though symptoms improve.

Wash hands thoroughly before and after treatments.

Ask physician about specific procedure for cleansing the skin before medication is applied. Some clinicians prefer plain tap water, others recommend normal saline or washing with mild soap followed by thorough rinsing. Regardless of method used, dry skin thoroughly before drug application.

Advise patient to report skin irritation or other possible signs of sensitization: redness, swelling, burning or unusual discomfort, itching, blistering, oozing. A reaction suggestive of sensitization warrants drug discontinuation.

Caution patient not to use occlusive dressings or wrappings.

Warn patient to avoid contact of drug in or near the eyes.

In general, tinea versicolor responds to drug treatment in about 2 weeks. Tinea pedis ("athlete's foot"), tinea corporis (ringworm), tinea cruris ("jock itch"), and candidiasis (moniliasis) require about 4 weeks of therapy. If clinical improvement does not occur within time periods stated, diagnosis should be reevaluated.

Patient-Teaching Points Related to Antifungal Therapy:

- ✓ Inform patient that fungal infections are transmitted by direct and indirect contact.
- ✓ Fungi thrive best under conditions that favor a warm, moist, environment, e.g., hot humid weather, profuse sweating, prolonged wearing of wet bathing suit, prolonged contact with wool, nylon, or other synthetic fiber, tight nylon undergarments, or tight jeans.
- ✓ Advise patient to keep linen, towels, facecloths, and other articles of personal hygiene, clothing (including sports equipment) separate.
- ✓ Wash anything that has contacted affected area(s) after each treatment. Launder clothing and other contaminated linen daily in hot water and nonirritating soap or detergent.
- ✓ Wear light clothing and footwear that will allow ventilation. Loose-fitting cotton underwear or socks are ideal. For tinea pedis ("athlete's foot"), advise patient to wear leather shoes or sandals without rubber soles, and to alternate shoes and change socks daily.
- ✓ Emphasize importance of cleanliness and keeping skin clean and dry.

Be mindful of the possibility that resistant candidiasis may be a presenting sign of unrecognized diabetes mellitus. Also, recurrences are especially likely to occur in patients with diabetes or other predisposing illnesses.

Store preferably at 15° to 30°C (59° to 86°F), unless otherwise directed by manufacturer.

PROTOTYPE

CIMETIDINE

(Apo-Cimetidine, Novo-Cimetine, Peptol, Tagamet)

(sye-met′i-deen)
Antihistamine
H_2-receptor antagonist

ACTIONS AND USES. An imidazole derivative structurally similar to histamine. Belongs chemically to antihistamine group, but unlike classical antihistamines, e.g., chorpheniramine (Chlor-Trimeton) which block histamine at H_1 receptors, cimetidine competitively inhibits histamine at H_2 receptor sites on parietal cells. Reduces volume and hydrogen ion concentration of gastric acid secretion in the nocturnal basal (fasting) state and also when stimulated by food, caffeine, histamine, insulin, pentagastrin, and bethanechol. Demonstrates weak antiandrogenic action and some antiviral activity.

Used for short-term treatment of active duodenal ulcer, prophylaxis against duodenal ulcer recurrence, and in treatment of pathologic hypersecretory conditions (Zollinger-Ellison syndrome, systemic mastocytosis, and multiple endocrine adenomas). *Investigational Use:* treatment of gastric ulcer, stress ulcers, upper GI bleeding, pancreatic insufficiency, short-bowel syndrome, reflux esophagitis, herpes zoster, and to abort herpes labialis.

ABSORPTION AND FATE. About 70% absorbed from GI tract following oral administration. Blood concentrations peak in 1 to 1.5 hours. In fasting state gastric output is reduced about 90% for 4 hours; with food, output is reduced 66% for around 3 hours. Distributed widely to most tissues; passes blood–brain barrier in high doses. About 15 to 23% bound to plasma proteins. Half-life ranges from 1.5 to 2 hours (longer in patients with impaired renal function). Metabolized in liver. Most of drug eliminated within 24 hours, primarily in urine; approximately 40 to 60% of oral drug and 77% of parenteral drug excreted unchanged. Some excretion in bile and feces. Crosses placenta. Excreted in breast milk.

CONTRAINDICATIONS AND PRECAUTIONS. Safe use in women with childbearing potential, in nursing mothers, or during pregnancy, or in children younger than 16 years not determined. *Cautious Use:* elderly or critically ill patients; impaired renal or hepatic function; organic brain syndrome.

ADVERSE/SIDE EFFECTS. Most frequently reported: headache, tiredness, diarrhea, constipation, dizziness, rash, muscle pain, mild gynecomastia. **Cardiac:** bradycardia and other arrhythmias. **CNS:** dizziness, lightheadedness, headache, confusion, restlessness, disorientation, paranoid psychosis, focal twitching or tremor, ataxia, diplopia, transient apnea, seizures. **GI:** diarrhea or constipation, abdominal discomfort, paralytic ileus. **Hematologic:** increased prothrombin time; rare: neutropenia, leukopenia, agranulocytosis, thrombocytopenia, autoimmune hemolytic or aplastic anemia. **Hypersensitivity:** facial edema, rash, urticaria, Stevens-Johnson syndrome, exfoliative dermatitis, dyspnea, laryngospasm. **Reproductive:** gynecomastia (males), galactorrhea (females), impotence. **Other:** alopecia, profuse sweating, flushing, fever, interstitial nephritis (rare), slight increase in serum uric acid, transient pain at IM site. **Overdosage:** tachycardia, respiratory failure.

ROUTE AND DOSAGE. Adults: Oral: 300 mg four times a day and at bedtime. **Intramuscular, intravenous** (cimetidine hydrochloride): 300 mg every 6 hours. (No dilution necessary for IM.) **Direct intravenous injection:** Dilute dose in 0.9% sodium chloride injection or other compatible IV solution to total volume of 20 ml and inject over 1 to 2 minutes. **Intermittent intravenous infusion:** Dilute dose in 100 ml of 5% dextrose injection or other compatible diluent and infuse over 15 to 20 minutes. Daily dosage not to exceed 2400 mg. Patients with impaired renal function: 300 mg every 12 hours (oral or IV). If required, increase frequency to every 8 hours with caution. *Prophylaxis:* **Oral:** 400 mg at bedtime. Hemodialysis reduces cimetidine blood levels; adjust dosing schedule to permit dose at end of hemodialysis. **Pediatric:** doses of 20 to 40 mg/kg/day in divided doses at 6-hour intervals have been used, but risk-benefit must be carefully weighed.

NURSING IMPLICATIONS

Taken with or immediately after meals. Food delays absorption and thus prolongs drug effect; also peak blood level of cimetidine will coincide with peak food-induced gastric acid secretion.

Concurrent administration of antacid may be prescribed to control acute ulcer pain. Administer at least 1 hour before or 1 hour after cimetidine.

Oral administration is substituted for IV therapy when bleeding has been controlled for at least 48 hours.

Gastric pH may be determined periodically during therapy. Ideally dosage is adjusted to maintain an intragastric pH greater than 5.

C

Monitor intake and output particularly in the elderly, severely ill, and in patients with impaired renal function.

Paralytic ileus has been reported in patients who are receiving cimetidine to prevent stress ulcers. Report loss of bowel sounds, absence of bowel movement or flatus, vomiting, crampy pain, abdominal distention.

Periodic evaluations of blood count, renal and hepatic function are advised during therapy.

Therapy for active duodenal ulcer is continued until healing is demonstrated by endoscopy (usually 4 to 6 weeks, but not to exceed 8 weeks).

Advise patient to keep clinician informed of any unusual symptoms and the effect of drug therapy.

Relapse of duodenal ulcer occurs commonly following discontinuation of therapy. Frequency of recurrence is apparently reduced if cimetidine withdrawal is gradual and if a propylactic bedtime dose is given. Instruct patient undergoing withdrawal to report promptly the recurrence of abdominal pain, black stools, or any other suspicious symptom.

Gynecomastia may occur after a month or more of therapy. It may disappear spontaneously or remain throughout therapy. Instruct patient to report this symptom to physician. Adverse reproductive symptoms are most commonly seen in males with Zollinger-Ellison syndrome or other pathologic hypersecretory disorders that require prolonged high dose therapy.

Mental confusion, dizziness, focal twitching, and other CNS symptoms *(See Adverse/Side Effects),* are most likely to occur in the elderly (even with recommended doses), the severely ill, and in patients with impaired renal function. Report immediately; drug should be withdrawn.

Since dizziness, light-headedness, and mental confusion are possible side effects, caution patient to avoid driving and other potentially hazardous activities until reaction to drug is known.

Smoking–Drug Interactions: Research studies show that ulcer recurrence is greater in smokers than in nonsmokers. If abstinence is not possible, advise patient to at least refrain from smoking after taking evening dose of cimetidine to prevent interfering with drug control of nocturnal gastric acid secretion (contributes to more rapid ulcer healing).

Food–Drug Interactions: Although strict dietary control is no longer considered a necessary therapeutic adjunct to the antiulcer drug regimen, the patient should avoid:

- Known food intolerances
- Dietary stimulants of gastric acid secretion (gastric irritants): e.g., caffeine beverages, alcohol, black pepper, harsh spices, excessive intake of high calcium foods and beverages (e.g., milk and milk products), extremely hot/cold foods or liquids, pattern of frequent eating
- Overeating and not chewing food thoroughly before swallowing

Urge patient not to self-dose with OTC antacids, aspirin or aspirin products (ulcerogenic) or other analgesics unless advised to do so by physician.

Parenteral solutions are stable for 48 hours at room temperature when added to commonly used IV solutions for dilution: 0.9% sodium chloride injection, 5% or 10% dextrose injection, lactated Ringer's solution, 5% sodium bicarbonate injection. Follow manufacturer's directions.

Pertinent Patient-Teaching Points:

✓ Impress on patient and responsible family member(s) that duodenal or gastric ulcer is a chronic recurrent condition that requires long-term therapy to avoid relapses.

✓ The patient and responsible family members should receive advice about management of life style in general: e.g., (1) create a relaxed atmosphere at mealtimes; (2) control or avoid anxiety-provoking situations; (3) emphasize the benefits of adequate rest and relaxation and advise curtailment of unnecessary activities during ulcer healing stage; (4) inform patient that ulcers tend to recur in the spring and the fall and therefore particular caution about ulcerogenic factors at these times is prudent.

Store all forms of cimetidine preferably between 15° and 30°C (59° and 86°F) and protected from light unless otherwise directed by manufacturer.

C

Diagnostic Test Interferences. Cimetidine may cause transient increases in **alkaline phosphatase, serum transaminase** levels, and **plasma creatinine.** False-positive **test for gastric bleeding** reported with hemoccult if test is performed within 15 minutes of oral cimetidine administration.

Drug Interactions: Cimetidine

Plus	Interactions
Alcohol (Ethanol)	Ethanol effects may be increased. Patient should be informed of possible reaction
Antacids	Antacids may reduce GI absorption of cimetidine. Administer antacids one hour before or after cimetidine
Antidepressants, tricyclics	Pharmacologic effects of tricyclics may be increased with possibility of toxicity (cimetidine decreases clearance of tricyclics). Dosage adjustments of tricyclics may be required
Anticoagulants, oral	Increased action (hypoprothrombinemia) of anticoagulant. Cimetidine inhibits hepatic metabolism of oral anticoagulants. Concurrent use generally avoided
Carmustine (BiCNU)	Cimetidine may increase carmustine toxicity (bone marrow suppression). Combination avoided if possible
Lidocaine	Increased lidocaine effects with possibility of toxicity (cimetidine reduces renal clearance of lidocaine). Monitor lidocaine plasma levels
Procainamide	Increased procainamide effects with possibility of toxicity (cimetidine reduces renal clearance of procainamide. Monitor plasma levels of procainamide and NAPA (its active metabolite)
Benzodiazepines: alprazolam, chlordiazepoxide, diazepam (Valium), flurazepam, triazolam. Exceptions: lorazepam, oxazepam, temazepam (inactivated by glucuronidation) are not affected Metoprolol (Lopressor), propranolol (Inderal) and possibly other beta-adrenergic blockers metabolized by liver Phenytoin (Dilantin) and other hydantoins Quinidine Theophyllines	By inhibiting hepatic microsomal enzymes, cimetidine impairs metabolism and may lead to toxic accumulation of these drugs. Monitor plasma levels and clinical response when cimetidine is added to, discontinued, or dosage is altered

C

CINOXACIN

(sin-ox'a-sin)

(Cinobac)

Antiinfective (urinary tract)

ACTIONS AND USES. Bactericidal agent with properties similar to those of nalidixic acid (qv) but with fewer side effects. Effective against a wide variety of gram-negative pathogens, particularly most strains of *Escherichia coli, Klebsiella* and *Enterobacter* species, *Proteus mirabilis,* and *P. vulgaris.* Not active against staphylococci, enterococci, or *Pseudomonas.*

Used for treatment of initial and recurrent urinary tract infections caused by susceptible microorganisms.

ABSORPTION AND FATE. Rapidly absorbed following oral administration. Effective urine concentrations maintained for approximately 6 to 8 or more hours. Mean serum half-life: 1.5 hours; 60 to 80% protein bound. About 97% excreted in urine; 60% eliminated unchanged and the remainder as inactive metabolites. Cinoxacin is removed by hemodialysis, but extent is uncertain.

CONTRAINDICATIONS AND PRECAUTIONS. Hypersensitivity to cinoxacin or to nalidixic acid; anuria. Safe use during pregnancy (category B), in nursing mothers, and in children under 12 years not established. *Cautious Use:* impaired renal or hepatic function.

ADVERSE/SIDE EFFECTS. CNS: headache, dizziness, insomnia, tingling sensations. **EENT:** photophobia, tinnitus. **GI:** nausea, vomiting, anorexia, abdominal cramps, diarrhea. **Hypersensitivity:** urticaria, pruritus, rash, edema. **Other:** perineal burning. *See also Nalidixic acid.*

ROUTE AND DOSAGE. Oral: 1 Gm/day divided into 2 to 4 doses, for 7 to 14 days. For patients with impaired renal function: initial: 500 mg; maintenance doses based on creatinine clearance values.

NURSING IMPLICATIONS

Cinoxacin may be taken with food. Although presence of food in stomach may reduce peak serum concentrations, total amount absorbed is not affected.

Susceptibility tests should be performed before start of therapy and during therapy if response is not satisfactory.

Therapeutic effectiveness is enhanced by taking the drug at evenly spaced intervals throughout the 24-hour period so that urinary drug level is maintained.

Advise patient to take drug for the full course of therapy as prescribed.

Instruct patient to report to physician if symptoms do not improve within a few days or if they become worse.

Since cinoxacin may cause dizziness, caution patient to avoid driving and other potentially hazardous tasks until reaction to drug is known.

Photophobia may be relieved by wearing dark glasses.

See also Naladixic acid.

Diagnostic Test Interferences. Cinoxacin may cause elevations of **AST, ALT, alkaline phosphatase, BUN,** and **serum creatinine.**

Drug Interactions: Cinoxacin

Plus	Interactions
Probenecid	Increased half-life and serum concentration of cinoxacin, raising possibility of adverse effects

CISPLATIN

(sis'pla-tin)

(*cis*-DDP, *cis*-platinum II, Platinol)

Antineoplastic

ACTIONS AND USES. Inorganic complex with platinum as central atom surrounded by 2 chloride atoms and 2 ammonia molecules in the *cis* position. Biochemical properties similar to those of bifunctional alkylating agents. Produces interstrand and intrastrand crosslinkage in DNA of rapidly dividing cells, thus preventing DNA, RNA, and protein synthesis. Cell-cycle nonspecific, i.e., effective throughout the entire cell life cycle. Carcinogenicity has not been fully studied, but other compounds with similar action mechanisms and mutogenicity have been reported to be carcinogenic.

Used in established combination therapy (cisplatin, vinblastine, bleomycin) in patient with metastatic testicular tumors and with doxorubicin for metastatic ovarian tumors following appropriate surgical and/or radiation therapy. Has been used in treatment of carcinoma of endometrium, bladder, head, and neck.

ABSORPTION AND FATE. Following IV dose, widely distributed in body with highest concentrations in liver, large and small intestines, and kidneys. Poor penetration into CNS. Plasma levels decline in biphasic pattern: initial phase half-life: 25 to 49 minutes; later phase: 58 to 73 hours up to 10 days. More than 90% bound to plasma proteins. Partly excreted in urine (27 to 43% in 5 days). Platinum may be detected in tissues for 4 months or more after administration.

CONTRAINDICATIONS AND PRECAUTIONS. History of hypersensitivity to cisplatin or other platinum-containing compounds, impaired renal function, myelosuppression, impaired hearing, use of other ototoxic and nephrotoxic drugs, history of gout and urate renal stones. *Cautious Use:* previous cytoxic drug or radiation therapy.

ADVERSE/SIDE EFFECTS. Anaphylactoid reaction: facial edema, wheezing, tachycardia, hypotension, bronchoconstriction. **CNS:** ototoxicity (may be irreversible): tinnitus, bilateral or unilateral hearing loss in high frequency range (4000 to 8000 Hz) deafness; seizures, headache; peripheral neuropathies (may be irreversible): numbness or tingling of fingers, toes, or face; loss of taste. **GI:** marked nausea, vomiting, anorexia, stomatitis, xerostomia, diarrhea, constipation. **Hematologic:** myelosuppression (25 to 30% patients): leukopenia, thrombocytopenia; hemolytic anemia, hemolysis. **Renal** (dose-related cumulative): nephrotoxicity. **Other:** cardiac abnormalities, hyperuricemia, elevated SGOT.

ROUTE AND DOSAGE. Intravenous: *Metastatic testicular tumor* (combination therapy): cisplatin: 20 mg/m^2 for 5 days every 3 weeks for three courses; bleomycin: 30 units weekly (day 2 of each week for 12 consecutive doses); vinblastine: 0.15 to 0.2 mg/kg twice weekly (days 1 and 2) every 3 weeks for four courses (total of 8 doses). *Metastatic ovarian tumor* (combination therapy): cisplatin 50 mg/m^2 once every 3 weeks (day 1); doxorubicin: 50 mg/m^2 once every 3 weeks (day 1). The drugs are administered sequentially. Cisplatin as single agent: 100 mg/m^2 every 4 weeks.

NURSING IMPLICATIONS

Administered only under supervision of a qualified physician experienced in the use of antineoplastics and where adequate diagnostic and treatment facilities are available.

Patient should be closely monitored for dose-related adverse reactions. Since drug action is cumulative, severity of most adverse effects increases with repeated doses.

A single course of therapy is given no more frequently than once every 3 or 4 weeks. A repeat course should not be given until (1) serum creatinine is below 1.5 mg/dl; (2) BUN is below 25 mg/dl; (3) platelets $\geq$ 100,000 mm^3; (4) WBC $\geq$ 4000 mm^3; (5) audiometric test is within normal limits.

C

A pretreatment ECG and cardiac monitoring during induction therapy are indicated because of possible myocarditis or focal irritability.

Eight to 12 hours before the initial dose a Foley catheter is inserted and hydration is started with 1 to 2 liters IV infusion fluid to reduce risk of nephrotoxicity and ototoxicity. Drug is then diluted in 2 L 5% dextrose in one-half or one-third normal saline containing 37.5 Gm mannitol (an osmotic diuretic) and infused over a 6- to 8-hour period. Hydration and forced diuresis are continued for at least 24 hours following drug administration to ensure adequate urinary output.

Monitor urine output and specific gravity for 4 consecutive hours before treatment and for 24 hours after therapy. Report if output is less than 100 ml/hour or if specific gravity is more than 1.030. A urine output of less than 75 ml/hour necessitates medical intervention to avert a renal emergency.

Nephrotoxicity reported in 28 to 36% patients receiving a single dose of 50 mg/m^2 usually occurs in the second week after drug administration and becomes more severe and prolonged with repeated courses of cisplatin.

Advise patient to continue maintenance of adequate hydration (at least 3000 ml/24 hours oral fluid if physician agrees) and to report promptly the symptoms of nephrotoxicity: reduced urinary output, flank pain, anorexia, nausea, vomiting, dry mucosae, itching skin, urine odor on breath, fluid retention (edema of extremities and sacral area).

Intractable nausea and vomiting severe enough to warrant discontinuation of drug usually begin 1 to 4 hours after treatment and may last 24 hours or persist for up to 1 week after treatment is ended.

Usually a parenteral antiemetic agent is administered ½ hour before cisplatin therapy is instituted and given on a scheduled basis throughout day and night as long as necessary.

Although psychological support is always important, do not give false reassurance that vomiting will not occur. Assist the patient to maintain nutrient intake if possible by offering frequent light meals or clear liquids (cold foods are better tolerated than hot foods) and foods of particular interest.

Monitor and report abnormal electrolyte levels: sodium more than 145 or less than 135 mEq/L, and potassium more than 5 or less than 3.5 mEq/L.

The following tests should be done before initiating every course of therapy and repeated each week during treatment period: serum uric acid and creatinine, BUN, urinary creatinine clearance. A decline in creatinine clearance and elevation of other values is indicative of nephrotoxicity.

Liver function should also be checked periodically.

Complete blood and platelet counts are done weekly for 2 weeks following each course of treatment. The nadirs in platelet and leukocyte counts occur between days 18 and 23 (range 7.5 to 45) with most patients recovering in 13 to 62 days. A decrease in hemoglobin (more than 2 Gm/dl) occurs at approximately the same time and with the same frequency.

Check blood pressure, mental status, pupils, and fundi every hour during therapy. Hydration and mannitol may increase blood pressure which, combined with vomiting, increases the danger of elevated intracranial pressure.

Neurologic examinations at regular intervals should include tests of muscle strength, Romberg, vibratory and position sense, tests of sensation. Changes in these parameters may occur not only because of cisplatin but also as associated side effects of vincristine (qv).

Tingling, numbness, and tremors of extremities; loss of position sense and taste; and constipation are early signs of neurotoxicity associated with both cisplatin and vincristine. Warn patient to report their occurrence promptly to prevent irreversibility. Pain with heel walking and difficulty in getting out of bed or chair are late indicators of nerve damage.

Monitor and report abnormal bowel elimination pattern. Constipation and the possibility of fecal impaction may be caused by neurotoxicity; diarrhea may be the response to GI irritation. A laxative for constipation or an antispasmodic (such as diphenoxylate) for diarrhea may be prescribed.

Audiometric testing should be performed prior to the first dose of cisplatin and before each subsequent dose. Ototoxicity, due to destruction of hair cells in organ of corti and reported in 31% of patients, may occur after a single dose of 50 mg/m². Children who receive repeated doses are especially susceptible.

Suspect ototoxicity if patient manifests tinnitus and/or difficulty hearing in the high frequency range (4000 to 8000 Hz). Decreased ability to hear ordinary conversational tones occurs occasionally.

Auscultate breath sounds and assess respiratory status during combination therapy. Pulmonary fibrosis is a serious side effect of bleomycin; fluid accumulation in the lungs may be an adverse effect of cisplatin.

Inspect oral membranes daily for xerostomia, white patches and ulcerations, and tongue for signs of fungal overgrowth (black, furry appearance). Frequent rinses with warm water and avoidance of highly acid fluids and rough foods will decrease irritation.

It is important to alleviate dryness of mouth if possible. Deprivation of saliva hastens demineralization of tooth surfaces and mucosal erosion. Advise patient to carefully clean teeth (with fluoride toothpaste) with soft toothbrush or with moistened gauze over finger to avoid gingival trauma. Daily flossing with waxed floss is also important. Consult physician about use of saliva substitute such as Salivert, or Moi-stir (OTC drugs).

If patient's oral discomfort interferes with eating, report to physician. A swish of lidocaine to anesthetize oral mucosa before eating will provide relief.

Keep vestibular stimulation to the minimum to avoid dizziness or falling: avoid unnecessary turning of patient in bed, and warn ambulating patient to change position gradually and slowly.

Monitor needle puncture wounds and other areas of minor trauma, skin and body excretions for bleeding. Instruct patient to report promptly evidence of unexplained bleeding and easy bruising.

Advise patient to report unexplained fatigue, fever, sore mouth and throat, abnormal body discharges. Because of hematologic side effects of combination therapy, patient is highly susceptible to bacterial infection.

Infection precautions should be instituted promptly if a temperature increase of 0.6°F over the previous reading is noted. Use strict aseptic technique when caring for the patient to prevent superimposed infections.

The patient should be weighed under standard conditions (same time, clothing, scale) every day. A gradual ascending weight profile occurring over a period of several days should be reported.

Anaphylactoid reactions particularly in patient previously exposed to cisplatin may occur within minutes of drug administration. IV epinephrine, antihistamines, corticosteroids, and equipment to maintain respiratory function should be immediately available.

Hyperuricemia may occur 3 to 5 days after doses of cisplatin greater than 50 mg/m². Allopurinol is prescribed to reduce uric acid levels.

Aluminum reacts with cisplatin resulting in possible precipitation and loss of potency. Do not use needles or other equipment composed of aluminum for drug preparation or administration.

Use disposable gloves when preparing cisplatin solutions. If drug accidentally contacts skin or mucosa, wash immediately and thoroughly with soap and water.

Reconstituted drug with sterile water for injection (1 mg/ml dilution) should be clear and

C

colorless. Keep at room temperature; refrigeration will cause a precipitate to form. Since it lacks bacterial preservatives it should be used within 20 hours.
Unless otherwise specified by manufacturer, store unopened vial in refrigerator at 2° to 8°C (36° to 46°F). Stability with proper storage is 2 years. Check expiration date.

Drug Interactions. **Aminoglycoside antibiotics** increase risk of ototoxicity and nephrotoxicity; concurrent use not recommended. **Antigout agents** may require dosage adjustment since cisplatin raises blood uric acid levels. Pharmacologic effects of **phenytoin** (Dilanten) may be decreased.

CLEMASTINE FUMARATE

(Tavist, Tavist-1)

(klem′as-teen)
Antihistamine
H_1-receptor antagonist

ACTIONS AND USES. An ethanolamine derivative antihistamine (H_1-receptor antagonist) with prominent antipruritic activity and low incidence of unpleasant side effects. Anticholinergic effects are weak, and central sedative effects generally mild. Reportedly no more effective than chlorpheniramine for treatment of allergic disorders, but transient drowsiness occurs more frequently with clemastine.

Used for symptomatic relief of allergic rhinitis (sneezing, rhinorrhea, pruritus) and mild uncomplicated allergic skin manifestations such as urticaria and angioedema. Commercially available in combination with phenylpropanolamine (Tavist-D).

ABSORPTION AND FATE. Rapidly and almost completely absorbed from GI tract. Peak antihistaminic effect in 5 to 7 hours; duration of activity 10 to 12 hours or longer. Excreted chiefly in urine.

CONTRAINDICATIONS AND PRECAUTIONS. Hypersensitivity to clemastine or to other antihistamines of similar chemical structure; lower respiratory tract symptoms, including acute asthma; concomitant MAO inhibitor therapy; in children younger than 12 years. Safe use during pregnancy and in nursing mothers not established. *Cautious Use:* history of bronchial asthma, increased intraocular pressure, GI or GU obstruction, hyperthyroidism, cardiovascular disease, hypertension, elderly patients.

ADVERSE/SIDE EFFECTS. CNS: Sedation, transient drowsiness (most common side effects), headache, dizziness, weakness, fatigue, disturbed coordination; less frequent: confusion, restlessness, nervousness, hysteria, convulsions, tremors, irritability, euphoria, insomnia, paresthesias, neuritis. **CV:** hypotension, palpitation, tachycardia, extrasystoles. **GI:** dry mouth, epigastric distress, anorexia, nausea, vomiting, diarrhea, constipation. **GU:** urinary frequency, difficult urination, urinary retention, early menses. **Hematologic:** hemolytic anemia, thrombocytopenia, agranulocytosis. **Hypersensitivity:** urticaria, rash, photosensitivity, anaphylaxis. **Respiratory:** dry nose and throat, thickening of bronchial secretions, tightness of chest, wheezing, nasal stuffiness. **Other:** excess perspiration, chills.

ROUTE AND DOSAGE. Oral: Adults and children (over 12 years): 1.34 mg twice daily to 2.68 mg three times a day. Not to exceed 8.04 mg daily. The 2.68 mg dosage level only is indicated for dermatologic conditions.

C

NURSING IMPLICATIONS

May be administered with food, water, or milk to reduce possibility of gastric irritation.

Advise patient to check with physician before taking alcohol or another CNS depressant, since effects may be additive.

Elderly patients usually require less than average adult dose. Inform the patient that clemastine may make him or her feel less alert and sleepy.

Advise elderly patients to make position changes slowly and in stages, particularly from recumbent to upright posture since they are more likely to experience dizziness and hypotension than younger patients.

Caution patient not to drive and to avoid other potentially hazardous activities until response to the drug has been established.

Inform patient that clemastine should be discontinued about 4 days before skin testing procedures since it may prevent otherwise positive reactions.

Store preferably between 15° and 30°C (59° and 86°F) unless otherwise directed by manufacturer.

See also Diphenhydromine (prototype ethanolamine antihistamine).

CLIDINIUM BROMIDE

(Quarzan)

(kli-di'nee-um)

Anticholinergic (parasympatholytic)
Antimuscarinic
Antispasmodic

ACTIONS AND USES. Synthetic quaternary ammonium compound structurally related to belladonna alkaloids and with similar actions, adverse reactions, and precautions. Anticholinergic activity approximates that of atropine (qv). In common with atropine, exerts antimuscarinic action by competitive antagonism of acetylcholine at postganglionic parasympathetic neuroeffector sites, including smooth muscle and secretory glands, with resulting reduction in GI motility and gastric acid secretion. Unlike atropine, exerts minimal effect on CNS and on eye.

Used as adjunctive therapy in treatment of peptic ulcer. Commercially available in combination with chlordiazepoxide (Librax) for treatment of irritable bowel syndrome.

ABSORPTION AND FATE. Onset of antisecretory action within 1 hour, with duration up to 3 hours. Totally ionized. Poor lipid solubility therefore does not readily cross blood–brain barrier, placenta, or eye. Excreted chiefly in urine; some fecal elimination. Distribution into breast milk not known.

CONTRAINDICATIONS AND PRECAUTIONS. Hypersensitivity to clidinium or to other anticholinergic drugs; narrow-angle glaucoma, suspected or actual obstruction of GI or GU tracts, intestinal atony, paralytic ileus, severe ulcerative colitis, toxic megacolon; unstable cardiovascular status in acute hemorrhage; myasthenia gravis. Safe use during pregnancy, in women of childbearing potential, nursing women, and in children not established. *Cautious Use:* impaired renal or hepatic function, geriatric or debilitated patients, hyperthroidism, prostatic hypertrophy, hiatal hernia associated with reflux esophagitis, autonomic neuropathy, coronary artery disease, arrhythmias, congestive heart failure, hypertension.

C

ADVERSE/SIDE EFFECTS. CNS: drowsiness, dizziness, headache, weakness, confusion, nervousness, insomnia; overdosage: fever, restlessness, excitement, psychoses, respiratory failure, paralysis, coma. **CV:** tachycardia, palpitation; overdosage: flushing, fall in blood pressure, circulatory failure. **GI:** dry mouth, impaired taste, nausea, vomiting, bloated feeling, constipation, paralytic ileus. **GU:** urinary hesitancy, urinary retention, impotence. **Hypersensitivity:** severe allergic reactions, urticaria and other skin eruptions, anaphylaxis. **Ophthalmic:** blurred vision, mydriasis, photophobia, cycloplegia, increased intraocular tension. **Other:** decreased sweating, suppression of lactation.

ROUTE AND DOSAGE. Oral: Adults: 2.5 to 5 mg 3 or 4 times daily before meals and at bedtime. **Geriatric or debilitated patients:** 2.5 mg 3 times daily before meals.

NURSING IMPLICATIONS

Commonly prescribed ½ to 1 hour before meals and at bedtime.

Because clidinium may cause drowsiness, dizziness, and blurred vision, caution patient to avoid driving and other potentially hazardous activities until reaction to drug is established.

Inform patient that certain side effects such as dry mouth, blurred vision, drowsiness, decreased sweating, and constipation occur with relative frequency and to keep physician informed.

Constipation and dry mouth may be relieved by increasing noncaloric fluid intake. Frequent warm, clear water rinses or the use of sugarless chewing gum or lemon drops may help mouth to relieve dryness. Saliva substitutes, e.g., Xero-Lube, Moi-stir, Orex are available, OTC, if necessary (consult physician).

Advise patient that he or she will be more susceptible to the effects of heat (e.g., heat stroke) because of decreased sweating, and therefore to avoid high environmental temperatures.

Store preferably at 15 to 30°C (59 to 86°F) in tight light-resistant container unless otherwise directed by manufacturer.

See Atropine Sulfate (prototype anticholinergic).

CLINDAMYCIN HYDROCHLORIDE
(Cleocin Hydrochloride)
CLINDAMYCIN PALMITATE HYDROCHLORIDE
(Cleocin Pediatric)
CLINDAMYCIN PHOSPHATE
(Cleocin Phosphate, Cleocin T)

(klin-da-mye′sin)
Antiinfective
Antibiotic (macrolide)

ACTIONS AND USES. Semisynthetic derivative of lincomycin with which it shares neuromuscular blocking properties and other actions as well as uses, contraindications, precautions, and adverse reactions. Reported to have greater degree of antibacterial activity in vitro, better absorption, and lower incidence of GI side effects than lincomycin. Like lincomycin, suppresses protein synthesis by binding to 50 S subunits of bacterial ribosomes, and therefore inhibits other antibiotics (e.g., erythromycin) that act at this site.

Used for treatment of serious infections when less toxic alternatives are inappropriate. Particularly effective against susceptible strains of anaerobic streptococci, *Bacteroides* (especially *B. fragilis*), *Fusobacterium*, *Actinomyces israelii*, *Peptococcus* and *Clostridium* species.

Also effective against aerobic gram-positive cocci, including *Staphylococcus aureus, S. epidermidis, Streptococci* (except *S. faecalis*), and *Pneumococci.* Topical applications used in treatment of acne vulgaris.

ABSORPTION AND FATE. Almost complete (90%) absorption following oral administration. Peak plasma concentrations within 45 minutes following 150-mg oral dose; effective levels persist 6 hours. Following IM injection, peak levels within 3 hours; effective levels persist 8 to 12 hours. Steady state attained after third dose. Approximately 10% of topical application absorbed into skin. Widely distributed to body fluids and tissues, including saliva and bone. No significant concentrations in cerebrospinal fluid, even when meninges are inflamed. About 90% protein-bound. Average half-life 2.4 hours. Most of drug is inactivated by hepatic metabolism; metabolized more rapidly in children than in adults. Excreted in urine, bile, and feces as bioactive and inactive metabolites and about 10% unchanged drug. Not cleared from blood by hemodialysis or peritoneal dialysis. Readily crosses placenta and may appear in breast milk.

CONTRAINDICATIONS AND PRECAUTIONS. History of hypersensitivity to clindamycin or lincomycin; history of regional enteritis, ulcerative colitis, or antibiotic-associated colitis. Safe use during pregnancy and in nursing mothers not established. Not recommended for infants younger than 1 month of age. *Cautious Use:* history of GI disease, renal or hepatic disease, atopic individuals (history of eczema, asthma, hay fever), history of drug or other allergies; older patients.

ADVERSE/SIDE EFFECTS. GI: diarrhea, abdominal pain, flatulence, bloating, nausea, vomiting, pseudomembranous colitis (potentially fatal); esophageal irritation, loss of taste, medicinal taste (high IV doses). **Hematologic:** leukopenia (chiefly neutropenia), eosinophilia, agranulocytosis, thrombocytopenia. **Hepatic:** jaundice, abnormal liver function tests. **Hypersensitivity:** skin rashes, urticaria, pruritus, fever, erythema multiforme resembling Stevens-Johnson syndrome (rare), anaphylactoid reactions, serum sickness. **Local reactions:** pain, induration, sterile abscess (following IM injections); thrombophlebitis (IV infusion). **Other:** sensitization, swelling of face (following topical use); dizziness, headache, hypotension (following IM), cardiac arrest (rapid IV), generalized myalgia, superinfections, proctitis, vaginitis, urinary frequency.

ROUTE AND DOSAGE. Adults: Oral: 150 to 450 mg every 6 hours. **Intramuscular, intravenous** (clindamycin phosphate): 300 to 600 mg every 6 to 8 hours, up to 2400 mg daily, if necessary. **Pediatric (over 1 month): Oral:** 8 to 25 mg/kg/day divided into three or four equal doses. **Intramuscular, intravenous:** 15 to 40 mg/kg/day divided into three or four equal doses or 350 to 450 mg/m²/day. All dosages individualized according to severity of infection and renal status. **Topical solution:** apply to affected area twice daily.

NURSING IMPLICATIONS

Culture and susceptibility testing should be performed initially and periodically during therapy.

A careful history should be taken of any previous sensitivities to drugs, or other allergens, prior to initiation of therapy.

Advise patient to take clindamycin capsules with a full (8 oz) glass of water to prevent esophagitis. Absorption of oral clindamycin is not significantly affected by food, or gastric acid although peak serum levels may be somewhat delayed.

Instruct patient to take drug for the full course of therapy as prescribed. Drug therapy should continue for at least 10 days in patients with group A beta-hemolytic streptococcal infections to reduce possibility of rheumatic fever or glomerulonephritis.

Note expiration date of oral solution; retains potency for 14 days at room temperature. Do not refrigerate as chilling causes thickening and thus makes pouring difficult. A calibrated measuring device should be included when dispensed.

Deep IM injection is recommended to minimize complications of administration. Rotate injection sites, and observe daily for evidence of inflammatory reaction. Single IM doses should not exceed 600 mg.

IV clindamycin is never given as a bolus dose. The infusion should not exceed 1200 mg in one hour. Prescribed continuous flow rate is slow to minimize risk of cardiac arrhythmias. Example: 10 mg/min for 30 minutes followed by continuous IV infusion at rate of 0.75 mg/minute (to maintain serum clindamycin concentrations of 4 to 5 mcg/ml).

Monitor blood pressure and pulse in patients receiving drug parenterally. Hypotension has occurred following IM injection. Advise patient to remain recumbent following drug administration, until blood pressure has stabilized.

Severe diarrhea and colitis including pseudomembranous colitis, have been associated with oral (highest incidence), parenteral, and topical clindamycin. Report immediately the onset of watery diarrhea, with or without fever; passage of tarry or bloody stools, pus, intestinal tissue, or mucus; abdominal cramps, or ileus. Symptoms may appear within a few days to 2 weeks after therapy is begun, or up to several weeks following cessation of therapy.

Elderly and bedridden patients are at a higher risk of developing severe colitis and therefore should be closely observed.

Monitor bowel elimination pattern. Question patient about number and consistency of stools, during therapy and for at least 3 weeks after therapy is completed.

Drug therapy is stopped if patient develops significant diarrhea (more than 5 loose stools daily) and/or sigmoidoscopy or colonoscopy establishes the diagnosis of colitis.

Antiperistaltic agents such as opiates or diphenoxylate with atropine (Lomotil) may prolong and worsen diarrhea by delaying removal of toxins from colon. Advise patient not to self-medicate with antidiarrheal preparations. Medical management of severe diarrhea consists of fluids, electrolytes, protein supplements, and possibly corticosteroids. Oral vancomycin or cholestyramine has been prescribed for pseudomembranous colitis caused by *Clostridium difficile.*

Be alert to signs of superinfection: vaginal or anal irritation, itching, foul-smelling discharge, diarrhea (also a sign of drug-induced colitis), mouth lesions, sudden fever, cough.

During prolonged therapy, periodic liver and kidney function tests and complete blood cell counts are recommended.

Serum clindamycin levels are monitored during high-dose therapy, particularly in patients with renal or hepatic disease.

Anaphylactoid reactions require immediate attention. Have on hand epinephrine, oxygen, IV corticosteroids.

Capsule preparations contain FD&C Yellow No.5 (tartrazine) which may cause an allergic type reaction including asthma in certain susceptible individuals. The reaction occurs frequently in persons with aspirin sensitivity.

Follow manufacturer's directions for reconstitution of parenteral drug, storage time, compatible IV fluids, and IV infusion rates. Reportedly local reactions following IV administration can be minimized by avoiding prolonged use of indwelling catheters. Observe IV injection sites for evidence of inflammatory reaction.

Patients using topical preparation for acne should be instructed to discontinue other acne preparations unless otherwise directed by physician. Advise patient to keep medication away from eyes.

Since 10% absorption of topical medication is possible, instruct patient to report the onset of systemic reactions to physician.
Store in tight containers, preferably between 15° and 30°C (59° and 86°F) unless otherwise directed by manufacturer.

C

Diagnostic Test Interferences. Clindamycin may cause increases in: **serum alkaline phosphatase, bilirubin, creatine phosphokinase** (CPK) from muscle irritation following IM injection; **SGOT,** and **SGPT.**

Drug Interactions: Clindamycin

Plus	Interactions
Chloramphenicol Erythromycin	Possibility of mutual antagonism *(See Actions and Uses)*
Antiperistaltic compounds, e.g., diphenoxylate (Lomotil) and opiates	Reduces rate but not extent of GI absorption of oral clindamycin. May prolong diarrhea
Neuromuscular blocking agents (nondepolarizing muscle relaxants), e.g., ether, tubocurarine, pancuronium	Enhanced neuromuscular blocking action. Used with caution

---

CLOCORTOLONE PIVALATE

(Cloderm)

(kloe-kor'toe-lone)
Corticosteroid

ACTIONS AND USES. In common with other topical corticosteroids has antiinflammatory, antipruritic, and vasoconstrictor properties *(see Hydrocortisone).*

Used for relief of inflammatory and pruritic manifestations of corticosteroid-responsive dermatoses.

ABSORPTION AND FATE. Drug absorption is enhanced when skin is inflamed or otherwise diseased. Absorption can also occur to lesser extent through normal intact skin. Portions of drug that are systemically absorbed are metabolized in liver and excreted in urine.

CONTRAINDICATIONS AND PRECAUTIONS. Hypersensitivity to corticosteroids, or to components in commercial formulation, e.g., parabens. Pregnancy (category C). Dosage for children not established. *Cautious Use:* nursing women.

ADVERSE/SIDE EFFECTS. (Generally well tolerated) Burning, itching, irritation, folliculitis, dryness, acneiform eruptions, hypertrichosis, hypopigmentation, perioral dermatitis, allergic contact dermatitis, skin maceration and atrophy, striae, and miliaria, especially with occlusive dressings or wrappings.

ROUTE AND DOSAGE. Topical (0.1% cream in water-washable emollient base): applied in thin film one to four times daily, depending on severity of condition.

NURSING IMPLICATIONS

The commercial preparation Cloderm contains parabens (preservatives), which are known sensitizing agents.
Discuss with physician specific procedure for cleansing skin prior to each application and proper use of occlusive dressings.

Antipruritic and antiinflammatory effectiveness of drug is enhanced by occlusive dressings since percutaneous absorption is substantially increased.

Occlusive dressings should not be used on weeping or exudative lesions. Patients with this type of lesion should be advised not to wear tight-fitting clothing or wrappings that could act as an occlusive dressing.

If infection develops, occlusive dressing should be discontinued and appropriate antimicrobial treatment initiated.

Patients receiving prolonged therapy or applications to large areas or in whom occlusive dressings are being used should be closely observed for signs of systemic absorption.

Tests of urinary free cortisol, and ACTH stimulation tests are advised at regular intervals to evaluate hypothalmic–pituitary–adrenal (HPA) axis suppression.

Elderly patients with atrophic skin are more susceptible to systemic toxicity because they tend to absorb proportionately larger amounts than young adults. (Children also absorb high amounts because of larger skin surface area to body weight ratio.)

Advise patient to notify physician if local irritation, signs of infection, hypersensitivity, or systemic reaction develop.

Caution patient to use medication as directed and only for the disorder prescribed.

Avoid contact of drug in or near the eyes.

Store between 15° and 30°C (59° and 86°F) unless otherwise directed by manufacturer.

See Hydrocortisone: Nursing Implications: topical applications.

PROTOTYPE

CLOFIBRATE

(Atromid-S)

(kloe-fye′brate)

Antilipemic

ACTIONS AND USES. Aryloxisobutyric acid derivative structurally unrelated to other antilipemic agents. Reduces very low density lipoproteins (VLDL) rich in triglycerides to a greater extent than low density lipoproteins (LDL) rich in cholesterol. Mechanism of action is unclear; it appears to inhibit cholesterol biosynthesis prior to mevalonate formation and transfer of triglycerides from liver to serum. Interferes with binding of free fatty acids to albumin and increases fecal excretion of neutral sterols. Its ability to cause regression of xanthomatous lesions is thought to be due to mobilization of cholesterol from tissue. Reduces platelet adhesiveness, and increases release of antidiuretic hormone from posterior pituitary. Studies suggest that incidence of hepatic cancer may increase in patients on high doses of clofibrate. Effects of drug-induced lowering of serum cholesterol and other lipids on morbidity and mortality due to atherosclerosis or coronary heart disease have not been determined. Use of drug reportedly increases risk of cholelithiasis and cholecystitis requiring surgery to twice nonusers.

Used as adjunct to appropriate dietary regulation and other measures for reduction of serum lipids in patients with hypercholesterolemia and/or hypertriglyceridemia. Drug of choice for treatment of type III hyperlipoproteinemia. *Investigational Use:* in management of diabetes insipidus. Also used in treatment of xanthoma tuberosum associated with hyperlipidemia.

ABSORPTION AND FATE. Intestinal biotransformation to active form *p*-chlorophenoxyisobutyric acid (CPIB) occurs before absorption which is slow but complete. Peak plasma levels: 2 to 6 hours; approximately 96% plasma protein binding of CPIB (reduced in nephrotic syndrome, renal failure, and cirrhosis). Elimination half-life: 6 to 25 hours (in presence of renal impairment: 30 to 110 hours). Plasma clearance of unbound drug is reduced in renal failure, and cirrhosis. About 40 to 60% drug eliminated as metabolites of CPIB; remainder as unchanged CPIB.

CONTRAINDICATIONS AND PRECAUTIONS. Impaired renal or hepatic function, primary biliary cirrhosis, pregnancy, nursing mothers. Safe use in children younger than 14 years not established. *Cautious Use:* history of jaundice or hepatic disease, peptic ulcer, gout, patients receiving furosemide or oral anticoagulants: existing or suspected coronary artery disease.

ADVERSE/SIDE EFFECTS. **CV:** thrombophlebitis, pulmonary embolus, intermittent claudication, increase or decrease in angina, congestive failure, arrhythmias. **Dermatologic:** swelling and phlebitis at xanthoma sites, skin rash, dry skin, dry brittle hair, alopecia, allergy, urticaria, pruritus. **GI:** nausea (common), vomiting, loose stools, diarrhea, flatulence, bloating, abdominal distress, gastritis, polyphagia, weight gain or loss, stomatitis, hepatomegaly, cholelithiasis, pancreatitis. **GU:** impotence, decreased libido, renal dysfunction (dysuria, hematuria, proteinuria, decreased urinary output). **Hematologic:** leukopenia, anemia, eosinophilia, agranulocytosis, potentiation of anticoagulant effect. **Musculoskeletal:** flulike symptoms: myalgia, myositis, arthralgia. **Neurologic:** fatigue, weakness, drowsiness, dizziness, headache. **Other:** (direct relationship to drug action not known): peptic ulcer, GI hemorrhage, tremor, diaphoresis, systemic lupus erythematosus, rheumatoid arthritis, thrombocytopenic purpura, gynecomastia, malignancy, blurred vision, altered taste sensation (hypogensia).

ROUTE AND DOSAGE. **Oral:** **Adult:** 2 Gm/day in 2 to 4 divided doses.

NURSING IMPLICATIONS

If gastric distress is a problem, administer drug with meals.

Before initiation of therapy a complete health history should be obtained, including physical examination, appropriate laboratory determinations, and personal family and dietary history.

Serum cholesterol and triglyceride levels should be determined initially and evaluated every 2 weeks during first few months of therapy, and then at monthly intervals. If tests show a steady rise or are otherwise abnormal, clofibrate should be withdrawn.

Since hyperlipoproteinemia is frequently genetically determined, family members especially children, should be screened for abnormal lipid levels.

Clofibrate is not generally prescribed until every effort is made to lower serum cholesterol and triglycerides by dietary regulations, weight control, and exercise.

Reduction to ideal weight, correction of sedentary habits, and control of smoking are applicable to all patients with hyperlipoproteinemia. Collaborate with dietitian in planning with the patient how to coordinate new adjustments to life-style and diet. Stress importance of adhering to diet.

Therapeutic response is indicated by reduction of lipid levels; this generally occurs during the first or second month of therapy. Rebound may occur in second or third month, followed by a further decrease; and may also occur with sudden withdrawal of drug.

Clofibrate therapy for increased serum cholesterol and triglycerides is generally withdrawn after 3 months if the response is not adequate. When used for xanthoma, therapy may be continued even up to 1 year, provided there is some reduction in size of lesions.

Flulike symptoms (malaise, muscle soreness, aching, weakness) should be reported promptly to the physician. Other reportable symptoms include: fever, chills, sore throat (leukopenia); gastric pain, nausea, vomiting (pancreatitis, cholecystitis); chest pain, dyspnea (pulmonary edema); dysuria, hematuria, lower leg edema (renal toxicity).

Since alcohol is a source of carbohydrate, its use may be restricted. Check with physician.

Women of childbearing years should be on birth control regimen. If pregnancy is desired, clofibrate therapy should be discontinued at least 2 months before conception (discuss with physician). If patient becomes pregnant while on clofibrate treatment, the risk to the fetus should be fully understood.

Advise patient to adhere to drug regimen as established. Instruct patient not to alter the dose or dose intervals and to not stop taking the drug without consulting the physician.

Caution patient about self-dosing with OTC drugs without the approval of the physician.

Frequent serum transaminase and other liver tests are advocated, as well as periodic complete blood counts, renal function tests, and determinations of plasma and urine steroid levels, serum electrolyte levels, and blood sugar.

Preserved in closed, light-resistant containers at temperature between 15° and 30°C (59° and 86°F), unless otherwise directed by manufacturer.

See Cholestyramine (prototype antilepemics).

C

Diagnostic Test Interferences. Clofibrate therapy may lead to increased **BSP** retention, **thymol** turbidity; increased **serum creatine phosphokinase (CPK), SGOT, SGPT** levels; **proteinuria,** parodoxical increase in **LDL** or **cholesterol** levels (if there is a large decrease in VLDL level); decreased **plasma fibrinogen** levels. Lower fasting **blood glucose** and **serum insulin** levels in patients with diabetes mellitus.

Drug Interactions. Clofibrate increases effects of **oral anticoagulants** by decreasing plasma protein binding. Concomitant use of clofibrate and **furosemide** may result in enhanced effect of both drugs. Clofibrate may enhance hypoglycemic effect of **tolbutamide** and other **sulfonylureas. Oral contraceptives** may antagonize the actions of clofibrate. Pharmacologic effect of clofibrate may be increased by **probenecid.**

CLOMIPHENE CITRATE

(Clomid, Serophene)

(kloe'mi-feen)
Ovulation stimulant
Antiestrogenic

ACTIONS AND USES. Nonsteroidal compound related to chlorotrianisene. Used to induce ovulation in anovulatory women. Has both estrogenic and antiestrogenic properties but lacks clinical evidence of androgenic or progestational effects. Competes for and diminishes available cytoplasmic estrogen receptors for endogenous estrogens. Subsequent reduction in "feedback" inhibition of hypothalamic-pituitary control of estrogen synthesis results in increased secretion of luteal and follicular hormones and gonadotropins. Increased gonadotropins lead to formation of large cystic ovaries, maturation of ovarian follicle, ovulation, and development and function of corpus luteum. Increases plasma progesterone levels in the luteal phase. Ineffective in presence of panhypopituitarism, endometrial carcinoma, ovarian failure or tubal nonpatency in the wife, azoospermia in the husband. A single ovulation is induced by a single course of therapy; normal ovulatory function does not usually resume after treatment or after pregnancy.

Used for treating infertility in appropriately selected women desiring pregnancy and in the management of idiopathic postpill amenorrhea. Investigational use: treatment of male infertility.

ABSORPTION AND FATE. Readily absorbed from GI tract. Detoxified in liver; 50% of dose is excreted in feces after 5 days; the remaining metabolites and drug are excreted from enterohepatic pool or are stored in body fat for later release.

CONTRAINDICATIONS AND PRECAUTIONS. Pregnancy, fibroid tumor, ovarian cyst, hepatic disease or dysfunction, abnormal and unexplained bleeding, visual abnormalities, mental depression, thrombophlebitis. *Cautious Use:* enlarged ovaries, pelvic discomfort, sensitivity to pituitary gonadotropins.

C

ADVERSE/SIDE EFFECTS. (Dose related). **Dermatologic:** skin rash, urticaria, allergic dermatitis. **GI:** nausea, vomiting, increased appetite, constipation. **GU:** urinary frequency, polyuria. **Ophthalmic:** (reversible and of short duration): transient blurring, diplopia, scintillating scotomata, photophobia, floaters, photopsia, decreased visual acuity (rare). **Reproductive:** spontaneous abortion, multiple ovulations, birth defects, ovarian failure, acute (irreversible) transition to menopause (rare). *Hyperstimulation of ovaries:* (mild) ovarian enlargement, abdominal distention, weight gain; (severe) ascites, pleural effusion, electrolyte imbalance, hypovolemia with hypotension and oliguria, tremendously enlarged ovaries with multiple follicular cysts. Also, hot flashes, breast discomfort, abdominal pain, pain of mittelschmerz, heavy menses, unfavorable cervical mucus, exacerbation of endometriosis. **Other:** dryness and loss of hair, nervous tension, depression, headache, fatigue, restlessness, insomnia, dizziness, vertigo, cholestatic jaundice. The following have been reported but causal relationships have not been established: detachment of posterior vitreous, posterior capsular cataract, thrombosis of temporal arteries of retina; hydatidiform mole.

ROUTE AND DOSAGE. Oral: *First course of therapy:* 50 mg/day for 5 days beginning on 5th day of cycle following spontaneous or induced bleeding (with progestin) or at any time in the patient who has had no recent uterine bleeding. *Second course of therapy:* (ovulation without conception) repeat first cycle until conception or for 3 to 4 cycles; *no ovulation:* 100 mg daily for 5 days. Usual dose limit: 100 mg/day for 5 days. Some patients need larger doses to induce ovulation but incidence of side effects increases with dose.

NURSING IMPLICATIONS

The importance of properly timed coitus must be understood by the patient and husband. Each course of therapy should start on or about the 5th cycle day once ovulation has been established.

A complete history, physical examination, thyroid, adrenal and pituitary disorders, diagnosed endometrial biopsy and liver function tests are checked before therapy begins.

Determine level of understanding of patient and her husband; reinforce teaching already begun. They should have a full understanding of frequency and potential hazards of multiple pregnancy before treatment is started.

Incidence of multiple pregnancy with clomiphene use is as high as 20% and appears to increase with dose increases.

A pelvic examination should be performed before initiation of each cycle of therapy and immediately, if abdominal pain occurs.

Patient who is going to respond usually ovulates after the first course of therapy (within 5 to 14 days).

The likelihood of conception diminishes with each succeeding course of therapy. If pregnancy is not achieved after 3 or 4 ovulatory responses, further treatment with clomiphene is not recommended.

A single injection of 5000 to 10,000 USP units of human chorionic gonadotropin (HCG) is given to some patients 5 to 7 days after the last dose of clomiphene to simulate the midcycle LH surge which results in ovulation.

Encourage patient to establish a flow chart for recording basal body temperatures (BBT) (indirect confirmatory evidence of ovulation) to determine day of ovulation.

To begin BBT record start on day 1 of menstrual period. Take temperature every morning upon awakening and before arising. Counsel patient to avoid all activity before taking BBT (e.g., smoking, intercourse, brushing teeth, drinking coffee).

C

The BBT is approximately 97.5°F for 2 weeks after menstruation and approximately 98.5°F during luteal phase (ovulation followed by menstruation). When menstruation begins or just before, BBT drops to 97.5°F.

During the "follicular period" (ovum maturation period immediately after menstruation) BBT is relatively low and stable; at time of ovulation there is a slight decrease, followed the next day by a sharp increase. This increase is maintained if progesterone levels are normal (luteal phase). Just before menstruation, BBT drops. If it does not decline, patient may be pregnant.

If the BBT is biphasic and not followed by menses after a cycle of clomiphene therapy, the next course of drug will be delayed until it is confirmed that patient is not pregnant.

A special thermometer which measures 96° to 100°F and is easy to read is available for oral temperatures. Some physicians prefer rectal temperatures for BBT record.

Physiologic release of the ovum is thought to occur on the day prior to the time of the first temperature elevation (BBT chart). The egg remains in fallopian tube 4 to 5 days before entering uterus.

Properly timed coitus is essential and is based on the estimation that sperm retain their ability to fertilize for 24 to 48 hours and that an ovum is fertilizable for 12 to 24 hours; therefore, conception occurs only during a period of 3 to 5 days each month.

If ovulation can be determined from the BBT chart, couple is instructed to attempt coitus every other day for 3 to 4 days before expected ovulation and for 2 or 3 days after ovulation.

The matching of times for apparent ovulation, viability of sperm, and fertilizability of the ovum is crucial. If timing is off it can take months for a woman to become pregnant. Review treatment regimen with patient to test understanding.

Symptoms that should be reported if they continue and are distressing: hot flashes resembling those associated with menopause; nausea, vomiting, headache. Appropriate drug therapy may be prescribed. Symptoms disappear after drug is discontinued.

Yellowing of eyes, light-colored stools, yellow, itchy skin and fever symptomatic of jaundice should be reported promptly.

If abnormal bleeding occurs, full diagnostic measures are crucial.

Instruct patient to stop taking clomiphene if she suspects pregnancy and to contact physician for a confirmatory examination.

Visual symptoms due to intensification and prolongation of after images are accentuated on exposure to a more brightly lit environment. If patient needs to wear dark glasses even inside, or if she has blurred or decreased vision or scotomatas (signs of ocular toxicity), she should promptly report for a complete ophthalmic examination. Drug will be stopped until symptoms subside (usually in a few weeks).

If clomiphene is continued more than one year, ophthalmic examination should be performed (including slit-lamp exam).

Because of the possibility of lightheadedness, dizziness, and visual disturbances, caution the patient against performing hazardous tasks requiring skill and coordination in an environment with variable lighting.

Warn patient to report excessive weight gain, signs of edema, bloating, decreased urinary output (signs of ovarian overstimulation). Hospital care is necessary to prevent ovarian rupture and to restore electrolyte balance.

Maximum enlargement of the ovary does not occur until several days after clomiphene is discontinued; enlargement and cyst formation then regress spontaneously within a month.

Pelvic pain indicates the need for immediate pelvic examination for diagnostic purposes. If pain is due to abnormal enlargement of the ovary or to polycystic ovary syndrome, medication will be stopped until pretreatment size is attained—usually in a few days. During next course of treatment, dosing regimen will be reduced.

Large doses of an oral contraceptive will cause rapid regression of ovarian enlargement.
Many monitoring procedures are important during clomiphene therapy. Help patient to understand importance of her cooperation and strict adherence to the therapeutic plan.
Advise patient to take the medicine at same time every day. This helps to maintain drug levels and prevents forgetting a dose.
Missed dose: instruct patient to take drug as soon as possible. If not remembered until time for next dose, take both doses together, then resume regular dosing schedule. If more than one dose is missed, patient should check with physician.
Store at temperature between 15° and 30°C (59° and 86°F) in tightly capped, light-resistant container.

Diagnostic Test Interferences. Clomiphene may increase **BSP** retention; **plasma transcortin, thyroxine,** and **sex hormone binding globulin** (TBG) levels. Also increases **follicular-stimulating** and **luteinizing hormone** secretion in most patients.

CLONAZEPAM
(Clonopin)

(kloe-na'zi-pam)
Anticonvulsant
Benzodiazepine derivative
C IV

ACTIONS AND USES. Benzodiazepine derivative with strong anticonvulsant activity and several other pharmacologic properties characteristic of the drug class. Suppresses spike and wave discharge in absence seizures (petit mal) and decreases amplitude, frequency, duration, and spread of discharge in minor motor seizures.

Used alone or with other drugs in absence, myoclonic, and akinetic seizures, Lennox-Gastaut syndrome, and in patients with absence seizures resistant to succinimide treatment. Also effective in infantile spasms, restless legs, photosensitivity epilepsy, and generalized tonic-clonic convulsions. *Investigational Use:* treatment of tardive dyskinesia.

ABSORPTION AND FATE. Maximal plasma levels reached in 1 to 2 hours after oral administration. Therapeutic serum concentrations: 20 to 80 ng/ml. Plasma protein binding: 82%. Half-life: 18 to 50 hours. Excreted in urine as metabolites (less than 2% excreted unchanged).

CONTRAINDICATIONS AND PRECAUTIONS. Hypersensitivity to benzodiazepines, liver disease, acute narrow-angle glaucoma, breast feeding. Safe use in pregnancy and in women of child-bearing potential not established. *Cautious Use:* renal disease, COPD, drug-controlled open-angle glaucoma, addiction-prone individuals; children (because of unknown consequences of long-term use on growth and development); patient with several coexisting seizure disorders.

ADVERSE/SIDE EFFECTS. CV: palpitations, bradycardia. **Dermatologic:** hirsutism, hair loss, skin rash, ankle and facial edema. **GI:** xerostomia, sore gums, anorexia, increased salivation, increased appetite, nausea, constipation, diarrhea. **GU:** dysuria, enuresis, nocturia, urinary retention. **Hematologic:** agranulocytosis, anemia, leukopenia, thrombocytopenia, eosinophilia. **Neurologic:** drowsiness (common), ataxia, insomnia, nystagmus, abnormal eye movements, aphasia, choreiform movements, coma, dysarthria, dysdiadochokinesia, "glassy-eyed" appearance, headache, hemiparesis, hypotonia, slurred speech, tremor, vertigo. **Psychiatric:** confusion, depression, hallucinations, aggressive behavior, hysteria, increased libido, suicide attempt. **Respiratory:** chest congestion, respiratory depression, rhinorrhea, dyspnea, hypersecretion in upper respiratory passages. **Other:** hepatomegaly, drug fever, hypersensitivity reaction, muscular weakness, dehydration, lymphadenopathy, changes in weight.

C

ROUTE AND DOSAGE. Highly individualized. **Oral: Adults:** 1.5 mg/day divided into 3 doses. Dose increased by increments of 0.5 to 1 mg every 3 days until seizures are controlled or until side effects preclude further increases. Maximum recommended dose: 20 mg/day. **Children (up to 10 years of age):** 0.01 to 0.03 mg/kg/day not to exceed 0.05 mg/kg/day in three divided doses. Increments of 0.25 to 0.5 mg every third day. *Maintenance:* 0.1 to 0.2 mg/kg/day divided into three doses. All doses should be equal; if one is larger it should be given at bedtime.

NURSING IMPLICATIONS

Anticonvulsant activity is often lost after 3 months of therapy; dosage adjustment may reestablish efficacy. Patient should be aware of necessity to report loss of seizure control promptly.

Counsel patient to take drug as prescribed and not to alter dosing regimen or stop medication without consulting physician. Additionally the patient should not give any of it to another person.

If a new anticonvulsant is to be substituted, it is usually added to the drug regimen as the former medication is gradually withdrawn. Slow tapering of dose over several days' time is imperative. Abrupt withdrawal in patient on high doses and long-term therapy can precipitate status epilepticus. Other withdrawal symptoms: convulsion, tremor, abdominal and muscle cramps, vomiting, sweating.

Caution patient not to self-medicate with OTC drugs before consulting the physician.

Monitor intake–output ratio and other indicators of renal function. Excess accumulation of metabolites because of impaired excretion leads to toxicity.

If multiple anticonvulsants are being given, watch patient carefully for signs of overdosage and/or drug interaction, i.e., increased depressant adverse effects.

If used as treatment for restless legs, suggest the following supportive measures (with physician approval):

- Avoid use of caffeine beverages at dinner and during evening
- Bed cradle to keep bedding off legs
- Support hose
- Stretch exercises for calf muscles
- Silk pajamas
- Ice bag or heat; aspirin

Alcohol and CNS depressants should be avoided during therapy with clonazepam.

Advise patient not to drive a car or engage in other activities requiring mental alertness and physical coordination until reaction to the drug is known. Drowsiness occurs in approximately 50% of patients.

Liver function tests, platelet counts, blood counts, and clinical evaluation of drug efficacy should be a part of the follow-up care of the patient on clonazepam.

Patient should carry identification (e.g., Medic Alert) bearing information about medication in use and the diagnosis.

Overdosage symptoms: somnolence, confusion, diminished reflexes, coma. Treatment includes: monitoring of vital signs, immediate gastric lavage, IV fluids, maintenance of open airway, vasopressors, CNS antidepressants.

Both psychological and physical dependence may occur in the patient on long-term, high-dose therapy. Watch patient to see that he or she does not cheek the tablet. Limit availability of large amounts of drug in the addiction-prone individual.

Classified as Schedule IV substance under Federal Controlled Substances Act.
Store in tightly closed container protected from light, at temperature between 15° and 30°C (59° and 86°F) unless otherwise specified by the manufacturer.

C

Diagnostic Test Interferences. Clonazepam causes transient elevation of **serum transaminase** and **alkaline phosphatase.**

Drug Interactions: Clonazepam

Plus	Interactions
Alcohol, barbiturates, antianxiety agents, antipsychotics, MAO inhibitors, tricyclic antidepressants, other anticonvulsants	Potentiate CNS depressant effect of clonazepam
Carbamazepine	Increases metabolism, and therefore reduces effects of clonazepam
Valproic acid	May produce absence (petit mal) status

CLONIDINE HYDROCHLORIDE

(Catapres, Dixarit)

(kloe'ni-deen)
Alpha-adrenergic agonist (centrally-acting)
Antihypertensive

ACTIONS AND USES. Centrally acting sympatholytic imidazoline derivative chemically related to tolazoline. Stimulates α_2-adrenergic receptors in CNS to produce inhibition of sympathetic vasomotor centers. Central actions result in reduced peripheral sympathetic nervous system activity, reduction in systolic and diastolic blood pressure, and decrease in heart rate. Orthostatic effects tend to be mild and occur infrequently. Initial dose is followed by enhanced tubular reabsorption of sodium and chloride; after 3 to 4 days sodium retention is reversed and natriuresis occurs. Other possible effects: inhibition of centrally induced salivation, decreased GI secretions and motility, decreased intraocular pressure, prolonged circulation time and inhibition of renin release from kidneys. Reportedly minimizes or eliminates many of the common clinical signs and symptoms associated with withdrawal of heroin, methadone, or other opiates. This action is believed to be related to stimulation of inhibitory receptors in locus coeruleus, a major noradrenergic nucleus in brain.

Used as step 2 drug in stepped care treatment of hypertension, either alone or with diuretic or other antihypertensive agents. *Investigational Use:* prophylaxis for migraine, treatment of dysmenorrhea, menopausal flushing, paroxysmal localized hyperhidroses; smoking and opiate withdrawal and in the clonidine suppression test for diagnosis of pheochromocytoma. Available in fixed-dose combination with chlorthalidone e.g., Combipres.

ABSORPTION AND FATE. Well absorbed from GI tract. Plasma drug level peaks in 3 to 5 hours; plasma half-life: 12 to 14 hours (25 to 37 hours in patients with impaired renal function). Duration of hypotensive effect is 8 hours in normotensive individuals and 4 to 24 hours or more in hypertensive patients. Believed to be widely distributed in body tissues. Metabolized in liver; 65% of dose is excreted by kidneys as unchanged drug (about 32%) and metabolites; about 20% is excreted through enterohepatic route in feces. Approximately 85% of single dose is eliminated within 72 hours; excretion completed after 5 days. Crosses blood–brain barrier.

CONTRAINDICATIONS AND PRECAUTIONS. Safe use during pregnancy and in women of childbearing potential and children not established. *Cautious Use:* severe coronary insufficiency, recent myocardial infarction, cerebrovascular disease, chronic renal failure, Raynaud's disease, thromboangiitis obliterans, history of mental depression.

ADVERSE/SIDE EFFECTS. Most frequent: dry mouth, drowsiness, sedation, constipation, dizziness, headache, weakness, sluggishness, fatigue, slight transient bradycardia. **CV:** postural hypotension (mild), Raynaud's phenomenon, congestive heart failure, ECG changes, bradycardia, palpitation, flushes, paradoxical increase in blood pressure (gross overdosage). **CNS:** vivid dreams, nightmares, insomnia, behavior changes, nervousness, restlessness, anxiety, mental depression. **Dermatologic:** rash, angioneurotic edema, urticaria, pruritus, thinning of hair. **GI and metabolic:** anorexia, nausea, vomiting, parotid pain, hepatitis, hyperbilirubinemia, weight gain (sodium retention). **GU:** impotence, urinary retention. **Other:** dry, itchy, and burning eyes, retinal degeneration (animal studies); constricted pupils (overdosage), dry nasal mucosa, pallor, increased sensitivity to alcohol, gynecomastia, bone pain.

ROUTE AND DOSAGE. Oral: *Antihypertensive:* Initial: 0.1 mg twice daily; increments of 0.1 or 0.2 mg/day may be made until desired response is achieved. Maintenance: 0.1 to 0.2 mg 2 to 4 times daily. (Studies have indicated that 2.4 mg is the maximun effective daily dose). *Severe dysmenorrhea:* 0.025 mg twice daily for 14 days before and during menses. *Menopausal flushing:* 0.025 to 0.075 mg twice daily. *Migraine supplement:* 0.025 mg two to four times daily, up to 0.05 mg three times daily. *Opiate withdrawal:* test dose: 0.005 mg/kg, then 0.010 to 0.017 mg/kg in divided doses for 7 to 14 days. If strength prescribed is not commercially available, contact pharmacist.

NURSING IMPLICATIONS

Consult physician regarding schedule of blood pressure determinations. Hypotensive response begins within 30 to 60 minutes after drug administration. Maximum decrease in blood pressure usually occurs in 2 to 4 hours. Antihypertensive effect lasts approximately 6 to 8 hours.

Last dose is commonly administered immediately before retiring to ensure overnight blood pressure control and to minimize daytime drowsiness.

Dosage is increased gradually over a period of weeks so as not to lower blood pressure abruptly (especially important in the elderly). Follow-up visits should be scheduled every 2 to 4 weeks until BP stabilizes, then every 2 to 4 months.

For patients undergoing surgery, clonidine is usually given 4 to 6 hours before scheduled surgery. Patient may be given a parenteral antihypertensive until oral medication can be resumed.

Dry mouth may be relieved by frequent rinses with clear water, increase in (noncaloric) fluid intake, or by sugarless gum or lemon drops. Saliva substitutes, e.g. Moi-stir, Xero-Lube, Orex are available OTC, if necessary.

Side effects that occur most frequently *(see Adverse/Side Effects)* tend to diminish with continued therapy, or they may be relieved by dosage reduction.

Although postural hypotension occurs infrequently, advise patient to make position changes slowly, and in stages, particularly from recumbent to upright position, and to dangle legs a few minutes before standing. Caution patient to lie down immediately if he or she feels faint.

Monitor intake and output during period of dosage adjustment. Report change in intake–output ratio or change in voiding pattern.

Determine weight daily. Patients not receiving a concomitant diuretic agent may gain weight, particularly during first 3 or 4 days of therapy, because of marked sodium and water retention. Consult physician regarding allowable sodium intake.

Patients with history of mental depression require close supervision, as they may be subject to further depressive episodes.

Tolerance sometimes develops in some patients. Physician may increase dosage or prescribe concomitant administration of a diuretic to enhance antihypertensive response.

Inform patient of the possible sedative effect of clonidine and caution against potentially hazardous activities such as operating machinery or driving until reaction to drug has been determined.

Blood pressure should be closely monitored whenever a drug is added to or withdrawn from therapeutic regimen.

If drug is to be discontinued, it is withdrawn over a period of 2 to 4 days. Abrupt withdrawal, particularly after long-term therapy, may result in restlessness and headache 2 to 3 hours after a missed dose and hypertensive crisis within 8 to 24 hours. Other symptoms associated with sudden withdrawal include anxiety, sweating, palpitation, increased heart rate, insomnia, tremors, muscle and stomach pain, and salivation; rarely, hypertensive encephalopathy and death may ensue.

It is recommended that patient be monitored for at least one month after clonidine is withdrawn.

Warn patient of the danger of omitting doses or stopping the drug without consulting the physician.

Periodic eye examination is advised (based on animal studies).

Advise patient to carry Medic Alert or other appropriate medical identification card or jewelry.

Caution patient not to take OTC medications without prior approval of physician.

Symptoms of clonidine overdosage usually respond to supportive treatment. Severe poisoning can be reversed by administration of tolazoline hydrochloride (Prescoline).

Store in well-closed container, preferably between 15° and 30°C (59° and 86°F) unless otherwise directed by manufacturer.

Diagnostic Test Interferences. Possibility of decreased urinary excretion of **aldosterone, catecholamines,** and **VMA** (however, sudden withdrawal of clonidine may cause increases in these values); transient increases in blood glucose; weakly positive direct antiglobulin (Coombs') tests.

Drug Interactions: Clonidine

Plus	Interactions
Beta adrenergic blocking agents e.g., propranolol (Inderal)	Paradoxical hypertension with combination therapy and following clonidine withdrawal. If withdrawal hypertension occurs discontinued drug is reinstituted. Withdrawal of beta adrenergic before clonidine suggested
CNS depressants (e.g., alcohol, barbiturates, sedatives, tranquilizers)	Enhanced CNS depression
Digitalis glycosides, guanethidine, propranolol, and other drugs that may decrease heart rate	Possibility of additive bradycardic effect
Levodopa	Clonidine may inhibit antiparkinson action
Tricyclin antidepressants	Possibility of rise in blood pressure. Concomitant use generally avoided

C

CLORAZEPATE DIPOTASSIUM

(Tranxene, Tranxene-SD)

(klor-az′e-pate)
Psychotropic
Anxiolytic
Anticonvulsant
Benzodiazepine
C IV

ACTIONS AND USES. Psychotherapeutic agent with actions, uses, and interactions qualitatively similar to those of chlordiazepoxide (qv) but with less unwanted side effects, e.g., sedation.

Used for the management of anxiety disorders, for short-term relief of anxiety symptoms, as adjunct in management of partial seizures, and for symptomatic relief of acute alcohol withdrawal.

ABSORPTION AND FATE. Decarboxylated in stomach; absorbed as active metabolite, desmethyldiazepam. Peak serum levels in about 1 hour; duration of action about 24 hours. Half-life approximately 48 hours. Metabolized in liver; excreted primarily in urine. Crosses placenta; excreted in breast milk.

CONTRAINDICATIONS AND PRECAUTIONS. Hypersensitivity to clorazepate and other benzodiazepines, patients under 9 years of age, acute narrow-angle glaucoma, depressive neuroses, psychotic reactions, drug abusers, pregnancy, lactation. *Cautious Use:* elderly, debilitated patients; hepatic disease; kidney disease. *See also Chlordiazepoxide.*

ADVERSE/SIDE EFFECTS. Drowsiness, GI disturbances, xerostomia, diplopia, blurred vision, dizziness, headache, ataxia, mental confusion, insomnia, hypotension; abnormal liver and kidney function tests, decreased Hct. *See also Chlordiazepoxide.*

ROUTE AND DOSAGE. Oral: Adults: Maximum recommended total daily dose: 90 mg. *Anxiety:* dose adjusted gradually within range of 15 to 60 mg/day in divided doses, or 15 mg initially as single bedtime dose with gradual increases as needed. *Acute alcohol withdrawal:* Day 1: 30 mg initially followed by 30 to 60 mg in divided doses. Day 2: 45 to 90 mg in divided doses. Day 3: 22.5 to 45 mg in divided doses. Day 4: 15 to 30 mg in divided doses. Thereafter reduce daily dose to 7.5 to 15 mg. Discontinue drug when patient's condition is stable. *Partial seizures:* 7.5 mg three times daily. **Children 9 to 12 years:** 7.5 mg two times daily. Dose increases no greater than 7.5 mg/week. Maximum recommended total daily dose: 60 mg.

NURSING IMPLICATIONS

Antacids delay absorption of drug. If patient has gastric distress, advise taking drug with food or milk. If necessary to use an antacid (with approval) it should be taken no less than 1 hour before or 1 hour after drug ingestion.

Effectiveness of clorazepate for long-term use (more than 4 months) has not been determined. Usefulness of drug should be periodically reassessed.

Drowsiness, a common side effect, is more likely to occur at initiation of therapy and with dose increments on successive days.

Counsel patient to take drug as prescribed: patient should not change dose or abruptly stop taking the drug without physician's approval. Additionally, patient should not "lend" or offer any of it to another person, or use it for a self-diagnosed problem.

Caution patient not to self-dose with OTC drugs (cold remedies, sleep medications, antacids) without consulting physician.

Patients most susceptible to side effects: elderly, debilitated, and patients with renal or hepatic disease.

Periodic blood counts and tests of liver and kidney function should be performed throughout therapy.
Caution patient to avoid potentially hazardous activities until reaction to drug is known.
Warn patient not to use alcohol and other CNS depressants while on clorazepate therapy.
Patient should be advised that if she becomes pregnant during therapy or intends to become pregnant she should communicate with her physician about the desirability of discontinuing the drug.
Patient with history of or actual cardiovascular disease should be monitored in early therapy for drug-induced responses. If systolic blood pressure drops more than 20 mm Hg or if there is a sudden increase in pulse rate, withhold drug and notify physician.
Alert responsible family member(s) to report signs of possible drug abuse and dependence to physician: nervousness, insomnia, memory impairment, diarrhea.
Drug dose should be decreased gradually over several day's time when regimen is to be discontinued. Abrupt termination may lead to memory impairment, severe GI symptoms, and muscle pain.
Classified as Schedule IV drug under the Federal Controlled Substances Act.
Store in light-resistant container at temperature between 15° and 30°C (59° and 86°F) unless otherwise specified by the manufacturer.
See Chlordiazepoxide (prototype anxiolytic) for Diagnostic Test Interferences and Drug Interactions.

C

CLOTRIMAZOLE

(kloe-trim'a-zole)

(Gyne-Lotrimin, Lotrimin, Mycelex, Mycelex-G)

Antiinfective
Antibiotic
Antifungal

ACTIONS AND USES. Imidazole derivative closely related chemically to miconazole. Broad spectrum of antifungal activity essentially identical to that of miconazole, but is reportedly less effective than miconazole for epidermophytoses and for candidiasis. Acts by damaging fungal cell membrane thereby altering its permeability which permits loss of potassium and other cellular constituents. Also active against some gram-negative bacteria.

Used topically in treatment of tinea pedis, cruris, and corporis due to *Trichophyton rubrum, T. mentagrophytes, Epidermophyton floccosum,* and *Microsporum canis,* and for tinea versicolor due to *Malassezia furfur,* and vulvovaginal and oropharyngeal candidiasis (moniliasis) caused by *Candida albicans.*

ABSORPTION AND FATE. Negligible amounts appear to be absorbed systemically following topical or intravaginal administration.

CONTRAINDICATIONS AND PRECAUTIONS. History of hypersensitivity to clotrimazole; use for systemic mycoses. Safe use during pregnancy (category C), in nursing mothers, and in children under 3 years not established.

ADVERSE/SIDE EFFECTS. Skin: stinging, erythema, edema, vesication, desquamation, pruritus, urticaria. **Vaginal:** mild burning sensation, lower abdominal cramps, bloating, cystitis, urethritis, mild urinary frequency, vulval erythema and itching and skin rash, abnormal liver function tests; occasional nausea and vomiting (with oral troche).

ROUTE AND DOSAGE. Topical (skin): cream 1%; solution 1%: gently massage small amount (of cream or solution) into affected and surrounding skin areas twice daily (morning and evening). **Vaginal:** vaginal cream 1%: 1 applicatorful daily for 7 to 14 consecutive days preferably at bedtime. Vaginal tablet 100 mg: using applicator supplied, insert 1 tablet intravaginally daily for 7 consecutive days, preferably at bedtime. Alternatively, 2 tablets daily for 3 consecutive days. **Oropharyngeal:** 1 troche (lozenge) 5 times a day for 14 consecutive days. Allow to dissolve slowly in mouth.

NURSING IMPLICATIONS

Skin cream and solution preparations should be applied sparingly. Protect hands with plastic gloves when applying medication.

Avoid contact of clotrimazole preparations with the eyes.

Occlusive dressings should not be applied unless otherwise directed by physician.

Consult physician for procedure to use for cleansing skin before applying medication. Some physicians recommend just plain tap water, others prefer use of a mild soap with thorough rinsing. Regardless of procedure used, dry skin thoroughly.

Diagnosis of superficial fungal infections can be determined by potassium hydroxide (KOH) smears and/or cultures. Since vaginal preparations have been shown to be effective only for candidiasis (moniliasis), diagnosis should be confirmed before initiation of therapy.

Advise patient to use clotrimazole as directed and for the length of time prescribed by physician.

Generally, clinical improvement is apparent during first week of therapy. Keep physician informed.

Urine and blood glucose studies and microbacteriologic analysis are indicated in patients who show no response to therapy.

Hepatic function tests should be performed periodically during therapy with clotrimazole troches (lozenges), particularly in patients with impaired renal function.

Resistant candidiasis may be a presenting sign of unrecognized diabetes mellitus.

Inform patient receiving the drug vaginally that sexual partner may experience burning and irritation of penis or urethritis and therefore to refrain from sexual intercourse during therapy, or advise sexual partner to wear a condom.

Consult physician regarding use of vaginal douche and sitz baths for patients receiving vaginal therapy.

Advise patient to report to physician if condition worsens or if signs of irritation or sensitivity develop, or if no improvement is noted after 4 weeks of therapy.

Review patient's hygienic practices for possible sources of infection.

Recurrence of vulvovaginal candidiasis occurs frequently. Discontinuation of systemic antibiotics and oral contraceptives have helped some patients.

General Patient-Teaching Points for Tinea Corporis (Ringworm of Body):

- ✓ Advise patient to keep linen, clothing, towels, facecloths, and other toilet articles separate.
- ✓ Wash anything that contacts affected areas, after each treatment.
- ✓ Launder clothing daily in hot water and nonirritating soap or detergent.
- ✓ Wear light clothing (or footwear) that will allow ventilation.
- ✓ Loose-fitting cotton underwear (and socks) are ideal.
- ✓ Keep skin clean and dry.
- ✓ For patients with tinea pedis (athlete's foot), leather shoes or sandals are best; avoid plastic footwear and sneakers. Advise patient to put on socks before underwear.

Store cream and solution formulations preferably between 2° and 30°C (35° and 86°F); do not store troches or vaginal tablets above 35°C (95°F) unless otherwise directed by manufacturer.

CLOXACILLIN, SODIUM

(Bactopen, Cloxapen, Cloxilean, Novocloxin, Orbenin, Tegopen)

(klox-a-sill'in)
Antiinfective
Antibiotic
Penicillin

ACTIONS AND USES. Semisynthetic, acid-stable, penicillinase-resistant, isoxazolyl penicillin. Mechanism of bactericidal action, contraindications, precautions, and adverse reactions as for penicillin G (qv). In common with other isoxazolyl penicillins (dicloxacillin, oxacillin) is highly active against most penicillinase-producing staphylococci, but less potent than penicillin G against penicillin-sensitive microorganisms, and is generally ineffective against gram-negative bacteria and methicillin-resistant staphylococci.

Used primarily in treatment of infections caused by penicillinase-producing staphylococci and penicillin-resistant staphylococci. May be used to initiate therapy in suspected staphylococcal infections pending culture and susceptibility test results. As with other penicillins, serum concentrations are enhanced by concurrent use of probenecid.

ABSORPTION AND FATE. Peak serum levels within 1 hour; effective levels maintained 4 to 6 hours after single dose. Distributed throughout body with highest concentrations in kidney and liver; cerebrospinal fluid penetration is low. Almost 90 to 98% protein bound. Half-life: 30 to 60 minutes. Excreted primarily in urine as active metabolite and intact drug; significant hepatic elimination through bile. Crosses placenta. Excreted in breast milk.

CONTRAINDICATIONS AND PRECAUTIONS. Sensitivity to penicillins or cephalosporins. Safe use during pregnancy and in neonates not established. *Cautious Use:* history of or suspected atopy or allergy (asthma, eczema, hives, hay fever), renal or hepatic function impairment.

ADVERSE/SIDE EFFECTS. Nausea, vomiting, flatulence, diarrhea. **Hypersensitivity reactions** *(see Penicillin G):* pruritus, urticaria, wheezing, sneezing, chills, drug fever, anaphylaxis; eosinophilia, leukopenia, agranulocytosis (malaise, elevated temperature, sore throat, adenopathy); elevated SGOT, SGPT, jaundice (rare), superinfections. *See also Penicillin G.*

ROUTE AND DOSAGE. Oral: Adults and children (weighing 20 kg or more): 250 to 500 mg or more every 6 hours. **Infants and children (up to 20 kg):** 12.5 to 25 mg/kg every 6 hours.

NURSING IMPLICATIONS

Before treatment is initiated, a careful inquiry should be made concerning patient's previous exposure and sensitivity to penicillins and cephalosporins, and other allergic reactions of any kind.

Best taken on an empty stomach (at least 1 hour before or 2 hours after meals), unless otherwise advised by physician. Food reduces rate and extent of drug absorption.

Instruct patient to take medication around the clock, not to miss a dose, and to continue taking the medication until it is all gone, unless otherwise directed by physician.

Inform patient to report to physician the onset of hypersensitivity reactions (such as hives, pruritus, rash, wheezing), and superinfections: black or white patchy tongue, anal or vaginal itching, loose, foul smelling stools.

Advise patient to check with physician if GI side effects (nausea, vomiting, diarrhea) appear.

Periodic assessments of renal, hepatic, and hematopoietic function are advised in patients on long-term therapy.

Following reconstitution (by pharmacist), oral solution retains potency for 14 days if refrigerated (container should be so labeled and dated). Shake well before pouring. A calibrated

C

measuring device should be dispensed with the preparation. Household teaspoons vary in measure and therefore are not advised.

Unless otherwise advised by manufacturer, store capsules at temperatures between 15° and 30°C (59° and 86°F).

See Penicillin G (prototype for penicillins).

COCAINE
COCAINE HYDROCHLORIDE

(koe-kane′)
Anesthetic (local)
C II

ACTIONS AND USES. Alkaloid obtained from leaves of *Erythroxylon coca.* Topical application blocks nerve conduction and produces surface anesthesia accompanied by local vasoconstriction. Exerts adrenergic effect by potentiating action of endogenous (and injected) epinephrine and norepinephrine possibly by inhibiting reuptake of catecholamines into sympathetic nerve terminals. Effective nasal decongestant, but rarely used for this purpose because of abuse potential. Systemic absorption produces descending CNS stimulation, with intense, short-lived euphoria accompanied by indifference to pain or hunger and with illusions of great strength, endurance, and mental capacity, all the bases for drug abuse.

Used for surface anesthesia of ear, nose, throat, rectum, and vagina. Ophthalmic use largely abandoned because of its tendency to cause corneal sloughing. Sometimes used as ingredient in Brompton's cocktail (qv).

ABSORPTION AND FATE. Readily absorbed through mucous membranes; rate of absorption is limited by vasoconstrictive action of cocaine. Absorption is enhanced in presence of inflammation. Onset of action within 1 minute, with duration up to 2 hours, depending on dose and concentration used. Plasma half-life approximately 1 hour. Slowly detoxified by liver. Excreted primarily in urine as metabolites and some unchanged drug.

CONTRAINDICATIONS AND PRECAUTIONS. Hypersensitivity to local anesthetics; sepsis in region of proposed application. Safe use in women of childbearing potential or during pregnancy not established. *Cautious use:* history of drug sensitivities, history of drug abuse.

ADVERSE/SIDE EFFECTS. Perforated nasal septum (prolonged application); clouding, pitting, and ulceration of cornea (direct application). Systemic absorption (CNS stimulation): euphoria, excitement, nervousness, pallor, insomnia, restlessness, tremors, hyperreflexia, convulsions, chills, fever, nausea, vomiting, anorexia, abdominal pain, mydriasis, exophthalmos, formication ("cocaine bugs"), pressure, tachycardia, ventricular fibrillation, tachypnea; (CNS depression): respiratory and circulatory failure. Hypersensitivity reactions.

ROUTE AND DOSAGE. Topical: *Surface anesthesia:* 1 or 2% solution applied as a spray or on a tampon. (Range: 1 to 10%.)

NURSING IMPLICATIONS

Administration of a test dose has been suggested.

When used for anesthesia of throat, cocaine causes temporary paralysis of cilia of respiratory tract cells reducing protection against aspiration. It also may interfere with pharyngeal stage of swallowing. Give nothing by mouth until sensation returns.

Continued use can result in psychologic dependence and a certain amount of tolerance particularly to euphoric effects. A true withdrawal syndrome has not been described, but heavy users may manifest irritability or depression ("cocaine blues") if deprived of the drug.

To discourage illegal use, cocaine solutions for topical application are often tinted with an antiseptic dye such as methylene blue. This dye also inhibits mold growth in the solution.

Cocaine has been abused for its cortical stimulant effect. Addicts take cocaine intranasally by "snorting" it ("snow") or by injection mixed with morphine or other opiates ("speed-ball"). "Street cocaine" is often adulterated with lidocaine or procaine, among other substances. Other names applied by drug abusers: "C," "coke," "girl," "lady," "happy dust," "gold dust," "stardust."

Some abusers remove the hydrochloride salt and inert adulterants from cocaine to derive "freebase," a more potent and potentially dangerous form of cocaine.

Treatment of acute toxicity: If taken orally induce emesis, gastric lavage. Have on hand propranolol (Inderal) to control tachycardia; short-acting barbiturate or diazepam (Valium) to control excessive CNS stimulation. Oxygen, respiratory, and circulatory support as indicated.

Classified as Schedule II drug under the Federal Controlled Substances Act.

Preserved in tightly closed, light-resistant containers.

Drug Interactions: Cocaine

Plus	Interactions
Epinephrine (Adrenalin)	Risk of severe hypertension and arrhythmias
Guanethidine (Ismelin)	Cocaine may reduce antihypertensive response to guanethidine
Norepinephrine (Levarterenol, Levophed)	Prolongs local action of norepinephrine
MAO inhibitors	Cocaine potentiates hypertension, tachycardia. Concomitant use generally avoided

---

CODEINE
(Methylmorphine)
CODEINE PHOSPHATE
(Paveral)
CODEINE SULFATE

(koe'deen)
Narcotic analgesic
Opiate agonist
Antitussive
C II

ACTIONS AND USES. Phenathrene derivative of opium made by methylation of morphine. Similar to morphine (qv) in actions, uses, contraindications, precautions, and adverse reactions. Not as potent as morphine and has shorter duration of action, thus produces less severe adverse reactions. However, in equianalgesic doses parenteral codeine produces similar degree of respiratory depression as does morphine. In contrast to morphine, orally administered codeine is about 60% as potent as the parenteral form. Histamine-releasing action appears to be more potent than that of morphine and may result in hypotension, flushing and rarely, bronchoconstriction. Analgesic potency is about one-sixth that of morphine; antitussive activity is also a little less than that of morphine. Oral codeine 65 mg is approximately equivalent to aspirin 650 mg (analgesic property). Reportedly not as effective for uterine or dental pain as are prostaglandin inhibitors such as aspirin.

Used for symptomatic relief of mild to moderately severe pain, when control cannot be obtained by nonnarcotic analgesics, and to suppress hyperactive or nonproductive cough. Commonly used in antitussive mixtures with guaifenesin, e.g., Cheracol, Nortussin with codeine, Robitussin A-C, Tolu-Sed, and in combination with aspirin and/or phenacetin for additive analgesic effect.

C

ABSORPTION AND FATE. Following oral or parenteral administration, onset of action occurs in 15 to 30 minutes and peaks in 1 to 1½ hours; duration of action 4 to 6 hours. Half-life: 2.5 to 4 hours. About 7% protein bound. Metabolized primarily in liver. Excreted chiefly in urine as norcodeine and free and conjugated morphine. Negligible amounts of codeine and metabolites excreted in feces. Crosses placenta and appears in breast milk.

CONTRAINDICATIONS AND PRECAUTIONS. Hypersensitivity to codeine or other morphine derivatives, acute asthma, chronic obstructive lung disease, increased intracranial pressure, head injury, acute alcoholism, hepatic or renal dysfunction, hypothyroidism. *Cautious Use:* prostatic hypertrophy, debilitated patients, very young and very old patients; history of drug abuse. *See also Morphine Sulfate.*

ADVERSE/SIDE EFFECTS. CNS: dizziness, lightheadedness, drowsiness, sedation, lethargy, euphoria, agitation. **CV:** palpitation, orthostatic hypotension, bradycardia. **GI:** nausea, vomiting, constipation. **GU:** urinary retention, difficult urination. **Other:** fixed-drug eruption; histamine-releasing effects: urticaria, pruritus, excessive perspiration (hyperhidrosis), facial flushing, shortness of breath, bronchoconstriction (rare). **Overdosage:** restlessness, exhilaration, convulsions, tachycardia, bradycardia, hypotension, miosis, narcosis, respiratory paralysis, circulatory collapse. *See also Morphine Sulfate.*

ROUTE AND DOSAGE. Oral, subcutaneous, intramuscular: Adults: *Analgesic:* 15 to 60 mg four times a day. *Antitussive:* 10 to 20 mg orally every 4 to 6 hours, if necessary. Not to exceed 120 mg/24 hours. **Children:** *Analgesic:* oral, SC, IM 0.5 mg/kg every 4 to 6 hours if necessary. *Antitussive:* **(6 to 12 years):** 5 to 10 mg every 4 to 6 hours. Not to exceed 60 mg/24 hours. **(2 to 6 years):** 2.5 to 5 mg every 4 to 6 hours; not to exceed 30 mg/24 hours.

NURSING IMPLICATIONS

Administer oral codeine with milk or other food to reduce possibility of GI distress.

Narcotics should not be administered routinely. Patient's individual need for medication should be evaluated before each administration.

Record relief of pain and duration of analgesia.

Since orthostatic hypotension is a possible side effect, instruct patient to make position changes slowly and in stages particularly from recumbent to upright posture. Also advise patient to lie down immediately if lightheadedness or dizziness occurs.

Nausea appears to be aggravated by ambulation. Advise patient to lie down when feeling nauseated and to notify physician if this symptom persists.

Inform patient that codeine may impair ability to perform tasks requiring mental alertness and therefore to avoid driving and other potentially hazardous activities until reaction to drug is known.

Advise patient not to take alcohol or other CNS depressant unless approved by physician.

Treatment of cough is directed toward decreasing frequency and intensity of cough without abolishing protective cough reflex, which serves the important function of removing bronchial secretions.

Excessive nonproductive cough tends to be self-perpetuating because it causes irritation of pharyngeal and tracheal mucosa.

Inform patient that hyperactive cough may be lessened by voluntary restraint and by avoid ing irritants such as smoking, dust, fumes, and other air pollutants. Humidification of ambient air may provide some relief. *See Nursing Interventions: Inhalation therapy.*

Locally acting sialagogues, e.g., hard candy (sugarless), may help to relieve cough due to irritation of pharyngeal mucosa. Adequate hydration (at least 1500 to 2000 ml/day) helps to liquefy sputum.

Cough syrups are commonly misused by drug abusers for their codeine and/or alcohol content. Terpin hydrate and codeine elixir known by abusers as "GI Gin" contains 10 mg of codeine per 5 ml and 39 to 44% alcohol.

Although codeine has less abuse liability than morphine, dependence is a major unwanted effect.

Classified as a Schedule II drug under the Federal Controlled Substances Act. Combination capsule formulations containing codeine are included under Schedule III; combination liquid or syrup preparations are classified under Schedule V.

Preserved in tight, light-resistant containers preferably between 15° and 30°C (59° and 86°F) unless otherwise directed by manufacturer.

See Morphine Sulfate [prototype narcotic analgesic (opiate agonist)].

C

Drug Interactions: Codeine

Plus	Interactions
Alcohol (ethanol), barbiturates and other CNS depressants	Additive CNS depression. Used concomitantly with caution if at all

PROTOTYPE

COLCHICINE

(Novocolchine)

(kol'chi-seen)

Antigout agent

ACTIONS AND USES. Alkaloid of the autumn crocus *Colchicum autumnale* with antimitotic and indirect antiinflammatory properties. Binds to microtubular protein, thereby arresting spindle formation in metaphase, and interfering with movement of mobile cells. Selective action in gouty arthritis believed to be related to inhibition of microtubule formation in leukocytes thus interfering with their migration and phagocytosis in gouty joints. Lactic acid produced by phagocytosis is reduced, and crystal deposition fostered by acid pH is decreased. The net effect is inhibition of inflammation and reduction of pain and swelling. Colchicine is nonanalgesic and nonuricosuric. Direct action on bone marrow produces temporary leukopenia later replaced by leukocytosis. Stimulates prostaglandin synthesis which may be one of the reasons for GI side effects. Tends to increase fecal excretion of Na, K, fat, nitrogen, and carotene and in large doses may reduce serum cholesterol and interfere with absorption of vitamin B_{12} (cyanocobalamin). Tolerance to colchicine does not develop.

Used prophylactically for recurrent gouty arthritis and as specific for acute gout, either as single agent or in combination with a uricosuric such as probenecid, allopurinol, or sulfinpyrazone. *Investigational Use:* in treatment of sarcoid arthritis, chondrocalcinosis (pseudogout), leukemia, adenocarcinoma, acute calcific tendonitis, familial Mediterranean fever, mycosis fungoides, and in experimental studies of normal and abnormal cell division. Available in fixed combination with probenecid (Colabid, ColBENEMID, Proben-C).

ABSORPTION AND FATE. Following oral administration, rapidly absorbed from GI tract and partially metabolized in liver. Metabolites and active drug recycled to intestinal tract via biliary and intestinal secretions. Plasma levels peak in 0.5 to 2 hours then decline for 1

C

to 2 hours before increasing again because of recycling. High concentrations appear in leukocytes, kidney, liver, spleen, and intestinal tract. Plasma half-life is 20 minutes; half-life in leukocytes is about 60 minutes. Drug concentrations in leukocytes may persist 9 days after single IV dose. Partly deacetylated in liver. Metabolites and active drug excreted primarily in feces; 10 to 20% (variable) excreted in urine.

CONTRAINDICATIONS AND PRECAUTIONS. Hypersensitivity to colchicine; blood dyscrasias; severe GI, renal, hepatic, or cardiac disease. Severe local irritation can result from subcutaneous or intramuscular use. Safe use during pregnancy, and in nursing mothers and children not established. *Cautious Use:* elderly and debilitated patients, early manifestations of GI, renal, hepatic, or cardiac impairment.

ADVERSE/SIDE EFFECTS. Dose-related: **CNS:** mental confusion, peripheral neuritis (numbness, tingling, pain, or weakness of hands or feet); loss of deep tendon reflexes, ascending CNS paralysis, respiratory failure, fever, delirium, convulsions. **GI:** nausea, vomiting, diarrhea, abdominal pain, anorexia, hemorrhagic gastroenteritis, steatorrhea, hepatotoxicity, pancreatitis, paralytic ileus (overdosage). **Hematologic:** severe neutropenia (with IV use), bone marrow depression (leukopenia followed by leukocytosis), thrombocytopenia, agranulocytosis, aplastic anemia. **IV extravasation:** pain, vein sclerosis, thrombophlebitis, necrosis of local tissues including nerves. **Renal:** azotemia, proteinuria, hematuria, oliguria. **Other:** burning sensations of throat, stomach, skin (overdosage), malabsorption syndrome, alopecia, bladder spasms, muscular weakness, hypothyroidism; arrhythmias, respiratory arrest (rapid IV) hypotension (large doses).

ROUTE AND DOSAGE. Oral: *Acute gouty attack:* Initial: 0.5 or 1.2 mg, followed by 0.5 or 0.6 mg every hour, or every 1 to 2 hours until pain is relieved or GI symptoms (nausea, vomiting, diarrhea, abdominal pain) appear. *Prophylaxis* (mild to moderate cases): 0.5 or 0.6 mg every night or every other night as required; (severe cases): 0.5 to 1.8 mg daily. **Intravenous:** *Acute gouty attack:* Initial: 2 mg followed by 0.5 mg every 6 hours until satisfactory response is obtained or GI symptoms intervene. Maximum 4 mg/24 hours. *Prophylaxis:* 0.5 to 1 mg once or twice daily. *For patients undergoing surgery:* 0.5 or 0.6 mg three times daily for 3 days before and 3 days after surgery.

NURSING IMPLICATIONS

Administer oral drug with milk or food to reduce possibility of GI upset.

IV preparation: Do not dilute colchicine with 5% dextrose injection, or other fluids that may change pH of colchicine solution, since a precipitate may form. Use 0.9% sodium chloride injection which does not contain a bacteriostatic agent for dilutions. Discard turbid solutions. Discard needle after withdrawing solution from vial and replace with fresh sterile needle for injection procedure to avoid tissue irritation. Injection should be made over a 2 to 5 minute period by direct IV injection or into tubing of free-flowing IV with compatible fluid.

Care must be taken to prevent extravasation of IV colchicine because severe tissue irritation including nerve damage can result.

Baseline and periodic determinations of serum uric acid are advised, as well as complete blood count, including hemoglobin. *Normal serum uric acid* is approximately 3 to 7 mg/dl.

Side effects (dose-related) are most likely to occur during the initial course of treatment. A latent period of several hours between drug administration and onset of toxic symptoms is usual.

Early signs of colchicine toxicity include weakness, abdominal discomfort, anorexia, nausea, vomiting, and diarrhea, regardless of administration route. Report to physician. To avoid more serious toxicity, drug should be discontinued promptly until symptoms subside. Diarrhea may require treatment with an antidiarrheal agent.

Monitor intake and output (during acute gouty attack). High fluid intake promotes urate excretion and reduces danger of crystal formation in kidneys and ureters; intake is usually prescribed to maintain urinary output of at least 2000 ml/day.

Since acute gout can be precipitated by even minor surgical procedures, the patient is usually given colchicine before and after surgery.

To avoid cumulative toxicity, a given course of colchicine therapy for acute gout is generally not repeated within 3 days.

During an acute attack, weight-bearing and heat to involved joint should be avoided. Bed cradle to keep off weight of bedclothes and elevation of gouty foot may provide relief. Mobilization is permitted when joint is no longer painful. Physical therapy and self-help devices may be indicated for patients with residual disability.

Gout commonly occurs in the great toe; however, the instep, ankle, and knee are also common sites. Wrist, finger, or elbow may be affected with recurrent attacks.

Keep physician informed of patient's progress. Drug should be stopped when pain of acute gout is relieved. Therapeutic response: articular pain and swelling generally subside within 8 to 12 hours and usually disappear in 24 to 72 hours after oral therapy, and 6 to 12 hours after IV administration.

Patients taking colchicine at home should be advised to withhold drug and report to the physician the onset of GI symptoms or signs of bone marrow depression (nausea, sore throat, bleeding gums, sore mouth, fever, fatigue, malaise, unusual bleeding or bruising).

Patients with gout should be instructed to keep colchicine at hand at all times so they can start therapy or increase dosage, as prescribed by physician, at the first suggestion of an acute attack. An attack can be aborted or reduced in severity by early recognition of prodromal signs: local pruritus or discomfort in joint, mood changes, diuresis.

Food–Drug Interactions:

- Long-term dietary management for patients with gout includes gradual weight reduction for obese patients (no more than 2 to 2½ lb/week). Sudden weight loss can precipitate a gouty attack. Physician may prescribe a diet high in carbohydrate, with moderate protein and low fat. To potentiate action of colchicine, some physicians advise increased intake of alkaline ash foods: milk, most fruits and vegetables, with the exception of corn, lentils, plums, prunes, cranberries. (Marked urinary acidity tends to occur during acute gout.)
- A low-purine diet contains almost no meat and therefore is unpleasant for most patients (seldom prescribed today since the use of a gout suppressant obviates the need for strict diet therapy). Some physicians merely advise patient to limit intake of high purine foods such as organ meats (liver, kidney, sweetbreads). Other foods high in purine content include wild game, goose, pork, caviar, anchovies, herring, sardines, mackerel, scallops, broth, meat extracts, gravy. Foods containing moderate amounts of purines include other meats, fish, seafood, fowl, asparagus, spinach, peas, and dried legumes.

Physician may prescribe sodium bicarbonate, or sodium or potassium citrate, to maintain alkaline urine and thus prevent formation of urate stones.

In addition to diet prescription:

Teaching Plan for Patients with Chronic Gout:

✓ Nature and volume of fluid intake
✓ How to test urine pH with reagent strip (e.g., N-Multstix C)
✓ Importance of early recognition of prodromal symptoms of an acute attack
✓ Importance of keeping drug at hand at all times and of initiating prescribed drug regimen when prodromal symptoms appear

C

- ✓ Adverse drug reactions that should be reported
- ✓ Medical follow-up appointment schedule
- ✓ Etiologic factors in acute gout: (a) trauma, e.g., poor-fitting shoes and socks, (b) overindulgence of food or alcohol, (c) fatigue, (d) emotional or physical stress, (e) infections, (f) surgery
- ✓ Confer with physician for specific guidelines.

Fermented beverages such as beer, ale, and wine may precipitate gouty attack and therefore should be avoided. The physician may allow distilled alcoholic beverages in moderation. Large amounts of alcohol reportedly can reduce the effects of colchicine.

Preserved in tight, light-resistant containers preferably between 15° and 30°C (59° and 86°F) unless otherwise directed by manufacturer.

Diagnostic Test Interferences. Possible interference with **urinary steroid (17-OHCS)** determinations when done by modifications of Reddy, Jenkins, Thorn procedure. Colchicine tends to reduce **serum cholesterol,** and **serum carotene** and may elevate **alkaline phosphatase, SGOT,** and **SGPT.** False-positive **urine tests for RBC's and hemoglobin** reported.

Drug Interactions: Colchicine

Plus	Interactions
Alcohol, ethyl	Large amounts may decrease effects of colchicine
CNS depressants	Colchicine may sensitize patients to these drugs
Sympathomimetic agents	Enhanced response to these drugs (based on animal studies)
Vitamin B_{12} (cyanocobalamin)	Colchicine can cause malabsorption of vitamin B_{12}
Acidifying agents; alkalinizing agents	Colchicine action is inhibited by acidifying agents and potentiated by alkalinizing agents

---

COLESTIPOL HYDROCHLORIDE
(Colestid)

(koe-les'ti-pole)
Resin exchange agent (anion)
Anion exchange resin, bile acid sequestrant, antihyperlipidemic
Antilipemic

ACTIONS AND USES. Insoluble chloride salt of a basic anion exchange resin, with high molecular weight. Binds with bile acids in intestinal tract to form an insoluble complex that is excreted in the feces resulting in reduced circulating cholesterol and increased serum LDL removal rate. Serum triglycerides are not affected or are minimally increased. Absorption and fate, contraindications, adverse reactions, interactions are similar to those of cholestyramine (qv).

Used to treat pruritus associated with partial biliary obstruction. Also used as an adjunct to diet therapy of patient with primary hypercholesterolemia (type IIa hyperlipoproteinemia) or with coronary artery disease unresponsive to diet or other measures alone. Used to treat digitoxin overdose and hyperoxaluria, and to control postoperative diarrhea caused by excess bile acids in colon.

CONTRAINDICATIONS AND PRECAUTIONS. Complete biliary obstruction, hypersensitivity to bile acid sequestrants; safe use by pregnant women, nursing mothers and children not established. *Cautious Use:* hemorrhoids, bleeding disorders, malabsorption states, the elderly. *See also Cholestyramine.*

ADVERSE/SIDE EFFECTS. CNS: headache, dizziness, anxiety, fatigue, drowsiness, weakness. **GI:** Constipation, abdominal pain or distention, belching, flatulance, nausea, vomiting, diarrhea, hemorrhoids, fecal impaction, perianal irritation. **Other:** dermatitis, urticaria, joint and muscle pain, arthritis, shortness of breath, transient increases in liver function tests, serum phosphorous, and chloride; decreases in serum sodium and potassium; vitamin A, D, E, K deficiency. *See also Cholestyramine.*

ROUTE AND DOSAGE. Oral: Adult: 15 to 30 Gm/day in 2 to 4 doses before meals. (Packets contain 5 Gm.) *Digitalis toxicity:* 10 Gm, followed by 5 Gm every 6 to 8 hours as needed.

NURSING IMPLICATIONS

Drugs given concomitantly should be scheduled at least 1 hour before or 4 hours after ingestion of colestipol to reduce interference with their absorption.

To prevent accidental inhalation or esophageal distress with dry form, always mix with liquids, soups, cereals, or pulpy fruits. Add powder to at least 90 ml fluid. When carbonated drink is used, slowly stir in a large glass because excess foaming may occur. Rinse glass with small amount extra fluid to be sure all of the drug is taken.

Watch for changes in bowel elimination pattern. Constipation should not be allowed to persist without medical attention. A stool softener may be prescribed, especially patients with coronary artery disease and for the elderly patient, as prophylaxis. Encourage dietary intake of high fiber foods if allowed, and adequate fluids.

Be sure patient understands importance of established regimens for colestipol and another concomitantly administered drug such as warfarin, thyroid hormone, or digitoxin. Patient should not change the times for taking each drug, nor omit or increase doses. Any change in established regimens should be approved by the physician.

Patients receiving prolonged colestipol therapy should be advised to report unusual bleeding (vitamin K deficiency). Colestipol prevents absorption of fat soluble vitamins (A, D, E, K). Supplemental vitamin A and D may be prescribed for these patients.

Urge patient not to use OTC drugs unless physician has given approval.

Check with physician regarding permitted amount of alcohol intake.

Store at temperature between 15° and 30°C (59° and 86°F) in well-closed container unless otherwise instructed by the manufacturer.

See Cholestyramine (prototype resin exchange agent).

Drug Interactions. **Oral hypoglycemic agents** may antagonize the action of colestipol. Pharmacologic effects of **digitalis glycosides** and **thiazide diuretics** may be reduced. (Colestipol impairs absorption of these drugs). Monitor clinical response.

COLISTIMETHATE SODIUM

(Coly-mycin M)

(koe-lis-ti-meth′ate)
Antiinfective
Antibiotic (polypeptide)
Polymyxin

ACTIONS AND USES. Polymyxin (E) antibiotic, sulfamethylated form of colistin. Similar to polymycin B in structure and actions, but about one-third to one-fifth as potent. Antibacterial activity and overall toxicity are less, but nephrotoxic potential is almost identical with that of polymycin B (qv). Bactericidal against most gram-negative organisms including *Pseudomonas aeruginosa, Escherichia coli, Enterobacter aerogenes, Klebsiella pneumoniae, Bru-*

cella. Complete cross-resistance and cross-sensitivity to polymycin B reported, but not to broad-spectrum antibiotics.

Used particularly in treatment of severe acute and chronic urinary tract infections caused by susceptible strains of gram-negative organisms resistant to other antibiotics. Has been used with carbenicillin for Pseudomonas sepsis in children with acute leukopenia.

ABSORPTION AND FATE. Peak plasma concentrations within 1 to 2 hours following IM injection, detectable for 8 to 12 hours; peak plasma levels following IV dose occur within 10 minutes, are higher, but decline more rapidly. Serum half-life: 2 to 3 hours. No distribution to cerebrospinal fluid even when meninges are inflamed. About 66 to 75% of dose excreted in urine within 24 hours, primarily as active metabolite. Crosses placenta and appears in breast milk.

CONTRAINDICATIONS AND PRECAUTIONS. Hypersensitivity to polypeptide antibiotics; concomitant use of drugs that potentiate neuromuscular blocking effect (aminoglycoside antibiotics, other polymyxins, anticholinesterases, curariform muscle relaxants, ether, sodium citrate), nephrotoxic and ototoxic drugs. Safe use during pregnancy not established. *Cautious Use:* impaired renal function, myasthenia gravis, elderly patients, infants.

ADVERSE/SIDE EFFECTS. Respiratory arrest following IM injection. **Hypersensitivity:** drug fever, pruritus, urticaria, dermatoses. **Nephrotoxicity:** albuminuria, cylinduria, azotemia, oliguria. **Neurotoxicity:** circumoral, lingual, and peripheral paresthesias; visual and speech disturbances, ototoxicity (impaired hearing, ataxia, dizziness, vertigo), neuromuscular blockade (generalized muscle weakness, dyspnea, respiratory depression or paralysis). **Other:** GI disturbances, pain at IM site, agranulocytosis, leukopenia, superinfections.

ROUTE AND DOSAGE. Intramuscular, intravenous: Adults and children: 2.5 to 5 mg/kg daily divided into 2 to 4 doses. Maximum daily dose should not exceed 5 mg/kg in patients with normal renal function. Dose and interval modified according to serum creatinine determinations. *For direct intermittent IV:* ½ daily dose injected over 3 to 5 minutes every 12 hours. *For continuous IV infusion:* ½ daily dose is slowly injected over 3 to 5 minutes; add remaining half to compatible infusion solution recommended by manufacturer and administer slowly 1 to 2 hours after initial dose.

NURSING IMPLICATIONS

Respiratory arrest has been reported following IM administration. Resuscitative equipment, oxygen, and IV calcium chloride should be immediately available. Report restlessness or dyspnea promptly.

IM injection should be made deep into upper outer quadrant of buttock. Patients commonly experience pain at injection site. Rotate sites.

IV infusion rate is prescribed by physician. (Rate of 5 to 6 mg/hour is recommended for patients with normal renal function.)

Infusion solution should be freshly prepared and used within 24 hours.

Culture and sensitivity tests should be performed initially and periodically during therapy to determine susceptibility of causative organisms.

Baseline renal function tests should be performed prior to therapy; frequent monitoring of renal function and urine drug levels is advisable during therapy. Impaired renal function increases the possibility of nephrotoxicity, apnea and neuromuscular blockade.

Monitor intake and output. Decrease in urine output or change in intake and output ratio, and rising BUN, serum creatinine, and serum drug levels (without dosage increase) are indications of renal toxicity. If they occur, withhold drug and report to physician. (*Normal BUN:* 10 to 20 mg/dl.)

Drug administration should be based on serum drug levels in patients with renal impairment.
Elderly patients and infants are particularly prone to develop renal toxicity because they tend to have inadequate renal reserves. Close monitoring is essential.
Be alert to changes in speech and hearing, visual changes, drowsiness, dizziness, and transient paresthesias and report them to the physician. Symptoms may be alleviated by reduction of dosage. Supervision of ambulation may be indicated.
Because of the possibility of transient neurologic disturbances such as dizziness, ataxia, weakness, caution ambulatory patient to avoid operating a vehicle or other activities requiring mental alertness and coordination while on drug therapy.
Postoperative patients who have received curariform muscle relaxants, ether, or sodium citrate should be closely monitored for signs of neuromuscular blockade (delayed recovery, muscle weakness, depressed respiration).
Reconstituted with sterile water for injection. Swirl vial gently during reconstitution to avoid bubble formation. Reconstituted solution may be stored in refrigerator at 2° to 8°C (36° to 46°F) or at controlled room temperature of 15° to 30°C (59° to 86°F). Use within 7 days. Store unopened vials at controlled room temperature.
See also Polymyxin B Sulfate (prototype polymyxin).

Drug Interactions. Nephrotoxic effects of colistimethate may be increased by **cephalothin.** *See also Polymyxin B.*

COLISTIN SULFATE

(Coly-Mycin S, Polymyxin E)

(koe-lis'tin)
Antiinfective
Antibiotic (polypeptide)
Polymyxin

ACTIONS AND USES. Polymyxin (E) antibiotic derived from *Bacillus polymyxa* var. *colistinus.* Similar to polymyxin B (qv) in actions, contraindications, precautions, and adverse reactions. Antibacterial potency appears to be equal to that of polymyxin B. Bactericidal against most gram-negative enteric pathogens especially *Escherichia coli, Shigella, Pseudomonas aeruginosa, Klebsiella pneumoniae,* and *Aerobacter aerogenes.* Not effective against *Proteus* or gram-positive microorganisms.

Used to treat diarrhea in infants and children, caused by susceptible organisms. Commercially available in fixed-dose combination with hydrocortisone and neomycin (Coly-Mycin S Otic) for treatment of ear infections.

ABSORPTION AND FATE. May be slightly absorbed from GI tract (degree of absorption in infants is unpredictable). Serum half-life: 2 to 3 hours. Excreted mainly in urine.

CONTRAINDICATIONS AND PRECAUTIONS. Hypersensitivity to colistin derivatives. *Cautious Use:* renal impairment. *See also Polymyxin B.*

ADVERSE/SIDE EFFECTS. Infrequent within recommended dosage range: nausea, vomiting, hypersensitivity reactions, superinfections. Same potential for nephrotoxicity and neurotoxicity as polymyxin B (qv).

ROUTE AND DOSAGE. Oral: Infants and children: 5 to 15 mg/kg/day divided into 3 doses and administered at 8-hour intervals. Each 5 ml of suspension contains the equivalent of 25 mg colistin base.

C

NURSING IMPLICATIONS

Renal function should be assessed prior to initiation of therapy and frequent measurements should be made during therapy in patients with impaired renal function.

Monitor intake and output. Bear in mind that urine output alone is not a reliable index of renal toxicity. Hematuria and proteinuria (cloudy urine), and increases in BUN and serum creatinine (signs of nonoliguric renal failure) can occur without oliguria.

Superinfections (due to change in intestinal flora) may occur with prolonged use. Report worsening of diarrhea, anal itching, and discharge, and sore tongue.

To protect the family members from causative agents of diarrhea, stress importance of hand washing particularly after handling patient and fomites, and before eating. Advise refrigeration of perishable foods and protection of food from flies. Airborne (dust) transmission may be a factor.

Separate isolation facilities for infected patient is advisable. Concurrent disinfection of all discharges and soiled articles is essential.

Oral suspension is prepared by reconstituting powder with 37 ml distilled water. Slowly add one-half of the diluent to bottle, replace cap, and shake well. Add remaining diluent and repeat shaking. Indicate expiration date on label.

Following reconstitution, solution is stable for 2 weeks when kept below 15°C (59°F). Store in tightly covered container; protect from light. Unopened bottles may be stored at controlled room temperature 15° to 30°C (59° to 86°F) unless otherwise directed by manufacturer.

See Polymyxin B (prototype polymixins).

COLLAGENASE

(Biozyme-C, Santyl)

(kol′la-je-nase)
Debriding agent
Enzyme

ACTIONS AND USES. Enzymatic debriding agent derived from fermentation of *Clostridium histolyticum.* Possesses specific ability to hydrolyze (digest) peptide bonds of denatured and undenatured collagen. Action results in liquefaction of necrotic tissue without affecting collagen in newly-formed granulation tissue or other healthy tissue, facilitation of tissue granulation, and subsequent wound epithelialization. Although it lacks direct antiinfective properties, it discourages bacterial growth by removing debris that might invite bacterial proliferation.

Used to debride necrotic tissue of severe burns or dermal ulcers including decubiti and stasis ulcers.

CONTRAINDICATIONS AND PRECAUTIONS. Local or systemic hypersensitivity to collagenase. *Cautious Use:* debilitated patients.

ADVERSE/SIDE EFFECTS. Local: pain, burning, redness, irritation. **Other:** hypersensitivity reactions reported following long-term use in combination with cortisone; bacteremia.

ROUTE AND DOSAGE. Topical: apply ointment once daily (or more frequently), or every other day, as directed. (Ointment is prepared in a white petrolatum base.)

NURSING IMPLICATIONS

Prior to each collagenase application, necrotic debris should be removed by gently cleansing lesion with cotton or gauze saturated with hydrogen peroxide or Dakin's solution, followed by sterile normal saline. Consult physician about specific procedure.

If lesion has had prior treatment with incompatible topical agent, site should be carefully cleansed by repeated washings with normal saline before applying collagenase.

Patient may require concomitant application of a topical antibacterial agent (prescribed) if infection is present. (Neomycin, bacitracin, polymyxin B are reportedly compatible with collagenase.)

Advise patient to avoid contact of drug in or near eyes. If contact occurs, irrigate immediately with copious amounts of water.

Irritation or redness of surrounding skin can be prevented by confining ointment to lesion being treated and by applying a protectant such as zinc oxide paste (Lassar's paste) to skin.

There is some risk of bacteremia associated with the use of debriding enzymes, particularly in debilitated patients. Monitor vital signs.

Complete wound debridement generally occurs in about 7 to 14 days. Collagenase should be discontinued when necrotic tissue has been debrided and healthy granulation tissue is present.

Optimal collagenase activity occurs in the pH range of 6 to 8. Collagenase is rendered irreversibly inactive at pH levels below 5 and reversibly inactive at pH 8.5 or above.

Action of collagenase can be stopped by application of aluminum acetate solution (Burow's solution), which has pH of 3.6 to 4.4 (aluminum ions may also inhibit enzymatic action).

The following agents reportedly do not interfere with collagenase activity: normal saline, hydrogen peroxide, 70% ethyl alcohol, modified Dakin's solution (diluted sodium hypochlorite solution), neomycin, bacitracin, polymyxin B, and streptomycin (unless antibodies are formulated as acid salts).

Store ointment at temperatures not exceeding 37°C (98.6°F), unless otherwise directed by manufacturer.

Drug Interactions: Collagenase

Plus	Interactions
Benzalkonium chloride Hexachlorophene Nitrofurazone (Furacin) Tincture of iodine Preparations containing heavy metal ions such as silver or mercury (e.g., sulfadiazine silver, silver nitrate, thimerosal), and aluminum ions (e.g., Burow's solution)	Reduce collagenase enzymatic activity

C

CORTICOTROPIN
(ACTH, Acthar)

CORTICOTROPIN REPOSITORY
(ACTH Gel, Acthron, Cortigel, Cortrophin-Gel, Cotropic Gel, H.P. Acthar Gel)

CORTICOTROPIN ZINC HYDROXIDE
(Cortrophin-Zinc)

(kor-ti-koe-troe'pin)
Hormone
Glucocorticoid

ACTIONS AND USES. Adrenocorticotropic hormone extracted from pituitary of domestic animals (usually pigs). Stimulates functioning adrenal cortex to produce and secrete corticosterone, cortisol (hydrocortisone), several weak androgens and limited amounts of aldosterone. Therapeutic effects appear more rapidly than do those of hydrocortisone (qv). Suppresses further release of corticotropin by negative feedback mechanism. Chronic administration of exogenous cortico steroids decreases ACTH store and causes structural changes in pituitary. Lack of ACTH stimulation can lead to adrenal cortex atrophy.

Used for diagnostic test of adrenocortical function and to treat adrenal insufficiency produced by cortisone, hydrocortisone, prednisone, and other corticosteroids by direct stimulation of atrophic adrenal gland. Used for its antiinflammatory and immunosuppressant properties and its effect on blood and lymphatic systems. Also used in the symptomatic treatment of acute exacerbation of multiple sclerosis and to increase muscle strength in patients with severe myasthenia gravis that is refractory to treatment with anticholinesterases. *See also Hydrocortisone.*

ABSORPTION AND FATE. Rapid absorption with onset of action within 6 hours following injection. Duration of action about 2 to 4 hours; half-life less than 20 minutes. (Repository preparations: absorption over an 8- to 16-hour period; duration of effect: 18 to 72 hours.) Binds to plasma proteins and concentrates in many tissues. Excreted in urine. Probably does not cross placenta.

CONTRAINDICATIONS AND PRECAUTIONS. Ocular herpes simplex, recent surgery, congestive heart failure, scleroderma, osteoporosis, systemic fungoid infections, hypertension, sensitivity to porcine proteins, conditions accompanied by primary adrenocortical insufficiency or hyperfunction. Use during pregnancy (category C), in lactating women or women in childbearing years requires evaluation of expected benefits against possible hazards to mother and child. *Cautious Use:* patients with latent tuberculosis or those reacting to tuberculin; hypothyroiditis, impaired hepatic function. *See also Hydrocortisone.*

ADVERSE/SIDE EFFECTS. (Usually reversible with discontinuation of treatment.) Hypersensitivity, Na and water retention, increased K excretion, calcium loss, impaired wound healing, reactivation of tuberculosis. With prolonged use: antibody production, loss of stimulating effect of ACTH, post-subcapsular cataracts, glaucoma, possible damage to optic nerve, pancreatitis. *See also Hydrocortisone.*

ROUTE AND DOSAGE. *Diagnosis:* Corticoptropin Injection only: **Intravenous infusion:** 10 to 25 units in 500 ml 5% dextrose injection, infused over 8 hours. *Deficiency states:* Corticotropin injection: **Intramuscular, subcutaneous:** 20 units four times daily. Repository: **Intramuscular, subcutaneous:** 40 to 80 units every 24 to 72 hours. Zinc hydroxide: **Intramuscular only:** 40 units every 12 to 24 hours. *Myasthenia gravis:* Corticotropin injection: **Intravenous:** 100 units/day to total of 1000 units for over 8-hour period for 10 days.

NURSING IMPLICATIONS

Verification tests (for adrenal responsiveness to corticotropin) are recommended prior to treatment using the route of administration proposed for treatment (IM or SC).

Before giving corticotropin to patient with suspected sensitivity to porcine proteins, hypersensitivity skin testing should be performed.

Dosage is individualized according to disease being treated and medical condition of patient. Changes in dosage regimen are gradual and only after full drug effects have become apparent.

Observe patient closely for 15 minutes for hypersensitivity reactions during IV administration or immediately after SC or IM injections. Epinephrine 1:1000 should be readily available for emergency treatment.

Adrenal response to corticotropin is measured against a baseline plasma cortisol level 1 hour before the 8-hour test. Another plasma level is determined after at least 1 hour of the infusion (before the end). When other test methods are used, plasma cortisol levels are determined at intervals during and/or after the test.

If patient has limited adrenal reserves, 1 mg dexamethasone may be given at midnight before the corticotropin test and 500 mcg at start of test.

To test for adrenal function: 10 to 25 units corticotropin injection (further diluted in 500 ml) is given by IV infusion over 8-hour period. In the normal individual and those with primary adrenal insufficiency one 8-hour infusion is adequate. To evaluate adrenocortical reserve with secondary adrenocortical insufficiency or hypopituitarism, an 8 hour infusion on each of 4 or 5 successive days may be required.

Test results: Patient with normal adrenal reserve: an increase in plasma cortisol levels of 15 to 40 mcg/dl by the eighth hour of the 8-hour corticotropin infusion (plasma cortisol levels more than 45 mcg/dl by 8 hours, urinary 17-OHCS increase to 12 to 25 mg/Gm creatinine; 17-KS increase by 1.5 to 2.5 times control level). Patient with complete primary adrenal suppression: no change from baseline plasma cortisol or urinary 17-OHCS or 17-KS excretion levels. Patient with hypopituitarism: plasma cortisol levels and urinary 17-OHCS increase in subnormal increments after the 8-hour test daily for 5 days.

Corticotropin Repository is quite viscid at room temperature.

Corticotropin zinc hydroxide and corticotropin repository forms are not suitable for IV use.

Shake zinc hydroxide bottle well before injecting drug deep into gluteal muscle.

Follow manufacturer's instructions for reconstitution and storage of drugs.

Normal baseline plasma cortisol levels: 8 AM: 10 to 25 mcg/dl; less than 10 mcg/dl late in evening.

Normal 17-OHCS: male, 5 to 12 mg/24 hours; female, 3 to 10 mg/24 hours.

Before, during, and after an unusual stressful event, rapidly acting corticosteroids may be given to supplement activity of corticotropin.

Corticotropin does not alter natural course of disease but may only suppress signs and symptoms of chronic disease.

Prolonged use increases risk of hypersensitivity reaction (skin reactions, dizziness, nausea, vomiting, mild fever, anaphylactic shock, wheezing, circulatory failure, death).

New infections, e.g., fungal or virus infection of eye, can appear during treatment. Because of decreased resistance and inability to localize the infection, it may be severe. Report immediately. Antiinfective therapy is indicated.

Eye examinations should be done before expected long-term therapy and periodically during treatment. Instruct patient to report to physician if blurred vision occurs.

Growth and development of a child receiving this drug should be carefully monitored.

Dietary salt restriction and K supplementation may be necessary to minimize edema caused by overstimulation of the adrenal cortex by corticotropin. Facilitate information-exchange conferences related to patient's diet-drug therapies with nutritionist, physician, patient, and responsible family member.

Patient should not be vaccinated while receiving corticotropin.

Administration of the hormone at high dosage levels is tapered rather than withdrawn suddenly. A 2- to 5-day period of adrenocortical hypofunction follows discontinuation of corticotropin.

See also Hydrocortisone.

CORTISONE ACETATE

(Cortoneacetate)

(kor'ti-sone)
Corticosteroid
Glucocorticoid
Mineralocorticoid

ACTIONS AND USES. Short-acting synthetic steroid with prominent glucocorticoid actions and in high doses, mineralocorticoid properties. Therapeutic activity depends on in vivo conversion to hydrocortisone (qv), with which it shares uses, absorption, fate, contraindications, adverse/side effects, and interactions.

ABSORPTION AND FATE. Rapid onset after oral administration but slow (24 to 48 hours) after IM administration. Peak effect (oral): 2 hours; (IM), 20 to 48 hours. Duration of action: 1.25 to 1.5 days. Half-life (plasma): 0.5 hours. HPA (hypothalamic–pituitary–adrenal) axis suppression: 8 to 12 hours.

CONTRAINDICATIONS AND PRECAUTIONS. Safe use in pregnancy (category C), during lactation, or by children not established. *See Hydrocortisone.*

ROUTE AND DOSAGE. Highly individualized. **Adults: Oral, Intramuscular:** Initial: 25 to 300 mg daily, as single or divided doses. Dose is reduced by periodic decrements of 10 to 25 mg/day to lowest effective amount. Oral dose lower than 25 mg may be adequate. **Pediatric: Oral:** 2.5 to 10 mg/kg body weight or 20 to 300 mg/m^2 body surface/day in 4 divided doses. **Intramuscular:** 200 mcg to 1.25 mcg/kg or 7 to 37.5 mg/m^2 one or two times daily.

NURSING IMPLICATIONS

Sodium chloride and a mineralocorticoid are usually given with cortisone as part of replacement therapy.

Parenteral cortisone is a suspension and therefore should not be used intravenously. Shake bottle well before withdrawing dose.

Admixtures with other parenteral medications are not recommended because of state of suspension and altered absorption rate.

Alternate-day therapy *(see Index)* with an oral intermediate acting glucocorticoid may decrease growth retardation effect in children.

Store at temperature between 15° and 30°C (59° and 86°F) in well-closed container, unless otherwise directed by manufacturer.

See Hydrocortisone (prototype glucocorticoid) for additional Nursing Implications and Drug Interactions.

COSYNTROPIN

(koe-sin-troe'pin)

(Cortrosyn, Synacthen Depot)

Diagnostic agent

C

ACTIONS AND USES. Synthetic polypeptide resembling corticotropin (ACTH) in the first 24 of the 39 amino acids in naturally occurring ACTH. Has less immunologic activity and less risk of sensitivity than corticotropin. In patient with normal adrenocortical function, stimulates adrenal cortex to secrete corticosterone, cortisol (hydrocortisone), several weak androgenic substances and limited amounts of aldosterone (steroidogenic activity). Extraadrenal actions include melanotropic and adipokinetic effects and increased secretion of growth hormone. Not used therapeutically.

Used as a diagnostic tool to differentiate primary adrenal from secondary (pituitary) adrenocortical insufficiency. *Investigational Use:* patient with normal adrenocortical function for the long-term treatment of chronic inflammatory or degenerative disorders responsive to glucocorticoids.

ABSORPTION AND FATE. In normal individual, following IM or rapid IV infusion, plasma cortisol levels begin to rise in 5 minutes and are doubled in 15 to 30 minutes. Peak levels in 1 hour are maintained about 2 to 4 hours. Precise distribution and metabolic fate unknown; bound to plasma proteins and rapidly removed from plasma by many tissues. Does not cross placenta.

CONTRAINDICATIONS AND PRECAUTIONS. Known hypersensitivity to cosyntropin; hydrocortisone on day of testing, history of allergic reactions to corticotropin.

ADVERSE/SIDE EFFECTS. Hypersensitivity reactions (rare); pruritus.

ROUTE AND DOSAGE. *Rapid screening test:* **Intramuscular, intravenous:** injection over 2 minute period: **Adults:** 0.25 mg. **Children (younger than 2 years):** 0.125 mg. For greater stimulation to adrenal cortex: **Intravenous infusion:** 0.125 mg administered over 4- to 8-hour period at rate of approximately 0.04 mg/hour over 6-hour period.

NURSING IMPLICATIONS

Reconstitute cosyntropin powder by adding 1 ml 0.9% NaCl injection to vial labeled 0.25 mg to provide solution containing 0.25 mg cosyntropin/ml.

Reconstituted solutions have pH of 5.5 to 7.5 and remain stable 24 hours at room temperature or 21 days at 2° to 8°C. Following further dilution, drug remains stable 12 hours at room temperature if pH is 5.5 to 7.5.

Cosyntropin should not be added to blood or to plasma infusions.

Screening test for adrenocortical insufficiency: Plasma cortisol levels are determined prior to and 30 or 60 minutes after administration of 250 mcg IM or IV. If patient has normal adrenocortical function, baseline plasma cortisol levels are greater than 5 mcg/dl; 30 minute levels are greater than 18 mcg/dl with an increase of at least 7 mcg/dl above control level. At end of 60 minutes a normal response is a doubling of the baseline level with an increase of 11 mcg/dl above base plasma cortisol levels.

Subnormal test results differentiate adrenal insufficiency of either adrenal (primary) or pituitary (secondary) origin. To distinguish between primary and secondary insufficiency, a second test is run: 40 units repository corticotropin injection IM two times daily for 4 days, or 60 units two times daily for 3 days, or 8 hours corticotropin infusion on each of 4 to 5 successive days, all followed by second cosyntropin test. Test results: *Patient with primary insufficiency:* little or no increase in plasma cortisol levels following second cosyntropin test. *Patients with secondary insufficiency;* normal or higher plasma cortisol levels after second cosyntropin test.

Although plasma cortisol levels are better indicators of adrenal function, the response can also be measured by 24 hour urinary 17-KS or 17-OHCS excretion before and at end of IV infusion.

Normal 17-KS levels: men, 10 to 25 mg/24 hours; women (under 50 years): 5 to 15 mg/24 hours; (over 50 years): 4 to 8 mg/24 hours.

17-OHCS levels: men: 5 to 12 mg/24 hours; women: 3 to 10 mg/24 hours; children 8 to 12 years: less than 4.5 mg/24 hours; younger children: 1.5 mg/24 hours. May be slightly higher in obese or muscular individuals.

Urine collection for study of 17-KS excretion may have to be postponed if female patient is menstruating.

If patient is on prednisone, dexamethasone, or betamethasone, therapy can continue through the test period, because these drugs do not interfere with analysis of serum cortisol.

Cortisone, hydrocortisone, or spironolactone should not be administered on the test day.

CROMOLYN SODIUM

(Disodium Cromoglycate, DSCG, Fivent, Intal, Nalcrom, Nasalcrom, Opticrom, Rynacrom, Sodium Cromoglycate)

(kroe'moe-lin)
Antiasthmatic
Mast cell stabilizer

ACTIONS AND USES. Synthetic asthma-prophylactic agent with unique action. Inhibits release of bronchoconstrictors—histamine and SRS-A (slow-reacting substance of anaphylaxis)—from sensitized pulmonary mast cells, thereby suppressing an allergic response. Has no direct bronchodilator, antihistaminic, or antiinflammatory properties. Particularly effective for IgE-mediated or "extrinsic asthma" (precipitated by exposure to specific allergen, e.g., pollen, dust, animal dander). Has also benefited many patients with nonatopic or "intrinsic asthma" which is triggered by nonallergic factors such as infections, irritants, emotions. Patient response is reportedly unpredictable. Believed to act by interfering with calcium transport across mast cell membrane and by promoting phosphorylation of mast cell protein.

Used prophylactically as adjunct in management of severe perennial bronchial asthma, and allergic ocular disorders. Of no value in acute asthmatic attack, especially status asthmaticus. Cromolyn does not obviate the need for usual therapy with bronchodilators, expectorants, antibiotics or corticosteroids, but the amount and frequency of use of these agents may be appreciably reduced.

ABSORPTION AND FATE. Peak plasma concentrations within 15 minutes, following inhalation. Duration of action: 4 to 6 hours but carryover effect (unexplainable) may be as long as 2 to 3 weeks. About 8% of dose reaches lungs and is readily absorbed into systemic circulation. The rest is deposited in mouth and back of throat and is then swallowed, and excreted unchanged in bile (feces) and urine in approximately equal amounts. Elimination half-life: 80 minutes. Small amounts exhaled.

CONTRAINDICATIONS AND PRECAUTIONS. Hypersensitivity to cromolyn or lactose; acute asthma, status asthmaticus, dyspnea; children younger than 5 years of age; patients unable to coordinate actions or follow instructions. Safe use during pregnancy and in nursing women not established (category B). *Cautious Use:* renal or hepatic dysfunction, long-term use.

ADVERSE/SIDE EFFECTS. Generally well tolerated. **CNS:** headache, dizziness, vertigo, peripheral neuritis. **ENT:** irritation of throat, trachea; cough, hoarseness; nasal congestion, bronchospasm, wheezing, laryngeal edema (rare). **GI:** swelling of parotid glands, dry mouth, slightly bitter after taste, nausea, vomiting, esophagitis. **Hypersensitivity:** erythema, urticaria, contact dermatitis, exfoliative dermatitis, photodermatitis, peripheral eosinophilia, angioedema, eosinophilic pneumonia, polymyositis, anaphylaxis (rare). **Nephrotoxicity:** dysuria, urinary frequency, nephrosis. **Opthalmic:** itchy, puffy eyes, lacrimation, transient burning, stinging. **Other:** joint swelling and pain, myalgia, periarteritis vasculitis, pericarditis with cardiac tamponade, fever, hemoptysis, anemia. Related to the delivery system: inhalation of gelatin particles, mouthpiece, or propeller.

ROUTE AND DOSAGE. Oral Inhalation: Adults and children (6 years or older): *Powder for inhalation:* contents of one capsule inhaled 4 times daily at regular intervals, using special accompanying inhaler. Each capsule (for inhalation only) contains 20 mg cromolyn as micronized powder in lactose powder vehicle. **Nasal Inhalation** (Administered by special nasal metered spray device. Each actuation delivers 5.2 mg cromolyn): 1 spray in each nostril 3 to 6 times daily, at regular intervals. **Ophthalmic** (solution 4%): 1 or 2 drops in each eye 4 to 6 times/day at regular intervals. One drop contains 1.6 mg cromolyn.

NURSING IMPLICATIONS

Pulmonary function test recommended prior to initiation of therapy. (Candidate for therapy must have a significant bronchodilator-reversible component to the airway obstruction.)

Patient should receive detailed instructions for loading the turbo-inhaler and administering preparation (see manufacturer's instructions) and must demonstrate correct use of apparatus. Therapeutic effect is largely dependent on proper scheduling of treatments and use of inhaler.

Advise patient to clear as much mucus as possible before inhalation treatments.

Instruct patient to exhale as completely as possible before placing inhaler mouthpiece between lips, tilt head backwards and inhale rapidly and deeply with steady, even breaths. Remove inhaler from mouth, hold breath for a few seconds then exhale into the air. Repeat until entire dose is taken.

Caution patient not to exhale into inhaler, because moisture from breath will interfere with its proper operation. Also inform patient that capsule is intended for inhalation only and is ineffective if swallowed because it is not absorbed from GI tract.

One or two inhalations of an immediate acting sympathomimetic bronchodilator, e.g., isoproterenol (Isuprel) or metaproterenol (Alupent), 15 minutes prior to cromolyn therapy may be prescribed for patients who develop cough or wheezing (bronchospasm) associated with inhalation of dry powder. This practice also enhances delivery of drug within tracheobronchial tree.

Throat irritation, cough, and hoarseness, possible adverse effects from inhaling cromolyn, can be minimized by gargling with water, drinking a few swallows of water or by sucking on a lozenge after each treatment. Esophageal irritation manifested as substernal burning sensation may be prevented by prophylactic administration of an antacid (consult physician) or a glass of milk before each cromolyn treatment.

Exacerbation of asthmatic symptoms including breathlessness and cough, may occur in patients receiving cromolyn during corticosteroid withdrawal. The same is true of patients on maintenance steroid therapy when cromolyn is withdrawn. Withdrawal of either agent should be accomplished gradually and under close supervision.

Patient should be provided with specific instructions regarding what to do in the event of an acute asthmatic attack.

Advise patient to report any unusual signs or symptoms. Hypersensitivity reactions can be severe and life-threatening. Eosinophil count is a reliable indicator of developing allergy and therefore should be monitored. Drug should be discontinued if an allergic reaction occurs.

Instruct patient to pay careful attention to general health and to protect against colds and flu.

Prior treatment with cromolyn 15 minutes before doing protracted exercise (e.g. jogging) reportedly blunts the effects of vigorous exercise as well as cold air.

Therapeutic effects may be noted within a few days but generally not until after 2 to 4 weeks of therapy: reduced number of asthmatic attacks; decreased cough, sputum, wheezing, and breathlessness; increased exercise tolerance; decreased requirement for concomitant drug (e.g., bronchodilators, corticosteroids) therapy. Keep physician informed.

Patient should be advised not to wear soft contact lenses during ocular therapy. They may be worn within a few hours after therapy is terminated.

Protect cromolyn from moisture and heat. Store at room temperature in well-closed, light-resistant container preferably between 15° and 30°C (59° and 86°F) unless otherwise directed by manufacturer.

CROTAMITON

(kroe-tam'i-tonn)

(Eurax)

Scabicide

ACTIONS AND USES. Used for eradication of scabies *(Sarcoptes scabiei)* and for symptomatic treatment of pruritus.

CONTRAINDICATIONS AND PRECAUTIONS. Should not be applied to acutely inflamed skin, raw or weeping surfaces, eyes, or mouth or used by patients with history of previous sensitivity to crotamiton.

ADVERSE/SIDE EFFECTS. Skin irritation (particularly with prolonged use), skin rash, erythema, sensation of warmth, allergic sensitization.

ROUTE AND DOSAGE. Topical: 10% in vanishing cream base; 10% lotion in an emollient base.

NURSING IMPLICATIONS

Preliminary bathing of skin is not essential, but if it is done, the skin must be thoroughly dry before applying medication.

Treatment for scabies: Thoroughly massage medication into skin on all parts of body from chin downward, paying particular attention to body folds and creases, hands, and feet. Caution patient to avoid contact with eyes, mouth, or urethral meatus. A second application 24 hours later is advised. Clothing and bedding should be changed the next morning, machine washed in hot water and dried in hot drier for at least 20 minutes or be dry-cleaned. Cleansing bath should follow 48 hours after last application.

Contaminated bed linen and washable clothing may be washed in the hot cycle of the washing machine or clothing can be dry cleaned.

Treatment for pruritus: Massage medication gently into affected areas until it is completely absorbed. Repeat as needed (usually effective for 6 to 10 hours).

Instruct the patient to discontinue medication and report to physician if irritation or sensitization develops.

See Lindane for additional points on management of scabies.

PROTOTYPE

CYANOCOBALAMIN

(sye-an-oh-koe-bal'a-min)
Vitamin B_{12}
Antianemic

(Anacoben, Bedoz, Berubigen, Betalin 12, Cabadon M, Cobalamin, Cobex, Crystimin, Cyanabin, Cyanoject, Kaybovite, Nova-Rubi, Pernavit, Redisol, Rubesol, Rubion, Rubramin PC, Sytobex, Vitamin B_{12}, Vi-Twel)

C

ACTIONS AND USES. Vitamin B_{12} is a cobalt-containing substance produced by *Streptomyces griseus.* Essential for normal growth, cell reproduction, maturation of RBC's, nucleoprotein synthesis, maintanance of nervous system (myelin synthesis), and believed to be involved in protein and carbohydrate metabolism. Also acts as coenzyme in various biologic reactions. Stimulates reticulocytes and together with folic acid is involved in formation of oxyribonucleotides from ribonucleotides. Vitamin B_{12} deficiency results in megaloblastic anemia, dysfunction of spinal cord with paralysis, GI lesions.

Used in treatment of vitamin B_{12} deficiency due to malabsorption syndrome as in pernicious (Addison's) anemia, sprue; GI pathology, dysfunction, or surgery; fish tapeworm infestation, and gluten enteropathy. Also used in B_{12} deficiency caused by increased physiologic requirements or inadequate dietary intake, and in vitamin B_{12} absorption (Schilling) test.

ABSORPTION AND FATE. Intestinal absorption requires presence of gastric "intrinsic factor" (lacking in pernicious anemia) to transfer drug across intestinal mucosa. Absorbed from terminal ileum in presence of calcium and bound to plasma proteins. With large oral doses, some absorption by diffusion. Converted in tissues to active coenzymes methylcobalamin and deoxyadenosylcobalamin. Small injected doses almost completely retained. Excreted in bile but then undergoes enterohepatic recycling. Widely distributed in most tissues. Principal storage site is in liver; also stored in kidneys and adrenals. Crosses placenta. When given in doses of 100 mcg or more, 50 to 95% is excreted in urine within 48 hours; most is eliminated during first 8 hours. Enters breast milk.

CONTRAINDICATIONS AND PRECAUTIONS. History of sensitivity to vitamin B_{12}, other cobalamins, or cobalt; early Leber's disease (hereditary optic nerve atrophy), indiscriminate use in folic acid deficiency. Safe use during pregnancy, in nursing women, and in children not established. *Cautious Use:* heart disease, history of gout, anemia, pulmonary disease; concomitant use with cardiac glycosides.

ADVERSE/SIDE EFFECTS. Mild transient diarrhea, itching, rash, flushing, feeling of swelling of body, peripheral vascular thrombosis, pulmonary edema, congestive heart failure, hypokalemia, sudden death. Severe optic nerve atrophy (in patients with Leber's disease), anaphylactic shock. Also reported: unmasking of polycythemia vera with correction of vitamin B_{12} deficiency; precipitation of gout.

ROUTE AND DOSAGE. Highly individualized dosage schedules. *Vitamin B deficiency:* **Intramuscular, deep subcutaneous: Adults:** 30 mcg daily for 5 to 10 days; maintenance: 100 to 200 mcg monthly. **Children:** 100 mcg doses to total of 1 to 5 mg over 2 or more weeks; maintenance: 60 mcg/month. *Pernicious anemia:* Initial: 100 mcg daily for 2 to 3 weeks; maintenance: 100 mcg IM every 2 to 4 weeks for life. *Diagnosis of megaloblastic anemia:* 1 mcg IM for 10 days while maintaining a low folate and vitamin B_{12} diet. Appearance of reticulocytes in 3 to 10 days of therapy confirms diagnosis of vitamin B_{12} deficiency. *Schilling test:* 1000 mcg flushing dose IM. *Nutritional supplement:* **Oral:** 1 to 25 mcg/day.

NURSING IMPLICATIONS

Oral preparations may be mixed with fruit juices, if patient prefers. However, administer promptly since ascorbic acid affects the stability of vitamin B_{12}.

C

Administration of oral vitamin B_{12} with meals increases its absorption presumably by stimulating production of intrinsic factor.

Bowel regularity is essential for consistent absorption of oral preparations.

Prior to initiation of therapy, reticulocyte and erythrocyte counts, Hgb, Hct; vitamin B_{12} and serum folate levels should be determined; these studies should be repeated between 5 and 7 days after start of therapy and at regular intervals during therapy. In some cases bone marrow studies, tests for gastric free acid, and GI series will be performed.

Normal serum vitamin B_{12} is 200 to 800 picograms (pg)/ml. Serum levels below 100 pg/ml usually result in megaloblastic anemia and/or neurologic damage and psychiatric manifestations.

A careful history of previous sensitivities should be obtained. An intradermal test dose is recommended in patients suspected of being sensitive to cyanocobalamin. Reportedly sensitization to cyanocobalamin can take as long as 8 years to develop.

Potassium levels should be monitored during the first 48 hours particularly in patients with Addisonian pernicious anemia or megaloblastic anemia, with supplementation if necessary. Conversion to normal erythropoiesis increases erythrocyte potassium requirement and can result in fatal hypokalemia in these patients.

Monitor vital signs in patients with cardiac disease and in those receiving parenteral cyanocobalamin, and be alert to symptoms of pulmonary edema, which generally occur early in therapy.

A complete diet and drug history and an inquiry into alcohol drinking patterns should be done on all patients receiving cyanocobalamin to identify and correct poor habits. Single deficiency of one vitamin is rare; generally patients will have multiple vitamin deficiency. Collaborate with physician, dietitian, patient, and responsible family member in constructing a teaching plan.

The Schilling test for pernicious anemia measures vitamin B_{12} absorption: Patient fasts 12 hours and drinks no water 4 hours before test. Radioactive $^{57}Co\text{-}B_{12}$ (0.5 to 1.0 mcg) is given by mouth; 2 hours later urine sample is collected and discarded, and an IM flushing dose (1000 mcg) of nonradioactive B_{12} is administered. Urine is accurately collected for a 24-hour period, and radioactivity is measured. Impaired absorption: less than 5% urinary excretion (normal is 7 to 30%).

Parenteral therapy is the preferred treatment for patients with pernicious anemia, since oral administration may be unreliable. In the presence of neurologic complications, prolonged inadequate oral therapy may lead to permanent spinal cord damage. However, oral therapy may be used when the condition is mild and is without neurologic signs, or in rare patients who are sensitive to the parenteral form or who refuse it.

Therapeutic response to drug therapy is usually dramatic, occurring within 48 hours. Effectiveness is measured by laboratory values and improvement in manifestations of vitamin B_{12} deficiency: fatigue, GI symptoms, anorexia, pale pallor, yellow complexion, glossitis, distaste for meat, dyspnea on exertion, palpitation, nervous system degeneration (paresthesias, loss of vibratory and position sense and deep reflexes, incoordination), psychotic behavior, anosmia, visual disturbances.

Characteristically, reticulocyte concentration rises in 3 to 4 days, peaks in 5 to 8 days, and then gradually declines as erythrocyte count and hemoglobin rise to normal levels (in 4 to 6 weeks).

Instruct patient to notify physician if an intercurrent disease or infection occurs. Increase in cyanocobalamin dosage may be required.

Patients with mild peripheral neurologic defects may respond to concomitant physical therapy. Usually, demonstrable neurologic damage is considered irreversible if there is no improvement after 1 to 1½ years of adequate therapy. Severe vitamin B_{12} deficiency that is allowed to progress 3 months or longer may cause permanent degenerative lesions

C

of spinal cord; this is generally observed when folic acid is used as the sole hematopoietic agent.

It is imperative for the patient with pernicious anemia to understand that parenteral drug therapy must be continued throughout life to prevent irreversible neurologic damage.

Smoking–Drug Interaction: Smokers appear to have increased requirements for vitamin B_{12}.

The RDA for adults and children over 7 years is 3 mcg; during pregnancy (category C) and lactation 4 mcg; infants up to 6 months: 0.5 mcg; 6 months to 1 year: 1.5 mcg. The average diet in most Western countries supplies 5 to 30 mcg daily.

Dietary deficiency of vitamin B_{12} alone is rare; however, it has been observed in vegetarians and their breast-fed infants. Rich food sources: organ meats, clams, oysters; good sources: egg yolk, crabs, salmon, sardines, muscle meat, milk and dairy products.

Preserved in light-resistant containers at room temperature preferably between 15° and 30°C (59° and 86°F) unless otherwise directed by manufacturer.

Diagnostic Test Interferences. Most antibiotics, methotrexate, and pyrimethamine may produce invalid diagnostic blood assays for vitamin B_{12}. Possibility of false-positive test for **intrinsic factor antibodies** in blood.

Drug Interactions: Cyanocobalamin

Plus	Interactions
Alcohol, ethyl (excessive intake); Aminoglycoside antibiotics; Aminosalicylic acid (PAS) and its salts; Anticonvulsants; Cobalt irradiation of small bowel; Colchicine; Potassium, extended release preparations	Absorption of vitamin B_{12} from GI tract may be decreased by these drugs
Chloramphenicol (chloromycetin)	Interferes with erythrocyte maturation and thus may cause poor therapeutic response to vitamin B_{12}
Prednisone	May increase absorption of vitamin B_{12}

CYCLACILLIN

(Cyclapen-W)

(sye-kla-sill′in)

Antiinfective (beta-lactam)

Antibiotic

Penicillin

ACTIONS AND USES. Acid stable, semisynthetic aminopenicillin derivative with broad antibacterial spectrum almost identical to that of ampicillin. Like ampicillin, it is also penicillinase-sensitive. Reported to have no appreciable advantage over ampicillin except that it is more completely absorbed and may have lower incidence of GI side effects and skin rash.

Used for treatment of urinary tract infections caused by *Escherichia coli* and *Proteus mirabilis;* otitis media and respiratory tract infections caused by *Streptococcus pneumonia, Haemophilus influenzae,* and group A beta-hemolytic streptococci; skin and soft tissue infections caused by group A beta-hemolytic streptococci and nonpenicillinase producing staphylococci.

C

ABSORPTION AND FATE. Rapidly and well absorbed from GI tract following oral administration. Serum levels peak in about 40 to 60 minutes in the fasting state. Approximately 20% protein bound (least protein bound of all the penicillins). Half-life: 30 to 40 minutes. Excreted rapidly in urine; about 80 to 85% of dose eliminated, mostly as unchanged drug.

CONTRAINDICATIONS AND PRECAUTIONS. History of penicillin allergy, or hypersensitivity to cephalosporins or penicillamine. Safe use during pregnancy, in nursing mothers, and in children under 2 months not established. *Cautious Use:* history of or suspected atopy or allergy (hay fever, asthma, hives, eczema); impaired renal function.

ADVERSE/SIDE EFFECTS. Diarrhea, nausea, vomiting, abdominal pain, dizziness, headache, hypersensitivity reactions (rash, urticaria, pruritus, anaphylaxis); superinfections. Infrequent: anemia, thrombocytopenia with or without purpura, leukopenia, neutropenia, eosinophilia.

ROUTE AND DOSAGE. Oral: Adults: 250 to 500 mg every 6 hours. **Children (up to 20 kg):** 125 mg every 8 hours; **(more than 20 kg):** 250 mg every 8 hours. For more severe infections: up to 100 mg/kg/day. Maximum daily dose not to exceed 2 Gm/day.

NURSING IMPLICATIONS

Absorption is faster and more complete if taken on an empty stomach (either 1 hour before or 2 hours after meals).

Shake suspension form well before pouring.

Culture and susceptibility tests should be performed before and during therapy. Therapy may be initiated pending test results.

Before therapy is initiated, a careful inquiry should be made concerning previous hypersensitivity to penicillins, cephalosporins, or other drugs.

For patients with impaired renal function, dosage intervals may be adjusted on basis of creatinine clearance values. When creatinine clearance is 10 ml/minute or less or serum creatinine is 10 mg% or more, evaluations of serum cyclacillin levels are recommended for determining subsequent dosage intervals.

For treatment of urinary tract infections, baseline and regularly scheduled bacteriologic and clinical evaluations may be required for several months.

Instruct patient to take medication at equally spaced intervals and to continue medication for the full course of therapy as prescribed by physician.

Advise patient to keep physician informed of progress and adverse reactions and also to report symptoms of superinfection (e.g., furry black tongue, perianal itching or irritation, foul-smelling vaginal discharge, loose stools).

Drug therapy for beta-hemolytic streptococcal infections should continue for at least 10 days to guard against risk of rheumatic fever and glomerulonephritis.

After reconstitution, suspension retains potency for 7 days at room temperature and for 14 days under refrigeration. Expiration date should appear on label. A calibrated measuring device should be dispensed with suspension.

Tablets are stored in a tight container at room temperature, preferably 25°C (77°F) unless otherwise directed by manufacturer.

See also Ampicillin (prototype broad-spectrum penicillin).

Diagnostic Test Interferences. As with other semisynthetic penicillins, cyclacillin may cause elevations of **SGOT.**

Drug Interactions. In common with other penicillins, concurrent use of bacteriostatic agents such as **chloramphenicol, erythromycins, sulfonamides,** or **tetracyclines** may interfere with the bactericidal effect of cyclacillin; penicillins should be administered a few hours or longer before these agents. **Probenicid** may cause increased and prolonged cyclacillin blood levels.

CYCLANDELATE

(sye-klan'de-late)

(Cyclan, Cyclospasmol, Cydel)

Vasodilator, peripheral

ACTIONS AND USES. Produces vasodilation by exerting papaverinelike relaxation of peripheral vascular smooth muscle by direct action. Principle effect is on vascular smooth muscle. Has no significant adrenergic stimulating or blocking actions.

Used as adjunctive therapy in arteriosclerosis obliterans, intermittent claudication, thrombophlebitis (to control associated vasospasm and muscular ischemia), nocturnal leg cramps, Raynaud's phenomenon, and in selected cases of ischemic cerebrovascular disease. Clinical effectiveness not confirmed.

ABSORPTION AND FATE. Readily absorbed from GI tract. Effects appear in 15 minutes, with maximum response in about 1 to 1½ hours. Duration of action approximately 3 to 4 hours. Metabolic fate unknown.

CONTRAINDICATIONS AND PRECAUTIONS. Known hypersensitivity to cyclandelate. Safe use during pregnancy and in nursing mothers not established. *Cautious Use:* severe obliterative coronary artery or cerebrovascular disease, recent myocardial infarction, bleeding tendencies, active bleeding, glaucoma, hypertension.

ADVERSE/SIDE EFFECTS. Reported to be relatively nontoxic. Infrequent: dizziness, facial flushing, sweating, tingling sensation in face, fingers, toes; tachycardia, weakness, headache; GI disturbances: heartburn (pyrosis), eructation, stomach pain, possible prolongation of bleeding time (high doses).

ROUTE AND DOSAGE. Oral: Initial: 200 to 400 mg four times daily, before meals and at bedtime. Once clinical response has occurred, dosage may be reduced by 200 mg decrements to maintenance dosage of 400 to 800 mg/day in two to four divided doses.

NURSING IMPLICATIONS

GI distress may be relieved by taking medication with meals, milk, or an antacid (if prescribed).

Some patients experience mild flushing, headaches, weakness, and tachycardia during the first week of therapy, requiring dosage reduction.

Cyclandelate can cause dizziness in some patients. Caution patient to make position changes slowly particularly from recumbent to upright posture and to dangle legs over bed for a few minutes before ambulating. Also instruct patient to lie down if feels faint or dizzy, and to notify physician if these symptoms persist.

Patient should be informed that improvement usually occurs gradually and that prolonged therapy may be necessary.

Therapeutic effect on peripheral circulation may be manifested by: slight rise in skin temperature, increased pulse volume, the ability to walk longer distances without discomfort, and lessened pain.

Meticulous hygiene is an important adjunct in treatment of peripheral vascular problems. *See Isoxuprine Hydrochloride for additional patient teaching points.*
Since nicotine constricts blood vessels, patient should be advised to stop smoking.
Store in well-closed container preferably between 15° and 30°C (59° and 86°F) unless otherwise directed by manufacturer.

CYCLIZINE HYDROCHLORIDE
(Marezine Hydrochloride)
CYCLIZINE LACTATE
(Marezine Lactate, Marzine)

(sye'kli-zeen)
Antihistamine
H_2-receptor antagonist
Antiemetic
Antivertigo

ACTIONS AND USES. Piperazine derivative antihistamine (H_1-receptor blocking agent) structurally and pharmacologically related to other cyclizine compounds (e.g., buclizine, hydroxyzine, meclizine). In common with these agents, it exhibits CNS depression and anticholinergic, antispasmodic, local anesthetic, and to antihistaminic activity. Has prominent depressant action on labyrinthine excitability and on conduction in vestibular-cerebellar pathways, thus producing marked antimotion and antiemetic effects. Precise mechanism of action not known.

Used chiefly for prevention and treatment of motion sickness and postoperative nausea and vomiting. Available in fixed-dose combination with ergotamine tartrate and caffeine (Migral) for treatment of migraine.

ABSORPTION AND FATE. Rapid onset of action, with duration of 4 to 6 hours. Metabolic fate unknown.

CONTRAINDICATIONS AND PRECAUTIONS. Hypersensitivity to cyclizine; pregnancy, women of childbearing potential, nursing mothers, children under 6 years of age. *Cautious Use:* narrow-angle glaucoma, prostatic hypertrophy, obstructive disease of GU and GI tracts; postoperative patients.

ADVERSE/SIDE EFFECTS. Usually dose-related: **CV:** hypotension, palpitation, tachycardia. **CNS:** drowsiness, vertigo, dizziness, restlessness, excitement, insomnia, euphoria, auditory and visual hallucinations, hyperexcitability alternating with drowsiness, convulsions, respiratory paralysis. **EENT:** dry mouth, nose and throat; blurred vision, diplopia, tinnitus. **GI:** anorexia, nausea, vomiting, diarrhea or constipation. **GU:** difficult or painful urination, urinary retention or frequency. **Hypersensitivity:** urticaria, rash, cholestatic jaundice, anaphylaxis (inadvertent IV administration). **Other:** pain at IM injection site.

ROUTE AND DOSAGE. Adults: Oral (hydrochloride): 50 mg every 4 to 6 hours as needed; not to exceed 200 mg daily. **Intramuscular (lactate):** 50 mg every 4 to 6 hours as needed. **Children (6 to 12 years): Oral:** 25 mg every 4 to 6 hours, as needed. **Intramuscular:** 1 mg/kg 3 times a day. Total daily dose not to exceed 75 mg.

NURSING IMPLICATIONS

Advise patient to take cyclizine with food or a glass of milk or water to minimize GI irritation.
Aspirate carefully before injecting IM to avoid entry into a blood vessel. Anaphylactic reactions following inadvertent IV have been reported.
Forewarn patient about side effects of drowsiness and dizziness and advise not to drive a

car or engage in other potentially hazardous activities until reaction to the drug is known.

Caution patient that sedative action may be additive to that of alcohol, barbiturates, narcotic analgesic, and other CNS depressants.

Recommended dosage when used to prevent motion sickness: 1 tablet (50 mg) ½ hour before anticipated departure, repeated in 4 to 6 hours if required. No more than 4 tablets should be taken in 1 day. For succeeding days of travel, 50 mg 3 or 4 times daily before meals. Continued administration after first 2 or 3 days of extended travel may be unnecessary.

Advise patient taking cyclizine to relieve motion sickness by positioning him- or herself during travel where there is least motion (e.g., over wing of plane, or amidships), to avoid reading, and to refrain from excessive eating or drinking while traveling.

For prophylaxis of postoperative nausea and vomiting, cyclizine is usually prescribed with preoperative medication or is administered 20 to 30 minutes before expected termination of surgery.

Since cyclizine can cause hypotension, the postoperative patient receiving the drug will require close monitoring of vital signs.

Dry mouth may be relieved by rinsing mouth with clear water or by sugarless gum or lemon drops.

Store tablets in tight, light-resistant container, preferably between 15° and 30°C (59° and 86°F) unless otherwise directed by manufacturer. Store parenteral form in a cold place preferably between 5° and 10°C (41° and 50°F). When parenteral solution is stored at room temperature for prolonged periods it may become slightly yellow, but this does not indicate loss of potency.

Diagnostic Test Interferences. Since cyclizine is an antihistamine, inform patient that **skin testing** procedures should not be scheduled for about 4 days after drug is discontinued or false-negative reactions may result.

Drug Interactions. Cyclizine may have additive effects with **alcohol, barbiturates, CNS depressants** (i.e., hypnotics, sedatives, tranquilizers, and anxiolytic agents), and it may mask signs of ototoxicity produced by **aminoglycoside antibiotics, aspirin,** or other **salicylates.**

PROTOTYPE

CYCLOBENZAPRINE HYDROCHLORIDE

(Flexeril)

(sye-kloe-ben'za-preen)
Skeletal muscle relaxant (centrally acting)

ACTIONS AND USES. Structurally and pharmacologically related to tricyclic antidepressants. Relieves skeletal muscle spasm of local origin without interfering with muscle function. Believed to act primarily within CNS at brain stem; some action at spinal cord level is also probable. Depresses somatic motor activity although both gamma and alpha motorneurons are affected. In common with other tricyclic compounds, it potentiates norepinephrine, and has sedative effects and potent central and peripheral anticholinergic (atropinelike) activity.

Used as short-term adjunct to rest and physical therapy for relief of muscle spasm associated with acute musculoskeletal conditions. Not effective in treatment of spasticity associated with cerebral palsy or cerebral or cord disease.

ABSORPTION AND FATE. Well absorbed following oral administration. Onset of action usually within 1 hour; duration: 12 to 24 hours. Peak plasma levels in 3 to 8 hours (wide interpatient variations in plasma levels). Highly bound (about 93%) to plasma proteins. Half-life: 1 to

3 days. Eliminated slowly primarily by kidneys, mostly as inactive metabolites. Some excretion of unchanged drug by feces via bile. Probably excreted in breast milk.

CONTRAINDICATIONS AND PRECAUTIONS. Hypersensitivity to cyclobenzaprine; acute recovery phase of myocardial infarction, patients with cardiac arrhythmias, heart block or conduction disturbances, congestive heart failure, hyperthyroidism; concomitant use of MAO inhibitors or within 14 days of their discontinuation. Use for periods longer than 2 or 3 weeks not recommended by manufacturer. Safe use during pregnancy and in nursing mothers and children under 15 years not established. *Cautious Use:* patients receiving anticholinergic medications; history of urinary retention; angle closure glaucoma, increased intraocular pressure, seizures, cardiovascular disease, hepatic impairment; elderly, debilitated patients; history of psychiatric illness.

ADVERSE/SIDE EFFECTS. **Allergic:** pruritus, urticaria, skin rash, edema of face and tongue. **CV:** increased heart rate, tachycardia, syncope, palpitation, vasodilation, chest pain, orthostatic hypotension, dyspnea; with high doses, possibility of severe arrhythmias and other adverse cardiac effects. **CNS:** drowsiness (common), dizziness, weakness, fatigue, paresthesias, tremors, muscle twitching, insomnia, depressed mood, euphoria, nervousness, disorientation, confusion, agitation, hallucination, headache, ataxia. **GI:** dry mouth, nausea, indigestion, unpleasant taste, coated tongue, tongue discoloration, vomiting, anorexia, abdominal pain, flatulence, diarrhea, constipation, paralytic ileus. **GU:** urinary retention or frequency, decreased bladder tonus. **Other:** sweating, myalgia, blurred vision, tinnitus, possibility of jaundice, hepatitis, alopecia, increased or decreased libido, impotence. Shares toxic potential of the tricyclic antidepressants *(see Imipramine).*

ROUTE AND DOSAGE. Oral: Usual dosage range is 20 to 40 mg daily in two to four divided doses. Not to exceed 60 mg daily.

NURSING IMPLICATIONS

Forewarn patient about side effects of drowsiness (occurs in about 40% of patients) and dizziness (11%) and advise to avoid driving and other potentially hazardous activities until reaction to drug is known.

Advise patient to avoid alcohol and other CNS depressants (unless otherwise directed by physician) because cyclobenzaprine enhances their effects.

Inform patient that dry mouth (anticholinergic effect) may be relieved by frequent rinses with clear water or by increasing (noncaloric) fluid intake, if allowed, or by sugarless gum or lemondrops. For more complete discussion, *see Nursing Intervention: dry mouth.*

Cyclobenzaprine is intended for short-term (2 or 3 weeks) treatment because risk-benefit associated with prolonged use is not known. Additionally, muscle spasm accompanying acute musculoskeletal conditions is generally of short duration.

Keep physician informed of therapeutic effectiveness. Spasmolytic effect usually begins within 1 or 2 days and may be manifested by lessening of pain and tenderness, increase in range of motion and ability to perform activities of daily living.

Treatment of overdosage is symptomatic and supportive: emesis, then gastric lavage, followed by 20 to 30 Gm activated charcoal every 4 to 6 hours during first 24 to 48 hours postingestion. Arrhythmias may be controlled by physostigmine IV, neostigmine, pyridostigmine, or propranolol. Short-acting digitalis may be used for signs of cardiac failure. Close monitoring of cardiac function should be maintained for at least 5 days if patient has had dysrythmia.

Store in well closed container preferably between 15° and 30°C (59° and 86°F) unless otherwise directed by manufacturer.

C

Drug Interactions: Cyclobenzaprine

Plus	Interactions
Alcohol, ethyl; barbiturates and other CNS depressants	Enhanced CNS depressant effects. Used with caution if at all
Anticholinergics	Potentiation of anticholinergic effects
Epinephrine (Adrenalin) Norepinephrine (Levarterenol, Levophed)	Increased pressor response
Guanethidine (Ismelin)	Cyclobenzaprine may block antihypertensive action of guanethidine and related drugs
MAO inhibitors	Hypertensive crisis, severe convulsions. Avoid concomitant use or use within 14 days following discontinuation of MAO inhibitor

---

CYCLOMETHYCAINE SULFATE

(Surfacaine)

(sye-kloe-meth'i-caine)

Anesthetic, local

ACTIONS AND USES. Synthetic benzoic ester but unlike most members of this group does not hydrolyze to *p*-aminobenzoic acid. Acts by inhibiting conduction of nerve impulses from sensory nerve endings in skin and mucous membranes.

Used as local anesthetic and lubricant on nontraumatized, accessible mucous membranes prior to clinical examination and instrumentation, and for symptomatic relief of anal fissures, fistulas, chafing, pruritus ani or vulvae, and various other skin conditions associated with pain, irritation, and itching of mucous membranes.

ABSORPTION AND FATE. Onset of action in 5 to 10 minutes.

CONTRAINDICATIONS AND PRECAUTIONS. Idiosyncrasy or allergy to any of the ingredients; use of ointment form on vesicular lesions. *Cautious Use:* history of drug sensitivities, allergic asthma, rhinitis, urticaria.

ADVERSE/SIDE EFFECTS. Stinging, burning sensation. **Allergic reactions:** pruritus, increased redness, papules, vesicles, contact dermatitis, anaphylactoid reaction.

ROUTE AND DOSAGE. Topical: Available as cream 0.5%; ointment 1%; jelly 0.75%.

NURSING IMPLICATIONS

Avoid applications to extensive skin areas or for prolonged periods.

Do not use in or near the eyes.

Cyclomethycaine should be discontinued if stinging or burning sensation persists or if signs of irritation, infection, or allergy appear.

Store preferably between 15° and 30°C (59° and 86°F) unless otherwise directed by manufacturer.

C

CYCLOPENTOLATE HYDROCHLORIDE

(Ak-Pentolate, Cyclogyl, Mydplegic)

(sye-kloe-pen′toe-late)
Anticholinergic
Cycloplegic
Mydriatic

ACTIONS AND USES. Tertiary amine compound with similar systemic side effects and CNS toxicity as atropine (qv). Acts by blocking response of iris sphincter muscle and muscle of accommodation in ciliary body to cholinergic stimulation with resulting dilation (mydriasis) and paralysis of accommodation (cycloplegia). Binds to melanin in pupil; thus highly pigmented eyes (brown eyes) may be less responsive to cycloplegic and mydriatic actions.

Used to produce mydriasis and cycloplegia as an aid in refraction and for diagnostic ophthalmoscopic procedures. Available in combination with phenylephrine (e.g., Cyclomydril) to produce more rapid and profound mydriasis.

ABSORPTION AND FATE. Maximal cycloplegic and mydriatic effects within 25 to 75 minutes with recovery in about 24 hours.

CONTRAINDICATIONS AND PRECAUTIONS. Narrow-angle glaucoma, excessively increased intraocular pressure. *Cautious Use:* elderly patients, brain damage (in children), Down's syndrome (mongolism), spastic paralysis in children, blue-eyed individuals.

ADVERSE/SIDE EFFECTS. Blurred vision, temporary burning sensation on instillation, eye dryness, photophobia, conjunctivitis, contact dermatitis, increased intraocular pressure. *Systemic absorption:* **CNS:** psychotic reaction, behavior disturbances, ataxia, incoherent speech, restlessness, hallucinations, somnolence, disorientation as to time and place, failure to recognize people, grand mal seizures. **GI:** abdominal distention, vomiting, adynamic ileus. **Other:** dry mouth, flushing, fever, thirst, rash, tachycardia, urinary retention. *See also Atropine Sulfate.*

ROUTE AND DOSAGE. Topical: Adults: *Cycloplegic refraction:* 1 drop of 0.5% solution instilled into eye. The 1% or 2% solution is recommended for use in individuals with darkly pigmented eyes. **Children:** 1 drop of 0.5%, 1%, or 2% solution instilled into eye, followed 5 minutes later by second instillation, if necessary.

NURSING IMPLICATIONS

Tonometric examination is advised in patients past middle age and in patients with increased intraocular pressure, prior to drop instillation.

Systemic absorption may be minimized by depressing lacrimal duct (inner canthus) for 1 or 2 minutes following instillation of drug. This is especially advisable in children and when the 2% solution is used. *See Index: Drug administration: eye drops.*

Forewarn patient that drug will cause disabling blurring of vision and advise against driving and other potentially hazardous activities until reaction to drug is known.

Physician may prescribe pilocarpine 1% or 2% (1 or 2 drops) to hasten recovery time from cycloplegia to 3 to 6 hours (normal recovery time is about 24 hours).

Wearing dark glasses may relieve sensitivity to light (photophobia). However, if this symptom persists for more than 36 hours after drug is discontinued, notify physician.

Store in well-closed containers preferably between 15° and 30°C (59° and 86°F) unless otherwise directed by manufacturer.

CYCLOPHOSPHAMIDE

(Cytoxan, Neosar, Procytox)

(sye-kloe-foss′fa-mide)
Antineoplastic
Alkylating agent
Immunosuppressant
Nitrogen mustard

ACTIONS AND USES. Cell-cycle nonspecific alkylating agent chemically related to the nitrogen mustards. Action mechanism unknown, but thought to be the result of cross-linkage of DNA strands thereby blocking synthesis of DNA, RNA, and protein. Has pronounced immunosuppressive activity and is a highly toxic drug; thus therapeutic effects are usually accompanied by evidence of toxicity. Associated with increased risk of development of secondary malignancies, including urinary bladder, myeloproliferative and lymphoproliferative malignancies. These may be detected several years after cyclophosphamide has been discontinued. Paternal use of drug in combination therapy prior to conception has been associated with cardiac and lymph abnormalities in the infant. Advantages over other nitrogen mustards include oral effectiveness and the possibility of giving fractional doses over long periods of time.

Used as single agent or in combination with other chemotherapeutic agents in treatment of malignant lymphoma, multiple myeloma, leukemias, mycosis fungoides (advanced disease), neuroblastoma, adenocarcinoma of ovary. Carcinoma of breast or malignant neoplasms of lung are infrequently responsive. *Investigational Use:* to control rejection following kidney, heart, liver and bone marrow transplants; to treat severe active and progressive rheumatoid disorders; to treat glomerular and nephrotic syndrome (especially in children); to treat bleeding syndrome in patient with acquired antibodies to clotting factors.

ABSORPTION AND FATE. Completely absorbed from GI tract and parenteral sites. Disappears rapidly from plasma, with peak concentration 1 hour after oral dose. Hepatic metabolism. Following IV administration, half-life is 4 to 6 hours, but drug and metabolites may be detected in plasma up to 72 hours. Distributed throughout body including brain and CSF. Protein binding: 10 to 56%. Excreted in urine as metabolites; less than 25% as unchanged drug. Crosses blood–brain barrier and is excreted in breast milk.

CONTRAINDICATIONS AND PRECAUTIONS. Men and women in childbearing years, serious infections (including chicken pox, herpes zoster); myelosuppression, pregnancy (category C), lactation. *Cautious Use:* history of radiation or cytotoxic drug therapy, hepatic and renal impairment, recent history of steroid therapy, varicella-zoster and other infections, bone marrow infiltration with tumor cells, history of urate calculi and gout, patients with leukopenia, thrombocytopenia.

ADVERSE/SIDE EFFECTS. **Dermatologic:** alopecia, transverse ridging and darkening of nails and skin, nonspecific dermatitis. **GI:** nausea, vomiting, mucositis, anorexia, hepatotoxicity, diarrhea. **GU:** sterile hemorrhagic and nonhemorrhagic cystitis, bladder fibrosis, nephrotoxicity, gonadal suppression (amenorrhea, azoospermia, oligospermia possibly irreversible). **Metabolic:** severe hyperkalemia, SIADH, hyponatremia, weight gain (but without edema) or weight loss, hyperuricemia. **Myelosuppression:** leukopenia, thrombocytopenia, anemia, thrombophlebitis, suppression of positive reactions to skin tests, interference with normal healing. **Pulmonary:** pulmonary emboli and edema, interstitial pulmonary fibrosis. **Other:** transient dizziness, fatigue, facial flushing, diaphoresis, fever, anaphylaxis, cardiotoxicity.

ROUTE AND DOSAGE. **Oral:** **Adults:** 1 to 5 mg/kg daily. **Pediatric:** *Induction:* 2 to 8 mg/kg or 60 to 250 mg/m^2 daily in divided doses for 6 or more days. *Maintenance:* 2 to 5 mg/kg twice a week. **Intravenous:** **Adults:** *Induction:* 40 to 50 mg/kg in divided doses over 2- to 5-day period. *Maintenance:* 10 to 15 mg/kg every 7 to 10 days or 3 to 5 mg/kg twice a week. **Pediatric:** *Induction:* 2 to 8 mg/kg or 60 to 250 mg/m^2 daily in divided doses for 6 or more days. Maintenance: 10 to 15 mg/kg every 7 to 10 days or 30 mg/kg at 3- or 4-week intervals, or when bone marrow recovery occurs. Solutions for injection may be given intramuscularly, intraperitoneally, intrapleurally or infused IV in Dextrose 5% Injection or Dextrose 5% and NaCl Injection 0.9%.

NURSING IMPLICATIONS

Liquid oral cyclophosphamide may be prepared by dissolving powder for injection in Aromatic Elixir to a concentration of 1 to 5 mg cyclophosphamide/ml. Store in refrigerator 2° to 8°C (36° to 46°F) and use within 14 days.

Administer oral drug on empty stomach. If nausea and vomiting are severe, however, take drug with food. An antiemetic medication given before this drug may control GI reactions.

IV solution: To reconstitute add Sterile Water for Injection or Bacteriostatic Water for Injection (paraben preserved only) to vial and shake vigorously to dissolve (5 ml to 100 mg vial). Should be used within 24 hours if stored at room temperature, or within 6 days if refrigerated.

Cyclophosphamide is dialysable; doses are greater during dialysis.

Unless the disease is unusually sensitive to cyclophosphamide, the largest maintenance dose that can be tolerated is the rule. Ordinarily a leukopenia of 3000 to 4000 cells/mm^3 can be maintained without risk of serious complications.

Usually extravasation does not cause local irritation, unlike other nitrogen mustards.

Total WBC and thrombocyte counts are determined at least twice a week during maintenance period. Periodic determinations of liver and kidney function and serum electrolytes should be made.

Thrombocytopenia is rare, but if thrombocyte count is 100,000/mm^3 or lower, watch for signs of unexplained bleeding or easy bruising. If count continues to descend or if symptoms are manifest, drug will be discontinued.

Marked leukopenia is the most serious side effect. Nadir may occur in 2 to 8 days after first dose, but may be as late as 1 month after a series of several daily doses. Leukopenia usually reverses 7 to 10 days after therapy is discontinued. Has been fatal.

Check leukocyte count. During severe leukopenic period, protect the patient from infection and trauma, and from visitors and medical personnel who have colds or other infections.

Report onset of unexplained fever, chills, sore throat, tachycardia.

During period of neutropenia, purulent drainage may become serosanguinous because there are not enough WBC to result in pus. Monitor temperature carefully and report elevation of 100°F or higher. Observe and report character of wound drainage.

The immunosuppressive property of cyclophosphamide makes the patient particularly susceptible to varicella-zoster infections (chicken pox, herpes zoster).

Because of suppressed immune mechanisms wound healing may be prolonged or incomplete.

Untreated stomatitis is not only uncomfortable, it also interferes with drinking and eating. *See Mechlorethamine for nursing implications.*

Anorexia should not be ignored. Plan with patient, dietitian, and physician a nutritional regimen, especially for leukopenic period.

Report any sign of overgrowth with opportunistic organisms (black furry or white, patchy appearance of tongue and oral membranes; diarrhea, foul-smelling stools; vulvar itching and vaginal discharge, cough) especially if patient is also receiving corticosteroids or has recently been on steroid therapy.

Maintenance of nutrition may depend as much on taste as on any other one factor. Discuss changing preferences for foods with patient and family member. When the patient experiences decreased (but not absent) taste (hypogeusia), cold foods high in protein with added flavorings may be liked best (e.g., ice cream, gelatin salad with cream or cottage cheese, fruit stuffed with peanut butter, puddings, custards). Increased sugar added to foods, and highly seasoned foods also seem to be tolerated and preferred. Meat is frequently rejected, but alternative protein sources (eggs, fish, milk) may be accepted. Consult dietitian for suggestions.

If a pattern to nausea and vomiting can be detected, an attempt should be made to plan the treatment/meals/antiemetic so as not to confront patient with food or start therapy when nausea is at its peak.

If a strong emetic is given only once a day, administering it late in the evening with a sedative may help the patient tolerate nausea.

Nausea has a strong suggestive component; the public is becoming increasingly aware that nausea and vomiting often accompany cancer chemotherapy. The patient needs to believe that antiemetic therapy will help. Listen, however, to patient's or family's suggestions about what might also help and if possible implement these suggestions. Vomiting can be the strongest reason for refusing further treatment. *See Estramustine for additional notes.*

Diarrhea may signal onset of hyperkalemia, particularly if accompanied by colicky pain, nausea, bradycardia, and skeletal muscle weakness. These symptoms warrant prompt reporting to physician.

CBC, uric acid, serum electrolytes, and renal and hepatic function should be monitored. *Normal serum potassium:* 3.6 to 5.5 mEq/L; *serum sodium:* 135 to 145 mEq/L; *serum uric acid:* 3 to 7 mg/dl.

Promptly report hematuria or dysuria. Drug schedule is usually interrupted and fluids are forced. Alert patient to the fact that hematuria may resolve spontaneously, or it may persist several months. In some cases, it has been serious enough to require transfusions.

Hyperuricemia occurs commonly during early treatment period in patients with leukemias or lymphoma. Report edema of lower legs and feet, joint, flank, or stomach pain. Alkalinization of urine, hydration, and allopurinol may prevent this side effect.

Intake and output ratio should be monitored. Since drug is a chemical irritant, fluid intake is generally increased to prevent renal irritation. Paradoxically, in patients with SIADH (a rare side effect) fluid intake may be restricted. Consult physician.

When fluid intake is to be pushed, encourage the patient to start increased intake early in the day to reduce night voiding.

Since patients are usually well hydrated as part of the therapy, watch for symptoms of dilutional hyponatremia (excess body Na with low serum Na): lethargy, confusion, headache, decreased skin turgor, tremors, convulsions. Should this condition occur, fluid intake may be reduced.

Report fever, dyspnea, and nonproductive cough. Pulmonary toxicity is not usual but the already debilitated patient is particularly susceptible.

Record body weight at least twice weekly (basis for dose determination). Alert physician to sudden change or slow, steady weight gain or loss over a period of time that appears inconsistent with caloric intake.

Observe and report signs of hepatotoxicity (frothy dark urine, light-colored stools, jaundice, pruritus) most apt to appear in the patient with liver impairment prior to institution of cyclophosphamide therapy.

Because of mutagenic potential, adequate means of contraception should be employed during and for at least 4 months after termination of drug treatment. Breast feeding should be discontinued before cyclophosphamide therapy is initiated.

Skin and nails may become darker during therapy and nonspecific dermatitis has been reported. These side effects are usually reversible.

Alopecia occurs in about 33% of patients on cyclophosphamide therapy. Discuss the possibility with the patient early in therapy. Hair loss may be noted 3 weeks after therapy begins; regrowth (may differ in texture and color) usually starts 5 to 6 weeks after drug is withheld and may occur while patient is on maintenance doses. This side effect, related

C

as it is to sexuality and self-image, requires much understanding. Help the patient to plan for cosmetic substitution if desired.

Amenorrhea may last up to 1 year after cessation of therapy in 10 to 30% of women receiving cyclophosphamide (due to lack of follicular maturation).

Urge patient to adhere to dosage regimen: he or she should not omit, increase, decrease, or delay doses; if for any reason the drug cannot be taken, notify the physician.

Cyclophosphamide may be carcinogenic; therefore, prolonged follow-up of patient following cyclophosphamide treatment is important; reportedly many years may elapse between treatment and development of bladder cancer.

Consult physician about plans for disclosure of diagnosis, prognosis and particulars about treatment so that discussions with patient and family are supportive and nonconflicting.

Store at temperature between 2° and 30°C (36° and 90°F) unless otherwise recommended by the manufacturer.

Diagnostic Test Interferences. Cyclophosphamide increases **blood** and **urine uric acid,** decreases **serum pseudocholinesterase,** and suppresses positive reactions to **Candida, mumps, trichophyta, tuberculin PPD.** May cause a false-positive **Papanicolaou (PAP) test.**

Drug Interactions: Cyclophosphamide

Plus	Interactions
Allopurinol (Zyloprim)	May inhibit hepatic microsomal enzyme activity, leading to enhanced pharmacologic effects of cyclophosphamide and bone marrow toxicity
Antigout agents	Elevates serum and urine uric acid levels necessitating dose adjustment of antigout agent
Chloramphenicol (Chloromycetin), Chloroquine (Aralen), Corticosteroids	*See Allopurinol (above)*
Daunorubicin (Cerubidine), Doxorubicin (Adriamycin)	May increase potential for cardiotoxicity
Imipramine (Toframil)	*See Allopurinol (above)*
Phenobarbital	Increases rate of drug metabolism and leukopenic activity of cyclophosphamide
Phenothiazines, Potassium chloride, Sex hormones	*See Allopurinol (above)*
Succinylcholine	Inhibits metabolism of succinylcholine leading to prolonged neuromuscular blocking activity (apnea). Used with caution
Vitamin A	*See Allopurinol (above)*

CYCLOSERINE

(Seromycin)

(sye-kloe-ser'een)

Antiinfective

Antituberculosis agent

ACTIONS AND USES. Broad-spectrum antiinfective derived from strains of *Streptomyces orchidaceus* or *S. garyphalus;* also produced synthetically. Structural analog of the amino acid D-alanine. Inhibits cell wall synthesis in susceptible strains of gram-positive and gram-negative bacteria and in *Mycobacterium tuberculosis* by competitively inhibiting the incorporation of D-alanine into the bacterial cell wall. May be bacteriostatic or bactericidal depending on concentration at site of infection and susceptibility of organism.

Used in conjunction with other tuberculostatic drugs in treatment of active pulmonary and extrapulmonary tuberculosis (including renal disease) when primary agents isoniazid, rifampin, ethambutol, streptomycin have failed. Also used in treatment of acute urinary infections caused by *Enterobacter* and *Escherichia coli* that are unresponsive to conventional treatment.

C

ABSORPTION AND FATE. About 70 to 90% of dose readily absorbed from GI tract. Serum levels peak within 3 to 4 hours. Not bound to plasma proteins. Concentrations in lung, ascitic, pleural, and synovial fluids approximately equal to plasma drug levels. Cerebrospinal fluid levels are about 50 to 80% of plasma levels when meninges are normal and 80 to 100% when meninges are inflamed. About 60 to 70% of drug is eliminated unchanged in urine within 72 hours. Small amounts excreted in feces. Readily crosses placenta and may appear in breast milk.

CONTRAINDICATIONS AND PRECAUTIONS. Hypersensitivity to cycloserine; epilepsy, depression, severe anxiety, history of psychoses; severe renal insufficiency, chronic alcoholism. Safe use during pregnancy and safe pediatric use not established.

ADVERSE/SIDE EFFECTS. **Allergic:** dermatitis; photosensitivity. **CV:** arrhythmias, congestive heart failure. **Hematologic:** vitamin B_{12} and/or folic acid deficiency, megaloblastic or sideroblastic anemia. **Neurotoxicity:** drowsiness, anxiety, headache, tremors, myoclonic jerking, convulsions, vertigo, visual disturbances, speech difficulties (dysarthria), lethargy, depression, disorientation with loss of memory; confusion, nervousness, psychoses (possibly with suicidal tendencies), character changes, hyperirritability, aggression, hyperreflexia, peripheral neuropathy, paresthesias, paresis, dyskinesias. **Ophthalmic:** blurred vision, loss of vision, eye pain (optic neuritis), photophobia. **Other:** abnormal liver function tests, jaundice, superinfections.

ROUTE AND DOSAGE. **Oral:** *Tuberculosis:* initially 250 mg twice daily at 12-hour intervals for first 2 weeks. Usual dosage: 500 mg to 1 Gm daily in divided doses, monitored by blood levels. Daily dosage should not exceed 1 Gm. *Urinary tract infection:* 250 mg every 12 hours.

NURSING IMPLICATIONS

Advise patient to take cycloserine after meals to prevent GI irritation.

Culture and bacterial susceptibility tests should be done prior to initiation of therapy and periodically thereafter to detect possible bacterial resistance.

Monitoring of blood–drug levels, hematologic, renal, and hepatic function at regular intervals is advised.

Stress importance of compliance in following medication regimen as prescribed and in keeping follow-up appointments.

Maintenance of blood–drug level below 30 mcg/ml considerably reduces incidence of neurotoxicity. Possibility of neurotoxicity increases when dose is 500 mg or more, when renal clearance is inadequate, or when patient shows signs suggestive of toxicity. Blood–drug levels should be determined at least weekly in these patients.

Some physicians prescribe large doses of pyridoxine (vitamin B_6) concomitantly to prevent neurologic reactions, but its value as a prophylactic has not been proved.

Neurotoxic effects generally appear within first 2 weeks of therapy and disappear after drug is discontinued.

C

Advise patient/responsible family member to notify physician immediately about onset of skin rash and early signs of neurotoxicity: drowsiness, confusion, headache, vertigo, anxiety, tremors, paresthesias, behavior changes.

Drug should be discontinued or dosage reduced if symptoms of neurotoxicity or allergy develop.

Advise patient to avoid potentially hazardous tasks such as driving until reaction to cycloserine has been determined.

Caution patient to avoid alcoholic beverages. Ingestion of alcohol increases the risk of convulsive seizures.

Cycloserine overdosage is treated with pyridoxine (vitamin B_6), anticonvulsants for seizure control, tranquilizers or sedative to control anxiety and tremors, and symptomatic and supportive therapy such as gastric lavage, oxygen, artificial respiration, measures for shock, and maintenance of body temperature.

Store in well-closed container preferably between 15° and 30°C (59° and 86°F) unless otherwise directed by manufacturer.

Diagnostic Test Interferences. **SGOT** and **SGPT** levels may be increased.

Drug Interactions: Cycloserine

Plus	Interactions
Alcohol, ethyl	Increased risk of seizures especially with chronic alcohol abuse
Ethionamide, Isoniazid	Potentiate neurotoxic effects of cycloserine
Phenytoin	Possibility of phenytoin toxicity (cycloserine inhibits hepatic metabolism of phenytoin)

CYCLOSPORINE

(sye'kloe-spor-een)

(Cyclosporin A, Sandimmune)

Immunosuppressant

ACTIONS AND USES. Immunsuppressant agent derived from an extract of soil fungi. Action appears to be due to selective and reversible inhibition of helper-T lymphocytes (which normally stimulate antibody function), creating an imbalance in favor of suppressor T-lymphocytes (which inhibit antibody production), thus immune response is subdued. Does not cause significant bone marrow depression. Believed to have antimalarial, antischistosomal, as well as antifungal activity.

Used in conjunction with adrenal corticosteroids to prevent organ rejection after kidney, liver, and heart transplants (allografts). Has had limited use in pancreas, bone marrow, and heart/lung transplantations. Also used for treatment of chronic transplant rejection in patients previously treated with other immunosuppressants. Used prophylactically in selected patients to reduce severity of graft-vs-host reaction after bone marrow transplantation.

ABSORPTION AND FATE. Following oral administration, GI absorption is variable and incomplete (about 40% of dose is absorbed). Bioavailability may increase with dosage increments and longer duration of therapy. Peak plasma concentrations in 3 to 4 hours. Widely distributed to body tissues and fluids. Approximately 90% bound, primarily to lipoproteins. Biphasic half-life: 1.2 hours; 19 to 27 hours. Extensively metabolized in liver on first pass. Primarily eliminated in bile via feces. About 6% excreted in urine (0.1% as unchanged drug). Crosses placenta. Excreted in breast milk.

CONTRAINDICATIONS AND PRECAUTIONS. Hypersensitivity to cyclosporine or to ingredients in commercially available formulations, e.g., Cremophor (polyoxyl 35 castor oil) in parenteral preparation. Safe use during pregnancy (category C), in nursing women, and in children not established. *Cautious Use:* renal and hepatic function impairment, hypertension, infection, malabsorption problems.

ADVERSE/SIDE EFFECTS. CV: hypertension, myocardial infarction (rare). **Dermatologic:** hirsutism, oily skin, acne, brittle fingernails, hair breaking, pruritus, ecchymoses or bruises (due to increased capillary permeability). **ENT:** sinusitis, tinnitus, hearing loss, sore throat. **Eye:** visual disturbances, conjunctivitis (rare). **GI:** gum hyperplasia, diarrhea, nausea, vomiting, abdominal discomfort, hepatotoxicity; infrequent: anorexia, gastritis, peptic ulcer, hiccoughs, mouth sores, swallowing difficulty, upper GI bleeding, pancreatitis, constipation. **Hematologic:** leukopenia, anemia, thrombocytopenia, elevated hepatic function tests (hepatotoxicity), abnormal renal function tests (nephrotoxicity), hyperkalemia, hyperuricemia, decreased serum bicarbonate, hyperglycemia. **Hypersensitivity:** anaphylaxis associated with polyoxyl 35 castor oil (Cremophor) in IV formulation (flushing, dyspnea, wheezing, hypotension, tachycardia, respiratory arrest). **Neurologic:** tremor, convulsions, headache, paresthesias, hyperesthesia, flushing, night sweats, confusion, anxiety, flat affect, depression, lethargy, weakness, quadriparesis, paraparesis, ataxia, amnesia. **Renal:** urinary retention, frequency, hematuria, nephrotoxicity, hemolytic–uremic syndrome (microangiopathic hemolytic anemia, thrombocytopenia, hypertension, renal failure). **Other:** benign fibroadenoma of breasts, lymphoma (causal relationships not established); gynecomastia, chest pain, muscle and joint pain, leg cramps, edema, fever, chills, weight loss, infections possibly due to concomitant corticosteroid therapy.

ROUTE AND DOSAGE. Highly individualized. **Oral:** 15 mg/kg beginning 4 to 12 hours before surgery. Same daily dose continued for 1 to 2 weeks postoperatively, then reduced by 5%/week to maintenance dose: 5 to 10 mg/kg/day. **Intravenous infusion (parenteral dose is usually ⅓ the oral dose):** 5 to 6 mg/kg given 4 to 12 hours prior to surgery. Same daily dose continued postoperatively until patient can tolerate oral administration. Reportedly, children have tolerated the same oral and IV dose as for adults.

NURSING IMPLICATIONS

Recipients of cyclosporine therapy should be under supervision of a physician experienced in immunosuppressive therapy and management of organ transplants.

Patient should be informed of the potential benefits and risks associated with the use of cyclosporine.

Patients receiving the drug parenterally should be observed continuously for at least 30 minutes after start of IV infusion and at frequent intervals thereafter to detect allergic or other adverse reactions. Equipment for maintaining airway, epinephrine, and oxygen should be immediately available.

Hypersensitivity reactions have been associated with Cremophor emulsifying agent in the parenteral formulation, but not with the oral solution, which does not contain this ingredient. (Cremophor can cause phthalate stripping from PVC tubing.)

Monitor intake and output ratio and pattern. Nephrotoxicity has been reported in about ⅓ of transplant patients. It has occurred in mild forms as late as 2 to 3 months after transplantation. In severe form it can be irreversible and therefore early recognition is critically important.

Signs and symptoms suggestive of nephrotoxicity: oliguria, urinary frequency, hematuria,

C

cloudy urine, elevated BUN and serum creatinine associated with high trough drug levels. Laboratory values respond to dosage reduction.

Signs of rejection in patients with renal transplant can be almost indistinguishable from nephrotoxicity. Indicators of graft rejection include low blood or plasma cyclosporine concentrations occurring with rapid rise in serum creatinine, fever, graft tenderness or enlargement. Laboratory values do not respond to dosage reduction.

Monitor vital signs. Be alert to indicators of local or systemic infection which can be fungal, viral, or bacterial. Also report significant rise in blood pressure.

Immunosuppression can occur with cyclosporine alone or in combination with corticosteroids. Although no causal relationship has been established, it appears that patients receiving cyclosporine may be more susceptible to infection and to development of lymphoma.

Lymph glands and breasts should be gently palpated at periodic intervals (consult physician) to detect abnormalities. Patients who have received T-cell globulin appear to be particularly prone to develop these complications.

Periodic tests should be made of neurologic function. Neurotoxic effects generally occur over 13 to 195 days after initiation of cyclosporine therapy. Signs and symptoms are reportedly fully reversible with dosage reduction or discontinuation of drug. Symptoms appear to occur most commonly in cancer patients who have received prior intrathecal methotrexate, cyclophosphamide, or total body irradiation.

Baseline and periodic tests are advised for (1) renal function (BUN, serum creatinine), (2) liver function (SGOT, SGPT, serum amylase, bilirubin, and alkaline phosphatase), and (3) serum potassium.

Blood or plasma drug concentrations should be monitored at regular intervals particularly in patients receiving the drug orally for prolonged periods since drug absorption is erratic. Patients with hepatic transplants should also be closely monitored because they tend to absorb drug with difficulty.

Although no fixed figures have been established, optimum trough values, as determined by RIA, for blood appear to be 250 to 800 ng/ml; trough values for plasma: 50 to 300 ng/ml. Trough levels are taken just prior to next dose, i.e., 24 hours after previous dose.

Advise patient to practice good oral hygiene: use soft tooth brush; brush gently (teeth and tongue); floss at least once daily; rinse or brush after food or sweet drinks; keep dental appointments. Some patients require gingivectomy for gingival hyperplasia.

Reassure patient that hirsutism is reversible with discontinuation of drug.

Before use, inspect concentrate for injection and diluted parenteral preparations for particulate matter and discoloration. Cyclosporine concentrate must be diluted immediately before administration: dilute each ml in 20 to 100 ml of 0.9% sodium chloride or 5% dextrose injection. Administered by slow infusion over approximately 2 to 6 hours, as prescribed by physician. Rapid IV can result in nephrotoxicity.

Patient Instructions Regarding Taking Oral Cyclosporine:

- ✓ take medication at same time each day to maintain therapeutic blood levels
- ✓ use the specially calibrated pipette provided to measure dose
- ✓ palatability of oral solution may be enhanced by mixing it with milk, chocolate milk, or orange juice, preferably at room temperature. Mix in glass rather than plastic container (minimal sticking to sides of container). Stir well, drink immediately, and rinse glass with small quantity of diluent to assure getting entire dose
- ✓ medication may be taken with meals or milk to reduce nausea or GI irritation
- ✓ keep scheduled follow-up appointments

Store preferably between 15° and 30°C (59° and 86°F) in well-closed containers. Do not refrigerate. Protect ampules from light. Once opened, oral solution should be dated and contents used within 2 months.

Diagnostic Test Interferences. **Hyperlipidemia** and abnormalities in **electrophoresis** reported; believed to be due to polyoxyl 35 castor oil (Cremophor) in IV cyclosporine.

C

Drug Interactions: Cyclosporine

Plus	Interactions
Acyclovir (Zovirax) Aminoglycosides	Additive nephrotoxic effects. Concurrent use generally avoided
Amphotericin B (Fungizone) Ketoconazole (Nizoral)	May increase plasma or blood cyclosporine levels, with possibility of additive nephrotoxicity. Used concomitantly only with great caution
Cimetidine (Tagamet)	Possibility of increased plasma or blood cyclosporine levels (by decreasing hepatic metabolism). Close monitoring advised
Immunosuppressants, other (e.g., corticosteroids)	Increased risk of infection and lymphoproliferative diseases. With exception of corticosteroids, concurrent use generally avoided
Phenobarbital Phenytoin and possibly other hydantoins Rifampin (Rifadin, Rimactane)	May cause decrease in blood or plasma cyclosporine concentrations (possibly by increasing hepatic metabolism). Monitor cyclosporine levels

---

CYCLOTHIAZIDE
(Anhydron, Fluidil)

(sye-kloe-thye'a-zide)
Diuretic
Antihypertensive
Thiazide
Sulfonamide derivative

ACTIONS AND USES. Benzothiadiazine (thiazide) derivative. Similar to chlorothiazide (qv) in actions and uses, contraindications, precautions, adverse reactions, and interactions.

Used to treat hypertension as sole agent or to enhance the effectiveness of another antihypertensive, and as adjunct in treatment of edema associated with hepatic cirrhosis, congestive heart failure, nephrotic syndrome.

ABSORPTION AND FATE. Diuretic effect begins within 6 hours of initial dose; peaks in 7 to 12 hours and lasts 18 to 24 hours. Excreted by kidneys; crosses placental barrier, appears in breast milk.

CONTRAINDICATIONS AND PRECAUTIONS. Hypersensitivity to thiazides and sulfonamides; anuria, hypokalemia, pregnancy, lactation, renal decompensation. *Cautious Use:* history of renal and hepatic disease, diabetes mellitus, gout, SLE. *See also Chlorothiazide.*

ADVERSE/SIDE EFFECTS. Orthostatic hypotension, hypokalemia, hypovolemia, dehydration, hyperglycemia, asymptomatic hyperuricemia, aplastic anemia, thrombocytopenia, GI irritation, exacerbation of gout (rare), paresthesias, vasculitis, photosensitivity. *See also Chlorothiazide.*

ROUTE AND DOSAGE. Oral: Adult: *Diuretic:* Initial: 1 to 2 mg daily; maintenance 1 to 2 mg on alternate days or two or three times weekly. *Antihypertensive:* 2 mg once daily; up to 2 mg two or three times daily. Highly individualized according to patient's requirements and response. **Pediatric:** 0.02 to 0.04 mg/kg daily.

C

NURSING IMPLICATIONS

Antihypertensive effects may be noted in 3 to 4 days; maximal effects usually require 3 to 4 weeks of therapy.

Give diuretic dose early in the morning to prevent interrupted sleep due to diuresis. Administer with food to reduce GI upset.

The elderly are especially sensitive to excessive diuresis. Monitor blood pressure and intake–output ratio to anticipate clinical problems of orthostatic hypotension, hyponatremia, hypokalemia.

Be alert for signs of hypokalemia (especially in the elderly): muscle cramps, weakness, mental confusion, polyuria, xerostomia, anorexia. Report to the physician.

Hypokalemia may be prevented if the daily diet contains potassium rich foods (e.g., banana, fruit juices, apricots, potatoes, beef, chicken, whole grain cereals, skim milk). Urge patient to eat a banana (about 370 mg potassium) and to drink at least 6 ounces of orange juice (about 330 mg potassium) every day. Collaborate with dietitian and physician.

If hypokalemia develops, dietary potassium supplement of 1000 to 2000 mg (25 to 50 mEq) is usually an adequate treatment.

Warn patient about the possibility of photosensitivity reaction and to notify physician if it occurs. Thiazide-related photosensitivity is considered a photoallergy (ultraviolet radiation changes drug structure and makes it allergenic for some individuals); it occurs 1½ to 2 weeks after initial sun exposure.

Monitor prediabetic and diabetic patient for signs of hyperglycemia: glycosuria, acute fatigue, mental changes, restlessness, drowsiness, flushed dry skin, fruitlike breath odor, polyuria, polydipsia. These symptoms are slow to develop and recognize. Notify physician and question need to adjust insulin dosage.

Encourage patient to keep a record of weights. If a 2-pound or more weight gain is noted in 2 to 3 days in addition to ankle and hand edema, the physician should be notified.

Compliance with diuretic therapy may be erratic and associated with omitted doses or altered dosage regimen. Urge patient on maintenance therapy not to change doses or intervals between doses.

Store medication in tightly closed container at 15° to 30°C (59° to 86°F) unless otherwise directed by manufacturer.

See Chlorothiazide (prototype thiazide diuretic).

CYPROHEPTADINE HYDROCHLORIDE

(Cyprodine, Periactin)

(si-proe-hep'ta-deen)

Antihistaminic

Antipruritic

H_2-receptor antagonist

ACTIONS AND USES. Potent antihistamine with pharmacologic actions similar to those of azatadine (qv). Structurally similar to phenothiazine derivative antihistame drugs. Mechanism of action is uncertain. Produces mild central depression and weak peripheral anticholinergic effects and has significant antipruritic, local anesthetic, and antiserotonin activity. Also stimulates appetite, perhaps by activation of hypothalamic appetite-regulating center.

Used for symptomatic relief of various allergic conditions, including hay fever, vasomotor rhinitis, allergic conjunctivitis, urticaria caused by cold sensitivity, pruritus of allergic dermatoses, migraine; and to ameliorate drug, blood, and plasma reactions. Effective in treatment of anaphylactoid reactions as adjunct to epinephrine and other standard measures, after acute symptoms have been controlled. *Investigational Use:* Cushing's disease. Use as appetite stimulant in children has been questioned.

ABSORPTION AND FATE. Duration of action approximately 4 to 6 hours. Small amount appears in breast milk.

CONTRAINDICATIONS AND PRECAUTIONS. Elderly and debilitated patients, patients predisposed to urinary retention, glaucoma, asthma; concurrent use of MAO inhibitors; pregnancy, nursing mothers, newborns, and prematures. *See also Azatadine.*

ADVERSE/SIDE EFFECTS. Drowsiness (common), dizziness, faintness, headache, jitteriness, disturbed coordination, dry mouth, nose, and throat, thickened bronchial secretions, urinary frequency, retention, and difficult urination, skin rash, nausea, epigastric distress, appetite stimulation, weight gain accompanied in children by increased rate of growth. Rarely, CNS stimulation: toxic psychosis, agitation, confusion, visual hallucinations, ataxia, tremors especially in children; transient decrease in fasting blood sugar level, increased serum amylase level, cholestatic jaundice (abdominal discomfort, dark urine, clay-colored stools, pruritus, abnormal liver function tests). *See also Azatadine.*

ROUTE AND DOSAGE. Adults: Oral: 4 mg three to four times daily. Therapeutic dose range is 4 to 20 mg/day. Total daily dose should not exceed 0.5 mg/kg. **Children:** approximately 0.25 mg/kg/24 hours divided into 3 or 4 doses. **Children: (2 to 6 years):** not to exceed 12 mg daily: **(7 to 14 years):** not to exceed 16 mg daily. Available in tablet and syrup forms.

NURSING IMPLICATIONS

GI side effects may be minimized by administering drug with food or milk.

Warn the patient to avoid activities requiring mental alertness and physical coordination, such as driving a car, until reaction to the drug is known.

Cyproheptadine is most likely to cause sedation, dizziness, and hypotension in the elderly. Advise patient to report these symptoms. Children are more apt to manifest CNS stimulation, e.g., confusion, agitation, tremors, hallucinations. Reduction in dosage may be indicated.

In some patients, the sedative effect disappears spontaneously after 3 or 4 days of drug administration.

Patient should know that cyproheptadine may increase and prolong the effects of alcohol, barbiturates, narcotic analgesics, tranquilizers, and other CNS depressants.

Monitor weight and keep physician informed of any significant weight gain.

For treatment of dry mouth (xerostomia), *see Azatadine.*

Store in tightly covered containers at room temperature, preferably between 15° and 30°C (59° and 86°F) unless otherwise directed by manufacturer.

Diagnostic Test Interferences. As a general rule, antihistamines are discontinued about 4 days before **skin testing** procedures are to be performed since they may produce false-negative results.

C

CYTARABINE

(ARA-C, Cytosar-U, Cytosine Arabinoside)

(sye-tare'a-been)
Antineoplastic
Antimetabolite

ACTIONS AND USES. Pyrimidine analogue with cell phase specificity affecting rapidly dividing cells in S-phase (DNA synthesis). In certain conditions prevents progress of cell development from G_1 to S-phase. Interferes with DNA synthesis by blocking conversion of cytidine to deoxycytidine and may be incorporated into RNA molecule. Has strong myelosuppressant activity. Immunosuppressant properties are exhibited by obliterated cell-mediated immune responses, such as delayed hypersensitivity skin reactions.

Used primarily to induce and maintain remission in acute myelocytic leukemia, acute lymphocytic leukemia, and meningeal leukemia in adults and children. Also used in combination with other antineoplastics in established chemotherapeutic protocols.

ABSORPTION AND FATE. Incompletely (less than 20%) absorbed from GI tract. After IV dose, drug is rapidly cleared from blood. Half-life: distribution phase, 10 minutes; elimination phase, 1⅓ hours. With intrathecal administration, half-life: 2 hours. Metabolized in liver, excreted in urine (about 80% total dose in 24 hours). Crosses blood–brain barrier.

CONTRAINDICATIONS AND PRECAUTIONS. Known hypersensitivity to cytarabine, drug-induced myelosuppression, infants; during pregnancy (category C) particularly during first trimester, women of childbearing age. *Cautious Use:* impaired renal or hepatic function, gout, drug-induced myelosuppression.

ADVERSE/SIDE EFFECTS. GI: nausea, vomiting, stomatitis, esophagitis, anorexia, diarrhea, anal inflammation or ulceration, abdominal pain, hemorrhage. **Hematologic:** myelosuppression (reversible): leukopenia, thrombocytopenia, anemia, megaloblastosis, reduced reticulocytes (rare). **Integument:** freckling, rash, keratitis, alopecia (rare), skin ulcerations. **Other:** weight loss, sore throat, fever, dizziness, cellulitis, thrombophlebitis and pain at injection site; pericarditis, hepatic and renal dysfunction, jaundice, urinary retention, transient hyperuricemia, bleeding (any site), chest pain, pneumonia, conjunctivitis, photophobia, headache, neurotoxicity, neuritis, lethargy, confusion, anaphylaxis; "flu"-like syndrome (infrequent): fever, malaise, myalgia, bone pain, chest pain, maculopapular rash. Potentially carcinogenic and mutagenic.

ROUTE AND DOSAGE. All doses highly individualized on basis of hematologic response. **Intravenous (injection or infusion): Adults and children:** *Acute myelocytic and other leukemias:* 200 mg/m^2/day by continuous infusion for 5 days to give total dose of 1000 mg/m^2. Course is repeated about every 2 weeks. **Intrathecal:** 5 to 75 mg/m^2 or 30 to 100 mg once every 2 to 7 days to once daily for 4 or 5 days. Maintenance: 1 to 1.5 mg/kg SC at 1 to 4 week intervals or 70 to 200 mg/m^2 daily by rapid IV injection or continuous IV infusion for 2 to 5 days at monthly intervals.

NURSING IMPLICATIONS

Toxicity necessitating dosage alterations almost always occurs.

Report adverse reactions immediately.

Leukocyte and platelet counts should be evaluated daily during initial therapy. Blood uric acid and hepatic function tests should be performed at regular intervals throughout treatment period.

Monitor blood reports for indicated adaptations of drug regimen and nursing intervention.

Nausea and vomiting of several hours' duration complicate rapid IV injection. Effects are less severe with IV infusion. Administration of cytarabine one hour before meals, or giving an antiemetic prior to cytarabine may reduce these side effects.

Noncontinuous dosage schedules may permit the patient to tolerate larger amounts of drug.

Hyperuricemia due to rapid destruction of neoplastic cells may accompany cytarabine therapy. (*Normal serum uric acid:* 3 to 7 mg/dl.) A regimen that includes a uricosuric agent such as allopurinol, urine alkalinization, and adequate hydration may be started. To reduce potential for urate stone formation, fluids are forced in excess of 2 L if tolerated. Consult physician.

"Flu"-like syndrome occurs usually within 6 to 12 weeks after drug administration and may recur with successive therapy.

Monitor intake–output ratio and pattern. Advise patient to report promptly protrated vomiting or signs of nephrotoxicity.

During the granulocytic periods, development of usual signs of inflammation may be inhibited. Monitor body temperature. Be alert to the most subtle signs of infection especially low-grade fever and report promptly.

When platelets decrease to below 50,000/mm^3 and polymorphonuclear granulocytes to below 1000/mm^3, therapy may be suspended. WBC nadir is usually reached in 5 to 7 days after therapy has been stopped. Therapy is restarted with appearance of bone marrow recovery and when above cell counts are reached.

Combined therapy with thioguanine usually results in hypoplastic bone marrow in 7 to 10 days. After a 10- to 20-day rest period, cytarabine may be repeated.

Courses of therapy with the combination of cytarabine, cyclophosphamide, vincristine, and prednisone are initiated at 2-week intervals. Intervals are shortened if there is rapid recovery of blast cells in the peripheral blood. If severe infection or hemorrhage develops, therapy is interrupted.

Combination therapy is continued until patient is in complete remission or until apparent failure of response after a minimum of 5 courses.

Inspect injection sites for signs of cellulitis.

Provide good oral hygiene to diminish side effects and chance of superinfection. Stomatitis and cheilosis usually appear 5 to 10 days into therapy *(see Mechlorethamine for nursing implications).*

Equipment and facilities for treatment of myelosuppressive emergencies (hemorrhage, granulocytopenia, and other impaired body defenses) should be readily available at all times.

Store cytarabine in refrigerator until reconstituted. The 100-mg and 500-mg vials are reconstituted with 5 ml and 10 ml, respectively, of bacteriostatic water for injection with benzyl alcohol 0.9%. Reconstituted solutions may be stored at room temperature preferably between 15 and 30°C (59 and 86°F) for 48 hours. Solutions with a slight haze should be discarded.

For IV infusion, the reconstituted solution may be further diluted with 5% dextrose or 0.9% sodium chloride injection.

For intrathecal injection, reconstitute with an isotonic, buffered diluent without preservatives. Follow manufacturer's recommendations. Solution should be administered as soon as possible after preparation.

See Mechlorethamine for nursing implications of antineoplastic therapy.

D

DACARBAZINE
(DTIC-Dome, DTIC, Imidazole carboxamide)

(da-kar′ba-zeen)
Antineoplastic
Alkylating agent

ACTIONS AND USES. Cytotoxic triazine with alkylating properties. Cell-cycle nonspecific. Interferes with purine metabolism and with RNA and protein synthesis in rapidly proliferating cells. Has minimal immunosuppressive activity; reportedly carcinogenic, mutagenic, and teratogenic.

Used as single agent or in combination with other antineoplastics in treatment of metastatic malignant melanoma, Hodgkin's disease, various sarcomas, and neuroblastoma. *Investigational Use:* soft tissue carcinoma and malignant glucagonoma.

ABSORPTION AND FATE. Only slightly (approximately 5%) protein-bound. Biphasic half-life: initial phase about 20 minutes; terminal phase: 5 hours. Localizes primarily in liver; concentration in CSF about 14% of that in plasma. 35 to 50% of dose eliminated by renal tubule secretion within 6 hours as unchanged drug and metabolite in approximately equal amounts.

CONTRAINDICATIONS AND PRECAUTIONS. Hypersensitivity to dacarbazine. Safe use in pregnancy (category C) not established.

ADVERSE/SIDE EFFECTS. CNS: confusion, headache, seizures, blurred vision. **Dermatologic:** erythematosus, urticarial rashes; hepatotoxicity, photosensitivity. **GI:** anorexia, nausea, vomiting, diarrhea (rare). **Hematologic:** severe leukopenia and thrombocytopenia, mild anemia. **Other:** alopecia, facial paresthesia and flushing, flu-like syndrome, myalgia, malaise, anaphylaxis, pain along injected vein.

ROUTE AND DOSAGE. Intravenous: 2 to 4.5 mg/kg daily for 10 days; repeated at 4-week intervals. Alternate recommended dosage: 250 mg/m^2/day for 5 days; repeated at 3-week intervals if necessary.

NURSING IMPLICATIONS

Should be administered to hospitalized patients because close observation and frequent laboratory studies are required during and after therapy.

Administer by IV push 1 minute or by IV infusion over a 30-minute period. Monitor BP and vital signs.

Monitor injection site. Subcutaneous extravasation causes severe pain and tissue damage. Treat infiltrated area with ice compresses.

Hematopoietic toxicity usually appears about 4 weeks after first dose. Generally a leukocyte count of less than 3000/mm^3 and a platelet count of less than 100,000/mm^3 require suspension or cessation of therapy.

Leukopenia and thrombocytopenia may be severe enough to cause death.

During platelet nadir avoid if possible all tests and treatments (e.g., IM) requiring needle punctures. Observe carefully and report evidence of unexplained bleeding: ecchymosis, petechiae, epistaxis, melena, or bruising.

Protect patient from excess expenditure of energy, and from infection, especially during leukocyte nadir (screen visitors and personnel that may enter patient's room).

Severe nausea and vomiting (over 90% of patients) begins within 1 hour after drug administration and may last for as long as 12 hours.

Restriction of oral fluids and food for 4 to 6 hours prior to treatment may prevent vomiting.

Palliation and prevention of vomiting may be provided also by administration of an antiemetic (e.g., dexamethasone, prochloperazone). *See Index: Nursing Interventions: nausea and vomiting.*

Most patients develop tolerance to vomiting and diarrhea after the first 1 or 2 days. If vomiting persists, discontinuation of therapy with dacarbazine may be necessary.

Monitor intake-output ratio and pattern and daily temperature. Renal impairment extends the half-life and increases danger of toxicity. Report symptoms of renal dysfunction and even a slight elevation of temperature.

"Flu"-like syndrome (fever, myalgia, malaise) may occur during or even a week after treatment is terminated and last 7 to 21 days. Symptoms frequently recur with successive treatments.

Caution patient to avoid prolonged exposure to sunlight or to ultraviolet light during treatment period and for at least 2 weeks after last dose. Protect exposed skin with sun screen lotion (SPF 15 or higher) and avoid exposure in midday.

Warn patient to report promptly if blurred vision or paresthesia (sensation of prickling, tingling, heightened sensitivity, or numbness) occurs.

Follow agency protocol for handling antineoplastic drug, for precautions to be taken if there is spillage, and for protection of personnel during preparation of solutions or during cleanup of spilled drug. There should be specific directions about:

- Protective covering for face, hands, eyes
- What to do when eyes are contaminated
- How and in what container to dispose of spilled drug
- Where to take container for disposal
- How to prevent further spillage

All handlers of dacabazine should wear gloves. If solution gets into the eyes, wash with soap and water immediately then irrigate with water or isotonic saline.

Reconstitute drug with sterile water for injection to make a solution containing 10 mg/ml dacarbazine (pH 3.0 to 4.0). Resulting solution is administered IV with 5% dextrose injection or sodium chloride injection for administration by IV infusion. The reconstituted solution may be further diluted.

Extravasation: Monitor injection site frequently (instruct patient to do so if able):

- Give prompt attention to patient's complaint of swelling, stinging and burning sensation around injection site. Perivenous extravasation can occur painlessly and without visual signs. Sometimes demonstrated blood return is from a leak around the venipuncture site; this is a particular possibility in the elderly.
- Full skin damage by dacarbazine can lead to deep necrosis requiring surgical debridement, skin grafting and even amputation. At risk are the elderly, very young (who cannot communicate the associated pain), comatose, and debilitated patients. Other risk factors include establishing an IV line in a vein previously punctured several times and non-plastic catheters.
- *Danger areas for extravasation:* dorsum of hand or ankle (especially if peripheral arteriosclerosis is present), joint spaces and previously irradiated areas. If possible avoid using antecubital vein or veins on dorsum of hand or wrist where extravasation could damage underlying tendons and nerves leading to loss of mobility of entire limb. Avoid veins in extremity with compromised venous or lymphatic drainage and veins near joint spaces.
- If extravasation is suspected, stop infusion immediately and restart in another vein. Report to the physician. Prompt institution of local treatment is imperative: infiltration of the area with SC corticosteroid and application of ice compresses. (Aspiration of extravasated drug may be attempted by physician.)

Store reconstituted solution up to 72 hours at 4°C (39°F) or at room temperature for up to 8 hours. Store diluted reconstituted solution for 24 hours at 4°C or at room temperature for up to 8 hours. Protect from light.

DACTINOMYCIN

(Actinomycin, Cosmegen, Lyovac)

(dak-ti-noe-mye′sin)
Antineoplastic
(Antibiotic)

ACTIONS AND USES. Potent cytotoxic antibiotic derived from mixture of actinomycins produced by *Streptomyces parvullus.* Toxic properties precludes its use as antibiotic. Complexes with DNA, thereby inhibiting DNA, RNA, and protein synthesis. Causes delayed myelosuppression; is strongly tissue corrosive and has a low therapeutic index. Potentiates effects of x-ray therapy; the converse also appears likely. Recent reports indicate increased potential for secondary primary tumors following treatment with x-ray and dactinomycin.

Used as single agent or in combination with other antineoplastics and/or radiation to treat Wilms' tumor, rhabdomyosarcoma, carcinoma of testes and uterus, Ewing's sarcoma, and sarcoma botroides.

ABSORPTION AND FATE. Very little active drug is detected in plasma 2 to 5 minutes after IV injection. Concentrates in liver, spleen, and kidneys but does not cross blood–brain barrier. Plasma half-life: 36 hours. About 50% of dose is excreted unchanged in bile and 10% in urine.

CONTRAINDICATIONS AND PRECAUTIONS. Chicken pox, herpes zoster, and other viral infections; patients of childbearing age, pregnancy (category C), lactation, infants under 6 months of age. *Cautious Use:* previous therapy with antineoplastics or radiation within 3 to 6 weeks, bone marrow depression, infections, history of gout, impairment of kidney or liver function, obesity.

ADVERSE/SIDE EFFECTS. Dermatologic: acne, hyperpigmentation and reactivation of erythema especially over previously irradiated areas, alopecia (reversible). **GI:** cheilitis, ulcerative stomatitis, esophagitis, dysphagia, pharyngitis, hepatomegaly, proctitis, anorexia, nausea, vomiting, abdominal pain, diarrhea, GI ulceration. **Hematologic:** anemia (including aplastic anemia), agranulocytosis, leukopenia, thrombocytopenia, pancytopenia, reticulopenia. **Other:** malaise, fatigue, lethargy, fever, myalgia, anaphylaxis, gonadal suppression, hypocalcemia, hyperuricemia, thrombophlebitis; necrosis, sloughing and contractures at site of extravasation. *Following isolation-perfusion administration:* hematopoietic depression, increased susceptibility to infection, impaired wound healing, edema of extremity involved, damage to soft tissues, venous thrombosis.

ROUTE AND DOSAGE. (Highly individualized) **Intravenous:** dose should not exceed 15 mcg/kg or 400 to 600 mcg/m² daily for 5 days. (Dosage for obese or edematous patient is on basis of surface area in order to relate dosage to lean body mass.) **Adults:** 0.5 mg/day for maximum of 5 days every 4 to 6 weeks. **Children:** 0.015 mg/kg/day for 5 days. *Alternate schedule:* total dosage of 2.5 mg/m² in divided doses over 7 day period. Second course in both adult and child may be given after at least 3 weeks have elapsed if toxicity is absent. **Isolation-perfusion:** 0.05 mg/kg body weight for lower extremity or pelvis; 0.035 mg/kg body weight for upper extremity.

NURSING IMPLICATIONS

Dactinomycin is reconstituted by adding 1.1 mg sterile water for injection (without preservative); the resulting solution will contain approximately 0.5 mg/ml. Other solvents may cause precipitation.

Once reconstituted, dactinomycin may be added directly to infusion solutions of 5% dextrose injection or sodium chloride injection, or into tubing or side arm of a running IV infusion, and administered over a 10- to 15-minute period. Because there is no preservative in the solution, discard unused portion.

If direct IV injection is given, the two-needle technique is used to prevent tissue irritation: the needle used to withdraw dose from vial after reconstitution is discarded; a fresh sterile needle is used for direct injection into vein.

Following IV injection, some clinicians recommend injecting 5 to 10 ml IV solution into the side arm or flushing the vein with running IV infusion for 2 to 5 minutes to remove any remaining drug from tubing.

Drug handling precautions: Manufacturer advises use of gloves and eye shield to protect the person making the solution. If skin is contaminated, rinse with running water for 10 minutes; then rinse with buffered phosphate solution. If solution gets into the eyes, wash with water immediately, then irrigate with water or isotonic saline for 10 minutes.

Particular care should be taken to avoid extravasation. Palpate injection site frequently; if extravasation occurs, stop infusion immediately and restart in another vein. Report to physician. Prompt institution of local treatment to prevent thrombophlebitis and necrosis is imperative: aspiration of as much drug solution as possible, infiltration of the area with hydrocortisone, sodium thiosulfate, or with ascorbic acid solution, and application of ice compresses. *(See Dacarbazine.)*

Follow institution protocol for precautions to be taken if there is spillage, and for protection of personnel during cleanup of spilled drug. There should be specific directions about:

- Protective covering for face, hands, eyes
- What to do when eyes are contaminated
- How and in what container to dispose of spilled drug
- Where to take container for disposal
- How to prevent further spillage

Dactinomycin may be given by the isolation-perfusion technique as palliative treatment or as an adjunct to tumor resection. This technique permits drug contact with the tumor for duration of treatment.

The dose for isolation-perfusion technique may be increased well over dose used by the systemic route without causing toxicity. Since the drug is confined to an isolated part, it should not interfere with patient's defense mechanisms.

The perfusate is removed following administration by isolation–perfusion to prevent systemic absorption of toxic products from neoplastic tissue.

Severe, sometimes fatal, toxic effects occur with high frequency in patients receiving dactinomycin. Effects usually appear 2 to 4 days after a course of therapy is stopped and may reach maximal severity 1 to 2 weeks following discontinuation of therapy.

Nausea and vomiting usually occur a few hours after drug administration and are generally controlled by an antiemetic drug (e.g., dexamethasone). Vomiting may be severe enough to require intermittent therapy. Observe patient daily for signs of drug toxicity.

Frequent determinations of renal, hepatic, and bone marrow function are advised. White blood cell counts should be performed daily and platelet counts every 3 days to detect hematopoietic depression. Check laboratory values for indicated adaptations to nursing care.

Some physicians reduce dosage of dactinomycin by ⅓ to ½ if *serum bilirubin* is elevated (normal: direct: 0.1 to 0.4 mg/dl).

D

Monitor temperature and inspect oral membranes daily. *See Mechlorethamine for nursing care of stomatitis, xerostomia.*

The combination of stomatitis, diarrhea, and severe hematopoietic depression (leukopenia or thrombocytopenia) usually requires prompt interruption of therapy until drug toxicity subsides (leukocyte and platelet recovery and improved clinical condition).

Be alert to signs of agranulocytosis (which may develop abruptly especially when dactinomycin and radiation are combined): extreme weakness and fatigue, sore throat, stomatitis, fever, chills. Report to physician. Antibiotic therapy, reverse precautions, and discontinuation of the antineoplastic are indicated.

Dactinomycin is usually given no later than the first 5 to 7 days of radiation therapy because of risk of severe drug-induced skin reactions (erythema, desquamation, pigmentation).

Radiation therapy is generally continued despite the occurrence of drug-induced skin reactions and the side effects of radiation (gastric distress, and severe mucositis near site of radiation).

Discuss possibility of gonadal suppression (amenorrhea or azoospermia) with patient before therapy is instituted. This may be an irreversible side effect.

The obese or edematous patient is given a lower dose of dactinomycin *(see Route and Dosage).* Monitor daily for symptoms of toxicity from overdosage.

Observe and report symptoms of hyperuricemia: swelling of lower legs and feet, flank, stomach, and joint pain. Urge patient to increase fluid intake up to 3000 ml/day if allowed. Treatment with allopurinol and alkalinization of urine may be instituted.

Report onset of unexplained bleeding (ecchymosis, melena, epistaxis, petechiae or easy bruising), jaundice, and wheezing.

Store drug at temperature between 15° and 30°C (59° and 86°F), unless otherwise advised by manufacturer. Protect from heat and light.

Diagnostic Test Interferences. Dactinomycin may increase **serum** and **urine uric acid** levels.

Drug Interactions: Dactinomycin

Plus	Interactions
Antigout agent	Elevated uric acid level produced by dactinomycin may necessitate dose adjustment of the antigout agent
Myelosuppressants, other	Potentiation of effects of both dactinomycin and other myelosuppressant
Radiation	Potentiated effects of both. Dactinomycin may reactivate erythema from previous radiation therapy
Vitamin K	Decreased vitamin K effects (antihemorrhagic) leading to prolonged clotting time and potential hemorrhage

---

DANAZOL

(da'na-zole)

(Cyclomen, Danocrine)

Androgen

ACTIONS AND USES. Synthetic androgen steroid; derivative of alpha-ethinyl testosterone with dose-related mild androgenic effects but no estrogenic or progestational activity. Suppresses pituitary output of follicle-stimulating hormone and luteinizing hormone, resulting in anovulation and associated amenorrhea. Interrupts progress and pain of endometriosis by causing atrophy and involution of both normal and ectopic endometrial tissue. Has no effect on large endometriomas or on anatomic deformities associated with pain of dysmenorrhea.

Used for palliative treatment of endometriosis when alternative hormonal therapy is ineffective, contraindicated, or intolerable. Reportedly has restored fertility in female made infertile by mild to moderate endometriosis. Also used to treat fibrocystic breast disease and severe acne in the post pubertal male. *Investigational Use:* to treat precocious puberty, gynecomastia, menorrhagia, hereditary angioedema, and hemophilia.

ABSORPTION AND FATE. Metabolized to 2-hydroxymethylethisterone, which attains plasma levels 5 to 10 times higher than that of parent drug. Distribution and elimination data not available.

CONTRAINDICATIONS AND PRECAUTIONS. Pregnancy, nursing mothers, undiagnosed abnormal genital bleeding; impaired renal, cardiac, or hepatic function. *Cautious Use:* migraine headache, epilepsy. *See also Testosterone.*

ADVERSE/SIDE EFFECTS. **Allergic:** skin rashes, nasal congestion. **Androgenic side effects (virilization):** acneiform lesions, oily skin and hair, edema, weight gain, clitoral enlargement, mild hirsutism, deepening of voice, increased hoarseness, decrease in breast size. **CNS:** dizziness, headache, sleep disorders, fatigue, tremor, paresthesias in extremities (rare), irritability, visual disturbances, changes in appetite, chills. **GI:** gastroenteritis; rarely, nausea, vomiting, and constipation. **GU:** hematuria (rare). **Hypoestrogenic effects:** flushing; sweating; emotional lability; nervousness; vaginitis with itching, drying, burning, or bleeding; amenorrhea. Causal relationship of danazol to the following reactions has been neither confirmed nor refuted: **Musculoskeletal:** muscle cramps or spasms in back, neck, or legs. **Other:** hair loss, decreased libido, elevated blood pressure, pelvic pain, conjunctival edema, possibility of cholestatic jaundice, acne vulgaris; carpal tunnel syndrome.

ROUTE AND DOSAGE. **Oral:** *Endometriosis:* 400 mg twice daily for 3 to 6 months. Started during menstruation or if pregnancy test is negative. Therapy may be extended 9 months if necessary. If symptoms recur after termination of therapy, drug regimen can be reinstituted. *Fibrocystic breast disease:* 100 to 400 mg in 2 doses daily as tolerated (regimen started as with endometriosis).

NURSING IMPLICATIONS

Inform patient that drug-induced amenorrhea (due to anovulation) is reversible. Ovulation and cyclic bleeding usually return within 60 to 90 days after therapeutic regimen is discontinued. Advise patient that potential for conception may also be restored at that time.

A nonhormonal contraceptive should be used during danazol treatment (if the patient wishes birth control) because ovulation may not be suppressed.

Routine breast examinations should be carried out during therapy. Advise patient to report to physician if any nodule enlarges or becomes tender or hard during therapy.

In fibrocystic breast disease, inform patient that pain and discomfort may be relieved in 2 to 3 months; the nodularity in 4 to 6 months. Menses may be regular or irregular in pattern during therapy.

Because danazol may cause fluid retention, patients with cardiac or renal problems, epilepsy, or migraine should be observed closely during therapy. Also, drug-induced edema may cause compression on median nerve producing symptoms of carpal tunnel syndrome. If patient complains of wrist pain that worsens at night, paresthesias in radial palmer aspect of the hand and fingers, consult physician. Condition is reversible within a few weeks with discontinuation of the drug.

Baseline and periodic liver function tests should be performed in all patients.

Advise patient to report voice changes promptly. Drug should be stopped to avoid permanent damage to voice. Although the side effects usually disappear when drug therapy is terminated, continue to observe patient for signs of virilization (sometimes irreversible).
Danazol is very expensive.
Store capsules between 15° and 30°C (59° and 86°F) in a well-closed container.
See Testosterone (prototype androgen).

D

DANTHRON

(dan'thron)

(Akshun, Dorbane, Dorbantyl, Modane, Roydan)

Laxative (stimulant)
Anthraquinone

ACTIONS AND USES. Synthetic anthraquinone similar to the natural anthraquinones, e.g., cascara sagrada (qv) in pharmacologic properties, uses, adverse reactions, contraindications, and precautions. Suitable for patients on low sodium diets, and at recommended dosage, claimed to produce overnight relief of constipation without straining, griping, or cramping. Contains 5% ethyl alcohol.

Used for temporary management of constipation particularly in geriatric, cardiac, and surgical patients. Available in fixed-dose combination with doxinate sodium (Dorbantyl) and with doxinate calcium (Doxidan).

ABSORPTION AND FATE. Acts in about 6 to 12 hours following oral administration. Metabolized in liver. Excreted in urine. Appears in breast milk.

CONTRAINDICATIONS AND PRECAUTIONS. Nausea, vomiting, abdominal pain, or other symptoms of acute surgical abdomen; fecal impaction; intestinal obstruction or perforation; rectal bleeding; nursing mothers.

ADVERSE/SIDE EFFECTS. Usually dose-related: nausea, vomiting, diarrhea, abdominal cramps, perianal irritation. With prolonged use: discoloration of rectal mucosa (melanosis coli), hypokalemia, dehydration, elevation of blood glucose, hepatic injury (when used repeatedly with an emollient laxative).

ROUTE AND DOSAGE. Oral: 37.5 to 150 mg with or 1 hour after the evening meal.

NURSING IMPLICATIONS

Administration of danthron with the evening meal usually produces evacuation of a soft stool the next morning.
Modane contains tartrazine which may cause allergic reactions including bronchial asthma in certain susceptible individuals. This reaction frequently occurs in patients with aspirin hypersensitivity.
Not to be confused with Modane Bulk (a mixture of psyllium and dextrose) or Modane Soft (doxinate sodium).
Prolonged use may lead to laxative dependence.
Pink to red coloration of urine is harmless and usually indicates that urine is alkaline.
Melanosis coli is a benign pigmentation of the colonic mucosa that occurs with prolonged use. It is usually reversible within 4 to 12 months after danthron is discontinued.
Store in tightly-closed container preferably between 15° and 30°C (59° and 86°F), unless otherwise directed by manufacturer.
See Cascara sagrada (prototype anthraquinone) for patient teaching points.

Diagnostic Test Interferences. Danthron may cause an apparent increase in urinary excretion of **PSP** due to urine discoloration.

DANTROLENE SODIUM

(Dantrium)

(dan′troe-leen)
Skeletal muscle relaxant
Hydantoin

ACTIONS AND USES. Hydantoin derivative, structurally related to phenytoin, with peripheral skeletal muscle relaxant action. Directly relaxes the spastic muscle by interfering with Ca ion (contraction activator) release from sarcoplasmic reticulum. Clinical doses produce about a 50% decrease in contractility of skeletal muscles but no effect on smooth or cardiac muscles. Relief of spasticity may be accompanied by muscle weakness, sufficient to affect overall functional capacity of the patient. Reduces spastic or reflex contractions more than voluntary activity.

Used orally for the symptomatic treatment of skeletal muscle spasms secondary to spinal cord injury, stroke, cerebral palsy, multiple sclerosis. Used intravenously for the management of malignant hyperthermia. Oral dantrolene has been used prophylactically (2 or 3 days before anesthesia) for patients with malignant hyperthermia or with a family history of the disorder.

ABSORPTION AND FATE. Absorption from GI tract is slow and incomplete, but rate is consistent. Significant amounts bound to plasma proteins, mostly albumin; binding is readily reversible. Mean half-life: 8.7 hours after 100 mg oral dose, and about 5 hours following IV administration. Slowly metabolized by liver. About 25% excreted in urine chiefly as metabolites and small amount of unchanged drug. About 45 to 50% eliminated in bile.

CONTRAINDICATIONS AND PRECAUTIONS. Active hepatic disease; when spasticity is necessary to sustain upright posture and balance in locomotion or to maintain increased body function; spasticity due to rheumatic disorders. Safe use during pregnancy, in women of childbearing potential, in nursing mothers and in children under 5 years not established. *Cautious Use:* impaired cardiac or pulmonary function, patients over 35 years, females.

ADVERSE/SIDE EFFECTS. CNS: drowsiness, muscle weakness, dizziness, light-headedness, unusual fatigue, speech disturbances, headache, confusion, nervousness, mental depression, insomnia, euphoria, seizures. **CV:** tachycardia, erratic blood pressure, phlebitis (IV extravasation). **GI:** diarrhea, constipation, nausea, vomiting, anorexia, swallowing difficulty, alterations of taste, gastric irritation, abdominal cramps, GI bleeding. **GU:** bloody or dark urine, crystalluria with pain or burning with urination, urinary frequency, urinary retention, nocturia, enuresis, difficult erection. **Hepatotoxic (prolonged use of high doses):** hepatitis, jaundice, hepatomegaly. **Hypersensitivity:** pruritus, urticaria, eczematoid skin eruption, photosensitivity, pleural effusion (with shortness of breath, dry cough, fever, chest pains, eosinophilia). **Ophthalmic:** blurred vision, diplopia, changes in vision, photophobia. **Other:** general malaise, myalgia, backache, pulmonary effusion, feeling of suffocation, increased salivation, lacrimation, or sweating; chills, fever, acnelike rash, abnormal hair growth.

ROUTE AND DOSAGE. Oral: *Relief of spasticity:* **Adults:** Initial: 25 mg once daily; increased to 25 mg two to four times daily, then by increments of 25 mg up to 100 mg two to four times daily, if necessary. Each dosage level should be maintained for 4 to 7 days to determine patient's response. **Children:** Initial: 0.5 mg/kg twice daily; increased to 0.5 mg/kg three or four times daily, then by increments of 0.5 mg/kg up to 3 mg/kg two to four times daily, if necessary. Not to exceed 100 mg four times daily. **Intravenous:** *Malignant hy-*

perthermia: **Adults, children:** 1 mg/kg by rapid IV push, repeated as necessary up to cumulative dose of 10 mg/kg. (It may be necessary to give oral dose of 1 to 2 mg/kg four times daily for 1 to 3 days to prevent recurrence.) Each vial is reconstituted with 60 ml sterile water for injection *without* a bacteriostatic agent. Shake until solution is completely clear.

D

NURSING IMPLICATIONS

If necessary, an oral suspension for a single dose may be made by emptying contents of capsule(s) into fruit juice or other liquid. Pharmacist can prepare a multiple dose suspension on request. Suspension should be shaken well before pouring. Since it will not contain a preservative, avoid contamination, keep refrigerated, and use within several days.

Prior to initiation of therapy, an assessment should be made of patient's neuromuscular function as a baseline for comparison: posture, gait, coordination, ROM, muscle strength, and tone, presence of abnormal muscle movements, reflexes.

Supervise ambulation until patient's reaction to drug is known. Relief of spasticity may be accompanied by some loss of voluntary strength, which may impede patient's ability to maintain balance and an upright posture.

The most common side effects of dantrolene are drowsiness, dizziness, fatigue, muscular weakness (which may be manifested by slurred speech, drooling, and enuresis), general malaise, headache, diarrhea. Symptoms are generally transient, lasting up to 14 days after initiation of therapy. Keep physician informed. Reduction in dosage or discontinuation of dantrolene may be necessary if symptoms persist.

Patients with impaired cardiac or pulmonary function should be closely monitored for cardiovascular or respiratory symptoms such as tachycardia, blood pressure changes, feeling of suffocation.

Because of the possibility of hepatic injury, it is recommended that drug be discontinued if improvement is not evident within 45 days.

Keep physician informed of therapeutic effectiveness. Improvement may not be apparent until a week or more of drug therapy.

Baseline and regularly scheduled hepatic function tests (alkaline phosphatase, SGOT (AST), SGPT (ALT), total bilirubin), blood cell counts, and renal function tests should be performed.

Risk of hepatotoxicity appears to be greater in females, patients over 35 years, patients taking other medications in addition to dantrolene, and in patients taking high dantrolene doses (400 mg or more daily) for prolonged periods.

Instruct patient to report promptly the onset of jaundice: yellow skin or sclerae, dark urine, clay-colored stools; itching, abdominal discomfort. Hepatotoxicity more frequently occurs between 3rd and 12th month of therapy.

IV extravasation should be avoided. Solution has a high pH and therefore is extremely irritating to tissue. Observe and palpate entry site frequently during therapy.

During IV infusion, monitor vital signs. EKG, central venous pressure, and serum potassium should also be monitored.

Malignant hyperthermia usually appears during anesthesia, but it has also occurred several hours postoperatively. It is an inherited susceptibility and most commonly is seen in patients receiving potent inhalation anesthetics (cyclopropane, ethyl ether, halothane, methoxyflurane), succinylcholine (Anectine), curare, and pancuronium (Pavulon). It may also occur solely from the stress of surgery. A past history of no reaction is no guarantee of safety with subsequent exposure to these agents.

In addition to dantrolene, malignant hyperthermia requires intensive symptomatic treatment such as continual monitoring of body temperature, management of fever (sponges or hypothermia blanket, as ordered), correction of acidosis, maintenance of fluid and electrolyte balance, adequate oxygenation, seizure precautions, monitoring of intake and output ratio.

Clinical signs of malignant hyperthermia include skeletal muscle rigidity (often the first sign), sudden tachycardia, cardiac arrhythmias, cyanosis, tachypnea, unstable blood pressure, rapidly rising temperature, acidosis, shock.

Some clinicians recommend that family members submit to a muscle biopsy to test their susceptibility to malignant hyperthermia.

Patients with malignant hyperthermia should be advised to wear medical identification (e.g., Medic Alert) indicating diagnosis, physician, telephone number, and drug.

Advise patient to report symptoms of allergy (rash, erythema, pruritus, urticaria) and allergic pleural effusion (shortness of breath, pleuritic pain, dry cough).

Monitor bowel function. Persistent diarrhea may necessitate drug withdrawal. Severe constipation with abdominal distention and signs of intestinal obstruction have been reported.

Forewarn patient of the possibility of dizziness and drowsiness and advise to avoid driving and other potentially hazardous activities until reaction to drug is known.

Since hepatotoxicity occurs more commonly when other drugs are taken concurrently with dantrolene, advise patient not to take OTC medications, alcoholic beverages, or other CNS depressants unless otherwise advised by physician.

Because of the possibility of photosensitivity reactions, advise patient to avoid unnecessary exposure to sunlight and to use physical protection such as a hat, protective clothing, and a sunscreen agent (SPF 12 or above).

Treatment of overdosage: immediate gastric lavage. General supportive measures include maintaining airway, monitoring cardiac and renal function. Large quantities of fluids are given to prevent crystalluria.

Store capsules in tightly-closed light-resistant container. Contents of vial (for IV use) must be protected from direct light and used within 6 hours after reconstitution, since it does not contain a preservative. Both oral and parenteral forms are stored preferably between 15° and 30°C (59° and 86°F), unless otherwise directed by manufacturer.

Drug Interactions. Alcohol and other CNS depressants may cause additive CNS depression. Concurrent use of **estrogens** in females over 35 years reportedly associated with a relatively higher frequency of hepatotoxicity

---

DAPSONE

(Avlosulfon, DDS)

(dap'sone)
Antiinfective
Leprostatic
Sulfone

ACTIONS AND USES. Sulfone derivative chemically related to sulfonamides, with bacteriostatic rather than bactericidal action. Spectrum of activity includes *Mycobacterium leprae* (Hansen's bacillus), *M. tuberculosis,* and non-acid-fast organisms such as *Streptococci.* Mechanism of antibacterial action thought to be competitive inhibition of bacterial synthesis of folic acid from para-aminobenzoic acid (PABA). Also causes fragmentation of bacilli in lesions by unknown mechanism and is thought to increase host resistance.

Used in treatment of all types of leprosy (Hansen's disease) and to control symptoms of dermatitis herpetiformis (Duhring's disease). *Unlabeled Use:* relapsing polychondritis, and prophylaxis and treatment of chloroquine-resistant falciparum malaria.

D

ABSORPTION AND FATE. Almost completely absorbed from GI tract, mainly from upper part of small intestines. Peak plasma levels in 4 to 8 hours. Distributed to all body tissues, with high concentrations in kidney, liver, muscle, and skin. About 50% bound to plasma proteins. Half-life: 10 to 50 hours (with mean of 28 hours). Acetylated in liver (degree of acetylation is genetically determined). Enters enterohepatic circulation following biliary excretion. Approximately 70 to 80% of dose is excreted slowly in urine, primarily as water soluble metabolites, with some free drug; a small percentage is excreted in feces. Traces may be found in blood 8 to 12 days after single 200-mg dose and for 35 days following discontinuation of repeated doses. Small amounts excreted in sweat, tears, saliva, sputum, and breast milk.

CONTRAINDICATIONS AND PRECAUTIONS. Hypersensitivity to sulfones or its derivatives; advanced renal amyloidosis, severe anemia, methemoglobin reductase deficiency. Safe use during pregnancy (category A) not established. *Cautious Use:* chronic renal, hepatic, pulmonary, or cardiovascular disease, refractory anemias, albuminuria, G6PD deficiency.

ADVERSE/SIDE EFFECTS. CNS: headache, giddiness, dizziness, lethargy, malaise, nervousness, insomnia, tinnitus, blurred vision, reversible peripheral neuropathy (especially thenar muscles of thumbs), paresthesias, motor neuropathy (muscle weakness), neuralgic pain, psychosis. **Hematologic:** methemoglobinemia (common); hemolytic-type anemia, macrocytic anemia, aplastic anemia, leukopenia, agranulocytosis, pancytopenia (infrequent). **Hypersensitivity:** hypermelanotic macules (fixed eruptions), pruritus, erythema multiforme (erythematous, edematous, or bullous lesions of skin or mucous membranes), exfoliative dermatitis (dry, itchy, red, scaly skin), loss of hair, toxic epidermal necrolysis ("scalded skin syndrome"), drug fever, allergic rhinitis, hepatitis, hepatic necrosis. **Lepra reaction (erythema nodosum leprosum):** malaise, fever, painful indurations of skin and mucosa, arthralgia, lymphadenitis, orchitis, peripheral neuritis, iridocyclitis, iritis, swelling of hands and feet, nephropathy, hepatomegaly. **Usually dose-related. GI:** anorexia, nausea, vomiting, abdominal colic. **Other:** tachycardia, hematuria, proteinuria.

ROUTE AND DOSAGE. Oral: Adult: *Leprosy:* 6 to 10 mg/kg weekly (50 to 100 mg daily); correspondingly smaller doses for children. *Tuberculoid and indeterminate type leprosy:* 50 mg daily for a minimum of 3 years. *Dermatitis herpetiformis:* 50 mg daily. May be increased by 50 mg/day up to 300 mg daily or higher if necessary. Not to exceed 500 mg daily. *Lepromatous leprosy and borderline patients:* dapsone administered in full dosage for at least 10 years. **Children:** *Leprostatic:* ¼ to ½ the adult dosage.

NURSING IMPLICATIONS

Administer with food to reduce possibility of GI distress.

Patients with lepromatous leprosy tend to be sensitive to dapsone and therefore may require dosage reduction to control adverse reactions.

Complete blood counts are performed prior to initiation of therapy, weekly during the first month of therapy, at monthly intervals for at least 6 months, and semi-annually thereafter. Periodic determinations of dapsone blood levels are also recommended. Dapsone blood levels of 0.1 to 7 mcg/dl reflect safe dosage.

Mild decrease in hemoglobin level may occur during the first few weeks of therapy. If hemoglobin falls below 9 Gm/dl, dosage should be reduced or drug temporarily discontinued. Drug therapy is usually terminated if RBC count falls below 2.5 million/mm^3 or remains persistently low after 6 weeks of therapy, or if leukocyte count falls below 5000/mm^3.

Monitor temperature during first few weeks of therapy. If fever is frequent or severe, dosage should be reduced or therapy interrupted.

Instruct patient to report to physician if symptoms of leprosy do not improve within 3 months or if they get worse. Bacterial resistance to dapsone has been reported.

Lepra reaction *(see Adverse Side Effects)* is believed to be a response to circulating antigens from disintegrating *Mycobacterium leprae* and not a specific drug reaction. It may be precipitated by infection, fever, vaccinations, or other stress, and has occurred 7 to 14 days postpartum in some patients. Dosage adjustment or temporary interruption of therapy (1 to 2 weeks) may be required.

Suspect methemoglobinemia if patient appears cyanotic and mucous membranes have a brownish hue. Report to physician. Usually, discontinuation of therapy is not required unless anoxemia is present.

The appearance of a skin rash should be reported promptly because it may signify developing sensitization which can lead to potentially fatal complications. Allergic skin reactions occur most frequently before the tenth week of therapy and indicate that drug should be discontinued. Interruption of therapy is usually not necessary for hypermelanotic, macular-type localized lesions which may develop 1 week to 1 year after treatment begins.

Patients who complain of loss of appetite, nausea, and vomiting should have liver function tests performed (urine bilirubin, AST).

Because of cumulative effects patient should be carefully taught to report the onset of adverse reactions.

Therapeutic effects in leprosy may not appear until after 3 to 6 months of therapy. Skin lesions respond well; recovery from nerve involvement is usually limited.

Deformities such as contractures may be prevented by physical therapy, careful positioning of anesthetic limbs or application of casts. Other disfigurements may necessitate reconstructive surgery.

Lepromatous eye lesions sometimes develop or progress during treatment, since the drug does not appreciably penetrate ocular tissues.

Optimum duration of therapy has not been determined. Some authorities recommend continuing treatment for lepromatous leprosy at least 10 years or more; current thinking seems to favor maintenance therapy for life. For the indeterminate and tuberculoid types, treatment may be continued for at least 3 years after disease is clinically quiescent. Leprosy is considered inactive when skin scrapings and/or biopsy are negative for bacteria, and there is no evidence of clinical activity for at least a year.

Hospitalization is advised during initial therapy for leprosy, but thereafter ambulatory treatment is sufficient. No special isolation procedures are necessary when patient is hospitalized but nasal discharge and discharge from lesions must be carefully disinfected.

Leprosy is transmitted by active skin lesions or nasal discharge of infected persons, but only susceptible people develop the disease. According to recent evidence most people have partial or complete resistance to leprosy.

There are no restrictions in employment or attending school in patients with inactive leprosy.

Scheduled follow-up is critical to detection of possible relapse. Examination of close contacts at 6- to 12-month intervals for at least 10 years is recommended.

Many clinicians believe that infants should not be separated from leprous mothers receiving therapy and that breast feeding should be encouraged as a means of providing chemoprophylaxis for the infant.

Infants fed breast milk containing dapsone may develop methemoglobinemia. This is reversible and reportedly is not serious except in infants with G6PD deficiency.

Food-Drug Interactions:

- Physician may prescribe a gluten-controlled diet in patients with dermatitis herpetiformis because the disease is usually accompanied by gluten sensitive lesions of the jejunum. Gluten control may improve intestinal inflammation and skin lesions to some extent and thus allow for reduction in dapsone dosage.

- Foods rich in gluten include the cereal grains, such as wheat, barley, oats, rye, bran, graham, millet, wheat germ, bulgur, durham, and malt. (Corn and rice cereals are allowed.) Foods that may contain cereals should also be avoided, e.g., certain coffees, root beer, meat loaf, pasta and macaroni products. Advise patient to read product labels carefully and to avoid commercially prepared foods containing gluten.

Preserved in tightly covered, light-resistant containers at 15° to 30°C (59° to 86°F). Drug discoloration apparently does not indicate a chemical change.

Drug Interactions. **Probenecid** may cause elevated dapsone blood levels (by inhibiting renal excretion of dapsone).

DAUNORUBICIN HYDROCHLORIDE

(Cerubidine, DNR)

(daw-noe-roo'bi-sin)
Antineoplastic
Antibiotic

ACTIONS AND USES. Cytotoxic and antimitotic anthracycline glycoside antibiotic; cell-cycle specific for S-phase of cell division. Toxic properties preclude its use as an antibiotic. Action mechanism unclear, but may be due to rapid intercalating of DNA molecule resulting in inhibition of DNA, RNA, and protein synthesis. A potent bone marrow suppressant, with immunosuppressive properties. Induces cardiac toxicity and may be mutagenic carcinogenic (development of secondary carcinomas).

Used as single agent or in combination with cytarabine to induce remission in acute nonlymphocytic leukemia (myelogenous, monocytic, erythroid) in adults. Also used to treat solid tumors of childhood and non-Hodgkin's lymphoma.

ABSORPTION AND FATE. Rapid disappearance from plasma following IV administration indicates rapid distribution to tissues. Thereafter, plasma levels slowly decline with a half-life of 18.5 hours. Hepatic metabolism within 1 hour. Active metabolite, daunorubicinol, predominates in plasma and maintains a half-life of 26.7 hours. About 25% administered dose excreted as metabolite in urine; 40% excreted in bile. Does not cross blood–brain barrier. Probably crosses placenta. Distribution to breast milk not known.

CONTRAINDICATIONS AND PRECAUTIONS. Severe myelosuppression, pregnancy (especially in first trimester), and preexisting cardiac disease unless risk-benefit is evaluated; lactation, uncontrolled systemic infection. *Cautious Use:* history of gout, urate calculi, hepatic or renal function impairment, elderly patients with inadequate bone reserve due to age or previous cytotoxic drug therapy, tumor cell infiltration of bone marrow, patient who has received potentially cardiotoxic drugs or related antineoplastics.

ADVERSE/SIDE EFFECTS. Cutaneous: generalized alopecia (reversible), rash (rare). **CV:** pericarditis, myocarditis, arrhythmias, congestive heart failure. **GI:** acute nausea and vomiting (mild), anorexia, mucositis, diarrhea (occasionally). **Hematopoietic:** thrombocytopenia, leukocytopenia, anemia. **Other:** hyperuricemia, fever, chills (rare), gonadal suppression, severe cellulitis or tissue sloughing at site of drug extravasation.

ROUTE AND DOSAGE. (Representative dose schedule for nonlymphocytic leukemia): **Intravenous: Adults:** 60 $mg/m^2/day$ on days 1, 2, 3, every 3 or 4 weeks. In combination: 45 $mg/m^2/day$ on days 1, 2, 3, of first course and on days 1 and 2 of subsequent courses with 100 $mg/m^2/day$ cytarabine by IV infusion daily for 7 days for first course, and for 5 days for subsequent courses. Dosage modifications are based on serum bilirubin and creatinine values.

NURSING IMPLICATIONS

Not to be confused with doxorubacin.

Use of gloves during preparation of the solution for infusion is recommended to prevent skin contact with the drug. If this occurs, decontaminate with copious amounts of water with soap. *(See Index: Antineoplastics: handling drug solutions.)*

Reconstitute vial contents with 4 ml sterile water for injection. Concentrations of the solution will be 5 ml daunorubicin/ml. Withdraw dose into syringe containing 10 to 15 ml normal saline and inject into the tubing or side arm of a rapidly flowing IV infusion of 5% glucose or normal saline solution.

Extravasation can cause severe tissue necrosis and therefore must be avoided.

Daunorubicin should never be administered IM or SC, and it should never be mixed with heparin or other drugs.

Hepatic and renal function tests should be performed prior to and during each course of treatment. If function is impaired therapeutic dosage levels are reduced to prevent toxicity.

If serum bilirubin is 1.2 to 3.0 mg/dl, the recommended dose of daunorubicin is ¾ normal dose; if serum bilirubin is more than 3 mg/dl ½ normal dose is recommended (*normal serum bilirubin:* 0.7 mg/dl).

When serum creatinine is more than 3 mg/dl the dose is reduced to ½ normal value (*normal serum creatinine:* 0.7 to 1.5 mg/dl).

Prior to each course of therapy an ECG and/or determination of systolic ejection fraction is performed to recognize patients at greatest risk for development of acute congestive heart failure (CHF).

Monitor blood pressure, temperature, pulse and respiratory function during daunorubicin treatment. Acute CHF can occur suddenly, especially when total dosage exceeds 550 mg/m^2, or in patients with compromised heart function because of previous radiation therapy in heart area.

Report immediately breathlessness, orthopnea, change in pulse and blood pressure parameters. Early clinical diagnosis of drug-induced CHF is essential for successful treatment (digitalis, diuretics, sodium restriction, bed rest).

A profound suppression of bone marrow is required to induce a complete remission. Peripheral blood and bone marrow studies are essential to treatment plans.

Nadirs for thrombocytes and leukocytes usually reached in 10 to 14 days after drug administration.

Myelosuppression imposes risk of superimposed infection. Promptly report elevation of temperature, chills, symptoms of upper respiratory tract infection, tachycardia, symptoms of overgrowth with opportunistic organisms (red or furry tongue, sore mouth, diarrhea with foul-smelling stools, vaginal itching, and discharge, sudden fever, cough).

Be alert to significance of immunosuppressive activity: reduced capacity to resist and overcome inflammatory conditions, slower wound healing, long periods of low-grade chronic infections. Protect patient from contact with persons with infections. The most hazardous period is during nadirs of thrombocytes and leukocytes.

Drug-induced hyperuricemia may occur because of rapid lysis of leukemic cells. Monitor *serum uric acid levels* (normal: 3 to 7 mg/dl).

The attainment of a normal bone marrow after daunorubicin administration may require as many as three courses of induction therapy.

A regimen of encouraged increase in oral fluid intake, alkalinization of urine, and allopurinol

D

may reduce incidence of hyperuricemia. Report pain in flank, stomach, or joints, and changes in intake and output ratio and pattern.

Nausea and vomiting are usually mild and may be controlled by antiemetic therapy.

Inspect oral membranes daily. Mucositis may occur 3 to 7 days after drug is administered. Institute appropriate nursing measures to reduce interference with adequate nutritional intake because of oral discomfort. *See Mechlorethamine for nursing care of stomatitis, xerostomia.*

Discuss probability of onset of alopecia with patient but inform patient that recovery is usual in 6 to 10 weeks.

Discuss possibility of gonadal suppression (amenorrhea or azoospermia) with patient before treatment begins. Patient should understand that usually it is an irreversible side effect.

Advise against conception during daunorubicin treatment period because of teratogenic properties of the drug. Advise patient to report to the physician should she become pregnant.

Daunorubicin may impart a red color to urine (a transient effect).

Reconstituted solution is stable 24 hours at room temperature and 48 hours under refrigeration between 2° and 8°C (36° and 46°F) protected from light.

Diagnostic Test Interferences. Daunorubicin may elevate serum and urine **uric acid** levels.

Drug Interactions: Daunorubicin

Plus	Interactions
Antigout agent	Increases uric acid level; dose adjustment of antigout agent may be necessary
Cyclophosphamide (Cytoxan, Neosar), doxorubicin (Adriamycin), radiation	Prior treatment with any of these modalities increases cardiac toxicity potential from daunorubicin therapy
Hepatotoxic drugs	Concurrent use increases risk of toxicity

DEFEROXAMINE MESYLATE

(Desferal Mesylate)

(de-fer-ox'a-meen)
Chelating agent
Antidote

ACTIONS AND USES. Chelating agent isolated from *Streptomyces pilosus* with specific affinity for ferric ion and low affinity for calcium. Binds ferric ions to form ferrioxamine complex, a stable water-soluble chelate readily excreted by kidneys. Main effect is removal of iron from ferritin, hemosiderin, and transferrin. Does not affect hemoglobin or cytochromes or increase excretion of electrolytes and other trace elements. Has histamine-releasing properties when administered rapidly by IV route. Theoretically, 100 mg of deferoxamine can chelate 8.5 mg of ferric iron.

Used as adjunct in treatment of acute iron intoxication. Has been used in management of hemochromatosis and hemosiderosis secondary to increased iron storage as from multiple transfusions used in treatment of congenital anemias, e.g., thalassemia (Cooley's or Mediterranean anemia), sickle cell anemia and other chronic anemias. *Unlabeled Use:* removal of aluminum from water used during dialysis to prevent aluminum toxicity; used during first 2 hours of dialysis.

ABSORPTION AND FATE. Widely distributed in body tissues following administration. Rapidly forms nontoxic complex with iron (complex is dialyzable). Metabolized primarily by plasma enzymes by unknown mechanism. Excreted rapidly in urine as iron chelate (ferrioxamine) and unchanged drug. Some is also excreted in feces via bile.

CONTRAINDICATIONS AND PRECAUTIONS. Severe renal disease, anuria, pregnancy, women of childbearing potential, and children under 3 years of age. *Cautious Use:* history of pyelonephritis.

ADVERSE/SIDE EFFECTS. Pain and induration at injection site; generalized erythema, urticaria, pruritus, fever, hypotension, shock (most commonly with rapid IV injection). Long-term therapy particularly: allergic-type reactions (pruritus, urticaria, rash, anaphylactoid reactions), blurred vision, cataracts, abdominal discomfort, dysuria, diarrhea, leg cramps, tachycardia, fever, exacerbation of pyelonephritis.

ROUTE AND DOSAGE. Adults and children: *Acute iron intoxication:* **Intramuscular (preferred route), intravenous infusion:** 1 Gm followed by 500 mg at 4-hour intervals for two doses. Depending on clinical response, subsequent doses of 500 mg every 4 to 12 hours. Maximum dose 6 Gm in 24 hours. Infusion rate should not exceed 15 mg/kg/hour. *Chronic iron overload:* **Intramuscular:** 500 mg to 1 Gm daily. In addition, 2 Gm IV with each unit of blood transfused. (Administered separately from blood). **Subcutaneous:** 1 to 2 Gm (20 to 40 mg/kg/ day administered over 8 to 24 hours using a continuous infusion pump. **Children:** 50 mg/ kg/dose IM or IV every 6 hours or up to 15 mg/kg/hour to a maximum of 6 Gm/24 hours or 2 Gm/dose.

NURSING IMPLICATIONS

Baseline tests of kidney function should be performed.

Reconstituted by adding 2 ml sterile water for injection to each 500-mg vial. Make certain that drug is completely dissolved before withdrawing from vial. Rotate injection sites.

IV route is used only for patients in shock. For IV administration, reconstitute as for IM or SC use. After drug is completely dissolved, withdraw prescribed amount from vial and add to 0.9% sodium chloride, 5% dextrose in water, or lactated Ringer's solution.

Physician will prescribe specific infusion flow rate (should not exceed 15 mg/kg of body weight per hour). Monitor vital signs.

Monitor intake and output ratio. Report any change. Observe stools for blood (iron intoxication frequently causes necrosis of GI tract).

Deferoxamine is used as adjunct to standard treatment for acute iron intoxication: emesis with syrup of ipecac, gastric lavage with 5% sodium bicarbonate, suction and maintenance of airway, control of shock (IV fluids, blood, oxygen, vasopressors), correction of acidosis. Speed is essential to prevent absorption of iron from GI tract.

Deferoxamine chelate imparts a characteristic reddish color to urine (presumptive evidence of elevated serum iron and indication for further therapy). Keep physician informed.

Periodic ophthalmoscopic examinations are advisable for patients on prolonged therapy for chronic iron overload.

Solutions reconstituted with sterile water may be stored at room temperature for not longer than 1 week. Protect from light.

DEHYDROCHOLIC ACID

(Cholan-DH, Decholin, Dycholium, Hepahydrin)

(dee-hye-droe-koe'lik)
Laxative (stimulant)
Hydrocholeretic

ACTIONS AND USES. Unconjugated oxidized acid made synthetically from cholanic acids (chiefly cholic acid) found in natural bile. Increases volume and flow of low-viscosity water-diluted bile by hydrocholeretic action and thus facilitates biliary tract drainage. Doubtful effect on production of bile salts. Probably much less effective than natural bile salts in lowering surface tension and hence emulsification or in promoting absorption of fats or fat-soluble vitamins. Exerts laxative action by inducing secretion of water and electrolytes from colon.

Used for temporary relief of constipation; as adjunct, primarily for flushing action, in management of chronic and recurring biliary tract disorders. Used prophylactically following biliary tract surgery to prevent accumulation of debris and bacteria in common bile duct and biliary drainage tube. Commercially available in combination with docusate sodium, e.g., Bilax, Neolax.

ABSORPTION AND FATE. Absorbed from intestines. Extensively metabolized by liver to cholic acid. Undergoes enterohepatic circulation. Excreted in feces via bile.

CONTRAINDICATIONS AND PRECAUTIONS. Cholelithiasis, jaundice, marked hepatic insufficiency, partial or complete obstruction of common or hepatic bile ducts, GI or GU tracts; use for critically or terminally ill patients; in presence of nausea, vomiting, or abdominal pain. *Cautious Use:* history of asthma or allergy, prostatic hypertrophy, acute hepatitis, acute yellow atrophy of liver, children under 12 years of age, the elderly.

ADVERSE/SIDE EFFECTS. Toxic effects not reported with recommended use.

ROUTE AND DOSAGE. Oral: 250 to 500 mg three times a day.

NURSING IMPLICATIONS

Administered with or after meals.

Frequent use may result in laxative dependence.

Therapy for biliary tract disorders usually is discontinued if no clinical improvement is noted within 4 to 6 weeks.

Patients with biliary fistula may require simultaneous administration of bile salts to promote normal digestion and absorption.

See Bisacodyl for patient teaching points concerning constipation.

Store at room temperature, preferably between 15° and 30°C (59° and 86°F), unless otherwise directed by manufacturer.

Diagnostic Test Interferences. Dehydrocholic acid may interfere with hepatic uptake or biliary excretion of **sulfobromophthalein (BSP).**

DEMECARIUM BROMIDE

(Humorsol)

(dem-e-kare′ee-um)

Cholinergic (parasympathomimetic)

Cholinesterase inhibitor

Miotic

ACTIONS AND USES. Potent, indirect-acting quaternary ammonium compound with prolonged effect. Action attributed to reversible cholinesterase inhibition, which permits accumulation and sustained action of endogenous acetylcholine at cholinergic synapses. Local application to conjunctiva produces intense miosis by contraction of iris sphincter and increased accommodation by contraction of ciliary muscle. The resultant widening of the trabecular network decreases intraocular pressure by facilitating aqueous humor outflow. Also enhances resorption of aqueous humor by increasing permeability and dilation of conjunctival vessels.

Used in treatment of open-angle glaucoma and in selected cases of glaucoma due to synechial formation. Also used following iridectomy and in management of accommodative esotropia (convergent strabismus) when less potent miotics have failed. Carbonic anhydrase inhibitor may be used concomitantly to enhance action. Reduces amount of convergence in accommodative esotropia by inducing peripheral accommodation.

ABSORPTION AND FATE. Absorbed through conjunctiva and intact skin. Miosis begins within 1 hour and reaches maximum in 2 to 4 hours. Reduction of intraocular pressure occurs in 12 hours and is maximal in 24 hours. Residual miosis and decreased intraocular pressure may persist 7 days or more following single instillation.

CONTRAINDICATIONS AND PRECAUTIONS. Narrow-angle glaucoma, history of retinal detachment, ocular hypertension accompanied by inflammation, active uveitis, glaucoma associated with iridocyclitis, bronchial asthma, spastic GI conditions, peptic ulcer, marked vagotonia, pronounced bradycardia or hypotension, recent myocardial infarction, parkinsonism, epilepsy. Safe use in pregnancy not established. *Cautious Use:* myasthenia gravis, corneal abrasion, individuals exposed to organophosphate insecticides or pesticides.

ADVERSE/SIDE EFFECTS. Local effects: stinging, burning, lacrimation, ciliary spasm with eye and brow pain, photophobia, frontal headache, myopia with visual blurring, twitching of eyelids, conjunctival and ciliary hyperemia, iris cysts (particularly in children following prolonged use), activation of latent iritis or uveitis, retinal detachment (occasionally), conjunctival thickening and obstruction of nasolacrimal canals (prolonged use), lens opacity, contact dermatitis. **Systemic effects *(parasympathetic stimulation)*:** nausea, vomiting, abdominal pain, diarrhea, urinary frequency or incontinence, excessive salivation, nasal congestion, rhinorrhea, profuse sweating, flushing, muscular weakness, paresthesias, bronchospasm, hypotension, shock, bradycardia, depression of serum cholinesterase and erythrocytes.

ROUTE AND DOSAGE. Topical: Adults: *Glaucoma:* 1 or 2 drops of 0.125 or 0.25% solution twice weekly up to twice daily. Intervals determined by intraocular pressure (IOP) evaluations. **Children:** *Accommodative esotropia* (convergent strabismus): 1 drop of 0.125% solution instilled into each eye daily for 2 to 3 weeks, reduce to 1 drop every 2 days for 3 to 4 weeks. Then 1 drop twice a week. If patient continues to improve dosage may be reduced to 1 drop weekly and then eventually discontinued. Highly individualized dosages.

NURSING IMPLICATIONS

Physician may prescribe schedule so that drug is instilled at bedtime in order to minimize disturbing visual effects.

Demecarium bromide is a dangerous drug capable of producing cumulative systemic effects. It is essential to adhere precisely to prescribed drug concentration, dosage schedule, and technique of administration. Closely observe patient during initial period.

Before initiation of therapy tonometric readings are determined, and usually gonioscopy is performed in patients with glaucoma to confirm that angle of the eye is open.

The first instillation will be made by physician. Since a transient paradoxic increase in intraocular pressure may occur initially, tonometric readings should be made at least hourly for 3 or 4 hours after first instillation.

Procedure for instilling eye drop to minimize overflow of solution into nasal and pharyngeal spaces, and possibly systemic absorption: Patient should be in supine position. After drop is instilled into lower conjunctiva gentle digital pressure is applied to inner canthus against nose (lacrimal duct). Maintain pressure for 1 or 2 minutes after drop is instilled. Instruct patient to avoid squeezing lids together. Blot excess medication with a clean tissue. Wash hands immediately after administration.

Always wash hands before and after the procedure.

D

Avoid prolonged contact of drug with skin. If solution contacts skin, wash promptly with large volumes of water.

Maintain sterility of dropper. If it becomes contaminated it should be sterilized before being returned to bottle.

Supervise ambulation. Inform patient that difficulty in accommodating to degree of light, blurred distant vision (ciliary or accommodative spasm), and miosis with dimmed vision and eyelid twitching may persist for a week or more.

Advise patient to avoid driving, particularly at night, and other potentially hazardous activities until side effects have disappeared.

Pain in affected eye is more intense with accommodative effort to near objects and with exposure to light. These effects appear more frequently in younger patients than in older patients.

Advise patient to report promptly to the physician the onset of excessive salivation, diaphoresis, urinary incontinence, diarrhea, muscle weakness, respiratory problems, cardiac irregularities or symptoms of shock (cold clammy skin, weak, rapid pulse). Drug should be discontinued.

Patients receiving demecarium should remain under constant medical supervision. Those being treated for accomodative esotropia should be evaluated every 4 to 12 weeks. If after 4 months of therapy, patient still requires every other day dosage, drug should be discontinued. All patients should be examined for lenticular opacities at intervals of 6 months or less.

In the event of systemic toxicity, atropine sulfate is used as antidote. Also have on hand pralidoxime (a cholinesterase reactivator) as an adjunct to atropine. Artificial respiration, oxygen, and other supportive measures may be necessary.

If possible demecarium bromide should be discontinued 2 to 6 weeks prior to surgery.

Caution patient of possible added systemic effects from skin contact or inhalation of organophosphate-type insecticides or pesticides while receiving demecarium. Persons who may be exposed should protect themselves by use of a respiratory mask and by frequent washing and clothing changes.

Preserved in tight, light-resistant containers, preferably between 15° and 30°C (59° and 86°F) unless otherwise directed by manufacturer.

Drug Interactions: Demecarium

Plus	Interactions
Cholinesterase inhibitors (systemic), e.g., ambenonium edrophonium, neostigmine, physostigmine, pyridostigmine	Additive systemic effects
Pilocarpine	Competitively inhibits miotic effect of demecarium
Succinylcholine	Concomitant use may cause prolonged apnea and cardiovascular collapse

DEMECLOCYCLINE HYDROCHLORIDE

(Declomycin, DMCT)

(dem-e-kloe-sye'kleen)
Antiinfective
Antibiotic
Tetracycline

ACTIONS AND USES. Tetracycline antibiotic isolated from mutant strain of *Streptomyces aureofaciens.* Similar to other tetracycline antibiotics in actions, uses, contraindications, precautions, and adverse reactions. Excreted more slowly than other tetracyclines and is more frequently associated with photosensitivity reactions. Promotes water diuresis in patients with water intoxication due to inappropriate secretion of antiduretic hormone (ADH) by antagonizing the action of ADH on renal tubules.

In addition to use in treatment of infections caused by susceptible organisms, also used investigationally as a diuretic in patients with syndrome of inappropriate antidiuretic hormone (SIADH) secretion.

ABSORPTION AND FATE. Peak serum concentrations within 3 to 6 hours; effective serum levels may persist 48 to 72 hours after last dose. About 40 to 90% is bound to serum proteins. Half-life: 10 to 17 hours. Concentrates in liver and is excreted in bile. Enterohepatic cycle maintains serum levels and delays ultimate removal. Approximately 40 to 50% of dose is excreted in urine and feces in 24 hours. Crosses placenta. Excreted in breast milk.

CONTRAINDICATIONS AND PRECAUTIONS. Hypersensitivity to any of the tetracyclines; use during period of tooth development (e.g., last half of pregnancy, infancy, and childhood to the age of 8 years). *Cautious Use:* impaired renal or hepatic function. *See also Tetracycline.*

ADVERSE/SIDE EFFECTS. Photosensitivity, urticaria, pruritus, erythematous eruptions, edema, increased pigmentation of skin, mucous membranes, and nails; loosening or softening of nails (onycholysis), GI disturbances (nausea, vomiting, diarrhea, abdominal cramps, anorexia), superinfections, blood dyscrasias, acute renal failure (in patients with Laennec's cirrhosis). Following long-term therapy: diabetes insipidus syndrome. *See also Tetracycline.*

ROUTE AND DOSAGE. Oral: Adults: *Antiinfective:* 150 mg every 6 hours or 300 mg every 12 hours. *Gonorrhea:* Initial: 600 mg followed by 300 mg every 12 hours for 4 days to a total of 3 Gm. *Diuretic (for SIADH):* 300 to 1200 mg daily in divided doses. **Children (over 8 years):** 6 to 12 mg/kg/day divided into two to four doses.

NURSING IMPLICATIONS

Check expiration date before administering drug. Renal damage (Fanconi syndrome) and death have resulted from use of outdated tetracyclines.

Demeclocycline should be taken on an empty stomach to enhance absorption. Because esophageal ulceration has been reported with oral tetracyclines, administer with a full glass of water and advise patient to avoid taking drug within 1 hour of bedtime.

If gastric distress is a problem, physician may prescribe taking drug with a light meal even though absorption may be reduced.

Food–Drug Interactions: Demeclocycline absorption may be impaired by food, milk, or other calcium-containing foods; iron salts; antacids containing aluminum, calcium, magnesium (or other divalent, or trivalent cations); and sodium bicarbonate. Administer demeclocycline not less than 1 hour before nor sooner than 2 hours after the above. Exception: iron preparations should be administered 3 hours before or 2 hours after demeclocycline.

Culture and susceptibility testing is recommended prior to initiation of therapy and at periodic intervals during prolonged therapy.

For most infections, therapy is usually continued 24 to 48 hours after fever and other symptoms have subsided. Therapy should continue for at least 10 days for streptococcal infections, to reduce resk of rheumatic fever or glomerulonephritis.

If drug therapy is prolonged, periodic evaluations of serum drug levels, and renal, hepatic, and hematopoietic systems are recommended..

Instruct patient to report symptoms of superinfections: black, furry tongue; oral lesions (stomatitis, glossitis); rectal or vaginal itching or discharge; loose, foul-smelling stools; diarrhea, unusual odor to urine, sudden fever, cough.

Caution patient to avoid exposure to sunlight or ultraviolet light during treatment and for several weeks after treatment so as to prevent severe burns (phototoxic reaction). Use of sun screen (SPF) above 12 is advisable.

Demeclocycline should be discontinued at first evidence of erythema.

Monitor intake and output ratio in patients with impaired kidney function or on prolonged therapy. Some patients develop diabetes insipidus syndrome (polydipsia, polyuria, weakness). It is usually dose-related and is reversible with discontinuation of therapy.

Preserved in tight, light-resistant containers, preferably between 15° and 30°C (59° and 86°F) unless otherwise directed by manufacturer.

See Tetracycline hydrochloride (prototype tetracyclines).

DESERPIDINE

(Harmonyl)

(de-ser'pi-deen)
Antihypertensive
Antipsychotic
Rauwolfia alkaloid

ACTIONS AND USES. Rauwolfia alkaloid almost identical to reserpine (qv) in actions, contraindications, precautions, adverse reactions and interactions. Incidence of dizziness and lethargy reportedly lower than produced by reserpine.

Used in treatment of mild essential hypertension and as adjunctive therapy with other antihypertensive agents in the more severe forms. Also has been used for relief of symptoms in agitated psychotic states, e.g., schizophrenia in patients unable to tolerate phenothiazines or in patients who also require antihypertensive medication. Available in fixed-dose combination with hydrochlorothiazide (Oreticyl), and with methyclothiazide (Enduronyl).

ABSORPTION AND FATE. Crosses placenta; appears in breast milk. *See Reserpine.*

CONTRAINDICATIONS AND PRECAUTIONS. Hypersensitivity to rauwolfia alkaloids; mental depression, acute peptic ulcer, acute ulcerative colitis, patients receiving electroconvulsive therapy, bronchial asthma, or other allergies or respiratory problems, pheochromocytoma. Safe use during pregnancy, in women of childbearing potential, in nursing mothers, and in children not established. *Cautious Use:* hypertension with renal insufficiency; epilepsy, gallstones, severe cardiac or cardiovascular disease, history of peptic ulcer, ulcerative colitis.

ADVERSE/SIDE EFFECTS. CNS: mental depression, confusion, drowsiness, nervousness, anxiety, lethargy, headache, vivid dreams, nightmares, increased appetite; with large doses: extrapyramidal symptoms, convulsions. **CV:** bradycardia, edema; excessive hypotension, anginalike symptoms, cutaneous flushing (overdosage). **EENT:** nasal stuffiness, epistaxis, dry mouth, conjunctival congestion. **GI:** nausea, vomiting, reactivation of peptic ulcer. **Hypersensitivity:** pruritus, rash. **Other:** impotence, decreased sexual interest, gynecomastia. *See also Reserpine.*

ROUTE AND DOSAGE. Oral: *Hypertension:* Initial: 0.75 to 1 mg daily. (Some clinicians do not use large initial doses.) Maintenance (maximum): 0.25 mg daily. *Psychiatric disorders:* Initial: 0.5 mg daily (range 0.1 to 1 mg). Dosage adjusted according to patient's response.

NURSING IMPLICATIONS

Administer with meals or with milk or other food to minimize possibility of gastric irritation.

Based on recent studies, withdrawal of rauwolfia derivatives prior to surgery is no longer recommended. However, anesthesiologist should be informed that patient is receiving such therapy.

Record blood pressure and pulse at intervals prescribed by physician. Compare readings with baseline determinations and keep physician informed. Antihypertensive effect is commonly associated with bradycardia.

Because deserpidine is cumulative in action, dosage adjustments when necessary are usually made at 10- to 14-day intervals.

Mental depression is a serious side effect and may be sufficiently severe to lead to suicide. It may not appear until after 2 to 8 months of therapy and may last for several months after drug is withdrawn. Instruct patient and responsible family members to report beginning symptoms of depression: early morning insomnia, nightmares or vivid dreams, impotence or decreased sexual interest, self-deprecation, mood swings, despondency, loss of appetite. Hospitalization may be necessary.

The 0.1 mg dosage strength contains tartrazine which may cause allergic manifestations including asthma in susceptible individuals. The reaction frequently occurs in patients with hypersensitivity to aspirin.

Advise patient to record weight and to check for edema daily. A gain of 3 to 5 pounds in 1 week should be reported to physician.

Orthostatic hypotension occurs rarely with recommended doses. Instruct patient to report symptoms of dizziness, light-headedness to physician. Dosage reduction may be indicated. Advise patient to make position changes slowly, particularly from recumbent to upright posture and to lie down immediately if feeling faint. Also advise patient not to take hot showers or tub baths, to avoid hot environments, and not to stand still for prolonged periods.

Mouth dryness may be relieved by frequent rinsing with warm water, increase in noncaloric fluid intake, if allowed, and particularly if fluid intake has been inadequate, sugarless gum, or lemon drops. If these measures fail, a saliva substitute may help (e.g., Xero-Lube, Moi-stir). Discuss with physician.

Advise patient not to take OTC drugs without prior approval of physician. Many drugs that might relieve nasal congestion, colds, hay fever, or other allergies contain sympathomimetic agents that may interfere with the effects of deserpidine.

Infants born to rauwolfia alkaloid-treated mothers should be observed for increased respiratory secretions, nasal congestion, cyanosis, and anorexia.

Warn patient that deserpidine may enhance the depressant effects of alcohol, barbiturates, and other CNS depressants, and to consult physician before taking these agents.

Advise patient to avoid driving and other potentially hazardous activities until reaction to drug is determined.

Store in tightly covered light-resistant containers, preferably between 15° and 30°C (59° and 86°F), unless otherwise directed by manufacturer.

See Reserpine (prototype rauwolfia derivative)for patient teaching outline and for diagnostic test interferences and drug interactions.

DESIPRAMINE HYDROCHLORIDE

(Norpramin, Pertofrane)

(dess-ip'ra-meen)
Psychotropic
Antidepressant
Tricyclic

D

ACTIONS AND USES. Dibenzazipine tricyclic antidepressant (TCA). Active metabolite of imipramine (qv) with similar pharmacologic actions, uses, limitations, and interactions. Onset of action is more rapid than that of imipramine; has mild sedative and anticholinergic actions.

Used to treat endogenous depression and various depression syndromes. *Unlabeled Use:* attention deficit disorder in children.

ABSORPTION AND FATE. Well-absorbed from GI tract. Hepatic metabolism. Half-life: 12 to 76 hours; effective therapeutic plasma levels: 150 to 300 ng/ml. Steady state reached in 2 to 11 days. Excreted in urine; crosses placenta.

CONTRAINDICATIONS AND PRECAUTIONS. Safe use during pregnancy (category C) and lactation not established. Acute recovery period of myocardial infarction, concomitant use or within 2 weeks of use of MAO inhibitors, convulsions, children under 12 years of age. *Cautious Use:* prostatic hypertrophy, narrow angle glaucoma, epilepsy, alcoholism; children, adolescents, elderly; thyroid, cardiovascular, renal and hepatic disease. *See also Imipramine.*

ADVERSE/SIDE EFFECTS. Drowsiness, dizziness, xerostomia, blurred vision, urinary retention, constipation, hypertension, orthostatic hypotension, tachycardia, confusional state (especially in the elderly and with high dosage), agranulocytosis, eosinophilia, decreased libido, exacerbation of psychosis in schizophrenia. *See also Imipramine.*

ROUTE AND DOSAGE. Oral: Adults: 75 to 150 mg/day in divided doses or as a single dose. **Elderly, Adolescents:** 25 to 50 mg/day (doses above 100 mg not recommended). Maintenance: lowest effective dose once a day continued for at least 2 months after a satisfactory response has been achieved.

NURSING IMPLICATIONS

Tablet may be crushed prior to administration and taken with fluid of patients' choice. Capsule may be emptied and contents swallowed with water or mixed with food.

Full therapeutic effect usually requires at least 2 weeks of therapy.

Careful observation for desired effects is important during early therapy. Drug metabolism may vary as much as 36-fold among users of desipramine, leading to wide differences in dose requirements.

Monitor blood pressure and pulse rate during early phase of therapy particularly in the elderly, debilitated, and cardiovascular patients. If BP falls more than 20 mm Hg or if there is a sudden increase in pulse rate, withhold drug and inform physician.

When desipramine is substituted for a MAO inhibitor, at least 2 weeks should elapse between treatments.

Drowsiness, dizziness, and orthostatic hypotension in patient on long-term, high dosage are signs of impending toxicity. Prepare for ECG study: prolonged QT or QRS intervals substantiate the danger. Report to physician.

Orthostatic hypotension may be controlled if patient moves from recumbent to standing position slowly and in stages. Consult physician about use of support hose.

Observe patient with history of glaucoma. Symptoms that may signal acute attack (severe headache, eye pain, dilated pupils, halos of light, nausea, vomiting) should be reported promptly.

Fine tremors, a distressing extrapyramidal side effect, may be reduced or alleviated by propranolol. Report symptom to physician.

Monitor bowel elimination pattern and intake–output ratio. Severe constipation and urinary retention are potential problems of desipramine treatment especially in the elderly patient, and during long-term high dosage treatment. Consult physician about increasing fluid intake, bulk and fiber in diet, and use of a stool softener.

Caution patient to avoid potentially hazardous activities such as driving until reaction to drug is known.

The effects of barbiturates and other CNS depressants are intensified by desipramine.

The actions of both alcohol and desipramine are potentiated when used together during therapy and for up to 2 weeks after the drug is discontinued. Consult physician about safe amount of alcohol, if any, that can be taken.

If a patient uses excessive amounts of alcohol it should be borne in mind that the potentiation of drug effects may increase the danger of overdosage or suicide attempt.

Smoking–Drug Interaction. Smoking may increase the metabolism of desipramine thereby diminishing its therapeutic action. Advise patient to stop or at least limit smoking.

Suicide is an inherent risk with any depressed patient and may remain until there is significant improvement. Supervise patient closely.

Smoking reduces desipramine antidepressant effects.

Caution patient to avoid prolonged exposure to the sun, until possibility of photosensitivity has been ruled out.

Instruct patient to take medication exactly as ordered: not to change the dose or dose intervals. Tell patient not to give any of it to another person, or use it for treatment of a self-diagnosed problem.

OTC drugs should not be taken unless the physician has approved their use.

Norpramin tablets contain *tartrazine* which may cause allergic-type reactions including bronchial asthma in susceptible individuals. Such individuals are frequently also sensitive to aspirin.

Store drug in tightly closed container at temperature between 15° and 30°C (59° and 86°F), unless otherwise specified by manufacturer.

See Imipramine (prototype psychotropic).

DESLANOSIDE

(Cedilanid-D, Desacety-anatoside C)

(des-lan'oh-side)
Antiarrhythmic
Cardiac glycoside

ACTIONS AND USES. Rapid-acting parenteral digitalis glycoside obtained by alkaline hydrolysis of lanatoside C, a glycoside of *Digitalis lanata.* Shares actions, contraindications, and adverse reactions of digitalis leaf (qv).

Used for rapid digitalizing effect in emergency treatment of congestive heart failure and cardiac arrhythmias such as atrial fibrillation or flutter, and paroxysmal atrial tachycardia, and cardiogenic shock.

ABSORPTION AND FATE. Onset of action within 10 minutes following IV or IM dose. Peak effect in 20 minutes; duration: 2 to 4 hours. Action usually regresses over 16 to 36 hours, but may persist for 2 to 5 days. Approximately 25% protein bound. Half-life: 33 to 36 hours. Approximately 20% excreted daily in urine, primarily as unchanged drug.

CONTRAINDICATIONS AND PRECAUTIONS. Hypersensitivity to digitalis preparations; patients with digitalis toxicity; loading dose to patients who have received a digitalis preparation within previous 2 to 3 weeks; ventricular tachycardia or fibrillation. Severe pulmonary disease, idiopathic hypertrophic subaortic stenosis, in presence of hypokalemia or hypercalcemia. Safe use during pregnancy (category C) not established. *Cautious Use:* elderly patients, acute myocardial infarction, electrical conversion of arrhythmias, incomplete AV block, constrictive pericarditis, hypothyroidism, impaired renal function, nursing mothers.

ADVERSE/SIDE EFFECTS. Anorexia, nausea, vomiting, diarrhea, headache, weakness, fatigue, apathy, visual disturbances, arrhythmias, gynecomastia (uncommon). *See also Digitalis.*

ROUTE AND DOSAGE. Highly individualized. **Intravenous: (preferred route): Adults:** *Loading dose:* 1.6 mg as single injection or divided into two injections and given 4 hours apart. **Intramuscular:** 1.6 mg divided into 0.8 mg portions and injected into each of two sites.

NURSING IMPLICATIONS

Patient must be closely observed during deslanoside therapy with monitoring of ECG, serum electrolytes, and renal function.

Maintenance therapy with an oral digitalis glycoside is preferred and may be instituted within 12 to 24 hours after digitalization with deslanoside.

Deslanoside should be protected from light. Store preferably between 15° and 30°C (59° and 86°F), unless otherwise directed by manufacturer.

See Digitalis (prototype cardiac glycoside).

DESMOPRESSIN ACETATE

(DDAVP, Stimate)

(des-moe-press'in)
Antidiuretic agent
Antienuretic

ACTIONS AND USES. Synthetic analogue of the natural human posterior pituitary (antidiuretic) hormone, arginine vasopressin. Has more specific and longer duration of action than antidiuretic hormone and lower incidence of allergic reactions. Also, oxytoccic and vasopressor actions are not apparent at therapeutic dosages. Unlike vasopressin, it does not stimulate release of adrenocorticotropic hormone nor does it increase plasma cortisol, growth hormone, prolactin, or luteinizing hormone levels. Reduces urine volume and osmolality in patients with central diabetes insipidus by increasing reabsorption of water by kidney collecting tubules. Produces a dose-related increase in factor VIII levels. Not effective in treatment of nephrogenic diabetes insipidus. Tolerance to drug effect rarely develops during prolonged therapy.

Used to control and prevent symptoms and complications of central (neurohypophyseal) diabetes insipidus, and to relieve temporary polyuria and polydipsia associated with trauma or surgery in the pituitary region. *Investigational Use:* to increase factor VIII activity in selected patients with mild to moderate hemophilia A and in some types of von Willebrand's disease, uremia, and to control enuresis.

ABSORPTION AND FATE. Slowly absorbed from nasal mucosa. Onset of antidiuretic effect occurs within 1 hour, peaks in 1 to 5 hours, and persists 8 to 20 hours. Biphasic half-life: 8 and 76 minutes. Drug is excreted in milk, otherwise distribution and metabolic fate unknown.

CONTRAINDICATIONS AND PRECAUTIONS. Hypersensitivity to desmopressin acetate; nephrogenic diabetes insipidus; safe use during pregnancy (category B) and in nursing mothers not established. *Cautious Use:* coronary artery insufficiency, hypertensive cardiovascular disease.

ADVERSE/SIDE EFFECTS. Dose-related: **CNS:** transient headache, drowsiness, listlessness. **ENT:** nasal congestion, rhinitis, nasal irritation. **GI:** nausea, heartburn, mild abdominal cramps. **Other:** vulval pain, shortness of breath, slight rise in blood pressure, flushing.

ROUTE AND DOSAGE. Intranasally: Adults: 0.1 to 0.4 ml daily in a single dose or divided into two or three doses. **Children (3 months to 12 years):** 0.05 to 0.3 ml daily in one or two doses. **Intravenous infusion:** 3 mcg/kg; infuse slowly over 15 to 30 minutes. **Intravenous (direct), subcutaneous:** 0.5 ml (2 mcg) to 1 ml (4 mcg) daily in 2 divided doses.

NURSING IMPLICATIONS

Check expiration date on label.

Initial dose usually administered in the evening and antidiuretic effect observed. Dose is increased each evening until uninterrupted sleep (free of nocturia) is obtained. If daily urine volume is more than 2 L after nocturia is controlled, morning dose is started and adjusted daily until urine volume does not exceed 1.5 to 2 L/24 hours.

Monitor intake and output ratio and pattern (timing). Fluid intake must be carefully controlled particularly in the elderly and in the very young to avoid water retention and sodium depletion. Symptoms suggestive of water intoxication; subtle changes in mental status, confusion, lethargy, neuromuscular excitability.

Weigh patient daily and observe for edema.

Monitor vital signs during dosage regulating period and whenever drug is administered parenterally.

Severe water retention may require reduction in dosage and use of a diuretic such as furosemide.

Therapeutic effectiveness is judged by adequacy of urine volume (control of polyuria and nocturia), relief of polydipsia, increased urine osmolality (concentration).

Report upper respiratory tract infection or nasal congestion. Although manufacturer states that drug effectiveness should not be affected some patients may require increased dosage.

Demonstrate administration technique to patient. Follow manufacturer's instructions to insure delivery of drug high into nasal cavity and not down throat. A flexible calibrated plastic tube (rhingle) is provided.

Nasal solution has an expiration date of 1 year following date of manufacture.

Store desmopressin parenteral solution and nasal spray in refrigerator preferably at 4°C (39.2°F) unless otherwise directed by manufacturer. Discard solutions that are discolored or contain particulate matter.

Drug Interactions: Desmopressin

Plus	Interactions
Alcohol Demeclocycline Epinephrine (large doses) Heparin Lithium carbonate	May decrease antidiuretic response. Used with caution
Carbamazepine (Tegretol) Chlorpropamide Clofibrate (Atromid-S) Fludrocortisone Urea	May potentiate antidiuretic response. Used with caution

DESONIDE

(Tridesilon)

(dess'oh-nide)
Corticosteroid
Glucocorticoid

ACTIONS AND USES. Synthetic nonfluorinated corticosteroid with antiinflammatory, antipruritic, and vasoconstrictive activity.

Used to relieve inflammatory symptoms of a variety of skin disorders responsive to corticosteroids. *See Hydrocortisone for absorption, fate, contraindications, and interactions.*

ADVERSE/SIDE EFFECTS. Dermatologic: burning sensation, pruritus, acneiform eruptions, hypopigmentation, hypertrichosis, folliculitis. With occlusive dressing: maceration of skin, atrophy, striae, secondary infection, miliaria. *See also Hydrocortisone for systemic effects.*

ROUTE AND DOSAGE. Topical: Apply thin layer of cream or ointment (0.05%) two or three times daily.

NURSING IMPLICATIONS

Avoid putting medication in or near eyes.

Before application of topical medication, cleanse skin area, dry thoroughly, then gently rub in a thin layer of the drug.

If signs of systemic absorption, skin irritation or ulceration, hypersensitivity, or infection occurs, patient should notify the physician.

Caution patient to apply medication as scheduled and not to change intervals or amount.

Inform patient not to use the preparation for any other skin disorder, and not to share the topical drug with anyone else.

Bandage or wrap treated area only if prescribed.

Inspect skin for infection, striae, atrophy. If present, patient should stop the drug and notify the physician.

Store drug in cool place, temperature less than 30°C (86°F), and protect from light and heat.

See Hydrocortisone (prototype corticosteroid) for nursing implications of topical medications.

DESOXIMETASONE

(Topicort)

(des-ox-i-met'a-sone)
Corticosteriod
Glucocorticoid

ACTIONS AND USES. Synthetic fluorinated adrenal steroid preparation with antiinflammatory, antipruritic, and vasoconstrictive activity.

Used to relieve inflammatory and pruritic symptoms of a variety of skin disorders responsive to corticosteroids. *See Hydrocortisone for absorption, fate, contraindications, and interactions.*

ADVERSE/SIDE EFFECTS. Dermatologic: pruritus, acneiform eruptions, burning sensation, hypopigmentation, hypertrichosis, folliculitis. With occlusive dressing: maceration of skin, atrophy, striae, secondary infection, miliaria. *See also Hydrocortisone for systemic effects.*

ROUTE AND DOSAGE. Topical: Apply small amount cream (0.25%; 0.05%), gel (0.05%), ointment (0.25%) twice daily.

NURSING IMPLICATIONS

Not for ophthalmic use; avoid putting medication near eyes. Do not apply to vulvovaginal or perianal areas.

Before application of topical medication, cleanse skin area, dry thoroughly, then gently rub in a thin layer of the drug.

If signs of systemic absorption, skin irritation, or ulceration, hypersensitivity, or infection occur, patient should notify physician.

Caution patient to apply medication as scheduled and not to change intervals or amount. Patient should be told not to use the preparation for any other skin disorder, and not to share the topical drug with anyone else.

Bandage or wrap treated area only if prescribed.

Inspect skin for infection, striae, atrophy; if present, patient should stop the drug and notify the physician.

Store drug preferably between 15° to 30°C (59° to 86°F) and protect from light and heat unless otherwise directed by manufacturer.

See Hydrocortisone (prototype corticosteroid)for nursing implications of topical medications.

DESOXYCORTICOSTERONE ACETATE (DOCA)
(Doca Acetate, Percorten Acetate)
DESOXYCORTICOSTERONE PIVALATE
(Percorten Pivalate)

(des-ox-i-kor-ti-koe-ster′one)
Corticosteroid
Mineralocorticoid

ACTIONS AND USES. Potent synthetic steroid. Acts on distal renal tubule to promote sodium reabsorption and hydrogen and potassium excretion. Lacks glucocorticoid (antiinflammatory and immunosuppressant) properties of hydrocortisone (qv). Has no effect on skin pigmentation, allergy, hypoglycemic tendency, circulating eosins or on the ability to excrete excess water or to withstand stress.

Used only in conjunction with other supplementary measures (glucocorticoids, glucose, control of infection, fluid and electrolytes) as partial replacement therapy for adrenocortical insufficiency. Also used for treatment of salt-losing forms of congenital adrenogenital syndrome after restoration of electrolyte balance. Available only in parenteral forms.

ABSORPTION AND FATE. Half-life: 70 minutes. Duration of action: *Injection:* 24 to 48 hours; *Repository form:* 4 to 6 weeks; *Pellet form:* 8 to 12 months, then effects begin to fade. *See also Hydrocortisone.*

CONTRAINDICATIONS AND PRECAUTIONS. Hypersensitivity to desoxycorticosterone; hypertension, cardiac disease, congestive heart failure. Safe use during pregnancy (category C) or lactation not established. *Cautious Use:* Addison's disease, infection. *See also Hydrocortisone.*

ADVERSE/SIDE EFFECTS. Hypersensitivity, hypertension, hypokalemia, edema, headache, arthralgia. *See also Hydrocortisone.*

ROUTE AND DOSAGE. Intramuscular *(pivalate repository):* 25 to 100 mg every 4 weeks; *(acetate in sesame oil):* 2 to 5 mg daily. **Subcutaneous implantation:** one pellet implanted for each 0.5 mg of the daily injected maintenance dose (each pellet contains 125 mg desoxycorticosterone).

D

NURSING IMPLICATIONS

Inject desoxycorticosterone acetate (DOCA) deep into upper outer quadrant of buttock; alternate injection sites. Avoid injecting into deltoid muscle because of high incidence of SC atrophy. A 19-gauge needle will facilitate withdrawal of medication from vial, but a 23-gauge needle is recommended for the injection. Aspirate carefully before injection to avoid inadvertent entry into blood vessel.

Desoxycorticosterone pivalate, the repository form, should be administered no more than once a month. Dose is determined after daily requirement for maintenance has been established with the acetate formulation. Inject into upper outer quadrant of one or both buttocks. A 20-gauge needle is recommended for administration because solution is viscous.

The patient with insufficiency may become hypoglycemic during the dose regulation period if without food more than 4 to 5 hours. Schedule laboratory tests so as to prevent long periods without nourishment.

Infrascapular region is most frequently used area for pellet implant.

Sodium intake may or may not require regulation, depending on individual needs and clinical situation. In general, a high intake of salt accelerates loss of K and retention of Na. Teach the patient that salt intake is a significant regulator of drug efficacy. Signs of edema should be reported immediately.

Alert patient to signs of potassium depletion (hypokalemia) associated with high sodium intake: muscle weakness, paresthesias, circumoral numbness; fatigue, anorexia, nausea, mental depression, polyuria, delirium, diminished reflexes, arrhythmias, cardiac failure, ileus, ECG changes.

Establish baseline and continuing data regarding blood pressure, intake and output ratio and pattern, and weight. Start flow chart as reference for planning individual patient care indicated by drug response. During period of dosage adjustment, blood pressure should be checked every 4 to 6 hours and weight at least every other day.

The patient maintained on pellets should be weighed under standard conditions every other day and keep a record for the physician. Patient should understand the significance of weight changes and other symptoms of overdosage and underdosage.

Signs of overdosage (hypercortisolism): Psychosis, excess weight gain, edema, congestive heart failure, ravenous appetite, severe insomnia, increase in blood pressure.

Signs of insufficient dosage (hypocortisolism): loss of weight, anorexia, nausea, vomiting, diarrhea, muscular weakness, increased fatigue, hypotension.

Implant dosage (highly individualized) is based on the maintenance dosage established during 2 to 3 months with desoxycorticosterone acetate injection.

Signs of insufficient pellet-supplied dosage may begin about 8 months after implant and should be reported promptly to the physician. Daily supplementary injections of desoxycorticosterone may be necessary for the next 4 to 6 weeks until the maintenance dose is reestablished. Reimplant then follows.

Caution the patient with a pellet implant to notify physician if patient anticipates vacationing in a climate warmer than that of home environment or if planning to do heavy physical labor in the heat (both changes may produce salt loss through excess sweating). Dose reevaluation may be necessary.

Intercurrent infection, trauma, or unexpected stress of any kind should be reported promptly by the patient on maintenance therapy. A supplementary rapid-acting corticosteroid before, during, and after the stressful situation may be ordered, as well as other measures such as change in amount of salt intake (tablet or diet).

After the initial period of healing following pellet implant, there should be no soreness or inflammation over implant site; however, if these symptoms are present, consult physician.

Desoxycorticosterone is not withdrawn from a patient undergoing major surgery if he or she has been on long-term therapy, but the surgeon should be aware of the history. Advise the patient to wear or carry medical identification card or jewelry stating drug being used and physician's identity.

Pellets are preserved in tight containers suitable for maintaining sterile contents; injectable forms are preserved in light-resistant containers. Store at 15° to 30° (59° to 86°F). Do not freeze.

See also Hydrocortisone (prototype glucocorticoid/mineralocorticoid) for additional nursing implications and drug interactions.

D

DEXAMETHASONE

(Decadern, Decadron, Decaspray, Deronil, Dexameth, Dexasone, Dexone, Dezone, Hexadrol, Maxidex, SK-Dexamethasone)

(dex-a-meth'a-sone)
Corticosteroid
Glucocorticoid
Antiemetic

DEXAMETHASONE ACETATE

(Dalalone-LA, Decadron-LA, Decaject-LA, Decameth-LA, Dalalone D.P., Dexasone-LA, Dexon LA Dexone LA, LA Dezone, Solurex-LA)

DEXAMETHASONE SODIUM PHOSPHATE

(Dalalone, Decadrol, Decadron Phosphate, Decaject, Decameth, Dexacen-4, Dexasone, Dexon, Dexone, Hexadrol Phosphate, Savacort-D, Solurex, Wexaphos "4")

ACTIONS AND USES. Long-acting synthetic adrenocorticoid with intense antiinflammatory activity and minimal mineralocorticoid properties. May promote potassium and nitrogen loss, and exacerbation of glycosuria in diabetic patient. *See also Hydrocortisone.*

Used as an immunosuppressant, antiinflammatory, and antiemetic agent. *Principal Use:* treatment of bronchial asthma and other bronchospastic states nonresponsive to conventional treatment and to treat life-threatening shock. Also used to treat cerebral edema and to relieve nausea and vomiting caused by cancer chemotherapy. Used as a diagnostic test for Cushing's syndrome, to distinguish adrenal tumor from adrenal hyperplasia, and in the differential diagnosis and clinical management of depression.

ABSORPTION AND FATE. Rapid onset of action after administration. Peak effect: oral, 1 or 2 hours; IM, 8 hours. Duration of effect: oral, 2.75 days; IM, 6 days; intralesional, soft tissue, intraarticular, 1 to 3 weeks. Half-life (plasma): 3 to 4.5 hours; HPA axis suppression: 36 to 54 hours.

CONTRAINDICATIONS AND PRECAUTIONS. Hypersensitivity; systemic fungal infection, acute infections, active or resting tuberculosis, vaccinia, varicella, positive sputum culture of *Candida albicans,* viral diseases. Ophthalmic use: primary open-angle glaucoma, eye infections, superficial ocular herpes simplex, keratitis and tuberculosis of eye. Perforated ear drum (otic use). Safe use during pregnancy (category C) and lactation has not been established. *Cautious Use:* stromal herpes simplex, keratitis, GI ulceration, renal disease, diabetes mellitus, myasthenia gravis, congestive heart failure. *See also Hydrocortisone.*

ADVERSE/SIDE EFFECTS. Aerosol therapy: nasal irritation, dryness, epistaxis, rebound congestion, bronchial asthma, anosomia, perforation of nasal septum, allergic and hypersensitivity reactions. **Systemic use:** slow healing, masked infections, perforation of small and large bowel (patients with inflammatory bowel disease); salt and water retention, GI irritation, hypertension, hypokalemia; perianal burning and itching with rapid IV administration.

See also Hydrocortisone. **Topical use:** burning sensations, itching, irritation, dryness, folliculitis, hypertricosis, acneiform eruptions, hypopigmentation.

ROUTE AND DOSAGE. *Dexamethasone:* (available in dose-pack with enough drug for 7 days) **Oral:** 0.75 to 9 mg daily divided into two to four doses. **Ophthalmic (suspension 1%):** Initial: 1 or 2 drops into conjunctival sac every hour during day and every 2 hours during night; with favorable response dosage is reduced to 1 drop every 3 to 4 hours.

D

Dexamethasone acetate (repository form): **Intramuscular (only):** 8 to 16 mg every 1 to 3 weeks, if necessary. **Intraarticular:** 4 to 16 mg every 1 to 3 weeks if needed. **Intralesional:** 0.8 to 1.6 mg. *Dexamethasone sodium phosphate:* **Intramuscular, intravenous:** 0.5 to 9 mg daily. **Intraarticular, intralesional:** 0.8 to 4 mg depending on size of affected part. **Topical (cream 0.1%):** apply sparingly to affected part 2 or 3 times/day. **Ophthalmic:** apply thin coating in lower conjunctival sac.

Intranasal: Adults: 2 metered sprays into each nostril two or three times daily; maximum 12 sprays. **Children (6 to 12 years):** 1 metered spray into each nostril two times/day; maximum 8 sprays. **Oral inhalation: Adults:** 3 inhalations three or four times/day. **Children:** 2 inhalations three or four times/day. **Ophthalmic:** Ointment 0.05%; solution 0.1%.

NURSING IMPLICATIONS

See manufacturer's instructions for teaching patient how to schedule dose-pack therapy.

Because dexamethasone causes prolonged HPA axis suppression, alternate day therapy (ADT) is not recommended.

As with other corticosteroids, dose changes up or down are made gradually.

Dexamethasone sodium phosphate with lidocaine hydrochloride (Decadron with Xylocaine) combines a local anesthetic with the steroid. (Used by physician for soft tissue injection as for bursitis, synovitis.) Onset of action is rapid and lasts 45 minutes to 1 hour. Steroid activity begins by the time the anesthetic wears off.

Dexamethasone with lidocaine for soft-tissue injection should not be administered intravenously.

Systemic effect of dexamethasone may follow topical, intralesional, or intraarticular use, particularly with long-term use and high dosage.

Effects of local injections persist about 24 hours. Injections may be repeated from once every 3 days to once every 3 weeks.

Diuresis may follow transfer from another steroid preparation to dexamethasone.

Since dexamethasone has minimal sodium- and water-retaining activity, symptom development of overadministration may be quite subtle.

Nonoperative cases of cerebral edema may be responsive to continuous therapy with dexamethazone to remain free of symptoms of increased intracranial pressure.

Ophthalmic preparations: Warn patient to consult physician promptly and to interrupt treatment with ophthalmic preparation if changes in visual acuity or diminished visual fields occur. Frequent measurement of intraocular pressure, slit-lamp microscopy, and examination of optic nerve head should accompany long-term therapy with ophthalmic formulation. An eye pad may be prescribed with ointment use to enhance effect of drug on corneal surface.

Wash hands thoroughly before and after treatments.

Observe eyelids and eye surfaces being treated with solution or ointment. If irritation develops, stop the treatment and consult physician.

See Index: Drug administration: eye drops.

Ophthalmic solution may also be instilled into the clean aural canal for treatment of inflammatory conditions. Consult physician regarding preparation of aural canal before instillation of medication. If gauze wick is used, it should be kept moist with medication while in place and removed after 12 to 24 hours.

Aerosol preparations: The order should be specific as to number of sprays for each nostril, for each administration.

If inhalant bronchodilator is used concurrently, it is usually administered a few minutes before dexamethasone to maximize penetration.

Rinse mouth with warm water after each inhalation treatment to prevent excessive drying of oral and pharyngeal membranes (prevent cough, hoarseness, sore throat) and to prevent development of superinfections (white patches, sore oral membranes and tongue).

To administer topical spray to skin, hold aerosol container upright approximately 6 inches from area being treated. Shake well before spraying. Usual dosage regimen: spray each 4-inch square of affected area for 1 to 2 seconds, two or three times daily.

If spray is to be applied about the face, the eyes should be protected, and spray should not be inhaled. If eyes are accidentally exposed to the aerosol, flush thoroughly and promptly with water and contact physician at once.

Dexamethasone is discontinued gradually to avoid consequences of hypocortisolism. Continuous supervision of patient after corticosteroid is stopped is necessary because there may be sudden reappearance of severe symptoms of the disease for which patient is being treated.

If the patient is being withdrawn from systemic corticosteroid to aerosol treatment, watch for symptoms of withdrawal (lassitude, depression, joint, muscle pain, hypoglycemia, hypotension, fever).

The dexamethasone dose regimen may need to be altered if patient is subjected to stress: e.g., surgery, infections, emotional stress, illness, acute bronchial attacks, trauma. It may also be indicated if there are extreme changes in patient's environment (stress on thermoregulation).

Consult physician if change in living or working environment is anticipated.

The neonate born to a mother who has been receiving a corticosteroid during pregnancy should be monitored for symptoms of hypocortisolism.

Dexamethasone Suppression Test:

- A baseline 24-hour urine specimen for 17-ketosteroids should be collected before the suppression test.
- 1.0 mg dexamethasone is administered orally between 11 PM and midnight; serum concentration of cortisol is measured at 8 AM the following morning. In the normal individual, the medication should depress the HPA axis and plasma 17-OHCS to less than 5 mcg/dl. When used to diagnosis depression, nonsuppression indicates HPA axis dysfunction and it occurs in a significant proportion of patients with psychiatric disorders, particularly those with affective disorders.

Caution patient on prolonged therapy not to self medicate with OTC medications unless the physician has approved.

Inform new physician or dentist that a corticosteroid drug is being used.

Patient should carry or wear medical identification card or jewelry with diagnosis, physician's name and telephone number, and drug being used.

Patient-Teaching Points:

- ✓ Remind patient that corticosteroid therapy is not curative but preventive.
- ✓ The prescribed regimen should be strictly adhered to, i.e., dose intervals should not be increased, decreased, interrupted or discontinued.
- ✓ Instruct patient about symptoms of hypocortisolism and hypercortisolism.
- ✓ Urge patient to report exacerbation of symptoms and onset of side effects promptly.

✓ Emphasize the implications of immunosuppression with regard to prevention of exposure to infection, trauma, and to sudden changes in environmental factors.

Repository acetate (for IM or local injection only) is a white suspension that settles on standing; mild shaking will resuspend the drug. Protect from heat.

Do not store or expose aerosol to temperature above 120°F; do not puncture or discard into a fire or an incinerator.

Stored at temperature between 15° and 30°C (59° and 86°F), unless otherwise directed by manufacturer.

See Hydrocortisone (prototype glucocorticoid) for additional Nursing Implications and Drug Interactions.

DEXCHLORPHENIRAMINE MALEATE

(Dexchlor, Poladex T.D., Polaramine)

(dex-klor-fen-eer'a meen)
Antihistamine
H_1-receptor antagonist

ACTIONS AND USES. Alkylamine antihistamine, derived from chlorpheniramine (qv) with which it shares actions, uses, contraindications, precautions, and adverse reactions. In common with other antihistamines also has anticholinergic properties and produces mild-to-moderate sedative effects.

Used in treatment of perennial and seasonal allergic rhinitis, other manifestations of allergy, and in vasomotor rhinitis. Also used as adjunct to epinephrine in treatment of anaphylactic reactions. Commercially available in combination with pseudoephedrine and guaifenesin (e.g., Polaramine Expectorant).

ABSORPTION AND FATE. Well absorbed from GI tract. Acts within 15 to 30 minutes. Effects peak in about 3 hours and persist 3 to 6 hours. Extensively metabolized, primarily by liver. Excreted in urine within 24 hours as inactive metabolites; negligible amounts eliminated unchanged. Small quantities appear in breast milk.

CONTRAINDICATIONS AND PRECAUTIONS. Hypersensitivity to antihistamines of similar class; acute asthmatic attack, lower respiratory tract symptoms, in patients receiving MAO inhibitors, newborns, premature infants, nursing mothers. Safe use during pregnancy not established. *Cautious Use:* increased intraocular pressure, prostatic hypertrophy, hyperthyroidism, renal and cardiovascular disease, elderly patients. *See Chlorpheniramine maleate.*

ADVERSE/SIDE EFFECTS. CNS: drowsiness, dizziness, weakness, tinnitus. **GI:** nausea, vomiting, anorexia, constipation, diarrhea. **GU:** difficulty in urinating, urinary retention, urinary frequency. **Other:** dry mouth, blurred vision, skin eruptions, photosensitivity. *See also Chlorpheniramine maleate.*

ROUTE AND DOSAGE. Oral: Adults and children (12 years and over): to 2 mg three or four times daily at 4- to 6-hour intervals; 4- to 6-mg or timed-release tablets every 8 to 10 hours as needed. **Children (under 12 years):** 0.15 mg/kg daily, divided into four doses. Timed-release tablet not recommended for use in children younger than 6 years.

NURSING IMPLICATIONS

Advise patient to take medication with food, water, or milk to lessen GI distress.

Instruct patient to swallow timed-release tablet whole. It should not be broken, crushed, or chewed. Regular tablet may be crushed and taken with fluid or mixed with food.

Because of the possibility of drowsiness, dizziness, and blurred vision, caution patient to avoid driving and other potentially hazardous activities until reaction to drug is known.

Advise patient to ask physician about the use of alcohol, tranquilizers, sedatives, or other CNS depressants because the effects of dexchlorpheniramine will be additive.
Dry mouth may be relieved by frequent rinses with water, increasing non-caloric fluid intake if it is low, or by sugarless gum or lemon drops.
Dexchlorpheniramine should be discontinued about 4 days before skin tests for allergies since test results may be inaccurate.
Stored preferably between 15° and 30°C (59° and 86°F), unless otherwise directed by manufacturer.
See Chlorpheniramine (prototype alkylamine antihistamine).

D

DEXPANTHENOL

(Ilopan, Panol, Panthoderm)

(dex-pan'the-nole)
Cholinergic (parasympathomimetic)
Vitamin B complex

ACTIONS AND USES. Alcohol analogue of the coenzyme vitamin, pantothenic acid, to which it is readily converted. A member of the B-complex group and precursor of coenzyme A, which is essential to normal epithelial function and biosynthesis of fatty acids, amino acids, and acetylcholine. Increases GI peristalsis and intestinal tone by stimulating acetylation of choline to acetylcholine. Topical application reportedly relieves itching and may aid healing of skin lesions by stimulating epithelialization and granulation. Also has antibacterial activity.

Used in prevention or treatment of postoperative abdominal distention, intestinal atony, and paralytic ileus. Used topically to relieve itching and to promote healing in minor skin lesions. Commercially available in combination with choline bitartrate (e.g., Ilopan-Choline).

ABSORPTION AND FATE. Well absorbed; very little is metabolized in body. Excreted as pantothenic acid, mostly in urine; small amounts excreted in feces and breast milk.

CONTRAINDICATIONS AND PRECAUTIONS. Hemophilia, ileus due to mechanical obstruction. Safe use during pregnancy (category C) and in children not established. *Cautious Use:* nursing mothers.

ADVERSE/SIDE EFFECTS. Generally well tolerated. Rare: allergic manifestations, hyperperistalsis, diarrhea, prolonged bleeding time.

ROUTE AND DOSAGE. Adults: Intramuscular: 250 to 500 mg repeated in 2 hours, then at 4- to 6-hour intervals, if necessary. **Intravenous:** 500 mg mixed with IV infusion solutions such as glucose or lactated Ringer's and administered by slow infusion. **Children:** 11 to 12.5 mg/kg (same schedule as for adults). **Topical (2% cream):** applied directly to affected area once or twice daily, or more often as needed.

NURSING IMPLICATIONS

Observe for and report bleeding tendency. Dexpanthenol may prolong bleeding time in some patients.
Report immediately any evidence of allergic reaction; drug should be discontinued.
Therapeutic results may not be obtained in patients with hypokalemia.
Observe for relief of abdominal distention. Keep physician informed concerning (1) passage of flatus or stool (character and amount); (2) bowel sounds (present? absent? frequency?

pitch?); (3) presence of pain or discomfort; (4) abdomen hard? soft?; (5) intake and output ratio and pattern.
Physician may prescribe insertion of rectal tube and also measurements of abdominal girth.
Manufacturer recommends waiting for 12 hours after neostigmine or other enterokinetic drugs and 1 hour after succinylcholine before starting dexpanthenol.
Store at room temperature preferably between 15° and 30°C (59° and 86°F); protect from freezing and excessive heat.

Drug Interactions. Concomitant use of dexpanthenol with **antibiotics, narcotics,** and **barbiturates** have caused allergic reactions in some patients (mechanism unknown).

DEXTRAN 40

(Gentran 40, 10% LMD, Rheomacrodex)

(dex'tran)
Replacement solution
Plasma volume expander

ACTIONS AND USES. Low molecular weight polysaccharide formed by the action of *Leuconostoc mesenteroides* on sucrose. Average molecular weight is approximately 40,000 (range 10,000 to 90,000). As a hypertonic colloidal solution, produces immediate and short-lived expansion of plasma volume by increasing colloidal osmotic pressure and drawing fluid from interstitial to intravascular spaces. Cardiovascular response to volume expansion includes increased blood pressure, pulse pressure, central venous pressure, cardiac output, venous return to heart, and urinary output. In addition to plasma volume expansion, it improves microcirculation, possibly by decreasing blood viscosity (lower hematocrit) and by retarding RBC sludging that may accompany shock. Reduces possibility of deep venous thrombosis and pulmonary embolism primarily by inhibiting venous stasis and platelet adhesiveness. Lower incidence of allergic reactions than with higher molecular weight products.

Used adjunctively to expand plasma volume in shock or impending shock caused by hemorrhage, burns, surgery, or other trauma. Also used in prophylaxis and therapy of venous thrombosis and pulmonary embolism. Used as priming fluid or as additive to other primers during extracorporeal circulation.

ABSORPTION AND FATE. Produces rapid expansion of plasma volume, generally 1 to 2 times the volume of dextran 40 infused, within minutes after end of infusion; gradually reverses over succeeding 12 hours, depending on renal clearance rate. About 75% is excreted in urine within 24 hours. Dextran molecules of higher molecular weights (50,000 or greater) are degraded to glucose and metabolized to carbon dioxide and water over a period of a few weeks. Small amounts are also excreted in GI tract and eliminated in feces.

CONTRAINDICATIONS AND PRECAUTIONS. Hypersensitivity to dextran, renal failure, hypervolemic conditions, severe congestive heart failure, thrombocytopenia, significant anemia, hypofibrinogenemia or other marked hemostatic defects including those caused by drugs, e.g., heparin, warfarin. Safe use during pregnancy and in women of child-bearing age not established. *Cautious Use:* active hemorrhage, severe dehydration, chronic liver disease, impaired renal function, patients susceptible to pulmonary edema or congestive heart failure.

ADVERSE/SIDE EFFECTS. Hypersensitivity: mild to generalized urticaria, pruritus, angioedema, nasal congestion, wheezing, tightness in chest, nausea, vomiting, fever, arthralgia, anaphylactic shock: flushing, angioneurotic edema, bronchospasm, hypotension, chills, fever, respiratory and cardiac arrest. Renal tubule vacuolization (osmotic nephrosis), stasis, and blocking; renal failure; increased SGOT (AST) and SGPT (ALT) (specific connection with dextran not established). **With high doses:** prolonged bleeding and coagulation times; decreased hematocrit and plasma protein levels, pulmonary edema.

ROUTE AND DOSAGE. Available as 10% dextran 40 in 5% dextrose or in 0.9% sodium chloride. **Intravenous infusion:** *Adjunctive therapy for shock:* total dosage during first 24 hours should not exceed 20 ml/kg body weight. First 500 ml may be administered rapidly (over 15 to 30 minutes), with central venous pressure monitoring. Repeated doses given more slowly. Succeeding doses for maximum of 4 additional days should not exceed 10 mg/kg/day. *Prophylaxis for thromboembolic complications:* 500 to 1000 ml (approximately 10 ml/kg) on day of operation. Continue 500 ml daily for additional 2 to 3 days. If necessary, 500 ml every second or third day during risk period for up to 2 weeks. *Priming fluid for extracorporeal circulation* (dosage varies with volume of pump oxygenator): generally 10 to 20 ml/kg added to perfusion circuit.

NURSING IMPLICATIONS

Not to be confused with dextran 70 or other dextrans.

Use only if seal is intact, vacuum is detectable, and solution is absolutely clear.

When stored for long periods, dextran flakes may form. To dissolve flakes, place unopened bottle in warm water bath until solution clears.

Baseline hematocrit should be taken prior to initiation of dextran and after administration (dextran usually lowers hematocrit). Notify physician if hematocrit is depressed below 30% by volume.

If blood is to be administered, a cross-match specimen should be drawn prior to dextran infusion *(see Diagnostic Test Interferences).*

Specific flow rate should be prescribed by physician.

A small percentage of individuals who have never received dextran develop an allergic reaction having been sensitized by dextrans present in commercial sugars and dextran-producing organisms found in human GI tract.

Hypersensitivity reaction is most likely to occur during the first few minutes of administration. Monitor vital signs and observe patient closely for at least the first 30 minutes of infusion. Therapy should be terminated at the first sign of a reaction. Other means of sustaining circulation should be immediately available. Have on hand resuscitative equipment, epinephrine, ephedrine, steroids, and antihistamines.

Monitoring of central venous pressure is advised as an estimate of blood volume status and as a guide for determining dosage. *Normal CVP:* 5 to 10 cm H_2O.

Observe patient for clinical signs of circulatory overload (shortness of breath, wheezing, coughing, marked increase in pulse and respiratory rate, sensation of chest pressure).

In patients for whom sodium restriction is indicated, it should be noted that 500 ml of dextran 40 in 0.9% normal saline contains 77 mEq of both sodium and chloride.

For patients in shock, monitor pulse, blood pressure, and urine output every 5 to 15 minutes for the first hour and hourly thereafter or more frequently as indicated. Report oliguria, anuria, or lack of improvement in urinary output (dextran usually causes an increase in urinary output).

Dextran should be discontinued at the first indication of renal dysfunction.

Monitor intake–output ratio and check *urine specific gravity* at regular intervals *(normal: 1.005 to 1.025).* Renal excretion of dextran produces minor elevations of urine viscosity and specific gravity in patients with adequate urine flow, but marked elevations occur in patients with diminished urine flow. Low urine specific gravity may signify failure of renal dextran clearance and is an indication for discontinuing therapy.

State of hydration is assessed by intake–output ratio and by determinations of urine and serum osmolarity.

In poorly hydrated patients dextran may attract water from extravascular spaces and cause dehydration (elevated temperature, dry skin and mucous membranes; dry, furrowed tongue; scant urinary output, urine specific gravity above 1.030, elevated Hgb). Renal damage can occur from precipitation of dextran in renal tubules.

Transient prolongation of bleeding time and interference with normal blood coagulation may occur when high doses are administered. Patients who have had major surgery or trauma are particularly susceptible to increased blood loss.

Hepatitis virus is not transmitted by dextran.

Dextran should be stored at a constant temperature, preferably 25°C (77°F). It has a tendency to crystallize when subjected to temperature variations or when stored for prolonged periods at elevated temperatures. Once opened, unused portion should be discarded because dextran contains no preservative.

Diagnostic Test Interferences. When blood samples are drawn for study, notify laboratory that patient has received dextran. Dextran may cause false increases in **blood glucose** values (ortho-toluidine methods or determinations employing sulfuric or acetic acid hydrolysis), and false increases in **urinary protein** determinations (utilizing Lowry method), **bilirubin** assays (when alcohol is used), and **total protein** assays (using biuret reagent). May interfere with **Rh testing, blood typing** and **cross-matching** procedures (by inducing rouleaux formation) when proteolytic enzyme techniques are used (saline agglutination and indirect antiglobulin methods reportedly not affected).

DEXTRAN 70
(Macrodex)
DEXTRAN 75
(Gentran 75)

(dex'tran)
Replacement solution
Plasma volume expander

ACTIONS AND USES. High molecular weight polysaccharides. Dextran 70 has an average molecular weight of 70,000; that of dextran 75 is 75,000 (molecular weight range for both: 20,000 to 200,000). Colloidal properties approximate those of serum albumin. Differs from dextran 40 in molecular weight, and in having less effect on rouleaux formation and sludging of red blood cells and higher incidence of severe allergic reactions.

Used primarily for emergency treatment of hypovolemic shock or impending shock caused by hemorrhage, burns, surgery, or other trauma. Intended for emergency treatment only when whole blood or blood products are not available or when haste precludes cross-matching of blood. *Investigational Use:* nephrosis, toxemia of pregnancy, and prophylaxis of deep-vein thrombosis. Dextran 75 is commercially available in 10% invert sugar–fructose/dextrose (Gentran 75 and 10% Travert).

ABSORPTION AND FATE. Produces plasma volume expansion slightly in excess of volume infused, approximately 1 hour after infusion; decreases over succeeding 24 hours, depending on renal clearance rate. Dextran molecules with molecular weights less than 50,000 are excreted by kidneys (approximately 40% of dose within 24 hours in patients with normal renal function). Molecules with molecular weights of 50,000 or greater are slowly degraded to dextrose and eliminated as carbon dioxide and water.

CONTRAINDICATIONS AND PRECAUTIONS. Known hypersensitivity to dextran, severe bleeding disorders, severe congestive failure, renal failure. *See Dextran 40.*

ADVERSE/SIDE EFFECTS. Allergic reactions, severe and fatal anaphylactoid reaction, lowered plasma protein levels (high doses). *See also Dextran 40.*

ROUTE AND DOSAGE. **Intravenous infusion:** 500 ml. Total daily dosage should not exceed 20 ml/kg body weight during first 24 hours. If therapy continues beyond 24 hours, total daily dosage should not exceed 10 ml/kg body weight.

NURSING IMPLICATIONS

Do not interchange with Dextran 40.

Use only if seal is intact, vacuum is detectable, and solution is absolutely clear.

Specific flow rate should be prescribed by physician. (For emergency treatment of shock, rate of administration for first 500 ml may be 20 to 40 ml/minute. In normovolemic patients flow rate should not exceed 4 ml/minute.)

Bleeding time may be temporarily prolonged in patients receiving more than 1000 ml of dextran 70 or 75.

Patient should be observed closely for symptoms of anaphylaxis especially during first 30 minutes of infusion. Severe reactions occasionally have resulted in fatalities.

Monitor intake and output.

Store at a constant temperature preferably at 25°C (77°F)

See Dextran 40.

DEXTRANOMER

(dex-tran'oh-mer)

(Debrisan)

Debriding agent

ACTIONS AND USES. Consists of small, spherical, dry, hydrophilic beads of a dextran polymer which when applied to secreting wound surface absorbs exudate and tissue debris. Also effective in removing bacteria and protein particularly fibrin/fibrinogen degradation products. Shortens healing time by retarding scab formation and by reducing inflammation and edema. Each gram of dextranomer absorbs about 4 ml of exudate. Dextranomer beads are made up of cross-linked dextran arranged in a 3-dimensional network large enough to allow low molecular weight substances (e.g., exudates) to be absorbed readily into beads; high molecular weight substances (such as plasma proteins, fibrinogen) remain in bead interspaces. Not effective for cleansing nonsecreting wounds. Systemic absorption does not occur; drug appears to have low sensitizing potential.

Used to cleanse exudating wounds such as venous stasis ulcers; decubitus ulcers; infected burns; and infected, traumatic and surgical wounds.

ADVERSE/SIDE EFFECTS. Reportedly well-tolerated. Erythema, pain, irritation, bleeding, blistering, usually associated with dressing changes.

ROUTE AND DOSAGE. **Topical:** Apply to affected area once or twice a day. For profusely draining wounds, more frequent changes may be required.

NURSING IMPLICATIONS

Content of container should be reserved for use in a single patient, to avoid possibility of cross contamination.

Before application, cleanse wound with sterile water, saline, or other cleansing agent prescribed by physician (hydrogen peroxide or povidone-iodine has been used). Leave wound surface moist. Ask physician if petroleum jelly can be applied to wound margin as a protectant, if indicated. Pour dextranomer into wound to depth of 3 mm (⅛ to ¼ inch). Cover with sterile gauze pad and tape in place (without occlusion) so as to contain medication but loose enough to allow for expansion of beads.

Do not use occlusive dressings because maceration of tissue surrounding wound may result.

For reapplication, beads should be removed before becoming fully saturated and dried out, to prevent difficult removal from wound surface. When saturated, beads appear grayish-yellow.

Beads can be removed by irrigating with sterile water, saline, or other cleansing solution. Removal should be as complete as possible. Soaking or whirlpool may be required to remove stubborn patches of beads.

For wounds in hard-to-reach body areas, a freshly-prepared paste of 4 parts dextranomer and 1 part sterile glycerine may be easier to apply. Consult physician.

Reduction of wound edema, which occurs during first few days of therapy, may make wound appear larger.

Dextranomer should be discontinued when wound is no longer draining and healthy granulation tissue is established.

Avoid contact with eyes.

If beads fall to floor, surface will be dangerously slippery. Thorough cleaning and drying of floor is essential.

Store in well-closed container in a dry place at a constant temperature, preferably 25°C (77°F) unless otherwise directed by manufacturer.

DEXTROAMPHETAMINE SULFATE

(dex-troe-am-fet′a-meen)

(Dexampex, Dexedrine, Ferndex, Oxydess, Spancap No. 1 and No. 4, Tidex)

Central stimulant, (sympathomimetic)
Anorexigenic agent
Amphetamine
C II

ACTIONS AND USES. Dextrorotatory isomer of amphetamine (qv), with which it shares actions, uses, contraindications, precautions, and adverse reactions. On a weight basis, has less pronounced action on cardiovascular and peripheral nervous systems and is a more potent appetite suppressant. CNS stimulating effect approximately twice that of racemic amphetamine.

Used as adjunct in short-term treatment of exogenous obesity, narcolepsy, and attention deficit disorder in children. Also used as adjunct in epilepsy to control ataxia and drowsiness induced by barbiturates, and to combat sedative effects of trimethadione in absence seizures. Commercially available in combination with amphetamine (e.g., Amphaplex, Biphetamine).

CONTRAINDICATIONS AND PRECAUTIONS. Hypersensitivity to sympathomimetic amines, glaucoma, agitated states, psychoses (especially in children), advanced arteriosclerosis, symptomatic heart disease, moderate to severe hypertension, hyperthroidism, history of drug abuse, during or within 14 days of MAO inhibitor therapy, use as anorexiant in children under 12 years, use for attention deficit disorder in children under 3 years. *See also Amphetamine.*

ADVERSE/SIDE EFFECTS. Allergic: rash, urticaria. **CNS:** nervousness, restlessness, hyperactivity, insomnia, euphoria, dizziness, headache; with prolonged use: severe depression, psychotic reactions. **CV:** palpitation, tachycardia, chest pains, elevated blood pressure. **GI:** dry mouth, unpleasant taste, anorexia, weight loss, diarrhea, constipation, abdominal cramps. **Other:** impotence, changes in libido, unusual fatigue; marked dystonia of head, neck, extremities; sweating. *See also Amphetamine.*

ROUTE AND DOSAGE. Oral: *Narcolepsy:* **Adults:** 5 to 20 mg one to three times daily at 4 to 6 hour intervals. **Children (12 years and over):** 10 mg daily, increased by 10 mg at weekly intervals, if necessary; **Children (6 to 12 years):** Initial: 5 mg daily, increased by 5 mg at weekly intervals, if necessary. *Attention deficit disorders:* **Children (6 years and older):** Initial: 5 mg one or two times daily, increased by 5 mg at weekly intervals, if necessary; **Children (3 to 5 years):** Initial: 2.5 mg daily, increased by 2.5 mg at weekly intervals, if necessary. *Anorexiant:* **Adults:** 5 to 10 mg, one to three times daily or sustained release form 10 to 15 mg once daily.

D

NURSING IMPLICATIONS

Administered 30 to 60 minutes before meals for treatment of obesity. Long-acting form is administered in the morning.

To avoid insomnia, administer last dose no later than 6 hours before patient retires (10 to 14 hours before bedtime for sustained-release form).

Instruct patient to swallow sustained-release capsule whole with a liquid and not to chew or crush it.

Dexedrine contains tartrazine which can cause allergic type reactions including bronchial asthma in susceptible individuals. Frequently such persons are also hypersensitive to aspirin.

Inform patient that drug may impair ability to drive or perform other potentially hazardous activities.

Because effect of prolonged use in children is not known, and because dextroamphetamine may depress growth by causing loss of appetite, growth rate should be closely monitored.

Periodic interruption of therapy or reduction in dosage is recommended to assess effectiveness of therapy in behavior disorders.

Tolerance to anorexiant effects may develop after a few weeks; however, tolerance does not appear to develop when used in treatment of narcolepsy.

Discontinuation of drug following prolonged use should be accomplished gradually to avoid extreme fatigue and mental depression that follows abrupt withdrawal.

Classified as Schedule II drug under Federal Controlled Substances Act. Has high abuse potential in common with other amphetamines.

Store in well-closed containers preferably between 15° and 30°C (59° and 86°F), unless otherwise directed by manufacturer.

See Amphetamine Sulphate (prototype amphetamine).

Diagnostic Test Interferences. Dextroamphetamine may cause significant elevation of plasma **corticosteroids** (evening levels are highest) and increases in **urinary epinephrine** excretion (during first 3 hours after drug administration).

DEXTROMETHORPHAN HYDROBROMIDE

(dex-troe-meth-or'fan)
Antitussive

(Balminil D.M. Syrup, Congespirin, Delsym, D.M. Syrup, Hold, Koffex Syrup, Robidex, Romilar CF, Romilar Children's Cough Syrup, Sedatuss, Sucrets, and others)

ACTIONS AND USES. Nonnarcotic derivative of levorphanol. Chemically related to morphine, but without its hypnotic or analgesic effect, or capacity to cause tolerance or addiction. Controls cough spasms by depressing cough center in medulla. Does not depress respiration or inhibit ciliary action. Antitussive activity comparable to that of codeine but is less likely than codeine to cause constipation, drowsiness or GI disturbances.

Used for temporary relief of cough spasms in nonproductive coughs due to colds, pertussis, and influenza. A common ingredient in many OTC cough mixtures.

ABSORPTION AND FATE. Antitussive action begins in 15 to 30 minutes and lasts 3 to 6 hours.

CONTRAINDICATIONS AND PRECAUTIONS. Sensitivity, children under 2 years of age, during or within 14 days of MAO inhibitor therapy. *Cautious Use:* productive cough, asthma.

ADVERSE/SIDE EFFECTS. Rare: dizziness, drowsiness, GI upset; CNS depression with very large doses.

ROUTE AND DOSAGE. Oral: Adults: 10 to 20 mg every 4 hours or 30 mg every 6 to 8 hours. **Children (6 to 12 years):** 5 to 10 mg every 4 hours or 15 mg every 6 to 8 hours; **Children (2 to 6 years):** 2.5 to 5 mg every 4 hours or 7.5 mg every 6 to 8 hours. *Controlled-release suspension:* (30 mg dextromethorphan 5 ml). **Adults:** 60 mg twice daily; **Children (6 to 12 years):** 30 mg twice daily; **(2 to 6 years):** 15 mg twice daily.

NURSING IMPLICATIONS

Although soothing local effect of the syrup may be enhanced if administered undiluted, depression of cough center depends upon systemic absorption of drug. Increasing fluid intake may help to liquefy tenacious mucus.

Excessive, nonproductive cough tends to be self-perpetuating because it causes irritation of pharyngeal and tracheal mucosa.

Unnecessary cough may be lessened by voluntary restraint and by avoiding irritants such as smoking, dust, fumes, and other air pollutants. Humidification of ambient air may provide some relief.

Locally acting sialogogues (e.g., sugarless hard candy) may help to relieve cough produced by irritation of pharyngeal mucosa.

Treatment is directed toward decreasing the frequency and intensity of cough without completely eliminating protective cough reflex.

Dextromethorphan may be purchased over the counter. Persons who self-medicate should be advised that symptom suppression does not mean cure of the underlying problem. Any cough persisting longer than 1 week or 10 days should be medically diagnosed.

See Benzonatate for patient-teaching points about cough.

Drug Interactions. Concurrent administration of dextromethorphan and **MAO inhibitors** has resulted in nausea, coma, hypotension, hyperpyrexia, and death.

DEXTROTHYROXINE SODIUM

(dex-troe-thye-rox'een)

(Choloxin)

Antilipemic agent

ACTIONS AND USES. Sodium salt of dextrorotatory isomer of thyroxine. Reduces serum cholesterol and LDL levels in hyperlipidemia; triglycerides, and beta lipoproteins may also be lowered from previously elevated levels. By an unclear mechanism, liver is stimulated to increase catabolism and excretion of cholesterol and its degradation products via the biliary route into feces. Greatest decrease in serum cholesterol occurs in patients with highest baseline concentrations, with maximum therapeutic effects in 1 or 2 months. Cholesterol synthesis is increased, but metabolic end products do not accumulate in the blood. It has not been determined whether drug-induced lowering of serum cholesterol or other lipids has beneficial, detrimental, or no effects on morbidity or mortality due to atherosclerosis or coronary heart disease.

Used as adjunct to diet and other measures to lower elevated serum cholesterol and LDL concentrations in the treatment of primary type II hyperlipoproteinemia, particularly type IIa, in euthyroid patients with no known evidence of cardiac disease.

ABSORPTION AND FATE. Absorbed from GI tract. Loosely bound to plasma proteins; metabolized in liver. Rapidly excreted in urine and feces in approximately equal amounts as intact drug and metabolites. Small amounts excreted in breast milk.

CONTRAINDICATIONS AND PRECAUTIONS. In euthyroids: known organic heart disease including angina pectoris, arrhythmias, decompensated or borderline compensated cardiac states; history of myocardial infarction or congestive heart failure; rheumatic heart disease, hypertension, advanced liver or kidney disease; history of iodism; pregnancy, nursing mothers; at least 2 weeks prior to elective surgery. *Cautious Use:* hypothyroid patients with concomitant coronary artery disease; women of childbearing age with familial hypercholesterolemia; diabetes mellitus; liver and kidney impairment; children.

ADVERSE/SIDE EFFECTS. Low incidence in euthyroid patients without cardiac disease; higher in hypothyroid patients, especially if organic heart disease is present. **CV:** angina pectoris, cardiac arrhythmia, ECG evidence of ischemic myocardial changes, increase in heart size; myocardial infarction (relationship to drug effect not known). **Iodism:** acneiform rash, pruritus, coryza, conjunctivitis, stomatitis, brassy taste, laryngitis, bronchitis. **Signs of hypermetabolism:** nervousness, weakness, insomnia, tremors, twitching, intolerance to heat, hyperpyrexia, flushing, sweating, palpitation, tachycardia, weight loss, altered taste sensation, anorexia, nausea, vomiting, diarrhea, constipation, menstrual irregularities, exophthalmos. **Other:** dizziness, tinnitus, vertigo, ptosis, malaise, fatigue, headache, hoarseness, visual disturbances, changes in libido, hair loss, psychic changes, paresthesias, muscle pain, gallstones and cholestatic jaundice (casual relationship not established); diuresis, peripheral edema; worsening of peripheral vascular disease and retinopathy.

ROUTE AND DOSAGE. Oral: Adult: *(euthyroid hypercholesterolemia):* Initial: 1 to 2 mg/day increased by 1 or 2 mg increments at intervals of not less than 1 month. Maintenance: 4 to 8 mg/day. **Pediatric:** *(hypercholesterolemia):* initial: 0.05 mg/kg/day increased by 0.05 mg/kg increments at monthly intervals to maximum level of 4 mg daily, if necessary.

NURSING IMPLICATIONS

Goal of therapy in hyperlipoproteinemia is to prevent further atherosclerosis, not merely to lower serum lipids. Encourage patient to adhere to diet regimen, an important adjunct to therapeutic plan.

Before initiation of therapy, a complete health history (personal, family, dietary) as well as physical examination and appropriate laboratory studies should be obtained.

D

Since hyperlipoproteinemia is frequently genetically determined, family members of patient, especially children 5 years and older, should be screened for abnormal lipid values to permit early treatment if indicated.

Serum lipids should be determined initially and evaluated at monthly intervals during therapy. Patient should be on a normal diet for several days prior to the test.

Cholesterol and triglyceride values are age-related: *average normal total cholesterol is 150 to 250 mg/dl; triglycerides, 30 to 190 mg/dl.*

Initial decrease in cholesterol levels may not occur until 2 weeks to 1 month after initiation of therapy. Maximum decrease usually occurs during second or third month of therapy.

Elevation of serum protein-bound iodine (PBI) levels in patients receiving dextrothyroxine is evidence of drug absorption and transport rather than hypermetabolism. A *PBI range* of 10 to 25 mcg/dl in treated patients is common *(normal: 4 to 8 mcg/dl).*

Use of drugs having thyroid hormone activity for treatment of obesity is not advised.

Patients with diabetes should be closely monitored. Dosage adjustment of insulin or oral antidiabetic agent may be required on initiation and on withdrawal of dextrothyroxine. Advise patient to report diminishing control of diabetes (glycosuria, hyperglycemic episode, polydipsia, diuresis).

Patients with cardiac disease should be observed closely in early therapy and seen at frequent intervals throughout the treatment period.

During period of coordination between dose regimens of digitalis and dextrothyroxine, carefully monitor effects of both drugs.

No more than 4 mg/day dextrothyroxine should be given to a patient already receiving digitalis because of danger of excess stimulation of myocardium (potentiation of digitalis effect).

Report immediately new signs and symptoms of cardiac disease or increased decompensation in the borderline compensated patient, e.g., dyspnea, pain on exercise, nocturnal cough, increased use of nitroglycerin to relieve angina, edema, palpitation, arrhythmias. Dose adjustment of dextrothyroxine may be indicated.

Teratogenic studies have been inconclusive; thus strict birth control measures are advised for the woman of childbearing potential who is receiving dextrothyroxine.

Advise patient to report promptly the onset of iodism *(see Adverse Reactions).* If iodism is developing, the drug will be withdrawn.

Other symptoms that should be promptly reported include: headache, chest pain, palpitation, sweating, diarrhea, skin rash.

Drug therapy in children with familial hypercholesterolemia should continue only if a significant serum cholesterol lowering effect is achieved.

Instruct patient not to self-dose with OTC medications unless physician's approval is obtained.

Advise patient not to change dose regimen in any way (dose or dose intervals) without consulting the physician.

Dextrothyroxine should be discontinued at least 2 weeks before surgery to reduce possibility of precipitating cardiac arrhythmias during surgery.

Patient should inform physician or dentist in an emergency situation that he or she is taking dextrothyroxine before any surgery is performed.

The 2-mg and 6-mg tablets of choloxin contain tartrazine which may cause an allergic-type reaction including bronchial asthma in susceptible individuals. These persons are also often sensitive to aspirin.

Store medication in light and moisture proof container at temperature between 15° and 30°C (59° and 86°F), unless otherwise specified by the manufacturer.

Diagnostic Test Interferences. Dextrothyroxine causes increased **blood sugar** level (in diabetic patient), increased **PBI** and a depressed **I-131 uptake.**

Drug Interactions: Dextrothyroxine

Plus	Interactions
Coumarin anticoagulants	Potentiated anticoagulation effect (requiring decrease in anticoagulant dose)
Digitalis	Enhanced digitalis effect
Epinephrine (in patient with coronary artery disease)	Enhanced danger of coronary insufficiency episode
Insulin and oral hypoglycemics	Decreased diabetes control (hypoglycemic dose may have to be increased)
Thyroid preparations	Increased sensitivity to dextrothyroxine effects

DIAZEPAM

(Apo-Diazepam, Meral, Neo-Calme, Novodipam, Rival, Serenack, Stress-Pam, Valium, Valrelease)

(dye-az'e-pam)
Psychotropic: anxiolytic
Anticonvulsant
Benzodiazepine
C IV

ACTIONS AND USES. Anxiolytic agent related to chlordiazepoxide (qv); reportedly superior in antianxiety and anticonvulsant activity, with somewhat shorter duration of action. Like chlordiazepoxide, appears to act at both limbic and subcortical levels of CNS. Shortens REM and stage 4 sleep, but increases total sleeptime. Causes transient analgesia after IV administration.

Used for management of anxiety disorders, for short-term relief of anxiety symptoms, to allay anxiety and tension prior to surgery, cardioversion and endoscopic procedures, as an amnesic, and treatment for restless legs. Also used to alleviate acute withdrawal symptoms of alcoholism and adjunctively for relief of skeletal muscle spasm associated with, e.g., cerebral palsy, paraplegia, voiding problems in the elderly, athetosis, stiff-man syndrome, tetanus. Effective when used adjunctively in status epilepticus and severe recurrent convulsive seizures.

ABSORPTION AND FATE. Onset of action 30 to 60 minutes after oral administration; 15 to 30 minutes after IM injection (absorption is erratic); 1 to 5 minutes following IV injection. Plasma levels decline rapidly following IV administration; duration of action 15 minutes to 1 hour. Effects may persist up to 3 hours following oral administration. Following absorption from GI tract, peak plasma concentrations occur in 1 to 2 hours. Metabolized in liver; elimination half-life: 20 to 50 hours (increased in the elderly and in renal and hepatic dysfunction). Excreted as metabolites in urine; small amount in feces. Crosses placenta and appears in breast milk.

CONTRAINDICATIONS AND PRECAUTIONS. Hypersensitivity to diazepam; use of injectable form to patients in shock, coma, or in acute alcoholic intoxication with depressed vital signs to obstetrical patients, to infants 30 days of age or less or tablet form in children under 6 months of age; acute narrow-angle glaucoma; untreated open-angle glaucoma, during or within 14 days of MAO inhibitor therapy; shock, coma, acute alcoholic intoxication. Safe use during pregnancy (category D), lactation, and in women of childbearing age not established. *Cautious Use:* epilepsy, psychoses, mental depression, myasthenia gravis, impaired hepatic or renal function, drug abuse, addiction-prone individuals. Injectable diazepam used with extreme caution in the elderly, the very ill, and patients with COPD.

ADVERSE/SIDE EFFECTS. CNS: drowsiness (common), fatigue, ataxia, confusion, paradoxic rage, dizziness, vertigo, amnesia, vivid dreams, headache, slurred speech, tremor, muscle weakness; EEG changes (low-stage; fast activity), tardive dyskinesia. **CV:** hypotension, tachycardia, edema, cardiovascular collapse. **GI:** xerostomia, nausea, constipation. **GU:** incontinence, urinary retention, gynecomastia (prolonged use) changes in libido, menstrual irregularities. **Ophthalmic:** blurred vision, diplopia, nystagmus. **Other:** hiccups, coughing, throat and chest pain, laryngospasm, ovulation failure, neutropenia, hepatic dysfunction including jaundice; pain, venous thrombosis, phlebitis at injection site.

ROUTE AND DOSAGE. Oral: *Anxiety, muscle spasm, convulsive disorders:* **Adult:** 2 to 10 mg, two to four times daily. *Sustained-release capsule (15 mg):* individualized dosage. **Children (over 6 months):** 1 to 2.5 mg, three to four times daily. **Elderly, debilitated:** 2 to 2.5 mg, one or two times daily. **Intramuscular, intravenous:** *Anxiety disorders, muscle spasm:* 2 to 10 mg. Repeat if necessary in 3 to 4 hours. **Elderly, debilitated:** 2 to 5 mg. *Status epilepticus:* **Adult:** Initial: 5 to 10 mg; repeat if necessary at 10- to 15-minute intervals up to 30 mg, repeated if necessary in 2 to 4 hours. **Children (under 5 years):** 0.2 to 0.5 mg slowly every 2 to 5 minutes up to maximum of 5 mg. **Children (over 5 years):** 1 mg every 2 to 5 minutes up to maximum of 10 mg. Repeat if necessary in 2 to 4 hours with EEG monitoring.

NURSING IMPLICATIONS

Tension and anxiety associated with stress of everyday life usually do not require treatment with an anxiolytic agent.

Most adverse reactions of diazepam are dose-related. Physician will rely on accurate observations and reporting of patient's response to the drug to determine lowest effective maintenance dose.

Maximum effect with steady state plasma levels may require 1 to 2 weeks; patient tolerance to therapeutic effects may develop after 4 weeks of treatment.

Tablet may be crushed before administration and taken with fluid or mixed with food.

Supervise oral ingestion of drug. The drug abuser or addiction-prone patient may "cheek" the pill, a maneuver to hoard or avoid medication.

Suicidal tendencies may be present in anxiety states accompanied by depression. Observe necessary preventive precautions.

Parenteral preparation:

- Do not mix or dilute with other drugs or solutions in same syringe or infusion flask.
- Avoid IV infusion of diazepam; it may precipitate in IV fluids. Also, diazepam interacts with plastic IV administration sets and containers with significant reduction in availability of drug.
- To prevent swelling, irritation, venous thrombosis, phlebitis, inject slowly taking at least 1 minute for each 5 mg (1 ml) given to adults, and taking at least a 3-minute period to inject 0.25 mg/kg body weight of children.
- If injection cannot be made directly into vein, manufacturer suggests making injection slowly through infusion tubing as close as possible to vein insertion. Check needle site frequently to prevent extravasation.
- Avoid small veins (e.g., dorsum of hand or wrist) and intraarterial administration.

IM administration should be made deep into large muscle mass. Aspirate for back flow. If present, remove needle, select another site. Inject slowly. Rotate injection sites.

When given parenterally, hypotension, muscular weakness, tachycardia, and respiratory depression may occur, particularly if barbiturates, or narcotics are used concomitantly. Observe patient closely and monitor vital signs. Resuscitative equipment should be readily available.

When used with a narcotic analgesic, the narcotic dose is reduced by at least ⅓ and given in small increments. In some cases, especially in the elderly, the narcotic is unnecessary.

Diazepam is used to diminish recall of a distressful procedure such as peroral endoscopy. It does not alter the potential for symptoms related to the procedure such as increase in cough reflex, laryngospasm, and hyperventilation.

Warn patient to avoid use of alcohol and other CNS depressants during therapy with diazepam, unless otherwise advised by physician. Concomitant use of these agents can cause severe drowsiness, respiratory depression and apnea.

Periodic blood cell counts and liver function tests are recommended during prolonged therapy.

Adverse reactions such as drowsiness, ataxia, constipation and urinary retention are more likely to occur in the elderly and debilitated or in those receiving larger doses. Dosage adjustment may be necessary. Supervise ambulation.

Monitor intake and output ratio and bowel elimination.

Because of possible sedation during early therapy, avoid activities requiring mental alertness and precision until reaction to diazepam has been evaluated.

Smoking–Drug Interaction. Smoking increases metabolism of diazepam, therefore clinical effectiveness is lowered. Heavy smokers may need a higher dose than the nonsmoker.

Abrupt discontinuation of diazepam should generally be avoided. Doses should be tapered to termination. If patient stops drug suddenly after long-term use, withdrawal symptoms (unusual irritability, mental confusion, tremulousness, paranoia, marked photophobia, ataxia, visual hallucinations, vomiting, sweating, abdominal and muscle cramps), may occur and persist for several weeks.

The patient should be advised that if she becomes pregnant during therapy or intends to become pregnant she should communicate with her physician regarding desirability of discontinuing drug.

Psychic and physical dependence may occur in patients on long-term high dosage therapy, in those with histories of alcohol or drug addiction, or in those who self-medicate.

Close supervision should be maintained over the amount of drug dispensed to the patient at one time.

Caution patient to take drug as prescribed, and not to change dose or dose intervals; also not to offer any of it to another person, or use it to treat a self-diagnosed problem.

Tell patient to check with physician before taking any OTC drug while on diazepam therapy.

Diazepam is classified as a Schedule IV drug under the Federal Controlled Substances Act.

Preserved in tight, light-resistant containers at temperature between 15° and 30°C (59° and 86°F), unless otherwise specified by manufacturer.

Drug Interactions. Patients receiving diazepam and nondepolarizing neuromuscular blocking agents, e.g., **pancuronium, succinylcholine** should be closely observed for increase in intensity and duration of respiratory depression. *See also Chlorodiazepoxide (prototype benzodiazepine).*

DIAZOXIDE

(Hyperstat I.V., Proglycem)

(dye-az-ox'ide)
Antihypertensive
Vasodilator
Hyperglycemic
Thiazide

D

ACTIONS AND USES. Rapid-acting benzothiadiazine (thiazide) nondiuretic hypotensive agent. In contrast to thiazide diuretics, causes sodium (Na) and water retention and decreased urinary output, probably because of increased proximal tubular reabsorption of Na and decreased glomerular filtration rate. Like thiazide diuretics, it produces hyperglycemia by inhibiting pancreatic insulin secretion and by stimulating endogenous catecholamine release. Reduces peripheral vascular resistance and blood pressure by direct vasodilatory effect on peripheral arteriolar smooth muscles, perhaps by direct competition for calcium receptor sites. Hypotensive effect may be accompanied by marked reflex, increase in heart rate, cardiac output, and stroke volume; thus cerebral and coronary blood flow are usually maintained. Renal blood flow initially decreases then increases. Oral drug has more prominent hyperglycemic action and less marked antihypertensive effect than parenteral drug. Diazoxide may inhibit ureteral and GI motility, and is a powerful uterine relaxant.

Used intravenously for emergency lowering of blood pressure in hospitalized patients with malignant hypertension, particularly when associated with renal impairment. Not effective in pheochromocytoma. Commonly used with a diuretic such as furosemide (Lasix) to counteract diazoxide-induced Na and water retention. Used orally in treatment of various diagnosed hypoglycemic states due to hyperinsulinism when other medical treatment or surgical management has been unsuccessful or is not feasible.

ABSORPTION AND FATE. Rapid IV injection of 300-mg bolus dose produces fall in blood pressure in 30 to 60 seconds, with maximal effect within 5 minutes; duration (unpredictable) 2 to 12 hours or longer. Following oral administration, hyperglycemic effect begins within 1 hour and may last up to 8 hours if renal function is normal. Plasma half-life: 20 to 36 hours in adults, 9 to 24 hours in children. More than 90% protein bound. Approximately 50% excreted by kidney unchanged. Crosses blood–brain barrier and placenta.

CONTRAINDICATIONS AND PRECAUTIONS. Hypersensitivity to diazoxide or other thiazides; eclampsia; aortic coarctation; AV shunt, significant coronary artery disease. Safe use during pregnancy (category C), in nursing mothers, and safety of parenteral drug for children not established. Use of oral diazoxide for functional hypoglycemia or in presence of increased bilirubin in newborns. *Cautious Use:* diabetes mellitus, impaired cerebral or cardiac circulation, impaired renal function, patients taking corticosteroids or estrogen–progestogen combinations, hyperuricemia, history of gout.

ADVERSE/SIDE EFFECTS. CNS: tinnitus, momentary hearing loss, headache, dizziness, polyneuritis, sleepiness, euphoria, anxiety, cerebral ischemia, (confusion, unconsciousness, convulsions, paralysis), paresthesias, extrapyramidal signs (oculogyrus, rigidity, trismus, tremor). **CV:** palpitations, atrial and ventricular arrhythmias, flushing, shock; orthostatic hypotension, myocardial ischemia and infarction, angina, congestive heart failure, transient hypertension. **Dermatologic:** pruritus, flushing, skin rash, monilial dermatitis, herpes, excessive hair growth (especially in children), loss of scalp hair, sweating, sensation of warmth, burning, or itching. **GI:** nausea, vomiting, abdominal discomfort, diarrhea, constipation, ileus, anorexia, transient loss of taste, parotid swelling, dry mouth. **Hematologic:** thrombocytopenia with or without purpura, transient neutropenia, eosinophilia. **Hypersensitivity:** rash, fever, leukopenia. **Ophthalmic:** blurred vision, transient cataracts, subconjunctival hemorrhage, ring scotoma, diplopia, lacrimation, papilledema. **Renal:** decreased urinary output, nephrotic syndrome (reversible), hematuria, increased nocturia, proteinuria, azotemia. **Other:** impaired hepatic function, chest and back pain, muscle cramps; acute pancreatitis; advance in bone age (children); sodium and water retention, edema, hyperuricemia, hyperglycemia, glycosuria, diabetic ketoacidosis and nonketotic hyperosmolar coma; inhibition of labor, enlargement of breast lump, galactorrhea; decreased immunoglobinemia. Injection site reactions: warmth or pain along injected vein; with extravasation: severe local pain, cellulitis, phlebitis.

ROUTE AND DOSAGE. *Hypertension:* **Intravenous: Adults only:** 300 mg administered undiluted over 30 seconds or less. Additional dose if no response within 30 minutes. Subsequent doses at 4- to 24-hour intervals depending on patient's response. Alternatively, administration of minibolus dose of 1 to 3 mg/kg up to maximum of 150 mg, repeated at 5- to 15-minute intervals, if necessary, or IV infusion of 15 mg/minute over 20 to 30 minutes. *Hypoglycemia:* **Oral: Adults and children:** 3 mg/kg/day divided into 2 or 3 equal doses every 8 or 12 hours. **Infants and newborns: Oral:** 8 to 15 mg/kg/day divided into 2 or 3 equal doses every 8 or 12 hours. Highly individualized.

NURSING IMPLICATIONS

Treatment of hypertension (intravenous preparation):

Blood glucose, serum electrolytes, and complete blood counts should be determined at start of therapy and regularly thereafter in patients receiving multiple doses.

Patient should be recumbent while receiving IV diazoxide and should remain in bed for at least 30 minutes following administration.

Monitor blood pressure every 5 minutes for the first 15 to 30 minutes or until stabilized, then hourly for balance of drug effect. In ambulatory patients, blood pressure measurement should be made with patient in standing position, before ending surveillance.

If blood pressure continues to fall 30 minutes or more after drug administration, suspect cause other than drug effect. Notify physician immediately.

A precipitous drop in blood pressure is especially dangerous for the elderly because they are less capable of adapting to the stress of compromised circulation to vital organs.

Monitor pulse: tachycardia has occurred immediately following IV; palpitation and bradycardia have also been reported.

Have on hand norepinephrine (levaterenol) for treatment of severe hypotension.

Since diazoxide causes Na and water retention, a diuretic is generally prescribed to avoid congestive heart failure and drug resistance, and to maximize hypotensive effect.

When a diuretic, e.g., furosemide (Lasix), is prescribed it is generally given 30 to 60 minutes prior to diazoxide. Patient should remain recumbent 8 to 10 hours because of possible additive hypotensive effect.

Intake and output should be monitored. Report promptly any change in intake and output ratio, constipation, abdominal distention, or absence of bowel sounds.

If feasible, daily weight provides another objective measure of fluid retention or mobilization.

Observe patient closely for signs and symptoms of congestive heart failure (distended neck veins, rales at bases of lungs, dyspnea, orthopnea, cough, fatigue, weakness, dependent edema).

Diazoxide may cause hyperglycemia and glycosuria in diabetic and diabetic-prone individuals. Blood and urine glucose should be closely monitored. Temporary dosage adjustment of antidiabetic drugs may be required.

Check IV injection sites daily. Solution is strongly alkaline. Extravasation of medication into subcutaneous or intramuscular tissues can cause severe inflammatory reaction *(see Index: Nursing Interventions: Extravasation)*. Diazoxide is administered only by peripheral vein.

Alternate oral antihypertensive therapy should be started as soon as possible after emergency is controlled. It is rarely necessary to give IV diazoxide therapy for more than 4 or 5 days.

D

Treatment of hypoglycemia (oral preparation):

During initial therapy, patient should be closely supervised, with blood glucose, serum electrolytes, and clinical response being carefully monitored until condition stabilizes satisfactorily on minimum dosage.

Blood glucose level should be determined periodically thereafter to evaluate need of dosage adjustment. Serum electrolyte levels should be evaluated at regular intervals particularly in patient with impaired renal function. (Hypokalemia potentiates hyperglycemic effect of diazoxide.)

Patients on prolonged therapy should have periodic determinations of Hct, Hgb, platelets, and total and differential leukocyte counts.

In contrast to IV administration of diazoxide, oral administration usually does not produce marked effects on blood pressure. However, periodic measurements of blood pressure and vital signs should be made.

Monitor intake and output ratio, and also weight. Diazoxide promotes Na and water retention, most commonly in young infants and in adults, and may precipitate congestive failure in patients with compromised cardiac reserve.

Patient should be taught to monitor urine regularly for sugar and ketones, especially during stress conditions, and instructed to report abnormal findings and unusual symptoms to physician. Hyperglycemia may require reduction in dosage or treatment with a hypoglycemic agent to avoid progression to ketoacidosis.

Ketoacidosis and hyperosmolar coma have been reported in patients treated with recommended doses, usually during an intercurrent illness. Emphasize importance of early recognition and reporting of symptoms: increased thirst, acetone (fruity) breath odor, nausea, vomiting, abdominal tenderness, confusion, air hunger. Insulin therapy and restoration of fluid and electrolyte balance are usually effective if instituted promptly.

Prolonged surveillance is essential because of long half-life of diazoxide (for both oral and parenteral forms). In the event of overdosage, surveillance as long as 7 days may be required.

Lanugo type hirsutism (mainly on forehead, back, limbs) occurs frequently and is most common in children and women (reversible with discontinuation of drug).

In some patients, higher diazoxide levels are attained with liquid than with capsule formulation. Dosage may require adjustment if patient is changed from one formulation to another.

Diazoxide is discontinued if not effective in 2 or 3 weeks. Therapy may be continued for several years, until insulin response to presumptive tests are normal.

Suspension formula should be shaken well before use.

Protect diazoxide from light, heat, and freezing.

Darkened solutions may have lost potency and therefore should not be administered.

Diagnostic Test Interferences. Diazoxide can cause elevations of **blood glucose, serum bilirubin, renin and uric acid,** and decreases in **plasma free fatty acids, creatinine,** and **PAH acid clearance, Hgb, Hct.**

Drug Interactions: Diazoxide

Plus	Interactions
Alpha adrenergic blocking agents (e.g., ergotamine, phentolamine)	May antagonize hyperglycemic action of diazoxide
Anticoagulants, oral	Diazoxide enhances anticoagulant effect
Antihypertensives (e.g., hydralazine, methyldopa, reserpine)	Potentiates antihypertensive effect. Use before, during or following diazoxide may result in profound drop in BP

Plus (cont.)	Interactions (cont.)
Corticosteroids Estrogen-progestogen combinations	Potentiate hyperglycemic effect of diazoxide
Oral antidiabetic agents	Pharmacologic effects of diazoxide and these agents may be reduced. Monitor blood glucose
Phenothiazines Thiazides and other diuretics	May intensify hyperglycemic, hyperuricemic, and antihypertensive effects of diazoxide. Monitor blood pressure, and blood glucose and serum uric acid levels
Phenytoin (Dilantin) and other hydantoins	Diazoxide may enhance phenytoin metabolism with possible loss of seizure control. Monitor phenytoin plasma levels
Vasodilators (e.g., nitrates, papaverine)	Risk of severe hypotension

D

DIBUCAINE

(dye'byoo-kane)
Anaesthetic, local

(Nupercainal)

DIBUCAINE HYDROCHLORIDE

(Nupercaine)

ACTIONS AND USES. Long-acting anesthetic of the amide type, and reportedly one of the most potent and most toxic. Duration of action is about 3 times longer than that of procaine, and it is approximately 15 times more toxic.

Parenteral dosage form is used only for spinal anesthesia. Topical forms are used for fast, temporary relief of pain and itching due to hemorrhoids, nonpoisonous insect bites, sunburn, minor burns, cuts, and scratches.

ABSORPTION AND FATE. Poorly absorbed from intact skin, but readily absorbed from mucous membranes, abraded, and ulcerated skin. Onset of local anesthetic action within 10 minutes; duration of action: 2 to 4 hours. Onset of spinal anesthesia within 10 to 15 minutes; duration 3 to 4 hours without epinephrine, and 6 hours by addition of epinephrine. Metabolized primarily in liver and excreted by kidneys.

CONTRAINDICATIONS AND PRECAUTIONS. Hypersensitivity to local anesthetics. When used for spinal anesthesia: diseases of cerebrospinal system, pernicious anemia with cord symptoms, diseases of spinal column (e.g., arthritis, spondylitis), septicemia, skin or tissue infection adjacent to point of puncture. Obstetrical contraindications: pelvic disproportion, placenta praevia, abruptio placenta, unengaged head, intrauterine manipulation. *Cautious Use:* debilitated or acutely ill patients, elderly patients, children, history of drug hypersensitivities; hysteria, excessive nervous tension, chronic backache, headaches; migraine, hypotension, cardiac decompensation, increased intraabdominal pressure, hemorrhagic spinal fluid.

ADVERSE/SIDE EFFECTS. Hypotension, temporary or permanent transverse myelitis, meningitis, transient nerve palsies, nausea, vomiting, CNS stimulation followed by depression, respiratory arrest; postanesthetic ("spinal") headache, hypersensitivity reactions.

ROUTE AND DOSAGE. *Isobaric spinal anesthesia: 1:200 (0.5%) solution:* perineum and lower limbs: 2.5 to 5 mg (0.5 to 1 ml); lower abdomen: 5 to 7.5 mg (1 to 1.5 ml); upper abdomen: 10 mg (2 ml). *Hypobaric spinal anesthesia: 1:1500 solution (0.067%):* simple caudal block:

4 mg (6 ml); lower abdomen: 6.67 to 10 mg (10 to 15 ml); upper abdomen: 10 to 12 mg (15 to 18 ml). *Hyperbaric spinal anesthesia (Heavy solution): 0.25% with 5% dextrose:* saddle block for obstetric, rectal, or urologic surgery not involving abdominal incision: 2.5 to 5 mg (1 to 2 ml). **Topical:** *Skin:* (0.5% cream; 1% ointment): apply gently to affected area. Cover with light dressing if necessary for protection. Do not exceed 1 ounce of ointment in 24 hours for adults or more than ¼ ounce/24 hours for children. **Rectal suppository 2.5 mg. (0.25%) or ointment 1%:** insert morning and night and after each bowel movement. (Special applicator is included for inserting ointment into rectum.)

NURSING IMPLICATIONS

Spinal anesthesia:

A careful drug history should be taken to determine drug hypersensitivities. An intradermal test is advisable for patients with a positive history.

In general patient should remain flat in bed for 6 to 8 hours following spinal (subarachnoid) or saddle block anesthesia to reduce risk of postanesthetic (spinal) headache. (Time period prescribed varies with individual physician.) Keeping head and spinal puncture site at same level helps to prevent escape of spinal fluid through puncture site, one of the presumed causes of "spinal headache."

Postanesthetic headache is less likely to occur as a consequence of caudal or epidural block unless dura has been punctured inadvertently.

Physician may prescribe hydration prophylactically as well as for treatment of "spinal headache." Other treatment measures may include tight abdominal binder, pituitrin 1 ml, ephedrine 100 mg. Reportedly, rapid relief may be obtained by intraspinal or caudal injection of 30 ml sterile saline.

Monitor blood pressure, pulse, and respirations, every 10 to 15 minutes during recovery period until stable, then every hour for 4 hours, then every 4 hours.

Resuscitative equipment and emergency drugs should be immediately available. Have on hand ephedrine, oxygen, a quick-acting barbiturate, suction, equipment for intubation, artificial respiration.

Note return of motor function (wearing off of motor blockade) and return of sensation (wearing off of autonomic blockade). Patients experiencing autonomic blockade tend to be more susceptible to hypotension.

Patient should not ambulate until motor functions and sensations return completely and vital signs are stabilized.

In obstetrical anesthesia, dibucaine is not used until cervix is 5 to 6 cm dilated and 60 to 80% effaced. Injection should not be made during a uterine contraction because solution could be carried toward head (cephalad) and result in higher spinal anesthesia than intended.

Some patients develop transient nerve palsies, particularly of eye muscles and legs about 2 weeks after spinal anesthesia. Symptoms usually do not last more than 1 to 2 weeks. Report to physician.

Because dibucaine hydrochloride precipitates in presence of even minute amounts of alkali, manufacturer recommends that syringes and needles used for spinal anesthesia be rinsed in slightly acidified distilled water.

Solutions of dibucaine hydrochloride without dextrose can be autoclaved up to 3 times at 120°C for 30 minutes. Solutions of dibucaine hydrochloride with dextrose should not be autoclaved more than once.

Partially used ampuls should be discarded.

Discard any solution that appears discolored. Protect dibucaine hydrochloride from light.

Topical Application:

The cream preparation is water washable and therefore should be applied after bathing or swimming.

Avoid contact of drug with or near eyes.

Instruct patient to use OTC preparations as directed. Review package label with patient.

Caution patient to discontinue medication if irritation or rectal bleeding (following use of rectal preparations) develops, and to consult physician.

Patient-Teaching for Administration of Rectal Suppository:

- ✓ Remove foil wrapper. (If suppository is too soft, rewrap it in foil and hold it under cold running water or refrigerate it for several minutes.)
- ✓ Moisten with water to facilitate insertion.
- ✓ Have patient lie on side. Gently insert suppository, rounded end first, directing it along rectal wall toward umbilicus until it passes internal anal sphincter (if other than patient inserts suppository use finger cot or glove).

Remind patient that hemorrhoids can be caused or worsened by constipation, excessive straining at stool, and excessive standing, sitting, and coughing.

Physician may prescribe Sitz baths three or four times daily to reduce the swelling and pain of hemorrhoids.

Patient should be informed that medication is intended only for temporary relief of mild to moderate itching or pain. Anesthetic formulations can mask symptoms and delay diagnosis of serious disorders.

Instruct patient to seek medical advice if he or she experiences continuing discomfort, severe pain or bleeding, or sensation of rectal pressure.

Suppositories should be stored below 30°C (86°F).

DICHLORPHENAMIDE

(Daranide, Oratrol)

(dye-klor-fen'a-mide)
Carbonic anhydrase inhibitor
Diuretic
Sulfonamide derivative

ACTIONS AND USES. Nonbacteriostatic sulfonamide derivative similar to acetazolamide, except that chloride excretion is increased, and thus potential for significant metabolic acidosis is less. Contraindications, precautions, and adverse reactions are the same as for acetazolamide (qv).

Used in adjunctive treatment of open-angle glaucoma and preoperatively in narrow-angle glaucoma when delay of surgery is desired in order to lower intraocular pressure. Commonly used in conjunction with a miotic; an osmotic agent may also be used to enhance reduction of intraocular pressure in acute-angle closure glaucoma.

ABSORPTION AND FATE. Onset of action within 1 hour; peaks in 2 to 4 hours and lasts 6 to 12 hours.

ADVERSE/SIDE EFFECTS. Paresthesias, drowsiness, headache, fatigue, dizziness, depression, visual disturbances, anorexia, nausea, vomiting, abdominal discomfort, rise in BUN, hyperchloremic acidosis, hypokalemia, asymptomatic hyperuricemia. *See also Acetazolamide.*

ROUTE AND DOSAGE. Oral: Initial: 100 to 200 mg followed by 100 mg every 12 hours until desired response is obtained. Maintenance: 25 to 50 mg 1 to 3 times daily.

NURSING IMPLICATIONS

Teach patient not to accept brand interchange as it is not recommended for carbonic anhydrase inhibitor products.

See Acetazolamide (prototype carbonic anhydrase inhibitor).

DICLOXACILLIN SODIUM

(Dycill, Dynapen, Pathocil, Veracillin)

(dye-klox-a-sill'in)
Antiinfective
Antibiotic (beta-lactam)
Penicillin

ACTIONS AND USES. Semisynthetic, acid-stable, penicillinase-resistant isoxazolyl penicillin. Mechanism of bactericidal action, contraindications, precautions, and adverse reactions similar to those of penicillin G (qv). However, platelet dysfunction not reported for dicloxacillin. Reportedly the most active of the isoxazolyl penicillins (cloxacillin, oxacillin) against penicillinase-producing staphylococci. Less potent than penicillin G against penicillin-sensitive microorganisms and generally ineffective against methicillin-resistant staphylococci, and gram-negative bacteria. Contains 12 mg Na 250 mg.

Used primarily in treatment of infections caused by penicillinase-producing staphylococci and penicillin-resistant staphylococci. May be used to initiate therapy in suspected staphylococcal infections pending culture and sensitivity test results. As with other penicillins, serum concentrations are enhanced by concurrent use of probenecid.

ABSORPTION AND FATE. Peak plasma levels in 1 hour; effective levels maintained 4 to 6 hours. Distributed throughout body with highest concentrations in kidney and liver. CSF penetration is low. Half-life: 30 to 60 minutes. Almost 90 to 96% protein bound. Excreted rapidly, primarily in urine; significant amounts eliminated by liver through bile. Crosses placenta. Excreted in breast milk.

CONTRAINDICATIONS AND PRECAUTIONS. Hypersensitivity to penicillins or cephalosporins. Safe use during pregnancy and in neonates not established. *Cautious Use:* history of or suspected atopy or allergy (asthma, eczema, hives, hay fever). *See Penicillin G.*

ADVERSE/SIDE EFFECTS. GI: Nausea, vomiting, flatulence, diarrhea, GI bleeding. **Hypersensitivity:** pruritus, urticaria, rash, wheezing, sneezing, anaphylaxis; eosinophilia. **Other:** transient elevations of SGPT (ALT), positive cephalin flocculation tests, jaundice (rare), superinfections. Generally well tolerated but carries same potential for adverse effects as other penicillins. *See Penicillin G.*

ROUTE AND DOSAGE. Oral: Adults; children (weighing 40 kg or more): 125 to 250 mg or higher every 6 hours. **Children (under 40 kg):** 3 to 6 mg/kg every 6 hours.

NURSING IMPLICATIONS

Careful inquiry should be made concerning patient's previous exposure and sensitivity to penicillins and cephalosporins, and other allergic reactions of any kind.

Best taken on an empty stomach (at least 1 hour before or 2 hours after meals), unless otherwise advised by the physician. Food reduces drug absorption.

Instruct patient to take medication around the clock, not to miss a dose, and to continue taking the medication until it is all gone, unless otherwise directed by physician.

Advise patient to check with physician if GI side effects appear.

Inform patient to report the onset of hypersensitivity reactions and superinfections: black furry tongue, anal or vaginal itching, vaginal discharge, loose foul-smelling stools.

Periodic assessment of renal, hepatic, and hematopoietic functions are advised in patients in prolonged therapy.

Following reconstitution (by pharmacist), oral suspensions are stable for 14 days under refrigeration (container should be so labeled and dated). Shake well before pouring; some preparations have a tendency to clump. A calibrated measuring device should be dispensed with the preparation. Household teaspoons vary in measure and therefore are not recommended.

See Penicillin G (prototype penicillin).

DICUMAROL

(Bishydroxycoumarin)

(dye-koo'ma-role)
Anticoagulant
Coumarin

ACTIONS AND USES. Long-acting coumarin derivative. Similar to other drugs of this series in actions, uses, contraindications, precautions, and adverse effects. *See Warfarin.*

ABSORPTION AND FATE. Slowly and incompletely absorbed from GI tract. Peak effect 1 to 4 days; duration 2 to 10 days. Half-life: 1 to 2 days (dose dependent); 99% protein bound. Metabolized by hepatic microsomal enzymes. Excreted in urine largely as inactive metabolites; excreted in stool as unchanged drug. Crosses placenta; enters breast milk.

ROUTE AND DOSAGE. Oral: First day, 200 to 300 mg; on subsequent days, 25 to 200 mg daily if prothrombin activity is 25% or more of normal.

NURSING IMPLICATIONS

Frequent dosage adjustment may be necessary during first 1 or 2 weeks of therapy because drug absorption is so variable. Administration with food enhances drug absorption.

During period of dosage adjustment, prothrombin activity should be checked daily and dose order obtained. Follow agency policies regarding administration of anticoagulants.

When patient is controlled on maintenance dose, prothrombin times may be checked semiweekly, weekly, or at 2- to 4-week intervals, depending on stability of patient's response.

Caution patient not to take or stop taking any other medication without approval of physician.

Counsel patient not to engage in contact sports or activities with high risk of injuries.

Advise patient to tell all doctors and dentists who may administer care about taking an anticoagulant.

Stress importance of avoiding unusual changes in diet or life-style without consulting physician.

Store in well-closed container in temperature between 15° and 30°C (59° and 86°F).

See Warfarin (prototype coumarin anticoagulant).

Diagnostic Test Interferences. May cause increase in **T3 uptake** (not reported with other coumarins), and decrease in **plasma uric acid.**

Drug Interactions: Dicumarol

Plus	Interactions
Milk of magnesia (Magnesium hydroxide)	Forms magnesium chelate of dicumarol which is readily absorbed and can cause earlier and higher dicumarol blood levels. Not reported with aluminum hydroxide or with other anticoagulants.
Oral hypoglycemics	Dicumarol appears to increase effects of oral hypoglycemics by inhibiting hepatic metabolism. Hypoglycemic drugs may cause initial increase then decrease in anticoagulant effect. (Interaction not reported with Warfarin.)
Phenytoin (Dilantin)	Dicumarol inhibits hepatic breakdown of phenytoin (increases phenytoin effect). Phenytoin causes transient initial increase in anticoagulant effect (by displacement from plasma protein-binding sites), then decreases (possibly by stimulating hepatic metabolism).

See also Warfarin.

D

DICYCLOMINE HYDROCHLORIDE

(dye-sye'kloe-meen)

(A-spas, Antispas, Baycyclomine, Bentyl, Bentylol, Byclomine, Cyclocen, Dibent, Dicen, Dilomine, Di-Spaz, Formulex, Lomine, Neoquess, Nospaz, Or-Tyl, Protylol)

Anticholinergic (parasympathomimetic)
Antimuscarinic
Antispasmodic

ACTIONS AND USES. Synthetic tertiary amine with antispasmodic properties. Effect on smooth muscle appears to be more musculotropic than anticholinergic; thus atropinelike (antimuscarinic) side effects on salivary and sweat glands, gastric secretions, eye, and cardiovascular system are generally slight with average dosage. Relieves smooth muscle spasm in GI and biliary tracts, uterus, and ureters by nonspecific direct relaxant action. Exhibits local anesthetic properties.

Used adjunctively in treatment of irritable bowel syndrome, neurogenic bowel disturbances, and infant colic. There are varied opinions about its value in treatment of peptic ulcer because of uncertainty as to its specific action.

ABSORPTION AND FATE. Readily absorbed after oral administration. Onset of action in 1 to 2 hours; duration: about 4 hours. Almost completely metabolized and eliminated in urine; small percentage excreted unchanged.

CONTRAINDICATIONS AND PRECAUTIONS. Obstructive diseases of GU and GI tracts, paralytic ileus, intestinal atony, biliary tract disease, unstable cardiovascular status, severe ulcerative colitis, toxic megacolon, myasthenia gravis. Safe use during pregnancy and in nursing mothers not established. *Cautious Use:* glaucoma, prostatic hypertrophy, autonomic neuropathy, ulcerative colitis, hyperthyroidism, coronary heart disease, congestive heart failure, arrhythmias, hypertension, hepatic or renal disease, hiatal hernia associated with esophageal reflux, infants 6 weeks of age and under.

ADVERSE/SIDE EFFECTS. Dose-related: transient dizziness, brief euphoria, headache, fever, confusion and excitement (especially elderly patients), drowsiness, insomnia, palpitation, tachycardia, constipation, paralytic ileus, dry mouth, nausea, vomiting, diminished sense of taste, bloated feeling, decreased sweating, allergic reactions. Overdosage: curarelike effect. *See Atropine Sulfate.*

ROUTE AND DOSAGE. Oral: Adults: 10 to 20 mg 3 or 4 times daily. **Children:** 10 mg 3 or 4 times daily. **Infants:** 5 mg 3 or 4 times daily. **Intramuscular (only): Adults:** 20 mg every 4 to 6 hours. Available in capsule, tablet, syrup, injection forms.

D

NURSING IMPLICATIONS

Usually administered before meals and at bedtime. Antacid may be prescribed to be given concurrently.

If necessary tablet can be crushed, or capsule may be emptied before administration and mixed with fluid or food of patient's choice.

Syrup formulation may be diluted with equal volume of water.

Advise patient to avoid hot environments. Dicyclomine may increase risk of heatstroke by decreasing sweating. This is a particular problem of the elderly because of age-related reduction in sweating response to heat.

Since dicyclomine may produce drowsiness and blurred vision, caution patient to avoid activities requiring mental alertness, such as operating a motor vehicle or dangerous machinery, until reaction to drug is known.

Instruct the patient to report changes in urinary volume or voiding pattern.

Infants 6 weeks and under have developed respiratory symptoms as well as seizures, fluctuations in heart rate, weakness, and coma within minutes after taking syrup formulation. Symptoms generally last 20 to 30 minutes and are believed to be due to local irritation.

See Atropine Sulfate (prototype anticholinergic).

DIENESTROL

(DV, Estraguard, OrthoDienestrol)

(dye-en-ess'trole)
Hormone
Estrogen

ACTIONS AND USES. Synthetic nonsteroidal estrogen structurally related to diethylstilbestrol. Shares actions of estradiol (qv).

Used for treatment of atrophic vaginitis and kraurosis vulvae associated with the menopause. Available in combination with sulfanilamide and aminacrine (AVC/Dienestrol).

ABSORPTION AND FATE, CONTRAINDICATIONS, PRECAUTIONS, ADVERSE SIDE EFFECTS. *See Estradiol.*

ROUTE AND DOSAGE. Intravaginal: cream (0.01%): one or 2 applicatorsful daily for 1 to 2 weeks. Dosage then reduced to half of initial dose for another 1 to 3 times weekly for 1 or 2 weeks. Vaginal suppository (0.7 mg): one or 2 daily for 1 to 2 weeks then one suppository every other day for a similar period.

NURSING IMPLICATIONS

Administration at bedtime increases absorption and thus effectiveness.

Intravaginal dienestrol is readily absorbed from the vaginal mucosa and reaches blood levels approaching those of orally administered estrogens. Systemic hyperestrogenic effects (reportable) include uterine bleeding, edema, reactivation of endometriosis and mastalgia and may result from overdosage of intravaginal drug or from overexposure of denuded or abraded skin surfaces of hands to estrogen.

D

Intravaginal administration of medication: Have patient in recumbent position, draped, with knees flexed and legs spread apart. Put on sterile gloves before inspecting perineal area. If discharge is present gently wash area with soap (if allowed) and warm water. Spread labia and slowly insert cream applicator (or suppository inserter) approximately 2 inches (5 cm) directing it slightly back toward sacrum. Patient should remain in recumbent position about 30 minutes to prevent losing the medication (no sphincter in vagina). Observe perineal area before each administration: if mucosa is red, swollen, or excoriated, or if there is a change in vaginal discharge, report to physician before giving the medication.

If patient is to administer medication to herself, instruct her to wash her hands well before and after the procedure; also tell her not to use tampons while on vaginal therapy. She may wish to wear a sanitary napkin to protect clothing.

DV suppositories contain tartrazine which may cause allergic-type reaction (including bronchial asthma) in certain susceptible persons. This sensitization is also frequently seen in aspirin-sensitive individuals.

Ordinarily a suppository inserter (or cream applicator) is dispensed with the medication.

Review package insert with patient to assure understanding of estrogen therapy.

Protect suppositories and cream from light. Store between 8° and 15°C (46° and 59°F) in a tight container, unless otherwise directed by manufacturer.

See Estradiol (prototype estrogen).

DIETHYLPROPION HYDROCHLORIDE

(Depletite, Dietic, Nobesine, Propion, Regibon, Tenuate, Tepanil)

(dye-eth-il-proe'pee-on)
Central stimulant
Anorexigenic agent
C IV

ACTIONS AND USES. Amphetamine congener with lower incidence of amphetamine-type adverse effects, but reportedly also less effective as an appetite suppressant. Anorexigenic action probably secondary to CNS stimulation.

Used solely in management of exogenous obesity as short-term (a few weeks) adjunct in a regimen of weight reduction based on caloric restriction.

ABSORPTION AND FATE. Readily absorbed from GI tract. Effects persist about 4 hours for regular tablet, and for 10 to 14 hours for controlled-release formulations. (Bioavailability may not be uniform.) Excreted in urine.

CONTRAINDICATIONS AND PRECAUTIONS. Known hypersensitivity or idiosyncrasy to sympathomimetic amines, severe hypertension, advanced arteriosclerosis, hyperthyroidism, glaucoma, agitated states, history of drug abuse, during or within 14 days following use of MAO inhibitors, concomitant use of CNS stimulants. Safe use during pregnancy (category C) and in children under 12 years of age not established. *Cautious Use:* hypertension, arrhythmias, symptomatic cardiovascular disease, epilepsy, diabetes mellitus.

ADVERSE/SIDE EFFECTS. CNS: restlessness, nervousness, dizziness, headache, insomnia, drowsiness, psychotic episodes. **CV:** palpitation, tachycardia, precordial pain, elevated blood pressure. **GI:** nausea, vomiting, diarrhea, constipation, dry mouth, unpleasant taste. **Hypersensitivity:** urticaria, rash, erythema. **Other:** muscle pain, dyspnea, hair loss, polyuria, dysuria, increased sweating, impotence, changes in libido, gynecomastia, menstrual irregularities, bone marrow depression, increase in convulsive episodes in patients with epilepsy. *See also Amphetamine.*

ROUTE AND DOSAGE. Oral: 25 mg 3 times daily, 1 hour before meals. Alternatively, sustained-release preparation: 75 mg daily in midmorning.

NURSING IMPLICATIONS

Additional dose sometimes prescribed in midevening to control nighttime hunger. Rarely causes insomnia except in high doses.

Sustained-release tablets should be swallowed whole and not chewed.

Dosage should be carefully titrated in patients with diabetes.

Patients with epilepsy should be observed closely for reduction in seizure control.

Anorexigenic effect seldom lasts more than a few weeks. If tolerance develops, drug should be discontinued.

Dry mouth may be relieved by frequent rinses with warm clear water, sugarless gum, or lemon drops, increasing noncaloric fluid intake (if allowed).

Classified as Schedule IV drug under the Federal Controlled Substances Act.

Varying degrees of psychologic and rarely physical dependence can occur. Drugs related to amphetamines are frequently misused by emotionally unstable individuals.

Because diethylpropion may mask fatigue and may cause dizziness, caution patient to avoid operating machinery or driving a car or other hazardous activities, until reaction to drug is determined.

See Amphetamine Sulfate (prototype anorexigenic).

D

DIETHYLSTILBESTROL

(Stilbestrol, DES)

(dye-eth-il-stil-bess′trole)

Hormone
Estrogen
Contraceptive (postcoital)
Antineoplastic

ACTIONS AND USES. Reportedly the most potent nonsteroidal synthetic estrogen compound. Has strong teratogenic potential; may cause vaginal or cervical cancer in offspring if mother is treated with diethylstilbestrol (DES) during pregnancy. Interferes with implantation of fertilized ovum in uterus by unclear mechanism; does not terminate pregnancy. Suppresses lactation. Excessive or prolonged use may inhibit anterior pituitary secretions. Long-term therapy with 5 mg/daily for prostatic carcinoma reportedly associated with increased risk of cardiovascular deaths.

Used in treatment of estrogen deficiency states, including menopausal symptoms, atrophic vaginitis, kraurosis vulvae, for palliative treatment of advanced metastatic carcinoma of the breast in men and postmenopausal women, and inoperable carcinoma of prostate. *Unlabeled Use:* emergency postcoital contraception ("morning after" pill); not used routinely as a contraceptive. Combined with methyltestosterone in several formulations for additive effects.

ABSORPTION AND FATE. *See Estradiol.*

CONTRAINDICATIONS AND PRECAUTIONS. Birth control, except emergency postcoital contraception; malignancies or precarcinomatous lesions (vagina, vulva, or breasts), pregnancy, blood clotting disorders, hepatic dysfunction, undiagnosed vaginal bleeding, long-term use during menopause. *Cautious Use:* hypertension, migraine, diabetes mellitus, asthma. *See also Estradiol.*

ROUTE AND DOSAGE. Oral (cyclic regimen) *Estrogen deficiency:* 0.2 to 0.5 mg daily. *Carcinoma palliation* (breast) 15 mg daily; (prostate) 1 to 3 mg daily, increased in advanced cases; later may be reduced to average 1 mg daily. *Postcoital contraception:* 25 mg twice daily for 5 days. **Intravaginal suppository:** 0.1 to 0.5 mg 1 or 2 times daily for 10 to 14 days as supplement to oral dose or as single drug source.

NURSING IMPLICATIONS

Cyclic therapy consists of 3 weeks on diethylstilbestrol (once daily), followed by 1 week without the drug (the usual regimen for prolonged treatment of menopausal symptoms).

Enteric-coated tablets should be swallowed whole.

Nausea and vomiting are common in the menopausal group of patients receiving 1 mg or more daily and relatively uncommon in men and nonpregnant women even when doses are 3 to 5 mg daily.

Reassure the male patient that drug-induced loss of libido and development of feminine characteristics will disappear with termination of therapy.

Women should have breasts and pelvic organs examined before treatment begins and at intervals throughout therapy. Teach the patient self-examination of breasts, and encourage her to do so on a regular monthly basis. Urge her to keep check-up appointments.

A pregnancy test is advised before the patient is started on therapy with DES.

Estrogen in the suppository is readily absorbed from the vaginal mucosa and reaches blood levels approaching those of parenteral or orally administered estrogen. Systemic hyperestrogenic effects (uterine bleeding, edema, mastalgia, reactivation of endometriosis) may result from overdosage of intravaginal drug or from overexposure of denuded or abraded skin surfaces of hands to estrogen.

To administer the vaginal suppository: Have patient in recumbent position, draped, with knees flexed and legs spread apart. Put on sterile gloves before inspecting perineal area. If discharge is present, gently wash area with soap (if allowed) and warm water. Spread labia and slowly insert suppository into vagina approximately 5 cm (2 in) directing it slightly back toward sacrum. Patient should remain in recumbent position about 30 minutes to prevent losing the medication (no sphincter in vagina). Observe perineal area before each administration: If mucosa is red, swollen or excoriated, or if there is a change in vaginal discharge, withhold medication and report to physician.

If patient is to administer suppository to herself, instruct her to wash her hands well before and after the procedure. Tell her not to use tampons while on vaginal suppository therapy. She may wish to wear a sanitary napkin to protect clothing.

If the patient who has been taking DES becomes pregnant, she should be informed of the teratogenic potential of this drug.

When used as an emergency postcoital contraceptive (such as for rape or for incest), drug is started within 24 hours and not later than 72 hours after sexual exposure. Although this dose will prevent conception, it will not terminate pregnancy. Full course of drug must be taken in spite of severe nausea if unwanted pregnancy is to be prevented. An antiemetic may be administered concurrently.

Dosage reduction or discontinuation of therapy is generally attempted at 3- to 6-month intervals.

Urge patient to maintain established regimen, i.e., the dose should not be increased, decreased, or omitted, without physician's advice.

Review package insert with patient to assure complete understanding about diethylstilbestrol therapy.

Store tablets at temperature between 15° and 30°C (59° and 86°F) in a well-closed container, and suppositories between 8° and 30°C (46° and 86°F) in a tight container, unless otherwise directed by manufacturer.

See Estradiol (prototype estrogen).

DIETHYLSTILBESTROL DIPHOSPHATE

(Honvol, Stilphostrol)

(dye-eth-il-stil-bess'trole)
Hormone
Estrogen
Antineoplastic

ACTIONS AND USES. Nonsteroidal synthetic estrogen with same actions, uses, absorption, fate, contraindications, and precautions as estradiol (qv). Exerts significant cytolytic action in treatment of prostatic carcinoma. Well tolerated in large doses; side effects are considerably less severe than those of diethylstilbestrol.

Used in advanced stages of prostatic cancer, especially when tolerance to other estrogenic regimens has developed.

ADVERSE/SIDE EFFECTS. Nausea, vomiting, dizziness. Temporary: burning and local pain in perineal and sacral regions and at metastasis sites; abdominal cramps, gynecomastia, anemia, increased prothrombin time. *See Estradiol.*

ROUTE AND DOSAGE. Oral: 50 to 200 mg three times daily depending on patient's tolerance. **Intravenous:** Initial: 0.5 Gm first day, then 1 Gm/daily for 5 or more days (depending on patient's response). Maintenance: 0.25 to 0.5 Gm once or twice weekly. Highly individualized regimens.

NURSING IMPLICATIONS

IV flow rate is usually adjusted so that after the first 10 to 15 minutes at 20 to 30 drops/minute the subsequent rate permits remainder to be administered in 1-hour period.

Patient should be lying down during infusion in order to reduce the incidence of dizziness.

Review package insert with patient to assure understanding about estrogen therapy.

Store tablets between 15° and 30°C (59° and 86°F) in tightly-covered container; injection solution: below 21°C (70°F) and protect from freezing.

See Estradiol (prototype estrogen).

DIFLORASONE DIACETATE

(Florone, Flutone, Maxiflor)

(dye-flor'a-sone)
Corticosteroid
Glucocorticoid

ACTIONS AND USES. Topical synthetic fluorinated corticosteroid with antiinflammatory, antipruritic, and vasoconstrictive activity.

Used to relieve inflammatory symptoms of a variety of skin disorders responsive to corticosteroids. *See Hydrocortisone for absorption, fate, limitations, and interactions.*

ADVERSE/SIDE EFFECTS. Dermatologic: acneiform eruptions, burning sensation, pruritus, hypertrichosis, hypopigmentation, folliculitis. With occlusive dressing: maceration of skin, atrophy, striae, secondary infection, miliaria. *See also Hydrocortisone for systemic effects.*

ROUTE AND DOSAGE. Topical: Apply small amount cream (ointment 0.05%) 1 to 3 times daily.

D

NURSING IMPLICATIONS

Before application of topical medication, cleanse skin area, then lightly rub in a thin layer of the drug.

If signs of systemic absorption, skin irritation or ulceration, hypersensitivity or infection occur, patient should notify physician.

Caution patient to apply medication as scheduled and not to change intervals or amount. Advise patient not to use the preparation for any other skin disorder, nor share the drug with anyone else.

Bandage or wrap treated area only if prescribed.

Inspect skin for infection, striae, atrophy. If present, patient should stop the drug and notify the physician.

Avoid contact of drug in or near eye.

Store drug in cool place and protect from light and heat.

See Hydrocortisone (prototype corticosteroid)for nursing implications of topical medications.

DIFLUNISAL

(Dolobid)

(dye-floo'ni-sal)
Analgesic
NSAID
Antirheumatic

ACTIONS AND USES. Long-acting nonsteroidal antiinflammatory drug (NSAID) with analgesic properties. Derived from salicylic acid, but is not hydrolyzed to salicylate in the body. Precise mode of action not known but appears to be related to inhibition of prostaglandin synthesis. Comparable to aspirin and acetaminophen in equianalgesic doses but has longer duration of effect. However, onset of analgesic action may be delayed unless loading dose is used. Unlike aspirin, inhibition of platelet function and effect on bleeding time are dose-related and reversible, lasting only about 24 hours after drug is discontinued. Reportedly has lower incidence of gastric erosion and significant fecal blood loss than aspirin. Exerts very mild antipyretic effect; therefore is not clinically useful for this purpose. Habituation, tolerance, or addiction have not been reported.

Used for acute and long-term relief of mild to moderate pain, and for symptomatic treatment of osteoarthritis and rheumatoid arthritis.

ABSORPTION AND FATE. Onset of analgesia usually within 1 hour, peak effect within 2 to 3 hours, and duration 12 hours. Peak plasma levels: 2 to 3 hours. Plasma protein binding: 98 to 99%. Half-life: 10 to 12 hours (longer in patients with renal insufficiency). Steady-state plasma levels achieved in several days following multiple doses. Metabolized in liver. Excreted in urine within 72 to 96 hours, about 90% of dose as glucuronide conjugates and 3% as unchanged drug. Less than 5% eliminated in feces. Probably crosses placenta. Excreted in breast milk (in concentrations 2 to 7% of that in plasma).

CONTRAINDICATIONS AND PRECAUTIONS. Hypersensitivity to diflunisal, patients in whom aspirin, other salicylates, or other NSAIDs precipitate an acute asthmatic attack, urticaria, angioedema, or severe rhinitis; active peptic ulcer, GI bleeding. Safe use during pregnancy (category C), in nursing mothers, children, and infants not established. Use during 3rd trimester of pregnancy specifically contraindicated because NSAIDs are known to cause premature closure on ductus arteriosus in fetus. *Cautious Use:* history of upper GI disease, impaired renal function, compromised cardiac function and other conditions predisposing to fluid retention; hypertension, patients who may be adversely affected by prolonged bleeding time (BT).

ADVERSE/SIDE EFFECTS. CNS: drowsiness, insomnia, dizziness, headache, fatigue, nervousness, vertigo, asthenia, disorientation, stupor (overdosage). Causal relationships not established—depression paresthesias, malaise. **Dermatologic:** rash, erythema multiforme, Stevens–Johnson syndrome, pruritus, sweating, dry mucous membranes. **ENT:** tinnitus, hearing loss. **GI:** nausea, vomiting, dyspepsia, GI pain, diarrhea, constipation, flatulence, GI bleeding, stomatitis, peptic ulcer, anorexia, eructation, cholestatic jaundice, severe hepatic dysfunction. **Hematolgic:** prolonged BT, anemia, thrombocytopenia, elevation of liver function tests. **Ophthalmic:** blurred vision, reduced visual acuity, changes in color vision, scotomata, corneal deposits, retinal disturbances. **Other:** peripheral edema, weight gain; causal relationships not established: dysuria, dyspnea, palpitation, syncope, muscle cramps, fever, hypersensitivity reactions including interstitial nephritis with renal failure; anaphylactic reactions with bronchospasm.

D

ROUTE AND DOSAGE. Oral: *Pain relief* (loading dose) 1000 mg, followed by maintenance doses of 500 mg every 8 to 12 hours. *Osteoarthritis:* 500 to 1000 mg in two divided doses twice daily; maintenance: up to 1500 mg daily. Lower dosages and/or longer intervals for patients with impaired renal function.

NURSING IMPLICATIONS

Diflunisal may be taken with water, milk, or food. Taking medication with food may help to reduce GI irritation. Food may cause slight reduction in absorption rate, but does not affect amount absorbed.

Instruct patient to swallow tablet whole. It should not be crushed or chewed.

Caution patient to take drug as prescribed. Doubling of dosage can produce greater than doubling of drug accumulation (concentration-dependent pharmacokinetics), particularly in patients receiving repetitive doses.

Full antiinflammatory effect for arthritis may not occur until after 8 days to several weeks of therapy in some patients.

Since eye complications have been associated with the use of NSAIDs, advise patient to report the onset of eye problems immediately to physician. Ophthalmologic studies are indicated.

Patients with impaired renal function should be closely monitored for drug effect to avoid excessive drug accumulation and toxicity. Instruct patient to be aware of intake–output ratio and pattern and to observe for peripheral edema and unusual weight gain.

Patients presenting signs of hepatic dysfunction (persistent abnormally high elevation of SGPT (ALT), SGOT (AST), eosinophilia, jaundice or rash) should be evaluated for hepatic reaction.

Advise all patients and particularly those with history of GI problems to promptly report to physician the onset of melena (bloody or tarry stools), hematemesis, severe stomach pain.

Caution patient about the possibility of drug-induced drowsiness and dizziness with respect to driving and other potentially hazardous activities.

Although the antipyretic effect of diflunisal is mild, be mindful of the possibility that in chronic or high doses it may mask fever in some patients.

If used concomitantly with an anticoagulant, close monitoring of PT is advised during and for several days after concomitant use.

Treatment of overdosage: empty stomach immediately by inducing emesis or by gastric lavage. Treatment is symptomatic and supportive.

Store between 15° and 30°C (59° and 86°F) in well-closed containers, unless otherwise directed by manufacturer.

Diagnostic Test Interferences. Diflunisal can cause lowering of **serum uric acid** concentrations by as much as 1.4 mg% and increased renal clearance of uric acid.

Drug Interactions: Diflunisal

Plus	Interactions
Acetaminophen (Tylenol, etc.)	Acetaminophen plasma levels may increase by about 50%. Used concomitantly with caution and careful monitoring of hepatic function
Antacids	Significant reduction of diflunisal absorption, particularly if antacids are used routinely
Anticoagulants, oral	Increased anticoagulant (hypoprothrombinemic) effect and prothrombin time (PT)
Aspirin	Small decreases in diflunisal plasma levels. Increased risk of GI irritation and bleeding
Furosemide (Lasix)	Decreased hyperuricemic effects of furosemide
Hydrochlorothiazide	Significant increases in hydrochlorothiazide plasma levels, and decrease in hyperuricemic effect
Indomethacin (Indocin)	Increased indomethacin plasma levels. Severe GI hemorrhage reported in some patients. Concomitant use not recommended
Lithium (Eskalith)	Increased steady-state plasma lithium levels
Naproxen (Anaprox, Naprosyn)	Significant decrease in urinary excretion of naproxen
Sulindac (Clinoril)	Lowering of active sulindac metabolite plasma levels by about ⅓

PROTOTYPE

DIGITALIS LEAF

(Digifortis, Pil-Digis)

(di-ji-tal'iss)
Antiarrhythmic
Cardiac glycoside

ACTIONS AND USES. Long-acting preparation derived from dried leaves of *Digitalis purpurea.* Consists primarily of three glycosides: digitoxin (which is responsible for most of its pharmacologic action), gitoxin, and gitalin. Mechanism of action unknown, but studies suggest that glycosides affect ATPases that promote passage of calcium, sodium, and potassium ions across sarcolemma. In the steady state, concentration in myocardium is 15 to 20 times that of plasma. Chief effect is increased force of cardiac contraction by direct action on myocardium (positive inotropic effect). In congestive heart failure, digitalis increases stroke volume and cardiac output, reduces residual diastolic volume, decreases heart size, improves systemic and pulmonary circulation, and results in diuresis and reduction of venous pressures. Heart rate is slowed by direct action and by vagal action (negative chronotropic effect). Bases for use in supraventricular tachyarrhythmias include reflex vagal stimulation, depression of impulse formation at sinoatrial (SA) node, and decreased conduction rate through atrioventricular (AV) nodal and bundle tissues (negative dromotropic effect) with lengthening of refractory period.

Used in treatment and prophylaxis of congestive heart failure and supraventricular tachycardias (atrial fibrillation, atrial flutter, paroxysmal atrial tachycardia).

ABSORPTION AND FATE. About 40% absorbed following oral administration. Action begins in 2 to 4 hours, peaks in 12 to 14 hours, and diminishes over next 48 to 72 hours. Some activity persists for about 2 weeks. Approximately 97% bound to plasma proteins. Half-life: 5 to 9 days. Wide body distribution, with high concentrations in myocardium, skeletal muscles, pancreas, red blood cells, intestines, liver, and kidney. Minimal distribution to fat. Metabolized by liver; unchanged drug and metabolites excreted slowly in urine. Crosses placenta and may appear in breast milk.

CONTRAINDICATIONS AND PRECAUTIONS. Hypersensitivity to digitalis preparations; full digitalizing doses to patients on long-acting digitalis preparations during preceding 2 weeks or digoxin within 1 week; ventricular tachycardia or fibrillation, severe myocarditis, heart failure from thyrotoxicosis, diphtheria, or shock; use in treatment of obesity; use of digitalis leaf in children. Safe use during pregnancy (category C) and in nursing mothers not established. *Cautious Use:* hypothyroidism, impaired renal or hepatic function, hypokalemia, hypercalcemia, acute myocardial infarction, Stokes-Adams syndrome, recent cardiac surgery, hypersensitive carotid sinus, chronic constrictive pericarditis, idiopathic subaortic stenosis, severe pulmonary disease, elderly or debilitated patients, coronary artery disease, rheumatic carditis.

ADVERSE/SIDE EFFECTS. CNS: extreme fatigue, mental depression, lethargy, apathy, headache, drowsiness or insomnia, mood changes, restlessness, disorientation, confusion, nightmares, agitation, delirium, hallucinations, convulsions (rare), facial and lumbar neuralgia, paresthesias of hands and feet, generalized weakness. **CV:** hypotension (all types of arrhythmias and all grades of impaired conduction possible), ectopic beats (most common): premature ventricular contractions (PVCs) including multifocal PVCs, bigeminy and trigeminy; premature nodal and atrial contractions; paroxysmal atrial tachycardia with AV block, sinus bradycardia, SA block, and SA arrest; ventricular tachycardia, ventricular fibrillation, thromboembolism (particularly in atrial fibrillation with congestive failure). **GI:** anorexia, nausea, vomiting, salivation, diarrhea, abdominal pain, bowel necrosis (rare). **Hypersensitivity:** pruritus, urticaria, facial edema, fever, joint tenderness, eosinophilia, thrombocytopenia. **Ophthalmic:** disturbed color perception (objects appear yellow or green or, less frequently, red, brown, or blue), hazy vision, flickering dots, halos on dark objects, diplopia, amblyopia, scotomata, retrobulbar and optic neuritis. **Other:** gynecomastia (uncommon), fixed drug eruption.

ROUTE AND DOSAGE. Oral: Loading dose *(rapid digitalization):* 1.2 to 1.8 Gm divided into 4 or more doses and administered at 4- to 6-hour intervals over 24 to 48 hours until therapeutic response or toxic effects occur. *Slow digitalization:* 100 mg 3 times daily (usually for 4 to 7 days). Maintenance 100 mg daily. Highly individualized according to individual requirements.

NURSING IMPLICATIONS

Read label carefully. Digitalis glycosides have similar names, but they differ widely in strengths and dosages.

A careful medication history should be taken before initiation of therapy regarding any prior or recent use of digitalis glycosides.

Be familiar with the patient's baseline data (quality of peripheral pulses, blood pressure, clinical symptoms, serum electrolytes, creatinine clearance), and with blood digitoxin levels as a foundation for making sensitive assessments.

For dosage regulation the physician will rely on accurate observations and prompt reporting of signs and symptoms of toxicity and therapeutic response. Digitalis is cumulative in action.

ECG, determinations of serum electrolytes (especially potassium, calcium, and magnesium), and liver and kidney function tests should be performed prior to and periodically during digitalis glycoside therapy.

D

The following suggested guidelines (also check agency policy) are especially important during the digitalization period and whenever dosage regimen is altered. Before administering digitalis preparation: (1) Check laboratory reports; know what the physician regards as acceptable parameters for blood levels of digitalis (digitoxin), potassium, magnesium, and calcium. (2) Take apical pulse for 1 full minute noting rate, rhythm, and quality. If changes are noted, withhold digitalis, take rhythm strip, if patient is on ECG monitor; notify physician promptly. Blood digitoxin level may be ordered if toxicity is suspected. (3) Check for signs and symptoms of toxicity.

Although a fall in ventricular rate to 60/minute or below in adults (70/minute in children) is used as one criterion for withholding medication and reporting to physician, actually any change in pulse rate or rhythm should be interpreted as a sign of digitalis intoxication and should be reported (e.g., a sudden increase or decrease in rate, irregular rhythm, regularization of a chronic irregular pulse).

Some physicians prescribe apical–radial pulse determinations in patients with atrial fibrillation to determine pulse deficit (apical pulse minus radial pulse).

If patient's cardiac problem does not require immediate digitalis effect, physician may initiate therapy with maintenance dose.

Intake–output ratio and daily weight are excellent indicators of fluid mobilization or retention. Weigh the patient each day under standard conditions (before breakfast and defecation, after voiding, same scale, similar type clothing).

Report any changes in weight and intake–output ratio. Weight gain in excess of 1 or 2 pounds/day usually indicates fluid retention. Digitalis dosage should be reduced if renal function is impaired.

The elderly appear to be more sensitive to the actions of digitalis. Incidence of toxicity is high in this group. Monitor these patients closely.

A dose of digitalis that was once tolerated may produce toxicity if the patient is experiencing conditions that sensitize the myocardium to cardiotonic glycosides (e.g., hypokalemia, hypomagnesemia, hypercalcemia, hypoxia due to pulmonary dysfunction).

Manifestations of hypokalemia: anorexia, paresthesias, drowsiness, mental depression, polyuria, cardiac irritability with PVCs, hypoperistalsis, weakness of large muscle group, hypoactive reflexes, postural hypotension, dyspnea.

Intracellular potassium depletion may be induced by an inadequate potassium intake, e.g., anorexia, poor dietary habits *(see Index: Food sources, potassium),* prolonged nasogastric suction, diarrhea, indiscriminate use of laxatives, persistent vomiting. *(See also Drug Interactions.)*

The margin between therapeutic and toxic effect is extremely narrow for the digitalis glycosides.

Instruct patient to report any of the following early indications of *digitalis intoxication:* unusual fatigue, weakness, anorexia, nausea, vomiting, diarrhea for more than 1 day, headache, visual disturbances, facial neuralgia; unusually slow or irregular pulse (PVCs) may be experienced in some patients as palpitation, choking sensation, sinking feeling in pit of stomach, precordial pain, dizziness, faintness, confusion, hallucinations (particularly in the elderly), mental depression.

In patients with atrial fibrillation, slowing of ventricular rate may be used as a guide in digitalization. Generally the patient is considered digitalized when the apical rate is reduced to between 60 and 80 beats/minute at rest and 80 to 100 beats/minute with exertion. These patients tend to tolerate large doses of digitalis; however, with resumption of sinus rhythm the same digitalis level may produce serious arrhythmias.

Observe for and report therapeutic response to digitalis in congestive heart failure: relief of nausea, vomiting, anorexia, weakness, and fatigue; diuresis, with relief of dyspnea, productive cough, distended neck veins, rales, and edema; improved pulse rate and rhythm;

improved peripheral pulses; increased tolerance to mild exertion. Persistence of symptoms may indicate underdigitalization.

Rigid sodium restriction generally is not required except in severe forms of congestive failure. The physician will, however, usually prescribe reduction of salt intake.

The average American diet contains approximately 110 to 260 mEq (2500 to 6000 mg) sodium which is equivalent to 6 to 15 Gm of sodium chloride/day. By eliminating salt-rich foods and not adding salt to served foods this amount can be reduced to 90 to 150 mEq or 2000 or 3500 mg sodium. (1 teaspoon of salt contains 2.3 Gm sodium.)

Salt substitutes should be prescribed by a physician. The main ingredient is potassium chloride, e.g., Adolph's Salt Substitute, No-Salt, Nu-Salt, Neocurtasal. Not advised for patients with impaired renal function, because they tend to retain potassium.

Foods high in sodium include the following: luncheon meats; canned, salted, or smoked meats and fish; "instant" or "quick" cooked foods, canned foods, commercial frozen dinners, tomato juice, bouillon, soy sauce, Chinese foods (high in monosodium glutamate), processed cheese and cheese spreads, salted snack foods. OTC drugs high in sodium: Alka-Seltzer, Bisodol, Bromo Seltzer, Fizrin, Sal Hepatica, Soda Mints, Fleet enema.

In communities where drinking water is high in sodium, patient should be advised to use bottled water. (The public health department will supply information concerning sodium content in water.)

Licorice in large quantities can induce salt and water retention, hypokalemia, hypertension, paresthesias, and symptoms of congestive failure. (Licorice contains glycyrrhizic acid, which resembles mineralocorticoids in chemical structure.)

Advise patient not to take OTC medications (especially those for coughs, colds, allergy, constipation, diarrhea, GI upset or obesity) without prior approval of physician.

Keep digitalis preparations out of the reach of children.

Treatment of toxicity: stop digitalis and diuretic. Have on hand: potassium salts, chelating agent to bind calcium, e.g., EDTA; atropine (to reverse heart block), antiarrhythmics: procainamide, phenytoin, lidocaine, quinidine, propranolol or other adrenergic blocking agent; binding resins, e.g., cholestyramine, colestipol; ECG monitor.

Patient-Teaching Points:

Since most patients on digitalis glycosides will continue therapy for a lifetime, it is important to design a comprehensive teaching plan in collaboration with physician, patient, and responsible family members. Instructions (verbal and written) should cover the following points:

- ✓ The medical problem; drug action, and dosage regimen. Take medication at the same time each day and in relation to some daily activity or habit as a reminder. Do not skip, reduce, or double a dose.
- ✓ Keep record of drug administration by check-off calendar.
- ✓ Count pulse for 1 full minute before taking digitalis and again around peak drug action (omit if it causes anxiety). If rate or rhythm has changed significantly, withhold medication and notify physician promptly.
- ✓ Reportable signs and symptoms.
- ✓ Daily weight under standard conditions. Report weight gain of more than 4 to 5 pounds/week ("1 pint is a pound the world around"). Also report other indicators of fluid retention such as tightness of rings or shoes, puffiness or pitting edema of ankles or legs.
- ✓ Diet and fluid restrictions if any, amount of salt (sodium), coffee, tea, alcohol allowed. Weight control to reduce myocardial work load.
- ✓ Graduated physical activity program, planned relaxation time.
- ✓ Emphasize importance of maintaining daily dietary potassium intake (orange juice, bananas). *See Index: Food sources: potassium.*

✓ Consult physician before taking OTC medications.
✓ Follow-up plans.
✓ VNA referral.
✓ Medical identification, e.g., Medic Alert.

Pamphlets supplied by the American Heart Association (contact local chapter) are excellent teaching aids. Free copies are available for professional and lay use.

Digitalis preparations are preserved in tightly covered, light-resistant containers. Store preferably at 15° to 30°C (59° to 86°F), unless otherwise directed by manufacturer.

D

Diagnostic Test Interferences. Digitalis may produce false-positive **exercise tolerance** ECG test results.

Drug Interactions: Digitalis (cardiac glycosides)

Plus	Interactions
Amphotericin B (Fungizone)	Increases digitalis toxicity (arrhythmias) by inducing hypokalemia
Antacids	May impair GI absorption of digitalis glycosides; space as far apart as possible
Calcium salts, parenteral	Hypercalcemia enhances digitalis toxicity (arrhythmias)
Cholestyramine and other anionic exchange resins Colestipol (Colestid)	May impair GI absorption of digitalis glycosides; space as far apart as possible
Corticosteroids Diuretics, potassium depleting, e.g., chlorthalidone, ethacrynic acid, (Edecrin), furosemide (Lasix), thiazides	Facilitate digitalis toxicity (arrhythmias) by inducing hypokalemia and hypomagnesemia
Edrophonium (Tensilon)	Additive bradycardia effect
Glucose infusion (large amounts)	Large amounts may facilitate digitalis toxicity by inducing hypokalemia (causes intracellular shift of K)
Kaolin-pectin mixtures	May impair GI absorption of digitalis glycosides; space at least several hours apart
Neomycin	Appears to inhibit GI absorption of digoxin and possibly other digitalis glycosides; spacing doses will not prevent interaction; monitor plasma digoxin levels
Phenobarbital and other barbiturates Phenylbutazone Phenytoin (Dilantin) Rifampin (Rifadin, Rimactane)	Increase hepatic metabolism of digitoxin (also in digitalis leaf) with resulting decreased plasma digitoxin levels
Propranolol (Inderal)	Possibility of profound bradycardia
Reserpine and other rauwolfia alkaloids Succinylcholine Sympathomimetics (e.g., ephedrine, epinephrine, isoproterenol)	Increased risk of cardiac arrhythmias

DIGITOXIN

(Crystodigin, Purodigin)

(di-ji-tox'in)
Antiarrhythmic
Cardiac glycoside

D

ACTIONS AND USES. Long-acting glycoside of *Digitalis purpurea* with same actions, uses, precautions, and adverse reactions as digitalis (qv). Has slowest onset of action, slowest peak-effect time, and longest half-life of all digitalis glycosides. Therefore, generally considered more desirable for maintenance therapy rather than for rapid digitalization in emergency situations. Usually preferred over digoxin for patients with actual or suspected renal disease.

ABSORPTION AND FATE. Onset of action following IV administration occurs in ½ to 2 hours; maximum effect in 4 to 12 hours; half-life: 5 to 7 days. About 90 to 100% absorbed following oral administration; effects are noticeable in 2 to 4 hours and peak in 12 to 24 hours. Action begins to regress in 2 or 3 days; almost completely absent in 2 to 3 weeks, although ECG effects may persist 6 weeks after single dose. About 97% protein-bound. Primarily metabolized in liver to inactive metabolites (92%) and to digoxin and other active metabolites (8%), which are excreted in urine. Small amounts of inactive metabolites are also excreted in bile and feces. Active metabolites may persist in urine 4 to 12 weeks. Only 11.4% of total body store is eliminated daily.

CONTRAINDICATIONS AND PRECAUTIONS. Full digitalizing doses in patients who have received digitalis preparations during preceding 3 weeks. *Cautious Use:* pregnancy (category C), nursing women, neonates, children, the elderly. *See also Digitalis.*

ADVERSE/SIDE EFFECTS. Fatigue, generalized weakness, hallucinations, agitation, confusion, paresthesias, arrhythmias, visual disturbances, nausea, vomiting, anorexia, diarrhea, thrombocytopenic purpura (rarely). *See also Digitalis.*

ROUTE AND DOSAGE. Since distribution to body fat is minimal, dosage is usually based on ideal body weight. **Oral, intravenous, and intramuscular:** *Total digitalizing dosage:* **Adults:** 1.2 to 1.6 mg in divided doses. **Children (2 to 12 years):** 0.03 mg/kg in divided doses; **Children (1 to 2 years):** 0.04 mg/kg in divided doses; **Infants and children (2 weeks to 1 year):** 0.045 mg/kg in divided doses. **Premature, newborn, and older infants:** with reduced renal function, myocarditis: 0.022 mg/kg in divided doses. **Adults and children:** total digitalizing dosage may be divided as follows: Initial: 30 to 50% of total dosage, followed by ⅛ to ⅓ of total dosage at 4- to 6-hour intervals. Maintenance: **Adults:** 0.05 to 0.2 mg daily; most commonly 0.15 mg daily. Maintenance dosage regardless of age is usually 10% of total digitalizing dosage.

NURSING IMPLICATIONS

Not to be confused with digoxin or other digitalis glycosides.

A careful medication history should be taken to determine prior or recent use of digitalis.

Dosage must be carefully titrated. Close observation of patient, ECG monitoring, and determinations of serum electrolytes and digitoxin levels are essential to avoid toxicity.

Serum digitoxin levels exceeding 40 to 45 ng/ml support clinical diagnosis of toxicity. Therapeutic serum level ranges from 20 to 35 ng/ml.

The following suggested guidelines (also check agency policy) are especially important during digitalization period or whenever dosage regimen is altered. *Before administering digitoxin:*

- Check laboratory reports if available. (Know what the physician regards as acceptable parameters for serum levels of digitoxin, potassium, magnesium, and calcium.)
- Take apical pulse for 1 full minute noting rate, rhythm and quality. If changes are noted withhold digitalis, take rhythm strip if patient is on ECG monitor; notify physician promptly. Blood digitoxin level may be ordered if toxicity is suspected.
- Check for signs and symptoms of digitoxin toxicity *(see Digitalis).*

Digitoxin is rarely given by the IM route because it may cause painful local reaction. If prescribed, inject deep into gluteal muscle. No more than 0.4 mg should be given into any single site.

Oral digitoxin therapy should replace parenteral administration as soon as possible.

Digitoxin is slowly eliminated; it has the greatest cumulative effects of all cardiotonic glycosides. Symptoms of toxicity must be reported immediately.

Maintenance dose is generally taken in the morning. Teach the patient the importance of taking the drug at the same time each day to avoid forgetting. Taking an extra dose of digitoxin poses more danger than omitting a dose.

Stored in airtight containers protected from light preferably at 15° to 30°C (59° to 86°F), unless otherwise directed by manufacturer.

See Digitalis (prototype cardiac glycoside).

DIGOXIN

(Lanoxin, Masoxin, Novodigoxin, SK-Digoxin)

(di-jox'in)
Antiarrhythmic
Cardiac glycoside

ACTIONS AND USES. Widely used glycoside of *Digitalis lanata.* Shares actions, uses, contraindications, and adverse reactions of digitalis and other cardiotonic glycosides. Action is more prompt and less prolonged than that of digitalis and digitoxin. Also, it is less likely to give rise to cumulative effects because it is more readily absorbed and exchanged in the body and is rather rapidly excreted in urine.

Used for rapid digitalization and for maintenance therapy in congestive heart failure, atrial fibrillation, atrial flutter, paroxysmal atrial tachycardia.

ABSORPTION AND FATE. Absorption of oral liquid preparation is virtually complete (80 to 90%); absorption of tablets may vary (50 to 85%) depending upon brand. Onset of effects occurs in 1 to 2 hours; peak effects in 6 to 8 hours. Wide interindividual variation. After IM administration, action begins in 30 minutes and peaks in 4 to 6 hours (erratic absorption patterns). Action following IV dose begins within 5 to 30 minutes and peaks in 1½ to 2 hours; action regresses in 8 to 10 hours. Duration of action regardless of route: 3 to 4 days. Half-life: 34 to 44 hours. Approximately 23% protein-bound. High concentrations in myocardium, skeletal muscle, and kidney. Minimal distribution to body fat. Only 14% eliminated by hepatic metabolism; 80 to 90% of dose excreted via kidneys primarily as unchanged drug and small amounts of active metabolites. Small amounts excreted in bile via feces. Crosses placenta and may appear in breast milk (but not in toxic amounts).

CONTRAINDICATIONS AND PRECAUTIONS. Digitalis hypersensitivity, ventricular fibrillation, ventricular tachycardia unless due to congestive heart failure. Full digitalizing dose not given if patient has received digoxin during previous week or if slowly excreted cardiotonic glycoside has been given during previous 2 weeks. *Cautious Use:* renal insufficiency, hypokalemia, advanced heart disease, acute myocardial infarction, incomplete AV block, cor pulmonale, hypothyroidism, lung disease, pregnancy (category A), nursing women, premature and immature infants, children, elderly, or debilitated patients. *See also Digitalis.*

ADVERSE/SIDE EFFECTS. CNS: fatigue, muscle weakness, headache, facial neuralgia, mental depression, paresthesias, hallucinations, confusion, drowsiness, agitation, dizziness. **CV:** arrhythmias, hypotension. **GI:** anorexia, nausea, vomiting, diarrhea. **Ophthalmic:** visual disturbances. **Other:** diaphoresis, recurrent malaise, dysphagia, gynecomastia (uncommon). *See also Digitalis.*

ROUTE AND DOSAGE. Dosage is highly individualized, based upon age, renal function, and lean body weights. *Rapid digitalization:* **Oral.** *Digitalizing dose:* **Adults and Children over 10 years:** 10 to 15 mcg/kg; **Children 5 to 10 years:** 20 to 35 mcg/kg. **2 to 5 years:** 30 to 40 mcg/kg; **1 to 24 months:** 35 to 60 mcg/kg; **Neonates:** 35 to 60 mcg/kg. **Intravenous.** *Digitalizing dose:* **Adults and children older than 10 years:** 8 to 12 mcg/kg; **Children 5 to 10 years:** 15 to 30 mcg/kg; **2 to 5 years:** 25 to 30 mcg/kg; **1 to 24 months:** 30 to 50 mcg/kg; **Neonates:** 20 to 30 mcg/kg. Maintenance: 25 to 35% of digitalizing dose. *Slow digitalization:* Steady-state serum digoxin concentration is usually achieved in 5 half-lives of the drug (requires about 1 to 3 weeks). Maintenance: **Adults and children over 10 years:** 100 to 375 mcg/day. **Children under 10 years:** 25 to 35% of total calculated daily dose of digoxin for rapid digitalization. **Elderly:** (creatinine clearance (Cr) 10 to 25 ml/minute): 0.125 mg/day; (26 to 49 ml/minute): 0.1875 mg/day; (50 to 79 ml/minute): 0.25 mg/day.

NURSING IMPLICATIONS

Not to be confused with digitoxin or other digitalis glycosides.

Digoxin may be given without regard to food unless otherwise directed by physician. Administration of digoxin after meals or food may slightly delay rate of absorption but total amount absorbed is not affected.

Tablet may be crushed and mixed with fluid or food if patient cannot swallow it whole.

A careful medication history should be taken before initiation of therapy regarding any prior or recent use of digitalis glycosides.

Be familiar with patient's baseline data: (e.g., quality of peripheral pulses, blood pressure, clinical symptoms, serum electrolytes, creatinine clearance) as a foundation for making sensitive assessments. Evaluations of these data guide dosage titration.

The following suggested guidelines (also check agency policy) are especially important during digitalization period or whenever dosage regimen is altered. Before administering digoxin:

- ✓ Check laboratory reports (know what the physician regards as acceptable parameters for serum levels of digoxin, potassium, magnesium, and calcium).
- ✓ Take apical pulse for 1 full minute noting rate, rhythm, and quality. If changes are noted, withhold digoxin, take rhythm strip if patient is on ECG monitor, notify physician promptly. Blood digoxin levels may be ordered if toxicity is suspected.
- ✓ Check for signs and symptoms of digoxin toxicity.

Although a fall in ventricular rate to 60/minute in adults (70/minute in children) is used as one criterion for withholding medication and reporting to physician, actually any change in pulse rate or rhythm should be interpreted as a sign of digitalis intoxication and should be reported promptly, e.g., sudden increase or decrease in heart rate, irregular rhythm, regularization of a chronically irregular pulse.

In children cardiac arrhythmias are usually more reliable signs of early toxicity. Early indicators of toxicity in adults (anorexia, nausea, vomiting, diarrhea, paresthesias, facial neuralgia, headaches, hallucinations, confusion, visual disturbances) occur rarely as initial signs in children.

Therapeutic range of serum digoxin is 0.8 to 2 ng/ml; toxic levels: > 2 ng/ml. Blood samples for determining plasma digoxin levels should be drawn at least 5 to 6 hours after daily dose and preferably just before next scheduled daily dose.

When patient is controlled on maintenance doses, generally radial pulse is taken for 1 full minute before drug administration. If abnormalities are detected, check apical pulse for 1 full minute and notify physician.

When digoxin is prescribed for atrial fibrillation, patient should be advised to report to physician if pulse falls below 60 or rises above 110 or if he or she detects skipped beats or other changes in rhythm.

D

The IM route is infrequently used because injection causes intense pain that may last for several days; it is also associated with erratic absorption patterns. Use in diabetics or in patients with poor tissue perfusion not advised.

If prescribed, make IM injection deep into large muscle mass and follow by massage. No more than 0.5 mg should be injected into a single IM site.

Direct IV injection of digoxin may be administered undiluted or diluted in dextrose 5% in water or sodium chloride 0.9% (if prescribed).

Infiltration of parenteral drug into subcutaneous tissue can cause local irritation and sloughing.

Monitor intake–output ratio during digitalization period particularly in patients with impaired renal function. Delayed or diminished renal excretion of drug can lead to toxicity. Observe for edema daily and auscultate chest for rales. Note patient's food intake. Anorexia is an early sign of toxicity.

Alterations of digoxin absorption may occur in patients with hypermotility secondary to laxative abuse and in patients with malabsorption syndrome.

Diarrhea from any cause leads to potassium loss and increased risk of digitalis toxicity. If it is a problem consult physician regarding an antidiarrheal medication.

Concurrent antibiotic/digoxin therapy could precipitate toxicity because of altered intestinal flora. Monitor serum digoxin levels closely to determine reduced bioavailability.

Creatinine clearance may be used to determine the need for dosage adjustment particularly in the elderly and other patients with impaired renal function. (Renal excretion of digoxin is reduced in proportion to creatinine clearance.) *Normal creatinine clearance:* males: 110 to 150 ml/minute; females: 105 to 132 ml/minute.

Instruct patient to weigh him- or herself each day under standard conditions: before breakfast and defecation, after voiding; same scale; similar type clothing. Advise patient to report weight gain in excess of 2 pounds a day.

If quinidine is to be added to treatment regimen, digoxin dose should be reduced by 30 to 50% to prevent digoxin toxicity *(see Drug Interactions).* Patient should be monitored for clinical and ECG indications of toxicity, and serum digoxin levels. Because syncope is a side effect of quinidine, observe necessary safety precautions. When quinidine is discontinued, serum digoxin concentrations may fall below therapeutic levels.

Although the FDA has recently established bioavailability standards for all marketed digoxin, patient should be informed that it is advisable to continue with the same brand originally prescribed unless otherwise directed by physician.

Dosage should be carefully titrated and patient closely observed when being transferred from one preparation (tablet, elixir, or parenteral) to another. For example, when tablet is replaced by elixir, potential for toxicity is increased because approximately 30% more of drug is absorbed.

Advise patient to reduce total daily salt intake by omitting obviously salty foods and table salt. *See Digitalis.*

Instruct patient to take digoxin precisely as prescribed, not to skip or double a dose or change dose intervals and to take it at the same time each day. Suggest taking drug in relation to some daily activity as a reminder and to keep a diary of drug administration such as a check-off calendar.

Caution patient not to remove digoxin from original container and not to mix it with other tablets in a pillbox.

When using elixir formulation, measure dose with specially calibrated dropper supplied.

Advise patient to keep digoxin out of reach of children.

Caution patient not to take OTC medications, especially those for coughs, colds, allergy, GI upset, or obesity without prior approval of physician.

Do not use parenteral solution if a precipitate or discoloration is present.
Preserved in airtight containers protected from light preferably at 15° to 30°C (59° to 86°F), unless otherwise directed by manufacturer.
See also Digitalis (prototype cardiac glycoside).

D

Diagnostic Test Interferences. Significant elevations of **creatinine phosphokinase (CPK)** may follow IM administration.

Drug Interactions: Digoxin

Plus	Interactions
Antacids, Cholestyramine	May decrease absorption of digoxin
Metoclopramide (Reglan)	May reduce digoxin absorption by increasing GI tract motility
Neomycin	Inhibits GI absorption of digoxin; spacing will not prevent interaction; monitor serum digoxin levels
Propantheline (Pro-Banthine)	May increase GI absorption of digoxin (by decreasing GI motility). Reportedly digoxin elixir not affected as much as tablet form
Quinidine	Increased risk of digoxin toxicity; (reduces renal clearance of digoxin)
Spironolactone (Aldactone)	Decreases renal tubular elimination of digoxin leading to toxicity
Sulfasalazine	May reduce bioavailability of digoxin
Thyroid preparations	Increases risk of digoxin toxicity
See also Digitalis	

DIHYDROERGOTAMINE MESYLATE

(D.H.E. 45, Hydergine)

(dye-hye-droe-er-got'a-meen)
Alpha-adrenergic blocking agent
Antimigraine agent
Ergot alkaloid

ACTIONS AND USES. Alpha-adrenergic blocking agent and dihydrogenated ergot alkaloid with direct constricting effect on smooth muscle of peripheral and cranial blood vessels. Has somewhat weaker vasoconstrictor action than ergotamine (qv), but greater adrenergic blocking activity. Toxicity potential is about one-tenth that of parent drug. Lacks uterine stimulating action in therapeutic dose. Offers no advantage if equipotent doses are compared with ergotamine.

Used to prevent or abort vascular headache (e.g., migraine or histaminic cephalalgia) when rapid control is desired or other routes are not feasible. *Unlabeled Use:* with low dose heparin therapy to prevent postoperative deep vein thrombosis.

ABSORPTION AND FATE. Onset of action in 15 to 30 minutes following IM injection, less than 5 minutes following IV; duration 3 to 4 hours. Half-life: 1.3 to 3.9 hours.

CONTRAINDICATIONS AND PRECAUTIONS. History of hypersensitivity to ergot preparations; presence of peripheral vascular disease, coronary heart disease, hypertension, peptic ulcer, impaired hepatic or renal function, sepsis. Safe use during pregnancy (category X), in nursing women, and in children not established. *See also Ergotamine.*

ADVERSE/SIDE EFFECTS. Numbness and tingling in fingers and toes, muscle pains and weakness of legs, precordial distress and pain, transient tachycardia or bradycardia, nausea, vomiting, localized edema and itching; ergotism (excessive doses). *See Ergotamine.*

ROUTE AND DOSAGE. Intramuscular, intravenous: 1 mg, may be repeated at 1-hour intervals to a total of 3 mg. Not to exceed 6 mg/week.

D

NURSING IMPLICATIONS

Drug is given at first warning of migraine headache. Optimum results are obtained by titrating the doses required to give relief for several headaches to determine the minimal effective dose. This dose is used for subsequent attacks.

Onset of action after IM injection is delayed about 20 minutes; therefore, when more rapid relief is required, the IV route is prescribed.

Protect ampuls from heat and light; do not freeze. Discard ampul if solution becomes discolored.

Store preferably at 15° to 30°C (59° to 86°F), unless otherwise directed by manufacturer.

See Ergotamine Tartrate (prototype ergot alkaloid).

DIHYDROTACHYSTEROL

(DHT, Hytakerol)

(dye-hye-droe-tak-iss′ter-ole)
Vitamin
Regulator, blood calcium

ACTIONS AND USES. Oil-soluble reduction product of ergocalciferol (vitamin D_2) with pharmacologic actions similar to those of both ergocalciferol and parathyroid hormone. In comparison with ergocalciferol, dihydrotachysterol has weak antirachitic activity, promotes less intestinal absorption of calcium but almost equal phosphate diuresis. In equivalent high doses has shorter duration of action and thus less potential hazards of hypercalcemia than ergocalciferol, and is more effective in mobilization of calcium from bone. (1 mg = 120,000 units of ergocalciferol.) Acts like parathyroid hormone in ability to raise serum calcium concentrations rapidly; also reported to increase intestinal absorption of sodium, potassium, and magnesium.

Used in treatment of hypocalcemia associated with hypoparathyroidism, both postoperative and idiopathic, and in pseudohypoparathyroidism. Also used for prophylaxis of hypocalcemic tetany following thyroid surgery. *Investigational Use:* treatment of vitamin-D-resistant rickets (familial hypophosphatemia), osteoporosis, and renal osteodystrophy.

ABSORPTION AND FATE. Maximum hypercalcemic effects occur within 2 weeks (within 1 week following loading doses). Following withdrawal, calcium blood levels decrease markedly within 4 or 5 days; hypercalcemic effects can persist up to 9 weeks. Metabolized by liver only; major metabolite 40% more active than parent drug. Probably secreted into bile and excreted in feces as active and inactive metabolites. Excreted in breast milk.

CONTRAINDICATIONS AND PRECAUTIONS. Sensitivity to vitamin D; hypercalcemia and hypocalcemia associated with renal insufficiency and hyperphosphatemia; renal stones, hypervitaminosis D. Safe use during pregnancy and in nursing mothers not established.

ADVERSE/SIDE EFFECTS. Overdosage: (hypercalcemia): drowsiness, anorexia, nausea, vomiting, headache, weakness, diarrhea, constipation, abdominal pain, vertigo, ataxia, atonia, mental depression, tinnitus, dry mouth, thirst, metallic taste, nocturia, polyuria, renal calculi. *See Ergocalciferol.*

ROUTE AND DOSAGE. **Oral:** Initial: 0.8 to 2.4 mg once daily for several days. Maintenance: 0.2 to 1 mg daily as required for normal serum calcium levels (average dose is 0.6 mg daily). Usually supplemented with 10- to 15-Gm per day of calcium lactate or gluconate by mouth. Available in capsule, tablet, and solution forms.

D

NURSING IMPLICATIONS

Careful monitoring of serum and urinary calcium levels is essential. The margin between a therapeutic dose and one causing hypercalcemia is very small. Serum calcium level should be maintained between 8.5 and 10.5 mg/dl.

Adequate calcium intake is necessary for clinical response to dihydrotachysterol therapy. Consult physician regarding allowable dietary calcium.

Patients with hyperphosphatemia as in renal osteodystrophy will require dietary restriction of phosphate and/or administration of aluminum gels to bind intestinal phosphates in order to prevent metastatic calcification.

Hypoparathyroid patients receiving thiazide diuretics are prone to develop hypercalcemia and therefore require close monitoring.

Withhold drug if symptoms of hypercalcemia appear *(see Adverse/Side Effects)* and report to physician.

Preserved in tightly closed, light-resistant glass containers. Store at 15° to 30°C (59° to 86°F), unless otherwise directed by manufacturer.

See Ergocalciferol.

DIHYDROXYALUMINUM SODIUM CARBONATE *Antacid*

(Rolaids)

ACTIONS AND USES. Combines antacid properties of sodium bicarbonate (as sodium carbonate) and aluminum hydroxide and therefore has systemic and nonsystemic effects. Has rapid onset of action due to sodium carbonate; prolonged action is attributed to aluminum hydroxide. Each tablet contains 53 mg of sodium.

CONTRAINDICATIONS AND PRECAUTIONS. Aluminum sensitivity, severe renal disease, patients on sodium-restricted diets, dehydration. *Cautious Use:* elderly patients, history of congestive heart failure.

ADVERSE/SIDE EFFECTS. Constipation, intestinal concretions.

ROUTE AND DOSAGE. **Oral:** 1 or 2 tablets 4 or more times daily, as required.

NURSING IMPLICATIONS

Instruct patient to chew tablet thoroughly before swallowing and to take it with water or milk.

Constipation occurs commonly and may be managed by alternating with a magnesium containing antacid.

Inform patient that Rolaids are not suitable for long-term or frequent use.

In common with other antacids, this drug can cause premature disintegration and absorption of enteric-coated tablets and may interfere with absorption of oral tetracyclines and other oral medications. In general, it is advisable not to take other oral drugs within 1 or 2 hours of an antacid.

Store in airtight containers.

See Aluminum hydroxide (prototype antacid).

DILOXANIDE FUROATE

(Entamide, Furamide)

(dye-lox'a-nide)
Antiinfective
Amebicide

ACTIONS AND USES. Investigational acetanilide with direct amebicidal action and low degree of toxicity. Mechanism of action not established. Acts principally in bowel lumen in cyst-carrier and cyst-passing states. Reportedly not effective for use alone in patients with acute amebic dysentery or who are passing trophozoites; also of no value in extraintestinal amebiasis.

Used for treatment of intestinal amebiasis particularly in asymptomatic cyst-passers. Has been used as supplement with chloroquine, oxytetracycline, and tetracycline in treatment of acute and chronic intestinal amebiasis.

ABSORPTION AND FATE. About 90% absorbed from GI tract. Blood concentrations peak within 1 hour following administration, but decline quickly over 6-hour period. Rapidly excreted in urine largely as glucuronide. Some excretion in feces.

CONTRAINDICATIONS AND PRECAUTIONS. Safe use during pregnancy and in children under 2 years not established.

ADVERSE/SIDE EFFECTS. Infrequent: nausea, vomiting, esophagitis, persistent or recurrent diarrhea, abdominal cramps, flatulence, pruritus, urticaria, albuminuria, tingling sensations.

ROUTE AND DOSAGE. Oral: Adults: 500 mg three times daily for 10 days. **Children:** 20 mg/kg daily divided into three doses, for 10 days. A course of treatment may be repeated, if necessary.

NURSING IMPLICATIONS

This investigational agent may be requested from Parasitic Division Drug Service, Bureau of Epidemiology, Centers for Disease Control, by calling 404–329–3670 (8:00 AM to 4:30 PM Monday through Friday); after hours call 404–329–3644.

Administer drug with meals to reduce risk of GI irritation.

Inform patient that absence of symptoms is not an indication of cure. Amebiasis is considered cured when no cysts or trophozoites of *Entamoeba histolytica* are found in repeated stool specimens at 6-month intervals.

Urge patient to remain under medical supervision until discharged by physician.

Household members and other suspected contacts should have microscopic examination of feces.

Review with patient and contacts preventive measures for controlling spread of amebiasis:

- sanitary disposal of feces
- boil drinking water when necessary (chlorination does not generally destroy cysts; diatomaceous earth filters remove them completely, and filtration removes nearly all cysts)

- personal hygiene such as handwashing after defecation and before preparing or eating food; risks of eating raw foods
- fly control

Incubation period is commonly 3 to 4 weeks (range 5 days to several months).
Store medication in well-covered container. Protect from light.
See metronidazole (prototype amebicide).

D

DILTIAZEM
(Cardizem)

(dil-tye'a-zem)
Antianginal
Antiarrhythmic
Vasodilator
Calcium channel blocking agent

ACTIONS AND USES. Slow channel blocker (class 4 antiarrhythmic agent) with pharmacologic actions similar to those of others in this class (verapamil, nefedipine). Antianginal action and increased exercise tolerance result from potent coronary dilatation effects and increased availability of oxygen for myocardial work. Diltiazem prevents transmembrane influx of extracellular calcium ions (Ca) during depolarization of cardiac and vascular smooth muscle without affecting serum calcium levels. Exact mechanism is not clear but it appears that the membrane slow channels may be deformed or the ion-control gating mechanism may be inhibitied so that Ca cannot enter the cell. It may also interfere with release of intracellular Ca from the sarcoplasm reticulum. Deprivation of free intracellular Ca ions prevents contraction, thereby dilating the main coronary and systemic arteries. Inhibition of coronary artery spasm increases oxygen delivery to myocardial tissue while dilatation of systemic vasculature results in decreased total peripheral resistance, afterload, and systemic blood pressure. Slightly decreases myocardial contractility; prolongs AV nodal refractory period.

Used in management of spontaneous coronary artery spasm (Printzmetal's variant angina), and chronic stable (classic effort-associated) angina. *Unlabeled Use:* essential hypertension, and refractory migraine headache.

ABSORPTION AND FATE. Approximately 80% of oral dose rapidly absorbed from GI tract. Extensive first-pass metabolism in liver resulting in low bioavailability with first dose (40%). Detectable plasma levels in 30 minutes; peak concentration in 2 to 3 hours; 70 to 85% protein bound. Half-life: about 3.5 to 9 hours at steady state (may increase in the elderly, but only slight increase in renal impairment). 2 to 4% drug eliminated in urine unchanged; remainder eliminated in urine and bile as metabolites.

CONTRAINDICATIONS AND PRECAUTIONS. Known hypersensitivity to the drug; sick sinus syndrome (unless pacemaker is in place and functioning); second- or third-degree AV block; severe hypotension (systolic less than 90 mm Hg or diastolic less than 60 mm Hg). Safety and efficacy in children not established; pregnancy (category C). *Cautious Use:* congestive heart failure (especially if patient is also receiving beta blocker), renal or hepatic impairment, the elderly, nursing mothers.

ADVERSE/SIDE EFFECTS. CV: Second- or third-degree AV block, bradycardia, congestive heart failure, asymptomatic systole, flushing, hypotension, syncope, palpitation, arrhythmias. **Dermatologic:** rash, photosensitivity, petechiae, urticaria, pruritus. **GI:** anorexia, nausea, vomiting, diarrhea, constipation, pyrosis. **Neurologic:** headache, fatigue, nervousness, depression, drowsiness, insomnia, confusion. **Other:** edema, acute renal failure.

ROUTE AND DOSAGE. Oral: 30 mg four times/day; dose is increased at 1- to 2-day intervals until optimal antianginal effect obtained (usually no more than 240 mg/day). Geriatric patient: lower doses.

D

NURSING IMPLICATIONS

Administer before meals and at bedtime. Tablet may be crushed if necessary and administered with a liquid of patient's choice.

Therapeutic blood level: 0.025 to 0.1 mcg/ml.

If patient is also receiving digoxin, serum digoxin concentration should be determined and patient should be monitored for signs and symptoms of digitalis toxicity.

Has been used concomitantly with short- or long-acting nitrates, but antianginal effectiveness needs to be studied further.

See Verapamil, prototype calcium channel blocking agent, for additional Nursing Implications, Drug Interactions.

DIMENHYDRINATE

(dye-men-hye'dri-nate)

(Dimentabs, Dinate, Dommanate, Dramaban, Dramilin, Dramamine, Dramocen, Dramoject, Dymenate, Hydrate, Marmine, Motion-Aid, Nauseatol, Reidamine, Travamine, Wehamine)

Antihistamine, H_1-receptor antagonist
Antiemetic, antivertigo agent

ACTIONS AND USES. Ethanolamine derivative and chlorotheophylline salt of diphenhydramine (qv), with which it shares similar properties. Precise mode of antinauseant action not known, but thought to be due to ability to inhibit cholinergic stimulation in vestibular and associated neural pathways.

Used chiefly in prevention and treatment of motion sickness. Also has been used in management of vertigo, nausea, and vomiting associated with radiation sickness, labyrinthitis, Meniere's syndrome, stapedectomy, anesthesia, and various medications.

ABSORPTION AND FATE. Duration of action approximately 3 to 6 hours. Small amounts excreted in breast milk. *See also Diphenhydramine.*

CONTRAINDICATIONS AND PRECAUTIONS. History of hypersensitivity to dimenhydrate or its components; narrow-angle glaucoma, prostatic hypertrophy. Safe use during pregnancy, in nursing women, and in neonates not established. *Cautious Use:* convulsive disorders.

ADVERSE/SIDE EFFECTS. CNS: drowsiness, headache, incoordination, dizziness, nervousness, restlessness, insomnia (especially children); hypotension, palpitation, blurred vision, dry mouth, nose, throat. Less frequently: anorexia, constipation or diarrhea, urinary frequency, dysuria. *See also Diphenhydramine.*

ROUTE AND DOSAGE. Adults: Oral: 50 to 100 mg every 4 to 6 hours. Not to exceed 400 mg/24 hours. **Intramuscular, intravenous:** 50 mg. For intravenous use, each 50 mg (1 ml) should be diluted in 10 ml of 0.9% sodium chloride injection; rate of administration, 2 minutes for each 50 mg. **Children: Intramuscular:** 1.25 mg/kg 4 times daily up to maximum of 300 mg daily. IV dosage not established for children. **Oral: Children (up to 12 years):** 25 to 50 mg every 6 to 8 hours. Not to exceed 150 mg/24 hours. **Children (2 to 6 years):** up to 25 mg every 6 to 8 hours. Not to exceed 75 mg/24 hours. Available in tablets, liquid, injection.

NURSING IMPLICATIONS

High incidence of drowsiness; this is often a desirable reaction for some patients. Bedsides and supervision of ambulation may be advisable. Caution ambulatory patient not to drive or operate dangerous machinery until drowsiness has passed.

To prevent radiation sickness, drug is usually administered 30 to 60 minutes before treatment, then repeated 1½ hours after treatment and again in 3 hours.
To prevent motion sickness, dimenhydrinate should be taken 30 minutes before departure and should be repeated before meals and upon retiring.
Some claim that motion sickness can largely be prevented by (1) avoiding fatty food intake before the trip; (2) eating lightly prior to and during travel; (3) munching on crackers or other complex carbohydrate during the trip. An empty stomach may actually contribute to the feeling of nausea. Other steps that may be taken: do not drink alcohol on day of travel; travel at night so as to eliminate visual causes of motion sickness.
Tolerance to CNS depressant effects usually occurs after a few days of drug therapy. Some decrease in antiemetic action may result with prolonged use.
Avoid mixing parenteral preparation with other drugs. Dimenhydrinate is incompatible with many solutions.
Store preferably between 15° and 30°C (59° and 86°F), unless otherwise directed by manufacturer. Examine parenteral preparation for particulate matter and discoloration. Do not use unless absolutely clear.

D

Drug Interactions. Dimenhydrinate may mask ototoxic symptoms associated with **aminoglycoside antibiotics.** Enhanced CNS depression (drowsiness) may occur when antihistamines are used concurrently with **alcohol, barbiturates,** and other **CNS depressants.** *See Diphenhydramine hydrochloride (prototype ethanolamine antihistamine).*

DIMERCAPROL

(BAL in Oil, British Anti-Lewisite)

(dye-mer-kap'role)
Antidote
Chelating agent

ACTIONS AND USES. Dithiol compound originally developed as antidote for Lewisite, an arsenic-containing chemical warfare agent. Combines with ions of various heavy metals to form relatively stable, nontoxic, soluble complexes called chelates (mercaptides), which can be excreted; inhibition of sulfhydryl enzymes by toxic metals is thus prevented. May also reactivate affected enzymes, but most effective when administered prior to enzyme damage.

Used in treatment of acute poisoning by arsenic, gold, and mercury; as adjunct to edetate calcium disodium in treatment of lead encephalopathy and as adjunct to penicillamine to increase rate of copper excretion in Wilson's disease. *Investigational Use* (topical): to treat chromium dermatitis; ocular and dermatologic manifestations of arsenic poisoning.

ABSORPTION AND FATE. Peak blood levels in 30 to 60 minutes. Distributed mainly in intercellular spaces including brain; highest concentrations in liver and kidneys. Short half-life. Free dimercaprol (uncomplexed) is rapidly metabolized to inactive products and excreted in urine and feces via bile. Metabolic degradation and urinary excretion essentially complete within 4 hours.

CONTRAINDICATIONS AND PRECAUTIONS. Hepatic insufficiency (with exception of postarsenical jaundice); pregnancy; severe renal insufficiency; concurrent iron therapy; treatment of poisoning due to cadmium, iron, selenium. Safe use during pregnancy and lactation not established. *Cautious Use:* hypertension, patients with G6PD deficiency.

ADVERSE/SIDE EFFECTS. Listed in approximate order of frequency, high doses are associated with: elevated blood pressure, tachycardia, nausea, vomiting, headache; burning sensation of lips, mouth, throat; feeling of constriction and pain in throat, chest, or hands; conjunctivitis, lacrimation, rhinorrhea, blepharospasm, salivation, paresthesias, burning sensation in penis, sweating, abdominal pain; local pain, sterile abscess at injection site; anxiety, weakness, restlessness, reduction in polymorphonuclear leukocytes; transient fever (in children). Toxic doses: tremors, convulsions, shock, metabolic acidosis with elevated serum lactate levels.

ROUTE AND DOSAGE. Intramuscular: *Mild arsenic or gold poisoning:* 2.5 mg/kg body weight four times a day for first 2 days, two times on third day, then once daily for 10 days. *Severe arsenic or gold poisoning:* 3 mg/kg body weight every 4 hours for first 2 days, then four times a day on third day, then twice daily thereafter for 10 days. *Mercury poisoning:* initial: 5 mg/kg body weight, followed by 2.5 mg/kg one or two times daily for 10 days. *Acute lead encephalopathy:* 4 mg/kg (first dose), thereafter every 4 hours with edetate calcium disodium (EDTA). Use separate sites. For less severe poisoning, 3 mg/kg after first dose. Treatment continued 2 to 7 days depending upon response.

NURSING IMPLICATIONS

Because irreversible tissue damage may occur quickly, particularly in mercury poisoning, dimercaprol therapy must be initiated as soon as possible (within 1 or 2 hours) after ingestion.

Usual emergency treatment for the particular poison should be instituted, as well as maintenance of body heat, fluids, electrolytes, and other supportive measures.

Administered only by deep IM injection. Local pain, gluteal abscess, and skin sensitization reported. Rotate injection sites and observe daily. If EDTA is to be given note that it should be administered in a separate site.

Monitor vital signs. Elevations of systolic and diastolic blood pressures accompanied by tachycardia frequently occur within a few minutes following injection and may remain elevated up to 2 hours. Degree of blood pressure elevation is roughly proportional to dose administered.

Fever occurs in approximately 30% of children receiving treatment and may persist throughout therapy (reaction is apparently peculiar to children).

Intake and output should be monitored. Drug is potentially nephrotoxic. Report oliguria or change in intake and output ratio. If renal insufficiency develops, drug should be discontinued or used with extreme caution, since toxic serum concentrations may result.

Urine should be kept alkaline (e.g., with acetazolamide, sodium citrate) to reduce possibility of renal damage during elimination of dimercaprol chelate. In acid medium, chelate rapidly dissociates and releases bound metal.

Daily urine examinations should be made for albumin, blood, casts, and pH. Blood and urinary levels of the metal serve as guides for dosage adjustments.

Minor adverse reactions usually reach maximum 15 to 20 minutes after drug administration and generally subside in 30 to 90 minutes. Ephedrine or an antihistamine is sometimes administered to prevent symptoms.

Contact of drug with skin may produce erythema, edema, dermatitis. Handle with caution.

Dimercaprol may impart an unpleasant garliclike odor to patient's breath. Inform patient.

Presence of sediment in ampul reportedly does not indicate drug deterioration.

Diagnostic Test Interferences. **^{131}I thyroidal uptake** values may be decreased if test is done during or immediately following dimercaprol therapy.

Drug Interactions. Dimercaprol forms toxic complexes with **iron, cadmium, selenium,** and **uranium.**

DIMETHYL SULFOXIDE

(DMSO, Kemsol, Rimso-50)

(dye-meth'il sul-fox'ide)
Antiinflammatory

ACTIONS AND USES. Mechanism of action not known. Reported actions attributed to dimethyl sulfoxide (DMSO) include antiinflammatory effects, membrane penetration, collagen dissolution, peripheral nerve blockade (local analgesia), vasodilation, muscle relaxation, diuresis, weak bacteriostatic and antifungal actions, initiation of histamine release at administration site, cholinesterase inhibition. Enhances percutaneous absorption of many drugs by increasing permeability of skin. Lens opacities have been observed in certain mammalian test animals receiving high doses for prolonged periods.

Used for symptomatic treatment of interstitial cystitis. *Investigational Use:* topical treatment of a variety of musculoskeletal disorders, arthritis, scleroderma, and other related collagen diseases, and as a carrier to enhance penetration and absorption of other drugs. Also used to protect living cells and tissues during cold storage (cryoprotection). Widely used as an industrial solvent (paint remover; antifreeze), and in veterinary medicine for treatment of musculoskeletal injuries, particularly in bones.

ABSORPTION AND FATE. Rapidly absorbed and widely distributed in tissues and body fluids. Peak serum levels in 4 to 8 hours following topical application. Penetrates blood–brain barrier. Small amount metabolized to dimethyl sulfide which is eliminated through lungs and skin. Also metabolized to dimethyl sulfone which may remain in serum for longer than 2 weeks; this metabolite is slowly excreted in urine and feces. Some unchanged drug is also eliminated in urine and feces. May be excreted in breast milk.

CONTRAINDICATIONS AND PRECAUTIONS. Hypersensitivity to dimethyl sulfoxide; urinary tract malignancy. Safe use during pregnancy, in nursing mothers, and in children not established. *Cautious Use:* hepatic or renal dysfunction.

ADVERSE/SIDE EFFECTS. Dermatologic: following instillation: garliclike odor on skin; following topical application: erythema, itching, and burning sensation; maceration (prolonged use of high concentration). **Hypersensitivity:** pruritus, urticaria, skin rash, swelling of face, dyspnea (anaphylactoid reaction). **Ophthalmic:** transient disturbances in color vision, photophobia. **Other:** nasal congestion, shortness of breath, garliclike odor on breath, garliclike taste; discomfort during administration; following topical application to skin: headache, nausea, diarrhea.

ROUTE AND DOSAGE. Intravesical instillation: 50 ml of a 50% solution instilled slowly into urinary bladder and retained for 15 minutes. Treatment repeated every 2 weeks until maximum relief obtained, then intervals between treatment may be increased.

NURSING IMPLICATIONS

Manufacturer suggests application of analgesic lubricant such as lidocaine jelly to urethra to facilitate insertion of catheter.

Instruct patient to retain instillation for 15 minutes and then to expel it by spontaneous voiding (unless otherwise prescribed by physician).

Discomfort associated with instillation usually becomes less prominent with repeated administration. Physician may prescribe an oral analgesic or suppository containing belladonna and an opiate prior to instillation to reduce bladder spasm. In patients with severely sensitive bladders, first few treatments may be done under saddle block anesthesia.

Inform patient that a garliclike taste may be experienced within minutes after drug instillation which may last for several hours. Garliclike odor on breath and skin may last 72 hours.

Complete blood cell counts, and liver and renal function tests are recommended, initially and at 6-month intervals.
Complete eye evaluation including slit-lamp examination is recommended prior to and at regular intervals during therapy.
Caution patient not to use OTC topical medications without consulting physician.
Patient should be informed that FDA has approved DMSO as being safe and effective only for symptomatic relief of interstitial cystitis and not for any other indication.
Preferably stored between 15° and 30°C (59° and 86°F), unless otherwise directed by manufacturer. Protect from strong light, and avoid contact with plastics.

D

Drug Interactions. DMSO may potentiate actions of other concomitantly administered medications.

PROTOTYPE

DINOPROST TROMETHAMINE

(dye'noe-prost)

($PGF_{2\alpha}$, Prostaglandin F_2 Alpha Tromethamine, Prostin F_2 Alpha)

Abortifacient
Oxytocic
Prostaglandin
Hormone

ACTIONS AND USES. Salt of naturally occurring hormone in the prostaglandin F series. Abortifacient action imitates and augments contractions of the nonpregnant and pregnant uterus. Unlike ergot alkaloids and other oxytocics, dinoprost ($PGF_{2\alpha}$) can induce labor anytime during pregnancy. Sensitivity of the gravid uterus to prostaglandins increases as gestation progresses: i.e., rate of success of abortifacient action in first trimester is low, but increases during second and third trimesters. Physiologic response of the uterus in late pregnancy to $PGF_{2\alpha}$ is reportedly similar to that of oxytocin. Contractions are usually sufficient to evacuate uterus; mean abortion time, about 20 hours. Stimulates smooth muscle of GI tract and bronchi (cause of several troublesome side effects); also constricts arteries and veins perhaps by increasing norepinephrine output. Blood pressure may be elevated with use of large doses; however, with dose used for terminating pregnancy, this effect is not clinically significant. Various administration routes have been used investigationally, but accompanying adverse reactions resulting from circulating prostaglandins have been unacceptably intense.

Used to terminate second-trimester pregnancy, between 16th- and 20th-week of gestation, as calculated from first day of last menstrual period. Often used in conjunction with dilation and curettage, oxytocin, or suction curettage to assure complete abortion.

ABSORPTION AND FATE. Acts directly on myometrium; onset of uterine contractions in 10 to 15 minutes following administration. Half-life in amniotic fluid: 3 to 6 hours; in plasma: less than 1 minute; maximum plasma levels occur about 2 hours after administration. Widely distributed in maternal and fetal tissues. Metabolized rapidly in most tissues but especially in maternal lungs and liver. Metabolites completely excreted within 24 hours, chiefly in urine; about 5% excreted in feces.

CONTRAINDICATIONS AND PRECAUTIONS. Hypersensitivity to dinoprost; acute pelvic inflammatory disease; history of cesarean section, or other major uterine surgery, uterine fibroids, cervical stenosis; ruptured membranes. *Cautious Use:* history of asthma, glaucoma, hypertension, cardiovascular or renal disease, epilepsy.

ADVERSE/SIDE EFFECTS. CNS: headache, dizziness, paresthesias, anxiety, drowsiness, seizures. **CV:** hypotension, syncope, flushing, hypertension, bradycardia and other arrhythmias, second degree heart block. **GI:** vomiting, nausea, diarrhea, epigastric pain, abdominal cramps. **Musculoskeletal:** pain (substernal, legs, shoulder, back). **Renal:** urine retention, hematuria, dysuria. **Reproductive:** cervical laceration or perforation, uterine rupture, endometritis, hot flashes, breast tenderness, burning sensation, lactation. **Respiratory:** bronchoconstriction, bronchospasm (wheezing), cough, chest rales, dyspnea, hyperventilation, sensation of chest constriction. **Other:** fever, chills, diaphoresis, polydipsia, burning sensation in eyes, diplopia, hiccoughs, malaise.

ROUTE AND DOSAGE. **Intraamniotic instillation (transabdominal tap):** 40 mg or 8 ml (5 mg/ml). If abortion process is not established or completed within 24 hours and if membranes are intact, patient is given an additional 10 to 40 mg (2 to 8 ml). **Extraamniotic (extraovular) instillation:** Investigational; various dose regimens are being studied.

NURSING IMPLICATIONS

Drug should be used only by qualified personnel in hospital setting with facilities that are immediately available for intensive care and surgery. Patient is usually hospitalized 1 to 4 days.

Incidence of incomplete abortion is higher with use of extraovular than intraamniotic route of administration. Both routes are associated with higher risk of incomplete abortion than with use of hypertonic saline.

Patient should be well aware of benefits and risks of dinoprost-induced abortion, and the nurse should be aware that the patient is in a life crisis.

A complete medical history and physical examination should be performed before starting therapy with dinoprost.

Instruct patient to empty her bladder before the transabdominal tap.

Intraamniotic instillation: An amniocentesis with removal of 1 ml fluid is performed before drug is instilled to verify presence of amniotic fluid. If fluid is bloody needle should be repositioned. Instillation of dinoprost begins with first milliliter given very slowly over a 1- to 2-minute period via transabdominal intraamniotic catheter. If no adverse effects present, remainder of dose is given over next 5 minutes. Contractions usually begin within first 15 minutes after injection and continue 20 to 30 minutes after drug is stopped. Catheter may be left in place for repeat administration, if necessary. During administration, patient is closely observed for signs of sensitivity and for signs that may indicate inadvertent systemic injection (e.g., vomiting, bronchoconstriction, tetanic uterine contractions, blood pressure changes, shock).

Extraamniotic instillation: If the uterus is too small for amniocentesis or if intraamniotic instillation procedure failed, the extraamniotic route may be selected. (This method is not widely used in the U.S.). A 14 or 16 Foley catheter with a 30-ml balloon is placed into lower uterine segment posteriorly in extraovular space. Instillation of prostaglandin through this route carries a high risk of uterine infection.

If membranes rupture during drug instillation, the procedure is terminated.

Adverse effects of prostaglandin administration, such as nausea and vomiting, seldom last longer than 15 to 20 minutes because drug is rapidly metabolized.

Monitor blood pressure, pulse, respirations, and uterine activity following drug administration. Report significant signs: pulse and blood pressure changes may signal hemorrhage; hypertonic uterine contractions can promote hemorrhage and cervical trauma. Save all clots and tissue for physician inspection and laboratory analysis.

Promptly report vasovagal symptoms (pallor, nausea, vomiting, bradycardia, rapid fall in arterial blood pressure). Instruct patient to remain in recumbent position.

The primipara may experience cervical laceration, particularly if oxytocin has been given before uterine response to dinoprost has ceased, and when cervix is poorly dilated.

D

Since lacerations may be asymptomatic, a careful vaginal examination should be done postabortion to determine condition of the cervix. (Depending on agency policy, may be done by the nurse if there is no bleeding.)

Failure to pass placenta within 1 hour after fetus is delivered may require use of oxytocin or curettage. Oxytocin should not be used until cervix is dilated and uterine response to dinoprost has stopped, to avoid cervical injury and uterine rupture.

Late postabortion hemorrhage can result from retained placental tissue, infection, or subinvolution of placental site. Note and report character and quantity of blood passed through birth canal. Emergency measures performed by the physician (including placental expression) and blood transfusions may be necessary.

Differentiation between drug-induced pyrexia and endometritis pyrexia is difficult but essential. Pyrexia is defined as at least 38°C (100.4°F). Observations and appropriate reporting by the nurse can be based upon the following criteria:

Drug-induced pyrexia:

Time of onset: Within 1 to 16 hours after first injection.

Duration: Temperature reverts to pretreatment level with discontinuation of therapy without further treatment.

Retention: Temperature elevation occurs whether or not tissue is retained.

Uterus: Normal uterine involution and no tenderness.

Discharge: Lochia normal.

Endometritis pyrexia:

Time of onset: Third day postabortion.

Duration: If untreated and infection continues, other pelvic infections may follow.

Retention: Products of conception often retained in cervical or uterine cavity.

Uterus: Often remains soft and boggy with tenderness over fundus; subinvolution and tenderness on palpation of round ligaments; pain on moving cervix and sensitivity over parietal peritoneum on bimanual examination.

Discharge: Foul-smelling lochia and leukorrhea.

Forcing fluids may be sufficient for drug-induced fever, if there is no clinical or bacterial evidence of intrauterine infection. Other more rigorous measures to reduce fever are not necessary because prostaglandin-induced elevated temperature is transient and self limiting.

Lactation of several days' duration may occur following successful termination of pregnancy.

Dinoprost does not seem to affect integrity of fetal–placental unit; thus, a live-born fetus may be delivered, particularly if abortion is accomplished at end of second trimester. If drug fails to terminate pregnancy another method is usually employed. Hypertonic saline may be utilized after cessation of uterine contractions.

Dinoprost ampuls should be stored at 2° to 8°C (36° to 46°F) and should be discarded 24 months following date of manufacture.

DINOPROSTONE

(PGE$_2$, Prostaglandin E$_2$, Prostin E$_2$)

(dye-noe-prost'one)
Abortifacient
Oxytocic
Prostaglandin
Hormone

ACTIONS AND USES. Synthetically prepared member of the prostaglandin E$_2$ series that appears to act directly on myometrium and on gastrointestinal, bronchial, and vascular smooth muscle. Stimulation of gravid uterus in early weeks of gestation more potent than that of oxytocin. Contractions are qualitatively similar to those that occur during term labor. Vaginal administration has the advantages of concentrated drug action on the target tissue and of being noninvasive. Like dinoprost (member of prostaglandin F series), dinoprostone can produce uterine contractions when given orally, intramuscularly, intravenously, or intra- and extraamniotically but use of these routes is investigational in the U.S. Has high success rate when used as abortifacient before 20th week and for stimulation of labor in cases of intrauterine fetal death. In addition to oxytocic action, dinoprostone enhances edema formation and pain-producing actions of bradykinin and other autocoids associated with the inflammatory process. May have teratogenic potential.

Used to terminate pregnancy from 12th week through second trimester as calculated from first day of last regular menstrual period; to evacuate uterine content in management of missed abortion or intrauterine fetal death up to 28 weeks gestational age, and to manage benign hydatidiform mole.

D

ABSORPTION AND FATE. Slowly absorbed following insertion of vaginal suppository. Widely distributed in body. Onset of uterine contractions within 10 minutes and may continue 2 to 3 hours. Rapidly metabolized in lungs, kidney, spleen, and other tissues. Excreted mainly in urine. Small amounts eliminated in feces.

CONTRAINDICATIONS AND PRECAUTIONS. Hypersensitivity to dinoprostone, acute pelvic inflammatory disease, history of uterine surgery, fibroids, cervical stenosis. *Cautious Use:* history of hypertension, hypotension, asthma, epilepsy, anemia, diabetes mellitus; jaundice; history of hepatic, renal and cardiovascular disease; cervicitis, acute vaginitis, infected endocervical lesion.

ADVERSE/SIDE EFFECTS. CNS: headache, tremor, tension. **CV:** transient hypotension (possibly with dizziness, fainting), flushing, cardiac arrhythmias, myocardial infarction, vascular collapse (rare). **ENT:** pharygitis, laryngitis, hearing impairment. **GI:** nausea, vomiting, diarrhea. **Musculoskeletal:** paresthesias, backache, joint inflammation or pain, arthralgia, stiff neck, nocturnal leg cramps, muscle cramps or pain. **Ophthalmic:** eye pain, blurred vision. **Reproductive:** vaginal pain, endometritis, vaginitis, vulvitis, vaginismus, breast tenderness, uterine rupture. **Respiratory:** bronchospasm (wheezing), dyspnea, pain or tightness of chest, cough. **Other:** fever, chills, dehydration, diaphoresis, rash, skin discoloration, urine retention. (Not all reactions listed are clearly drug-related).

ROUTE AND DOSAGE. Intravaginal: one suppository (20 mg) inserted high into vagina; additional suppositories at 3- to 5-hour intervals until abortion occurs or membranes rupture, but not to exceed total dose of 240 mg. (Mean total doses: elective abortion 90 mg; intrauterine fetal death 60 mg; benign hydatidiform mole 70 mg.)

NURSING IMPLICATIONS

Dinoprostone is to be used only by trained personnel in hospital settings with intensive care and operating room facilities.

A complete medical history and physical examination should be performed before drug is administered. Patient should be informed of potential risks associated with dinoprostone.

Antiemetic and antidiarrheal medications may be prescribed before dinoprostone to minimize GI side effects.

The foil-wrapped suppository should be warmed to room temperature prior to use.

Remove wrapper carefully; avoid contact because of risk of absorption. Wash hands carefully before and after preparing medication for administration.

Patient should remain in supine position for 10 minutes after administration of dinoprostone to prevent expulsion of the suppository and to enhance absorption.

D

Although rupture of the membranes is not a contraindication to use of dinoprostone, be aware that profuse bleeding may result in expulsion of the suppository. Observe patient carefully, after insertion of the drug.

Prepare for the possible administration of a blood transfusion to the patient aborting a benign hydatidiform mole: high blood loss is usual.

Monitor uterine contractions (frequency, duration, intensity) and observe for and report excessive vaginal bleeding and cramping pain. Save all clots and tissues for physician inspection and laboratory analysis.

Monitor vital signs. Fever is a physiologic response of the hypothalamus to use of dinoprostone and occurs within 15 to 45 minutes after insertion of suppository. Temperature elevation of 1.1°C (2°F) has been observed in about 50% of patients. The temperature returns to normal within 2 to 6 hours after discontinuation of medication or removal of the suppository.

Monitor and record vital signs for about 3 days after discontinuation of dinoprostone administration. Chills, shivering, or fever greater than 2°F above normal may signal onset of sepsis and should be reported.

A differential diagnosis must be made between drug-induced fever and endometritis pyrexia especially in intrauterine fetal death, which is associated with high risk of sepsis. Dinoprostone-induced fever usually occurs 1 to 16 hours following drug administration. It is self-limiting and defervesces after drug is stopped; lochia is not foul-smelling.

Observe patient closely during entire period of drug action: report wheezing, chest pain, dyspnea, and significant changes in blood pressure and pulse to the physician.

Approximately 10% of patients using dinoprostone have demonstrated a transient diastolic blood pressure decrease greater than 20 mm Hg.

Check vaginal discharge daily. Report change in quantity and foul-odor, and an unusual increase in bleeding.

Because lacerations may be asymptomatic, a careful vaginal examination should be done postabortion to determine condition of the cervix. (Depending on agency policy, may be done by nurse if there is no bleeding.)

Fetal death is confirmed by a negative pregnancy test for chorionic gonadotropic activity. Test is performed prior to dinoprostone treatment for diagnosed late fetal intrauterine death, and after elective interruption of diagnosed missed abortion.

Dinoprostone administration does not appear to have a direct effect on the fetoplacental unit; thus the possibility of a live-born fetus exists especially if treatment occurs at the end of second trimester. Because of possible teratogenic effects, failed termination should be completed by other means.

If patient has had a joint disorder, dinoprostone may exacerbate pain and limitation because of its effect on the inflammatory process. Consult physician concerning use of appropriate antiinflammatory medication.

Advise patient to continue taking her temperature (late afternoon) for a few days after she is discharged from hospital. Advise her to contact physician with onset of fever, bleeding, abdominal cramps, abnormal or foul-smelling vaginal discharge.

Having an abortion is an emotion-laden experience. It is important not to introduce one's moral values about the issue.

Follow-up counseling is indicated for the patient who experiences grief reaction, depression, or feelings of guilt. These responses are not unusual postabortion.

Patient should be advised to avoid douches, tampons, intercourse, and tub baths for at least 2 weeks. Clarify with physician.

In some women, ovulation may be established as early as 2 weeks postabortion. Patient should be advised about appropriate contraception.

Store suppositories at 4°C (39°F), unless otherwise specified by manufacturer. Do not freeze.

PROTOTYPE

DIPHENHYDRAMINE HYDROCHLORIDE

(dye-fen-hye'dra-meen)

(Allerdryl, BayDryl, Belix, Bena-D, Benadryl, Benahist, Benaphen, Bendylate, Benoject, Benylin, Compoz, Diahist, Dihydrex, Diphen, Diphenacen, Fenylhist, Fynex, Hydril, Hyrexin, Insomnal, Noradryl, Nordryl, Nytol with DPH, Tusstat, Twilite, Valdrene, Wehdryl)

Antihistamine (H_1-receptor antagonist); antivertigo agent, antiemetic, antitussive, antiparkinsonian agent

D

ACTIONS AND USES. Ethanolamine antihistamine with significant anticholinergic activity. High incidence of drowsiness, but GI side effects are minor. Like other antihistamines, competes for H_1-receptor sites on effector cells, thus blocking histamine release. (Histamine promotes capillary permeability and edema formation, and constriction of respiratory, GI, and vascular smooth muscle.) Effects in parkinsonism and drug-induced extrapyramidal symptoms are apparently related to its ability to suppress central cholinergic activity and to prolong action of dopamine by inhibiting its reuptake and storage. Does not inhibit gastric secretion, but has prominent antiemetic effect. Also has central antitussive action and some local anesthetic properties.

Used for symptomatic relief of various allergic conditions and to treat or prevent motion sickness, vertigo, and reactions to blood or plasma in susceptible patients. Also used in anaphylaxis as adjunct to epinephrine and other standard measures after acute symptoms have been controlled, and in treatment of parkinsonism and intractable insomnia. Occasionally used as a sedative in pediatric practice. Has been used as local anesthetic in dentistry and for treatment of canker sores. Incorporated in elixirs and syrups as an antitussive, and other antihistaminic-decongestant preparations to relieve symptoms of coughs due to colds and allergies. Available in combination with calamine (Caladryl) for topical use.

ABSORPTION AND FATE. Readily absorbed from all routes. Maximal antihistamine and sedative effects within 1 to 3 hours; duration 4 to 7 hours. About 90 to 95% plasma bound. Half-life 2 to 7 hours. Metabolized primarily by liver; some degradation by lung and kidney. Most of dose excreted in urine within 24 to 48 hours, chiefly as metabolites; small portion excreted as unchanged drug. Probably crosses placenta. Appears in breast milk.

CONTRAINDICATIONS AND PRECAUTIONS. Hypersensitivity to antihistamines of similar structure, lower respiratory tract symptoms (including acute asthma), narrow-angle glaucoma, prostatic hypertrophy, bladder neck obstruction, GI obstruction or stenosis, pregnancy, nursing mothers, prematures and newborns. *Cautious Use:* history of asthma, convulsive disorders, increased intraocular pressure, hyperthyroidism, hypertension, cardiovascular disease, diabetes mellitus, elderly patients.

ADVERSE/SIDE EFFECTS. CNS (common): drowsiness, dizziness, headache, fatigue, disturbed coordination, tingling, heaviness and weakness of hands, tremors, euphoria, nervousness, restlessness, insomnia; confusion; (especially in children): hallucinations, excitement, fever, ataxia, athetosis, convulsions, coma, cardiovascular collapse. **CV:** palpitation, tachycardia, mild hypotension or hypertension. **ENT:** tinnitus, acute labyrinthitis, vertigo, dry mouth, nose, throat, nasal stuffiness. **GI:** epigastric distress, anorexia, nausea, vomiting, constipation or diarrhea. **GU:** urinary frequency or retention, dysuria. **Hematologic:** leukopenia, agranulocytosis, hemolytic anemia. **Hypersensitivity:** skin rash, urticaria, photosensitivity, anaphylactic shock. **Ophthalmic:** blurred vision, diplopia, dry eyes. **Respiratory:** thickened bronchial secretions, wheezing, sensation of chest tightness.

ROUTE AND DOSAGE. Adults: Oral, intramuscular, intravenous: 25 to 50 mg three or four times a day (at 4- to 6-hour intervals). Maximum daily dosage is 400 mg. **Children: Oral, intravenous, intramuscular:** 5 mg/kg/24 hours in four divided doses as required. Not to exceed 300 mg/24 hours. Available in capsules, tablets, elixir, syrup, and sterile solution for injection.

D

NURSING IMPLICATIONS

GI side effects may be lessened by administration of drug with meals or with milk.

Capsule may be emptied and contents swallowed with water or mixed with food.

When used for motion sickness, the first dose is given 30 minutes before exposure to motion. For duration of exposure it is given before meals and on retiring.

Administer IM injection deep into large muscle mass; alternate injection sites. Avoid perivascular or subcutaneous injections of the drug because of its irritating effects. Hypersensitivity reactions (including anaphylactic shock) are more likely to occur with parenteral injections than with oral administration.

In patients taking diphenhydramine for allergic manifestations, a careful history should be taken that includes change from usual pattern of recently ingested foods and drugs, as well as social or emotional stress.

Patients with blood pressure problems receiving the drug parenterally should be closely observed, with blood pressure being monitored.

Drowsiness, the principal side effect, is most prominent during the first few days of therapy and often disappears with continued therapy. Elderly patients are especially likely to manifest dizziness, sedation, and hypotension. Bedsides and supervision of ambulation may be advisable for some patients.

Caution the patient against activities requiring alertness and coordination until drug response has been evaluated.

Warn the patient about possible additive CNS depressant effects with concurrent use of alcohol and other CNS depressants (such as sedatives, hypnotics, and antianxiety agents) while taking antihistamines.

Urge the patient on continuing therapy to report any unusual signs or symptoms to physician. Most mild reactions can be alleviated by decreasing dosage; however, a change to another preparation may be necessary.

Patients receiving long-term therapy should have periodic blood counts.

Elixir or syrup formulations are used for relief of cough.

Bear in mind that the drug has an atropinelike drying effect (thickens bronchial secretions) that may make expectoration difficult.

If mouth dryness is a problem, the following measures may provide relief: rinse mouth with clear warm water; increase noncaloric fluid intake (if allowed) and particularly if it has been inadequate; sugarless gum or lemon drops. If these measures fail, a saliva substitute may help, e.g., Xero-Lube, Moi-stir (available OTC). Consult physician.

Antihistamines have no therapeutic effect on the common cold. Their continued popularity, despite being debunked as cures for the common cold, apparently stems from their drying effect.

Caution the patient to store antihistamines out of reach of children. Fatalities have been reported.

Patients with allergies should be advised to carry medical information card or jewelry indicating type allergy, medication, physician's name, address, and telephone number.

Stored in tightly covered containers at 15° to 30°C (59° to 86°F), unless otherwise directed by manufacturer. Injection and elixir formulations should be stored in light-resistant containers and protected from light.

Diagnostic Test Interferences. In common with other antihistamines, diphenhydramine should be discontinued 4 days prior to **skin testing** procedures for allergy because it may obscure otherwise positive reactions.

Drug Interactions. Concurrent administration of antihistamines and **barbiturates, alcohol,** and **antianxiety agents** may enhance CNS depression caused by either drug. **MAO inhibitors** may prolong and intensify the anticholinergic (drying) effects of antihistamines and can cause severe hypertension (concurrent use avoided).

D

DIPHENIDOL HYDROCHLORIDE

(Vontrol)

(dye-fen'i-dole)

Antiemetic, antivertigo

ACTIONS AND USES. Agent with strong antivertigo and antiemetic effects structurally related to trihexyphenidyl. Mechanism of action is unknown; it appears to have direct depressant action on labyrinthine excitability and on conduction in vestibular-cerebellar pathways; it may also depress the CTZ in the medulla. Exhibits weak anticholinergic, CNS depressant, and antihistaminic activity.

Used in management of nausea and vomiting associated with infectious diseases, radiation sickness, antineoplastic therapy, general anesthesia; management of vertigo in labyrinthitis, following middle and inner ear surgery; Meniere's disease.

ABSORPTION AND FATE. Onset of action within 30 to 45 minutes after oral administration. Duration of action 3 to 6 hours. Readily metabolized in liver; approximately 90% excreted in urine.

CONTRAINDICATIONS AND PRECAUTIONS. Known hypersensitivity to diphenidol; anuria, hypotension, use of diphenidol in infants under 6 months of age or in those weighing less than 12 kg; use in patients with history of sinus tachycardia. Safe use during pregnancy or lactation or in women of childbearing potential not established. *Cautious Use:* glaucoma, pyloric stenosis, pylorospasm, prostatic hypertrophy, other obstructive lesions of GI tract or genitourinary tract.

ADVERSE/SIDE EFFECTS. Auditory and visual hallucinations, disorientation, confusion; drowsiness, overstimulation, depression, sleep disturbances, dry mouth, nausea, indigestion, blurred vision. Rarely: dizziness, skin rash, malaise, headache, heartburn, mild jaundice; slight transient lowering of blood pressure.

ROUTE AND DOSAGE. Adults: Oral: 25 to 50 mg every 4 hours as needed. **Children (for nausea and vomiting only): Oral:** 0.88 mg/kg, not to exceed 5.5 mg/kg/24 hours. Children's doses are not given more often than every 4 hours; if symptoms persist after first dose, however, physician may order repeat dose after 1 hour.

NURSING IMPLICATIONS

Diphenidol may cause hallucinations, disorientation, or confusion. For this reason, use is limited to hospitalized patients or to patients under comparable close, professional supervision.

Notify physician of side effects. Auditory and visual hallucinations, disorientation, and confusion usually occur within 3 days after initiation of drug therapy and usually subside spontaneously within 3 days after drug is discontinued. Observe appropriate safety precautions.

Monitor intake and output. Report oliguria or change in intake-output ratio.

Because of possible drowsiness and dizziness, caution patient against performing hazardous activities requiring mental alertness and physical coordination. Supervision of ambulation may be indicated.

Blood dyscrasias have not been reported, but since diphenidol is a comparatively new drug, manufacturer recommends regularly scheduled blood studies.

Bear in mind that antiemetic effect of diphenidol may obscure signs of overdosage of concomitant drug therapy or underlying pathology.

There is a possibility of additive effects with concurrent administration of CNS depressants.

Protect drug from exposure to light. Store preferably at 15° to 30°C (59° to 86°F), unless otherwise directed by manufacturer.

PROTOTYPE

DIPHENOXYLATE HYDROCHLORIDE WITH ATROPINE SULFATE

(Diphenatol, Enoxa, Latropine, Lofene, Lomotil, Lonox, Lo-Trol, Low-Quel, Nor-Mil, Sk-Diphenoxylate)

(dye-fen-ox′i-late)
Opiate agonist
Antidiarrheal agent
C v

ACTIONS AND USES. Diphenoxylate is a synthetic narcotic and phenylpiperidine analog structurally related to meperidine. Commercially available only with atropine sulfate, added in subtherapeutic doses to discourage deliberate overdosage. Inhibits mucosal receptors responsible for peristaltic reflex thereby reducing GI motility. Has little or no analgesic activity or risk of dependence, except in high doses.

Used as adjunct in symptomatic management of diarrhea.

ABSORPTION AND FATE. Well-absorbed after oral administration; onset of action within 45 to 60 minutes, with duration of 3 to 4 hours. Peak plasma levels reached in 2 hours; plasma half-life 2.5 hours. Rapidly metabolized to active metabolite diphenoxylic acid (plasma half-life 4.4 hours) and inactive metabolites. Excreted slowly, primarily in feces via bile. About 14% eliminated in urine; less than 1% as unchanged drug. Appears in breast milk.

CONTRAINDICATIONS AND PRECAUTIONS. Hypersensitivity to diphenoxylate or atropine; severe dehydration or electrolyte imbalance, advanced liver disease, obstructive jaundice, diarrhea caused by pseudomembranous enterocolitis associated with use of broad-spectrum antibiotics; diarrhea associated with organisms that penetrate intestinal mucosa; diarrhea induced by poisons until toxic material is eliminated from GI tract; glaucoma; children less than 2 years of age. Safe use during pregnancy, lactation, or in women of childbearing potential not established. *Cautious Use:* advanced hepatic disease, abnormal liver function tests; renal function impairment, patients receiving addicting drugs, addiction-prone individuals or whose history suggests drug abuse; ulcerative colitis; young children (particularly patients with Down's syndrome).

ADVERSE/SIDE EFFECTS. CNS: headache, sedation, drowsiness, dizziness, lethargy, numbness of extremities; restlessness, euphoria, mental depression, weakness, general malaise. **CV:** flushing, palpitation, tachycardia. **GI:** nausea, vomiting, anorexia, dry mouth, abdominal discomfort or distention, paralytic ileus, toxic megacolon. **Hypersensitivity:** pruritus, angioneurotic edema, giant urticaria, rash. **Ophthalmic:** nystagmus, mydriasis, blurred vision, miosis (toxicity). **Other:** urinary retention, swelling of gums. **Overdosage:** hypotonia, loss of reflexes, fever, seizures, respiratory depression, coma.

ROUTE AND DOSAGE. Adults: Oral: Initial: 5 mg 3 or 4 times a day. Commercial tablet (Lomotil) contains 2.5 mg diphenoxylate hydrochloride with 0.025 mg atropine sulfate; liquid preparation contains same amount per 5 ml. **Children (2 to 12 years) (use liquid form only):** Initial: 0.3 to 0.4 mg/kg/day in divided doses. Dosage may be reduced to as low as one-quarter dose as soon as symptoms are controlled.

NURSING IMPLICATIONS

A careful history will usually reveal probable cause of acute diarrhea.

Use only the plastic calibrated dropper supplied by manufacturer for measuring liquid preparation.

If necessary, tablet may be crushed and taken with fluid of patient's choice.

Dosage should be reduced as soon as initial control of symptoms occurs. Instruct patient to note time and number of stools as well as color, odor, consistency, presence of blood, pus, mucus or other foreign matter. Also note color, amount and frequency of urine (rough index of dehydration).

Report signs of atropine poisoning (atropinism): dry mouth, flushing, hyperthermia, tachycardia, urinary retention; may occur even with recommended doses in children, particularly those with Down's syndrome.

Dehydration occurs more rapidly in the younger child and may further influence variability of response to diphenoxylate and predispose patient to delayed toxic effects. Close monitoring is essential.

Drug should be withheld in presence of severe dehydration or electrolyte imbalance until appropriate corrective therapy has been initiated.

Observe for and report abdominal distention. In ulcerative colitis, diphenoxylate-induced delay of intestinal motility may cause toxic megacolon. As a result fluid is retained in colon and thus further aggravates dehydration and electrolyte imbalance. Distention is an ominous sign in patients with ulcerative colitis.

Magnitude of fluid and electrolyte deficits can be estimated by the following signs of dehydration: weakness, lethargy, confusion, postural hypotension, increased pulse, scanty concentrated urine, decreased sweating, increased temperature; tongue and mucosal dryness, poor skin turgor (gently pinch up skin over chest or forehead; if dehydrated, pinched appearance remains for several minutes), decreased eyeball tension (sunken eyeballs).

Further gross calculations of fluid loss can be made by careful measurements of body weight and intake and output. Note frequency, color, odor, and consistency of stools; presence of blood, pus, mucus, or other foreign matter; note color, amount and frequency of urine.

Serial measurements of body weight, serum electrolytes, BUN, creatinine, hemoglobin and serum albumin are essential for determining degree of dehydration and adequacy of fluid and electrolyte balance.

Consult physician regarding management of oral fluids and electrolytes. *(See Index: Rehydration.)* For acute diarrhea, food is generally withheld 24 to 48 hours to reduce bowel stimulation, or patient is restricted to only clear liquids such as broth, bouillon, weak tea, ginger ale, gelatin. Some clinicians allow simple foods such as plain toast, crackers, biscuits, banana. Ice-cold liquids, spicy foods, caffeine, beverages, milk and milk products, and concentrated sweets are usually avoided. Bland diet with frequent small meals is then added as tolerated, gradually progressing to normal diet.

Rehydration is an important adjunct to diarrhea treatment. Caffeine beverages and alcohol should be avoided as both increase peristalsis. Gatorade, caffeine-free soft drinks and fruit juices are adequate for mild cases; if more severe, oral electrolyte mixtures may be prescribed (e.g., Pedialyte). Example of home prepared solution: ½ tsp salt, ½ tsp baking soda, ¼ tsp salt substitute, 8 Tbsp sugar; dissolve in 1 quart of water.

Advise patients who are traveling to places where sanitation may be questionable to drink only boiled water or commercially bottled water, soft drinks, beer or wine. Also caution patient not to brush teeth or rinse mouth with "raw" water and to avoid ice cubes, salads, uncooked vegetables, and unpeeled fruit.

Counsel patient to take medication only as directed by physician.

Instruct patient to notify physician if diarrhea persists or if fever, palpitation, or other adverse reactions occur.

Since drug may cause dizziness and drowsiness, advise patient to use caution when driving or performing other activities requiring coordination and alertness.

Caution patients to keep drug out of reach of children. Fatalities have been reported.

Overdosage treatment: induction of emesis or gastric lavage (effective even several hours after drug ingestion). Facilities for resuscitation and a narcotic antagonist (e.g., naloxone) should be readily available. Bladder catheterization may be necessary. (Atropine causes urinary retention.) Respiratory depression may occur 12 to 30 hours after overdose. Because duration of diphenoxylate action exceeds that of naloxone, extend period of observation over at least 48 hours until diphenoxylate effect on respiratory system is passed.

Addiction to diphenoxylate is possible at high dosages and prolonged use. Classified as Schedule V drug under the Federal Controlled Substances Act.

Stored in tightly covered, light-resistant container, preferably between 15° and 30°C (59° and 86°F), unless otherwise directed by manufacturer.

Drug Interactions. Concomitant use of **MAO inhibitors** with diphenoxylate may precipitate hypertensive crisis. Diphenoxylate may potentiate action of **alcohol, barbiturates,** and **anxiolytic agents** and other **CNS depressants.** Patient should be observed closely if these drugs are used concomitantly.

DIPHENYLPYRALINE HYDROCHLORIDE

(Hispril)

(dye-fen-il-peer'a-leen)
Antihistamine
H_1-receptor antagonist

ACTIONS AND USES. Ethanolamine derivative antihistamine with properties similar to those of other antihistamines. *See Diphenhydramine.*

Used for symptomatic treatment of seasonal hay fever, perennial allergic rhinitis, vasomotor rhinitis, and various other allergic manifestations.

ABSORPTION AND FATE. Acts within 15 to 30 minutes. Peak effect in 1 to 2 hours; duration 3 to 6 hours for regular tablet and 8 to 12 hours for timed release form.

CONTRAINDICATIONS AND PRECAUTIONS. Hypersensitivity to diphenylpyraline; lower respiratory tract symptoms including acute bronchial asthma; concomitant use or within 2 weeks of MAO inhibitors, GU or GI obstruction. Safe use in newborns, premature infants, children under 6 years, nursing women, and during pregnancy not established. *Cautious Use:* increased intraocular pressure, cardiovascular or renal disease, hypertension, prostatic hypertrophy, hyperthyroidism, diabetes mellitus, elderly patients.

ADVERSE/SIDE EFFECTS. CNS: drowsiness, sedation, headache, dizziness, impaired coordination, confusion, lassitude, apathy, excitement particularly in children. **CV:** hypotension or hypertension, palpitation, tachycardia, extrasystoles. **ENT:** tinnitus, nasal stuffiness, dry nose and throat. **GI:** dry mouth, anorexia, nausea, vomiting, diarrhea, constipation. **Ophthalmic:** blurred vision, diplopia. **Other:** facial flushing, thickening of bronchial secretions, urinary frequency or retention, difficult urination, hypersensitivity reactions.

ROUTE AND DOSAGE. Oral (time-release capsule): Adults: 2 mg every 4 hours or 5 mg every 12 hours. **Children (over 6 years):** 5 mg once daily.

NURSING IMPLICATIONS

Advise patient to take drug with food, water, or milk to minimize GI distress.
Time-release form should be swallowed whole and not crushed or chewed.
Sedation and drowsiness may be pronounced in some individuals. Advise patient to avoid driving and other potentially hazardous activities until reaction to drug is known.
Because of the possibility of additive CNS depression, caution patient not to take alcohol or other CNS depressants, e.g., tranquilizers, antidepressants, sedatives, sleep medications without consulting physician.
Elderly patients are most likely to experience sedation, dizziness, light-headedness, and confusion. Observe necessary safety precautions.
Mouth dryness may be relieved by frequent rinses with warm water, by increasing noncaloric fluid intake (if allowed) or by sugarless gum or lemon drops. If these measures fail, a saliva substitute may help, e.g., Xero-Lube, Moi-Stir, Orex (all available OTC).
Bear in mind that antihistamines may mask ototoxic and other adverse effects of drugs taken concurrently.
Antihistamines may prevent positive reactions to skin tests for allergy if taken within 4 days of such tests.
Store preferably at 15° to 30°C (59° to 86°F), unless otherwise directed by manufacturer.
See also Diphenhydramine (prototype ethanolamine antihistamine).

D

DIPIVEFRIN
(Propine)

(dye-pi've-frin)
Adrenergic agonist (sympathomimetic)
Antiglaucoma agent

ACTIONS AND USES. Formed by diesterification of epinephrine in pivalic acid which enhances lipophilic and penetrating properties. Classified as a prodrug of epinephrine. (Prodrugs are compounds that are therapeutically inactive until biotransformed to parent compound.) Converted to epinephrine inside the eye by enzymatic hydrolysis. Ability to penetrate cornea is reportedly about 17 times that of epinephrine. Intraocular pressure (IOP) lowering effect is approximately equal to that of epinephrine, but believed to be associated with lower incidence of adverse effects. Appears to lower intraocular pressure by reducing production of aqueous humor and by enhancing its outflow. Does not produce miosis or accommodative spasms, blurred vision, or night blindness associated with miotic agents.

Used alone or in combination with other antiglaucoma agents to control intraocular pressure in chronic open-angle glaucoma.

ABSORPTION AND FATE. Onset of action in about 30 minutes. Maximal effect in about 1 hour.

CONTRAINDICATIONS AND PRECAUTIONS. Hypersensitivity to any component, narrow-angle glaucoma. Safe use in women of childbearing potential, during pregnancy (category B), in nursing mothers, and in children not established. *Cautious Use:* patients with aphakia (absence of crystalline lens).

ADVERSE/SIDE EFFECTS. CV: tachycardia, palpitation, arrhythmias, hypertension. **Ophthalmic:** mydriasis, local reactions (burning or stinging on instillation), conjunctival injection, photophobia (glare and light sensitivity), adrenochrome deposits on conjunctiva and cornea, macular edema (aphakic patients).

ROUTE AND DOSAGE. Topical: Adults: (0.1% solution) one drop in eye every 12 hours.

D

NURSING IMPLICATIONS

Apply light finger pressure to lacrimal duct during and for 1 or 2 minutes following instillation. Blot excess medication with clean tissue. *(See Index: Drug Administration: Eye drops, for more complete description of this technique.)*

Inform patient that he or she may experience a temporary stinging and burning sensation with initial instillation.

IOP determinations should be performed at regular intervals throughout therapy.

Store preferably at 15° to 30°C (59° to 86°F), unless otherwise directed by manufacturer.

DIPYRIDAMOLE

(Persantine)

(dye-peer-id'a-mole)
Vasodilator
Antiangina
Antiplatelet agent

ACTIONS AND USES. Nonnitrate coronary vasodilator with many properties similar to those of papaverine. Increases oxygen saturation in coronary sinus without coincident elevation in myocardial oxygen consumption. Also increases coronary blood flow, decreases coronary vascular resistance, and reportedly promotes development of collateral circulation in the diseased heart. Has little effect on blood pressure and blood flow in peripheral arteries. Inhibits ADP-induced platelet aggregation. Does not affect prothrombin activity.

Used for long-term management of chronic angina pectoris, but not useful for relieving acute anginal attacks. Also used in treatment regimen following myocardial infarction. *Investigational Use:* in combination with aspirin and oral anticoagulants to decrease platelet aggregation in various thromboembolic disorders; with aspirin alone to prevent coronary by-pass graft occlusion; with thallium imaging to determine cardiac risk prior to peripheral vascular surgery.

ABSORPTION AND FATE. Readily absorbed from GI tract. Plasma levels in 2 to 2½ hours following administration. Concentrates in liver where it is metabolized. Protein binding: 91 to 97%. Mainly excreted in feces via bile as intact drug or as glucuronide. Small amounts cross placenta.

CONTRAINDICATIONS AND PRECAUTIONS. Acute myocardial infarction. Safe use in pregnancy and nursing mothers not established. *Cautious Use:* hypotension, anticoagulant therapy.

ADVERSE/SIDE EFFECTS. Usually dose-related, minimal and transient: gastric distress, diarrhea, headache, dizziness, faintness, weakness, aggravation of angina pectoris (rarely); peripheral vasodilation, flushing, hypotension (excessive dosage), skin rash.

ROUTE AND DOSAGE. Oral: *Antiangina:* 50 mg 3 times daily. *Thromboembolic disorders:* 150 to 400 mg daily (in combination with another antiplatelet drug or an anticoagulant).

NURSING IMPLICATIONS

Administer at least 1 hour before or 2 hours after meals, preferably with a full glass of water. Physician may prescribe it to be taken with food if gastric distress persists.

If necessary, tablet may be crushed and mixed with liquid or soft food.

Counsel patient to notify physician of any side effects.

Some products (e.g., Persantine 25 mg tablets) contain tartrazine which may cause an allergic type reaction in susceptible individuals. It is frequently seen in persons with aspirin hypersensitivity.

Monitor blood pressure during period of dosage adjustment and in patients receiving high dosages.

If postural hypotension is a problem advise patient to make all position changes slowly and in stages, especially from recumbent to upright posture.

Clinical response may not be evident before second or third month of continuous therapy.

Expected therapeutic effects: reduced frequency or elimination of anginal episodes, improved exercise tolerance, reduced requirement for nitrates.

Store in well-closed container preferably at 15° to 30°C (59° to 86°F), unless otherwise directed by manufacturer.

See Nitroglycerin prototype vasodilator (coronary) for patient teaching points.

Drug Interactions. Dipyridamole inhibits platelet aggregation and thus increases the danger of hemorrhage in patients receiving **heparin. Aspirin** enhances dipyridamole absorption.

DISOPYRAMIDE PHOSPHATE

(DSP, Norpace, Norpace CR, Rythmodan)

(dye-soe-peer'a-mide)
Antiarrhythmic

ACTIONS AND USES. Class I antiarrhythmic agent with pharmacologic actions similar to those of quinidine and procainamide, although chemically unrelated. Reduces rate of spontaneous diastolic depolarization in pacemaker cells, thereby suppressing ectopic focal activity. In usual doses, retards upstroke velocity, lengthens action potential of normal cardiac cells, and reduces differences in duration of action potential between normal and infarcted tissue. Disopyramide shortens sinus node recovery time and increases atrial and ventricular effective refractory period, but has minimal effect on refractoriness and conduction time of AV node or on conduction time of His–Purkinje system or QRS duration. Has prominent atropine-like (anticholinergic) effects particularly on GI and urogenital systems.

Used to suppress and prevent recurrence of premature ventricular contractions (unifocal, multifocal, paired), and ventricular tachycardia not severe enough to require cardioversion. Has been used in combination with propranolol, phenytoin, and other antiarrhythmic drugs to treat serious refractory arrhythmias.

ABSORPTION AND FATE. Approximately 70 to 90% rapidly absorbed from GI tract. Onset of action in 30 minutes to 3.5 hours; duration 1.5 to 8.5 hours. Peak plasma concentration in 1 to 2 hours. About 50 to 65% bound to plasma proteins. Half-life: 4 to 10 hours (prolonged in patients with decreased cardiac output, recent MI, ventricular arrhythmias, renal or hepatic insufficiency). Primarily metabolized by liver. Approximately 80% of dose eliminated by kidney: 40 to 60% as unchanged drug and remainder as partially active metabolites. The major metabolite has considerably more anticholinergic activity than parent drug. About 10% excreted in feces. Crosses placenta. Appears in breast milk.

CONTRAINDICATIONS AND PRECAUTIONS. History of hypersensitivity to disopyramide; cardiogenic shock, preexisting 2nd or 3rd degree AV block (if no pacemaker is present); uncompensated or inadequately compensated congestive heart failure; hypotension (unless secondary to cardiac arrhythmia), hypokalemia. Safe use in women of childbearing potential and during pregnancy, or in nursing women and in children not established. *Cautious Use:* sick sinus syndrome (bradycardia–tachycardia); Wolff-Parkinson-White (WPW) syndrome or bundle branch block, myocarditis or other cardiomyopathy, underlying cardiac conduction abnormalities, hepatic or renal impairment, urinary tract disease (especially prostatic hypertrophy), myasthenia gravis, narrow-angle glaucoma, family history of glaucoma.

ADVERSE/SIDE EFFECTS. **Anticholinergic:** dry mouth, urinary hesitancy, urinary retention, constipation, blurred vision, dry eyes, nose and throat. **CNS:** dizziness, headache, fatigue, muscle weakness, paresthesias, peripheral neuropathy, nervousness, depression, acute psychosis. **CV:** hypotension, chest pain, dyspea, syncope, bradycardia, tachycardia, excessive widening of QRS complex or prolongation of QT interval; worsening of CHF; heart block; rarely: increased PVC's, ventricular tachycardia or fibrillation, cardiac arrest; edema with weight gain. **GI:** cholestatic jaundice; infrequent: nausea, vomiting, anorexia, bloating, gas, diarrhea, epigastric or abdominal pain. **GU:** urinary frequency, urgency, hesitancy, dysuria (rare), impotence. **Hypersensitivity:** pruritus, urticaria, rash, photosensitivity, anaphylactoid reaction (rare). **Ophthalmic:** precipitation of acute angle-closure glaucoma. **Other:** hypoglycemia, hypokalemia, agranulocytosis, drying of bronchial secretions, initiation of uterine contractions (in pregnant patients), muscle aches, precipitation of myasthenia gravis.

ROUTE AND DOSAGE. **Oral: Adults (weighing over 50 kg):** Initial loading dose: 300 mg (when rapid control is required), then 150 to 200 mg every 6 hours. Hospitalized patients with *refractory ventricular tachycardia* have received up to 400 mg every 6 hours. **Adults (weighing less than 50 kg):** Initial loading dose: 200 mg, then 100 mg every 6 hours. For patients with *cardiomyopathy or congestive failure:* Initial dosage limited to 100 mg every 6 hours. *Renal failure:* Creatinine clearance (Ccr) greater than 40 ml/min: loading dose 200 mg, then 100 mg every 6 hours. Ccr 40 to 30 ml/min: loading dose 150 mg, then 100 mg every 8 hours. Ccr 30 to 15 ml/min: loading dose 150 mg, then 100 mg every 12 hours. Ccr less than 15 ml/min: loading dose 150 mg, then 100 mg every 24 hours.

NURSING IMPLICATIONS

Check apical pulse before administering drug. Withhold drug and notify physician if pulse rate is slower than 60 beats/minute, faster than 120 beats/minute, or if there is any unusual change in rate, rhythm or quality.

ECG should be closely monitored, especially in patients with severe heart disease, hypotension, or hepatic or renal dysfunction. The following signs are indications for drug withdrawal: prolongation of QT interval and worsening of arrhythmia interval, QRS widening (more than 25%).

Monitor blood pressure during therapy in patients with myocarditis, uncompensated heart failure, and in those receiving other cardiac depressants.

Therapeutic plasma levels generally required to control ventricular tachycardia reportedly range between 2 and 4 mcg/ml. Refractory patients may require up to 7 mcg/ml.

For patients who have been receiving either quinidine or procainamide, manufacturer suggests starting disopyramide 6 to 12 hours after last quinidine dose and 3 to 6 hours after last procainamide dose.

Patients with atrial flutter or fibrillation are usually digitalized prior to initiation of therapy to ensure that disopyramide-induced improvement in AV conduction does not lead to a dangerously rapid ventricular rate.

Monitor intake and output particularly in patients with impaired renal function or prostatic hypertrophy. Persistent urinary hesitancy or retention may necessitate discontinuation of drug. Patients with renal dysfunction should be observed closely for toxic symptoms.

Instruct patient to weigh daily under standard conditions and to check ankles and tibiae daily for edema. Report to physician a weekly weight gain of 2 to 4 pounds or more.

Baseline and periodic determinations should be made of hepatic and renal function, and serum potassium. Patients with family history of glaucoma should have measurement of intraocular pressure before initiation of therapy.

Toxic effects are enhanced by hyperkalemia. Report symptoms promptly. *See Index.*

Blood glucose levels should be monitored in patients with congestive heart failure, hepatic or renal disease, and in patients taking beta adrenergic blocking agents (e.g., metoprolol, propranolol). Observe for and report symptoms of hypoglycemia: cold sweats, excessive hunger, nervousness, tremulousness, weakness, palpitation. (Symptoms may not be prominent.)

Patients with history of heart disease should be checked for symptoms of congestive heart failure: orthopnea, shortness of breath with exertion, paroxysmal nocturnal dyspnea, pulmonary rales, weight gain, distended neck veins.

Disopyramide should be discontinued promptly if symptoms of agranulocytosis (unusual fatigue, fever, malaise, sore mouth or throat) or jaundice appear.

Because of the possibility of hypotension, advise patient to make position changes slowly particularly from recumbent posture, to dangle legs for a few minutes before ambulating, and not to stand still for prolonged periods. Instruct patient to lie down or sit down (in head low position) if he or she feels faint or light-headed.

Dry mouth occurs in about 12% of patients receiving disopyramide, but frequently becomes less prominent with continued therapy. Symptom may be relieved by sugarless gum or lemon drops, frequent clear warm water rinses, increase in noncalorie fluid intake (if allowed), use of saliva substitute (available OTC) such as Xero-lube, Moi-stir (discuss physician).

If patient uses a large quantity of sugarless hard candy, urge brushing of teeth three or four times daily because most contain some sugar.

Instruct patient that in order to maintain regularity of heartbeat, drug must be taken precisely as prescribed. Emphasize importance of not skipping, stopping medication, or changing dose without consulting physician.

Urge patient to keep appointments for periodic clinical evaluation.

Advise patient not to take OTC medications unless approved by physician.

Inform patient that disopyramide may cause photosensitivity and therefore to avoid exposure to sunlight or ultraviolet light.

Since drug may cause dizziness and blurring of vision, caution patient to avoid driving and other potentially hazardous activities until reaction to drug effects is known.

Warn patient not to drink alcoholic beverages while taking disopyramide *(see Drug Interactions).*

Physician may prescribe a laxative to prevent constipation and straining.

Management of overdosage is largely supportive. Treatment may include administration of isoproterenol, dopamine, cardiac glycoside, diuretic, activated charcoal, hemoperfusion, hemodialysis, intraaortic balloon, counterpulsation, mechanically assisted respiration. ECG monitoring is essential.

Diagnostic Test Interferences. **Blood glucose** levels may be increased; **liver enzymes, triglycerides, cholesterol, BUN, creatinine** may be elevated and **hemoglobin** and **hematocrit** may be lowered.

Drug Interactions: Disopyramide

Plus	Interactions
Alcohol, ethyl	Additive hypoglycemia and hypotension
Antiarrhythmic drugs (e.g., Lidocaine, Phenytoin, Procainamide, Propranolol, Quinidine)	May enhance effect of disopyramide
Anticoagulants, oral	Elevation of warfarin serum levels by inhibiting warfarin metabolism
Anticholinergic drugs	Additive atropinelike effects

DISULFIRAM

(Antabuse, Cronetal, Ro-sulfiram)

(dye-sul'fi-ram)
Enzyme inhibitor
Alcohol deterrent

D

ACTIONS AND USES. Aldehyde dehydrogenase inhibitor. Blocks alcohol oxidation at the acetaldehyde level. When a small amount of alcohol is introduced into the system sensitized by disulfiram action, acetaldehyde concentration of blood rises 5 to 10 times above normal. A complex of highly unpleasant symptoms is produced and is referred to as the disulfiram reaction. This reaction persists as long as alcohol is being metabolized and serves as a deterrent to further drinking. Disulfiram possesses antithyroid and sedative actions usually unimportant unless alcohol is ingested. Does not produce tolerance and is not a cure for alcoholism.

Used as adjunct in treatment of the patient with chronic alcoholism who sincerely wants to maintain sobriety.

ABSORPTION AND FATE. Rapidly and completely absorbed from GI tract. Full action may require 12 hours because initially drug is deposited in fat. Greater part of drug is oxidized largely by liver. 5 to 20% of dose excreted unchanged in feces; about 20% remains in body for 1 to 2 weeks. Some may be excreted in the breath as carbon disulfide.

CONTRAINDICATIONS AND PRECAUTIONS. Hypersensitivity to disulfiram; severe myocardial disease; psychoses; pregnancy; patients receiving or patients who have recently received alcohol, metronidazole, paraldehyde, multiple drug dependence. *Cautious Use:* diabetes mellitus, epilepsy, hypothyroidism, cerebral damage, chronic and acute nephritis, hepatic cirrhosis or insufficiency.

ADVERSE/SIDE EFFECTS. Mild GI disturbances, garliclike or metallic taste, headache, allergic or acneiform dermatitis; urticaria, fixed-drug eruption, drowsiness, fatigue, restlessness, tremor, impotence, psychoses (usually with high doses); polyneuritis, peripheral neuritis, optic neuritis; hepatotoxicity. *Disulfiram reaction:* flushing of face, chest, arms, pulsating headache, nausea, violent vomiting, thirst, sweating, marked uneasiness, confusion, weakness, vertigo, blurred vision, palpitation, hyperventilation, abnormal gait, slurred speech, disorientation, confusion, personality changes, bizarre behavior, psychoses, tachycardia, chest pain, hypotension to shock level, arrhythmias, acute congestive failure, marked respiratory depression, unconsciousness, convulsions, sudden death.

ROUTE AND DOSAGE. Oral: initial: 250 mg daily in single dose for 1 to 2 weeks. Maintenance: 250 to 500 mg daily. Should not exceed 500 mg daily.

NURSING IMPLICATIONS

Daily dose should be taken in the morning when the resolve not to drink may be strongest. Tablets may be crushed and well mixed with liquid beverage if compliance is a problem.

To minimize sedative effect the drug may be prescribed to be taken at bedtime. Decrease in dose may also reduce sedative effect.

Patient should be completely aware of and should consent to therapy with disulfiram. Patient and family should be fully informed of possible danger to life if alcohol is ingested during disulfiram treatment.

Disulfiram therapy is attempted only under careful medical and nursing supervision. It is used as an adjunct to supportive and psychiatric therapy and only in patients who are motivated and fully cooperative.

Therapy is not initiated until patient has abstained from alcohol and alcohol-containing preparations for at least 12 hours and preferably 48 hours.

D

Complete physical examination, especially of circulatory and nervous systems, and careful drug history are advised prior to therapy. Baseline and follow-up transaminase tests every 10 to 14 days are suggested to detect hepatic dysfunction. In addition, complete blood count and sequential multiple analysis (SMA-12) tests should be performed every 6 months.

External application of solutions, creams, lotions that contain alcohol may be sufficient to produce a reaction. Teach patient to read labels and avoid use of anything that contains alcohol. Examples of unusual sources of alcohol: liniments; shaving, face, or body lotions; colognes, backrub solutions; elixirs, fluid extracts, tinctures (e.g., cough medicines, Geritol, paregoric); vanilla, vinegars.

Patient should be informed that prolonged administration of disulfiram does not produce tolerance; the longer one remains on therapy, the more sensitive one becomes to alcohol.

Disulfiram reaction *(see also Adverse Reactions):* occurs within 5 to 10 minutes following ingestion of alcohol and may last 30 minutes to several hours. When blood alcohol concentration is as little as 5 to 10 mg% patient may experience a mild reaction. Symptoms are fully developed with 50 mg% concentration and unconsciousness results when level reaches 125 to 150 mg%. When symptoms subside, patient may sleep for several hours after which patient is well again.

Intensity of reaction varies with each individual, but it is generally proportional to amount of alcohol ingested.

Warn patient that alcohol sensitivity may last as long as 2 weeks after disulfiram has been discontinued.

Patient may have disagreeable breath because of one of the metabolites, carbon disulfide.

Psychotic responses (usually associated with high dosages) may unmask underlying psychosis in some patients stressed by alcohol withdrawal.

During first 2 weeks of therapy, patient may experience side effects of disulfiram itself *(see Adverse Reactions).* These symptoms usually disappear with continued therapy or with dose reduction.

Advise patient to carry an identification card stating that patient is on disulfiram therapy and describing the symptoms of disulfiram reaction. The names of the physician or institution to contact in an emergency should also be provided. Cards may be obtained from Ayerst Laboratories. Ask pharmacist for nearest address.

During early therapy when drowsiness may be a problem, the patient should avoid driving or performing other tasks requiring alertness.

The disulfiram test is seldom used but if given patient must be under close supervision. When employed it serves as a guide to proper dosage level, and it permits the patient to experience under controlled conditions what happens when alcohol is ingested during disulfiram treatment. It is not administered to a person over 50 years of age. A clear detailed description of the reaction as an alternative to the test is felt to be sufficient in most cases.

Supervised disulfiram test: After first 1 to 2 weeks of therapy with 500 mg/day, a drink of 15 ml of 100 proof whiskey or equivalent is taken slowly. Test dose may be repeated only once.

During treatment of severe disulfiram reaction, treat patient as though in shock: oxygen or carbogen (O_2, 95% and CO_2, 5%); large doses of intravenous vitamin C; ephedrine sulfate; antihistamines. Monitor potassium levels, especially if patient has diabetes mellitus.

Maintenance therapy with disulfiram may be required for months or even years. Compliance should be determined periodically.

Physician may prescribe pyridoxine (vitamin B_6) for patients on long-term therapy to reduce cholesterol elevating effect of disulfiram.

Narcotic or sedative dependence may accompany or follow alcoholism. Thus, if either type

D

of medication is indicated during time patient is on disulfiram treatment, the family as well as prescriber should be alert to signs of drug abuse.

If a limited course of an antianxiety agent is indicated, discuss its use with patient from point of view of drug abuse. Patient should be warned not to change established dosing schedule and not to take a double dose (to make up for a missed dose).

Behavior modification has been achieved for many patients through *Alcoholics Anonymous, Al-Anon* (for relatives and friends), and *Alateen* (for teenage children of the alcoholic parent).

Patient Teaching Points. (Reenforcement of preliminary information given to secure consent to therapy with disulfiram.) Disulfiram reaction:

- ✓ begins within 5 to 15 minutes after ingestion of as little as 7 ml of 100 proof whiskey or equivalent
- ✓ persists 30 minutes to several hours
- ✓ can occur up to 2 weeks after discontinuation of therapy
- ✓ is not only unpleasant but can threaten life
- ✓ may require medical attention

Protect tablets from light. Store between 15° and 30°C (59° and 86°F).

Diagnostic Test Interferences. Disulfiram reduces **uptake of I-131;** decreases **PBI** test results; decreases **urinary VMA;** increases urinary concentrations of **homovanillic acid;** increases **serum cholesterol** (occurs 3 to 6 weeks after initiation of therapy).

Drug Interactions: Disulfiram

Plus	Interactions
Alcohol	Increased toxicity of alcohol
Antidepressants, tricyclic	Enhance reaction between alcohol and disulfiram
Chlorodiazepoxide (Librium)	Exaggerated clinical effects of chlorodiazepoxide
Diazepam (Valium)	Exaggerated clinical effects of diazepam
Isoniazid (INH)	Unsteady gait, incoordination, or marked behavioral changes
Metronidazole (Flagyl)	Confusional states and psychotic episodes
Oral anticoagulants	Prolonged prothrombin time
Paraldehyde	Increased toxicity of paraldehyde
Phenytoin (Dilantin) and congeners	Phenytoin intoxication

DOBUTAMINE HYDROCHLORIDE

(Dobutrex)

(doe-byoo'ta-meen)
Beta-adrenergic agonist
Sympathomimetic
Cardiac inotropic

ACTIONS AND USES. Direct-acting adrenergic (sympathomimetic) amine with electrophysiologic effects on heart similar to those of isoproterenol and dopamine. Produces inotropic effect by acting primarily on myocardial adrenergic $beta_1$ receptors with less prominent action on $beta_2$ and alpha receptors. In comparison with other catecholamines, a given increase in cardiac output is accompanied by a comparatively mild increase in heart rate and blood pressure. Also the occurrence of arrhythmias, vasodilation, and fall in peripheral vascular resistance is reportedly less except at higher doses. In patients with congestive heart failure, dobutamine increases myocardial contractility and usually stroke volume with resulting increase in cardiac output, and possibly in coronary blood flow and myocardial oxygen consumption.

Used for inotropic support in short-term treatment of adults with cardiac decompensation due to depressed myocardial contractility, as an adjunct in cardiac surgery. *Investigational Use:* to augment cardiovascular function in children undergoing cardiac catheterization. Commonly used with nitroprusside for additive effects *(see Drug Interactions).*

D

ABSORPTION AND FATE. Onset of action within 1 to 10 minutes. Peak effect within 10 minutes. Plasma half-life: 2 minutes. Rapidly metabolized in liver to inactive metabolites. Excreted primarily in urine.

CONTRAINDICATIONS AND PRECAUTIONS. History of hypersensitivity to other sympathomimetic amines, ventricular tachycardia, idiopathic hypertrophic subaortic stenosis. Safe use during pregnancy, in nursing mothers and children, or following acute myocardial infarction not established. *Cautious Use:* preexisting hypertension.

ADVERSE/SIDE EFFECTS. CV (dose related): increased heart rate and blood pressure, ventricular ectopic activity, premature ventricular beats, ventricular tachycardia (rare), palpitation, anginal pain. **Other:** nausea, vomiting, nonspecific chest pain, shortness of breath, headache, paresthesias, mild leg cramps; nervousness, fatigue (with overdosage); local pain (with infiltration).

ROUTE AND DOSAGE. Intravenous infusion rate: 2.5 to 10 mcg/kg/min. Rarely, up to 40 mcg/kg/min may be required. Concentration of dobutamine depends on dosage and fluid requirements of patient. Infusions have been given up to 72 hours.

NURSING IMPLICATIONS

Therapeutic plasma level: 40 to 190 ng/ml.

ECG and BP should be monitored continuously during administration of dobutamine.

IV infusion rate and duration of therapy are determined by heart rate, blood pressure, ectopic activity, urine output, and whenever possible, by measurements of cardiac output and central venous or pulmonary wedge pressures.

Patients are usually managed with a Swan-Ganz catheter so that pulmonary artery wedge pressure (PAWP) and cardiac output can be monitored during drug administration.

PAWP reflects left atrial pressure and left ventricular end-diastolic pressure (LVEDP). An elevated PAWP also indicates an increase in LVEDP and signifies left ventricular dysfunction: a low PAWP may indicate that volume replacement is needed. *(Normal PAWP:* 6 to 12 mm Hg. *Normal cardiac output:* 4 to 6 L/min.)

Since dobutamine enhances atrioventricular conduction, patients with atrial fibrillation are generally given a digitalis preparation prior to initiation of dobutamine therapy, to reduce risk of ventricular tachycardia.

Marked increases in blood pressure (systolic pressure is the most likely to be affected) and heart rate, or the appearance of arrhythmias or other adverse cardiac effects are usually reversed promptly by reduction in dosage.

Patients with preexisting hypertension must be closely observed for exaggerated pressor response.

Most patients have a 10 to 20 mm Hg increase in systolic pressure (rise may be as high as 50 mm Hg in some patients), and an increase in heart rate of 5 to 15 beats/min (as high as 30 beats in some patients).

Hypovolemia should be corrected by administration of appropriate volume expanders prior to initiation of therapy.

D

Monitor intake and output. Urine output and sodium excretion generally increase because of improved cardiac output and renal perfusion.

Dobutamine may be reconstituted by adding 10 ml sterile water for injection or 5% dextrose injection to 250 mg vial. If not completely dissolved additional 10 ml of diluent may be added.

For IV infusion, reconstituted solution must be further diluted before administration to at least 50 ml with 5% dextrose, 0.9% sodium chloride, or sodium lactate injection. IV solutions should be used within 24 hours.

Solutions containing dobutamine may exhibit color changes due to slight oxidation of drug. This does not affect potency.

Dobutamine is incompatible with sodium bicarbonate and other alkaline solutions.

Reconstituted solution may be stored under refrigeration at 2°C to 15°C (36° to 59°F) for 48 hours or for 6 hours at room temperature.

Drug Interactions

Plus	Interactions
Anesthetics, general (especially cyclopropane and halothane)	May sensitize myocardium to effects of catecholamines such as dobutamine and lead to serious arrhythmias
Beta adrenergic blocking agents: e.g., metoprolol, propranolol	May make dobutamine ineffective in increasing cardiac output, but total peripheral resistance may increase
MAO inhibitors Tricyclic antidepressants	Potentiation of pressor effects
Nitroprusside, sodium	Concomitant use produces greater increase in cardiac output and usually lower pulmonary wedge pressure
Oxytocic drugs	Combined use may cause severe persistent hypertension

---

DOCUSATE CALCIUM
(Dioctyl calcium sulfosuccinate, DCS, Pro-Cal-Sof, Surfak)

DOCUSATE POTASSIUM
(Dialose, Diocto-k, Kasof)

DOCUSATE SODIUM
(Afko-Lube, Bu-Lax, Colace, Dilax, Diocto, Disonate, D-S-S, Duosol, Lax-gel, Modane Soft, Molatoc, Regulex, Regutol, Stulex)

(dok'yoo-sate)
Laxative
Emollient
Stool softener, surfactant

ACTIONS AND USES. Anionic surface-active agent with emulsifying and wetting properties. Lowers surface tension, permitting water and fats to penetrate and soften stools for easier passage.

Used in treatment of constipation associated with hard, dry stools; used for painful anorectal conditions and in cardiac or other patients who should avoid straining during defecation.

CONTRAINDICATIONS AND PRECAUTIONS. Atonic constipation, nausea, vomiting, abdominal pain, fecal impaction, intestinal obstruction or perforation; use of sodium salts in patients on sodium restriction; use of potassium salts in patients with renal dysfunction; concomitant use of mineral oil.

ADVERSE/SIDE EFFECTS. Rare: occasional mild abdominal cramps, bitter taste, throat irritation (liquid preparation), nausea, rash.

ROUTE AND DOSAGE. Oral: Adults and children (over 12 years): 50 to 200 mg/day. **Children (6 to 12 years):** 40 to 120 mg; **Children (3 to 6 years):** 20 to 60 mg; **Children (under 3 years):** 10 to 40 mg. High doses recommended for initial therapy, then adjusted according to individual response. **Rectal (retention enema; suppository): Adults and older children:** *docusate sodium, docusate potassium:* 50 to 100 mg (5 to 10 ml of solution added to retention or flushing enema). Available as capsule, tablet, syrup, and solution.

D

NURSING IMPLICATIONS

Advise patient to take sufficient liquid with each dose and to increase fluid intake during the day if allowed. Oral solution (not syrup) may be administered in one-half glass of milk or fruit juice to mask bitter taste.

Docusate enhances systemic absorption of mineral oil and may result in tumorlike deposits; therefore, concomitant use is not recommended.

Effect on stools is usually apparent 1 to 3 days after first dose.

Docusate should not be administered for prolonged period in treatment of constipation in lieu of proper dietary management or other treatment of underlying causes. *See Bisacodyl.*

FDA Panel on Laxatives recommends against daily use of docusate for longer than 1 week. If prescribed by physician for chronic use, patient should be monitored for hepatotoxicity. There is a possibility that it increases intestinal absorption or hepatic uptake of other concomitantly administered drugs and thus may enhance their toxicity.

Some preparations, e.g., Comfolax, contain tartrazine which may cause an allergic-type response including bronchial asthma in susceptible individuals. This reaction is frequently seen in patients with aspirin hypersensitivity.

Docusate sodium is available in fixed combination with casanthranol (Peri-Colace), with senna concentrate (Senokap), and with phenolphthalein (Correctol).

Stored in tightly covered containers. Syrup formulations should be stored in light-resistant containers at 15° to 30°C (59° to 86°F), unless directed otherwise by manufacturer.

DOPAMINE HYDROCHLORIDE

(Intropin, Revimine)

(doe'pa-meen)

Adrenergic agonist (sympathomimetic)

Catecholamine

ACTIONS AND USES. Naturally occurring neurotransmitter and immediate precursor of norepinephrine. Major cardiovascular effects produced by direct action on alpha- and beta-adrenergic receptors and on specific dopaminergic receptors in mesenteric and renal vascular beds. Positive inotropic effect on myocardium produces increased cardiac output with increase in systolic and pulse pressure and little or no effect on diastolic pressure. Improves circulation to renal vascular bed by decreasing renal vascular resistance with resulting increase in glomerular filtration rate and urinary output. Blood flow to peripheral vascular bed may decrease while mesenteric flow increases. Less prone to cause substantial decrease in systemic vascular resistance, tachyarrhythmias, or increased myocardial oxygen consumption than are other catecholamines. More effective when therapy is started shortly after signs and symptoms of shock appear and before urine flow has decreased to approximately 0.3 ml/minute.

Used to correct hemodynamic imbalance in shock syndrome due to myocardial infarction (cardiogenic shock), trauma, endotoxic septicemia (septic shock), open heart surgery, and renal and congestive failure. *Investigational Use:* treatment of children with congenital heart disease.

ABSORPTION AND FATE. Onset of action within 5 minutes; duration less than 10 minutes. Widely distributed in body, but does not cross blood–brain barrier. About 75% of dose is inactivated, chiefly by monoamine oxidase (MAO) in liver, kidney, and plasma. Approximately 25% of dose is metabolized to norepinephrine within adrenergic nerve terminals. Plasma half-life: 2 minutes. Excreted in urine primarily as metabolites; small portion excreted unchanged.

CONTRAINDICATIONS AND PRECAUTIONS. Pheochromocytoma; tachyarrhythmias or ventricular fibrillation. Safe use during pregnancy, lactation, and in pediatric patients not established. *Cautious Use:* within 14 days before or after MAO inhibitor therapy; during pregnancy; patients with history of occlusive vascular disease (e.g., Buerger's or Raynaud's disease), cold injury, diabetic endarteritis, arterial embolism.

ADVERSE/SIDE EFFECTS. Most frequent: ectopic beats, nausea, vomiting, tachycardia, anginal pain, palpitation, dyspnea, headache, hypotension, vasoconstriction (indicated by disproportionate rise in diastolic pressure). Less frequent: piloerection, aberrant conduction, bradycardia, widening of QRS complex, azotemia, elevated blood pressure, necrosis, tissue sloughing with extravasation, gangrene.

ROUTE AND DOSAGE. Intravenous infusion: Initial: 2 to 5 mcg/kg/minute; may be increased gradually up to a rate of 20 to 50 mcg/kg/minute, if necessary. Must be first diluted with appropriate sterile solution recommended by manufacturer. *See package insert.*

NURSING IMPLICATIONS

Therapeutic plasma level: 40 to 190 ng/dl.

Before initiation of dopamine therapy, hypovolemia should be corrected, if possible, with either whole blood or plasma.

Dilution should be made just prior to administration, although reportedly the solution may remain stable for 24 hours after dilution.

IV infusion rate and guidelines for adjusting rate of flow in relation to changes in blood pressure will be prescribed by physician. Microdrip or other reliable metering device should be used for accuracy of flow rate.

Monitor blood pressure, pulse, peripheral pulses, and urinary output at intervals prescribed by physician. Precise measurements are essential for accurate titration of dosage.

Indicators for decreasing or temporarily suspending dose (report promptly to physician): reduced urine flow rate in absence of hypotension; ascending tachycardia; dysarrhythmias; disproportionate rise in diastolic pressure (marked decrease in pulse pressure); signs of peripheral ischemia, pallor, cyanosis, mottling; complaints of tenderness, pain, numbness, or burning sensation. (Presence of peripheral pulses is not always indicative of adequate circulation.)

Monitor for cold extremities (fingers, toes) and report if present. Reportedly nitroglycerin ointment (2 inch strip) applied to warmest areas of chest or abdominal wall is effective in increasing peripheral blood flow in the hypotensive patient with dopamine-induced peripheral ischemia. (Blood pressure is not affected, however.)

Signs and symptoms of overdosage generally respond to dosage reduction or temporary discontinuation of drug, since dopamine has short duration of action. However, if these measures fail, a short-acting alpha-adrenergic blocking agent (e.g., phentolamine) may be given to antagonize peripheral vasoconstriction.

Infusion rate must be continuously monitored for free flow, and care must be taken to avoid extravasation, which can result in tissue sloughing and gangrene. For this reason, infusion is made preferably into a large vein of the antecubital fossa.

Antidote for extravasation: infiltration of ischemic area should be made as soon as possible with 10 to 15 ml of normal saline containing 5 to 10 mg phentolamine (Regitine), using syringe and fine needle. *See Index: Nursing Interventions: extravasation.*

Dopamine is a potent drug. Patient must be under constant observation.

In addition to improvement in vital signs and urine flow, other indices of adequate dosage and perfusion of vital organs include loss of pallor, increase in toe temperature, adequacy of nail bed capillary filling, and reversal of confusion or comatose state.

Protect dopamine from light. Discolored solutions should not be used. Reconstituted solution is stable for 48 hours when stored at 2° to 15°C (36° to 59°F) or for 6 hours at room temperature 15° to 30°C (59° to 86°F).

Drug Interactions. Administration of **MAO inhibitors** within previous 2 or 3 weeks may cause hypertensive crisis since they prolong and intensify pressor effects of dopamine. (Initial dose of dopamine should be reduced by at least one-tenth the usual dose in these patients.) A similar reaction may occur with concomitant use of **furazolidone** since it reportedly may cause dose-related inhibition of MAO. Concomitant use with **ergot alkaloids** may result in excessive vasoconstriction. Possibility of enhanced response to dopamine in patients receiving or patients who have recently received **guanethidine.** Concurrent administration of dopamine and **diuretic agents** may produce additive or potentiating effect; **phenytoin** may cause hypotension and bradycardia. **Cyclopropane** and related anesthetics may sensitize myocardium to action of dopamine. Dopamine should be used with extreme caution in these patients.

DOXAPRAM HYDROCHLORIDE

(dox'a-pram)

(Dopram)

Central stimulant (respiratory)

ACTIONS AND USES. Short-acting analeptic capable of stimulating all levels of the cerebrospinal axis. Actions similar to those of nikethamide, but reported to have greater margin of safety because of minor effect on cortex. Respiratory stimulation by direct medullary action or possibly by indirect activation of peripheral chemoreceptors produces increased tidal volume and slight increase in respiratory rate. Decreases P_{CO_2} and increases P_{O_2} by increasing alveolar ventilation; may elevate blood pressure and pulse rate by stimulation of brainstem vasomotor areas. Also increases salivation, and release of gastric acids and epinephrine.

Used as short-term adjunctive therapy to alleviate postanesthesia and drug-induced respiratory depression and to hasten arousal and return of pharyngeal and laryngeal reflexes. Also used as temporary measure (approximately 2 hours) in hospitalized patients with chronic pulmonary disease associated with acute respiratory insufficiency as an aid to prevent elevation of arterial CO_2 tension during administration of oxygen (not used in conjunction with mechanical ventilation).

ABSORPTION AND FATE. Onset of respiratory stimulation following a single IV injection occurs in 20 to 40 seconds and peaks in 1 or 2 minutes, with duration rarely more than 5 to 12 minutes. Rapidly metabolized. Believed to be excreted in urine as metabolites within 24 to 48 hours after administration.

CONTRAINDICATIONS AND PRECAUTIONS. Known hypersensitivity to doxapram; epilepsy and other convulsive disorders; incompetence of ventilatory mechanism due to muscle paresis, pulmonary fibrosis, flail chest, pneumothorax, airway obstruction, extreme dyspnea, acute bronchial asthma; severe hypertension, coronary artery disease, uncompensated heart failure, cerebrovascular accident. Safe use during pregnancy and in children 12 years of age or younger not established. *Cautious Use:* cerebral edema, history of bronchial asthma, chronic obstructive pulmonary disease (COPD), cardiac disease, severe tachycardia, arrhythmias, hyperthyroidism, pheochromocytoma, hypertension, head injury, increased intracranial pressure, peptic ulcer, patients undergoing gastric surgery, acute agitation.

ADVERSE/SIDE EFFECTS. CNS: dizziness, sneezing, apprehension, confusion, involuntary movements, hyperactivity, paresthesias; feeling of warmth and burning, especially of genitalia, perineum; flushing, sweating, hyperpyrexia, headache, pilomotor erection, pruritus, muscle tremor, spasms, rigidity, convulsions (rarely), increased deep-tendon reflexes, bilateral Babinski sign, carpopedal spasm, pupillary dilation, mild delayed narcosis. **CV:** mild to moderate increase in blood pressure, sinus tachycardia, bradycardia, extrasystoles, lowered T waves, PVCs, chest pains, tightness in chest. **GI:** nausea, vomiting, diarrhea, salivation, sour taste. **GU:** urinary retention, frequency, incontinence. **Respiratory:** dyspnea, tachypnea, cough, laryngospasm, bronchospasm, hiccups, rebound hypoventilation, hypocapnia with tetany. **Other:** local skin irritation, thrombophlebitis with extravasation (cause-effect relationship not established): decreased hemoglobin, hematocrit, and RBC count; elevated BUN; albuminuria.

ROUTE AND DOSAGE. *Postanesthesia:* **Intravenous injection:** 0.5 to 1 mg/kg body weight; single injection not to exceed 1.5 mg/kg body weight or 2 mg/kg when repeated at 5-minute intervals. **Intravenous infusion:** 1 to 3 mg/minute. Recommended maximum dose 4 mg/kg; not to exceed 3 Gm/day. Compatible with 5 or 10% dextrose in water or normal saline. *Drug-induced CNS depression:* priming dose: 2.0 mg/kg. **Intermittent injection:** repeat priming dose in 5 minutes; then every 1 to 2 hours until patient awakens. If relapse occurs: resume 1 to 2 hourly injections until arousal is sustained or until maximum dose of 3 Gm is given. **Intermittent infusion** (if no response after priming dose): 1 to 3 mg/minute (1 mg/ml solution) until patient awakens or maximum dose of 3 Gm is given. *COPD:* **IV infusion:** 1 to 3 mg/minute (2 mg/ml solution) for maximum of 2 hours.

NURSING IMPLICATIONS

Adequacy of airway and oxygenation must be assured before initiation of doxapram therapy.

IV flow rate is prescribed by physician. Infusion rate may start at 1 mg/minute until satisfactory respiratory response is observed. It should then be maintained at 1 to 3 mg/minute and be adjusted to maintain desired respiratory response. An infusion pump is advisable for regulatory flow rate.

Extravasation or use of same IV site for prolonged periods can cause thrombophlebitis or tissue irritation. *(See Index: Nursing Interventions: Extravasation.)*

Careful monitoring and accurate observations of blood pressure, pulse, deep tendon reflexes, airway, and arterial blood gases are essential guides for determining minimum effective dosage and preventing overdosage.

Determinations of blood gases, Po_2, Pco_2, and O_2 saturation are important for assessing effectiveness of respiratory stimulation. In patients with chronic obstructive pulmonary disease, arterial blood gases should be drawn prior to initiation of doxapram infusion and oxygen administration and then at least every ½ hour during infusion. Infusion should not be administered for longer than 2 hours.

Doxapram should be discontinued if arterial blood gases show evidence of deterioration and mechanical ventilation is initiated.

Postoperative patients or patients in a state of narcosis with chronic pulmonary insufficiency should receive oxygen concomitantly. Respiratory stimulation produced by doxapram increases the work of breathing and thus increases oxygen consumption and CO_2 production.

Observe patient continuously during therapy and maintain vigilance until patient is fully alert (usually about 1 hour) and protective pharyngeal and laryngeal reflexes are completely restored.

Notify physician immediately of any side effects. Be alert for early signs of toxicity: tachycardia, muscle tremor, spasticity, hyperactive reflexes.

A mild to moderate increase in blood pressure commonly occurs; this is a matter of concern in patients with preexisting hypertension.

If sudden hypotension or dyspnea develops, doxapram should be discontinued.

Doxapram generally produces increased alertness in postoperative patients and earlier perception of pain than usual. Because the action of doxapram is short, however, keep in mind that poststimulation narcosis may occur.

Oxygen, resuscitative equipment, and IV barbiturates should be readily available in the event of excessive CNS stimulation.

Store drug at 15° to 30°C (59° to 86°F), unless directed to do otherwise by manufacturer.

D

Drug Interactions. Synergistic pressor effects (increase in blood pressure, arrhythmias) may occur in patients receiving **sympathomimetic agents** or **MAO inhibitors.** Initiation of doxapram should be delayed for at least 10 minutes following discontinuation of anesthetics that sensitize myocardium to catecholamines, such as **cyclopropane, enflurane,** and **halothane.**

DOXEPIN HYDROCHLORIDE

(Adapin, Sinequan)

(dox'e-pin)
Psychotropic
Antidepressant
Tricyclic

ACTIONS AND USES. Dibenzoxepin tricyclic antidepressant (TCA). Actions, limitations and interactions are similar to those of imipramine (qv). Reportedly one of the most sedative of the tricyclic antidepressants.

Used to treat psychoneurotic anxiety and/or depressive reactions, mixed symptoms of anxiety and depression, anxiety and/or depression associated with alcoholism, organic disease, psychotic depressive disorders. *Investigational Use:* treatment of peptic ulcer disease.

ABSORPTION AND FATE. Average serum half life: 17 ±6 hours; effective plasma concentration: 100 to 150 ng/ml. Hepatic metabolism; excretion largely by kidneys; crosses placenta and enters breast milk.

CONTRAINDICATIONS AND PRECAUTIONS. Prior sensitivity to any TCA; use during acute recovery phase following myocardial infarction; glaucoma, prostatic hypertrophy, tendency toward urinary retention; concurrent use of MAO inhibitors. Safe use during pregnancy, in nursing women, and in children under 12 years not established. *Cautious Use:* patients receiving electroshock therapy, patient with suicidal tendency; renal, cardiovascular or hepatic dysfunction. *See also Imipramine.*

ADVERSE/SIDE EFFECTS. Anticholinergic: blurred vision, xerostomia, sour or metallic taste, epigastric distress, constipation, urinary retention. **CNS:** drowsiness, dizziness, weakness, fatigue, hypomania, confusion, paresthesias. **CV:** orthostatic hypotension, tachycardia. **Other:** tinnitus, weight gain, photosensitivity reaction, agranulocytosis. *See also Imipramine.*

ROUTE AND DOSAGE. (Highly individualized). **Oral: Adult:** *Mild to moderate anxiety and/or depression:* 25 to 150 mg daily. *Mild symptomatology* or *emotional symptoms accompanying organic disease:* 25 to 50 mg/daily. *Severe anxiety and/or depression:* 50 mg three times daily; gradually increased to 300 mg/day if necessary. (Oral concentrate): Contains equivalent to 10 mg doxepin per ml.

NURSING IMPLICATIONS

Oral concentrate must be diluted with approximately 120 ml water, milk or fruit juice just prior to administration. (Not physically compatible with carbonated beverages.)

Capsule may be emptied and contents swallowed with fluid or mixed with food.

If daytime sedation is pronounced, inform physician. Since doxepin is long-acting, entire daily dose (up to 150 mg) may be prescribed for bedtime administration.

If patient is also receiving methadone, it can be mixed with the oral concentrate of doxepin. Dilute with Gatorade, Tang, sugar water, or orange juice. Avoid grape juice for this combination. Do not prepare and store bulk dilutions.

Supervise drug ingestion. Be sure patient does not "cheek" the capsule. Teach the necessity to maintain established dosage regimen and to avoid change of intervals, doubling, reducing or skipping doses. Tell patient not to give any of the medication to another person.

Antianxiety effect usually precedes antidepressant effect. Optimum antidepressant response may require 2 to 3 weeks of therapy.

The activities of both alcohol and doxepin are potentiated when used together during therapy and for up to 2 weeks after doxepin is discontinued. Consult physician about safe amount of alcohol, if any, that can be taken.

If a patient uses excessive amounts of alcohol it should be borne in mind that the potentiation of doxepin effects may increase the danger of overdosage or suicide attempt.

Suicide is an inherent risk with any depressed patient and may remain a possibility until there is significant improvement. Supervise patient closely during early course of therapy.

Doxepin has moderate to strong anticholinergic effects. Be alert to changes in intake–output ratio and check patient for constipation and abdominal distention.

Be suspicious of xerostomia if patient keeps dentures out except at meal time. Inspect oral membranes and institute measures to give symptomatic relief if necessary. Alert physician. Dose adjustment or change in medication may be indicated.

Caution patient to avoid driving and other potentially hazardous activities until reaction to drug is known. Doxepin has a pronounced sedative effect; symptom tends to disappear with continued therapy.

Note that Adapin contains tartrazine which may evoke an allergic response including asthma in susceptible individuals. Frequently such persons are also sensitive to aspirin.

Store drug at room temperature (59° to 86°F) in tightly closed light-resistant container.

See Imipramine (prototype antidepressant psychotropic).

Drug Interactions. At dosages of 300 mg/day or higher, doxepin antagonizes antihypertensive effects of **guanethidine.** *See also Imipramine.*

DOXORUBICIN HYDROCHLORIDE

(Adriamycin, ADR)

(dox-oh-roo'bi-sin)
Antineoplastic (antibiotic)
Immunosuppressant

D

ACTIONS AND USES. Cytotoxic anthracycline antibiotic isolated from *Streptomyces peucetius,* with wide spectrum of antitumor activity and strong immunosuppressive properties. Intercalates with preformed DNA residues, blocking effective DNA and RNA transcription. Highly destructive to rapidly proliferating cells and slow-developing carcinomas; selectively toxic to cardiac tissue. A potent radiosensitizer capable of enhancing radiation reactions. No clinical cross-resistance to standard antineoplastics; therefore, it may be especially effective in patients with less advanced disease. Cytotoxicity precludes its use as antiinfective agent. Tests on experimental models have shown mutagenic and carcinogenic properties.

Used to produce regression in neoplastic conditions, including acute lymphoblastic and myeloblastic leukemias, Wilms' tumor neuroblastoma, soft tissue and bone sarcomas, breast and ovary carcinomas, lymphomas, bronchogenic carcinoma. Generally used in combined modalities with surgery, radiation, and immunotherapy. Also effective pretreatment to sensitize superficial tumors to local radiation therapy.

ABSORPTION AND FATE. IV administration followed by rapid plasma clearance and significant tissue binding. Half-life: 0.6 hours; 3.3 hours for metabolites. Metabolized in liver and other tissues to both active and inactive metabolites. Does not cross blood–brain barrier or achieve significant level in CSF. Excreted mainly in bile; 40 to 50% of administered dose recovered in bile and feces in 7 days. Less than 5% excreted in urine after 5 days, primarily as unchanged drug.

CONTRAINDICATIONS AND PRECAUTIONS. Myelosuppression, impaired cardiac function, obstructive jaundice, previous treatment with complete cumulative doses of doxorubicin and/or daunorubicin. Safe use in patients of childbearing potential or during pregnancy not established. *Cautious Use:* impaired hepatic or renal function, patients having had radiotherapy to areas surrounding heart, history of atopic dermatitis.

ADVERSE/SIDE EFFECTS. CV: serious, irreversible myocardial toxicity with delayed congestive heart failure, acute left ventricular failure, and hypotension. **Dermatologic:** hyperpigmentation of nail beds and buccal mucosa (especially in blacks); hyperpigmentation of dermal creases (especially in children), rash, complete alopecia, recall phenomenon (skin reaction due to prior radiotherapy). **GI:** stomatitis and esophagitis (common) with ulcerations, nausea, vomiting, anorexia, inanition, diarrhea. **Hematopoietic:** severe myelosuppression (60 to 85% of patients); leukopenia (principally granulocytes), thrombocytopenia, anemia. **Other:** conjunctivitis (rare), lacrimation, drowsiness, fever, facial flush with too rapid IV infusion rate, hyperuricemia, hypersensitivity, anaphylaxis. *With extravasation:* severe cellulitis, vesication, tissue necrosis, lymphangitis, phlebosclerosis.

ROUTE AND DOSAGE. (Dose regimens highly individualized) **Intravenous: Adults:** 60 to 75 mg/m^2 as single dose at 21-day intervals. Alternate dose schedule: 30 mg/m^2 on each of 3 successive days, repeated every 4 weeks. Total cumulative dose not to exceed 550 mg/m^2. Reconstituted by adding 5 ml of 0.9% sodium chloride for injection to the 10-mg vial, or 25 ml to the 50-mg vial to give final concentration of 2 mg/ml doxorubicin.

NURSING IMPLICATIONS

Not to be confused with daunorubicin.

It is recommended that patient be hospitalized during the first phase of treatment to permit both medical and nursing surveillance, and extensive laboratory monitoring.

Caution should be observed in preparing doxorubicin solution. Wear gloves. If powder or solution contacts skin or mucosa, wash copiously with soap and water. For more detailed information *see Index: Antineoplastics: handling vesicant drugs.*

Administered slowly into side arm of freely running IV infusion of sodium chloride injection or 5% dextrose injection. Tubing should be attached to a Butterfly needle inserted into a large vein.

Do not mix this drug with other drugs.

Infusion rate usually permits administration of the dose in a 3- to 5-minute period. Rate will be specifically ordered. Facial flushing and local red streaking along the vein may occur if drug is administered too rapidly. Urticaria around injection site (due to histamine release) is usually self-limiting.

If possible avoid using antecubital vein or veins on dorsum of hand or wrist where extravasation could damage underlying tendons and nerves leading to loss of mobility of entire limb. Also avoid veins in extremity with compromised venous or lymphatic drainage.

Care should be taken to avoid extravasation. Examine the injection site frequently during infusion. Provide meticulous site care to prevent infection.

Give prompt attention to patient's complaint of a stinging or burning sensation around injection site; stop infusion immediately, even though blood return can be demonstrated, and restart in another vein. Apply cold (ice) compresses.

Perivenous extravasation can occur painlessly. If it is suspected, local infiltration with injectable corticosteroid and flooding the site with normal saline may lessen local reaction. To insure that these agents follow the same path as the doxorubicin, they may be given through the original needle left in place.

Monitor area of extravasation frequently. If ulceration begins (usually 1 to 4 weeks after extravasation), a plastic surgeon should be consulted. Early wide excision of the area with skin grafting may be necessary.

Begin a flow chart to establish baseline data for reference purposes. Include temperature, pulse, respiration, BP, body weight, laboratory values, and intake and output ratio and pattern.

Evaluation of hepatic, renal, hematopoietic, and cardiac function (ECG) should be performed prior to initiation of therapy, at regular intervals thereafter, and at end of therapy.

Since congestive heart failure may occur several weeks to months after cessation of therapy, ECG and radionuclide scanning may be monitored at least monthly during this posttreatment period.

Dosage may be guided by serum bilirubin level: if it is 1.2 to 3.0 mg/dl, one-half normal dose is prescribed; if bilirubin is more than 3 mg/dl, one-fourth normal dose is given. *(Normal indirect serum bilirubin* [adult]: 0.1 to 0.4 mg/dl or less.)

Therapeutic response to doxorubicin is unlikely to occur without some evidence of toxicity.

Myocardial toxicity (irreversible) becomes more of a threat as cumulative dose approaches 550 mg/m^2 body surface and particularly if drug therapy is in conjunction with therapeutic radiation.

Doxorubicin cardiomyopathy is associated with persistent reduction of QRS wave, prolonged systolic (time) interval, and reduced ejection fraction (by echocardiography or radionuclide angiography).

Be alert to early signs of cardiotoxicity (dyspnea, steady weight gain, hypotension, rapid pulse, arrhythmias) to permit immediate medical treatment. Monitor pulse and blood pressure frequently. Acute life-threatening arrhythmias may occur within a few hours of drug administration.

Objective signs of hepatic dysfunction (jaundice, dark urine, pruritus) or kidney dysfunction (altered intake–output ratio and pattern, local discomfort with voiding) demand prompt attention, since both conditions cause delayed drug elimination. Report to physician.

Stomatitis, generally maximal in second week of therapy, frequently begins with a burning sensation accompanied by erythema of oral mucosa that may progress to ulceration and dysphagia in 2 or 3 days. Fastidious oral hygiene is required, especially before and after meals. Patient should be referred to a dentist if dental caries or periodontal disease is present. *See Mechlorethamine for mouth care.*

Immunosuppressive properties of doxorubicin require careful screening of visitors and attending personnel to shield the patient from infection, especially during leukopenic periods.

The nadir of leukopenia (an expected $1000/mm^3$) typically occurs 10 to 14 days after single dose with recovery occurring within 21 days. RBC and platelet levels may be depressed also.

Superinfections by microflora may result from antibiotic therapy during leukopenic period. Report black or furry tongue, diarrhea, and foul-smelling stools, or vaginal discharge and vulvar or anal itching.

Complete alopecia (reversible) is an expected side effect. Discuss this side effect with the patient so that plans for cosmetic substitution can be made if desired. An awareness of the impact of the loss of scalp and body hair on one's concept of sexuality should guide this discussion.

If patient at risk of losing scalp hair intends to wear a wig, suggest an early fitting and wearing it before a large amount of hair is lost.

Inform patient that alopecia may also involve eyelashes and eyebrows, beard and mustache, pubic and axillary hair. Regrowth of hair usually begins 2 to 3 months after drug is discontinued.

Prophylactic treatment (controversial) by use of scalp tourniquet and/or ice pack may be instituted. Temporary constriction of superficial scalp blood vessels by cold or pressure is thought to minimize drug contact with hair follicles. Scalp cap or ice pack is applied 5 minutes before, during, and for 15 minutes after IV bolus administration of short-acting chemotherapeutic agent that is cleared from the blood after injection.

Bloody diarrhea may result from an antiblastic effect on rapidly growing intestinal mucosal cells. The physician may prescribe an antidiarrheal medication. Avoid rectal medications and use of rectal thermometer in order to prevent trauma.

Hyperuricemia, due to rapid lysis of neoplastic cells, may be treated by increased hydration, alkalinization of urine, and allopurinol. Urge patient to increase fluid intake to 2500 to 3000 ml in 24-hour period, if allowed. Monitor *blood uric acid* (normal: 3 to 7 mg/dl).

Symptoms of hyperuricemia should be reported: edema of lower legs and feet; joint, flank, or stomach pain.

Advise patient that the drug imparts a red color to urine for 1 to 2 days after administration.

Increased lacrimation for 5 to 10 days after a single dose is a possibility. Caution patient to keep hands away from eyes to prevent conjunctivitis.

Consult the physician about plan for disclosure of diagnosis, expected results of therapy, and prognosis to the patient and family in order to facilitate better communication with the patient.

Collaborate with dietitian and patient's family to help the patient maintain optimum nutritional status. Determine dietary preferences; try to support and augment rather than reform eating patterns during period of discomfort. Space pain medication so that peak effect is at mealtime; appropriately schedule fatiguing treatments to avoid presenting food to a tired patient.

Reconstituted solution is stable for 24 hours at room temperature and for 48 hours under refrigeration (4° to 10°C). Protect from sunlight; discard unused solution.

DOXYCYCLINE HYCLATE

(dox-i-sye'kleen)

(Doxy-Caps, Doxychel, Doxy-Lemmon, Doxy-Tabs, Vibramycin, Vibra-Tabs)

Antiinfective
Antibiotic
Tetracycline

D

ACTIONS AND USES. Broad spectrum antibiotic synthetically derived from oxytetracycline. Similar to tetracycline (qv) in actions, uses, contraindications, precautions, and adverse reactions. Antibacterial spectrum includes a variety of gram-negative and gram-positive microorganisms. More completely absorbed, effective blood levels maintained for longer periods, and excreted more slowly than most tetracyclines; thus, it requires smaller and less frequent doses. Usual doses of doxycycline do not ordinarily lead to excessive blood accumulation in patients with renal impairment.

Used to treat acute pelvic inflammatory disease, primary and secondary syphilis, uncomplicated urethral, endocervical, or rectal infections caused by *Chlamydia trachomatis. Investigational Use:* short-term prophylaxis of traveler's diarrhea caused by enterotoxigenic *E. coli;* treatment of genital, inguinal, and anorectal infections caused by lymphogranuloma venereum.

ABSORPTION AND FATE. Almost completely absorbed following oral administration (in fasting adults). Absorption reduced up to 20% by food or milk, but this is usually of no clinical significance. Serum levels peak in 1.5 to 4 hours. Range of plasma protein binding 25 to 90%. Half-life about 15 hours after single dose and up to 22 hours after repeated doses (essentially the same for patients with normal and impaired renal function). Inactivated by intestinal chelation; excreted primarily in bile and feces (up to 90%).

CONTRAINDICATIONS AND PRECAUTIONS. Sensitivity to tetracyclines; use during pregnancy, in nursing women, and in children under 8 years of age. *See also Tetracycline.*

ADVERSE/SIDE EFFECTS. With oral drug: nausea, diarrhea, GI discomfort, esophagitis, esophageal ulcers. For all routes: renal impairment, hepatotoxicity with excessive dosage; increased intracranial pressure; discoloration of nails, onycholysis; permanent discoloration and inadequate calcification of deciduous and permanent teeth when used during period of tooth development (from fourth month of fetal development to 8 years of life); overgrowth of nonsusceptible organisms; photosensitivity. *See also Tetracycline.*

ROUTE AND DOSAGE. Adults: Oral: 100 mg every 12 hours on first day, followed by maintenance dose of 100 mg/day as single dose or 50 mg every 12 hours (for severe infections 100 mg every 12 hours is recommended). **Intravenous:** 200 mg on first day administered in one or two infusions; subsequent daily dosage: 100 to 200 mg depending on severity of infection. **Children (over 8 years) (45 kg and under): Oral, intravenous:** 4.4 mg/kg on first day of treatment as single dose or divided into two doses; subsequent daily dosage: 2.2 to 4.4 mg/kg as single dose or divided into two doses. Available in capsules, tablets, oral suspension (as the calcium salt), syrup, and sterile injection.

NURSING IMPLICATIONS

Check expiration date. Degradation products of tetracycline or its congeners are nephrotoxic and have caused Fanconi-like syndrome (renal injury; glycosuria, phosphatemia, aminoacidemia, patchy depigmentation of retina).

Note that usual dosage and frequency of administration differ from those of other tetracyclines. Dosages in excess of those recommended may result in increased incidence of side effects.

Oral doxycycline may be taken with food and/or milk to minimize nausea, without significantly affecting bioavailability of drug.

Iron preparations, sodium bicarbonate, and antacids containing aluminum, calcium, or magnesium may significantly interfere with absorption. Therefore, these medications should be spaced at least 3 hours after doxycycline.

Esophageal ulcerations with use of doxycycline capsules have been reported. (Drug is highly acidic.)

Instructions for patients taking capsule or tablet forms (to prevent esophageal ulceration):

✓ Take drug with plenty of water to assure passage into stomach.
✓ For 1 to 2 hours after taking medication, avoid lying down, straining, or bending over.
✓ Avoid taking capsule or tablet within 1 hour of retiring.

For traveler's diarrhea, some clinicians have prescribed 200 mg of doxycycline on the day of travel, followed by 100 mg capsule daily for 3 weeks.

Preparation and storage of solutions: all tetracycline solutions should be used before the manufacturer's stated expiration date. Reconstituted solutions may be stored up to 72 hours prior to start of infusion if refrigerated and protected from sun and artificial light.

For IV use, the reconstituted solution must be diluted further with NaCl, 5% dextrose, or other diluents (recommended by manufacturer) before administration. Infusion must be completed within 12 hours of dilution. During infusion, solution must be protected from direct sunlight.

When diluted with lactated Ringer's or dextrose 5% in lactated Ringer's injection, infusion must be completed within 6 hours to ensure adequate stability.

IV infusion rate will be prescribed by physician. Duration of infusion will vary with dose, but it is usually 1 to 4 hours. Recommended minimum infusion time for 100 mg of 0.5 mg/ml solution is 1 hour.

Solutions of doxycycline hyclate containing 10 mg/ml sterile water may be frozen immediately after reconstitution and are stable for 8 weeks at −20°C. If solutions are warmed to thaw, care should be taken to prevent heating after thawing is completed. Do not refreeze.

Refer to manufacturer's information regarding storage of other reconstituted solutions.

Therapy should be continued at least 24 to 48 hours after symptoms have subsided.

Caution patient to avoid exposure to direct sunlight and ultraviolet light while taking doxycycline and for 4 or 5 days after therapy is terminated. Suggest use of a sunscreen agent (SPF above 12) when sun exposure is unavoidable.

In common with other tetracyclines, doxycycline may interfere with urine glucose determinations using either cupric sulfate method (Benedict's, Clinitest) or glucose oxidase reagent (Clinistix, Tes-Tape).

See Tetracycline hydrochloride (prototype tetracycline).

Drug Interactions. **Barbiturates, carbamazepine,** and **phenytoin** may hasten metabolism of doxycycline by inducing microsomal enzyme activity thereby decreasing antibiotic activity. *See also Tetracycline.*

DOXYLAMINE SUCCINATE

(Decapryn, Unisom)

(dox-il'a-meen)
Antihistamine
H_1-receptor antagonist
Antiemetic
Sedative

ACTIONS AND USES. Ethanolamine derivative with pronounced antinauseant and antiemetic and sedative effects. Mechanisms of action not known but thought to be related to central anticholinergic and CNS depressant actions. Similar to diphenhydramine (qv) in actions, uses, contraindications, precautions, and adverse reactions.

Used for treatment of seasonal and perennial rhinitis and as a nighttime sleep aid. Doxylamine is an ingredient in Nyquil and Vicks Formula 44.

CONTRAINDICATIONS AND PRECAUTIONS. Acute asthma, GI or GU obstruction, narrow-angle glaucoma. *Cautious Use:* cardiovascular disease, hypertension, elderly patients. *See also Diphenhydramine.*

ADVERSE/SIDE EFFECTS. Drowsiness, dizziness, headache, nervousness, palpitation, diarrhea or constipation, epigastric pain, thickening of bronchial secretions, dry mouth, nose, throat, blurred vision, difficulty in urination; disorientation, irritability, insomnia, tremor, vertigo (especially in the elderly); excitement, hallucinations (in children).

ROUTE AND DOSAGE. **Oral: Adults:** 12.5 to 25 mg every 4 to 6 hours if necessary. **Children (6 to 12 years):** 6.25 to 12.5 mg every 4 to 6 hours; not to exceed 75 mg daily. Available as tablets and syrup.

NURSING IMPLICATIONS

High incidence of drowsiness. Caution patient to avoid driving and other potentially hazardous activities until reaction to drug is determined.

Instruct patient not to drink alcoholic beverages while taking this medication. Patient should also be informed that other CNS depressants, e.g., antianxiety agents, sedatives, pain or sleeping medicines, will add to the CNS depressant effect of doxylamine.

Stored in tightly covered, light-resistant container, preferably at 15° to 30°C (59° to 86°F), unless otherwise directed by manufacturer.

See also Diphenhydramine hydrochloride (prototype ethanolamine antihistamine).

DROMOSTANOLONE PROPIONATE
(Drolban)

(droe-moe-stan'oh-lone)
Antineoplastic
Hormone
Androgen

ACTIONS AND USES. Synthetic steroid hormone chemically and pharmacologically related to testosterone (qv). Has lower incidence of androgenic side effects than parent compound. In advanced carcinoma, promotes weight gain and feeling of well-being, even though objective remission may not be obtained.

Used palliatively in advanced inoperable metastatic carcinoma of breast in women who are 1 to 5 years postmenopause.

CONTRAINDICATIONS AND PRECAUTIONS. Carcinoma of male breast; premenopausal women. *Cautious Use:* during pregnancy, liver disease, cardiac decompensation, nephritis, nephrosis, carcinoma of prostate. *See Testosterone.*

ADVERSE/SIDE EFFECTS. Virilism; hypercalcemia; edema (occasionally); severe, reversible CNS side effects (rare); local reaction at injection site (rare). *See Testosterone.*

ROUTE AND DOSAGE. **Intramuscular (in sesame oil):** 100 mg 3 times weekly.

NURSING IMPLICATIONS

At least 8 to 12 weeks of therapy may be necessary to produce satisfactory results. If disease being treated progresses significantly during first 6 to 8 weeks of treatment, another form of therapy may be indicated.

Treatment is generally continued as long as satisfactory results are obtained.

Patients with edema may require diuretic therapy before and during treatment with dromostanolone. Monitor weight and inspect dependent areas for signs of fluid retention. Report significant weight changes to physician.

In patients with bone metastasis, serum calcium and alkaline phosphatase levels should be determined before and periodically during therapy.

Advise patient to report symptoms of hypercalcemia: deep bone and flank pain, thirst, polyuria, renal calculi, muscle weakness, nausea, vomiting, anorexia, constipation, lethargy, psychosis. Dromostanolone should be discontinued if severe hypercalcemia occurs.

Product should not be refrigerated since a precipitate may form. Store preferably at 15° to 30°C (59° to 86°F), unless otherwise directed by manufacturer.

See Testosterone (prototype androgen).

DROPERIDOL

(Inapsine)

(droe-per'i-dole)
Psychotropic
Antipsychotic (neuroleptic)
Antiemetic
Butyrophenone

ACTIONS AND USES. Butyrophenone derivative structurally and pharmacologically related to haloperidol (qv). Antagonizes emetic effects of morphinelike analgesics and other drugs that act on CTZ. Mild alpha-adrenergic blocking activity and direct vasodilator effect may cause hypotension. Reduces anxiety and motor activity without necessarily inducing sleep; patient remains responsive. Potentiates other CNS depressants. Reduces pressor effects of epinephrine, and decreases epinephrine-induced arrhythmias, but does not prevent cardiac arrhythmias. May decrease pulmonary arterial pressure. Has greater tendency to produce extrapyramidal symptoms than haloperidol.

Used to produce tranquilizing effect and to reduce nausea and vomiting during surgical and diagnostic procedures. Also used for premedication, during induction, and as adjunct in maintenance of general or regional anesthesia. Principally used in fixed combination with a potent narcotic analgesic such as fentanyl (Innovar) to produce neuroleptanalgesia (quiescence, reduced motor activity, and indifference to pain and environmental stimuli) to permit carrying out a variety of diagnostic and minor surgical procedures. *Unlabeled Use:* IV antiemetic in cancer chemotherapy.

ABSORPTION AND FATE. Onset of action within 3 to 10 minutes; peaks in about 30 minutes following single IM or IV dose. Duration of sedative and tranquilizing effects (ataraxia) is generally 3 to 6 hours, but may persist 6 to 24 hours. Metabolized in liver and excreted primarily in urine. About 10% eliminated in urine as unchanged drug. Crosses placenta.

CONTRAINDICATIONS AND PRECAUTIONS. Known intolerance to droperidol; pregnancy, in women of childbearing potential, and children younger than 2 years of age. *Cautious Use:* elderly, debilitated, and other poor-risk patients; Parkinson's disease, hypotension; liver, kidney, cardiac disease; cardiac bradyarrhythmias.

ADVERSE/SIDE EFFECTS. Most frequent: hypotension, tachycardia, drowsiness. Chills, shivering, dizziness, restlessness, anxiety, hallucinations, mental depression, laryngospasm, bronchospasm. Extrapyramidal symptoms: dystonia, akathisia, oculogyric crisis. *See Haloperidol.*

ROUTE AND DOSAGE. *Premedication:* **Adults: Intramuscular:** 2.5 to 10 mg 30 to 60 minutes before the procedure. **Children (2 to 12 years):** 1 to 1.5 mg per 20 to 25 lb body weight. **Elderly, debilitated patients:** initial dose less than for adult. Maintenance: 1.25 to 2.5 mg. *For induction:* **Adults: Intravenous:** 2.5 mg per 9 to 11 kg (20 to 25 lbs) with an analgesic and/or general anesthetic.

NURSING IMPLICATIONS

FDA approval is granted for use only as adjunct to preanesthesia and during anesthetic period.

Monitor vital signs closely. Hypotension (possibly due to hypovolemia) and tachycardia are common side effects of droperidol. Fluids and pressor agents (other than epinephrine which causes a paradoxical lowering of blood pressure) should be immediately available.

Because of possibility of severe orthostatic hypotension, always exercise care in moving and positioning the medicated patient. Avoid abrupt changes in position.

Consult anesthesiologist concerning advisability of placing the immediate postoperative patient in head-low position. In patients who have had spinal or peridural anesthesia this position may result in a higher level of anesthesia and enhanced sympathetic blockade.

Patient who receives a narcotic analgesic (opiate agonist), e.g., fentanyl, concurrently should be observed carefully for signs of impending respiratory depression (restlessness, apnea, rigidity). A narcotic antagonist and resuscitative equipment, including oropharyngeal airway or endotracheal tube, suction, and oxygen, should be readily available.

Elevated blood pressure has been reported following administration of droperidol with parenteral analgesics (perhaps due to respiratory or surgical stimulation during light anesthesia).

During the postoperative period, EEG patterns are slow to return to normal.

When patient is under the effect of another CNS depressant, the required dose of droperidol may be less than usual. Postoperative narcotics or other CNS depressants are prescribed in reduced doses (as low as 25 or 30% of those usually recommended), since they have additive or potentiating effects with droperidol.

Extrapyramidal symptoms may occur within 24 to 48 hours postoperatively. Observe patient carefully for early signs of acute dystonia: facial grimacing, restlessness, tremors, torticollis, oculogyric crisis. Report promptly. Anticholinergic antiparkinsonian drugs produce dramatic relief (e.g., atropine, benztropine, or diphenhydramine).

Droperidol may aggravate symptoms of acute depression.

Drug incompatibilities: do not mix with parenteral barbiturates, since a precipitate may occur.

Protect from light. Store at temperature between 15° and 30°C (59° and 86°F), unless otherwise directed by manufacturer.

See Haloperidol (prototype butyrophenone antipsychotic).

DYCLONINE HYDROCHLORIDE

(dye-kloe-neen)

(Dyclone)

Anesthetic, local

ACTIONS AND USES. Organic ketone, synthetic local topical anesthetic agent. Produces local anesthesia by blocking impulses at peripheral nerve endings in skin and mucous membranes.

Used for topical anesthesia of mucous membranes preparatory for endoscopic examinations and gynecologic and proctologic procedures. Also used to suppress gag reflex, to relieve pain of minor burns or trauma, and to alleviate itching of pruritus ani or vulvae. *Unlabeled Use:* to provide relief from discomfort of fever blisters.

ABSORPTION AND FATE. Absorbed through skin and mucous membranes. Onset of anesthetic action within 2 to 10 minutes; duration: up to 1 hour.

CONTRAINDICATIONS AND PRECAUTIONS. Cystoscopic procedures following IV pyelography (because contrast media containing iodine may precipitate and interfere with visualization); applications to extensive areas or to bleeding surfaces. Safe use during pregnancy not established. *Cautious Use:* debilitated or elderly patients, children, patients with drug sensitivities, or family history of allergies severe trauma or sepsis in region of application.

ADVERSE/SIDE EFFECTS. Allergic: urticaria, edema, contact dermatitis. **Local:** burning, tenderness, swelling, irritation, urethritis. **Systemic absorption:** nervousness, dizziness, drowsiness, excitement or depression, tremors, blurred vision, hypotension, bradycardia, cardiac or respiratory arrest.

ROUTE AND DOSAGE. Topical: 0.5 to 1% solution. Methods of application: swabbing, gargle, spray, instillation, compress.

NURSING IMPLICATIONS

When applied orally, dyclonine may interfere with second stage of swallowing (pharyngeal stage). Do not give patient anything by mouth within 60 minutes (until return of gag reflex) following drug administration.

If necessary, gag reflex may be tested by gently touching back of pharynx on each side with a cotton swab (while holding tongue down with a depressor). If patient does not gag or swallow, give nothing by mouth. Suctioning of secretions may be necessary to prevent aspiration.

A sip of clean water should be the first thing swallowed when gag reflex returns.

Dyclonine 5 to 15 ml of 0.5% solution may be swallowed (prescribed) to relieve pain of esophageal lesions.

Avoid contact with eyes or eyelids. Applications to large areas should be avoided.

Instruct patient to discontinue medication and to contact physician if irritation, sensitization, or infection occurs.

Resuscitation equipment (e.g., for administration of oxygen, artificial respiration, cardiac massage) and drugs such as vasopressors and ultra short-acting barbiturates (e.g., thiopental) and muscle relaxants (e.g., succinylcholine) should be immediately available. This is a general rule to follow whenever a patient is receiving an anesthetic.

Protect drug from light. Store at 15° to 30°C (59° to 86°F), unless otherwise directed by manufacturer.

DYPHYLLINE

(Asminyl, Dilin, Dilor, Dyflex, Dylline, Lufyllin, Neothylline, Protophylline, and others)

(dye'fi-lin)
Smooth muscle relaxant
Bronchodilator
Xanthine

ACTIONS AND USES. Xanthine and derivative of theophylline (qv) with which it shares similar pharmacologic effects: (bronchodilation, myocardial stimulation, vasodilation, diuresis, and smooth muscle relaxation). Unlike other xanthines, dyphylline is not metabolized to theophylline in body; therefore serum theophylline levels are not useful. Claimed to cause less gastric distress than theophylline because of its neutral pH. Appears to be more uniformly and predictably absorbed than theophylline, but levels and activity are lower, and it has a short half-life; thus higher and more frequent dosing may be required to attain comparable sustained effects.

Used in treatment of acute bronchial asthma and for reversible bronchospasm associated with chronic bronchitis and emphysema. Available in several antiasthmatic preparations in combination with guaifenesin (Dilor-G, Dyflex-G, Dyline-GG, Neothylline-GG).

ABSORPTION AND FATE. Readily absorbed from GI tract and from IM sites. Peak plasma levels in 1 hour; half-life: 2 hours. Wide interindividual variations in blood levels and duration of action. Excreted by kidneys primarily as unchanged drug.

CONTRAINDICATIONS AND PRECAUTIONS. Hypersensitivity to xanthine compounds. Safe use during pregnancy and in nursing mothers not established. *Cautious Use:* severe cardiac disease, hypertension, acute myocardial injury, renal or hepatic dysfunction, glaucoma, hyperthyroidism, peptic ulcer, use in the elderly and in children; concomitant administration of other xanthine formulations or other CNS stimulating drugs.

ADVERSE/SIDE EFFECTS. CNS: headache, irritability, restlessness, dizziness, insomnia. **CV:** palpitation, tachycardia, extrasystoles, flushing, hypotension. **GI:** nausea, vomiting, epigastric distress. **Respiratory:** tachypnea. **Other:** albuminuria, fever, dehydration.

ROUTE AND DOSAGE. Adults: Oral: 15 mg/kg every 6 hours, up to 4 times a day. **Intramuscular:** 250 to 500 mg at 6-hour intervals, if necessary. **Children (6 years and older): Oral:** 4.4 to 6.6 mg/kg daily in divided doses. All dosages titrated to individual patient's requirements.

NURSING IMPLICATIONS

Absorption is enhanced by taking oral preparation with a full glass of water on an empty stomach, e.g., 1 hour before or 2 hours after meals. However, administration after meals may help to relieve gastric discomfort.

Care should be exercised in the amount of elixir given to children because it has a high alcohol content (18 to 20%).

For IM administration, aspirate carefully before injecting drug to avoid inadvertent intravascular injection. Inject drug slowly.

Do not use parenteral form if a precipitate is present.

Baseline and periodic pulmonary function tests may be done to assess therapeutic effectiveness of dyphylline.

Minimal effective therapeutic dyphylline blood level is reported to be 12 mcg/ml.

Caution patient to avoid alcohol, and also large amounts of coffee and other xanthine-containing beverages, e.g., tea, cocoa, colas during therapy.

Since many OTC drugs for coughs, colds, and allergies contain ephedrine or other sympathomimetics and xanthines (e.g., caffeine, theophylline, aminophylline), advise patient to consult physician before taking OTC preparations.

Store at room temperature preferably between 15° and 30°C (59° and 86°F), unless otherwise directed by manufacturer. Protect dyphylline solution from light.

Drug Interactions. Concurrent administration of dyphylline with **ephedrine** or other **sympathomimetic agents** can cause excessive CNS stimulation. *See also Theophylline (prototype xanthine).*

E

ECHOTHIOPHATE IODIDE

(Phospholine Iodide)

(ek-oh-thye'oh-fate)

Cholinergic (parasympathomimetic)
Cholinesterase inhibitor
Miotic
Organophosphate

ACTIONS AND USES. Extremely potent, long-acting cholinesterase inhibitors; quaternary organophosphorus compound. Similar to demecarium in actions, uses, contraindications, precautions, and adverse effects. In contrast to demecarium, the cholinesterase inhibition produced by echothiophate is relatively irreversible, i.e., cholinesterase activity returns only when new enzyme is formed.

Used particularly in treatment of chronic open angle glaucoma, conditions obstructing aqueous outflow such as synechia formation, following iridectomy or cataract surgery and for diagnosis and treatment of accommodative esotropia. Use is usually reserved for patients not satisfactorily controlled by less potent miotics.

ABSORPTION AND FATE. Absorbed through conjunctival sac. Miosis usually begins within 10 minutes following instillation, and is maximal within 30 minutes. Intraocular pressure (IOP) decreases within 4 to 8 hours; peak reduction within 24 hours. Miosis and IOP reduction may persist 1 to 4 weeks.

CONTRAINDICATIONS AND PRECAUTIONS. Hypersensitivity to drug ingredients; acute-angle closure glaucoma, history of or active uveitis. Safe use during pregnancy not established. *Cautious Use:* history of retinal detachment, corneal abrasion; disorders that may respond adversely to vagotonic action, e.g., bronchial asthma, spastic diseases of GI tract, bradycardia, epilepsy, Parkinson's disease; patients routinely exposed to organophosphate insecticides.

ADVERSE/SIDE EFFECTS. Browache, headache, lacrimation, stinging, dimness or blurring of vision, photosensitivity, ciliary or accommodative spasm, lid muscle twitching, iris cysts (especially in children), conjunctival redness and thickening, hyperactivity in children with Down's syndrome; reduced serum cholinesterases; decreased pseudocholinesterase activity. *Systemic reactions (cholinergic effects):* salivation, frequent urination or incontinence, diarrhea, abdominal cramps, nausea, vomiting, profuse sweating, muscle weakness, respiratory difficulties, nasal congestion, cardiac irregularities.

ROUTE AND DOSAGE. Topical: *Glaucoma:* 1 drop of 0.03 to 0.25% ophthalmic solution instilled into conjunctival sac once or twice daily (morning and before retiring). Not to exceed a twice-daily schedule. Highly individualized. *Accomodative esotropia* (Diagnosis): 1 drop of 0.125% solution instilled in both eyes once daily at bedtime for 2 to 3 weeks. (Treatment): 1 drop of 0.125% solution every other day or 1 drop of 0.06% daily. Usual maximum recommended dosage is 1 drop of 0.125% daily.

NURSING IMPLICATIONS

When possible, instillation of daily dose or one of the daily doses should be made at bedtime to minimize patient distress from blurred vision.

Administration technique: Gentle finger pressure should be applied against nasolacrimal

E

duct while drug is being instilled; maintain pressure for 1 or 2 minutes following instillation. This minimizes drainage into nose and throat and thus systemic absorption. Immediately blot excess solution around eye with tissue. Wash hands thoroughly before and after handling drug.

Generally advisable for patient to remove soft contact lenses before instilling eye drops. Soft lenses may absorb medication or may be stained or otherwise damaged by the drug itself or by preservatives in the medication. It is usually unnecessary to remove hard contact lenses before instilling eyedrops. Consult the patient's physician about this teaching point.

Gonioscopic examination is recommended prior to initiation of therapy for glaucoma to confirm that eye angle is open.

Drug concentration and frequency of instillation are determined by tonometric readings during therapy.

Slit lamp examinations and tonometric measurements are performed before and during therapy. Tonometric readings are generally taken at least hourly for the first 3 to 4 hours after the initial instillation to detect a rise in IOP (from unexpected angle closure) or a sudden drop in IOP (possibly from retinal detachment).

Browache, headache, dimness or blurring of vision may occur at onset of therapy, but these symptoms usually disappear within 5 to 10 days. Patient may require an analgesic for headache or browache (caused by miosis).

Inform patient that vision may be especially poor in dim light and at night. Advise patient to avoid night driving particularly.

Physician may prescribe concomitant instillation of phenylephrine or epinephrine hydrochloride to improve visual acuity (dilates miotic treated eye without increasing intraocular pressure) and to reduce conjunctival redness.

Since toxicity is cumulative, symptoms may not appear for several weeks after start of therapy. Advise patient to notify physician promptly of any unusual signs or symptoms, or any new or worsening visual problem.

A positive diagnosis of accommodative esotropia (convergent strabismus) is made if eyes appear straighter with therapy. (Response may begin within a few hours.)

Duration of echothiophate therapy for convergent strabismus may range from 1 to 5 years. If eyes deviate following drug withdrawal, surgery is usually considered.

Patient should be informed that alcoholic beverages may increase severity of systemic drug effects.

All patients should remain under close supervision while receiving echothiophate.

In most patients, serum pseudocholinesterase and erythrocyte cholinesterase levels will be depressed after a few weeks of eyedrop therapy.

Caution patient to report salivation, diarrhea, profuse sweating, urinary incontinence, or muscle weakness. These systemic effects indicate the need to terminate medication.

Warn patients of possible additive systemic effects from exposure to organophosphorus-type insecticides and pesticides, e.g., parathion, malathion. If exposure to these substances is unavoidable, advise the patient to wear a respiratory mask, and to wash and change clothing frequently.

Treatment of overdosage: systemic effects occurring after topical application, skin contact, or accidental ingestion can be antagonized by parenteral atropine sulfate or pralidoxime chloride (Protopam). Artificial respiration may be necessary.

Tolerance may develop after prolonged use, but the response is usually restored by a prescribed rest period from drug.

Aqueous solutions remain stable for 1 month at room temperature. Expiration date should appear on label. Stability time of solutions under refrigeration varies with manufacturer.

Protect powder and solutions from light.

Drug Interactions. Other cholinesterase inhibitors (e.g., **ambenonium, edrophonium, neostigmine, physostigmine, pyridostigmine**) potentiate the action of echothiophate. With prolonged use of echothiophate, severe reactions may follow injections of **procaine** or administration of **succinylcholine.** *See also Demecarium Bromide.*

ECONAZOLE NITRATE

(Ecostatin, Spectazole)

(e-kone'a-zole)
Antiinfective
Antibiotic
Antifungal

ACTIONS AND USES. Synthetic imidazole derivative with broad antifungal spectrum of activity similar to that of miconazole. Exerts fungistatic action but may be fungicidal for certain microorganisms or at high concentrations. Mechanism of action not known but appears to be related to altered cellular membrane permeability and to interference with RNA, protein, and lipid biosynthesis. Active against dermatophyes (including *Trichophyton mentagrophytes, T. rubrum, T. tonsurans, Epidermophyton floccosum, Microsporum audouini, M. canis*), yeasts, e.g., *Candida albicans, Pityrosporum obiculare* (tinea versicolor), and many other genera of fungi. Also appears to be active against some gram-positive bacteria (e.g., *Staphylococcus aureus, Streptococcus pyogenes,* and *Corynebacterium diphtheriae*).

Used topically for treatment of tinea pedis (athlete's foot: ringworm of foot), tinea cruris ("jock itch": ringworm of groin), tinea corporis (ringworm of body), and for treatment of tinea versicolor, and cutaneous candidiasis (moniliasis). Has been used for topical treatment of erythrasma, and with corticosteroids for fungal or bacterial dermatoses associated with inflammation.

ABSORPTION AND FATE. Minimal percutaneous absorption from intact skin; absorption somewhat increased from denuded skin. Inhibitory concentrations achieved in stratum corneum, epidermis, and middle region of dermis in ½ to 5 hours after topical application. Metabolic fate and complete excretory pattern not known. Less than 1% of applied dose eliminated in urine and feces.

CONTRAINDICATIONS AND PRECAUTIONS. Hypersensitivity to econazole nitrate or to any ingredients in the formulation. Safe use during pregnancy (category C) and in nursing women not established.

ADVERSE/SIDE EFFECTS. Burning, stinging sensation, pruritus, erythema.

ROUTE AND DOSAGE. Topical (1% cream in water-miscible base): *Tinea cruris, tinea corporis, tinea pedis, cutaneous candidiasis:* Apply sufficient amount and rub gently into affected areas twice daily, morning and evening. *Tinea versicolor:* Apply once daily to affected areas.

NURSING IMPLICATIONS

Consult physician regarding specific procedure for cleansing affected area(s) before applying medication.

Wash hands thoroughly before and after treatments.

Do not use occlusive dressings unless prescribed by physician.

Instruct patient to use medication for the prescribed time even if symptoms improve, and to report to physician skin reactions suggestive of irritation or sensitization.

Clinical improvement should occur within the first 1 or 2 weeks of therapy. Advise patient to notify physician if full course of therapy does not result in improvement. Diagnosis should be reevaluated.

To reduce possibility of recurrence, candidal infections, tinea corporis and tinea cruris should be treated for 2 weeks and tinea pedis for 1 month. Some patients require longer periods of treatment. Patients with tinea versicolor usually improve after 2 weeks of therapy.

Caution patient not to apply the topical cream in or near the eyes or intravaginally.

Store at temperature less than 30°C (86°F), unless otherwise directed by manufacturer.

See Index: Nursing Interventions: Fungal infections.

EDETATE CALCIUM DISODIUM

(Calcium Disodium Versenate, Calcium EDTA)

(ed′e-tate)
Chelating agent
Diagnostic agent

ACTIONS AND USES. Chelating agent that combines with divalent and trivalent metals to form stable, nonionizing soluble complexes that can be readily excreted by kidneys. Action is dependent on ability of heavy metal to displace the less strongly bound calcium in the drug molecule. Contains approximately 5.3 mEq of sodium per gram of drug.

Used principally as adjunct in treatment of acute and chronic lead poisoning (plumbism). Generally used in combination with dimercaprol (BAL) in treatment of lead encephalopathy and/or when blood lead level exceeds 100 mcg/dl. Reported to be of some value in treatment of poisoning from other heavy metals such as chromium, manganese, nickel, zinc, and possibly vanadium, and also in removal of radioactive and nuclear fission products such as plutonium, yttrium, uranium. Not effective in poisoning from arsenic, gold, or mercury. Also used to diagnose suspected lead poisoning.

ABSORPTION AND FATE. Plasma half-life: about 20 to 60 minutes following IV and 1½ hours after IM administration. Following IV administration distributed to extracellular fluid; does not enter CSF. Is not metabolized. Approximately 50% of chelated lead excreted within 1 hour. Over 95% of chelates excreted within 24 to 48 hours.

CONTRAINDICATIONS AND PRECAUTIONS. Severe renal disease, anuria, IV use in patients with lead encephalopathy not generally recommended (because of possible increase in intracranial pressure); during pregnancy or in women of childbearing potential. *Cautious Use:* renal dysfunction, active tubercular lesions, history of gout.

ADVERSE/SIDE EFFECTS. Numbness, tingling sensations (paresthesias), headache, muscle cramps, anorexia, nausea, vomiting, diarrhea, abdominal cramps, weakness, hypotension, cardiac arrhythmias, burning sensation at injection site, thrombophlebitis, hypercalcemia, gout. **With high doses or prolonged administration:** nephrotoxicity (usually reversible), transient bone marrow depression, cheilosis and other mucocutaneous lesions; depletion of blood metals. Febrile systemic reaction (malaise, fatigue, excessive thirst, fever, chills, severe myalgia, arthralgia, frontal headache, GI distress, nephrotoxicity) and accompanied by histaminelike reactions: flushing, throbbing headache, sweating, sneezing, nasal congestion, lacrimation, postural hypotension, tachycardia.

ROUTE AND DOSAGE. **Intravenous: Adults:** 1 Gm diluted in 250 to 500 ml 5% dextrose in water or isotonic sodium chloride injection. Administer over period of at least 1 hour if patient is asymptomatic and at least 2 hours if patient is symptomatic. Doses may be administered twice daily (12-hour intervals) for up to 5 days. Therapy should then be interrupted for 2 days, followed by additional 5 days of treatment, if indicated. **Intramuscular: Children**

(preferred route): not to exceed 35 mg/kg twice daily. In mild cases, not to exceed 50 mg/kg/day. In **young children** total daily dose may be given in divided doses every 8 to 12 hours for 3 to 5 days. Second course may be given after rest period of 4 or more drug free days.

NURSING IMPLICATIONS

Not to be confused with edetate disodium.

Adequacy of urinary output must be determined before therapy is initiated. This may be done by administering IV fluids before giving first dose of calcium EDTA.

Fluid intake is generally increased to enhance urinary excretion of chelates. Excess fluid intake, however, should be avoided in patients with lead encephalopathy because of the danger of further increasing intracranial pressure. Consult physician regarding allowable intake.

Procaine hydrochloride should be added to minimize pain at IM injection site (usually 1 ml of procaine 1% to each ml of concentrated drug). Consult physician.

Closely monitor infusion rate as prescribed by physician. Rapid IV infusion in a patient with cerebral edema can be lethal.

When dimercaprol (BAL) and calcium EDTA are given concurrently, each should be injected into separate IM sites.

Monitor intake and output. Since drug is excreted almost exclusively via kidneys, toxicity may develop if output is inadequate. Therapy should be stopped if urine flow is markedly diminished or absent. Report any change in output or intake–output ratio to physician.

Home-based patients and responsible family members should be instructed to adhere to prescribed dosage regimen, to report adverse reactions immediately to physician, and to keep scheduled follow-up appointments.

Calcium disodium edetate can produce potentially fatal effects when higher than recommended doses are used or when it is continued after toxic effects appear.

Routine urinalyses including tests for coproporphyrins should be performed prior to therapy and daily during entire course of therapy. Presence of large renal epithelial cells or increasing hematuria and proteinuria are indications to terminate drug immediately. BUN, serum creatinine, calcium, and phosphorous determinations should be done before and during each course of therapy.

Because edetate calcium disodium may chelate metals other than lead, patients on prolonged therapy should have periodic determinations of blood trace element metals (e.g., copper, zinc, magnesium).

Lead poisoning is a persistent problem in certain occupations (such as workers in storage-battery factories or in lead smelters), and in areas where older homes exist. Steps should be taken to identify and eliminate environmental sources of lead immediately after diagnosis of lead poisoning is made. In areas where lead poisoning is endemic, parents should be encouraged to take their children to lead-detection clinics.

Manifestations of lead poisoning (plumbism) include abdominal colic, pallor, anemia, blue-black pigmented line along gingival margins (in patients with poor oral hygiene), metallic taste, peripheral neuritis, encephalopathy (ataxia, vomiting, lethargy, stupor, followed by convulsions, mania, and coma).

Normal whole blood lead level: 0 to 40 mcg/dl. Clinical symptoms of lead poisoning occur with blood levels greater than 50 mcg/dl.

Calcium EDTA interferes with duration of action of zinc insulin preparations (forms chelate with zinc); therefore do not administer them concurrently.

Report cardiac rhythm abnormalities.

Be alert for occurrence of febrile systemic reaction that may appear 4 to 8 hours after drug infusion *(see Adverse/Side Effects).*

E

Diagnostic Test Interferences. Edetate calcium disodium may decrease **serum cholesterol, plasma lipid** levels (if elevated), and **serum potassium** values. **Glycosuria** may occur with toxic doses.

EDETATE DISODIUM

(Chealamide, Disotate, EDTA, Endrate, Sodium Versenate)

(ed'e-tate)
Chelating agent
Regulator: calcium

E

ACTIONS AND USES. Structurally distinct from edetate calcium disodium. Forms chelates with many bivalent and trivalent metals, e.g., magnesium, zinc, and other trace metals, but has particular affinity for calcium. Forms a stable, nonionizing soluble complex that can be readily excreted via kidneys. Does not chelate potassium but promotes its urinary excretion and may reduce serum potassium levels. Not recommended for treatment of lead toxicity because it may cause severe hypocalcemia. Exerts negative inotropic effect on heart and may antagonize the inotropic and chronotropic effects of digitalis glycosides. Topical applications to the eye can dissolve calcium deposits on cornea. Contains approximately 5.4 mEq of sodium per gram of drug.

Used in selected patients for emergency treatment of hypercalcemia, and to control ventricular arrhythmias and heart block associated with digitalis toxicity when other drugs, e.g., phenytoin and potassium are contraindicated or ineffective. *Investigational Use:* in ophthalmology to remove calcium deposits from corneal epithelium, either by topical use or by iontophoresis, and also for emergency treatment of lime (calcium oxide) burns to eye.

ABSORPTION AND FATE. Approximately 95% of dose excreted rapidly from urine following IV administration; eliminated primarily as calcium chelate.

CONTRAINDICATIONS AND PRECAUTIONS. Significant renal disease, anuria, hypocalcemia, history of seizure disorders or intracranial lesions, active or healed calcified tubercular lesions, generalized arteriosclerosis associated with advancing age, coronary or peripheral vascular disease. Safe use during pregnancy and in women of childbearing potential not established. *Cautious Use:* limited cardiac reserve, incipient congestive heart failure, potassium deficiency states.

ADVERSE/SIDE EFFECTS. CNS: transient numbness, circumoral paresthesias, muscle cramps, muscle weakness, back pain, lassitude, malaise, headache, fatigue, convulsions. **CV:** hypotension, thrombophlebitis. **Dermatologic:** exfoliative dermatitis and other skin and mucous membrane lesions resembling those of pyridoxine (vitamin B_6) deficiency. **GI:** nausea, vomiting, anorexia, diarrhea, abdominal cramps. **GU (with excessive dosage):** nephrotoxicity: urgency, dysuria, nocturia, oliguria, polyuria, proteinuria, tubular necrosis. **Local reactions:** pain, erythema, dermatitis at infusion site. **Other:** fever, chills, anemia, glycosuria, hyperuricemia, severe hypocalcemia (rapid IV or high dosages), hypomagnesemia (prolonged therapy), calcium embolization, damage to reticuloendothelial system with hemorrhagic tendencies (excessive dosage).

ROUTE AND DOSAGE. Intravenous: *Hypercalcemia:* **Adults:** 50 mg/kg/daily up to 3 Gm/day. Dose should be added to 500 ml of 5% dextrose or 0.9% sodium chloride injection and administered over 3 to 4 hours. **Children:** 40 mg/kg/daily not to exceed 70 mg/kg/day. Add to sufficient amount of 5% dextrose injection or 0.9% sodium chloride to make no greater than 30 mg/ml (3%) solution and administer over 3 to 4 hours. *Digitalis-induced ventricular arrhythmia.* **Adults and children:** 15 mg/kg/hour up to maximum of 60 mg/kg/day by IV infusion in 5% dextrose injection. *Investigational Use (by physician) for corneal calcium deposits:* 0.35 to 1.85% solution depending on density of deposit; diluted with 0.9% sodium chloride injection to desired concentration. After removal of corneal epithelium, applied topically or by iontophoresis, following which eye is irrigated with 0.9% sodium chloride injection or sterile balanced salt solution.

NURSING IMPLICATIONS

Not to be confused with *Edetate calcium disodium.* This preparation should not be used for treatment of lead poisoning because it causes hypocalcemia.

The commercially-available injection must be diluted before administration.

Drug is extremely irritating to tissue and therefore should be well diluted before infusion. Extravasation must be prevented. Rotate infusion sites.

Monitor IV infusion rate as prescribed by physician. Rapid IV infusion (or high serum drug levels) can result in hypocalcemic tetany, cardiac arrhythmias, seizures, and cardiac arrest.

Advise patient to remain in bed for about 20 to 30 minutes after infusion because of the possibility of postural hypotension. Check blood pressure and pulse before patient ambulates. Instruct patient to make position changes slowly, to dangle legs and move ankles and toes for a few minutes before getting out of bed, and to avoid standing still. Supervise ambulation.

Serum calcium levels should be determined after each administration. Observe for and report immediately early signs and symptoms of hypocalcemia: paresthesias of lips, tongue, fingers, feet; mental instability, stupor, seizures, carpopedal spasm, and positive Chvostek's and Trousseau's signs *(see Index).*

Keep calcium gluconate or other suitable IV calcium preparation immediately available for emergency use.

Cardiac function should be monitored, particularly in patients with arrhythmia and those with history of seizure disorders or intracranial lesions.

Monitor and report any significant change in intake–output ratio to physician.

Urinalyses should be done daily throughout therapy and renal function studies (BUN, serum creatinine) should be performed prior to initiation of therapy and at regular intervals during therapy. Nephrotoxicity is usually reversible if drug is stopped promptly at the first appearance of symptoms.

Insulin-dependent diabetic (IDDM) patients may require reduction of insulin dosage while receiving edetate disodium therapy *(see Drug Interactions).*

Diagnostic Test Interferences. Colorimetric method of determining **serum calcium** levels will not be accurate; oxalate method may yield artificially low serum calcium values. Greater accuracy may be possible by performing test immediately before due dose is administered, or by acidifying the sample (atomic absorption spectrometry reportedly not affected). **Serum alkaline phosphatase** may be decreased (thought to be induced by low **serum magnesium** levels).

Drug Interactions. Edetate disodium may lower **blood glucose** levels and thus reduce insulin requirements in (IDDM) diabetic patients; reaction is thought to be due to chelation of the **zinc in insulin** preparations.

E

EDROPHONIUM CHLORIDE

(Tensilon)

(ed-roe-foe'nee-um)

Cholinergic (parasympathomimetic), Cholinesterase inhibitor

Antidote, diagnostic agent

ACTIONS AND USES. Indirect-acting cholinesterase inhibitor (quaternary ammonium compound) similar to neostigmine (qv) in actions, contraindications, precautions, and adverse reactions. Acts as antidote to curariform drugs by displacing them from muscle cell receptor sites, thus permitting resumption of normal transmission of neuromuscular impulses. However, like neostigmine, it prolongs skeletal muscle relaxant action of succinylcholine chloride and decamethonium bromide.

Used for differential diagnosis and as adjunct in evaluation of treatment requirements of myasthenia gravis, for differentiating myasthenic from cholinergic crisis, and to reverse neuromuscular block produced by overdosage of curariform drugs, e.g., tubocurarine, gallamine. Not recommended for maintenance therapy in myasthenia gravis because of its short duration of action. *Investigational Use:* to terminate paroxysmal atrial tachycardia or as an aid in diagnosing supraventricular tacchyarrhythmias, and evaluating function of demand pacemakers.

ABSORPTION AND FATE. Onset of effects on skeletal muscle within 30 to 60 seconds after IV injection; duration 6 to 24 minutes. Onset of effects following IM: 2 to 10 minutes; duration 12 to 45 minutes. Passes blood–brain barrier only at extremely high doses.

CONTRAINDICATIONS AND PRECAUTIONS. Hypersensitivity to anticholinesterase agents; intestinal and urinary obstruction. Safe use in women of childbearing potential and during pregnancy and lactation not established. *Cautious Use:* bronchial asthma, cardiac arrhythmias, patients receiving digitalis.

ADVERSE/SIDE EFFECTS. Severe side effects uncommon with usual doses. **CNS:** weakness, muscle cramps, fasciculations, incoordination, respiratory paralysis. **CV:** bradycardia, irregular pulse, hypotension. **GI:** diarrhea, abdominal cramps, nausea, vomiting, excessive salivation. **Ophthalmic:** miosis, blurred vision, lacrimation. **Other:** excessive sweating, increased bronchial secretions, bronchospasm, pulmonary edema.

ROUTE AND DOSAGE. Adults: *Edrophonium test for myasthenia gravis:* **Intravenous:** (prepare 10 mg in tuberculin syringe): Initial: 2 mg injected within 15 to 30 seconds; needle is left in situ; if there is no reaction after 45 seconds, the remaining 8 mg is injected; test may be repeated after 30 minutes. **Intramuscular:** 10 mg; if cholinergic reaction occurs, retest after 30 minutes with 2 mg to rule out false-negative reaction. *Evaluation of myasthenic treatment:* 1 to 2 mg IV administered 1 hour after last oral dose of anticholinesterase medication used in treatment. *Myasthenic crisis evaluation* (prepare 2 mg in tuberculin syringe): initially 1 mg IV; if after an interval of 1 minute the patient's condition does not deteriorate, administer remaining 1 mg. *Curare antagonist:* 10 mg IV administered over 30 to 45 seconds; repeated every 5 to 10 minutes as necessary; maximal dose 40 mg. **Children:** *Edrophonium test for myasthenia gravis:* **Children weighing up to 75 lb:** 1 mg IV; if no response after 45 seconds, dose may be titrated up to 5 mg; alternatively, 2 mg IM. **Children over 75 lb:** 2 mg IV; if no response after 45 seconds, dose may be titrated up to 10 mg; alternatively, 5 mg IM. **Infants:** recommended dose is 0.5 mg.

NURSING IMPLICATIONS

Edrophonium is administered by a physician. Monitor vital signs. Observe for signs of respiratory distress. Patients over 50 years of age are particularly likely to develop bradycardia, hypotension, and cardiac arrest.

Some clinicians recommend giving a 1 to 2 mg test dose of edrophonium to elderly patients, to those with history of heart disease or who take digitalis, and possibly to all patients.

Antidote (atropine sulfate) and facilities for endotracheal intubation, tracheostomy, suction, assisted respiration, and cardiac monitoring should be immediately available for treatment of cholinergic reaction.

Edrophonium test for myasthenia gravis: All cholinesterase inhibitors (anticholinesterases) should be discontinued for at least 8 hours before test. Estimates of muscle strength should be made before and after administration of edrophonium, e.g., width of palpebral fissure before and after 1 minute of sustained upward gaze, range of extraocular movements, grip strength, vital capacity, ability to elevate head and extremities, ability to cough, swallow, and talk.

Positive response to edrophonium test consists of brief improvement in muscle strength unaccompanied by lingual or skeletal muscle fasciculations. In nonmyasthenic patients, edrophonium produces a cholinergic reaction (muscarinic side effects): skeletal muscle fasciculations, muscle weakness.

Evaluation of myasthenic treatment: Myasthenic response: immediate subjective improvement with increased muscle strength (improvement of ptosis, respiration, ability to speak, swallow, and talk), absence of fasciculations; generally indicates that patient requires larger dose of anticholinesterase agent or longer-acting drug. *Cholinergic response* (muscarinic side effects): lacrimation, diaphoresis, salivation, abdominal cramps, diarrhea, nausea, vomiting; accompanied by decrease in muscle strength. Muscle weakness may appear in the following order: muscles of neck, chewing, swallowing, shoulder girdle, upper extremities, pelvic girdle, extraocular muscles, legs; fasciculations may be present or absent. Usually indicates overtreatment with cholinesterase inhibitor. *Adequate response:* no change in muscle strength; fasciculations may be present or absent; minimal cholinergic side effects (observed in patients at or near optimal dosage level).

Test to differentiate myasthenic crisis from cholinergic crisis (same principle as for evaluation of myasthenic treatment): respiratory exchange must be adequate before test is performed. *Myasthenic crisis* may be secondary to sudden increase in severity of myasthenia gravis: edrophonium will cause improvement of respiration; indicates need for longer-acting anticholinesterase drug. *Cholinergic crisis* (caused by overstimulation by anticholinesterase drugs): edrophonium will produce increase in oropharyngeal secretions and further weakness of muscles of respiration; usually indicates need for discontinuing anticholinesterase drug.

When used as curare antagonist, the effect of each dose of edrophonium on respiration should be carefully observed before it is repeated, and assisted ventilation should always be employed.

Drug Interactions: Edrophonium

Plus	Interactions
Digitalis glycosides	Additive bradycardic effects
Procainamide Quinidine	Anticholinergic properties of these drugs may antagonize cholinergic effects of edrophonium.

E

E

EMETINE HYDROCHLORIDE

(em'e-teen)
Amebicide

ACTIONS AND USES. Natural or synthetic alkaloid of ipecac with direct lethal action on *Entamoeba histolytica* in tissues. More effective against motile forms (trophozoites) than cysts. Causes degeneration of nucleus and cytoplasm of amebae and eradicates parasites, possibly by interfering with multiplication of trophozoites. Also has adrenergic and neuromuscular blocking activities, expectorant, diaphoretic, and emetic actions, but not used clinically for these effects.

Used in combination with other amebicides in management of acute fulminating amebic dysentery (intestinal amebiasis) or for acute exacerbations of chronic amebic dysentery. Highly effective in treatment of extraintestinal amebiasis (amebic abscess, amebic hepatitis). Also used in certain cases of balantidiasis, fascioliasis, and paragonimiasis. *Investigational Use:* as irrigation solution (Emetine in NaCl Injection) used at site of amebic abscess (after pus aspiration).

ABSORPTION AND FATE. Readily absorbed and widely distributed in body. Highest concentration in liver; appreciable amounts also found in lung, kidney, and spleen. Appears in urine 20 to 40 minutes after injection; still present 40 to 60 days after being discontinued.

CONTRAINDICATIONS AND PRECAUTIONS. In patients who have received a course of emetine 6 weeks to 2 months previously; for treatment of mild symptoms or carriers of amebiasis; liver, heart, or kidney disease; pregnancy. Contraindicated in children except those with severe dysentery not controlled by other amebicides. Safe use in nursing mothers not established. *Cautious use:* debilitated or elderly patients, hypotension, patients about to have surgery.

ADVERSE/SIDE EFFECTS. CV (cardiotoxicity): hypotension, tachycardia, arrhythmias, myocarditis, pericarditis, precordial pain, dyspnea, ECG abnormalities, gallop rhythm, cardiac dilatation, congestive failure, death. **GI:** diarrhea; abdominal cramps; nausea and vomiting associated with dizziness, faintness, headache, epigastric burning and pain. **Injection site reactions:** (frequent): aching, tenderness, and local muscle weakness; eczematous, urticarial, or purpuric lesions, necrosis, cellulitis, abscess. **Large doses:** acute lesions in heart, liver, kidney, intestinal tract, skeletal muscle. **Neuromuscular:** skeletal muscle weakness, tenderness, stiffness, pain, tremors, peripheral neuropathy, loss of sense of taste. **Other:** decrease in serum potassium, thrombocytopenia.

ROUTE AND DOSAGE. Adults: Subcutaneous (deep), intramuscular: 65 mg daily or 32 mg twice daily (morning and evening). Dosage should not exceed 65 mg/day or a total of 650 mg in 10 days. For hepatic amebiasis or abscess, may be administered up to 10 days. For acute fulminating amebic dysentery, administered long enough to control diarrhea, usually 3 to 5 days. A course should not be repeated in less than 6 weeks. **Children (under 8 years of age):** no more than 10 mg daily; **(over 8 years):** no more than 20 mg daily.

NURSING IMPLICATIONS

Emetine is a potent drug. Patients should be hospitalized and on absolute bed rest during therapy and for several days thereafter. Tachycardia may occur in patients permitted to ambulate. It is also advisable for patients to remain sedentary for several weeks after drug is terminated.

Isolation precautions are not required. However, use meticulous technique in disposal of feces and collection of stool specimens.

Emetine is administered by deep subcutaneous or IM injection. Aspirate carefully after needle is introduced.

IV injection is dangerous and is specifically contraindicated.

Make a record of injection sites and observe these sites daily. Muscle ache and tenderness at area of injection occur frequently.

Emetine is very irritating to tissues. Avoid contact of drug with eyes and mucous membranes. Wash hands thoroughly after handling drug.

Cumulative toxic action may occur. The patient should be closely observed and advised to report any unusual symptom, no matter how minor it may seem.

Emetine is potentially toxic to the heart. An ECG should be taken before emetine is initiated, as well as after the fifth dose, on completion of therapy, and 1 week later. ECG changes usually appear about 7 days after drug is administered; they are generally reversible. Report their appearance immediately.

ECG alterations may persist in some patients 2 months or more after discontinuation of drug. Some patients experience dyspnea until drug is stopped.

Pulse (rate and quality) and blood pressure should be recorded at least 3 times daily. Tachycardia frequently precedes appearance of ECG abnormalities.

Emetine should be discontinued on the appearance of tachycardia, a precipitous fall in blood pressure, marked weakness or other neuromuscular symptoms, and severe GI effects. These adverse reactions should be reported promptly.

Monitor neuromuscular function, especially of neck and extremities (most likely involved). Report immediately any signs of weakness and complaints of fatigability, listlessness, muscular stiffness, tenderness, or pain. These symptoms usually appear before more serious symptoms and thus may serve as guides to avoid overdosage.

Monitor intake and output. Report oliguria or change in intake–output ratio. Record number, unusual odor, and consistency of stools, as well as the presence of mucus, blood, or other foreign matter. Stool specimens should be delivered to the laboratory while they are still warm to facilitate identification of amebae.

Suspect emetine-induced reaction if stools increase in number following improvement of diarrhea.

Restoration of body fluids and nutrients is an important adjunct to drug therapy.

Emetine for treatment of acute fulminating amebic dysentery is administered only long enough to control symptoms (usually 3 to 5 days). For extraintestinal amebiasis (amebic hepatitis or abscess) it is generally given for 10 days; another amebicide should be given simultaneously or as an immediate follow-up to guarantee eradication of *E. histolytica* from primary lesions in intestines.

Patients to be discharged should be instructed about the amount of activity allowed and urged to remain under medical supervision until otherwise advised.

Repeated fecal examinations at intervals of up to 3 months are necessary to assure elimination of amebae. Patients with acute amebic dysentery often become asymptomatic carriers, depending on the adequacy of concomitant amebicide therapy to remove intestinal cysts.

Microscopic examination of the feces of household members and other suspected contacts should be supplemented by a search for direct contamination of water or other possible sources of infection.

A health teaching plan for patients and family members should include personal hygiene, particularly regarding sanitary disposal of feces, handwashing after defecation and before preparing or eating food, the risks of eating raw food, and control of fly contamination. *See also Index: Nursing Interventions: amebiasis.*

Protect drug from light.

ENCAINIDE

(en-kay'nide)
Antiarrhythmic (class I)

ACTIONS AND USES. Antiarrhythmic agent (Class IC) with potent local anesthetic action. Action mechanisms are similar to those of Class IA antiarrhythmics (e.g., quinidine): slows upstroke velocity of the action potential (AP), but unlike Class IA drugs, does not significantly prolong AP duration. IV doses increase His-ventricle (HQ) and QRS intervals and slightly prolong QT interval. Sinus node function is not changed but blood pressure is moderately lowered; has mild negative inotropic effect and induces slight decrease in cardiac output. Oral doses produce little if any change in cardiac function or hemodynamics; more effective than quinidine in suppressing PVCs. Onset of malignant arrhythmias (new sustained ventricular tachycardia or fibrillation in patient who previously had only PVCs or nonsustained ventricular tachycardia) about 30 hours after a dose change or oral dose, has been reported.

Used in treatment of both atrial and ventricular arrhythmias; to prevent recurrence of reentrant tachycardias in patients with Wolff–Parkinson–White syndrome, and in management of PVCs.

ABSORPTION AND FATE. Well absorbed; half-life 2½ to 4 hours. Since therapeutic actions last longer, it appears that active metabolites with longer half-life than parent compound are responsible for actions. Wide individual differences in bioavailability.

ADVERSE/SIDE EFFECTS. CV: *electrophysiologic toxicity:* sustained ventricular tachycardia, irreversible ventricular fibrillation, and hypotension (with IV administration). **GI:** nausea, constipation. **Neurologic:** tremors, dizziness, ataxia. **Ophthalmic:** visual disturbances—diplopia, blurred vision. **Otic:** tinnitus.

ROUTE AND DOSAGE. Oral: 25 to 50 mg every 6 hours. **Intravenous:** 0.9 mg/kg over 15 minute period.

NURSING IMPLICATIONS

Effective serum concentration: 0.002 to 0.056 mcg/ml.

Electrophysiologic toxicity is severe because encainide is a potent blocker of the sodium influx current during the action potential.

Patient should remain hospitalized until firmly stabilized on oral dose.

See Tocainide for Nursing Implications and Drug Interactions.

PROTOTYPE

EPHEDRINE
(Gluco-Fedrin, *l*-Sedrin)
EPHEDRINE SULFATE
(Efedron, Vatronol)

(e-fed'rin)
Adrenergic agonist
Bronchodilator
Decongestant
Antieneuretic

ACTIONS AND USES. Both indirect and direct acting sympathomimetic amine. Pharmacologically similar to epinephrine (qv), but less potent, with slower onset and more prolonged action; effective by oral route. Causes less elevation of blood sugar than epinephrine and has more pronounced central stimulatory actions. Thought to act indirectly by releasing tissue stores of norepinephrine and directly by stimulation of α and β_1 and β_2 adrenergic receptors. Cardiovascular actions (positive inotropic and pressor effects) persist 7 to 10 times as long as those of epinephrine; although bronchodilation is less prominent, it is more sustained.

Like epinephrine, it contracts dilated arterioles of nasal mucosa, thus reducing engorgement and edema and facilitating ventilation and drainage. Local application to eye produces mydriasis without loss of light reflexes or accommodation or change in intraocular pressure. Its use in enuresis is based on its ability to contract urinary bladder sphincter and its central effects, which decrease depth of sleep. Potentiates action of acetylcholine at neuromuscular junctions; thus it may increase skeletal muscle tone in myasthenia gravis.

Used for temporary relief of congestion of hay fever, allergic rhinitis, and sinusitis; and in treatment and prophylaxis of mild cases of acute asthma and in patients with chronic asthma requiring continuing treatment. Also has been used for its CNS stimulant actions: in treatment of narcolepsy, to improve respiration in narcotic and barbiturate poisoning, to combat hypotensive states, especially those associated with spinal anesthesia; in management of enuresis or impaired bladder control; as adjunct in treatment of myasthenia gravis; as mydriatic; to relieve dysmenorrhea; and for temporary support of ventricular rate in Adams-Stokes syndrome; and for management of peripheral edema secondary to type I diabetic neuropathy. Available in fixed-dose combinations with theophylline and hydroxyzine (Marax, Hydromax, Hydrophed), and with theophylline and phenobarbital (Tedral, Thalfed, Theofedral, Theodrine) and with amobarbitol (Ephedrine and Amytal).

E

ABSORPTION AND FATE. Readily absorbed when given by oral and parenteral routes. Maximum bronchodilator effect occurs within 15 minutes to 1 hour and persists approximately 2 to 4 hours. Cardiac and pressor effects last up to 4 hours after oral administration and about 1 hour after IV. Widely distributed in body fluids; crosses blood–brain barrier. Small amounts slowly metabolized in the liver. About 60 to 75% excreted unchanged in urine within 24 hours; remainder eliminated as metabolite. Acidification of urine increases urinary excretion. Appears in breast milk. Probably crosses placenta.

CONTRAINDICATIONS AND PRECAUTIONS. History of hypersensitivity to ephedrine or other sympathomimetics; narrow-angle glaucoma; within 14 days before or after MAO inhibitor therapy; patients receiving tricyclic antidepressants, digitalis, oxytocics. Safe use during pregnancy (category C) not established. *Cautious Use:* Use with extreme caution if at all in hypertension, arteriosclerosis, angina pectoris, coronary insufficiency, chronic heart disease, diabetes mellitus, hyperthyroidism, prostatic hypertrophy.

ADVERSE/SIDE EFFECTS. **Systemic (usually with large doses): CNS:** headache, insomnia, nervousness, anxiety, tremulousness, giddiness. **CV:** palpitation, tachycardia, precordial pain, cardiac arrhythmias; difficult or painful urination, acute urinary retention (especially older men with prostatism. **GI:** nausea, vomiting, anorexia. **Other:** sweating, thirst, fixed-drug eruption. **Topical use:** burning, stinging, dryness of nasal mucosa, sneezing, rebound congestion. **Overdosage:** euphoria, confusion, delirium, convulsions, pyrexia, CNS depression (somnolence, coma), hypertension, rebound hypotension, respiratory depression, paranoid psychosis, visual and auditory hallucinations.

ROUTE AND DOSAGE. **Adults: Subcutaneous, intramuscular, intravenous (slowly):** 25 to 50 mg as necessary. Maximum total 24-hour dose should not exceed 150 mg. **Intranasal:** (0.5 to 3% solution): 2 to 4 drops or small amount of jelly in each nostril no more than four times a day for 3 or 4 consecutive days (do not repeat before 2 hours). **Children: Subcutaneous, intravenous:** 2 to 3 mg/kg/24 hours, divided into 4 to 6 doses.

NURSING IMPLICATIONS

Patients receiving ephedrine IV must be under constant supervision. Take baseline blood pressure and other vital signs. Check blood pressure repeatedly during first 5 minutes then every 3 to 5 minutes until stabilized.

E

Monitor intake–output ratio and pattern especially in older male patients. Encourage patient to void before taking medication *(see Adverse/Side Effects).*

When ephedrine is given IV it initially causes constriction of renal blood vessels and consequent reduction in urine formation. As blood pressure rises toward normal levels renal function is restored. However, if blood pressure increases toward hypertensive levels renal blood flow and urine output again decreases.

Frequent dosing in patients with hypertension can result in tachyphylaxis (diminution of response) to cardiac and pressor effects with resulting rebound hypotension. Monitoring of central venous pressure or left ventricular filling pressure is advisable in these patients.

Ephedrine is a commonly abused drug. Patients should be advised of side effects and dangers and should be cautioned to take medication only as prescribed.

Warn patient not to take OTC medications for coughs, colds, allergies, or asthma unless approved by physician. Ephedrine is a common ingredient in these preparations.

Insomnia is common, particularly with continued therapy. Timing of administration and size of dosage are important considerations. If possible, administer last dose a few hours before bedtime.

OR personnel are cautioned to avoid the dangerous practice of having syringes filled with ephedrine placed together with other syringes containing local anesthetics. Ephedrine has been mistakenly injected into the epidural space instead of the local anesthetic.

Intranasal administration: Have patient clear nose before instilling drops. Instruct patient to blow gently with both nostrils open. Generally, nose drops are instilled with head in lateral, head-low position to avoid entry of drug into throat. Check with physician.

Systemic effects can occur because of excessive dosage from rapid absorption of drug solution through nasal mucosa. These are most likely to occur in the elderly.

Instruct patient to rinse dropper or spray tip in hot water and shake dry after each use in order to prevent contamination of nasal solution.

Treatment of overdosages: Have on hand phentolamine mesylate IV or SC, or paraldehyde for hypotension; diazepam (Valium) for convulsions; cool applications and dexamethasone for pyrexia.

In general, topical treatment should not be continued for more than 3 to 5 consecutive days. Tachyphylaxis (diminution of response) with rebound congestion may occur if drug is administered in rapidly repeated doses or over prolonged period of time. Prescribed withdrawal of drug over several days frequently enables the patient to attain former responsiveness.

Preserved in well-closed, light-resistant containers preferably between 15° and 20°C (59° and 86°F) unless otherwise directed by manufacturer. Examine liquid preparation; do not administer unless absolutely clear.

Diagnostic Test Interferences: Ephedrine is generally withdrawn at least 12 hours before sensitivity tests are made, in order to prevent false-positive reactions.

Drug Interactions: Ephedrine

Plus	Interactions
Acetazolamide (Diamox); sodium bicarbonate, and other urinary alkalinizers	Increase effect of ephedrine (pH dependent decrease in urinary ephedrine excretion). Monitor for ephedrine toxicity
Ammonium chloride (and other urinary acidifiers)	Increase urinary excretion of ephedrine by acidification of urine. Therefore, decrease effects of ephedrine
Anesthetics, general (particularly Cylopropane or halogenated hydrocarbons)	Concurrent use may cause cardiac arrhythmias (these drugs sensitize heart to effects of ephedrine). Used with caution

Plus (cont.)	Interactions (cont.)
Corticosteroids	Ephedrine may reduce response to corticosteroids
Digitalis glycosides	Risk of cardiac arrhythmias (digitalis sensitizes heart to ephedrine). Combination used with caution
Guanethidine (Ismelin)	Ephedrine antagonizes antihypertensive action of guanethidine. Combination avoided, if possible
Methyldopa (Aldomet) Ranwolfia alkaloids	Reduce activity of ephedrine
MAO inhibitors, including drugs with significant MAOI activity, e.g., furazolidone	Use of ephedrine within 14 days of an MAO inhibitor can result in hypertensive crisis: additive alpha-adrenergic (pressor) effects. Combination generally avoided
Oxytocics	Concurrent use with ephedrine can cause severe hypertension: additive alpha-adrenergic (pressor) effects. Used concurrently with caution and only if BP does not exceed 130/80
Tricyclic antidepressants	May decrease pressor effects of ephedrine. Concurrent use generally avoided

PROTOTYPE

EPINEPHRINE

(Bronkaid Mist, EpiPen Auto-Injector Primatene Mist Solution, Sus-Phrine)

EPINEPHRINE BITARTRATE

(AsthmaHaler, Bronitin Mist, Suspension, Broncaid Mist Suspension, Epitrate, Medihaler-Epi, Primatene Mist Suspension)

EPINEPHRINE HYDROCHLORIDE

(Adrenalin Chloride, Dysne-Inhal, Epifrin, Glaucon, Sus-Phrine)

EPINEPHRINE, RACEMIC

(AsthmaNefrin, Dey-Dose Epinephrine, microNefrin, Vaponefrin)

EPINEPHRYL BORATE

(Epinal, Eppy/N)

(ep-i-nef'rin)
(ep-i-nef'rill bor'ate)
α-Adrenergic agonist (direct)
Bronchodilator

ACTIONS AND USES. Naturally occurring catecholamine obtained from animal adrenal glands; also prepared synthetically. Acts directly on both alpha and beta receptors; the most potent activator of alpha receptors. Imitates all actions of sympathetic nervous system except those on arteries of the face and sweat glands. Strengthens myocardial contraction; increases blood pressure, cardiac rate, and cardiac output. In common with other adrenergic antagonists, stimulates the enzyme adenyl cyclase and consequently enhances synthesis of cyclic AMP (cAMP), which mediates bronchial muscle relaxation. Also constricts bronchial arterioles and inhibits histamine release; thus reduces congestion and edema and increases tidal volume and vital capacity. Constricts arterioles, particularly in skin, mucous membranes, and kidneys, but dilates skeletal muscle blood vessels. Raises blood sugar by promoting conversion of glycogen reserves in liver to glucose and inhibits insulin release in pancreas. Relaxes uterine musculature and inhibits uterine contractions. CNS stimulation believed to result from peripheral effects. Topical applications to the eye lowers intraocular pressure possibly by decreasing aqueous humor formation and by increasing facility of aqueous outflow; produces brief mydriasis, and slight relaxation of ciliary muscle. Has only slight effect on normal eye, and reportedly is more effective in light-colored eyes than in dark eyes.

Used for temporary relief of bronchospasm, acute asthmatic attack, mucosal congestion, hypersensitivity, and anaphylactic reactions, syncope due to heart block or carotid sinus hypersensitivity, and to restore cardiac rhythm in cardiac arrest. Ophthalmic preparation is used in management of simple (open-angle) glaucoma, generally as an adjunct to topical miotics and oral carbonic anhydrase inhibitors; also used as ophthalmic decongestant. Used to relax myometrium and inhibit uterine contractions, to prolong action and delay systemic absorption of local and intraspinal anesthetics, and topically to control superficial bleeding.

ABSORPTION AND FATE. Rapid onset but brief duration of action. (Inactive when swallowed.) **Subcutaneous injection:** bronchodilation occurs within 3 to 5 minutes following administration of 1:1000 solution, with maximal effects in 20 minutes. **Parenteral suspension forms (1:200):** provides both rapid and sustained action that may persist 8 to 10 hours or more. **Oral inhalation:** bronchodilation occurs within 1 minute. **Topical application:** to conjunctiva reduces intraocular pressure within 1 hour; maximal effects in 4 to 8 hours; action may persist 12 to 24 hours or more. Mydriasis usually occurs within a few minutes and may last several hours. Pharmacologic actions terminated primarily by uptake and metabolism in sympathetic nerve endings. Circulating drug metabolized in liver and other tissues by MAO and *COMT* (C-methyl-o-transferase). Inactive metabolites (metanephrine and VMA) and small amount of unchanged drug excreted in urine. Crosses placenta but not blood–brain barrier; enters breast milk.

CONTRAINDICATIONS AND PRECAUTIONS. Hypersensitivity to sympathomimetic amines or to any ingredient in the formulation; narrow-angle glaucoma; hemorrhagic, traumatic, or cardiogenic shock; cardiac dilatation, cerebral arteriosclerosis, coronary insufficiency, arrhythmias, organic heart or brain disease; during second stage of labor; for local anesthesia of fingers, toes, ears, nose, genitalia. Safe use during pregnancy (category C), in nursing women, and in children not established. *Cautious Use:* elderly or debilitated patients; prostatic hypertrophy, hypertension; diabetes mellitus, hyperthyroidism, Parkinson's disease, tuberculosis, psychoneurosis, during pregnancy (category C), in patients with long-standing bronchial asthma and emphysema with degenerative heart disease, in children under 6 years of age.

ADVERSE/SIDE EFFECTS. **Nasal use:** burning, stinging, dryness of nasal mucosa, sneezing, rebound congestion. **Ophthalmic use:** transient stinging or burning of eyes, lacrimation, browache, headache, rebound conjunctival hyperemia, allergy, iritis; with prolonged use: melaninlike deposits on lids, conjunctiva, and cornea; corneal edema; loss of lashes (reversible); maculopathy with central scotoma in aphakic patients (reversible). **Systemic reactions:** nervousness, restlessness, sleeplessness, fear, anxiety, tremors, severe headache, cerebrovascular accident, weakness, dizziness, syncope, pallor, nausea, vomiting, sweating, dyspnea, precordial pain, palpitation, hypertension, myocardial infarction, tachyarrhythmias including fatal fibrillation; bronchial and pulmonary edema, urinary retention, tissue necrosis, metabolic acidoses, elevated serum lactic acid, transient elevations of blood glucose, altered state of perception and thought, psychosis.

ROUTE AND DOSAGE. **Parenteral:** **Adults:** *Anaphylaxis:* 0.1 to 0.5 ml of 1:1,000 SC or IM. SC doses may be repeated at 10 to 15 minute intervals as necessary. For *severe anaphylaxis:* 0.1 to 0.25 ml of 1:1,000 or 1 to 2.5 ml of 1:10,000 IV. *Asthma:* 0.1 to 0.5 ml SC or IM. SC doses may be repeated at 20 minute to 4 hour intervals. *For prolonged effect:* Sterile suspension 1:200 (Sus-Phrine): 0.1 to 0.3 ml SC *only;* repeat doses at 8 to 12 hour intervals, if necessary. **Parenteral:** **Children:** *Anaphylaxis, asthma:* 0.01 ml/kg of 1:1,000 SC. Repeat at 20 minute to 4 hour intervals if necessary; or 0.004 to 0.005 ml/kg of 1:200 sterile suspension (Sus-Phrine) SC. Subsequent doses as necessary at 6 to 8 hour intervals. **Cardiac**

arrest: Adults: 0.1 to 1 mg (1 to 10 ml of 1:10,000) IV repeated at 5 minute intervals if needed. *Intracardiac:* 0.3 to 0.5 mg (3 to 5 ml) of 1:10,000. **Children:** 0.01 mg (0.1 ml) 1 kg of 1:1,000 repeated every 5 minutes, if necessary. *Intracardiac:* 0.005 to 0.01 mg (0.05 to 0.1 ml)/kg of 1:10,000. **Inhalation: Adults and Children:** *Hand bulb nebulizer:* 1:100 or 2.25% racemic form. 1 or 2 inhalations at 1 to 5 minute intervals as prescribed, until relief obtained. *Metered dose aerosol:* 1 inhalation repeat after at least 1 minute. Subsequent doses after at least 4 hours, if necessary. **Topical:** Eye: *Glaucoma:* 1 or 2 drops of 0.25 to 2% ophthalmic solution instilled in conjunctival sac 1 or 2 times daily. Ocular mydriasis; hemostasis: 1 or 2 drops of 0.1% (1:1,000) ophthalmic solution. Nasal: 0.1% (1:1,000) solution. Hemostatic: 1:50,000 to 1:1,000 applied topically. With local anesthetic: 1:500,000 to 1:50,000 mixed with local anesthetic. **Intraspinal:** 0:2 to 0.4 ml of 1:1,000 added to anesthetic spinal fluid mixture.

NURSING IMPLICATIONS

Parenteral:

A tuberculin syringe may assure greater accuracy in measurement of parenteral doses.

Medication errors associated with epinephrine have resulted in fatalities. For example, injection of the 1:100 solution intended for inhalation has caused death when mistaken for the 1:1000 solution designed for parenteral administration. Be certain to check type of solution prescribed, concentration, dosage, and route.

Epinephrine injection should be protected from exposure to light at all times. Do not remove ampul or vial from carton until ready to use.

Before withdrawing epinephrine suspension into syringe, shake vial or ampul thoroughly to disperse particles; then inject promptly.

Carefully aspirate before injecting epinephrine. Inadvertent IV injection of usual subcutaneous or IM doses can result in sudden hypertension and possibly cerebral hemorrhage.

Drug absorption (and action) can be hastened by massaging the injection site.

Repeated injections may cause tissue necrosis due to vascular constriction. Rotate injection sites and observe for signs of blanching.

If IM route is prescribed, injection into buttocks should be avoided. Epinephrine-induced vasoconstriction reduces oxygen tension of tissues and thus favors growth of anaerobic *Clostridium welchii* (gas gangrene), which may be present in feces and on buttocks.

Monitor blood pressure, pulse, respirations, urinary output, and observe patient closely. Epinephrine may widen pulse pressure (elevate systolic with minimal rise or even decrease of diastolic). If disturbances in cardiac rhythm occur, withhold epinephrine and notify physician immediately. Keep physician informed of any changes in intake–output ratio.

Patients receiving epinephrine IV should be on cardiac monitor. Have full crash cart immediately available in the event the patient requires defibrillation or cardioversion. *(See General Discussion.)*

When administered IV, blood pressure should be checked repeatedly during first 5 minutes then checked every 3 to 5 minutes until stabilized.

When drug is given intracardially (by physician), it must be followed by external cardiac massage to permit drug to enter coronary circulation.

Consult physician for compatability information.

Inhalation:

Treatment should start with first symptoms of bronchospasm. The least number of inhalations that provide relief should be used. To prevent excessive dosage, at least 1 or 2 minutes should elapse before taking additional inhalations of epinephrine. Dosage requirements vary with each patient. Caution patient that overuse or too frequent use can result in severe adverse effects.

E

Instruct the patient to rinse mouth and throat with water immediately after inhalation to avoid swallowing residual drug (may cause epigastric pain and systemic effects from the propellant in the aerosol preparation) and to prevent dryness of oropharyngeal membranes.

If patient is also taking isoproterenol, it should not be used concurrently with epinephrine. An interval of 4 hours should elapse before changing from one drug to the other.

Patient should be advised to report to physician if symptoms are not relieved in 20 minutes or if they become worse.

Advise patient to report bronchial irritation, nervousness, or sleeplessness. Dosage should be reduced.

Nasal:

Nose drops should be instilled with head in lateral, head-low position to prevent entry of drug into throat. Discuss with physician.

Forewarn patient that intranasal application may sting slightly.

Instruct patients to rinse nose dropper or spray tip with hot water after each use to prevent contamination of solution with nasal secretions.

Inform patient that intranasal applications frequently cause rebound congestion and that prolonged use may result in drug-induced rhinitis. Caution patient to use medication as prescribed and to inform physician if drug is not effective. In general, nose drops should not be used for longer than 3 or 4 days.

Ophthalmic:

Ophthalmic preparation may cause mydriasis with blurred vision and sensitivity to light in some patients being treated for glaucoma. Drug is usually administered at bedtime or following prescribed miotic to minimize these symptoms.

It is generally advisable to remove soft lenses before instilling eye drops. Soft lenses may absorb medication or be stained or otherwise damaged by the medication or preservatives included.

To prevent excessive systemic absorption, instruct patient to apply gentle finger pressure against nasolacrimal duct immediately after drug is instilled for at least 1 or 2 minutes following instillation. For more complete description, *see Index: Drug administration: eye drops.*

Repeated tonometer readings are advised during continuous therapy, especially in elderly patients.

When separate solutions of epinephrine and a topical miotic are used, the miotic should be instilled 2 to 10 minutes prior to epinephrine because of the limited capacity of the conjunctival sac. Consult physician.

Inform patient that transitory stinging may follow initial administration and that headache and browache occur frequently at first, but usually subside with continued use. Advise patient to report to physician if symptoms persist. Local reactions are sometimes controlled by lower drug concentration.

Patient should be instructed to discontinue epinephrine and to consult a physician if signs of hypersensitivity develop (edema of lids, itching, discharge, crusting eyelids).

Treatment of overdosage: The cardiac and bronchodilating effects of epinephrine are antagonized by beta-adrenergic blocking agents such as propranolol; marked pressor effects are antagonized by alpha-adrenergic blocking agents such as phentolamine and trimethophan camsylate, a nondepolarizing ganglionic blocking agent. Treatment also consists of general supportive measures. Patient must be constantly attended.

General:

Patients subject to acute asthmatic attacks and responsible family members should be taught how to administer epinephrine subcutaneously. Medication and equipment should be available for home emergency. Confer with physician.

Epinephrine reduces bronchial secretions and thus may make mucus plugs more difficult to dislodge. Physician may prescribe bronchial hygiene program, including postural drainage, breathing exercises, and adequate hydration (3000 to 4000 ml) to facilitate expectoration. Spirometric measurements may be used to assess response to therapy.

Describe sputum color, consistency, and estimate amount.

Tolerance ("epinephrine fastness") can occur with repeated or prolonged use (effectiveness often returns if drug is withheld 12 hours to several days). Caution the patient to report to physician; continued use of epinephrine in the presence of tolerance can be dangerous.

Advise patient to report difficulty in voiding or urinary retention (especially male patients). It may be advisable to have patient void before taking drug.

Epinephrine may increase blood glucose levels. Patients with diabetes should be observed closely for loss of diabetes control.

Instruct patient to take medication only as prescribed and to report the onset of systemic effects of epinephrine. A decrease in frequency of administration or concentration of drug or temporary discontinuation of therapy may be indicated.

Epinephrine is destroyed by oxidizing agents, alkalies (including sodium bicarbonate), halogens, permanganates, chromates, nitrates, and salts of easily reducible metals such as iron, copper, and zinc.

Oxidation of epinephrine imparts a color ranging from pink to brown. Discard discolored or precipitated solutions.

Preserved in tight, light-resistant containers. Commercial preparations vary in stability; therefore, follow manufacturer's directions with respect to expiration date and storage requirements for each product.

Drug Interactions: Epinephrine and other adrenergics

Plus	Interactions
Anesthetics, general, e.g., cyclopropane, halothane and other halogenated anesthetics	Possibility of additive arrhythmic effects. These agents may sensitize heart to catecholamines. Concurrent use with cyclopropane avoided. Used with caution if at all with other agents
Antidiabetic agents	Epinephrine may increase blood glucose levels. Used concomitantly with caution
Digitalis glycozides (high doses)	May sensitize heart to epinephrine effects. Concurrent use generally avoided
Guanethedine (Ismelin)	Antihypertensive effects of guanethidine may be reversed resulting in severe hypertension and arrhythmias. Guanethidine may prolong mydriatic effects of epinephrine. Concurrent use generally avoided
Phentolamine (Regitine), Phenothiazines and other alpha-adrenergic blocking agents	Antagonize epinephrine pressor effects with possibility of additive hypotension. Used concurrently with caution
Propranolol (Inderal) and other beta-adrenergic blocking agents	Blockade of epinephrine beta effects causes domination of alpha effects with resulting hypertension and reflex bradycardia
Tricyclic antidepressants	Potentiation of epinephrine pressor response with possibility of severe hypertension. Concurrent use generally avoided

—PROTOTYPE

ERGOCALCIFEROL

(er-goe-kal-sif'e-role)
Antirachitic vitamin
Vitamin D

(Activated Ergosterol, Calciferol, Deltalin, Drisdol, Synthetic Oleo-vitamin D, Ostoforte, Viosterol, Vitamin D_2)

E

ACTIONS AND USES. The name vitamin D encompasses two related fat-soluble substances (sterols) that occur in nature and/or are synthetically prepared. One is cholecalciferol (vitamin D_3) formed by activation of provitamin 7-dehydrocholesterol in skin following exposure to ultraviolet irradiation; it is also found in fish liver oils and in livers of fish-eating animals. Cholecalciferol is commercially available only in combination products. (Cod liver oil contains about 2 mcg cholecalciferol per ml plus 780 units of vitamin A per ml.) The other, ergocalciferol, (vitamin D_2) is formed by ultraviolet irradiation of ergosterol, a provitamin found in yeasts and fungi. Each has essentially equal antirachitic and hypercalcemic potency. Vitamin D acts like a hormone in that it is distributed through the circulation and plays a major regulatory role. Maintains normal blood calcium and phosphate ion levels by enhancing their intestinal absorption and by promoting mobilization of calcium from bone and renal tubular resorption of phosphate. Essential for normal bone development; stimulates production and prolongs life span of osteoclasts, and promotes mineral resorption by bones. Functions in magnesium metabolism, and in maintenance of normal parathyroid activity and neuromuscular function. Vitamin D deficiency causes rickets in children and osteomalacia in adults. Activity of cholecalciferol and ergocalciferol may be expressed as USP units or IU (International Units) of vitamin D which are equivalent. (40 USP units or IU = biologic activity of 1 mcg of ergocalciferol or cholecalciferol.)

Used in treatment of familial hypophosphatemia (vitamin-D resistant rickets), osteomalacia (adult rickets), anticonvulsant-induced rickets and osteomalacia, osteoporosis, renal osteodystrophy hypocalcemia associated with hypoparathyroidism; and in prophylaxis and treatment of nutritional rickets. Also has been used to treat hypophosphatemia in Fanconi's syndrome and, with varying clinical results, in lupus vulgaris, psoriasis, and rheumatoid arthritis.

ABSORPTION AND FATE. Readily absorbed from GI tract (intestinal absorption requires adequate amount of bile). Most of drug appears first in lymph, then concentrates rapidly in liver. Inert until hydroxylated in liver and kidney to active metabolites: calcifediol and then to calcitriol (most active form) with half-life of 7 to 12 hours. Half-life of ergocalciferol about 12 to 24 hours, but may be stored in tissues for months. Stored chiefly in liver and to lesser extent in skin, brain, spleen, and bones. Has cumulative action. Peak hypercalcemic effect in about 4 weeks after daily, fixed doses; duration of activity: 2 months or more. About one-half oral dose eliminated (mostly as metabolites) via bile in feces; small amounts excreted slowly in urine.

CONTRAINDICATIONS AND PRECAUTIONS. Hypersensitivity to vitamin D, hypervitaminosis D, hypercalcemia, hyperphosphatemia, renal osteodystrophy with hyperphosphatemia, malabsorption syndrome, decreased renal function. Safe use of amounts in excess of 400 IU daily in pregnancy (category C) not established. *Cautious Use:* coronary disease; nursing women, arteriosclerosis (especially in the elderly), history of renal stones.

ADVERSE/SIDE EFFECTS. **Vitamin D toxicity (hypervitaminosis D)** produces symptoms of hypercalcemia: Initial: fatigue, weakness, headache, drowsiness, metallic taste, dry mouth, anorexia, nausea, vomiting, diarrhea, constipation, abdominal cramps, vertigo, tinnitus, ataxia, muscle and joint pain, hypotonia (infants), exanthema. *Later:* anemia, calcification of soft tissues (kidneys, blood vessels, myocardium, lungs, skin); nephrotoxicity: polyuria, hyposthenuria, polydipsia, nocturia, casts, albuminuria, hematuria; hypertension, conjunctivitis (calcific), photophobia, rhinorrhea, pruritus; overt psychosis (rare), mild acidosis, convulsions, cardiac arrhythmias, osteoporosis (adults), weight loss, renal failure. **Chronic hy-**

pervitaminosis D in children: mental and physical retardation, suppression of linear growth.

ROUTE AND DOSAGE. Oral, intramuscular: *Prophylaxis against rickets:* 400 IU daily. *Nutritional rickets or osteomalacia:* 1000 to 4000 IU daily. *Vitamin-D-resistant rickets:* 50,000 to 500,000 IU daily. *Hypoparathyroidism:* 50,000 to 400,000 IU daily (plus 4 Gm of calcium lactate, 6 times a day). Highly individualized dosages. Available in capsule, tablet, liquid, drops, and injection forms.

NURSING IMPLICATIONS

IM injection should be made deeply, preferably into gluteus maximus and injected slowly. Aspirate carefully to avoid inadvertent intravascular injection. Rotate injection sites.

Physician may prescribe ergocalciferol IM for patients with malabsorption syndrome or impaired hepatic or biliary function since bile is necessary for absorption of the oral form.

Patients receiving therapeutic doses of vitamin D must remain under close medical supervision. The margin of safety between therapeutic and toxic doses is extremely narrow.

Indiscriminate use of vitamin D is hazardous because of its cumulative action. Several weeks are required before the hypercalcemia and hypercalciuria that accompany overdosage are cleared.

When high therapeutic doses are used, progress is followed by frequent determinations (every 2 weeks or more often) of serum calcium, phosphorous, magnesium, alkaline phosphatase, BUN, and determinations of urine calcium (quantitative), casts, albumin, and red blood cells. Blood calcium concentration is generally kept between 9 and 10 mg/dl. (The product of serum calcium × phosphorous in mg/dl should not exceed 70.) Normal vitamin D blood levels range from 50 to 135 IU/dl.

Management of vitamin D therapy is predicated on normal serum calcium levels, maintained either by dietary intake or by calcium supplements.

A complete dietary and drug history should be taken. Therapeutic dosages are based on consideration of all sources of vitamin D, calcium, and phosphate.

Most foods contain little or no vitamin D. High concentrations are found in liver oil from cod, turbot, and halibut. Other good sources include salmon, sardines, herring, egg yolk, fortified milk, butter, and margarine. Most milk in the U.S. is fortified with 400 units of vitamin D per quart. Patients receiving therapeutic doses of vitamin D should be informed regarding allowable intake of these foods. Collaborate with dietitian.

Generally, vitamin D supplements are not required by the healthy individual who has access to sunlight and fortified food sources. The RDA of vitamin D for infants, children, and young adults under 19 years of age is 400 IU; for 19 to 22 years of age: 300 IU, and for 23 years and older: 200 IU. The RDA during pregnancy and lactation is +600 IU.

More than 85% of calcium is stored in bone and teeth during the last trimester of pregnancy; thus prematures require therapeutic doses of vitamin D.

Patients who develop hyperphosphatemia will require restriction of dietary phosphate and/or administration of aluminum gels to bind intestinal phosphate and thereby prevent metastatic calcification.

Magnesium-containing antacids and laxatives should be avoided in patients with chronic renal failure receiving vitamin D preparations since they are more prone to develop magnesium intoxication than other patients.

Patients with familial hypophosphatemia (vitamin D-resistant rickets) should receive daily supplements of oral phosphate to maintain serum phosphorus of at least 3 mg/dl.

Once symptoms of vitamin D deficiency are relieved, dosage should be reduced, to prevent hypercalcemia.

Advise patient not to use OTC medications unless approved by physician.

Treatment of vitamin D toxicity consists of prompt discontinuation of the vitamin, a low-calcium diet, generous fluid intake and acidification of urine (to prevent calculus formation and enhance urinary excretion of calcium), and general symptomatic and supportive treatment.

In patients with osteomalacia a decrease in serum alkaline phosphatase may signal the onset of hypercalcemia.

Preserved in tightly covered, light-resistant containers preferably between 15 to 30°C (59 to 86°F), unless otherwise directed by manufacturer. Decomposes on exposure to light and air.

E

Diagnostic Test Interferences. Vitamin D may cause false increase in **serum cholesterol** measurements (Zlatkis-Zak reaction).

Drug Interactions: Ergocalciferol

Plus	Interactions
Antacids containing magnesium Laxatives	Increased risk of hypermagnesemia especially in patients with chronic renal failure
Cholestyramine (Questran) Colestipol (Colestid) Mineral oil	May interfere with intestinal absorption of oral vitamin D (space doses as far apart as possible)
Digitalis glycosides	Vitamin D-induced hypercalcemia may precipitate cardiac arrhythmias
Phenobarbital Phenytoin (Dilantin)	By inducing hepatic enzymes, these drugs may increase metabolic inactivation of vitamin D
Thiazide diuretics	May cause hypercalcemia in patients with hypoparathyroidism

---

ERGOLOID MESYLATES

(er'goe-loid mess'i lates)

(Circanol, Deapril-ST, Dihydroergotoxine, Hydergine, Hydroloid, Niloric)

Cognition adjuvant
Ergot alkaloid

ACTIONS AND USES. Combination of three hydrogenated derivatives of ergot alkaloids. Produces peripheral vasodilation primarily by central action and may cause slight reduction in blood pressure and heart rate. Lacks vasoconstrictor and oxytocic properties of the natural ergot alkaloids. Reportedly relieves symptoms of cerebral arteriosclerosis possibly by increasing cerebral metabolism with consequent increase in blood flow. Conclusive evidence of therapeutic effectiveness for senile dementia is lacking. However, short-term clinical studies have demonstrated modest improvement in some patients. Each mg contains dihydroergocornine, dihydroergocristine, and dihydroergocryptine, 0.33 mg each as the mesylates.

Used for treatment of impaired mental function in the elderly and investigationally for Alzheimer's disease.

ABSORPTION AND FATE. Conventional tablets are rapidly but incompletely absorbed. Plasma levels peak in 1 hour. Undergoes rapid first-pass metabolism in liver; less than 50% bioavailability. Half-life: 3.5 hours.

CONTRAINDICATIONS AND PRECAUTIONS. Hypersensitivity to ergoloid mesylates; acute or chronic psychosis. *Cautious Use:* acute intermittent porphyria.

ADVERSE/SIDE EFFECTS. CV: orthostatic hypotension, lightheadedness, flushing, sinus bradycardia. **EENT:** blurred vision, nasal stuffiness, increased nasopharyngeal secretions. **GI:** sublingual irritation, transient nausea and vomiting, heartburn. **Other:** skin rash, precipitation of acute intermittent porphyria.

ROUTE AND DOSAGE. Sublingual, oral tablet: 1 mg, three times daily. Available also in capsule and liquid forms.

NURSING IMPLICATIONS

Establish baseline values of blood pressure and pulse; check at regular intervals throughout therapy.

Advise patient to make position changes slowly particularly from recumbent to upright posture and to move ankles and feet for a few minutes before ambulating.

Instruct patient to allow sublingual tablet to dissolve under tongue and not to drink, eat, or smoke while tablet is in place. Sublingual tablets should not be crushed.

Regular tablets may be crushed prior to administration and taken with fluid or mixed with food.

Sinus bradycardia (40 beats/min) has been reported in patients receiving 1.5-mg doses. Report to physician. Pulse rate usually returns to normal within 2 days after drug is discontinued.

Continuous clinical evaluations must be made to determine effect of therapy. The following items suggested by manufacturer might be used as guidelines for observations: mental alertness, emotional lability, ability to do self-care, improvement in depression, anxieties, fears, cooperativeness, sociability, appetite, fatigue, dizziness.

Deapril-ST contains tartrazine which may cause an allergic type reaction including asthma in susceptible individuals. Such reactions are frequently seen in patients with aspirin hypersensitivity.

Improvement may not be apparent until after 3 to 4 weeks of therapy.

Protect drug from light, moisture, or temperatures above 30°C (86°F).

ERGONOVINE MALEATE

(Ergotrate Maleate)

(er-goe-noe'veen)
α-Adrenergic blocking agent
Oxytocic
Ergot alkaloid

ACTIONS AND USES. Ergot alkaloid with slow but powerful oxytocic effect; less toxic and less prone to cause gangrene than other ergot derivatives. Exerts moderate cerebral vascular constriction, but is inferior to ergotamine (qv) as a migraine specific. Produces prolonged nonphasic uterine contractions. Like other oxytocics, may evoke severe hypertensive episodes in hypertensive or toxemic patients, or when regional anesthesia (caudal or spinal) containing vasoconstrictors has been used.

Used to prevent or reduce postpartum and postabortal hemorrhage due to uterine atony.

ABSORPTION AND FATE. Rapidly and completely absorbed by all routes. Onset of uterine contractions following oral administration; 5 to 15 minutes with duration of 3 hours or longer; onset following IM in 2 to 5 minutes with duration of 3 hours. Onset is almost immediate following IV; duration is about 45 minutes. Thought to be slowly metabolized in liver. Excreted in urine.

CONTRAINDICATIONS AND PRECAUTIONS. Hypersensitivity to ergot preparations, to induce labor, use prior to delivery of placenta, threatened spontaneous abortion, prolonged use, uterine sepsis, hypertension, toxemia.

ADVERSE/SIDE EFFECTS. Nausea, vomiting (especially with IV doses), severe hypertensive episodes, bradycardia, allergic phenomena including shock, ergotism. *See Ergotamine.*

ROUTE AND DOSAGE. Intramuscular or emergency intravenous: 0.2 mg (1 ml). *Postpartum hemorrhage:* every 2 to 4 hours up to maximum of five doses, if necessary. **Oral:** 0.2 to 0.4 mg every 6 to 12 hours until danger of atony passes (usually 48 hours).

E

NURSING IMPLICATIONS

Assess and record character of uterine contractions.

IM injection produces initial firm titanic contraction of the postpartum uterus; a succession of minor relaxations and contractions then occur with relaxation increasing over the next period of 1.5 hours. Vigorous rhythmic contractions continue for 3 hours or more after injection.

Desired oxytocic action of ergonovine may be antagonized by hypocalcemia. Treatment: cautious IV calcium gluconate (if patient is not also taking digitalis) before ergonovine administration.

Severe cramping following oral doses is evidence of effectiveness; however, it may also indicate need to reduce dose.

Monitor blood pressure, pulse, and uterine response following injection until postpartum condition is stabilized (about 1 or 2 hours).

Report sudden increase in blood pressure, pulse changes, and frequent periods of uterine relaxation. (Uterus may fail to respond in hypocalcemic patients.)

Patient may be more sensitive to cold. Avoid unnecessary or prolonged exposure.

High incidence of nausea and danger of hypertensive and cerebrovascular accident have limited the use of IV route for emergency treatment.

IV ergonovine given in second stage of labor as head is born induces contractions in 1 minute. IM injection as infant is being born produces, in 2 to 5 minutes, uterine contractions that separate placenta and prevent blood loss.

Oral tablets may also be administered on tongue (perlingually) or by rectum (suspended in water as retention enema).

Before labor is induced, consult with physician about route to be used for administration of ergonovine during delivery. Have drug prepared so that there is no delay.

If solution for injection is discolored or contains particles, do not use.

Store drug in cool place, below 8°C (46°F). However, delivery room stocks may be kept at room temperature for up to 60 days.

See also Ergotamine Tartrate.

PROTOTYPE

ERGOTAMINE TARTRATE

(Ergomar, Ergostat, Gynergen, Medihaler Ergotamine, Wigrettes)

(er-got'a-meen)

Alpha-adrenergic blocking agent (sympatholytic)
Vasoconstrictor
Antimigraine agent
Ergot alkaloid

ACTIONS AND USES. Natural amino acid alkaloid of ergot. Alpha-adrenergic blocking agent with direct stimulating action on cranial and peripheral vascular smooth muscles and depressant effect on central vasomotor centers. In vascular headache, exerts vasoconstrictive action on previously dilated cerebral vessels, reduces amplitude of arterial pulsations, and antagonizes effects of serotonin (implicated in etiology of vascular headaches). Does not demonstrate intrinsic sedative or analgesic actions. By unknown mechanism, ergotamine activity can lead to damage of vascular endothelium, with subsequent occlusion, thrombosis, and gangrene. Large doses may induce slight elevation of blood pressure and diminish arterial blood flow sufficiently to cause tissue ischemia. Myometrium stimulation (oxytocic effect) becomes more prominent with dose increases and as uterine sensitivity to ergot develops during adolescence and pregnancy. Small doses given in third stage of labor promote strong uterine response without significant side effects. Stimulates chemoreceptor trigger zone (CTZ) and therefore may cause nausea and vomiting. May inhibit prolactin secretion.

Used as single agent or in combination with caffeine (Cafergot, Cafetrate, Ercatal) to relieve pain of migraine, cluster headache (histamine cephalalgia), and other vascular headaches. Not recommended for migraine prophylaxis because of the possibility of adverse effects. Commercially available in combination with phenobarbitol and belladonna alkaloids (Belleragol-S, Cafergot P-B).

ABSORPTION AND FATE. Poorly and erratically absorbed from GI tract; response is delayed and unpredictable. Peak plasma levels in ½ to 3 hours. Rate and extent of absorption is enhanced by caffeine. Rapid and complete absorption following administration by inhalation. Crosses blood–brain barrier. Extensively metabolized in liver. About 90% of dose excreted as metabolites in bile via feces. Trace amounts of unchanged drug eliminated in urine and feces. Appears in breast milk.

CONTRAINDICATIONS AND PRECAUTIONS. Hypersensitivity, pregnancy (category X), use in children, sepsis, obliterative vascular disease, thromboembolic disease, prolonged use of excessive dosage, hepatic and renal disease, severe pruritus, marked arteriosclerosis, coronary heart disease, hypertension, infectious states, anemia, and malnutrition. *Cautious Use:* during lactation, elderly patients.

ADVERSE/SIDE EFFECTS. **Acute ergotism (rare):** vomiting, diarrhea, abdominal pain, unquenchable thirst, paresthesias, pain (spasms) of facial muscles, tongue, limbs and lumbar region with difficulty in walking; delirium, paresthesias, convulsive seizures, rapid or weak or irregular pulse, confusion, itching and cold skin; (occasionally): gangrene of nose, digits, ears. **Chronic ergotism:** intermittent claudication, muscle pains, weakness, numbness, coldness and cyanosis of digits (Raynaud's phenomenon). **Other:** complete absence of medium- and large-vessel pulsations in extremities; precordial distress and pain; transient bradycardia or tachycardia; elevated or lowered blood pressure; depression; drowsiness; mixed miosis (rare); kidney failure; fibrotic changes (long-term therapy), partial necrosis of tongue.

ROUTE AND DOSAGE. **Oral tablet, sublingual tablet:** Initial: 2 mg at start of migraine followed by 1 to 2 mg at 30 to 60 minute intervals until attack has abated. Dosage should not exceed 6 mg/24-hours or 10 mg/week. **Inhalation:** each spray delivers 0.36 mg dose. Start with one inhalation; repeat, if not relieved in 5 minutes. Space additional inhalations no less than 5 minutes apart. Not to exceed 6 inhalations in 24 hours or 15 inhalations/week. Available in tablets (1 mg), sublingual tablets (2 mg), and aerosol.

NURSING IMPLICATIONS

Oral doses are less effective than inhalation, but they usually relieve mild or incipient attacks of migraine.

Sublingual tablet is preferred early in the attack because of its rapid absorption and lower effective dose.

Since degree of pain relief is proportional to rapidity of treatment, drug therapy should begin as soon after onset of attack as possible, preferably during prodrome (scintillating scotomatas, visual field defects, paresthesias, usually on side opposite to that of the migraine, nausea).

Metered dose nebulizers administer an exact dose and are safe if used as directed. Review instructions with patient.

The patient's optimum dosage is determined by titrating the dose during several migraine attacks, and using the lowest effective dose for subsequent attacks.

If migraine attacks occur more frequently or are not relieved, advise patient to report to physician. Prophylactic therapy, e.g., propranolol (Inderal), or amitriptyline (Elavil) may be indicated.

Advise patient to lie down in a quiet, dark room for 2 to 3 hours after drug administration. Although caffeine increases ergotamine absorption, some clinicians question its value because it may keep the patient awake and sleep contributes to the relief of migraine.

Acute ergot poisoning is rare; but can result from overdosing or attempts at abortion.

Instruct patient to report claudication, muscle pain or weakness of extremities, cold or numb digits, irregular heartbeat, nausea, or vomiting. Dose adjustment is indicated. With avoidance of the drug for 1 to 3 days, vasoconstriction usually subsides. Carefully protect extremities from exposure to cold temperatures; provide warmth, but not heat, to ischemic areas. For severe peripheral vasoconstriction, IV sodium nitroprusside (Nipride) or intraarterial tolazoline (Priscoline) has been used in conjunction with heparin.

Food–Drug Interactions: Triggers to classic migraine headache:

- Caffeine withdrawal (therefore, avoid caffeine beverages, e.g., tea, coffee)
- Tyramine-containing foods, e.g., aged cheese especially portion close to rind, Chianti, broad beans, overripe avocado *(see also Index: Food sources)*
- Foods containing other vasopressors, chocolate (phenylethylamine), fava beans (dopamine)
- Food additives, e.g., preservatives in cured meats, monosodium glutamate (MSG)

Patients receiving high ergotamine doses for prolonged periods may experience increased frequency of headaches, fatigue, and depression. Discontinuation of the drug in these patients results in severe withdrawal headache that may last a few days.

Patients with migraine should be helped to identify underlying emotional and physical stresses that may precipitate attacks and should be assisted in learning how to deal with them. Adequate relaxation, recreation, and sleep may help to reduce severity and frequency of attacks.

Warn the woman of childbearing age to avoid use of ergotamine if she suspects she is pregnant because of its oxytocic effect.

Warn patients not to increase dosage without consulting physician; overdosage is the chief cause of untoward effects from the drug.

Keep drug out of reach of children. Fatalities have been reported.

Patient-Teaching Points: Patients with migraine should be helped to identify underlying emotional, physical and environmental stresses that may trigger an attack and should be assisted in learning how to deal with them:

- ✓ Precipitating factors vary from person to person but commonly involve fatigue, stress, sleep deprivation, ingestion of certain foods (see Food-drug interactions above); hormonal changes particularly those associated with menstruation, drugs such as oral contraceptives, vasodilators; the over-achiever personality.
- ✓ Emphasize that adequate relaxation, recreation, and sleep may help to reduce severity and frequency of attacks.

✓ Warn patients not to increase dosage without consulting physician; overdosage is the chief cause of untoward effects from the drug.

✓ Avoid self-dosing with OTC drugs without advice of physician.

Preserved in light-resistant container preferably between 15° and 30°C (59° and 86°F) unless otherwise directed by manufacturer.

Drug Interactions. Ergotamine tartrate

Plus	Interactions
Propranolol (Inderal) and possibly other beta-adrenergic blockers	Possibility of enhanced vasoconstrictor activity with high doses of ergot alkaloids. Used concomitantly with caution
Troleandomycin (Tao)	Possibility of severe peripheral vasospasm and hypertension (troleandomycin probably interferes with ergotamine metabolism). Used concomitantly with caution

E

ERYTHRITYL TETRANITRATE

(Cardilate)

(e-ri'thri-till)

Vasodilator (coronary)

ACTIONS AND USES. Similar to nitroglycerin (qv), but has slower onset and longer duration of action. *See Nitroglycerin for contraindications, precautions, and adverse reactions.*

Used in prophylaxis and long-term treatment of angina pectoris, rather than in acute attacks, in patients with frequent and recurrent anginal pain and reduced exercise tolerance. Available in combination with phenobarbital (Cardilate-P).

ABSORPTION AND FATE. Effects following administration of sublingual or chewable tablet occur after 5 to 10 minutes, with maximum action in 30 to 45 minutes. Following ingestion of oral tablet, effects appear in 30 minutes, with maximum effects in 60 to 90 minutes. Duration of action for all forms 2 to 4 hours.

ROUTE AND DOSAGE. *Anticipated emotional and physical stress:* **Sublingual:** Initial: 10 mg prior to anticipated stress and at bedtime, if necessary. *Long-term prophylactic* management: **Oral tablet:** 10 mg before meals and, if necessary, at midmorning, midafternoon, and at bedtime. Maximal optimum dose up to 100 mg daily.

NURSING IMPLICATIONS

The regular tablet may be taken orally or sublingually. Chewable tablets should be thoroughly chewed and wetted before swallowing.

Oral tablet is preferably taken with a glass of water on an empty stomach either 1 hour before or 2 hours after meals.

Note that onset of action varies with preparation and route of administration.

Because of its more rapid onset of action, the physician may prescribe additional sublingual doses, as is done with nitroglycerin, prior to contemplated exertion or anticipated stress.

Combined rapid action and slower action may be obtained by allowing the tablet to dissolve partially under the tongue for 2 or 3 minutes, then swallowing remaining portion; consult physician about teaching the patient.

Sublingual administration may produce a tingling sensation at points of drug contact with mucous membranes. If the patient finds this objectionable, tablet may be placed in buccal pouch.

Mild GI disturbances, fall in blood pressure (lightheadedness), and headache may occur with large doses and may be controlled by dosage reduction.
Vascular headaches are common during first week of therapy because of disturbed cerebral hemodynamics. Advise patient to report to physician. Temporary reduction of dosage and administration of analgesics generally provide relief.
Oral tablet is reported less likely to produce headaches than other forms.
Since the patient may misinterpret freedom from anginal attacks as an indication to drop all restrictions, guidelines should be provided regarding allowable activities.
Tolerance to drug effect may develop with extended use.
Stored in cool place in airtight containers. Protect from light.
See Nitroglycerin (prototype coronary vasodilator).

PROTOTYPE

ERYTHROMYCIN

(A/T/S, Eryc, EryDerm, E-Mycin, Erythrocin, Erythromid, Ilotycin, Robimycin, RP-Mycin, Staticin, T-Stat)

(er-ith-roe-mye'sin)
Antiinfective
Antibiotic (macrolide)
Erythromycin

ACTIONS AND USES. Macrolide antibiotic produced by a strain of *Streptomyces erythreus.* Considered one of the safest antibiotics in use today. Bacteriostatic or bactericidal, depending on nature of organism and drug concentration used. Antibacterial spectrum is similar to but broader than that of penicillin; commonly used as penicillin substitute in hypersensitive patients for infections not requiring high antibiotic blood levels. More active against gram-positive than gram-negative bacteria. Effective against *Chlamydia trachomatis* is basis for its topical use in prophylaxis of neonatal inclusion conjunctivitis. Acts by inhibiting protein synthesis of sensitive microorganisms. Resistant mutants are especially frequent among staphylococci.

Used in treatment of pneumococcal and diplococcal pneumonia, *Mycoplasma pneumoniae* (primary atypical pneumonia), acute pelvic inflammatory disease caused by *Neisseria gonorrhoeae* in females sensitive to penicillin, infections caused by susceptible strains of staphylococci, streptococci, and certain strains of *Haemophilus influenzae.* Also used in intestinal amebiasis, Legionnaires disease, uncomplicated urethral, endocervical, and rectal infections caused by *Chlamydia trachomatis,* for prophylaxis of ophthalmia neonatorum caused by *N. gonorrhoeae, C. trachomatis,* and for chlamydial conjunctivitis in neonates. Considered an acceptable alternative to penicillin for treatment of streptococcal pharyngitis for prophylaxis of rheumatic fever and bacterial endocarditis, and for treatment of diphtheria as adjunct to antitoxin and for carrier state, and as alternate choice in treatment of primary syphilis in patients allergic to penicillins. Topical applications used in treatment of pyodermas, acne vulgaris, and external ocular infections, including neonatal chlamydial conjunctivitis and gonococcal ophthalmia.

ABSORPTION AND FATE. Peak plasma concentrations in about 4 hours following oral administration (absorption is delayed by presence of food in stomach). Adequate blood levels maintained by administration every 6 hours. Diffuses readily into tissues and most body fluids, including pleural and peritoneal spaces and inflamed meninges. Concentrates in normal liver. Half-life: 0.8 to 3 hours. Excreted in active form primarily in bile and feces. About 2 to 5% of orally administered dose excreted in urine as active drug. Crosses placenta and is excreted in breast milk.

CONTRAINDICATIONS AND PRECAUTIONS. Hypersensitivity to erythromycins. Safe use during pregnancy not established. *Cautious Use:* impaired hepatic function.

ADVERSE/SIDE EFFECTS. Infrequent: nausea, vomiting, heartburn, anorexia, and hypersensitivity reactions: fever, eosinophilia, urticaria, skin eruptions, anaphylaxis (rare), ototoxicity (rare). Superinfections by nonsusceptible bacteria, yeasts, or fungi. **Most frequent:** abdominal cramping, discomfort, distention, diarrhea. **Topical:** erythema, desquamation, burning, tenderness, dryness or oiliness, pruritus.

ROUTE AND DOSAGE. Adults: Oral: 250 mg every 6 hours. For twice-a-day schedule, one-half total daily dose may be prescribed every 12 hours (usual dose range 1 to 4 Gm daily). **Ophthalmic:** *ointment* (5 mg/Gm): applied one or more times daily (see below). **Topical solution (1.5 to 2%):** applied to affected skin areas two or three times daily. **Children: Oral:** 30 to 50 mg/kg/day in four equally divided doses; for more severe infections dose may be doubled.

E

NURSING IMPLICATIONS

Culture and susceptibility testing should be done to determine organism susceptibility.

Activity of erythromycin may be decreased in acid medium and by the presence of food in the stomach. Therefore it is administered preferably on an empty stomach 1 hour before or 3 hours after meals. Do not give with, or immediately before or after, fruit juices and advise patient not to crush or chew tablets.

Manufacturers of enteric coated tablets state that they may be given without regard to meals.

GI symptoms following oral administration are dose-related. Report their onset to physician. If symptoms persist following dosage reduction, physician may prescribe drug to be given with meals in spite of impaired absorption.

Bear in mind that pseudomembranous colitis, a potentially life-threatening condition, may occur during or after antibiotic therapy.

Before receiving erythromycin for gonorrhea, patients suspected of having syphilis should have microscopic examination for *Treponema pallidum* and monthly serologic tests for a minimum of 4 months.

In treatment of primary syphilis, spinal fluid examination should be done before treatment and as part of follow-up after therapy.

Observe for symptoms of overgrowth of nonsusceptible bacteria or fungi (fever, black furry tongue, sore mouth, enteritis, perianal irritation or itching, vaginal discharge). Emergence of resistant staphylococcal strains is highly predictable during prolonged therapy.

In treatment of streptococcal infections, erythromycin therapy should be continued for at least 10 days.

Hepatic function tests should be performed periodically during prolonged drug regimens.

Hepatotoxicity is believed to be a hypersensitivity reaction. Premonitory signs and symptoms may include abdominal pain, nausea, vomiting, fever, leukocytosis, and eosinophilia. Jaundice (dark urine, light-colored stools, yellow skin, pruritus yellow sclerae and soft palate) may or may not be present.

Symptoms of hepatotoxicity may appear a few days after initiation of drug but usually occur after 1 to 2 weeks of continuous therapy. Symptoms are reversible with prompt discontinuation of erythromycin.

Strict adherence of patient to prescribed dosage regimen should be stressed.

Topical erythromycin ointment is used as an alternative to 1% silver nitrate topical solution for prevention of neonatal gonococcal ophthalmia. Reportedly it causes less irritation than the silver nitrate, and since it is also effective against chlamydial conjunctivitis it may become a preferred agent. In some states, the use of topical erythromycin ointment has legally replaced (by changes in public health law) the silver nitrate prophylactic procedure (Credé method).

Prophylaxis: neonatal eye infection: ribbon of ointment approximately 0.5 to 1 cm in length is placed into lower conjunctival sac of neonate shortly after birth.

Prophylaxis of neonatal chlamydial conjunctivitis or gonorrheal ophthalmia is used on neonates delivered by cesarean section as well as those delivered by vaginal route. Use a new tube of erythromycin for each neonate. Do not flush the ointment from the eyes following application.

For topical applications to skin: Consult physician about procedure to use for cleaning affected area prior to each application.

Ointment preparation for skin problems should not be used in eyes or in external ear if eardrum is perforated. Drug should be discontinued if signs of sensitivity or irritation appear.

For treatment of eye infections, use only preparations labeled for ophthalmic use.

Store in tightly capped containers preferably between 15° and 30°C (59° and 86°) unless otherwise directed by manufacturer.

E

Diagnostic Test Interferences. False elevations of **urinary catecholamines, urinary steroids,** and AST (SGOT), ALT (SGPT) (by colorimetric methods).

Drug Interactions: Erythromycins

Plus	Interactions
Anticoagulants, oral	Potentiation of anticoagulant (hypoprothrombinemic) effect. Monitor prothrombin time
Carbamazepine (Tegretol) Corticosteroids	Effects of these drugs may increase (erythromycin inhibits their hepatic metabolism). Reduced dosages of these drugs and close monitoring indicated
Clindamycin (Cleocin)	Antagonistic action. Concomitant use generally avoided
Digoxin (Lanoxin) and other Digitalis glycosides	Possibility of increased digitalis effect in some patients. Interaction may occur several months after discontinuation of erythromycin (erythromycin increases digitalis bioavailability in some patients). Reduction of digitalis dosage may be necessary
Penicillins	Erythromycin in low doses may antagonize antimicrobial action of penicillins. Combination used only when adequate amounts of each are given, administer penicillin at least a few hours before erythromycin
Theophyllines	Pharmacologic effects of theophyllines may increase (erythromycin inhibits their hepatic metabolism). Theophyllines may reduce erythromycin serum concentrations. Reduced dosage of theophyllines and close monitoring indicated

ERYTHROMYCIN ESTOLATE
(Ilosone)

Antiinfective
Antibiotic (macrolide)
Erythromycin

ACTIONS AND USES. Acid ester salt of erythromycin (qv). Reported to be acid-stable and thus less susceptible to action of gastric juices or food in stomach and to give higher, more predictable, and more prolonged antibiotic blood levels than other oral forms of erythromycin. Unlike other erythromycins it may produce hepatotoxicity.

ABSORPTION AND FATE. Peak blood levels in about 2 hours following oral administration. Serum half-life: approximately 3 to 5 hours. About 0.8% of dose excreted in urine in 6 hours. Primarily excreted in bile. *See Erythromycin.*

CONTRAINDICATIONS AND PRECAUTIONS. Hypersensitivity to erythromycins; hepatic dysfunction; treatment of skin disorders such as acne or furunculosis or prophylaxis of rheumatic fever. Safe use during pregnancy not established. *See also Erythromycin.*

ADVERSE/SIDE EFFECTS. *Cholestatic hepatitis syndrome* **(hypersensitivity reaction):** malaise, nausea, vomiting, heartburn, abdominal cramps, right upper quadrant pain or tenderness, jaundice, fever, disturbance in color vision, headache, myalgia, abnormal liver function tests, eosinophilia, leukocytosis, slight increase in prothrombin time. *See also Erythromycin.*

ROUTE AND DOSAGE. Oral: Adults: 250 mg every 6 hours; dosage may be increased up to 4 Gm or more per day according to severity of infection. **Children:** 30 to 50 mg/kg/day orally in divided doses; for more severe infections dosage may be doubled. For twice-a-day dosage, in both adults and children, one-half of total daily dose may be prescribed. Available forms: tablet, chewable tablet, capsule, drops, suspension.

NURSING IMPLICATIONS

Culture and sensitivity testing should be done before initiation of treatment.

Cholestatic hepatitis syndrome appears most frequently after 1 to 2 weeks of continuous therapy or following several repeated courses of the drug, but it has also occurred after a few days of treatment; this condition is generally reversible within 3 to 5 days after cessation of therapy.

Premonitory symptoms of hepatitis may include abdominal cramps, nausea, and vomiting, followed by fever, leukocytosis, and eosinophilia. Advise patients to report immediately the onset of adverse reactions and to be on the alert for signs and symptoms associated with jaundice: dark urine, light-colored stools, pruritus, yellow skin, sclerae, and soft palate.

Hepatic function tests and blood cell counts should be conducted periodically if therapy is prolonged 10 days or more.

Chewable tablets should be chewed or crushed, not swallowed whole.

Serum levels are comparable whether taken after food or in the fasting state.

Therapeutic dosage should be continued for at least 10 days in treatment of group A beta-hemolytic streptococcal infections.

After reconstitution, suspensions are stable for 14 days at room temperature; however, palatability is retained if kept refrigerated.Protect from light.

See Erythromycin (prototype erythromycins).

ERYTHROMYCIN ETHYLSUCCINATE

(E.E.S., E-Mycin E, Pediamycin, Wyamycin E)

Antiinfective
Antibiotic (macrolide)
Erythromycin

ACTIONS AND USES. Acid-stable ester salt of erythromycin. Intramuscular preparation is used only when administration by other routes is not practical. *See Erythromycin.*

ABSORPTION AND FATE. Usually readily and reliably absorbed after oral ingestion; however, individual variability has been reported. Following IM administration of 100 mg in adults, peak serum levels are attained in 1 hour, gradually falling to 0.1 mg/ml in 6 to 8 hours. In children, peak levels are produced within 2 hours, gradually falling to low levels by 6 hours. Half-life: 2 to 5 hours. Concentrates in liver; excreted primarily in bile. *See also Erythromycin.*

CONTRAINDICATIONS AND PRECAUTIONS. Hypersensitivity to erythromycins or to butyl aminobenzoate (local anesthetic used in commercial IM preparation); IM use in small children or in serious infections when high dosage and/or frequent or prolonged administration is required. Safe use during pregnancy not established. *Cautious Use:* impaired hepatic function.

ADVERSE/SIDE EFFECTS. Pain on injection and possible sterile abscess and necrosis, abdominal cramps, diarrhea, anorexia, nausea, vomiting, skin eruptions, superinfections. *See Erythromycin.*

ROUTE AND DOSAGE. Adults: Oral: 400 mg every 6 hours; may be increased up to 4 Gm or more per day according to severity of infection. **Children: Oral:** 30 to 50 mg/kg/day in four equally divided doses; dosage may be doubled in more severe infections. For twice-a-day schedule in both adults and children, one-half the total daily dose may be prescribed every 12 hours. Available oral forms: tablet, chewable tablet, suspension.

NURSING IMPLICATIONS

Culture and sensitivity testing should be done.

Oral formulations may be administered without regard to meals in patients 2 years of age or older. Drug should be administered on empty stomach in patients under 2 years of age pending results of bioavailability studies in this age group.

Commercially available chewable tablets should be chewed and not swallowed whole.

Oral suspensions are stable for 10 days under refrigeration. Note expiration date.

In treatment of group A β-hemolytic streptococcal infections, therapeutic oral dosage should be continued for at least 10 days.

See Erythromycin (prototype erythromycins).

ERYTHROMYCIN GLUCEPTATE

(Ilotycin Gluceptate)

Antiinfective: antibiotic
Erythromycin

ACTIONS AND USES. Soluble salt of erythromycin indicated for use when oral or rectal administration is not possible or the severity of infection requires immediate high serum levels. *See Erythromycin.*

ABSORPTION AND FATE. Peak serum level of 3 to 4 mcg/ml achieved in 1 hour following administration of 200 mg IV; falls to 0.5 mcg/ml at 6 hours. Principally eliminated via bile. Approximately 12 to 15% of dose is excreted in urine in active form. *See Erythromycin.*

CONTRAINDICATIONS AND PRECAUTIONS. Hypersensitivity to erythromycins. Safe use during pregnancy not established. *Cautious Use:* impaired hepatic function.

ADVERSE/SIDE EFFECTS. Pain and venous irritation following IV injection; allergic reactions, anaphylaxis (rare); superinfections and variations in liver function tests following prolonged or repeated therapy.

ROUTE AND DOSAGE. Adults and children: Intravenous: 15 to 20 mg/kg body weight daily. Up to 4 Gm/day may be given in very severe infections. Continuous infusion is preferable, but may also be administered in divided doses by intermittent infusion, over 20 to 60 minutes, and no less frequently than every 6 hours.

NURSING IMPLICATIONS

Culture and susceptibility testing should be done.

Initial solution is prepared by adding sterile water for injection *without preservatives* to the vial (see manufacturer's directions for dilution). Shake vial until drug is completely dissolved. Saline or other solutions may cause gel formation and therefore should not be used in this initial step. Stable up to 7 days if refrigerated preferably between 2° to 8°C (36° to 46°F).

Prior to administration, initial solution as prepared above may then be diluted with 0.9% sodium chloride injection or 5% dextrose in water, and buffered to neutrality (see manufacturer's directions). Stability of solution is dependent on pH and is optimal at pH 6 to pH 8.

Continuous infusion is administered slowly within 24 hours after dilution.

A physician will prescribe specific IV infusion rate. Rate should be sufficiently slow to avoid pain along course of vein.

IV infusion of large doses reported to be associated with thrombophlebitis.

Since hearing impairment has been associated with large IV doses of erythromycin lactobionate, it is possible that it may occur with large doses of erythromycin gluceptate (it has occurred as early as the second day and as late as the third week of therapy and has been completely reversible after discontinuation of drug).

Periodic hepatic function tests are advised in patients receiving daily high doses or prolonged therapy.

Oral therapy should replace IV administration as soon as possible.

Store sterile powder preferably between 15° and 30°C (59° and 86°F) unless otherwise directed by manufacturer.

See Erythromycin (prototype erythromycins).

E

ERYTHROMYCIN LACTOBIONATE

(Erythrocin Lactobionate-I.V., Erythrocin Piggyback)

Antiinfective
Antibiotic (macrolide)
Erythromycin

ACTIONS AND USES. Lactobionate salt of erythromycin. Indicated for use when oral or rectal administration is not possible or severity of infection requires immediate high serum levels.

ABSORPTION AND FATE. Rapid IV infusion of 200 mg produces peak serum levels of 3 to 4 mcg/ml almost immediately; levels gradually reduce to 0.5 mcg/ml at 6 hours. Approximately 12 to 15% of dose is excreted in urine in active form. Primarily excreted in bile. *See Erythromycin.*

CONTRAINDICATIONS AND PRECAUTIONS. Hypersensitivity to erythromycins. Safe use during pregnancy not established. *Cautious Use:* impaired hepatic function.

ADVERSE/SIDE EFFECTS. Anorexia, abdominal discomfort, diarrhea, nausea, vomiting, allergic reactions, thrombophlebitis at injection site, impaired hearing associated with IV infusions of 4 Gm/day or more (reversible). *See also Erythromycin.*

ROUTE AND DOSAGE. Adults and children: Intravenous: 15 to 20 mg/kg body weight daily. Higher doses may be given in very severe infections (up to 4 Gm/day). Continuous infusion is preferable, but may be administered in divided doses by intermittent infusion, giving one-fourth total daily dose over 20 to 60 minutes, at intervals not greater than every 6 hours. Drug should be administered by direct IV injection (IV push).

NURSING IMPLICATIONS

Culture and susceptibility tests should be done.

Initial solution is prepared by adding 10 ml sterile water for injection *without preservatives* to the 200 or 500 mg vial or at least 20 ml to the 1 Gm vial. Shake vial until drug is completely dissolved. Saline or other solutions may cause precipitation and therefore should not be used in this initial step. Stable up to 2 weeks if refrigerated.

For continuous IV infusion, initial solution as prepared above may then be added to 0.9% sodium chloride injection, lactated Ringer's, or other IV fluids recommended by manufacturer, and buffered to neutrality (see manufacturer's directions). The final diluted solution (1 mg/ml) should be administered within 24 hours.

IV infusion rate will be prescribed by physician. Rate should be sufficiently slow to avoid pain along course of vein.

IV infusions of large doses reportedly are associated with thrombophlebitis at injection site and hearing difficulty. Hearing defects have appeared as early as the second day of therapy and as late as the third week; these are completely reversible after discontinuation of drug.

Periodic hepatic function tests are advised in patients receiving daily high doses or prolonged therapy.

Store sterile powder preferably between 15° to 30°C (59° and 86°F) unless otherwise directed by manufacturer.

IV therapy should be replaced by oral dosage form as soon as possible.

See Erythromycin (prototype erythromycins).

ERYTHROMYCIN STEARATE

(Eramycin, Erypar, Ethril, SK-Erythromycin, Wyamycin S)

Antiinfective
Antibiotic (macrolide)
Erythromycin

ACTIONS AND USES. Acid-labile stearic acid salt of erythromycin (qv). Reportedly one of the most completely and reliably absorbed forms of erythromycin.

ABSORPTION AND FATE. Readily absorbed, especially on empty stomach; but individual variations have been observed. Oral dose of 250 mg produces average serum level of at least 0.6 mcg/ml in 2 hours. Peak serum levels rise with repeated administration. Average half-life is approximately 5.5 hours. Excreted primarily in bile. *See Erythromycin.*

CONTRAINDICATIONS AND PRECAUTIONS. Hypersensitivity to erythromycins. Safe use during pregnancy not established. *Cautious Use:* impaired hepatic function.

ADVERSE/SIDE EFFECTS. Abdominal cramps, diarrhea, nausea, vomiting, urticaria, skin eruptions, superinfections. *See Erythromycin.*

ROUTE AND DOSAGE. Adults: Oral: 250 mg every 6 hours; dosage may be increased up to 4 Gm/day or more according to severity of infection. **Children:** 30 to 50 mg/kg/day orally in four equally divided doses. For more severe infections, dosage may be doubled. For twice-a-day schedule in both adults and children, one-half of total daily dose may be prescribed every 12 hours.

NURSING IMPLICATIONS

Optimum blood levels are obtained when drug is given on empty stomach (preferably 1 hour before or 3 hours after meals).
Culture and sensitivity testing should be done.
Instruct patient not to chew or crush film coated tablet.
In treatment of group A β-hemolytic streptococcal infections, therapeutic dosage should be administered for at least 10 days.
Ethril '500' contains tartrazine which may cause an allergic reaction, including bronchial asthma, in susceptible persons, who frequently are also sensitive to aspirin.
Protect tablets from light.
See Erythromycin (prototype erythromycins).

ESSENTIAL AMINO ACID INJECTION

Caloric agent

(Aminosyn-RF, Nephramine, Renamin)

ACTIONS AND USES. Contains only essential amino acids prepared to be diluted with hypertonic dextrose solution and administered by central vein. By supplying patient with sufficient essential amino acids and calories, excess nitrogen in patient's body can be used up in manufacture of nonessential acids for anabolism. Since the mixture reduces rate of blood urea production and minimizes serum potassium, magnesium, and phosphorous imbalances, it is appropriate for use in patients with potentially reversible renal decompensation when oral nutrition is not possible or impractical.

See Amino Acid Injection for adverse reactions and for information concerning TPN (total parenteral nutrition or hyperalimentation).

CONTRAINDICATIONS AND PRECAUTIONS. Severe uncorrected electrolyte and acid-base imbalances; hyperammonemia, decreased circulating blood volume, inborn errors of amino acid metabolism. *Cautious Use:* pediatric patients, especially low birth-weight infants.

ADVERSE/SIDE EFFECTS. Hyperammonemia, hyperglycemia, electrolyte imbalances, circulatory overload. *See also Amino Acid Injection.*

ROUTE AND DOSAGE. Intravenous (central venous catheter): 250 to 500 ml containing approximately 1.6 to 3.2 Gm nitrogen in 14 to 27 Gm of essential amino acids daily. Each 250 ml is usually mixed with 500 ml of 70% dextrose. Electrolytes and vitamins may be added, if needed.

NURSING IMPLICATIONS

Hyperglycemia is a frequent complication, particularly in low-birth-weight or infants with sepsis, and uremic patients. Urine and blood glucose must be closely monitored. Exogenous insulin may be required.
Electrolytes, calcium, phosphorous, and magnesium should be checked daily.
Serum concentrations of potassium, phosphorous, and magnesium may decrease dramatically during therapy. Supplements may be required. Observe for signs and symptoms of hypokalemia; muscular weakness, paresthesias, polyuria, polydipsia, gastric distention, arrhythmias; also hypomagnesemia: nausea, vomiting, personality changes, tetany, muscle fasciculations.

Hyperammonemia commonly occurs in infants. Observe for and report promptly: vomiting, lethargy, irritability.

Monitor intake and output. Observe patient for signs of circulatory overload: rapid and shallow breathing, cyanosis, rapid pulse, falling blood pressure.

Initial infusion rate generally does not exceed 20 to 30 ml/hour. Increases by increments of 10 ml/hour each 24 hours are recommended up to maximum of 60 to 100 ml/hour.

See Amino Acid Injection.

E

PROTOTYPE

ESTRADIOL

(Estrace)

(ess-tra-dye'ole)
Hormone
Estrogen

ACTIONS AND USES. Natural or synthetic steroid hormone produced by ovaries. Essential for normal maturation of the female and for maintenance of normal menstrual cycles during reproductive years. Promotes endometrial lining development and increases volume, acidity, and glycogen content of vaginal secretions. Weakly anabolic; large doses induce sodium and fluid retention. Decreases intestinal motility but stimulates uterine motility. By unclear mechanism, contributes to molding of body contours, shaping the skeleton and acceleration of epiphyseal closure of long bones. Decreases bone resorption rate which is accelerated at time of menopause. Estrogen therapy increases risk of thrombosis in women receiving hormone for postpartum breast engorgement and in men receiving estrogens for prostatic cancer; also increases risk of endometrial carcinoma and gallbladder disease in postmenopausal women. May mask onset of climacteric. Men receiving large doses of estrogens are more prone than nonusers to nonfatal myocardial infarction, pulmonary embolism, and thrombophlebitis. There is no evidence that estrogen therapy for postmenopausal women increases risk of breast cancer; furthermore, recent studies support the position that the healthy postmenopausal woman need not fear thrombosis or hypercoagulation from combination estrogen/progesterone therapy.

Used to treat natural or surgical menopausal symptoms (except nervous symptoms or depression), kraurosis vulvae, atrophic vaginitis, primary ovarian failure, female hypogonadism, and castration. Also used to prevent and treat postmenopausal osteoporosis and as palliative for advanced prostatic carcinoma and inoperable breast cancer in women at least 5 years postmenopause. Combined with progestins in many oral contraceptive formulations.

ABSORPTION AND FATE. Readily absorbed from GI tract. Half-life: 50 minutes. 50 to 80% binding with plasma proteins. Enters cells of estrogen responsive tissues (female genital organs, breasts, pituitary and hypothalamus) and by unknown mechanism is transported to the nucleus where it stimulates DNA, RNA and protein synthesis. (The palliative response to estrogen treatment in women with metastasic cancer of breast results from the presence of these receptor proteins.) Large amounts of free estrogen excreted into bile, reabsorbed from GI tract and recirculated through liver, principle site of degradation. Excretion primarily in urine as sulfates and glucuronides; small amounts present in feces. Crosses placenta and appears in breast milk.

CONTRAINDICATIONS AND PRECAUTIONS. Estrogen hypersensitivity, known or suspected pregnancy, estrogenic-dependent neoplasms, breast cancer (except in selected patients being treated for metastatic disease). History of active thromboembolic disorders, arterial thrombosis, or thrombophlebitis; undiagnosed abnormal genital bleeding; history of cholestatic disease; thyroid dysfunction, blood dyscrasias. *Cautious Use:* Adolescents with incomplete bone growth; endometriosis, lactation, hypertension, cardiac insufficiency, diseases of calcium and phosphate metabolism, cerebrovascular disease, mental depression, benign breast disease, family history of breast or genital tract neoplasm; diabetes mellitus, gallbladder disease, preexisting leiomyoma, abnormal mammogram, history of idiopathic jaundice of pregnancy; varicosities, asthma, epilepsy, migraine headaches, hepatic or renal dysfunction; jaundice, acute intermittent porphyria, pyridoxine deficiency.

ADVERSE/SIDE EFFECTS. **Dermatologic:** skin rash, photosensitivity, pruritus, acne, chloasma, melasma, loss of scalp hair, hirsutism, chorea, scotomata, steepening of corneal curvature, intolerance to contact lenses. **GI:** nausea, vomiting, anorexia, diarrhea, abdominal cramps, bloating, cholestatic jaundice, thirst, benign hepatoadenoma. **Reproductive:** mastodynia, breast secretion, changes in vaginal bleeding pattern, spotting, changes in menstrual flow, vaginal candidiasis, reactivation of endometriosis, increased size of preexisting fibromyomata. *In males:* gynecomastia, testicular atrophy, feminization, impotence (reversible). **Other:** thromboembolic disorders, reduced carbohydrate tolerance, hypercalcemia, hypertension, leg cramps, edema, weight gain or loss, aggravation of porphyria, abdominal pain, changes in libido, fatigue, backache, cystitislike syndrome.

ROUTE AND DOSAGE. (Generally, lowest effective dosage for shortest possible time to decrease adverse effects; highly individualized.) **Oral:** *Menopause, kraurosis vulvae, female castration, primary ovarian failure:* 1 to 2 mg daily (cyclic regimen). Adjusted to minimal requirements by titration. *Prostatic cancer:* 1 to 2 mg three times daily. *Breast cancer:* 10 mg 3 times daily for at least 3 months.

NURSING IMPLICATIONS

To avoid overstimulation of estrogen-activated tissues and to mimic natural menses, estrogens are usually administered on a cyclic dosage regimen: 3 weeks on and 1 week off medication. This schedule may not be used, however, for male or hysterectomized patients.

Take oral medication with or immediately after solid food to reduce nausea.

Nausea, frequently at breakfast time, seldom interferes with eating or causes weight loss and usually disappears after 1 or 2 weeks of drug use.

In some cases, a progestational agent is added to the last 5 days of each cycle of estrogen therapy to produce more regularity.

A complete history (including menstrual pattern) and physical examination with particular reference to blood pressure, eyes, breasts, abdomen and pelvic organs, and including Pap smear should precede initiation of estrogen therapy and be repeated every 6 to 12 months during treatment.

Urge patient to read the patient package insert (PPI) carefully then discuss it with patient to assure complete understanding about estrogen therapy.

Attempts to discontinue or taper estrogen therapy should be made at 3- to 6-month intervals.

Estrogen primed endometrium may bleed 48 to 72 hours after dose is discontinued. In cyclic therapy, estradiol is resumed on schedule before induced vaginal bleeding stops.

Withdrawal bleeding may occur even after oophorectomy and after menopause. Inform postmenopausal women that such bleeding is pseudomenstruation and does not indicate return of fertility.

If a patient has intermittent bleeding or begins to bleed without having previously done so, she should promptly report to her physician for an evaluation. Breakthrough bleeding may be stopped by increasing estrogen dose; however if bleeding persists, the physician may recommend curettage.

Spotting or breakthrough bleeding occurring when a barbiturate and estradiol are taken concurrently indicates reduced availability of the estrogen.

Estrogen stimulation in women sterilized because of endometriosis may cause serious bleeding in remaining foci of endometrial tissues. Report unexplained and sudden pain.

Advise patient to report abdominal pain and tenderness or abdominal mass, possible symptoms of hepatic adenoma and/or hepatic hemorrhage.

If user suspects she is pregnant, she should stop taking the estrogen immediately and inform the physician. She should be apprised of the potential risk of masculinization of female fetus.

Cyclic fluid retention should be reported. A low-salt diet and diuretic may be prescribed.

During intensive therapy with estrogens, monitor vital signs and chart for comparison purposes. A gradual increase in blood pressure and pulse readings over time is reportable.

Be alert to the possibility of behavior changes or increasing mental depression, symptoms that may suggest recurrence of pretreatment psychic disorders. Report to physician; drug will usually be discontinued.

Instruct patient to report the following symptoms of thromboembolic disorders immediately: tenderness, swelling, and redness in extremity; sudden, severe headache or chest pain; sudden slurring of speech; sudden change in vision; tenderness, pain, sudden shortness of breath. If physician is not available, patient should go to the nearest hospital emergency room.

Teach patient how to elicit Homan's sign: pain in calf and popliteal region with forced dorsiflexion of foot (early sign of thrombosis).

Symptoms of vaginal candidiasis (thick, white, curdlike secretions and inflamed congested introitus) should be reported to permit appropriate treatment.

Reassure male patients that estrogen-induced feminization and impotence are reversible with termination of therapy.

Since estradiol decreases free thyroxine, patient on therapy for a nonfunctioning thyroid may need an increase in thyroid replacement agent while also receiving an estrogen.

History of jaundice in pregnancy increases the possibility of estrogen-induced jaundice. Instruct patient to report yellow skin and sclera, pruritus, dark urine, and light-colored stools. Estrogen therapy is usually interrupted pending clinical investigation.

Advise patient to determine weight under standard conditions 1 or 2 times/week and to report sudden weight gain or other signs of fluid retention.

Menopausal symptoms in well-controlled patients on estrogens begin to return in full intensity by end of rest period without estrogen.

Advise diabetic users to report positive urine tests promptly. Dosage adjustment of antidiabetic drug may be indicated. Stress necessity of periodic clinical evaluation for the potential diabetic (family history).

Smoking–Drug Interactions: Recent studies suggest that smoking increases serum estradiol and estrone concentrations. Since incidence of heart attack in men treated with estrogen is known to increase, smoking behavior should be discussed with patient on estrogen therapy.

Food–Drug Interactions:

- Estrogenic depression of caffeine metabolism may cause caffeinism. Urge patient to decrease caffeine intake from sources such as tea, coffee, cola.
- Pyridoxine (Vitamin B_6) levels are lowered by estrogens. A supplement may be ordered for the patient on long-term therapy, especially if undernourished.

Emphasize need for compliance with established dosage schedule which should not be altered unless physician prescribes a change.

If patient forgets a dose, she should take it as soon as remembered, unless it is near the time for the next dose. In that case, she should take it on time and without doubling the amount.

Teach self-examination of breasts, emphasizing a monthly schedule.

Long-term or high-dosage therapy with estrogens is reduced or terminated gradually.

When hypercalcemia (*normal serum calcium:* 8.5 to 10.5 mg/dl) occurs in patient with breast cancer, it usually indicates progression of bone metastasis; estrogen treatment is usually terminated.

Severe hypercalcemia (above 15 mg/dl) may be caused by estradiol therapy in patients with breast cancer and bone metastasis. Monitor carefully in order to identify symptoms promptly: hypotonicity of muscles, deep bone and flank pain, polyuria, extreme thirst, GI symptoms, mental confusion, lethargy, cardiac arrhythmia. Discontinuation of estrogen is indicated with institution of measures to encourage calcium excretion.

Caution patient to be careful about exposure to sun lamps and to sun. Estrogen users sometimes sunburn more easily and develop brown, blotchy spots on exposed skin (reversible with termination of therapy).

Acute overdosage of an estrogen does not have serious effects even in small children. Nausea may occur and withdrawal bleeding may result. Notify physician.

Estrace tablet contains tartrazine which may cause allergic-type reactions (including bronchial asthma) in certain susceptible persons. This sensitivity is also frequently seen in aspirin-sensitive persons.

Cosmetic use: Systemic effects have followed excessive use of estrogen creams in cosmetic preparations (edema, vaginal bleeding, nausea, vomiting).

Dermal thickness may be slightly increased by estrogen cosmetic cream, but usually without altering facial appearance.

There is no scientific evidence that estrogen creams as cosmetics are more effective than simple emolients in relieving dry skin.

The pathologist should be advised of estrogen therapy when relevant specimens are submitted; the dentist should know if extraction or periodontal surgery is anticipated and in an emergency, the attending physician should be informed.

Estrogen treatment is usually interrupted at least 4 weeks before surgery that may be associated with a prolonged period of immobilization or with vascular complications.

If liver or endocrine function tests are abnormal, they should be repeated after estrogen has been withdrawn for two cycles.

Protect tablets from light and moisture in well-closed container. Store between 15° and 30°C (59° and 86°F) and protect from freezing, unless otherwise directed by manufacturer.

Diagnostic Test Interferences. Estradiol reduces response of **metyrapone** test and excretion of **pregnanediol.** *Increases:* **BSP** retention, norepinephrine-induced **platelet aggregability, hydrocortisone, PBI, T_4, sodium, thyroxine-binding globulin** (TBG), **prothrombin and factors VII, VIII, IX** and **X; triglyceride** and **lipoprotein** (especially HDL) concentrations, **renin** substrate. *Decreases:* **antithrombin III, pyridoxine** and **serum folate** concentrations, serum **cholesterol,** values for the **T_3 resin uptake** test, **glucose tolerance.** May cause false-positive test for **LE cells** and/or **antinuclear antibodies** (ANA).

Drug Interactions: Estradiol (estrogens)

Plus	Interactions
Anticoagulants, oral	Estradiol decreases anticoagulant activity by increasing action of selected clotting factors
Antidiabetic agents	Decreases glucose tolerance

Plus (cont.)	Interactions (cont.)
Anticonvulsants Barbiturates Carbamazepine (Tegretol) Phenylbutazone Primidone Rifampin (Rifadin, Remactane)	Decrease estrogen effect by increasing rate of hepatic breakdown of estrogen
Corticosteroids	Potentiates antiinflammatory and glycosuric effects of hydrocortisone
Meperidine (Demerol)	Increases narcotic effect by depressing hepatic breakdown of meperidine
Tricyclic antidepressants	Increases toxicity of antidepressants

E

ESTRADIOL CYPIONATE

Hormone
Estrogen

(Cypionate, Depo-Estradiol Depogen, Dura-Estrin, E-Ionate PA, Estra-D, Estro-Cyp, Estroject-LA, Hormogen Depot)

ACTIONS AND USES. *See Estradiol for action, absorption, fate, contraindications, and adverse reactions.* Average duration of effects 3 to 8 weeks.

ROUTE AND DOSAGE. Intramuscular (cottonseed oil vehicle): *Menopause:* 1 to 5 mg, repeated in 3 to 4 weeks. *Female hypogonadism:* 1.5 to 2 mg at monthly intervals.

NURSING IMPLICATIONS

Discuss package insert with patient to assure understanding of estrogen therapy.
Store drug at controlled room temperature; protect from light.
See Estradiol (prototype estrogen).

ESTRADIOL VALERATE

Hormone
Estrogen

(Delestrogen, Dioval, Duragen, Estraval-PA, Femogex, Valergen)

ACTIONS AND USES. Provides 2 to 3 weeks of estrogen effects from single IM injection. *See Estradiol for absorption fate and limitations.*

ROUTE AND DOSAGE. Intramuscular (sesame or castor oil vehicle): *Female castration, menopausal syndrome, atrophic vaginitis:* 10 to 20 mg every 4 weeks. *Prostatic carcinoma:* 30 mg or more every 1 or 2 weeks. *Prevention of postpartum breast engorgement:* 10 to 25 mg as single injection at end of first stage of labor.

NURSING IMPLICATIONS

Discuss package insert with patient to assure understanding of estrogen therapy.
Store drug at controlled room temperature; protect from light.
See Estradiol (prototype estrogen).

ESTRAMUSTINE PHOSPHATE SODIUM

(Emcyt)

(ess-tra-muss′teen)
Antineoplastic
Hormone
Estrogen

ACTIONS AND USES. Conjugate of estradiol and the carbamate of nitrogen mustard. Extent of antitumor activity contributed by each, as well as precise mechanisms of action unknown. Appears to act as a relatively weak alkylating agent and estrogen. Major effectiveness reported to be in patients who have been refractory to estrogen therapy alone. Contains 0.5 mEq (12.5 mg) of sodium per capsule.

Used in palliative treatment of metabolic and/or progressive carcinoma of prostate.

E

ABSORPTION AND FATE. Well absorbed from GI tract. Peak plasma concentration in 2 to 3 hours. Rapidly dephosphorylated in intestines; ultimately oxidized and hydrolyzed to estramustine, estradiol, estrone, and nitrogen mustard. Elimination appears to be multiphasic. Half-life of terminal phase approximately 20 hours. Metabolized in liver. Most of drug excreted in bile via feces.

CONTRAINDICATIONS AND PRECAUTIONS. Hypersensitivity to either estradiol or nitrogen mustard; active thrombophlebitis, or thromboembolic disorders. *Cautious Use:* history of thrombophlebitis, thromboses, or thromboembolic disorders, cerebrovascular or coronary artery disease, gallstones, or peptic ulcer; impaired liver function, metabolic bone diseases associated with hypercalcemia; diabetes mellitus, hypertension, conditions that might be aggravated by fluid retention (e.g., epilepsy, migraine, renal dysfunction); elderly patients.

ADVERSE/SIDE EFFECTS. CV: hypertension, cerebrovascular accident, myocardial infarction, thrombophlebitis, congestive heart failure, peripheral edema. **Dermatologic:** rash, pruritus, urticaria, dry skin, easy bruising, flushing, peeling skin and fingertips, thinning hair. **GI:** nausea, diarrhea, anorexia, flatulence, vomiting, thirst, GI bleeding. **Hematologic:** leukopenia, thrombocytopenia, hypercalcemia, abnormalities in liver function tests. **Neurologic:** lethargy, emotional lability, insomnia, headache, anxiety, epilepsy. **Respiratory:** hoarseness, burning sensation in throat, dyspnea, upper respiratory discharge, pulmonary emboli. **Other:** tearing of eyes, gynecomastia, breast tenderness, impotence, renal dysfunction, leg cramps, decrease in glucose tolerance, bone marrow toxicity (uncommon).

ROUTE AND DOSAGE. Oral: 14 mg/kg/day in three or four divided doses. Dosage range: 10 to 16 mg/kg/day.

NURSING IMPLICATIONS

Note expiration date on product label.

Drug can be taken with meals to reduce incidence of GI side effects. Physician may prescribe an antacid or antiemetic if GI symptoms persist. Some patients require drug withdrawal.

Patient-Teaching Points Related to Drug Induced Nausea:

- ✓ Eat small feedings at frequent intervals; eat slowly.
- ✓ Keep physically quiet when nauseated and keep upper torso elevated (for about 2 hours after eating).
- ✓ Drink liquids 1 hour before or 1 hour after rather than with meals; clear liquids may be more palatable.
- ✓ Control odors and avoid foods known to patient that precipitate or aggravate nausea.
- ✓ Avoid fried, greasy, spicy, and overly sweet foods.
- ✓ Cold foods may be less offensive than hot foods because they are generally almost odorless.

✓ If nausea occurs on awakening, eat dry foods such as a cracker or dry toast before activity.
✓ Cleanse mouth after each meal; sour balls, breath fresheners, or ice chips may help.
✓ Inspect oral cavity after vomiting for retained food/vomitus (debilitated patients or severely depressed patients may be unaware of their presence.) Cleanse mouth if necessary.
✓ Patient may be reassured if emesis basin is kept handy but not visible.
✓ Eliminate smoking by caretaker in presence of sick person.

Elderly patients who have nausea and vomiting should be kept turned on side with head of bed raised to prevent aspiration. Suction equipment should be readily available.

Check blood pressure at regular intervals throughout therapy. Report significant elevations to physician.

Keep track of weight and examine daily for peripheral edema. Be mindful that drug can cause congestive heart failure.

Monitor intake–output ratio and pattern to prevent dehydration and electrolyte imbalance.

Patient with diabetes should be closely observed because of possibility of estramustine-induced reduction in glucose tolerance. Baseline and periodic glucose tolerance tests are advised.

Patient should be advised to use a barrier contraceptive. (Drug has mutagenic and teratogenic properties.) Some patients formerly impotent have regained potency while taking estramustine.

Advise patient who experiences thinning of hair to avoid vigorous treatment of scalp and to wash and comb hair gently.

Baseline and periodic hepatic enzymes and bilirubin tests should be performed, then repeated after drug has been discontinued for 2 months.

Patient should receive therapy for 30 to 90 days before evaluations are made to determine adequacy or response and possible benefits of continuing treatment.

Some patients have received therapy more than 3 years. Therapy is usually continued as long as patient demonstrates a favorable response.

Treatment of overdosage: stomach contents evacuated by gastric lavage. Therapy is symptomatic and supportive. Hematologic and hepatic studies should be done for at least 6 weeks after drug ingestion.

Store in refrigerator at 2° to 8°C (38° to 46°F) in tight, light-resistant containers, unless otherwise directed by manufacturer.

ESTROGENS, CONJUGATED

(Estrocon, Evestrone, Premarin)

(ess'tro-jenz)

Estrogen, postcoital contraceptive (emergency), systemic hemostatic

ACTIONS AND USES. Short-acting estrogen preparation. Contains mixture of conjugated estrogens, including sodium estrone sulfate (50 to 65%) and sodium equilin sulfate (20 to 35%).

Used for atrophic vaginitis and kraurosis vulvae and to arrest abnormal uterine bleeding due to hormonal imbalance;also used to treat hypogonadism, primary ovarian failure, moderate to severe vasomotor symptoms associated with menopause; to prevent postpartum breast engorgement, to retard progression of osteoporosis, and as palliative therapy of mammary and prostatic carcinomas. *See Estradiol for absorption, fate, contraindications, precautions, adverse/side effects, and drug interactions.*

ROUTE AND DOSAGE. Oral: *Menopause:* 0.3 to 1.25 mg daily given cyclically; adjusted up or down for maintenance at lowest level that provides effective control (usually 0.625 mg or less). *Female hypogonadism:* 0.625 to 1.25 mg one to three times daily for 20 days followed by 10-day rest period; if there is no bleeding at end of this cycle, same dosage is repeated. If bleeding occurs before end of 10-day period, begin a 20-day estrogen-progestin regimen. If bleeding occurs before the regimen is concluded, discontinue therapy. Resume on day 5 of bleeding in next cycle. *Atrophic vaginitis; kraurosis vulvae:* 0.3 to 1.25 mg daily. *Breast cancer* (palliation): 10 mg three times daily for at least 3 months. *Prostatic cancer* (palliation): 1.25 to 2.5 mg three times daily. Prophylaxis for *postpartum breast engorgement:* 3.75 mg every 4 hours for 5 doses or 1.25 mg every 4 hours for 5 days. **Intravenous, intramuscular:** 25 mg repeated in 6 to 12 hours if necessary. **Intravaginal cream** (cyclic regimen), e.g., 3 weeks on and 1 week off): (0.625%) ½ to 1 applicatorful (2 to 4 Gm) daily, intravaginally or topically.

NURSING IMPLICATIONS

Given cyclically except when used for treatment of postpartum breast engorgement and for palliation of cancer.

To reconstitute parenteral preparation, add diluent to ampul and agitate gently; use within a few hours.

If reconstituted solution is stored in refrigerator and protected from light, it will remain stable for 60 days. Discard precipitated or discolored solution.

Rapid IV injection may cause skin flushing.

Estrogen in the cream preparation is readily absorbed and reaches blood levels approaching those of parenteral or orally administered estrogen. Systemic hyperestrogenic effects (uterine bleeding, edema, mastalgia, reactivation of endometriosis) may result from overdosage of intravaginal cream or from overexposure of denuded or abraded skin surfaces of hands to estrogen.

Intravaginal administration: Have patient in recumbent position, draped, with knees flexed and legs spread apart. Put on sterile gloves before inspecting perineal area. If discharge is present, gently wash area with soap (if allowed) and warm water. Spread labia and slowly insert calibrated dosage applicator approximately 5 cm (2 in) directing it slightly back toward sacrum. Instill medication by pushing plunger. If applicator is reusable, wash well with warm water and soap before replacing in its container. Patient should remain in recumbent position about 30 minutes to prevent losing the medication (no sphincter in vagina). Observe perineal area before each administration: if mucosa is red, swollen or excoriated, or if there is a change in vaginal discharge, report to physician before giving the medication.

If patient is to administer medication to herself, instruct her to wash her hands well before and after the application, and to avoid contact of denuded areas with the cream. Also tell her not to use tampons while on vaginal cream therapy. She may wish to wear a sanitary napkin to protect clothing.

Caution patient to adhere to prescribed regimen and to report adverse symptoms of estrogen therapy to the physician promptly.

Large doses of conjugated estrogens as used in treatment of cancer of breast or prostrate have been shown to increase risk of nonfatal myocardial infarction, pulmonary embolism, and thrombophlebitis.

Note that esterified estrogens (qv) combine the same estrogenic substances that are in conjugated estrogens but in different proportions.

Combined estrogens (Hormonen) is a mixture of estriol, estradiol, and estrone but does not conform to USP definitions of each conjugated or esterified estrogen. Has same uses and adverse reactions as estradiol.

Conjugated estrogens solution is compatible with dextrose, normal saline and invert sugar solutions, and incompatible with any solution with an acid pH (below 7.0).

A calibrated dosage applicator should be dispensed with the drug. Inform the patient.

Review package insert with patient to assure understanding of estrogen therapy.

Store vaginal cream at temperature between 15° and 30°C (59° and 86°F); protect from light and from freezing.

See Estradiol (prototype estrogens).

E

ESTROGENS, ESTERIFIED

(Estratab, Evex, Menest, Zeste)

Hormone
Estrogen

ACTIONS AND USES. Combination of same estrogens as found in conjugated estrogens but in different proportions: 75 to 85% sodium estrone sulfate and 6.5 to 15% sodium equilin sulfate.

Used for symptomatic treatment of menopause; to treat primary ovarian failure, female gonadism and castration, and as palliation for cancer of female breast and prostate. *See Estradiol for absorption, fate, and limitations.*

ROUTE AND DOSAGE. Oral: *Menopause:* 0.3 to 1.25 mg daily (cyclic regimen). Dosage may be increased to 2.5 or 3.75 mg daily if satisfactory response not obtained in 3 to 4 days. *Female hypogonadism:* 2.5 to 7.5 mg daily in divided doses for 20 days followed by 10-day rest period. If bleeding does not occur, repeat same dosage schedule. If bleeding occurs before end of 10-day period, begin a 20-day estrogen-progestin cyclic regimen. *Prostatic carcinoma:* 1.25 to 2.5 mg three times a day for several weeks. *Breast cancer:* 10 mg three times daily for 2 to 3 months for subjective response and total of 3 months for objective response.

NURSING IMPLICATIONS

Given cyclically, except when used for palliation of cancer.

Review package insert with patient to assure understanding of estrogen therapy.

Store tablets between 15° and 30°C (59° and 86°F) in a tightly closed container.

See Estradiol (prototype estrogen).

ESTRONE

ESTRONE AQUEOUS SUSPENSION

(Estronol, Kestrone-5, Theelin Aqueous)

ESTROGENIC SUBSTANCE AQUEOUS SUSPENSION

(Estaqua, Estrofol, Estroject-2, Foygen Aqueous, Gravigen, Gynogen, Kestrin, Unigen Aqueous, Wehgen)

ESTROGENIC SUBSTANCE IN OIL

(Gravigen in Oil, Kestrin in Oil)

(ess′trone)
Hormone
Estrogen

ACTIONS AND USES. First sex hormone isolated in pure form; present in urine of pregnant mares along with other estrogens. Synthetic estrone has same actions absorption, fate, contraindications, precautions, and adverse reactions as estradiol (qv).

Used in estrogen substitution therapy following cessation of ovarian function, x-ray or radium treatment, and natural menopause; and to provide palliation to patients with inoperable carcinoma of prostate.

ROUTE AND DOSAGE. **Intramuscular:** *Menopausal symptoms:* 0.1 to 0.5 mg two or three times weekly. *Female hypogonadism, castration, primary ovarian failure:* 0.5 to 2 mg weekly in single or divided doses. *Inoperable prostatic cancer:* 2 to 4 mg two or three times weekly. If response is to occur, it will be evident within 3 months of started regimen. If response does occur, therapy is continued until disease is again progressive.

NURSING IMPLICATIONS

IM preparations have either water or oil for the base. Oily preparation may become cloudy on chilling because of drug precipitation. Warm solution to room temperature until it is clear before administration.

Note that several types of estrone preparations are available and that the classification nomenclature is confusing.

Review package insert with patient to assure understanding of estrogen therapy.

Stored preferably between 15° and 30°C (59° and 86°F) unless otherwise directed by manufacturer. Protect from light and from freezing.

See Estradiol (prototype estrogen).

ESTROPIPATE

(ee-troe-pi′pate)

(Ogen, Piperazine Estrone Sulfate)

Hormone

Estrogen

ACTIONS AND USES. Water-soluble preparation of pure crystalline estrone (responsible for therapeutic actions conjugated as the sulfate and stabilized with piperazine). Has same actions, absorption, fate, contraindications, precautions, and adverse reactions as Estradiol (qv).

Used in estrogen substitution therapy.

ROUTE AND DOSAGE. **Oral:** *Menopausal symptoms:* The equivalent of 0.625 to 5 mg of estrone sulfate daily, cyclically each month. *Female hypogonadism, castration, primary ovarian failure:* the equivalent of 1.25 to 7.5 mg of estrone sulfate daily for 21 days, followed by 8 to 10 days drug-free period. Cycle repeated if no withdrawal bleeding by 10th day. If satisfactory withdrawal bleeding does not occur, an oral progestin may be added to regimen during 3rd week of cycle. **Intravaginal:** (vaginal cream contains 1.5 mg estropipate/Gm): *Atrophic vaginitis* and *kraurosis vulvae:* Usually, 1 or 2 applicatorfuls (2 to 4 Gm) daily; cyclic regimen.

NURSING IMPLICATIONS

Vaginal cream is dispensed with a calibrated dosage applicator. Squeeze tube of cream to force sufficient amount into applicator so that number on plunger indicating prescribed dose is level with top of barrel.

To administer intravaginal medication: have patient in recumbent position, draped, with knees flexed and legs spread apart. Put on sterile gloves before inspecting perineal area. If discharge is present, gently wash area with soap (if allowed) and warm water. Spread labia and slowly insert applicator approximately 5 cm (2 inches) directing it slightly back toward sacrum. Push plunger all the way down into barrel to expell cream. Patient should remain in recumbent position about 30 minutes to prevent losing the medication (no sphincter in vagina). Observe perineal area each time before vaginal medication is given: if mucosa is red, swollen or excoriated, or if there is a change in vaginal discharge, report to physician before giving the medication.

Between uses, pull plunger out of barrel and wash applicator in warm soapy water. Do not place plunger in hot or boiling water.

Warn patient not to use tampons while on vaginal cream therapy. She may wish to wear a sanitary napkin to protect clothing.

If patient is to administer medication to herself, instruct her to wash her hands well before and after the procedure.

Estrogen in cream is readily absorbed from the vaginal mucosa and reaches blood levels approaching those of parenteral or orally administered estrogen. Systemic hyperestrogenic effects (reportable) (uterine bleeding, edema, mastalgia, reactivation of endometriosis) may result from overdosage of intravaginal drug or from overexposure of denuded or abraded skin surfaces of hands to estrogen.

Cytologic study or D and C may be required to differentiate the bleeding that follows estrone absorption from ovarian carcinoma.

Sudden discontinuation of vaginal cream after high dosage or prolonged use may evoke withdrawal bleeding.

Review patient package insert (PPI) with patient.

Stored in tightly closed containers preferably between 15° and 30°C (59° and 86°F) unless otherwise directed by manufacturer.

See Estradiol (prototype estrogen).

PROTOTYPE

ETHACRYNIC ACID
(Edecrin)

ETHACRYNATE SODIUM
(Sodium Edecrin)

(eth-a-krin'ik)
(eth-a-kri'nate)
Diuretic (loop)

ACTIONS AND USES. Unsaturated ketone derivative of phenoxyacetic acid with rapid and potent diuretic action. Action mechanism is unclear, but it may involve blocking of sulfhydryl-catalyzed enzyme systems. Inhibits sodium and chloride reabsorption in proximal tubule and most segments of loop of Henle, promotes potassium and hydrogen ion excretion, and decreases urinary ammonium ion concentration and pH. Appears to have little effect on bicarbonate excretion but chloruretic effect may foster bicarbonate retention. Promotes calcium loss in hypercalcemia and nephrogenic diabetes insipidus. Paradoxic decrease in urine volume may follow drug-induced sodium loss. Fluid-electrolyte loss may exceed that produced by thiazides, but the effect on carbohydrate metabolism and blood glucose is less. Tends to promote urate excretion at high doses and retention at low doses; does not inhibit carbonic anhydrase. Action is independent of systemic acid–base balance. Appears to have little or no direct effect on renal blood flow or glomerular filtration rate. Aldosterone secretion may be increased, thus contributing to hypokalemia. Hypotensive effect may be due to hypovolemia secondary to diuresis, and in part to decreased vascular resistance.

Used in treatment of severe edema associated with congestive heart failure, hepatic cirrhosis, ascites of malignancy, renal disease, nephrotic syndrome, lymphedema. *Unlabeled Use:* treatment of nephrogenic diabetes insipidus and hypercalcemia. *Investigational Use:* treatment of mild to moderate hypertension and as adjunct to therapy of hypertensive crisis complicated by pulmonary edema or renal failure.

ABSORPTION AND FATE. Diuretic effect occurs within 30 minutes following oral administration, peaks in 2 hours, and lasts 6 to 8 hours, possibly up to 12 hours. Following IV injection, diuresis is apparent within 5 minutes; it reaches maximum within 15 to 30 minutes and persists approximately 2 or more hours. About 95% protein bound. Half-life: 30 to 70 minutes. Accumulates in liver. Metabolized to active cysteine conjugate; approximately one-half to two-thirds of dose is excreted in urine; remainder is eliminated in bile. Rate of urinary excretion increases as pH increases. It is not known whether it crosses placenta or enters breast milk.

CONTRAINDICATIONS AND PRECAUTIONS. History of hypersensitivity to ethacrynic acid; anuria, hepatic coma, advanced hepatic cirrhosis, severe diarrhea, dehydration, electrolyte imbalance, hypotension, pregnancy, lactation, women of childbearing age, infants, parenteral use in pediatric patients. *Cautious Use:* hepatic cirrhosis, elderly cardiac patients, diabetes mellitus; history of gout; pulmonary edema associated with acute myocardial infarction, nephrotic syndrome.

ADVERSE/SIDE EFFECTS. CV: postural hypotension, thrombophlebitis, emboli. **Dermatologic:** skin rash, pruritus. **Electrolyte imbalance:** hyponatremia, hypokalemia, hypochloremic alkalosis, hypomagnesemia, hypocalcemia, hypercalciuria, hypovolemia, hyperuricemia. **GI:** anorexia, nausea, vomiting, dysphagia, abdominal discomfort or pain, malaise, diarrhea, GI bleeding (IV use), acute pancreatitis (increased serum amylase), abnormal liver function tests, jaundice, hepatic damage, hypoproteinemia. **Hematologic:** thrombocytopenia, agranulocytosis, severe neutropenia, Henoch's purpura (in patients with rheumatic fever). **Other:** tetany, acute gout, elevated BUN, hematuria, hyperglycemia, acute hypoglycemia (rare), gynecomastia, headache, fever, chills, blurred vision, fatigue, weakness, apprehension, confusion, local irritation of IV site, vertigo, tinnitus, sense of fullness in ears, temporary or permanent deafness.

ROUTE AND DOSAGE. Adults: Oral: Initial: 50 to 100 mg (single dose); maintenance (following diuresis) consists of minimal effective dose (50 to 100 mg once or twice daily after meals) administered on continuous or intermittent dosage schedule. Dosage adjustments are usually made in increments of 25 to 50 mg. Total daily dosage should not exceed 400 mg. **Children: Oral:** Initial: 25 mg followed by 25 mg increments to level of maintenance dose. **Adults only: Intravenous (ethacrynate sodium):** 0.5 to 1 mg/kg body weight. Administered by direct IV over at least 5 minutes, or through tubing of running infusion of compatible IV fluid. Usually one dose is sufficient. If second dose is necessary, select new injection site to avoid possibility of thrombophlebitis. Single doses should not exceed 100 mg.

NURSING IMPLICATIONS

Follow manufacturer's directions for reconstitution of sodium ethacrynate. Solution should be used within 24 hours; discard solution if it is cloudy or opalescent.

Baseline and periodic determinations should be made of blood count, serum electrolytes, CO_2, BUN, creatinine, blood sugar, uric acid, and liver function. Frequent WBC determinations and liver function tests are advised during prolonged therapy.

Schedule doses to avoid nocturia and thus sleep interference.

Explain diuretic effect (increased volume and frequency of voiding) to the patient.

Diuretic effect tends to diminish with continuous therapy.

Administer oral drug after a meal or food to prevent gastric irritation.

Parenteral drug is given by direct IV injection or into tubing of a running infusion, slowly over a few minutes. Usually one dose is sufficient. If a second dose is required select another site to prevent thrombophlebitis.

Monitor blood pressure during initial therapy. Since orthostatic hypotension sometimes

E

occurs, supervision of ambulation is advisable. Caution the patient to make position changes slowly, particularly from recumbent to upright position.

Patient should be observed closely when receiving the drug by IV infusion. Rapid, copious diuresis following IV administration can produce hypotension and peripheral vascular collapse. Check infusion site frequently. Extravasation causes local pain and tissue irritation.

Monitor intake–output ratio as an important measure of drug action. Drug should be discontinued if excessive diuresis, oliguria, hematuria, or sudden profuse diarrhea occurs. Report signs to physician.

Establish baseline weight prior to start of therapy; weigh patient under standard conditions. To initiate diuresis, the smallest dose required to produce weight loss of 1 to 2 lb per day is recommended. Report weight gain in excess of 2 lb/day.

Once "dry weight" has been achieved, drug dosage and frequency of administration should be reduced.

Observe for and report warning signs and symptoms of electrolyte imbalance: anorexia, nausea, vomiting, thirst, dry mouth, polyuria, oliguria, weakness, fatigue, dizziness, headache, muscle cramps, paresthesias, drowsiness, mental confusion.

Fluid and electrolyte depletion is most apt to occur in patients on large doses or salt-intake restriction. Consult physician regarding allowable salt and fluid intake. Generally, salt intake is liberalized.

Elderly and debilitated patients require close observation. Excessive diuresis promotes dehydration and hypovolemia, both of which often precede circulatory collapse, cerebrovascular thrombosis, and pulmonary emboli, especially in these patients.

Report immediately possible signs of thromboembolic complications: pain in chest, back, pelvis, legs.

Monitor blood pressure and pulse of patients with impaired cardiac function. Diuretic-induced hypovolemia may reduce cardiac output, and electrolyte loss promotes cardiotoxicity in those receiving digitalis or other cardiac glycosides.

To reduce or prevent potassium depletion, the physician may prescribe daily ingestion of potassium-rich foods (banana, orange, peach, dried dates, milk, yogurt), potassium supplement, and intermittent dosage schedule.

GI side effects occur most frequently after 1 to 3 months of therapy or in patients on high dosage. Loose stools or other GI symptoms at any time during therapy should be reported in order to permit dosage adjustment or discontinuation of drug if indicated.

In patients receiving aminoglycoside antibiotics concurrently with ethacrynic acid, renal status, audiograms, and vestibular function tests are advised before initiation of therapy and regularly throughout therapy.

Report immediately any evidence of impaired hearing. Ototoxicity has been associated with renal insufficiency, concomitant administration of aminoglycoside antibiotics, and rapid IV administration. Hearing loss may be preceded by vertigo, tinnitus, or fullness in ears; it may be transient, lasting 1 to 24 hours, or it may be permanent.

Impaired glucose tolerance with hyperglycemia and glycosuria may occur in diabetic and diabetic-prone individuals and in patients with decompensated hepatic cirrhosis. Watch for signs of hypoglycemia when ethacrynic acid is withdrawn.

Acute hypoglycemia with convulsions reportedly has been associated with use of large doses in patients with uremia.

Drug Interactions: Ethacrynic acid

Plus	Interactions
Aminoglycosides	Additive ototoxic effects. Used concomitantly with caution if at all. Monitor 8th nerve function

Plus (cont.)	Interactions (cont.)
Anticoagulants	Potentiation of anticoagulant (hypoprothrombinemic) effect. Increased possibility of GI bleeding. Used concomitantly with caution
Cisplatin (Platinol)	Additive ototoxic effects. Concurrent use generally avoided, if possible
Digitalis glycosides	Increased incidence of arrhythmias (hypokalemia, induced by ethocrynic acid, sensitizes myocardium to effects of digitalis). Monitor serum potassium
Lithium	Increases risk of lithium toxicity (lithium excretion decreases with sodium depletion). Used concurrently with caution if at all

ETHAMBUTOL HYDROCHLORIDE

(e-tham′byoo-tole)

(Etibi, Myambutol)

Antiinfective: tuberculostatic

ACTIONS AND USES. Synthetic antituberculosis agent with bacteriostatic action. Mode of action not completely understood, but it appears to inhibit RNA synthesis and thus arrests multiplication of tubercle bacilli. Not recommended for use as sole agent. The emergence of resistant strains is delayed by administering ethambutol in combination with other antituberculosis drugs.

Used in conjunction with at least one other antituberculosis agent in treatment of pulmonary tuberculosis. Also used in treatment of diseases caused by other mycobacteria.

ABSORPTION AND FATE. Approximately 70 to 80% readily absorbed from GI tract following oral administration. Absorption is not significantly affected by presence of food. Peak serum levels within 2 to 4 hours; 50% of peak level remains at 8 hours and 10% at 24 hours. Plasma half-life: 3 to 4 hours (up to 8 hours in patients with impaired renal function); 20 to 30% protein bound. Widely distributed to most body fluids and tissues. Highest concentrations in erythrocytes, kidneys, lungs, saliva. Lowest concentrations in ascitic and pleural fluid, brain, and cerebrospinal fluid. Detoxified in liver. Approximately 50% of drug is excreted unchanged in urine within 24 hours; 8 to 15% appears as inactive metabolites and 20 to 22% excreted in feces as unchanged drug.

CONTRAINDICATIONS AND PRECAUTIONS. Hypersensitivity to ethambutol; patients with optic neuritis, children under 13 years of age. Safe use during pregnancy not established. *Cautious Use:* patients with renal impairment, gout, ocular defects, e.g., cataract, recurrent ocular inflammatory conditions, diabetic retinopathy.

ADVERSE/SIDE EFFECTS. CNS: headache, dizziness, confusion, hallucinations, peripheral neuritis (rare), joint pains and weakness of lower extremities. **GI:** anorexia, nausea, vomiting, abdominal pain. **Hypersensitivity:** pruritus, dermatitis, anaphylaxis. **Ophthalmic** *(ocular toxicity):* optic neuritis with decrease in visual acuity, temporary loss of vision, constriction of visual fields, red-green color blindness, central and peripheral scotomata, eye pain, photophobia. **Other:** fever, malaise, leukopenia (rare), bloody sputum, transient impairment of liver function, nephrotoxicity, hyperuricemia, acute gouty arthritis, ECG abnormalities.

ROUTE AND DOSAGE. Oral: *Initial treatment:* 15 mg/kg once every 24 hours. *Retreatment:* 25 mg/kg once every 24 hours for 60 days, with at least one other antitubercular drug; then 15 mg/kg daily in single doses.

NURSING IMPLICATIONS

Ethambutol may be taken with food if GI irritation occurs. Absorption is reportedly not significantly affected by food in stomach.

Culture and susceptibility tests should be performed prior to initiation of therapy and repeated periodically throughout therapy.

Ocular toxicity generally appears within 1 to 7 months after start of therapy. Symptoms usually disappear within several weeks to months after drug is discontinued, depending on degree of ocular damage.

Advise patient to report promptly to physician the onset of blurred vision, changes in color perception, constriction of visual fields, or any other visual symptoms. Patient should be questioned periodically about eyes.

Ophthalmoscopic examination including tests of visual fields (finger perimetry), tests for visual acuity using a Snellen eye chart, and tests for color discrimination should be performed prior to start of therapy and at monthly intervals during therapy. Eyes should be tested separately as well as together.

If detected early, visual defects generally disappear over several weeks to months. In rare instances, recovery may be delayed for a year or more or defect may be irreversible.

Monitor intake and output ratio in patients with renal impairment. Report oliguria or any significant changes in intake–output ratio or in laboratory reports of renal function. Systemic accumulation with toxicity can result from delayed drug excretion.

In general, therapy may continue for 1 to 2 years or longer although shorter treatment regimens have been used with success.

Hepatic and renal function tests, blood cell counts, and serum uric acid determinations should be performed at regular intervals throughout therapy.

Emphasize importance of adhering to drug regimen and of keeping follow-up appointments.

If patient becomes pregnant during therapy, advise her to notify physician immediately. Drug should be withdrawn.

Protect ethambutol from light, moisture, and excessive heat.

Diagnostic Test Interferences. Ethambutol may increase **serum uric acid** levels and may cause elevations in **liver function tests.**

ETHAVERINE HYDROCHLORIDE

(Circubid, Ethaquin, Ethatab, Ethavex, Isovex-100)

(eth'a-ver-een)
Antispasmodic
Vasodilator (peripheral)

ACTIONS AND USES. Non-narcotic derivative of isoquinoline. Closely related chemically to papaverine (qv) and with similar actions and uses. Direct relaxant effect on vascular smooth muscle claimed to be 2 to 4 times greater than that of papaverine and associated with fewer adverse effects.

Used for treatment of peripheral and cerebral vascular insufficiency associated with arterial spasm and to relieve spasms of GI and GU tracts.

CONTRAINDICATIONS AND PRECAUTIONS. Complete AV dissociation, serious arrhythmias, severe hepatic disease. Safe use in women of childbearing potential, during pregnancy, and in nursing mothers not established. *Cautious Use:* glaucoma, pulmonary embolism.

ADVERSE/SIDE EFFECTS. CV: hypotension, flushing, sweating, arrhythmias, cardiac depression. **CNS:** headache, vertigo, drowsiness, lassitude. **GI:** anorexia, nausea, abdominal distress, constipation or diarrhea. **Hypersensitivity (hepatic):** jaundice, GI symptoms, alterations of liver function tests, eosinophilia. **Other:** malaise, dry throat, skin rash, respiratory depression.

ROUTE AND DOSAGE. Oral: 100 to 200 mg three times daily. Alternatively, 150 to 300 mg of timed release capsule every 12 hours.

NURSING IMPLICATIONS

Administration with or directly after meals may reduce incidence of nausea.

Instruct patient to swallow timed-release capsule whole and not to crush or chew it.

Caution patient to avoid driving and other potentially hazardous activities until reaction to drug is known.

Problems related to peripheral and cerebral vascular insufficiency require long-term therapy.

Inform patient that alcohol may intensify dizziness and lightheadedness.

ETHCHLORVYNOL

(Placidyl)

(eth-klor-vi'nole)
Sedative/Hypnotic
C IV

ACTIONS AND USES. Tertiary acetylenic alcohol with CNS depressant effects similar to those of chloral hydrate and barbiturates. Mechanism of action not known. Hypnotic doses produce cerebral depression and quiet, deep sleep; sedative doses reduce anxiety and apprehension. Also exhibits anticonvulsant and muscle relaxant activity. Has no analgesic properties. Effect on REM sleep not known.

Used for short-term therapy of simple insomnia and as daytime sedative in mild anxiety or tension states.

ABSORPTION AND FATE. Rapidly absorbed from GI tract. Hypnotic dose induces sleep within 15 to 30 minutes. Maximal blood levels in 1 to 1.5 hours; duration of action about 5 hours. Half-life (biphasic): initial phase 10 to 20 hours; terminal phase 21 to 100 hours. Localizes in adipose tissue, liver, kidney, spleen, brain, cerebrospinal fluid, bile. Extensively metabolized, probably by liver. Approximately 10% of dose is excreted unchanged in urine within 24 hours. Removed by resin or charcoal hemoperfusion, hemodialysis, and peritoneal dialysis.

CONTRAINDICATIONS AND PRECAUTIONS. Known hypersensitivity to ethchlorvynol, porphyria, patients with uncontrolled pain, first and second trimesters of pregnancy. Safe use in children not established. *Cautious Use:* third trimester of pregnancy; patients with mental depression or suicidal tendencies, addiction-prone individuals, impaired hepatic or renal function, elderly or debilitated patients; 14 days before and after MAO inhibitor therapy, tricyclic antidepressants; patients who respond unpredictably to alcohol or barbiturates.

ADVERSE/SIDE EFFECTS. Hypotension, nausea, vomiting, aftertaste, blurred vision, dizziness, facial numbness, urticaria, headache, mild hangover. In susceptible patients: giddiness, ataxia, prolonged hypnosis, profound muscular weakness, excitement, hysteria, syncope. Rare: hypersensitivity reactions (urticaria, thrombocytopenia), cholestatic jaundice. **Chronic abuse:** tremors, incoordination, slurred speech, nystagmus, toxic amblyopia, permanent visual defects, peripheral neuropathy. **Overdosage:** stupor, coma, bradycardia, hypotension, respiratory failure.

ROUTE AND DOSAGE. Oral: *sedative,* 100 to 200 mg two or three times a day; *hypnotic,* 500 mg to 1 Gm at bedtime.

NURSING IMPLICATIONS

Ethchlorvynol produces transient giddiness and ataxia in some patients who apparently absorb the drug very rapidly. Symptoms may be minimized by administering the drug with milk or other food.

Capsule may be emptied and contents swallowed with a fluid or mixed with food.

Report the appearance of mental confusion, hallucinations, or drowsiness in patients receiving daytime sedation; dosage should be decreased, or drug should be discontinued.

The elderly may not tolerate average adult doses. Observe intensity and duration of drug action.

Report to physician if pain is present. Pain should be controlled before administration of ethchlorvynol.

The 750-mg dosage strength contains tartrazine which may cause allergic-type reactions in susceptible patients. Reactions frequently occur in individuals who also have aspirin hypersensitivity.

Caution the patient to avoid driving a motor vehicle or engaging in other activities requiring mental alertness and physical coordination for at least 5 hours after taking drug.

Psychologic and physical dependence is possible; therefore, prolonged administration is not recommended. Urge patient to adhere to established drug regimen.

Classified as Schedule IV drug under Federal Controlled Substances Act.

Severe withdrawal symptoms may occur if drug is discontinued abruptly in patients taking regular doses (unusual anxiety, tremors, ataxia, irritability, slurred speech, memory loss, hallucinations, delirium, convulsions).

Preserved in tight, light-resistant containers (darkens on exposure to light; slight darkening does not affect potency). Store preferably at 15° to 30°C (59° to 86°F), unless otherwise directed by manufacturer.

Drug Interactions. Dosage of ethchlorvynol should be reduced in patients receiving **MAO inhibitors** (concurrent use may enhance the effects of either). Transient delirium has been reported when **ethchlorvynol** and **tricyclic antidepressants** especially **amitriptyline** have been used concurrently. Additive CNS depression may occur when ethchlorvynol is administered concomitantly with **alcohol, barbiturates,** or other **CNS depressants;** caution the patient. Ethchlorvynol may decrease hypoprothrombinemic effects of **oral anticoagulants.**

ETHINAMATE

(Valmid)

(e-thin'a-mate)
Sedative/Hypnotic
C IV

ACTIONS AND USES. Carbamic acid derivative with central depressant effects similar to those produced by barbiturates, but with shorter duration of action. Also exhibits anticonvulsant activity.

Used chiefly as rapid-acting hypnotic in simple insomnia.

ABSORPTION AND FATE. Rapidly and almost completely absorbed from GI tract. Induces sleep in about 20 minutes; effects last 3 to 5 hours. Half-life: 2.5 hours. Rapidly metabolized, primarily in liver; metabolites excreted in urine.

CONTRAINDICATIONS AND PRECAUTIONS. Known hypersensitivity to ethinamate; patients with uncontrolled pain. Safe use during pregnancy, lactation, and in pediatric patients not established. *Cautious Use:* elderly, debilitated patients; patients with mental depression or suicidal tendencies; addiction-prone individuals.

ADVERSE/SIDE EFFECTS. *Infrequent:* mild GI symptoms, skin rash, paradoxical excitement (especially in children), thrombocytopenic purpura and drug idiosyncrasy with fever (rare). **Overdosage:** hypotension, respiratory depression, coma.

ROUTE AND DOSAGE. Oral: 500 mg to 1 Gm 20 minutes before retiring.

NURSING IMPLICATIONS

Lower doses are generally prescribed for elderly and debilitated patients.

Psychic and physical dependence may occur with chronic use of large doses. For this reason, prolonged therapy is not recommended. Urge patient to adhere to established regimen.

Gradual withdrawal in a controlled hospital setting and psychiatric follow-up are recommended after prolonged overdosage. Abrupt withdrawal can precipitate severe reactions (tremulousness, hyperactive reflexes, agitation, disorientation, severe insomnia, syncopal episodes, hallucinations, convulsions).

Caution the patient to avoid driving and other dangerous activities for at least 4 or 5 hours after taking ethinamate.

Patients should be informed that additive CNS effects may occur with concomitant administration of alcohol, barbiturates, or other CNS depressants.

Classified as Schedule IV drug under Federal Controlled Substances Act.

Store preferably at room temperature 15° to 30°C (59° to 86°F), unless otherwise directed by manufacturer.

Diagnostic Test Interferences. Falsely high **urinary 17-ketosteroid** levels (Holtorff-Koch modification of Zimmerman reaction) reported.

ETHINYL ESTRADIOL

(Estinyl, Feminone)

(eth'in-il ess-tra-dye'ole)
Hormone
Estrogen

ACTIONS AND USES. Oral estrogen with actions similar to those of estradiol (qv). *See Estradiol for absorption, fate, contraindications, precautions, and adverse/side effects.* Given cyclically for short-term use only.

Used in combination with progestins to control ovulation, also used to treat spontaneous or clomiphene-associated hostile cervical mucus, the excessive bleeding of endometrial hyperplasia, and to control severe vasomotor symptoms of menopause and to inhibit postmenopausal bone loss.

ROUTE AND DOSAGE. Oral: *Menopause:* 0.02 to 0.05 mg daily given cyclically; dosage adjusted to minimal effective level. *Postpartum breast engorgement:* 0.5 to 1 mg daily for 3 days, then gradually decreased to 0.1 mg after 7 days; therapy then discontinued. *Female hypogonadism:* 0.05 mg one to three times daily for 2 weeks, followed by 2 weeks of a progestin; regimen is continued 3 to 6 months. Patient then allowed to go untreated for 2 months to determine whether or not she can maintain the menstrual cycle without hormone therapy. *Breast cancer:* 1 mg 3 times daily. *Prostatic cancer:* 0.15 to 0.2 mg daily.

NURSING IMPLICATIONS

Given cyclically, except when used for treatment of postpartum breast engorgement and palliation of carcinoma. Usual cyclic regimen: once daily for 3 weeks, followed by 1 week without the drug; then repeat this regimen.

Food–Drug Interactions: High vitamin C intake (e.g., 1 Gm/day) may increase ethinyl estradiol levels. Abrupt withdrawal of vitamin C may lead to break through bleeding.

Urge patient to read package insert to assure understanding about estrogen therapy.

Store between 15° and 30°C (59° and 86°F) in well-closed, light-resistant container.

See Estradiol (prototype estrogen).

E

ETHIONAMIDE

(Trecator-SC)

(e-thye-on-am′ide)
Antiinfective
Antituberculosis agent

ACTIONS AND USES. Thiomide derivative of isonicotinic acid chemically related to isoniazid. Bacteriostatic or bactericidal depending on concentration used and susceptibility of organisms. Mechanism of action not known, but believed to act by inhibiting bacterial peptide synthesis. Effective against human and bovine strains of *Mycobacterium tuberculosis* and against *M. kansasii* and some strains *M. avium* and *M. intracellular.* Emergence of resistant strains may be delayed or prevented when administered concurrently with other antituberculosis drugs; cross resistance not reported.

Used for any form of active tuberculosis when treatment with primary tuberculostatic drugs (e.g., isoniazid, streptomycin, ethambutol, rifampin) has failed. Must be given with at least one other effective antituberculosis agent. *Investigational Use:* in treatment of other mycobacterial diseases including dapsone-resistant lepromatous leprosy.

ABSORPTION AND FATE. Approximately 80% of oral dose readily absorbed following oral administration. Widely distributed to most tissues and body fluids. Concentrations in CSF and in organs approximately equal to that of plasma. Peak plasma levels within 3 hours; duration about 9 hours. Plasma half-life: about 3 hours; 10% bound to plasma proteins. Metabolized slowly, probably in liver. Excreted in urine, approximately 1 to 5% as unchanged drug and active metabolites and the remainder as inactive metabolites. Readily crosses placenta.

CONTRAINDICATIONS AND PRECAUTIONS. Hypersensitivity to ethionamide and chemically related drugs, e.g., isoniazid, niacin (nicotinamide), pyrazinamide; severe hepatic damage. Safe use during pregnancy and in women of childbearing potential not established. *Cautious Use:* diabetes mellitus, hepatic dysfunction.

ADVERSE/SIDE EFFECTS. CNS: headache, restlessness, psychotic disturbances including mental depression, hallucinations; drowsiness, dizziness, ataxia, weakness, peripheral neuritis, paresthesias, tremors, convulsions, optic neuritis (blurred vision, diplopia), olfactory disturbances. **GI:** (Dose related and frequent; symptoms may be due to CNS stimulation rather than to GI irritation): anorexia, nausea, vomiting, metallic taste, upper abdominal discomfort, diarrhea, stomatitis, sialorrhea. **Hypersensitivity (rare):** skin rash, exfoliative dermatitis, photosensitivity, thrombocytopenia, purpura. **Other:** menorrhagia, gynecomastia, impotence, acne; goiter; cold, dry, puffy skin; alopecia, jaundice, hepatotoxicity, pellagra-like syndrome, severe postural hypotension, superinfections, joint pains, acute rheumatic symptoms, hypoglycemia.

ROUTE AND DOSAGE. Oral: Adults: 0.5 up to 1 Gm daily in one to three equally divided doses at 8- to 12-hour intervals. **Pediatric:** 12 to 15 mg/kg in three or four equally divided doses. Maximum daily dosage not to exceed 750 mg.

NURSING IMPLICATIONS

GI side effects may be minimized by taking drug with or after meals. Some patients tolerate ethionamide best when taken as a single dose after the evening meal or as a single dose at bedtime.

About 50% of patients cannot tolerate a single dose larger than 500 mg because of GI side effects. Dosage may be reduced as much as ⅓ to ½ for these patients. An antiemetic is sometimes prescribed, but if symptoms persist drug should be discontinued.

Physician may prescribe pyridoxine (vitamin B_6) concurrently to prevent or relieve peripheral neuritis and other neurotoxic effects.

Culture and susceptibility tests should be made prior to start of therapy.

Liver function tests: serum transaminases: SGOT (AST), SGPT (ALT), CBC, and renal function tests including urinalysis should be done prior to and at regular intervals during therapy. Manufacturer recommends repeating liver function tests every 2 to 4 weeks.

Report onset of skin rash. Progression to exfoliative dermatitis can occur if drug is not promptly discontinued.

Patients with diabetes mellitus must be closely monitored for untoward symptoms. These patients appear to be especially prone to hepatotoxicity.

Hepatotoxicity is generally reversible if drug is promptly withdrawn. Instruct patient to report onset of dark urine, light-colored stools, yellow skin, sclerae, or hard palate; itchy skin, abdominal cramps, nausea, vomiting, and fever.

If patient complains of optic symptoms, ophthalmoscopic examination is advised promptly and then periodically thereafter during therapy.

Caution patient to make position changes slowly particularly from recumbent to upright posture and to dangle legs and move feet and ankles a few minutes before ambulating. Instruct patient to lie down or sit down in head low position immediately if feeling faint or dizzy and not to stand still for prolonged periods, or take very hot baths or showers.

Advise patient not to drink alcoholic beverages. *See Drug Interactions.*

Emphasize importance of adhering to established drug regimen.

Drug has a faint sulfide odor.

Store in a cool, dry place preferably between 8° and 15°C (46° and 59°F), unless otherwise directed by manufacturer.

Diagnostic Test Interferences. Ethionamide may cause transient increases in **liver function tests** and may depress serum **PBI** and **thyroxine (T_4)** values.

Drug Interactions. Increased neurotoxic effects may occur with **cycloserine,** and **ethyl alcohol.** Ethionamide may intensify adverse effects of other **tuberculostatic agents.**

ETHOPROPAZINE HYDROCHLORIDE

(Parsidol, Parsitan)

(eth-oh-proe′pa-zeen)
Anticholinergic
Antimuscarinic
Antiparkinsonian

E

ACTIONS AND USES. Phenothiazine derivative with prominent atropine-like blocking action. In addition to centrally-acting anticholinergic (parasympatholytic) effects, also exhibits some antihistaminic, local anesthetic, ganglionic blocking and adrenergic blocking actions. Differs from other phenothiazines in that it is used to control extrapyramidal reactions caused by drugs of this class, and it has no antiemetic activity. Mode of action not known but believed to be related to ability to block both muscarinic and nicotinic actions of acetylcholine.

Used as adjunctive therapy in all forms of parkinsonism (arteriosclerotic, idiopathic, postencephalitic), and to control drug-induced extrapyramidal reactions. Also being used for symptomatic treatment of hepatolenticular degeneration and for congenital athetosis.

ABSORPTION AND FATE. Onset of effects in about ½ to 1 hour after oral administration; duration: 4 hours. Metabolic fate not known.

CONTRAINDICATIONS AND PRECAUTIONS. Hypersensitivity to ethopropazine; glaucoma, prostatic hypertrophy or bladder neck obstruction, pyloric or duodenal obstruction. Safe use during pregnancy (category C), in nursing women, and in children not established. *Cautious Use:* tardive dyskinesia, hepatic, renal, or cardiac disease, myasthenia gravis, elderly patients, achalasia, chronic pulmonary disease.

ADVERSE/SIDE EFFECTS. *Generally dose-related.* **CNS:** drowsiness, cerebral reaction (fogginess, inability to think, lassitude, forgetfulness, confusion), dizziness, headache, paresthesias, ataxia, toxic psychosis, accentuation of parkinsonism. **CV:** hypotension, tachycardia. **GI:** nausea, vomiting, epigastric distress, dry mouth, constipation. **GU:** urinary retention. **Ophthalmic:** blurred vision, diplopia, mydriasis. **Other:** muscle cramps; sensation of heaviness of extremities; rash; theoretically possible for all phenothiazines: jaundice, ECG abnormalities, hematologic reactions (agranulocytosis, pancytopenia, purpura), endocrine disturbances, jaundice, pigmentation of cornea, lens, retina, skin, visual hallucinations.

ROUTE AND DOSAGE. Oral: Initial: 50 mg once or twice daily; increased gradually if necessary until optimum effect or limit of tolerance is reached. Maintenance: 100 to 400 mg daily in divided doses. Some patients require 500 to 600 mg or more daily.

NURSING IMPLICATIONS

High incidence of side effects in therapeutic dosage range. Close medical supervision is necessary, especially of the elderly since they are more prone to develop adverse effects.

Elderly patients should be examined periodically for glaucoma.

Mentally ill patients require close observation for worsening of mental symptoms, particularly when drug therapy is initiated and whenever dosage adjustments are made.

Caution patient to avoid driving and other potentially hazardous activities until reaction to drug is known. Drowsiness usually disappears after a few days of therapy.

Since transient hypotension is a potential side effect, advise patient to make position changes slowly, particularly from recumbent to upright position, and to lie down or sit down if lightheadedness or dizziness occurs.

Caution patient to keep cool during hot weather and to avoid strenuous exercise. Ethopromazine can interfere with normal body temperature regulation by diminishing sweat secretion. Bear in mind that risk of hyperthermia is increased in patients with fever and in the elderly.

Dry mouth may be a distressing side effect for some patients. It may be relieved by frequent sips of water, sugarless chewing gum, or sour balls. If severe enough to interfere with eating, talking, or swallowing, report to physician. Artificial saliva, Moi-Stir, Zero-Lube, may provide relief.

Observe for and report therapeutic drug effects: reduction in severity of rigidity, tremor, spasms, drooling (sialorrhea), forward-leaning walking gait (festination), and abnormal fixation of eyeballs (oculogyric crisis).

Transfer to or from ethopromazine should be done gradually to avoid aggravation of symptoms.

Urge patient to keep follow-up appointments.

Store preferably between 15° to 30°C (59° to 86°F) in well-closed container, unless otherwise specified by manufacturer. Protect from light.

PROTOTYPE

ETHOSUXIMIDE

(Zarontin)

(eth-oh-sux'i-mide)
Anticonvulsant
Succinimide

ACTIONS AND USES. Succinimide anticonvulsant. Reduces frequency of epileptiform attacks, apparently by depressing motor cortex and by elevating CNS threshold to stimuli. Usually ineffective in management of psychomotor or major motor seizures.

Used in management of absence (petit mal) seizures, partial seizures with complex symptomology (psychomotor seizures) and tonic–clonic (grand mal) seizures. May be administered in combination with other anticonvulsants when other forms of epilepsy coexist with petit mal.

ABSORPTION AND FATE. Essentially completely absorbed from GI tract. Peak plasma concentrations in 1 to 7 hours; however, 4 to 7 days are required for steady-state plasma concentrations. Plasma half-life 24 to 60 hours. No significant degree of plasma protein binding. Metabolized by liver. Excreted slowly in urine, about 50% as metabolites and 10 to 20% as unchanged drug. Small amounts excreted in bile and feces.

CONTRAINDICATIONS AND PRECAUTIONS. Hypersensitivity to succinimides; severe liver or renal disease; use alone in mixed types of epilepsy (may increase frequency of grand mal seizures). Safe use in women of childbearing potential or during pregnancy not established.

ADVERSE/SIDE EFFECTS. CNS: hiccups, ataxia, dizziness, drowsiness, headache, euphoria, restlessness, irritability, anxiety, hyperactivity, aggressiveness, depression, inability to concentrate, lethargy, confusion, sleep disturbances, night terrors, hypochondriacal behavior; rarely: psychosis, increased depression with overt suicidal intentions, auditory hallucinations. **Dermatologic:** Stevens-Johnson syndrome, pruritic erythematous skin eruptions, exfoliative dermatitis, systemic lupus erythematosus. **GI:** nausea, vomiting, anorexia, weight loss, epigastric distress, abdominal pain, diarrhea, constipation. **GU:** frequency, hematuria, albuminuria, renal damage. **Hematologic:** eosinophilia, leukopenia, thrombocytopenia, agranulocytosis, pancytopenia, aplastic anemia, positive direct Coombs' test. **Ophthalmic:** blurred vision, myopia, photophobia, periorbital edema. **Other:** increased libido, hirsutism, alopecia, vaginal bleeding, swelling of tongue, gum hypertrophy, muscle weakness.

ROUTE AND DOSAGE. Highly individualized. **Oral: Adults and children (6 years and older):** 250 mg two times daily. **Children (3 to 6 years):** 250 mg/day. Dosage increases are made in small increments. One recommended method is to increase daily dose by 250 mg every 4 to 7 days until control is achieved with minimal side effects. A total daily dose exceeding 1.5 Gm for adults or 1 Gm for children up to 6 years should be administered only under strict medical supervision.

NURSING IMPLICATIONS

Baseline and periodic hematologic studies and tests of liver and renal function should be made.

Since ethosuximide may impair mental and physical abilities, caution the patient to avoid driving a motor vehicle and other hazardous activities.

GI symptoms, drowsiness, ataxia, dizziness, and other neurologic side effects occur frequently and indicate the need for dosage adjustment.

Close observation is required during the period of dosage adjustment and whenever other medications are added to or eliminated from the drug regimen. Therapeutic serum levels: 40 to 100 mcg/ml.

Behavioral changes are most likely to occur in the patient with a prior history of psychiatric disturbances. Close supervision is indicated. Drug should be withdrawn slowly if these symptoms appear.

Abrupt withdrawal of ethosuximide (whether used alone or in combination therapy) may precipitate seizures or petit mal status.

Since long-term drug therapy is generally required, the occurrence of adverse drug effects is a possibility. Caution the patient and responsible family members to report any unusual sign or symptom to the physician. Stress the importance of follow-up visits.

Advise the patient to carry a wallet identification card or jewelry (e.g., Medic Alert) indicating that he or she has epilepsy, is taking medication, and the physician's name and telephone number.

Store capsules in tight containers, and syrup in light-resistant containers at 15° to 30°C (59° to 86°F); avoid freezing.

Drug Interactions: Ethosuximide

Plus	Interactions
Antipsychotics e.g., haloperidol (Haldol), pimozide (Orap)	May decrease anticonvulsant effect and augment CNS depression
Estrogens Contraceptives, oral (OC) (except progestogen-only agents)	Decreased effectiveness of estrogen and 25-fold increased risk of unplanned pregnancy in women taking OCs
Phenothiazines (e.g., chlorpromazine)	*See Antipsychotics (above)*
Tricyclic antidepressants (TCA), e.g., imipramine (Tofranil), doxepin (Adapin, Sinequan)	Mutually antagonistic; TCAs can decrease effect of an anticonvulsant; ethosuximide can decrease antidepressant effect of TCA; possible additive CNS effect on anticonvulsant activity

See also Phenytoin (prototype anticonvulsant).

ETHOTOIN

(Peganone)

(eth'oh-toyin)
Anticonvulsant
Hydantoin

ACTIONS AND USES. Hydantoin derivative structurally similar to phenytoin (qv). Reported to be less toxic but less effective than phenytoin and lacks its antiarrhythmic properties.

Used for management of tonic–clonic (grand mal) seizures and partial seizures with complex symptomology (psychomotor seizures). Usually an adjunct to other anticonvulsant medications.

E

ABSORPTION AND FATE. Probably metabolized by liver. Excreted in urine and bile as unchanged drug and metabolites; small quantities excreted in saliva.

CONTRAINDICATIONS AND PRECAUTIONS. Hypersensitivity to hydantoins; hepatic abnormalities; hematologic disorders. Risk potential during pregnancy and in women of childbearing age. Safe use in women of childbearing age and pregnancy not assured (teratogenic effects on fetus have been reported). *Cautious Use:* elderly or gravely ill patients.

ADVERSE/SIDE EFFECTS. *Common:* anorexia, nausea, vomiting, drowsiness, skin rash. *Infrequent:* lymphadenopathy, ataxia, gingival hyperplasia. *See also Phenytoin Sodium.*

ROUTE AND DOSAGE. Adults: Oral: Initial: 1 Gm or less daily, in four to six divided doses. Subsequent dosage gradually increased over period of several days; maintenance: 2 to 3 Gm daily in four to six divided doses. **Children:** initial dose should not exceed 750 mg daily; maintenance: 500 mg to 1 Gm daily. Optimum dosage determined on basis of individual response.

NURSING IMPLICATIONS

Doses should be spaced as evenly as practicable. Administer with or immediately after food to reduce incidence of gastric irritation.

Dosage reduction, or substitution or discontinuation of other anticonvulsant medications should be accomplished gradually and with close observation of patient.

Blood counts and urinalyses are advised at start of therapy and at monthly intervals thereafter.

Patients with psychomotor epilepsy should be closely observed for symptoms of depression or other changes of behavior.

If drug is discontinued, withdrawal should be done slowly to prevent precipitating seizures or status epilepticus.

Ethotoin darkens on exposure to light and extreme heat. Store at 15° to 30°C (59° to 86°F).

See Phenytoin sodium (prototype anticonvulsant).

Drug Interactions. Concurrent administration of ethotoin and **phenacemide** may cause paranoid symptoms. *See also Phenytoin sodium.*

PROTOTYPE

ETHYLESTRENOL

(Maxibolin)

(eth-il-ess'tre-nole)
Anabolic

ACTIONS AND USES. Synthetic steroid hormone with relatively more anabolic than androgenic activity. Promotes body tissue-building and inhibits tissue-depleting processes; supports nitrogen, potassium, chloride, and phosphorus conservation. Enhances weight gain and combats depression and weakness in debilitating conditions. Stimulates bone growth, aids in bone matrix reconstitution, and may support calcification of metastatic lesions of breast cancer. Prevents or reverses profound nitrogen loss associated with corticosteroid therapy without compromising antiinflammatory activity. Mechanism of action in refractory anemias is unclear, but may be due to direct stimulation of bone marrow or protein anabolic activity, or to androgenic stimulation of erythropoiesis. Suppresses pituitary gonadotropic functions, and may exert direct effect on testes. Potentially has all the side effects of testosterone.

Used to reverse catabolic effects of prolonged immobilization and debilitative states (severe burns, paraplegia, extensive surgery) and to control pain of metastasis in female breast cancer. Probably effective as adjunctive therapy for osteoporosis, pituitary dwarfism, and marked maturational delay and in selected types of refractory anemias and arthritis. Will not enhance athletic ability.

E

ABSORPTION AND FATE. Well-absorbed from GI tract; metabolized in liver, and excreted in urine. Crosses placenta; appears in breast milk.

CONTRAINDICATIONS AND PRECAUTIONS. Hypersensitivity to drug; nephrosis; cardiac, hepatic, or renal decompensation; hypercalcemia; infancy. **Males:** known or suspected prostatic cancer, benign prostatic hypertrophy with obstruction, carcinoma of breast. **Females:** lactation, pregnancy, menstrual disorders. *Cautious Use:* prepubertal males; patients easily stimulated sexually; concomitant ACTH, corticosteroid, or anticoagulant therapy; diabetes mellitus, history of coronary disease or myocardial infarction.

ADVERSE/SIDE EFFECTS. Both sexes: nausea, vomiting, diarrhea, gastric irritation, burning of tongue, hypersensitivity, anaphylactoid reaction (rare), habituation, excitation, insomnia, increased or decreased libido, skin flushing, acne (especially females and prepubertal males), hypercalcemia, leukopenia, hepatocellular carcinoma (rare), chills, sodium and water retention, edema, jaundice. **Females:** virilism (hoarseness, acne, oily skin, hirsutism, enlarged clitoris, stimulation of libido, menstrual irregularities, male-pattern baldness, decrease in breast size, edema. **Males:** *(prepubertal):* premature epiphyseal closure, acne, priapism, growth of facial and body hair, phallic enlargement; *(postpubertal):* inhibition of testicular function, testicular atrophy, impotence, epididymitis, gynecomastia, bladder irritability.

ROUTE AND DOSAGE. Oral: Adults: 4 to 8 mg/day, reduced to minimum levels at first evidence of clinical response (daily dosage usually does not exceed 0.1 mg/kg body weight). **Children:** 1 to 3 mg/day; highly individualized. A single course of therapy for adults and children should not exceed 6 weeks. If necessary, treatment may be restarted after interval of 4 weeks.

NURSING IMPLICATIONS

Administer drug immediately before or with meals to diminish GI distress.

Reportedly, anabolic drugs are most effective when combined with a therapeutic dietary regimen (high in calories, protein, vitamins, and minerals), physical therapy, and optimum health-promoting habits. All these measures require the patient's understanding and cooperation.

Reinforce adherence to scheduled appointments for physical therapy (if prescribed) and laboratory tests. Stress importance of good personal hygiene, including meticulous skin care (females and prepubertal males are especially likely to develop acne).

Elicit support of responsible family member and nutritionist in development of dietary regimen that satisfies the anorexic debilitated patient. Diet may be tolerated better if given in frequent small feedings.

Baseline and periodic determinations of liver function and serum electrolytes are indicated (drug may cause retention of sodium, chloride, water, potassium, and inorganic phosphates). Serial determinations of serum cholesterol are advised in patients with history of myocardial infarction or coronary artery disease. *(Normal total cholesterol:* 150 to 280 mg/dl.)

Teach patient to note and report symptoms of jaundice (dark urine, pruritus, yellow skin, or sclerae) to physician. Dose adjustment may reverse the condition; however, if liver function tests are abnormal, therapy will be discontinued.

Monitor intake–output ratio and pattern and weight, and check for edema; report significant changes. Edema is generally controllable with salt restriction and/or diuretic therapy.

Hypercalcemia symptoms (lassitude, anorexia, nausea, vomiting, constipation, dehydration, polyuria, polydipsia, asthenia, loss of muscle tone) may be difficult to distinguish from symptoms associated with condition being treated unless they are anticipated and thought of as a symptom cluster. Hypercalcemia is particularly likely to occur in patients with metastatic breast carcinoma and may indicate bone metastases. Anabolic therapy will be stopped if it develops; consult physician about hydration and activity of patient.

Be alert for voice changes in female patient. Onset of hoarseness or deepening of voice can easily be overlooked if its significance as an early sign of virilism is not appreciated. Virilism may be irreversible even after prompt discontinuation of therapy. Unless the benefits of the drug are considered to outweigh its distressing side effects, therapy will be discontinued.

Instruct female patient to report menstrual irregularities. Usually the physician will discontinue medication pending determination of etiology.

Record beneficial effects of anabolic therapy, such as stimulation of appetite, euphoria, and general feeling of renewed vigor and well-being.

When used in pediatrics, therapy is preceded by x-ray of wrist bones to establish level of bone maturation. During treatment, bone maturation may proceed more rapidly than linear growth; therefore intermittent dosage schedule and periodic x-rays are usual.

Since skeletal stimulation continues about 6 months after treatment has been stopped, x-rays are used as determinants for discontinuing therapy well before bone maturation reaches the norm for chronologic age. Teach parents the importance of keeping child's appointments for bone maturation studies (usually every 3 to 6 months) in order to prevent compromised adult height.

Children under 7 years of age are particularly sensitive to androgenic effects and therefore should be closely observed for precocious development of male sexual characteristics or masculinization; they should be questioned about the presence of priapism (inappropriate and frequent erections). These symptoms may necessitate drug withdrawal.

Patient with congenital aplastic anemia usually requires continued maintenance doses and supplementary iron.

Anabolic treatment may cause reduction of blood glucose in some diabetic patients. Watch closely for symptoms of hypoglycemia and report to physician. Change in dosage of antidiabetic drug may be required.

Anabolic steroids do not enhance athletic ability. Their use for this purpose is hazardous and has been condemned by medical experts.

Observe patient on concomitant anticoagulant therapy for ecchymotic areas, petechiae, or abnormal bleeding from any site. Close monitoring or prothrombin time is essential.

Since anabolic steroids may alter many laboratory tests, inform pathologist when tissues or body fluids are submitted for study. Several values remain altered for 2 to 3 weeks after discontinuation of drug.

Diagnostic Test Interferences. The following laboratory tests may be altered: metyrapone test; fasting blood sugar and glucose tolerance tests; thyroid function tests; blood coagulation tests (increased factors II, V, VII, X); decreased creatinine and creatinine excretion; increased 17-ketosteroid excretion; elevated BSP, transaminase, bilirubin, serum cholesterol.

Drug Interactions. Anabolic steroids may potentiate **oral anticoagulants,** enhance hypoglycemic response to **antidiabetic drugs,** and increase **oxyphenbutazone** and **phenylbutazone** plasma levels. **Barbiturates** decrease the effect of androgens by increasing their hepatic breakdown.

E

ETHYLNOREPINEPHRINE HYDROCHLORIDE

(Bronkephrine)

(eth-il-nor-ep-i-nef'rin)
Beta-adrenergic agonist (sympathomimetic)
Smooth muscle relaxant (respiratory)
Bronchodilator

ACTIONS AND USES. Synthetic, direct-acting sympathomimetic amine. Primarily a beta-adrenergic agonist but also has mild alpha-adrenergic activity. Similar to epinephrine (qv) in bronchodilating activity, but unlike epinephrine lacks significant pressor effects and therefore may be safer for hypertensives and severely ill patients. Also reportedly suitable for use in children because it generally does not produce CNS stimulation, and for diabetic asthmatics because it lacks glycogenolytic activity.

Used as bronchodilator in bronchial asthma, and for bronchospasm associated with bronchitis and emphysema.

ABSORPTION AND FATE. Onset of action in 6 to 12 minutes following either IM or SC injection. Duration of action 1 to 2 hours.

CONTRAINDICATIONS AND PRECAUTIONS. Hypersensitivity to adrenergic agents or to any ingredients in the formulation. Safe use during pregnancy (category C), in nursing women, or in children not established. *Cautious Use:* cardiovascular disease, history of coronary artery disease or stroke.

ADVERSE/SIDE EFFECTS. CNS: anxiety, trembling, headache, weakness, insomnia, dizziness, seizures. **CV:** palpitation, irregular or pounding heartbeat, extremes in heart rate, elevation or depression of blood pressure, chest pains. **GI:** severe nausea, vomiting. **Other:** pale cold skin, chills, fever, mydriasis.

ROUTE AND DOSAGE. Intramuscular, subcutaneous: Adults: 0.5 to 1 ml. **Children:** 0.1 to 0.5 ml. Each ml contains 2 mg ethylnorepinephrine.

NURSING IMPLICATIONS

Carefully select injection site. Aspirate to avoid inadvertent intravascular injection.

Elderly patients tend to be more sensitive to sympathomimetic drugs than younger patients and therefore should be closely observed for adverse effects.

Monitor blood pressure and pulse for duration of drug action (1 to 2 hours).

During acute episodes of respiratory deficit limit the patient's activity to prevent physical fatigue. This is especially important in the elderly patient.

Store preferably between 15° and 30°C (59° and 86°F) in light-resistant container unless otherwise directed by manufacturer.

See Epinephrine (prototype bronchodilators).

ETIDRONATE DISODIUM

(Didronel)

(e-ti-droe′nate)

Regulator (calcium)

ACTIONS AND USES. Diphosphate preparation with primary action on bone. Slows rate of bone turnover (bone resorption and new bone accretion) in pagetic bone lesions and in normal remodeling process. Lowers serum alkaline phosphatase and urinary hydroxyproline levels and reduces elevated cardiac output by decreasing vascularity of bone. Induces reversible hyperphosphatemia without adverse effects.

Used to treat symptomatic polyostotic Paget's disease and heterotopic ossification due to spinal cord injury. Also used to prevent and treat heterotopic ossification following total hip replacement. *Unlabeled Use:* to prevent parathyroid hormone-induced bone resorption.

E

ABSORPTION AND FATE. Absorption is dose-dependent. Etidronate is not metabolized and is cleared from blood in 6 hours. Within 24 hours, half of absorbed dose is excreted by kidneys; the remainder is chemically adsorbed on bone and slowly eliminated. Unabsorbed drug excreted in feces.

CONTRAINDICATIONS AND PRECAUTIONS. Enterocolitis, children, pathologic fractures. *Cautious Use:* renal impairment, pregnancy, lactation, patients on restricted calcium and vitamin D intake.

ADVERSE/SIDE EFFECTS. Nausea, loose bowel movements, diarrhea; increased risk of fractures in patient with Paget's disease, increased or recurrent bone pain in Pagetic sites, onset of bone pain in previously asymptomatic sites, hypocalcemia, suppressed mineralization of uninvolved skeleton.

ROUTE AND DOSAGE. Oral: *(Paget's disease):* Initial: 5 mg/kg/day for no more than 6 months. (Doses above 10 mg/kg/day for no more than 3 months reserved for use when prompt reduction of elevated cardiac output or suppression of bone turnover are required.) Retreatment after drug-free period of at least 3 months: *heterotopic ossification due to spinal cord injury:* Initial: 20 mg/kg/day for 2 weeks followed by 10 mg/kg/day for 10 weeks; heterotopic ossification complicating total hip replacement: 20 mg/kg/day for 1 month preoperatively; then 20 mg/kg/day for 3 months postoperatively.

NURSING IMPLICATIONS

Take as single dose on empty stomach 2 hours before meals with full glass of water or juice to reduce gastric irritation.

Therapeutic response to this drug may be slow (1 to 3 months) and may continue for months after treatment has been discontinued.

Maintenance of optimum nutritional status, especially adequate intake of calcium and vitamin D, is an important adjunct to effective therapy. Advise patient to include milk, dairy products, and leafy vegetables in diet.

GI side effects may interfere with adequate nutritional status and should be treated promptly. Persistent nausea or diarrhea should be reported.

Monitor intake–output ratio of patient with impaired renal function.

Hypocalcemia is a theoretical possibility. Symptoms should be reported at onset: skeletal muscle spasms, facial muscle twitching, carpopedal spasm, laryngospasm, paresthesias, intestinal colic.

Latent tetany (hypocalcemia) may be detected by Chvostek's and Trousseau's signs *(see Index)* and a serum calcium value of 7 to 8 mg/dl.

The risk of pathologic fractures increases when daily dose of 20 mg/kg is taken longer than 3 months. Instruct patient to report promptly the sudden onset of unexplained pain.

Laboratory test values that may suggest clinical progress: e.g., decreased urinary excretion of hydroxyproline reflects decreased bone resorption; decreased serum alkaline phosphatase level indicates decreased bone formation. *(Normal urinary hydroxyproline:* 15 to 50 mg/24 hours; *serum alkaline phosphatase:* 1.4 to 4.1 Bodansky units.)

Serum phosphate levels generally return to normal 2 to 4 weeks after medication is discontinued.

Retreatment should not be instituted prematurely or before symptoms return. Instruct patient to report promptly if bone pain, restricted mobility, heat over involved bone site occur.

Urge patient to keep appointments for periodic evaluation of clinical tests.

E

ETOMIDATE

(e-tom'i-date)

(Amidate)

Anesthetic, general

ACTIONS AND USES. Nonbarbiturate intravenous anesthetic induction agent with hypnotic but no analgesic action. Lowers cerebral blood flow and causes slight decrease in intracranial pressure and moderate decrease in intraocular pressure. Lacks cardiovascular depressant activity. These characteristics and associated low incidence of cardiovascular and respiratory effects assign an advantage to the agent for anesthetic induction in high risk patients (e.g., patients with asthma, drug allergy, cardiovascular disease, or those undergoing neurosurgery). Prolonged administration may suppress cortisol secretion, an effect that may be apparent within several hours or not for days.

Used for induction of general anesthesia, to supplement subpotent anesthetic agents (e.g., nitrous oxide), and for anesthesia maintenance during brief operative procedures.

ABSORPTION AND FATE. Hypnotic action characterized by rapid onset; peak action in 1 minute, duration 3 to 5 minutes. Rapidly metabolized in liver. Plasma levels of unchanged drug decrease rapidly over 30-minute period following injection and slowly thereafter. Half-life: 75 minutes. Approximately 75% dose excreted in urine during the first day after IV injection.

CONTRAINDICATIONS AND PRECAUTIONS. Sensitivity to etomidate; during labor and delivery; as sedation for patient on respirator; in pregnancy unless clearly needed and when potential benefit outweighs unknown risk to fetus. Safe use during lactation and in children under 10 years of age not established.

ADVERSE/SIDE EFFECTS. CV: hypertension, hypotension, tachycardia, bradycardia, and other arrhythmias. **GI:** postoperative nausea and vomiting. **Neurologic:** myoclonus, averting and tonic movements; uncontrolled eye movements. **Respiratory:** hypo- or hyperventilation, transient apnea, laryngospasm, hiccups, snoring. **Other:** Addisonian crisis (rare), hyperkalemia and/or hyponatremia, oliguria; fever, then hypothermia; profound weakness.

ROUTE AND DOSAGE. Intravenous injection: *Induction:* 0.2 to 0.6 mg/kg (individualized); usual: 0.3 mg/kg injected over 30- to 60-minute period.

NURSING IMPLICATIONS

Transient muscular movements can be reduced, and the recovery period shortened, by giving fentanyl IV 1 to 2 minutes before anesthesia induction.

Etomidate is compatible with all commonly used preanesthetic medications.

When drug is administered over a several hour period, the potential for an antisteroidogenic effect is magnified. Plasma cortisol levels will be monitored to detect a sudden fall leading to hypotension. *(Normal free plasma cortisol range:* 5 to 20 mcg/100 ml).

During recovery period, monitor blood pressure, pulse, and respirations every 10 to 15 minutes until stable, then every hour for 4 hours. Continue checking vital signs every 4 hours for 12 to 24 hours.
Severe drug-induced hypotenstion is rapidly reversed by a corticosteroid but not by catecholamines.
Monitor intake–output ratio and pattern, and serum K during recovery period; be prepared to intervene if symptoms of Addisonian crisis occur.
Store drug at 2° to 8°C (36° to 46°F). Avoid exposure to extreme heat; do not freeze.

ETOPOSIDE

(e-toe-poe'side)

(VP-16, VP-16-213, VePesid)

Antineoplastic (class I)

ACTIONS AND USES. Semisynthetic podophyllin derivative of the mandrake or May apple plant. Produces cytotoxic action by unclear mechanism. Primary effect is on G_2 (resting or premitotic) phase of cell cycle; also acts on S (DNA synthesis) phase. High doses cause lysis of cells entering mitotic phase, and lower doses inhibit cells from entering prophase.

Used in treatment of refractory testicular neoplasms, usually in combination with other chemotherapeutic agents, in patients who have already received appropriate surgery, chemotherapy, and radiation therapy. Has also been used in treatment of choriosarcoma in women, small cell carcinoma of the lung, malignant lymphomas, Hodgkin's disease, acute myelogenous (nonlymphocytic) leukemia.

ABSORPTION AND FATE. Variable degree of penetration into CSF, generally about 1%. Distribution into other body fluids and tissues not known. Probably metabolized in liver. Extensively (94%) bound to plasma proteins. Biphasic half-life: initial phase about 3 hours; terminal phase, 15 hours. Approximately 44 to 60% of dose excreted in urine within 48 to 72 hours, about ⅔ as unchanged drug and remainder as metabolites. Variable amounts eliminated in feces (2 to 16%) over 3 days.

CONTRAINDICATIONS AND PRECAUTIONS. Hypersensitivity to etoposide or to formulation ingredients; severe bone marrow depression, severe hepatic or renal impairment, existing or recent viral infection, bacterial infection, intraperitoneal, intrapleural, or intrathecal administration. Safe use during pregnancy (category D), in fertile women, nursing mothers, and in children not established. *Cautious Use:* impaired renal or hepatic function, gout.

ADVERSE/SIDE EFFECTS. CV: hypotension, palpitation, tachycardia, hypertension; myocardial infarction, pulmonary edema (causal relationship not established). **Dermatologic:** reversible alopecia (can progress to total baldness); nail pigmentation, radiation recall dermatitis, severe pruritus (rare), Stevens–Johnson syndrome. **GI:** nausea, vomiting, dyspepsia, anorexia, diarrhea, constipation, stomatitis, aftertaste. **Hematologic:** severe myelosuppression: leukopenia (principally granulocytopenia), thrombocytopenia, hyperuricemia, anemia, pancytopenia, neutropenia. **Hypersensitivity:** sweating, chills, fever, coryza, tachycardia, throat, back and general body pain; abdominal cramps, high-frequency deafness, pulmonary edema, anaphylactoid reaction. **Neurologic:** peripheral neuropathy, paresthesias, CNS toxicity: somnolence, unusual tiredness, weakness, depression, headache, ataxia (rare), transient vertigo (rare). **Respiratory:** pleural effusion, bronchospasm. **Other:** necrosis, thrombophlebitis (with extravasation), pain at IV site; sepsis (immunosuppression), intermittent muscle cramps, gonadal suppression; nephrotoxicity, hepatotoxicity, and hematotoxicity with overdosage; possibility of carcinogenesis.

ROUTE AND DOSAGE. *Highly individualized* according to clinical response, hematology, and tolerance. **Intravenous infusion:** 50 to 100 mg/m²/day for 5 consecutive days every 3 or 4 weeks for three or four courses of therapy, or 100 mg/m²/day on days 1, 3, and 5 every 3 or 4 weeks for three or four courses of therapy. Administered over 30 to 60 minutes. Not to be given by rapid IV push.

E

NURSING IMPLICATIONS

Etoposide should be administered under the supervision of a qualified physician experienced in the use of antineoplastic therapy.

Before treatment begins, patient and responsible family members should be informed of the possible adverse effects of etoposide, such as blood dyscrasias, alopecia, carcinogenesis.

Etoposide concentrate must be diluted before administration with either 5% dextrose injection or 0.9% sodium chloride injection to produce final concentrations of 0.2 to 0.4 mg/ml. Higher concentrations than 0.4 mg/ml tend to crystallize. Diluted solutions with concentration of 0.2 mg/ml are stable for 96 hours, and the 0.4-mg/ml solutions are stable for 48 hours at room temperature, under normal room fluorescent light in glass or plastic (PVC) containers.

Wear disposable surgical gloves when preparing or disposing of etoposide. Unused solution and equipment or materials used in its preparation should be properly disposed of to prevent contamination of the work environment. Follow agency policy. *See Index: Antineoplastics: handling vesicants.*

Etoposide is administered by slow IV infusion over 30 to 60 minutes to reduce risk of hypotension and bronchospasm. These symptoms can occur with rapid injection or following slow infusion of higher than recommended dosages.

Be prepared to treat an anaphylactoid reaction (sense of uneasiness, agitation, flushing, palpitation, coughing, difficulty in breathing, primary cardiovascular collapse); can develop in 1 to 2 minutes; can culminate in shock and death.

Have readily available: pressor agents, e.g., epinephrine, corticosteroid, and antihistamine, plasma volume expander oxygen, and equipment for maintaining airway. If the reaction occurs, infusion should be stopped immediately.

Most patients will manifest some evidence of toxicity, therefore, constant vigilance is essential. Adverse effects are generally reversible with reduction of dosage or discontinuation of drug. Physician may reinstitute therapy following drug withdrawal, but it must be done with extreme caution.

Check IV site during and after infusion. Extravasation can cause thrombophlebitis and necrosis.

Monitor vital signs during and after infusion. If hypotension occurs, infusion should be stopped immediately.

Since transient hypotension after therapy is a possible side effect, caution patient to make position changes slowly, particularly from recumbent to upright position. Be mindful of the possibility that geriatric patients are prone to manifest transient decreases or increases in blood pressure.

Patients who develop severe toxic reactions to etoposide should be closely monitored for 3 to 4 weeks because the drug is extensively bound to plasma proteins.

Women of childbearing potential should be advised to avoid pregnancy because of possible harm to fetus. Facilitate discussion with physician regarding appropriate contraceptive measures.

The following laboratory tests are advised before initiating therapy, at regular intervals during therapy, and before each subsequent treatment course: CBC (including platelet count, Hgb, Hct, WBC and differential); hepatic and renal function tests: SGOT (AST), SGPT (ALT), serum bilirubin, LDH, BUN, serum creatinine.

Bone marrow depression, notably leukopenia and thrombocytopenia, is used as an index for dosage regulation. White blood cell counts reach their lowest point (nadir) over 7 to 14 days, and platelet nadirs occur over 9 to 16 days after drug administration. An absolute neutrophil count below 500/mm³ or a platelet count below 50,000/mm³ signifies need to withhold therapy until counts return to acceptable limits. A WBC count between 2000 to 3000/mm³ or a platelet count between 75,000 to 100,000/mm³ generally suggests that dosage can be reduced by 50%. Bone recovery is usually complete by 20 days.

Be alert to evidence of patient complaints that might suggest development of leukopenia (fever, chills, sore mouth or throat), infection (immunosuppression), and bleeding (thrombocytopenia).

During period of platelet nadir particularly, protect patient from any trauma that might precipitate bleeding. If possible, invasive procedures such as rectal temperatures, enemas, catheterizations, IMs, and IVs should be withheld until platelet count has recovered sufficiently.

Inspect patient's mouth (inside cheeks, tongue, gums, throat, lips) daily for ulcerations and bleeding. Stomatitis is especially likely to occur in patients who have had prior radiation therapy of head and neck. Patients with stomatitis should be advised to avoid obvious irritants such as extremely hot foods, spicy and rough foods, smoking, alcohol, strong commercial mouth washes, and irritating tooth pastes.

GI side effects are generally mild and do not appear to be dose related. Some patients may require an antiemetic.

Before administration, inspect solution for particulate matter and discoloration. Solution should be clear and yellow in color. If crystals are present, discard.

Store preferably between 15° and 30°C (59° and 86°F) unless otherwise directed by manufacturer.

F

F

FACTOR IX COMPLEX

Hemostatic (systemic)

(Konyne, Profilnine, Proplex, Proplex SX)

ACTIONS AND USES. Dried, purified concentrate of vitamin K-dependent blood coagulation factors II, VII, IX, and X derived from fresh pooled plasma of healthy donors. Although tested for presence of hepatitis virus, some risk of transmitting hepatitis exists. Possibility of developing hepatitis is small in patients with severe hemophilia since they have received numerous transfusions and, therefore, have developed hepatitis antibodies. Factor IX complex contains only traces of blood groups A and B isohemagglutins; however, when large doses are administered, the amount of isohemagglutins becomes significant and can cause intravascular hemolysis. Congenital deficiency of any one of the four blood coagulation factors present in factor IX complex can result in a hemorrhagic problem. Factor VII (proconvertin or serum prothrombin conversion accelerator), factor IX (Christmas factor or plasma thromboplastin component), and factor X or Stuart–Prower factor (resembles factor VII) are all essential for conversion of factor II prothrombin to thrombin. Note that some products are heparin free (Konyne, Profilnine), others contain heparin as a stabilizing agent (Proplex, Proplex SX).

Used primarily to control bleeding in patients with factor IX deficiency, i.e., hemophilia B (Christmas disease). Also used to reverse effects of coumarin anticoagulants. Proplex is used to control bleeding in patients with hemophilia A (who have factor VIII inhibitors).

ABSORPTION AND FATE. Rapidly cleared from plasma following IV administration. Biplasic half-life: first phase, 4 to 6 hours; terminal phase, 22.5 hours.

CONTRAINDICATIONS AND PRECAUTIONS. Liver disease or suspicious signs of disseminated intravascular coagulation (DIC) or fibrinolysis; patients with mild factor IX deficiency who could be treated effectively with fresh-frozen plasma; patients who have had little exposure to blood products (at high risk of developing viral hepatitis); patients undergoing elective surgery (risk of thromboses). Safe use during pregnancy not established.

F

ADVERSE/SIDE EFFECTS. Generally well tolerated. **With large doses:** chills, fever (pyrogenic reaction), disseminated intravascular clotting (DIC), thromboses, myocardial infarction. **With rapid infusion:** vasomotor reactions (flushing, changes in blood pressure, or pulse rate), transient fever, chills, headache, tingling, urticaria, nausea, vomiting, somnolence, lethargy. **Other:** severe hypersensitivity reactions including anaphylactic shock (rare) viral hepatitis.

ROUTE AND DOSAGE. Highly individualized according to coagulation studies and nature of factor deficiency, factor level desired, weight of patient, and severity of bleeding. Dosage expressed in terms of units of factor IX activity: one unit contains the factor IX activity of 1 ml of normal fresh plasma (1 U/kg increases factor IX activity by 1%). Formula for approximating desired number of units required = body weight in kg × 0.8 to 1.0 × factor IX increase desired in percentage of normal.

NURSING IMPLICATIONS

Check expiration date. Typing and crossmatching should be done to reduce risk of intravascular hemolysis in patients with type A, B, or AB blood, and for general emergency purposes.

Patients should be informed of the potential risk of viral hepatitis associated with the use of factor IX complex. Some physicians propose active immunization with hepatitis B vaccine if multiple administrations of factor IX complex is planned.

Coagulation assays should be performed prior to initiation of therapy and at regular intervals during therapy to individualize dosage.

Monitor vital signs and intake–output.

Rate of flow is prescribed (generally not to exceed 3 ml/minute).

Be alert to signs of disseminated intravascular coagulation (DIC), e.g., oliguria, mucosal bleeding, ecchymoses, abnormal coagulation tests and hypersensitivity reactions.

Risk of (DIC) increases with repeated administrations since unnecessarily high levels of factors II, IX, and X, which have a particularly long half-life, are produced. The possibility of DIC is reportedly reduced by avoiding elevations of the patient's factor IX levels to more than 50% of normal.

Patients with hemophillia A (classic hemophilia) commonly have hemarthrosis: e.g., bleeding into joints causing swelling, pain, and immobility. Bleeding into soft tissues and muscle causes hematomas that compress nerves, blood vessels, and even the airway. Prompt treatment and physicial therapy can prevent irreversible joint damage and muscle atrophy.

Hemophiliac patients are usually credible informers. Patients with severe hemophilia have been known to sense the onset of a bleeding episode long before it can be detected objectively.

Most large cities now have hemophilia diagnostic and treatment centers that provide comprehensive care for adults and children with hemophilia.

Before reconstitution, warm diluent (sterile water for injection) to room temperature. After diluent is added, vial should be gently agitated to assure complete dissolution of powder. After reconstitution, solution should be administered within 3 hours to avoid possibility of microbial contamination. It should not be refrigerated because precipitation may occur. Refrigerate unopened vials between 2° and 8°C (35 and 46°F) until reconstituted, unless otherwise directed by manufacturer. Do not freeze.

FAT EMULSION, INTRAVENOUS

Caloric agent (fatty acids)

(Intralipid, Liposyn, Soyacal, Travamulsion)

ACTIONS AND USES. Intralipid (available in 10 and 20% concentrations) is a soybean oil in water emulsion containing egg yolk phospholipids and glycerin. Liposyn 10% is a safflower oil in water emulsion containing egg phosphatides and glycerin. Caloric value per ml of Intralipid 10% and Liposyn 10% is 1.1, and for Intralipid 20% it is 2. Fat emulsions contain a mixture of neutral triglycerides, mostly unsaturated fatty acids, the majority of which include linoleic, oleic and palmitic acids. Intralipid also contains linolenic acid, and Liposyn also contains stearic acid. Emulsified fat particles are approximately 0.4 to 0.5 μ in diameter, similar in size to chylomicrons (naturally occurring fat molecules). Fatty acids are essential for normal structure and function of cell membranes. They are also utilized by body as a source of energy and may cause an increase in heat production, decrease in respiratory quotient (ratio of $CO_2:O_2$), and an increase in oxygen consumption. When used as a source of calories in patients receiving amino acid-dextrose infusions, fat emulsion should supply no more than 60% of total caloric input for adults and children and 40% in newborns (remainder is supplied by amino acid-dextrose mixture). When used to prevent or correct fatty acid deficiency, 8 to 10% of total calories should be supplied by fat emulsion. Fat emulsion preparations are isotonic and may be given by central or peripheral venous routes.

Used in treatment of fatty acid deficiency. Also used to supply fatty acids and calories in high density form to patients receiving prolonged TPN therapy who cannot tolerate high dextrose concentrations or when fluid intake must be restricted as in renal failure, congestive heart disease, ascites.

CONTRAINDICATIONS AND PRECAUTIONS. Hypersensitivity to any components, hyperlipemia, bone marrow dyscrasias, impaired fat metabolism as in pathologic hyperlipemia, lipoid nephrosis, acute pancreatitis accompanied by hyperlipemia. *Cautious Use:* severe hepatic or pulmonary disease, coagulation disorders, anemia, newborns, prematures, infants with hyperbilirubinemia, when danger of fat embolism exists, diabetes mellitus, thrombocytopenia, history of gastric ulcer.

ADVERSE/SIDE EFFECTS. Acute reactions: fever, chills, flushing, sweating, pain in back and chest, dyspnea, cyanosis, pressure sensation over eyes, nausea, vomiting, headache, dizziness, sleepiness, neurologic symptoms, hypersensitivity reactions (to egg protein), hyperlipemia, hypercoagulability, transient increases in liver function tests, thrombocytopenia in neonates, irritation at infusion site. **Long-term administration:** sepsis, jaundice (cholestasis), hepatomegaly, kernicterus (infants with hyperbilirubinemia); rarely: thrombophlebitis, leukopenia, anemia; "overloading syndrome" (focal seizures, lethargy, delayed clotting, fever, leukocytosis, impaired liver function, splenomegaly, shock), gastroduodenal ulcer, hemorrhagic diathesis; fat deposits in lungs, IV fat pigment (brown pigmentation in reticuloendothelial system).

ROUTE AND DOSAGE. Intravenous: via peripheral or central venous infusion: *Intralipid 10%:* **Adults:** 1 ml/minute for first 15 to 30 minutes. If no adverse reactions, rate is increased so that 500 ml (maximum dosage first day), are infused over 4 to 6 hours. Not to exceed 2.5 Gm/kg daily. **Pediatric:** 0.1 ml/minute for first 10 to 15 minutes. If no adverse reactions, may be increased to 1 Gm/kg over 4 hours. Daily dose not to exceed 4 Gm/kg. *Intralipid 20%:* **Adults:** 0.5 ml for first 15 to 30 minutes. If no adverse reactions, increase rate so that 500 ml is infused over 8 hours. **Pediatric:** 0.05 ml/minute for first 10 to 15 minutes. If no adverse reactions, rate is increased to 1 Gm/kg in 4 hours. Not to exceed 100 ml/hour or 4 Gm/kg/24 hours. *Liposyn 10%:* **Adults:** 500 ml twice weekly. Infuse initially at rate of 1 ml/minute for 30 minutes. If no adverse reactions, rate may be increased to maximum of 500 ml over 4 to 6 hours. **Pediatric:** 5 to 10 ml/kg daily at initial rate of 0.1 ml/minute over first 30 minutes. May be increased to maximum of 100 ml/hour.

NURSING IMPLICATIONS

Prior to initiation of therapy, a comprehensive individualized nutrition plan should be established.

If possible, allow preparations that have been refrigerated to stand at room temperature for about 30 minutes before using.

Do not use if emulsion appears to be "oiling out."

Note expiration date on bottle label.

Acute reactions tend to occur within the first 2½ hours of therapy. Observe patient closely, especially during this time.

In adults, fat emulsion is usually delivered during waking hours so as not to interrupt patient's sleep. Since newborns and prematures tend to metabolize fat slowly, it is usually administered at a constant rate over 20 to 24 hours to reduce risk of hyperlipemia.

The following baseline determinations are recommended: hemogram, platelet count, blood coagulation, liver function tests, plasma lipid profile (especially serum triglycerides and cholesterol, free fatty acids in plasma). These tests are usually repeated one or two times weekly during therapy in adults, and more frequently in children since they do not readily eliminate fat from circulation. Significant alterations in any of these parameters should be reported promptly.

Triglyceride values are age-related: 0 to 29 years: 10 to 140 mg/dl; 30 to 39 years: 10 to 150 mg/dl; 40 to 49 years: 10 to 160 mg/dl; 50 to 59 years: 10 to 190 mg/dl. *Serum cholesterol* also varies with age and may range from 120 to 220 mg/dl.

Since newborns are prone to develop thrombocytopenia, daily platelet counts are advised during first week of therapy then every other day during second week and three times weekly thereafter.

Lipemia must clear after each daily infusion. Degree of lipemia is measured by serum triglycerides and cholesterol levels 4 to 6 hours after infusion has ceased or by turbidity check of plasma 8 to 12 hours after infusion.

Fat emulsions may be administered via a separate peripheral site or by piggyback into same vein receiving amino acid injection and dextrose mixtures. Administered by piggyback through a Y connector near infusion site so that the two solutions mix only in short piece of tubing proximal to needle.

Since fat emulsions have lower specific gravity, container must be hung higher than hyperalimentation solution bottle to prevent back up of fat emulsion into primary line.

An in-line filter is not recommended because size of fat particles is larger than pore size.

Flow rate of each solution should be controlled by separate infusion pumps.

Do not mix fat emulsions with electrolytes, vitamins, drugs, or other nutrient solutions.

Observe and report effect of therapy on clinical manifestations of essential fatty acid deficiency (EFAD) syndrome: scaly dermatitis, growth retardation, poor wound healing, sparse hair growth, thrombocytopenia.

It is reported that lipid-containing fluids may extract phthalates from phthalate-plasticized polyvinyl chloride (PVC). A nonphthalate infusion set is considered advisable.

Unless otherwise directed by manufacturer, the 10% solutions Intralipid 10% and Liposyn 10% may be stored at room temperature (25°C or below). Intralipid 20% should be stored under refrigeration. Do not freeze.

Contents of partly used containers should not be stored for later use.

Diagnostic Test Interferences. Blood samples drawn during or shortly after fat emulsion infusion may produce abnormally high **hemoglobin MCH and MCHC** values. Fat emulsions may cause transient abnormalities in **liver function tests** and may interfere with estimations of **serum bilirubin** (especially in infants).

F

FENFLURAMINE HYDROCHLORIDE

(Pondimin, Ponderal)

(fen-flure'a-meen)
Anorexigenic
C IV

ACTIONS AND USES. Indirect-acting sympathomimetic amine related to amphetamine. Differs pharmacologically from amphetamine in that it generally produces CNS depression more often than stimulation. Exact mechanism of appetite-inhibiting action not clearly defined, but may be due to stimulation of hypothalamus. Believed to have intrinsic hypoglycemic activity; appears to increase glucose uptake by skeletal muscles, thus reducing glucose available for conversion to lipid.

Used as short-term (a few weeks) adjunct in treatment of exogenous obesity.

ABSORPTION AND FATE. Readily absorbed from GI tract. Onset of action 1 to 2 hours; duration of anorexigenic effect 4 to 6 hours. Widely distributed to most body tissues. Considerable individual variation in drug metabolism and elimination. Slowly excreted in urine, primarily as metabolites; small quantities excreted as unchanged drug. Rate of urinary excretion is increased in acid urine. Excreted in saliva and sweat in small amounts.

CONTRAINDICATIONS AND PRECAUTIONS. Hypersensitivity to sympathomimetic amines; hyperthyroidism; severe hypertension; glaucoma; symptomatic cardiovascular disease including arrhythmias; history of drug abuse; agitated states; during or within 14 days following administration of MAO inhibitors; concomitant use of CNS depressants or CNS stimulants. Safe use during pregnancy, in women of childbearing age, and in children under 12 years of age not established. *Cautious Use:* mental depression, hypertension, diabetes mellitus.

ADVERSE/SIDE EFFECTS. CNS: drowsiness, dizziness, confusion, incoordination, headache, elevated mood, dysphoria, mental depression, anxiety, nervousness, psychotic episodes, tremors, agitation, weakness, fatigue, dysarthria, insomnia, vivid dreams, nightmares. **CV:** palpitation, tachycardia, chest pain, arrhythmias, hypotension, hypertension, fainting. **Dermatologic:** skin rashes, urticaria, ecchymosis, erythema, burning sensation of skin, hair loss. **GI:** dry mouth, diarrhea, nausea, vomiting, unpleasant taste, abdominal pain, constipation. **Ophthalmic:** blurred vision, mydriasis, eye irritation. **Reproductive:** increased or decreased libido, impotence, menstrual irregularities. **Other:** myalgia, edema, dysuria, urinary frequency, grinding teeth during sleep (bruxism), sweating, fever, chills, myalgia, edema, dysuria. **Overdosage:** confusion, agitation, hyperventilation, exaggerated or depressed reflexes, convulsions, hyperpyrexia, dilated nonreactive pupils, rotatory nystagmus, coma, cardiac arrest.

ROUTE AND DOSAGE. Oral: Initial: 20 to 40 mg three times daily before meals. May be increased at weekly intervals by 20 mg daily to maximum of 40 mg three times daily. Not to exceed 120 mg/day.

NURSING IMPLICATIONS

Dose increase should be made gradually to minimize possibility of side effects.

Diarrhea may occur during first week of therapy; report it to physician; dose reduction or termination of therapy may be required.

Patients with diabetes maintained on insulin or other antidiabetic drugs should be observed for excessive hypoglycemic activity when fenfluramine is added to the therapeutic regimen.

If fenfluramine is prescribed for patients with hypertension, blood pressure should be monitored.

Mentally depressed patients may become more depressed during therapy and/or following withdrawal of fenfluramine.

Warn patient that fenfluramine may impair ability to perform hazardous tasks such as driving a motor vehicle.

If tolerance to anorexigenic effect develops, drug should be discontinued.

To achieve and maintain loss of weight, patient should be adequately instructed in dietary management.

Following excessive use, abrupt discontinuation of fenfluramine may be associated with irritability and mental depression.

Classified as Schedule IV substance under Federal Controlled Substances Act.

Store in well-closed container preferably between 15° and 30°C (59° and 86°F), unless otherwise directed by manufacturer.

Drug Interactions. Use of fenfluramine during or within 14 days following administration of **MAO inhibitors** may result in hypertensive crisis. Fenfluramine reportedly may alter the effects of **hypotensive drugs,** e.g., **guanethidine, methyldopa, reserpine.** Effects of **CNS depressants** or **stimulants** may be additive (caution patient).

FENOPROFEN CALCIUM

(Nalfon)

(fen-oh-proe'fen)

Analgesic/Antipyretic, NSAID
Antirheumatic agent

ACTIONS AND USES. Propionic acid derivative chemically and pharmacologically similar to ibuprofen and naproxen. In common with these drugs, exhibits antiinflammatory, analgesic, and antipyretic properties. Exact mode of antiinflammatory action not known, but believed to be related to ability to inhibit prostaglandin synthesis. Serum uric acid lowering and suppression of platelet aggregation reportedly less than that of aspirin. May prolong bleeding time, but prothrombin time, whole blood clotting time, and platelet counts are usually not affected. Claimed to be comparable to aspirin in antiinflammatory activity and to be associated with lower incidence of adverse GI symptoms. Studies suggest that fenoprofen may prolong labor by reducing uterine contractility. Cross-sensitivity to other nonsteroidal antiinflammatory drugs (NSAID) has been reported.

Used for antiinflammatory and analgesic effects in the symptomatic treatment of acute and chronic rheumatoid arthritis and osteoarthritis. *Investigational Use:* management of acute gout and fever.

ABSORPTION AND FATE. Rapidly and almost completely absorbed from upper GI tract. Peak plasma levels within 2 hours. Plasma half-life: approximately 3 hours; 99% protein bound. Metabolized in liver; appears to undergo enterohepatic recirculation. About 90% of single dose excreted in urine within 24 hours primarily as metabolites and about 3% as unchanged drug. Small amounts excreted in feces. Does not cross placenta (preliminary studies); excreted in breast milk.

CONTRAINDICATIONS AND PRECAUTIONS. History of hypersensitivity to fenoprofen calcium; history of hypersensitivity or nephrotic syndrome associated with aspirin or other nonsteroidal antiinflammatory agents; significant renal or hepatic dysfunction. Safe use during pregnancy, in nursing mothers, and in children not established. *Cautious Use:* history of upper GI tract disorders, hemophilia or other bleeding tendencies, compromised cardiac function, hypertension, impaired hearing.

ADVERSE/SIDE EFFECTS. CNS (also see EENT): headache, drowsiness, dizziness, fatigue, lassitude, tremor, confusion, insomnia, nervousness, depression. **CV:** palpitation, tachycardia, peripheral edema. **Dermatologic:** (may or may not be hypersensitivity reaction): pruritus, rash, purpura, increased sweating, urticaria. **ENT:** tinnitus, decreased hearing, deafness. **GI:** indigestion, nausea, vomiting, anorexia, constipation, diarrhea, flatulence, abdominal pain, dry mouth; infrequent: gastritis, peptic ulcer, jaundice, cholestatic hepatitis. **GU:** nephrotoxicity (rare): dysuria, cystitis, hematuria, oliguria, azotemia, anuria, allergic nephritis, papillary necrosis. **Hematologic (infrequent):** thrombocytopenic, hemolytic anemia, agranulocytosis, pancytopenia. **Other:** blurred vision, dyspnea, asthenia, fatigue, malaise, anaphylaxis.

ROUTE AND DOSAGE. Oral: *Analgesic:* 200 mg every 4 to 6 hours, as needed. *Antirheumatic:* 300 to 600 mg four times a day. Not to exceed 3.2 Gm daily.

NURSING IMPLICATIONS

For rapid absorption, best taken on an empty stomach 30 minutes to 1 hour before or 2 hours after meals. May be administered with meals, milk, or antacid (prescribed), however, if patient experiences GI disturbances. Peak plasma levels may be delayed by food or antacids, but total amount absorbed is not affected.

Tablet may be crushed and capsule may be emptied and contents swallowed with fluid or mixed with food.

Important to take a detailed drug history prior to initiation of therapy. *See Contraindications and Precautions.*

Because fenoprofen may cause dizziness and drowsiness, advise patient to exercise caution when driving or performing other potentially hazardous activities.

Baseline and periodic evaluations of hemoglobin, renal and hepatic function, and auditory and ophthalmic examinations are recommended in patients receiving prolonged or high dose therapy.

Although eye changes have not been reported, since they have been observed with other nonsteroidal antiinflammatory agents, manufacturer warns of possible occurrence with fenoprofen. An ophthalmologic examination is recommended if patient has eye complaints.

Instruct patient to report immediately the onset of unexplained fever, rash, arthralgia, oliguria, edema, weight gain. Possible symptoms of nephrotic syndrome, rapidly reversible if drug is promptly withdrawn.

Therapeutic effectiveness of fenoprofen in patients with arthritis may be evidenced within a few days to peak effect in 2 to 3 weeks (relief of joint pains and stiffness, reduction in joint swelling, increase in grip strength, and improved mobility).

Inform patient that alcohol and aspirin may increase risk of GI ulceration and bleeding tendencies and, therefore, unless otherwise advised by physician should be avoided.

Fenoprofen may prolong bleeding time; therefore, advise patients to inform dentist or surgeon that they are taking this drug.

Drug Interactions: Fenoprofen

Plus	Interactions
Anticoagulants (coumarins)	Prolongation of prothrombin time
Aspirin (in multiple doses), Phenobarbital	Decrease effect of fenoprofen by hepatic enzyme induction
Phenytoin (Dilantin) and other hydantoin anticonvulants, Sulfonamides, Sulfonylureas (oral hypoglycemics)	Action of these drugs may be increased by being displaced from plasma protein sites

F

FENTANYL CITRATE

(Sublimaze)

(fen′ta-nil)

Narcotic analgesic, opiate agonist

C II

ACTIONS AND USES. Synthetic phenylpiperidine derivative. Pharmacologic actions qualitatively similar to those of morphine and meperidine, but action is more prompt and less prolonged, and fentanyl appears to have less emetic activity. On a weight basis, it is estimated to be about 80 times more potent than morphine. Histamine release occurs rarely.

Used for analgesic action of short duration preoperatively, during surgery, and in immediate postoperative period. Also used as a supplement to general or regional anesthesia, often in combination with a neuroleptic. Commercially available combination of fentanyl with the neuroleptic drug droperidol (Innovar) is used to produce tranquilization and analgesia for surgical and diagnostic procedures.

ABSORPTION AND FATE. Onset of action is almost immediate following IV administration, with peak analgesic effect in 3 to 5 minutes; duration 30 to 60 minutes. Onset of action following IM injection occurs in 7 to 15 minutes; duration 1 to 2 hours. Metabolized primarily in liver. Excreted in urine chiefly as metabolites; about 10% excreted as unchanged drug.

CONTRAINDICATIONS AND PRECAUTIONS. Patients who have received MAO inhibitors within 14 days; myasthenia gravis. Safe use in women of childbearing potential, during pregnancy, and in children younger than 2 years of age not established. *Cautious Use:* head injuries, increased intracranial pressure; elderly, debilitated, poor-risk patients; chronic obstructive pulmonary disease and other respiratory problems; liver and kidney dysfunction; bradyarrhythmias.

ADVERSE/SIDE EFFECTS. Euphoria, miosis, blurred vision, nausea, vomiting, dizziness, diaphoresis, delirium, hypotension; muscle rigidity (especially muscles of respiration) following rapid IV infusion; laryngospasm, bronchoconstriction, respiratory depression, respiratory arrest, bradycardia, circulatory depression, cardiac arrest.

ROUTE AND DOSAGE. Highly individualized. **Adults: Intramuscular, intravenous (slow):** 0.05 to 0.1 mg. **Children (2 to 12 years):** 0.02 to 0.03 mg per 10 kg.

NURSING IMPLICATIONS

Monitor vital signs and observe patient for signs of skeletal and thoracic muscle (depressed respirations) rigidity and weakness.

Instructions should be given preoperatively regarding deep breathing, turning, and moving of extremities to reduce possibility of complications.

Duration of respiratory depressant effect may be considerably longer than analgesic effect. Have immediately available: oxygen, resuscitative equipment, endotracheal tube, suction, narcotic antagonist such as naloxone, and skeletal muscle relaxant, e.g., succinylcholine.

Physician will rely on accurate reporting of drug effect following initial dose to estimate effects of subsequent doses if needed.

Narcotics and other CNS depressants have additive or potentiating effects. If prescribed, initial dosage of narcotic analgesic should be reduced to one-fourth or one-third of those usually employed.

Fentanyl can produce dependence of the morphine type and therefore has abuse potential.

Classified as Schedule II drug under Federal Controlled Substances Act.

Store at room temperature, preferably between 15° and 30°C (59° and 86°F), unless otherwise directed by manufacturer. Protect drug from light.

FERROUS FUMARATE

(foo'ma-rate)
Antianemic agent

(Feco-T, Feostat, Fersamal, Fumasorb, Fumerin, Hemocyte, Ircon, Neo-Fer, Novofumar, Palafer, Palmiron)

ACTIONS AND USES. Comparable to ferrous sulfate in actions, uses, contraindications, and adverse reactions. Contains 33% elemental iron. Available in fixed-dose combination with vitamin C, which may facilitate absorption of iron.

ROUTE AND DOSAGE. Oral: Adults and children (over 6 years): 200 mg (equivalent to 66 mg elemental iron) 1 to 4 times daily. **Infants and children (under 6 years):** 100 to 300 mg daily in 3 to 4 divided doses. Dosage depends on severity of anemia. Available in tablets, capsules, timed release tablets, chewable tablets, and suspension.

NURSING IMPLICATIONS

See Ferrous sulfate (prototype antianemic agent).

FERROUS GLUCONATE

(gloo'koe-nate)
Antianemic agent

(Fergon, Ferralet, Fertinic, Novoferrogluc, Simron)

ACTIONS AND USES. Claimed to cause less gastric irritation and to be better tolerated than ferrous sulfate. Has same actions, uses, contraindications, and adverse reactions as ferrous sulfate. Contains 11.6% ferrous iron.

ROUTE AND DOSAGE. Oral: Adults: 300 to 600 mg daily (equivalent to 24 to 72 mg elemental iron). **Children (6 to 12 years):** 100 to 300 mg 3 times daily. **Infants and children (under 6 years):** 100 to 300 mg/day in divided doses. Dosage depends on severity of anemia. Available in tablets, capsules, and elixir.

NURSING IMPLICATIONS

See Ferrous sulfate (prototype antianemic agent).

PROTOTYPE

FERROUS SULFATE

Antianemic agent

(Feosol, Fer-in-Sol, Fer-Iron, Fero-Gradumet, Ferospace, Fesofar, Hematinic, Mol-Iron, Novoferrosulfa, Slow-Fe)

F

ACTIONS AND USES. Standard iron preparation against which other oral preparations are usually measured. Reportedly the cheapest form of supplemental iron and as effective as other more expensive iron salts. Corrects erythropoietic abnormalities and may reverse gastric, esophageal, and other tissue changes caused by lack of iron. Ferrous sulfate contains 20% elemental iron; ferrous sulfate exsicated contains 29.7% iron.

Used to correct simple iron deficiency and to treat iron deficiency (microcytic, hypochromic) anemias. Also may be used prophylactically during periods of increased iron needs, as in infancy, childhood, and pregnancy.

ABSORPTION AND FATE. Absorbed into mucosal cells of small intestines (primarily duodenum) where a small fraction is changed to ferric iron, and subsequently incorporated into ferritin; lost into feces when mucosal cells are shed at end of 5-day life cycle. When iron presented to gut is in excess of need, mucosal cell uptake is minimal ("mucosal block"). Larger fraction enters bloodstream and bound to transferrin. Distributed to functional and storage sites in bone marrow, spleen, liver, hemoglobin, myoglobin, metalloenzymes. Plasma iron concentration and total iron-binding capacity vary with disease states and physiologic conditions (higher in men than in women and higher in morning than in evening); regulated principally by hemoglobin synthesis. Major excretion route in feces via shedding of mucosal cells; also lost in epithelial cells of skin, nails, hair, and in sweat, urine, and breast milk.

CONTRAINDICATIONS AND PRECAUTIONS. Peptic ulcer, regional enteritis, ulcerative colitis, hemolytic anemias (in absence of iron deficiency), hemochromatosis, hemosiderosis, patients receiving repeated transfusions, pyridoxine responsive anemia, cirrhosis of liver.

ADVERSE/SIDE EFFECTS. Generally minimal: nausea, heartburn, anorexia, constipation, diarrhea, epigastric pain, abdominal distress, headache, yellow-brown discoloration of eyes, teeth; iron-overload hemosiderosis (rare). **Large chronic doses in infants:** rickets (due to interference with phosphorous absorption). **Massive overdosage:** lethargy, drowsiness, nausea, vomiting, abdominal pain, diarrhea, local corrosion of stomach and small intestines, pallor or cyanosis acidosis, shock, cardiovascular collapse, convulsions, liver necrosis, coma, death.

ROUTE AND DOSAGE. Oral: Adults: 300 mg to 1.2 Gm (the equivalent of 60 to 240 mg elemental iron) daily. Therapeutic dosages depend on severity of iron deficiency. Preferably given in divided doses rather than in single large daily doses. **Children (6 to 12 years):** 120 to 600 mg (24 to 120 mg elemental iron) daily in divided doses. **Children (under 6 years):** 75 to 225 mg (15 to 45 mg elemental iron) daily in divided doses. Available in tablets, timed-release capsules and tablets, syrup liquid, elixir.

NURSING IMPLICATIONS

Oral iron preparations are best absorbed when taken on an empty stomach (i.e., between meals). However, to minimize gastric distress it may be necessary to administer the drug with or immediately after meals; or the physician may prescribe smaller doses.

If an antacid is prescribed it should be taken at least 1 hour before or 1 hour after the iron preparation.

Food-Drug Interactions:

- Tannins in tea can block absorption of inorganic (but not organic) iron. However, addition of cream or lemon binds the tannins so they cannot interact.
- Ascorbic acid increases absorption of iron; consuming citrus fruit or tomato juice with iron preparation (except the elixir) may increase its availability.
- In patients with uncomplicated iron deficiency, there is little therapeutic indication for concurrent administration of ascorbic acid, since these patients are able to absorb oral iron adequately. However, ascorbic acid may be prescribed in patients who have difficulty in absorbing adequate quantities or iron, such as infants and young children with severe anemia.
- Iron absorption may be inhibited if the iron preparation is taken with milk, eggs, or caffeine beverage (e.g., coffee, tea).

Since iron is potentially corrosive, tablets or capsules should not be taken within 1 hour of bedtime, and adequate liquid should accompany ingestion of medication to assure passage into stomach. Instruct patient *not* to crush tablet or empty contents of capsule prior to administration.

If the patient experiences difficulty in swallowing tablet or capsule, consult physician about prescribing a liquid formulation or a less corrosive form, such as ferrous gluconate. (Sustained contact of iron with esophageal mucosa can cause ulceration.)

Sustained-release preparations are generally not preferred over ferrous sulfate tablets because they tend to transport iron beyond sites of optimal absorption. Also, they are more expensive.

In general, liquid preparations should be well diluted and administered through a straw or placed on the back of tongue with a dropper to prevent staining of teeth and to mask taste. Instruct the patient to rinse mouth with clear water immediately after ingestion.

Feosol elixir may be mixed with water, but it is not compatible with milk, fruit juice, or wine vehicles. However, the preparation Fer-In-Sol drops may be given in water or in fruit or vegetable juice, according to manufacturer.

Therapeutic dosages are prescribed only if indicated by appropriate diagnostic procedures. If hemoglobin and hematocrit determinations suggest anemia, a complete blood count, reticulocyte count, and serum bilirubin determination are usually obtained; bone marrow examination may also be done.

In addition to iron replacement, an important therapeutic goal is to determine underlying cause of iron loss and to remedy or alleviate causative factors.

A complete health history should be recorded to determine, among other things, dietary iron intake, adequacy of diet, in general, and possible drug-induced causes of anemia, such as aspirin in high dosages, sulfonamides, quinidine, antimalarial drugs, and phenylbutazone.

Inform patient that iron preparations cause dark green or black stools. Advise patient to report constipation or diarrhea. These symptoms may be relieved by adjustments in dosage or diet or by change to another iron preparation.

Simple iron deficiency may be asymptomatic, but it is usually associated with ill-defined symptoms such as anorexia, easy fatigability, headache, dizziness, tinnitus, and sensitivity to cold. As iron depletion becomes more severe, signs and symptoms may include dyspnea on exertion, palpitation, menstrual disturbances, decreased libido, waxy pallor, paresthesias, epithelial changes including itchy skin, brittleness of hair and nails and ridging, flattening, or concavity of nails, and Plummer-Vinson syndrome (severe anemia): dysphagia, stomatitis, atrophic glossitis.

Therapeutic response may be experienced within 48 hours as a sense of well-being, increased vigor, improved appetite, and decreased irritability (in children). Reticulocyte response may begin in 4 days; it usually peaks in 7 to 10 days (reticulocytosis) and returns to normal after 2 or 3 weeks. Hemoglobin generally increases by 2 Gm/dl and hematocrit by 6% in 3 weeks.

Hemoglobin and reticulocyte values should be monitored during therapy. In the absence of satisfactory response after 3 weeks of drug treatment, possible reasons for failure warrant investigation: e.g., noncompliance, inadequate dosage, occult blood loss, malabsorption, infection, presence of other anemias.

RDA for iron in children 4 to 6 years: 10 mg; for adult males: 10 mg; adult females: 18 mg. In pregnancy requirement cannot be met by ordinary diets, so 30 to 60 mg supplemental iron is recommended during pregnancy and for 2 or 3 months after parturition. lactation: 18 mg.

The average American diet provides approximately 6 mg of iron per 1000 calories. Foods high in iron content (> 5 mg/100 Gm): organ meats (liver, heart, kidney), brewer's yeast, wheat germ, egg yolk, dried beans, dried fruits, oysters. Other good sources (1 to 5 mg/100 Gm): most muscle meats, fish, fowl, most cereals and green vegetables, dark molasses.

Facilitate development of a dietary teaching plan for patient and family.

At present there is no convincing evidence that iron utilization is influenced by concomitant administration of copper, molybdenum, magnesium, calcium, or chlorophyll.

As a general rule, iron should not be administered for longer than 6 months except in repeated pregnancies, persistent bleeding, or menorrhagia.

Iron therapy is usually continued for 2 to 3 months after the hemoglobin level has returned to normal (roughly twice the period required to normalize hemoglobin concentration). Replenishment of iron stores is a slow process, because the rate of iron absorption decreases as hemoglobin approaches normal levels.

Ingested overdoses of iron preparations in children may be fatal. Caution patients to store these drugs out of reach of children (at least one death per month is reported).

Treatment of overdosage: Vomiting should be induced quickly, and eggs and milk should be fed to form iron complexes until gastric lavage can be done (within first hour of ingestion). Lavage solution: 1% sodium bicarbonate or 5% phosphate solution; iron chelating agent (e.g., deferoxamine mesylate) should be administered. Measures to combat shock, dehydration, blood loss, and respiratory failure may be necessary. (Gastric lavage should not be performed after the first hour because of danger of perforation due to gastric necrosis. Dimercaprol should not be used because it may form toxic complexes.)

Preserve in well-closed containers. Protect from moisture. Do not use discolored tablets.

Diagnostic Test Interferences. Large iron doses may cause false-positive tests for **occult blood** with *o*-toluidine (Hematest, Occultest, Labstix) and guaiac reagent; benzidine test is reportedly not affected.

Drug Interactions. Absorption of oral iron is inhibited by **antacids, cholestyramine, cimetidine,** and **pancreatic extracts** (space doses as far apart as possible). There may be delayed or impaired hematologic response to iron therapy with **chloramphenicol** or **vitamin E** (in children). Simultaneous administration of oral iron interferes with absorption of **oral tetracyclines** and vice versa; if concurrent administration is necessary, patient should receive tetracycline 3 hours after or 2 hours before iron administration. Oral iron decreases action of **doxycycline,** and **penicillamine;** separate doses by at least 2 hours. Concurrent administration of **ascorbic acid** (> 200 mg orally) increases GI absorption of elemental iron. Studies in humans do not support findings from earlier animal studies that **allopurinol** may increase hepatic iron stores.

FIBRINOLYSIN AND DESOXYRIBONUCLEASE

(Elase)

(fye-bri-noe-lye'sin)
Debriding agent
Enzymes

ACTIONS AND USES. Combination of two bovine proteolytic enzymes: fibrinolysin extracted from bovine plasma acts primarily on fibrin in blood clots and exudates, and desoxyribonuclease derived from beef pancreas attacks DNA in devitalized tissue and disintegrating cells. Enzymatic debridement is directed primarily against denatured proteins in dead tissue; normal tissue remains relatively unaffected. Lacks antiinfective activity, but debriding action reduces necrotic material that tends to favor bacterial growth. Commercial formulation is prepared with a small amount of sodium chloride, sucrose, and thimerosal.

Used as debriding agent in a variety of inflammatory and infected lesions such as general surgical wounds, abscesses, fistulae, and sinus tracts; ulcerative lesions, second-and third-degree burns, circumcision and episiotomy, cervicitis, and vaginitis. Available in fixed combination with chloramphenicol (Elase-Chloromycetin).

F

CONTRAINDICATIONS AND PRECAUTIONS. Hypersensitivity to bovine products or to mercury derivatives (e.g., thimerosal): not recommended for parenteral use except for conditions indicated under route and dosage; hematomas adjacent to or within adipose tissue.

ADVERSE/SIDE EFFECTS. With higher than recommended dosage: local hyperemia.

ROUTE AND DOSAGE. Topical: *Intravaginal: Vaginitis, cervicitis:* 5 Gm ointment deposited deep into vagina (using supplied disposable applicator) once nightly at bedtime for approximately 5 nights or until 30-Gm tube has been used. For severe conditions physician may instill 10 ml of solution into vagina and insert a cotton tampon after waiting 1 or 2 minutes for solution to disperse. Tampon is removed the next day and therapy continued with ointment. *Irrigation: Infected wounds, empyema cavities, fistulae, sinus tracts, subcutaneous hematomas:* solution should be drained and replaced every 6 to 10 hours. Wound dressing: *See Nursing Implications.* Vials of 30-ml capacity contain 25 units of fibrinolysis and 15,000 units of desoxyribonuclease. The ointment contains 1 unit of fibrinolysin and 666.6 units of desoxyribonuclease per gram.

NURSING IMPLICATIONS

Reconstitute contents of vial with 10 ml sterile isotonic sodium chloride solution.

Solution must be freshly prepared before use. Loss of potency is delayed somewhat by refrigeration; however, solution must be used within 24 hours.

For maximal effectiveness: (1) dense eschars should be removed surgically before therapy is initiated; (2) accumulated necrotic debris must be removed periodically to ensure contact of medication with substrate; (3) dressing should be changed at least once daily, preferably two or three times daily.

Wound-dressing procedure requires careful aseptic technique.

Application of ointment: flush away necrotic debris and exudates with hydrogen peroxide, sterile warm water, or normal saline (as prescribed), and gently dry area. Apply thin layer of ointment and cover with vaseline gauze or other nonocclusive dressing (as prescribed).

Application of solution (wet-to-dry dressing method): (1) Mix vial of powder with 10 to 50 ml of saline. (2) Saturate fine mesh gauze or unfolded sterile gauze sponge with the solution. (3) Carefully pack ulcerated area with the saturated gauze. (4) Allow gauze to dry in contact with wound for 6 to 8 hours (as prescribed). (5) Wound is mechanically debrided when dried gauze is removed. (6) Repeat three or four times daily (as prescribed). After a few days, area usually begins to fill in with granulation tissue.

Solution may be applied as a gentle spray using a sterile conventional atomizer.
Note quality and amount of wound drainage and keep physician informed.
Manufacturer states that Elase is compatible with chloramphenicol, penicillin, streptomycin, and tetracycline. It is inactivated by plasma, serum, urea, and heat.
The dry powder is stable at room temperature (59 to 86°F). Note expiration date printed on package.

F

FLAVOXATE HYDROCHLORIDE

(Urispas)

(fla-vox'ate)
Smooth muscle relaxant, urinary antispasmodic

ACTIONS AND USES. Exerts spasmolytic (papaverinelike) action on smooth muscle. Reported to produce an increase in urinary bladder capacity in patients with spastic bladder, possibly by direct action on detrusor muscle.

Used for symptomatic relief of dysuria, frequency, urgency, nocturia, incontinence, and suprapubic pain associated with various urologic disorders.

ABSORPTION AND FATE. Following oral administration of a single 100-mg dose, 10 to 30% is excreted in urine within 6 hours.

CONTRAINDICATIONS AND PRECAUTIONS. Pyloric or duodenal obstruction, obstructive intestinal lesions, ileus, achalasia, GI hemorrhage, obstructive uropathies of lower urinary tract, use in children younger than 12 years of age, use during pregnancy and in women of childbearing potential. *Cautious Use:* suspected glaucoma.

ADVERSE/SIDE EFFECTS. CNS: headache, vertigo, drowsiness, mental confusion (especially in the elderly), difficulty with concentration, nervousness. **CV:** palpitation, tachycardia. **EENT:** blurred vision, increased intraocular tension, disturbances of eye accommodation, dry mouth and throat. **GI:** nausea, vomiting, abdominal pain, constipation (with high doses). **Skin:** dermatoses, urticaria. **Other:** dysuria, hyperpyrexia, eosinophilia, leukopenia.

ROUTE AND DOSAGE. Oral: 100 to 200 mg three or four times a day.

NURSING IMPLICATIONS

Because of the possibility of drowsiness, mental confusion, and blurred vision, advise patients to avoid driving or performing tasks that require mental alertness and physical coordination until reaction to drug is known.
Advise patient to report to physician adverse reactions and the lack of a favorable response.

FLECAINIDE

(Tambocor)

(fle-kay'nide)
Antiarrhythmic
Anesthetic (local)

ACTIONS AND USES. Local (membrane) anesthetic and antiarrhythmic with electrophysiologic properties similar to other Class I drugs (e.g., quinidine, procainamide, tocainide). Slows conduction velocity throughout myocardial conduction system, increases ventricular refractoriness but has little effect on repolarization. Prolongs His-ventricular (HQ) and QRS intervals at therapeutic doses. Clinically, flecainide causes both hypotension and negative inotropy (in higher dose ranges) and is an effective suppressant of PVCs and a variety of atrial and ventricular arrhythmias. Generally dose not alter cardiac function, but with IV administration, pulmonary capillary wedge pressure may be increased in patient with coronary disease.

Used in treatment of PVCs; atrial tachycardia and other arrhythmias unresponsive to standard agents (e.g., quinidine), Wolff–Parkinson–White syndrome, and recurrent ventricular tachycardias.

ABSORPTION AND FATE. Absorbed promptly and almost completely with 95% bioavailability. Peak plasma concentration after oral dose reached in 1½ to 3 hours. Minimal first-pass effect. Half-life: 7 to 22 hours, increased in patients with congestive heart failure or renal failure. 40% protein bound. Approximately 30% drug excreted in urine unchanged.

F

CONTRAINDICATIONS AND PRECAUTIONS. Compromised ventricular function congestive heart failure. *See also Tocainide.*

ADVERSE/SIDE EFFECTS. **After IV:** chest discomfort and tinnitus. *Also:* ataxia, leg cramps; blurred vision, transient conjunctival infection; nasal congestion; dizziness, sense of warmth, headache; nausea, oral paresthesia, dry mouth.

ROUTE AND DOSAGE. **Oral:** 200 to 300 mg every 12 hours. **Intravenous:** Initial: 1 mg, followed by 0.5 mg/kg every 30 to 60 minutes. Maximum dose: 2 mg/kg.

NURSING IMPLICATIONS

Effective serum concentration: 0.4 to 1.0 mcg/ml.

Food does not affect bioavailability.

Monitor closely for cardiac side effects during intravenous therapy.

In prolonged therapy, serum alkaline phosphatase may be mildly elevated *(normal serum alkaline phosphatase:* 1 to 4 Bodansky units/dl). Clinical significance unknown.

See Tocainide for additional Nursing Implications.

Drug Interactions: Flecainide

Plus	Interactions
Digoxin (Lanoxin) Propranolol (Inderal)	Increased serum levels of both drugs leading to increased toxicity potential, or more intensive drug effects

---

FLOXURIDINE

(FUDR)

(flox-yoor'i-deen)

Antineoplastic

Antimetabolite

ACTIONS AND USES. Pyrimidine antagonist and cell-cycle nonspecific. Catabolized to fluorouracil in vivo thus producing same systemic effects as fluorouracil (qv).

Used as palliative agent in management of selected patients with GI metastasis to liver. *See Fluorouracil.*

ADVERSE/SIDE EFFECTS. **CV:** myocardial ischemia, angina. **Dermatologic:** alopecia, dermatitis, pruritic ulcerations, rash. **GI:** stomatitis, diarrhea, enteritis, gastritis, esophagopharyngitis.

Other: ataxia, blurred vision, nystagmus, vertigo, convulsions, depression, euphoria, fever, hemiplegia, hiccups, renal insufficiency, gonadal suppression, photophobia, epistaxis. *See Fluorouracil.*

ROUTE AND DOSAGE. Intraarterial infusion (continuous): 0.1 to 0.6 mg/kg/day. Given by intraarterial infusion with appropriate infusion pump to overcome large artery pressure and to assure uniform rate of infusion. Higher dosages (0.4 to 0.6 mg/kg/day) required for hepatic artery infusion because of hepatic degradation of drug.

NURSING IMPLICATIONS

F

Drug is reconstituted with 5 ml sterile distilled water for injection.

Patient should be hospitalized at least during the initial course of therapy.

Examine infusion site frequently for signs of extravasation. If this occurs, stop infusion and restart in another vessel.

Therapeutic response will likely be accompanied by some evidence of toxicity. Supervise patient carefully to note onset of serious side effects, particularly those in the mouth. *See Mechlorethamine for nursing care of stomatitis and xerostomia.*

Therapy should be discontinued promptly with onset of any of the following: stomatitis, esophagopharyngitis, intractable vomiting, diarrhea, leukopenia (WBC under 3500/mm^3), or rapidly falling WBC count, thrombocytopenia (platelets 100,000 mm^3), GI bleeding, hemorrhage from any site.

Reconstituted solutions are stable at 2° to 8°C (36° to 46°F) for no more than 2 weeks.

Store drug at temperature between 15° and 30°C (59° and 86°F) unless otherwise directed by manufacturer.

Diagnostic Test Interferences. Floxuridine increases **serum alkaline phosphatase, bilirubin, SGOT, SGPT, LDH** levels. *See Fluorouracil for Drug Interactions.*

FLUCYTOSINE

(Ancobon, Ancotil, 5-FC, 5-Fluorocytosine)

(floo-sye'toe-seen)
Antiinfective
Antibiotic
Antifungal

ACTIONS AND USES. Fluorinated pyrimidine structurally related to fluorouracil. Precise mechanism of action poorly understood. Selectively enters fungal cell and is converted to fluorouracil, an antimetabolite believed to be responsible for antifungal activity. Conversion to fluorouracil in body of host is considerably less than in fungi.

Used in treatment of serious systemic infections caused by susceptible strains of *Cryptococcus* and *Candida. Unlabeled Use:* Treatment of chromomycosis.

ABSORPTION AND FATE. Rapidly and well absorbed from GI tract; widely distributed in body tissues and fluid, including aqueous humor and cerebrospinal fluid. Peak serum levels in 2.5 to 6 hours. Half-life: 3 to 6 hours (may be as long as 200 hours in renal failure). Slightly bound to plasma proteins. Minimally metabolized. Approximately 80% of dose is excreted unchanged in urine.

CONTRAINDICATIONS AND PRECAUTIONS. Safe use in women of childbearing potential, during pregnancy, and lactation not established. Extreme caution in impaired renal function, bone marrow depression, hematologic disorders, patients being treated with or having received radiation or bone marrow depressant drugs.

ADVERSE/SIDE EFFECTS. Hypoplasia of bone marrow: anemia, leukopenia, thrombocytopenia, agranulocytosis (rare); nausea, vomiting, diarrhea, abdominal bloating, enterocolitis, bowel perforation (rare); rash; elevated levels of serum alkaline phosphatase, SGOT, SGPT, BUN, and serum creatinine. Less frequently: confusion, hallucinations, headache, sedation, vertigo, hepatomegaly, eosinophilia.

ROUTE AND DOSAGE. Oral: Adults, children (weighing more than 50 kg): 50 to 150 mg/kg/day at 6-hour intervals (dosage modified in patients with renal dysfunction). **Children (weighing less than 50 kg):** 1.5 to 4.5 Gm/m² body surface in four divided doses/day.

NURSING IMPLICATIONS

Not to be confused with 5-FU.

Incidence and severity of nausea and vomiting may be decreased by giving capsules a few at a time over a 15-minute period.

Culture and susceptibility tests should be performed before initiation of therapy and at weekly intervals during therapy. Organism resistance has been reported.

Hematologic, renal, and hepatic function tests should be performed on all patients prior to and at frequent intervals during therapy.

Instruct patient to report fever, sore mouth or throat, and unusual bleeding or bruising tendency.

Frequent assays of blood drug level are recommended especially in patients with impaired renal function to determine adequacy of drug excretion (therapeutic range reported to be 25 to 120 mcg/ml).

Lower dosages and longer dosage intervals are recommended in patients with serum creatinine of 1.7 mg/dl or higher.

Monitor intake and output. Report change in intake–output ratio. Since most of drug is eliminated unchanged by kidneys, compromised function can lead to drug accumulation.

Duration of therapy is generally 4 to 6 weeks, but it may continue for several months.

Flucytosine is preserved in light-resistant containers at temperature between 15° and 30°C (59° and 86°F).

FLUDROCORTISONE ACETATE

(Florinef)

(floo-droe-kor'ti-sone)
Corticosteroid
Mineralocorticoid

ACTIONS AND USES. Long-acting synthetic steroid with potent mineralocorticoid and moderate glucocorticoid activity. Small doses produce marked sodium retention, increased urinary potassium excretion, and elevated blood pressure. If protein intake is inadequate, fludrocortisone induces negative nitrogen balance. Contraindications and adverse/side effects are same as for hydrocortisone (qv).

Used as partial replacement therapy for adrenocortical insufficiency and for treatment of salt-losing forms of congenital adrenogenital syndrome. *Investigational Use:* to increase systolic and diastolic blood pressure in patients with severe hypotension secondary to diabetes mellitus or to levodopa therapy.

ABSORPTION AND FATE. Has short duration of action. Half-life: 30 minutes.

ROUTE AND DOSAGE. Oral *(Addison's disease):* 0.1 mg daily (dosage may range from 0.1 mg three times a week to 0.2 mg daily). *Salt-losing adrenogenital syndrome:* 0.1 to 0.2 mg/day.

NURSING IMPLICATIONS

Concomitant oral cortisone or hydrocortisone therapy may be advisable to provide substitute therapy approximating normal adrenal activity.

Periodic checking of serum electrolyte levels is usual during prolonged therapy. Supplemental calcium and potassium chloride, as well as restricted salt intake, may be necessary during long-term therapy.

Monitor weight and intake–output ratio to observe onset of fluid accumulation, especially if patient is on unrestricted salt intake and without potassium supplement.

Instruct patient to report signs of potassium deficit (anorexia, paresthesias, drowsiness, muscle weakness, nausea, polyuria, postural hypotension, mental depression).

Patient may be advised to eat foods with high potassium content *(see Index: Food sources).* Consult with physician and dietician. A potassium supplement may be necessary.

Monitor and record blood pressure daily. If transient hypertension develops as a consequence of therapy, report to physician. Usually the dose will be reduced to 0.05 mg daily.

Store in airtight containers at temperature 15° to 30°C (59° to 86°F). Protect from light.

See Hydrocortisone (prototype glucocorticoid/mineralocorticoid)for additional nursing implications and drug interactions.

FLUNISOLIDE

(floo-niss'oh-lide)

(AeroBid, Nasalide, Rhinalar)

Corticosteroid
Glucocorticoid

ACTIONS AND USES. Modified steroid preparation with topical antiinflammatory and vasoconstrictor activity, structurally related to hydrocortisone. Exact mechanism of action not known. Glucocorticoid activity is more potent than mineralocorticoid action. Does not suppress hypothalamus–pituitary–adrenal function (HPA) except in excessive doses. Commercial preparations contain no propellant (fluorocarbon), which has been associated with excessive dryness of nasal mucosa.

Used for symptomatic relief of seasonal and perennial rhinitis in patients who have developed tolerance or poor response to conventional therapy. Also has been used for treatment of serous otitis media in children.

ABSORPTION AND FATE. Rapidly absorbed following nasal inhalation; about 50% reaches systemic circulation. Approximately 50% bound to plasma proteins. Biphasic half-life: initial: about 6 minutes; terminal: 1.8 hours. Rapidly metabolized in liver to active metabolites, 50% of which are excreted in urine and 50% in feces. Distribution to placenta and breast milk not known.

CONTRAINDICATIONS AND PRECAUTIONS. Hypersensitivity to any ingredients in the formulation: patients receiving systemic corticosteroids; use in children under 6 years. Safe use during pregnancy (category C) and in nursing women not established. *Cautious Use:* recent nasal ulcers, nasal surgery or trauma, active or latent tuberculosis (respiratory tract); untreated fungal, bacterial, or systemic viral infection; ocular herpes.

ADVERSE/SIDE EFFECTS. CNS: headache, dizziness. **ENT:** mild transient sensation of nasal burning or stinging (common), nasal congestion, sneezing, epistaxis or bloody nasal discharge, nasal irritation or dryness, sore throat, hoarseness, bitter taste, loss of taste or smell. **GI:** nausea, vomiting, abdominal bloating. **Hypersensitivity:** HPA suppression with excessive dosages, increase in SGOT (AST). **Other:** watery eyes; nasal septal perforation (rare; causal relationships not established), localized candidal infections.

ROUTE AND DOSAGE. Topical (intranasal): Adults: Initial: 2 sprays in each nostril twice daily. If needed, dosage increased to 2 sprays in each nostril three times daily. Maintenance: smallest effective dosage. **Children (6 to 14 years):** Initial: 1 spray in each nostril three times daily or 2 sprays in each nostril twice daily. Amount of drug delivered with each actuation of metered dose spray: 25 mcg. Maximum recommended dose also varies with product.

NURSING IMPLICATIONS

Topical nasal spray preparations of flunisolide are not intended for oral inhalation since safety of ingredients for use in mouth has not been determined.

Inform patient that maximum therapeutic effects are achieved by taking medication specifically as directed (prescribed dosage, intervals, and procedure). Review patient instructions provided by manufacturer with patient.

Have patient clear nasal passages of secretions before administering medication. Physician may prescribe supplemental therapy with a topical nasal decongestant and oral antihistamine for patients with blocked nasal passages, until symptomatic relief is provided by flunisolide.

Mild transient nasal burning or stinging occurs commonly (almost 45% of patients). If symptoms persist or increase in severity, notify physician. Discontinuation of therapy may be necessary.

Advise patient to notify physician if condition worsens, if sneezing, nasal irritation, or infection develops, or if no improvement is noted within 3 weeks.

Patients being transferred from prolonged systemic steroid therapy to flunisolide should be closely monitored. If done too rapidly, symptoms of cortiosteroid withdrawal (joint or muscle pain, lassitude, depression), acute adrenal insufficiency, or exacerbation of asthma may occur.

No clinically significant drug interactions or diagnostic test interferences reported.

Stored preferably between 15° and 30°C (59° and 86°F) in light-resistant containers, unless otherwise directed by manufacturer. Opened containers of flunisolide should be discarded after 3 months.

FLUOCINOLONE ACETONIDE

(floo-oh-sin′oh-lone)
Corticosteroid
Glucocorticoid

(Dermalar, Dermophyl, Fluoderm, Fluolar, Fluonid, Flurosyn, Synalar, Synalar-HP, Synemol, and others)

ACTIONS AND USES. Synthetic fluorinated steroid with strong antiinflammatory, antipruritic, and vasoconstrictive actions, but negligible mineralocorticoid effects. More effective than hydrocortisone (qv).

Used to relieve inflammatory manifestations of corticosteroid-responsive dermatoses.

CONTRAINDICATIONS AND PRECAUTIONS. Infants under 2 years of age; ophthalmic use. *See also Hydrocortisone.*

ADVERSE/SIDE EFFECTS. *See Hydrocortisone.*

ROUTE AND DOSAGE. Topical: applied in thin layer over affected area two to four times daily. Supplied as cream, ointment, and solution in 0.025% and 0.01% strengths. 0.2% cream should be used only for restricted periods, and quantity used per day should not exceed 2 Gm.

NURSING IMPLICATIONS

Protect drug from light.
See Hydrocortisone for nursing implications related to topical application.

FLUOCINONIDE

(Lidermol, Lidex, Lidex-E, Lyderm, Topsyn)

(floo-oh-sin′oh-nide)
Corticosteroid
Glucocorticoid

ACTIONS AND USES. Synthetic fluorinated glucocorticoid used only topically for antiinflammatory effects in glucocorticoid-responsive dermatoses. *See Hydrocortisone for absorption, fate, limitations, interactions.*

ADVERSE/SIDE EFFECTS. Burning, itching, hypertrichosis, dermatitis. *See also Hydrocortisone.*

ROUTE AND DOSAGE. Topical: apply thin layer of ointment, cream, or gel (0.05%) to affected area three or four times daily, or as needed.

NURSING IMPLICATIONS

See Hydrocortisone for nursing implications of topical application.

FLUORESCEIN SODIUM

(AK-Fluor, Fluorescite, Fluor-I-Strip, Fluor-I-Ful-Glo, Funduscein, Strip A.T.)

(flure′e-seen)
Diagnostic agent

ACTIONS AND USES. Mildly antiseptic fluorescent dye related chemically to phenolphthalein. Used as an aid in fitting hard contact lenses, applanation tonometry, detecting corneal epithelial defects, and testing potency of lacrimal system. Used intravenously as a diagnostic aid in retinal angiography. Also used as an antidote for aniline dye. Available in combination with benoxinate (Fluress).

CONTRAINDICATIONS AND PRECAUTIONS. Hypersensitivity to any component in the formulation; topical use in patients with soft contact lenses not recommended. *Cautious Use:* history of hypersensitivity, allergies, bronchial asthma.

ADVERSE/SIDE EFFECTS. *Topical use:* temporary stinging, burning sensation, conjunctival redness. *IV administration:* **CNS:** headache, paresthesias, dizziness, pyrexia, convulsions. **CV:** hypotension, transient dyspnea, acute pulmonary edema, basilar artery ischemia, syncope, severe shock, cardiac arrest. **GI:** nausea, vomiting. **Hypersensitivity:** urticaria, pruritus, angioneurotic edema, anaphylactic reaction. **Other:** thromobophlebitis at injection site, temporary discoloration of skin and urine following IV use, strong metallic taste following high dosage.

ROUTE AND DOSAGE. Topical: Solution (2%): instill 1 drop; have patient keep lids closed for 60 seconds. Manufacturer recommends irrigating to remove excess stain before observation. Strips: moisten strip with sterile water. Touch conjunctiva or fornix with moistened tip. Have patient blink eyes to distribute stain. **Intravenous:** *Retinal angiography:* **Adults:** 5

ml of 10% solution (500 mg) or 3 ml of 25% solution (750 mg) injected rapidly into antecubital vein. (Usually preceded by a test dose.) Drug should appear in central retinal artery in 9 to 14 seconds. **Children:** dose calculated on basis of 35 mg/10 pounds of body weight.

NURSING IMPLICATIONS

Surface eye defects absorb more fluorescein than intact tissue. Thus corneal abrasions or ulcerations appear green under normal light or bright yellow under cobalt blue illumination. Foreign bodies are surrounded by a green ring. Similar lesions in conjunctiva will appear orange-yellow. Aqueous humor (being more alkaline) will cause bright green fluorescence (useful for detecting wound leaks).

Fluorescein inactivates preservatives commonly used in ophthalmic preparations; therefore, solutions can be easily contaminated, particularly with pseudomonas. Unit-dose containers or individually wrapped filter paper strips impregnated with fluorescein offer greater assurance of sterility.

Avoid touching eyelids of surrounding area with eyedropper when instilling medication.

To fit hard contact lenses: Fluorescein is instilled with contact lenses in place. Patient should be instructed to blink several times to distribute dye. Under blue light, areas that lack fluorescein will appear black indicating that contact lens is touching cornea at these points.

To test for potency of lacrimal system: 1 drop of 2% solution is instilled into conjunctival sac. Instruct patient to blink at least 4 times. After 6 minutes nasal secretions are examined under blue light. Traces of dye in secretions indicate that nasolacrimal drainage system is open.

As an antidote for aniline dye (in indelible pencils): Following removal of pencil point, eye is irrigated with 2% solution every 10 minutes until visible precipitate is no longer present. Irrigations are repeated every 30 minutes for 12 to 24 hours.

Facilities for treatment of anaphylactic reaction should be immediately available, e.g., epinephrine 1:1000 for IV or IM use, an antihistamine, and oxygen.

IV administration may impact a yellowish-orange discoloration to skin and to urine. Skin discoloration usually fades in 6 to 12 hours; urine clears in 24 to 36 hours.

Fluorescein should be discontinued immediately if signs of sensitivity develop.

Solution container should be kept tightly closed when not in use.

Store at temperature below 80°F. Protect from light and freezing.

F

FLUOROMETHOLONE

(FML Liquifilm Ophthalmic)

(flure-oh-meth'oh-lone)
Corticosteroid
Glucocorticoid

ACTIONS AND USES. Adrenal cortical steroid with actions, contraindications, and adverse/side effects similar to those of hydrocortisone (qv).

Used topically in management of glucocorticoid-responsive ocular inflammations.

ADVERSE/SIDE EFFECTS. Ophthalmic: increased intraocular pressure, especially in the elderly patient, corneal pathology; with excessive use: diminished visual field, optic nerve damage, cataracts, glaucoma exacerbation.

ROUTE AND DOSAGE. Ophthalmic: 1 to 2 drops 0.1% ophthalmic suspension three to four times daily.

NURSING IMPLICATIONS

Eye drops are not to be used for extended period of time.

Depress lacrimal duct after instilling eye drops. *See Index: Drug administration: eye drops.*

Caution patient to follow established dose regimen.

If visual acuity decreases or visual field diminishes, the patient should stop the drug and notify the physician.

See also Hydrocortisone (prototype corticosteroid).

FLUOROURACIL

(Adrucil, Efudex, 5-Fluorouracil, 5-FU, Fluoroplex)

(flure-oh-yoor'a-sil)
Antineoplastic
Antimetabolite

ACTIONS AND USES. Pyrimidine antagonist and cell-cycle nonspecific. Blocks action of enzymes essential to normal DNA and RNA synthesis, and may become incorporated in RNA to form a fraudulent molecule; unbalanced growth and death of cell follow. Has higher affinity for tumor tissue than normal tissue. Highly toxic, especially to proliferative cells in neoplasms, bone marrow, and intestinal mucosa. Low therapeutic index with high potential for severe hematologic toxicity. Both local and systemic administration cause increases in skin pigmentation. Is not intended as adjuvant to surgery, or for prophylaxis.

Used as single agent and in combination with other antineoplastics for palliative treatment of carefully selected patients with inoperable neoplasms of breast, colon or rectum, stomach, pancreas, urinary bladder, ovary, cervix, liver. Has been used orally in a small number of patients. Also used topically for solar or actinic keratoses and superficial basal cell carcinoma. *Unlabeled Use:* to induce repigmentation in vitiligo.

ABSORPTION AND FATE. Minimal absorption from topically applied preparation if skin is intact. Following rapid infusion, drug leaves plasma within 3 hours. Metabolized in liver; half-life (alpha phase): 10 to 20 minutes; (beta phase): up to 20 hours. 15% of unchanged drug is excreted in urine in 6 hours; 60 to 80% as respiratory carbon dioxide in 8 to 12 hours. Crosses blood–brain barrier. Distribution to placenta and into breast milk not known.

CONTRAINDICATIONS AND PRECAUTIONS. Poor nutritional status, pregnancy, myelosuppression. *Cautious Use:* major surgery during previous month, history of high-dose pelvic irradiation, metastatic cell infiltration of bone marrow, previous use of alkylating agents, men and women in childbearing ages, hepatic and renal impairment.

ADVERSE/SIDE EFFECTS. **GI:** anorexia, nausea, vomiting, stomatitis, esophagopharyngitis, medicinal taste, diarrhea, proctitis, paralytic ileus, GI hemorrhage. **Hematologic:** leukopenia, thrombocytopenia, anemia (common), eosinophilia. **Topical use:** local pain, pruritus, hyperpigmentation, burning at site of application, dermatitis, suppuration, swelling, scarring, toxic granulation. **Other:** (may be evidenced with parenteral and topical preparations): alopecia, nail changes or loss (rare); pruritic maculopapular rash (extremities and occasionally trunk); cardiotoxicity, mild angina to crushing central chest pain with ECG changes; photosensitivity, erythema, increased pigmentation, skin dryness and fissuring, epistaxis, photophobia, lacrimation, euphoria, insomnia, acute cerebellar syndrome (dysmetria, nystagmus, ataxia), severe mental deterioration.

ROUTE AND DOSAGE. Highly individualized. **Intravenous:** initially 12 mg/kg body weight daily for 4 successive days; not to exceed 800 mg. If no toxicity develops, 6 mg/kg on 6th, 8th,

10th, and 12th days, unless toxicity occurs. (Dosage is reduced for severely debilitated patients.) Discontinue at end of 12th day. *Maintenance:* If no toxicity, courses may be repeated at 1-month intervals following last IV dose. If toxicity occurs, single weekly dose of 10 to 15 mg/kg (no more than 1 Gm/week) may be given after toxicity has subsided. **Topical:** (solution: 1%, 2%, 5%; cream: 1%, 5%): *Actinic and solar keratosis:* apply twice daily for 2 to 4 weeks. *Superficial basal cell carcinoma:* apply two times daily for 3 to 6 weeks. (Only the 5% strength is recommended.)

NURSING IMPLICATIONS

Fluorouracil is to be administered only by or under the direct supervision of a physician experienced in cancer chemotherapy.

Hospitalization and strict supervision during the first course of therapy with 5-FU is necessary.

Avoid skin exposure and inhalation of drug particles.

Dose is determined by actual weight unless patient is obese, in which case ideal weight is used. Weigh patient under standard conditions and record weight every 3 or 4 days. Report unexplained gradual increase in weight.

Total and differential leukocyte counts should be determined before each dose is administered. Drug should be discontinued if leukopenia occurs (WBC below 3500/mm³) or if patient develops thrombocytopenia (platelet count below 100,000 mm³). Baseline and periodic checks of hematocrit and liver and kidney function test are also advised.

A dose sufficient to create mild toxicity (anorexia, vomiting) may be necessary to produce antineoplastic effects.

Establish a reference data base for body weight, intake–output ratio and pattern, food preferences and dietary habits, bowel habits, and condition of mouth.

This drug may be given without dilution by direct IV injection or by IV infusion with Dextrose 5% in Water and Sodium Chloride 0.9% as infusion vehicles. Rapid injections are more effective, but administration over a 2- to 8-hour period appears to reduce onset of toxicity.

Inspect injection site frequently; avoid extravasation. If it occurs, stop infusion and restart in another vein. Ice compresses may reduce danger of local tissue damage from infiltrated solution.

Commonly, leukopenic nadir is between 9 and 14 days after initial dose, but may be delayed as long as 20 days. Usually count is in normal range by 30th day. Monitor blood counts as indicators for design of patient care.

During leukopenic period (WBC below 3500/mm³) patient should be in protective isolation. Restrict visitors and personnel with colds or infections. Plan care so that patient's energy expenditure is at minimum.

Protect patient from trauma, unnecessary injections, and use of rectal thermometer or invasive tubing.

During thrombocytopenic period (7th to 17th day), watch for and report signs of abnormal bleeding from any source; inspect skin for ecchymotic and petechial areas.

Antiemetics may be ordered to alleviate nausea and vomiting. Monitor patient carefully if vomiting is intractable, and report to physician.

Indications for drug discontinuation: severe stomatitis, leukopenia (WBC below 3500/mm³ or rapidly decreasing count), intractable vomiting, diarrhea, thrombocytopenia (below 100,000/mm³), hemorrhage from any site.

Inform the patient of the importance of prompt reporting of the first signs of toxicity: anorexia, vomiting, nausea, stomatitis, diarrhea, GI bleeding.

F

Poor-risk patients and occasionally patients in fairly good condition may die from the severe toxicity characteristic of this drug.

Remissions are often short, lasting no longer than 5 to 6 months; some patients have received 9 to 45 courses of treatment over periods of time ranging from 12 to 60 months.

The maculopapular rash usually responds to symptomatic treatment and is reversible.

A skin lesion treated with topical fluorouracil heals without scarring in 1 to 2 months after cessation of therapy. Expected response of lesion to topical 5-FU: erythema followed in sequence by vesiculation, erosion, ulceration, necrosis, epithelialization. Applications of drug are continued until ulcerative stage is reached (2 to 6 weeks after initial application) and then discontinued.

Consult physician about pretreatment preparation of lesion, i.e., should previous drug applications be removed? How?

Use nonmetallic applicator or gloved fingers to apply medication. If unprotected fingers are used, wash hands thoroughly.

Even if absorption is minimal, systemic toxicity may follow use on large ulcerated area. Report symptoms promptly.

If occlusive dressing is used there may be inflammatory reaction on adjacent normal tissue; however, use of a porous gauze dressing for cosmetic purposes does not cause inflammatory changes.

Avoid application of cream or solution near eyes, nose, and mouth.

If skin area treated with topical medication fails to respond to treatment, a biopsy is usually done to rule out frank neoplastic disease.

Report disorientation or confusion observed in a patient on 5-FU. The drug should be withdrawn immediately. Symptoms may occur earlier in each subsequent course of treatment and increase in severity.

Periodic checks on liver and kidney function will be scheduled.

Urge the ambulatory patient to keep appointments for clinical evaluation.

Help the patient to design drug regimen to fit life style, and other concurrent drug regimens. Involvement with reasonable planning supports compliance.

Caution patient not to change dosage regimen, i.e., not to increase, decrease, or omit doses or change dosage intervals.

Inspect pressure areas daily (coccyx region, elbows, heels). Danger of skin breakdown is greatly increased in a patient with immunosuppression, myelosuppression, and inanition.

Caution patient to avoid exposure to sunlight or to ultraviolet lamp treatments. Protect exposed skin; if it is necessary to go outdoors, apply sun-screen lotion (SPF 12 or above). Avoid midday exposure. Photosensitivity usually subsides 2 to 3 months after last dose of the antineoplastic.

Photophobia and lacrimation are frequent side effects. If bothersome, report to physician. Dark glasses may be helpful.

If patient manifests difficulty in balance while ambulating, give assistance, and report symptom to physician promptly.

Facilitate discussion with patient about problem of gonadal suppression (which may be irreversible), and potential change in sexuality.

Contraception is advisable during 5-FU treatment. Advise patient to report to physician if she suspects pregnancy.

Prepare patient for alopecia, an expected transient toxic effect. Discuss plans for cosmetic substitution if patient desires; new hair growth usually begins within 6 to 8 weeks. *See Index: Nursing Interventions: alopecia.*

Maintenance of adequate nutrition is imperative. Work with dietitian and family to provide adaptations in dietary habits and patterns called for by the mild but troublesome symptoms that must be tolerated (e.g., anorexia, nausea, sore mouth).

Stomatitis, a reliable early sign of toxicity, often precedes the leukopenic period by days. Inspect patient's mouth daily. Promptly report cracked lips, xerostomia, white patches, and erythema of buccal membranes.

To help patient eat with comfort, ask physician for anesthetic solution to be swished in mouth before eating. *See Mechlorethamine for nursing care of stomatitis, xerostomia.*

Fluorouracil solution is normally colorless to faint yellow. Slight discoloration during storage does not appear to affect potency or safety. Discard dark yellow solution. If a precipitate forms, redissolve drug by heating to 60°C (140°F) and shake vigorously. Allow to cool to body temperature before administration.

Store drugs at temperature between 15° and 30°C (59° and 86°F) unless otherwise directed by manufacturer. Protect from light and freezing.

Diagnostic Test Interferences. Fluorouracil may increase excretion of **5-hydroxyindoleacetic acid (5-HIAA)** and decrease **plasma albumin** (because of drug-induced protein malabsorption).

Drug Interactions: Fluorouracil

Plus	Interactions
Myelosuppressive agents, other Radiation therapy	May enhance total effects necessitating dose adjustments

FLUOXYMESTERONE

(Android-F, Halotestin, Ora-Testryl)

(floo-ox-ee-mess′te-rone)
Androgen
Anabolic

ACTIONS AND USES. Short-acting orally effective halogenated derivative of testosterone (qv) with up to five times the androgenic-anabolic activity of methyltestosterone. Has hypercholesterolemic effect; causes minimum retention of sodium; thus hypertension and edema rarely complicate therapy. Reduces nitrogen, potassium, and calcium excretion and promotes recalcification of osseous metastases and regression of soft-tissue lesions.

Used in both sexes to treat debilitating conditions (such as those associated with burns, paraplegia, prolonged corticosterone therapy, chronic malnutrition). In males, used as replacement therapy in conditions associated with testicular hormone deficiency. In females, used to antagonize effects of estrogen in androgen-responsive inoperable breast cancer. Available in fixed combination with ethinyl estradiol (Halodrin). *See Testosterone for absorption and fate.*

CONTRAINDICATIONS AND PRECAUTIONS. Severe cardiorenal disease or liver damage; nephrosis or nephrotic phase of nephritis; history of myocardial infarct; athletes; infants; women with advanced inoperable mammary cancer less than 1 year or more than 5 years postmenopause; pregnancy; lactation. *See also Testosterone.*

ADVERSE/SIDE EFFECTS. Jaundice (reversible), hepatocellular carcinoma, peliosis hepatitis, nausea, vomiting, diarrhea, symptoms resembling peptic ulcer, anaphylactic reactions (rare). *See also Testosterone.*

ROUTE AND DOSAGE. Oral: *(male hypogonadism and climacteric):* 2 to 10 mg daily (highly individualized); *Metastatic carcinoma of female breast:* 15 to 30 mg daily in divided doses; *(postpartum breast engorgement):* 2.5 mg when active labor has started, then 5 to 10 mg daily in divided doses for 4 to 6 days.

NURSING IMPLICATIONS

Administer drug with food to diminish GI distress.

Instruct patient to report priapism (symptom of overdosage) promptly; temporary interruption of regimen is indicated. Also advise patient to report persistent GI distress, diarrhea, or the onset of jaundice.

Explain to female patient on drug for palliation of mammary cancer that virilization usually occurs at dosage used. Give emotional support. Urge early reporting of voice change (hoarseness or deepening), increased libido (associated with clitoral enlargement), hirsutism. Usually, stopping therapy will end further development of symptoms but will not reverse hirsutism or voice change.

When used for palliation of mammary cancer, subjective effects of therapy may not be experienced for about 1 month; objective symptoms may be delayed for as long as 3 months.

Anabolic response may be evidenced by euphoria and gain in weight and appetite, especially in emaciated and debilitated patient.

Some products (e.g., Ora-Testryl) contain tartrazine which can cause allergic-type reactions including bronchial asthma in susceptible individuals. Frequently such persons are also hypersensitive to aspirin.

See also Testosterone (prototype androgen).

F

FLUPHENAZINE DECANOATE
(Prolixin Decanoate)
FLUPHENAZINE ENANTHATE
(Prolixin Enanthate, Modecate, Moditen Enanthate)
FLUPHENAZINE HYDROCHLORIDE
(Moditen Hydrochloride, Permitil, Prolixin)

(floo-fen'a-zeen)
Psychotropic
Antipsychotic; neuroleptic
Phenothiazine

ACTIONS AND USES. Potent piperazine derivative of phenothiazine. Similar to other phenothiazines, with the following exceptions: more potent on weight basis, higher incidence of extrapyramidal complications, and lower frequency of sedative and hypotensive effects. Has weak antiemetic and anticholinergic actions. The hydrochloride has more rapid action and shorter duration of action and thus may be used initially to determine the patient's response or to establish appropriate dosage. The decanoate and enanthate forms are indicated primarily for maintenance therapy in patients who cannot be relied on to take daily oral formulations. *See Chlorpromazine.*

Used for management of manifestations of psychotic disorders.

ABSORPTION AND FATE. Onset of action following subcutaneous or IM injection of fluphenazine decanoate or enanthate occurs in 24 to 72 hours; peak antipsychotic effect in 48 to 96 hours; duration of effect 4 weeks or longer for decanoate, 1 to 3 weeks for enanthate. Following oral or IM administration of the hydrochloride, onset of action occurs within 1 hour; duration of action is 6 to 8 hours. Metabolized in liver; crosses placenta; appears in breast milk.

CONTRAINDICATIONS AND PRECAUTIONS. Known hypersensitivity to fluphenazine; subcortical brain damage, comatose or severely depressed states, blood dyscrasias, or hepatic disease. Safe use in women of childbearing potential and during pregnancy or lactation not established. Parenteral form not recommended for children under 12 years of age. *Cautious Use:* hypersensitivity to other phenothiazines; use of anticholinergic agents, other CNS depressants; elderly patients, previously diagnosed breast cancer, cardiovascular diseases, pheochromocytoma, history of convulsive disorders, patients exposed to extreme heat or phosphorous insecticides, peptic ulcer, respiratory impairment. *See also Chlorpromazine.*

ADVERSE/SIDE EFFECTS. CV: tachycardia, hypotension. **GI:** xerostomia, nausea, epigastric pain, constipation, fecal impaction, cholecystatic jaundice. **GU:** urinary retention, polyuria, inhibition of ejaculation. **Hematologic:** transient leukopenia, agranulocytosis. **Neurologic:** drowsiness, dizziness, headache, mental depression, catatonic-like state, extrapyramidal symptoms, impaired thermoregulation, grand mal seizures. **Other:** SLE-like syndrome, contact dermatitis, peripheral edema, nasal congestion, blurred vision, increased intraocular pressure, photosensitivity, "silent pneumonia," hyperprolactinemia. *See also Chlorpromazine.*

ROUTE AND DOSAGE. Adult: Oral *(hydrochloride):* 0.5 to 2.5 mg one to four times daily, maximum 20 mg daily. **Intramuscular** *(hydrochloride):* 1.25 to 2.5 mg every 6 to 8 hours as necessary and tolerated. Usual upper limit: 10 mg daily. *(Decanoate, enanthate)* **Subcutaneous: 12.5 to 25 mg, repeated in 1 to 3 weeks. Usual upper limit: 100 mg/dose. Children (12 years and older):** adult dose. **Elderly, debilitated:** initial dose: 1 to 2.5 mg daily; increased gradually as needed and tolerated. **Elixir:** 2.5 mg/ml. **Oral solution:** 5 mg/ml.

F

NURSING IMPLICATIONS

Extended release tablet should be swallowed whole (not recommended for children).

Dilute oral concentrate in fruit juice, water, carbonated beverage, milk, soup; avoid coffee or tea as diluent.

Persons preparing oral concentrate or liquid preparations for injection should be careful not to contact skin or clothing with drug. Warn patient to avoid spilling drug. If skin is contacted it should be rinsed promptly with warm water.

Antacids diminish absorption, therefore, administer oral preparations at least 1 hour before or 1 hour after the antacid.

Advise patient not to alter dosage regimen or stop it abruptly. Caution not to give the drug to any other person.

Dry syringe and needle (at least 21 gauge) should be used when administering fluphenazine decanoate or enanthate (both are in a sesame oil vehicle). Moisture may cause solution to become cloudy.

Note that parenteral fluphenazine hydrochloride is given by IM route only.

Mental depression and extrapyramidal symptoms *(see Chlorpromazine)* occur with high frequency, particularly with long-acting forms (decanoate and enanthate). Be alert for appearance of acute dystonic reactions: abnormal posturing, torticollis, grimacing, fine tremor, oculogyric crisis.

The physician should give approval before patient self-doses with OTC drugs.

Since both decanoate and enanthate formulations have a long duration of action, early detection of adverse effects is critically important. Patient should inform the physician promptly if the following symptoms appear: light-colored stools, changes in vision, sore throat, fever, cellulitis, rash, any interference with volitional movement.

Control environment temperature; patient may be unable to adjust to extremes. If patient complains of being cold even at average room temperature, heed complaints and furnish additional clothing or blankets if necessary. Do not apply heating pad or hot water bottles. A severe burn may result because of depressed conditioned avoidance behaviors.

Extended exposure to high environmental temperature, to sun's rays, or to a high fever associated with serious illness places this patient at risk for heat stroke. Be alert to signs: red, dry, hot skin; full, bounding pulse, dilated pupils, dyspnea, mental confusion, elevated blood pressure, temperature over 40.6°C (105°F). Inform physician and institute measures to reduce body temperature rapidly.

Warn patient to avoid exposure to sun especially during hours of 10 AM to 2 PM: also, to wear protective clothing and cover exposed skin surfaces with sun screen lotion (SPF above 12). Photosensitivity is a fairly common side effect for the person on long-term therapy.

Renal function should be monitored in patients on long-term treatment. The drug should be discontinued if *BUN* is elevated (*normal:* 10 to 20 mg/dl). Blood studies, hepatic function tests, and ophthalmologic examinations should also be performed periodically.

Monitor blood pressure during early therapy. Hypotension is rarely a problem, however, fluctuations in BP have occurred in some patients. If systolic drop is more than 20 mm Hg, inform physician.

F

It has been reported that although the patient is not responsive during acute catatonia (side effect) everything that happens during the episode can be recalled.

Monitor intake–output ratio and bowel elimination pattern. Check for abdominal distention and pain. Encourage adequate food and fluid intake as prophylaxis for constipation and for xerostomia. The depressed patient may not seek help for either of these conditions, or for urinary retention.

Patients on large doses who undergo surgery, and those with cerebrovascular, cardiac, or renal insufficiency are especially prone to hypotensive effects.

Caution patient against driving motor vehicle or other hazardous activities until reaction to the drug is known.

Alcohol should be avoided while patient is on fluphenazine therapy.

Inform patient that fluphenazine may discolor urine pink to red or reddish brown.

Some products (e.g., Prolixin tablets) contain tartrazine which can cause an allergic reaction including bronchial asthma in susceptible individuals. Frequently such persons are also sensitive to aspirin.

All preparations of fluphenazine should be protected from light and from freezing. Solutions may safely vary in color from almost colorless to light amber. Discard dark or otherwise discolored solutions.

Store in tightly closed container at temperature between 15° and 30°C (59° and 86°F) unless otherwise specified by manufacturer.

See Chlorpromazine (prototype phenothiazine).

FLURANDRENOLIDE

(flure-an-dren'oh-lide)

(Cordran, Cordran SP, Drenison)

Corticosteroid
Glucocorticoid

ACTIONS AND USES. Topical fluorinated steroid with substituted 17-hydroxyl group. Crosses skin cell membranes, complexes with nuclear DNA, and stimulates synthesis of enzymes thought to be responsible for antiinflammatory effects. Also has antipruritic and vasoconstrictive properties. Systemic absorption leads to actions, limitations, and drug interactions of hydrocortisone, prototype for corticosteroids (qv).

Used for relief of pruritis and inflammatory manifestations of corticosteroid-responsive dermatoses.

ABSORPTION AND FATE. Resistant to metabolism by skin. Repeated applications lead to depot effects on skin, resulting in increased potential for systemic absorption and more severe side effects.

CONTRAINDICATIONS AND PRECAUTIONS. Hypersensitivity to any component, fungal infections, tuberculosis of skin, herpes simplex, vaccinia, varicella, in ear if drum is perforated, impaired circulation to the part being treated, ophthalmic use, application to face and intertriginous areas or to weeping or exudative surfaces; concomitant use with more potent steroids, pregnancy. *Cautious Use:* application to large surface areas, prolonged use, occlusive dressings, application to scrotal, vulval, perineal areas.

ADVERSE/SIDE EFFECTS. (Especially with occlusive dressings): burning, itching, irritation, dryness, folliculitis, hypertrichosis, hypopigmentation, allergic contact dermatitis, acneiform eruptions, perioral dermatitis, skin maceration and atrophy, secondary infection, striae, miliaria (cutaneous changes associated with sweat retention); cataracts and glaucoma (prolonged application around eyes); purpura (on diffusedly atrophied skin), photosensitivity. Adrenal suppression, in adults: Cushing's syndrome, hyperglycemia, glycosuria; in children (reversible): benign intracranial hypertension, development of Cushingoid features and edema, delayed linear growth and weight gain, low plasma cortisol, absence of response of ACTH.

F

ROUTE AND DOSAGE. Topical: Adults: Cream, lotion, ointment (0.025 to 0.05%): apply two or three times daily. Tape: (0.004 mg/cm^2): one or two times daily at 12-hour intervals. **Pediatric:** Ointment or cream: (0.025%) one or two times daily; 0.05%, once/day. Tape: once daily.

NURSING IMPLICATIONS

Discuss administration details with physician.

The ointment is usually indicated for dry, scaly skin, the cream and lotion are appropriate for moist lesions.

Always wash skin before applying flurandrenolide to prevent buildup of drug on skin surface. Do not use alcohol or alcohol base solutions to cleanse affected area. Lightly rub in the thin film of medication: avoid damage to skin surface. If area is hairy, shave or clip the hair and apply lotion or ointment directly to skin.

Occlusive dressings are not applied unless specifically prescribed.

If an occlusive dressing is to be used, apply a generous layer of cream or ointment, cover with a thin pliable plastic film then seal to skin with hypoallergenic tape.

Since a tight fitting diaper or one covered with plastic pants may serve as an occlusive dressing, it should be avoided if drug is to be applied to skin in diaper area.

Avoid use of occlusive dressing if skin surface is weeping or if exudative lesion is present.

Usually occlusive dressings are applied intermittently.

Use stockinette, elastic bandages, or gauze to hold dressing in place if adhesive materials are irritating.

Cordran tape is a flexible polyethelene film impregnated with flurandrenolide in the acrylic adhesive. It serves as an occlusive dressing and should not be applied to intertriginous areas or to exudative lesions.

Apply tape to clean and dry affected area. Remove carefully; it can strip the epidermis. It may also cause purpura in treated area.

Pediatric treatment for more than 2 weeks with tape, or with ointment or cream of potency of 0.05% should be evaluated carefully by the physician.

Children and infants are more susceptible to topical corticosteroid-induced adrenal suppression than adults because of a larger skin surface area to body weight ratio.

Close surveillance and periodic evaluation for evidence of systemic absorption are indicated when occlusive dressings are used, when patient is receiving long-term therapy, and when large areas of skin surface are covered with topical steroid.

If systemic absorption is noted, an attempt will be made to withdraw the drug by decreasing frequency of applications or by substituting a less potent steroid.

Topical corticosteroid therapy is terminated gradually to prevent withdrawal symptoms.

Occasionally steroid withdrawal symptoms (rebound inflammation, fainting, dyspnea, anorexia, hypoglycemia, hypotension, fever, weakness, arthralgia) develop even though medication dosage is gradually tapered.

Frequently inspect treated area for signs of exudation, infection, irritation, ulceration, hypersensitivity. If present, stop application of topical corticosteroid and notify physician.

If large surface area is covered with an occlusive dressing, check body temperature. (Thermoregulation may be impaired.) If temperature is elevated, discontinue use of topical corticosteroid.

The antiinflammatory action may mask signs of infection. Monitor treated areas carefully for presence of infection and apparent extention of inflammation. Report to physician. Usually the topical steroid will be withdrawn, and therapy with an appropriate antimicrobial agent will be started.

During long-term therapy because of danger of systemic effects it is advisable for patient to use contraceptive measures. If she suspects pregnancy, she should promptly consult the physician.

Advise patient to avoid exposure of affected areas to ultraviolet rays or to direct sunlight because of danger of photosensitivity.

Store formulations at temperature between 15° and 30°C (59° and 86°F). Protect from moisture, heat, freezing, or light.

F

FLURAZEPAM HYDROCHLORIDE

(Apo-Flurazepam, Dalmane, Novoflupam)

(flure-az′e-pam)
Psychotropic
Antianxiety (anxiolytic)
Hypnotic
Benzodiazepine
C IV

ACTIONS AND USES. Benzodiazepine derivative, with hypnotic activity equal to or greater than that produced by barbiturates or chloral hydrate. Mode and site of action not known but appears to act at limbic and subcortical levels of CNS to produce sedation, skeletal muscle relaxation, and anticonvulsant effects. Reduces sleep induction time; produces slight if any suppression of REM time (dream sleep) but marked reduction of stage 4 sleep (deepest sleep stage) while at the same time increasing duration of total sleep time. Significance of sleep alterations not understood.

Used as hypnotic in management of all kinds of insomnia; e.g., difficulty in falling asleep, frequent nocturnal awakening, and/or early morning awakening. Used also for treatment of poor sleeping habits.

ABSORPTION AND FATE. Rapidly absorbed from GI tract. Induces sleep within 20 to 30 minutes that lasts 7 to 8 hours. Widely distributed throughout body tissues. Elimination half-life of major metabolite 47 to 100 hours. Rapidly metabolized by liver. Excreted primarily in urine as active and inactive metabolites. Crosses placenta; appears in breast milk.

CONTRAINDICATIONS AND PRECAUTIONS. Known hypersensitivity to flurazepam; prolonged administration; intermittent porphyria, acute narrow-angle glaucoma, children under 15 years of age; pregnancy, lactation. *Cautious Use:* impaired renal or hepatic function, mental depression, psychoses, history of suicidal tendencies, addiction-prone individuals, elderly or debilitated patients, COPD.

ADVERSE/SIDE EFFECTS. CNS: residual sedation, drowsiness, lightheadedness, dizziness, ataxia, headache, nervousness, apprehension, talkativeness, irritability. Rarely: blurred vision, depression, hallucinations, nightmares, confusion, paradoxic reactions: excitement, euphoria, hyperactivity. **GI:** heartburn, nausea, vomiting, diarrhea, abdominal pain. Rarely: xerostomia, excessive salivation, bitter taste, swollen tongue. **Other:** chest pain, muscle and joint pain, genitourinary complaints. Rarely: granulocytopenia, leukopenia, shortness of breath, burning eyes, hypotension, sweating. **Overdosage:** severe sedation, disorientation, coma. *See also Chlordiazepoxide.*

ROUTE AND DOSAGE. Oral: Adult: 15 to 30 mg before retiring. **Elderly; debilitated patients:** 15 mg initially; increased as necessary and tolerated.

NURSING IMPLICATIONS

Capsule may be opened and contents swallowed with milk or water if patient cannot swallow it intact.

Hypnotic effect is apparent on second or third night of consecutive use and continues 1 or 2 nights after drug is stopped.

Excessive drowsiness, ataxia, vertigo, and falling occur more frequently in elderly or debilitated patients. Supervise ambulation. Bed rails may be advisable.

Warn patients that the drug may impair ability to perform hazardous activities such as driving a motor vehicle or operating machinery.

Advise patient to avoid alcohol. Concurrent ingestion with flurazepam causes an intensification of CNS depressant effects. Symptoms may occur even when alcohol is ingested as long as 10 hours after last flurazepam dose.

Caution patients about the possibility of additive depressant effects if combined with barbiturates, tranquilizers, or other CNS depressants.

Advise patient to seek approval from physician before self-dosing with OTC drugs.

The patient should understand that the drug is prescribed especially for patient. The patient should not change dose intervals or dosage. Instruct patient not to "loan" the drug, give it to another person, or use it for a self-diagnosed problem. Keep bottle out of the reach of children.

Discuss mental, physical, and environmental preparation for sleep with patient. Control sources of noise and remove cigarettes. Encourage patient to remain upright in bed (e.g., reading) for 20 to 30 minutes after taking the drug. This may help patient experience the onset of natural sleepiness.

Prolonged use of large doses can result in psychic and physical dependence. If patient has a history of drug abuse, monitor drug ingestion to prevent "cheeking," a maneuver to hoard or avoid drug ingestion.

Patient should be advised that if she becomes pregnant during therapy or intends to become pregnant she should communicate with her physician about the desirability of discontinuing the drug.

With repeated use, blood counts and liver and kidney function tests are advised.

Since insomnia is usually transient, the prolonged use of this hypnotic is inadvisable.

Subject to control under Federal Controlled Substances Act. Classified as Schedule IV drug.

Store in light-resistant container with child-proof cap at temperature between 15° and 30°C (59° and 86°F) unless otherwise specified by manufacturer.

See Chlordiazepoxide.

Diagnostic Test Interferences. Flurazepam may increase serum levels of total and direct **bilirubin** tests, **serum alkaline phosphatase, SGOT,** and **SGPT.** False-negative **urine glucose** reactions may occur with Clinistix and Diastix—no effect with Tes-Tape.

Drug Interactions. Concurrent use of flurazepam and **cimetidine** results in increased sedation. *See also Chlordiazepoxide (prototype benzodiazepine).*

FOLIC ACID

(Apo-Folic, Folacin, Folvite, Novofolacid, Pteroylglutamic Acid, Vitamin B_9)

Vitamin
Antianemic

FOLATE SODIUM

(Folvite Sodium)

F

ACTIONS AND USES. Member of vitamin B complex group essential for nucleoprotein synthesis and maintenance of normal erythropoiesis. Stimulates production of red blood cells, white blood cells, and platelets in patients with megaloblastic anemias. Folic acid is not metabolically active, but is reduced in body to the coenzyme tetrahydrofolic acid, which is involved in the 1-carbon transfer reactions in purine and thymidylate biosynthesis. In folic acid deficiency, impaired thymidylate synthesis results in the production of defective DNA that leads to megaloblast formation and arrest of bone marrow maturation.

Used in treatment of folate deficiency, macrocytic anemia, and megaloblastic anemias associated with malabsorption syndromes, alcoholism, primary liver disease, inadequate dietary intake, certain drugs, pregnancy, infancy, and childhood.

ABSORPTION AND FATE. Readily absorbed from small intestine (primarily proximal portion). Peak folate activity in 30 to 60 minutes, following oral administration. Largely reduced and methylated in liver to metabolically active folate forms. Distributed to all body tissues, with high concentration in cerebrospinal fluid. Enters enterohepatic cycle. Extensively bound to plasma proteins in patients with folic acid deficiency. Traces of unchanged drug excreted in urine with usual therapeutic doses, but large amounts eliminated following high doses. Excreted in breast milk.

CONTRAINDICATIONS AND PRECAUTIONS. Use of folic acid alone for treatment of pernicious anemia or other vitamin B_{12} deficiency states; use in normocytic, refractory, aplastic, or undiagnosed anemia.

ADVERSE/SIDE EFFECTS. Reportedly nontoxic. Rarely: allergic sensitization (rash, pruritus, general malaise, bronchospasm). Slight flushing and feeling of warmth following IV administration.

ROUTE AND DOSAGE. **Oral, subcutaneous (deep), intramuscular, intravenous:** *Therapeutic:* usual therapeutic dose for adults and children regardless of age: up to 1 mg daily. *Maintenance:* **Adults and children (over 4 years):** up to 0.1 mg daily; **children (under 4 years):** up to 0.3 mg daily. **Infants:** up to 0.1 mg daily. **Pregnant and lactating women:** 0.8 mg daily.

NURSING IMPLICATIONS

A careful history of dietary intake and drug and alcohol usage should be obtained prior to start of therapy. Drugs reported to cause folate deficiency include oral contraceptives, alcohol, barbiturates, methotrexate, phenytoin, primidone, and trimethoprim. Folate deficiency may also result from renal dialysis.

Folic acid can obscure diagnosis of pernicious anemia by alleviating hematologic manifestations of vitamin B_{12} deficiency while allowing irreparable neurologic damage to remain progressive.

Treatment of anemia with OTC vitamin preparations containing folic acid subject the patient with iron-deficiency anemia to needless expense and may delay early detection of pernicious anemia.

Normal serum folate levels have been reported to range from 6 to 15 mcg/ml.

Folates are present in a wide variety of foods; high sources include yeast, whole grain, bran, fresh leafy vegetables, asparagus, dried beans and lentils, nuts, and fruits. Approximately 50 to 90% of folate content is destroyed by long cooking or by canning.

The recommended daily allowances of folic acid are as follows: infants: 30 mcg; children: 100 to 300 mcg; adults: 400 mcg; during pregnancy 800 mcg; during lactation 500 mcg.

Therapeutic effects of folic acid therapy include a sense of well-being during first 24 hours of treatment, improvement in blood picture (reticulocytosis within 2 to 5 days, reversion to normoblastic hematopoiesis and eventually normal hemoglobin), gradual reversal of symptoms of folic acid deficiency (glossitis, diarrhea, constipation, weight loss, irritability, fatigue, restless legs, diffuse muscular pain, insomnia, forgetfulness, mental depression, pallor). Keep physician informed of patient's response.

Emphasize the need to remain under close medical supervision while receiving folic acid therapy. Adjustment of maintenance dose should be made if there is threat of relapse.

Folic acid injection should be protected from light.

Diagnostic Test Interferences. Falsely low serum erythrocyte **folate levels may occur with** *L. cassei* assay method in patients receiving antibiotics such as tetracyclines.

Drug Interactions. **Chloramphenicol** may antagonize hematologic response to folate therapy. Daily administration of 5 mg or more of folic acid may increase metabolism of **phenobarbitol** and also **phenytoin** and other **hydantoin** derivatives with resultant decrease in seizure control. Folic acid may inhibit antimicrobial effect of **pyrimethamine** and may worsen leukemic patients taking pyrimethamine.

FURAZOLIDONE

(Furoxone)

(fur-a-zoe'li-done)

Antiinfective, antiprotozoal
MAO inhibitor
Nitrofuran

ACTIONS AND USES. Synthetic nitrofuran with antibacterial and antiprotozoal properties. Acts by interfering with several bacterial enzyme systems. Bactericidal against majority of GI pathogens, including species of *Enterobacter aerogenes, Escherichia coli, Giardia lamblia, Proteus, Salmonella, Shigella, Staphylococcus,* and *Vibrio cholerae.* Also has MAO inhibitor action that is cumulative and dose-related (occurring after 4 or 5 days of therapy) and is thought to be due to a metabolite.

Used in treatment of bacterial or protozoal diarrhea and enteritis caused by susceptible organisms. Available in combination with nifuroxime (Tricofuron) for intravaginal treatment of vaginitis caused by *Trichomonas vaginalis, Candida albicans,* and *Haemophilus vaginalis.*

ABSORPTION AND FATE. Poorly absorbed from GI tract. Catabolic end products excreted in urine. About 5% excreted unchanged.

CONTRAINDICATIONS AND PRECAUTIONS. Hypersensitivity to furazolidone, concurrent use with alcohol, other MAO inhibitors, tyramine-containing foods, indirect-acting sympathomimetic amines; use in infants under 1 month of age. Safe use in women of childbearing age and during pregnancy or nursing mothers not established. *Cautious Use:* if at all, in patients with glucose-6-phosphate dehydrogenase (G6PD) deficiency.

ADVERSE/SIDE EFFECTS. GI: anorexia, nausea, vomiting, abdominal pain, diarrhea. **Hypersensitivity:** fever, arthralgia, hypotension, urticaria, angioedema, vesicular or morbilliform rash. **Other:** headache, malaise, hypoglycemia, intravascular hemolysis in patients with G6PD deficiency (reversible), agranulocytosis (rare).

ROUTE AND DOSAGE. Oral: Adults: 100 mg four times daily. **Children (5 years and older):** 25 to 50 mg four times daily; **(1 to 4 years):** 17 to 25 mg four times daily; **(1 month to 1 year):** 8 to 17 mg four times daily. Dosages should not exceed 8.8 mg/kg/day because of possibility of nausea and vomiting.

NURSING IMPLICATIONS

Nausea and vomiting occur commonly but may be relieved by reducing dosage. If symptoms persist, drug discontinuation may be necessary.

Bed rest and fluid and electrolyte replacement (as indicated) are important adjuncts to drug therapy. Consult physician regarding dietary allowances.

Advise patient and family member to record number of stools passed, fluid intake, and daily weight (useful criteria for determining fluid loss).

Examine patient and keep physician informed of signs of dehydration and electrolyte imbalance: decreased skin turgor, sunken eyes; dry, furrowed tongue, low blood pressure, diminished or irregular pulse, muscle or abdominal cramps.

Caution patient not to exceed prescribed dosage and to contact physician if diarrhea persists or worsens or if side effects develop. If satisfactory clinical response does not occur within 7 days, drug should be discontinued.

Since drug may cause hypoglycemia, diabetic patients will require close monitoring. Use glucose oxidase methods for urine testing, e.g., Clinistix, Diastix, Tes-Tape. *See Diagnostic Test Interferences.*

Faintness, weakness, and lightheadedness may be symptoms of hypersensitivity reaction or hypoglycemia and should be reported.

Food–Drug Interactions: Foods high in tyramine (e.g., aged and fermented food and drinks) may produce hypertensive reaction. Provide patient with list of high-tyramine foods *(see Index: Food sources).* Hypertensive crisis is most likely to occur when drug is continued beyond 5 days or when large doses are given.

Warn patients not to drink alcohol during furazolidone therapy and for at least 4 days after drug is stopped. Ingestion of alcohol may cause disulfiramlike reaction: nausea, sweating, fever, flushing, pounding headache, palpitation, tachycardia, drop in blood pressure, dyspnea, sense of chest constriction; symptoms may last up to 24 hours. If treatment of hypotension is required norepinephrine (levarterenol, Levophed) or other direct-acting adrenergic agent is used; indirect-acting agents, e.g., ephedrine, are contraindicated.

Drug history prior to therapy is advisable. Advise patient not to take OTC medications unless approved by physician. Nasal decongestants, cold and hay-fever remedies, appetite suppressants, and other medications containing indirect-acting amines expose patient to hazards of hypertensive reaction.

Patients with G6PD deficiency (e.g., patients of Mediterranean or Near East origin and blacks) should be closely followed by blood and urine studies for intravascular hemolysis: hematuria (pink or red urine), hemoglobinuria, hemoglobinemia.

Inform patients that drug may impart a harmless brown color to urine.

Possible causes of diarrhea should be investigated, e.g., contaminated foods or water, carriers, general sanitation. Fecal cultures from family members should be considered.

Preserved in tight, light-resistant containers (drug darkens on exposure to light). Protect from excessive heat.

Diagnostic Test Interferences. Furazolidone metabolite reportedly may cause false-positive reactions for **urine glucose** with copper sulfate reduction methods e.g., Benedict's reagent, Clinitest, and Fehling's solution.

Drug Interactions. A disulfiram like reaction may occur with **alcohol.** Concomitant use of **antihistamines,** other **MAO inhibitors, narcotics, sedatives, indirect-acting sympathomimetic amines** (e.g., amphetamines, cyclopentamine, dopamine, metaraminol, methylphenidate, pseudoephedrine), **ephedrine, phenylephrine,** and **tyramine** predispose to hypertensive reactions—combination generally avoided. Pharmacologic effects of levodopa (Dopar, Laradopa) may increase; combination generally avoided. Concomitant use with **tricyclic antidepressants** may cause toxic psychosis.

F

FUROSEMIDE

(Apo-Furosemide, Furoside, Lasix, Neo-Renal, Novosemide, Uritol)

(fur-oh'se-mide)
Diuretic (loop)
Sulfonamide derivative

ACTIONS AND USES. Rapid-acting potent sulfonamide "loop" diuretic and antihypertensive with pharmacologic effects and uses almost identical to those of ethacrynic acid (qv). Exact mode of action not clearly defined. As with ethacrynic acid, urinary pH falls after administration, but in some patients bicarbonate excretion may temporarily increase the pH. Renal vascular resistance decreases and renal blood flow may increase during drug administration. Inhibits reabsorption of sodium and chloride primarily in loop of Henle and also in proximal and distal renal tubules. Also enhances excretion of potassium, hydrogen, calcium, magnesium, ammonium, bicarbonate, and possibly phosphate. Reportedly less ototoxic than ethacrynic acid.

Used in treatment of edema associated with congestive heart failure, cirrhosis of liver, and renal disease, including nephrotic syndrome. May be used for management of hypertension, alone or in combination with other antihypertensive agents, and for treatment of hypercalcemia. Has been used concomitantly with mannitol for treatment of severe cerebral edema, particularly in meningitis.

ABSORPTION AND FATE. Well absorbed following oral administration; diuretic effect begins in 30 to 60 minutes, peaks in 1 to 2 hours, and persists 6 to 8 hours. Following IV injection, diuretic effect starts within 5 minutes (somewhat later after IM) and peaks in 20 to 60 minutes, with duration of 2 hours. Approximately 95% bound to plasma proteins. Small amount metabolized by liver. Rapidly excreted in urine, primarily as unchanged drug; approximately 50% of oral dose and 80% of IV dose are excreted within 24 hours. Small amounts excreted in feces. Crosses placenta; appears in breast milk.

CONTRAINDICATIONS AND PRECAUTIONS. History of hypersensitivity to furosemide or sulfonamides. Oliguria, anuria, fluid and electrolyte depletion states, hepatic coma; women of childbearing potential; pregnancy. *Cautious Use:* elderly patients, hepatic cirrhosis, nephrotic syndrome, cardiogenic shock associated with acute myocardial infarction, history of systemic lupus erythematosus (SLE), history of gout, patients receiving digitalis glycosides or potassium-depleting steroids.

ADVERSE/SIDE EFFECTS. CV: postural hypotension with excessive diuresis, acute hypotensive episodes, circulatory collapse, thromboembolic episodes. **Dermatologic:** pruritus, urticaria, exfoliative dermatitis, erythema multiforme (rare), purpura, photosensitivity, necrotizing angiitis (vasculitis). **Fluid and electrolyte imbalance:** hypovolemia, dehydration, hyponatremia, hypokalemia, hypochloremia, metabolic alkalosis, hypomagnesemia, hypocalcemia (tetany), hyperammonemia. **GI:** nausea, vomiting, oral and gastric burning, anorexia, diarrhea, constipation, abdominal cramping, acute pancreatitis, jaundice. **GU:** flank and loin pain, allergic interstitial nephritis, irreversible renal failure, bladder pressure or spasm, urinary frequency. **Hematologic:** anemia, leukopenia, aplastic anemia (rare), thrombocytopenic purpura, agranulocytosis (rare). **Ototoxicity:** tinnitus, feeling of fullness in ears, hearing loss (rarely permanent). **Other:** hyperglycemia, glycosuria, elevated BUN, hyperuricemia, acute gout (rare); increased perspiration; paresthesias; blurred vision, activation of SLE, muscle spasms, weakness; thrombophlebitis, pain at IM injection site.

ROUTE AND DOSAGE. *Edema:* **Adults: Oral:** 20 to 80 mg followed by second dose 6 to 8 hours later; if necessary, doses carefully titrated up to 600 mg daily. **Intramuscular, intravenous:** 20 to 40 mg, administered slowly over 1 to 2 minutes; may be increased by 20-mg increments every 2 hours, if necessary. High dose parenteral therapy is given by IV infusion at rate not exceeding 4 mg/minute. *Hypertension:* 40 mg twice daily PO. *Acute pulmonary edema:* 40 mg IV, slowly over 1 to 2 minutes; if necessary, increased to 80 mg within 1 hour. **Infants and Children: Oral:** 2 mg/kg body weight as single dose; if necessary, may be increased by 1 or 2 mg/kg not sooner than 6 to 8 hours after previous dose; maintenance dosage adjusted to minimum effective level. **Intramuscular, intravenous:** initially 1 mg/kg body weight; if necessary, dosage may be increased by 1 mg/kg not sooner than 2 hours after previous dose. Pediatric doses greater than 6 mg/kg by any route not recommended. Available in tablets, oral solution, injection forms.

NURSING IMPLICATIONS

Schedule doses to avoid nocturia and sleep disturbance (e.g., a single dose is generally administered in the morning; twice-a-day doses may be prescribed for 8 AM and 2 PM).

Intermittent dosage schedule is frequently used to allow time for natural correction of electrolyte and acid-base imbalance (e.g., drug is given for 2 to 4 consecutive days each week).

Hospitalization is recommended when therapy is initiated in patients with hepatic cirrhosis and ascites.

Frequent determinations should be made of blood count, serum and urine electrolytes, CO_2, BUN, blood sugar, and uric acid during first few months of therapy and periodically thereafter.

Patients receiving the drug parenterally should be observed carefully and blood pressure and vital signs closely monitored. Sudden death from cardiac arrest has been reported. Parenteral administration should be replaced by oral administration when practical.

Infusion rate will be prescribed by physician and should be checked frequently (generally the rate should not exceed 4 mg/minute to avoid ototoxicity).

Close observation of the elderly patient is particularly essential during period of brisk diuresis. Sudden alteration in fluid and electrolyte balance may precipitate adverse reactions: anorexia, nausea, vomiting, thirst, dry mouth, confusion, weakness, fatigue, lightheadedness, dizziness, perspiration, muscle cramps, bladder spasm, and urinary frequency. Report onset of these symptoms to physician. *See also Index: Nursing Interventions: for symptoms of specific electrolyte depletion state.*

Monitor intake–output ratio. Report decrease in output, excessive diuresis, or diarrhea.

The sorbitol (flavoring agent) used in oral preparations may cause diarrhea, especially in children receiving high doses.

Weigh patient daily under standard conditions. Rapid and excessive weight loss (from vigorous diuresis) can induce dehydration and acute hypotensive episodes.

Monitor blood pressure during periods of diuresis and through period of dosage adjustment.

Excessive dehydration is most likely to occur in the elderly, in those with chronic cardiac disease on prolonged salt restriction, or in those receiving sympatholytic agents. Resultant hypovolemia may lead to vascular thrombi and emboli (from hemoconcentration) or circulatory collapse.

Consult physician regarding allowable salt and fluid intake. To prevent hyponatremia and hypochloremia, salt intake is generally liberalized in most patients. Patients with cirrhosis usually require at least moderate salt restriction.

Patients receiving high doses or other antihypertensive drugs concurrently are subject to episodes of postural hypotension usually experienced as lightheadedness, dizziness, weakness, lethargy. (Dosage of other agents is generally reduced by at least 50% when furosemide is added to regimen.) Caution patient to make position changes slowly, particularly from recumbent to upright position. Also advise against prolonged standing in one position, very hot baths or showers, and strenuous exercise in hot weather. Instruct patient to lie down or sit down in head-low position if faint or lightheaded.

To reduce or prevent potassium depletion, the physician may prescribe daily ingestion of potassium-rich foods (e.g., bananas, oranges, peaches, dried dates), potassium supplement, and intermittent administration of furosemide.

Be alert to signs of hearing loss, complaints of fullness in ears and tinnitus. Ototoxicity is usually associated with renal insufficiency, uremia, rapid IV injection of large doses, or concomitant administration of other ototoxic drugs.

Furosemide may cause hyperglycemia. Diabetic and diabetic-prone individuals and patients with decompensated hepatic cirrhosis require careful monitoring of urine and blood glucose.

Acute gout can occur in susceptible patients. Advise patient to report onset of joint redness, swelling, or pain.

Oral solution contains *tartrazine* which may cause an allergic-type reaction including bronchial asthma in susceptible patients. The reaction occurs commonly in individuals with aspirin hypersensitivity.

Advise patient to avoid prolonged exposure to direct sunlight. A sunscreen agent may be advisable.

Oral furosemide should be discontinued 1 week and parenteral furosemide 2 days before elective surgery.

Slight discoloration of tablets reportedly does not alter potency; however, injection solutions having a yellow color should be discarded.

Infusion solutions in which furosemide has been mixed should be used within 24 hours. Reportedly compatible with dextrose 5% in water, sodium chloride 0.9%, and Ringer's injection, lactated.

Protect syringes from light once they are removed from package.

Store tablets and parenteral solution at controlled room temperature, preferably between 15° and 30°C (59° and 86°F) unless otherwise directed by manufacturer. Protect from light.

Store oral solution in refrigerator, preferably between 2° and 8°C (36° and 46°F). Protect from light and freezing.

Diagnostic Test Interferences. Furosemide may cause elevations in **BUN, serum amylase, cholesterol, triglycerides, uric acid** and **blood glucose** levels, and may decrease **serum calcium, magnesium, potassium,** and **sodium** levels.

Drug Interactions: Furosemide

Plus	Interactions
Aminoglycoside antibiotics	Potentiation of ototoxicity
Antidiabetic agents	Furosemide may antagonize hypoglycemic effect of antidiabetic agents
Antihypertensives	Additive hypotension
Cephaloridine	Enhanced nephrotoxicity
Chloral hydrate	Increased vasomotor instability with flushing, sweating, BP fluctuations
Clofibrate (Atromid-S)	In patients with nephrotic syndrome: muscular pain and marked diuresis
Corticosteroids	Excessive potassium loss
CNS depressants, e.g., alcohol, barbiturates, narcotics	Potentiate orthostatic hypotension
Digitalis glycosides	Increased risk of digitalis toxicity because of excess K, Ca, and Mg loss
Diuretics	Excessive potassium loss with other potent diuretics
Indomethacin (Indocin)	Response to both drugs may be impaired
Lithium	Increased risk of lithium toxicity
Norepinephrine (levarterenol, Levophed)	Arterial response to norepinephrine may be somewhat diminished
Phenytoin (Dilantin)	Reduced GI absorption of furosemide
Salicylates	Increased risk of salicylate toxicity with high doses
Skeletal muscle relaxants (surgical), e.g., Succinylcholine, Tubocurarine	Enhanced neuromuscular blockade

G

GALLAMINE TRIETHIODIDE
(Flaxedil)

(gal'a-meen)
Skeletal muscle relaxant (nondepolarizing)

ACTIONS AND USES. Synthetic, nondepolarizing neuromuscular blocking agent (curariform drug). Similar to tubocurarine (qv) in actions, uses, contraindications, precautions, and adverse reactions. About 20% as potent as tubocurarine; reported to produce less ganglionic blockade and to have no histamine-releasing properties except in very high doses. Has parasympatholytic effect on vagus, and may cause tachycardia and occasionally hypertension.

Used as preanesthetic and intraanesthetic medication, for treatment of GI disorders, and to reverse neuromuscular blockade.

ABSORPTION AND FATE. Muscle relaxation peaks within 3 minutes, with duration of 15 to 20 minutes. Significantly bound to serum albumin. Excreted primarily unchanged in urine. Crosses placenta.

CONTRAINDICATIONS AND PRECAUTIONS. Hypersensitivity to gallamine or iodides, myasthenia gravis, impaired pulmonary or renal function, shock; patients weighing less than 5 kg, hyperthyroidism, hypertension, tachycardia, cardiac insufficiency, hypoalbuminemia. *See also Tubocurarine.*

ROUTE AND DOSAGE. Intravenous: 1 mg/kg body weight. Single dose not to exceed 100 mg. Highly individualized. May be repeated after 30 minutes at dose of 0.5 to 1 mg/kg.

NURSING IMPLICATIONS

Tachycardia occurs almost immediately after administration, reaches maximum within 3 minutes, and declines gradually to premedication level.

Patients with electrolyte imbalance, dehydration, or elevated temperature may be more sensitive to the effects of gallamine.

May be stored at room temperature, protected from light and excessive heat.

See Tubocurarine chloride (prototype skeletal muscle relaxant).

G

GEMFIBROZIL
(Lopid)

(gem-fi'broe-zil)
Antilipemic

ACTIONS AND USES. Lipid lowering agent closely resembling clofibrate (qv) chemically, pharmacologically, and clinically. Lowers elevated serum lipids primarily by reducing serum triglycerides. Decreases occur chiefly in very low-density lipoproteins (VLDL); low-density lipoproteins (LDL) may also be lowered, but to a smaller extent. More effective than clofibrate in increasing serum levels of high-density lipoproteins (HDL). In theory HDLs help to inhibit the arteriosclerotic process by removing excess cholesterol from artery walls and transporting it to liver for catabolism and excretion. Mechanism of action, not completely known. Inhibits peripheral lipolysis, and by reducing hepatic extraction of free fatty acids interferes with production of triglycerides. Also appears to decrease hepatic production of VLDL by reducing incorporation of long-chain fatty acids into newly formed triglycerides and by inhibiting synthesis of VLDL carrier apoprotein. Gemfibrozil may not affect normally occurring seasonal variations in serum lipids (higher in midwinter and late summer; lower in fall and spring). Because gemfibrozil, like clofibrate, may increase cholesterol excretion into bile, the risk for developing cholelithiasis is believed to be the same for both. It is also possible that other complications associated with clofibrate may pertain to gemfibrozil. In common with clofibrate, inhibits platelet aggregation.

Used for patients with very high serum triglyceride levels (type IV hyperlipoproteinemia) who have not responded adequately to dietary control and who are at risk of pancreatitis and abdominal pain. Also has been used for severe familial hypercholesterolemia (type IIa or IIb) that developed in childhood and has not responded to dietary control or other cholesterol-lowering drugs.

ABSORPTION AND FATE. Well absorbed from GI track. Peak plasma levels in 1 to 2 hours. Half-life: 1.3 to 1.5 hours. Portion of drug undergoes enterohepatic circulation. About 75% of dose excreted in urine primarily as unchanged drug; 6% excreted in feces.

CONTRAINDICATIONS AND PRECAUTIONS. Hypersensitivity to gemfibrozil; gallbladder disease, hepatic or severe kidney dysfunction. Safe use during pregnancy (category B), in nursing mothers, and in children not established. *Cautious Use:* diabetes mellitus.

ADVERSE/SIDE EFFECTS. CNS: headache, dizziness, blurred vision. **Dermatologic:** rash, dermatitis, pruritus, urticaria. **GI:** abdominal or epigastric pain, diarrhea, nausea, vomiting, flatulence. **Hematologic:** anemia, eosinophilia, leukopenia, hyperglycemia. **Musculoskeletal:** painful extremities. **Other:** causal relationship not established (viral or bacterial infection, fatigue, malaise, syncope, vertigo, insomnia, paresthesias, tinnitus, dry mouth, constipation, anorexia, gas pain, dyspepsia, cholelithiasis, cholecystitis, malignancy, postcholecystectomy complications, pancreatitis; cardiac arrhythmias, intermittent claudication), back pain, muscle cramps, myalgia, arthralgia, swollen joints; hypokalemia, increases in liver function tests.

ROUTE AND DOSAGE. Oral: 1200 mg/day in two divided doses, 30 minutes before morning and evening meal. Usual dosage range 900 to 1500 mg/day.

NURSING IMPLICATIONS

Instruct patient to take drug ½ hour before breakfast and evening meal.

The following laboratory tests should be performed initially and at regular intervals throughout therapy: serum LDL and VLDL, triglycerides, total cholesterol, complete blood counts, blood glucose, liver function tests.

Mild decreases in WBC, Hgb, Hct may occur during early stage of treatment, but these values generally stabilize with continued therapy.

Weight loss, diet therapy specific to the type of hyperlipidemia involved, no smoking, exercise, and regulation of alcohol intake should be the initial interventions in treatment of lipid disorders and should be used as adjuncts when drug therapy is introduced.

Collaborate with physician and dietitian regarding appropriate dietary restrictions. Patients with high serum triglyceride levels are generally advised to lose excess weight and to restrict carbohydrate and alcohol intake. For hypercholesterolemia (type II): LDL level and hence cholesterol may be lowered by avoiding foods containing cholesterol and saturated fatty acids, (e.g., meats, especially organ meats, eggs, whole milk, cream, butter, lard), and replacing with foods low in cholesterol and saturated fats: fish, poultry, vegetables, polyunsaturated oils and margarines.

Gemfibrozil should be discontinued if lipids fail to show a favorable response after 3 months of therapy.

Gallbladder studies are indicated if patient presents signs and symptoms suggestive of cholelithiasis or cholecystitis (right upper quadrant and epigastric pain frequently radiating to right shoulder blade, and generally associated with nausea, vomiting, and flatulence. Symptoms often occur during the night or early morning; jaundice may or may not be present).

Since gemfibrozil may cause blurred vision and vertigo, caution patient to avoid driving and other potentially hazardous activities until reaction to drug is known.

Store preferably between 15° and 30°C (59° and 86°F), unless otherwise directed by manufacturer.

Drug Interactions: Gemfibrozil

Plus	Interactions
Anticoagulants	Potentiation of anticoagulant effect Close monitoring of prothrombin time recommended

PROTOTYPE

GENTAMICIN SULFATE

(Apogen, Bristagen, Cidomycin, Garamycin, Garamycin Ophthalmic, Genoptic, Jenamicin, U-Genicin)

(jen-ta-mye'sin)
Antiinfective
Antibiotic
Aminoglycoside

ACTIONS AND USES. Broad-spectrum aminoglycoside antibiotic derived from *Micromonospora purpurea,* an actinomyces organism. By acting directly on bacterial ribosome, inhibits protein biosynthesis. Active against a wide variety of gram-negative bacteria, including *Pseudomonas aeruginosa, Proteus* species (including indole-positive and -negative strains), *Escherichia coli,* and *Klebsiella, Enterobacter,* and *Serratia* species. Also effective against certain gram-negative organisms, particularly penicillin-sensitive and some methicillin-resistant strains of *Staphylococcus aureus.* Cross-resistance and allergenicity with other members of aminoglycoside group thought to be possible. Has neuromuscular blocking action, in common with other aminoglycoside antibiotics.

G

Parenteral use restricted to treatment of serious infections of GI tract, respiratory tract, urinary tract, CNS, bone, skin, and soft tissue (including burns), when other less toxic antimicrobial agents are ineffective or are contraindicated. May be used in combination with other antibiotics. Also used topically for primary and secondary skin infections and for infections of external eye and its adnexa. *Investigational Use:* to control Meniere's disease.

ABSORPTION AND FATE. Rapidly absorbed following IM injection. Peak serum concentrations in 30 to 90 minutes; effective serum levels persist 6 to 8 hours. Administration of IV infusion over 2-hour period produces similar concentrations. Serum levels higher and more prolonged in patients with impaired renal function. Widely distributed to extracellular fluids. Poorly distributed to adipose tissue and to CSF even when meninges are inflamed. However, high CSF concentrations attained by intraventricular or intrathecal routes. Approximately 25% loosely bound to plasma proteins. Serum half-life about 1 to 2 hours. Excreted primarily in urine, largely as unchanged drug (excretion correlates with creatinine clearance). Slight absorption may occur following topical applications, especially with cream formulations. Crosses placenta.

CONTRAINDICATIONS AND PRECAUTIONS. Known hypersensitivity to gentamicin, concomitant use with other neurotoxic (ototoxic) and/or nephrotoxic drugs; myasthenia gravis. Safe use during pregnancy not established. *Cautious Use:* impaired renal function; topical applications to widespread areas; elderly, infants, and children.

ADVERSE/SIDE EFFECTS. **Allergic reactions:** rash, pruritus, urticaria, eosinophilia, burning sensation of skin, fever, joint pains, laryngeal edema. **Hematologic:** granulocytopenia, agranulocytosis, thrombocytopenic purpura, anemia. **Nephrotoxicity:** proteinuria, cells or casts in urine, rising levels of BUN, nonprotein nitrogen, serum creatinine; oliguria, decreased creatinine clearance, renal damage. **Neurotoxicity:** ototoxicity (vestibular disturbances, impaired hearing), optic neuritis, peripheral neuritis, numbness, tingling of skin, muscle twitching, convulsions. **Topical use:** photosensitivity, erythema, pruritus; burning, stinging, and lacrimation with ophthalmic use. **Other:** increased SGOT, SGPT, and serum bilirubin; decreased serum calcium; hypomagnesemia, increased or decreased reticulocyte counts; transient hepatomegaly, splenomegaly; superinfections; anorexia, nausea, vomiting, weight loss, increased salivation; headache, drug fever, lethargy; loss of hair and eyebrows; pulmonary fibrosis, hypotension or hypertension; local irritation and pain following IM use; neuromuscular blockade and respiratory paralysis (with high doses).

ROUTE AND DOSAGE. **Intramuscular, intravenous: Adults:** 3 to 5 mg/kg/day in three equal doses every 8 hours. (IV dosage is based on estimate of ideal body weight. Single IV doses diluted in 50 to 200 ml of isotonic saline or 5% dextrose in water for injection (not to exceed 1 mg/ml concentration) and administered slowly over 30 minutes to 2 hours.)

Children: 6 to 7.5 mg/kg/day in three equal doses every 8 hours. **Infants and neonates:** 7.5 mg/kg/day in three equal doses every 8 hours. **Premature or full-term neonates (1 week of age or less):** 5 mg/kg/day in two equal doses every 12 hours. Dosages must be adjusted for patients with impaired renal function. **Intrathecal: Adults:** 4 to 8 mg once *daily*. **Children, infants 3 months and older:** 1 to 2 mg daily. Only the 2 mg/ml intrathecal preparation *without* preservatives is recommended. **Topical:** 0.1% cream or ointment, applied gently to lesions three or four times daily. **Ophthalmic solution (0.3%):** 1 or 2 drops in affected eye every 4 hours. **Ophthalmic ointment (0.3%):** applied in small amount to lower conjunctival sac two or three times daily.

NURSING IMPLICATIONS

G

Culture and sensitivity tests should be performed initially and periodically during continued therapy. Drug is generally given for 7 to 10 days.

Renal function and vestibular and auditory function should be determined before initiation of therapy and at regular intervals during treatment, especially in the elderly and other patients with impaired renal function and in those receiving higher doses or longer treatment. Vestibular and auditory function should also be checked 3 to 4 weeks after drug is discontinued.

Ototoxic effect is greatest on vestibular branch of 8th cranial nerve (symptoms: headache, dizziness, nausea, and vomiting with motion, ataxia, nystagmus); however, auditory branch damage (tinnitus, roaring noises) may also occur. Hearing loss occurs particularly in high tone range and can be detected only by audiometer. Generally, conversational hearing range is not affected. Prompt reporting is critically essential to prevent permanent damage.

Drug plasma concentrations should be determined at frequent intervals for patients with impaired renal function. When peak plasma concentrations are monitored, dosage is adjusted to prevent prolonged levels above 12 mcg/ml. When trough concentrations are monitored, dosage is usually adjusted so that levels above 2 mcg/ml are avoided.

Physician may use creatinine clearance rate and serum creatinine concentration as guides to dosage scheduling when serum levels are not feasible (frequency of administration in hours is approximated by multiplying serum creatinine by eight).

Intake and output should be monitored. Consult physician about desirable intake; generally, patient is kept well hydrated during gentamicin therapy to prevent chemical irritation of renal tubules. Report oliguria and unusual change in intake and output ratio.

Be alert for signs of bacterial overgrowth (superinfection) with nonsusceptible organisms (diarrhea, anogenital itching, vaginal discharge, stomatitis, glossitis).

In treatment of urinary tract infections, concomitant alkalinizing agent may be prescribed to raise urinary pH above 7, since gentamicin is less active in an acidic medium.

Topically treated lesions may be covered with gauze, if necessary.

Systemic absorption and toxicity are possible when topical applications, particularly cream preparations, are made to large denuded body surfaces.

In treatment of impetigo contagiosa, individual crusts should first be removed (gently) to allow topical medication to contact infected site. Removal may be facilitated by soaking crusts with warm soap and water or by application of wet compresses. Consult physician regarding specific procedure.

Caution patients using topical applications to avoid excessive exposure to sunlight because of danger of photosensitivity. Also advise patient to withhold medication and to notify physician if signs of irritation or sensitivity occur.

Gentamicin is incompatible in a syringe or in solution with any other drug.

Store preferably between 15° and 30°C (59° and 86°F) unless otherwise directed by manufacturer. Do not use solution if it is discolored or contains a precipitate.

Drug Interactions. Possibility of additive nephrotoxic effects with combined use of gentamicin and **cephalosporins. Ethacrynic acid** and **furosemide** may enhance ototoxicity of gentamicin (and other aminoglycoside antibiotics). Concurrent use is usually avoided. Combined or sequential use of **other aminoglycoside antibiotics** with gentamicin increases the probability of ototoxicity and nephrotoxicity. **Antimotion-sickness drugs** may mask symptoms of ototoxicity. There is enhanced neuromuscular blockade with neuromuscular blocking drugs (e.g., **decamethonium, ether, succinylcholine, tubocurarine,** and related anesthetics). Activity of gentamicin is diminished significantly by **carbenicillin.** If concurrent administration is prescribed, they should be given about 1 to 2 hours apart. **Carbenicillin** may inactivate gentamicin when mixed together for IV infusion.

PROTOTYPE

GLIPIZIDE
(Glucotrol)

(glip'i-zide)
Antidiabetic agent
Sulfonylurea (second generation)

G

ACTIONS AND USES. Second-generation sulfonylurea hypoglycemic agent structurally similar to acetahexamide (first generation). Potency is enhanced by as much as 200-fold over first generation agents i.e., therapeutic dosage equivalents are: glipizide 5 mg = chloropropamide = 250 mg = tolazamide 250 mg = acetohexamide = 500 mg = tolbutamide 1 Gm (sulfonylurea prototype, qv). Glipizide directly stimulates functioning pancreatic beta cells to secrete insulin, leading to an acute drop in blood glucose. Indirect action leads to altered numbers and sensitivity of peripheral insulin receptors resulting in increased insulin binding. It also causes inhibition of hepatic glucose production and reduction in serum glucagon levels. Fasting insulin levels are not increased by long-term glipizide therapy; however, a postprandial insulin response lasting through the meal challenge continues to be enhanced for at least 6 months. Glipizide has no antidiuretic activity and has no effect on plasma lipoproteins in patient being treated for type II non-insulin dependent diabetes mellitus (NIDDM). Since loss of control when patient is being treated by diet alone may be transient, a short course of glipizide therapy may be adequate to restore control. It has not been established that this drug will prevent long-term cardiovascular and neurologic complications of diabetes mellitus.

Used as adjunct to diet for control of hyperglycemia in patient with type II diabetes after dietary control alone has failed; also used to treat transient loss of control in patient usually controlled well on diet.

ABSORPTION AND FATE. Following oral administration drug is completely absorbed (with food, absorption is delayed by about 0.5 hours). Peak plasma concentration achieved in 1 to 3 hours after a single dose; duration of action (blood glucose control) up to 24 hours. 92 to 99% protein-bound by nonionic bonds; extensive hepatic metabolism (primary metabolites are inactive). Half-life: 2 to 4 hours. Excreted mainly by renal route but some excretion is via bile (feces).

CONTRAINDICATIONS AND PRECAUTIONS. Hypersensitivity to glipizide, diabetic ketoacidosis with or without coma; pregnancy (category B), nursing mothers. Safe use in children not established. *Cautious Use:* impaired renal and hepatic function, the elderly, debilitated, malnourished patient; patient with adrenal or pituitary insufficiency.

ADVERSE/SIDE EFFECTS. Dermatologic: erythema, morbilliform or maculopapular rash, pruritus, urticaria, eczema (transient), porphyria cutanea tarda, photosensitivity reactions. **GI:** nausea, diarrhea, constipation, gastralgia, cholestatic jaundice (rare). **Hematologic:** leukopenia, thrombocytopenia, hemolytic anemia, aplastic anemia, agranulocytosis, pancytopenia. **Metabolic:** hepatic porphyria; disulfiram-like reactions (rare). **Other** (transient): drowsiness, headache. **Overdosage:** hypoglycemia (mild): fatigue, drowsiness, hunger, GI distress (heartburn, abdominal pain, anorexia), headache, anxiety; (severe): visual disturbances, ataxia, confusion, tachycardia, seizures, coma.

ROUTE AND DOSAGE. (Regimen is individualized) **Oral:** recommended initial dose: 5 mg 30 minutes before breakfast (2.5 mg for geriatric patient or patient with hepatic disease). Dosage is adjusted with increments of 2.5 to 5 mg dependent on blood glucose response, but no sooner than 1 or 2 weeks to allow reaching steady-state serum levels and full pharmacologic effect. Maximum once-daily dose: 15 mg. Doses above 15 mg should ordinarily be divided and given before meals. Doses above 30 mg have been safely given on a twice-a-day schedule for long-term therapy. Maximum recommended total daily dose: 40 mg.

NURSING IMPLICATIONS

Glipizide is not effective as sole therapy for patients with type I diabetes mellitus; these patients require insulin.

Take ½ hour before a meal to give best protection against postprandial hyperglycemia.

Glipizide is prescribed after control of blood glucose by diet alone has failed. Inform the patient that glipizide treatment accompanies (does not substitute for) continued control of diet and (if patient is obese) a weight-loss program.

Urine testing: When diabetes is stabilized, patient is advised to test urine for glucose (using Chemstrip UG, or other similar test strip) 2 hours after each meal.

If urine test is positive for glucose for 2 or 3 days, then patient is usually advised to check for urine ketones (with Chemstrip UGK) and report to physician. Urine should be tested for ketones also, when patient has an illness or is subjected to stress such as surgery.

Capillary glucose testing is encouraged for the patient on a sulfonylurea.

At the beginning of the treatment program, the patient should be checked for cardiovascular risk factors, and if necessary corrective measures should be instituted.

Severe drug-induced skin rashes and pruritus may necessitate discontinuation of drug use. Symptoms usually subside rapidly when drug is withdrawn.

Inform patient about the importance of exercise as a part of the total control program. Plan this treatment adjunct specifically, with guidance from the physician.

The initial dose and establishment of a maintenance regimen in the elderly or debilitated patient is approached both conservatively and gradually. Close observation for early signs of hypoglycemia (easily overlooked—*see Adverse/Side Effects)* is paramount.

Usually 5 to 7 days are allowed to elapse between titration steps. If response to a single dose is unsatisfactory, the dose may be divided.

Advise patient on glipizide who wishes to become pregnant that a transfer to insulin for blood glucose control is recommended by many clinicians.

If glipizide is used during pregnancy, it is discontinued at least 1 month before the expected delivery date to prevent prolonged severe hypoglycemia (4 to 10 days) in the neonate.

The potential for hypoglycemia in nursing infants presents the necessity to decide whether to discontinue nursing or to temporarily transfer to insulin (if diet alone is inadequate for blood sugar control).

Transfer of a patient from insulin to glipizide: accomplished according to the following guidelines:

- If insulin daily requirement is 20 units or less: discontinue insulin and start glipizide at usual dosages with titration steps at intervals of 5 to 7 days.
- If insulin daily requirement is more than 20 units: reduce insulin dose by 50% and start glipizide at usual doses. (Subsequent reduction of insulin depends on patient response.) Titration steps as above.

During insulin withdrawal period, urine tests for sugar and ketone bodies should be checked at least three times daily. Advise patient to contact the physician if tests are abnormal.

The patient receiving insulin in doses more than 40 units/day is usually hospitalized during period of transfer to a sulfonylurea.

If the patient is being transferred from one to another sulfonylurea, no transition period is necessary. However, the patient who is transferred from one with a long half-life (e.g., chlorpropamide: half-life: 30 to 40 hours) must be observed for hypoglycemic responses for 1 to 2 weeks because of potential overlapping of drug effect.

When a drug that affects the hypoglycemic action of sulfonylureas *(see Drug Interactions)* is withdrawn or added to the glipizide regimen the patient should be alerted to the added danger of loss of control (hyperglycemia). Urine and blood glucose tests and test for ketone bodies should be carefully monitored and possibly increased in frequency for several days to determine if antidiabetic drug dose adjustment is indicated.

Keep in mind that if the patient is also receiving a beta adrenergic blocking agent (suppresses reflex tachycardia) or is elderly, the first signs of hypoglycemia may be hard to detect.

In the diabetic patient, hypoglycemia is a potential effect of the following situations: after severe or prolonged exercise, after alcohol ingestion, when caloric intake is deficient, when more than one glucose lowering drug is being used.

Be alert to the danger of loss of control of diabetes which may result from stress such as fever, surgery, trauma, infection. Blood and urine glucose and ketone body detection may need to be checked more frequently during these stress periods, and transfer from the sulfonylurea to insulin may be necessary.

Advise patient and/or primary care provider to observe for signs of cholestatic jaundice (yellow sclera, dark urine, pruritus). If they occur, inform the physician promptly. The drug may have to be discontinued and replaced by another antidiabetic agent.

Treatment of overdosage: Mild hypoglycemia (reaction without loss of consciousness of neurologic symptoms) is treated with oral glucose and adjustment of dosage and meal pattern. The patient should be closely monitored for at least 5 to 7 days to assure reestablishment of safe control. Severe hypoglycemia (reaction with coma, seizure or other neurological manifestations) requires emergency hospitalization to permit rapid IV injection of concentrated (50%) glucose solution. This will be followed by continuous infusion of 10% glucose solution at a rate adequate to maintain a blood glucose level above 100 mg/dl.

Monitor patient for 24 to 48 hours because hypoglycemia may recur after apparent clinical recovery.

Store in tightly closed light resistant container at a temperature 15° to 30°C (59° to 86°F).

See Tolbutamide (prototype sulfonylurea) for additional patient teaching points.

Drug Interactions: Glipizide

Plus	Interactions
Anticoagulants (coumarins) Beta adrenergic blocking agents (e.g., propranolol) Chloramphenicol (Chloromycetin) NSAIDs MAO inhibitors Probenecid (Benemid) Sulfonamides	May potentiate hypoglycemic action of sulfonylurea agent

Plus (cont.)	Interactions (cont.)
Adrenergics Calcium channel blocking agents (e.g., verapamil) Corticosteroids Estrogens Isoniazid (INH) Oral contraceptives Niacin (Nicobid) Phenothiazines Phenytoin (Dilantin) Thiazides and other diuretics Thyroid products	May cause loss of control and produce hyperglycemia

GLUCAGON

(gloo′ka-gon)
Antihypoglycemic
Glucose elevating agent
Diagnostic agent

ACTIONS AND USES. Polypeptide hormone produced by alpha cells of islets of Langerhans. Actions appear to be related to increased synthesis of cyclic adenosine monophosphate (cAMP) and phosphorylase activity resulting in increased hepatic gluconeogenesis. Stimulates uptake of amino acids and their conversion to glucose precursors; promotes lipolysis in liver and adipose tissue with release of free fatty acid and glycerol, which further stimulates ketogenesis and hepatic gluconeogenesis. Under normal conditions proper blood sugar level is maintained by homeostatic balance between glucagon and insulin. Intensity of glucose-elevating action is dependent on hepatic glycogen reserve and presence of phosphorylase. Glucagon is of little value in starvation, adrenal insufficiency, or chronic hypoglycemia; juvenile or unstable diabetics do not respond satisfactorily. Exerts positive inotropic and chronotropic action on heart similar to that produced by catecholamines, and a relaxant effect on smooth muscle.

Used in emergency treatment of severe hypoglycemic reactions in diabetic patients, and in psychiatric patients receiving insulin-shock therapy. Also used in radiologic studies of GI tract to relax smooth muscle and thereby allow finer detail of mucosa; and has been used to diagnose insulinoma. *Investigational Use:* to treat various hypoglycemic disorders, to stimulate growth hormone secretion, and to overcome excessive myocardial depressant effects of beta-blockers.

ABSORPTION AND FATE. Blood glucose level increases within 5 to 20 minutes after injection; falls to normal or hypoglycemic level within 1 to 1.5 hours. Half-life: 3 to 6 minutes. Metabolized primarily in liver, but also in plasma and kidneys.

CONTRAINDICATIONS AND PRECAUTIONS. Hypersensitivity to protein compounds. *Cautious Use:* insulinoma, pheochromocytoma.

ADVERSE/SIDE EFFECTS. Infrequent: nausea and vomiting, hypersensitivity reactions, anaphylaxis; hypotension, Stevens-Johnson syndrome (rare).

ROUTE AND DOSAGE. *Hypoglycemia:* **Subcutaneous, intramuscular, intravenous: Adults:** 0.5 to 1 mg. **Children:** 0.025 mg/kg. If no response occurs within 20 minutes, dose may be repeated once or twice. Depending on depth and duration of coma, failure to respond may necessitate immediate administration of IV glucose. *Insulin shock therapy:* 0.5 to 1 mg usually 1 hour after coma develops; if necessary, repeat dose within 25 minutes. *Diagnostic aid:* **Intramuscular, intravenous:** 0.25 to 2 mg (1 mg of glucagon is equivalent to 1 USP unit).

NURSING IMPLICATIONS

Check expiration date of glucagon vial and kit.

Hypoglycemic reactions require *immediate* treatment. Prolonged hypoglycemic coma can result in brain damage.

Patient usually awakens from hypoglycemic coma 10 to 20 minutes following glucagon injection. As soon as possible after patient regains consciousness, oral carbohydrate should be given to restore liver glycogen and to prevent secondary hypoglycemic episode. Physician may administer IV dextrose in cases of very deep coma or if patient fails to respond to glucagon within 20 minutes. The usual dietary regimen should be followed.

Vomiting sometimes occurs on awakening. Have emesis basin and suction equipment immediately available, and position patient on side to prevent aspiration.

Following recovery from hypoglycemic reaction, symptoms such as headache, nausea, and weakness may persist.

For patients with frequent or severe hypoglycemic reactions, physician may request that a responsible family member be taught how to administer glucagon SC or IM. Stress importance of notifying physician whenever a hypoglycemic reaction occurs so that reason for the reaction can be ascertained to prevent further episodes. Also review package insert with patient and family member.

A diabetic teaching plan should be reviewed for all patients and responsible family members. Commonly, hypoglycemic episodes follow too much insulin, delay of food intake, vomiting, or increased physical activity. Review the early symptoms of hypoglycemia (nausea, headache, weakness, hunger, tremor, irritability, unusual fatigue, lack of muscle coordination, weakness, apprehension, chills, diaphoresis), and emphasize the importance of routinely carrying lump sugar, candy, or other readily available carbohydrate to take at first warning of oncoming reaction.

Because glucagon is a protein, the possibility of a hypersensitivity should be borne in mind.

After reconstitution glucagon solution in vial remains potent for 3 months if kept refrigerated at 2° to 15°C (36° to 59°F). Use only special vehicle supplied by manufacturer for dilution. Indicate date on label. Lyophilized (dry powder) form is stable at room temperature.

Glucagon should be considered incompatible in syringe with any other drug.

Glucagon will form a precipitate in saline solutions and solutions with pH of 3 to 9.5 (pH of glucagon is 2.5 to 3).

Diagnostic Test Interferences. Glucagon may decrease **serum cholesterol,** and may increase or decrease **serum potassium** values.

Drug Interactions: Glucagon

Plus	Interactions
Anticoagulants, oral	Potentiates hypoprothrombinemic response to oral anticoagulants
Antidiabetic agents	Antagonizes hypoglycemic effect of antidiabetic drugs

Plus (cont.)	Interactions (cont.)
Diazoxide (Hyperstat, Proglycem) Phenytoin (Dilantin) Thiazides Tolbutamide (Orinase)	Additive hyperglycemic effect. These drugs inhibit insulin release from pancreatic islet cells
Propranolol (Inderal) and possibly other beta-blockers	Propranolol may partially inhibit hyperglycemic response to glucagon, and glucagon may reverse propranolol-induced cardiac depressant effects

G

GLUTAMIC ACID HYDROCHLORIDE

(Acidulin)

(gloo-tam'ik)
Acidifier (gastric)

ACTIONS AND USES. Amino acid chemically combined with hydrochloric acid that is released on contact with water. May be prescribed instead of diluted hydrochloric acid for treatment of hypochlorhydria and achlorhydria because it is convenient to carry and does not injure dental enamel. Also available in OTC preparations in combination with pepsin to aid in digestion, e.g., Glutasyn, Muripsin, Milco-Zyme.

CONTRAINDICATIONS AND PRECAUTIONS. Gastric hyperacidity, peptic ulcer.

ADVERSE/SIDE EFFECTS. Overdose: systemic acidosis.

ROUTE AND DOSAGE. Oral: 1 to 3 capsules or tablets three times daily before each meal. Each capsule contains 340 mg of glutamic acid hydrochloride (1.8 mEq HCl).

NURSING IMPLICATIONS

See Hydrochloric Acid, Diluted.

GLUTETHIMIDE

(Doriden)

(gloo-teth'i-mide)
Sedative
C III

ACTIONS AND USES. Piperidine derivative structurally related to methyprylon. Pharmacologic actions similar to those of barbiturates. Can induce hypnosis without producing reliable analgesic, antitussive, or anticonvulsant action. Produces less respiratory depression, but greater degree of hypotension, than barbiturates. Exhibits anticholinergic activity, especially mydriasis, and inhibits salivary secretions and intestinal motility. Significantly suppresses REM sleep (dreaming stage of sleep); but following drug withdrawal after chronic administration, REM rebound occurs, and patient may experience markedly increased dreaming, nightmares, and/or insomnia. Addiction liability similar to that of barbiturates. Stimulates hepatic microsomal enzymes and thus may alter metabolism of other drugs.

Used in treatment of temporary insomnia and for sedative effect preoperatively and during first stage of labor. Not indicated for routine sedation or persistent insomnia.

ABSORPTION AND FATE. Erratic absorption from GI tract. Sleep is usually induced within 30 minutes following hypnotic dose, lasting 4 to 8 hours. Serum level decline is biphasic: first phase about 4 hours, second phase 10 to 12 hours. Widely distributed to body tissues; localizes particularly in adipose tissue, liver, kidney, brain, and bile. About 50% bound to plasma proteins. Almost completely metabolized in liver by hydroxylation; conjugates with glucuronic acid. Glucuronides are excreted slowly in urine; less than 2% of dose excreted unchanged. About 1 to 2% excreted in feces. Crosses placenta; small quantities may appear in breast milk.

CONTRAINDICATIONS AND PRECAUTIONS. Known hypersensitivity to glutethimide; uncontrolled pain; intermittent porphyria; severe hepatic and renal impairment; prolonged administration; children younger than 12 years of age. Safe use in women of childbearing potential and during pregnancy (except with caution during first stage of labor) and in children younger than 12 years not established. *Cautious Use:* elderly or debilitated patients, prostatic hypertrophy, bladder neck obstruction, pyloroduodenal obstruction, stenosing peptic ulcer, narrow-angle glaucoma, hypotension, cardiac arrhythmias, mental depression (particularly in patients with suicidal tendencies), history of alcoholism, or drug abuse.

G

ADVERSE/SIDE EFFECTS. Generally infrequent: gastric irritation, nausea, hiccups, drug "hangover," dry mouth, blurred vision, generalized skin rash (occasionally, purpuric or urticarial), exfoliative dermatitis, paradoxic excitement, headache, vertigo, acute hypersensitivity reactions, porphyria, jaundice, blood dyscrasias (thrombocytopenic purpura, aplastic anemia, leukopenia), CNS depression in fetus. **Acute overdosage (CNS depression):** coma; depressed reflexes, including corneal reflex; dilated, fixed pupils; hypotension; hypothermia followed by hyperpyrexia; tachycardia; respiratory depression; cyanosis; sudden apnea; urinary bladder atony; decreased intestinal motility; adynamic ileus; facial twitching; intermittent spasticity; flaccid paralysis; pulmonary and cerebral edema; renal tubular necrosis; severe infections. **Chronic toxicity (toxic psychosis):** slurred speech, impaired memory, inability to concentrate, mydriasis, dry mouth, nystagmus, ataxia, hyporeflexia, tremors, peripheral neuropathy, osteomalacia (rare).

ROUTE AND DOSAGE. Oral: *(for insomnia)* 250 to 500 mg at bedtime, repeated if necessary, but not less than 4 hours before arising; *(preoperatively)* 500 mg the night before surgery and 500 mg to 1 Gm 1 hour before anesthesia; *(first stage of labor)* 500 mg at onset of labor, repeated once if necessary. **Elderly or debilitated patient:** Initial: total daily dose should not exceed 500 mg at bedtime.

NURSING IMPLICATIONS

Tablet may be crushed before administration and taken with fluid of patient's choice.

Capsule may be emptied and contents swallowed with water or mixed with food.

If administered for insomnia, glutethimide should be given 4 hours or more before the usual time of arising in order to avoid residual daytime effects.

Sedative-hypnotic effect of glutethimide is counteracted by pain. Consult physician about prescribing an analgesic for pain, if required.

Keep physician informed of patient's response to drug. Smallest effective dosage should be used for the shortest period of time compatible with patient's needs.

Advise patient to report onset of rash or any other unusual symptoms. Discontinuation of drug is indicated if a rash occurs.

Caution patient to avoid driving a motor vehicle or engaging in other activities requiring mental alertness for 7 to 8 hours following drug ingestion.

Warn patient about possible adverse reactions when glutethimide is combined with alcohol or other CNS depressants *(see Drug Interactions)*.

Prolonged use of moderate to high doses of glutethimide can produce tolerance and psychologic and physical dependence.

Abrupt withdrawal following regular use may produce nausea, vomiting, nervousness, tremors, abdominal cramps, nightmares, insomnia, tachycardia, chills, fever, numbness of extremities, dysphagia, delirium, hallucinations, or convulsions. Withdrawal should be gradual, with stepwise dose reduction over a period of several days or weeks.

Overdosage of glutethimide is difficult to treat. Patients tend to go in and out of toxicity, possibly due to delayed absorption of the drug.

Treatment of acute overdosage: gastric lavage, regardless of time that has elapsed since drug ingestion. Some physicians lavage with a 1:1 mixture of castor oil and water (glutethimide is lipid-soluble). Supportive treatment is based on presenting signs and symptoms.

Classified as Schedule III drug under Federal Controlled Substances Act.

Drug Interactions. Possibility of increased CNS depression with concomitant administration of **alcohol** (also enhances glutethimide absorption), **barbiturates,** and other **CNS depressants.** Additive anticholinergic effects may occur with **tricyclic antidepressants.** There is decreased anticoagulant response in patients receiving **oral anticoagulants.** Anticoagulant dosage may require adjustment during treatment and on cessation of glutethimide.

GLYBURIDE

(DiaBeta, Euglucon, Micronaise)

(glye'byoor-ide)
Antidiabetic agent
Sulfonylurea (second generation)

ACTIONS AND USES. One of the most potent of the sulfonylurea hypoglycemic agents. Second-generation sulfonylurea closely related in actions, uses, and limitations to glipizide (qv). Potency is enhanced by as much as 200-fold over first generation agents e.g., therapeutic dosage equivalents are glyburide 5 mg = glipizide 5 to 10 mg = chlorpropamide 250 to 275 mg = acetohexamide 500 to 750 mg = tolbutamide 1 to 1.5 mg. Lowers blood sugar concentration in both diabetic and nondiabetic individuals by stimulating insulin release from functioning pancreatic beta cells. Blood glucose lowering effect persists during long-term glyburide treatment, but there is a gradual decline in meal-stimulated secretion of endogenous insulin toward pretreatment levels. Extrapancreatic effects are thought to augment drug effect on the beta cells; i.e., enhanced peripheral sensitization to insulin, decrease in hepatic glucose production, and increased insulin binding to cell membrane receptors. Produces mild diuresis by enhanced free water clearance, perhaps by inhibiting reabsorption of Na in the proximal renal tubule or by blocking nonvasopressor-dependent reabsorption of water in the distal renal tubules.

Used as adjunct to diet to lower blood glucose in patients with type II (NIDDM) diabetes mellitus after dietary control alone has failed.

ABSORPTION AND FATE. Following oral administration drug is well absorbed within 1 hour, with peak concentration reached in 2 to 8 hours. Blood glucose lowering effect persists for 24 hours. Plasma insulin concentration begins to increase within 15 to 60 minutes after a single dose and is maximal in 1 to 2 hours; in a diabetic patient plasma insulin may persist for up to 24 hours. Distributed in highest concentrations to liver, kidneys and intestines. Metabolized in liver; more than 99% protein bound. Half-life of drug and its metabolites: about 10 hours (may be prolonged in patient with severe renal impairment). Excreted as metabolites in urine and feces in approximately equal proportions. Appears to cross placenta but distribution into milk is not known. Minimally removed by hemodialysis.

CONTRAINDICATIONS AND PRECAUTIONS. *See Glipizide.*

ADVERSE/SIDE EFFECTS. Hypoglycemia (may be fatal in patient receiving as little as 2.5 to 5 mg glyburide/day); epigastric fullness, heartburn, nausea, paresthesia, joint pain, nocturia. *See also Glipizide.*

ROUTE AND DOSAGE. (Dosage regimen is individualized to establish the minimum effective dose.) Recommended initial dose: **Oral:** 2.5 to 5 mg daily given with breakfast or first main meal. Usual maintenance dose: 1.25 to 2.0 mg daily as single or divided doses. Dose adjustment is accomplished by increments of 2.5 mg depending on blood glucose response, but no sooner than 1 or 2 weeks to allow reaching steady-state serum levels and full pharmacologic effect.

NURSING IMPLICATIONS

The elderly patient is especially vulnerable to glyburide-induced hypoglycemia. Urine and blood glucose levels should be monitored carefully during the dangerous early treatment period when dosage is being individualized.

Keep in mind that if the patient is also receiving a beta-adrenergic blocking agent (suppresses reflex tachycardia) or if the patient is elderly, the first signs of hypoglycemia may be hard to detect.

In the diabetic patient, hypoglycemia is a potential effect of the following situations: after severe or prolonged exercise, after alcohol ingestion, when caloric intake is deficient, when more than one glucose lowering drug is being used.

Be alert to the danger of loss of control of diabetes which may result from stress such as fever, surgery, trauma, infection. Blood and urine glucose and ketone body detection may need to be checked more frequently during these stress periods, and transfer from the sulfonylurea to insulin may be necessary.

Urine testing: When diabetes is stabilized, patient is advised to test urine for glucose (using Chemstrip UG, or other similar test strip) 2 hours after each meal. If urine is positive for glucose for 2 or 3 days, then patient is usually advised to check for urine ketones (with Chemstrip UGK) and report to physician. Urine should be tested for ketones also, when patient has an illness or is subjected to stress such as surgery.

Capillary glucose testing is encouraged for the patient on a sulfonylurea.

During conversion period when both insulin and glyburide are being used, instruct patient to test urine for ketone bodies and glucose at least three times daily and to report promptly abnormal findings to the physician.

Persistence of acetonuria with glycosuria, indicates that the patient is a type I (IDDM) diabetic who requires insulin therapy.

Store in tightly closed, light resistant container at a temperature 15° to 30°C (59° to 86°F).

See Glipizide for additional Nursing Implications and for Drug Interactions.

GLYCERIN

(gli′ser-in)

(Fleet Babylax, Glycerol, Glyrol, Osmoglyn, Sani Supp)

Laxative (hyperosmotic)

GLYCERIN ANHYDROUS

(Ophthalgan)

ACTIONS AND USES. Trihydric alcohol. When administered orally raises plasma osmotic pressure by withdrawing fluid from extravascular spaces; lowers ocular tension by decreasing volume of intraocular fluid. Also may decrease cerebrospinal fluid pressure and produce slight diuresis. Topical application to eye reduces edema by hygroscopic effect. Glycerin suppositories apparently work by causing dehydration of exposed tissue which produces an irritant effect and by absorbing water from tissues thus creating more mass. Both actions stimulate peristalis. Available in combination with alcohol as skin lotion (Corn Husker's Lotion).

Used orally to reduce elevated intraocular pressure in patients with acute narrow-angle glaucoma prior to or following surgery, retinal detachment, or cataract extraction and to reduce elevated CSF pressure. Sterile glycerin (anhydrous) is used topically to reduce superficial corneal edema resulting from trauma, surgery, or disease and to facilitate ophthalmoscopic examination. Used rectally (suppository or enema) to relieve constipation.

ABSORPTION AND FATE. Rapidly absorbed from GI tract following oral administration and distributed through blood. Intraocular pressure begins to decline within 10 minutes; maximal effect occurs in 30 minutes to 2 hours and may persist 4 to 8 hours. Metabolized in liver to CO_2 and water, or utilized in glucose or glycogen synthesis. Approximately 7 to 14% excreted unchanged in urine.

G

CONTRAINDICATIONS AND PRECAUTIONS. Hypersensitivity to any of the ingredients. Safe use during pregnancy (category C) and in nursing women not established. *Cautious Use:* cardiac, renal, or hepatic disease; diabetes mellitus; dehydrated or elderly patients.

ADVERSE/SIDE EFFECTS. Headache, dizziness, nausea, vomiting, thirst, diarrhea, hyperglycemia, glycosuria, dehydration, hyperosmolar nonketotic coma, irregular heartbeat, disorientation, convulsive seizures (rare). Suppository form: abdominal cramps, rectal discomfort.

ROUTE AND DOSAGE. **Oral (50% to 75% solution):** 1 to 1.5 Gm/kg body weight 1 to 1½ hours prior to ocular surgery; repeated at approximately 5-hour intervals. **Rectal suppository:** *Constipation:* **Adults and children:** 1 suppository inserted high into rectum and retained for 15 minutes (laxative action does not require melting of suppository). **Enema: Adults:** 5 to 15 ml; **Children (1 to 6 years):** 2 to 5 ml. **Topical ophthalmic** (sterile anhydrous glycerin 0.5%): 1 or 2 drops instilled into eye every 3 to 4 hours for reduction of corneal edema. A local anesthetic should be instilled shortly before use.

NURSING IMPLICATIONS

Commercially available flavored solution may be poured over crushed ice and sipped through a straw. Lemon juice and 0.9% sodium chloride (if allowed) may be added to unflavored solution for palatability.

Headache (from cerebral dehydration) may be prevented or relieved by having patient lie down during and after administration of oral drug.

Consult physician regarding fluid intake in patients receiving drug for elevated intraocular pressure. Although hypotonic fluids will relieve thirst and headache caused by the dehydrating action of glycerin, these fluids may nullify its osmotic effect.

Slight hyperglycemia and glycosuria may occur with oral use. Patients with diabetes may require adjustment in insulin dosage.

Glycerin is used as a vehicle for many drugs applied to the skin. Undiluted glycerin (95 to 99%) adsorbs moisture and hence is somewhat dehydrating and irritating when applied to skin and mucous membranes. When diluted with water, it acts as an emollient and humectant.

Many dentists discourage use of glycerin and lemon for mouth care because of its drying effect on mucous membranes. *See Index for mouth care procedure.*

GLYCOPYRROLATE

(glye-koe-pye'roe-late)

(Robinul, Roninul Forte)

Anticholinergic

ACTIONS AND USES. Synthetic anticholinergic (antimuscarinic) quaternary ammonium compound with pharmacologic effects similar to those of atropine (qv). In contrast to atropine, glycopyrrolate is highly polar and therefore does not easily penetrate lipid membranes such as the blood–brain barrier. Has lower incidence of CNS-related side effects than atropine, and reportedly has longer vagal blocking and antisialogogue effects. Inhibits motility of GI tract and genitourinary tract and decreases volume of gastric and pancreatic secretions, saliva, and perspiration. Also antagonizes muscarinic symptoms (e.g., excessive tracheal or bronchial secretions, bronchospasm, bradycardia, intestinal hypermotility) induced by cholinergic drugs, such as anticholinesterases, and anesthetic agents.

Used in adjunctive management of peptic ulcer and other GI disorders associated with hyperacidity, hypermotility, and spasm. Also used parenterally as preanesthetic and intraoperative medication and to reverse neuromuscular blockade. Commercially available in combination with phenobarbital (Robinul-PH).

ABSORPTION AND FATE. Poorly and irregularly absorbed following oral administration; peak effects appear in about 1 hour and may persist 6 hours. Following sc or IM administration, peak effects occur in 30 to 45 minutes; vagal blocking effects may last 2 to 3 hours, and antisialogogue effects may persist up to 7 hours. Action following IV dose begins in 10 to 15 minutes; duration of action shorter than with other routes. Thought to be excreted primarily in urine and bile and as unchanged drug in feces.

CONTRAINDICATIONS AND PRECAUTIONS. Hypersensitivity to glycopyrrolate; glaucoma, asthma, prostatic hypertrophy, obstructive uropathy, obstructive lesions or atony of GI tract; severe ulcerative colitis, myasthenia gravis, tachycardia, during cyclopropane anesthesia, children under age 12 (except parenteral use in conjunction with anesthesia). Safe use during pregnancy or lactation not established. *See also Atropine.*

ADVERSE/SIDE EFFECTS. Xerostomia, decreased sweating, urinary hesitancy or retention, blurred vision, mydriasis, constipation, palpitation, tachycardia, drowsiness, weakness, dizziness. **Overdosage:** neuromuscular blockade (curarelike action) leading to muscular weakness and paralysis is theoretically possible. *See also Atropine.*

ROUTE AND DOSAGE. Oral: Adults; Children above 12 years: Initial: 1 mg 3 times daily in morning, early afternoon, and evening. Alternatively, 2 mg two or three times daily at equally spaced intervals. Dosage adjusted to needs of individual patient. Recommended maximum daily dosage is 8 mg. Maintenance: 1 mg 2 times daily. **Intramuscular, intravenous (without dilution):** 0.1 to 0.2 mg as single dose. *Reversal of neuromuscular blockade:* 0.2 mg IV for each 1 mg of neostigmine or 5 mg pyridostigmine administered. Glycopyrrolate is prescribed to be given concurrently in same syringe with or a few minutes before the anticholinesterase agent.

NURSING IMPLICATIONS

Incidence and severity of side effects are generally dose related. Caution patient to avoid high environmental temperatures. (Heat prostration can occur due to decreased sweating.)

Since glycopyrrolate may produce dizziness and blurred vision, warn patient not to engage in activities requiring mental alertness, such as operating a motor vehicle or performing other hazardous tasks.

There are no known drug interactions.

Do not combine glycopyrrolate in same syringe with chloramphenicol, diazepam, sodium

pentobarbitol, sodium bicarbonate, or other drugs capable of raising the pH above 6.0. A precipitate and gas will be formed.
Inspect parenteral products for cloudiness and discoloration. Discard such solutions.
See Atropine Sulfate (prototype anticholinergic).

GOLD SODIUM THIOMALATE

(thye-oh-mah′late)

(Myochrysine)

Antirheumatic

ACTIONS AND USES. Water-soluble gold compound similar to aurothioglucose (qv) in actions and uses. Contains approximately 50% gold.

Used in treatment of selected patients (adults and juveniles) with acute rheumatoid arthritis.

ABSORPTION AND FATE. Readily absorbed following IM injection. Peak plasma concentrations reached in 4 to 6 hours. Thought to be highly concentrated in kidney, liver, spleen, and synovial fluid. Bound to plasma proteins. Half-life lengthens with successive injections. Excreted primarily in urine; appreciable amounts also eliminated in feces. After a course of treatment, traces may be found in urine for 6 months or more.

CONTRAINDICATIONS AND PRECAUTIONS. History of severe toxicity from previous exposure to gold or other heavy metals, severe debilitation, systemic lupus erythematosus, Sjögren's syndrome in rheumatoid arthritis, renal disease, hepatic dysfunction, history of infectious hepatitis or hematologic disorders, uncontrolled diabetes, or congestive heart failure. Safe use during pregnancy not established. *Cautious Use:* history of drug allergies or hypersensitivity, hypertension.

ADVERSE/SIDE EFFECTS. Allergic (nitritoid-type reactions): flushing, fainting, dizziness, fall in blood pressure, sweating, nausea, vomiting, weakness. Less frequently: anaphylactic shock, bradycardia, edema of tongue, angioneurotic edema. **Hematologic (rare):** leukopenia, agranulocytosis, thrombocytopenia, hypoplastic and aplastic anemia, eosinophilia. **Renal:** nephrotic syndrome, glomerulitis with hematuria, proteinuria. **Skin and mucous membranes:** transient pruritus, erythema, dermatitis (common), fixed drug eruption, alopecia, shedding of nails, gray to blue pigmentation of skin (chrysiasis), stomatitis (common), glossitis, bronchitis, pharyngitis, pneumonitis, gastritis, colitis, vaginitis, conjunctivitis (rare). **Other:** gold deposits in ocular tissues, photosensitivity, hepatitis with jaundice, bilirubinemia, peripheral neuritis, encephalitis.

ROUTE AND DOSAGE. Highly individualized. **Adults: Intramuscular** (weekly injections): 1st injection, 10 mg; 2nd injection, 25 mg; then 25 to 50 mg weekly until toxicity intervenes or clinical improvement occurs or cumulative dose administered totals 1 Gm. If no improvement occurs after this amount, treatment is generally discontinued. If improvement occurs, patient is placed on maintenance schedule: 25 to 50 mg at 2-week intervals for 2 to 20 weeks. **Pediatric:** Initial test dose: 10 mg, then 1 mg/kg/week. Alternatively 2.5 to 5 mg for the first and second weeks followed by 1 mg/kg/week or at 3 to 4 week intervals (depending on patient response) indefinitely. No more than 25 mg in a single dose should be given to children under 12 years of age.

NURSING IMPLICATIONS

Agitate vial before withdrawing dose to assure uniform suspension.
Baseline hemoglobin and erythrocyte determinations, WBC count, differential count, platelet

count, and urinalysis should be obtained before initiation of therapy and at regular intervals thereafter.

Rapid reduction in hemoglobin level, WBC count below 4000/mm^3, eosinophil count above 5%, and platelet count below 100,000/mm^3 signify possible toxicity.

Prior to each injection, urine should be analyzed for protein, blood, and sediment. Drug should be discontinued promptly if proteinuria or hematuria develops.

Patient should be interviewed and examined before each injection to detect occurrence of transient pruritus or dermatitis (both are common early indications of toxicity), stomatitis (sore tongue, palate, or throat), metallic taste, indigestion, or other signs and symptoms of possible toxicity. Treatment should be interrupted immediately if any of these reactions occurs.

Drug is usually administered deep into upper outer quadrant of gluteus with patient lying down. Patient should remain recumbent for at least 30 minutes after injection because of the danger of "nitritoid reaction" (transient giddiness, vertigo, facial flushing, fainting). Observe for allergic reactions.

Allergic reaction may occur almost immediately after injection, 10 minutes after injection, or at any time during therapy. If it is observed, treatment should be discontinued. At time of injection have antidote dimercaprol (BAL) on hand.

Therapeutic effects may not appear until after 3 months of therapy. This may be a basis for noncompliance.

Rapid improvement in joint swelling usually indicates that patient is closely approaching drug tolerance level; report to physician.

Patients who develop gold dermatitis should be warned that exposure to sunlight may aggravate the problem.

The appearance of purpura or ecchymoses is always an indication for doing a platelet count; report to physician.

Patients should be informed about possible adverse reactions and warned to report any symptom suggestive of toxicity as soon as it appears. Adverse reactions may occur at any time during drug therapy or even a few months after drug is discontinued; most reactions occur during second or third month of treatment (usually after the amount injected has reached about 250 to 500 mg).

Preserved in tight, light-resistant containers at room temperature preferably between 15° and 30°C (59° and 86°F). Drug should not be used if it is any darker than pale yellow.

See Aurothioglucose.

G

GONADORELIN HYDROCHLORIDE

(goe-nad-oh-rell'in)

(Factrel)

Diagnostic agent

ACTIONS AND USES. Synthetic luteinizing hormone-releasing hormone (LH-RH) with stucture identical to the natural hormone; also referred to as gonadotropin-releasing hormone (GnRH). Stimulates anterior pituitary to release the gonadotropin, LH. Range for normal baseline LH levels: 5 to 25 mIU/ml in postpubertal males, postpubertal and premenopausal females. Tests are performed during early follicular phase of the menstrual cycle (days 1 and 7).

Used to evaluate functional capacity and response of the gonadotropes of anterior pituitary and in suspected gonadotropic deficiency. Also used to evaluate residual gonadotropic function of the pituitary following surgical or radiologic removal of a pituitary tumor. *Unlabeled Use:* induction of ovulation IV, nasal routes, ovulation inhibition (contraceptive effect), treatment of precocious puberty.

CONTRAINDICATIONS AND PRECAUTIONS. Hypersensitivity to gonadorelin or to any of the components. Safe use in pregnancy (category B) not established; concurrent use of other drugs having effect on pituitary–gonadotropic function.

ADVERSE/SIDE EFFECTS. GI: nausea, abdominal discomfort. **Neurologic:** headache, light-headedness. **Other:** flushing, local inflammation at injection site if given SC; allergic or hypersensitivity reactions (rare); rash (rare).

ROUTE AND DOSAGE. Subcutaneous, intravenous: Adult: 100 mcg.

NURSING IMPLICATIONS

Test procedure is according to established protocol (see manufacturer's information).

Interpretation of test:

- In menopausal and postmenopausal women, baseline LH levels are elevated.
- Patient clinically diagnosed or suspected pituitary or hypothalamus dysfunction often demonstrates subnormal or absent LH response following test dose.
- The normal response indicates presence of functional pituitary gonadotropes.
- The single dose does not determine pathologic cause for the subnormal response and does not measure pituitary gonadotropic reserve.

Preparation of the solution: reconstitute 100 mcg vial with 1.0 ml sterile diluent (supplied by manufacturer), and the 500 mcg vial with 2.0 ml. Solution should be used immediately after preparation.

Overdosage has not been reported. Doses as high as 3 mg twice daily for 28 days have been used without signs of toxicity.

Repetitive, high doses of gonadorelin may cause inhibition of spermatogenesis, and luteolysis.

After reconstitution, store drug at room temperature and use within 24 hours. Discard unused diluted solution and diluent. Store ampule at room temperature.

Drug Interactions: Gonadorelin

Plus	Interactions
Androgens, estrogens, progestins, glucocorticoids	Production of false test results (all these agents also affect pituitary secretion of gonatotropins)
Digoxin, Oral Contraceptives	Suppress gonadotropin levels
Spironolactone, Levodopa	Elevate gonadotropin levels
Dopamine antagonists, phenothiazines	Increase prolactin and blunt reponse of pituitary to gonadorelin

---

GRISEOFULVIN MICROSIZE

(gri-see-oh-ful′vin)

(Fulvicin-U/F, Grifulvin V, Grisactin, Grisovin-FP)

GRISEOFULVIN ULTRAMICROSIZE

(Fulvicin P/G, Grisactin Ultra, Gris-PEG)

Antiinfective
Antibiotic
Antifungal

ACTIONS AND USES. Fungistatic antibiotic derived from species of *Penicillium.* Deposits in keratin precursor cells and has special affinity for diseased tissue. Tightly bound to new keratin of skin, hair, and nails, which becomes highly resistant to fungal invasion. Effective against various species of *Epidermophyton, Microsporum,* and *Trichophyton* (has no effect on other fungi, including candida, bacteria, and yeasts). Exerts fungistatic action primarily by arresting metaphase of cell division. Also has some direct vasodilatory activity. Efficacy of GI absorption of ultramicrosize formulation reported to be twice that of microsize griseofulvin. Theoretically cross-sensitivity with penicillin is a possibility.

Used in treatment of mycotic disease of skin, hair, and nails not amenable to conventional topical measures. Concomitant use of appropriate topical agent may be required, particularly for tinea pedis. *Investigational Use:* treatment of Raynaud's disease, angina pectoris, and gout.

ABSORPTION AND FATE. Absorbed primarily from duodenum (extent varies among individuals). Absorption of microsize griseofulvin is variable and unpredictable; ultramicrosize is almost completely absorbed. Single 500-mg dose of microsize and 250-mg dose of ultramicrosize form produce roughly comparable peak plasma levels in about 4 hours. Concentrates in skin, hair, nails, liver, fat, and skeletal muscle. Can be detected in outer layers of stratum corneum soon after absorption. Elimination half-life is 9 to 24 hours. Metabolized in liver. Excreted in urine and feces chiefly as inactive metabolites and small amounts of unchanged drug. Also excreted in perspiration.

G

CONTRAINDICATIONS AND PRECAUTIONS. History of sensitivity to griseofulvin, porphyria, hepatic disease, systemic lupus erythematosus. Safe use during pregnancy, for children 2 years of age and younger, or for prophylaxis against fungal infections not established. *Cautious Use:* penicillin-sensitive patients (possibility of cross-sensitivity with penicillin exists; however, reportedly penicillin-sensitive patients have been treated without difficulty).

ADVERSE/SIDE EFFECTS. Low incidence of side effects. **GI:** heartburn, nausea, vomiting, diarrhea, flatulence, dry mouth, thirst, decreased taste acuity, anorexia, unpleasant taste, furred tongue, oral thrush. **Hematologic:** leukopenia, neutropenia, granulocytopenia, punctate basophilia, monocytosis. **Hypersensitivity:** urticaria, photosensitivity, lichen planus, skin rashes, fixed drug eruption, serum sickness syndromes, severe angioedema. **Neurologic:** severe headache, insomnia, peripheral neuritis, paresthesias, fatigue, mental confusion, impaired performance of routine functions, vertigo, blurred vision, diminished hearing (rare). **Renal (nephrotoxicity):** proteinuria, cylinduria. **Other:** hepatotoxicity, estrogenlike effects (in children), aggravation of systemic lupus erythematosus, overgrowth of nonsusceptible organisms, candidal intertrigo, elevated porphyrins in feces and erythrocytes.

ROUTE AND DOSAGE. Oral: Adults: 250 to 500 mg of ultramicrosize griseofulvin (Gris-PEG) or 500 mg to 1 Gm of microsize griseofulvin per day (best results reportedly obtained when calculated dose is divided into 4 equal parts and given at 6-hour intervals). **Pediatric:** 5.5 to 7.3 mg/kg daily of ultramicrosize or 30.0 mg/m² daily of microsize. All dosages highly individualized.

NURSING IMPLICATIONS

Accurate laboratory identification of infecting organism is essential prior to initiation of treatment.

Giving the drug with or after meals may allay GI disturbances.

Serum levels may be increased by giving the microsize formulations with a high fat content meal (increases drug absorption rate). Consult physician.

Monitor food intake. Griseofulvin may alter taste sensations and thus may cause appetite suppression and inadequate nutrient intake.

Headaches often occur during early therapy but frequently disappear with continued drug administration.

Blood studies should be performed at least once weekly during first month of therapy or longer. Periodic tests of renal and hepatic function are also advised.

Patient may experience symptomatic relief after 48 to 96 hours of therapy. Stress the importance of continuing treatment as prescribed to prevent relapse.

Treatment should be continued until there is clinical improvement, as well as negative potassium hydroxide amounts of lesion scrapings, or until 2 or 3 consecutive weekly cultures are negative.

Duration of treatment depends on time required to replace infected skin, hair, or nails and thus varies with infection site. Average duration of treatment for tinea capitis (scalp ringworm) is 4 to 6 weeks; tinea corporis (body ringworm), 2 to 4 weeks; tinea pedis (athlete's foot), 4 to 8 weeks; tinea unguium (nail fungus), at least 4 months for fingernails, depending on rate of growth, and 6 months or more for toenails.

Caution patient to avoid exposure to intense natural or artificial sunlight, because photosensitivity-type reactions may occur.

Warn patient of possible reaction (tachycardia, flushing) on ingestion of alcohol during therapy.

Emphasize importance of cleanliness and keeping skin dry (moist skin favors growth of fungi). For athlete's foot, advise patient to wear well-ventilated shoes without rubber soles, to alternate shoes, and to change socks daily. Physician may prescribe a drying powder as necessary. *See Index: Nursing Interventions: fungal infection.*

G

Drug Interactions. Griseofulvin may potentiate the effects of **alcohol.** Activity of griseofulvin may be diminished by **barbiturates** (cause reduction of griseofulvin serum levels). In some patients, griseofulvin may decrease the hypoprothrombinemic effects of **warfarin** and possibly other **oral anticoagulants.** Close monitoring of prothrombin time is advised when griseofulvin is added to or withdrawn from anticoagulant drug regimen.

GUAIFENESIN

(gwye-fen'e-sin)
Expectorant

(Anti-Tuss, Baytussin, Colrex, Dilyn, Gee-Gee, GG-CEN, Glyceryl Guaiacolate, Glytuss, Glycotuss, Hytuss, Malotuss, Neo-Spec, Resyl, Robitussin)

ACTIONS AND USES. Enhances reflex outflow of respiratory tract fluids by irritation of gastric mucosa and aids in expectoration by reducing adhesiveness and surface tension of respiratory tract fluid.

Used to combat dry, productive cough associated with colds and bronchitis. A common ingredient in cough mixtures.

ADVERSE/SIDE EFFECTS. Low incidence: GI upset, nausea, drowsiness.

ROUTE AND DOSAGE. Oral: Adults: 100 to 400 mg every 4 hours, not to exceed 2.4 Gm daily. **Children (6 to 11 years):** 100 to 200 mg every 4 hours, not to exceed 1.2 Gm daily. **(2 to 5 years):** 50 to 100 mg every 4 hours as required, not to exceed 600 mg daily. Available forms: **tablets, capsules, syrup.**

NURSING IMPLICATIONS

See Benzonatate for patient teaching points.

Diagnostic Test Interferences. Guaifenesin may produce color interferences with certain laboratory determinations of urinary 5-hydroxyindoleacetic acid (**5-HIAA**) and vanillylmandelic acid (**VMA**).

Drug Interactions. By inhibiting platelet function, guaifenesin may increase risk of hemorrhage in patients receiving **heparin** therapy.

GUANABENZ ACETATE

(Wytensin)

(gwan'a-benz)
Alpha-adrenergic agonist, sympathomimetic
Antihypertensive

ACTIONS AND USES. Centrally acting alpha-2 adrenergic agonist. A derivative of guanethidine, but pharmacologic actions more closely resemble those of clonidine. Lowers blood pressure primarily by stimulating central alpha adrenergic receptors which results in reduction of sympathetic outflow from brain. Reduces both supine and standing blood pressures usually without producing postural hypotension and causes slight lowering of pulse rate (about 5 beats/minute). Peripheral resistance lowers with long-term therapy, but cardiac output and left ventricular ejection fraction are unaffected. Also has no effect on exercise tolerance or on potassium levels. May cause slight reduction in serum cholesterol and total triglycerides but does not affect HDL cholesterol fraction. Tolerance to antihypertensive actions not reported. Given the fact that central adrenergic hyperactivity causes symptoms of narcotic withdrawal, guanabenz appears to help control abstinence symptoms by reducing norepinephrine output.

Used in treatment of hypertension alone or in combination with a thiazide diuretic (stepped-care approach: step 2.) Also has been used for opiate detoxification.

ABSORPTION AND FATE. About 75% of dose rapidly absorbed from GI tract. Onset of antihypertensive action within 60 minutes after administration. Peak effect in 2 to 4 hours; duration 6 to 12 hours. Average half-life: approximately 6 hours. Metabolic fate unknown. About 80% of dose excreted in urine, chiefly as metabolites. Distribution to placenta and breast milk not known.

CONTRAINDICATIONS AND PRECAUTIONS. History of hypersensitivity to guanabenz. Safe use during pregnancy (category C), in nursing mothers, and in children not established. *Cautious Use:* severe coronary insufficiency, recent myocardial infarction, cerebrovascular disease, severe hepatic or renal failure.

ADVERSE/SIDE EFFECTS. CNS: drowsiness or sedation, dizziness, weakness, headache, anxiety, ataxia, depression, sleep disturbances. **CV:** chest pain, edema, arrhythmias, palpitation. **GI:** dry mouth, nausea, epigastric pain, diarrhea, vomiting, constipation, abdominal discomfort, taste disorders. **GU:** urinary frequency, sexual dysfunction. **Hematologic:** decreases in serum cholesterol, triglycerides, norepinephrine, dopamine, beta hydroxylase, renin; increase in hepatic enzymes (rare). **Other:** gynecomastia, blurred vision, nasal congestion, dyspnea, muscle aches, aches in extremities, rash, pruritus. **Overdosage:** hypotension, somnolence, lethargy, irritability, miosis, bradycardia, unusual fatigue or weakness, nervousness.

ROUTE AND DOSAGE. Oral: Initial: 4 mg twice daily. Increased if necessary by increments of 4 to 8 mg/day every 1 to 2 weeks, depending upon patient's response, to maximum of 32 mg twice daily.

NURSING IMPLICATIONS

One dose is usually prescribed for bedtime administration to ensure overnight control and to reduce possibility of daytime drowsiness or sedation.

Baseline and periodic tests should include blood chemistry (serum potassium, CBC, creatinine, uric acid, cholesterol, glucose), urinalysis for protein and sugar, and ECG.

Geriatric patients tend to be more sensitive to normal adult doses of antihypertensive drugs because of deficient baroreceptor reflexes. Therefore, although orthostatic hypotension is not an expected guanabenz effect, caution patient to make all position changes slowly and in stages.

Dry mouth, a common side effect, may be relieved by frequent rinses with water, and use of sugar-free gum or sour balls. Advise edentulous patients to remove dentures at least two or three times a day when rinsing so that all oral tissues are moistened. Review good oral hygiene: daily flossing; use of soft toothbrush to brush teeth and tongue; use of fluoride toothpaste. Avoid overuse of commercial mouthwashes; most contain alcohol which tends to cause even more dryness. If relief is not provided by these measures, a saliva substitute may help, e.g., Moi-Stir, Salivart, Xero-Lube. All are available OTC.

Dry mouth requires early attention and specific treatment because: (1) it can interfere with patient's food and fluid intake; (2) deprivation of normal salivary flow is a potential dental hazard since it favors demineralization of teeth; and (3) it can be a factor in noncompliance.

Warn patient not to omit dosage and not to stop drug therapy without consulting the physician. Abrupt discontinuation of guanabenz may cause sympathetic overactivity: anxiety, nervousness, palpitation, chest pain, fast or irregular heartbeat, trembling, flushing, headache, increased sweating and salivation, elevation of blood pressure (usually above basal level).

As a general rule, antihypertensive medications are not discontinued in patients undergoing surgery. Consult physician. Anesthesiologist should be informed that patient is receiving antihypertensive therapy.

Since guanabenz can cause drowsiness and dizziness, advise patient to use caution when driving or performing other potentially hazardous activities until reaction to drug is determined. Also warn patient that tolerance to alcohol and other CNS depressants may be reduced by guanabenz.

See Guanethidine: Patient teaching plan (for patients with hypertension).

Store preferably between 15° and 30°C (59° and 86°F) in tightly closed containers, unless otherwise directed by manufacturer. Protect from light.

Drug Interactions: Guanabenz

Plus	Interactions
Alcohol (Ethanol) Barbiturates Benzodiazepines Phenothiazines Other CNS depressants	Potentiation of CNS depression. Used concurrently with caution

---

GUANADREL SULFATE

(Hylorel)

(gwahn'a-drel)

Ganglionic blocking agent

Antihypertensive

ACTIONS AND USES. Adrenergic ganglionic blocking agent structurally and pharmacologically related to guanethidine. Not as potent as guanethidine and onset of action and duration of effects are shorter. Less apt to cause morning orthostatic hypotension than guanethidine and incidence of diarrhea is less. Acts as a false neurotransmitter without adrenergic activity because it blocks the release of norepinephrine from adrenal medulla and adrenergic nerve endings that normally follows sympathetic nerve stimulation. The net effect is catecholamine depletion with resulting relaxation of vascular smooth muscle, reduction of peripheral vascular resistance, lowering of systolic and diastolic blood pressures, and a relative increase in parasympathetic tone. Unlike several other step-2 drugs, hypotensive effect is not related to CNS activity and therefore produces less sedation and depression; may cause sodium and water retention and consequent expansion of plasma volume which generally requires use of a diuretic to maintain hypotensive effect. Decreases standing (orthostatic) more than supine blood pressure and is more effective in lowering systolic than diastolic blood pressure.

Used in stepped-care approach: step-2 treatment of hypertension, usually with a diuretic.

ABSORPTION AND FATE. Rapidly and almost completely absorbed from GI tract. Onset of hypotensive effect in ½ to 2 hours, peaks in 4 to 6 hours; duration 4 to 14 hours. Widely distributed to most body tissues and fluid. Little if any crosses blood–brain barrier. About 20% protein bound. Plasma half-life appears to be biphasic (wide interindividual variation): Initial: 1 to 4 hours; terminal: 5 to 45 hours. Approximately 85% of dose excreted in urine within 24 hours, about 40 to 50% as unchanged drug, and the remainder as metabolites. Distribution to placenta and breast milk not known.

CONTRAINDICATIONS AND PRECAUTIONS. History of hypersensitivity to guanadrel, pheochromocytoma, congestive heart failure, patients taking MAO inhibitors. Safe use during pregnancy (category B), in nursing women, and in children not established. *Cautious Use:* cerebrovascular, coronary artery, or peripheral vascular disease, bronchial asthma, history of peptic ulcer, diarrhea, elderly patients.

ADVERSE/SIDE EFFECTS. Generally dose related. **CNS:** tiredness, headache, drowsiness, paresthesias, tremors, confusion, depression or other psychologic problems, sleep disorders. **CV:** orthostatic hypotension, palpitation, chest pain. **GI:** diarrhea, or increased number of stools, indigestion, constipation, dry mouth and thirst, anorexia, glossitis, nausea, vomiting, abdominal distress or pain. **GU:** nocturia, urinary urgency or frequency, hematuria, retrograde ejaculation, impotence. **Other:** visual disturbances; musculoskeletal aches, pains, or inflammation; excessive weight gain or loss, peripheral edema, nasal stuffiness, cough, shortness of breath at rest or with exercise.

ROUTE AND DOSAGE. Oral: Initial: 5 mg twice daily. Dosage range for most patients is 20 to 75 mg, usually twice daily. Larger doses may require three or four times daily dosing. Highly individualized.

NURSING IMPLICATIONS

Since serum half-life of guanadrel averages about 10 hours, dosage adjustments are generally made weekly or monthly.

Dosage adjustments should be based on blood pressure response in supine position and after standing 2 to 20 minutes. Record baseline measurements for future comparison purposes.

The full effect of guanadrel on standing (orthostatic) blood pressure should be carefully evaluated before the hospitalized patient is discharged. For ambulatory patient, blood pressure measurements should also be taken following exercise for complete assessment.

Inform patient about the possibility of orthostatic hypotension. Hypotensive effect of guanadrel is most prominent in the standing position or with prolonged standing, following exercise, and with vasodilation effects associated with fever, hot shower, or tub bath, hot environment, or with ingestion of alcohol.

Patients with cerebrovascular or coronary artery, or peripheral vascular disease are particularly prone to orthostatic hypotension and therefore should be closely monitored.

Caution elderly patients particularly not to get out of bed without assistance during initial dosage adjustment period.

Warn patient to make position changes slowly and in stages, especially from recumbent to upright posture. These precautions should be observed throughout drug therapy. Some clinicians prescribe surgical support hose and advise patient to flex arms and legs prior to standing to augment venous return.

Advise patient to lie down immediately at first hint of faintness, dizziness, weakness, or lightheadedness. All are possible manifestations of orthostatic hypotension.

Teach patient to monitor weight and to check legs and ankles for edema, and in particular to note if rings or shoes suddenly seem too tight. Advise patient to notify physician of peripheral edema or unexpected weight gain of 2 pounds or more per day.

Guanadrel tends to enhance sodium and water retention, but these effects are generally controlled by concurrent diuretic therapy. Consult physician regarding allowable salt intake. Patients are usually advised to omit obviously salty foods and to avoid adding salt to served foods.

To encourage patient compliance in taking guanadrel at the same time(s) each day, suggest that it be taken in relation to a daily routine activity.

Most side effects disappear or at least diminish in intensity after about 8 weeks of therapy.

Dry mouth may be relieved by frequent rinsing with water and use of sugar-free gum or sour balls. Advise patient against overuse of commercial mouthwashes. Most contain alcohol which tends to cause even more dryness. *See Index: Nursing Interventions: dry mouth,* for more complete discussion.

Manufacturer recommends discontinuing guanadrel 48 to 72 hours before elective surgery to reduce risk of vascular collapse and cardiac arrest during anesthesia. If elective or emergency surgery is to be performed, anesthesiologist should be informed that patient is receiving guanadrel therapy.

Some patients develop tolerance to hypotensive effect of guanadrel following long-term therapy and require careful and gradual dosage increases.

Patient should be specifically cautioned not to use OTC drugs for treatment of colds, allergy, asthma, or appetite suppressants without consulting the physician or pharmacist. Many of these products contain adrenergic (sympathomimetic) amines which may interfere with hypotensive action of guanadrel.

Management of overdosage: Emesis or gastric lavage, symptomatic and supportive treatment. Keep patient supine. Have on hand phenylephine for excessive hypotension (used with caution and in small doses).

See Guanethidine: Patient teaching plan (for patients with hypertension).

Store preferably between 15° and 30°C (59° and 86°F) unless otherwise directed by manufacturer.

Drug Interactions: Guanadrel

Plus	Interactions
Alcohol (Ethanol)	Additive orthostatic hypotension and sedative effects. Avoid or limit intake
Alpha or beta adrenergic blocking agents, reserpine and other rauwolfia alkaloids	Possibility of excess orthostatic hypotension and bradycardia. Used concurrently with caution
MAO inhibitors	Antagonize hypotensive effect of guanadrel. Not used concurrently or within 1 week of MAO inhibitors

Plus (cont.)	Interactions (cont.)
Phenothiazines Tricyclic antidepressants Indirect-acting sympathomimetic amines e.g., ephedrine, phenylpropanolamine	These drugs may decrease hypotensive effect of guanadrel (by blocking its neuronal uptake). Concurrent use generally avoided
Direct-acting sympathomimetic amines e.g., epinephrine, norepinephrine, methoxamine	Guanadrel may enhance pharmacologic action of these drugs (by inhibiting their neuronal uptake). Concurrent use generally avoided

G

GUANETHIDINE SULFATE

(Ismelin)

(gwahn-eth'i-deen)
Adrenergic blocking agent
Antihypertensive

ACTIONS AND USES. Potent, long-acting, postganglionic adrenergic blocking agent. Competes with norepinephrine for reuptake into adrenergic neurons; displaces stored norepinephrine thus exposing it to degradation by MAO. Guanethidine slowly accumulates in storage granules and is released by nerve stimulation as a "false neurotransmitter" that effectively blocks adrenergic actions of norepinephrine. Produces gradual prolonged fall in blood pressure, usually associated with bradycardia and decreased pulse pressure. Antihypertensive effect results from venous dilatation with peripheral pooling, decreased venous return, and decreased cardiac output. Drug-induced sodium retention and expansion of plasma volume, with resulting tolerance to antihypertensive effect, may occur unless concomitant diuretic therapy is administered. Renal blood flow and glomerular filtration rate may decrease during early therapy. Guanethidine also causes decreased plasma renin activity. It diminishes or eliminates cardiovascular reflexes and is therefore more effective in lowering orthostatic than supine blood pressure. Marked increase in GI motility is thought to be partly due to unopposed parasympathetic activity, but mechanism is poorly understood. Has weak local anesthetic effect, and appears to have some antidiabetic action. Local instillation in eye causes miosis and reduces intraocular pressure in glaucomatous eyes.

Used in stepped care approach to treatment of moderate to severe hypertension either alone or in conjunction with a thiazide diuretic and/or hydralazine (step 4). *Investigational Use:* to treat glaucoma and to increase finger capillary blood flow in patients with Raynaud's phenomenon. Commercially available in combination with hydrochlorothiazide (Esimil).

ABSORPTION AND FATE. Irregularly absorbed from GI tract (3 to 30% variability in absorption rate, but rate remains constant for each individual). Peak antihypertensive effect in 6 to 8 hours; duration: 24 to 48 hours. Half-life: 5 days. Partially metabolized by hepatic microsomal enzymes. Highly concentrated in cells of kidney, liver, and lungs. Does not readily cross blood–brain barrier. Excreted in urine as active drug and less active metabolites; some excretion via feces. Small amounts may remain in body up to 14 days or longer. Appears in breast milk in negligible amounts.

CONTRAINDICATIONS AND PRECAUTIONS. Hypersensitivity to guanethidine; pheochromocytoma, frank congestive heart failure (not due to hypertension). Safe use during pregnancy and in women of childbearing potential not established. *Cautious Use:* diabetes mellitus, impaired renal or hepatic function, sinus bradycardia, limited cardiac reserve, coronary disease with insufficiency, recent myocardial infarction, cerebrovascular insufficiency, febrile illnesses, use in the elderly; history of peptic ulcer, colitis, or bronchial asthma.

ADVERSE/SIDE EFFECTS. CV: marked orthostatic and exertional hypotension with dizziness, light-headedness, fainting, bradycardia, angina, edema with weight gain, dyspnea, congestive heart failure, complete heart block. **Dermatologic:** skin eruptions, loss of scalp hair. **EENT:** blurred vision, ptosis of eyelids, parotid tenderness, nasal congestion. **GI:** severe diarrhea, nausea, vomiting, constipation, dry mouth. **GU:** nocturia, urinary retention, incontinence, inhibition of ejaculation, psychological impotence. **Other:** psychic depression, weakness, fatigue, myalgia, tremor, chest paresthesias, asthma, rise in BUN, polyarteritis nodosa. Reported, but causal relationship not established: anemia, thrombocytopenia, leukopenia, priapism.

ROUTE AND DOSAGE. Adults: Oral: *Ambulatory patients:* Initial: 10 mg daily, depending on patient's response; incremental increases of 10 mg no more often than every 5 to 7 days; maintenance: 25 to 50 mg once daily. *Hospitalized patients:* 25 to 50 mg daily, increased by 25 or 50 mg daily or every other day as indicated. **Pediatric:** 0.2 mg/kg or 6 mg/m^2 daily. If necessary, increased gradually every 1 to 3 weeks in increments of 0.2 mg/kg/24 hours, up to maximum dose: 3 mg/kg/24 hours. All dosages highly individualized.

G

NURSING IMPLICATIONS

Tablet may be crushed before administration and taken with fluid of patient's choice.

Some products (e.g., Ismelin 10 mg tablets) contain *tartrazine* which can cause allergic type reactions including bronchial asthma in susceptible individuals, such as persons with aspirin hypersensitivity.

To reinforce patient compliance in taking drug regularly at the same time each day, suggest that it be taken to coincide with some routine activity such as brushing teeth in the morning. Stress importance of not stopping drug without advice of physician.

During period of dosage adjustment, doses must be carefully titrated on the basis of orthostatic and supine blood pressures. The hypotensive effect of guanethidine is greater with patient in orthostatic position as opposed to supine position. Take readings before initiation of therapy as baseline for comparison.

Physician generally prescribes taking blood pressure first in supine position and then again after patient has been standing for 10 minutes. Some physicians also request that it be taken immediately after mild exercise.

Since hospitalized patients are given higher initial doses than ambulatory patients, standing blood pressure determinations should be made regularly during the day, if possible. The full effect of guanethidine on standing blood pressure should be carefully evaluated before patient is discharged.

Caution patient not to get out of bed without assistance. Supervise ambulation particularly in the elderly since they are prone to develop orthostatic hypotension.

Patients should be informed that orthostatic hypotension is most prominent shortly after arising from sleep and when too rapid changes are made to sitting or upright positions. Warn patients to move gradually to sitting position. Some physicians advise patient to apply elastic stockings and/or flex arms and legs slowly prior to standing to augment venous return. These precautions should be observed throughout drug therapy and for several days after drug is withdrawn.

Patients should also be informed that orthostatic hypotension is intensified by prolonged standing, hot baths or showers, hot weather, alcohol ingestion, and strenuous physical exercise (particularly if followed by immobility).

Warn patients to lie down or sit down (in head-low position) immediately at the onset of dizziness, weakness, or faintness. Fainting or blackout occurs when such symptoms are ignored. To control these symptoms, the physician may reduce dosage of guanethidine.

Intake and output should be monitored especially in the elderly and in patients with limited cardiac reserve or impaired renal function. Report changes in intake–output ratio.

Advise the patient to report character and frequency of stools. Diarrhea due to accelerated GI motility may be manifested by increased frequency of bowel movements rather than loose stools and may be explosive and embarrassing to patient. Physician may prescribe an anticholinergic agent (e.g., atropine), paregoric, or a kaolin-pectin preparation. Dosage adjustment or discontinuation of drug may be required. State of hydration and electrolyte levels should be checked in patients with severe and persistent diarrhea.

Patients with limited cardiac reserve are particularly susceptible to guanethidine-induced sodium and water retention, with resulting edema, congestive failure, and drug resistance (a thiazide diuretic is generally prescribed to reduce the possibility of these effects).

Observe for evidence of edema, and weigh patients daily (or as prescribed) under standard conditions: same time (preferably in the morning before breakfast and after voiding), same weight of clothing, same scale. Sudden weight gain of 2 lb or more should be reported to physician.

Consult physician regarding allowable salt intake. Generally, patients are advised to omit obviously salty foods and to avoid adding salt to served foods. Physician may prescribe greater restriction of sodium-containing foods for patients with limited cardiac reserve.

Because guanethidine has prolonged onset and duration of action and since its effects are cumulative, dosage should be increased slowly (at intervals of no less than 5 to 7 days for adults and 1 to 3 weeks in children) and only if there has been no reduction in standing blood pressure from previous levels. Blood pressure should be monitored during dosage adjustment period.

A limited degree of tolerance may develop early in therapy. Dosage plateau is usually reached in 2 weeks.

Ideal dosage is that which reduces orthostatic blood pressure to within normal range without faintness, dizziness, weakness, or fatigue.

Dosage requirements may be reduced in presence of febrile illnesses. Advise patient to report fever to physician.

Guanethidine may sensitize the patient to some sympathomimetic agents found in OTC cold remedies and cause hypertensive crisis. Caution patient to consult physician or pharmacist before taking any OTC drug.

Guanethidine is reported to have antidiabetic activity (mechanism unknown). Patients on antidiabetic therapy should be observed closely for signs of hypoglycemia.

Candidates for home blood pressure measurements are selected on the basis of ability to follow directions, emotional stability, cooperation, and normal hearing.

Assist the patient to develop a record system for sitting and standing blood pressures (as prescribed) so as to provide physician with information on degree of control achieved.

Patient must understand that although hypertension is usually an asymptomatic disease, it can result in a variety of serious complications if untreated.

Periodic blood counts and liver and kidney function tests are advised during prolonged therapy.

In patients undergoing elective surgery, manufacturer recommends that if possible guanethidine be withdrawn 2 weeks prior to surgery to reduce the possibility of vascular collapse and cardiac arrest during anesthesia. (This point is controversial. Some clinicians believe it is both unnecessary and potentially dangerous to withdraw antihypertensives before anesthesia.) If emergency surgery is indicated, preanesthetic and anesthetic agents should be administered cautiously in reduced dosages.

Patient-Teaching Plan for Patient with Hypertension:

✓ knowledge of the medical problem

✓ drug action (reason for taking drug)
✓ dosage regimen
✓ importance of keeping follow-up appointments
✓ symptoms to be reported
✓ diet restrictions, if prescribed (e.g., salt regulation)
✓ weight control plans
✓ importance of limiting alcohol intake and avoiding tobacco, and excessive caffeine (coffee, tea, and colas), as well as emotionally charged situations
✓ dangers of self-medication
✓ importance of planned graduated exercise program
✓ importance of hobbies and regular vacations
✓ continual reinforcement of the potential need for life-long therapy

Store in well closed container at room temperature unless otherwise directed by manufacturer.

Diagnostic Test Interferences. Guanethidine may increase **BUN,** decrease **blood glucose** (in patients with diabetes mellitus), and may decrease **urinary norepinephrine** excretion and **urinary VMA** excretion.

Drug Interactions: Guanethidine

Plus	Interactions
Alcohol, ethyl Levodopa Methotrimeprazine (Levoprome) Rauwolfia derivatives Thiazides and related diuretics	Enhance hypotensive effects of guanethidine. Used with caution
Amphetamines Antidepressants, tricyclic Cocaine Diethylpropion Doxepin (Sinequan) Ephedrine Haloperidol (Haldol) MAO inhibitors Methylphenidate (Ritalin) Oral contraceptives Phenothiazines Thiothixene (Navane)	Inhibit antihypertensive effect of guanethidine
Dopamine (Intropin) Epinephrine Norepinephrine (Levarterenol, Levophed) Metaraminol (Aramine) Methoxamine Phenylephrine	Guanethidine may augment pressor response to direct-acting alpha-adrenergic sympathomimetic amines
Anesthetics, general	Increased risk of cardiovascular collapse and cardiac arrest
Antidiabetic agents	Enhanced hypoglycemic effect
Digitalis glycosides	Additive bradycardic effect

H

HALAZEPAM

(Paxipam)

(hal-az'e-pam)
Psychotropic
Anxiolytic
Benzodiazepine
C IV

ACTIONS AND USES. Psychotropic drug that shares antianxiety actions of other short-term benzodiazepine derivatives. Exact mechanism of action is unknown but clinically, it produces dose-related CNS depressant effect ranging from mild improvement of psychomotor activity to hypnosis. Clinical efficacy in long-term use (i.e., more than 4 months) has not been evaluated. Animal studies suggest that drug induces activity of hepatic microsomal enzymes, therefore metabolism of other drugs given concurrently may be increased.

Used to manage anxiety disorders or for short-term relief of anxiety symptoms.

ABSORPTION AND FATE. Rapidly and almost completely absorbed following oral dose. Peak plasma concentrations reached 1 to 3 hours after 40-mg dose, with peak concentrations of major metabolite (*N*-desmethyldiazepam) reached in 3 to 6 hours. Hepatic biotransformation (probable enterohepatic recycling in patient with uremia). Half-life: halazepam, about 14 hours; metabolite, 50 to 100 hours. Plasma protein binding is high, therefore is affected by plasma albumin concentration. Excreted in urine. May cross placenta barrier; appears in breast milk.

CONTRAINDICATIONS AND PRECAUTIONS. Pregnancy (category D); safe use and effectiveness in children under age 18 not established. *See also Chlordiazepoxide.*

ADVERSE/SIDE EFFECTS. *See Chlordiazepoxide.*

ROUTE AND DOSAGE. Individualized. **Oral: Adults:** 20 to 40 mg three or four times daily. (Daily doses up to 600 mg have been given.) **Elderly, debilitated patient:** Initial: 20 mg once or twice a day.

NURSING IMPLICATIONS

Note that an antianxiety agent is not indicated as treatment for anxiety or tension associated with stress of everyday life.

If patient becomes pregnant or plans on pregnancy, she should discuss with physician desirability of discontinuing drug because of its potential hazard to the fetus.

Ataxia, confusion, or oversedation (sleeping in daytime) may be symptoms of overdosage and can occur at relatively low dosage in the elderly or debilitated patient.

Smoking–Drug Interaction. Smoking decreases sedative effects of benzodiazepines, including halazepam. This is especially true if patient is a heavy smoker.

Psychic and/or physical dependence can develop, especially in addiction-prone patient, who should be under careful surveillance while on this drug.

Warn patient not to alter drug regimen (dose or interval) and not to stop taking drug suddenly. Barbiturate-like withdrawal symptoms may occur. Dosage is tapered after long-term use to discontinue its use.

Halazepam is classified as Schedule IV drug under Federal Controlled Substances Act.

See Chlordiazepoxide (prototype benzodiazepine) for additional Nursing Implications and Drug Interactions.

HALCINONIDE

(Halciderm, Halog)

(hal-sin′oh-nide)
Corticosteroid
Glucocorticoid

ACTIONS AND USES. Fluorinated steroid with substituted 17-hydroxyl group. Crosses cell membranes, complexes with nuclear DNA and stimulates synthesis of enzymes thought to be responsible for antiinflammatory effects. Systemic absorption leads to actions, limitations and drug interactions observed with use of hydrocortisone (qv). Topical action, and limitations are similar to those of flurandrenolide (qv).

Used for relief of pruritic and inflammatory manifestations of corticosteroid-responsive dermatoses.

ROUTE AND DOSAGE. **Topical:** **Adult:** Cream, ointment (0.025 or 0.1%), solution (0.1%) applied two or three times daily. **Pediatric:** medication applied once daily.

NURSING IMPLICATIONS

Check with physician regarding specific procedure. Generally, skin is gently washed and thoroughly dried before each application.

Selection of medication vehicle depends on condition of lesions. Ointment is usually preferred for dry scaly lesions. Moist lesions are appropriately treated with solution.

Medication should be discontinued if signs of infection or irritation occur.

Not to be applied in or around the eyes.

Systemic corticosteroid effects may be produced when occlusive dressings are used and when topical application covers large areas of skin.

Occlusive dressings should not be applied over areas covered with halcinonide unless specifically prescribed.

See also Flurandrenolide (prototype topical corticosteroid).

H

PROTOTYPE

HALOPERIDOL

(Haldol, Peridol)

(ha-loe-per′i-dole)
Antipsychotic
Neuroleptic
Butyrophenone

ACTIONS AND USES. Potent, long-acting butyrophenone derivative with pharmacologic actions similar to those of piperazine phenothiazines but with higher incidence of extrapyramidal effects, less hypotensive, and relatively low sedative activity. Exerts strong antiemetic effect, and impairs central thermoregulation. Produces weak central anticholinergic effects and transient orthostatic hypotension. Actions thought to be due to blockade of dopamine activity.

Used for management of manifestations of psychotic disorders and for control of tics and vocal utterances of Gilles de la Tourette's syndrome; for treatment of agitated states in acute and chronic psychoses. Used for treatment of hyperactive children, and for severe behavior problems in children of combative, explosive hyperexcitability. *Investigational Use:* as an effective antiemetic in doses smaller than those required for antipsychotic effects.

ABSORPTION AND FATE. Well absorbed from GI tract. Peak plasma levels: 2 to 6 hours following oral administration and 20 minutes following IM administration. Blood levels may plateau for as long as 72 hours, with detectable levels persisting for weeks. Metabolized in liver to inactive metabolites. Serum protein binding more than 90%. Elimination half-life: 13 to 35 hours. Approximately 40% excreted in urine during first 5 days; about 15% excreted in bile (then feces). Small amounts continue to be excreted for 28 days. Crosses placenta; appears in breast milk.

CONTRAINDICATIONS AND PRECAUTIONS. Hypersensitivity to haloperidol, Parkinson's disease, seizure disorders, coma, alcoholism, severe mental depression, CNS depression, thyrotoxicosis. Safe use during pregnancy and in women of childbearing potential, in nursing mothers, and in children under 3 years not established. *Cautious Use:* history of drug allergies, elderly or debilitated patients, urinary retention, glaucoma, severe cardiovascular disorders; patients receiving anticonvulsant, anticoagulant or lithium therapy.

ADVERSE/SIDE EFFECTS. Autonomic: dry mouth; hypersalivation, "drooling," constipation, diarrhea, urinary retention, diaphoresis, blurred vision. **CNS:** extrapyramidal reactions: parkinsonlike symptoms, dystonia, akathisia, tardive dyskinesia (rarely); insomnia, restlessness, anxiety, euphoria, agitation, drowsiness, mental depression, lethargy, headache, confusion, vertigo, hyperthermia, grand mal seizures, exacerbation of psychotic symptoms. **CV:** tachycardia, hypotension, hypertension (with overdosage). **Dermatologic:** maculopapular and acneiform rash, alopecia; (rarely), photosensitivity. **Endocrine:** menstrual irregularities, galactorrhea, lactation, gynecomastia, impotence, increased libido, hyperglycemia, hypoglycemia. **Hematologic:** mild and usually transient leukopenia, leukocytosis, anemia, tendency toward lymphomonocytosis, agranulocytosis (rarely). **Respiratory:** laryngospasm, bronchospasm, increased depth of respiration, bronchopneumonia, respiratory depression. **Other:** anorexia, nausea, vomiting, jaundice (occasionally), ocular and cutaneous changes, variations in liver function tests, decreased serum cholesterol, "therapeutic window" effect.

ROUTE AND DOSAGE. *Highly individualized.* Maintenance dose established at lowest effective level. **Oral: Adult:** *Moderate symptoms:* 0.5 to 2 mg two to three times daily; *severe symptoms,* 3 to 5 mg two to three times daily. Higher doses may be required for prompt control. **Geriatric:** lower dose range. **Chronic or resistant patients:** higher dose range. *Severely disturbed:* up to 100 mg per day may be necessary. Safety of long-term therapy in excess of 100 mg/day not established. **Pediatric (3 to 12 years):** 0.05 to 0.15 mg/kg/day. **Intramuscular: Adult:** Initial: 2 to 5 mg. Subsequent doses (if necessary) usually at 4 to 8 hour intervals until oral form is feasible. Oral concentrate contains 2 mg/ml.

NURSING IMPLICATIONS

Preliminary reports suggest that haloperidol concentrate may precipitate when mixed with coffee or with tea; avoid these beverages as diluents and administer oral forms of the drug with some other fluid.

Because of long half-life of haloperidol, therapeutic effects are slow to develop in early therapy or when established dosing regimen is changed.

Once the neuroleptic plan is established, monitor patient's mental status daily: appearance and general behavior, thought content, affect and mood, sensorium.

Target symptoms expected to decrease with successful haloperidol treatment include: hallucinations, insomnia, hostility, agitation, and delusions. If no improvement in 2 to 4 weeks, medication may be increased.

Psychotic exacerbation at the beginning of therapy has been reported. Increasing the dosage may produce improvement.

"Therapeutic window" effect (point at which increased dose or concentration actually decreases therapeutic response) may occur after long period of high doses. Close observation is imperative when doses are changed.

Although orthostatic hypotension is not common, take necessary safety precautions. Have patient recumbent at time of parenteral administration and for about 1 hour following injection (levarterenol or phenylephrine is prescribed when a vasopressor is indicated; epinephrine is contraindicated).

Extrapyramidal reactions *(see Chlorpromazine)* occur frequently during first few days of treatment. Symptoms are usually dose-related and are controlled by dosage reduction or concomitant administration of antiparkinsonian drugs. Discontinuation of therapy may be necessary. Reactions appear to be more prominent in younger patients.

Be alert for behavioral changes in patients who are concurrently receiving antiparkinsonian drugs (e.g., benztropine, trihexyphenidyl). Such medication may have to be continued beyond termination of haloperidol therapy to prevent extrapyramidal symptoms which may appear during the period when haloperidol levels are decreasing (3 to 4 days).

Haloperidol is administered cautiously to patients receiving anticonvulsant medication because it may lower the convulsant threshold. The established dose of the anticonvulsant is not changed.

When haloperidol is used to control mania or cyclic disorders, the patient should be closely observed for rapid mood shift to depression. Depression may represent a drug side effect or a reversion from a manic state.

Differential diagnosis between extrapyramidal side effects and psychotic reaction requires sensitive observation and prompt reporting.

Fatal bronchospasm associated with use of antipsychotics has been postulated to result from drug-induced lethargy, reduced sensation of thirst, dehydration, hemoconcentration, and reduced ventilation. Adequate fluid intake and regularly scheduled breathing exercises may help to prevent its occurrence.

Protect patient from extremes in environmental temperature.

Alcohol should be avoided during haloperidol therapy.

Caution against use of OTC drugs without physician's approval.

Patient should not change dosing regimen. Tell patient not to give drug to any other person.

Ambulatory patients and responsible family members should be completely informed about what symptoms to report and the importance of follow-up appointments.

Advise patient not to drive a car or engage in other activities requiring mental alertness and physical coordination until drug response is known.

Dosing regimen should be tapered when therapy is to be discontinued. Abrupt termination of treatment can initiate extrapyramidal symptoms.

If patient suspects pregnancy or wants to be pregnant, she should discuss drug regimen with her physician. Sporadic case reports suggest that haloperidol is teratogenic during the first trimester.

Haldol tablets contain **tartrazine** which can cause allergic reactions including bronchial asthma in susceptible persons. Such individuals are also frequently sensitive to aspirin.

Xerostomia may promote dental problems. Deprivation of saliva fosters demineralization of normal tooth surfaces and loosening of dentures. Discuss oral hygiene with patient. *(See Chlorpromazine.)* Encourage adequate fluid intake.

Patient on home therapy should be told what laxative may be used if necessary.

Periodic blood studies and liver function tests are advised in patients on prolonged therapy.

Discard darkened solutions; slight yellowing does not affect potency, however.

Store in light-resistant container at temperature between 15° and 30°C (59° and 86°F) unless otherwise specified by manufacturer.

See Chlorpromazine (prototype antipsychotic).

Drug Interactions: Haloperidol

Plus	Interactions
Alcohol	Enhanced CNS depressant effects; hypotension
Amphetamines	Haloperidol antagonizes effects of amphetamines
Anticholinergic agents	Increased intraocular pressure and may inhibit haloperidol effects
Anticonvulsants	Haloperidol lowers convulsive threshold
Anticoagulants	Interference with anticoagulant activity (based on limited data)
Antiparkinson agents	Increased intraocular pressure
CNS depressants	Additive depressant activity
Guanethidine (Ismelin)	Reversal of hypotensive action
Lithium	Possibility of encephalopathy (extrapyramidal symptoms, fever, confusion)
Methyldopa (Aldomet)	Possibility of dementia
See also Chlorpromazine	

HALOPROGIN
(Halotex)

(ha-loe-proe'jin)
Antiinfective
Antifungal

ACTIONS AND USES. Synthetic iodinated phenolic ether. Fungicidal or fungistatic against various species of *Trichophyton, Epidermophyton, Microsporum, Malassezia,* and *Candida.* Also active in vitro against *Staphylococcus aureus* and *Streptococcus pyogenes.*

Used for treatment of superficial fungal infections such as tinea pedis, tinea cruris, tinea corporis, and tinea manus. Also used in treatment of tinea versicolor caused by *Malassezia furfur.* May be used in combination with antiinfective therapy for mixed infections.

ABSORPTION AND FATE. Poorly absorbed through skin. Converted to trichlorophenol in body if systemically absorbed.

CONTRAINDICATIONS AND PRECAUTIONS. Hypersensitivity to any component in formulation. Safe use during pregnancy not established.

ADVERSE/SIDE EFFECTS. Local irritation, burning sensation, vesiculation, increased maceration, exacerbation of preexisting lesions, sensitization, pruritus. Low incidence of systemic toxicity.

ROUTE AND DOSAGE. Topical: 1% cream, 1% solution: Apply liberally to affected area twice daily for 2 to 3 weeks. Interdigital lesions may require up to 4 weeks of therapy.

NURSING IMPLICATIONS

Avoid contact of medication with eyes.

Advise patient to discontinue medication if condition worsens, or if burning, irritation, or signs of sensitization occur, and consult physician.

Therapy should be reevaluated if no improvement is noted after 2 to 3 weeks.

Patients with tinea pedis (athlete's foot) should be advised not to wear occlusive footwear because it tends to promote systemic drug absorption and enhance fungal growth.

To avoid spread of infection to others, instruct patient to keep facecloth, towels, and other articles of personal hygiene separate.
Advise patient to wear freshly laundered clothes daily.
See Tolnaftate for other patient teaching points.

HEMIN

(hee'min)

[Panhematin (formerly Hematin)]

Enzyme inhibitor
Blood derivative

H

ACTIONS AND USES. Sterile, nonpyrogenic ferric iron complex of protoporphyrin IX; derived from processed red blood cells. Represses synthesis of porphyrin precursors probably by blocking production of delta-aminolevulinic acid (ALA) synthetase, an essential enzyme in the porphyrin/heme biosynthetic pathway. Each vial contains hemin 313 mg with sodium carbonate 215 mg, sorbitol 300 mg (no preservatives).

Used in treatment of recurrent attacks of acute intermittent porphyria (AIP) only after an appropriate period of alternate therapy has been tried (i.e., 400 Gm glucose/day for 1 to 2 days).

ABSORPTION AND FATE. Highly bound to plasma proteins. Can be detected in plasma up to 5 days postinfusion. Amounts in excess of capacity for hepatocellular uptake and plasma binding are eliminated in bile and urine.

CONTRAINDICATIONS AND PRECAUTIONS. History of hypersensitivity to hemin; use for porphyria cutanea tarda. Safe use during pregnancy (category C), in nursing women and in children not established.

ADVERSE/SIDE EFFECTS. Phlebitis (when administrated into small veins); anticoagulant effect: prolonged PT, thromboplastin time, thrombocytopenia, hypofibrinogenemia, decreased hematocrit; reversible renal shutdown (with excessive doses).

ROUTE AND DOSAGE. Intravenous: 1 to 4 mg/kg/day administered over 10 to 15 minutes for 3 to 14 days. For severe conditions, dose may be repeated no earlier than every 12 hours. Not to exceed 6 mg/kg in any 24-hour period.

NURSING IMPLICATIONS

Hemin is administered only by physicians experienced in the management of porphyria, in hospitals equipped to perform the recommended clinical and laboratory monitoring.
Before therapy is initiated, the following diagnostic measures should have been done to confirm diagnosis of acute prophyria: identification of clinical symptoms; positive Watson–Schwartz or Hoesch test. If further confirmation is needed, quantitative tests of ALA and porphobilinogen in serum and urine are performed.
Hemin should be administered via a large arm vein or central venous catheter to reduce risk of phlebitis. Terminal filtration through a sterile 0.45 μ or smaller filter is recommended to assure that no undissolved particles are injected into patient.
The following laboratory values are monitored throughout hemin therapy (decrease in these values is an indication of a favorable clinical response): ALA, UPG (uroporphyrinogen), PBG (porphobilinogen or corproporphyrin).
In order to monitor clinical effect of drug therapy, be aware of the patient's symptoms and complaints associated with acute porphyria including: mental disturbances: depres-

sion, insomnia, anxiety, disorientation, hallucinations, psychoses; dark urine, nausea, vomiting, abdominal pain, low back and leg pain, pareses (neuropathy), seizures.

Monitor intake–output ratio and pattern particularly in patients receiving high doses. Promptly report the onset of oliguria or anuria.

Since many drugs have been implicated in precipitating attacks of acute porphyria, questions regarding drug safety should be referred to a pharmacist who has access to special references.

Because hemin contains no preservatives, it should be reconstituted immediately before use. Reconstitute by aseptically adding 43 ml sterile water for injection to vial. Shake well for 2 or 3 minutes to dissolve all particles.

Freeze and store lyophilized powder until time of use.

Drug Interactions: Hemin

Plus	Interactions
Anticoagulants	Potentiation of anticoagulant effect. Combination generally avoided
Barbiturates Estrogens Sulfonamides	These drugs increase ALA enzyme activity and therefore counteract hemin effect. Combination should be avoided

H

HEPARIN CALCIUM
(Calciparine)

HEPARIN SODIUM
(Hepalean, Lipo-Hepin, Liquaemin Sodium)

(hep'a-rin)
Anticoagulant

ACTIONS AND USES. Strongly acidic, high molecular weight mucopolysaccharide with rapid anticoagulant effect, prepared from bovine lung tissue or porcine intestinal mucosa. Exerts direct effect on blood coagulation (clotting) by enhancing the inhibitory actions of antithrombin III (heparin cofactor) on several factors essential to normal blood clotting, thereby blocking the conversion of prothrombin to thrombin and fibrinogen to fibrin. Does not lyse already existing thrombi, but may prevent their extension and propagation. Inhibits formation of new clots. Prolongs whole blood clotting time, thrombin time, partial thromboplastin time and prothrombin time, but bleeding time (test of platelet function) is usually unaffected except with high doses. Reduces plasma triglycerides (antilipemic action), exhibits antiinflammatory and diuretic effects, and may suppress aldosterone secretion. Reportedly enhances potassium retention and possibly plays a role in immunologic reactions. The calcium salt is derived from porcine intestinal mucosa; the sodium salt is prepared from either porcine intestinal mucosa or bovine lung tissue.

Used in the prophylaxis and treatment of venous thrombosis and pulmonary embolism, and to prevent thromboembolic complications arising from cardiac and vascular surgery, frostbite, and during acute stage of myocardial infarction. Also used in treatment of disseminated intravascular clotting syndrome (DIC), atrial fibrillation with embolization, and as anticoagulant in blood transfusions, extracorporeal circulation, and dialysis procedures.

ABSORPTION AND FATE. Peak effects within minutes following direct IV injection; clotting time returns to normal within 2 to 6 hours. Onset of action following SC occurs within 20 to 60 minutes, (wide interpatient variation), duration of effects: 8 to 12 hours (dose dependent). Absorption following IM is unpredictable. Plasma half-life: 1½ hours (possibly shorter in patients with pulmonary embolism infections, or malignancy and longer in hepatic or renal dysfunction, and obesity). About 95% bound to plasma proteins. Some uptake and storage in mast cells. Believed to be partially metabolized by reticuloendothelial system and heparinase in liver. Excreted slowly in urine as partially degraded heparin; 20 to 50% of single dose excreted unchanged. Unlike oral anticoagulants, heparin does not cross the placenta (because of its large molecular size) and does not appear in breast milk.

CONTRAINDICATIONS AND PRECAUTIONS. Hypersensitivity to heparin, active bleeding, bleeding tendencies (hemophilia, purpura, thrombocytopenia), jaundice, ascorbic acid deficiency, inaccessible ulcerative lesions, visceral carcinoma, open wounds, extensive denudation of skin, suppurative thrombophlebitis, advanced kidney, liver or biliary disease, active tuberculosis, subacute bacterial endocarditis, continuous tube drainage of stomach or small intestines, threatened abortion, suspected intracranial hemorrhage, severe hypertension, recent surgery of eye, brain or spinal cord, spinal tap, shock. Teratogenic potential or safe use in persons of childbearing age not established. *Cautious Use:* alcoholism, history of atopy or allergy (asthma, hives, hay fever, eczema), during menstruation, during pregnancy (category C), especially the last trimester, immediate postpartum period, patients with indwelling catheters, the elderly, use of ACD-converted blood (may contain heparin), patients in hazardous occupations.

ADVERSE/SIDE EFFECTS. Spontaneous bleeding, injection site reactions: pain, itching, ecchymoses, tissue irritation and sloughing, cyanosis and pains in arms or legs (vasospasm), diarrhea, transient thrombocytopenia, hypofibrinogenemia. Rarely, frequent and persistent erections (priapism), hypersensitivity reactions: fever, chills, urticaria, pruritus, skin rashes, itching and burning sensations of feet, numbness and tingling of hands and feet, elevated blood pressure, headache, reversible transient alopecia (usually around temporal area), nasal congestion, lacrimation, conjunctivitis, chest pains, arthralgia, bronchospasm, anaphylactoid reactions. Large doses for prolonged periods: osteoporosis (back or rib pain, decrease in height, spontaneous fractures), hypoaldosteronism, suppressed renal function, hyperkalemia. Rebound hyperlipemia (following termination of heparin therapy).

ROUTE AND DOSAGE. Adult: [Based on 150-pound (68 kg) patient. For accuracy, dosage should be expressed in standard USP units and not in milligrams or International Units (IU), neither of which is equivalent:] **Deep subcutaneous (intrafat):** Initial: 10,000 to 20,000 U (usually preceded by bolus dose of 5000 U IV); *maintenance:* 8000 to 10,000 U every 8 hours, or 15,000 to 20,000 U every 12 hours. *Postoperative thromboembolism* (low dose prophylaxis): 5000 U by deep SC (intrafat) 2 hours prior to surgery, then every 8 to 12 hours, postoperatively for 7 days or until patient is fully ambulatory, which ever is longer. **Continuous intravenous infusion:** Initial bolus dose of 5000 U by direct IV, then 20,000 to 40,000 U daily added to 1000 ml isotonic sodium chloride injection or in compatible solution for infusion. **Intermittent intravenous injection:** Initial: 10,000 U followed by 5000 to 10,000 U every 4 to 6 hours. *Open heart surgery:* 150 to 400 U/kg. *Extracorporeal dialysis:* follow equipment manufacturer's instructions. *Test dose* (in patients with history of allergy): 1000 U. **Pediatric:** Initial: 50 U/kg IV; maintenance: 50 to 100 U/kg every 4 hours, or 20,000 U/m^2/kg/24 hours by continuous IV infusion.

NURSING IMPLICATIONS

Read label carefully. Heparin comes in various strengths.

Baseline blood coagulation tests, HCT, Hgb, red blood cell, and platelet counts should be performed before therapy is initiated, at regular intervals throughout therapy, and whenever patient shows signs of bleeding. Some physicians make periodic tests of urine for hematuria and stools for occult blood.

The activated partial thromboplastin time (APTT) and the activated coagulation time (ACT) are coagulation tests commonly used to monitor heparin therapy. In general, dosage is adjusted to keep APTT between 1½ and 2½ times normal control level, and the ACT at approximately 2 to 3 times the control value in seconds. (Values may vary in different laboratories.)

During dosage adjustment period, blood is drawn for coagulation test one-half hour before each scheduled SC or intermittent IV dose, and approximately every 4 hours for patients receiving continuous IV heparin. After dosage is established tests may be done once daily.

Before administering heparin, coagulation (clotting) test results must be checked by physician; if results are not within therapeutic range, dosage adjustment is made. Because heparin has short half-life it must be given on time to maintain anticoagulant effect. Follow agency protocol for administration of heparin.

Suggested technique and general guidelines for deep SC intrafat injection:

(1) Injections are made preferably into the fatty layer of the abdomen or just above the iliac crest. Shallow SC injection should be avoided because it is more painful and is associated with higher risk of hematoma and shorter duration of effect. (2) Use tuberculin syringe for accuracy in measuring dose, and a 25 or 26 gauge, ½ to ⅝ inch needle to make injection. (3) Discard needle used to withdraw heparin from vial. (4) Sponge selected site with alcohol and allow to dry. Do not massage (rubbing can rupture small blood vessels). (5) Avoid injecting within 2 inches of umbilicus, or any scar or bruise. Gently bunch up a defined roll of tissue without pinching, and insert needle into tissue roll at a 90° angle to skin. Still maintaining hold of tissue but with slightly less pressure, and keeping needle steady, slowly inject drug. To avoid possibility of tissue injury and hematoma *do not withdraw plunger to check entry into blood vessel.* (6) Hesitate for a few seconds before withdrawing needle to prevent trailing drug through needle tract. Withdraw needle rapidly in same direction as introduced while sumultaneously releasing tissue hold. (7) Apply gentle pressure to puncture site for about 1 minute, but do not massage. Application of ice following injection may help the patient who bruises easily. Discuss with physician. (8) Systematically rotate injection sites and keep record.

When heparin is added to an infusion solution (by authorized person), manufacturer recommends inverting container at least 6 times to insure adequate mixing and to prevent pooling of heparin.

Continuous IV infusion of heparin requires close monitoring to assure accuracy in dosage. A constant infusion pump or other approved volume control unit should be used to regulate flow rate and fluid volume. Gravity flow is not recommended because it is difficult to regulate and is subject to significant variations in flow rate when patient changes position.

When a roller pump is used, care should be taken to avoid negative pressure at infusion site which may increase rate of heparin administered into the system. Check at least hourly for signs of infiltration, see that tubing is not kinked, that it is properly positioned on pump rollers, and check all connections for leakage. Pump should be out of the reach of patient. Follow agency policy for daily care and how frequently to change infusion site.

Observe all needle sites daily for hematoma and signs of inflammation (swelling, heat, redness, pain).

Administration of heparin or any other drug IM is usually not prescribed because of risk of hematoma. If an IM drug is ordered, its administration should be timed when patient has minimal prolongation of coagulation time. This also pertains to invasive procedures, e.g., catheterizations, enemas.

Construct a flow chart indicating dates, coagulation time determinations, Hct, leukocyte and platelet counts, heparin doses, urine and stool tests for occult bleeding.

It is critically important to make accurate observations of clinical response.

Patients vary widely in their reaction to heparin and no test can reliably predict bleeding.

H

The risk of hemorrhage appears to be greatest in women, all patients 70 years of age or older, patients receiving heparin prophylactically following surgery, and patients with renal insufficiency.

Monitor vital signs. Report fever, drop in blood pressure, rapid pulse, and other signs and symptoms of hemorrhage. *Inform patient without frightening him to protect himself from injury and to report:* pink, red, dark brown, or cloudy urine (hematuria); red or dark brown vomitus (hematemesis); constipation (paralytic ileus, intestinal obstruction); red or black stools, bleeding gums or oral mucosa; petechiae of soft palate, conjunctiva, and retina (characteristic signs of thrombocytopenia); ecchymoses, hematoma, purpura, epistaxis, bloody sputum; chest pain (hemipericardium), abdominal or lumbar pain or swelling (retroperitoneal bleeding); unusual increase in menstrual flow, pelvic pain (corpus luteum hemorrhage); severe or continuous headache, faintness, or dizziness (intracranial bleeding). *Antidote:* have on hand protamine sulfate (1% solution), specific heparin antagonist. Because heparin has a short half-life, mild overdosage can frequently be controlled by merely withdrawing heparin. In some cases, however, whole blood or plasma transfusion may be necessary.

H

Menstruation may be somewhat increased and prolonged. Usually this is not a contraindication to continued therapy if bleeding is not excessive, and patient has no underlying pathology.

Monitor intake and output during early therapy. Inform patient that heparin may have a diuretic effect beginning 36 to 48 hours after initial dose and lasting 36 to 48 hours after termination of therapy.

In the absence of a low platelet (thrombocyte) count, patient may carry out normal activities such as shaving with a safety razor. Usually, heparin does not affect bleeding time.

Transient alopecia sometimes occurs several months after heparin therapy. Reassure patient that condition is reversible.

Smoking and alcohol consumption may alter response to heparin and, therefore, are not advised. Also, caution patient not to take aspirin, antihistamines, cough preparations containing guaifenesin (glyceryl guaiacolate), or any other OTC medication without physician's approval.

"Heparin resistance" has occurred in conditions associated with large amounts of fibrin deposition, such as early stage of thrombophlebitis, peritonitis, fever, pleurisy, cancer, myocardial infarction, extensive surgery.

Abrupt withdrawal of heparin may precipitate increased coagulability; generally, full dose heparin is followed by oral anticoagulant prophylactic therapy.

Administration of an oral anticoagulant usually overlaps that of heparin for 3 to 5 days while heparin is being tapered off. To obtain valid prothrombin time, a period of at least 4 to 6 hours after last IV dose, and 12 to 24 hours after the last SC (intrafat) dose of heparin should elapse before blood is drawn. Blood samples are usually drawn at any time when heparin is administered by continuous IV infusion.

Heparin Lock Flush Solution (e.g., Hep-Lock) is a sterile heparin-saline solution for intravenous flush only. It is *not intended for therapeutic purposes.* Follow agency policy regarding its use. In general, heparin lock care procedure reflects the following:

- A physician's order is required for use of Heparin Lock Flush Solution and the order must be renewed according to a specific policy.
- Heparin Lock Flush Solution is commonly used to maintain the patency of central venous catheters, femoral, and dialysis catheters. Heparinized flushing is not indicated when patency is maintained by continuous IV drip, nor is it generally used to maintain patency of short catheters as used in primary line or intermittent infusion sets.
- Each injection part of a multiple lumen catheter should be treated and recorded as a separate procedure.

- Refer to literature issued by manufacturer of the particular heparin lock set being used for detailed instructions.
- It is generally considered good practice to flush a heparin-lock set with 1 or 2 ml of normal saline before and after a medication is administered to avoid the possibility of drug interactions. If Heparin Lock Flush Solution is prescribed it is introduced following the second saline flush.
- A baseline activated partial thromboplastin time (APTT) is recommended when Heparin Lock Flush Solution is to be used.

Since heparin is strongly acidic, it is incompatible with many drugs; therefore, avoid mixing any drug with heparin unless specifically advised by physician or pharmacist.

Heparin is stable at room temperature 15° to 30°C (59° to 86° F). Protect from freezing. Inspect all preparations for discoloration and particulate matter prior to administration.

Diagnostic Test Interferences. (Notify laboratory that patient is receiving heparin, if a laboratory test is to be performed.) Possibility of: false-positive rise in **BSP** test; reduction in **serum cholesterol;** significant elevations of **SGOT** (AST), **SGPT** (ALT);false increase in **plasma corticosteroids** (with heparin containing benzyl alcohol); reportedly may increase **blood glucose;** may decrease urinary excretion of **5-HIAA;** and may interfere with thyroid function tests (elevations of **serum free thyroxine** and **resin T_3** uptake), **LE cell test,** and **direct Coombs' test** (in patients with hemolytic anemia).

Drug Interactions: Heparin Sodium

Plus	Interactions
Anticoagulants, oral	Heparin (especially IV bolus doses) may prolong prothrombin time used to monitor oral anticoagulant therapy
Antihistamines Aspirin other NSAIDs, and selected salicylates	May partially antagonize anticoagulant action of heparin; increased risk of hemorrhage due to inhibition of platelet adhesiveness and aggregation; potentially ulcerogenic
Contraceptives, oral	Estrogen-containing contraceptives may reduce concentration of antithrombin III and thus paradoxically may increase thrombotic tendency
Corticotropin	Potentially ulcerogenic; increased risk of hemorrhage
Digitalis glycosides	May partially antagonize anticoagulant action of heparin
Dextran Dipyridamole (Persantine) Ethacrynic acid (Edecrin) Glucocorticoids Guaifenesin (glyceryl guaiacolate) Hydrochloroquine (Plaquenil) Indomethacin (Indocin) Ibuprofen (Motrin) Mefenamic acid (Ponstel) Oxyphenbutazone Phenylbutazone Probenecid	Increased risk of hemorrhage due to inhibition of platelet adhesiveness and aggregation; potentially ulcerogenic

Plus (cont.)	Interactions (cont.)
Methinazole, Propylthiouracil	Enhanced anticoagulant effect because of hypoprothrombinemic effect of thiomide antithyroid agents
Protamine	Antagonizes anticoagulant action of heparin; used as heparin antidote
Quinine	Increased risk of hemorrhage due to inhibition of platelet aggregation
Streptokinase, Tetracyclines, Urokinase	May partially antagonize anticoagulant action of heparin

HEPATITIS B IMMUNE GLOBULIN

(HBIG, H-BIG, Hep-B-Gammagee, HyperHep)

Serum product
Immunizing agent

H

ACTIONS AND USES. Sterile solution of immunoglobulins, i.e., antibodies (10 to 18%) prepared by a special process using pooled human plasma, obtained from a small group of well monitored individuals hyperimmunized with hepatitis B virus (HBV). The preparation contains a high antibody titer specific to hepatitis B surface antigen (HBsAg) thereby causing neutralization of HBV and thus inhibiting its infectious or pathogenic properties. Since testing of preparation does not show serologic evidence of HBsAg, the possibility of transmitting hepatitis B is considered remote.

Used prophylactically to provide passive immunity in individuals exposed to HBV through pipetting, "needlesticks," or splash accidents with HBsAg = positive materials. Also has been used as prophylactic measure for susceptible individuals in close association with persons who are HBsAg-positive, for neonates born to HBsAg-positive women, and for dialysis patients.

ABSORPTION AND FATE. Slowly absorbed for IM site. Antibody (anti-HBs) appears in serum within 1 to 6 days; peak serum levels occur within 3 to 11 days and persist about 2 to 6 months. Serum half-life: 21 days. Distribution to placenta and breast milk not known.

CONTRAINDICATIONS AND PRECAUTIONS. *Cautious Use:* history of systemic allergic reactions to immune globulin, thrombocytopenia or bleeding disorders, HBsAg-positive individuals, patients with specific immunoglobulin A (IgA) deficiency.

ADVERSE/SIDE EFFECTS. Usually infrequent and mild. **Dermatologic/Hypersensitivity:** urticaria, rash, angioedema, pruritus, erythema, sensitization (following large or repeated doses), anaphylaxis (rare). **Local:** pain, muscle stiffness, tenderness, swelling, erythema of injection site. **Other:** nausea, faintness, fever, dizziness, malaise, lassitude, body and joint pain, leg cramps.

ROUTE AND DOSAGE. **Intramuscular: Adults and Children:** 0.06 ml/kg as soon as possible after exposure, preferably within 24 hours, but not later than 7 days, and again 28 to 30 days after exposure. (Usual adult dose is 3 to 5 ml.) **Newborn exposure (neonates born to HBsAG-positive women):** 0.5 ml administered as soon as possible after birth, but no later than 24 hours. Dose repeated 3 months and 6 months later.

NURSING IMPLICATIONS

Not to be confused with Immune Globulin IV. Hepatitis B immune globulin (HBIG) is not intended for IV administration.

Skin testing with HBIG is not advised because the concentration of the solution itself can cause a localized inflammatory reaction easily mistaken for a positive reaction.

IM injections should be made preferably into deltoid muscle or anterolateral aspect of thigh. Because of risk of injury to the sciatic nerve, injections into the gluteus are not advised routinely except when large volumes must be given or large doses must be divided into multiple injections. This route is used only for adults. Carefully select injection site in upper outer quadrant of gluteal muscle.

For all IM injections, aspirate carefully to avoid entry into a blood vessel. If blood is seen, withdraw needle, prepare another dose using a new syringe and needle, and administer into a different site. Inadvertent IV administration can cause a precipitous fall in blood pressure and an anaphylactic reaction.

Hypersensitivity reactions are most likely to occur in patients receiving large doses or repeated injections. Have epinephrine 1:1000 readily available.

Another name for hepatitis B virus (HBV) infection is serum hepatitis. Incubation period following exposure ranges from 40 to 180 days (average 90 days).

Although most patients recover from hepatitis B infection, about 10% may become chronic carriers and therefore a potential source of infection to others. Patients at high risk of becoming carriers include parenteral drug abusers, male homosexuals, chronic hemodialysis patients, patients with leukemia, Hodgkins disease, Down's syndrome, or polyarteritis nodosa.

Health care professionals are especially at risk of contracting hepatitis B because of their potential exposure to blood and secretions of asymptomatic carriers.

Serologic screening for hepatitis B surface antigen (HBsAg) is commonly done by solid phase radioimmunoassay (RIA). The antigen can be detected 1 to 7 weeks before onset of clinical hepatitis and remains for 1 to 6 weeks afterward. The passive hemagglutination test or RIA may be used to confirm recent HBV infection. These tests detect changes in level of antibody to antigen.

Hepatitis B virus infection usually spreads by parenteral means, as from contaminated blood, plasma serum, needles, contamination of cuts or mucous membranes with the virus, and by oral ingestion, e.g., pipetting accident. It has also been reported that HBsAg may be present in many body fluids (e.g., saliva, tears, urine, feces, pleural effusions, semen). Although the clinical significance of this finding has not been determined, all body fluids should be considered contaminated pending full study.

Presence of HBsAg in serum indicates active hepatitis B infection or that the person is a chronic carrier. Care providers should be aware that this *serum is highly infective.*

Care providers should use gloves and if necessary a gown when handling contaminated materials. Disposable formites should be placed in impermeable bags and clearly labelled for incineration.

Hepatitis B virus transmission can be prevented in part by needle–blood precautions, meticulous hygiene, e.g., keeping articles of personal hygiene separate (washcloth, towel, shaving equipment, toothbrush). Articles in close patient contact should first be mechanically cleaned and then sterilized either by autoclave, ethylene oxide gas, sodium hypochlorite solution (e.g., Clorox) 0.05 to 0.5%, or by boiling for 30 minutes.

Store preferably between 2° and 8°C (36° and 46°F) unless otherwise directed by manufacturer. Avoid freezing. Solution should be clear, very slightly amber, and moderately viscous. Do not mix with other medications.

Drug Interactions: Hepatitis B Immune Globulin

Plus	Interactions
Live virus vaccine e.g., measles, mumps, rubella, poliovirus, vaccines	Antibody in HBIG preparations may interfere with immune response to live virus vaccine. Administration within 3 months after HBIG not advised

HEPATITIS B VACCINE

(Heptavax-B)

Vaccine
Immunizing agent

ACTIONS AND USES. Suspension of inactivated and purified hepatitis B surface antigen (HBsAg) derived from human plasma of screened asymptomatic HBsAg-positive carriers of hepatitis B virus. (Purification process also removes or inactivates representatives of all other known groups of animal viruses.) The recommended 3-dose regimen produces active immunity against hepatitis B infection by inducing protective antibody (anti-HBs) formation. Children respond with a higher titer of anti-HBs than adults; response tends to be less in immunodeficient patients than healthy individuals, lower in males than in females, and lower in older than young adults. For most healthy persons, immunity (i.e., protective anti-HBs titer) appears to persist for about 5 years. Hepatitis B vaccine will not prevent infection if it is administered during the incubation period. There is no evidence to date that suggests transmission of acquired immune deficiency syndrome (AIDS) by this vaccine.

Used to promote active immunity in individuals at high risk of potential exposure to hepatitis B virus or HBsAg-positive materials. Has been used simultaneously (into different sites) with hepatitis B immune globulin (HBIG) for postexposure prophylaxis in selected patients, and in infants born to HBsAg-positive mothers.

H

ABSORPTION AND FATE. Following IM injection, anti-HBs appears in serum in about 2 weeks; peak concentration occurs after 6 months and persists at least 3 years. Distribution to placenta and breast milk not known.

CONTRAINDICATIONS AND PRECAUTIONS. History of allergic reaction to hepatitis B vaccine or to any ingredient in the formulation (Heptavax-B contains alum and thimerosal, a mercury derivative, as a preservative); for HBsAg carriers. Safe use during pregnancy (category C) and in nursing mothers not established. *Cautious Use:* compromised cardiopulmonary status, serious active infection or fever.

ADVERSE/SIDE EFFECTS. Mild local tenderness at injection site (common), local inflammatory reaction (swelling, heat, redness, induration, pain, fever, malaise, fatigue, headache, dizziness, myalgia, arthralgia, nausea, vomiting) uncommon; diarrhea, rash, pruritus; possibility of subcutaneous nodules following SC injections. Causal relationship not established: tremors, recurrent Bell's palsy, transverse myelitis, seizures, paresthesias, Guillain–Barré syndrome, acute radiculoneuropathy, aseptic meningitis, flu-like symptoms, joint inflammation, chest pain, hives, herpes zoster infection, psoriasis, skin and mucous membrane eruptions, erythema multiforme.

ROUTE AND DOSAGE. **Intramuscular: Adults and older children:** Initial: 1 ml; same dose 1 month later, same dose 6 months after first dose. **Children (birth to 10 years):** Initial: 0.5 ml; same dose 1 month later; same dose 6 months after first dose. **Dialysis and immunodeficient patients:** Initial: 2 ml; same dose 1 month later; same dose 6 months after first dose. Contains 20 mcg hepatitis B surface antigen per ml.

NURSING IMPLICATIONS

Check expiration date on label.

Not to be administered IV or intradermally. Hepatitis B vaccine is intended for IM use; however, it may be administered SC in patients (e.g., hemophiliacs) at risk of hemorrhage from IM injection.

IM injection should be made preferably into the deltoid, and in neonates into the anterolateral thigh, avoiding blood vessels and nerves. Carefully aspirate to prevent inadvertent intravascular injection.

The manufacturer, The American Hospital Association, and the Advisory Committee on Immunization Practices (ACIP) of the USPHS currently recommend preexposure prophylaxis for persons at high risk of coming in contact with hepatitis B infection or virus.

The ACIP recommends serologic confirmation of postvaccination immunity in patients undergoing dialysis and in immunodeficient patients.

Monitor temperature. Some patients develop a temperature elevation of 38.3°C (101°F) following vaccination that usually lasts 1 or 2 days.

Following the 5-year period of immunity conferred by hepatitis B vaccine, a single booster is presently suggested to maintain immunity.

It is a general rule that whenever a vaccine is to be administered, epinephrine should be immediately available to treat anaphylaxis.

It is estimated that the incidence of hepatitis B infection in the U.S. is about 200,000. Vaccination is not advised for the general public, but is strongly recommended for high-risk groups including health care personnel, selected patients and patient contacts (e.g., hemophilia, thalassemia, hemodialysis patients, the mentally handicapped, spouses of chronic carriers), Alaskan Eskimos, Indochinese and Haitian refugees, sexually-active homosexual males, prostitutes, prisoners, morticians, embalmers, users of ilicit injectable drugs, and blood bank personnel.

Shake vial well before withdrawing dose to assure uniform suspension. Use dry, sterile needle and syringe.

Store unopened and opened vials at 2° to 8°C (36° to 46°F), unless otherwise directed by manufacturer. Avoid freezing (freezing destroys potency).

H

HETACILLIN
(Versapen)
HETACILLIN POTASSIUM
(Versapen-K)

(het-a-sill'in)
Antiinfective
Antibiotic
Penicillin

ACTIONS AND USES. Penicillinase-sensitive, acid-stable, semisynthetic penicillin with extended antibacterial spectrum. Has no activity itself until it is hydrolyzed to ampicillin (and acetone) in body. Thus, actions, antibacterial spectrum, uses, contraindications, precautions, and adverse reactions are essentially identical to those of ampicillin (qv).

ABSORPTION AND FATE. Well-absorbed from GI tract. Serum levels peak in about 2 hours; significant concentrations persist even after 8 hours. Diffuses into most body tissues and fluids. Penetrates cerebrospinal fluid only when meninges are inflamed. Partially metabolized in liver. Excreted unchanged in urine and bile (drug levels in urine and bile may exceed those in blood). Crosses placenta. Appears in breast milk.

CONTRAINDICATIONS AND PRECAUTIONS. Hypersensitivity to penicillins or cephalosporins, infectious mononucleosis. Safe use during pregnancy not established. *Cautious Use:* history of or suspected allergy or atopy (eczema, hives, hay fever, asthma); severe renal impairment. *See Ampicillin.*

ADVERSE/SIDE EFFECTS. Nausea, vomiting, diarrhea, flatulence, hypersensitivity reactions, superinfections: stomatitis, glossitis, black, hairy tongue; crystalluria. *See also Ampicillin.*

ROUTE AND DOSAGE. Oral: Patients weighing 40 kg or more: 225 to 450 mg every 6 hours. **Patients weighing less than 40 kg:** 22.5 to 45 mg/kg/day in 4 equally-divided doses. Available as capsules (hetacillin potassium) and as oral suspension, and pediatric drops (hetacillin).

NURSING IMPLICATIONS

Before treatment is initiated, a careful inquiry should be made concerning history of sensitivity to penicillins, cephalosporins, or other allergies.

Check expiration date.

Best taken on an empty stomach (at least 1 hour before or 2 hours after meals). Although drug is acid-stable, food retards absorption. Absorption is enhanced by taking drug with a full glass of water.

Inform patient that in order to maintain a constant blood level, hetacillin should be given around the clock at specific intervals. If it is not prescribed in this way, physician should be asked to clarify the order.

Instruct patient not to miss any doses and to continue taking medication until it is all gone, unless otherwise directed by physician.

Infections due to group A beta-hemolytic streptococci should be treated for a minimum of 10 days.

Patients with urinary or GI tract infections may require therapy for several weeks and bacteriologic and/or clinical follow-up for several months after drug is discontinued.

Reconstituted oral liquid formulation is stable for 14 days under refrigeration. Date and time of reconstitution and discard date should appear on containers. Shake well before pouring.

See Ampicillin.

H

HETASTARCH

(HES, Hespan, Volex)

(het'a-starch)
Replacement solution
Plasma volume expander

ACTIONS AND USES. Synthetic hydroxyethyl starch closely resembling human glycogen. Has an average molecular weight of about 450,000 (range 10,000 to 1 million). Colloidal osmotic properties are approximately equal to those of human serum albumin. Acts much like dextran, but claimed to be less likely to produce anaphylaxis or to interfere with crossmatching or bloodtyping procedures. Expansion of plasma volume is slightly greater than amount of hetastarch administered. Not a substitute for blood or plasma. Commercially available as 6% hetastarch in 0.9% Sodium Chloride in 500 mg infusion bottle; contains 77 mEq each of sodium and chloride/500 ml.

Used to expand plasma volume during cardiopulmonary bypass, and in treatment of shock caused by hemorrhage, burns, surgery, sepsis, or other trauma. Also used as sedimenting agent in preparation of granulocytes by leukopheresis. *Investigational Use:* as a cryoprotective agent for long-term storage of whole blood.

ABSORPTION AND FATE. Plasma volume expansion lasts approximately 24 to 36 hours. Molecules of low molecular weight (below 50,000) are readily eliminated via kidneys; approximately 40% of dose excreted within 24 hours. Remaining heavier molecules are metabolized slowly to molecules small enough to be excreted over 2 to 3 weeks.

CONTRAINDICATIONS AND PRECAUTIONS. Severe bleeding disorders, congestive heart failure, renal failure with oliguria and anuria, treatment of shock not accompanied by hypovolemia. Safe use during pregnancy and in children not established. *Cautious Use:* hepatic insufficiency, pulmonary edema in very young or the elderly, patients on sodium restriction.

ADVERSE/SIDE EFFECTS. Allergic: pruritus, anaphylactoid reactions (periorbital edema, urticaria, wheezing). **CV:** peripheral edema, circulatory overload, heart failure. **Hematologic:** with large volumes: prolongation of: prothrombin time (PT), partial prothrombin time (PPT), clotting time (CT), and bleeding time (BT); decreased: hematocrit, hemoglobin, platelets, calcium, and fibrinogen; dilution of plasma proteins, hyperbilirubinemia. **Other:** vomiting, mild fever, chills, influenzalike symptoms, headache, muscle pains, submaxillary and parotid glandular swelling.

ROUTE AND DOSAGE. Intravenous infusion (only): *Plasma volume expansion:* 500 to 1000 ml; not to exceed 1500 ml/day. Maximum infusion rate for hemorrhagic shock is 20 ml/kg/hour; slower rates advised for patients with burns or septic shock. *Leukopheresis:* in continuous flow centrifugation (CFC) procedures: 250 to 700 ml infused at a constant fixed ratio usually 8:1 to venous whole blood. Multiple CFC procedures of up to 2 weeks to total of 7 to 10 procedures reportedly safe and effective.

NURSING IMPLICATIONS

Specific flow rate is prescribed by physician.

Measure and record intake and output. Report oliguria or significant changes in intake–output ratio.

Monitor blood pressure and vital signs and observe patient for unusual bruising or bleeding.

Observe for signs of circulatory overload: shortness of breath, wheezing, coughing, marked increase in pulse and respiration, pulmonary rales, sensation of chest pressure, elevation of central venous pressure.

Check laboratory reports of hematocrit (Hct) values. Notify physician if there is an appreciable drop in Hct or if value approaches 30% by volume. Hct should not be allowed to drop below 30%.

Recommended laboratory determinations for donors undergoing repeated leukopheresis procedures: (in addition to regular and frequent clinical evaluation) close monitoring of the following values are essential: CBC, total leukocyte and platelet counts, leukocyte differential count, Hgb, Hct, PT, and PTT.

Partially used bottles should be discarded. Hetastarch solution contains no preservatives.

H

HEXACHLOROPHENE

(hex-a-klor'oh-feen)
Antiinfective (topical)

(Germa-Medica, pHisoHex, pHisoScrub, Septi-Soft, Septisol, Soy-Dome Cleanser, WescoHEX)

ACTIONS AND USES. Polychlorinated phenol derivative. Bacteriostatic against gram-positive bacteria, especially strains of staphylococci. Less active against gram-negative organisms; has little effect on spores. Effectiveness depends on absorption of antibacterial residue on skin that resists removal by water, soaps, and detergents for several days. Cumulative antibacterial action develops with repeated use.

Used for surgical scrub and as bacteriostatic skin cleanser. May also be used, only as long as necessary, to control an outbreak of gram-positive infection when other procedures have been unsuccessful.

CONTRAINDICATIONS AND PRECAUTIONS. Sensitivity to any of its components, primary light sensitivity to halogenated phenol derivatives, use with premature infants, use on open cuts, burns, wounds, use as occlusive dressing, wet pack, or lotion, use for vaginal pack or tampon;

application to any mucous membranes, to large surface areas, or for prophylactic total body bathing; multiple daily handwashing with hexachlorophene during pregnancy.

ADVERSE/SIDE EFFECTS. **Accidental ingestion:** cramping, diarrhea, abdominal distention and pain, anorexia, nausea, vomiting, hypotension, shock. **Sensitization** (photosensitivity, dermatitis, erythema, scaling). **Systemic toxicity** (from absorption or accidental ingestion): **CNS:** irritation manifested by dizziness, headache, confusion, diplopia, miosis, twitching, irritability, convulsions, respiratory arrest.

ROUTE AND DOSAGE. **Topical (3% emulsion, liquid soap):** Surgical wash or scrub (as indicated). Bacteriostatic cleansing: Squeeze ½ to 1 teaspoon into palm; add water; work up into lather; apply to area to be cleansed. Rinse thoroughly after each washing.

NURSING IMPLICATIONS

A single application has little more effect than nonmedicated soaps. Regular and repeated applications are required to build up antibacterial residue (maximal concentration reached in 2 to 4 days).

Presence of organic matter (e.g., pus, serum) reduces activity of hexachlorophene, but activity is retained in the presence of soaps, oils, and vehicles for topical application.

Infants, especially premature infants or those with dermatoses, are particularly susceptible to hexachlorophene absorption leading to systemic toxicity and brain abscess.

Hexachlorophene should be rinsed thoroughly with clear water, especially from sensitive areas such as scrotum, to prevent possibility of systemic absorption. Do not use alcohol or alcohol-containing products, since they remove the antibacterial residue.

Hexachlorophene may produce erythema, dryness, and scaling in patients with sensitive skin, especially when combined with excessive rubbing or exposure to heat or cold.

Discontinue immediately if signs of cerebral irritability or other adverse reactions (suggestive of absorption) occur.

If suds enters eyes accidentally, rinse out promptly and thoroughly with water.

Accidental ingestion: If patient is seen early, stomach is evacuated by emesis or gastric lavage. Olive oil or vegetable oil (60 ml) may then be given to delay drug absorption, followed by a saline cathartic to hasten removal. IV fluids, electrolyte replacement; vasopressors for marked hypotension; opiates if necessary for severe GI symptoms.

Do not pour hexachlorophene into a medicine cup, medicine bottle, or similar container, since it may be mistaken for baby formula or other medication.

Preserved in tightly covered, light-resistant containers.

HEXAFLUORENIUM BROMIDE

(Mylaxen)

(hex-a-flure-en′ee-um)
Cholinesterase inhibitor

ACTIONS AND USES. Reversible inhibitor of plasma cholinesterase. Unlike other drugs of this class (e.g., edrophonium or neostigmine) hexafluorenium does not appear to inhibit intracellular cholinesterases and therefore cholinergic (muscarinic) actions are not as potent. Suppresses enzymatic hydrolysis of succinylcholine and thus prolongs its actions. Also may help to reduce succinylcholine-induced muscle fasciculations and associated pain. Has mild nondepolarizing neuromuscular blocking activity (curarelike effect) at myoneural function but this is evident only when high doses or other neuromuscular blocking agents are used.

Used during anesthesia only in conjunction with succinylcholine to prolong its neuromuscular blocking activity and thereby reduce amount of drug required.

ABSORPTION AND FATE. In anesthetized adults, IV administration followed in 3 minutes by succinylcholine injection produces apnea and skeletal muscle relaxation within 3 to 4 minutes. Muscle relaxation lasts 20 to 30 minutes. Biphasic half-life: first phase, 10 to 20 minutes; second phase (elimination), 2 to 4 hours. About 5 to 10% excreted in urine during first 18 hours, 27 to 45% eliminated in bile.

CONTRAINDICATIONS AND PRECAUTIONS. Hypersensitivity to hexafluorenium or to bromides, history of bronchial asthma. Safe use in women of childbearing potential or during pregnancy not established. *Cautious Use:* patients with cardiovascular, renal, hepatic, pulmonary, or metabolic disorders; during ocular surgery, patients with severe burns, fractures, muscle spasms or any type of neuromyopathy, e.g., myasthenia gravis, muscular dystrophy.

ADVERSE/SIDE EFFECTS. CNS: profound and prolonged muscle spasm, muscle paralysis, respiratory depression, apnea, hyperthermia. **CV:** bradycardia, tachycardia, hypertension, hypotension, cardiac arrest. **Other:** bronchospasm, salivation, abdominal cramps, increased intraocular pressure, hypersensitivity reactions (rare).

ROUTE AND DOSAGE. Intravenous: 0.4 mg/kg (not to exceed 36 mg) followed in 3 minutes by succinylcholine 0.2 mg/kg (not to exceed 18 mg). If necessary, relaxation may be sustained by giving repeat doses of 0.15 mg/kg of succinylcholine at 15- to 30-minute intervals.

H

NURSING IMPLICATIONS

Serum cholinesterase levels are evaluated prior to administration. If low, drug is not used.

Facilities for intubation, artificial respiration and administration of oxygen must be immediately available.

Position patient to facilitate drainage of excessive oropharngeal secretions.

Monitor vital signs closely until recovery from drug effects is complete.

Since hexafluorenium is always used to prolong the relaxant effects of succinylcholine, be familiar with actions, precautions, and adverse reactions of the latter drug.

HEXOBARBITAL
(Sombulex)

(hex-oh-bar′bi-tal)
Sedative
Hypnotic
Barbiturate
C III

ACTIONS AND USES. Rapidly acting barbiturate with ultrashort duration of action. Produces sleep within 15 to 30 minutes; completely metabolized and cleared from plasma in 4 to 5 hours. *See Phenobarbital for absorption and fate, adverse reactions and interactions.*

Used to treat simple insomnia and as a preanesthetic, preoperative, and postoperative sedative. Also used for short-term sedation in minor diagnostic procedures.

CONTRAINDICATIONS AND PRECAUTIONS. Hypersensitivity to barbiturates, history of drug abuse, porphyria, uncontrolled severe pain, respiratory disease with dyspnea. *Cautious Use:* renal or hepatic impairment. *See also Phenobarbital.*

ROUTE AND DOSAGE. Oral: *Hypnotic:* 250 to 500 mg at bedtime. If sleep is interrupted, one tablet (250 mg) may be taken. *Sedative:* 250 mg repeated every 2 or 3 hours as necessary.

NURSING IMPLICATIONS

May be used in obstetrics with scopolamine, and preoperatively with atropine when morphine contraindicated.

Supervise the sedated patient's physical activity, especially if patient is elderly or debilitated.

Observe to see that the patient does not hoard or "cheek" the drug.

Since hexobarbital has a short duration of action, inadvertent overdosage in an attempt to assure sleep is possible. The patient with a history of addiction should not have easy access to this drug.

Classified as Schedule III drug under Federal Controlled Substances Act.

See Phenobarbital.

HEXOCYCLIUM METHYLSULFATE

(Tral)

(hex-oh-sye'klee-um)
Anticholinergic
(Parasympatholytic)
Antispasmodic

ACTIONS AND USES. Synthetic quaternary ammonium compound with antisecretory and antispasmodic effects qualitatively similar to those of atropine. Contraindications, precautions, and adverse effects essentially as for atropine (qv).

Used in adjunctive management of peptic ulcer and other GI disorders associated with hyperacidity, hypermotility, and spasm.

ABSORPTION AND FATE. Degree of absorption varies among individuals. Onset of action in about 1 hour; effects persist 3 to 4 hours (approximately 10 hours with sustained-release tablet). Excreted primarily in urine and bile; some unchanged drug eliminated in feces.

CONTRAINDICATIONS AND PRECAUTIONS. Safe use during pregnancy or lactation and in children not established. *Cautious Use:* cardiac disease, prostatic hypertrophy, pylorospasm or cardiospasm. *See also Atropine.*

ADVERSE/SIDE EFFECTS. Blurred vision, dry mouth, urinary hesitancy or retention, drowsiness, constipation, palpitation, tachycardia, headache, mental confusion and/or excitement, especially in the elderly. *See also Atropine.*

ROUTE AND DOSAGE. Oral: 25 mg four times daily, before meals and at bedtime. Sustained-release tablet: 50 mg two times daily, before lunch and at bedtime or before breakfast and before evening meal. Highly individualized.

NURSING IMPLICATIONS

Because of the possibility of drowsiness and blurred vision, caution the patient to avoid driving and other potentially hazardous activities until response to drug is known. Also advise elderly patients to be careful when climbing or descending stairs and when getting out of bed.

First signs of overdosage may be flushing of skin and increased intensity of mouth dryness.

Tral tablets contain *tartrazine* that may cause allergic-type reaction including bronchial asthma in susceptible patients. The reaction is frequently seen in individuals who also have aspirin hypersensitivity.

Sustained-release tablet should be swallowed whole.

Caution patient to avoid high environmental temperature; heat prostration can occur because of drug-induced depression of sweating.
See Atropine sulfate (prototype anticholinergic)

HOMATROPINE HYDROBROMIDE

(Homatrocel, Isopto Homatropine, Murocoll Homatropine)

(hoe-ma'troe-peen)
Anticholinergic (ophthalmic)
Antimuscarinic
Mydriatic, cycloplegic

ACTIONS AND USES. Synthetic alkaloid with actions, contraindications, precautions, and adverse reactions similar to those of atropine (qv). Preferred to atropine for certain ophthalmologic purposes because its mydriatic and cycloplegic actions occur more rapidly and are less prolonged. Cycloplegia is usually incomplete unless applications are made repeatedly.

Used as mydriatic for ocular examination and as cycloplegic to measure errors of refraction. Also used in treatment of inflammatory conditions of uveal tract, ciliary spasm and as cycloplegic and mydriatic in preoperative and postoperative conditions.

H

ABSORPTION AND FATE. Following instillation, maximal paralysis of accommodation and mydriatic effects occur in 30 to 60 minutes, with recovery in 1 to 3 days.

CONTRAINDICATIONS AND PRECAUTIONS. Hypersensitivity; narrow-angle glaucoma; children under 6 years of age. *Cautious Use:* increased intraocular pressure, infants, children, the elderly, hypertension, hyperthyroidism, diabetes. *See also Atropine.*

ADVERSE/SIDE EFFECTS. Increased intraocular pressure. *With prolonged use:* local irritation, congestion, edema, eczema, follicular conjunctivitis. *Excessive dosage:* symptoms of atropine poisoning. *See Atropine.*

ROUTE AND DOSAGE. Topical: 1 or 2 drops of 1 to 5% solution instilled in eye up to every 3 or 4 hours. For refraction: 1 or 2 drops of 2 to 5% solution; repeat in 5 to 10 minutes if necessary.

NURSING IMPLICATIONS

Determinations of intraocular pressure and width of anterior chamber angle (gonioscopy) are advised before and during drug use, particularly if therapy is intensive or prolonged. Drug may increase intraocular pressure even in the normal eye.

Systemic absorption may be minimized by applying pressure against inner canthus of eye (lacrimal duct) during and for 1 or 2 minutes after each instillation. This is particularly advisable when stronger solutions are used. *See Index: Drug Administration: eye drops.*

Recommended dosage should not be exceeded.

Frequent and continued use or overdosage may produce symptoms of atropine poisoning.

Advise the patient to report immediately the onset of eye pain, changes in visual acuity, rapid pulse, or dizziness. Drug should be discontinued if these symptoms occur.

Advise the patient to report dryness of mouth. This symptom may be relieved by reduction in dosage.

Photophobia associated with mydriasis may require patient to wear dark glasses.

Since the drug produces blurred vision, advise the patient against driving and other hazardous activities until effect disappears.

See Atropine sulfate (prototype anticholinergic).

HOMATROPINE METHYLBROMIDE

(Homapin, Ru-Spas No. 2, Sed-Tens SE)

(hoe-ma'troe-peen)
Anticholinergic
Antispasmodic

ACTIONS AND USES. Semisynthetic quaternary ammonium derivative of belladonna alkaloids. Actions, contraindications, precautions, and adverse reactions as for atropine (qv). Has less antimuscarinic activity than atropine, but is reported to be four times more potent as a ganglionic blocking agent, and has no CNS action.

Used adjunctively in treatment of peptic and duodenal ulcer, pylorospasm, functional diarrhea, hypermotility states, spasticity of colon and biliary tract.

ADVERSE/SIDE EFFECTS. Xerostomia, urinary hesitancy and retention, blurred vision, tachycardia, palpitation, headache. *See also Atropine.*

ROUTE AND DOSAGE. Oral: 10 mg ½ hour before meals and at bedtime.

H

NURSING IMPLICATIONS

Elderly patients may react with symptoms of excitement, agitation, drowsiness, and other untoward reactions even if doses are small.

Investigate tachycardia before giving medication; if other atropine-like side effects are present, consult physician.

Because of drug-induced depression of sweating, patient may be susceptible to heat prostration in a high environmental temperature.

Since the drug may produce dizziness and blurred vision, advise the patient against driving and other hazardous activities until reaction to the drug has been determined.

Preserved in tight, light-resistant containers at temperature between 15° and 30°C (59° and 86°F). Prevent freezing.

HYALURONIDASE

(Wydase)

(hye-al-yoor-on'i dase)
Enzyme

ACTIONS AND USES. Mucolytic enzyme prepared from purified bovine testicular hyaluronidase. Hydrolyzes hyaluronic acid, which normally obstructs intercellular diffusion of invasive substances. Promotes diffusion and consequently absorption of transudates, exudates, and injected fluids.

Used to enhance dispersion and absorption of other injected drugs; used for hypodermoclysis, and as adjunct in subcutaneous urography for improving resorption of radiopaque agents.

CONTRAINDICATIONS AND PRECAUTIONS. Injection into or around inflamed, infected, or cancerous areas; congestive heart failure; hypoproteinemia.

ADVERSE/SIDE EFFECTS. Infrequent: sensitivity, spread of infectious processes, overhydration.

ROUTE AND DOSAGE. *For absorption and dispersion of injected drugs:* 150 U added to other drug solution. *Hypodermoclysis:* 150 U added to clysis (injected into rubber tubing, close to needle) or injected subcutaneously prior to clysis (150 N.F. units will facilitate absorption of 1000 ml or more of solution). *Subcutaneous urography:* with patient prone, 75 U is injected SC over each scapula, followed by injection of contrast medium at same sites.

NURSING IMPLICATIONS

Preliminary skin test for sensitivity is advised. Approximately 0.02 ml of 150 U/ml solution (3 U) is injected intradermally by physician; positive reaction consists of wheal with pseudopods and localized itching within 5 minutes, persisting 20 to 30 minutes. Erythema alone is not a positive reaction.

Addition of hyaluronidase to hypodermoclyses may promote overhydration because it speeds water absorption. Infusion flow rate should be prescribed by physician. Patient should be closely monitored.

When it is used to increase diffusion of a drug, bear in mind that absorption will be enhanced. Therefore, watch for adverse reactions and expect a shorter duration of drug action.

Lyophilized form is unstable in solution and therefore is reconstituted with sodium chloride injection just before use (usually in the proportion of 1 ml per 150 U of hyaluronidase).

Hyaluronidase for injection is reportedly stable for up to 3 months when stored at 2° to 8°C (36° to 46°F). Consult pharmacist.

HYDRALAZINE HYDROCHLORIDE

(Apresoline, Dralzine, Hydrallazine Hydrochloride, Hydralyn, Rolazine)

(hye-dral'a-zeen)
Antihypertensive
Vasodilator, peripheral

ACTIONS AND USES. The only phthalazine used clinically in North America. Reduces blood pressure by direct relaxation of vascular smooth muscles, with greater effect on arterioles than on veins. Diastolic response is often greater than systolic. Resulting vasodilation reduces peripheral vascular resistance and increases renal and cerebral blood flow. Has little effect on capacitance blood vessels. Antihypertensive effect may be limited by sympathetic reflexes, which cause increased heart rate, stroke volume, and cardiac output. Postural hypotensive effect is reportedly less than that produced by ganglionic blocking agents. Usually increases plasma renin activity.

Used most commonly in stepped care approach to treat moderate hypertension (step 3 agent). Also used in early malignant hypertension and in hypertension that persists after sympathectomy. Has been used to improve heart function in patients with congestive heart failure. Commercially available in fixed-dose combination with hydrochlorothiazide (e.g., Apresazide), and with both hydrochlorothiazide and reserpine (e.g., Hydropres, Unipres).

ABSORPTION AND FATE. Following oral administration, onset of action in 20 to 30 minutes. Peak plasma concentration within 2 hours; duration: 2 to 4 hours. Antihypertensive effect occurs within 10 to 30 minutes following IM injection and lasts 2 to 6 hours. Blood pressure begins to fall within 5 to 20 minutes following IV injection; maximal effect in 10 to 80 minutes, and lasts 2 to 6 hours. Approximately 85% bound to plasma proteins. Half-life: 2 to 8 hours. Extensively metabolized in intestinal wall and liver primarily by acetylation (rate of which is genetically determined). Rapidly excreted in urine, primarily as metabolites. Excretion rate greatest between 2 and 10 hours. About 10% of oral dose excreted in feces.

CONTRAINDICATIONS AND PRECAUTIONS. Hypersensitivity to hydralazine, coronary artery disease, mitral valvular rheumatic heart disease, myocardial infarction, tachycardia, lupus erythematosus. Safe use during pregnancy not established. *Cautious Use:* cerebrovascular accident, advanced renal impairment, use with MAO inhibitors.

ADVERSE/SIDE EFFECTS. CNS: headache, dizziness, peripheral neuritis, paresthesias, tremors, psychotic reactions (depression, anxiety, disorientation). **CV:** (common): palpitation, angina, tachycardia; less frequent: flushing, orthostatic hypotension, paradoxical pressor response, arrhythmias, profound shock (overdosage). **EENT:** lacrimation, conjunctivitis, nasal congestion. **GI (common):** anorexia, nausea, vomiting, diarrhea; less frequent: constipation, paralytic ileus. **GU:** difficulty in urination, impotence (rare). **Hematologic:** reduced hemoglobin and RBCs, leukopenia, agranulocytosis, purpura. **Hypersensitivity:** rash, urticaria, pruritus, fever, chills, arthralgia, eosinophilia, hepatitis (rare), obstructive jaundice. **Other:** muscle cramps, lymphadenopathy, splenomegaly; sweating (common), rheumatoid or SLE-like syndrome, fixed drug eruption, sodium retention and edema (long-term therapy).

ROUTE AND DOSAGE. Adults: Oral: Initial: 10 mg four times daily for 2 to 4 days, increased to 25 mg four times daily for balance of first week; for second and subsequent weeks, 50 mg four times daily. For maintenance, dosage is adjusted to lowest effective level. *Highly individualized.* **Intramuscular, intravenous:** 10 to 40 mg repeated as necessary (generally every 4 to 6 hours. **Pediatric: Oral:** Initial: 0.75 mg/kg or 25 mg/m² in 4 divided doses daily. If necessary, dosage may be increased gradually over 3 to 4 weeks, up to 7.5 mg/kg daily. **Parenteral:** Initial: 1.7 to 3.5 mg/kg daily or 50 to 100 mg/m² daily divided into 4 to 6 doses.

H

NURSING IMPLICATIONS

Reportedly two to three times as much hydralazine enters the general circulation when it is taken with food (food reduces first-pass metabolism of drug in the intestinal wall). It is advisable to be consistent in taking drug either with meals or on an empty stomach to minimize fluctuations in blood levels.

Some products (e.g., Apresoline 10 and 100 mg tablets) contain *tartrazine* which can cause allergic type reactions including asthma in susceptible individuals. It is frequently seen in patients with aspirin hypersensitivity.

Complete blood count, LE cell preparation, and antinuclear antibody titer determinations are advised before initiation of therapy and periodically during prolonged therapy.

Observe mental status; note anxiety, depression, obtundation (signs of cerebral ischemia from too rapid reduction in blood pressure).

Blood pressure should be closely monitored in patients receiving parenteral hydralazine. Check every 5 minutes until stabilized at desired level, then every 15 minutes thereafter throughout hypertensive crisis.

A marked fall in blood pressure may further compromise renal blood flow in patients with renal damage and result in reduced urinary output.

Intake and output should be monitored when drug is given parenterally and in those with renal dysfunction. Output may be increased in some patients because of improved renal blood flow.

Instruct patient to monitor weight and to check for edema. Advise patient to report sudden gain or apparent slow increase in weight, and the onset of edema. Sodium retention has occurred with long-term use.

Consult physician regarding dietary management: allowable salt intake; weight control.

Most patients receiving parenteral hydralazine are transferred to oral form within 24 to 48 hours.

Some patients experience headache and palpitation within 2 to 4 hours after first oral dose. Symptoms usually subside spontaneously. Advise patients to inform physician of adverse reactions; most can be controlled by dose reduction.

Physician may prescribe pyridoxine (vitamin B_6) prophylactically or when patient develops symptoms of peripheral neuritis (paresthesias, numbness). This complication is believed to result from antipyridoxine effect of hydralazine.

Because of the possibility of postural hypotension, caution patients to make position changes slowly, particularly from lying to sitting position and from sitting to standing, and to avoid standing still, taking hot baths and showers, strenuous exercise, and excessive alcohol intake.

Caution patient to lie down or sit down (in head-low position) if feels faint or dizzy. Patients who engage in potentially hazardous activities such as driving or operating machinery should be advised of the possibility of these symptoms.

Withdrawal of hydralazine should be accomplished gradually to avoid sudden rise in pressure and heart failure. Patients should be informed of the dangers of sudden withdrawal.

An LE cell preparation is indicated if patient manifests arthralgia, fever, chest pain, malaise, or other unexplained signs and symptoms.

Reportedly, hydralazine-induced systemic lupus erythematosus (SLE) is associated with high dosages (more than 200 mg/day) and occurs almost exclusively in Caucasians who are slow acetylators.

Manifestations of SLE usually regress after drug is withdrawn; however, some residual effects may continue 7 to 8 years and require steroid therapy.

Stress the importance of follow-up care. Some patients develop tolerance during chronic drug administration requiring higher dosages or a change in drug regimen.

Store preferably at 15° to 30°C (59° to 86°F) in tight, light-resistant containers, unless otherwise directed by manufacturer. Avoid freezing.

See Guanethidine for summary of teaching points for patients with hypertension.

H

Diagnostic Test Interferences. Positive **direct Coombs' tests** in patients with hydralazine-induced SLE. Hydralazine interferes with urinary **17-OHCS** determinations (modified Glenn-Nelson technique)

Drug Interactions: Hydralazine

Plus	Interactions
Diazoxide and other potent antihypertensives	Severe additive hypotensive effect
Diuretics MAO inhibitors	Potentiation of antihypertensive action

HYDROCHLORIC ACID, DILUTED

Acidifer (gastric)
Digestant

ACTIONS AND USES. Gastric hydrochloric acid is essential for conversion of pepsinogen to active pepsin (important for protein digestion), activation of pancreatic and hepatic secretions, stimulation of secretin, and neutralization of bicarbonates of intestinal secretions, thus helping to maintain electrolyte balance. It also has germicidal effects on numerous bacteria.

Used in hydrochloric acid deficiency states, as in pernicious anemia, gastric carcinoma, chronic gastritis, and idiopathic achlorhydria. Largely replaced by other sources of Hcl e.g., glutamic acid hydrochloride.

CONTRAINDICATIONS AND PRECAUTIONS. Gastric hyperacidity, peptic ulcer.

ADVERSE/SIDE EFFECTS. Damage to tooth enamel. Prolonged use of high doses, depletion of bicarbonate and rise of serum chloride; metabolic acidosis.

ROUTE AND DOSAGE. Oral: 2 to 8 ml (10% solution) three times daily.

NURSING IMPLICATIONS

Administer well diluted (at least 150 to 250 ml of water) through glass drinking tube in order to prevent damage to tooth enamel. Inform patient that the taste is sour, and instruct patient to place the tube well back into mouth and to sip slowly.

Hydrochloric acid may be prescribed to be taken during meals or immediately after meals. If taken after meals, follow immediately with alkaline mouthwash.

Observe and record therapeutic effects. Symptoms of achlorhydria are poorly defined, but may consist of vague epigastric distress after meals, belching, abdominal distention, coated tongue, nausea, vomiting, and morning diarrhea.

Physician may prescribe high-alkaline diet consisting of citrus fruits and green vegetables or alkalinizing salts to help maintain acid-base balance.

With large doses, acid-base status should be checked every few days after start of therapy and periodically during therapy.

HYDROCHLOROTHIAZIDE

(hye-droe-klor-oh-thye'a-zide)

(Apo-Hydro, Chlorzide, Diaqua, Diu-Scrip, Esidrix, Hydro-Chlor, HydroDiuril, Hydromal, Hydro-T, Hydro-Z, Nefrol, Oretic, SK-Hydrochlorothiazide, Thiuretic, HCTZ, Urozide, Zide)

Diuretic
Antihypertensive
Thiazide
Sulfonamide derivative

ACTIONS AND USES. Benzothiadiazine (thiazide) derivative. Similar to chlorothiazide (qv) in actions, uses, contraindications, precautions, adverse reactions, and interactions.

Used as adjunct in treatment of edema associated with congestive heart failure, hepatic cirrhosis, renal failure, and in the management of hypertension (step 1 agent). Available in fixed combination with methyldopa (Aldoril) with reserpine (Hydro-serp); with triamterene (Dyazide); with propranolol (Inderide), with hydralazine (Apresazide), and with guanethidine (Esimil).

ABSORPTION AND FATE. Diuretic effect begins in 2 hours, peaks in 4 hours, and lasts 6 to 12 hours. Half-life: normal kidneys, 2 hours; anuria, 15 hours. Excreted unchanged by kidneys within 24 hours. Crosses placenta; found in breast milk.

CONTRAINDICATIONS AND PRECAUTIONS. Hypersensitivity to thiazides or other sulfonamides; anuria, pregnancy (category B), lactation. *Cautious Use:* bronchial asthma, allergy, hepatic cirrhosis, renal dysfunction; history of gout, SLE. *See also Chlorothiazide.*

ADVERSE/SIDE EFFECTS. Nausea, vomiting, orthostatic hypotension, unusual fatigue, photosensitivity, exacerbation of gout, lupus erythematosus, hyperglycemia, agranulocytosis, hypokalemia. *See also Chlorothiazide.*

ROUTE AND DOSAGE. Oral: Adults: *Edema:* Initial: 25 to 100 mg one or two times daily until dry weight attained; maintenance: 25 to 100 mg daily or intermittently according to patient's response. *Antihypertensive:* Initial: 75 mg daily as single dose in AM; maintenance 25 to 100 mg daily (determined by patient response). **Pediatric:** 2.2 mg/kg/day in two divided doses. A liquid formulation (Hydrochlorothiazide Intensol Solution) is available (100 mg hydrochlorthiazide/ml).

NURSING IMPLICATIONS

Tablet may be crushed and mixed with a full glass of fluid or with food before swallowing.

Schedule doses to avoid nocturia and interrupted sleep. Administer oral drug early in AM after eating to prevent gastric irritation. If given in 2 doses, schedule second dose no later than 3 PM.

Thiazides are used as step 1 agents in treatment of hypertension. The *stepped care approach* (a gradual progressive drug regimen) treats various levels of severity of the disease with "stepping up" occurring at 2 to 3 month intervals (thus allowing enough time for a predictable clinical response). *A typical stepped-care protocol:*

- step 1 (mild hypertension) thiazide-type diuretic and/or beta blocker
- step 2 (mild to moderate hypertension): add an adrenergic inhibiting agent, e.g., clonidine (Catapres), quanadrel (Hylorel), prozosin (Minipress).
- step 3 (moderate hypertension): add vasodilator, e.g., hydralazine (Apresoline), captopril (Capoten).
- step 4 (severe hypertension): add guanethidine (Ismelin), minoxidil (Loniten).

Calcium channel blocker may be substituted in steps 2 or 3 and captopril may be substituted in steps 2 to 4. Reduction of drug dosage or "step down" is usually attempted after patient's blood pressure has been controlled for 6 to 8 months.

H

Hypertension is commonly classified according to diastolic (mm/Hg) values: i.e., mild, 90 to 104; moderate, 105 to 114; severe, higher than 115.

Antihypertensive effects may be noted in 3 to 4 days; maximal effects may require 3 to 4 weeks.

Hypokalemia is rarely severe in most patients on prolonged therapy with thiazides, if present at all. To prevent onset, urge patient to eat a normal diet (usually includes K-rich foods such as potatoes, fruit juices, cereals, skim milk) and to include a banana (370 mg K) and at least 6 ounces orange juice (330 mg K) every day.

If hypokalemia develops, dietary K supplement of 1000 to 2000 mg (25 to 50 mEq) is usually an adequate treatment.

Be alert for signs of hypokalemia (especially in the elderly): muscle cramps, weakness, mental confusion, polyuria, dry mouth, anorexia. Report to the physician.

Instruct patient with orthostatic hypotension to change from recumbent to upright positions slowly and in stages; to avoid hot baths or showers, extended exposure to sunlight, and sitting or standing still for long periods. Provide assistance if necessary to prevent falling. Consult physician about use of support hose or knee socks.

Baseline and periodic determinations of serum electrolytes, blood counts, BUN, blood glucose, uric acid, CO_2 are recommended.

Warn patient about the possibility of photosensitivity reaction and to notify the physician if it occurs (like an exaggerated sun burn). Thiazide-related photosensitivity is considered a photoallergy (ultraviolet radiation changes drug structure and makes it allergenic for some individuals). It usually occurs 1½ to 2 weeks after initial sun exposure.

Instruct patient to weigh him- or herself daily. Consult physician about acceptable range of weight change. Report sudden weight gain.

Advise patient to consult physician before using OTC drugs. Many contain large amounts of sodium as well as potassium.

Store tablets in tightly closed container between 15° and 30°C (59° and 86°F) unless otherwise directed by manufacturer.

See Chlorothiazide (prototype thiazide diuretic).

HYDROCODONE BITARTRATE

(Corutol DH, Dihydrocodeinone Bitartrate, Robidone)

(hye-droe-koe'done)
Antitussive (narcotic)
C II

ACTIONS AND USES. Morphine derivative similar to codeine, but more addicting and with slightly greater antitussive activity. Available in the U.S. only in combination with other drugs. The above trade names are Canadian.

Used for symptomatic relief of hyperactive or nonproductive cough, and for relief of moderate to moderately severe pain. A common ingredient in a variety of proprietary mixtures. Available in fixed combination with homatropine (Hycodan); with phenylpropanolamine (Hycomine); with guaifenesin (Hycotuss); with pseudoephedrine and guaifenesin (Tussend Liquid); and with acetaminophen (Vicodin).

ABSORPTION AND FATE. Onset of action in 10 to 20 minutes; duration 3 to 6 hours. Plasma half-life: 3.8 hours. Metabolized in liver. Excreted primarily in urine. Crosses placenta.

CONTRAINDICATIONS AND PRECAUTIONS. *Cautious Use:* asthma, emphysema, history of drug abuse or dependence, postoperative patients, debilitated patients, children under 1 year of age. *See Morphine.*

ADVERSE/SIDE EFFECTS. Dry mouth, constipation, nausea, vomiting, dizziness, drowsiness. *See also Morphine.*

ROUTE AND DOSAGE. Oral: **Adults and children over 12 years:** 5 mg every 4 hours, as needed; **2 to 12 years:** 1.25 to 5 mg every 4 hours as needed. A single dose should not exceed 15 mg in adults; 10 mg in children 2 to 12 years old; 1.25 mg in children 1 to 2 years old.

NURSING IMPLICATIONS

May be taken with food or milk to prevent GI irritation.

Since hydrocodone may cause dizziness and drowsiness, caution patient to avoid driving and other potentially hazardous activities until response to drug is determined.

Warn patient that alcohol and other CNS depressants may cause additive depression.

Treatment for cough is directed toward decreasing the frequency and intensity of nonproductive cough without abolishing the protective cough reflex.

Adequate hydration (at least 1500 to 1800 ml/day) may help to liquefy tenacious sputum. *See Index: Nursing Interventions: cough for other patient teaching points regarding cough therapy.*

Caution patient not to take larger doses than prescribed. Psychic and physical dependence and tolerance may develop with repeated administration.

Classified as Schedule II drug under Federal Controlled Substances Act.

Preserved in tight, light-resistant containers.

See Morphine Sulfate.

PROTOTYPE

HYDROCORTISONE (CORTISOL)

(Aeroseb, Barseb, Cort-Dome, Cortef, Cortenema, DermaCort, Dermolate and others)

HYDROCORTISONE ACETATE

(Biosone, CaldeCort, Carmol, Cortate, Cortef Acetate, Cortifoam, Cortril Acetate, Epifoam, Fernisone, Hydrocortone Acetate, and others)

HYDROCORTISONE CYPIONATE

(Cortef Fluid)

HYDROCORTISONE SODIUM PHOSPHATE

(Hydrocortone Phosphate)

HYDROCORTISONE SODIUM SUCCINATE

(A-hydroCort, Solu-Cortef)

HYDROCORTISONE VALERATE

(Westcort)

(hye-droe-kor′ti-sone)
Corticosteroid
Glucocorticoid
Mineralocorticoid

H

ACTIONS AND USES. Short-acting synthetic steroid with strong glucocorticoid actions and, in high doses, mineralocorticoid properties. Action mechanism: corticosteroids cross cell membranes to complex with specific cytoplasmic receptors. The resulting complexes enter the nucleus, bind to DNA thereby initiating cytoplasmic synthesis of enzymes responsible for systemic effects of adrenocorticoids. *Metabolic effects:* promotes hepatic gluconeogenesis but decreases peripheral utilization of glucose thus predisposing patient on high doses to diabetes mellitus. Promotes protein catabolism, lipolysis, and, with high doses, redistribution of body fat. Interrupts normal linear growth in children. Displays antivitamin D activity leading to interference with calcium (Ca) absorption from GI tract; promotes gastroduodenal ulceration, and enhances peripheral vascular responsiveness to catecholamines. *Antiinflammatory effects (glucocorticoid):* prevents or suppresses clinical phenomena of inflammation including inhibition of phagocytosis, histamine activity and release of kinins; decreased complement components, reduced proliferation of fibroblasts and collagen deposition resulting in suppressed healing and scar tissue formation. *Immunosuppressive effects:* modified immune response to various stimuli with consequent decreased number of circulating eosinophils and lymphocytes decreased passage of immune complexes through basement membranes, reduction in antibody titers, and suppressed cell-mediated hypersensitivity reactions. *Mineralocorticoid effects:* sodium (Na) retention and potassium (K) excretion, preservation of normal water and increased glomerular filtration rate (GFR). High doses may lead to depression, disorientation, euphoria. Prolonged hypothalamic–pituitary–adrenal (HPA) axis suppression, promotes adrenal cortex atrophy with development of Cushingoid (hypercorticism) features; response to stress as in primary adrenocortical insufficiency (hypocorticism), depending on dosage and duration.

Used as replacement therapy in hypocorticism (adrenocortical insufficiency); to reduce serum calcium in hypercalcemia associated with vitamin D intoxication, sarcoidosis, multiple myelomas and breast cancer in premenopausal women; to suppress undesirable inflammatory or immune responses, to produce temporary remission in nonadrenal disease, and to block ACTH production in diagnostic tests. Specific indications include: rheumatic disorders and collagen diseases; dermatologic diseases, alopecia areata, shock unresponsive to conventional therapy; oral, otic, and ocular inflammatory conditions; neoplastic disease of lymphatic system, severe allergic states, chronic ulcerative colitis, respiratory diseases, hematologic disorders, cerebral edema, nephrotic syndrome, acute exacerbation of multiple sclerosis, thyroiditis, tuberculosis, meningitis, acute status asthmaticus; to decrease bleeding tendencies and normalize blood counts; aplastic anemia.

ABSORPTION AND FATE. Rapid absorption from GI tract. 90 to 95% protein bound. Onset of action: oral: 1 to 2 hours; parenteral, rapid; rectal, 3 to 5 days. Peak effect: oral, 1 hour; IM, 4 to 8 hours. Duration of action: oral, IM: 1 to 1½ days; intraarticular, intralesional, soft tissue injection: 3 days to 4 weeks. Half-life: plasma: 1.5 to 2 hours; HPA suppression: 8 to 12 hours. Metabolized in liver. Excreted in urine principally as 17-hydroxysteroids (17-OHCS) and 17-ketosteroids (17-KS). Crosses placenta.

CONTRAINDICATIONS AND PRECAUTIONS. Hypersensitivity to glucocorticoids, idiopathic thrombocytopenic purpura, psychoses, acute glomerulonephritis, viral or bacterial diseases of skin, infections not controlled by antibiotics, active or latent amebiasis, hypercorticism (Cushing's syndrome), small pox vaccination or other immunologic procedures. (Topical steroids contraindicated in presence of varicella, vaccinia, on surfaces with compromised circulation, and in children less than 2 years old.) Safe use in women of childbearing potential, nursing mothers, during pregnancy (category C) not established. *Cautious Use:* children, diabetes mellitus; chronic active hepatitis positive for hepatitis B surface antigen, hyperlipidemia, cirrhosis, stromal herpes simplex, glaucoma, tuberculosis of eye, osteoporosis, convulsive disorders, hypothyroidism, diverticulitis, nonspecific ulcerative colitis, fresh intestinal anastomoses, active or latent peptic ulcer, gastritis, esophagitis, thromboembolic disorders, congestive heart failure, metastatic carcinoma, hypertension, renal insufficiency, history of allergies, active or arrested tuberculosis, systemic fungal infection, myasthenia gravis.

H

ADVERSE/SIDE EFFECTS. (Dose and treatment-duration dependent.) **CV:** syncopal episodes, thrombophlebitis, thromboembolism or fat embolism, palpitation, tachycardia, necrotizing angiitis. **Dermatologic:** skin thinning and atrophy, acne, impaired wound healing, petechiae, ecchymosis, easy bruisings, suppression of skin test reaction; hypo- or hyperpigmentation, hirsutism, acneiform eruptions, subcutaneous fat atrophy; allergic dermatitis, urticaria, angioneurotic edema, increased sweating. **Endocrine:** suppressed linear growth in children, decreased glucose tolerance; hyperglycemia, manifestations of latent diabetes mellitus, secondary pituitary and adrenocortical unresponsiveness especially in stress; amenorrhea and other menstrual difficulties. **Fluid and electrolyte disturbances:** hypocalcemia, Na and fluid retention, hypokalemia and hypokalemic alkalosis; congestive heart failure, hypertension. **GI:** nausea, increased appetite, ulcerative esophagitis, pancreatitis, abdominal distention, peptic ulcer with perforation and hemorrhage, melena. **Hematologic:** thrombocytopenia. **Musculoskeletal:** osteoporosis, compression fractures, muscle wasting and weakness, tendon rupture, aseptic necrosis of femoral and humeral heads. **Neurologic:** vertigo, headache, nystagmus, ataxia (rare), increased intracranial pressure with papilledema (usually after discontinuation of medication), mental disturbances, aggravation of preexisting psychiatric conditions, insomnia. **Ophthalmic:** posterior subcapsular cataracts (especially in children), glaucoma, exophthalmus, increased intraocular pressure with optic nerve damage, perforation of the globe, fungal infection of the cornea, decreased or blurred vision. **With parenteral therapy:** IV site: pain, irritation, necrosis, atrophy, sterile abscess; Charcot-like arthropathy; following intraarticular use, burning and tingling in perineal area (after IV injection). **Other:** negative nitrogen balance, anaphylactoid or hypersensitivity reactions; aggravation or masking of infections; malaise, hiccoughs, hoarseness, dry mouth, sore throat (with inhalation therapy), weight gain, obesity; increased or decreased motility and number of spermatozoa, decreased serum concentration of vitamins A and C; urinary frequency and urgency, enuresis. **Overdosage (hypercorticism):** anxiety, mental confusion, depression, hyperglycemia, hypokalemia, hypernatremia, polycythemia, hypertension, edema, GI cramping or bleeding, ecchymoses, "moon" facies.

ROUTE AND DOSAGE. Adults: all doses vary according to condition being treated; **Pediatric:** doses, if available, usually governed more by severity of condition and clinical response of patient than by age or body weight. **Oral** (hydrocortisone and cypionate): 10 to 320 mg daily (single or divided doses). **Intramuscular** (hydrocortisone, sodium phosphate, sodium succinate): one-third to one-half oral dose every 12 hours. **Intravenous** (sodium phosphate, sodium succinate): 20 to 240 mg daily. **Subcutaneous** (sodium phosphate): 20 to 240 mg daily (single or divided doses). **Intralesional, intraarticular, soft tissue injection (acetate):** 25 to 75 mg. **Retention enema:** 100 mg nightly for 21 days or until clinical and proctologic remission occurs. **Rectal suppository:** one suppository inserted in rectum two or three times daily or 2 suppositories twice daily. Duration of treatment: 2 to up to 8 weeks. **Topical:** Apply thin film or spray to affected area two to four times daily. **Ophthalmic (suspension):** Initial: instill 1 or 2 drops into conjunctival sac every hour during day and every 2 hours during night. With favorable response: reduce dosage to 1 drop every 4 hours; later: 1 drop three or four times/day. **Otic:** Initial: (into aural canal): 3 or 4 drops two or three times daily. Dosage reduced gradually according to response.

NURSING IMPLICATIONS

Carefully check manufacturer's label for recommended route of administration.

Before systemic corticosteroid therapy is started, a skin test for tuberculosis may be done.

The initial suppressive dosing regimen should be brief, especially if alternate-day therapy is anticipated. Usually 4 to 10 days is sufficient for satisfactory clinical response in many allergic and collagen diseases.

Alternate-day therapy (See Index) single dose administered every other day is used when long-term oral glucocorticoid treatment is anticipated.

Inject *IM preparation* deeply into upper outer quadrant of buttock to avoid local atrophy. Avoid using deltoid muscle. Rotate injection site.

Avoid *SC injection;* may produce sterile abscess or pseudoatrophy with persistent depression of overlying dermis lasting several weeks or months.

Cortisol plasma levels are maximal between 2 AM and 8 AM and minimal between 4 PM and midnight (normal: 7 to 28 mcg/dl in AM and 2 to 18 mcg/dl in afternoon). Exogenous corticosteroids suppress adrenal cortex activity less when given in the morning. To minimize HPA axis suppression, replacement steroid should be given before 9 AM.

Take oral drug at mealtimes or with a (low-salt) snack to reduce gastric irritation.

Counsel patient to take drug as prescribed and not to alter dosing regimen or stop medication without consulting physician. Additionally, patient should not give any of the drug to another person.

Establish baseline and continuing data regarding blood pressure, intake and output ratio and pattern, weight, and sleep pattern. Start flow chart as reference for planning individualized pharmacotherapeutic patient care.

Check and record blood pressure during dose stabilization period at least two times daily. Report an ascending pattern.

24-hour urine specimens for studies of 17-KS may be prescribed to rule out Cushing's syndrome (hypercorticism). Normal 17-KS values: men, 10 to 25 mg/24 hours; women under 50 years: 5 to 15 mg/24 hours; women over 50 years; 4 to 8 mg/24 hours.

During long-term therapy, patient should be monitored for evidence of HPT axis suppression by determining plasma cortisol levels at weekly intervals.

Two-hour postprandial blood glucose, serum K, chest x-ray, and routine laboratory studies are performed at regular intervals during long-term steroid therapy.

The elderly patient and the patient with low serum albumen are especially susceptible to adverse/side effects because of excess circulating free glucocorticoids.

If patient has a history of diabetes mellitus, urine should be tested for glycosuria daily.

Report positive findings; dietary and antidiabetic medication dose adjustments may be indicated.

Be alert to signs of hypocalcemia: muscle twitching, cramps, carpopedal spasm, positive Trousseau's and Chvostek's signs; and of hypokalemia: muscle twitching, flaccid paralysis, postural hypotension, tetany, polydipsia, polyurea, cardiac dysrhythmias. Patients with hypocalcemia have increased requirements for pyridoxine (vitamin B_6), vitamin C and D, and folates.

Ophthalmoscopic examinations including tonometry are recommended every 2 to 3 months, especially if patient is receiving ophthalmic steroid therapy.

Monitor patient's weight under standard conditions. Inform patient that a slight weight gain with improved appetite is expected, but after dosage stabilization has been achieved, a sudden slow but steady weight increase (5 lb/week) should be reported.

A salt-restricted diet (unless otherwise contraindicated) and one rich in vitamin D and K and protein, is usually prescribed.

Facilitate collaboration with dietitian and patient to plan diet. Teach food sources of K (leafy vegetables, potato, avocado, wheat, citrus fruit, melon, bananas, whole grains) as well as foods to avoid in order to decrease Na intake (snack foods, prepared luncheon meats, bouillon, sauces, processed cheese).

Because of immunosuppression and the possibility of masked infection, warn patient to report incidence of slow healing or persistent inflammation in an abrasion, wound, or joint or any vague feeling of being sick without clear etiologic definition, or return of pretreatment symptoms.

The immunocompromised patient should be fastidious about personal hygiene, give special attention to foot care, and be particularly cautious about bruising or abrading the skin.

To continue beneficial effect of *intraarticular injection,* teach the patient proper joint alignment, appropriate posttreatment exercise, when to begin the exercises, and how long to avoid weight-bearing activities.

Exaggerated sense of well-being and analgesic effects (painless joints) may encourage patient to increase physical activity even if acute disease process still exists. Discuss with physician and work with patient/family to plan reasonable and safe range of activities of daily living.

Intraarticular injections can lead to systemic effects.

Compression and spontaneous fractures of long bones and vertebrae present hazards particularly in long-term corticosteroid treatment of rheumatoid arthritis or diabetes, in immobilized patients, and the elderly. Supervise getting out of bed or chair. Report persistent backache or chest pain (possible symptoms of vertebral or rib fracture). Patient's mattress should be firm or supported by a bedboard.

Be aware of previous history of psychotic tendencies. Watch for changes in mood and behavior, emotional stability, sleep pattern, or psychomotor activity especially with long-term therapy, that may signal onset of recurrence. Report symptoms to physician.

Dose adjustment may be required if patient is subjected to severe stress (serious infection, surgery, or injury) or if a remission or disease exacerbation occurs.

Dyspepsia with hyperacidity should not be ignored. Encourage patient to report symptoms to physician and not to self-medicate in order to find relief.

If a patient is receiving aspirin concomitantly with a corticosteroid, salicylism may be induced when the corticosteroid dosage is decreased or discontinued.

Warn patient not to use aspirin or other OTC drugs unless prescribed specifically by the physician.

Steroid ulcers with long-term therapy are frequently treated with an antacid. Encourage patient to avoid alcohol and caffeine (secretagogues).

When corticosteroid is given for rheumatoid arthritis, complete relief is not sought because of the hazards of continuous treatment. A regimen of rest, physical therapy, and salicylates continues during steroid therapy.

Observe newborn infant born of mother on substantial doses of corticosteroid during pregnancy for signs of hypoadrenalism.

The *retention enema* preparation (Cortenema) produces the same systemic effects as other formulations of hydrocortisone. Administer preferably after a bowel movement. Advise patient to lie on left side at least 30 minutes, but if given at bedtime, the enema should be retained at least 1 hour or all night if possible. This route is usually used for 21 days then withdrawn gradually if intestinal symptoms do not abate. Report rectal infection or irritation.

Topical Applications: (hydrocortisone, and its esters):

- Warn patient not to use OTC topical preparations of a corticosteroid more than 7 days. They should not be used for children less than 2 years old. If symptoms do not abate, consult physician.
- Wash hands before and after application of medication.
- Usually topical preparations are applied to hydrated skin, i.e., after a shower or bath when skin is damp or wet.
- Cleansing and application of prescribed preparation should be done with extreme gentleness because of easy bruisability and poor healing. Do not apply thick layers of medication or an occlusive dressing unless specifically prescribed.
- A light film of the topical preparation should be massaged into affected area gently and thoroughly until it disappears. If an *occlusive dressing* is to be used, apply medication sparingly, rub until it disappears, and then reapply, leaving a thin coat over lesion. Completely cover area with transparent plastic or other occlusive device or vehicle. Consult physician about frequency of dressing change.
- Occlusive vehicles or transparent plastic enhance absorption. Greasy ointments are more occlusive than gels and seem to be the preferred preparation for dry scaly skin. Other preparations for topical application include solutions, aerosols, and lotions for use on hairy areas, and steroid impregnated tape.
- If lesion is essentially dry, make dressing as airtight and water tight as possible. Prevent evaporation by sealing dressing to adjacent skin. Discuss with physician.
- Avoid covering a weeping or exudative lesion.
- If treated area is large, a sequential approach may be used with treatment of only a portion of the total area at a time.
- An occlusive dressing over a large area should be removed if a patient has a fever to avoid interference with thermostatic defense mechanisms.
- An occlusive dressing increases percutaneous penetration as much as 10%. Discomfort and warmth may be troublesome. Inspect skin carefully between applications for ecchymotic, petechial and purpuric signs, maceration, secondary infection, skin atrophy, striae or miliaria; if present, stop medication and notify physician. Antifungal or antimicrobial treatment may be instituted.
- Rates of penetration of topical corticosteroid differ in various anatomic sites: thus comparatively small doses are used on face, scalp, scrotum, axilla, and groin. Usually occlusive dressings are not applied to these areas.
- Advise patient to avoid exposure of treated skin to temperature extremes.
- Caution should be used when a plastic film dressing is used on children to avoid possibility of accidental suffocation. Also warn patient to exercise great precaution when smoking while plastic is in use.
- Instruct patient to report promptly if initial therapeutic response is followed by relapse.

Contact sensitivity or sensitivity to corticosteroid impurities may be presenting. The medication will be changed in kind or in dose.

- Although adrenal suppression from topical therapy infrequently occurs, whole-body applications of potent corticosteroid, occlusion, and stress may present a hazard. Replacement therapy before surgery may be given to prevent adrenal crisis.
- Urge patient on long-term therapy with topical corticosterone to check shelf-life date. (Full potency is supposed to be maintained to end of shelf-life.) Application of an old preparation with loss of potency may simulate sudden withdrawal of medication.
- Determine need for continued therapy with topical preparation. Since absorption of corticosteroid through abraded skin is greater than through normal skin, a healed area can simulate sudden withdrawal of medication by causing withdrawal symptoms with continued application.

Abrupt discontinuation of corticosteroids after long-term therapy may result in *withdrawal syndrome* (myalgia, fever, arthralgia, malaise) and hypocorticism (anorexia, vomiting, nausea, fatigue, dizziness, hypotension, hypoglycemia, myalgia, arthralgia).

H

Single doses of corticosteroids or use for a short period (less than 1 week) do not produce withdrawal symptoms when discontinued, even with moderately large doses precautions should be taken when a patient is transferred from systemic to oral or nasal inhalation therapy (e.g., beclomethasone, flunisolide) as well as at time of discontinuing long-term therapy.

To prevent withdrawal symptoms and permit adrenals to recover from drug-induced partial atrophy, doses are gradually reduced by scheduled decrements (various regimes).

If during withdrawal, the disease flares up, a dosage increase followed by a more gradual withdrawal may be necessary.

Patient is supervised about 1 year after withdrawal from systemic corticosteroids, or until HPA axis function is restored. During period of HPA suppression, severe stress (trauma, surgery, infections) may induce symptoms of adrenal insufficiency necessitating reinstitution of glucocorticoid and mineralocorticoid treatment.

Patient/family should be advised to tell a dentist or new physician about recently prolonged corticosteroid treatment.

Ordinarily long-term corticosteroid therapy is not interrupted when patient undergoes major surgery, but dosage may be increased.

Advise patient receiving corticosteroid to carry a medical identification card or jewelry with recorded diagnosis, drug therapy, and name of physician.

Urge patient to adhere to scheduled appointments for regimen reevaluation.

Store medication between 15° and 30°C (59° and 86°F); unless otherwise directed by manufacturer. Protect drug from light and freezing.

Diagnostic Test Interferences. Hydrocortisone (corticosteroids) may increase serum **cholesterol, blood glucose,** serum **Na, uric acid** (in acute leukemia) and **Ca** (in bone metastasis). It may decrease serum **Ca, K, PBI, thyroxin (T_4), triiodothyronine (T_3)** and reduce **thyroid I 131** uptake. It increases **urine glucose** level and **calcium** excretion; decreases **urine 17-OHCS** and **17-KS** levels. May produce false-negative results with nitroblue tetrazolium test for systemic bacterial infection, and suppress reactions to skin tests.

Drug Interactions: Hydrocortisone (corticosteroids)

Plus	**Interactions**
Alcohol and ulcerogenic drugs (e.g., aspirin, indomethacin, salicylates, corticosteroids)	Increased risk of GI ulceration

Plus (cont.)	Interactions (cont.)
Amphotericin B, K-depleting diuretics (e.g., thiazides, furosamide (Lasix), ethacrynic acid (Edecrin)	Increased hypokalemic effect of hydrocortisone
Anion exchange resins, (Questran), e.g., cholestyramine, colestipol (Colestid)	Decreased pharmacologic effects of corticosteroids (interference with absorption)
Anticoagulants, oral, e.g., coumarins	May decrease anticoagulant effect of coumarins
Anticonvulsants, e.g., phenytoin (Dilantin)	Corticosteroids lower seizure threshold requiring close monitoring of anticonvulsant activity
Antidiabetic agents (oral and insulin)	Decreased hypoglycemic effect of antidiabetic agents
Barbiturates, ephedrine, phenytoin, rifampin	Decreased glucocorticoid response
Cholinesterase inhibitors, e.g., ambenonium (Mytelase), neostigmine (Prostigmin)	Decreased effect of cholinesterase
Digitalis glycosides	Increased risk of digitalis toxicity and arrhythmias due to hypokalemic effect of corticosteroids
Estrogens, indomethacin, nicotine, salicylates, pyrazolones	Increased antiinflammatory activity of corticosteroids
Isoniazid (INH)	Antitubercular effectiveness may be decreased
Salicylates	Decreased serum levels of salicylates (decreased pharmacologic effects)
Oral contraceptives, erythromycins, troleandomycin (TAO)	Increased or prolonged corticosteroid activity
Theophyllines	Decreased glucocorticosteroid response
Vaccines, toxoids	Diminished response to toxoids, live and inactivated vaccines

HYDROFLUMETHIAZIDE
(Diucardin, Saluron)

(hye-droe-floo-meth-eye'a-zide)
Diuretic
Antihypertensive
Thiazide
Sulfonamide derivative

ACTIONS AND USES. Benzothiadiazine (thiazide) derivative. Similar to chlorothiazide (qv) in actions, uses, contraindications, precautions, adverse reactions, and interactions. Available in fixed combination with reserpine (Salutensin).

ABSORPTION AND FATE. Diuretic effect begins in 1 to 2 hours, peaks in 3 to 4 hours and lasts 18 to 24 hours. Presumed to be distributed and excreted similarly to other thiazides. *See Chlorothiazide.*

CONTRAINDICATIONS AND PRECAUTIONS. Hypersensitivity to other thiazides or sulfonamide derivatives; anuria; pregnancy (category B), lactation, hypokalemia. *See Chlorothiazide.*

ADVERSE/SIDE EFFECTS. Postural hypotension, photosensitivity hypokalemia, hyperglycemia, hyponatremia, asymptomatic hyperuricemia, agranulocytosis. *See also Chlorothiazide.*

ROUTE AND DOSAGE. Oral: Adult: *Edema:* Initial 50 mg one or two times daily. Maintenance: 25 to 200 mg in divided doses daily or on alternate days, or 3 to 5 days a week. *Hypertension:* Initial 50 mg twice daily; dose adjusted according to blood pressure response. Maintenance: 50 to 100 mg daily. Dosage not to exceed 200 mg/day. **Pediatric:** 1 mg/kg body weight or 30 mg/m² body surface area once daily.

NURSING IMPLICATIONS

Elderly patients are especially susceptible to the hypotensive effects that may accompany excessive diuresis.

Schedule diuretic dose early in the morning to prevent interrupted sleep because of diuresis. (If two doses are taken each day, schedule second dose no later than 3 PM.)

H

Antihypertensive effects may be noted in 3 to 4 days, maximal effects may require 3 to 4 weeks.

Baseline and periodic determinations should be made for serum electrolytes, blood counts, BUN, blood glucose, uric acid, and CO_2.

Monitor patient for hypokalemia: dry mouth, anorexia, thirst, paresthesias, muscle cramps, cardiac arrhythmias. Report promptly. Physician may change dose and institute replacement therapy.

Hypokalemia is rarely severe in most patients even on long-term therapy with thiazides. To prevent onset, urge patient to eat a normal diet (usually includes K-rich foods such as potatoes, fruit juices, cereals, skim milk) and to include a banana (about 370 mg K) and at least 6 ounces orange juice (about 330 mg K) every day.

If hypokalemia develops, dietary K supplement of 1000 to 2000 mg (25 to 50 mEq) is usually an adequate treatment.

Dietary management is important in thiazide treatment for hypertension. The physician will specifically order goals of the diet: electrolyte, weight, or fluid control. Collaborate with dietitian and arrange for patient-dietitian planning for an individualized diet.

Asymptomatic hyperuricemia can be produced because of interference with uric acid excretion although thiazides rarely precipitate acute gout. Report onset of joint pain and limitation of motion. Patient with history of gout may be continued on a thiazide with adjusted doses of uricosuric agent.

The prediabetic or diabetic mellitus patient should be watched carefully for loss of control of diabetes or early signs of hyperglycemia: drowsiness; flushed, dry skin; fruit-like breath odor, polyuria, polydipsia, anorexia. These symptoms are slow to develop and to recognize. Notify physician and question need to adjust insulin dosage.

Warn patient about the possibility of photosensitivity reaction and to notify the physician if it occurs (like an exaggerated sun burn). Thiazide-related photosensitivity is considered a photoallergy (ultraviolet radiation changes drug structure and makes it allergenic for some individuals on thiazide therapy). It occurs 1½ to 2 weeks after initial sun exposure.

Notify the anesthetist that patient is on thiazide therapy.

Counsel patient to avoid use of OTC drugs unless approved by the physician. Many preparations contain both potassium and sodium and if misused, or if patient overdoses, electrolyte side effects may be induced.

Store tablets in tightly closed container at 15° to 30°C (59° to 86°F), unless otherwise directed by manufacturer.

See Chlorothiazide (prototype thiazide diuretic).

HYDROGEN PEROXIDE

(H_2O_2)

(hye'droe-jen per-ox'ide)
Antiinfective, topical
Oxidizing agent

ACTIONS AND USES. Comparatively weak, short-acting antibacterial agent with oxidizing properties and acidic pH. Effective as wound cleanser and deodorant. Slowly releases nascent oxygen and water on contact with catalase, an enzyme found in blood and most other tissue fluids. Effervescence caused by release of oxygen mechanically loosens wound debris and pockets of bacteria. Reduction in bacteria is believed to be more a factor of mechanical action than antibacterial activity. Each ml of 3% hydrogen peroxide releases about 10 ml of molecular oxygen.

Used as cleansing agent for wounds and suppurating ulcers, as mouthwash or gargle as in Vincent's stomatitis. Also has been used to remove ear wax in patients with ceruminosis.

ABSORPTION AND FATE. Duration of action: period of active oxygen release (visual evidence: during bubbling action).

CONTRAINDICATIONS AND PRECAUTIONS. Instillation into closed body cavities or into abscesses. *Cautious Use:* deep wounds, serious burns.

H

ADVERSE/SIDE EFFECTS. Irritation of skin or mucous membranes; superinfections (black hairy tongue), decalcification of tooth enamel (overuse as mouthwash); systemic oxygen emboli with instillation into closed body cavities.

ROUTE AND DOSAGE. **Topical:** 1.5 to 3% solution for cleansing wounds, mouthwash, or gargle. Available as 3% solution for uses described.

NURSING IMPLICATIONS

Note expiration date on label.

Point bottle away from face when removing screw cap. Release of oxygen which occurs with decomposition may cause pressure build-up within bottle.

May be diluted with water or normal saline. Use immediately after diluting; solution loses oxygen with storage and therefore is ineffective.

H_2O_2 should never be instilled into closed body cavities or into abscesses which do not allow the liberated free oxygen escape, nor should bandages be applied too soon following its use for wound cleansing. Wound irrigation with H_2O_2, even when diluted, has caused near-fatal systemic oxygen microemboli by passage of oxygen into the vascular system.

If redness, swelling, pain, or irritation in or around wound increases or persists, or if infection occurs, discontinue use and notify physician.

When used as a mouthwash, H_2O_2 should be diluted with at least 1 or more parts of water or saline. Dilutions may range from 2 to 8 parts of water or saline. Discontinue promptly if irritation of tongue or buccal mucosa occurs or if tongue appears black and furry (hypertrophy of papillae of tongue also called lingua nigra, possibly from fungal overgrowth). Full-strength H_2O_2 can harm the gums.

Overuse of H_2O_2 as mouthwash (i.e., too frequent use even if diluted) decreases oral pH (normally, oral cavity is alkaline), creating an acid environment that can support superinfections, enamel decalcification, and dental caries.

Warn patient not to use peroxide for bleaching hair as a substitute since it is considerably more concentrated (e.g., 20 to 30% as compared to antiinfective preparation which is 3%), and can be caustic.

Patients with intact eardrums who have hard but not impacted ear wax are advised by some clinicians to instill H_2O_2 occasionally into affected ear(s) to facilitate natural wax removal. Professional cleansing is required when wax is excessive, or impacted, or if inflammation or infection is present.

Ear wax is believed to be bacterial and fungistatic and therefore protective. In most patients the ear canal is self-cleaning. However, cerumen may harden and accumulate if there is insufficient environmental humidity or if ear canals are narrow or tortuous, or hair in ears is excessive. Warn patient not to attempt wax removal with a swab or any other instrument.

H_2O_2 decomposes with age, agitation, and with exposure to heat, light, air, and organic material. Decomposition is accelerated by metals and metallic salts.

Store preferably between 15° and 30°C (59° and 86°F) in tightly-covered, light-resistant container, unless otherwise directed by manufacturer. Protect from heat and light.

H

HYDROMORPHONE HYDROCHLORIDE

(Dilaudid)

(hye-droe-mor′fone)
Narcotic analgesic
C II

ACTIONS AND USES. Semisynthetic phenanthrene derivative structurally similar to morphine (qv), but with eight to ten times more potent analgesic effect. Has more rapid onset and shorter duration of action that morphine, and reported to have less hypnotic action and less tendency to produce nausea and vomiting.

Used for relief of moderate to severe pain.

ABSORPTION AND FATE. Onset of analgesic effect in 15 to 30 minutes; peaks in 30 to 90 minutes, and lasts 4 to 5 hours. Metabolized primarily in liver. Excreted chiefly in urine as glucuronide conjugate.

ROUTE AND DOSAGE. **Oral, subcutaneous, intramuscular, intravenous (slowly):** 2 mg every 4 to 6 hours. For severe pain, parenteral dose may be increased to 3 to 4 mg every 4 to 6 hours. **Rectal suppository (3 mg):** one every 6 to 8 hours.

NURSING IMPLICATIONS

When sleep follows administration of hydromorphone, it is usually due to relief of pain rather than hypnosis.

Produces physical dependence after prolonged administration.

Withdrawal symptoms are similar to those of morphine dependence but occur sooner.

High drug abuse potential. Very high "street demand."

Classified as Schedule II drug under Federal Controlled Substances Act.

Preserved in tight, light-resistant containers.

See Morphine Sulfate.

HYDROQUINONE

(Eldopaque, Eldoquin, Melanex, Mercolized Cocrema, Pabaquinone, Porcelana, Quinnone, Solaquin)

(hye′droe-kwin-one)
Depigmenting agent
Enzyme inhibitor

ACTIONS AND USES. Topical agent that causes reversible bleaching of hyperpigmented skin due to increased melanin. Interferes with formation of new melanin, but does not destroy existing pigment. Believed to act by inhibiting tyrosinase in melanocytes, thereby depressing melanin synthesis and melanocytic growth, and possibly by increasing excretion of melanin from melanocytes.

Used for gradual bleaching of hyperpigmented skin conditions such as chloasma or melasma, severe freckling, senile lentigines (age spots or liver spots). Also used as an antioxidant in topical preparations. Some formulations include a sunscreening agent (e.g., Porcelana with Sunscreen, Mercolized Cocrema, Pabaquinone, and Solaquin).

CONTRAINDICATIONS AND PRECAUTIONS. History of sensitivity or allergic reaction to hydroquinone or to any ingredient in the formulation. Safe use during pregnancy (category C), in nursing women, and in children 12 years and younger not established.

ADVERSE/SIDE EFFECTS. Dryness and fissuring of paranasal and infraorbital areas, inflammatory reaction, erythema; stinging, tingling, burning sensations; irritation, sensitization and contact dermatitis.

ROUTE AND DOSAGE. Topical (2 to 4%): Apply thin layer and rub into depigmented area(s) (unless otherwise directed by manufacturer), twice daily, morning and evening. Available in cream, lotion, and solution.

NURSING IMPLICATIONS

Skin should be tested for sensitivity before treatment is initiated. Apply small amount of drug (about 25 mm in diameter) to an unbroken patch of skin and check in 24 hours. Some clinicians recommend preparing 1% hydroquinone in petrolatum for patch testing. If vesicle formation, itching, or excessive inflammation occurs, drug should not be used. Minor redness is not a contraindication.

Hydroquinone acts faster and more dependably if skin is protected from sunlight or ultraviolet (UV) light. Advise patient to use a sunscreening agent or a hydroquinone formulation containing a sunscreen for day time applications. Unnecessary or excessive exposure to the sun or to UV light should be avoided to prevent stimulation of melanocyte activity.

Inform patient that sensitization and contact dermatitis have been reported. Advise using only the smallest quantity of medication necessary to cover affected part and to wash and dry hands thoroughly before and after application.

Applications should be limited to an area no larger than that of face and neck.

If rash or irritation develops, instruct patient to wash drug off, withhold further treatment, and consult physician.

Avoid contact of hydroquinone with the eyes and do not use on open lesions, sunburned, irritated or otherwise damaged skin.

Pregnant patients should be advised to wait for several months after delivery before contemplating use of a depigmentation agent. Chloasma or melanasma gravidarum ("mask of pregnancy") disappears or at least regresses without treatment after pregnancy.

In general, complete depigmentation occurs in 1 to 4 months and lasts 2 to 6 months after hydroquinone is discontinued. Once desired results are obtained, amount and frequency of applications should be reduced to the very least that will maintain depigmentation.

Patient should be advised to continue use of protective clothing and sunscreening agent after treatment is terminated to reduce possibility of repigmentation.

Some hydroquinone preparations are available OTC without sunscreen agent, e.g., Eldopaque, Eldoquin, Porcelana, and with a sunscreen, e.g., Porcelana with Sunscreen, Mercolized Cocrema, Solaquin, and Pabaquinone.

HYDROXOCOBALAMIN

(hye-drox-oh-koe-bal'a-min)
Vitamin
Antianemic

(Acti-B_{12}, Alphamin, AlphaRedisol, CoDROXOMIN, Droxomin, Hybalamin, Hydrobexan, Hydroxo-12, LA-12, Vibal L.A., Vitamin $B_{12\alpha}$)

ACTIONS AND USES. Cobalamin derivative similar to cyanocobalamin (vitamin B_{12}) in actions, uses, contraindications, precautions, and adverse reactions. More slowly absorbed from injection site than cyanocobalamin, and may be taken up by liver in larger quantities. Results in higher and more sustained serum cobalamin levels and significantly less urinary excretion of cobalamin than produced by similar doses of cyanocobalamin; however, some patients reportedly develop an antibody to the plasma B_{12}-binding protein. *Investigational Use:* in treatment of cyanide poisoning and tobacco amblyopia.

ROUTE AND DOSAGE. Intramuscular (only): Adults: doses as low as 30 mcg daily for 5 to 10 days, followed by 100 to 200 mcg once monthly, and doses as high as 1000 mcg on alternate days until remission, then 1000 mcg monthly. **Children:** 100 mcg over 2 or more weeks to total dosage of 1 to 5 mg. Maintenance: 30 to 50 mcg/month.

H

NURSING IMPLICATIONS

Some patients experience mild pain at injection site following administration.
See Cyanocobalamin.

HYDROXYAMPHETAMINE HYDROBROMIDE

(hye-drox-ee-am-fe'ta-meen)
Adrenergic (ophthalmic)
(Sympathomimetic)
Mydriatic

(Paredrine)

ACTIONS AND USES. Sympathomimetic amine similar to ephedrine in many actions, but almost lacking in CNS stimulant activity. Indirectly stimulates alpha- and beta-adrenergic receptors by releasing catecholamine stores. Topical application to eye produces mydriasis without cycloplegia, thus sparing patient of long-lasting residual blurred vision.

Used topically to produce mydriasis and vasoconstriction for diagnostic eye examinations; used during surgery, and used to prevent synechiae in uveitis.

ABSORPTION AND FATE. Produces mydriasis in 45 to 60 minutes, with recovery in about 6 hours following topical application to eye.

CONTRAINDICATIONS AND PRECAUTIONS. Hypersensitivity or idiosyncrasy to sympathomimetic amines, narrow-angle glaucoma. *Cautious Use:* diabetes mellitus, hypertension, hyperthyroidism, the elderly.

ROUTE AND DOSAGE. Topical: 1% ophthalmic solution: 1 or 2 drops into the conjunctival sac.

NURSING IMPLICATIONS

This agent or its preservative may stain soft contact lenses; therefore, remove them before drug instillation. Consult physician about necessity to remove hard lenses.

Patient may be more comfortable with dark glasses after drug instillation, because of photophobia.

Warn patient to avoid driving until after recovery from mydriasis.
Recovery from mydriasis will be prolonged in the elderly, because of normal change with aging in the eye musculature.
Preserved in tightly closed, light-resistant containers.
See Index: Drug administration: eye drops.

HYDROXYCHLOROQUINE SULFATE

(Plaquenil Sulfate)

(hye-drox-ee-klor′oh-kwin)
Antiinfective
Antimalarial, suppressant (lupus erythematosus)
Antirheumatic

ACTIONS AND USES. 4-Aminoquinoline derivative closely related to chloroquine and with similar actions, uses, contraindications, precautions, adverse reactions, and interactions.

Used for suppressive prophylaxis and for treatment of acute malarial attacks due to all forms of susceptible malaria. Used adjunctively with primaquine for eradication of *P. vivax* and *P. malariae.* More commonly prescribed than chloroquine for treatment of rheumatoid arthritis and lupus erythematosus (usually in conjunction with salicylate or corticosteroid therapy).

CONTRAINDICATIONS AND PRECAUTIONS. Known hypersensitivity to 4-aminoquinoline compounds; psoriasis, porphyria, long-term therapy in children, pregnancy. Safe use in juvenile arthritis not established. *Cautious Use:* hepatic disease, alcoholism, with hepatotoxic drugs, impaired renal function, metabolic acidosis, patients with tendency toward dermatitis. *See also Chloroquine.*

ADVERSE/SIDE EFFECTS. GI distress, visual disturbances, retinopathy, muscle weakness, vertigo, tinnitus, nerve deafness, dermatologic and hematologic reactions. With overdosage: respiratory depression, cardiovascular collapse, shock. *See also Chloroquine.*

ROUTE AND DOSAGE. Oral: *Acute malaria:* **Adults:** Initial: 800 mg, followed by 400 mg after 6 to 8 hours, then 400 mg on each of next 2 days to total of 2 Gm. **Children (11 to 15 years):** 600 mg, then 2 doses of 200 mg after 8 and 24 hours; **(6 to 10 years):** 400 mg, then 2 doses of 200 mg at 8-hour intervals; **(2 to 5 years):** 400 mg then 200 mg 8 hours later; **(1 year and under):** 100 mg, then 3 doses of 100 mg every 6 to 8 hours. *Malaria suppression:* **Adults:** 400 mg once weekly on same day of each week. If possible, suppressive therapy should begin 2 weeks prior to exposure and continued for 8 weeks after leaving endemic area; failing this, an initial double (loading) dose of 800 mg in adults or 10 mg base/kg in children administered in 2 divided doses 6 hours apart. *Lupus erythematosus:* **Adults:** 400 mg once or twice daily for several weeks or months, depending on patient response; maintenance 200 to 400 mg daily. *Antirheumatic:* **Adults:** Initial: 400 to 600 mg daily; dosage increased gradually to optimum response level, then reduced slowly to maintenance level: 200 to 400 mg daily.

NURSING IMPLICATIONS

Administration of drug immediately before or after meals may reduce incidence of GI distress.
All patients on long-term therapy should have baseline and periodic (every 3 months) ophthalmoscopic examinations (including visual acuity, slit lamp, fundoscopy, and visual fields), and blood cell counts.

Hydroxychloroquine has cumulative actions. In patients requiring long-term therapy, therapeutic effect may not appear for several weeks, and maximal benefit may not occur for 6 months.

Patients receiving prolonged therapy should be informed about adverse symptoms and advised to report their onset immediately. Patients should be questioned about possible symptoms and examined periodically (include tests for muscle weakness, knee and ankle reflexes, and opthalmoscopic examinations). Drug should be discontinued if weakness, visual symptoms, or skin eruptions occur.

Counsel patient to follow drug regimen as prescribed by the physician.

Caution patients to keep drug out of reach of children. Children are especially sensitive to 4-aminoquinoline compounds (chloroquine, hydroxychloroquine). A number of fatalities have been reported.

Store preferably between 15° and 30°C (59° and 86°F) unless otherwise directed by manufacturer.

See Chloroquine (prototype antimalarial drug).

HYDROXYPROGESTERONE CAPROATE

(hye-drox-ee-proe-jess'te-rone)

(Delalutin, Duralutin, Gesterol L.A., Hydrosterone, Hydroxon, Hylutin, Hyprogest 250, Hyproval PA, Pro-Depo)

Progestin

ACTIONS AND USES. Long-acting synthetic progestational hormone. Has slower onset and longer action than progesterone (qv). Lacks estrogenic and androgenic activity. Not approved as a single agent contraceptive.

Used to treat amenorrhea, abnormal uterine bleeding, advanced uterine cancer, and as "medical D and C" (conversion of proliferative endometrium to secretory endometrium and desquamation). Has been used as test for endogenous estrogen production.

ADVERSE/SIDE EFFECTS. Coughing, dyspnea, chest constriction, allergylike reactions (especially at high doses), female fetus masculinization. *See also Progesterone.*

ROUTE AND DOSAGE. **Intramuscular (in sesame oil or castor oil vehicle):** *Amenorrhea, primary and secondary:* 375 mg anytime. After 4 days of desquamation or if no bleeding 21 days after hydroxyprogesterone alone, start cyclic therapy *(see Nursing Implications).* Repeat cyclic therapy every 4 weeks; stop after four cycles. *Advanced uterine adenocarcinoma:* 1 Gm or more at once; repeat one or more times each week. (1 to 7 Gm/week). Stop drug at time of relapse or, if no desirable results obtained after a total of 12 weeks of therapy. *Test for endogenous estrogen production:* 250 mg any time. Repeat for confirmation 4 weeks after first injection; stop after second injection.

NURSING IMPLICATIONS

Before hormone therapy is begun genital malignancy should be excluded.

Test for endogenous estrogen production: If patient is not pregnant and has a responsive endometrium, i.e., produces estrogen, bleeding (progesterone withdrawal sign) occurs 7 to 14 days after injection indicating endogenous estrogen.

Hydroxyprogesterone "cyclic therapy": a 28-day cycle repeated every 4 weeks. Administer estradiol valerate 20 mg on day 1 of each cycle; 2 weeks after day 1, administer hydroxyprogesterone 250 mg and estradiol valerate 5 mg. Four weeks after day 1 is day 1 of next cycle.

Teach patient self-breast examination (SBE).
Counsel patient that onset of normal menstrual cycles may not occur for 2 or 3 months after cessation of cyclic therapy.
Hydroxyprogesterone may be used concurrently with other anticancer modalities (surgery, radiation, chemotherapy).
Review package insert with patient to assure understanding of progestin therapy.
Protect drug preparation from light; store at room temperature.
See Progesterone (prototype progestin).

HYDROXYUREA

(Hydrea)

(hye-drox'ee-yoo-ree-ah)
Antineoplastic

ACTIONS AND USES. Synthetic analogue of urea with antimetabolite activity. Blocks incorporation of thymidine into DNA and may damage already formed DNA molecules; does not affect synthesis of RNA or protein. Cytotoxic effect limited to tissues with high rates of cell proliferation. May reduce iron utilization by erythrocytes; has no effect on erythrocyte survival time. No cross resistance with other antineoplastics has been demonstrated.

Used in palliative treatment of metastatic melanoma, chronic myelocytic leukemia; recurrent metastatic, or inoperable ovarian cancer. Also used as adjunct to X-ray therapy for treatment of advanced primary squamous cell (epidermoid) carcinoma of head (excluding lip), neck, lungs. *Investigational Use:* in treatment of psoriasis.

ABSORPTION AND FATE. Readily absorbed from GI tract; peak serum concentrations in 2 hours. Undetectable in blood after 24 hours. Degraded in liver. Over 80% recovered as respiratory CO_2 and as urea in urine, within 12 hours; remainder excreted unchanged. No cumulative effect. Passes blood–brain barrier.

CONTRAINDICATIONS AND PRECAUTIONS. Pregnancy, patients of childbearing age, children, myelosuppression. *Cautious Use:* following recent use of other cytotoxic drugs or irradiation; renal dysfunction, elderly patients, history of gout.

ADVERSE/SIDE EFFECTS. Dermatologic: maculopapular rash, facial erythema, postirradiation erythema, alopecia (rare). **GI:** (occasional): stomatitis, anorexia, nausea, vomiting, diarrhea, constipation. **Hematologic:** leukopenia, thrombocytopenia, megaloblastic erythropoiesis, anemia. **Neurologic (rare):** headache, dizziness, disorientation, drowsiness (large doses), hallucinations, convulsions. **Other:** renal tubular dysfunction, dysuria (rare), elevated BUN, serum uric acid, creatinine levels; hyperuricemia; abnormal BSP retention.

ROUTE AND DOSAGE. Oral (individualized on basis of patient's actual or ideal weight, whichever is less): *Intermittent therapy:* 80 mg/kg body weight as single dose every third day. *Continuous therapy:* 20 to 30 mg/kg body weight as single daily dose.

NURSING IMPLICATIONS

If patient cannot swallow capsule, contents may be emptied into glass of water and taken immediately. Small amounts of inert material used as drug vehicle may not dissolve, but can be ingested.
Toxicity incidence with use of hydroxyurea is as high as 66% with doses of 40 mg/kg body weight. Inform patient of potential side effects and of importance of reporting symptoms promptly.

Status of kidney, liver, bone marrow functions should be determined prior to and periodically during therapy. Hemoglobin, WBC, platelet counts are monitored at least once weekly while patient is taking hydroxyurea.

If WBC drops to 2500/mm^3 or platelets to 100,000/mm^3, therapy will be interrupted. Values are rechecked after 3 days; if significant recovery is manifest, therapy may be resumed. Drug-induced anemia is usually treated by whole blood replacement without interrupting drug therapy.

Monitor body weight and report steady, slow change or precipitous change to physician.

Monitor intake and output. Patients with high serum uric acid levels particularly should be advised to drink at least 10 to 12 (8 ounce) glasses of fluid daily to prevent uric acid nephropathy. Physician may also prescribe alkalinization of urine and administration of allopurinol for patients with hyperuricemia.

Patients with marked renal dysfunction may rapidly develop visual and auditory hallucinations and hematologic toxicity. Changes in intake–output ratio or pattern may be significant indicators of impending nephrotoxicity and are reportable.

Adequate trial period for antineoplastic efficacy (tumor shrinking or growth arrest) is 6 weeks. If satisfactory, therapy may be continued indefinitely (with weekly monitoring of leukocytes).

Advise patient to use barrier contraceptive during therapy. Drug is teratogenic.

Stored in tightly covered container at room temperature, or preferably between 15° and 30°C (59° and 86°F) unless otherwise directed by manufacturer.

See Fluorouracil.

H

HYDROXYZINE HYDROCHLORIDE

(Anxanil, Atarax, Atozine, Durrax, E-Vista, Hyzine-50, Orgatrax, Quiess, Vistaril Intramuscular, Vistacon, Vistaject)

HYDROXYZINE PAMOATE

(Hy-Pam, Vamate, Vistaril Oral)

(hye-drox'i-zeen)
Psychotropic
Anxiolytic
Antihistamine
H_2-receptor agonist

ACTIONS AND USES. Piperazine derivative of diphenylmethane, structurally and pharmacologically related to other cyclizines (e.g., buclizine, chlorcyclizine). In common with such agents, it causes CNS depression and has anticholinergic, antiemetic, bronchodilator and antihistaminic activity. Its ataractic effect is produced primarily by depression of hypothalamus and brain-stem reticular formation, rather than cortical areas. Also has skeletal muscle relaxant effect and mild antisecretory and analgesic activity. The hydrochloride is available in both intramuscular and oral preparations.

Used for treatment of emotional or psychoneurotic states characterized by anxiety, tension, or psychomotor agitation; to relieve anxiety, control nausea and emesis, and reduce narcotic requirements prior to or following surgery or delivery. Also used in management of pruritus due to allergic conditions, e.g., chronic urticaria, atopic and contact dermatoses, and in treatment of acute and chronic alcoholism with withdrawal symptoms or delirium tremens. Available in fixed combination with pentaerythritol (Cartrax) and with oxyphencyclimine (Enarax, Vistrax).

ABSORPTION AND FATE. Rapidly absorbed from GI tract. Onset of effects within 15 to 30 minutes following oral administration; duration of action 4 to 6 hours. Metabolic fate not known.

CONTRAINDICATIONS AND PRECAUTIONS. Known hypersensitivity to hydroxyzine; use as sole treatment in psychoses or depression. Safe use during early pregnancy or in nursing mothers not established; lactation.

ADVERSE/SIDE EFFECTS. Drowsiness, sedation, dizziness, injection site reactions, dry mouth, headache. Rarely: involuntary motor activity, tremor, convulsions. Hypersensitivity reactions: urticaria, erythematous macular eruptions, erythema multiforme.

ROUTE AND DOSAGE. Oral (hydrochloride or pamoate): **Adults:** 25 mg to 100 mg three or four times daily. **Children (under 6 years):** 50 mg daily in divided doses; **(over 6 years):** 50 to 100 mg daily in divided doses. **Intramuscular** (hydrochloride): **Adults:** 25 to 100 mg; dose repeated in 4 to 6 hours, as needed. **Children:** 1.1 mg/kg every 4 to 6 hours as needed.

NURSING IMPLICATIONS

Tablets may be crushed before administration and taken with fluid of patient's choice. Capsule may be emptied and contents swallowed with water or mixed with food.

The IM preparation (hydrochloride) does not need to be diluted.

IM administration should be made deep into body of a relatively large muscle. In adults, the preferred site is the upper outer quadrant of buttock or the midlateral thigh. In children, the recommended site is the midlateral muscle of thigh. *Infants and small children:* periphery of upper outer quadrant of gluteal region should be used only if necessary (e.g., in burn patient with limited injection sites). The deltoid muscle should be used only if well developed; avoid lower and mid-third of arm to prevent radial nerve injury.

Carefully aspirate to check back flow. If present, remove needle and select another site. Hydroxyzine must not be administered by SC, intraarterial, or IV injections. Inadvertent injection by these routes may cause painful site, tissue damage, and may lead to thrombosis or phlebitis.

Rotate injection sites and observe daily.

Drowsiness may occur, but it usually disappears with continued therapy or following reduction of dosage.

Forewarn the patient about the possibility of drowsiness and dizziness, and caution against driving a car or performing hazardous tasks requiring mental alertness and physical coordination while taking hydroxyzine.

Alcohol and hydroxyzine should not be taken at the same time. Concomitant use enhances the effects of both agents. When CNS depressants are prescribed concomitantly, dosage of the depressant is reduced up to 50%.

Patient should be advised that if she becomes pregnant during therapy or intends to become pregnant she should communicate with her physician about the desirability of discontinuing the drug.

Xerostomia is uncomfortable and sets the stage for potential loss of taste and other serious clinical problems. If patient is on high dosage of hydroxyzine, monitor condition of oral membranes daily.

Dry mouth may be relieved by frequent warm water rinses, increasing fluid intake an by use of a salivary substitute (e.g., Moi-stir, Xero-Lube) if necessary. Avoid freque use of commercial mouth rinses. They may change normal flora of the mouth and perm onset of a superinfection.

Urge patient to give scrupulous care to teeth: use unwaxed dental floss and floss th daily, brush gently with a soft small tooth brush after meals, and use a fluoride paste at least once a day. Avoid irritation or abrasion of tissues.

Effectiveness of use longer than 4 months should be reassessed on basis of indi al's response to the drug.

Advise patient to consult physician before self-dosing with OTC medications.

Protect hydroxyzine from light. Store at temperature between 15° and 30°C (59° 86°F) unless otherwise specified by the manufacturer.

H

Diagnostic Test Interferences. Possibility of false-positive **urinary 17-hydroxycorticosteroid** determinations (modified Glenn-Nelson technique).

Drug Interactions: Hydroxyzine

Plus	Interactions
Alcohol Analgesics, nonnarcotic Antipsychotics, other Barbiturates and other sedatives Narcotics	Mutual potentiation of CNS depressant effects

HYOSCYAMINE SULFATE

(Anaspaz, Bellaspaz, Cytospaz, Levsin, Levsinex, Neoques)

(hye-oh-sye'a-meen)
Anticholinergic
Antispasmodic
Belladonna alkaloid

ACTIONS AND USES. Extremely potent, belladonna alkaloid with anticholinergic and antispasmodic activity. Said to be twice as potent as atropine (qv), four times as potent as methantheline bromide, and 20 times as potent as homatropine methylbromide. Anticholinergic effect chiefly related to the levo isomer. Action is produced by competitive inhibition of acetylcholine at the parasympathetic neuroeffector junctions.

Used to treat GI tract disorders caused by spasm and hypermotility, as conjunct therapy with diet and antacids for peptic ulcer management, and as an aid in the control of gastric hypersecretion and intestinal hypermotility. Also in symptomatic relief of biliary and renal colic as a "drying agent" to relieve symptoms of acute rhinitis, and to control preanesthesia salivation and respiratory tract secretions. Used to treat symptoms of parkinsonism and to reduce pain and hypersecretion in pancreatitis. Available in fixed combinations with atropine, butabarbital, and phenobarbital.

ABSORPTION AND FATE. Duration of effect, 4 to 6 hours. Metabolized by the liver; half-life 13 to 38 hours; protein binding 50%. Excreted in urine.

CONTRAINDICATIONS AND PRECAUTIONS. Hypersensitivity to belladonna alkaloids. Narrow-angle glaucoma, prostatic hypertrophy. *Cautious Use:* diabetes mellitus, cardiac disease. *See also Atropine.*

ADVERSE/SIDE EFFECTS. Confusion, excitement in elderly patients; palpitations, blurred vision, xerostomia, constipation, paralytic ileus, urinary retention, anhidrosis. *See also Atropine.*

ROUTE AND DOSAGE. Highly individualized. **Oral, sublingual: Adults:** 0.125 to 0.25 mg three or four times daily as needed. **Children:** proportionately less according to weight. **Intramuscular, intravenous, subcutaneous: Adults:** 0.25 to 0.5 mg (1 or 2 ml) every 6 hours. Available in tablets, sustained-release capsules, elixir, injection.

RSING IMPLICATIONS

ninister oral preparation about one hour before meals and at bedtime (at least 2 hours er last meal).

e patient on hyoscyamine therapy to avoid excessive exposure to a high temperature nvironment; drug-induced heat stroke can develop.

Monitor urinary output. If changes in intake–output ratio and/or voiding pattern occur, notify physician.
Dose for the elderly patient should be less than the standard adult dose. Observe patient carefully for signs of paradoxic reactions.
This drug may cause drowsiness. Advise patient to be cautious while driving a car until response to drug is known.
See Methchlorethamine for discussion about care of dry mouth.
If patient complains about blurred vision, suggest use of dark glasses; but if this side effect persists, advise patient to report to physician for dose adjustment or possible change of drug.
See Atropine sulfate (prototype belladonna alkaloid).

I

IBUPROFEN

(Advil, Amersol, Motrin, Nuprin, Rufen)

(eye-byoo′proe-fen)
NSAID
Antirheumatic

ACTIONS AND USES. Propionic acid derivative with nonsteroid antiinflammatory activity and significant antipyretic and analgesic properties. Comparable to aspirin in analgesic action, but higher doses are required for antiinflammatory effect; also reported to cause fewer GI symptoms than aspirin in equieffective doses. Antiinflammatory action postulated to be due to inhibition of prostaglandin synthesis and/or release. Antipyretic effect is thought to result from action on hypothalamus; heat dissipation accompanies vasodilation and peripheral blood flow. Inhibits platelet aggregation and prolongs bleeding time, but does not affect prothrombin or whole blood clotting times. Cross-sensitivity with aspirin and other nonsteroidal antiinflammatory drugs has been reported.

Used in chronic, symptomatic treatment of active rheumatoid arthritis and osteoarthritis; and as analgesic for dysmenorrhea, postextraction dental pain, postoperative pain, and musculoskeletal pain. *Unlabeled Use:* gout, juvenile rheumatoid arthritis.

ABSORPTION AND FATE. Rapidly absorbed. Peak plasma levels occur in 1 to 2 hours and decline to about one-half peak level in 4 hours. Approximately 90 to 99% bound to plasma proteins; plasma half-life: 2 to 4 hours. Metabolized by oxidation to inactive metabolites. Excretion almost complete within 24 hours after last dose. About 50 to 60% excreted in urine as inactive metabolites and less than 10% as unchanged drug. Some biliary excretion occurs.

CONTRAINDICATIONS AND PRECAUTIONS. History of hypersensitivity to ibuprofen; patients with syndrome of nasal polyps, rhinitis, and asthma associated with aspirin (aspirin triad) or other nonsteroidal antiinflammatory drugs; active peptic ulcer; children 14 years of age or younger; pregnancy, nursing mothers. *Cautious Use:* history of GI ulceration, impaired hepatic or renal function, cardiac decompensation, patients with SLE.

ADVERSE/SIDE EFFECTS. CNS: headache, dizziness, nystagmus, lightheadedness, tinnitus, deafness (rare), fatigue, malaise, drowsiness, anxiety, confusion, depression. **Dermatologic:** maculopapular and vesicobullous skin eruptions, erythema multiforme, pruritus, rectal itching, acne. **GI (most common):** dyspepsia, heartburn, nausea, vomiting, anorexia, diarrhea, constipation, bloating, flatulence, stomatitis, epigastric or abdominal pain, GI ulceration, bleeding. **Hematologic:** leukopenia; decreased hemoglobin and hematocrit; transitory rise in SGOT, SGPT, serum alkaline phosphatase; rise in (Ivy) bleeding time. **Ophthalmic:** toxic amblyopia (rare), blurred vision, visual-field defects. **Other:** sore throat, epistaxis, flushing, fluid retention with edema, Stevens-Johnson syndrome, toxic hepatitis, nephrotoxicity, aseptic meningitis.

ROUTE AND DOSAGE. Oral: *Rheumatoid arthritis:* 300 to 600 mg three or four times a day. *Mild to moderate pain:* 200 to 400 mg every 4 to 6 hours, as necessary. *Primary dysmenorrhea:* 400 mg every 4 hours, as necessary. Total daily dosage not to exceed 2400 mg. Highly individualized.

NURSING IMPLICATIONS

Absorption rate is slower and drug plasma level is reduced when ibuprofen is administered with food; therefore it is usually given on an empty stomach, e.g., 1 hour before or 2 hours after meals.

Tablet may be crushed if patient is unable to swallow it whole and mixed with food or liquid before swallowing.

If GI intolerance occurs, physician may prescribe administration of drug with food or milk or may decrease dosage.

It is important to take a detailed drug history prior to initiation of therapy. *See Contraindications and Precautions.*

Patients with history of cardiac decompensation should be observed closely for evidence of fluid retention and edema.

Baseline and periodic evaluations of hemoglobin, renal, and hepatic function, and auditory and ophthalmic examinations are recommended in patients receiving prolonged or high dose therapy.

Side effects appear to be dose-related. Physician will rely on accurate observation and reporting to estimate lowest effective dosage level.

Inform patients about possible CNS effects (lightheadedness, dizziness, drowsiness), and caution them to avoid dangerous activities until their reactions to the drug have been determined.

Patients should be advised to report immediately to physician the onset of GI disturbances, skin rash, blurred vision or other eye symptoms.

Patients who experience any visual disturbances should have ophthalmoscopic evaluation, including examination of visual fields.

Optimum therapeutic response generally occurs within 2 weeks (e.g., relief of pain, stiffness, or swelling or improved joint flexion and strength). When satisfactory response occurs, dosage should be reviewed by physician and adjusted as required.

If patient is self-medicating with ibuprofen, advise discontinuing drug and consulting physician if pain persists beyond 10 days or fever persists more than 3 days, or if joint swelling develops or if pain and fever worsen.

Advise patient not to self-medicate with ibuprofen if taking prescribed drugs, without physician approval.

Inform patient that alcohol and aspirin may increase risk of GI ulceration and bleeding tendencies and therefore should be avoided, unless otherwise advised by physician.

Since ibuprofen may prolong bleeding time, advise patient to inform dentist or surgeon that he or she is taking drug.

Store preferably between 15° and 30°C (59° and 86°F) in well-closed, light-resistant container unless otherwise directed by manufacturer.

Drug Interactions. Ulcerogenic effect may be potentiated by concomitant administration of ibuprofen and **indomethacin, phenylbutazone,** or **salicylates.** There is also the possibility (based on animal studies) that **aspirin** may cause lower blood levels and decrease the antiinflammatory activity of ibuprofen. Although ibuprofen has not been shown to enhance the hypoprothrombinemic effects of **oral anticoagulants,** cautious use is advised if they are given concurrently, since ibuprofen inhibits platelet aggregation.

IDOXURIDINE (IDU)

(Dendrid, Herplex, Herplex Liquifilm, IDU, Stoxil)

(eye-dox-yoor′i-deen)
Antiinfective
Antiviral

ACTIONS AND USES. Topical antiviral agent. Pyrimidine nucleoside structurally related to thymidine, a metabolite essential for synthesis of DNA. Antiviral activity is primarily due to a substitution process. During viral replication, idoxuridine complexes with viral DNA by substituting for thymidine. The DNA–drug complex is more susceptible to breakage than normal DNA, resulting in increased number of errors in protein formation and inhibition of viral replication. Idoxuridine (IDU) is also incorporated into host DNA; large IV doses of the drug may adversely affect rapidly dividing host cells, e.g., in GI tract, bone marrow, and epidermal cells. Inhibits growth of herpes simplex types I and II, varicella–zoster, vaccinia, cytomegalovirus, and small animal viruses containing DNA. Not effective against RNA viruses. Epithelial viral infections characterized by a dendritic figure respond well to the antiviral activity especially during initial attacks. Chronic or recurrent viral infections that involve deep stromal structures (e.g., herpetic iritis) respond less well and do not heal. Idoxuridine has no effect on accumulated scarring, vascularization, or consequent progressive loss of vision. Some resistant strains of herpes simplex have been reported. Potentially carcinogenic. Squamous cell carcinoma at site of topical treatment has been reported.

Used in treatment of herpes simplex keratitis as single agent or conjunctively with a corticosteroid. *Investigational Use:* to treat cutaneous herpes simplex.

ABSORPTION AND FATE. Poorly absorbed following instillation into eyes. Tissue uptake of drug (a function of cellular metabolism) is reportedly less with increasing drug concentrations, higher concentrations. Slowly degraded when instilled in eye permitting long enough contact with eye surface for antiviral action. Following IV administration, metabolized to iodouracil and iodine in liver and excreted in urine. Crosses placental barrier.

CONTRAINDICATIONS AND PRECAUTIONS. Hypersensitivity to idoxuridine, iodine or iodine containing preparations, or to any components in the formulation. *Cautious Use:* women of childbearing potential, during pregnancy and lactation; corticosteroids.

ADVERSE/SIDE EFFECTS. Local: (occasionally) local irritation, pain, burning, lacrimation, pruritus, inflammation, or edema of eyes, lids, and surrounding face; follicular conjunctivitis, photophobia; local allergic reaction (rare); corneal clouding, stippling, and small punctate defects; corneal ulceration and swelling; delayed healing. **Systemic absorption:** stomatitis, anorexia, nausea, vomiting, alopecia, leukopenia, thrombocytopenia, iodism, hepatotoxicity. **Overdosage (local):** small defects in corneal epithelium.

ROUTE AND DOSAGE. Topical: *Ophthalmic solution 0.1%:* Initial: 1 drop instilled in conjunctival sac of each infected eye every hour during the day and every 2 hours at night until improvement occurs. Dosage may then be reduced to 1 drop every 2 hours during the day and every 4 hours at night. *Ophthalmic ointment 0.5%:* 5 instillations daily into conjunctival sac of infected eye; given approximately every 4 hours, with last dose at bedtime.

NURSING IMPLICATIONS

Boric acid should not be used during therapy with idoxuridine, since irritation may occur.

To prevent the possibility of systemic absorption, apply light finger pressure to head of lacrimal duct for 1 minute when eyedrop is instilled. *See Index: Drug administration: eye drops.*

If photosensitivity is troublesome, advise patient to wear sunglasses.

Idoxuridine should not be mixed with other medications.

The recommended frequency and duration of therapy must not be exceeded.

Patients should be closely supervised by ophthalmologist.

To prevent recurrence, instillations are usually continued for at least 3 to 5 days after corneal healing appears complete, as demonstrated by loss of staining with fluorescein.

Epithelial infections usually improve within 7 or 8 days. If patient continues to improve, therapy is generally continued up to 21 days. If no improvement is noted after 7 or 8 days, physician may institute another form of therapy. In some cases, physician may continue therapy using fresh solution.

Topical corticosteroids may be used with idoxuridine for herpes simplex with stromal lesions, corneal edema or iritis. Idoxuridine therapy should continue a few days after the steroid is discontinued.

Do not mix idoxuridine with any other drug. Antibiotics and atropine may be given concurrently if necessary.

Follow manufacturers directions regarding storage. Decomposed idoxuridine not only has reduced antiviral activity but also may be toxic.

Store at controlled room temperature.

PROTOTYPE

IMIPRAMINE HYDROCHLORIDE

(im-ip′ra-meen)

(Impril, Janimine, Novopramine, SK-Pramine, Tipramine, Tofranil)

IMIPRAMINE PAMOATE

(Tofranil-PM)

Psychotropic
Antidepressant
Antineuritic
Tricyclic

ACTIONS AND USES. Dibenzazepine derivative and tertiary amine. Tricyclic antidepressant (TCA), structurally related to the phenothiazines. In contrast to phenothiazines which act on dopamine receptors, TCAs block reuptake of serotonin and norepinephrine by presynaptic neurones in CNS. Resulting increase in concentration in synaptic cleft enhances activity at receptor site, thought to be the basis for antidepressant effects. Imipramine appears to be a more active inhibitor of norepinephrine than serotonin reuptake. Exhibits anticholinergic, antihistaminic, hypotensive, sedative and mild peripheral vasodilator effects. Decreases number of awakenings from sleep, markedly reduces time in REM sleep, and increases stage 4 sleep. Prolongs myocardial repolarization time and may produce quinidinelike conduction abnormalities (arrhythmias, heart block, bundle branch block). Relief of nocturnal enuresis perhaps due to nervous system stimulation resulting in earlier arousal to sensation of full bladder.

Used in endogenous depression; occasionally used for reactive depression. Less effective in presence of organic brain damage or schizophrenia. *Investigational Use:* in certain syndromes that mimic depression or overlap diagnostically with depression: alcoholism, phobic-anxiety syndromes, obsessive-compulsive neurosis, chronic pain. Imipramine is the only TCA used for temporary adjuvant treatment of enuresis in children over 6 years old.

ABSORPTION AND FATE. Well absorbed from GI tract and highly bound to plasma proteins; wide distribution, including CNS. Hepatic metabolism with possible enterohepatic cycling. Principle active metabolite: desipramine. Plasma half-life: 6 to 20 hours; wide interpatient plasma level variation due to differences in first-pass (hepatic) metabolism, perhaps a genetic effect. (In general, the elderly metabolize TCAs more slowly than young adults.) Excreted primarily as inactive metabolite in urine; small amount in feces. Crosses placental barrier and may be secreted in breast milk.

CONTRAINDICATIONS AND PRECAUTIONS. Sensitivity to other dibenzazepines; acute recovery period following myocardial infarction; severe renal or hepatic impairment; use of hydrochloride in children under 12 except to treat enuresis; use of pamoate in children of any age; concomitant use of MAO inhibitors; pregnancy (category C) lactation (may be teratogenic). *Cautious Use:* children, adolescents; elderly especially with cardiac disorder; respiratory difficulties, cardiovascular, hepatic or GI diseases; increased intraocular pressure, narrow angle glaucoma, schizophrenia, hypomania or manic episodes, patient with suicide tendency, seizure disorders; prostatic hypertrophy, urinary retention, alcoholism, hyperthyroidism, concomitant use of thyroid medication, electroshock therapy.

ADVERSE/SIDE EFFECTS. Allergic: skin rash, petechiae, urticaria, pruritus, photosensitivity, edema (face, tongue, generalized); drug fever. **Anticholinergic:** xerostomia, blurred vision, disturbance of accommodation, mydriasis, constipation, paralytic ileus, urinary retention, delayed micturition. **CV:** orthostatic hypotension, hypertension or hypotension, palpitation, myocardial infarction, congestive heart failure, arrhythmias, heart block, cardiotoxicity, ECG changes, stroke, shock. **Endocrinologic:** testicular swelling, gynecomastia (males), galactorrhea and breast enlargement (females), increased or decreased libido, ejaculatory and erectile disturbances, delayed orgasm (male and female); elevation or depression of blood glucose levels. **GI:** nausea, vomiting, diarrhea, slowed gastric emptying time, flatulence, abdominal cramps, esophageal reflux, anorexia, stomatitis, increased salivation, black tongue, peculiar taste. **Hematologic:** bone marrow depression: agranulocytosis, eosinophilia, purpura, thrombocytopenia. **Most common:** orthostatic hypotension, tachycardia, arrhythmias, blurred vision, constipation, xerostomia, impaired micturition. **Neurologic:** dizziness, tinnitus; numbness, tingling and paresthesias of extremities; incoordination, ataxia, tremors, peripheral neuropathy, extrapyramidal symptoms, lowered seizure threshold, altered EEG patterns, delirium. **Psychiatric:** disturbed concentration, confusion, hallucinations, anxiety, restlessness, agitation, insomnia, nightmares; shift to hypomania, mania; exacerbation of psychoses. **Other:** cholestatic jaundice, precipitated acute intermittent porphyria, nasal congestion, excessive perspiration, flushing, paradoxic urinary frequency, nocturia, drowsiness, fatigue, weakness, headache, proneness to falling, alopecia, excessive appetite, changes in heat and cold tolerance.

ROUTE AND DOSAGE. Oral: Adult: *Endogenous depression* **(hospitalized patient):** 50 mg 2 times daily; gradually increased to 200 mg daily as required; if no response after 2 weeks, increased gradually to 250 to 300 mg/day. **(Outpatients):** Initial: 75 mg/day, gradually increased to 150 mg/day, as required; maximum dose 200 mg/day. **Adolescent, elderly:** Initial: 30 to 40 mg/day; rarely exceeds 100 mg/day. Maintenance: 50 to 150 mg/day. *Enuresis* (hydrochloride only): **Oral:** Initial: 25 mg/day 1 hour before bedtime. If response is unsatisfactory within 1 week, dose is increased to 50 mg nightly in children under 12 years; children 12 years and older may receive up to 75 mg nightly. Dose limit for children: 2.5 mg/kg/day. **Intramuscular: Adults** (Used only for starting therapy in patients unable or unwilling to use oral medication): Initial: 100 mg/day in divided doses.

NURSING IMPLICATIONS

Before treatment starts, patient should have a complete assessment of physical pathology with special attention to GI and cardiac status (including ECG), eyes, and hematology.

Administer drug with or immediately after food to reduce gastric irritation.

Administer single daily dose at bedtime if dizziness and drowsiness are bothersome and dangerous during the day. If insomnia and stimulation are problems, administer drug in the AM.

Crystals may form in some ampuls of injectable imipramine. To dissolve, immerse intact ampul in warm water for about 1 minute.

Dose sensitivity and side effects are most likely to occur in adolescents and the elderly. A lower initial dose should be used for these patients.

Supervise drug ingestion. Be sure patient does not "cheek" the dose. When patient is discharged from medical management, instruct patient and family members not to double or skip doses, change dose interval, or combine dose with another nonprescribed drug.

To minimize possibility of suicide attempt, only a small amount of drug should be dispensed to patient at a time.

I J

Risk of suicide is particularly great when patient nears the end of a depressive cycle. Be alert to sudden improvement in mood and behavior, which may signify patient has finally come to an "acceptable" solution: to commit suicide.

Accurate early reporting to physician about patient's response to drug therapy is essential to prevent serious adverse effects, and to the design of an individualized therapeutic regimen.

Signs of therapeutic effectiveness of tricyclic antidepressants (TCAs): renewed interest in surroundings and personal appearance, mood elevation, increased physical activity and energy, improved appetite and sleep patterns, reduction in morbid preoccupations.

A trial of therapy with adequate dose is not judged a failure for at least a month: with no improvement, drug is discontinued. With apparent improvement, maintenance dosage can be instituted. Therapeutic plasma level: 150 to 300 mg/ml.

Some patients on TCA therapy experience complete recovery within 4 to 6 weeks; others may require drug therapy several years, or for life.

Because of long serum half-life, dose adjustments are not made more frequently than every 4 days.

Advise patient not to use OTC drugs while on a TCA, without physician's approval. Many preparations contain sympathomimetic amines and concomitant administration with imipramine could precipitate hypertensive crisis.

The actions of both alcohol and imipramine are potentiated when used together during therapy and for up to 2 weeks after TCA is discontinued. Consult physician about safe amount of alcohol, if any, that can be taken.

If a patient uses excessive amounts of alcohol it should be borne in mind that the potentiation of TCA effects may increase the danger of overdosage or suicide attempt.

Smoking–Drug Interaction: Imipramine metabolism may be increased by smoking, thus changing dose requirements.

Elderly patients are apt to develop "confusional reaction" (restlessness, disturbed sleep, forgetfulness) during first 2 weeks of therapy. Symptoms last 3 to 20 days. Report to physician.

Warn patient to avoid hazardous tasks such as driving a motor vehicle or operating machinery until drug response is known.

Exposure to strong sunlight should be avoided because of potential photosensitivity. Advise use of sun screen lotion (SPF 12 to 15), if allowed. Remind patient that ultraviolet radiation is present even on dark days and that danger from sun is less when it is closest to horizon (before 10 AM and after 1 PM).

Report promptly early signs of agranulocytosis (fever, malaise, sore throat). Need to stop drug and appropriate treatment will depend upon evaluation of WBC and differential.

Report signs of cholestatic jaundice: flulike symptoms (general malaise, nausea, vomiting, fever, upper abdominal pain), yellow skin or sclerae, dark urine, light-colored stools, pruritus.

Observe patient with history of glaucoma. The onset of a severe headache, halos of light, dilated pupils, eye pain, nausea, vomiting, may signal acute attack. Notify physician.

TCAs may cause grand mal seizures in susceptible patients e.g., those with seizure disorders, organic brain disease, alcoholism, barbiturate withdrawal, and those receiving high doses of TCA.

Monitor blood pressure, and pulse rate for tachycardia and other arrhythmias. Withhold drug if systolic BP falls more than 20 mm Hg or if there is a sudden increase in pulse rate, and notify physician.

If patient has cardiovascular disease or its history, cardiac surveillance by ECG is necessary during period of dose adjustment and periodically during maintenance treatment.

Orthostatic hypotension tends to be mild in normotensive individuals, but may be marked in pretreatment hypertensive or cardiac patients.

Instruct patient to change position slowly and in stages especially from recumbency to upright posture; dangle legs over bed for a few minutes before ambulation. Caution against standing still for prolonged periods, taking hot showers or baths, or exposure for prolonged periods to the sun.

Sitting with legs elevated and wearing support hose or socks may prevent orthostatic hypotension. Consult physician.

Extrapyramidal symptoms (tremors, twitching, ataxia, incoordination, hyperreflexia, drooling) may occur in patients receiving large doses and especially in the elderly. Fine tremors may be alleviated by small doses of propranolol. The physician may change dosage, or drug.

Promptly report appearance of psychogenic reactions: transition from depression to hypomania or mania, hallucinations, delusion (especially apt to occur in patients with organic brain damage or history of psychosis). TCA therapy will be discontinued.

Monitor intake–output ratio and bowel elimination, at least until maintenance dosage is stabilized, to detect urinary retention or frequency, constipation or paralytic ileus. Palpate for bladder distention and auscultate for peristalsis as indicated. Notify physician if patient is unable to void. A cholinergic drug may be ordered.

Note depressed patient's interest in food and fluids. Some patients may require increases in bulk foods (such as whole grain cereals) or fluids and a laxative to overcome drug-induced constipation.

Drug-induced *xerostomia* is frequently an anticholinergic overlay of a chronically dry mouth in the depressed person.

Xerostomic condition is characterized by sore mouth, crusting of oral mucosa, repeated clicking of tongue as patient attempts to lubricate the mouth, pebbly tongue surface (leads to decreased taste perception). Alert physician.

Frequently inspect oral mucosa, especially gingival surfaces under dentures. Dry mouth promotes tissue erosion and shrinkage, leading to poor adhesion of dentures to bony ridges.

Discomfort from oral dryness interferes with speech, mastication, and swallowing and is a potential dental hazard: deprivation of normal saliva favors demineralization of tooth surfaces.

Relief of xerostomia may result from (1) frequent warm clear water rinses, (2) use of a saliva substitute (such as Xero-Lube, Moi-stir) which when sprayed onto oral surfaces provides lubrication effect for 1 to 3 hours; (3) avoidance of hard, rough food, (4) increased noncaloric fluid intake.

If salivary flow responds to stimulation, relief may be provided by chewing sugarless gum. Dip gum in a droplet of cooking oil to reduce force of mastication and to make gum very slippery.

Urge patient to floss teeth daily with waxed floss and to brush gently with a small soft tooth brush after eating. A fluoride tooth paste helps to restore mineralization of tooth surface.

Persistence of xerostomia may cause reduction in food and liquid intake and is a known factor in noncompliance. It should be brought under control before patient is discharged. A consult with a dentist may be indicated.

Weigh patients under standard conditions at least biweekly. A gain of 1½ to 2 pounds within 2 to 3 days and frank edema should be reported.

Tricyclic therapy should be discontinued as long as possible before elective surgery because of possibility of a hypertensive episode.

If patient is on electroshock therapy, question whether to administer doses of TCA.

Hyperglycemia or hypoglycemia may occur in some patients. Diabetic patients should be monitored, particularly during early therapy.

TCA may cause a change in tolerance to heat and cold. Regulate environmental temperature, personal clothing, and bed-covers accordingly. Protect patient from inadvertent contact with uncontrolled hot objects (e.g., radiators, heating pads).

The severely depressed patient may need assistance with personal hygiene because of excessive sweating produced by the drug.

Overdosage onset may be sudden and is manifested by anticholinergic, extrapyramidal, and cardiac symptoms. Physostigmine salicylate by slow IV reverses TCA effects. (There is no specific antidote.) Additionally, aggressive supportive therapy includes: gastric lavage, active charcoal slurry, anticonvulsant, cardiac monitor, resuscitation equipment. Keep patient in quiet darkened environment. Observe closely for at least 72 hours and monitor by ECG for at least 5 days. Relapse may occur after apparent recovery.

Coma in the patient with an overdose of TCA has accompanying symptoms of warm skin, dilated pupils, and tachycardia ("atropine syndrome"). Hypertension and hypereflexia may also be present.

Drug withdrawal should be gradual. Abrupt termination of therapy, especially in patients receiving high doses for 2 months or more may result in nausea, headache, vertigo, malaise, insomnia, nightmares.

Tofranil and Janimine contain *tartrazine* which can cause allergic reactions (including bronchial asthma) in susceptible individuals. Frequently such persons are also sensitive to aspirin.

Education of patient/family in collaboration with physician from start of therapy may help to promote patient compliance.

Enuresis Patient-Teaching Points: (Imipramine is the only TCA used for enuresis)

- ✓ Early evening bedwetters are usually given 25 mg in midafternoon and a repeat dose at bedtime.
- ✓ With adequate dosage, positive results generally occur in 1 to 2 weeks. Maintenance dosage is continued until the child is dry every night for 3 months.
- ✓ A drug-free period following adequate response to drug therapy is sometimes instituted. When imipramine is to be withdrawn dosage is tapered to reduce possibility of relapse.
- ✓ Children who relapse when drug is withheld do not always respond to restart of therapy. In some patients, effectiveness decreases with continued drug administration. Counsel parent to inform physician if this occurs.

✓ Most frequent side effects in children: fatigue, nervousness, sleep disorders, mild GI symptoms. Others include: constipation, convulsions, emotional instability, syncope, collapse. Parent should report these symptoms; termination of therapy may be indicated.
✓ Enuresis is generally associated with an emotional component, such as guilt feelings and anxiety, even when it is not primarily psychogenic in origin; ample time should be given to parent and child to discuss problems of management.

Summary of Patient-Teaching Points Pertinent to Therapy with an Antidepressant:
✓ Stress biochemical theory of endogenous depression.
✓ Permanent remission occurs in most cases (75 to 80%).
✓ Symptom relief may require as long as 21 days.
✓ Side effects may occur that have to be "lived with"; tolerance develops however to most of them, or there are medications that help to reduce discomfort. Keep physician informed.
✓ Maintain dosage schedule until advised otherwise by physician.
✓ Keep follow-up appointments throughout maintenance therapy.
✓ Advise significant others to encourage physical and diversional activities. Do not let patient "vegetate."

Counsel parent regarding the proper use and physical security of imipramine. Poisoning in children is an emerging public health problem. A dose as low as 15 mg/kg can be lethal.

Store oral and parenteral solution at temperature between 15° and 30°C (59° and 86°F) unless advised differently by manufacturer.

Diagnostic Test Interferences. Imipramine elevates **serum bilirubin, alkaline phosphatase** and may elevate **blood glucose.** It decreases **urinary 5-HIAA** and **VMA** excretion and may falsely increase excretion of **urinary catecholamines.**

Drug Interactions: Imipramine: Tricyclic antidepressants (TCAs)

Plus	Interactions
Acetazolamide (Diamox)	Increased TCA effects
Alcohol (Ethanol)	Mutual potentiation of effects
Ammonium chloride	Decreased TCA effects
Amphetamines	Enhanced amphetamine effects
Anticholinergics	Mutual potentiation of atropine-like effects
Anticoagulant, oral	Increased hypoprothrombinemia
Anticonvulsants	Anticonvulsant effect may be reduced by TCA
Antihistamines	Additive anticholinergic effects of TCA
Ascorbic acid	Decreased TCA effects
Barbiturates	Potentiated adverse effects of toxic dose of TCA; decreased TCA serum levels and thus TCA effectiveness. Potentiated action of barbiturates
Beta-adrenergic blockers	Actions antagonized by TCA
Chlordiazepoxide (Librium)	Additive sedative effect of TCA
Clonidine (Catapres)	Decreased antihypertensive effect of clonidine
Diazepam (Valium)	Additive atropinelike and sedative effects of TCA
Epinephrine (Adrenalin)	Increased pressor response to epinephrine
Ethychlorvynol (Placidyl)	Transient delirium
Fenfluramine (Pondimine)	Potentiates sedative action of TCA
Furazolidone (Furoxone)	Toxic psychosis with concomitant administration
Glutethimide	Additive anticholinergic effects of TCA

Plus (cont.)	Interactions (cont.)
Guanethidine (Ismelin)	Decreased antihypertensive effect of guanethidine
MAO inhibitors	Hyperpyretic crises, convulsions, hypertensive episodes, death
Methyldopa (Aldomet)	Blocked hypotensive effect of methyldopa
Methylphenidate (Ritalin)	Enhanced effect of TCA
Narcotic analgesics	Increased narcotic-induced respiratory depression
Norepinephrine (Levarterenol, Levophed)	Increased pressor response to levarterenol
Oral contraceptives	May inhibit TCA effects
Oxazepam (Serax)	Additive sedation and atropinelike side effects
Phenothiazines	Additive effects of TCA
Phenylbutazone (Oxalid, Tandearil)	Desipramine inhibits GI absorption of phenylbutazone
Phenylephrine	Increased pressor response to phenylephrine
Phenytoin (Dilantin) Procainamide (Procan, Pronestyl)	Possibility of decreased phenytoin seizure control
Quinidine	Potentiated cardiovascular effects of TCA
Reserpine	Decreases hypotensive action of reserpine; reserpine may exert stimulating effect in depressed patient
Sodium bicarbonate	Increased TCA effects
Sympathomimetics	Increased hypertensive and cardiac arrhythmic effects of sympathomimetics
Thyroid preparations	Mutually potentiating effects
Vasodilators	Additive hypotensive effect of TCA

IMMUNE GLOBULIN (INTRAMUSCULAR)

(Gamma Globulin, Gamastan, Gammar, IG, Immuglobin, Immune Serum Globulin, ISG, IGIM)

IMMUNE GLOBULIN (INTRAVENOUS)

(Gamimune, IGIV, Sandoglobulin)

Serum
Immunizing agent

ACTIONS AND USES. Sterile concentrated solution containing globulin (primarily IgG) prepared from large pools of normal human plasma of either venous or placental origin, and processed by a special fractionating technique. Like hepatitis B immune globulin (HBIG), contains antibody specific to hepatitis B surface antigen but in lower concentrations. Therefore, not considered treatment of first choice for postexposure prophylaxis against hepatitis B but usually an acceptable alternative when HBIG is not available. Also much less expensive than HBIG. Nonreactive when tested for hepatitis B.

The IM preparation is used in susceptible persons to provide passive immunity or to modify severity of certain infectious diseases, e.g., rubeola (measles), rubella (German measles), varicella-zoster (chickenpox), type A (infectious) hepatitis, and as replacement therapy in congenital agammaglobulinemia or other immunoglobin (IgG) deficiency diseases. May be used as an alternative to hepatitis B immune globulin (HBIG) to provide passive immunity in hepatitis B infection (serum hepatitis). Also has been used for postexposure prophylaxis of hepatitis non-A, non-B and nonspecific hepatitis. Immune globulin IV is used principally as maintenance therapy in patients unable to manufacture sufficient quantities of IgG antibodies, in patients requiring an immediate increase in immunoglobulin levels, and when

IM injections are contraindicated as in patients with bleeding disorders or who have small muscle mass. The IV preparation has been used also in treatment of chronic autoimmune thrombocytopenia or neutropenia, and idiopathic thrombocytopenic purpura (ITP).

ABSORPTION AND FATE. Following administration of IM preparation, serum levels of IgG peak within 2 days. Rapidly and evenly distributed to intravascular and extravascular fluid compartments. Half-life: about 23 days. Following administration of IV preparation, serum concentrations of IgG rise immediately. Half-life: 21 days, however interindividual variations reported.

CONTRAINDICATIONS AND PRECAUTIONS. History of anaphylaxis or severe reaction to immune globulin (IG) or to any ingredient in the formulation such as thimerosal (mercury derivative) preservative in IM formulations, and maltose (stabilizing agent) in IV formulations; persons with clinical hepatitis A. Use of IGIV for patients with class-specific anti-IgA deficiencies; use of IGIM in severe thrombocytopenia or other bleeding disorders. Safe use during pregnancy not established.

ADVERSE/SIDE EFFECTS. IGIM: pain, tenderness, muscle stiffness of IM site; local inflammatory reaction, erythema, urticaria, angioedema, headache, malaise, fever, arthralgia, nephrotic syndrome, hypersensitivity (fever, chills, anaphylactic shock). **IGIV (mostly related to rate of administration):** nausea, flushing, chills, headache, chest tightness, wheezing, skeletal pain, back pain, abdominal cramps, anaphylaxis.

I J

ROUTE AND DOSAGE. Intramuscular *(IGIM only):* **Adults and children:** Type A (infectious) hepatitis exposure: 0.02 ml/kg as single dose before or soon after exposure. When period of exposure is 3 months or more: 0.05 to 0.06 ml/kg once every 4 to 5 months. *Hepatitis B:* 0.06 ml/kg preferably within 7 days after exposure; repeat 25 to 30 days after exposure. *Measles:* 0.25 ml/kg within 6 days after exposure. *German measles:* 20 ml in susceptible women. *Varicella-Zoster:* 0.6 to 1.2 ml/kg promptly. *Immunoglobulin deficiency:* Initial: 1.3 ml/kg IM followed in 2 to 4 weeks by 0.66 ml/kg given every 2 to 4 weeks; or IV infusion (IGIV only) of 100 mg/kg monthly; if clinical response is not adequate increased to 200 mg/kg or usual dose given more frequently than monthly.

NURSING IMPLICATIONS

Note that immune globulin IM (IGIM) is intended only for IM use. Immune globulin IV (IGIV) is meant only for IV use. They are not interchangeable.

For adults and older children, IM injections are made preferably into deltoid or anterolateral aspect of thigh; in neonates and small children into anterolateral aspect of thigh.

Gluteal injections are generally avoided because of risk of injury to sciatic nerve. However, when large volumes of immune globulin are prescribed or when large doses must be divided into several injections, the upper outer quadrant of the gluteus may be used in adults.

Aspirate carefully after introducing needle into muscle to avoid inadvertent injection into blood vessel. If blood is seen, withdraw needle, and discard needle and syringe. Prepare another dose using a new syringe and needle, and select a different site.

Bear in mind that some viral diseases may only be attenuated by immune globulin and therefore remain infectious (e.g., if it is given later than recommended after exposure).

Hepatitis A (infectious hepatitis): Immune globulin is most effective when given before or as soon as possible after exposure, but not more than 2 weeks after (incubation period for hepatitis A is 15 to 50 days). Persons who are already presenting clinical manifestations of hepatitis A should not receive immune globulin.

Hepatitis B (serum hepatitis): Immune globulin is administered preferably within 24 hours and not less than 7 days after exposure. *See Hepatitis B Immune Globulin, Nursing Implications, for management of patients with hepatitis B.*

Measles (rubeola): Following immune globulin administration, passive immunity lasts about 3 to 4 weeks. In general, patients who are at least 15 months of age should receive measles virus vaccine 3 months after having immune globulin.

Immunodeficiency diseases: To prevent serious infections, serum concentrations of immune globulin are commonly kept above 200 mg/dl.

Epinephrine, other emergency drugs, and appropriate facilities should be immediately available for treatment of anaphylaxis or sensitization.

Hypersensitivity reactions are most likely to occur in patients receiving large IM doses, repeated injections, or rapid IV infusion of immune globulin.

When patient is receiving immune globulin IV (IGIV) monitor vital signs continuously and keep close watch over infusion rate.

Infusion flow rate should be prescribed by physician. For example, IGIV is generally started at 0.01 to 0.02 ml/kg/minute for 30 minutes; if tolerated, rate is increased to 0.02 to 0.04 ml/kg/minute.

Refer to manufacturer's directions for information on reconstitution, dilution, and flow rates.

Immune globulin IV may have a mild diuretic effect on some patients due to the presence of maltose in the formulation.

Store preferably at 2° to 8°C (36° to 46°F), unless otherwise directed by manufacturer. Avoid freezing. Do not use if turbidity has occurred or if product has been frozen. Do not mix with other drugs. Discard partially used vial.

I J

Drug Interactions: Immune globulin

Plus	Interactions
Live virus vaccine (e.g., for measles, mumps, poliovirus, rubella)	Antibodies in immune globulin may interfere with patient's response to live virus vaccines; these vaccines should not be administered within 3 months of immune globulin

---

Rh_o(D) IMMUNE GLOBULIN

(Gamulin Rh, HypRho-D, Rhesonativ, RhoGAM, Win Rho)

Serum
Immunizing agent

Rh_{uo}(D) IMMUNE GLOBULIN MICRO-DOSE

(MICRhoGAM, Mini-Gamulin Rh)

ACTIONS AND USES. Sterile nonpyrogenic gamma globulin solution containing immunoglobulins (IgG). Prepared from a human plasma or serum pool with high titer of anti-Rh_o(D) antibody (anti-Rh antibody) and confirmed nonreactivity for hepatitis B surface antigen (HBsAg). The solution is at least 90% IgG; thiomerosol (a mercury derivative) is the preservative. The globulin provides passive immunity by supressing active antibody response and formation of anti-Rh_o(D) (isoimmunization) in Rh-negative (Rh_o(D)-negative, D^u-negative) individuals previously exposed to Rh-positive (Rh_o(D)-positive, D^u-positive) blood. Such exposure occurs in Rh-negative women when Rh-positive fetal RBC enter maternal circulation: during third stage labor, fetal–maternal hemorrhage (as early as second trimester), amniocentesis, or other trauma during pregnancy, termination of pregnancy, and following transfusion with Rh-positive RBC, whole blood, or components (platelets, WBC) prepared from Rh-positive blood. Although the mechanism of action is unclear, it is hypothesized that anti-Rh antibody in the immune globulin solution binds to the Rh antigen on fetal RBC that have entered maternal circulation, thus suppressing a maternal primary immune response with its production of anti-Rh$_o$(D).

Used to prevent isoimmunization in Rh-negative individuals exposed to Rh-positive RBC (see above). Rh$_o$(D) Immune Globulin Micro-dose is for use only after spontaneous or induced abortion, or termination of ectopic pregnancy up to and including 12 weeks of gestation.

CONTRAINDICATIONS AND PRECAUTIONS. Rh$_o$(D)-positive or D^u-positive patient; person previously immunized against Rh$_o$(D) factor.

ADVERSE/SIDE EFFECTS. (Infrequent); injection site irritation, slight fever, myalgia, lethargy.

ROUTE AND DOSAGE. Intramuscular: *Antepartum prophylaxis:* One vial (300 mg) at approximately 28 weeks; followed by one vial within 72 hours of delivery if infant is Rh-positive. *Postpartum prophylaxis:* one vial within 72 hours of delivery. Suspected large *fetal–maternal hemorrhage:* dose based on estimated volume of Rh-positive RBC in maternal circulation (Kleihauer-Betke technique). Following *amniocentesis, miscarriage, abortion, ectopic pregnancy* (at or beyond 13th week of gestation): one vial (preferably within 3 hours, but may be given up to 72 hours after event). If products of conception are passed before 13th week: one vial micro-dose. *Transfusion accident:* (Rh-positive RBC to Rh-negative recipient): one vial protects against each 15 ml of transfused RBC.

I J

NURSING IMPLICATIONS

Before administration of Rh$_o$(D) immune globulin and immediately after delivery, send sample of newborn's cord blood to laboratory for cross-match and typing. Confirm that mother is Rh$_o$(D) and D^u-negative. Infant must be Rh-positive.

Lot numbers of drug used for the cross-match and the drug to be administered must be the same.

Rh$_o$(D) immune globulin is administered IM to the mother.

Use the deltoid muscle. Be sure that needle is not in a blood vessel. If blood is drawn back, withdraw needle and discard it and syringe, then administer a new dose into a different site with a new syringe and needle.

The IM may be given in divided doses at different sites, all at once or at intervals, as long as the entire dose is given within 72 hours after delivery or termination of pregnancy.

Each vial of Rh$_o$(D) immune globulin contains enough anti-Rh$_o$(D) to suppress the immunizing potential of 15 ml Rh-positive packed RBC. Each vial of micro-dose contains enough anti-Rh$_o$(D) to suppress the immune response to 2.5 ml of Rh-positive packed RBC.

All pregnant women should be tested for presence or absence of Rh$_o$(D) antigen on their RBCs. If there is doubt about the test, Rh$_o$(D) immune globulin should be given.

Rh antigens are inherited independently of all other blood group antigens. Many have been identified, but Rh$_o$(D) is the most antigenic and when present, the patient type is Rh-positive. Approximately 13% of white Americans lack Rh$_o$(D) completely and therefore are Rh-negative. Other racial differences in Rh antigen occurrence: about 1% of American Indians, Chinese, and other Asians are Rh-negative; about 7 to 10% American blacks are Rh-negative.

Ordinarily Rh antigens lack their corresponding antibodies in the serum; thus when antibodies appear, they result from sensitization caused by Rh stimulation following receipt of another person's RBCs, as from transfusion or in pregnancy (i.e., mother develops antibodies against fetal Rh antigen).

Administration of Rh$_o$(D) immune globulin (antibody) prevents hemolytic disease of the newborn in a subsequent pregnancy.

The infant born of a woman treated with Rh immune globulin antepartum, may have a weakly positive direct Coombs' test on cord and infant blood.

Passively acquired immunity may be detected in maternal serum if antibody screening tests are performed after ante- or postpartum administration of Rh immune globulin.

Store preferably at 2° to 8°C (36° to 46°F), unless otherwise directed by manufacturer. Avoid freezing.

INDAPAMIDE

(Lozol)

(in-dap'a-mide)
Antihypertensive
Diuretic
Sulfonamide derivative
Indoline

ACTIONS AND USES. First member of new class of antihypertensive/diuretic agents, the indolines. Has both diuretic and direct vascular effects; action mechanism is similar to that of the thiazide diuretics. Principal site of action is on the proximal portion of the distal renal tubules. Enhances excretion of Na, K and water by interfering with Na transfer across renal epithelium. Like the thiazides, indapamide increases Ca reabsorption without causing important changes in serum Ca concentration. Free water clearance during hydration is decreased. Hypotensive activity in the hypertensive patient appears to result from a decrease in plasma and extracellular fluid volume, decreased peripheral vascular resistance, direct arteriolar dilation, and calcium channel blockade. Has little effect on cardiac output, rate, or rhythm, and, unlike the thiazides, does not increase serum cholesterol. Augments the action of other hypotensive agents.

Used alone or with other antihypertensives as step 1 agent (stepped-care approach) in the management of hypertension in patients who have failed to respond to diet, exercise, or weight reduction. Also used in treatment of edema associated with congestive heart failure.

ABSORPTION AND FATE. Rapidly and completely absorbed from GI tract. Peak blood concentration of 230 to 260 ng/ml achieved 2 to 2½ hours after single 5-mg dose; 71 to 79% protein bound. Half-life: 14 to 18 hours; not prolonged by impaired renal function. Extensive hepatic metabolism with production of glucuronide and sulfate conjugates. About 60% of dose excreted in urine in 48 hours; only 7% of dose excreted unchanged. 16 to 23% excreted in feces via bile.

CONTRAINDICATION AND PRECAUTIONS. Hypersensitivity to indapamide or other sulfonamide derivatives, anuria. Safe use during pregnancy (category B), lactation, and in children not established. *Cautious Use:* electrolyte imbalance, severe renal disease, impaired hepatic function or progressive liver disease, hypokalemia, prediabetic and type II diabetic patient, hyperparathyroidism, thyroid disorders, SLE, sympathectomized patient, history of gout.

ADVERSE/SIDE EFFECTS. CV: orthostatic hypotension, PVCs, dysrhythmias, palpitation. **CNS/neuromuscular:** headache, dizziness, fatigue, weakness, loss of energy, muscle cramps or spasm, paresthesia, tension, anxiety, agitation, vertigo, insomnia, depression, blurred vision. **Dermatologic:** rash, hives, pruritus, vasculitis. **GI:** dry mouth, anorexia, nausea, vomiting, diarrhea, constipation, abdominal cramps or pain. **GU:** urinary frequency, nocturia, polyuria. **Other:** impotence or reduced libido, rhinorrhea, flushing, dilutional hyponatremia, hyperuricemia, hyperglycemia, hypochloremia, increased BUN or creatinine, glycosuria, weight loss, tingling of extremities. **Overdosage:** nausea, vomiting, weakness, electrolyte balance disturbance, hypotension, depressed respirations.

ROUTE AND DOSAGE. *Hypertension and edema of congestive heart disease:* **Oral:** 2.5 mg as a single daily dose. If response is inadequate after 1 (edema) to 4 (hypertension) weeks, daily dose is increased to 5.0 mg once daily. Doses of 5.0 mg or higher provide little additional therapeutic benefit in hypertension or edema, but do increase degree of hypokalemia.

NURSING IMPLICATIONS

Administer in morning to prevent nocturia. Urge patient to take at least 8 ounces of fluid (if allowed) with the medication.

Laboratory tests to monitor serum electrolytes should be evaluated periodically during treatment. Individuals at particular risk for electrolyte imbalance during indapamide therapy include: those receiving a digitalis preparation or on salt-restricted diet or low (voluntary or prescribed) dietary K intake or who have diseases subject to electrolyte disturbance (e.g., hepatic cirrhosis, ascites, renal disease). Also those with history of ventricular arrhythmias, patients receiving K-depleting drugs (corticosteroids, corticotropin) elderly patients who are especially sensitive to both diuretic action and the effects of K deficit.

Side effects of indapamide are mild and transient; however drug-induced potential or weak electrolyte imbalance may become clinically serious in the following situations: protracted vomiting and diarrhea, excessive sweating, GI drainage and parencentesis (lead to serious deficits in K, Cl causing hypochloremic alkalosis and contraction of extracellular fluid volume). Restoration of electrolyte and fluid volume may be indicated.

Fluid and salt intake are generally not altered during treatment with indapamide. However, the elderly patient is especially vulnerable to fluid volume changes. If diuresis has been brisk (characteristic of the response in an older person), be alert to sudden appearance of symptoms of hypovolemia (profound weakness, dizziness, perspiration, vomiting) and hypokalemia (dry mouth, nausea, vomiting, thirst, muscle cramps, confusion, paresthesias, abdominal distention, tachycardia, hypoactive reflexes).

Report promptly when signs of electrolyte imbalance are observed. K supplements or K-rich foods may be prescribed *(See Index: Food sources).*

An elderly patient may have a severe potassium deficit before it is diagnosed if the early symptoms of weakness, confusion, easy fatiguability are attributed to old age alone. Correlation of serum K levels with alerted observation is especially important in prevention of diuretic-induced hypokalemia in this age group.

Moderate hyperuricemia with exacerbation of gout symptoms (tender, reddened, painful joints) may be promoted by indapamide and should be reported. If dose adjustment does not reduce symptoms or serum uric acid level, probenecid or sulfinpyrazone may be prescribed, or drug may be discontinued.

Instruct patient to report promptly to the physician symptoms of developing renal impairment (urinary frequency, altered input–output ratio and pattern, painful urination, weight change, edema). Withholding or discontinuation of diuretic may be considered. Periodic renal function tests are indicated throughout therapy with indapamide.

Advise patient to report unexplained, progressive weight gain (e.g., 2 to 3 pounds in 2 to 3 days). Discuss salt and fluid intake parameters with physician and be certain these guidelines are fully understood by the patient.

Keep in mind that if the patient is receiving a cardiac glycoside, hypokalemia increases the risk of digitalis intoxication (cardiac arrhythmia).

If patient has hepatic dysfunction, even minor changes in fluid–electrolyte balance can precipitate hepatic coma. Instruct patient to report promptly the onset of symptoms suggestive of decreasing hepatic function (jaundice, dyspepsia, darkened urine, pruritus).

Routine examination for blood glucose level changes or for glycosuria should continue throughout indapamide treatment period. The drug may alter insulin requirements and cause borderline diabetes to manifest.

Since indapamide may cause hypercalcemia (and hypophosphatemia), it is withheld before tests for parathyroid function are performed.

Monitor elimination pattern since constipation may be a side effect. Advise patient to consult physician for a laxative if needed and not to self-dose with an OTC product. Discuss prevention of constipation with patient, e.g., adding more bulk to diet, increased exercise and fluid intake (if allowed).

A diuretic regimen may be sufficient therapy for reducing mild hypertension. Urge patient to keep scheduled appointments so that hypotensive response can be monitored. Lack of optimum clinical response may indicate changing the stepped-care regimen to step 2 (i.e., addition of an adrenergic drug).

Store drug in tightly closed, light-resistant container at controlled room temperature less than 40°C, preferably 15° to 30°C (59° to 86°F) unless otherwise directed by manufacturer.

Drug Interactions: Indapamide

Plus	Interactions
Antihypertensives, other	Potentiated hypotensive action
Alcohol, barbiturates, narcotic analgesics	Increased risk of orthostatic hypotension
Cardiac glycosides (e.g., digoxin)	Increased risk of digitalis toxicity (because of hypokalemic effect of indapamide)
Corticosteroids, corticotropin, amphotericin B	Enhanced hypokalemic effect of indapamide
Insulins, oral hypoglycemics (e.g., tolbutamide)	Increased hypoglycemic effect of antidiabetic agents
Lithium (Eskalith)	Decreased renal clearance of lithium; increased risk of lithium toxicity. Concomitant use should be avoided
Tubocurarine, other nondepolarizing skeletal muscle relaxants	Increased skeletal muscle relaxation
Vasopressors (e.g., norepinephrine)	Decreased responsiveness to vasopressor activity. Use of indapamide only with extreme caution

INDOMETHACIN

(Indocin, Novomethacin)

(in-doe-meth'a-sin)
NSAID

ACTIONS AND USES. Potent nonsteroid arylacetic acid compound with antiinflammatory, analgesic, and antipyretic effects similar to those of aspirin. Antipyretic and antiinflammatory actions may be related to ability to inhibit prostaglandin biosynthesis. Uncouples oxidative phosphorylation in cartilaginous and hepatic mitochondria. Appears to reduce motility of polymorphonuclear leukocytes, development of cellular exudates, and vascular permeability in injured tissue. Apparently has no uricosuric action. Inhibits platelet aggregation but effect is of shorter duration than that of aspirin (effect usually disappears within 24 hours after drug is discontinued). Enhances effect of ADH and therefore promotes sodium and water retention.

Used for palliative treatment in active stages of moderate to severe rheumatoid arthritis, ankylosing rheumatoid spondylitis, acute gouty arthritis, and osteoarthritis of hip in patients intolerant to or unresponsive to adequate trials with salicylates and other therapy. *Investigational Use:* to relieve biliary pain, dysmenorrhea, and to close patent ductus arteriosus in the premature infant.

ABSORPTION AND FATE. Promptly and almost completely absorbed from GI tract. Onset of action in 1 to 2 hours. Peak plasma levels within 3 hours following single oral dose; duration of action 4 to 6 hours. Approximately 90% bound to plasma protein, and also extensively bound in tissues; low concentrations in cerebrospinal fluid. Half-life: about 4½ hours. Largely metabolized in liver and kidneys. Excreted primarily in urine, mainly as glucuronide and about 10 to 20% as unchanged drug. Some elimination in bile and feces. Crosses placenta; appears in breast milk.

CONTRAINDICATIONS AND PRECAUTIONS. Allergy to indomethacin, aspirin, or other nonsteroidal antiinflammatory agents; nasal polyps associated with angioedema, history of GI lesions; pregnancy, nursing mothers, children (14 years of age or younger). *Cautious Use:* history of psychiatric illness, epilepsy, parkinsonism; impaired renal or hepatic function, controlled infections, coagulation defects, congestive heart failure, elderly patients, persons in hazardous occupations.

I J

ADVERSE/SIDE EFFECTS. **Altered laboratory findings:** Increased SGOT, SGPT, bilirubin, BUN; positive direct Coombs' test. **CV:** elevated BP, palpitation, chest pains, tachycardia. **CNS:** headache (common), dizziness, vertigo, lightheadedness, syncope, fatigue, muscle weakness, ataxia, insomnia, nightmares, drowsiness, narcolepsy, confusion, coma, convulsions, peripheral neuropathy, psychic disturbances (hallucinations, depersonalization, depression), aggravation of epilepsy, parkinsonism. **Eye and ear:** blurred vision, lacrimation, eye pain, visual field changes, corneal deposits, retinal disturbances including macula, tinnitus, hearing disturbances, deafness (rarely). **GI:** (common): nausea, vomiting, diarrhea, anorexia, bloating, abdominal distention, ulcerative stomatitis, proctitis, rectal bleeding, GI ulceration, hemorrhage, perforation. **Hematologic:** hemolytic anemia, aplastic anemia (sometimes fatal), agranulocytosis, leukopenia, thrombocytopenic purpura. **Hypersensitivity:** rash, purpura, pruritus, urticaria, angioedema, angiitis, rapid fall in blood pressure, dyspnea, asthma syndrome (in aspirin-sensitive patients). **Renal:** hematuria, urinary frequency, renal failure (causal relationships not established). **Other:** epistaxis, hair loss, exfoliative dermatitis, erythema nodosum, vaginal bleeding, breast changes, hyperglycemia and glycosuria (rare), toxic hepatitis, edema, weight gain, flushing, sweating.

ROUTE AND DOSAGE. **Oral:** *Rheumatoid arthritis:* 25 mg two or three times daily; if tolerated, may be increased by 25 mg at weekly intervals until satisfactory response is obtained or total daily dosage of 150 to 200 mg is reached. *Acute gouty arthritis:* 50 mg three times daily until pain is tolerable; then dose is rapidly reduced to complete termination of drug therapy. *Bursitis:* 75 to 150 mg daily in 3 or 4 divided doses as needed. **Sustained-release form:** 75 mg sustained-release capsule once daily is an alternate dosage form for 25 to 50 mg capsules 3 times daily. One 75 mg sustained-release capsule twice daily can be substituted (by prescription) for the 50 mg capsule three times daily.

NURSING IMPLICATIONS

Indomethacin is contraindicated in patients allergic to aspirin. Question patient carefully regarding aspirin sensitivity prior to initiation of therapy.

Administer immediately after meals, or with food, milk, or antacid (if prescribed) to minimize

GI side effects. Food or antacid may cause somewhat delayed and reduced absorption, but advantage of safety outweighs risk of impaired absorption.

Incidence of adverse reactions is high (especially in elderly patients) and is dose-related in most patients. Physician will rely on accurate and prompt reporting of patient's response and tolerance to establish lowest possible effective dosage.

Indomethacin can cause severe GI complications (reported to be among the most common side effects). Be alert to suspicious signs and symptoms and report immediately.

Patient should be carefully observed and should be instructed to report adverse reactions in order to prevent serious and sometimes irreversible or fatal effects.

In patients with underlying cardiovascular disease, the potential for sodium and water retention should be anticipated. Monitor weight and observe dependent areas for signs of edema.

Frontal headache is the most frequent CNS side effect; it should be reported. If it persists, dosage reduction or cessation of drug may be indicated. Usually it is more severe in the morning, but it may occur within 1 hour after drug ingestion. A dose scheduled at bedtime, with milk, may reduce the incidence of morning headache.

Complete blood counts, renal and hepatic function tests, ophthalmoscopic examinations, and hearing tests should be performed periodically during prolonged therapy.

Following control of acute flairs of chronic rheumatoid arthritis, physician may make repeated attempts to reduce daily doses until drug is finally discontinued.

Expected therapeutic effects in rheumatoid arthritis are reduced fever, increased strength, reduced stiffness, and relief of pain, swelling, and tenderness. If improvement is not noted in 2 to 3 weeks, alternate therapy is generally prescribed.

Therapeutic effect in acute gouty attack (relief of joint tenderness and pain) is usually apparent in 24 to 36 hours; swelling generally disappears in 3 to 5 days. Keep physician informed; dosage should be reduced once pain is tolerable.

Bear in mind that indomethacin may mask signs and symptoms of latent infections.

Because of the possibility of dizziness and lightheadedness, caution the patient to avoid activities requiring mental alertness and motor coordination.

Advise the patient not to take aspirin, because it may potentiate the ulcerogenic effects of indomethacin. *See also Drug Interactions.*

Green coloration of urine has been reported in patients who develop indomethacin-induced hepatitis.

Preserved in tight, light-resistant containers.

Drug Interactions. Ulcerogenic effects of indomethacin may be potentiated by concomitant administration of **corticosteroids, phenylbutazone,** or **salicylates;** concurrently administered **aspirin** may delay or decrease indomethacin absorption and thus may interfere with its therapeutic effectiveness. Recent reports indicate that indomethacin does not enhance the hypoprothrombinemic effects of **oral anticoagulants;** however, since indomethacin inhibits platelet aggregation and may cause GI ulceration and bleeding, cautious use is advised. Concomitant use with **furosemide:** response to both drugs may be inhibited. Indomethacin may cause slight increase in **penicillin G** half-life. **Probenecid** may increase indomethacin serum levels. Possibility of impaired antihypertensive response to **propranolol** and other **beta adrenergic blockers.** Indomethacin may predispose patients to severe reactions from **smallpox vaccine.**

INSULIN, HUMAN

(Human insulin, Humulin, Novolin)

Antidiabetic
Hypoglycemic

ACTIONS AND USES. Biosynthetic human insulin is derived not from human pancreas but from cultures of genetically modified *Escherichia coli* by recombinant DNA technology. Contains less than 4 ppm of immunoreactive *E. coli* polypeptides (ECPs). Semisynthetic human insulin is prepared from pork insulin by an enzymatic process that substitutes an alanine residue of pork insulin with threonine, resulting in an insulin molecule with the amino acid sequence indentical to that of human insulin. Manufacturer claims that these products are devoid of the following insulin contaminants: proinsulin, glucagon, vasoactive intestinal polypeptide, pancreatic polypeptide, somatostatin. Biological potency of one mg insulin human: not less than 26 USP human insulin units.

Regular Human Insulin is a rapid-acting clear, colorless aqueous solution of antidiabetic principle of the pancreas containing 100 U/ml. The biosynthetic preparation (Humulin-R) contains 10 to 40 mcg zinc/100 U/ml. The semisynthetic preparation (Novolin-R) contains only trace amounts of zinc (10 to 20 mcg/100 U/ml). Both biosynthetic and semisynthetic preparations also contain glycerin and cresol as preservatives. The only form of human insulin that can be administered intravenously.

NPH Human Insulin Isophane (Humulin-N, Novolin-N) is an intermediate-acting cloudy or milky suspension of zinc insulin crystals and protamine sulfate in buffered water. Each 100 USP units contains 10 to 40 mcg zinc and 0.15 to 0.25% dibasic sodium phosphate, glycerin, cresol and phenol.

I J

Lente Human Insulin (zinc suspension) (Novolin-L) is an intermediate-acting cloudy or milky suspension of insulin modified by addition of zinc chloride in buffered water. Each 100 USP units contains approximately 150 mcg zinc; also contains sodium acetate, sodium chloride and methylparaben.

Human insulin may be preferred over pork, beef, or mixed species insulins because it theoretically is less likely to elicit formation of insulin antibodies than animal insulins. *See Insulin Injection for actions.*

Used as replacement therapy in the management of the newly diagnosed patient with type I (IDDM) diabetes and for patient currently receiving pork, beef, or mixed species insulin. Also used in some patients with history of insulin allergy or resistance.

ABSORPTION AND FATE. Regular Human Insulin appears to be absorbed more rapidly than purified pork insulin (regular). In patient with diabetes, the human insulin appears to have a slightly faster onset and slightly shorter duration of action than purified pork insulin. *See Insulin Injection.*

CONTRAINDICATIONS AND PRECAUTIONS. *See Insulin Injection.*

ADVERSE/SIDE EFFECTS. Generalized and cutaneous allergic reactions in patient who is also allergic to animal insulins. *See Insulin Injection.*

ROUTE AND DOSAGE **Subcutaneous, intramuscular, intravenous:** Individualized dosage.

NURSING IMPLICATIONS

Human insulin (regular) is given SC, IM, and IV. The IV preparation usually is diluted in 0.9% sodium chloride injection. NPH Human Insulin Isophane and Lente Human Insulin are usually given SC; never IV.

Any changes in purity, strength, brand, type, and/or species should be made under medical surveillance. Monitor patient closely. Adjustments in dosage may be needed with the first dose and even with subsequent doses for a period of several weeks.

Active principle is in the milky white precipitate. To assure complete dispersion, mix thoroughly, gently rotating vial between palms and inverting it end to end several times. Do not shake; frothing will interfere with accurate measurement. If suspension or vial walls display granules or clumps after mixing or if solution is clear and remains clear after rotating vial, discard vial.

For information about transfer of patient from Lente Human Insulin to NPH Human Insulin Isophane and visa versa, or from Regular Human Insulin to either of these insulins see monographs on Insulin, Isophane and Insulin Zinc Suspension.

Avoid use of solution that is discolored, turbid or has unusual viscosity.

Human insulin preparations should be dispensed in original unopened multidose containers; they have an expiration date of not later than 24 months after vial was filled.

Discard partially empty vial if it has not been used for several weeks.

Available OTC.

Store unopened vial at 2° to 8°C (36° to 46°F) and vial-in-use at room temperature 15° to 30°C (56° to 89°F). Avoid freezing, exposure to extremes in temperature, or to direct sunlight.

See also Insulin Injection (prototype insulin).

PROTOTYPE

INSULIN INJECTION

(in'su-lin)
Antidiabetic
Hypoglycemic

(*Lilly Co:* Regular Iletin I, Regular Iletin II)
(*Squibb-Novo Co:* Regular Purified Pork, Regular Standard Pork)
(*Nordisk Co:* Velosulin)

ACTIONS AND USES. Short-acting, clear, colorless solution of exogenous unmodified insulin extracted from beta cells in beef and/or pork pancreas (as labelled). Enhances transmembrane passage of glucose into most body cells and by unknown mechanism may itself enter the cell to activate selected intermediary metabolic processes. Promotes conversion of glucose to glycogen, inhibits fatty acid mobilization from fat depots, promotes triglyceride synthesis, stimulates protein production, and promotes intracellular shift of K and Mg (magnesium). In the diabetic, insulin temporarily restores proper utilization of glucose and fat thereby preventing glycosuria, diabetic ketoacidosis, and coma. (Regular purified pork insulin was formerly called Actrapid.) Insulin Injection is the only form of insulin that can be given IV.

Used in the emergency treatment of diabetic ketoacidosis or coma, to initiate therapy in patient with insulin-dependent diabetes mellitus (type I, IDDM), and in combination with intermediate-acting or long-acting insulin to provide better control of blood glucose concentrations in the diabetic patient. Used IV to stimulate growth hormone secretion (by producing hypoglycemia) to evaluate pituitary growth hormone reserve in patient with known or suspected growth hormone deficiency. Other uses include: promotion of intracellular shift of K in treatment of hyperkalemia (IV); to induce hypoglycemic shock as therapy in psychiatry.

ABSORPTION AND FATE. Following administration, absorbed directly into blood, circulated widely in extracellular fluid as free hormone. After SC injection, action begins in ½ hour, effects: (Lilly products): 2 to 4 hours; (Squibb-Novo): 2.5 to 5 hours; (Nordisk): 2 to 3 hours. Duration of effect: 6 to 8 hours. Following IV injection, action begins in 10 to 30 minutes, peaks in ½ to 1 hour and lasts 1 to 2 hours. Plasma half-life following IV injection, 3 to 5 minutes. Half-life after SC injection, 4 hours and after IM, 2 hours. Metabolized primarily in liver and to lesser extent in kidney and muscle. Less than 2% of dose eliminated in urine.

CONTRAINDICATIONS AND PRECAUTIONS. Hypersensitivity to insulin animal protein.

ADVERSE/SIDE EFFECTS. **Hypersensitivity (usually occurs when insulin is at peak action point):** localized allergic reactions at injection site; generalized urticaria or bullae, lymphadenopathy, anaphylaxis (rare). **Hypoglycemia (hyperinsulinism):** profuse sweating, hunger, headache, nausea, tremulousness, tremors, palpitation, tachycardia, weakness, fatigue, nystagmus, circumoral pallor; numb mouth, tongue, and other paresthesias; visual disturbances (diplopia, blurred vision, mydriasis), staring expression, confusion, personality changes, ataxia, incoherent speech, apprehension, irritability, inability to concentrate, personality changes, uncontrolled yawning, loss of consciousness, delirium, hypothermia, convulsions, Babinski reflex, coma. (Urine glucose tests will be negative.) **Other:** posthypoglycemic or rebound hyperglycemia (Somogyi effect), lipoatrophy and lipohypertrophy of injection sites; insulin resistance. **Overdosage:** psychic disturbances, i.e., aphasia, personality changes, maniacal behavior.

ROUTE AND DOSAGE. Initial (new diabetic, unstable diabetes or for diabetes with complications): **Subcutaneous: Adult:** 5 to 10 units; **Children:** 2 to 4 units, 15 to 30 minutes before meals and at bedtime. Dosage highly individualized according to blood and urine glucose concentrations. *Ketoacidosis, coma:* Appropriate dosage highly individualized and often depends on patient's weight. Some physicians prescribe **Intramuscular or Intravenous bolus:** 10 to 20 units Regular insulin followed by an **Intravenous infusion:** 2 to 12 units of insulin solution (50 units Regular insulin/500 ml normal saline). *Infusion rate:* determined by blood glucose levels. Subsequent doses based on therapeutic response and blood glucose, acetone or ketone concentrations at 1 to 2 hour intervals. *Provocative test for growth hormone secretion:* 0.05 to 0.15 units/kg by rapid IV injection.

NURSING IMPLICATIONS

Insulin Injection (variously called "regular," "neutral," "plain," "ordinary," "unmodified," or just "insulin") should not be confused with the modified insulins.

All insulins are available OTC with the exception of Insulin Injection, concentrated (U-500) which requires a prescription.

Regular insulin is often mixed with intermediate acting insulins to attain good control. When Regular insulin is used alone, multiple injections are required.

Regular insulin may be adsorbed to the container or tubing when added to an IV infusion solution. Amount lost is variable and depends on concentration of insulin, infusion system, contact duration, and flow rate. The less the concentration of insulin in the solution and the slower the rate of flow, the greater the percentage absorbed.

To reduce the potential for loss of insulin, Normal Serum Albumin can be added to the insulin solution, or insulin may be added from a syringe directly into vein or IV tubing.

Any change in the strength (U-40,U-100, etc.), brand (manufacturer), purity, type (regular, etc.), species (beef, pork, human), or sequence of mixing two kinds of insulin is made by the physician only, since a simultaneous change in dosage may be necessary.

In general, dosage is adjusted to maintain postprandial blood glucose below 160 mg/dl. *Normal fasting blood sugar:* 60 to 100 mg/dl; *normal 2-hour postprandial blood sugar:* 70 to 130 mg/dl.

During early period of dosage regulation, some patients experience visual difficulties. Advise patient to delay changing prescription lenses until vision stabilizes (usually 3 to 6 weeks).

In the event of unavoidable insulin shortage, advise patient to reduce dosage temporarily, decrease food intake by one-third of usual quantity, and drink generous amounts of liquids with little or no caloric value (water, coffee, tea, clear soup, broth).

The amount and distribution of food throughout the day is determined by the physician and should not be changed unless prescribed.

Storage, Preparation, and Administration:

- Insulin may be purchased OTC; however, a prescription may be needed for the syringe and needle, depending on state law.
- Advise patient to keep an extra vial of insulin, syringe, and needle on hand.
- Insulin in use is stable at room temperature up to 1 month. Avoid exposure to temperature extremes or to direct sunlight. Refrigerate stock supply.
- Avoid injection of cold insulin; it can lead to lipodystrophy, reduced rate of absorption, and local reactions.
- VNA nurses sometimes prepare a week's supply of daily insulin doses for select patients. The prepared syringes are refrigerated until ready for use. Patient should be instructed to remove syringe from refrigerator about 1 hour before administration time.
- Examine vial before preparing dose. Do not use if solution is discolored, cloudy, or contains a precipitate.
- Check expiration date on label. Discard outdated vials and partially used vials that have not been in use for several weeks.
- Insulins should not be mixed unless prescribed by physician. In general regular insulin is drawn up into syringe first to avoid contaminating it with the second insulin.
- Always use a syringe that coordinates with strength of insulin to be administered. Standardized color code for cap and syringe markings are as follows: red for U-40, orange for U-100.
- Insulin is generally administered 15 to 30 minutes before a meal so that peak action will coincide with postprandial hyperglycemia.
- Eliminate air bubble within syringe and hub of needle (dead space) for accurate dosage. In syringes with detachable needles, dead space may be equivalent to 0.1 ml. Some disposable syringes with permanently attached needles have no dead space and thus provide more accurate measurement.
- Before introducing needle, wipe top of bottle and skin with an alcohol swab. Allow skin to dry (alcohol precipitates insulin), and inject insulin into area that has a substantial layer of fat and is free of large blood vessels and nerves.
- Commonly used injection sites: upper arms, thighs, abdomen (avoid area over urinary bladder and 2 inches around navel), buttocks, and upper back (if fat is loose enough to pick up).
- Some physicians favor varying the injection site within a given anatomic area; others stress importance of varying sites among widely different body areas. Clarify this issue with physician before patient teaching.
- Superficial subcutaneous injection may cause local allergic reaction or irritation and therefore should be avoided.
- For self-injection of an arm, instruct patient to press back of upper arm against a chair back so that tissue is "bunched up," making needle insertion easier.
- If patient is engaged in active sports it has been suggested that injection of insulin be made into the abdomen rather than into a muscle that will be heavily taxed, since this may speed up insulin absorption.
- Available injection sites are lost when lipodystrophy (dimpling or atrophy of adipose tissue seen predominantly in women and children) and hypertrophy or thickening develops. Lipodystrophy has been associated with inadequate rotation of injection sites, use

of cold insulin, and intrafat insulin injections. (Reportedly, injection of purified insulins directly into lesions may correct lipodystrophy.)

- Allow approximately 1 inch between injection sites and avoid reuse of a site for 6 to 8 weeks, if possible.
- Maintain an injection record or chart to assure systematic site rotation.
- Special equipment is available for patients who are visually impaired or who have other handicaps. Contact local chapter of the American Diabetes Association.

Care of Reusable Equipment:

- Reusable syringe and needle may be sterilized by boiling (in a strainer) for 10 minutes. If a strainer is not used fold a clean cloth in bottom of pan to protect syringe. Avoid heavily chlorinated water; use soft tap water, distilled water, or clean rainwater. Advise patient to keep pan, strainer, or cloth separate for this purpose.
- If reusable syringe and needle cannot be boiled for whatever reason, sterilize by immersing them in ethyl alcohol 70% or isopropyl alcohol 90% for at least 5 minutes. Do not use bathing, rubbing, or medicated alcohol for this purpose.
- Use dry syringe and needle to administer insulin. After administration rinse syringe thoroughly with water and clean needle with wire.
- If there appears to be a precipitate on the inner surface of the syringe; remove, by use of a vinegar-soaked cotton swab. Rinse thoroughly before sterilization.

I J

Special Points on Adverse Reactions:

- Local reactions at injection site sometimes develop 1 to 3 weeks after therapy starts appearing 1 to 12 hours after an injection. Symptoms may last several hours to days, but usually disappear with continued use. Advise patient to report symptoms; physician may prescribe an antihistamine. Zinc senstivitiy has been implicated. Injection technique should be checked.
- Generalized allergic reaction (sensitivity to species source of insulin) may be reversed by substituting insulin from another source.
- Patients highly sensitive to insulin who cannot be maintained on oral hypoglycemics may be rapidly desensitized with subcutaneous administration of small and frequent doses of insulin. Observe patient closely for anaphylaxis and onset of hypoglycemia during desensitization period.
- Topical applications of insulin reportedly stimulate healing of small uncomplicated decubiti. Use specific dosage ordered and do not apply insulin to large surfaces, since systemic absorption with consequent hypoglycemia is possible.
- *Hypoglycemic reaction* (insulin shock) may occur from excess insulin, insufficient food intake, e.g., skipped or delayed meals, vomiting, diarrhea, unaccustomed exercise (burns up sugar and thus adds to insulin effect of lowering blood sugar), infection or illness or nervous or emotional tension, overindulgence in alcohol.
- Symptomatic hypoglycemia occurs when blood sugar drops to 50 mg/dl or when fall is sudden and rapid. Onset generally corresponds to peak action of insulin.
- Somogyi effect develops when patient chronically receives unnecessarily large doses of insulin with resulting unrecognized or uncorrected hypoglycemia. The body attempts to compensate by accelerating release of hormones concerned with plasma glucose regulation (e.g., glucagon, catecholamines, somatropin, adrenal corticosteroids) with resulting rebound hyperglycemia. Suspect Somogyi effect if evening blood or urine glucose levels are low followed by morning hyperglycemia, or if patient appears to require increasingly more insulin.
- Restlessness and diaphoresis occurring during sleep are suggestive of hypoglycemia in the diabetic patient.
- Instruct patient and responsible family members to respond promptly to beginning

symptoms of hypoglycemia (often vague): profuse sweating, hunger, fatigue, inability to concentrate, lassitude, depression, early morning headache, drowsiness, anxiety *(see Adverse/Side Effects).*

- Hypoglycemic reaction occurs suddenly (in minutes to hours) and is an emergency situation, since prolonged hypoglycemia can cause irreversible brain damage. Advise patient to take 4 ounces of orange juice (1.5 to 3 ounces for child) followed by a meal of 1 glass milk with crackers or a sandwich (or other longer-acting carbohydrate or protein food). Other emergency sources of fast-acting carbohydrate include 4 ounces of a sugar sweetened soft drink, 2 sugar cubes, 2½ teaspoons of sugar, 2 teaspoons of honey or corn syrup, 5 Life-Savers. Failure to show signs of recovery within 30 minutes indicates necessity for emergency treatment.
- Patients with severe hypoglycemia may receive glucagon, epinephrine, or IV glucose 10 to 50%. As soon as patient is fully conscious, oral carbohydrate, e.g., dilute corn syrup or orange juice with sugar, Gatorade or Pedialyte should be given to prevent secondary hypoglycemia.
- Since severe hypoglycemia develops suddenly in some patients, physician may advise patient to keep a supply of glucagon on hand for home emergency use; a responsible family member may be taught how to administer it.
- Glutose, and Instant Glucose are commercial concentrated glucose products for emergency use particularly when patient in hypoglycemia is unconscious. Prescribed amount squeezed into buccal cavity adheres to mucous membrane and is absorbed directly through cheek membrane or swallowed by reflex action.
- Advise patient to carry some form of rapid-acting carbohydrate (e.g., lump sugar, Life-Savers or other candy) at all times to treat hypoglycemia.
- *Diabetic ketoacidosis* as a sequel to insulin deficiency or resistance is a medical emergency that appears over a period of weeks in controlled diabetics or in a few hours in noncontrolled patients. Blood sugar levels may rise as high as 300 to 800 mg/dl or higher. Precipitating factors: omission of insulin, improperly balanced diet, overeating, failure to increase insulin dosage during times of increased need, such as rapid growth in juveniles, fever, infection, or other illness, emotional stress, surgery, trauma, pregnancy. Patient/family education is critically important.
- *Symptoms of diabetic ketoacidosis:* drowsiness, nausea, diarrhea, abdominal pain, intense thirst (polydipsia); polyuria, dry mouth, dry flushed skin, poor skin turgor, soft eyeballs, low BP, weak rapid pulse, fruity (acetone) breath, Kussmaul's respirations (air hunger), inattention, weakness, drowsiness, coma. Elevated laboratory values: urine glucose, urine ketones, blood glucose, serum ketoacids; decreased blood pH, and sodium bicarbonate.
- Severe ketoacidosis is treated with insulin injection IV, large amounts of IV fluids. When blood glucose falls to approximately 250 mg/dl, 5% Dextrose is added to IV solution. Potassium and an alkalinizing agent (sodium bicarbonate) are sometimes necessary. Blood sugar is monitored hourly at bedside until values improve, then every 2 to 4 hours, as prescribed.
- During treatment for ketoacidosis with IV insulin, check blood pressure, intake and output ratio, and urine glucose and ketones every hour.
- Observe level of consciousness; be alert for signs of hypoglycemia (patient may pass from hyperglycemia into insulin shock without regaining consciousness). Also observe for signs of hyperkalemia *(see Index: Clinical signs and symptoms).*
- The juvenile diabetic generally is more prone to hypoglycemia and ketoacidosis than the mature diabetic. Both child and parent must know signs of impending complications *(see Adverse Effects).* Short-term weight loss provides an accurate assessment of dehydration.

- Loss of diabetes control (hyperglycemia or hypoglycemia) occurs commonly at the beginning of a menstrual period. Advise patient to test urine regularly during this time and to adjust insulin dosage accordingly, as prescribed by physician.
- Activity and insulin requirement vary inversely; thus insulin requirements of the normally active diabetic child tend to decrease in the summer (when activity increases) and increase in the fall. The abnormally active child with diabetes requires added food before and during anticipated activity.
- In the event of an illness, advise patient to continue taking insulin, go to bed, and drink liberally (every hour if possible) of noncaloric liquids. Do not force liquids if nauseated or vomiting. If unable to eat prescribed diet, replace with liquid or semiliquid carbohydrate according to food exchange list. Test urine for sugar and acetone four times a day, before meals and at bedtime. Consult physician for insulin regulation if unable to eat prescribed diet, or if 4 meals of liquid or semiliquid carbohydrates have been taken or if urine tests are unusual (e.g., high sugar, sugar with acetone).
- Hyperosmolar nonketotic diabetic coma most frequently occurs in type II diabetic patients who receive insufficient insulin to prevent advancing hyperglycemia.

Glucose Urine Testing, Glucose Blood Testing:

- Check patient's ability to match colors on urine chart. Diastix (a dip and read strip) rather than Clinitest (tablet for solution) may be preferable for patients who are red-green color blind. Other available test strips include Chemstrip uG (urine glucose test), Chemstrip-K (urine ketone test) or Chemstrip uGK (test for both glucose and ketones).
- For reliability of results, advise patient to use only the prescribed type of urine test. Review the instructions on the package insert with the patient.
- Test of first voiding reflects a summation of blood sugars; test of second voiding (preferred and usually prescribed) reflects an instantaneous measurement of sugar in the blood.
- Check with physician about frequency of urine testing, and urine glucose values that suggest need for insulin and/or diet adjustments. In the labile diabetic, urine may be tested four times daily, before meals and at bedtime to determine the pattern of urine sugars. Occasionally, tests are done at times of peak and minimum insulin effects.
- In general, glycosuria indicates unsuitable insulin dosage or dietary imbalance or indiscretion and a renal threshold exceeding 180 mg/dl. Some physicians prefer to have their patients show an occasional trace or positive reading to prevent Somogyi effect *(see above)*.
- Usually urine test for ketones is not done routinely in stabilized diabetics. It is checked routinely in new, unstable, and juvenile diabetes and if patient has lost weight, exercises vigorously, has an illness, and whenever urine contains glucose.
- Presence of acetone without sugar usually signifies insufficient carbohydrate intake. Acetone with sugar may indicate onset of ketoacidosis. Notify physician promptly.
- Since women in third trimester of pregnancy and nursing mothers may have lactose in urine, cupric sulfate reagents such as Benedict's test or Clinitest should not be used. Glucose oxidase reagents, e.g., Chemstrip uG, Clinistix, Diastix, Tes-Tape may be used.
- Caution patients to avoid OTC medications (which may have high sugar content) unless approved by physician. Aspirin or ascorbic acid in large doses may cause positive urine glucose test.
- Blood (capillary) glucose test kits, including lancet or monolet for finger or ear lobe prick, are now available for home use, e.g., Chemstrip bG. Other self-monitoring kits (e.g., Dextrostix) require a special instrument for accurate interpretation of test readings.
- Physician may have patient supplement urine testing with blood glucose tests to improve diabetic control. The patient may be instructed to do the test before a meal or 2 hours after a meal (or more frequently, if indicated), during infection, unusual stress, any

illness, pregnancy, when urine tests for ketones are positive and urine glucose shows 5% for 3 or 4 tests; before and immediately following a new exercise program. During pregnancy, tests are done more routinely (at least 4 or 5 times a week).

Smoking–Drug Interaction:

- Insulin absorption is decreased during the first 30 minutes after smoking. This interaction combined with a known increase in catecholamine release during smoking may have significant clinical effects. A heavy smoker may require up to 30% more insulin than the non-smoker.

Other:

- The American Diabetes Association supports use of the FDA approved sweetening ingredient aspartame (in Equal, NutraSweet) by diabetic patients.
- Emphasize need for maintaining optimum skin care and foot care to prevent vascular-related complications and infection.
- Hypoglycemic reaction is sometimes the first indication of pregnancy in the diabetic woman. Patient should report promptly to physician.
- Insulin requirements during first trimester of pregnancy frequently decrease by one-third (utilization of glucose by fetus). During second and third trimesters, hormonal changes induced by pregnancy and action of placental insulinase may necessitate increased dosage (decreased insulin requirement during this period suggests a failing placenta). On day of delivery, physician may omit insulin dose and administer IV glucose.
- After delivery, maternal insulin requirements usually are less than prepregnant dosage. Observe patient closely for hypoglycemia. Insulin requirement gradually returns to prepregnancy level within 1 to 6 weeks.
- During lactation, frequent blood glucose determinations are advised. Both Benedict's test and Clinitest give positive readings for lactose; therefore, they should not be used during this period. Greater reliance will be placed on blood glucose analyses.
- When the patient plans to travel, advise patient to carry ample insulin (in event of delay in flight), at least 2 or 3 syringes and needles, and an adequate supply of emergency carbohydrate in hand luggage or handbag (travel kits are available).
- Insulin dosage adjustment when traveling requires preplanning with physician, particularly when changes in time zones are involved.
- If foreign languages are spoken in countries to be visited, advise the patient to learn emergency vocabulary: "Sugar." "May I have orange juice?" "I am a diabetic." "I need a doctor."
- For information about diabetic care in foreign countries, patients can write to International Diabetes Foundation, 3–6 Alfred Place, London WC1, England.
- Advise patient to wear medical identification bracelet, necklace, or card (available in local pharmacies, or from Medic Alert; *see Index)* with patient's and physician's names addresses, and telephone numbers, as well as diagnosis, dosage, and type of antidiabetic agent being taken.
- A high fiber diet may help to lower plasma glucose in some patients. Remind patient that dietary changes must be prescribed by physician.
- Advise patient to avoid alcohol, since it may reduce gluconeogenesis and thus precipitate hypoglycemic crisis.
- Suicidal overdosing with SC injection has been successfully managed by excision of injection site.
- Be familiar with the information on insulin package insert, which is also available to the patient, and consult with physician for directions the patient is to follow. Prepare a teaching plan in collaboration with physician, dietitian, patient, and responsible family members.

Summary of Patient/Family Teaching Plan:

- ✓ Nature of diabetes mellitus.
- ✓ Review patient instruction sheet (package insert).
- ✓ Insulin: action, administration, storage, syringe-insulin coordination.
- ✓ What to do in the event of unavoidable insulin shortage.
- ✓ Adjustments of insulin dosage (as prescribed) in relation to urine tests, illness, changes in activity, diet, travel; pregnancy.
- ✓ Urine and blood testing and recording, how and when to test.
- ✓ Cause, symptoms, prevention, and treatment of hypoglycemia and ketoacidosis.
- ✓ Importance of adhering to prescribed diet and maintaining optimal body weight.
- ✓ Planned, graded exercise schedule (approved by physician). Personal hygiene: foot care, skin and dental care, prevention of infection.
- ✓ OTC medications and alcohol.
- ✓ Referral to VNA to assure continued health supervision.
- ✓ Importance of regular follow-up visits for check of blood sugar and adjustment of insulin dosage and diet, if necessary.
- ✓ Educational resources: American Diabetes Association (contact local chapter).

Diagnostic Test Interferences. Large doses of insulin may increase urinary excretion of **VMA.** Insulin may cause alterations in **thyroid function tests,** and **liver function tests,** and may decrease **serum potassium,** and **serum calcium.**

Drug Interactions: Insulin

Plus	Interactions
Alcohol, ethyl (Ethanol)	Excessive alcohol intake can precipitate hypoglycemic crisis
Anabolic steroids	Additive hypoglycemic effects
Chlorthalidone (Hygroton)	Antagonizes hypoglycemic effects of insulin
Clonidine (Catapres)	Inhibits normal catecholamine response to insulin-induced hypoglycemia, also suppresses signs and symptoms of hypoglycemia
Contraceptives, oral Corticosteroids Dextrothyroxine (Choloxin) Diazoxide (Hyperstat) Epinephrine (Adrenalin) Estrogens Ethacrynic acid (Edecrin)	Hyperglycemic action of these drugs may increase insulin requirements
Fenfluramin (Pondimin)	Additive hypoglycemic effects
Furosemide (Lasix)	Hyperglycemic action may increase insulin requirements
Glucagon	Antagonizes hypoglycemic effects of insulin
Guanethidine (Ismelin) Hypoglycemics, oral	Additive hypoglycemic effects
Lithium	Hyperglycemic action may increase insulin requirements

Plus (cont.)	Interactions (cont.)
MAO inhibitors	May enhance hypoglycemic action of insulin
Marijuana	Hyperglycemic action may impair glucose tolerance
Oxytetracycline	Possibility of additive hypoglycemic effects
Phenothiazines, Phenytoin (Dilantin)	Hyperglycemic action may increase insulin requirements
Propranolol (Inderal)	Interferes with carbohydrate metabolism with risk of prolonged hypoglycemia; also may blunt warning signs of hypoglycemia, e.g., palpitation, tachycardia
Salicylates (large doses), Sulfinpyrazone (Anturane)	Possibility of additive hypoglycemic effects
Tiazide diuretics, Thyroid preparations, Triamterene (Dyrenium)	Hyperglycemic action may increase insulin requirements

I J

INSULIN INJECTION CONCENTRATED

[Regular (Concentrated) Iletin II]

Antidiabetic
Hypoglycemic

ACTIONS AND USES. Concentrated purified insulin from pork pancreas unmodified by any agent that might prolong its action. Because of its high concentration, duration of action is similar to that of an intermediate-acting insulin. *See Insulin Injection for contraindications, precautions, and adverse reactions.*

Used for the occasional patient who develops insulin resistance and requires daily doses greater than 200 U (even as high as several thousand units).

ABSORPTION AND FATE. May show activity over 24-hour period. *See Insulin Injection.*

ROUTE AND DOSAGE. Subcutaneous, intramuscular: one to three times daily. Highly individualized dosage. Concentration available: U-500 (per ml).

NURSING IMPLICATIONS

Label on U 500 insulin is brown-and-white striped. Check expiration date. This preparation requires a prescription.

This preparation should not be administered IV.

Discard solution that is not absolutely clear and colorless.

Use a tuberculin syringe for accuracy in measurement. Even a slight variation can mean a large overdose or underdose.

There seems to be no condition of absolute resistance. All insulin-resistant patients will respond if dose is large enough.

Patients receiving concentrated insulin are kept under close surveillance until dosage is established. Close monitoring of water and electrolyte balance is essential.

Severe secondary hypoglycemia reactions may develop 18 to 24 hours after administration of drug. Have on hand glucagon, IV dextrose, epinephrine.

Frequently, responsiveness to insulin effect is regained after a short period of therapy concentrated insulin.

See also Insulin Injection (prototype insulin).

INSULIN, ISOPHANE

Antidiabetic
Hypoglycemic

(Insulatard NPH, NPH, NPH Iletin I, NPH Iletin II, NPH Purified Beef, NPH Purified Pork)

ACTIONS AND USES. Intermediate-acting cloudy suspension of zinc insulin crystals (derived from beef or pork pancreas, or both) and modified by protamine, in a neutral buffer. NPH Iletin II (beef or pork), and Insulatard are "purified" or "single component" insulins that have been purified and are less likely to cause allergic reactions than nonpurified preparations. Combines some of the advantages and eliminates some of the disadvantages of both very short-acting and very long-acting preparations. Therapeutic effect is prompt enough to control postprandial hyperglycemia, which formerly called for supplemental doses of Insulin Injection. *See Insulin Injection for actions, contraindications, and adverse reactions.*

Generally considered drug of choice to control hyperglycemia in the diabetic patient. Mixtard is a fixed combination of purified regular pork insulin 30% and 70% NPH.

ABSORPTION AND FATE. Action onset: 1 to 2 hours, peak effect: 4 to 12 hours; duration of action: about 24 hours. *See Insulin Injection.*

ROUTE AND DOSAGE. Subcutaneous (individualized): Usual dose: 7 to 26 units as single dose. Dose may be increased by increments of 2 to 10 units at daily or weekly intervals. Concentrations available are U-40, and U-100 (per ml).

NURSING IMPLICATIONS

This preparation should never be administered IV; it is not suitable for emergency use.

Usually given 30 to 60 minutes before first meal of the day. If necessary a second smaller dose may be prescribed 30 minutes before supper or at bedtime.

Active principal is in the milky white precipitate. To assure complete dispersion, mix thoroughly by gently rotating vial between palms and inverting it end to end several times. Do not shake; frothing will interfere with accurate measurement. If suspension or vial walls display granules or clumps after mixing, or if solution is clear and remains clear after mixing, discard vial.

Isophane insulin may be mixed with Insulin Injection without altering either solution.

Isophane insulin should not be mixed with lente forms.

Patient receiving Insulin Injection (regular) may be transferred directly to Isophane insulin on unit-for-unit basis: initial dose of Isophane should be about two-thirds to three-fourths total daily dose of regular insulin. Monitor patient closely.

If dosage is very high, physician may prescribe divided doses; two-thirds in morning and one-third 30 minutes before supper or at bedtime.

Insulins should not be mixed unless prescribed by physician. In general, when Insulin Injection (regular insulin) is to be combined, it is drawn first. For example, to give 5-U Insulin Injection and 10-U Isophane Insulin: using aseptic technique, inject 10-U air into Isophane Insulin bottle. Withdraw needle. Inject 5-U air into Insulin Injection bottle, and withdraw 5-U. Eliminate all air bubbles from hub of needle and syringe barrel. Insert needle into bottle of Isophane Insulin (make sure needle tip is below level of liquid), withdraw 10-U. Important to follow the same order of sequence with the same stock bottles every day.

Suspect hypoglycemia if patient complains of fatigue, weakness, sweating, tremor or nervousness. *See Insulin Injection for complete description.*

If insulin was given before breakfast, a hypoglycemic episode is most likely to occur between midafternoon and dinnertime, when insulin effect is peaking. Patient should be told to eat a snack in midafternoon and to carry sugar or candy to treat a reaction. A snack at bedtime will prevent insulin reaction during the night.

The patient should always consult his or her physician before making changes in dosage to accommodate anticipated stress or exercise.

The initials NPH stand for Neutral Protamine Hagedorn.

Available OTC.

Isophane insulin should be dispensed in original unopened multidose container with expiration date of not later than 24 months after vial was filled.

Discard partially empty vial if it has not been used for several weeks.

Store unopened vial at 2° to 8°C (36° to 46°F); store vial in use at room temperature, i.e., 15° to 30°C (59° to 86°F). Avoid freezing, exposure to extremes in temperature or to direct sunlight.

See also Insulin Injection for nursing implications, diagnostic test interferences and drug interactions.

INSULIN, PROTAMINE ZINC

Antidiabetic
Hypoglycemic

(Beef Protamine, Zinc and Iletin II; Pork Protamine, Zinc and Iletin II; Protamine, Zinc and Iletin I; Protamine Zinc Insulin; PZI)

ACTIONS AND USES. Long-acting, cloudy suspension of insulin modified by addition of zinc chloride and protamine sulfate which has poor solubility and thus delays absorption. Derived from beef or pork pancreas, or both. May be used in combination with a shorter-acting form. *See Insulin Injection for actions, contraindications, precautions, and adverse/side effects.* (PZI is rarely used.)

Used to treat diabetes mellitus in patients who are not adequately controlled by unmodified insulin.

ABSORPTION AND FATE. Action onset: effects in 4 to 8 hours; peak effect: 14 to 24 hours; duration of action in excess of 36 hours. *See Insulin Injection.*

ADVERSE/SIDE EFFECTS. Lymphedema around injection site, hypoglycemia, hypersensitivity reactions. *See also Insulin Injection.*

NURSING IMPLICATIONS

Should not be administered IV. Not suitable for emergency use.

Usually administered 30 to 60 minutes before breakfast.

Active principal is in the milky white precipitate. To assure complete dispersion, mix thoroughly by gently rotating vial between palms and inverting it end to end several times. Do not shake; frothing will interfere with accurate measurement. If suspension or vial walls display granules or clumps after mixing, or if solution is clear and remains clear after mixing, discard vial.

Teach patient that prolonged insulin effect requires careful distribution of carbohydrates in a balanced diet. Patient should not redistribute food or alter dose or time of taking insulin, unless advised by physician.

If one dose of insulin has controlled diabetes for some time, the patient may test urine and blood for glucose once a day or two or three times weekly. In the event of infection, emotional stress, or change in activity, patient should increase number of tests per day.

When mixing insulin injection with PZI, prepare solution immediately before administration. Withdraw Insulin Injection into syringe before PZI so that vial of insulin injection will not be contaminated with excess protamine. *See Isophane Insulin for procedure for mixing insulins.*

The usual proportion of PZI to Insulin Injection prescribed is 1:2 or 1:3, in order to provide a preparation with both rapid onset and prolonged duration of action.

If injection is given in the morning, hypoglycemia is most likely to occur during the night or early morning.

Blood sugar levels fall slowly after injection of PZI; thus, marked hypoglycemia may develop without producing an apparent cluster of symptoms. Teach patient and a responsible other to be alert to the significance of sweating or fatigue unwarranted by patient's activities, as well as other vague symptoms such as lassitude, drowsiness, tremulousness. The physician should be notified immediately. Without prompt and adequate treatment, patient may become unconscious.

Treatment of PZI-induced hypoglycemia requires both fast-acting and slowly digestible carbohydrate: e.g., corn syrup or honey with bread, followed in 1 or 2 hours by additional "slow" carbohydrates, such as milk and crackers. Emergency treatment: 10 to 20 Gm glucose IV followed later by food.

Between meal snacks may be necessary; bedtime snacks are essential.

Full therapeutic effect of PZI may be delayed several days following institution of treatment. During this interval, small supplemental doses of insulin injection are often necessary.

Available OTC.

Protamine zinc insulin should be dispensed in original unopened multidose container with expiration date of not later than 24 months after vial was filled.

Discard partially empty vial if it has not been used for several weeks.

Store unopened vial at 2° to 8°C (36° to 46°F); store vial in use at room temperature (15° to 30°C) (59° to 86°F). Avoid freezing, exposure to extremes in temperature or to direct sunlight.

See also Insulin Injection (prototype insulin) for nursing implications, diagnostic test interferences, drug interactions.

INSULIN ZINC SUSPENSION

Antidiabetic
Hypoglycemic

(*Squibb-Novo Co:* Lente Insulin Zinc Suspension (beef), Lente Purified Pork)
(*Lilly Co:* Lente Iletin I (beef and pork), Lente Iletin II (purified beef), Lente Iletin II (purified pork)

ACTIONS AND USES. Intermediate-acting cloudy insulin suspension, equivalent to a mixture of 30% prompt insulin zinc (Semilente) and 70% extended zinc insulin (Ultralente) suspensions. Obtained from beef or pork pancreas or both.

Because insulin zinc suspension contains no modifying foreign protein (protamine or globin), allergic reactions are rare. Time action is intermediate between those of prompt and extended insulins and is so close to that of isophane (NPH) insulin that the two forms may be used interchangeably. *See Insulin Injection for contraindications, precautions, and adverse/side effects.*

Used for treatment of hypoglycemia in diabetic patients allergic to other preparations of insulin. Also used for patients with evidence pointing toward thrombotic phenomena in which protamine may be a factor. *See Insulin Injection.*

ABSORPTION AND FATE. Action onset: 1 to 3 hours; peak effect: (Lilly products): 6 to 12 hours; (Squibb-Novo): 7 to 15 hours. Duration of action: (Lilly): 18 to 26 hours; (Squibb-Novo): 18 to 24 hours. *See Insulin Injection.*

ROUTE AND DOSAGE. Subcutaneous (individualized): concentrations available: U 40, and U 100 (per ml).

NURSING IMPLICATIONS

Usually administered 30 to 60 minutes before breakfast. Some patients require another injection 30 minutes before suppertime or at bedtime.

Should not be administered IV. This preparation is not suitable for emergency treatment.

Zinc insulin preparations (Ultralente, Lente, Semilente) can be mixed with one another if prescribed by physician, but they must not be mixed with other modified insulins.

Active principal is in the milky white precipitate. To assure complete dispersion, mix thoroughly by gently rotating the vial between the palms and by inverting it end-to-end several times. Do not shake; frothing will interfere with accurate measurement. If the suspension or vial walls display granules or clumps of precipitate after mixing, or if solution is clear and remains clear after rotating, discard vial.

Symptoms of hypoglycemia are most apt to occur between midafternoon and dinner time (an early symptom may be a sense of extreme fatigue). Notify the physician promptly and give patient emergency soluble carbohydrate (e.g., orange juice, honey, corn syrup). If the period of time between the midday and evening meal is prolonged, an afternoon snack may be ordered.

The possibility of nocturnal hypoglycemia should not be overlooked, especially during dose adjustment. Watch the sleeping patient carefully for signs of restlessness or profuse sweating.

Since time action of insulin zinc suspension (Lente) approximates that of isophane insulin suspension (NPH), the patient can usually be transferred directly to the latter on a unit-for-unit basis. Transfer from regular insulin to Insulin Zinc Suspension: initial dose of Insulin Zinc should be two-thirds to three-fourths total daily dose of regular insulin.

Available OTC.

Insulin Zinc Suspension should be dispensed in original unopened multidose container with expiration date of not later than 24 months after vial was filled.

Discard partially empty vial if it has not been used for several weeks.

Store unopened vial at 2° to 8°C (36° to 46°F); store vial in use at room temperature (15° to 30°C) (59° to 86°F). Avoid freezing, exposure to extremes in temperature or to direct sunlight.

See also Insulin Injection (prototype insulin).

I J

INSULIN ZINC SUSPENSION, EXTENDED

Antidiabetic, hypoglycemic

(Ultralente Iletin I, Ultralente Insulin, Ultralente Purified Beef)

ACTIONS AND USES. Long-acting cloudy suspension of insulin modified by addition of zinc chloride. Large particle size and high zinc content delay absorption and prolong action. Obtained from beef or pork pancreas or both. No modifying protein (protamine or globin) is added; therefore, incidence of allergic reactions is low. Similar to protamine zinc insulin suspension

(PZI) in actions and indications. Usually administered in combination with a shorter acting insulin preparation. *See Insulin Injection for actions, uses, contraindications, and adverse/side effects.*

ABSORPTION AND FATE. Action onset: within 4 to 8 hours. Peak action: (Ultralente Iletin): 14 to 24 hours; (Other preparations): 10 to 30 hours. Duration of action: 28 to 36 hours. *See Insulin Injection.*

ROUTE AND DOSAGE. Subcutaneous (individualized): concentrations available: U 40 and U 100 (per ml).

NURSING IMPLICATIONS

This drug is not to be used IV, and it is not suitable for emergency situations.

Administered 30 to 60 minutes before breakfast by deep subcutaneous injection.

Active principal is in the milky white precipitate. To assure complete dispersion, mix thoroughly by gently rotating vial between palms and by inverting it end to end several times. Do not shake; frothing will interfere with accurate measurement. Discard vial if suspension on vial walls displays granules or clumps of precipitate or if solution is clear and remains clear after mixing.

May be mixed with Lente and Semilente, but must not be mixed with other modified insulin preparations.

When switching from a standard insulin to one of the purified insulins, dosage should be reduced initially and patient closely monitored. Usually dosage reduction is about 20%.

Hypoglycemia is most apt to occur during the night or early morning. Notify physician promptly if it occurs (watch sleeping patient carefully for signs of restlessness or profuse sweating). Hypoglycemia is treated by administering soluble carbohydrate (orange juice, sugar, honey) plus a slowly digestible carbohydrate (bread, crackers). Supplemental feedings may be prescribed.

Available OTC.

Should be dispensed in original unopened multidose container with expiration date of not later than 24 months after vial was filled.

Discard partially empty vial if it has not been used for several weeks.

Store unopened vial at 2° to 8°C (36° to 46°F); store vial in use at room temperature (15° to 30°C) (59° to 86°F). Avoid freezing, exposure to extremes in temperature or to direct sunlight.

See also Insulin Injection (prototype insulin).

I J

INSULIN ZINC, PROMPT

(Semilente Iletin I, Semilente Insulin, Semilente Purified Pork)

Antidiabetic
Hypoglycemic

ACTIONS AND USES. Rapid-acting cloudy suspension of insulin modified by addition of zinc chloride so that solid phase of suspension is amorphous and therefore more quickly absorbed. Obtained from beef or pork pancreas or both. No modifying protein (protamine or globin) is added; therefore, incidence of allergic reactions is low. *See Insulin Injection for actions, contraindications, precautions, and adverse reactions.*

Used most commonly to supplement intermediate and long-acting insulins. Also used for routine management of diabetes, especially for patients allergic to other types of insulin, and for patients with evidence pointing toward thrombotic phenomena in which protamine may be a factor.

ABSORPTION AND FATE. Action onset: within 1 to 2 hours; peak effect: 3 to 10 hours; duration of effect; 10 to 16 hours. *See Insulin Injection.*

ROUTE AND DOSAGE. **Subcutaneous (individualized):** Initial (newly diagnosed, mild diabetics): 10 to 20 units (usually 2 doses/day are required). Concentrations available are U 40 and U 100 (per ml).

NURSING IMPLICATIONS

Should never be administered IV. Preparation is not suitable for emergency use.

Usually administered once daily, 30 minutes before breakfast. Additional doses may be required for some patients, 30 minutes before a meal or at bedtime.

Active principal is in the milky white precipitate. To assure complete dispersion, mix thoroughly by gently rotating vial between palms and by inverting it end to end several times. Do not shake; frothing will interfere with accurate measurement. If the suspension on vial walls displays granules or clumps of crystalline precipitate after mixing, or if solution is clear and remains clear after vial is rotated, discard vial.

Symptoms of hypoglycemia are most apt to appear before lunch; glycosuria is most apt to appear during the night.

The zinc insulin preparations (Ultralente, Lente, Semilente) can be mixed with one another, but they must not be mixed with other modified insulin.

This preparation should not be substituted for another insulin preparation without direction by a physician.

Should be dispensed in original unopened multidose container with expiration date of not later than 24 months after vial was filled.

Discard partially empty vial if it has not been used for several weeks.

Store unopened vial at 2° to 8°C (36° to 46°F); store vial in use at room temperature (15° to 30°C) (59° to 86°F). Avoid freezing, exposure to extremes in temperature or to direct sunlight.

See also Insulin Injection (prototype insulin).

IODINATED GLYCEROL

(Organidin)

(eye'oh-di-nay-ted gli'ser-ole)
Expectorant

ACTIONS AND USES. Stable complex of iodine and glycerol. Liquefies thick, tenacious respiratory tract fluid and facilitates expectoration. Contains approximately 50% organically bound iodine, little or no inorganic iodine, and no free iodine. Does not appreciably raise protein bound iodine values.

Used as adjunctive treatment in bronchial asthma, bronchitis, emphysema, and other respiratory disorders and after surgery to help prevent atelectasis.

CONTRAINDICATIONS AND PRECAUTIONS. History of marked sensitivity to inorganic iodides; hypersensitivity to iodinated glycerol (or any of its ingredients) and related compounds; hypothyroidism.

Used with extreme caution if at all during pregnancy.

ADVERSE/SIDE EFFECTS. Rarely: GI irritation, rash, hypersensitivity, iodism (dose-related and reversible): coryza, headache, parotitis, ulcerations of mouth and throat, metallic taste, salivation.

ROUTE AND DOSAGE. Oral: Adults: 60 mg 4 times a day. **Children:** up to one-half the adult dosage, based on child's weight. Available as tablets (30 mg each), 5% solution (50 mg/ml), and elixir (60 mg/5 ml).

NURSING IMPLICATIONS

All preparations should be administered with liquid.

Drug should be discontinued if skin rash or other evidence of hypersensitivity occurs.

See Benzonatate for patient teaching points regarding cough therapy.

Diagnostic Test Interferences. Iodinated glycerol may depress **RAI uptake** values.

IODOCHLORHYDROXYQUIN

(Clioquinol, Quin III, Torofor, Vioform)

(eye-oh-doe-klor-hye-drox′ee-kwin)

Antiinfective (topical)

Antifungal

ACTIONS AND USES. Halogenated hydroxyquinoline with broad spectrum of antifungal and antibacterial activity. Available OTC.

Used topically for treatment of inflamed cutaneous conditions such as eczema, athlete's foot, and other fungal conditions. Available in fixed combination with nystatin (Nystaform).

ABSORPTION AND FATE. May be absorbed through skin. Some is excreted rapidly in urine in conjungated form; remainder is excreted slowly, persisting in body for 1 month or more.

CONTRAINDICATIONS AND PRECAUTIONS. Hypersensitivity to iodine or iodine-containing preparations; tuberculosis; vaccinia, varicella, or other viral skin conditions; severe renal disease; hepatic damage; thyroid disorder.

ADVERSE/SIDE EFFECTS. Infrequent: local burning, irritation, redness, swelling, itching, rash, staining of hair and skin. Systemic reactions (if used on large skin areas); iodism (furunculosis, dermatitis, chills, fever, sore throat, brassy taste, stomatitis, coryza, swelling of salivary glands), diarrhea, constipation, abdominal discomfort, slight enlargement of thyroid gland, hair loss, agranulocytosis, subacute myeloptic neuropathy.

ROUTE AND DOSAGE. Topical (3% cream, or ointment): apply thin layer to affected areas two or three times daily, for one week only.

NURSING IMPLICATIONS

Area to be treated is generally washed with soap and water, and dried thoroughly before each application. Consult physician.

Do not apply an occlusive dressing without a physician's order.

Systemic absorption may result from applications to widespread areas and use of occlusive dressings.

Inform patients that the drug may stain fabric, skin, or hair yellow on contact.

Warn patients to avoid contact of drug in or around eyes.

Drug should be discontinued if skin irritation, rash, or other signs of sensitivity, and systemic absorption develop.
Caution patient to apply the drug as directed and only for the period of time prescribed.
Preserved in tightly covered, light-resistant containers.

Diagnostic Test Interferences. Possibility of elevated **PBI** and decreased **I-131 thyroidal uptake.** False-positive ferric chloride test for phenylketonuria (**PKU**) may result if iodochlorhydroxyquin is present on diaper or in urine.

IODOQUINOL

(eye-oh-do-kwin′ole)

(Diiodohydroxyquin, Diiodhydroxyquinoline, Moebiquin, Sebaquin, Yodoxin)

Antiprotozoal, antiamebic

I J

ACTIONS AND USES. Dihalogenated derivative of 8-hydroxyquinoline chemically and pharmacologically related to Clioquinol (iodochlorhydroxyquin; not currently available in U.S.). Iodoquinol is a direct-acting (contact) amebicide effective against both trophozoites and cyst forms of *Entameba histolytica* in intestinal lumen. Not useful for extraintestinal amebiasis. Range of antiprotozoal action includes *Trichomonas vaginalis* and *Balantidium coli;* also has some antibacterial and antifungal properties. Contains approximately 64% organically bound iodine.

Used for treatment of intestinal amebiasis and for asymptomatic passers of cysts. Commonly used either concurrently or in alternating courses with another intestinal amebicide. Also used in treatment of balantidiasis and for *Acrodermatitis enteropathica,* and *Trichomonas vaginalis* vaginitis. Used in combination with hydrocortisone for treatment of various subacute and chronic dermatoses, e.g., Vytone.

ABSORPTION AND FATE. Small amount may be absorbed following oral administration evidenced by increase in blood iodine levels. Distribution and fate not known but believed drug is excreted in feces and urine.

CONTRAINDICATIONS AND PRECAUTIONS. Hypersensitivity to any 8-hydroxyquinoline or to iodine-containing preparations or foods; hepatic or renal damage, preexisting optic neuropathy, severe thyroid disease, use in treatment of nonspecific or "traveler's" diarrhea or minor self-limiting problems, prolonged high dosage therapy. Safe use during pregnancy and in nursing mothers not established.

ADVERSE/SIDE EFFECTS. CNS: headache, vertigo, ataxia. Associated with prolonged high dosages particularly in children: subacute myelo-optic neuropathy (SMON). Muscle pain, weakness usually below T_{12} vertebrae, dysesthesias especially of lower limbs, paresthesias, ataxia, blurred vision, optic atrophy, permanent loss of vision, psychological changes, greenish discoloration of tongue. **Dermatologic:** discoloration of hair and nails, acne, alopecia, urticaria, pruritus, various forms of skin eruptions. **GI:** nausea, vomiting, abdominal cramps, diarrhea, constipation, rectal irritation and itching. **Hypersensitivity:** urticaria, pruritus. **Other:** increased sense of warmth, thyroid hypertrophy, agranulocytosis, iodism: generalized furunculosis (iodine toxiderma), dermatitis, rhinitis, ptyalism, frontal headache, sore throat, chills, fever.

ROUTE AND DOSAGE. Oral: *Intestinal amebiasis:* **Adults:** 650 mg three times daily for 20 days. Course may be repeated after drug-free interval of 2 to 3 weeks. **Children:** 30 to 40 mg/kg divided into 2 or 3 doses for 20 days. Not to exceed 2 Gm/day.

NURSING IMPLICATIONS

Administer drug after meals to reduce GI irritation. If patient has difficulty swallowing tablet, it may be crushed and mixed with applesauce or chocolate syrup.

Monitor intake–output ratio. Record characteristics of stools: color, odor, consistency, frequency, presence of blood, mucus or other material.

Treatment also includes replacement of fluid and electrolytes as indicated by laboratory determinations.

It is advisable for patient to have ophthalmologic examinations at regular intervals during prolonged therapy.

If possible, stool specimens should be sent promptly to medical laboratory while still warm. Viability of parasite may be affected by urine, antacids, antidiarrheals, antibiotics, temperature change.

Family members and other suspected contacts should also have microscopic examination of feces.

Ideally, patient is discharged when three stool specimens repeated daily for 3 consecutive days are negative of parasites. Stool should be examined again in 1, 3, and 6 months after termination of treatment.

Instruct patient to report unexplained fever, sore mouth or throat, malaise, swollen glands (possible symptoms of agranulocytosis).

Intestinal amebiasis is spread mainly by contaminated water, raw fruits or vegetables, flies, roaches, and hand-to-mouth transfer of infected feces. Emphasize importance of handwashing after defecation and before eating.

Patient should be instructed not to prepare, process, or serve foods until treatment is completed.

Store preferably between 15° and 30°C (59° and 86°F) unless otherwise directed by manufacturer.

See Index: Nursing Interventions: amebiasis.

Diagnostic Test Interferences. Iodoquinol can cause elevations of **PBI** and decrease of **I-131 uptake** (effects may last for several weeks to 6 months after discontinuation of therapy). Ferric chloride test for **PKU** (phenylketonuria) may yield false-positive results if iodoquinol is present in urine.

IPECAC SYRUP

(ip′e-kak)
Emetic

ACTIONS AND USES. Derived from dried rhizomes and roots of *Cephaelis ipecacuanha.* Contains several alkaloids including cephaeline and emetine (methylcephaeline), of which emetine comprises over 50%. Acts locally on gastric mucosa and centrally on chemoreceptor trigger zone (CTZ) to induce vomiting. Also has expectorant action that is thought to result from increased bronchial secretions resulting from reflex stimulation of gastric mucosa.

Used as emergency emetic to remove unabsorbed ingested poisons. An ingredient in many OTC expectorant mixtures.

CONTRAINDICATIONS AND PRECAUTIONS. Comatose, semicomatose, inebriated, convulsing, deeply sedated patients; patients in shock; patients with depressed gag reflex; when danger of convulsions is present; impaired cardiac function; arteriosclerosis; for treatment of ingested strong alkalis, acids, or other corrosives; strychnine, petroleum distillates, volatile oils, or rapidly-acting CNS depressants; pregnancy (category C), during breast feeding.

ADVERSE/SIDE EFFECTS. *If drug is not vomited but absorbed, or for overdosage:* persistent vomiting, bloody diarrhea, shock, cardiac arrhythmias, cardiotoxicity, atrial fibrillation, fatal mycarditis, convulsions, coma.

ROUTE AND DOSAGE. Oral: Adults and children (over 1 year of age): 15 ml (3 teaspoonsful). Dose may be repeated once in 20 to 30 minutes, if vomiting has not occurred. **Children (less than 1 year of age):** 5 to 10 ml (1 to 2 teaspoonsful). Syrup contains alcohol.

NURSING IMPLICATIONS

Not to be confused with ipecac fluid extract, which is 14 times stronger and has caused deaths when mistakenly given at the same dosage as ipecac syrup.

Action of ipecac is facilitated by following the dose with 1 or 2 glasses of tepid water (adults), ½ to 1 glass for children. Avoid milk or carbonated beverages since they may delay emesis.

Emetic effect occurs in 15 to 30 minutes and continues for 20 to 25 minutes. If vomiting does not occur in 20 to 30 minutes, dose may be repeated once.

Activated charcoal should not be given simultaneously with ipecac because charcoal absorbs ipecac and renders it completely ineffective.

In small children, emetic effect is reportedly enhanced by gently bouncing the child.

Available without prescription in quantity of 30 ml for emergency use as emetic. Food and Drug Administration requires labeling to include the following cautions before use: call a physician, a poison control center, or a hospital emergency room immediately for advice before administering drug.

Keep the drug out of reach of children.

Ipecac may be ineffective if patient is also taking a drug with antiemetic action.

If vomiting does not occur within 15 to 20 minutes after the second dose, contact physician or emergency room immediately. Dosage should be recovered by gastric lavage, and activated charcoal, if necessary.

Stored in tight containers, preferably at temperature not exceeding 25°C (77°F).

IRON DEXTRAN

Antianemic

(Feostat, Feronim, Hematran, Hydextran, I.D. 50, Imferon, Irodex, K-Feron, Nor-Feran, Proferdex, Rocyte)

ACTIONS AND USES. A dark-brown slightly viscous liquid complex of ferric hydroxide with dextran in 0.9% sodium chloride solution for injection. Reticuloendothelial cells of liver, spleen, and bone marrow dissociate iron from iron dextran complex; the released ferric ion combines with transferrin, and is transported to bone marrow, where it is incorporated into hemoglobin.

Used only in patients with clearly established iron deficiency anemia when oral administration of iron is unsatisfactory or impossible. Each milliliter of iron dextran contains 50 mg elemental iron.

ABSORPTION AND FATE. Following IM administration, most of drug is absorbed from injection site through lymphatic system. The remainder (10 to 50%) becomes fixed locally and is gradually absorbed over several months or longer. Slowly cleared from plasma by reticuloendothelial system. Small amounts of iron dextran cross the placenta. Traces are excreted in breast milk, urine, bile, and feces.

CONTRAINDICATIONS AND PRECAUTIONS. Hypersensitivity to the product; all anemias except iron-deficiency anemia. Safe use during pregnancy and childbearing period not established. *Cautious Use:* rheumatoid arthritis, ankylosing spondylitis, impaired hepatic function, history of allergies and/or asthma.

ADVERSE/SIDE EFFECTS. CNS: headache, shivering, transient paresthesias, syncope, dizziness. **CV:** peripheral vascular flushing (rapid IV), hypotension, precordial pain or pressure sensation, tachycardia, fatal cardiac arrhythmias, circulatory collapse. **GI:** nausea, vomiting, metallic taste, abdominal pain. **Hypersensitivity:** urticaria, skin rash, pruritus, fever, chills, dyspnea, arthralgia, myalgia; fatal anaphylaxis. **Other:** sterile abscess and brown skin discoloration (IM site), local phlebitis (IV site), lymphadenopathy, hemosiderosis, risk of carcinogenesis at injection site associated with IM administration, reactivation of quiescent rheumatoid arthritis, exogenous hemosiderosis.

ROUTE AND DOSAGE. Iron dextran contains the equivalent of 50 mg elemental iron per ml. *Maximum recommended adult daily dose: 2 ml (100 mg) IM or IV.* Dosage determined from a table of correlations between patient's weight, hemoglobin and (ml) requirements for iron, or by an appropriate formula. For example,

$$0.3 \times \text{weight (lb)} \times \left(100 - \frac{\text{Hgb (Gm/dl)} \times 100}{14.8}\right) = \text{mg of iron}$$

To calculate dose in ml: divide by 50. Requirements of individuals weighing 30 lb or less should be reduced to 80% of the amount calculated by this formula. **Intramuscular:** Daily doses ordinarily do not exceed 0.5 ml (25 mg iron) for infants under 10 lb; 1.0 ml (50 mg iron) for children under 20 lb; 2.0 ml (100 mg iron) for other patients. **Intravenous (intermittent):** 2 ml or less daily.

NURSING IMPLICATIONS

Oral iron should be discontinued prior to iron dextran administration.

Diagnosis of iron-deficiency anemia should be corroborated by appropriate laboratory investigations, with the cause being determined and if possible corrected, before therapy is initiated.

Anticipated response to parenteral iron therapy is an average weekly hemoglobin rise of about 1 Gm/dl. As with oral therapy, peak levels are generally reached in about 4 to 8 weeks.

Regardless of route used, a test dose of 0.5 ml is given over a 5 minute period prior to the first IM or IV therapeutic dose to observe patient's response to the drug. If no reaction to the IM test dose occurs, after at least 1 hour, the remaining portion of initial dose is administered. If no reaction occurs after the IV test dose, the therapeutic regimen is started in 2 to 3 days. Fatal anaphylactic reactions have occurred. Epinephrine (0.5 ml of a 1:1000 solution) should be immediately available for hypersensitivity emergency.

Although anaphylactic reactions usually occur within a few minutes after injection, it is recommended that 1 hour or more elapse before giving remainder of initial dose following test dose.

IM injections should be given only into the muscle mass in upper outer quadrant of buttock (never in the upper arm or other exposed area). Use a 2- or 3-inch, 19- or 20-gauge needle. The Z-tract technique is recommended to prevent drug leakage along the needle track and brown staining of subcutaneous tissue. Staining of skin may also be minimized by using one needle to withdraw drug from container and another needle for injection. Brown staining of skin may persist 1 to 2 years, since drug is absorbed slowly from subcutaneous tissue.

Z-track technique: Firmly displace skin laterally prior to injection. After needle is inserted, withdraw plunger carefully to check that there is no entry into a blood vessel. Inject slowly. Rotate injection sites. No more than 5 ml should be injected into a single IM site.

If patient is receiving IM in standing position, patient should be bearing weight on the leg opposite the injection site; if in bed, patient should be in the lateral position with injection site uppermost.

The multiple-dose vial is used *only* for IM injections. Since it contains a preservative (phenol), it is not suitable for IV use.

Mixing any other drug in syringe or solution with iron dextran is not advised.

The IV route is preferred and recommended for patients with insufficient muscle mass, those with impaired absorption (as in edema), when uncontrolled bleeding is a possibility, or when massive and prolonged parenteral therapy is indicated.

If the IV injection does not exceed 100 mg, it is administered undiluted at a prescribed rate (usually no more than 50 mg or less per minute).

The diluent for IV infusion is 0.9% NaCl injection. (5% dextrose solution is associated with a higher incidence of phlebitis and local pain.) Increased frequency of adverse effects may be expected with large IV doses, particularly delayed reactions (arthralgia, myalgia, fever).

Following IV administration, the patient should remain in bed for at least 30 minutes to prevent orthostatic hypotension. Monitor blood pressure and pulse.

IV administration may exacerbate acute joint pain in patients with rheumatoid arthritis or ankylosing spondylitis. For this reason, the IM route is generally preferred in these patients.

Systemic reactions may occur over a 24-hour period after parenteral iron has been administered. Instruct patient to report any unusual symptoms.

Clinical response to iron dextran may be delayed if patient is also receiving chloramphenicol.

Periodic determinations of hemoglobin, hematocrit, and reticulocyte count should be made as a guide to therapy. Oral iron therapy should replace parenteral therapy as soon as feasible.

Blood typing and cross matching are reportedly not affected by iron dextran.

Diagnostic Test Interferences. Falsely elevated **serum bilirubin** and falsely decreased **serum calcium** values may occur. Large doses of iron dextran may impart a brown color to serum drawn 4 hours after iron administration. **Bone scans** involving Tc-99m diphosphonate have shown dense areas of activity along contour of iliac crest 1 to 6 days after IM injections of iron dextran.

ISOCARBOXAZID

(Marplan)

(eye-soe-kar-box'a-zid)
Psychotropic
Antidepressant
MAO inhibitor
Hydrazine

ACTIONS AND USES. MAO inhibitor of the hydrazine group. Similar in actions, uses, contraindications, precautions, and adverse reactions to phenelzine (qv).

Recommended only for treatment of depressed patients refractory to or intolerant to tricyclic antidepressants or to electroconvulsive therapy.

CONTRAINDICATIONS AND PRECAUTIONS. Children (under 16); elderly (over 60 years of age). *Cautious Use:* hypertension, hyperthyroidism, parkinsonism, renal impairment, cardiac arrhythmias. *See also Phenelzine.*

ROUTE AND DOSAGE. Oral: Initial: 30 mg daily in single or divided doses; maintenance: 10 to 20 mg (or less) daily. Doses larger than 30 mg daily not recommended.

NURSING IMPLICATIONS

A complete review of prior drug therapy is advised before initiation of isocarboxazid.

Most adverse reactions occur because of failure to recognize cumulative effects of isocarboxazid *(see Phenelzine sulfate).*

Therapeutic effects may be apparent within a week or less, but in some patients there may be time lag of 3 to 4 weeks before improvement occurs.

Dosage is individually adjusted on basis of careful observations of patient.

Physician will reduce dosage to maintenance level as soon as improvement is observed, because drug has a cumulative effect.

Advise patient to avoid alcoholic beverages.

Warn patient to adhere to established drug regimen, i.e., not to omit, increase, or decrease doses.

Although therapeutic effect is delayed, toxic symptoms from overdosage or from ingestion of contraindicated substances (e.g., foods high in tyramine) may occur within hours.

Store in a well closed, light-resistant container at temperature between 15° and 30°C (59° and 86°F).

See also Phenelzine sulfate (prototype MAO inhibitor).

I J

PROTOTYPE

ISOETHARINE HYDROCHLORIDE

(Arm-a-Med, Beta-2, Bronkosol, Dey-Lute, Dispos-a-Med)

ISOETHARINE MESYLATE

(Bronkometer)

(eye-soe-eth'a-reen)

Smooth muscle relaxant (respiratory)

Beta-adrenergic agonist

Bronchodilator

ACTIONS AND USES. Synthetic adrenergic stimulant with relatively rapid onset and long duration of action. Has selective affinity for $beta_2$ adrenoceptors on bronchial and selected arteriolar musculature, and a lower order of affinity for $beta_1$ receptors. Produces few cardiac side effects. Relieves reversible bronchospasm and by bronchodilation, facilitates expectoration of pulmonary secretions. Increases vital capacity and decreases airway resistance. May inhibit antigen-induced release of histamine.

Used as bronchodilator for bronchial asthma and for reversible bronchospasm occurring with bronchitis and emphysema.

ABSORPTION AND FATE. Onset of action, immediately after oral inhalation; peak effect in 5 to 15 minutes. Duration of action: 1 to 4 hours. Metabolized in lungs, liver, GI tract, and other tissues. Excreted by kidneys; about 10% as unchanged drug.

CONTRAINDICATIONS AND PRECAUTIONS. Known hypersensitivity to sympathomimetic amines and to bisulfites; concomitant use with epinephrine or other sympathomimetic amines; patients with preexisting cardiac arrhythmias associated with tachycardia. Use during pregnancy (category C), lactation, or by women of childbearing age requires judgment of risk/benefit ratio. *Cautious Use:* elderly patients; hypertension, acute coronary artery disease, congestive heart failure, cardiac asthma, hyperthyroidism, diabetes mellitus, tuberculosis; history of seizures.

ADVERSE/SIDE EFFECTS. Tachycardia, palpitations, changes in blood pressure, nausea, headache, anxiety, tension, restlessness, insomnia, tremor, weakness, dizziness, excitement, cardiac arrest.

ROUTE AND DOSAGE. Treatments are usually not repeated more often than every 4 hours, except in severe cases. **Inhalation (Hydrochloride):** *Hand nebulizer:* 3 to 7 inhalations undiluted. *Oxygen aerolization; IPPB:* 0.25 to 1 ml diluted 1:3 with sterile normal saline or other prescribed sterile diluent. *Metered dose nebulizer* (Mesylate): 1 or 2 inhalations every 4 hours if necessary. (Bronkometer delivers 340 mcg per metered dose.)

NURSING IMPLICATIONS

The preservative sodium bisulfite is in the hydrochloride formulation. If patient has an allergic history to sulfiting agents, this product should be avoided. Symptoms of throat irritation, chest tightness and wheezing following nebulized drug suggest an allergy.

Oxygen aerosolization: Special recommendations for administration: Oxygen flow rate: 4 to 6 L/minute over period of 15 to 20 minutes. *IPPB:* inspiratory flow rate of 15 L/minute at cycling pressure of 15 cm water. Highly individualized.

Administer therapy on arising in morning and before meals to reduce fatigue from activity by improving lung ventilation.

Instruct patient to wait 1 full minute after initial 1 to 2 inhalations (Bronkometer) to be sure of necessity for another dose. Action should begin immediately and peak within 5 to 15 minutes.

Caution patient to keep spray away from eyes.

Urge patient to increase daily fluid intake to aid in liquefaction of bronchial secretions. In addition to coughing and breathing exercises, physician may prescribe postural drainage, and chest vibration and percussion to promote mobilization of secretions.

Caution patient to use inhalation therapy according to prescribed regimen. If symptoms being treated fail to respond, consult physician. Overuse because of inadequate relief, may decrease desired effect and cause symptoms including tachycardia, palpitations, headache, nausea, dizziness.

For unknown reasons, paradoxical airway resistance (manifested by sudden increase in dyspnea) may occur with repeated excessive use. Should this occur, instruct patient/family to discontinue isoetharine and report to physician for alternative therapy (such as epinephrine).

Isoetharine inhalation may be alternated with epinephrine administration if necessary, but not administered simultaneously because of danger of excessive tachycardia.

Elderly patients may be especially sensitive to adrenergic drug effects.

Remind patient not to discard drug applicator. Refill units are available.

Information and instructions are furnished with the aerosol form of isoetharine. Urge patient to read and ask questions if necessary.

Do not use discolored or precipitated solutions.

Protect solutions from light, freezing, and heat. Store at controlled room temperature.

See Isoproterenol for additional nursing points related to aerosol therapy.

Drug Interactions: Isoetharine

Plus	Interactions
Propranolol (Inderal)	May antagonize bronchodilation effect of isoetharine
Sympathomimetics (epinephrine and others)	Increased drug effects and possibility of toxicity of both isoetharine and the sympathomimetic agent

PROTOTYPE

ISONIAZID

(INH, Isonicotinic Acid Hydrazide, Isotamine, Laniazid, Nydrazid, Rimifon, Teebaconin)

(eye-soe-nye'a-zid)
Antiinfective
Antituberculosis agent

ACTIONS AND USES. Hydrazide of isonicotinic acid with highly specific action against *Mycobacterium tuberculosis.* Exerts bacteriostatic action against actively growing tubercle bacilli; may be bactericidal in higher concentrations. Postulated to act by interfering with biosynthesis of bacterial proteins, nucleic acid, and lipids. Reported to have some MAO-inhibiting properties and to act as a competitive antagonist of pyridoxine (vitamin B_6).

Used in treatment of all forms of active tuberculosis caused by susceptible organisms and as preventive in high-risk persons (e.g., household members, persons with positive tuberculin skin test reactions). May be used alone or with other tuberculostatic agents. Available in fixed combination with pyridoxine (P-I-N Forte and others), and with rifampin (Rifamate).

I J

ABSORPTION AND FATE. Peak blood levels in 1 to 2 hours following oral administration and sooner following IM injection. Levels decline to 50% or less within 6 hours. Diffuses readily into body tissues, organs and fluids, notably saliva, bronchial secretions, and pleural, ascitic, and cerebrospinal fluids. Metabolized in liver primarily by acetylation and dehydrazination (rate of acetylation is genetically determined). Half-life 2 to 5 hours in hepatic insufficiency and in "slow" inactivators, and 0.5 to 1.6 hours in fast inactivators. About 75 to 95% of dose is excreted in urine within 24 hours as metabolites; small amounts executed in saliva and feces. Crosses placenta and passes into breast milk.

CONTRAINDICATIONS AND PRECAUTIONS. History of isoniazid-associated hypersensitivity reactions, including hepatic injury; acute liver damage of any etiology; pregnancy (unless risk is warranted). *Cautious Use:* chronic liver disease, renal dysfunction, history of convulsive disorders.

ADVERSE/SIDE EFFECTS. Usually dose-related. **GI:** nausea, vomiting, epigastric distress, constipation. **Hematologic:** agranulocytosis, hemolytic or aplastic anemia, thrombocytopenia, eosinophilia, methemoglobinemia. **Hepatotoxicity:** elevated SGOT and SGPT, bilirubinemia, jaundice, fatal hepatitis. **Hypersensitivity:** fever, chills, skin eruptions (morbiliform, maculopapular, purpuric, urticarial), lymphadenitis, vasculitis, keratitis. **Metabolic and endocrine:** decreased vitamin B_{12} absorption, pyridoxine (vitamin B_6) deficiency, pellagra, gynecomastia, hyperglycemia, glycosuria, hyperkalemia, acetonuria, metabolic acidosis, proteinuria. **Neurologic:** paresthesias, peripheral neuropathy, visual disturbances, optic neuritis and atrophy, tinnitus, vertigo, ataxia, somnolence, excessive dreaming, insomnia, amnesia, euphoria, toxic psychosis, changes in affect and behavior, depression impaired memory, hyperreflexia, muscle twitching, convulsions. **Other:** headache, tachycardia, dyspnea, dry mouth, urinary retention (males), postural hypotension, rheumatic and lupus-erythematosus-like syndromes, irritation at injection site. **Overdosage:** dizziness, nausea, vomiting, slurred speech, visual hallucinations, blurred vision, respiratory distress, CNS depression, convulsions, stupor.

ROUTE AND DOSAGE. Oral, intramuscular: (dosages are identical). Administered in single or divided doses. *Treatment:* **Adults:** 5 mg/kg body weight (up to 300 mg) daily. **Infants and children:** 10 to 20 mg/kg (up to 300 to 500 mg) daily. *Preventive therapy:* **Adults:** 300 mg daily. **Infants and children:** 10 mg/kg (up to 300 mg) daily.

NURSING IMPLICATIONS

Oral isoniazid is best taken on an empty stomach since food interferes with its absorption. However, if GI irritation occurs, drug may be taken with meals.

Isoniazid in solution tends to crystallize at low temperatures; if this occurs, solution should be allowed to warm to room temperature to redissolve crystals prior to use.

Local transient pain may follow IM injections. Massage injection site following drug administration. Rotate injection sites.

Appropriate mycobacteriologic studies and susceptibility tests should be performed before initiation of therapy and periodically thereafter to detect possible bacterial resistance.

Vision testing and ophthalmoscopic examinations are recommended initially, periodically during drug therapy, and whenever visual symptoms appear. Early cessation of therapy usually results in resolution of ocular reactions.

Adverse reactions occur most frequently in malnourished patients, the elderly, and in "slow" isoniazid inactivators (acetylators). Rate of acetylation (a metabolic process) is genetically determined and affects plasma drug concentration. Slow acetylation leads to high plasma drug levels and thus to increased risk of toxicity. Approximately 50% of blacks and Caucasians are "slow" inactivators; the majority of American Indians, Eskimos, and Orientals are "rapid" inactivators.

Food–Drug Interactions:

- Warn patient that concurrent ingestion of tyramine-containing foods (e.g., aged cheeses, smoked fish) may cause palpitation, flushing, and blood pressure elevation (possibly by isoniazid-induced MAO inhibition).
- Warn patient that histamine-containing foods (e.g., skipjack, tuna, sauerkraut juice, yeast extracts) may cause exaggerated drug response (headache, hypotension, palpitation, sweating, itching, flushing, diarrhea) possibly by isoniazid inhibition of diamine oxidase.
- Isoniazid-induced pyridoxine (vitamin B_6) depletion causes neurotoxic effects. B_6 supplementation usually accompanies isoniazid use.
- Niacin (vitamin B_3) and folate stores are also decreased during isoniazid therapy.

Peripheral neuritis, the most common vitamin B_{12} deficiency symptom, is usually preceded by paresthesias of feet and hands (numbness, tingling, burning). Patients particularly susceptible include malnourished patients, diabetics, adolescents, and "slow acetylators."

Monitor tuberculin precipitation reaction and blood pressure during period of dosage adjustment. Some patients experience orthostatic hypotension; therefore, caution against rapid positional changes. Supervision of ambulation may be indicated, particularly in the elderly.

Diabetic patients should be observed for loss of diabetes control. Both true glycosuria and false-positive Benedict's tests have been reported. *See Diagnostic Test Interferences.*

Isoniazid hepatitis (sometimes fatal) usually develops during the first 4 to 6 months of treatment, but it may occur at any time during drug therapy; it is most common in patients 50 years of age and older in those who ingest alcohol daily, and possibly in rapid acetylators.

Continuation of isoniazid therapy after the onset of hepatic dysfunction increases risk of severe liver damage.

Patients should be carefully interviewed and examined at monthly intervals for early detection of signs and symptoms of hepatotoxicity (loss of appetite, fatigue, malaise, nausea, vomiting, abdominal discomfort, dark urine, jaundice or scleral icterus). Instruct patient to withhold medication and report promptly to physician if any of these effects occur. Some physicians order monthly liver function tests throughout therapy.

Advise patient to reduce alcohol intake while on isoniazid therapy because of increased risk of hepatotoxicity *(see Drug Interactions).*

Hypersensitivity reactions should be reported immediately and all drugs withheld. Generally, they occur within 3 to 7 weeks following initiation of therapy.

Therapeutic effects of isoniazid usually become evident within the first 2 to 3 weeks of therapy and may include reduction of fever and night sweats, diminished cough and sputum, increased appetite and weight gain, reduction of fatigue, and sense of well-being. Over 90% of patients receiving optimal therapy have negative sputum by the 6th month.

Check weight at least twice weekly under standard conditions.

Isoniazid may produce a sense of euphoria, which tempts the patient to do more than he or she should. Stress the importance of planned rest periods.

Antituberculous agents permit therapy to continue on an outpatient basis after initial hospitalization. Patients and responsible family members must understand the importance of continuous medical supervision to follow course of disease, and uninterrupted drug therapy to prevent relapse and spread of infection to others.

In general, isoniazid therapy is continued for a minimum of 18 months to 2 years for original treatment of active tuberculosis. When used for preventive therapy, isoniazid is usually continued for 12 months. Duration of treatment is shorter (minimum of 9 months) when both isoniazid and rifampin are used.

Pyridoxine (IV) is a specific antidote for isoniazid overdosage.

Preserved in tightly closed, light-resistant containers at 15° to 30°C (59° to 86°F) unless otherwise directed by manufacturer.

I J

Diagnostic Test Interferences. Isoniazid may produce false-positive results using **Benedict's solution,** but usually not with Clinitest or glucose oxidase methods (e.g., Clinstix, Dextrostix, Tes-Tape); urinary excretion of **5-HIAA** may be decreased in patients with carcinoid syndrome.

Drug Interactions. Daily ingestion of **alcohol** may increase risk of isoniazid-induced hepatotoxicity. Simultaneous administration of large doses of **aluminum hydroxide** and other aluminum-containing antacids may delay or decrease absorption of isoniazid; to minimize risk of interaction, schedule isoniazid at least 1 hour prior to antacid and administration. **Aminosalicylic acid** (PAS) reduces rate of isoniazid acetylation and thus may result in higher blood levels. **Cycloserine** and **ethionamide** increase risk of CNS toxicity (dizziness, drowsiness). **Disulfiram:** concurrent use with isoniazid may result in changes in coordination, affect, and behavior. **Rifampin** increases risk of hepatotoxicity. Concurrent administration of isoniazid and **phenytoin** (and possibly other hydantoin derivatives) may result in a significant rise in serum phenytoin levels and toxicity (ataxia, drowsiness, nystagmus); reduced phenytoin dosage is recommended in "slow acetylators" particularly, with isoniazid is added to the therapeutic regimen.

ISOPROPAMIDE IODIDE

(Darbid)

(eye-soe-proe'pa-mide)
Anticholinergic
Antispasmodic

ACTIONS AND USES. Synthetic quaternary ammonium compound; long acting anticholinergic with actions similar to those of atropine (qv).

Used primarily for adjunctive treatment of peptic ulcer. Probably effective in irritable bowel syndrome (irritable colon, spastic colon, mucous colitis and functional GI disorders), and urinary spasm. *See Atropine.*

CONTRAINDICATIONS AND PRECAUTIONS. Hypersensitivity to iodine, tachycardia, obstructive uropathy, obstructive diseases of GI tract, paralytic ileus, myasthenia gravis, pregnancy (category C). *Cautious Use:* elderly patients, autonomic neuropathy, hepatic and renal disease, ulcerative colitis, hyperthyroidism, coronary disease, hypertension, cardiac arrhythmias, children under 12 years of age. *See also Atropine.*

ADVERSE/SIDE EFFECTS. Iodine skin rash (rare): acneiform eruptions, exfoliative dermatitis, drowsiness, headache, constipation, suppression of lactation. **Overdosage:** depression, circulatory collapse, curarelike action: weakness in short muscles (i.e., eye, eyelids, fingers and toes) and in muscles of jaw, neck, leg; hypotension. *See also Atropine.*

ROUTE AND DOSAGE. Oral: Adults and children (over 12 years): 5 to 10 mg every 12 hours.

NURSING IMPLICATIONS

Isopropamide may alter PBI level and suppress I-131 uptake; therefore drug is discontinued 1 week before these tests are made. Patient should inform a new physician that patient is taking this drug.

If patient is on continuous therapy, teach patient to check pulse periodically. Advise consultation with physician if pulse rate increases above 96 beats/minute.

Patient should understand importance of prompt reporting of the following symptoms: hazy vision, drooping of eyelids, weakness in hand muscles. While these curarelike symptoms seldom occur, their appearance necessitates discontinuation of the drug.

Preserve drug in well closed, light-resistant container.

See also Atropine sulfate (prototype antispasmodic).

ISOPROTERENOL HYDROCHLORIDE

(Aerolone, Dey-Dose, Dispos-a-Med, Isuprel, Norisodrine Aerotrol)

ISOPROTERENOL SULFATE

(Medihaler-Iso, Norisodrine Sulfate)

(eye-soe-proe-ter′e-nole)
Adrenergic agonist (beta)
Sympathamimetic
Bronchodilator

ACTIONS AND USES. Synthetic direct-acting sympathomimetic amine chemically and pharmacologically similar to epinephrine, but acts almost exclusively on beta-adrenergic receptors. Primary therapeutic effects include cardiac stimulation (positive inotropic and chronotropic actions), relaxation of bronchial tree, and peripheral vasodilation. Usually increases cardiac output and work, but may diminish efficiency. Lowers peripheral vascular resistance, and increases venous return to heart. Decreases both diastolic and mean pressures, but maintains or slightly increases systolic pressure, especially when patient is in shock. Large doses cause substantial drop in blood pressure, and repeated large doses may result in cardiac enlargement and focal myocarditis. Relaxes GI and uterine smooth muscles; inhibits histamine release. Increases hepatic glycogenolysis; but, unlike epinephrine, stimulates insulin secretion and thus rarely produces hyperglycemia. Can also cause central excitation.

Used as bronchodilator in acute and chronic asthma and other respiratory disorders and in bronchospasm induced by anesthesia. Effective as cardiac stimulant in cardiac arrest, carotid sinus hypersensitivity, cardiogenic and bacteremic shock, Stokes-Adams syndrome, or ventricular arrhythmias due to A-V block. Also may be used in treatment of shock which persists after adequate fluid replacement.

ABSORPTION AND FATE. Readily absorbed following parenteral injection and oral inhalation. Absorption following oral, sublingual, and rectal routes reportedly not as predictable. Bronchodilation occurs promptly and persists 1 to 2 hours following inhalation and sublingual tablet (variable), up to 2 hours following subcutaneous injection, and 2 to 4 hours following rectal administration. Pharmacologic action appears to terminate primarily by tissue uptake. Metabolized by conjugation in GI tract, liver, lungs, and other tissues. Metabolism in children may be more rapid and extensive. Secreted in urine within 24 to 48 hours. Small quantities of inactive metabolites excreted in feces.

CONTRAINDICATIONS AND PRECAUTIONS. Preexisting cardiac arrhythmias associated with tachycardia; central hyperexcitability, simultaneous use with epinephrine. Safe use in women of childbearing potential and during pregnancy (category C) and lactation not established. *Cautious Use:* sensitivity to sympathomimetic amines, elderly and debilitated patients, hypertension, coronary insufficiency and other cardiovascular disease, renal dysfunction, hyperthyroidism, diabetes, prostatic hypertrophy, glaucoma, tuberculosis.

ADVERSE/SIDE EFFECTS. CNS: headache, mild tremors, nervousness, anxiety, lightheadedness, vertigo, insomnia, excitement, weakness, fatigue. **CV:** flushing, palpitation, tachycardia, paradoxic Stokes-Adams seizure (rare), precordial pain or distress. **GI:** nausea, vomiting, swelling of parotids (prolonged use), bad taste, buccal ulcerations (sublingual administration). **Other:** severe prolonged asthma attack, sweating, bronchial irritation and edema (particularly with inhalations of powder). **Overdosage:** cardiac excitability, extrasystoles, arrhythmias, elevation followed by fall in blood pressure, severe bronchoconstriction, cardiac arrest, sudden death (especially following excessive use of aerosols).

ROUTE AND DOSAGE. Isoproterenol hydrochloride: Inhalation: *Metered-dose nebulizer* (120 to 250 mcg): Start with 1 inhalation; if no relief after 2 to 5 minutes, inhalation may be repeated. Maintenance: 1 or 2 inhalations four to six times daily at not less than 3- to 4-hour intervals. No more than 2 inhalations at any one time. *Hand-bulb nebulizer* (1:200 solution): 5 to 15 deep inhalations; (1:100 solution): 3 to 7 deep inhalations. If necessary, repeated once after 5 to 10 minutes. Treatment intervals not less than 3 to 4 hours up to five times daily. *Nebulization by oxygen, compressed air, or IPPB apparatus:* 0.5 ml of 1:200 solution diluted to 2 to 2.5 ml with water or isotonic saline. Flow rate regulated to administer over 10 to 20 minutes; may be repeated up to five times daily, if necessary. **Sublingual, rectal Adults:** 10 to 20 mg three or four times daily; maximum 60 mg/day; **(children):** 5 to 10 mg three or four times daily; maximum 30 mg/day. **Subcutaneous:** 0.15 to 0.2 mg. **Intramuscular:** 0.02 to 1 mg. **Intravenous infusion:** 5 mcg/minute, 1:250,000 solution. **Intravenous (direct):** 0.01 to 0.2 mg (0.5 to 1.0 ml) of 1:50,000 solution. **Intracardiac:** 0.02 mg. **Isoproterenol sulfate:** *Metered powder inhaler* (strength per inhalation is product-specific): 1 or 2 inhalations of normal depth; if necessary, second dose repeated in 5 minutes and third dose 10 minutes after second dose; not to exceed three doses for each attack. *Metered aerosol nebulizer* (1:800 to 1:1000): start with 1 inhalation; if necessary, repeat after 2 to 5 minutes; maintenance: 1 or 2 inhalations four to six times daily, not to exceed 2 inhalations at any one time or more than 6 inhalations in an hour.

NURSING IMPLICATIONS

IV administration is regulated by continuous ECG monitoring.

Patient must be observed constantly, and response to therapy must be carefully monitored by frequent determinations of heart rate, ECG pattern, blood pressure, and central venous pressure, as well as (for patients with shock) urine volume, blood pH, and Pco_2 levels.

IV infusion rate should be prescribed by physician, with specific guidelines for regulating flow or terminating infusion in relation to heart rate, premature beats, ECG changes, precordial distress, BP, and urine flow. Rate of infusion is generally decreased or infusion may be temporarily discontinued if heart rate exceeds 110 beats/minute because of the danger of precipitating arrhythmias.

Constant-infusion pump apparatus is recommended to prevent sudden influx of large amounts of drug.

Facilities for administration of oxygen mixtures and respiratory assistance should be immediately available.

High frequency of arrhythmias reported, particularly when administered IV to patients with cardiogenic shock or ischemic heart disease, digitalized patients, and those with electrolyte imbalance.

Intracardiac injection for cardiac standstill must be accompanied by cardiac massage to perfuse drug to myocardium.

Solutions intended for oral inhalation must not be injected.

Sublingual tablet: Patient should be forewarned of potential transient facial flushing, palpitation, and precordial discomfort. (Systemic effects reported to occur more frequently by this route than by inhalation.)

Sublingual tablet administration: Instruct patient to allow tablet to dissolve under tongue, without sucking, and not to swallow saliva (may cause epigastric pain) until drug has been completely absorbed.

Sublingual tablet may be administered rectally, if prescribed.

Prolonged use of sublingual tablets reportedly can damage teeth, possibly because of drug acidity. Patient should be advised to rinse mouth with water after medication has completely absorbed and between doses.

Patient-Teaching Instructions: Drug Inhalation

Note that dosage and recommended method of inhaling may vary with type of nebulizer and formulation used. Patient should be carefully instructed in use of nebulizer and cautioned to take the lowest effective dose necessary to obtain relief.

- ✓ Treatment should start with first symptoms of bronchospasm.
- ✓ *Administration by metered-dose nebulizers:* Shake cannister thoroughly to activate; place mouthpiece well into mouth, aimed at back of throat. Close lips and teeth around mouthpiece. Exhale through nose as completely as possible, then inhale through mouth slowly and deeply while actuating the nebulizer to release dose. Hold breath 10 seconds, (count 1 to 100, 2 to 100, 3 to 100 until 10 to 100 is reached); remove mouth piece, and then exhale slowly.
- ✓ *Administration by metered powder inhaler:* Caution patient *not* to take forced deep breathing, but to breathe with normal force and depth. Observe patient closely for exaggerated systemic drug action.
- ✓ Patients requiring more than 3 aerosol treatments within 24 hours should be under close medical supervision.
- ✓ *Administration by oxygen aerosolization:* Administered over 15- to 20-minute period, generally, with oxygen flow rate adjusted to 4 liters/minute. Turn on oxygen supply before patient places nebulizer in mouth. Lips need not be closed tightly around nebulizer opening. Placement of Y tube in rubber tubing permits patient to control administration.
- ✓ Advise patient to rinse mouth immediately after inhalation therapy to help prevent dryness and throat irritation.

✓ Rinse mouthpiece thoroughly with warm running water at least once daily to prevent clogging. (It is not dishwasher safe.) After cleaning, wait until mouthpiece is completely dry before storing. Do not place near artificial heat (dishwasher or oven). It is recommended that the reservoir bag be replaced every 2 or 3 weeks or as needed; replace mouthpiece every 6 to 9 months or as needed. Replacement of bags or mouthpieces may require a prescription.

✓ Check agency procedure for daily cleansing of IPPB nebulizer cup.

✓ Volume of solution placed in nebulizer should be sufficient for not more than 1 day's supply. Change solution daily.

✓ Inform patient that saliva and sputum may appear pink following inhalation treatment.

Tolerance to bronchodilating effect and cardiac stimulant effect may develop with prolonged or too frequent use, and rebound bronchospasm may occur when effects of drug end.

Caution patient to take medication as prescribed, and advise patient to report to physician if usual dosage does not produce expected relief. Once tolerance has developed, continued use can result in serious adverse effects.

Parotid swelling following prolonged use has been reported. Drug should be discontinued if this occurs.

Inform patient taking repeated doses (as well as responsible family members) about adverse reactions, and advise them to report onset of such reactions to physician.

Some isoproterenol products contain bisulfites or metabisulfites. These products should not be used by the patient with known allergy to sulfites. Check label.

Preserved in tight, light-resistant containers preferably between 15° and 30°C (59° and 86°F) unless otherwise directed by manufacturer. Isoproterenol solutions lose potency with standing, and solutions gradually become pink to brownish pink from exposure to air, light, or heat or contact with metal or alkali. Do not use if precipitate or discoloration is present.

Drug Interactions. Effects of isoproterenol are antagonized by **propranolol** and other beta-adrenergic blocking agents. Possibility of additive effects and increased cardiotoxicity when administered concomitantly with **epinephrine** and most other sympathomimetic bronchodilators (may be prevented if given at least 4 hours apart). Administration of isoproterenol in patients receiving **tricyclic antidepressants** may increase the possibility of arrhythmias.

ISOSORBIDE

(Ismotic)

(eye-soe-sor'bide)

Diuretic, osmotic

ACTIONS AND USES. Actions similar to those of other osmotic agents, e.g., mannitol, but produces greater diuresis and does not cause hyperglycemia. Reduces intraocular pressure by increasing plasma osmotic pressure. Commercial preparation contains sodium 105 mEq, and potassium 34 mEq.

Used for short-term emergency treatment of acute angle-closure glaucoma, and for reducing intraocular pressure prior to and after surgery for glaucoma and cataract.

ABSORPTION AND FATE. Rapidly absorbed following oral administration. Onset of action within 30 minutes. Peak effect in 1 to 1½ hours; duration up to 5 or 6 hours. Eliminated unchanged via kidneys.

CONTRAINDICATIONS AND PRECAUTIONS. Severe renal disease, anuria, severe dehydration, frank or impending pulmonary edema, hemorrhagic glaucoma. Safe use during pregnancy not established. *Cautious Use:* disease associated with salt retention.

ADVERSE/SIDE EFFECTS. CNS: headache, lethargy, vertigo, lightheadedness, syncope, irritability. **GI:** nausea, vomiting, diarrhea, anorexia, gastric discomfort. **Other:** thirst, hiccoughs, rash, hypernatremia, hyperosmolality.

ROUTE AND DOSAGE. Oral: Initial: 1.5 Gm/kg; usual range 1 to 3 Gm/kg two to four times a day.

NURSING IMPLICATIONS

Not to be confused with isosorbide dinitrate, an antianginal drug.

Isosorbide may be more palatable if poured over cracked ice and sipped.

Fluid and electrolyte balance should be carefully maintained during therapy.

Monitor intake and output. Report oliguria or significant changes in intake and output ratio.

ISOSORBIDE DINITRATE

(eye-soe-sor'bide)

(Apo-ISDN, Coronex, Iso-Bid, Isonate, Isordil, Isotrate, Novosorbide, Onset, Sorate, Sorbide, Sorbitrate)

Vasodilator (coronary)
Antianginal
Nitrate

ACTIONS AND USES. Organic nitrate with pharmacologic actions similar to those of nitroglycerin (qv). Mechanism of action not specifically understood. Relaxes vascular smooth muscle with resulting vasodilation. Dilation of peripheral blood vessels tends to cause peripheral pooling of blood, decrease in venous return to heart, decrease in left ventricular end-diastolic pressure, and consequent reduction in myocardial oxygen consumption. Cross tolerance with other nitrates possible.

Used for relief of acute anginal attacks and for management of long-term angina pectoris. Has been used alone or in combination with a cardiac glycoside or with other vasodilators, e.g., hydralazine, prazosin, for treatment of refractory congestive heart failure.

ABSORPTION AND FATE. Well absorbed from sublingual mucosa; onset of antianginal action in 2 to 5 minutes with duration of 1 to 2 hours. For conventional oral tablet onset of action in 15 to 30 minutes; duration 4 to 6 hours. For chewable tablet, onset of action is within 3 minutes, duration ½ to 3 hours. For sustained-action form duration of action is 6 to 12 hours. Approximately 80 to 100% of amount absorbed is excreted in urine within 24 hours, usually as metabolite.

CONTRAINDICATIONS AND PRECAUTIONS. Hypersensitivity to nitrates or nitrites; severe anemia, increased intracranial pressure. Safe use during pregnancy (category C) and in nursing mothers not established. *Cautious Use:* glaucoma, hypotension.

ADVERSE/SIDE EFFECTS. Flushing, headache, dizziness, weakness, postural hypotension sometimes accompanied by nausea, vomiting; restlessness, pallor, perspiration, palpitation, tachycardia, rash, exfoliative dermatitis, paradoxical increase in anginal pain. *See Nitroglycerin.*

ROUTE AND DOSAGE. Oral: *Conventional tablet:* 5 to 30 mg (average 10 to 20 mg) four times daily before meals and at bedtime; for prophylaxis only. *Sublingual tablet:* 2.5 to 10 mg every 2 to 3 hours as needed for prompt relief of acute anginal pain, or every 4 to 6 hours for prophylaxis. *Chewable tablet:* initially 5 mg. If significant hypotension does not occur dosage may be increased as necessary. For relief of acute attack take as needed. For prophylaxis take every 2 to 3 hours. *Sustained action form:* 40 mg every 6 to 12 hours (for prophylaxis only).

NURSING IMPLICATIONS

Not to be confused with isosorbide, an oral osmotic diuretic.

Best taken on an empty stomach (1 hour before or 2 hours after meals). If patient complains of vascular headache, however, it may be taken with meals.

Patient should be sitting when taking rapid acting forms of isosorbide dinitrate (sublingual and chewable tablets).

Advise patient not to eat, drink, talk, or smoke while sublingual tablet is under tongue.

Chewable tablet must be thoroughly chewed before swallowing.

Sustained release forms should be swallowed whole and not crushed or chewed.

Therapeutic effectiveness of isosorbide dinitrate may be evaluated by having patient keep a record of anginal attacks and the number of sublingual tablets required to provide relief.

Note that certain formulations of isosorbide dinitrate, e.g., Sorbitrate, contain *tartrazine* which can cause allergic response including bronchial asthma in susceptible individuals. The reaction is frequently seen in patients with aspirin hypersensitivity.

Caution patient to make position changes slowly, particularly from recumbent to upright posture, and to dangle and move feet and ankles for a few minutes before ambulating. Also advise patient to avoid very hot showers or tub baths, strenuous exercise in hot weather, and standing still.

Instruct patient to sit down at the first indication of lightheadedness or faintness. Deep breathing and movement of arms and legs may help to hasten recovery.

Headaches tend to decrease in intensity and frequency with continued therapy, but may require administration of analgesic (acetaminophen or aspirin) and reduction in dosage. If severe headaches persist, drug discontinuation may be necessary.

Chronic administration of large doses may produce tolerance and thus decrease effectiveness of nitrate preparations. Advise patient to report any reduction in drug effect.

Advise patient not to drink alcohol because it may increase possibility of lightheadedness and faintness.

Store in well-closed container in a cool dry place, preferably between 15° and 30°C (59° and 86°F) unless otherwise directed by manufacturer.

See Nitroglycerin (prototype nitrate).

Drug Interactions. Isosorbide dinitrate antagonizes the effects of **acetylcholine, histamine,** and **norepinephrine. Alcohol** may enhance hypotensive effect and lead to cardiovascular collapse. *See also Nitroglycerin.*

ISOTRETINOIN

(Accutane, 13-cis-Retinoic acid)

(eye-soe-tret′i-noyn)
Cell stimulant
Vitamin A isomer
Retinoid

ACTIONS AND USES. Highly toxic metabolite of retinol (vitamin A). Principal actions: regulation of cell (e.g., epithelial) differentiation and proliferation, and altered lipid composition on skin surface. Decreases sebum secretion by reducing sebaceous gland size, inhibits gland cell differentiation, and blocks follicular keratinization. Composition of liquid sebum is changed during treatment but restored to pretreatment composition at end of therapy. Prolonged clinical remissions that occur in many patients may be secondary to additional action mechanisms: antiinflammatory, antibacterial, antineoplastic. Shares with other retinoids immunoadjuvant activity which leads to increased production and cytotoxic effects of lymphocytes. Female patients with severe facial acne seem to respond to treatment better than males, especially if the latter have trunk acne.

Used for treatment of severe recalcitrant cystic and/or conglobate acne in patient unresponsive to conventional treatment, including systemic antibiotics. *Unlabeled Uses:* lamellar ichthyosis, hyperkeratosis, acne rosacea, scarring gram-negative folliculitis, and adjuvant therapy of basal cell carcinoma of the lung and cutaneous T-cell lymphoma (mycosis fungoides).

ABSORPTION AND FATE. Peak plasma concentration demonstrated in about 3 hours followed by a rapid decrease. Distributed to all tissues but is not stored. Steady state concentration averages 160 ng/ml on an 80-mg/day dose; 99.9% is protein bound. Major metabolite, 4-oxo-isotretinoin, exceeds isotretinoin concentration after 6 hours. Half-life of the metabolite: 11 to 50 hours. 65 to 85% of an 80-mg dose excreted in urine and feces (enterohepatic circulation probably occurs). Crosses placenta; enters milk.

CONTRAINDICATIONS AND PRECAUTIONS. Pregnancy (category X), sensitivity to parabens (preservatives in the formulation), nursing mothers. *Cautious Use:* coronary artery disease, diabetes mellitus, obesity, alcoholism, rheumatologic disorders, history of pancreatitis, hepatitis.

ADVERSE/SIDE EFFECTS. (Most are dose-related i.e., occurring at doses above 1 mg/kg/day; and reversible with termination of therapy.) **CNS:** lethargy, headache, insomnia, fatigue, paresthesias, dizziness, visual disturbances, papilledema. **Dermatologic:** cheilitis, skin fragility, dry skin, pruritus, peeling of palms and soles, photosensitivity (photoallergic and phototoxic), skin infections, nail brittleness, rash, thinning of hair, erythema nodosum; hypo- or hyperpigmentation (rare); urticaria, exaggerated healing response (painful exuberant granulation tissue with crusting). **GI:** dry mouth, anorexia, nausea, vomiting, abdominal pain, nonspecific GI symptoms, acute hepatotoxic reactions, inflammatory bowel disease including regional ileitis, mild GI bleeding, weight loss. **GU:** WBC in urine, proteinuria, hematuria, abnormal menses. **Musculoskeletal:** arthralgia; bone, joint, and muscle pain and stiffness; skeletal hyperostosis (especially in athletic people and with prolonged therapy). **Ophthalmic:** eye irritation, conjunctivitis, corneal opacities. **Other:** epistaxis, dry nose, mild bleeding and bruising, disseminated herpes simplex, edema, respiratory infections, hypertriglyceridemia often with decrease in HDL cholesterol.

ROUTE AND DOSAGE. Highly individualized according to body weight and disease severity. **Adult:** 1 or 2 mg/kg/day divided into two doses for 15 to 20 weeks. If total cyst count decreases by more than 70% beforehand, drug may be discontinued. Smaller doses may be effective; however, relapses are more frequent.

NURSING IMPLICATIONS

Take isotretenoin with meals once daily or in two doses.

Patients who have acne principally on chest and back and the patient who weighs more than 70 kg may need a dose at higher end of the dose range.

After 2 weeks of treatment, regimen is reassessed and dose adjusted as warranted.

A single course of therapy provides adequate control in many patients. If a second course is necessary it is delayed at least 8 weeks because improvement may continue without the drug.

Therapeutic effect: decreased erythema, tenderness, and oiliness of skin; decrease in number of comedones and noncystic lesions. Duration of remission and relapse rates have not been determined.

During the first few weeks, an exacerbation of acne may occur. Urge patient to maintain drug regimen, however, since recurring symptoms may signify response of deep unseen lesions to the drug.

Be certain that the patient fully understands that serious fetal abnormalities can be produced by this drug if it is continued through pregnancy.

Pregnancy should be ruled out by a pregnancy test 2 weeks prior to starting treatment. Patient should use a reliable contraceptive at least 1 month before and throughout treatment, and for 1 month after therapy has been discontinued.

The patient should discuss with her physician about continuing pregnancy if it occurs during therapy.

Baseline control values for blood lipids should be determined at outset of treatment with isotretinoin, then every 2 weeks, 1 month, and every month thereafter throughout course of therapy. If patient has consumed alcohol, test should be delayed for 36 hours (alcohol increases serum triglyceride).

Normal serum (total) cholesterol: 150 to 250 mg/100 ml; *triglyceride:* 30 to 190 mg/100 ml.

Persistence of hypertriglyceridemia (levels above 500 to 800 mg/100 ml) despite a reduced dose indicates necessity to stop drug to prevent onset of acute pancreatitis.

Weight reduction (if patient is obese), reduction of or abstinence from smoking, abstinence from alcohol, and decreased dietary fat intake are indicated if triglyceride levels climb, especially in patients at high risk *(see Cautious Use).* Facilitate patient–dietitian conference to design an appropriate diet (i.e., low fat, restricted concentrated sweets).

Drug therapy can be resumed when serum lipid levels normalize. Advise patient not to self-medicate with multivitamins, which usually contain vitamin A. Toxicity of isotretinoin is enhanced by vitamin A supplements. Discuss with physician.

Liver function tests are performed at 2- or 3-week intervals, then in 6 months and every month thereafter during treatment. Signs of liver dysfunction (jaundice, pruritus, dark urine) should be reported promptly. Since pruritus is a side effect of isotretinoin use, as well as of jaundice, differentiation between the side effect and hepatic disorder may rest upon observation of yellow sclera (symptom of jaundice).

Protect face from extremes in weather (e.g., wind, cold) to decrease stimuli to drug-induced dry skin and mucous membranes.

Warn patient to avoid or minimize exposure of the treated skin to sun or sunlamps. Photosensitivity (both photoallergic and phototoxic) *(see Index)* potential is high. The risk of skin cancer may be increased by this drug.

Although the FDA has not established that sun screening provides absolute protection against ultraviolet radiation, advise patient to use a sunscreen lotion (SPF of 15 or more) and to wear protective clothing if he or she must go out in the sun, until tolerance is established.

If sunscreen lotion contains PABA, it should be applied 1 to 2 hours before exposure to the sun and reapplied every 2 hours, particularly if there is profuse sweating.

If visual disturbances occur along with nausea, vomiting, and headache, instruct the patient to discontinue the medication at once and report to the physician to rule out benign intracranial hypertension (papilledema).

Consult physician about use of cosmetics.

Visual disturbances may also signify development of corneal opacities which should be ruled out by ophthalmic examination. If present, drug will be discontinued. Urge patient to return for a follow-up exam in 6 weeks; usually the opacities have resolved during that period.

Report abdominal pain, rectal bleeding, or severe diarrhea, possible symptoms of drug-induced inflammatory bowel disease. Drug treatment will be discontinued.

Dry mouth and cheilitis, frequent side effects of isotretinoin, are distressing and are potential preconditions conducive to infections. Urge patient to keep lips moist and softened (use thin layer of lubricant such as vaseline) and to rinse mouth with water as necessary for comfort. Commercial rinses should be avoided because of alcohol or other mucosal irritant components.

Although cheilitis is an expected side effect, its etiology should be differentiated from that related to a nutritional deficiency (e.g., folic acid, vitamin B_{12}, pyridoxine, riboflavin), all of which are associated with cheilitis and other oral signs. Collaborate with the dietitian in review of patient's daily diet and in the design of adjusted nutrient intake if necessary.

Advise patient to report joint pain, such as pain in the great toe (symptomatic of gout and hyperuricemia). Phenylbutazone may be prescribed without interrupting isotretinoin therapy.

Isotretenoin is photosensitive. Store in tight, light resistant container at 15° to 30°C (59° to 86°F). Stability of capsules continues 2 years.

See Tretinoin for additional teaching points.

Diagnostic Test Interferences. Isotretinoin may produce elevations of **erythrocyte sedimentation rate, platelet count, serum triglyceride, alkaline phosphatase, AST, ALT** (minimal and transient), **LDH, fasting serum glucose, cholesterol** (minimum), **uric acid;** and decreases in **HDL, RBC parameters,** and **WBC count.**

Drug Interactions: Isotretinoin

Plus	Interactions
Minocycline and other tetracyclines	May cause papilledema
Vitamin A supplements	Increased risk of toxicity. Concurrent use contraindicated

PROTOTYPE

ISOXSUPRINE HYDROCHLORIDE

(Vasodilan, Voxsuprine)

(eye-sox'syoo-preen)

Adrenergic agonist (beta)
Vasodilator
Tocolytic

ACTIONS AND USES. Sympathomimetic agent with beta-adrenergic stimulant activity and with slight effect on α-receptors. Action is not blocked by propranolol (a beta-adrenergic blocker) suggesting that isoxuprine acts directly on vascular smooth muscle. Vasodilating action on arteries within skeletal muscles is greater than on cutaneous vessels. Also causes cardiac stimulation (increases cardiac contractility, rate, and output) and may produce bronchodilatation, mild inhibition of GI motility, and uterine relaxation by direct action on smooth muscles. At high doses inhibits platelet aggregation and lowers blood viscosity.

Used as adjunctive therapy in treatment of cerebral vascular insufficiency and peripheral vascular disease, such as arteriosclerosis obliterans, thromboangiitis obliterans (Buerger's disease), and Raynaud's disease. *Investigational Use:* in treatment of dysmenorrhea, and threatened abortion and preterm labor, but efficacy has not been established.

ABSORPTION AND FATE. Well absorbed from GI tract. Therapeutic blood levels are achieved within 1 hour and persist for almost 3 hours. Mean plasma half-life: 1.25 hours. Partly conjugated in blood; excreted primarily in urine. Crosses placenta.

CONTRAINDICATIONS AND PRECAUTIONS. Immediately postpartum; in presence of arterial bleeding; parenteral use in presence of hypotension, tachycardia. Safe use in pregnancy not established. *Cautious Use:* bleeding disorders, severe cerebrovascular disease, severe obliterative coronary artery disease, recent myocardial infarction.

ADVERSE/SIDE EFFECTS. CV: flushing, orthostatic hypotension with lightheadedness, faintness; palpitation, tachycardia. **CNS:** dizziness, nervousness, trembling, weakness, **GI:** nausea, vomiting, abdominal distress, abdominal distention. **Other:** severe rash.

ROUTE AND DOSAGE. Oral: 10 to 20 mg three or four times daily. **Intramuscular:** 5 to 10 mg 2 or 3 times a day. Single IM doses exceeding 10 mg not recommended. *Preterm labor:* **Intravenous:** 0.2 to 1 mg/minute for 10 minutes followed by 0.1 to 3 mg/minute for 24 hours. *Maintenance:* **Oral:** 20 mg 4 times daily for 2 to 3 weeks.

NURSING IMPLICATIONS

Advise patient to report adverse reactions (skin rash, palpitation, flushing) promptly; symptoms are usually effectively controlled by dosage reduction or discontinuation of drug.

Parenteral administration may cause hypotension and tachycardia. Monitor blood pressure and pulse. Supervise ambulation.

To prevent orthostatic hypotension, instruct patient to make position changes slowly and in stages particularly from recumbent to upright posture and to avoid standing still.

Therapeutic response to isoxsuprine in treatment of peripheral vascular disorders may take several weeks. Evaluate clinical manifestations of arterial insufficiency: pain with walking (intermittent claudication), rest pain, sensations of numbness, coldness, burning; weak or absent peripheral pulses, rapid blanching when legs are elevated; rubor (cyanosis or dusky skin color) in dependent position, keep physician informed.

Patients should be completely informed about skin care of legs and feet and care of toenails. Properly fitted shoes and stockings and the importance of avoiding mechanical, chemical, and thermal trauma should be emphasized. Cessation of smoking and control of weight are crucial adjuncts to pharmacotherapeutic regimen.

If isoxsuprine has been used to delay premature labor, hyportension, irregular and rapid heart beat may be observed in both mother and baby.

Hypocalcemia, hypoglycemia, and ileus have been observed in babies born of mothers taking isoxsuprine.

Discuss with physician the rehabilitative management of the patient with peripheral vascular disease. Prescribed adjuncts to drug therapy may include the following: support hose, elevation of head of bed with 4- to 6-inch blocks to relieve rest pain (by enhancing blood flow to extremities); Buerger-Allen exercises; graduated exercise program to develop collateral blood supply.

For treatment of menstrual cramps, isoxsuprine is usually started 1 to 3 days before onset of menstruation and continued until pain is relieved or menstrual flow stops.

K

KANAMYCIN

(Anamid, Kantrex, Klebcil)

(kan-a-mye'sin)
Antiinfective
Antibiotic
Aminoglycoside

ACTIONS AND USES. Aminoglycoside antibiotic derived from *Streptomyces kanamyceticus* and similar to neomycin in chemical structure and antibacterial properties. Active against many gram-negative microorganisms, especially *Klebisella pneumoniae, Enterobacter aerogenes, Proteus* species, *E. coli, Serratia marcescens,* and *Acinetobacter.* Also effective against many strains of *Staphylococcus aureus,* but it is not the drug of choice. Cross-resistance between kanamycin and neomycin is complete. As with other aminoglycosides, exerts curarelike effect on neuromuscular junction. Oral kanamycin reportedly decreases serum cholesterol.

Used orally to reduce ammonia-producing bacteria in intestinal tract as adjunctive treatment of hepatic coma; also used for preoperative bowel antisepsis and for treatment of intestinal infections. Parenteral drug is used in short-term treatment of serious infections. Used intraperitoneally following fecal spill during surgery. Also used as irrigation solution and as aerosol treatment.

ABSORPTION AND FATE. Poorly absorbed from GI tract. Excreted in feces as unchanged drug; absorbed portion, if any, excreted unchanged in urine. Completely absorbed following IM injection in about 1.5 hours. Peak serum concentrations reached in about 1 hour, declining to very low levels by 12 hours. Serum half-life: 2 to 4 hours. Diffuses to most body fluids, including cerebrospinal fluid, but only if meninges are inflamed. Also readily absorbed from peritoneal cavity. Excreted by kidneys (mostly by glomerular filtration); 81% excreted in urine as unchanged drug. Approximately one-half of IM dose eliminated in 4 hours; excretion complete within 24 to 48 hours (prolonged in patients with renal impairment). Crosses placenta and appears in breast milk.

CONTRAINDICATIONS AND PRECAUTIONS. History of hypersensitivity to kanamycin or other aminoglycosides; history of drug-induced ototoxicity; long-term therapy; concurrent or sequential administration with other ototoxic, nephrotoxic, and/or neurotoxic agents; potent diuretics; oral use in intestinal obstruction; intraperitoneally to patients under effects of anesthetics or muscle relaxants; IV administration to patients with renal impairment. Safe use in pregnancy and in nursing women not established. *Cautious Use:* impaired renal function, myasthenia gravis.

ADVERSE/SIDE EFFECTS. GI: nausea, vomiting, diarrhea, appetite changes, abdominal discomfort, stomatitis, malabsorption syndrome (with prolonged oral administration). **Hematologic:** anemia, increased or decreased reticulocytes, decreased plasma fibrinogen, granulocytopenia, agranulocytosis, thrombocytopenia, purpura. **Hypersensitivity:** eosinophilia, maculopapular rashes, pruritus, anaphylaxis. **Nephrotoxicity:** hematuria, proteinuria; elevated serum creatinine and BUN, acute tubular necrosis (rare). **Neurologic:** circumoral and other paresthesias, optic neuritis, peripheral neuritis, headache, restlessness, acute brain syndrome, bulging fontanelles, arachnoiditis, convulsions; rarely: neuromuscular paralysis, respiratory depression, sensory involvement of glossopharyngeal (IX) cranial nerve. **Otic:** deafness (may be irreversible), vertigo, tinnitus. **Other:** superinfections; laryngeal edema; blurred vision; fever; joint pain; pulmonary fibrosis; hypotension; hypertension; tachycardia; increased salivation; weight loss; decreased serum calcium; increased SGOT, SGPT, and serum bilirubin; transient hepatomegaly; splenomegaly; local pain; nodular formation at injection site.

ROUTE AND DOSAGE. Oral: *Preoperative intestinal antisepsis:* 1 Gm every hour for 4 doses, then every 6 hours for 36 to 72 hours. *Intestinal infections:* **Adults:** 3 to 4 Gm/day in divided doses for 3 to 5 days. **Children:** 50 mg/kg daily in 4 to 6 equally divided doses, usually continued 5 to 7 days. *Hepatic coma:* 8 to 12 Gm/day in divided doses. **Intramuscular: Adults; children:** 15 mg/kg in 2 to 4 equally divided and spaced doses. Maximum daily dose is 1.5 Gm regardless of body weight. **Intravenous:** not to exceed 15 mg/kg body weight daily in 2 or 3 equal doses. **Intraperitoneal: Adults only:** 500 mg diluted in 20 ml sterile distilled water, instilled through wound catheter. **Inhalation (aerosol):** 250 mg diluted with 3 ml normal saline two to four times a day. **Irrigation solution:** (0.25%).

NURSING IMPLICATIONS

Culture and susceptibility studies should be performed at initiation of therapy and periodically thereafter (therapy may be started prior to return of results).

Administer IM injection deep into upper outer quadrant of buttock (often painful). Observe sites daily for signs of irritation; rotate injection sites.

Urinalysis and kidney function tests should be assessed before and at regular intervals during therapy.

Monitor intake and output. Report decrease in urine output or change in intake-output ratio.

Risk of ototoxicity is high in patients with impaired renal function, the elderly, poorly hydrated patients, and patients in whom therapy is expected to last 5 days or more. Close monitoring of kidney function and pretreatment and repeat audiograms are advised in these patients.

Lower than usual dosages are prescribed for patients with renal dysfunction. One suggested method of estimating dosage interval is to multiply serum creatinine value by 9 and to use resulting figure as interval in hours between doses: e.g., if creatinine level is 2 mg/dl ($2 \times 9 = 18$), dose should be administered every 18 hours.

Check reports of urinalysis and kidney function test and notify physician immediately of signs of renal irritation: albuminuria, casts, red and white cells in urine, increasing NPN, BUN, and serum creatinine and edema. Audiogram should be obtained if any of these signs are present. Physician may terminate kanamycin therapy.

Since parenteral kanamycin is highly concentrated in the urinary system, patient should be well hydrated to prevent chemical irritation of renal tubules. Fluid intake should be sufficient to produce output of at least 1500 ml/day. Consult physician.

Monitoring of peak and trough serum drug concentrations is advised in patients with impaired renal function. Generally desired peak concentration for systemic infection is 15 to 30 mcg/ml; trough concentrations should not exceed 5 to 10 mcg/ml. Risk of toxicity increases with prolonged peak concentrations > 30 to 35 mcg/ml.

Drug should be stopped if patient complains of tinnitus, dizziness or vertigo, sense of fullness in ears, or subjective hearing loss or if follow-up audiograms show loss of high-frequency perception. High-frequency deafness usually occurs first, but it can be detected only by audiometry (auditory toxicity occurs more commonly than vestibular toxicity).

In patients with impaired renal function, deafness has occurred 2 to 7 days after termination of therapy.

If no objective clinical response occurs within 3 to 5 days of parenteral therapy, sensitivity tests should be rechecked and therapy terminated.

Patients receiving kanamycin in the postoperative period should be closely monitored for neuromuscular and respiratory depression. Have on hand parenteral neostigmine, calcium gluconate, and sodium bicarbonate.

Some vials may darken with time, but this does not indicate loss of potency.

Kanamycin should not be mixed in the same syringe with other drugs. Discard partially used vials within 48 hours.
Advise home patients to discard remaining drug after therapy is completed.
Kanamycin is stable for 24 hours at 15° to 30°C (59° to 86°F) in most IV solutions. Consult manufacturer's literature for storage information.

Drug Interactions. It is possible for additive nephrotoxic effects to occur with **cephalosporins.** Combined or sequential use of kanamycin with other **aminoglycoside antibiotics** increases the possibility of nephrotoxicity and ototoxicity. Concurrent use with potent diuretics, e.g., **bumetanide** (Bumex) **ethacrynic acid, furosemide** potentiates ototoxicity. Enhanced neuromuscular blockade and respiratory depression may occur with **ether** and related **inhalation anesthetic agents,** and **skeletal muscle relaxants** e.g., **succinylcholine, tubocurarine.** *See Gentamicin for other possible interactions.*

KETAMINE HYDROCHLORIDE

(Ketalar)

(keet'a-meen)
Anesthetic (general)

K

ACTIONS AND USES. Rapid-acting phencyclidine derivative. Produces profound anesthesia that may be accompanied by increase in salivary secretions, depression of pharyngeal and laryngeal reflexes and slight stimulation of skeletal muscle tone, cardiovascular action, and increase in cerebral blood flow and intracranial pressure. Acts primarily on cortex and limbic system which probably accounts for emergence reactions of recovery period. (*See Nursing Implications*). Produces "dissociative anesthesia" which describes the feeling of separation from surroundings experienced by patient. Since it does not relax skeletal muscles effectively it is not used for intraabdominal or intrathoracic procedures unless supplemented with another inhalation anesthetic.

Used as sole anesthetic agent for diagnostic and surgical procedures of short duration that do not require skeletal muscle relaxation. Also used to induce anesthesia prior to administration of other general anesthetics or to supplement low potency anesthetics such as nitrous oxide.

ABSORPTION AND FATE. Rapidly absorbed from IV or IM injection sites and widely distributed in body. Relatively high concentrations in brain, lungs, liver, and body fat. Produces surgical anesthesia within 30 to 40 seconds following IV and in 3 to 8 minutes after IM administration; duration: 5 to 10 minutes (IV); 12 to 25 minutes (IM).

CONTRAINDICATIONS AND PRECAUTIONS. Hypersensitivity to ketamine, severe hypertension, severe coronary heart disease or cardiac decompensation, increased intracranial pressure, history of cerebrovascular accident, increased intraocular pressure, psychiatric disorders. Safe use during pregnancy including obstetrics not established. *Cautious Use:* patients on thyroid replacement therapy; chronic alcoholism, convulsive disorders.

ADVERSE/SIDE EFFECTS. CNS: emergence reactions (hallucinations, delirium, confusion, excitement, irrational behavior), polyneuropathy, athetoid movements of mouth and tongue, muscular rigidity, fasciculations, tremors, tonic and clonic movements resembling convulsions, increased intracranial pressure. **CV:** hypertension, hypotension, tachycardia, bradycardia, arrhythmias, cardiac arrest. **GI:** anorexia, nausea, vomiting. **Ophthalmic:** diplopia, nystagmus, slight increase in intraocular pressure, temporary loss of vision, lacrimation. **Respiratory:** respiratory depression, apnea, laryngospasm. **Other:** hypersalivation, transient erythema, skin rashes, local pain and irritation at injection site.

ROUTE AND DOSAGE. **Intravenous:** Initial: 1 to 4.5 mg/kg administered slowly over 1 minute period. Slow microdrip infusion reportedly allows administration of lowest effective dosage. **Intramuscular:** 6.5 to 13 mg/kg repeated as needed in increments of ½ to the full induction dose. Dosage based preferably on lean body mass rather than on total body weight.

NURSING IMPLICATIONS

Because ketamine tends to stimulate flow of saliva, an anticholinergic ("drying agent") should be included in premedication prior to anesthesia.

Intravenous thiopental or diazepam or a narcotic may be prescribed as premedication to control severity of symptoms associated with recovery phase.

Recovery (emergence) from ketamine anesthesia is frequently prolonged and may be accompanied by hallucinations, vivid imagery, delirium, and "dissociative anesthesia" (the feeling of separation from surroundings).

Emergence reactions occur most commonly in patients between the ages of 16 and 65 years receiving IV ketamine.

Severity of recovery symptoms may be reduced by allowing patient to awaken quietly with minimal amount of talking and touching during recovery period. (However, blood pressure and vital signs must still be taken as indicated.)

Hallucinations similar to "LSD flashbacks" have occurred days, weeks, or as long as a year after ketamine anesthesia. Reportedly, ketamine has been abused for its hallucinogenic properties.

Monitor blood pressure and vital signs. Ketamine tends to increase blood pressure, cardiac output, pulse rate, and can cause respiratory depression and apnea.

Resuscitative equipment should be immediately available.

Patients with history of convulsive disorders should be closely observed for apparent loss of seizure control.

Monitor airway. Aspiration is a possibility since hypersalivation occurs commonly and laryngeal and pharyngeal reflexes may be depressed.

If used in ambulatory services, patient should not be released until completely recovered from anesthesia and unless accompanied by a responsible adult.

Manufacturer cautions not to mix barbiturates in same syringe with ketamine because a precipitate will form.

Store preferably between 15° and 30°C (59° and 86°F) unless otherwise directed by manufacturer. Protect from heat and light.

Drug Interactions. **Atropine, meperidine, morphine** in large doses may increase depth and duration of ketamine-induced anesthesia. Ketamine may potentiate the neuromuscular blocking action of **tubocurarine.**

KETOCONAZOLE

(Nizoral)

(ke-to-con′a-zol)
Antiinfective
Antibiotic
Antifungal

ACTIONS AND USES. Broad-spectrum antifungal agent active against clinical infections with *Coccidioides immitis, Histoplasma capsulatum, Paracoccidioides brasiliensis, Phialophora,* and *Candida* species. In vitro studies suggest mode of action involves interference with synthesis of ergosterol, an essential component of fungal cell membranes.

Used for treatment of many oral and systemic fungal infections including candidiasis (chronic mucocutaneous candidiasis, oral thrush, candiduria) coccidioidomycosis, histoplasmosis, paracoccidioidomycosis, chromomycosis, and dermatophytoses.

ABSORPTION AND FATE. Following oral administration of single dose mean peak plasma levels (3.5 mcg/ml) reached within 1 to 2 hours. Plasma elimination is biphasic: half-life of 2 hours within first 10 hours and 8 hours thereafter. Poor penetration into CSF. Metabolized in liver; plasma protein binding about 99%. About 13% excreted in urine (2 to 4% unchanged drug); major excretory route through bile into intestinal tract.

CONTRAINDICATIONS AND PRECAUTIONS. Hypersensitivity to ketoconazole; use during pregnancy not advised (teratogenic and embryotoxic effects reported in animal studies); lactation, children under age 2, fungal meningitis. *Cautious Use:* drug-induced achlorhydria, hepatic impairment.

ADVERSE/SIDE EFFECTS. Usually well tolerated. Nausea, vomiting, abdominal pain, diarrhea pruritus, headache, dizziness, somnolence, fever, chills, photophobia, transient increases in serum liver enzymes.

ROUTE AND DOSAGE. Oral: Adults: Initial: 200 mg once daily. May be increased to 400 mg once daily for serious infection or to improve clinical response. **Children: older than 2 years:** 3.3 to 6.6 mg/kg/daily as single doses.

K

NURSING IMPLICATIONS

The infective organism should be identified but treatment may be started before obtaining lab results.

Ketoconazole requires an acid medium for dissolution; therefore administer it at least 2 hours before an antacid, anticholinergic, cimetidine, or ranitidine (agents that may elevate GI pH) is given.

Give drug with water, fruit juice, coffee, or tea. However, if patient has achlorhydria or reduced gastric acidity (as with surgical intervention, or in the elderly) the physician may prescribe drug to be given with diluted hydrochloric acid (HCl).

Instruct patient to dissolve each tablet in 4 ml aqueous solution of 0.2 N HCl solution and sip the solution through a glass or plastic straw to avoid contact of acid with teeth surfaces. Follow with a glass of tap water.

Advise patient to refrain from driving a car or using hazardous equipment until response to the drug is known. Drowsiness and dizziness are early and time-limited side effects.

Treatment is continued until all clinical and lab tests indicate that fungal infection has subsided.

Minimal treatment period for candidiasis is 1 to 2 weeks. Chronic mucocutaneous candidiasis may require maintenance therapy. Minimal treatment for systemic fungal infection is 6 months.

Instruct patient to avoid OTC drugs for gastric distress, such as Rolaids, Soda Mints, Tums, Gelusil, Alka-Seltzer. Consult physician before taking any nonprescribed medicines.

Caution patient not to alter the dose or dose interval and not to stop taking ketoconazole before consulting the physician. Poor response and recurrence of clinical symptoms are often related to an erratic dose regimen.

Store in tightly-covered container, preferably between 15° and 30°C (59° and 86°F) unless otherwise directed by manufacturer.

Drug Interactions. **Antacids, anticholinergics, antihistamines** (H_2-receptor antagonists) decrease absorption of ketoconazole leading to inadequate plasma level. Antifungal action of ketoconazole may be reduced by concurrent administration of **Isoniazid** and **rifampin** (effect of rifampin may also be reduced). Pharmacologic effects of **cyclosporine** may be increased; monitor cyclosporine serum levels and serum creatinine.

L

LABETALOL HYDROCHLORIDE

(Normodyne, Trandate)

(la-bet'a-lole)

Adrenergic blocking agent (alpha/beta)

(Sympatholytic)

Antihypertensive

ACTIONS AND USES. Adrenergic receptor blocking agent that combines selective alpha activity and nonselective beta adrenergic blocking actions. Both activities contribute to blood pressure reduction. Alpha blockade results in vasodilation, decreased peripheral resistance, and orthostatic hypotension, and only slightly affects cardiac output and coronary artery blood flow. Beta blocking effects on sinus node, AV node, and ventricular muscle lead to bradycardia, delay in AV conduction, and depression of cardiac contractility. Similar to propranolol and other nonselective beta blockers in ability to decrease resting and exercise-induced heart rate. Depresses plasma renin activity both at rest and during exercise. Also has weak membrane stabilizing properties at recommended doses. Does not abolish digitalis-induced inotropic action on heart muscle.

Used for treatment of mild, moderate, and severe hypertension, primarily as a step-2 drug. May be used alone or in combination with other antihypertensive agents, especially thiazide diuretics.

ABSORPTION AND FATE. Rapidly and completely absorbed following oral administration. Onset of hypotensive action usually within 1 to 2 hours; peak plasma levels in 2 to 4 hours. Duration of action: 8 to 12 hours (dose-dependent). Onset of action following IV administration: within 5 minutes; plasma levels peak in 20 to 40 minutes. Approximately 50% protein bound. Plasma half-life 3 to 8 hours. Steady-state plasma response in 24 to 72 hours. Undergoes extensive first-pass metabolism in liver. About 60% of dose excreted by kidneys as inactive metabolites and unchanged drug (5%); 40% of dose eliminated in feces via bile. Crosses placenta. Small amounts appear in breast milk.

CONTRAINDICATIONS AND PRECAUTIONS. Bronchial asthma, uncontrolled cardiac failure, heart block (greater than first degree), cardiogenic shock, severe bradycardia. Safe use during pregnancy (category C), in nursing women, and in children not established. *Cautious Use:* nonallergic bronchospastic disease (COPD), well compensated patients with history of heart failure, pheochromocytoma, impaired hepatic function, jaundice, diabetes mellitus.

ADVERSE/SIDE EFFECTS. CV: postural hypotension, light-headedness, angina pectoris, palpitation, bradycardia, syncope, pedal or peripheral edema, pulmonary edema, congestive heart failure, flushing, cold extremities, Raynaud's phenomenon, arrhythmias (following IV), paradoxical hypertension (patients with pheochromocytoma). **Dermatologic:** rashes of various types, reversible alopecia, increased sweating, pruritus. **GI:** nausea/vomiting, dyspepsia, constipation, diarrhea, taste disturbances, cholestasis with or without jaundice, increases in serum transaminases, dry mouth. **NS:** dizziness, fatigue/malaise (asthenia), headache, tremors, paresthesias (especially scalp tingling), hypoesthesia (numbness) following IV, mental depression, sleep disturbances, nightmares. **Ophthalmic:** dry eyes, activity disturbances. **Renal:** acute urinary retention, difficult micturition, transient rises in BUN and serum creatinine. **Reprod:** impotence, ejaculation failure, loss of libido, Peyronie's disease. **Respiratory:** dyspnea, bronchospasm. **Other:** nasal stuffiness, myalgia, muscle cramps, toxic myopathy, antimitochondrial antibodies, positive antinuclear factor (ANF), SLE syndrome, pain at IV injection site. For potential adverse effects listed for other beta blockers *see Propranolol.*

ROUTE AND DOSAGE. Oral: initially, 100 mg twice daily. After 2 or 3 days, dosage may be increased to 200 mg twice daily. *Usual maintenance dose:* 200 to 400 mg twice daily. Patients with severe hypertension may require 1200 to 2400 mg/day in two or three divided doses. Titrated increments not to exceed 200 mg twice daily. **Intravenous:** *Intermittent injections:* 20 mg slowly over 2 minutes. If necessary, additional doses of 40 to 80 mg given at 10 minute intervals until desired supine blood pressure is achieved or to total dose of 300 mg. *Continuous infusion:* 2 mg/minute of diluted solution until desired response obtained. Usual dose range 100 to 200 mg, up to 300 mg. See manufacturer's directions for dilutions, compatibility, and storage.

NURSING IMPLICATIONS

Administered oral preparation preferably with or immediately after food. Food increases drug bioavailability. Advise consistency.

Monitor blood pressure and pulse during dosage adjustment period. Standing blood pressure is used as indicator for making dosage adjustments.

Patient should be supine when receiving labetalol IV. Take blood pressure immediately before drug is administered, then 5 minutes and 10 minutes after injection.

Supine position should be maintained for at least 3 hours after IV administration. At the end of this time, determine patient's ability to tolerate elevated and upright positions before allowing ambulation.

Controller device is recommended for maintaining accurate flow rate during IV infusion. Physician should prescribe precise flow rate and adjustments to be made according to blood pressure response. (Usually administered at rate of 2 mg/ml.)

Caution patient that postural hypotension is most likely to occur during peak plasma levels, i.e., 2 to 4 hours after drug administration.

Instruct patient to adopt the habit of making position changes slowly and in stages, particularly from recumbent to upright position. Bear in mind that elderly patients are particularly sensitive to hypotensive effects.

Diabetic patients should be closely monitored. Inform patient that labetalol may mask usual cardiovascular response to acute hypoglycemia, e.g., tachycardia. Advise patient to be alert to possible signs of hypoglycemia, e.g., weakness, clammy skin, headache, confusion, visual disturbances.

Reassure patient that most adverse effects are transient and dose-related and occur early in therapy. Encourage patient to telephone any unusual symptoms or problems to clinician or responsible care provider.

Periodic ophthalmoscopic examinations are advised during prolonged therapy. Reportedly, labetalol may accumulate in tissues with high melanin content such as the choroid. This eye problem has not been reported in humans, but has occurred in laboratory animals.

Stress importance of keeping follow-up appointments. Tests of liver and renal function should be performed periodically during therapy.

Warn patient not to interrupt or discontinue drug therapy without consulting the physician.

Discontinuation of labetalol following chronic administration should be done by gradual reduction of dosage over a 1- to 2-week period. Patient should be closely monitored and advised to restrict physical activity during this time. Patients with coronary artery disease should be told beforehand by physician what to do if anginal pain is experienced. (Generally, labetalol is reinstituted promptly.) In addition to angina, abrupt discontinuation of labetalol can result in acute myocardial infarction.

Since labetalol can cause dizziness and light-headedness, advise patient to avoid driving and other potentially hazardous activities until reaction to drug is known.

Withdrawal of antihypertensive therapy before surgery remains controversial. Anesthetist should be informed of physician's decision.

Treatment of overdosage: induce emesis (syrup of ipecac) or gastric lavage. Keep patient supine with legs elevated if necessary. Have on hand atropine (3 mg) for excessive bradycardia, isoproterenol, digitalis glycoside, diuretic, norepinephrine; theophylline or a beta-2-stimulating agent for bronchospasm.

Store preferably between 2° to 30°C (36° to 86°F), unless otherwise advised by physician. Do not freeze. Protect tablets from excess moisture.

See Propranolol for patient teaching points regarding hypertensive therapy.

Diagnostic Test Interferences. False increases in **urinary catecholamines** when measured by nonspecific trihydroxyindole (THI) reaction (due to labetalol metabolites), but not with specific radioenzymatic or high performance liquid chromatography assay techniques.

Drug Interactions: Labetalol

Plus	Interactions
Beta-adrenergic agonist bronchodilators, e.g., ephedrine, metaproterenol, terbutaline	Labetalol may blunt bronchodilator effect requiring higher doses of these drugs
Cimetidine (Tagament)	Increases bioavailability of labetalol (by increasing its absorption or decreasing hepatic metabolism). May require lower doses
Halothane (Fluothane)	Additive hypotensive effects, especially with high concentrations (3% or above) of halothane
Insulins	Pharmacologic effects of insulins may be increased and symptoms of hypoglycemia may be obscured by labetalol
Nitroglycerin	Possibility of additive hypotensive effects. Labetalol blunts reflex tachycardia induced by nitroglycerin
Tricyclic antidepressants	Possibility of increased incidence of tremor

See also Propranolol for other possible drug interactions.

LACTULOSE

(lak'tyoo-lose)

(Cephulac, Chronulac)

Ammonia detoxicant

ACTIONS AND USES. An ammonia detoxicant that reduces blood ammonia levels by as much as 25 to 50%. Syrup preparation contains galactose (less than 2.2 Gm/15 ml) and lactulose (less than 1.2 Gm/15 ml). Action relies on environmental changes in the colon produced by bacterial degradation of lactulose. Resulting acidification of colon and osmotic fermentative diarrhea prevents absorption of ammonium ion (NH_4^+) while promoting migration of blood ammonia (NH_3) into the intestinal tract. Once in the acid colon, NH_3 is converted to the nonabsorbable NH_4^+ ion and lost to systemic circulation. Other lactulose metabolites with laxative properties, plus the osmotically increased water, stimulate expulsion of the trapped ammonia. Lactulose therapy is reported to improve protein tolerance.

Used for prevention and treatment of portal–systemic encephalopathy, including stages of hepatic precoma and coma, and for chronic constipation.

ABSORPTION AND FATE. Poorly absorbed. 97% reaches intestinal tract relatively unchanged where it is metabolized by resident bacteria to organic acids. Excretion (3% or less) in urine completed within 24 hours.

CONTRAINDICATIONS AND PRECAUTIONS. Low galactose diet; safe use in pregnancy and during lactation not determined. *Cautious Use:* diabetes mellitus, concomitant use with electrocautery procedures (proctoscopy, colonoscopy), elderly and debilitated patients, children.

ADVERSE/SIDE EFFECTS. *Initial dose:* flatulence, belching, intestinal cramps, abdominal pain, diarrhea (excessive dose), nausea, vomiting, colon accumulation of H_2 gas, hypernatremia.

ROUTE AND DOSAGE. (30 ml syrup contains approximately 20 Gm lactulose) **Oral: Adult:** Initial: 30 to 45 ml every hour until laxation effect is achieved (up to 48 hours), dosage is then reduced to 30 to 45 ml three to four times daily. Prophylaxis (long-term)—30 to 45 ml three to four times daily; adjusted every day or two to produce two to three soft stools daily. **Pediatric–Infant:** 2.5 to 10 ml daily in divided doses. **Child and Adolescent:** 40 to 90 mg/day in divided doses. **Rectal:** *retention enema:* (Chronulac): at least 100 ml lactulose solution; retained 30 to 60 minutes. Repeated in 4 to 6 hours if necessary.

L

NURSING IMPLICATIONS

Administer with fruit juice or other nonfat drink to increase palatability; avoid meal time.

Laxative action is not instituted until drug reaches the colon; therefore transit time before reaching the colon and during passage through colon affects response time. 24 to 48 hours (normally required for a bowel movement) is also required for drug-induced laxation.

Any factor that slows gastric or small intestine transit time may extend initial response time to oral lactulose therapy (e.g., food, constipation, hypercatabolic states, as with infection).

Therapeutic response (decreased blood ammonia) in patient with hepatic encephalopathy is marked by clearing of confusion, apathy, and irritation, and by improved mental state and EEG patterns. (*Normal blood ammonia:* 30 to 70 mcg/100 ml).

When endoscopic examination or intubation procedures are necessary or danger of aspiration exists, lactulose may be administered by retention enema. Dilute 300 ml lactulose in 700 ml water or normal saline; instill via a rectal balloon catheter. If enema is evacuated too soon after instillation, it may be promptly repeated.

If the initial dose for children causes diarrhea, the dose is reduced immediately. If diarrhea persists, lactulose is discontinued.

Advise patient on prolonged therapy to report to the physician if diarrhea (i.e., more than two soft stools daily) persists more than 24 to 48 hours. Dose adjustment may be indicated.

Following serious diarrhea, the patient is likely to be dehydrated. Consult physician about use of oral rehydration solutions, particularly since some contain proteins. *(See Index: Nursing Intervention: rehydration, oral).*

Warn patient who may be discouraged by slow onset of drug action not to self-medicate with another laxative.

Abuse of lactulose therapy for constipation should be prevented because of danger of electrolyte imbalance. Periodic lab evaluations of K, chlorides, CO_2 are indicated during chronic lactulose use.

Changes in aging retard and reduce capacity of the elderly to adjust to electrolyte imbalance.

Lactulose-induced osmotic changes in the bowel support intestinal water loss and potential hypernatremia. Fluid intake (often self-limited by the elderly) should be actively promoted (up to 1500 to 2000 ml/day) during drug therapy for constipation.

A potential therapeutic hazard with lactulose therapy is the accumulation of intestinal H_2 gas from bacterial degradation of the drug. Significant concentrations in presence of an electrical spark (a potential with electrocautery procedures) may result in explosive action. Preparation for colonoscopy or proctoscopy is thorough bowel cleansing with nonfermentable or nonfoaming solution (i.e., avoid alkaline or soapsuds solution).

Food–Drug Interactions:

- With improvement from hepatic coma during and following lactulose treatment, protein intake (which may have been drastically reduced with reliance on glucose and fat for energy) will be increased as tolerated.
- Transition from *low-protein foods* (to reduce intestinal ammonia) (e.g., bread, rusk, macaroni, noodles, hot cereals, gelatin) to more liberalized protein intake will be guided by lab evidence of improvement (e.g., serum ammonia levels). Collaborate with dietitian in the support of diet therapy during recovery period.

Avoid exposing lactulose solution to light. Normal darkening does not affect action. Discard solution that is very dark or cloudy.

If solution is refrigerated, it will be too viscous to pour. Store at room temperature (below 30°C, or 86°F), which will reduce viscosity; do not freeze.

See Bisocodyl for patient teaching regarding management of chronic constipation.

Drug Interactions: Lactulose

Plus	Interactions
Laxatives	Laxation may incorrectly suggest therapeutic action of lactulose
Neomycin and possibly other oral antiinfectives	May inhibit lactulose action by reduction or removal of resident colon bacteria

LEUCOVORIN CALCIUM

(Calcium Folinate, Citrovorum Factor, Folinic Acid)

(loo-koe-vor'in)
Antianemic
Antidote

ACTIONS AND USES. Tetrahydrofolic acid derivative and active metabolite of folic acid. Functions as an essential cell growth factor. When given during antineoplastic therapy, leucovorin prevents serious toxicity by preferentially protecting normal cells from the action of folic acid antagonists such as methotrexate. This process is called "leucovorin or folinic acid rescue." Reportedly superior to folic acid in this respect because folic acid antagonists interfere with conversion of folic acid to leucovorin, but do not affect action of leucovorin itself.

Used for treatment of folate deficient megaloblastic anemias due to sprue, pregnancy, and nutritional deficiency when oral therapy is not feasible. Also used to prevent or diminish toxicity of antineoplastic folic acid antagonists, particularly methotrexate. Also used as adjunct with antifols (e.g., pyrimethamine) in treatment of pneumocystosis or toxoplasmosis to prevent significant bone marrow toxicity.

CONTRAINDICATIONS AND PRECAUTIONS. Undiagnosed anemia, pernicious anemia, or other megaloblastic anemias secondary to vitamin B_{12} deficiency. *Cautious Use:* renal dysfunction.

ADVERSE/SIDE EFFECTS. Allergic sensitization (urticaria, pruritus, rash, wheezing).

ROUTE AND DOSAGE. *Megaloblastic anemias:* **Intramuscular:** no more than 1 mg daily. *Leukovorin rescue for methotrexate toxicity* (within 24 hours after methotrexate administration): **Oral, parenteral:** 10 mg/m^2 followed by 10 mg/m^2 orally every 6 hours for 72 hours. Further treatment determined by serum creatinine concentrations. *Leucovorin rescue for hematologic toxicity from other folic acid antagonists:* **Oral, parenteral:** 5 to 15 mg/day. *As adjunct in treatment of pneumocystosis or toxoplasmosis:* 3 to 6 mg three times daily.

NURSING IMPLICATIONS

Leucovorin calcium (folinic acid) is not to be confused with folic acid.

Leucovorin calcium is available in 1 ml ampuls containing 3 mg/ml. It is also available in vials containing 50 mg of leucovorin calcium in lyophilized form of lyophilized form.

For reconstitution, manufacturer recommends using Bacteriostatic Water for Injection, which contains benzyl alcohol. (Leucovorin calcium contains no preservatives). When reconstituted as directed, solution must be used within 7 days. If reconstituted with Sterile Water for Injection, use immediately.

Use of leucovorin alone in treatment of pernicious anemia or other megaloblastic anemias associated with vitamin B_{12} deficiency can result in an apparent hematological remission while allowing already present neurologic damage to progress.

To be effective as *antidote for overdosage of folic acid antagonists,* leucovorin must be administered within 1 hour if possible; usually ineffective if delayed more than 4 hours. Duration of treatment depends on hematologic response to leucovorin.

Plasma methotrexate levels may be used to determine dosage and duration of leucovorin rescue therapy. Creatinine clearance determinations prior to initiation of leucovorin rescue and daily serum creatinine levels are recommended to detect onset of renal function impairment.

Stored at controlled room temperature, preferably between 15 and 30°C (59 and 86°F) unless otherwise directed by manufacturer. Protect from light.

See Folic acid.

L

LEVALLORPHAN TARTRATE

(Lorfan)

(lev-al-or'fan)

Narcotic antagonist

ACTIONS AND USES. *N*-allyl analogue of levorphanol. Has both narcotic antagonist and agonist (morphinelike) effects. Antagonizes severe narcotic-induced respiratory depression, but exerts little action against mild respiratory depression and may even increase it, nor does it reverse opiate-induced excitation or convulsions. Largely replaced by naloxone, which has little or no agonistic activity. In the absence of a narcotic (or, in high doses), levallorphan can produce morphinelike effects, e.g., analgesia, sedation, miosis, respiratory depression.

Used in treatment of significant narcotic-induced respiratory depression.

ABSORPTION AND FATE. Acts within 1 to 2 minutes; effects last about 2 to 5 hours. Readily crosses blood–brain barrier and placenta.

CONTRAINDICATIONS AND PRECAUTIONS. Mild narcotic-induced respiratory depression; respiratory depression due to barbiturates or other sedatives and hypnotics, anesthetics, other nonnarcotic CNS depressants, or pathologic causes; narcotic addiction (may precipitate severe and possibly fatal withdrawal symptoms).

ADVERSE/SIDE EFFECTS. Dysphoria, miosis, pseudoptosis, sweating, pallor, lethargy, drowsiness, dizziness, agitation, restlessness, nausea, vomiting, sense of heaviness in limbs, hypertension, tachycardia, respiratory depression. High doses: weird dreams, visual hallucinations, disorientation, feelings of unreality. Neonates: irritability, increased crying.

ROUTE AND DOSAGE. **Intravenous: Adults:** 1 mg; if required, this may be followed by one or two additional doses of 0.5 mg at 10- to 15-minute intervals. Total dose not to exceed 3 mg. **Neonates** (approximately one-tenth adult dose): 0.05 to 0.1 mg diluted to 2 ml with 0.9% sodium chloride injection and injected into umbilical cord vein immediately after delivery. If vein cannot be used, injection may be given **subcutaneously** or **intramuscularly.**

NURSING IMPLICATIONS

Not to be confused with levorphanol tartrate, a narcotic analgesic.

Artificial respiration with oxygen and other resuscitative measures may accompany drug administration.

Monitor vital signs, blood pressure, and drug effect. Duration of narcotic action is often longer than that of levallorphan, therefore, observe patient closely for return of respiratory depression. Additional dose of levallorphan may be necessary.

Patient should be closely observed for a day or more, even if patient shows signs of apparent improvement.

Since levallorphan is capable of producing respiratory depression, it is generally given in small doses and drug effect observed carefully before subsequent doses are given.

L

PROTOTYPE

LEVODOPA

(lee-voe-doe'pa)

(Dopar, Larodopa)

Antiparkinsonian

ACTIONS AND USES. Metabolic precursor of dopamine, a catecholamine neurotransmitter. Unlike dopamine, levodopa readily crosses the blood–brain barrier. Precise mechanism of action unknown. It is hypothesized that levodopa is rapidly decarboxylated to dopamine and thus restores dopamine levels in extrapyramidal centers (believed to be depleted in parkinsonism). Cardiac stimulation may be produced by action of dopamine on β-adrenergic receptors. Also may augment secretion of growth hormone, which in turn is postulated to affect glucose utilization.

Used in treatment of idiopathic Parkinson's disease, postencephalitic and arteriosclerotic parkinsonism, and parkinsonian symptoms associated with manganese and carbon monoxide poisoning. Also commercially available in combination with carbidopa (e.g., as Sinemet), a decarboxylase inhibitor, to permit lower dosage range of levodopa and thus reduce incidence of adverse reactions.

ABSORPTION AND FATE. Rapidly and completely absorbed from GI tract. Peak plasma concentrations within 1 to 3 hours. Converted to dopamine by decarboxylation in GI tract and liver; small amount of levodopa reaches CNS, where it is metabolized to dopamine by dopa decarboxylase. Major metabolite is homovanillic acid; minute amounts of dopamine are converted to norepinephrine. About 80% of dose is excreted in urine within 24 hours; negligible amounts are eliminated in feces.

CONTRAINDICATIONS AND PRECAUTIONS. Known hypersensitivity to levodopa, narrow-angle glaucoma patients with suspicious pigmented lesion or history of melanoma, acute psychoses, severe psychoneurosis, within 2 weeks of MAO inhibitors. Safe use in women of childbearing potential, during pregnancy and lactation, and in children under 12 years of age not established. *Cautious Use:* cardiovascular, renal, hepatic, or endocrine disease, history of myocardial infarction with residual arrhythmias, peptic ulcer, convulsions, psychiatric disorders, chronic wide-angle glaucoma, diabetes, pulmonary diseases, bronchial asthma, patients receiving antihypertensive drugs.

ADVERSE/SIDE EFFECTS. Altered laboratory values: elevated BUN, SGOT, SGPT, alkaline phosphatase, LDH, bilirubin, protein-bound iodine, serum level of growth hormone; decreased glucose tolerance; hypokalemia. **CV (common):** orthostatic hypotension; (less frequent): palpitation, tachycardia, hypertension, phlebitis. **GI (common):** anorexia, nausea, vomiting, abdominal distress, flatulence, dry mouth, dysphagia, sialorrhea; (less frequent): burning sensation of tongue, bitter taste, diarrhea or constipation; (rarely): duodenal ulcer, GI bleeding. **Hematologic:** hemolytic anemia, agranulocytosis, reduced hemoglobin and hematocrit, leukopenia. **Neuropsychiatric (frequent):** choreiform and involuntary movements, increased hand tremor, bradykinetic episodes (on–off phenomena), trismus, grinding of teeth (bruxism), ataxia, muscle twitching, numbness, weakness, fatigue, headache, opisthotonos, confusion, agitation, anxiety, euphoria, insomnia, nightmares; (less frequent): psychotic episodes with paranoid delusions or hallucinations, severe depression, hypomania; (rare): convulsions. **Ophthalmic:** blepharospasm, diplopia, blurred vision, dilated pupils, widening of palpebral fissures, oculogyric crises (rare). **Other:** rhinorrhea, flushing, skin rashes, increased sweating, bizarre breathing patterns, urinary retention or incontinence, increased sexual drive, priapism, weight gain or loss, edema; (rarely): hiccups, loss of hair, and malignant melanoma.

ROUTE AND DOSAGE. Oral: Initial: 0.5 to 1 Gm daily divided into two or more equal doses; daily dosage increased gradually in increments of not more than 0.75 Gm every 3 to 7 days, as tolerated. Total daily dosage not to exceed 8 Gm. Highly individualized.

NURSING IMPLICATIONS

Food–Drug Interactions: Ingestion of l-dopa with meals, especially if high in protein, appears to interfere with plasma-to-CNS transport of the drug. Administration of drug between meals and with low protein snack (if desired) may decrease fluctuations in clinical response.

If patient is unable to swallow capsule or tablet form, consult pharmacist about preparing a liquid formulation.

Rate of dosage increase is determined primarily by patient's tolerance and response to levodopa. Make accurate observations and report promptly adverse reactions (generally dose-related and reversible) and therapeutic effects.

Monitor vital signs, particularly during period of dosage adjustment. Report alterations in blood pressure, pulse, and respiratory rate and rhythm.

Orthostatic hypotension is usually asymptomatic, but some patients experience dizziness and syncope. Caution patient to make positional changes slowly, particularly from recumbent to upright position, and to dangle legs a few minutes before standing. Supervision of ambulation is indicated. Tolerance to this effect usually develops within a few months of therapy. Elastic stockings may help some patients; consult physician.

Muscle twitching and spasmodic winking (blepharospasm) are *early signs of overdosage;* report them promptly.

All patients should be closely monitored for behavior changes. Patients in depression should be closely observed for suicidal tendencies.

Therapeutic effects: significant improvement usually appears during second or third week of therapy, but it may not occur for 6 months or more in some patients. Therapeutic effect on Parkinsons disease appears to decline after 6 to 8 years of therapy.

Elevation of mood and sense of well-being may precede objective improvement. Stress the importance of resuming activities gradually and observing safety precautions in order to avoid injury. The patient with a history of cardiac problems should be cautioned against overactivity.

Patients with chronic wide-angle glaucoma should be monitored during therapy for changes in intraocular pressure.

Patients with diabetes should be observed carefully for alterations in diabetes control. Frequent monitoring of blood sugar is advised.

All patients on extended therapy should be checked periodically for symptoms of diabetes and acromegaly and for functioning of hematopoietic, hepatic, and renal systems.

About 80% of patients on full therapeutic doses for 1 year or longer develop abnormal involuntary movements such as facial grimacing, exaggerated chewing, protrusion of tongue, rhythmic opening and closing of mouth, bobbing of head, jerky arm and leg movements, and exaggerated respiration. Symptoms tend to increase if dosage is not reduced.

Chronic management may be accompanied by the on-off phenomenon: rapid unpredictable swings in intensity of motor symptoms of parkinsonism evidenced by increase in bradykinesia (attacks of "leg freezing" or slow body movement). The patient is unable to perform ADL such as walking during the "off" periods as opposed to independent ability during "on" periods. Attacks develop within minutes, last 1 to 3 hours, usually appear at same time of day, and are due to excessive drug levels. The phenomenon may be precipitated by emotional stress.

Solicit help of family members to establish a baseline profile of the patient's disabilities. This information is essential for accurate differentiation between desired response to therapy and drug-induced neuropsychiatric adverse reactions.

Urge patient to maintain prescribed drug regimen. Sudden *withdrawal* of medication can lead to parkinsonian crisis with return of marked rigidity, akinesia, tremor, hyperpyrexia.

Inform patients that a metabolite of levodopa may cause urine to darken on standing and may also cause sweat to be dark-colored.

Caution patients not to take over-the-counter preparations or fortified cereals unless approved by physician. Multivitamins, antinauseants, and fortified cereals usually contain pyridoxine (vitamin B_6); 5 mg or more of pyridoxine daily may reverse the effects of levodopa.

Dopar contains *tartrazine* which may cause an allergic-type reaction including asthma in susceptible patients. The reaction is frequently seen in individuals with aspirin hypersensitivity.

In the event a patient requires general anesthesia, levodopa therapy is continued as long as patient is able to take fluids and medication by mouth (generally discontinued 6 to 24 hours prior to anesthesia). Therapy usually is resumed as soon as patient is able to take oral medication.

Patient and responsible family members require guidance and supervision of drug regimen.

Physical therapy is an important adjunct to drug therapy.

Stored in tight, light-resistant containers preferably between 15° and 30°C (59° and 86°F) unless otherwise directed by manufacturer.

L

Diagnostic Test Interferences. False-negative **urine glucose** tests may result with use of glucose oxidase methods (e.g., Clinistix, Tes-Tape) and false-positive results with the copper reduction method (e.g., Clinitest), especially in patients receiving large doses. It is reported that Clinistix and Tes-Tape may be used if reading is taken at margin of wet and dry tape. There is also possibility of false-positive tests for **urinary ketones** by dip-stick tests, e.g., Acetest (equivocal), Ketostix, Labstix, false elevations of **serum and urinary uric acid** levels by colorimetric methods, but not with uricase; false increases in **urinary protein** by Lowry method; false decreases in **urinary VMA** by Pisano method, and false increases in urinary catecholamine levels by Hingerty method.

Drug Interactions. Drugs that may inhibit or decrease therapeutic effects of levodopa include **anticholinergics, diazepam** (Valium) and possibly other **phenothiazines** (mutually antagonistic), **phenylbutazone phenytoin** (Dilantin) and other hydantoins, **pyridoxine,** (vitamin B_6) in doses of 5 mg or more, and **reserpine.** Levodopa may enhance the hypotensive effects of **guanethidine** (Ismelin) and **methyldopa** (Aldomet); methyldopa may enhance antiparkinsonian effects of levodopa (used therapeutically). Concomitant use of **MAO inhibitors** and drugs with MAO activity e.g., furazolidone (Furoxone) may produce hypertension (levodopa contraindicated with MAOIs, but may be used concurrently in carbidopa-levodopa combination product). **Propranolol** (Inderal) may enhance the therapeutic effect of levodopa and may also enhance levodopa-induced stimulation of growth hormone secretion.

LEVORPHANOL TARTRATE
(Levo-Dromoran)

(lee-vor′fa-nole)
Narcotic analgesic
C II

L

ACTIONS AND USES. Synthetic morphinan derivative with agonist activity only. Actions, uses, contraindications, precautions, and adverse reactions similar to those of morphine (qv). More potent as an analgesic and has somewhat longer duration of action than morphine. Reported to cause less nausea, vomiting, and constipation than equivalent doses of morphine, but may produce more sedation, smooth-muscle stimulation, and respiratory depression. Unlike morphine, can be given by mouth.

Used to relieve moderate to severe pain. Used also preoperatively to allay apprehension.

ABSORPTION AND FATE. Peak analgesia within 60 to 90 minutes following subcutaneous injection, and within 20 minutes following IV injection. Duration of action 4 to 5 hours. Half-life: 1.2 hours; 50% protein bound. Metabolized primarily in liver. Excreted in urine mainly as glucuronide conjugate.

ROUTE AND DOSAGE. Oral, subcutaneous: 2 to 3 mg, repeated in 4 to 6 hours, if necessary. Dosage is reduced in poor-risk patients, very young or very old patients and in patients receiving other CNS depressants. Has been used intravenously to supplement anesthesia.

NURSING IMPLICATIONS

Not to be confused with levallorphan tartrate, a narcotic antagonist, and sometimes used as an antidote for levorphanol.

Levorphanol should be given in the smallest effective dose and as infrequently as possible to minimize the possibility of tolerance and physical dependence.

Classified as Schedule II drug under the Federal Controlled Substances Act.

See Morphine Sulfate.

LEVOTHYROXINE SODIUM

(Eltroxin, Levothroid, L-Thyroxine, Noroxine, Synthroid, T_4)

(lee-voe-thye-rox'een)
Hormone, thyroid

ACTIONS AND USES. Synthetically prepared monosodium salt and levo isomer of thyroxine, with similar actions and uses: 0.1 mg is equivalent to 65 mg desiccated thyroid and is about 600 times more potent. *For contraindications, precautions, and adverse reactions, see Thyroid.*

Used as specific replacement therapy for diminished or absent thyroid function resulting from primary or secondary atrophy of gland, surgery, excessive radiation or antithyroid drugs, congenital defect. Administered orally for hypothyroid state; administered IV for myxedematous coma or other thyroid dysfunctions demanding rapid replacement, as well as in failure to respond to oral therapy.

ABSORPTION AND FATE. Following absorption, binds to plasma protein. Circulation half-life: 6 or 7 days. Distributed widely; gradually released into tissue cells, where it causes increased metabolic rate, usually after 12 to 48 hours. One mg of levothyroxine increases heat production about 1000 calories.

ROUTE AND DOSAGE. All doses individualized and initiated cautiously according to age, physical condition, severity, and duration of hypothyroidism. **Oral** (thyroid replacement): **Adults:** 0.1 mg daily, with gradual increments of 0.05 to 0.1 mg every 1 to 3 weeks until desired response; maintenance: 0.1 to 0.2 mg daily. **Elderly:** Initial: 0.025 mg/day with increments of 0.025 mg daily at 3- to 4-week intervals until desired response. **Children:** Initial: 0.025 to 0.05 mg daily, with increments of 0.05 to 0.1 mg at 2-week intervals until desired response; maintenance: 0.3 to 0.4 mg daily. **Intravenous** (myxedematous coma or stupor): 0.2 to 0.5 mg first day; 0.1 to 0.2 mg or more on second day if no evidence of progressive improvement; daily doses of lesser amounts are continued until patient can accept daily dose. **Intramuscular:** used when oral route is not feasible.

NURSING IMPLICATIONS

Administered as single dose, preferably before breakfast.

Parenteral preparation should be reconstituted with NaCl injection immediately before administration. Shake vial until solution is clear. Discard unused portion.

Transfer from levothyroxine to liothyronine: discontinue levothyroxine before starting small dose of liothyronine. Transfer from liothyronine to levothyroxine: start levothyroxine; then, after several days, discontinue liothyronine.

Monitor for adverse effects during early adjustment period. If metabolism is increased too rapidly, especially in the elderly and in patients with heart disease, symptoms of angina and/or cardiac failure may appear.

Levothyroxine may aggravate severity of previously obscured symptoms of diabetes mellitus, Addison's disease, or diabetes insipidus. Therapeutic measures directed at these disorders may require adjustment.

There is great urgency in achieving full thyroid replacement in infants or children because of the critical importance of the hormone in sustaining growth and development; therefore doses are generally higher than adult doses.

Therapy with levothyroxine results in euthyroidism, and a return to normal of laboratory values, e.g., free T_4, total T_4, free thyroxine index (FTI).

See also Thyroid (prototype for thyroid agents).

LIDOCAINE HYDROCHLORIDE

(lye'doe-kane)

(Anestacon, Baylocaine, BayCaine, Dilocaine, L-Caine, Lida-Mantle, LidoPen, Nervocaine, Nulicaine, Octocaine, Ultracaine, Xylocaine, Xylocard)

Antiarrhythmic (Class I)
Anesthetic (local)

ACTIONS AND USES. Aminoacyl amide with anesthetic, and antiarrhythmic (class I) properties. Cardiac actions similar to those of procainamide and quinidine, but has little effect on myocardial contractility, A-V and intraventricular conduction, cardiac output, and systolic arterial pressure in equivalent doses. Exerts antiarrhythmic action by suppressing automaticity in His-Purkinje system and by elevating electrical stimulation threshold of ventricle during diastole. Progressive depression of CNS occurs with increasing blood concentrations; produces anticonvulsant, sedative, and analgesic effects. Action as local anesthetic is more prompt, more intense, and longer lasting than that of procaine. Suppresses cough and gag reflexes.

Used for rapid control of ventricular arrhythmias occurring during acute myocardial infarction, cardiac surgery, and cardiac catheterization and those caused by digitalis intoxication. *Investigational Use:* to treat refractory status epilepticus. Preparations also available for surface and infiltration anesthesia and for nerve block, including caudal and spinal block anesthesia. Topical preparations are used to relieve local discomfort of skin and mucous membranes.

ABSORPTION AND FATE. Following IV bolus dose, action begins within 10 to 90 seconds and lasts up to 20 minutes. Following IM injection, effective antiarrhythmic blood levels occur within 5 to 15 minutes and persist 60 to 90 minutes. Duration of action: lumbar epidural block 100 minutes; spinal anesthesia: motor 100 minutes, sensory 140 minutes; caudal block: 75 to 135 minutes. Peak effect after local application to mucous membranes: 2 to 5 minutes; duration: 30 to 60 minutes. Rapidly distributed to most body tissues. Biphasic half-life: initial: 7 to 8 minutes; terminal 1 to 2 hours (longer in patients with renal or hepatic disease). About 50 to 75% bound to plasma proteins. Approximately 90% metabolized by liver and excreted in urine as metabolites; less than 3% excreted unchanged. Average duration of anesthetic action is 90 to 120 minutes. Crosses placenta.

CONTRAINDICATIONS AND PRECAUTIONS. History of hypersensitivity to amide-type local anesthetics; application or injection of lidocaine anesthetic in presence of severe trauma or sepsis, blood dyscrasias, supraventricular arrhythmias, Stokes-Adams syndrome, untreated sinus bradycardia, severe degrees of sinoatrial, atrioventricular, and intraventricular heart block. Safe use during pregnancy (category B), and in children not established. *Cautious Use:* liver or renal disease, congestive heart failure, marked hypoxia, respiratory depression, hypovolemia, shock, myasthenia gravis, debilitated patients, the elderly, family history of malignant hyperthermia (fulminant hypermetabolism).

ADVERSE/SIDE EFFECTS. CNS: drowsiness, dizziness, lightheadedness, restlessness, confusion, disorientation, irritability, apprehension, euphoria, wild excitement, tinnitus, decreased hearing, blurred or double vision, impaired color perception, numbness of lips or tongue and other paresthesias including sensations of heat and cold, chest heaviness, difficulty in speaking, difficulty in breathing or swallowing, muscular twitching, tremors, psychosis. With high doses: convulsions, respiratory depression and arrest. **CV (with high doses):** hypotension, bradycardia, conduction disorders including heart block, cardiovascular collapse, cardiac arrest. **Other reported:** anorexia, nausea, vomiting, excessive perspiration, soreness at IM site, local thrombophlebitis (with prolonged IV infusion), hypersensitivity reactions (urticaria, rash, edema, anaphylactoid reactions).

ROUTE AND DOSAGE. Intravenous bolus: 50 to 100 mg, administered at rate of 20 to 50 mg/minute; if indicated, may be repeated after 5 minutes. No more than 200 to 300 mg in a

1-hour period is advised. **Intravenous infusion:** 20 to 50 mcg/kg/minute for average 70-kg man (1 to 4 mg/minute); may be prescribed immediately after bolus dose. **Intramuscular:** 200 to 300 mg if necessary, may be repeated once after interval of 60 to 90 minutes. Anesthetic use: **Infiltration:** 0.5 to 1%. **Nerve block:** 1 to 2%; **Epidural:** 1 to 2%; **Caudal:** 1 to 1.5%; **Spinal:** 5% with glucose; **Saddle block:** 1.5% with dextrose. **Topical** (jelly, ointment, cream, solution): 2.5 to 5% (weaker concentrations used for the elderly, and debilitated patients).

NURSING IMPLICATIONS

Only lidocaine hydrochloride injection without preservatives or epinephrine that is specifically labeled for IV use should be used for IV injection or infusion.

For IV infusion, use microdropper and timer, or infusion pump. Physician will prescribe specific rate of flow, usually no more than 4 mg/minute. Rate must be closely monitored.

Lidocaine should not be added to transfusion assemblies.

Constant ECG monitoring and frequent determinations of blood pressure are essential to avoid potential overdosage and toxicity.

Ausculate lungs for basilar rales, especially in patients who tend to metabolize the drug slowly (e.g., congestive heart failure, cardiogenic shock, hepatic dysfunction).

In patients with sinus bradycardia or incomplete heart block administration of IV lidocaine to eliminate ventricular ectopic beats is usually preceded by prior acceleration of heart (e.g., by atropine, isoproterenol or electric pacing) to avoid provoking more frequent and serious ventricular arrhythmias or complete heart block.

Watch for neurotoxic effects, particularly in patients receiving IV infusions of lidocaine or those with high lidocaine blood levels (drowsiness, dizziness, confusion, paresthesias, visual disturbances, excitement, behavioral changes).

It is not known whether lidocaine can trigger malignant hyperthermia in patients with this genetic predisposition. Unexplained signs of tachycardia, rapid breathing, fluctuating blood pressure, and metabolic acidosis may precede temperature elevation and should be reported promptly. Prognosis is dependent on early diagnosis, immediate discontinuation of drug, oxygen therapy, supportive measures, and dantrolene. *See Index: Clinical signs and symptoms: malignant hyperthermia.*

IV infusion should be terminated as soon as patient's basic cardiac rhythm stabilizes or at earliest signs and symptoms of toxicity (infusions are rarely continued beyond 24 hours). An oral antiarrhythmic is used for maintenance therapy.

If ECG signs of excessive cardiac depression such as prolongation of PR interval or QRS complex and the appearance or aggravation of arrhythmias occur, infusion should be stopped immediately.

Reports of convulsions are common. Resuscitative equipment, oxygen, and emergency drugs including diazepam, ultrashort-acting barbiturate (Thiopental, Thiamylal), vasopressors (ephedrine or metaraminol) should be immediately available for management of convulsions and respiratory depression.

Deltoid muscle is recommended as the preferred IM site, since faster and higher peak blood levels are produced than by injection into gluteus or lateral thigh.

IM injection should be made with frequent aspirations to avoid inadvertent intravascular administration.

Lidocaine blood levels of approximately 1.5 to 6 mcg/ml are reported to provide "usually effective" antiarrhythmic activity. Blood levels greater than 7 mcg/ml are potentially toxic.

Anesthetic use: Lidocaine solutions containing preservatives should not be used for spinal or epidural (including caudal) block.

For positioning of patient following spinal anesthesia, *see Index: Nursing interventions: spinal anesthesia.*

Instruct patient using lidocaine for relief of oral discomfort to swish solution around in mouth. It can be swallowed, but patient should know that oral topical anesthetic (xylocaine viscous) may interfere with swallowing reflex. Food should not be ingested within 60 minutes following drug application, especially in pediatric, elderly, or debilitated patients. Also, warn against chewing gum while buccal and throat membranes are anesthetized to prevent biting trauma.

Partially used solutions of lidocaine without preservatives should be discarded after initial use.

Inspect solutions for particulate matter and discoloration prior to administration and discard if either is present.

Lidocaine injection and commercially prepared solutions containing the drug in 5% dextrose are stored preferably at 15 to 30°C (59 to 86°F) unless otherwise directed by manufacturer.

Diagnostic Test Interferences. Increases in **creatine phosphokinase** level may occur for 48 hours following IM dose and may interfere with test for presence in myocardial infarction.

Drug Interactions: Lidocaine

Plus	Interactions
Barbiturates	Decrease lidocaine action through enzyme induction
Cimetidine (Tagamet)	Increases pharmacologic effects of lidocaine. Monitor for lidocaine toxicity
Phenytoin (Dilantin)	Increases cardiac depressant effect of lidocaine
Procainamide	Additive neurologic effects
Propranolol (Inderal), quinidine	Increase cardiac depressant effect of lidocaine. Monitor for lidocaine toxicity
Succinylcholine, and other neuromuscular blocking agents	Enhance muscle relaxant effects. Monitor for respiratory depression

L

LINCOMYCIN HYDROCHLORIDE

(Lincocin)

(lin-koe-mye'sin)
Antiinfective
Antibiotic (macrolide)

ACTIONS AND USES. Derived from *Streptomyces lincolnensis.* Bacteriostatic or bactericidal depending on concentration used and sensitivity of organism. Acts by binding selectivity to 50S subunits of bacterial ribosomes, thus suppressing protein synthesis. Similar to erythromycin in antibacterial activity, and demonstrates some cross-resistance with it. Effective against most of the common Gram-positive pathogens, particularly streptococci, pneumococci, and staphylococci. Also effective against *Bacteroides* and other anaerobes; however, little activity against most gram-negative organisms, and ineffective against viruses, yeasts, or fungi. Resistance by *Staphylococcus* is acquired in stepwise manner. Lincomycin is reported to have neuromuscular blocking properties.

Use reserved for treatment of serious infections caused by susceptible bacteria in penicillin-allergic patients or patients for whom penicillin is inappropriate.

ABSORPTION AND FATE. Rapidly but only partially (20 to 35%) absorbed from GI tract. Peak plasma concentrations in 2 to 4 hours after oral dose; levels maintained above minimal inhibitory concentration (MIC) for 6 to 8 hours. IM injection produces maximal plasma concentrations within 30 minutes; effective levels persist 12 to 14 hours. IV infusion of

600 mg over a 2-hour period produces therapeutic levels that persist for 14 hours. Following subconjunctival injection, ocular fluid drug levels last 5 hours. Distributed to most body tissues and fluids. Significant concentrations in bone, aqueous humor, bile, peritoneal, pleural, and synovial fluids. Low concentrations have been attained in cerebrospinal fluid when meninges are inflamed. Half-life about 5 hours; 57 to 72% protein bound depending on plasma concentration. Partially metabolized in liver. Excreted in urine, bile, and feces mostly as unchanged drug and bioactive metabolite. Not cleared from blood by hemodialysis or peritoneal dialysis. Crosses placenta and may appear in breast milk.

CONTRAINDICATIONS AND PRECAUTIONS. Previous hypersensitivity to lincomycin and clindamycin; impaired hepatic function, known monilial infections (unless treated concurrently); use in newborns. Safe use in pregnancy and nursing mothers not established. *Cautious Use:* impaired renal function; history of GI disease, particularly colitis; history of liver, endocrine, or metabolic diseases; history of asthma, hayfever, eczema, drug or other allergies; elderly patients. *See also Drug Interactions.*

ADVERSE/SIDE EFFECTS. CV: hypotension, syncope, cardiopulmonary arrest (particularly after rapid IV). **GI:** glossitis, stomatitis, nausea, vomiting, anorexia, decreased taste acuity, unpleasant or altered taste, abdominal cramps, diarrhea, acute enterocolitis, pseudomembranous colitis (potentially fatal). **Hematopoietic:** neutropenia, leukopenia, agranulocytosis, thrombocytopenic purpura, and aplastic anemia and pancytopenia (rare). **Hypersensitivity:** pruritus, urticaria, skin rashes, exfoliative and vesiculobullous dermatitis, erythema multiforme resembling Stevens-Johnson syndrome (rare), angioedema, photosensitivity, anaphylactoid reaction, serum sickness. **Other:** superinfections (proctitis, pruritus ani, vaginitis), tinnitus, vertigo, dizziness, headache, generalized myalgia, thrombophlebitis following IV use (infrequent); pain at IM injection site (infrequent); jaundice and abnormal liver function tests (direct relationship to lincomycin not established).

L

ROUTE AND DOSAGE. Oral: Adults: 500 mg every 6 to 8 hours. **Pediatric (over 1 month of age):** 30 to 60 mg/kg divided into 3 or 4 equal doses. **Intramuscular: Adults:** 600 mg every 12 to 24 hours. **Pediatric (over 1 month of age):** 10 mg/kg every 12 to 24 hours. **Intravenous: Adults:** 600 mg to 1 Gm every 8 to 12 hours. Maximum recommended dose 8 Gm (1 Gm of lincomycin is diluted in not less than 100 ml of 5% dextrose in water or in saline or other appropriate solution recommended by manufacturer and infused over period of not less than 1 hour). **Pediatric (over 1 month of age):** 10 to 20 mg/kg/day divided equally and infused every 8 to 12 hours. Available as capsules, pediatric capsules, syrup, and injection. **Subjunctival injection:** 0.25 ml (75 mg).

NURSING IMPLICATIONS

A careful history should be taken of previous sensitivities to drugs or other allergens.

Culture and sensitivity tests should be performed initially and during therapy to determine continued microbial susceptibility.

Absorption is reduced and delayed by presence of food in stomach. Administer oral drug with a full glass (8 ounces) of water at least 1 to 2 hours before meals or 2 to 3 hours after meals.

Administer IM injection deep into large muscle mass; inject slowly to minimize pain. Rotate injection sites.

Monitor blood pressure and pulse in patients receiving parenteral drug. Have patient remain recumbent following drug administration until blood pressure stability is assured.

Relatively high incidence of diarrhea (20%) is associated with use of lincomycin. Monitor patients closely and report changes in bowel frequency. If significant diarrhea occurs, drug should be discontinued; large bowel endoscopy is recommended.

Antiperistaltic agents such as opiates or diphenoxylate with atropine (Lomotil) may prolong and worsen diarrhea by delaying removal of toxins from colon. Advise patient not to self-medicate. Medical management consists of fluid, electrolyte, and protein supplements, as indicated, and possibly corticosteroids. Oral vancomycin or cholestyramine has been prescribed for pseudomembranous colitis caused by *C. difficile.*

Diarrhea, acute colitis, or pseudomembranous colitis (suspect this if patient develops high temperature, diarrhea, or ileus) may occur up to several weeks following cessation of therapy. Advise patients to report promptly the onset of perianal irritation, diarrhea, or blood and mucus in stools.

Advise patients to report immediately symptoms of hypersensitivity. Drug should be discontinued.

Serum drug levels should be monitored closely in patients with severe impairment of renal function (levels tend to be higher). Recommended dosage for these patients is 25 to 30% of that for patients with normal renal function.

Periodic hepatic and renal function studies and complete blood cell counts are indicated during prolonged drug therapy.

Superinfections by nonsusceptible organisms are most likely to occur when duration of therapy exceeds 10 days.

Instruct patient to take drug for full course of therapy as prescribed. Drug therapy should continue at least 10 days in patients with group A β-hemolytic streptococcal infections to reduce the possibility of rheumatic fever or glomerulonephritis.

Follow manufacturer's directions for reconstitution, storage time, compatible IV fluids, and IV administration rates.

Store unopened vials and oral drug preferably between 15° and 30°C (59° and 86°F) unless otherwise directed by manufacturer.

L

Diagnostic Test Interferences. Lincomycin may cause increases in **serum alkaline phosphatase, bilirubin, CPK, SGOT,** and **SGPT,** and possibly **serum triglycerides.**

Drug Interactions: Lincomycin

Plus	Interactions
Chloramphenicol Erythromycin	Possibility of mutual antagonism
Kaolin antidiarrheal compounds (e.g., Kaopectate)	Reduce intestinal absorption of lincomycin by about 90%. If used, administer kaolin at least 12 hours before or 3 to 4 hours after lincomycin
Skeletal muscle relaxants (e.g., ether, tubocurarine, pancuronium)	Enhanced neuromuscular blocking action

PROTOTYPE

LINDANE

(lin-dane)

(Gamma Benzene Hexachloride, gBh, Kwell, Kwellada, Scabene)

Antiinfective
Pediculicide
Scabicide

ACTIONS AND USES. Synthetic chlorinated hydrocarbon chemically related to DDT.

Used for eradication of itch mite of scabies *(Sarcoptes scabiei)* and for infestations of head lice *(Pediculus capitis)* and crab lice *(Phthirus pubis)* and their nits.

CONTRAINDICATIONS AND PRECAUTIONS. Hypersensitivity to any component of the drug; application to eyes, face, acutely inflamed skin areas; prolonged or repeated applications (can be absorbed through skin, especially in the young). *Cautious Use:* infants, children, during pregnancy.

ADVERSE/SIDE EFFECTS. Skin irritation, erythema, pruritus, sensitization (eczematous eruptions). Highly toxic if absorbed through skin or ingested: vomiting; diarrhea; irritation of eyes, skin, and mucosa; paresthesias; vertigo; CNS stimulation (tremors, convulsions); aplastic anemia; ventricular fibrillation; liver and kidney damage.

ROUTE AND DOSAGE. Topical: 1% cream, lotion, or shampoo.

NURSING IMPLICATIONS

Cream or lotion (shake well): *Scabies:* If crusted lesions are present, take soapy bath or shower, rinse well, dry thoroughly, and allow skin to cool. Apply thin film of cream or lotion over entire body surface from neck down (avoid urethral meatus). Pay particular attention to intertriginous areas (finger webs and other body creases and folds), wrists, elbows, and belt line. After 8 to 12 hours, remove medication by thorough washing (shower or bath). Put on clean clothing; change bed linen. A second application is usually not needed. *Pediculosis:* After a bath or shower, apply to hairy infested areas and adjacent areas. Leave on for 8 to 12 hours. Wash thoroughly and put on clean clothing; change bed linen.

Shampoo: *Head and crab lice:* Pour about 1 ounce (2 tablespoonfuls) of shampoo onto affected area; being sure to wet all hairy areas with shampoo. Add small amount of warm water and work into thick lather; allow to remain in place for at least 4 minutes. For head lice, pay particular attention to areas above and behind ears and back of head. Rinse completely; dry thoroughly with towel. Use fine-tooth comb to remove remaining nit shells. If necessary, treatment may be repeated after 7 days, but not more than twice in 1 week. Inform patient that shampoo formulation is intended only for treatment of head and crab lice; it should not be used as a routine shampoo. Combs, brushes, and other washable items may be cleaned with the shampoo.

Advise patient to use medication only as directed by physician. Stress the importance of avoiding overdosage.

Shaving of hair is not necessary.

Instruct patient to discontinue medication and report to a physician if signs of irritation or sensitization occur. Medication should be removed by thorough washing.

Caution patient not to apply medication to face and to avoid contact with eyes. If accidental eye contact occurs, flush thoroughly with water.

Contaminated bed linen and clothing should be carefully washed (boiled if possible) or dry cleaned (if not washable) to prevent reinfestation. Particular attention should be paid to the seams of clothing. For dry cleaning, place clothing in a plastic bag, seal it carefully, and inform dry cleaner of contents.

Microscopic confirmation of scabies mites is recommended before treatment, if diagnosis is in doubt. Burrows occur in 15 to 18% of patients and can be seen by oblique light or hand lens.

Pruritic nodules sometimes develop after scabies infestation and may last for weeks, months, or years. Further scabicide treatment is not indicated; however, advise the patient to report to physician. Intralesional steroids or surgical excision are sometimes required.

Patients with crab lice should be examined for venereal disease. In addition to close body

contact, crab lice may also be transmitted by toilet seats, bedclothes, or clothing of infested persons. A careful history should be taken to identify the source of infestation.
Gamma benzene hexachloride is a highly toxic drug if topical applications are excessive or if taken internally. Caution patients to keep it out of reach of children. Accidental ingestion is treated by gastric lavage and saline cathartics. Oily liquids and epinephrine are contraindicated.
First infestations of scabies may exist 2 to 6 weeks before the patient becomes symptomatic. During this phase, scabies is highly contagious.
Case-finding efforts should include family members and other close-contact persons. Suspect scabies if a person complains of nocturnal itching (classic symptom).
Scabies is commonly called the 7-year itch, probably because reinfestations are common unless precautions are taken. Recurring, limited infestations of scabies may indicate a domestic animal source, especially dogs, cats, cattle, or poultry.

LIOTHYRONINE SODIUM

(Cytomel, Tertroxin, T_3)

(lye-oh-thye'roe-neen)
Hormone

L

ACTIONS AND USES. Synthetic form of natural thyroid hormone. Shares actions and uses of thyroid (qv), but has more rapid action and more rapid disappearance of effect, permitting quick dosage adjustment if necessary; 25 mcg are equivalent to approximately 65 mg of thyroid or thyroglobulin. May be used in T_3 suppression test to differentiate suspected hyperthyroidism from euthyroidism. *See Thyroid for absorption, fate, contraindications, precautions, and adverse reactions.*

ROUTE AND DOSAGE. All doses gradually increased from initial to maintenance levels with 12.5- to 25-mcg increments at 1- or 2-week intervals. **Oral: Adults:** *Hypothyroidism:* Initial: 25 mcg daily; maintenance: 25 to 75 mcg daily. *Myxedema:* Initial: 5 mcg daily; maintenance: 50 to 100 mcg daily. *Male infertility due to hypothyroidism:* Initial: 5 mcg; maintenance: 25 to 50 mcg daily. *Goiter:* Initial: 5 mcg daily; maintenance: 75 mcg daily. **Children:** *Cretinism:* Initial: 5 mcg daily, with a 5-mcg increment every 3 to 4 days until desired response is attained; **(1 year of age):** 50 mcg daily; **(more than 3 years):** full adult dosage. **Elderly:** same dosage as children.

NURSING IMPLICATIONS

Metabolic effects persist a few days after drug withdrawal.
Infants with thyroid dysfunction (mother provides little or no thyroid hormone to fetus) are started on replacement therapy as soon as possible to prevent permanent mental and physical changes.
When changing to liothyronine from thyroid, levothyroxine, or thyroglobulin, discontinue other medication, initiate liothyronine at low dosage, with gradual increases according to patient's response.
Residual actions of other thyroid preparations may persist for weeks; therefore, during early period of liothyronine substitution for another preparation, watch for possible additive effects, particularly if the patient is elderly, has cardiovascular disease, or is a child.
With onset of overdosage symptoms (hyperthyroidism), drug is withheld for 1 or 2 days; usually therapy can be resumed with lower dosage.
T_3 suppression test: when thyroid uptake of ^{131}I (radioactive iodine, RAI) is in borderline

high range, give 75 to 100 mcg liothyronine daily for 7 days, then repeat RAI uptake test. In hyperthyroidism, 24-hour RAI uptake will not be significantly affected; in euthyroid patient, 24-hour RAI uptake will decrease to less than 20%.

Depresses RAI uptake, especially when dose is above 75 mcg daily. This effect disappears in 2 weeks after drug withdrawal.

Advise patient not to take OTC medications unless approved by physician.

See also Thyroid (prototype thyroid agent).

LIOTRIX

(lye'oh-trix)

(Euthroid, Thyrolar, T_3, T_4)

Hormone, thyroid

ACTIONS AND USES. A mixture of synthetic levothyroxine (T_4) and liothyronine (T_3) combined in a constant 4:1 ratio by weight. Actions, uses, fate, precautions, and adverse reactions as for thyroid (qv). Products by different manufacturers differ in total amounts of each drug included in the formulation.

CONTRAINDICATIONS AND PRECAUTIONS. Thyrotoxicosis, acute myocardial infarction, morphologic hypogonadism, nephrosis, adrenal deficiency due to hypopituitarism. *Cautious Use:* concomitant anticoagulant therapy, myxedema, angina pectoris, hypertension, arteriosclerosis, renal dysfunction.

ADVERSE/SIDE EFFECTS. CV: palpitation, tachycardia, angina pectoris, cardiac arrhythmias, hypertension, congestive heart failure. **CNS:** nervousness, headache, tremors, insomnia. **GI:** nausea, abdominal cramps, diarrhea. **Other:** weight loss, heat intolerance, fever, sweating, menstrual irregularities.

ROUTE AND DOSAGE. Dosage individualized to approximate thyroid replacement need. **Oral: Adults and children:** Initial: 15 or 30 mg tablet daily, with gradual increases every 1 or 2 weeks for adults, every 2 weeks for children. Eventual maintenance dosage in growing child may be higher than in adult.

NURSING IMPLICATIONS

Usually administered as a single daily dose, preferably before breakfast.

Advise patient not to take OTC medications unless approved by physician.

Diabetic patients may require an increase in insulin or oral hypoglycemic dosage while taking liotrix. Decrease in dosage of antidiabetic drug may be necessary if liotrix dosage is reduced or if drug is withdrawn.

Report headache in euthyroid patient since this may indicate need for dosage adjustment or change to another thyroid preparation.

Available liotrix preparations contain variable amounts of T_3 and T_4; e.g., preparations said to be equivalent to desiccated thyroid may contain 60 mcg T_4 and 15 mcg T_3 (Euthroid-1) or 50 mcg T_4 and 12.5 mcg T_3 (Thyrolar-1). Instruct patients to have their prescriptions filled with the same brand currently being taken.

Changeover from another thyroid preparation can be made by direct substitution of liotrix for current dose of the other product, with gradual dose increase every 1 or 2 weeks.

Store in heat-, light-, and moisture-proof container. Shelf-life: 2 years.

See also Thyroid (prototype thyroid agent).

LITHIUM CARBONATE

(li'thee-um)
Antimanic agent

(Carbolith, Cibalith, Eskalith, Lithane, Lithizine, Lithobid, Lithonate, Lithotabs)

ACTIONS AND USES. Alkali metal salt which behaves in body much like sodium ion. Accumulates within neurons since Na pump is less efficient in transporting it out than Na, and thus alters electrophysiological characteristics of neurons. Introduction of lithium (Li) in body is followed by cation balance between Na, K, and Li. Subsequent lithium-induced increase in Na and K excretion places particular importance on Na and fluid balance. Enhances reuptake (thus inactivation) of biogenic amines, 5-HT and norepinephrine at nerve terminals, but apparently does not affect dopaminergic systems in brain. Specific relationship of these actions in treatment of mania not known. May induce several endocrinologic effects. Decreases amount of circulating thyroid hormones, but normal functioning usually returns through pituitary feedback. Other possible effects: blocking of renal response to ADH, elevation of serum growth hormone levels (clinical significance not determined); and decrease in glucose tolerance.

Used for control and prophylaxis of manic episodes in manic-depressive psychosis. May be given simultaneously with an antipsychotic agent during acute manic episode until clinical response to Li occurs. *Investigational Use:* to treat tardive dyskinesia, cluster headaches, SIADH, to prevent depression, and to increase leukocyte count in patient receiving cancer chemotherapy.

ABSORPTION AND FATE. Absorbed well from GI tract; peak serum levels reached ½ to 4 hours after a dose. Half-life adult: 24 hours; adolescent: 18 hours; elderly: 36 hours or more. No evidence of protein binding. Crosses blood–brain barrier slowly with appreciable amounts in cerebrospinal fluid, once steady state established. Approximately 50 to 75% of single dose excreted in urine within 24 hours followed by slower excretion over several days. Alkalinization of urine increases excretion. Less than 1% eliminated in feces and 4 to 5% in sweat. Crosses placenta; enters breast milk.

CONTRAINDICATIONS AND PRECAUTIONS. Significant cardiovascular or renal disease, brain damage, schizophrenia, organic brain syndrome, severe debilitation, dehydration or Na depletion; patients on low salt diet or receiving diuretics; pregnancy, especially first trimester (category D) nursing mothers, children under age 12. *Cautious Use:* elderly patients, thyroid disease, epilepsy, concomitant use with haloperidol and other antipsychotics, parkinsonism, diabetes mellitus, severe infections, urinary retention.

ADVERSE/SIDE EFFECTS. CNS: dizziness, headache, lethargy, drowsiness, fatigue, slurred speech, psychomotor retardation, giddiness, tinnitus, impaired vision, incontinence, restlessness, seizures, confusion, blackout spells, disorientation, recent memory loss, stupor, coma, EEG changes. **CV:** arrhythmias, hypotension, vasculitis, peripheral circulatory collapse, ECG changes. **Dermatologic** (thought to be toxicity rather than allergy): pruritus, maculopapular rash, hyperkeratosis, chronic folliculitis, transient acneiform papules (face, neck, intertriginous areas), anesthesia of skin, cutaneous ulcers, drying and thinning of hair, allergic vasculitis. **EENT:** impaired vision, transient scotomata, tinnitus. **GI:** nausea, vomiting, anorexia, abdominal pain, diarrhea, incontinence, dry mouth, metallic taste. **Endocrine:** diffuse thyroid enlargement, hypothyroidism, nephrogenic diabetes insipidus, transient hyperglycemia, glycosuria, hyponatremia. **Neuromuscular:** fine hand tremors (common), coarse tremors, choreoathetotic movements; fasciculations, clonic movements, incoordination including ataxia, muscle weakness, hyperreflexia, encephalopathic syndrome (weakness, lethargy, fever, tremors, confusion, extrapyramidal symptoms). **Other:** reversible leukocytosis (14,000 to 18,000/mm^3), albuminuria, oliguria, urinary incontinence, polyuria, polydipsia, increased uric acid excretion, edema, weight gain (common) or loss, exacerbation of psoriasis, flulike symptoms.

ROUTE AND DOSAGE. Individualized according to both serum lithium level and clinical condition *(see Nursing Implications).* **Oral: Adults:** *Acute mania:* 600 mg three times daily. *Maintenance:* 300 mg three or four times daily. Slow release form: 300 to 450 mg two or three times daily. (Available in capsules, tablets, controlled release tablets, syrup formulations.)

NURSING IMPLICATIONS

GI symptoms may be minimized by taking drug with meals. Transient nausea and general discomfort appear to coincide with peak rise in serum Li levels. Report persistent symptoms. Dosage may be adjusted to provide levels without high peaks.

Hospitalization is usually a necessity during initial treatment stage of daily serum lithium determinations until therapeutic dose is established.

Dose control: (1) generally dosage regimen is designed to maintain serum Li levels of 1.0 to 1.5 mEq/L in acute mania, and 0.6 to 1.6 mEq/L during maintenance treatment. (2) Blood sample for determining serum Li level is drawn prior to next dose (8 to 12 hours after last dose) when Li level is fairly stable. (3) If serum Li is above 1.5 mEq/L or if a clinical event has decreased patient's tolerance to Li (e.g., persistent vomiting or diarrhea, excessive sweating in hot weather, change in intake–output ratio, intercurrent infection, fever, noncompliance), consult physician before administering next dose. Timing of blood study and an accurate analysis of patient's condition will determine if next dose is to be changed or delayed.

Onset of therapeutic effects usually is preceded by a lag of 1 to 2 weeks. If drug control is not apparent within 1 to 3 weeks, drug is usually withdrawn.

Therapeutic response to Li therapy is evidenced by changed facial affect, improved posture, assumption of self-care, improved ability to concentrate, improved sleep pattern. Keep physician informed of patient's progress.

Urge patient to drink plenty of liquids (2 to 3 L/day) during stabilization period and at least 1 to 1½ L/day during remainder of therapy.

Instruct patient to be alert to increased output of dilute urine and persistent thirst. Chronic lithium therapy may be associated with diminished renal concentrating ability occasionally presenting as nephrogenic diabetes insipidus (with polydypsia and polyuria). Dose reduction may be indicated.

Teach patient to establish and adhere to a schedule for testing renal function by periodic evaluations of *urine specific gravity* (normal: 1.005 to 1.025).

Weigh patient daily: check ankles, tibiae, and wrists for edema. Report changes in intake–output ratio, sudden weight gain, or edema.

Reduced intake of fluid and sodium (Na) can accelerate Li retention with subsequent toxicity. Conversely, marked increase in Na intake can increase Li excretion and reduce drug effect.

Food-Drug Interactions: 6 to 10 Gm salt intake (average American intake) is required to keep serum lithium in the therapeutic range.

Normal dietary salt intake can be inadvertently compromised by lack of understanding. Caution patient to avoid self-prescribed low salt regimen, self-dosing with Rolaids, Sodamints, or other sodium antacids, high sodium foods, e.g., prepared meats, and drinks such as diet soda. Also warn against "crash" diets or diet pills that reduce appetite and food, salt and fluid intake.

Diffuse thyroid enlargement, generally without change in thyroid function, may occur in some patients (mostly women) after 5 months to 2 years of Li therapy. Lab studies of thyroid hormone and periodic palpation of the thyroid gland should be a part of preventive therapy. Be alert to and report symptoms of *hypothyroidism:* hoarseness, lethargy, fatigue, myxedema, headache, puffed face, weight gain, cold intolerance. Symptoms are reversible when Li is discontinued and supplemental thyroid is provided.

Contraceptive measures should be used during Li therapy but if the patient becomes pregnant she should be apprised of the potential risk to the fetus. If therapy is continued, serum Li levels must be closely monitored to prevent toxicity. Renal clearance of Li increases during pregnancy but reverts to lower rate immediately after delivery; dose, therefore, will be reduced to prevent toxicity.

Neonates born of mothers who took lithium during pregnancy may have high serum lithium level manifested by flaccidity, poor reflexes, cardiac dysrhythmia, and chronic twitching.

Li may impair both physical and mental ability. Caution against any activity demanding alertness (e.g., driving a car) until clinical response to drug has been established.

The elderly require special monitoring to prevent toxicity which may occur at serum levels ordinarily tolerated by other patients. Ability to excrete lithium decreases with aging, thus a smaller dose than usual may give desired control. Urinary creatinine clearance may be used as an index of patient's excretory function. Lithium clearance may be only one-fifth that of creatinine.

Polydipsia and polyuria, apparently not dose-related, are common early side effects particularly in the elderly. Symptoms may lessen but then reappear after several months or even years of maintenance therapy.

The encephalopathic syndrome may be induced when lithium is given concomitantly with haloperidol or with other antipsychotic medication, particularly in the elderly. Promptly report to the physician early signs of extrapyramidal reactions *(see Index: Clinical signs and symptoms).*

L

The fine tremor of hand or jaw, polyurea, mild thirst, transient mild nausea, and general discomfort that may occur in early treatment of mania sometimes persist throughout therapy. Usually, however, symptoms subside with temporary reduction of dose. If symptoms persist, drug is withdrawn.

Early signs of Li intoxication may occur several days after starting therapy and when Li levels are between 1.5 and 2.0 mEq/L: vomiting, diarrhea, lack of coordination, drowsiness, muscular weakness, slurred speech.

When Li levels are above 2.0 mEq/L: ataxia, blurred vision, giddiness, tinnitus, muscle twitching or coarse tremors, and a large output of dilute urine.

Warn patient not to switch brands of lithium carbonate. Because of varying fillers, a different brand may introduce a change in dose.

Urge patient to adhere to established dosage regimen, i.e., not to change or omit doses and not to change dose intervals.

Clinical follow-up and regular checks on serum Li levels are essential if treatment is to be safe and effective. Emphasize importance to family and patient of keeping all scheduled appointments for clinic visits.

Treatment of overdosage: induced vomiting, or gastric lavage if patient is conscious. Have available supportive measures for maintenance of airway and respiratory function and correction of fluid and electrolyte inbalance. Dialysis may be required for severe intoxication. Supportive therapy should continue for several days because of prolonged half-life and slow release of Li from brain tissue.

Store drug at temperature between 15° and 30°C (59° and 86°F) unless manufacturer directs otherwise. Protect from light and moisture.

Diagnostic Test Interferences. Lithium carbonate may cause **hypokalemia, glycosuria,** transient **hyperglycemia, proteinuria,** increased **VMA** excretion, increased serum **enzymes, BUN, FBS,**

and **magnesium** levels; lowered **serum T_3, T_4,** and **PBI** levels, elevated **I-131** uptake, leukocytosis, increased **uric acid** excretion.

Drug Interactions: Lithium (Li)

Plus	Interactions
Acetazolamide (Diamox), aminophylline, caffeine, mannitol, sodium chloride (excess), urinary alkalinizers (e.g., sodium bicarbonate), theophylline, urea	Increase Li excretion; lower serum Li and thus decrease therapeutic effects of Li
Amphetamines	Inhibit amphetamine activity
Antipsychotic agents, e.g., haloperidol (Haldol)	Augment potential Li toxicity: e.g., encephalopathic syndrome and brain damage
Carbamazepine (Tegretol)	
Chlorpromazine and other phenothiazines	Increase Li excretion; enhanced potential hyperglycemic effect of Li; reduced chlorpromazine serum and brain levels
Diazepam (Valium)	Monitor for hypothermia
Ethacrynic acid (Edecrin), furosemide (Lasix) Sodium chloride loss	Decrease Li excretion; increase serum Li level and thus enhance Li effects
Indomethacin (Indocin), methyldopa (Aldomet), Piroxicam (Feldene), spironolactone, tetracyclines	Increase risk of Li toxicity
Norepinephrine (Levarterenol, Levophed)	Decrease pressor effects of norepinephrine
Potassium iodide and other iodides; tricyclic antidepressants	Enhance hypothyroid effects of Li
Skeletal muscle relaxants	Increase neuromuscular blocking activity
Thiazide diuretics	Potentiate neurotoxic and cardiotoxic effects of Li

---

LOMUSTINE

(CeeNU, CCNU)

(loe-mus'teen)
Antineoplastic
Alkylating agent
Nitrosurea

ACTIONS AND USES. Lipid-soluble alkylating nitrosurea with actions like those of carmustine (qv).

Used as palliative therapy in addition to other modalities or with other chemotherapeutic agents in primary and metastatic brain tumors and as secondary therapy in Hodgkin's disease.

ABSORPTION AND FATE. Rapidly absorbed from GI tract. Serum half-life of drug and/or metabolites: 16 to 48 hours. About 50% protein bound. 50% of dose excreted in urine within 24 hours; 75% within 4 days. Because of high lipid solubility and relatively no ionization at physiologic pH, crosses blood–brain barrier readily. CSF levels are 50% greater than concurrent plasma levels. Rapidly and completely metabolized in liver. Excreted in urine as metabolites. Appears in breast milk.

CONTRAINDICATIONS AND PRECAUTIONS. History of hypersensitivity to lomustine. Safe use in pregnancy and in nursing mothers not established. Reported to be carcinogenic in laboratory animals. *Cautious Use:* patients with decreased circulating platelets, leukocytes, or erythrocytes, renal or hepatic function impairment, infection, previous cytotoxic or radiation therapy.

ADVERSE/SIDE EFFECTS. Delayed (cumulative) myelosuppression, stomatitis, alopecia (reversible), anemia, hepatotoxicity, nausea, vomiting; neurologic reactions (relationship to drug unclear): lethargy, ataxia, dysarthria.

ROUTE AND DOSAGE. **Oral:** **Adults and children:** 130 mg/m^2 as single dose, repeated in 6 weeks. Subsequent doses adjusted to patient's hematologic response.

NURSING IMPLICATIONS

Blood counts should be monitored weekly for at least 6 weeks after last dose. Liver and kidney function tests should be performed periodically.

Since hematologic toxicity is delayed and cumulative, a repeat course is not given before 6 weeks and not until platelets have returned to above 100,000 mm^3 and leukocytes to above 4000 mm^3.

Nausea and vomiting may occur 3 to 4 hours after drug administration, usually lasting less than 24 hours. Symptoms may be controlled by administering drug to fasting patient, or physician may prescribe an antiemetic prior to dosage.

L

Anorexia may persist for 2 or 3 days after a dose.

Thrombocytopenia occurs about 4 weeks and leukopenia about 6 weeks after a dose, persisting 1 to 2 weeks.

Inspect oral cavity daily for symptoms of superinfections and for signs of stomatitis or xerostomia. *See Meclorethamine for nursing care of oral lesions.*

Contraceptive measures are recommended during therapy.

Pharmacist will prepare prescribed dose by combining various capsule strengths. Explain to patient that a given dose may include capsules of different colors.

Store capsules away from excessive heat (over 40°C).

See Mechlorethamine (prototype alkylating agent).

LOPERAMIDE

(loe-per'a-mide)

(Imodium)

Antidiarrheal

C v

ACTIONS AND USES. Synthetic piperidine derivative chemically related to diphenoxylate and to meperidine. Reportedly as effective an antidiarrheal as diphenoxylate with longer duration of action. Inhibits GI peristaltic activity by direct action on circular and longitudinal intestinal muscles. Prolongs transit time of intestinal contents, increases consistency of stools, and reduces fluid and electrolyte loss.

Used to treat acute nonspecific diarrhea, chronic diarrhea associated with inflammatory bowel disease, and to reduce fecal volume from ileostomies.

ABSORPTION AND FATE. Poorly absorbed from GI tract. Onset of action in 30 to 60 minutes; duration: 4 to 5 hours. Approximately 97% protein bound. Half-life: 7 to 14 hours. Metabolized in liver. Less than 2% of dose excreted in urine; about 30% eliminated in feces as unchanged drug.

CONTRAINDICATIONS AND PRECAUTIONS. Hypersensitivity to loperamide, severe colitis, acute diarrhea caused by broad spectrum antibiotics (pseudomembranous colitis), or associated with microorganisms that penetrate intestinal mucosa, e.g., toxigenic *E. coli,* salmonella, or shigella. Safe use during pregnancy, in nursing mothers, and in children not established. *Cautious Use:* dehydration, diarrhea caused by invasive bacteria, impaired hepatic function.

ADVERSE/SIDE EFFECTS. CNS: drowsiness, dizziness, CNS depression (overdosage). **GI:** abdominal discomfort or pain, abdominal distention, bloating, constipation, nausea, vomiting, anorexia, dry mouth. **Hypersensitivity:** skin rash. **Other:** fatigue, fever, toxic megacolon (patients with ulcerative colitis).

ROUTE AND DOSAGE. Oral: *Acute diarrhea:* Initial: 4 mg followed by 2 mg after each unformed stool. Once diarrhea is controlled, dosage is reduced to maintenance level. Usual maintenance dose: 4 to 8 mg daily.

NURSING IMPLICATIONS

Since loperamide may cause drowsiness and dizziness, caution patient to avoid driving and other potentially hazardous activities until drug response is known.

In acute diarrhea, loperamide should be discontinued if there is no improvement after 48 hours of therapy. Advise patient to notify physician if diarrhea persists or if fever develops.

Patients with chronic diarrhea usually respond to loperamide therapy within 10 days. Loperamide may be continued if diarrhea cannot be controlled by diet or specific treatment, e.g., antibiotics.

Instruct patient to record number and consistency of stools. Fluids and electrolytes should be monitored especially in young children.

If the patient with ulcerative colitis develops abdominal distention or other GI symptoms, notify physician promptly (possible signs of toxic megacolon).

Inform patient that alcohol and other CNS depressants may enhance drowsiness and therefore should not be taken concomitantly unless otherwise advised by physician.

Classified as Schedule V drug under the Federal Controlled Substances Act. Animal studies indicate that loperamide in high doses can produce symptoms of physical dependence of the morphine type.

Treatment of overdosage: Slurry of activated charcoal; if vomiting does not occur, gastric lavage followed by activated charcoal slurry. Monitor patient for signs of CNS depression for at least 24 hours. Have naxolone on hand.

Dry mouth may be reduced by frequent rinsing with clear warm water and by increasing fluid intake. If these measures fail to provide relief a saliva substitute, e.g., Xero-Lube, Moi-stir, Orex may help (all are available OTC).

Store at room temperature preferably between 15° and 30°C (59° and 86°F) unless otherwise specified by manufacturer.

See Diphenoxylate Hydrochloride with Atropine Sulfate (prototype antidiarrheal agent).

L

LORAZEPAM

(Ativan)

(lor-a'ze-pam)
Psychotropic
Anxiolytic
Benzodiazepine
C IV

ACTIONS AND USES. Most potent of the available benzodiazepines with actions, uses, limitations, and interactions similar to those of chlordiazepoxide (qv).

Used for management of anxiety disorders, and for short-term relief of symptoms of anxiety. Also used for preanesthetic medication to produce sedation, and to reduce anxiety and recall of events related to day of surgery.

ABSORPTION AND FATE. Readily absorbed from GI tract and following IM administration. Peak concentrations in plasma in 2 hours after oral administration, and 60 to 90 minutes after IM injection. Approximately 85% bound to plasma proteins. Elimination half-life of oral drug: 10 to 15 hours; of parenteral drug: about 16 hours. Metabolized in liver and excreted in urine with no residual accumulation. Crosses placenta and enters breast milk.

CONTRAINDICATIONS AND PRECAUTIONS. Known sensitivity to benzodiazepines; acute narrow-angle glaucoma, primary depressive disorders or psychosis, children under 12 years of age (oral preparation) patients under 18 years of age (parenteral preparation); coma, shock, acute alcohol intoxication, pregnancy, lactation. *Cautious Use:* renal or hepatic impairment, narrow-angle glaucoma, suicidal tendency, GI disorders, elderly and debilitated patients; limited pulmonary reserve. *See also Chlordiazepoxide.*

L

ADVERSE/SIDE EFFECTS. (Usually disappear with continued medication or with reduced dosage): sedation, dizziness, weakness, unsteadiness, disorientation, depression, sleep disturbance, restlessness, confusion, hallucinations, hypertension or hypotension (occasionally) nausea, anorexia, blurred vision, diplopia, depressed hearing. *See also Chlodiazepoxide.*

ROUTE AND DOSAGE. *Highly individualized.* **Oral:** usual range: 2 to 6 mg/day in divided doses with largest dose at bedtime. *Anxiety:* 1 to 2 mg/day two to three times daily. *Insomnia:* single daily dose: 2 to 4 mg at bedtime. **Elderly, debilitated:** Initial: 1 to 2 mg individual doses, then adjusted as needed. **Intramuscular:** *Premedication* (at least 2 hours before anticipated surgery): 0.05 mg/kg up to maximum of 4 mg. **Intravenous:** *Sedation and relief of anxiety:* 2 mg total or 0.02 mg/lb whichever is smaller. *Reduction of recall:* 0.05 mg/kg up to total of 4 mg, administered 15 to 20 minutes before anticipated surgery.

NURSING IMPLICATIONS

The tension and anxiety associated with stresses of everyday living usually do not require treatment with an anxiolytic agent.

When high dosage is required, the evening dose should be increased before the daytime doses.

Watch to be sure patient does not "cheek" the tablet, a maneuver to hoard or avoid medication.

IM lorazepam is injected undiluted, deep into a large muscle mass.

Prepare lorazepam for IV administration immediately before use. Dilute with an equal volume of compatible solution. Do not use a solution that is discolored or that has a precipitate.

Diluted drug is injected directly into vein or into IV infusion tubing at rate not to exceed 2 mg/minute, and with repeated aspiration to confirm intravenous entry. Extreme precautions should be taken to prevent intraarterial injection and perivascular extravasation.

Inadvertant intraarterial injection may produce arteriospasm resulting in gangrene which may require amputation. *(See Index: Nursing Interventions: extravasation.)*

Patients over 50 years of age may have more profound and prolonged sedation with IV lorazepam. Usually an initial dose of 2 mg should not be exceeded.

When scopolamine is given concomitantly with injectable lorazepan, hallucinations, irrational behavior, and increased depth of sedation have been observed.

IM or IV lorazepam injection of 2 to 4 mg is usually followed by a depth of drowsiness or sleepiness that permits patient to respond to simple instructions whether patient appears to be asleep or awake.

The majority of patients will have difficulty recalling peri-operative events. This *retrograde amnesia* is optimum within 2 hours following the IM administration and 15 to 20 minutes after IV injection. Full recall and recognition may not return for about 8 hours. Inform patient of this possibility.

If a narcotic analgesic, another tranquilizer, or sedative is given with injectable lorazepam, lack of recall may extend for as long as 48 hours.

The elderly patient should be aware that he or she will be sleepy for a period longer than 6 to 8 hours after surgery. Supervise ambulation of patient for at least 8 hours after lorazepam injection to prevent falling and injury.

When lorazepam is given as a preoperative medication the narcotic analgesic should be administered at the usual preoperative time.

Equipment for maintaining patent airway should be immediately available before IV administration. Partial airway obstruction has occurred in the lorazepam medicated patient undergoing regional anesthesia.

Advise patient to refrain from any hazardous activity including dangerous sports and driving a car, for at least 24 to 48 hours after receiving IM injection of lorazepam. If patient is on oral drug therapy, patient should not drive until the sedative action of lorazepam has diminished. In time, patient may know how many hours he or she should wait before it is safe to drive.

When alcohol or a CNS depressant is combined with lorazepam the depressant effects of each agent are potentiated. Alcoholic beverages should not be consumed for at least 24 to 48 hours after receiving an injection and should be avoided when patient is on an oral regimen.

Food-Drug Interactions: Advise patient to avoid large volume intake of coffee. Anxiolytic effects of lorazepam can significantly be altered by 500 mg caffeine. (1 cup of coffee contains 125 to 250 mg caffeine.)

Frequent monitoring for symptoms of upper GI disease should be a part of the care of geriatric patients on long-term lorazepam therapy.

An individualized effective dose for treatment of insomnia should provide enforced sleepiness, deeper than usual, and with minimum "hangover." Discuss this with patient and keep physician informed to facilitate dose adjustment and/or discontinuation of drug therapy.

Habituation and dependence may be developed with use of this drug.

Closely supervise patient who exhibits depression with anxiety; the possibility of suicide should be borne in mind, particularly when there is apparent improvement in mood.

If daytime psychomotor function is impaired consult physician. A change in regimen or drug may be indicated.

When regimen is to be terminated, it should be done gradually over a period of several days. Warn patient on long-term therapy not to stop the drug abruptly because symptoms similar to those of barbiturate and alcohol withdrawal may be induced: feelings of panic, tonic-clinic seizures, tremors, abdominal and muscle cramps, sweating, vomiting.

Advise patient not to self-medicate with OTC drugs unless the physician approves.

Tell the patient that if she becomes pregnant or wishes to become pregnant, she should communicate with her physician about the desirability of continuing the drug.

Periodic blood counts and liver function tests are recommended for the patient on long-term therapy.

Lorazepam is subject to control under Federal Controlled Substances Act as a Schedule IV drug.

Keep parenteral preparation in refrigerator; do not freeze. Store tablets at temperature between 15° and 30°C (59° and 86°F) unless manufacturer specifies otherwise.

See Chlordiozepoxide.

Diagnostic Test Interferences. Lorazepam may increase **serum lactic dehydrogenase (LDH).** *See also Chlordiazepoxide.*

LOXAPINE HYDROCHLORIDE
(Loxitane C)
LOXAPINE SUCCINATE
(Loxapac, Loxitane)

(lox′a-peen)
Psychotropic
Antipsychotic
Neuroleptic

L

ACTIONS AND USES. Dibenzoxazepine antipsychotic, chemically distinct from other antipsychotics. Exact mode of action not established. Stabilizes emotional component of schizophrenia by acting on subcortical level of CNS. Sedative action is less than that produced by chlorpromazine (qv), but anticholinergic effects are comparable and extrapyramidal effects may be more intense. Also has antiemetic activity; lowers seizure threshold in patients with history of convulsive disorders.

Used to treat manifestations of psychotic disorders.

ABSORPTION AND FATE. Completely absorbed from GI tract; tranquilizing action begins in 20 to 30 minutes; peaks in 1½ to 3 hours and lasts about 12 hours. Wide distribution to most tissues. Serum levels decline in biphasic manner: first phase half-life: 5 hours; second phase half-life: 19 hours. Excreted in urine principally as glucuronides; about 50% of single dose excreted in urine and feces in 24 hours. Crosses placenta and is excreted in breast milk.

CONTRAINDICATIONS AND PRECAUTIONS. Known hypersensitivity to loxapine; severe drug-induced CNS depression; comatose states, children under age of 16. Safe use during pregnancy and by nursing mothers not established. *Cautious Use:* glaucoma, prostatic hypertrophy, urinary retention, history of convulsive disorders, cardiovascular disease. *See also Chlorpromazine.*

ADVERSE/SIDE EFFECTS. Drowsiness, sedation, dizziness, syncope, staggering gait, muscle weakness, extrapyramidal effects, akathisia, tachycardia, changes in blood pressure, dermatitis, facial edema, pruritus, photosensitivity, xerostomia, blurred vision, constipation, urinary retention. *See also Chlorpromazine.*

ROUTE AND DOSAGE. Oral: 10 mg twice daily; up to 50 mg daily. Usual therapeutic and maintenance range: 20 to 60 mg daily; doses higher than 250 mg daily not recommended. **Intramuscular:** 12.5 to 50 mg every 4 to 6 hours to control severely disturbed patient.

NURSING IMPLICATIONS

Dilute oral concentrate in about 2 to 3 ounces (60 to 90 ml) water, orange or grapefruit juice shortly before administration (do not store diluted solution). Measure with calibrated dropper dispensed with drug.

Caution patient not to change the dosage regimen in any way unless the physician approves.

The patient should be warned to avoid self-dosing with OTC drugs unless prescribed by the physician.

Drowsiness usually decreases with continued therapy. If it persists and interferes with ADL, consult physician. A change in time of administration or dose may help to prevent interference with normal physical activities.

Observe carefully for extrapyramidal effects *(see Index)* during early therapy with loxapine. Most symptoms disappear with dose adjustment or with antiparkinsonism drug therapy.

If a patient is on long-term treatment with this drug, be alert to first signs of impending tardive dyskinesia: fine vermicular movements of the tongue. Discontinue therapy and report promptly.

Instruct patient not to drive a car or engage in any activity that requires mental coordination and physical skill until drug response is known.

Monitor intake–output and bowel elimination patterns and check for bladder distention. The depressed patient often fails to report urinary retention or constipation.

Upon discharge, patient should be told what laxative may be used if necessary.

Determine blood pressure pattern: both hypotension and hypertension have been reported as adverse reactions.

Alcohol and other CNS depressants should be avoided during loxapine therapy.

Xerostomia discomfort should be attended to, since deprivation of saliva fosters tissue erosion and demineralization of tooth surfaces. Frequent warm water rinses and, if there is salivary response, sugarfree gum and candy may be helpful. Avoid commercial mouth rinses. Consult physician about use of saliva substitute if necessary (e.g., Moi-Stir, Zero-Lube).

If patient complains of blurred and/or colored vision report to physician. Facilitate periodic ophthalmologic examinations for patient on prolonged therapy. Ocular toxicity is possible.

Advise patient to withhold drug dose if the following appear: light-colored stools, bruising, unexplained bleeding, prolonged constipation, tremor, restlessness and excitement, sore throat and fever, rash.

Caution patient to stay out of bright sun. Exposed skin area should be covered with sunscreen lotion (SPF above 15).

Have available seizure precaution measures if patient has history of convulsive disorders.

When therapy is to be terminated, dosage should be gradually reduced over period of several days.

Protect medication from light. Intensification of straw color to light amber is acceptable. If noticeably discolored however, discard solution.

See Chlorpromazine (prototype antipsychotic).

L

LYPRESSIN

(Diapid)

(lye-press'in)
Hormone
Antidiuretic

ACTIONS AND USES. Lysine vasopressin; synthetic polypeptide with pharmacologic action similar to that of vasopressin (qv). Possesses antidiuretic activity, with very little oxytocic and minimal cardiovascular pressor activity in therapeutic doses.

Used to control or prevent complications of diabetes insipidus due to deficiency of endogenous posterior pituitary antidiuretic hormone. Particularly useful in patients who are nonresponsive to other forms of therapy and who experience allergic or other undesirable effects from vasopressin of animal origin.

ABSORPTION AND FATE. Following intranasal application of 1 or 2 sprays, onset of action in about 1 hour; antidiuretic effect lasts 3 to 8 hours. Plasma half-life about 15 minutes. Metabolized in kidney and liver and excreted in urine.

CONTRAINDICATIONS AND PRECAUTIONS. Pregnant women or women of childbearing potential. *Cautious Use:* patients for whom pressor effects would be undesirable, coronary artery disease, known sensitivity to antidiuretic hormone. *See also Vasopressin.*

ADVERSE/SIDE EFFECTS. *Infrequent and mild:* hypersensitivity, rhinorrhea, nasal congestion and irritation, pruritus and ulceration of nasal passages, headache, conjunctivitis, heartburn secondary to excessive nasal administration with postnasal drip, abdominal cramps, increased bowel movements. With inadvertent inhalation: substernal tightness, coughing, and transient dyspnea. *Overdosage:* marked but transient fluid retention. *See also Vasopressin.*

ROUTE AND DOSAGE. **Topical (intranasal): Adults and children:** 1 or 2 sprays in each nostril four times daily. One spray provides approximately 2 U.S.P. Posterior Pituitary (Pressor) Units.

NURSING IMPLICATIONS

Warn patient not to inhale the spray.

Instruct patient to clear nasal passages well before administering the spray.

Hold bottle upright and insert nozzle into nostril with patient's head in a vertical position.

If more than 2 sprays for each nostril are needed every 4 to 6 hours to give relief, the frequency of administration rather than number of sprays per dose should be increased. Large doses (excess) will drain posteriorly into digestive tract, where drug will be inactivated. Warn patients not to increase dosage without physician's order.

If nocturia is a problem, physician may prescribe an additional dose at bedtime.

If the patient develops a cold or allergy, absorption of lypressin will be diminished. Advise the patient to report to physician; adjustment of therapy may be required.

Lypressin dosage is individualized to control symptoms of diabetes insipidus: frequent urination and excessive thirst.

See also Vasopressin (prototype ADH).

M

MAFENIDE ACETATE
(Sulfamylon)

(ma'fe-nide)
Antiinfective
Antibacterial (topical)
Sulfonamide derivative

ACTIONS AND USES. Synthetic topical sulfonamide. Bacteriostatic against many gram-positive and gram-negative organisms, including *Pseudomonas aeruginosa,* and certain strains of anaerobes. Topical applications produce marked reduction of bacterial growth in avascular tissue. Active in presence of pus and serum, and not affected by changes in pH of tissue environment. Major metabolite of mafenide inhibits carbonic anhydrase, which may result in alkaline urine and metabolic acidosis when large amounts of drug are absorbed from application sites. Cross-sensitivity with other sulfonamides not established.

Used as adjunctive therapy in second- and third-degree burns to prevent sepsis.

ABSORPTION AND FATE. Rapidly absorbed from burn surface. Peak plasma concentrations in 2 to 4 hours following systemic absorption; rapidly eliminated through kidneys.

CONTRAINDICATIONS AND PRECAUTIONS. History of hypersensitivity to mafenide or to any ingredients in the formulation (e.g., bisulfite); respiratory (inhalation) injury, pulmonary infection, women of childbearing potential. Safe use during pregnancy not established. *Cautious Use:* impaired renal or pulmonary function.

ADVERSE/SIDE EFFECTS. Intense pain, burning, or stinging at application sites (common), bleeding of skin, excessive body water loss, delayed eschar separation, excoriation of new skin, superinfections (fungal colonization in and below burn eschar), allergic manifestations (pruritus, rash, urticaria, blisters, facial edema, eosinophilia), metabolic acidosis, fatal hemolytic anemia (rare); bone marrow suppression (rare).

ROUTE AND DOSAGE. **Topical (cream contains equivalent of 85 mg of mafenide base per gram):** applied aseptically to burn areas to thickness of approximately ¹⁄₁₆ inch once or twice daily. (Formulation contains sodium bisulfite as preservative.)

NURSING IMPLICATIONS

It is frequently difficult to distinguish between adverse reactions to mafenide and the effects of severe burns. Accurate observations are critically important.

Wound cleaning and removal of debris should be carried out before each reapplication of mafenide cream.

Mafenide cream is applied aseptically to cleansed, debrided burn areas with sterile gloved hand.

To aid in debridement, patient should be bathed daily by whirlpool bath (preferable) or shower or in bed.

Dressings are not usually required, but if they are necessary, only a thin layer should be used. Some physicians prescribe dressings when eschar begins to separate (about 16 to 20 days) to expedite its removal.

Burn areas must be covered with cream at all times. When necessary, reapplications should be made to areas from which cream has been removed (e.g., by patient's activity).

Intensity of local pain caused by mafenide may require administration of analgesic. Report to physician.

Monitor vital signs. Report immediately changes in blood pressure, pulse, and respiratory rate and volume.

Monitor intake and output. Report oliguria or changes in intake–output ratio. Physician may request urinary pH determinations (excessive renal alkaline loss can result in metabolic acidosis).

Acid–base balance should be monitored in patients with extensive burns and in those with pulmonary or renal dysfunction. Be alert to signs and symptoms of *metabolic acidosis:* dull headache, weakness, abdominal pain, nausea, vomiting, diarrhea, stupor, disorientation, Kussmaul respirations, reduced Pco_2 and blood pH.

In patients with extensive burns, it is advisable to maintain a flow chart to monitor mental status, vital signs, intake and output, weight, burn wound care, medications, and laboratory data.

Allergic reactions have reportedly occurred 10 to 14 days following initiation of mafenide therapy. Temporary discontinuation of drug may be necessary.

Mafenide therapy is usually continued until healing is progressing well (usually up to 60 days) or site is ready for grafting (after about 35 to 40 days). It is not withdrawn while there is a possibility of infection, unless adverse reactions intervene.

MAGALDRATE

(mag'al-drate)

(Hydromagnesium aluminate, Lowsium, Riopan)

Antacid

ACTIONS AND USES. Complex of aluminum and magnesium hydroxides. Nonsystemic antacid with true buffering action and high acid-consuming capacity. Reportedly does not produce alkalosis or acid rebound and not as likely to produce alterations of bowel function that occur with either aluminum or magnesium hydroxide alone. Low sodium content (not more than 0.3 mg of sodium per 400 mg tablet or 5 ml of suspension).

Used for symptomatic relief of hyperacidity associated with peptic ulcer, gastritis, peptic esophagitis, and hiatal hernia, particularly in patients who need to restrict sodium. Available in combination with simethicone (Riopan Plus).

ABSORPTION AND FATE. Minimal absorption from GI tract. Buffering action may persist for about 60 minutes.

CONTRAINDICATIONS AND PRECAUTIONS. Sensitivity to components. *Cautious Use:* impaired renal function.

ADVERSE/SIDE EFFECTS. Infrequent: constipation or diarrhea (with prolonged use), hypermagnesemia (in patients with impaired renal function). *See Magnesium Hydroxide.*

M

ROUTE AND DOSAGE. Oral: 480 to 960 mg (5 to 10 ml of suspension or 1 or 2 tablets) four times daily (not to exceed 20 tablets or 100 ml/day). Physician may prescribe hourly administration initially to control severe symptoms. Available as suspension, chewable tablets, and swallow tablets.

NURSING IMPLICATIONS

Shake suspension vigorously before pouring. Preferably administered between meals and at bedtime.

Suspension should be taken with sufficient water to ensure passage of drug into stomach.

Chewable tablet should be chewed thoroughly before swallowing. Swallow tablet should be taken with enough water to ensure prompt swallowing without chewing.

Serum magnesium levels should be monitored in patients with impaired renal function.

In common with other antacids, magaldrate may cause premature dissolution and absorption of enteric-coated tablets, and may interfere with the absorption of oral tetracyclines and other oral medications. In general it is advisable not to take other oral drugs within 1 or 2 hours of an antacid.

MAGNESIUM CARBONATE

Antacid
Laxative

ACTIONS AND USES. Nonsystemic antacid and saline laxative with properties similar to those of magnesium hydroxide (qv). Has high neutralizing capacity, and intermediate onset of action. Converted to magnesium chloride and carbon dioxide in stomach; in intestines, magnesium salts act as saline laxative.

Used for temporary relief of hyperacidity and constipation.

ABSORPTION AND FATE. Small amount of magnesium may be absorbed. Excreted in urine.

CONTRAINDICATIONS AND PRECAUTIONS. Severe renal disease. *See Magnesium Hydroxide.*

ADVERSE/SIDE EFFECTS. Diarrhea, belching, distention, abdominal pain, flatulence; hypermagnesemia (prolonged use). *See Magnesium hydroxide.*

ROUTE AND DOSAGE. Oral: *Antacid:* 0.5 to 2 Gm between meals and at bedtime, if necessary. *Laxative:* 8 Gm at bedtime. Available as powder and chewable tablet.

NURSING IMPLICATIONS

Instruct patient to chew tablet thoroughly before swallowing. Administer antacid dose with a half glass of water. Taken with a full glass of water for maximum laxative effect.

Inform patient that frequent or long-term use of magnesium carbonate is inadvisable without medical supervision.

Note frequency and consistency of stools. If stools are loose, magnesium carbonate may be alternated with an antacid with constipating action, e.g., aluminum hydroxide or calcium carbonate.

In common with other antacids, magnesium carbonate can cause premature disintegration and absorption of enteric-coated tablets and may interfere with absorption of oral tetracyclines and other oral medications. In general, it is advisable not to take other oral drugs within 1 or 2 hours of an antacid.

See Magnesium hydroxide (prototype saline laxative).

M

MAGNESIUM CITRATE

Laxative (saline)

(Citrate of Magnesia, Citroma, Citro-Nesia, Evac-Q-Mag)

ACTIONS AND USES. Contains magnesium carbonate, citric acid, potassium or sodium bicarbonate for added effervescence, in a lemon oil or cherry-flavored base. Magnesium content approximately 140 mEq per 200 ml.

Used to evacuate bowel prior to certain surgical and diagnostic procedures and to help eliminate parasites and toxic materials following treatment with a vermifuge.

CONTRAINDICATIONS AND PRECAUTIONS. Renal disease, nausea, vomiting, diarrhea, abdominal pain, acute surgical abdomen; intestinal impaction, obstruction or perforation; rectal bleeding; use of solutions containing sodium bicarbonate in patients on sodium restricted diets.

ADVERSE/SIDE EFFECTS. Abdominal cramps, nausea, fluid and electrolyte imbalance, hypermagnesemia (prolonged use). *See Magnesium Hydroxide.*

ROUTE AND DOSAGE. Oral: Adult: 200 ml. **Children (up to 2 years):** only as directed by physician; **(2 to 6 years):** 4 to 12 ml; **(6 to 12 years):** 50 to 100 ml.

NURSING IMPLICATIONS

Most effective when taken on an empty stomach with a full (240 ml) glass of water. Time dosing so that it does not interfere with sleep. Produces a watery or semifluid evacuation in 2 to 6 hours.

To increase palatability manufacturer suggests chilling the solution by pouring over ice, or refrigerate until ready to use.
Once container is opened, magnesium citrate will lose some of its effervescence. This may affect palatability somewhat, but not quality of preparation.
Store in tightly-covered containers between 2° and 30°C (36° and 86°F).
See Magnesium hydroxide (prototype saline laxative).

PROTOTYPE

MAGNESIUM HYDROXIDE

(Magnesia, Magnesia Magma, Milk of Magnesia, M.O.M.)

Antacid
Laxative (saline)

ACTIONS AND USES. Milk of magnesia is an aqueous suspension of magnesium hydroxide with rapid and long-acting neutralizing action. Although classified as nonsystemic antacid, 5 to 10% of the magnesium may be absorbed to produce alkaline urine. Also may cause slight acid rebound. Acts as antacid in low doses and as mild saline laxative at higher doses. Reacts with hydrochloric acid in stomach to form magnesium chloride, which has neutralizing action. Magnesium chloride causes osmotic retention of fluid which distends colon resulting in mechanical stimulation of peristaltic activity. Each milliliter of magnesium hydroxide contains about 2.4 to 2.9 mEq of magnesium and reportedly is capable of neutralizing approximately 2.7 mEq of gastric acid. Commercially available in combination with aluminum hydroxide, e.g., Aludrox, Kolantyl, Maalox. Also available as emulsion combined with mineral oil: Haley's M-O.

Used for short-term treatment of occasional constipation, for relief of GI symptoms associated with hyperacidity, and as adjunct in treatment of peptic ulcer. Also has been used in treatment of poisoning by mineral acids and arsenic, and as mouthwash to neutralize acidity.

M

ABSORPTION AND FATE. Absorbed magnesium ions are usually excreted rapidly by kidney. Laxative action occurs in about 4 to 8 hours, depending on dosage. Crosses placenta. Excreted in breast milk.

CONTRAINDICATIONS AND PRECAUTIONS. Abdominal pain, nausea, vomiting, diarrhea, severe renal dysfunction, fecal impaction, intestinal obstruction or perforation, rectal bleeding, colostomy, ileostomy. Safe use during pregnancy and in children under 2 years of age not established.

ADVERSE/SIDE EFFECTS. *Excessive dosage:* nausea, vomiting, abdominal cramps, diarrhea, alkalinization of urine, dehydration. **Hypermagnesemia:** weakness, nausea, vomiting, lethargy, mental depression, hyporeflexia, hypotension, bradycardia, complete heart block and other ECG abnormalities, respiratory depression, coma. *Prolonged Use:* rectal concretions (rare), electrolyte imbalance.

ROUTE AND DOSAGE. Oral: Adults: *Antacid:* 5 to 10 ml, or 1 or 2 tablets 1 to 3 hours after meals and at bedtime. *Laxative:* 15 to 30 ml at bedtime (up to 60 ml if necessary). **Pediatric: Infants:** *Laxative:* 5 ml added to morning feeding; **(2 to 6 years):** 5 to 15 ml; **(6 years and over):** 15 to 30 ml. Administer with 1 glass of water.

NURSING IMPLICATIONS

Shake bottle well before pouring to assure administration of suspension and not supernatant liquid.

For antacid action, usually given 20 minutes to 1 hour before meals and at bedtime. Mix suspension with water or follow with sufficient water to assure that it reaches the stomach.

When intended for antacid use, laxative effect of milk of magnesia can be minimized by coadministering or alternating with an antacid with constipating effects, e.g., calcium carbonate or aluminum hydroxide. Consult physician.

For laxative effect, follow the drug with at least a full glass of water to enhance drug action. Administer in the morning or at bedtime. Most effective when taken on an empty stomach.

Evaluate the patient's continued need for drug. Prolonged and frequent use of laxative doses may lead to dependence and tends to reinforce neurotic preoccupation with bowels. Additionally, even therapeutic doses can raise urinary pH and thereby predispose susceptible patients to urinary infection and urolithiasis, or elevate serum magnesium concentrations and cause bradycardia and other symptoms of hypermagnesemia.

Inform patient that the cause of persistent or recurrent constipation should be investigated by physician.

Teaching Outline for Laxative Users: Correct patient's misconceptions about constipation. Inform patient that constipation is defined as infrequent or difficult passage of stools. The omission of one day's evacuation is not constipation and will not cause accumulation of poisons in the body. Functional constipation can be corrected by:

- ✓ regularity of meals
- ✓ addition of bulk and fiber to diet (if allowed) such as raw and cooked vegetables and fruits, whole grain cereals, and bread (some physicians recommend 4 to 6 tablespoonfuls of whole bran daily)
- ✓ adequate daily fluid intake (at least 6 to 8 full glasses of liquid). Drinking a large glass of warm water flavored with lemon or orange juice, immediately on arising is helpful
- ✓ planned exercise program
- ✓ unhurried defecation time at approximately the same time each day (duodenocolic and defecation reflexes are most active following a meal, especially breakfast).

Stored at room temperature in tightly covered container. Slowly absorbs carbon dioxide on exposure to air. Avoid freezing.

Diagnostic Test Interferences. Magnesium antacids cause significant elevations in **urinary pH** that may persist for 1 or more days after drug is withdrawn. Decreased **serum potassium** levels and elevated **blood glucose** with prolonged use of high doses.

Drug Interactions: Magnesium hydroxide

Plus	Interactions
Chlordiazepoxide (Librium)	Antacids reduce absorption and therefore decrease chlordiazepoxide effect
Chlorpromazine and other phenothiazines	Lower phenothiazine serum levels by decreasing GI absorption
Dicumarol	Milk of magnesia may increase serum dicumarol levels by enhancing its absorption if given concurrently
Digoxin (Lanoxin) Iron salts Isoniazid (INH)	Antacids reduce effects of these drugs by reducing absorption

Plus (cont.)	Interactions (cont.)
Nitrofurantoin (Furadantin) Pencillamine (Cuprimine) Salicylates	Magnesium-containing drugs may enhance muscular relaxation effect (theoretical possibility)
Neuromuscular blocking agents Gallamine (Flaxedil) Succinylcholine Tubocurarine and others	Coadministration may cause metabolic alkalosis in patients with renal dysfunction
Sodium polystyrene sulfonate Tetracylines (oral)	Concurrent use of antacid results in formation of insoluble complex

In common with other antacids, magnesium hydroxide may cause premature dissolution and absorption of enteric-coated tablets and may interfere with the absorption of other oral medications. In general it is advisable not to take other oral drugs within 1 or 2 hours of an antacid.

MAGNESIUM OXIDE

(Mag-Ox, Maox, Par-Mag, Uro-Mag)

Antacid
Laxative (saline)

ACTIONS AND USES. Nonsystemic antacid with high neutralizing capacity, and relatively long duration of action. Its action and uses are essentially the same as those of magnesium hydroxide (qv).

ADVERSE/SIDE EFFECTS. Diarrhea, abdominal cramps, nausea; hypermagnesemia, renal stones (chronic use). *See Magnesium Hydroxide.*

M

ROUTE AND DOSAGE. Oral: *Antacid:* 250 mg to 1.5 Gm with water or milk, four times a day, after meals and at bedtime. *Laxative:* 2 to 4 Gm usually at bedtime; administered with full glass of water.

NURSING IMPLICATIONS

As with other antacids, the liquid preparation is reportedly more effective than tablet form.

In common with other antacids, magnesium oxide can cause premature dissolution and absorption of enteric-coated and sustained release tablets and also may complex with and thus reduce absorption of oral tetracyclines and other oral drugs. In general, it is advisable not to take other oral medications within 1 or 2 hours of an antacid.

Store in airtight containers. On exposure to air it rapidly absorbs moisture and carbon dioxide.

See Magnesium hydroxide (prototype saline laxative).

MAGNESIUM SALICYLATE

(Doan's Pills, Durasal, Efficin, Magan, Mobidin)

NSAID
Salicylate
Antirheumatic

ACTIONS AND USES. Sodium-free salicylate derivative with low incidence of GI irritation. In equal doses, less potent than aspirin as an analgesic and antipyretic. Unlike aspirin (qv) is not associated with asthmatic reactions, and does not inhibit platelet aggregation or increase bleeding time. 1 Gm magnesium salicylate is equivalent to 1 Gm aspirin. Available in fixed combination with choline salicylate (Trilisate).

Used for relief of pain and inflammation in rheumatoid arthritis, osteoarthritis, bursitis, and other musculoskeletal disorders.

CONTRAINDICATIONS AND PRECAUTIONS. Hypersensitivity to salicylates, erosive gastritis, peptic ulcer, advanced renal insufficiency, liver damage, bleeding disorders, before surgery. Safe use in children under 12 years not established. *See also Aspirin.*

ADVERSE/SIDE EFFECTS. Salicylism: dizziness, drowsiness, tinnitus, hearing loss, nausea, vomiting, hypermagnesemia (with high doses in patients with renal insufficiency). *See also Aspirin.*

ROUTE AND DOSAGE. Oral: *Analgesic, antipyretic:* 600 mg three or four times daily; may be increased to 3.6 to 4.8 Gm daily in divided doses, at 3- to 6-hour intervals. *Rheumatic fever:* up to 9.6 Gm daily in divided doses.

NURSING IMPLICATIONS

Administer with a full glass of water or with food or milk.
See Aspirin (prototype salicylate and NSAID).

M

MAGNESIUM SULFATE

(Epsom Salt)

Anticonvulsant
Laxative (saline)
Tocolytic Replenisher (magnesium)

ACTIONS AND USES. When taken orally, acts as laxative by osmotic retention of fluid, which distends colon, increases water content of feces, and causes mechanical stimulation of bowel activity. When given parenterally, acts as CNS depressant and also depressant of smooth, skeletal, and cardiac muscle. Anticonvulsant properties believed to be produced by CNS depression, principally by decreasing the amount of acetylcholine liberated from motor nerve terminals, thus producing peripheral neuromuscular blockade. Believed to act on myocardium by slowing rate of S-A node impulse formation and prolonging conduction time. In excessive doses, produces vasodilation by ganglionic blockade and direct action on blood vessels.

Used orally to relieve acute constipation and to evacuate bowel in preparation for x-ray of intestines. Used parenterally to control seizures in toxemia of pregnancy, epilepsy, acute nephritis, hypomagnesemia, and hypothyroidism, as well as to counteract muscle stimulating effects of barium poisoning. Used topically to reduce edema, inflammation, and itching. *Unlabeled Use:* To inhibit premature labor (tocolytic action), and pregnancy (category A) as replacement therapy in acute magnesium deficiency; and as adjunct in hyperalimentation.

ABSORPTION AND FATE. Following oral administration, cathartic action within 1 to 2 hours; excreted primarily in feces. Absorbed magnesium (20%) is rapidly eliminated by kidney. Immediate action following IV injection; duration about 30 minutes. Following IM administration, acts in approximately 1 hour and lasts 3 to 4 hours.

CONTRAINDICATIONS AND PRECAUTIONS. Myocardial damage; heart block; IV administration during the 2 hours preceding delivery; oral use in patients with abdominal pain, nausea, vomiting, fecal impaction, or intestinal irritation, obstruction, or perforation. *Cautious Use:* impaired renal function, digitalized patients, concomitant use of other CNS depressants or neuromuscular blocking agents.

ADVERSE/SIDE EFFECTS. **Hypermagnesemia:** flushing, sweating, extreme thirst, hypotension, sedation, confusion, depressed reflexes or no reflexes, muscle weakness, flaccid paralysis, hypothermia, depressed cardiac function, complete heart block, circulatory collapse, respiratory paralysis; hypocalcemia. **Repeated laxative use:** dehydration, electrolyte imbalance, including hypocalcemia.

ROUTE AND DOSAGE. *Laxative:* **Oral: Adult:** 10 to 15 Gm. **Pediatric:** 5 to 10 Gm. *Anticonvulsant:* **Intravenous: Adult:** 1 to 4 Gm of 10 to 20% solution not exceeding 1.5 ml/minute. **Intramuscular: Adult:** 1 to 5 Gm of 25 to 50% solution 6 times daily as necessary. **Pediatric:** 20 to 40 mg/kg in a 20% solution; repeated as necessary. *Hyperalimentation:* (1 Gm magnesium sulfate provides 8.12 mEq/magnesium.) **Adult:** 8 to 24 mEq/day. *Hypomagnesemia (mild):* **Intramuscular:** 1 Gm, or **Oral:** 3 Gm-every 6 hours for 4 doses. *(severe)* **Intravenous:** 5 Gm/1000 ml dextrose 5% in water or normal saline infused over 3 hours.

NURSING IMPLICATIONS

For laxative action, magnesium sulfate is best administered in the morning or midafternoon in a glass of water. Bitter, salty taste may be disguised by chilling medication or adding ice chips. It may be flavored with lemon or orange juice.

Sufficient water should be taken during the day when drug is administered orally to prevent net loss of body water.

When magnesium sulfate is given intravenously, patient requires constant observation. Check blood pressure and pulse every 10 to 15 minutes or more often if indicated.

Monitoring of plasma magnesium levels is advised in patients receiving drug parenterally (normal: 1.8 to 3.0 mEq/L). Plasma levels in excess of 4 mEq/L are reflected in depressed deep tendon reflexes and other symptoms of Mg intoxication. Cardiac arrest occurs at levels in excess of 25 mEq/L.

Early indicators of *magnesium toxicity* (hypermagnesemia) include profound thirst, feeling of warmth, sedation, confusion, depressed deep tendon reflexes, and muscle weakness.

Before each repeated parenteral dose, knee jerks (patellar reflex) should be tested. Depressed reflexes or absence of patellar reflexes is a useful, objective index of early magnesium intoxication. Also check respiratory rate and character, and urinary output, especially in patients with impaired renal function. Therapy is generally not continued if urinary output is less than 100 ml during the 4 hours preceding each dose.

Monitor intake and output (in patients receiving drug parenterally). Report oliguria and changes in intake–output ratio.

Resuscitation equipment and facilities for maintaining artificial respiration must be immediately available, as well as specific antidote: calcium gluconate or calcium gluceptate.

Newborns of mothers who have received parenteral magnesium sulfate within a few hours of delivery should be observed for signs of magnesium toxicity, including respiratory and neuromuscular depression.

Patients receiving the drug for treatment of hypomagnesemia should be observed for improvement in these signs of deficiency: irritability, choreiform movements, tremors, tetany, twitching, muscle cramps, tachycardia, hypertension, psychotic behavior. (Hypomagnesemia is usually associated with other electrolyte deficiencies, especially calcium and potassium.)

Recommended daily allowances of magnesium (350 mg/day for men; 300 mg/day for women; 450 mg/day during pregnancy and lactation) are obtained in a normal diet. Rich sources are found in whole-grain cereals, legumes, most green leafy vegetables, and bananas.

Drug Interactions. Additive CNS depression may occur when magnesium sulfate is administered with CNS depressants, e.g., **barbiturates, narcotics, general anesthetics** (dosage of these agents should be adjusted). Excessive neuromuscular blockade has occurred in patients receiving magnesium sulfate and another **neuromuscular blocking agent** concomitantly.

MALATHION

(Prioderm)

(mal-a-thye'on)
Cholinesterase inhibitor
Antiinfective
Pediculocide
Organophosphate

ACTIONS AND USES. Highly purified derivative of the crude organophosphate insecticide, Malathion, which is a weak cholinesterase inhibitor (indirect cholinergic). Prioderm which contains only 0.5% malathion reportedly has no effect on red blood cell cholinesterase levels and has not been associated with sensitization or contact dermatitis. Pediculocidal and ovicidal activity is thought to result from conversion of malathion in the insect to a highly active metabolite that causes massive paralysis and death and prevents eggs (nits) from hatching. Resistance to malathion has not been reported.

Used for topical treatment of pediculosis capitis (head lice).

M

ABSORPTION AND FATE. Percutaneous absorption of Prioderm has not been studied. Malathion in higher concentrations (than 0.5% as in Prioderm) can be absorbed systemically through skin and mucous membranes. Systemic absorption can also occur following accidental ingestion. Following absorption, distributed into many tissues, especially liver and bone. Oxidizes to active metabolite (malaoxon) and inactive metabolites. Probably excreted via kidney.

CONTRAINDICATIONS AND PRECAUTIONS. Hypersensitivity to malathion or to any ingredient in the formulation. Safe use during pregnancy (category B) and in nursing women not established.

ADVERSE/SIDE EFFECTS. Low order of toxicity when used as directed. **Skin:** irritation, stinging or burning sensation of scalp, pruritis, dryness of hair, increase in dandruff. *Accidental ingestion* (signs and symptoms of cholinergic intoxication): light-headedness, dizziness, headache, weakness, excessive sweating, nausea, blurred vision, lacrimation, nasal congestion, increased salivation and bronchial secretions, bronchospasm, severe respiratory distress, bradycardia, GI hypermotility, slow shallow breathing, sensory–motor disturbances (paralysis, neuropathy), seizures, coma, circulatory collapse.

ROUTE AND DOSAGE. **Topical (0.5% lotion):** (1) Sprinkle lotion on dry hair and rub gently until hair and scalp are thoroughly moistened. (2) Allow to dry naturally, use no heat or hair dryer and leave uncovered. (3) After 8 to 12 hours shampoo, rinse well. (4) Comb hair with fine toothed comb to remove dead lice and nits. Treatment may be repeated in 7 to 9 days if nits or lice are observed. Usually first treatment is successful.

NURSING IMPLICATIONS

Advise patient to use malathion precisely as directed. Residual pediculocidal and ovicidal effects result if drug is used according to directions, and may last up to 7 weeks even with shampooing. This protective effect is lost by applying lotion to wet hair or by shampooing before 8 hours, following application. It is also canceled by contact of hair with heat (e.g., hair dryer) or with chlorine (e.g., in swimming pools as in some community water supplies). Note that chlorine interferes with the protective residual effect, but not the initial pediculocidal or ovicidal activity.

The commercial preparation (Prioderm) contains 0.5% malathion in an isopropyl alcohol 78% vehicle and is scented with pine needle oil.

Malathion is very irritating to the eyes and mucous membranes. Caution patient to avoid contact with eyes and to wash hands thoroughly after treatment is completed. If drug accidentally enters the eye, flush immediately with water.

Secondary infections, usually from intensive scratching, should be treated by topical antibiotic therapy. If secondary lymphadenopathy is present, a systemic antibiotic may be indicated.

Keep drug out of the reach of children. Malathion is a potent poison if ingested.

Pertinent Patient/Responsibile Family Member Teaching Points:

- ✓ Contaminated bedlinen, wash cloths, towels, clothing, combs, and brushes should be carefully washed in hot water and detergent (boiled if possible or dry cleaned if not washable) to prevent reinfestation. Particular attention should be paid to seams of clothing. For dry cleaning, place clothing in a plastic bag, seal carefully, and inform dry cleaner of contents.
- ✓ Family members and close contacts should be examined for pediculi and nits. If infested, they should receive concurrent treatment.

Treatment for accidental ingestion: Treatment must be initiated promptly. Empty stomach by inducing emesis or by gastric lavage with 5% sodium bicarbonate. Have on hand equipment for artificial respiration and for maintenance of airway; oxygen, suction, and drugs to combat cholinesterase depletion: atropine, pralidoxime chloride, short-acting barbiturate (for convulsions). Diagnosis of overdosage is confirmed by repeated serum and RBC cholinesterase determinations. Keep patient quiet. Because absorption of malathion may be delayed, patient should be kept under surveillance for an adequate time period.

Malathion is flammable. Also, drug is inactivated by heat. Store away from heat and open flames, and caution patient not to smoke while using it.

Store preferably between 15° and 30°C (59° and 86°F) in well closed container. Protect from freezing.

M

PROTOTYPE

MANNITOL

(Osmitrol, Resectisol)

(man'i-tole)

Diuretic, osmotic

Diagnostic agent

ACTIONS AND USES. Hexahydric alcohol prepared commercially by reduction of dextrose. Induces diuresis by raising osmotic pressure of glomerular filtrate, thereby inhibiting tubular reabsorption of water and solutes. In large doses, may increase rate of electrolyte excretion, particularly sodium, chloride, and potassium. Reduces elevated intraocular and cerebrospinal pressures by increasing plasma osmolality, thus inducing diffusion of water from these fluids back into plasma and extravascular space. Rebound increase in intracranial pressure sometimes occurs about 12 hours following drug administration.

Used to promote diuresis in prevention and treatment of oliguric phase of acute renal failure following cardiovascular surgery, severe traumatic injury, surgery in presence of severe jaundice, hemolytic transfusion reaction. Also used to reduce elevated intraocular and intracranial pressures, to measure glomerular filtration rate (GFR), to promote excretion of toxic substances, to relieve symptoms of pulmonary edema, and as irrigating solution in transurethral prostatic reaction to minimize hemolytic effects of water. Commercially available in combination with sorbitol for urogenital irrigation.

ABSORPTION AND FATE. Diuresis occurs within 1 to 3 hours. Elevated intraocular pressure is lowered within 30 to 60 minutes for period of 4 to 6 hours; elevated cerebrospinal fluid pressure may be reduced within 15 minutes, with effect lasting 3 to 8 hours. Confined to extracellular space; does not cross blood–brain barrier, except with very high plasma concentrations or in the presence of acidosis. Half-life: about 100 minutes. Small quantity metabolized to glycogen in liver. Rapidly excreted by kidney. Approximately 80% of 100 Gm dose eliminated unchanged in urine within 3 hours.

CONTRAINDICATIONS AND PRECAUTIONS. Anuria, marked pulmonary edema or congestive heart failure, metabolic edema, organic CNS disease, intracranial bleeding, shock, severe dehydration, history of allergy. Safe use during pregnancy and in women of childbearing potential and children under 12 years of age not established.

ADVERSE/SIDE EFFECTS. Dry mouth, thirst, blurred vision, marked diuresis, urinary retention, edema, headache, circulatory overload with pulmonary congestion, congestive heart failure, fluid and electrolyte imbalance, dehydration, acidosis, nausea, vomiting, rhinitis, arm pain, anginalike pains, tachycardia, backache, transient muscle rigidity, tremors, convulsions, chills, fever, dizziness, hypotension, hypertension, allergic reactions, nephrosis, uricosuria, thrombophlebitis; with extravasation: local edema, skin necrosis.

ROUTE AND DOSAGE. **Intravenous infusion:** *Acute renal failure:* 50 to 100 Gm of a concentrated solution (5 to 25%). *Elevated intraocular and intracranial pressure:* 1.5 to 2 Gm/kg as a 15 to 25% solution, over 30 to 60 minutes. *Acute chemical toxicity:* 100 to 200 Gm (depending on urinary output). *Measurement of glomerular filtration rate:* 100 ml of 20% solution diluted with 180 ml NaCl Injection; infused at rate of 20 ml/minute. *Test dose* (patient with marked oliguria): 0.2 Gm/kg as a 15 or 20% solution infused over 3 to 5 minutes to produce a urine flow of at least 30 to 50 ml/hour. All doses highly individualized.

NURSING IMPLICATIONS

IV infusion flow rate (prescribed by physician) is generally adjusted to maintain urine flow of at least 30 to 50 ml/hour.

A test dose is given to patients with marked oliguria. Response is considered adequate if urine flow of at least 30 to 50 ml/hour is produced over 2 to 3 hours after drug administration.

Serum and urine electrolytes (particularly sodium, potassium, and chloride), central venous pressure, and renal function should be closely monitored during therapy.

Intake and output must be accurately measured and recorded to achieve proper fluid balance. Check output on the half-hour or hourly. Intake and output must be accurately measured and recorded to achieve proper fluid balance. Increasing oliguria is an indication to terminate therapy; report immediately. (If urinary output is not adequate, mannitol may accumulate and cause circulatory overload, with resulting pulmonary edema, water intoxication, and congestive heart failure.)

Consult physician regarding allowable oral fluid intake volume. In general, volume of total fluid intake (all sources) should be no more than 1 L in excess of urinary output.

Monitor vital signs, and be alert for indications of fluid and electrolyte imbalance (e.g., thirst, muscle cramps or weakness, paresthesias, and signs of congestive heart failure: distended neck veins, dyspnea, chest rales, tachycardia, blood pressure changes).

Accurate daily weight under standard conditions provides another reliable index of fluid balance.

Care should be taken to avoid extravasation. Observe injection site for signs of inflammation or edema.

To measure GFR, urine is collected by catheter for a specific time period and analyzed for amount of mannitol excreted (mg/minute). Blood samples are drawn at start and end of time period, and plasma concentrations of mannitol are determined (mg/ml). Normal rate for men is 125 ml/minute; for women, 116 ml/minute.

Parenteral mannitol may crystalize when exposed to low temperatures. If crystallization occurs, place bottle in hot water bath (approximately 50°C) and periodically shake vigorously. Cool to body temperature before administration. Do not use solution if crystals cannot be completely dissolved.

Concentrations higher than 15% have a greater tendency to crystallize. Administration set with an in-line IV filter should be used when infusing concentrations of 15% or above.

Mannitol should not be added to whole blood transfusion. However, if blood must be given simultaneously, at least 20 mEq of sodium chloride should be added to each liter of mannitol solution to avoid pseudoagglutination.

Patients receiving urologic irrigations of mannitol should be observed closely for systemic reactions.

Store preferably between 15° and 30°C (59° and 86°F) unless otherwise directed by manufacturer. Avoid freezing.

M

Diagnostic Test Interferences. Mannitol may interfere with blood **inorganic phosphorus** and **ethylene glycol** determinations.

Drug Interactions. Mannitol increases lithium excretion.

MAPROTILINE HYDROCHLORIDE

(Ludiomil)

(ma-proe'ti-leen)
Antidepressant
Tetracyclic

ACTIONS AND USES. Tetracyclic antidepressant pharmacologically and therapeutically similar to the tricyclic antidepressants. Has significant sedative effect and less prominent anticholinergic action; may lower seizure threshold. Useful in depression associated with anxiety and sleep disturbances.

Used for treatment of depressive neurosis (dysthymic disorder) and manic-depressive illness, depressed type (major depressive disorder). *See Imipramine.*

ABSORPTION AND FATE. Slow, complete absorption from GI tract; peak blood concentrations in 12 hours. Half-life: 51 hours; about 88% bound to plasma proteins. Hepatic metabolism. Excreted primarily in urine (70% of dose) also in feces (30%) as metabolites, within 21 days.

CONTRAINDICATIONS AND PRECAUTIONS. Patients under 18 years of age. *See Imipramine.*

ADVERSE/SIDE EFFECTS. Sedation, seizures. *Anticholinergic:* xerostomia, constipation, urinary retention, blurred vision. *See also Imipramine.*

ROUTE AND DOSAGE. Oral: Adult: (Outpatient): *Mild to moderate depression:* Initial: 75 mg/day with incremental increases as required to 150 mg/day. (Hospitalized): *Severe depression:* Initial: 100 to 150 mg/day; gradually increased to 300 mg/day if necessary. **Elderly:** 50 to 75 mg/day usually is satisfactory. Maintenance: during prolonged therapy dose is kept at lowest effect level; frequently at 75 to 150 mg/day.

NURSING IMPLICATIONS

Drug may be given as single dose or in divided doses. Risk of seizures is reduced by initiating therapy with low dosages.

Therapeutic effects are sometimes seen in 3 to 7 days; 2 to 3 weeks are usually necessary.

Assess level of sedative effect. If recovering patient becomes too lethargic to care for personal hygiene or to maintain food intake and interactions with others, report to physician.

The severely depressed patient may need assistance with personal hygiene particularly because of excessive sweating caused by the drug.

Monitor bowel elimination pattern and intake–output ratio. Severe constipation and urinary retention are potential problems, especially in the elderly. Advise increased fluid intake (at least 1500 ml daily); consult physician about stool softener (if necessary) and a high fiber diet.

Urge outpatient on high doses to report symptoms of stomatitis, sialoadenitis, xerostomia.

If xerostomia is a problem, institute symptomatic therapy *(see Imipramine).* Sore or dry mouth interferes with mastication and swallowing and can be a major cause of poor food intake, dental problems, and lack of compliance. Consult physician about use of a saliva substitute (e.g., Moi-Stir).

Caution patient that ability to perform tasks requiring alertness and skill may be impaired during early therapy.

Urge patient not to change dose or dose schedule without consulting physician. The patient should not give the medication to any other person, nor use it for a self-diagnosed problem.

Advise patient not to use OTC drugs unless physician approves.

The actions of both alcohol and maprotiline are potentiated when used together during therapy and for up to 2 weeks after maprotiline is discontinued. Consult physician about allowable amount of alcohol, if any, that can be taken.

If patient uses excessive amounts of alcohol it should be borne in mind that the potentiation of maprotiline effects may increase the danger of overdosage or suicide attempt.

Store drug at temperature between 15° and 30°C (59° and 86°F) unless otherwise specified by the manufacturer.

See Imipramine (prototype tricyclic antidepressant).

M

MAZINDOL

(Mazanor, Sanorex)

(may'zin-dole)
Anorexogenic
C IV

ACTIONS AND USES. Imidazoisoindole derivative with pharmacologic properties similar to those of amphetamines. Produces CNS and cardiac stimulation in addition to amphetaminelike effects. Appears to exert primary effects on limbic system; also appears to alter norepinephrine metabolism by inhibiting normal neuronal uptake mechanism.

Used in short-term management of exogenous obesity.

ABSORPTION AND FATE. Readily absorbed from GI tract. Onset of action in 30 to 60 minutes; duration 8 to 15 hours. Excreted primarily in urine as unchanged drug and conjugated metabolites.

CONTRAINDICATIONS AND PRECAUTIONS. Glaucoma; hypersensitivity to the drug; severe hypertension; symptomatic cardiovascular disease, including arrhythmias; agitated states; history of drug abuse; during or within 14 days following administration of MAO inhibitors; children under age 12. Safe use in women of childbearing potential or during pregnancy not established. *Cautious Use:* hyperexcitability states.

ADVERSE/SIDE EFFECTS. CNS: restlessness, dizziness, insomnia, dysphoria, depression, tremor, headache, drowsiness, weakness. **CV:** palpitation, tachycardia. **Dermatologic:** rash, excessive sweating, clamminess. **Endocrine:** impotence, changes in libido (rare). **GI:** dry mouth, unpleasant taste, diarrhea, constipation, nausea, vomiting.

ROUTE AND DOSAGE. Oral: 1 mg three times daily 1 hour before meals or 2 mg once daily 1 hour before lunch.

NURSING IMPLICATIONS

Drug may be taken with meals if GI discomfort occurs.

Possibility of abuse potential should be kept in mind.

Rate of weight loss is greatest during first few weeks of therapy and tends to decrease thereafter.

Tolerance may develop within a few weeks. When it occurs, drug should be discontinued.

Insulin requirements of patients with diabetes may be decreased in association with use of mazindol and concomitant caloric restriction and weight loss.

Caution patients that mazindol may impair ability to perform hazardous activities such as driving a car or operating machinery.

Classified as Schedule IV drug under the Federal Controlled Substances Act.

Drug Interactions. Mazindol may decrease the hypotensive effects of **guanethidine** and potentiate pressor amines, e.g., **norepinephrine, isoproterenol** (patient should be closely monitored if given concomitantly). Administration of mazindol with or within 14 days of **MAO inhibitors** can produce hypertensive crisis.

PROTOTYPE

MEBENDAZOLE

(Vermox)

(me-ben'da-zole)

Anthelmintic

ACTIONS AND USES. Carbamate with unusually broad spectrum of anthelmintic activity. Mechanism of action not known. Inhibits formation of worm's microtubules and inhibits glucose and other nutrient uptake by susceptible helminths.

Used in treatment of *Trichuris trichiura* (whipworm), *Enterobius vermicularis* (pinworm), *Ascaris lumbricoides* (roundworm), *Ancylostoma duodenale* (common hookworm), *Necator americanus* (American hookworm) in single or mixed infections. *Unlabeled Use:* beef, dwarf, pork tapeworm, threadworm infections.

ABSORPTION AND FATE. Only a small portion (5 to 10%) is absorbed from GI tract. Peak plasma levels in 2 to 4 hours. Most of dose excreted in feces; 5 to 10% of dose excreted in urine within 3 days, mainly as inactive metabolites.

CONTRAINDICATIONS AND PRECAUTIONS. Hypersensitivity to mebendazole. Safe use during pregnancy (category C), in nursing women, and in children under 2 years of age not established.

ADVERSE/SIDE EFFECTS. Transient abdominal pain, diarrhea, dizziness, fever (possibly due to tissue necrosis in cysts).

ROUTE AND DOSAGE. Oral: Adults and children over 2 years: *Whipworm* (trichuriasis); *roundworm* (ascariasis): *hookworm;* mixed infection: 100 mg two times daily (morning and evening) for 3 consecutive days. Second course in 3 weeks if cure is not achieved. *Pinworm* (enterobiasis): 100 mg as single dose. Second course 3 weeks later if necessary.

NURSING IMPLICATIONS

May be given without regard to food. Food in GI tract reportedly does not affect drug action.

Commercial chewable tablet may be chewed, crushed, mixed with food, or swallowed whole.

If cure does not occur within 3 weeks after initiation of therapy, second course of treatment is advised.

Fasting and purging are not required.

Because pinworms are readily transmitted from person to person all family members should be examined and treated simultaneously.

Patient Teaching During Period of Drug Therapy for Parasite Infestation

- ✓ Emphasize importance of washing hands thoroughly after toilet and before eating.
- ✓ Keep hands away from mouth; keep fingernails short
- ✓ Avoid walking barefoot (hookworm)
- ✓ Handle bedding carefully without shaking it to avoid dispersing ova into the air
- ✓ Advise patient to change underclothing, bedclothes, towels and facecloths daily and to bathe frequently, preferably by showering
- ✓ Disinfect toilet facilities daily
- ✓ Infected person should sleep alone
- ✓ House should be vacuum cleaned and damp mopped daily to reduce number of ova

Stools will be examined for ova and parasites to establish diagnosis and cure. Collect specimen in clean, dry container, e.g., bedpan. Then transfer to properly labeled container to be sent to laboratory. Parasites may be destroyed by water from toilet bowl, urine, or certain medications e.g., antibiotics, castor oil, mineral oil, antidiarrheal formulations.

To collect pinworm specimen: Female pinworms usually deposit their ova at night in patient's perianal area, rather than in feces. Wrap a strip of transparent cellophane, sticky side out, over end of throat stick. Press tape firmly against perianal area, then transfer tape, sticky side down, to a microscope slide. Collect specimen in early morning before patient arises for prescribed number of days.

MECAMYLAMINE HYDROCHLORIDE

(Inversine)

(mek-a-mill'a-meen)
Antihypertensive
Ganglionic blocking agent

ACTIONS AND USES. Potent, long-acting secondary amine nondepolarizing ganglionic blocking agent. Blocks neurotransmission at both sympathetic and parasympathetic ganglia by competing with ACh for cholinergic receptor sites on postsynaptic membranes. Reduces blood pressure in both normotensive and hypertensive individuals, generally with greater decrease in standing or sitting blood pressure than in supine blood pressures. Tolerance rarely develops; curare-like effects may be produced by large doses.

Used in treatment of moderately severe to severe hypertension and in uncomplicated malignant hypertension.

ABSORPTION AND FATE. Almost completely absorbed from GI tract. Effects appear gradually over 30 minutes to 2 hours; action peaks in 3 to 5 hours and lasts 6 to 12 hours or longer. Readily crosses blood–brain barrier; high concentrations accumulate in liver and kidney, spleen, lungs, heart. About 50% of dose excreted by kidney in unchanged form when urine is acidic (excretion promoted by acid urine and diminished in alkaline urine). Scant amounts excreted in feces and probably in milk. Crosses placenta.

CONTRAINDICATIONS AND PRECAUTIONS. Coronary insufficiency, pyloric stenosis, glaucoma, uremia, chronic pyelonephritis, recent MI; use in mild labile hypertension; unreliable uncooperative patients, pregnancy. *Cautious Use:* rising or elevated BUN; renal, cerebral, or coronary vascular pathology; recent CVA; prostatic hypertrophy, bladder neck obstruction, urethral stricture.

ADVERSE/SIDE EFFECTS. CNS: weakness, fatigue, sedation, headache, paresthesias, choreiform movements, tremor, nervousness, anxiety, insomnia, slurred speech, seizures, mental aberrations, confusion, mania, or depression. **CV:** orthostatic hypotension, changes in heart rate, dizziness, syncope, precipitation of angina. **EENT:** mydriasis, blurred vision, cyclopegia, nasal congestion, dry mouth with dysphagia, glossitis. **GI:** anorexia, glossitis, nausea, vomiting, constipation, diarrhea, adynamic ileus. **Other:** decreased libido, impotence, urinary retention, dysuria, malaise, hyperuricemia, interstitial pulmonary edema and fibrosis, anhidrosis, exacerbation of psoriasis, hyperuricemia (asymptomatic).

ROUTE AND DOSAGE. Oral: Initial: 2.5 mg two times daily, after meals; increased by increments of 2.5 mg at intervals of not less than 2 days until desired blood pressure response is attained. Maintenance: 2.5 mg daily to 25 mg, in 2 to 4 divided doses. Highly individualized.

NURSING IMPLICATIONS

Administration of drug after meals may result in more gradual absorption and smoother control of blood pressure. Timing of doses in relation to meals should be consistent.

Because of diurnal variations in blood pressure, physician may prescribe relatively small dose in the morning or omission of morning dose (morning BP usually lower) and larger doses for afternoon or evening administration.

Seasonal variations may alter the hypotensive effect, e.g., usually smaller doses are required in summer than in winter.

Initial regulation of dosage should be dictated by blood pressure readings in standing position at time of maximal drug effect, as well as symptoms of orthostatic hypotension (faintness, dizziness, lightheadedness). Also note any changes in pulse rate.

Some physicians direct their patients to check blood pressure before taking mecamylamine and to reduce or omit a dose if reading is below a previously designated figure.

Instruct patient to make position changes slowly and in stages, particularly from recumbent to upright posture, and to sit on edge of bed and move ankles and feet before ambulating.

Advise patient to lie down immediately if feeling lightheaded or dizzy. Adverse reactions should be reported immediately, since drug effects may last for hours to days after drug is discontinued.

Constipation, frequent loose stools with abdominal distention, or decreased bowel sounds may be the first signs of paralytic ileus (relatively frequent) and should be reported promptly. Paralytic ileus is sometimes preceded by small, frequent stools.

Physician may prescribe neostigmine concurrently or a laxative such as milk of magnesia, cascara sagrada, or magnesium sulfate if constipation is a problem. Bulk laxatives are not recommended.

Patients should be informed of factors that may potentiate the action of mecamylamine: excessive heat, fever, infection, alcohol, vigorous exercise, salt depletion (vomiting, diarrhea, excessive sweating, diuresis). Hypotensive action may also be prominent during pregnancy, anesthesia, or surgery.

Sodium intake is generally not restricted. Consult physician.

If mouth dryness is a problem, advise patient to: rinse mouth frequently with clear warm water; increase noncaloric intake, if allowed; try sugarless gum or lemon drops. If these measures fail, a saliva substitute, e.g., Xero-Lube, Moi-stir, may help (available OTC).

Partial tolerance may develop in some patients, necessitating dosage adjustment. Follow-up supervision is an essential part of therapy.

Caution patient to avoid driving and other potentially hazardous activities until reaction to drug is known.

Mecamylamine withdrawal should be accomplished slowly. Sudden discontinuation of drug can result in severe hypertensive rebound with CVA and acute congestive heart failure. Usually, other antihypertensive therapy must be substituted gradually, and patient must be supervised daily during period of dosage adjustment.

Store preferably between 15° and 30°C (59° and 86°F) unless otherwise directed by manufacturer.

Drug Interactions. Mecamylamine may potentiate **sympathomimetics** (use reduced dose). There may be potentiated hypotensive effects with **alcohol,** other **antihypertensive agents, bethanechol,** and **thiazide diuretics** (used therapeutically). Mecamylamine toxicity may result with agents that increase urine pH such as **acetazolamide** and **sodium bicarbonate.**

PROTOTYPE

MECHLORETHAMINE HYDROCHLORIDE

(Mustargen)

(me-klor-eth'a-meen)

Antineoplastic

Alkylating agent

Nitrogen mustard

ACTIONS AND USES. Analogue of mustard gas and standard of reference for nitrogen mustards. Forms highly reactive carbonium ion, which causes cross-linking and abnormal base-pairing in DNA thereby interfering with DNA replication and RNA and protein synthesis. Cell-cycle nonspecific, i.e., highly toxic to rapidly proliferating cells at any time during cell cycle. Actions simulate those of x-ray therapy, but nitrogen mustards produce more acute tissue damage and more rapid recovery. Has strong myelosuppressive and weak immunosuppressive activity and is a powerful vesicant. Therapy may be associated with incidence of a second malignant tumor particularly if mechlorethamine is combined with radiation therapy or with other antineoplastics.

Use generally confined to nonterminal stages of neoplastic disease. Employed as single agent or in combination with other agents in palliative treatment of Hodgkin's disease (stages III and IV), lymphosarcoma, mycosis fungoides, polycythemia vera, bronchogenic carcinoma, chronic myelocytic or chronic lymphocytic leukemia. Also used for intrapleural, intrapericardial and intraperitoneal palliative treatment of metastatic carcinoma resulting in effusion.

ABSORPTION AND FATE. Rapid transformation to metabolites; less than 0.01% of unchanged drug excreted in urine. Interruption of blood supply to given tissue a few minutes during and immediately after drug injection protects area from drug cytotoxic effects.

CONTRAINDICATIONS AND PRECAUTIONS. Pregnancy at least until third trimester, lactation, myelosuppression, infectious granuloma, known infectious diseases, acute herpes zoster, intracavitary use with other systemic bone marrow suppressants. *Cautious Use:* bone marrow infiltration with malignant cells, chronic lymphocytic leukemia, men or women in childbearing age, use with x-ray treatment or other chemotherapy in alternating courses.

ADVERSE/SIDE EFFECTS. CNS (neurotoxicity): vertigo, tinnitus, diminished hearing, headache, drowsiness, peripheral neuropathy, lightheadedness, paresthesias, cerebral deterioration, coma. **Dermatologic:** pruritus, hyperpigmentation, maculopapular skin eruptions (rare), herpes zoster, alopecia. **GI:** stomatitis, xerostomia, anorexia, nausea, vomiting, diarrhea, peptic ulcer, jaundice. **Hematopoietic:** leukopenia, thrombocytopenia, lymphocytopenia, agranulocytosis, anemia, hyperheparinemia. **Reproductive:** delayed catamenia, oligomenorrhea, amenorrhea, azoospermia, impaired spermatogenesis, total germinal aplasia, chromosomal abnormalities. **Other:** hyperuricemia, metallic taste immediately after dose, weakness, fever, hypersensitivity reactions. With extravasation: painful inflammatory reaction, tissue sloughing, thrombosis, thrombophlebitis.

ROUTE AND DOSAGE. Intravenous: Total dose 0.4 mg/kg body weight for each course of treatment as single dose or in divided doses of 0.1 to 0.2 mg/kg/day. **Intracavitary:** 0.2 to 0.4 mg/kg body weight.

NURSING IMPLICATIONS

Solution should be prepared and administered while wearing surgical gloves for protection of skin. Avoid inhalation of vapors and dust and contact of drug with eyes and skin.

If drug contacts the skin, flush contaminated area immediately with copious amounts of water for at least 15 minutes, followed by 2% sodium thiosulfate solution. Irritation may appear after a latent period.

If eye contact occurs, irrigate immediately with copious amounts of 0.9% sodium chloride, followed by ophthalmologic examination as soon as possible.

Prepare mechlorethamine solution immediately before administration by adding 10 ml Sterile Water for Injection or 0.9% NaCl injection to drug vial. With needle still in rubber stopper, shake vial several times to hasten dissolving. Solution will contain 1 mg mechlorethamine/ml solution.

Do not use discolored solution or contents of vial in which there are drops of moisture.

Reconstituted solution may be injected over a few minutes directly into any suitable vein. However, to reduce risk of severe infections from extravasation or high concentration of the drug, injection is made preferably directly into tubing or sidearm of freely flowing

IV infusion. Some clinicians flush vein with running IV solution for 2 to 5 minutes to clear tubing of any remaining drug.

If direct IV injection is to be made needle used to withdraw dose should be discarded and a fresh needle used to administer medication.

Rubber gloves, tubing, glassware, etc., used in the preparation and administration of mechlorethamine should be soaked in an aqueous solution of equal volumes of sodium thiosulfate 5% and sodium bicarbonate 5% for 45 minutes.

Any unused injection solution and mechlorethamine vials should also be treated (neutralized) with an equal volume of sodium thiosulfate/sodium bicarbonate solution for 45 minutes before disposal.

If drug extravasates, prompt subcutaneous or intradermal injection with isotonic sodium thiosulfate solution (1/6 molar) and application of ice compresses intermittently for a 6- to 12-hour period may reduce local tissue damage and discomfort. Tissue induration and tenderness may persist 4 to 6 weeks, and tissue may slough.

Begin flow chart with established baseline data relative to body weight, intake–output ratio and pattern, and blood picture as reference for design of drug and nursing care regimens.

Mechlorethamine dosage is determined on basis of ideal dry body weight, i.e., unaugmented by edema or ascites. Record daily weight. Alert physician to sudden or slow, steady weight gain.

Laboratory studies of peripheral blood are essential guides for determining when to give another course of therapy. Urge patient to keep appointments for clinical evaluation.

Give drug preferably late in the day to prevent interference with sleep by side effects.

Intracavitary administration is preceded by removal of most of the fluid in the cavity to be treated. Introduction of mechlorethamine into the nearly empty cavity produces a chemical poudrage effect.

Intrapleural or intrapericardial injection of nitrogen mustard is given directly through the thoracentesis needle.

Intraperitoneal injection is given through a rubber catheter inserted into the paracentesis trocar or through a No. 18 gauge needle inserted in another site.

Immediately after intracavitary administration, change the patient's position (prone, supine, right side, left side, knee-chest) every 5 to 10 minutes for an hour, to assure full contact of drug with all parts of the cavity. Paracentesis may be done 24 to 36 hours later to remove any remaining fluid.

Reaccumulation of fluid in the treated cavity is a possibility and requires careful monitoring by x-ray and clinical evaluation. Watch for signs of compromised vital functions because of fluid pressure.

Pain is rare with intrapleural injection but transient cardiac irregularities may occur. Monitor cardiac function during and after treatment until cardiac status is stable.

Pain is common with intraperitoneal injection and usually is associated with nausea, vomiting, and diarrhea of 2 to 3 days' duration.

Nausea and vomiting may occur 1 to 3 hours after drug injection; vomiting usually subsides within 8 hours, but nausea may persist. Chlorpromazine alone or with barbiturate may be prescribed before or at time of injection to help control nausea and vomiting. Attempt to schedule treatments, other drugs, and meals so as to avoid peak times of nausea.

Prolonged vomiting and diarrhea can produce blood volume depletion: signs: decreased skin turgor, shrunken and dry tongue, postural hypotension, weakness, confusion. Carefully monitor and record patient's fluid losses. Discuss with physician the supportive measures that will restore and maintain fluid balance.

Work with dietitian and patient's family to help patient maintain optimum nutritional status. Anorexia should not be ignored. Determine dietary preferences; support and augment (rather than attempt to reform) eating patterns during periods of discomfort and leukopenia.

Myelosuppressive symptoms appear by the fourth day after treatment begins and are maximal by tenth day. Generally, lymphocytopenia begins within 24 hours and is maximum in 6 to 8 days. Significant granulocytopenia usually occurs within 6 to 8 days, is maximum between 14 to 25 days with recovery complete within 2 weeks of its nadir.

Thrombocytopenia usually manifests 6 to 8 days after a treatment. Explain its significance to patient. Petechiae, ecchymoses, or abnormal bleeding from intestinal and buccal membranes should be reported immediately. Warn patient to prevent bruising or falls. During period of thrombocytopenia, injections and use of rectal thermometer or rectal tube, and other invasive procedures should be kept at a minimum.

Report symptoms of unexplained fever, chills, sore throat, tachycardia, and mucosal ulceration since they may signal onset of agranulocytosis (relatively infrequent incidence).

Symptoms of depression of leukopenic system may be evident up to 50 days or more from the start of therapy.

Profound immunosuppression places patient at risk for infections, poor healing and lowered defense mechanisms for combating stress. Prevent exposure of patient to persons with infection especially upper respiratory tract infections, and plan nursing interventions to keep patient's expenditure of energy at a minimum.

Rapid neoplastic cell and leukocyte destruction leads to elevated serum uric acid (hyperuricemia) and potential renal urate calculi. Studies reveal that the incidence of urate stones is about 22% with serum uric acid level of 8 to 8.9 mg/dl; 40% with 9 mg/dl (normal: 3 to 7 mg/dl).

Preventive measures against incidence of hyperuricemia include increased fluid intake, alkalinizing of urine, and administration of allopurinol.

Encourage patient to increase fluid intake up to 3000 ml/day if allowed. Urge prompt reporting of symptoms including: flank or joint pain, swelling of lower legs and feet, changes in voiding pattern.

M

Azoospermia and amenorrhea after a course of therapy may be irreversible. Occasionally spermatogenesis may return in patients in remission several years after intensive chemotherapy. This should be discussed with patient before therapy is started.

High doses and regional infusion of mechlorethamine increase incidence of tinnitus and deafness. Alert patient to report symptoms promptly.

Herpes zoster may be precipitated by mechlorethamine treatment and usually necessitates withdrawal of the drug. It occurs commonly in patients with lymphoma. Maculopapular skin eruptions usually do not necessitate stopping drug.

Discuss the problem of alopecia (reversible) with the patient. If desired, facilitate cosmetic substitution. Keep in mind the psychologic importance of hair to one's self-image and concept of sexuality. *(See Index: Nursing interventions: alopecia.)*

Mouth care: Cytoxic effects of antineoplastic therapy are reflected in oral membranes and structures and in salivary glands.

Establish baselines for oral care by inspecting oral cavity before chemotherapy begins. Note and record state of hydration of oral mucosa, condition of gingiva, teeth, tongue, mucosa, and lips. If prosthetic devices do not fit properly, record.

If patient has correctable oral problems, they should be treated before therapy with antineoplastics. Institute corrective measures to minimize possibility of irritation or infection after immunosuppression and myelosuppression has been established. Facilitate consultation with a dentist if necessary.

Stomatitis (muscositis): Continuous meticulous measures are important to prevent oral infection from superinfection or trauma, and to relieve discomfort, and to prevent demineralization of tooth surfaces because of saliva deprivation.

- Keep oral membranes well hydrated by frequent rinses with warm water or, if patient cannot do this, irrigate cavity with warm water at least every 2 hours.
- Brush teeth using soft-bristled toothbrush (softened with warm water); if gums are painful, use moistened cotton covered finger or rubber tip on toothbrush. Use fluoride toothpaste or medication at least once daily.
- Cleansing before and after meals is important. Encourage patient to floss teeth gently with waxed floss at least once daily. Do it for patient if necessary.
- As oral complications increase because of drug-induced cell destruction, the following guidelines are useful: discontinue flossing when platelet count decreases to between 15,000 and 10,000; discontinue brushing when count is between 10,000 and 5000. Maintain oral hygiene with wet cotton swabs and *gentle* stream of warm water. Consult physician about oral antiseptic and anesthetic agent.
- Apply thin film of petroleum jelly to cracked, dry lips. Avoid use of lemon and glycerin swabs, which irritate membranes, change consistency of saliva, and may promote decalcification of teeth.
- In presence of ulcerations or dysphagia, avoid hot or cold foods and drinks; avoid spicy, sour, dry, rough or chunky foods as well as smoking and alcoholic beverages.
- Xerostomia may be relieved by use of a saliva substitute (available OTC) such as Xero-Lube, Moi-stir, Salivart.

Dietary supplements may be indicated during period of oral complications. Facilitate patient-dietitian conferences.

Diagnostic Test Interferences. Mechlorethamine may increase **serum** and **urine uric acid** and decrease **serum cholinesterase.**

Drug Interactions. Mechlorethamine (nitrogen mustards) may reduce effectiveness of **antigout agents** necessitating dose adjustment. Other **myelosuppressants** augment action of mechlorethamine necessitating dose adjustment.

M

MECLIZINE HYDROCHLORIDE

(Antivert, Bonamine, Bonine, Dizmiss, Motion Cure, Wehvert)

(mek′li-zeen)
Antiemetic
Antivertigo
Antihistamine
H_1-receptor antagonist

ACTIONS AND USES. Long-acting piperazine derivative of diphenylmethane, structurally and pharmacologically related to cyclizine compounds. Has marked effect in blocking histamine-induced vasopressive response, but only slight anticholinergic action. In common with similar agents, also exhibits CNS depression, antispasmodic, antiemetic, and local anesthetic activity. Has marked depressant action on labyrinthine excitability and on conduction in vestibular-cerebellar pathways.

Used in management of nausea, vomiting, and dizziness associated with motion sickness and in vertigo associated with diseases affecting vestibular system.

ABSORPTION AND FATE. Slow onset of action; duration of action 8 to 24 hours. Plasma half-life: 6 hours. Metabolic fate unknown.

CONTRAINDICATIONS AND PRECAUTIONS. Hypersensitivity to meclizine; use during pregnancy and in women of childbearing potential; use in pediatric age group. *Cautious Use:* angle-closure glaucoma, prostatic hypertrophy. *See Diphenhydramine.*

ADVERSE/SIDE EFFECTS. Drowsiness, dry mouth, blurred vision, fatigue.

ROUTE AND DOSAGE. Oral: *Motion sickness:* 25 to 50 mg 1 hour before travel. Repeated every 24 hours, if necessary for duration of journey. *Vertigo:* 25 to 100 mg daily in divided doses. Available forms: tablets, chewable tablets.

NURSING IMPLICATIONS

Forewarn patients about side effects such as drowsiness, and advise patients not to drive a car or engage in other hazardous activities until their reactions to the drug are known.

Caution patients that the sedative action may be additive to that of alcohol, barbiturates, narcotic analgesics, or other CNS depressants.

See also Diphenhydramine (prototype ethanolamine antihistamine).

MECLOCYCLINE SULFOSALICYLATE

(Meclan)

(me-kloe-sye'kleen)
Antiinfective
Antibiotic
Tetracycline

ACTIONS AND USES. Synthetic derivative of oxytetracycline. Antibacterial action appears to be related to ability to suppress growth of susceptible organisms, principally *Propionibacterium acnes* an anaerobic organism in sebaceous glands and follicles. Another proposed mechanism of action is the reduction of free fatty acids in sebum. (Free fatty acids are believed to contribute to formation of inflammatory acne lesions and comedones.) Inactive against viruses and fungi. Sensitivity and contact dermatitis have not been demonstrated by patch testing. The commercial preparation Meclan contains sodium formaldehyde sulfoxylate.

Used for topical treatment of inflammatory acne vulgaris.

M

ABSORPTION AND FATE. Not absorbed systemically in measurable amounts.

CONTRAINDICATIONS AND PRECAUTIONS. Hypersensitivity to tetracyclines or to any ingredients in the formulation, e.g., formaldehyde. Safe use during pregnancy (category B), in nursing women, and in children below 11 years, not established.

ADVERSE/SIDE EFFECTS. Skin irritation; stinging, burning sensation; temporary yellow staining of skin around hair follicles (with excessive applications), superinfections.

ROUTE AND DOSAGE. Topical (1% cream): apply to affected areas twice daily, morning and evening. Less frequent application may be used depending on patient response.

NURSING IMPLICATIONS

Advise patient to apply medication as directed and to keep follow-up appointments. Overuse of tetracycline preparations can result in overgrowth of nonsusceptible organisms.

Inform patient that excessive applications of meclocycline may cause temporary staining around hair roots, and also can stain fabrics.

Avoid use of meclocycline near or in eyes, ears, nose, mouth, or other mucous membranes.

Advise patient to notify physician if noticeable improvement has not occurred by 6 to 8 weeks. Maximum benefit may not be apparent for up to 12 weeks.

Patients should be informed that skin areas treated with meclocycline will fluoresce under ultraviolet light.

Chronic acne can be a devastating and aggravating condition because it commonly occurs during personality development. In addition to drug therapy, most patients require psychologic support and counseling to put their skin problem into perspective, and to dispel some misconceptions about acne: e.g., (1) Acne is not caused by poor hygiene or by masturbating; it is generally genetic. (2) Diet is not a major influence in acne.

Pertinent Patient-Teaching Points Related To Acne Therapy:

- ✓ Skin hygiene: some clinicians advise thoroughly cleansing of skin with soap and water twice daily; a cosmetic scrubbing pad (e.g., Buf-Puf) facilitates removal of dry scales.
- ✓ Keep hands away from face and other affected parts. Do not finger or squeeze lesions.
- ✓ Choose cosmetics carefully. Avoid oily (comedogenic) preparations, particularly those containing wax esters, e.g., isopropyl myristate and its analogues (isopropyl palmitate, isostearyl neopentenate, butyl or isopropyl stearate, among others). Also avoid lanolin derivatives and D and C red dyes (used as blushing agents). Use water-based powder or foundation.
- ✓ Wash hair frequently, especially if oily, and keep off face.
- ✓ Eat a well-balanced diet.
- ✓ Get sufficient rest.

Store preferably at 15° to 30°C (59° to 86°F), unless otherwise directed by manufacturer.

Drug Interactions: Meclocycline

Plus	Interactions
Abrasive or medicated soaps and cleaners, other topical acne preparations, alcohol-containing preparations (e.g., after shave astringents, lotions), "cover-up" medications, peeling agents (e.g., benzoyl peroxide, resorcinal, sulfur, salicylic acid tretinoin	Possibility of cumulative drying or irritant effects

M

MECLOFENAMATE SODIUM

(Meclomen)

(me-kloe-fen-am'ate)
NSAID
Antirheumatic

ACTIONS AND USES. Halogenated anthranilic acid derivative with pharmacologic properties similar to those of aspirin. Has palliative antiinflammatory, analgesic, and antipyretic activity. Action mechanism unclear but animal studies suggest that effects may result from inhibition of prostaglandin synthesis and competition for binding at prostaglandin receptor sites. Does not appear to alter course of arthritis. Comparable to aspirin with respect to drug efficacy in rheumatoid arthritis and to GI side effects, but produces fewer reactions involving special senses and less fecal blood loss than aspirin. Transient inhibition of platelet aggregation has been reported; platelet count and bleeding time are not apparently affected. Each 100 mg meclofenamate sodium contains 0.34 mEq sodium (Na).

Used for symptomatic treatment of acute or chronic rheumatoid arthritis and osteoarthritis. Also used in combination with gold salts or corticosteroids in treatment of rheumatoid arthritis. *Investigational Use:* management of acute gouty arthritis.

ABSORPTION AND FATE. Rapidly and completely absorbed from GI tract. Peak plasma levels in 1 to 2 hours; duration of action: 2 to 4 hours. Half-life: 2 to 3.3 hours. Metabolized in liver; strongly bound (about 99%) to plasma albumin. Excreted in urine (⅔) as glucuronide conjugates and in feces (⅓). Crosses placenta.

CONTRAINDICATIONS AND PRECAUTIONS. Hypersensitivity to meclofenamate, patient in whom bronchospasm, urticaria, and allergic rhinitis are induced by aspirin or other nonsteroid antiinflammatory drugs; first and third trimester of pregnancy, nursing mothers, children under age of 14, patient designated as Functional Class IV rheumatoid arthritis (incapacitated, bedridden, or confined to wheelchair, little or no self care); active peptic ulcer. *Cautious Use:* history of upper GI tract disease, compromised cardiac and renal function or other conditions predisposing to fluid retention.

ADVERSE/SIDE EFFECTS. **Causal relationship unknown:** palpitations, malaise, fatigue, drowsiness, paresthesia, asthenia, myalgia, insomnia, depression, dyspnea, hot flashes, blurred vision, taste disturbances, nocturia, hematuria, renal calculi, leukopenia (rare), paralytic ileus. **CNS:** dizziness, vertigo, lack of concentration, confusion, headache, tinnitus, hearing loss (rare). **CV:** edema. **GI:** severe diarrhea (dose-related), peptic ulceration, GI bleeding, severe diarrhea (dose-related), dyspepsia, abdominal pain, nausea, vomiting (may be severe), flatulence, eructation, pyrosis, anorexia, constipation, stomatitis. **Skin:** rash, pruritus, urticaria.

ROUTE AND DOSAGE. **Oral:** 200 to 400 mg/day in 3 or 4 equally divided doses. (Initially, start with lower dose, then adjust dose as necessary at lowest clinically effective level.) Maximum recommended dose: 400 mg/day.

NURSING IMPLICATIONS

M

This drug is usually reserved for use in patient unresponsive to adequate trial therapy with salicylates and other measures such as appropriate rest.

If patient complains of GI distress, suggest administration with food, milk, or an aluminum and magnesium hydroxide antacid (Maalox) may be prescribed. If symptoms persist the physician should be consulted.

Clinical improvement in the rheumatoid patient is evidenced within 2 to 3 weeks with reduction in number of tender joints, severity of tenderness, and duration of morning stiffness.

Improvement in the osteoarthritic patient is reflected by reduced night pain and pain on walking, reduced degree of starting pain and pain with passive motion, and improved joint function.

Diarrhea is the most frequent adverse effect and is usually dose-related. Reportedly, the incidence of diarrhea is lower in patients with osteoroarthritis than in those with rheumatoid arthritis.

Instruct patient to stop taking this drug and promptly notify the physician if nausea, vomiting, severe diarrhea, and abdominal pain occur. Generally dose reduction or temporary withdrawal will control symptoms.

Although incidence of side effects related to special senses is low, instruct patient to report without delay if blurred vision, tinnitus, or taste disturbances occur.

Since visual disturbances have been reported with other nonsteroid antiinflammatory agents, ophthalmic examinations are recommended prior to and periodically during treatment, and whenever patient experiences visual disturbances.

If patient becomes pregnant while on meclofenamate therapy she should notify the physician promptly.

The patient should be weighed under standard conditions (similar clothing, same time of day) twice weekly. A weight gain of more than 3 to 4 pounds/week should be reported as well as signs of edema: swollen ankles, tibiae, hands, feet.

The Na content of meclofenamate tablets should be considered if the patient is on restricted Na intake.

Discourage use of OTC drugs without approval of physician. Many commonly used medications contain aspirin (increase potential for toxicity) and Na (augments Na component of the meclofenamate compound). Examples: *OTC drugs containing aspirin:* Anacin (400 mg), Arthritis Strength Bufferin (486 mg), Measurin (650 mg), Ecotrin (325 mg). *Na containing drugs:* Alka-Seltzer (296 mg), Rolaids (53 mg), Soda Mint (88.7 mg), Tums (2.7 mg).

Check patient's self medication habits. Many elderly persons use "Soda bicarb" routinely to "settle the stomach."

If patient is also receiving a corticosteroid, any reduction in steroid dosage should be gradual to avoid withdrawal symptoms.

The patient with renal damage should be closely monitored and perhaps given lower doses. Incidence of adverse reactions is potentially high because the drug is excreted primarily by the kidneys. Monitor intake–output ratio if patient has renal impairment. Encourage fluid intake of at least 8 glasses of liquid/day.

Dizziness, a troublesome side effect early in the course of treatment frequently disappears in time. Advise patient to avoid driving a car or using hazardous equipment until response to drug is known.

If patient is receiving an oral anticoagulant, patient should immediately report any sign of bleeding (e.g., melena, epistaxis, ecchymosis). Prothrombin times should be closely monitored.

Response to therapy should be periodically evaluated. Urge patient to keep appointments for clinical evaluation of drug effectiveness and for laboratory studies, hemoglobin, hematocrit (if anemia is suspected) and kidney function.

Advise patient to inform surgeon or dentist that patient is on meclofenamate therapy.

Overdosage treatment includes emesis or gastric lavage, and administration of activated charcoal. Support for vital functions should be readily available.

Drug should be stored in airtight, light-resistant container between 15° and 30°C (59° and 86°F) unless otherwise recommended by manufacturer.

M

Diagnostic Test Interferences. Meclofenamate increases **BUN** and serum levels of **alkaline phosphatase, creatinine, bilirubin, transaminase.** These changes often return to pretreatment levels with continuation of therapy.

Drug Interactions. Meclofenamate may increase hypoprothrombinemic effect of **warfarin;** carefully monitor prothrombin time. Administration with aspirin may cause greater fecal blood loss; concomitant use generally avoided.

MEDROXYPROGESTERONE ACETATE

(Amen, Curretab, Depo-Provera, Provera)

(me-drox'ee-proe-jess'te-rone)

Progestin

Antineoplastic

ACTIONS AND USES. Synthetic derivative of progesterone with prolonged, variable duration of action. Lacks estrogenic and androgenic properties and has no deleterious effects on lipid metabolism. Effective on estrogen-primed endometrium. Not approved by FDA as single agent contraceptive. Actions, uses, absorption, fate and limitations similar to those of progesterone (qv).

ADVERSE/SIDE EFFECTS. (Rare): hyperpyrexia, headache. *See also Progesterone.*

ROUTE AND DOSAGE. **Oral:** *Secondary amenorrhea:* 5 to 10 mg daily for 5 to 10 days beginning anytime if endometrium is adequately estrogen-primed. (Withdrawal bleeding occurs in 3 to 7 days after discontinuing therapy. *Abnormal bleeding due to hormonal imbalance:* 5 to 10 mg daily for 5 to 10 days beginning on the 16th and 21st day of menstrual cycle. If bleeding is controlled, administer 2 subsequent cycles. **Intramuscular:** *Endometrial carcinoma:* 400 to 1000 mg weekly; if improvement occurs and disease stabilizes; maintenance; 400 mg/month.

NURSING IMPLICATIONS

IM injection may be painful. Monitor sites for evidence of sterile abscess. A residual lump and discoloration of tissue may develop.

Following repeated IM injections, infertility and amenorrhea may persist for as long as 18 months.

Planned menstrual cycling with medroxyprogesterone may benefit the patient with a history of recurrent episodes of abnormal uterine bleeding.

Teach patient self-breast examination (SBE).

Discuss package insert with patient to assure complete understanding of progestin therapy.

Store drug at temperature between 15° and 30°C (59° and 86°F); protect from freezing.

See Progesterone (prototype progestin).

MEFENAMIC ACID

(Ponstel)

(me-fe-nam′ik)
NSAID

ACTIONS AND USES. Anthranilic acid derivative with analgesic, anti-inflammatory, and antipyretic actions similar to those of aspirin. Like aspirin, inhibits prostaglandin synthesis, and affects platelet function. No evidence that it is superior to aspirin. Associated with a number of serious adverse reactions, particularly when used for prolonged periods at high doses.

Used for short-term relief of mild to moderate pain including primary dysmenorrhea.

ABSORPTION AND FATE. Absorbed slowly from GI tract. Peak analgesic effect in 2 to 4 hours may persist up to 6 hours. Firmly bound to plasma proteins. Partly detoxified in liver. Excreted in urine and feces as free drug and conjugated metabolites. Approximately 50% of dose is excreted in urine within 48 hours.

CONTRAINDICATIONS AND PRECAUTIONS. Hypersensitivity to drug, GI inflammation, or ulceration. Safe use in women of childbearing potential, children under age 14, and during pregnancy or lactation not established. *Cautious Use:* history of renal or hepatic disease, blood dyscrasias, asthma, diabetes mellitus, hypersensitivity to aspirin. *See also Drug Interactions.*

ADVERSE/SIDE EFFECTS. **CNS:** drowsiness, insomnia, dizziness, vertigo, unsteady gait, nervousness, confusion, headache; status epilepticus with overdose. **Dermatologic:** urticaria, rash, facial edema. **GI:** severe diarrhea (common), GI inflammation, ulceration, and bleeding; nausea, vomiting, abdominal cramps, flatus, constipation. **Hematopoietic:** prolonged prothrombin time, severe autoimmune hemolytic anemia (long-term use), leukopenia, eosinophilia, agranulocytosis, thrombocytopenic purpura, megaloblastic anemia, pancytopenia, bone marrow hypoplasia. **Renal:** nephrotoxicity, dysuria, albuminuria, hematuria, elevation of BUN. **Other:** eye irritation, loss of color vision (reversible), blurred vision, ear pain, perspiration, increased need for insulin in diabetic patients, hepatic toxicity, palpitation, dyspnea; acute exacerbation of asthma; bronchoconstriction (in patients sensitive to aspirin).

ROUTE AND DOSAGE. Oral: Initial: 500 mg, followed by 250 mg every 6 hours, as needed.

NURSING IMPLICATIONS

Administer with meals, food, or milk to minimize GI adverse effects.

Use of drug for a period exceeding 1 week is not recommended (manufacturer's warning).

Mefenamic acid should be discontinued promptly if diarrhea, dark stools, hematemesis, ecchymoses, epistaxis, or rash occur, and not used thereafter. Advise patients to report these signs to the physician.

Also advise patient to notify physician if persistent GI discomfort, sore throat, fever, or malaise occurs.

Since the drug may cause dizziness and drowsiness, caution patients to avoid driving a car and other potentially hazardous activities until response to drug is known.

Diabetic patients may show increased need for insulin.

Diagnostic Test Interferences. False-positive reactions for **urinary bilirubin** (using diazo tablet test).

Drug Interactions: Mefanamic

Plus	Interactions
Oral anticoagulants	Increased hypoprothrombinemia; displaces anticoagulants from protein binding sites. Concomitant use generally avoided
Corticosteroids Indomethacin Phenylbutazone Salicylates	Ulcerogenic effects potentiated

M

MEGESTROL ACETATE

(Megace, Pallace)

(me-jess'trole)
Progestin
Antineoplastic

ACTIONS AND USES. Progestational hormone with antineoplastic properties. Mechanism of action unclear; however, an antiluteinizing effect mediated via the pituitary has been postulated. Has local effect when instilled directly into the endometrial cavity.

Used as palliative agent for treatment of advanced carcinoma of breast or endometrium.

CONTRAINDICATIONS AND PRECAUTIONS. Diagnostic test for pregnancy; use in neoplastic diseases other than cancer of endometrium and breast; first 4 months of pregnancy. *See also Progesterone.*

ADVERSE/SIDE EFFECTS. Carpal tunnel syndrome, alopecia, deep vein thrombophlebitis, breast tenderness, abdominal pain, nausea, vomiting, headache, allergic-type reactions (including bronchial asthma). *See also Progesterone.*

ROUTE AND DOSAGE. Oral: *Breast cancer:* 40 mg four times daily. *Endometrial cancer:* 40 to 320 mg daily in divided doses. Continue therapy at least 2 months as adequate period for determining efficacy of megestrol.

NURSING IMPLICATIONS

Contraception measures are recommended during therapy for carcinoma with megestrol.

Tartrazine used in the tablet formulation may produce sensitivity including bronchial asthma in susceptible individuals, especially those with aspirin hypersensitivity.

Monitor for breathing distress characteristic of asthma; rash, urticaria, anaphylaxis, tachypnea, anxiety. Stop medication if they appear and notify physician.

Teach patient self-breast examination (SBE).

Discuss package insert with patient to assure understanding of megestrol therapy.

Store tablets in a well-closed container at temperatures between 15° and 30°C (59° and 86°F) unless otherwise specified by manufacturer.

See Progesterone (prototype progestin).

MELPHALAN

(mel′fa-lan)

(Alkeran, Pam, L-Pam, Phenylalanine Mustard, L-Sarcolysin)

Antineoplastic
Alkylating agent
Nitrogen mustard

ACTIONS AND USES. Nitrogen mustard chemically and pharmacologically related to mechlorethamine (qv). Has strong immunosuppressive and myelosuppressive effects, but unlike mechlorethamine, lacks vesicant properties. Carcinogenic potential suspected.

Used chiefly for palliative treatment of multiple myeloma. Also used in treatment of many other neoplasms, including Hodgkin's disease and carcinomas of breast, and ovary. Regional perfusion alone or with other antineoplastics is investigational.

ABSORPTION AND FATE. Well absorbed from GI tract. Plasma half-life: about 90 minutes. Widely distributed to all tissues; metabolism and excretion not fully known. Approximately 10 to 15% excreted unchanged in urine.

CONTRAINDICATIONS AND PRECAUTIONS. Hypersensitivity to melphalan; use during pregnancy or in men and women of childbearing age not established. *Cautious Use:* recent treatment with other chemotherapeutic agent; concurrent administration with radiation therapy; severe anemia, neutrophilia, or thrombocytopenia, impaired renal function.

ADVERSE/SIDE EFFECTS. Hematologic: leukopenia, agranulocytosis, thrombocytopenia, anemia, acute nonlymphatic leukemia. **Other:** mild thrombophlebitis at site of infusion, uremia, angioneurotic peripheral edema, minor neurologic toxicity (rare), nausea, vomiting (with high doses); occasional stomatitis, diarrhea hypersensitivity reactions, temporary alopecia, skin rash, bronchopulmonary dysplasia (rare), pulmonary fibrosis, menstrual irregularities, hyperuricemia. *See Mechlorethamine.*

ROUTE AND DOSAGE. Oral: *Multiple myeloma:* 6 mg daily for 2 to 3 weeks; drug is then withdrawn for 4 to 5 weeks. When WBC and platelet counts start to rise, maintenance dose is instituted: 2 mg/day. *Epithelial ovarian cancer:* 0.2 mg/kg/day for 5 days as a single course. Courses repeated every 4 to 5 weeks depending on hematological tolerance.

NURSING IMPLICATIONS

Administer parenteral drug immediately after preparation of solution.

Administer oral drug with meals to reduce nausea and vomiting. An antiemetic may be ordered if dose is high and side effects are increased.

Leukocyte and platelet counts are done two to three times each week during dosage adjustment period; WBC is usually determined each 6 to 8 weeks during maintenance therapy.

Nadirs of platelets and leukocytes occur within a few weeks after therapy begins; recovery is rapid.

Dosage adjustment is primarily based on blood counts. Usually, drug is discontinued after 2 to 3 weeks' treatment for about 4 weeks. When WBC and platelet counts begin to rise, maintenance dose of 2 mg daily is instituted.

Monitor laboratory reports to anticipate leukopenic and thrombocytopenic periods in order to adapt nursing care accordingly.

A degree of myelosuppression is maintained during therapy so as to keep leukocyte count in range of 3000 to 3500/mm^3.

The combination of reduced capacity for normal antibody production (characteristic of multiple myeloma) and melphalan-induced toxic hematopoietic depression makes the patient particularly susceptible to infections and prolonged responses to trauma. Be alert to onset of fever, profound weakness, chills, tachycardia, cough, sore throat, changes in kidney function, or prolonged infections, and report them to physician.

Flank and joint pains may signal onset of hyperuricemia. Report to physician.

A favorable response to oral melphalan in patients with multiple myeloma may be very gradual over many months. Encourage patient not to abandon treatment too soon to receive maximum benefit.

Stored in light-resistant airtight containers at room temperature, preferably between 15 and 30°C (59 and 86°F) unless otherwise directed by manufacturer.

See Mechlorethamine (prototype alkylating agent).

M

MENADIOL SODIUM DIPHOSPHATE

(men-a-dye'ole)

(Synkayvite, Vitamin K_4)

Vitamin

ACTIONS AND USES. Synthetic, water-soluble vitamin K analog derived from menadione (qv). Has same actions, uses, contraindications, precautions and adverse reactions as menadione, but is about one-half as potent. Like menadione, it does not counteract action of heparin. Its use as a liver function test has generally been replaced by newer methods. In combination with radiotherapy it may selectively increase radiosensitivity of tumor cells through an unknown action. Also reported to reduce adenosine triphosphate level in tumor cells.

ABSORPTION AND FATE. Absorbed directly into bloodstream after oral administration, even in the absence of bile salts. Converted to menadione in body. Following SC or IM administration, bleeding may be controlled within 1 to 2 hours; prothrombin time usually returns to normal in 8 to 24 hours. Response after IV administration is more prompt, but action is less sustained.

ADVERSE/SIDE EFFECTS. Nausea, vomiting, allergic reaction; pruritus, urticaria, rash. *See also Menadione.*

ROUTE AND DOSAGE. Oral, subcutaneous, intramuscular, intravenous: 5 to 15 mg once or twice daily.

NURSING IMPLICATIONS

Dosage and duration of treatment are determined by prothrombin times and clinical response.

Concomitant administration of bile salts is not required for intestinal absorption since menadiol sodium diphosphate is water-soluble.

Solutions of menadiol sodium diphosphate may be irritating to skin.

Parenteral drug is incompatible with protein hydrolysate.

Stored in tight, light-resistant containers at room temperature, preferably between 15 and 30°C (59 and 86°F) unless otherwise directed by manufacturer.

See Menadione.

MENADIONE

(men-a-dye′one)

(Menaphthone, Vitamin K_3)

Vitamin

ACTIONS AND USES. Synthetic, fat-soluble vitamin K analog. Similar in activity to naturally occurring vitamin K, which is essential in hepatic biosynthesis of blood clotting factors II, VII, IX, X. Mechanism of action unknown.

Used in treatment of hypoprothrombinemia caused by vitamin K deficiency secondary to oral antibacterial therapy and salicylates. Also effective in prevention and treatment of hypothrombinemia resulting from inadequate absorption and synthesis of vitamin K, as in obstructive jaundice, biliary fistula, ulcerative colitis, celiac disease, intestinal resection, regional enteritis, cystic fibrosis of pancreas. Largely replaced by phytonadione (vitamin K_1) as an antidote for oral anticoagulant overdosage and in prophylaxis and treatment of hemorrhagic disease of newborns. Like other forms of vitamin K, ineffective in treatment of heparin overdosage.

M

ABSORPTION AND FATE. Adequately absorbed after oral administration. Limited storage in fat tissue for short time. Completely metabolized. Crosses placenta.

CONTRAINDICATIONS AND PRECAUTIONS. Hypersensitivity to menadione or its derivatives, severe liver disease, patients with G6PD deficiency, administration to mothers during last few weeks of pregnancy as prophylaxis against hemorrhagic disease of newborn; use in neonates. Effects on human fertility and teratogenic potential not known. *Also see Drug Interactions.*

ADVERSE/SIDE EFFECTS. Gastric upset, headache, allergic reactions (skin rash, urticaria); erythrocyte hemolysis (persons with G6PD deficiency and newborns). With large doses: BSP retention, prolonged prothrombin time, further depression of liver function (patients with hepatic disease). In infants, particularly prematures, or when administered to mother prior to delivery: hemolytic anemia, hemoglobinuria, hyperbilirubinemia, kernicterus, brain damage, death.

ROUTE AND DOSAGE. Oral: 2 to 10 mg daily.

NURSING IMPLICATIONS

Prothrombin times and clinical response are used as guides for dosage and duration of treatment.

Concomitant administration of bile salts is not essential for adequate absorption.

Consult physician regarding dietary vitamin K intake. Vitamin K-rich foods include: asparagus, broccoli, cabbage, lettuce, turnip greens, beef liver, green tea, spinach, watercress, tomatoes, coffee.

Therapeutic response to menadione is indicated by shortening of prothrombin, bleeding, and clotting times, and by a decrease in hemorrhagic tendencies.

Normal prothrombin time: 2 seconds deviation from control; *bleeding times* (Ivy): 1 to 6 minutes; *clotting time* (3 tubes): 5 to 15 minutes.

The minimum daily requirement of vitamin K has not been established, but is estimated to be about 0.03 mcg/kg for adults, and 1 to 5 mcg/kg for infants. A deficiency is not likely to occur in healthy individuals since the vitamin is found in many foods (vitamin K_1), and also is synthesized by intestinal bacteria (vitamin K_2).

Drug Interactions: Menadione

Plus	Interactions
Antibiotics, oral (broad spectrum), long-term therapy	Oral antibiotics enhance hypoprothrombinemia by suppressing vitamin K-producing intestinal bacteria
Anticoagulants, oral	Vitamin K significantly antagonizes effects of anticoagulants
Cholestyramine (Questran) Mineral oil	Inhibit GI absorption of vitamin K; space doses as far apart as possible

MENOTROPINS

(Pergonal)

(men-oh-troe'pins)
Ovulation stimulant
Gonadotropin

M

ACTIONS AND USES. Purified preparation of exogenous gonadotropins, extracted from human menopausal urinary gonadotropin and standardized biologically for follicle-stimulating hormone (FSH) and luteinizing hormone (LH) gonadotropic activities. Promotes growth of graafian follicles in women who do not have primary anovulation. Treatment usually results only in ovarian follicular growth and maturation. With clinical proof of follicular maturation, ovulation is induced by menotropins followed by administration of human chorionic gonadotropin (HCG). Stimulates spermatogenesis in men with primary or secondary hypogonado tropic hypogonadism after pretreatment with HCG.

Used with HCG (in sequence) to induce ovulation and pregnancy in the infertile woman with functional anovultion (i.e., secondary to pituitary insufficiency). Also used in conjunction with HCG to treat male infertility.

ABSORPTION AND FATE. Disposition factors following parenteral administration not known. Approximately 8% of dose is excreted unchanged in urine. Urinary estrogen excretion during treatment reflects level of follicular enlargement.

CONTRAINDICATIONS AND PRECAUTIONS. Pregnancy, primary anovulation, thyroid and adrenal dysfunction, organic intracranial lesion, infertility caused by factors other than anovulation, abnormal bleeding of unknown origin, ovarian cysts or enlargement not due to polycystic ovary syndrome; men with normal urinary gonadotropin concentrations, or primary testicular failure.

ADVERSE/SIDE EFFECTS. Dose related: mild to moderate ovarian enlargement, abdominal distention and pain, *ovarian hyperstimulation syndrome* (sudden ovarian enlargement accompanied by ascites with or without pain and/or pleural effusion), hemoperitoneum, fever, nausea, vomiting, diarrhea, arterial thromboembolism (rare), hypovolemia, multiple ovulations, follicular cysts, birth defects; gynecomastia (men).

ROUTE AND DOSAGE. Intramuscular (individualized): *Induction of ovulation and pregnancy:* Initial: 75 IU each of FSH and LH (1 ampul) daily for 9 to 12 days; followed by HCG (10,000 IU) one day after last dose of menotropins. Menotropins should not be given beyond 12 days. If ovulation occurs without pregnancy, regimen may be repeated at least twice at same dosage before increasing dosage to 150 IU each of FSH and LH daily for 9 to 12 days. As before, HCG (10,000 IU) is given 1 day after last dose of menotropins. If ovulation occurs without pregnancy, treatment may be repeated at monthly intervals for two more courses. *Stimulation of spermatogenesis:* (following pretreatment with HCG): 75 IU each of FSH and LH three times weekly (in conjunction with HCG) until detection of spermatozoa in the ejaculate (4 to 6 months).

NURSING IMPLICATIONS

Treatment with menotropins for women is preceded by a thorough gynecologic and endocrinologic examination to rule out early pregnancy, primary ovarian failure, neoplastic lesion; husband's fertility is also evaluated. Menotropins treatment for men is preceded by at least 4 to 6 months of HCG or until normal serum testosterone concentration is achieved.

Drug is prepared immediately before administration by dissolving ampul contents in 1 to 2 ml of sterile NaCl injection. Unused portion should be discarded.

Most reliable index of follicular maturation (estrogenic activity) is the rate of urinary estrogen excretion. Other indirect estimates include serial examination of vaginal smears and cervical mucus specimens, and changes in appearance (Spinnbarkeit, ferning) and volume.

Teach patient to recognize indirect indices of progesterone production: rise in basal body temperature (BBT), menstruation following shift in BBT, increased volume of thin and watery vaginal secretion, increased urinary pregnanediol levels, change of cervical mucus from "fern" to cellular pattern; vaginal cytology characteristic of luteal phase of menstrual cycle.

The couple should be encouraged to have intercourse daily beginning on day prior to administration of HCG until ovulation becomes apparent from indices of progestational activity. Care must be taken to insure insemination.

When total estrogen excretion level is more than 100 mcg/24 hours, HCG is not administered because hyperstimulation syndrome is more likely to occur.

Patient should be examined at least every other day and for 2 weeks following HCG injection to detect excessive ovarian stimulation. Examiner should proceed with caution in performing pelvic examination to avoid rupture of possible ovarian cysts and consequent hemoperitoneum.

If significant ovarian enlargement occurs after ovulation, patient should refrain from intercourse.

Warn patient to report immediately if symptoms of hyperstimulation syndrome occur: abdominal distention and pain, dyspnea, vaginal bleeding. Discontinuation of intercourse, as well as hospitalization, may be necessary.

Monitor intake–output ratio to indirectly monitor fluid loss into abdominal cavity during hyperstimulation syndrome.

Advise patient to weigh herself every other day to detect sudden weight gain (hyperstimulation syndrome develops rapidly over a 3- to 4-day period and usually occurs within 2 weeks following therapy). Patient should understand the range of weight gain that is unacceptable and that should be reported to physician.

Mild ovarian enlargement (with or without abdominal distention and pain) usually regresses without treatment in 2 to 3 weeks.
Patient and husband should be aware of statistics related to pregnancy after menotropins/ HCG treatment. Reportedly, there is a 20% frequency of multiple births, 15% of which may be twins; 5% of total pregnancies result in 3 or more fetuses, of which 20% are viable.
Generally, pregnancy occurs within four to six courses of therapy.
For the male receiving menotropins therapy, if there is no evidence of increased spermatogenesis after 4 months, therapy can continue with increased dosage of menotropins.

MEPENZOLATE BROMIDE

(Cantil)

(me-pen'zoe-late)
Anticholinergic
Antispasmodic

ACTIONS AND USES. Synthetic anticholinergic quaternary ammonium compound. Qualitatively similar to atropine in actions, contraindications, precautions, and adverse reactions. Acts predominantly on GI tract. Reduces motility of stomach, small intestine, and particularly colon. Large oral doses can reduce gastric secretion of hydrochloric acid. Also relaxes sphincter of Oddi. As with other quaternary anticholinergic agents, high doses may block ganglionic and skeletal neuromuscular transmission.

Used in adjunctive treatment of peptic ulcer, irritable bowel syndrome, neurogenic bowel disturbances, diverticulitis, and diarrhea.

ABSORPTION AND FATE. Irregular GI absorption. Onset of action in about 1 hour, lasting 3 to 4 hours. Excreted primarily in urine and bile and as unchanged drug in feces.

ROUTE AND DOSAGE. Oral: 25 to 50 mg three times a day and at bedtime. Low doses are used initially and are increased gradually until desired effects are obtained or side effects intervene.

NURSING IMPLICATIONS

Administered preferably before or with meals.
Caution patients not to engage in activities requiring mental alertness, such as driving a car, if drowsiness or blurred vision occurs.
See Atropine Sulfate (protype antispasmodic).

MEPERIDINE HYDROCHLORIDE

(Demerol, Pethadol, Pethidine Hydrochloride)

(me-per'i-deen)
Narcotic analgesic
C II

ACTIONS AND USES. Synthetic morphinelike compound (phenylpiperidine derivative). Chemically dissimilar to morphine, but in equianalgesic doses it is qualitatively comparable with regard to analgesic effects, sedation, euphoria, pupillary constriction, and respiratory depression. Reported to differ from morphine in having a somewhat more rapid onset and shorter duration of action and in producing less depression of cough reflex, constipation, urinary retention, and smooth muscle spasm. Usual doses produce either no pupillary change or slight miosis, but overdosage results in marked miosis or mydriasis. Also, unlike morphine, has little or no antidiarrheic or antitussive action and produces CNS stimulation in toxic doses. In common with morphine, it causes sensitization of labyrinthine apparatus, stimulation of chemoreceptor trigger zone, and depression of medullary vasomotor center; it also has vagolytic and anticholinergic actions and may inhibit release of ACTH and gonadotropic hormones. Promotes release of histamine and antidiuretic hormone, and elevation of blood sugar.

Used for relief of moderate to severe pain, for preoperative medication, for support of anesthesia, and for obstetric analgesia.

ABSORPTION AND FATE. Well absorbed from GI tract; analgesic effect following oral administration begins in 15 minutes, peaks in about 1 hour, and subsides over 2 to 4 hours. Onset of action following SC or IM administration occurs within 10 minutes; action peaks within 60 minutes, duration of action for both routes 2 to 4 hours. Onset of action following IV administration in about 5 minutes; duration approximately 2 hours. Half-life: 2.4 to 4 hours; 65 to 75% bound to plasma proteins. Metabolized chiefly in liver to active and inactive metabolites. Excreted in urine, mostly as metabolites and about 5% unchanged drug (excretion enhanced by acidification of urine). Crosses placenta and appears in breast milk.

CONTRAINDICATIONS AND PRECAUTIONS. Hypersensitivity to meperidine, convulsive disorders, acute abdominal conditions prior to diagnosis, pregnancy (prior to labor), nursing mothers. *Cautious Use:* head injuries, increased intracranial pressure, asthma and other respiratory conditions, supraventricular tachycardias, prostatic hypertrophy, urethral stricture, glaucoma, elderly or debilitated patients, impaired renal or hepatic function, hypothyroidism, Addison's disease.

ADVERSE/SIDE EFFECTS. Allergic: pruritus, urticaria, skin rashes, wheal and flare over IV site. **CNS:** dizziness, weakness, euphoria, dysphoria, sedation, headache, uncoordinated muscle movements, disorientation, decreased cough reflex, miosis, corneal anesthesia, respiratory depression. Toxic doses: muscle twitching, tremors, hyperactive reflexes, excitement, hypersensitivity to external stimuli, agitation, confusion, hallucinations, dilated pupils, convulsions. **CV:** facial flushing, lightheadedness, hypotension, syncope, palpitation, bradycardia, tachycardia, cardiovascular collapse, cardiac arrest (toxic doses). **GI:** dry mouth, nausea, vomiting, constipation, biliary tract spasm. **Other reported:** oliguria, urinary retention, profuse perspiration, respiratory depression in newborn, bronchoconstriction (large doses), phlebitis (following IV use), pain, tissue irritation and induration, particularly following subcutaneous injection; increased levels of serum amylase, BSP retention, bilirubin, SGOT, SGPT.

ROUTE AND DOSAGE. Oral, subcutaneous, intramuscular, intravenous (given slowly IV and as diluted solution): **Adults:** 50 to 150 mg every 3 or 4 hours as necessary; *preoperative:* 50 to 100 mg IM or subcutaneously 30 to 90 minutes before anesthesia; *obstetric analgesia:* 50 to 100 mg IM or subcutaneously when pains become regular; may be repeated at 1- to 3-hour intervals. **Children:** 1 mg/kg IM, subcutaneously, or orally up to 100 mg, every 4 hours as necessary.

NURSING IMPLICATIONS

Narcotic analgesics should be given in the smallest effective dose and for the least period of time compatible with patient's needs.

Evaluate the patient's need for p.r.n. medication; check time of last dose and validity of physician's order. Follow agency policy regarding time limit of narcotic orders. Record time of onset, duration, and quality of pain, preferably in patient's words.

In patients receiving repeated doses, note respiratory rate, depth, and rhythm and size of pupils. If respirations are 12 per minute or below and pupils are constricted or dilated *(see Actions and Uses)* or breathing is shallow, or if signs of CNS hyperactivity are present, consult physician before administering drug.

Carefully aspirate before giving IM injection in order to avoid inadvertent IV administration. IV injection of undiluted drug can cause a marked increase in heart rate and syncope.

Although the SC route is sometimes prescribed, it is painful and can cause local irritation. The IM route is generally preferred when repeated doses are required.

A high incidence of severe untoward effects is associated with IV use. Facilities for administration of oxygen and control of respiration should be immediately available, as well as a narcotic antagonist (e.g., naloxone, naltrexone).

Vital signs should be monitored closely. Heart rate may increase markedly, and hypotension may occur.

The syrup formulation should be taken in half a glass of water. Undiluted syrup may cause topical anesthesia of mucous membranes.

Before administering meperidine, provide maximum comfort measures and reduce environmental stimuli. Caution patient not to smoke and not to ambulate without assistance after receiving the drug. Bedsides are advisable.

Use of comfort measures, as well as displays of thoughtfulness and interest by those attending the patient, are as important as medication in control of pain.

Monitor vital signs, particularly in patients receiving repeated doses. Meperidine may cause severe hypotension in postoperative patients and those with depleted blood volume.

Deep breathing, coughing (unless contraindicated), and changes in position at scheduled intervals may help to overcome the respiratory depressant effects of meperidine.

Parenteral administration has caused corneal anesthesia and thus abolishment of corneal reflex in some patients. Be alert for this possibility.

Ambulatory patients are more likely than supine patients to manifest nausea, vomiting, dizziness, and faintness associated with fall in blood pressure (these symptoms may also occur in patients without pain who are given meperidine). Symptoms are lessened by the recumbent position and aggravated by the head-up position. Report to physician; dosage reduction or drug discontinuation may be indicated.

Caution ambulatory patients to avoid driving a car or engaging in other hazardous activities until any drowsiness and dizziness have passed.

Chart the patient's response to meperidine and evaluate continued need for the drug. Suggest to physician a change to a milder analgesic when in your judgment it is indicated.

Repeated use of meperidine can lead to tolerance and psychic and physical dependence of the morphine type. High abuse potential has been reported among nurses and physicians.

Abrupt discontinuation of meperidine following repeated use results in *morphinelike withdrawal symptoms.* Symptoms develop more rapidly (within 3 hours, peaking in 8 to 12 hours) and are of shorter duration than with morphine. Nausea, vomiting, diarrhea, and pupillary dilatation are less prominent, but muscle twitching, restlessness, and nervousness are greater than produced by morphine.

Classified as Schedule II drug under Federal Controlled Substances Act.

Preserved in tightly closed, light-resistant containers preferably between 15 to 30°C (59 to 86°F) unless otherwise directed by manufacturer.

Drug Interactions. CNS stimulation or depression induced by meperidine and its congeners may be potentiated by **amphetamines, barbiturates, cimetidine** (Tagamet), **MAO inhibitors** including drugs with significant MAOI activity e.g., **furazolidone** (Furoxone), **isoniazid** (INH) (concurrent use avoided); **phenothiazines** (concurrent use avoided); **phenytoin** (Dilantin) and other hydantoins; **tricyclic antidepressants, other CNS depressants,** including **alcohol.**

MEPHENTERMINE SULFATE
(Wyamine)

(me-fen′ter-meen)
Adrenergic agonist
(Sympathomimetic)

ACTIONS AND USES. Synthetic noncatecholamine with alpha- and predominant beta-adrenergic activity. Acts both directly and indirectly (by releasing norepinephrine from tissue storage sites). Elevation of blood pressure probably results primarily from positive inotropic action and increased cardiac output, and to lesser extent to increase in peripheral resistance caused by peripheral vasoconstriction. Heart rate may be reflexly slowed. Antiarrhythmic action results from decrease in A-V conduction time, atrial refractory period, and conduction time in ventricular muscle. CNS effects are usually not prominent except with large doses.

Used mainly as pressor agent in treatment of hypotension secondary to ganglionic blockade or spinal anesthesia. Also has been used as an emergency measure in therapy of shock secondary to hemorrhage until whole blood replacement is available; as adjunct in treatment of cardiogenic shock, and to abolish certain cardiac arrhythmias.

ABSORPTION AND FATE. Onset of pressor effect following IM injection in 5 to 15 minutes; duration 1 to 2 hours. Following IV administration, pressor response begins almost immediately and lasts 30 to 45 minutes. Rapidly metabolized. Excreted in urine. Alkaline urine favors drug retention and tends to produce higher plasma levels.

CONTRAINDICATIONS AND PRECAUTIONS. History of sensitivity to mephentermine; shock secondary to hemorrhage (except in emergency). Safe use in women of childbearing age and during pregnancy or lactation not established. *Cautious Use:* arteriosclerosis, cardiovascular disease, hypovolemia, hypertension, hyperthyroidism, patients with known hypersensitivities, chronically ill patients.

ADVERSE/SIDE EFFECTS. Infrequent: euphoria, anorexia, weeping, nervousness, anxiety, tremor. With large doses: cardiac arrhythmias, marked elevation of blood pressure, incoherence, drowsiness, convulsions.

M

ROUTE AND DOSAGE. Intramuscular, intravenous: 15 to 45 mg. Average dose to produce pressor response in **Adults:** 0.5 mg/kg, **Children:** 0.4 mg/kg. **Intravenous infusion:** *Hypotensive emergency:* 20 to 60 mg. Infusion solutions are usually prepared by adding 600 mg of mephentamine to 500 ml of 5% dextrose in water (solution will contain approximately 1.2 mg/ml).

NURSING IMPLICATIONS

Close observation of patient and monitoring of blood pressure, heart rate, ECG, and central venous pressure (CVP) are essential.

During IV administration, check blood pressure and pulse every 2 minutes until stabilized at prescribed level, then every 5 minutes thereafter during therapy. Continue monitoring vital signs for at least the duration of drug action *(see Absorption and Fate)* and longer if indicated.

IV flow rate should be prescribed by physician. Usual infusion rate is 1 to 5 mg/minute.

Tolerance may occur after repeated injections.

Preserved in tightly closed, light-resistant containers preferably at 15° to 30°C (59° and 86°F) unless otherwise directed by manufacturer.

Mephentermine is incompatible with epinephrine hydrochloride and hydralazine hydrochloride.

Drug Interactions. Mephentermine may be ineffective in patients receiving **reserpine** or **guanethidine;** these drugs reduce quantity of available norepinephrine in sympathetic nerve endings (combination avoided). Pressor response may be potentiated by other **sympathomimetic amines, MAO inhibitors,** or drugs with significant MAOI activity e.g., **furazolidone** (Furoxone), **isoniazid** (INH) (concurrent use and use within 2 weeks avoided);**methyldopa,** and **tricyclic antidepressants** (concomitant use generally avoided). Administration of mephentermine during **cyclopropane** or **halothane** anesthesia may result in serious arrhythmias (concurrent use generally avoided). Concomitant use with **digitalis** may increase possibility of arrhythmias (used only with caution).

MEPHENYTOIN
(Mesantoin)

(me-fen'i-toyn)
Anticonvulsant
Hydantoin

ACTIONS AND USES. Hydantoin derivative, with actions, contraindications, precautions, and adverse reactions similar to those of phenytoin (qv). Reported to have lower incidence of ataxia, gingival hyperplasia, gastric distress, and hirsutism, but produces more sedative and hypnotic action than phenytoin; causes serious toxic reactions, including fatal blood dyscrasias, more frequently. Relatively ineffective for petit mal seizures.

Used for control of grand mal, focal, jacksonian, and psychomotor seizures in patients refractory to less toxic anticonvulsants. Usually used concomitantly with other antiepilepsy agents.

ABSORPTION AND FATE. Rapidly absorbed following oral administration. Onset of action in 30 minutes; duration 24 to 48 hours. Demethylated in liver to phethenylate (nirvanol), an active metabolite believed to have both therapeutic and toxic properties. Excreted in urine. Half-life: 144 hours.

M

CONTRAINDICATIONS AND PRECAUTIONS. History of hypersensitivity to mephenytoin; use in conjunction with oxazolidinedione anticonvulsant agents, e.g., paramethadione, trimethadione (toxic synergism). Safe use during pregnancy not established. *Cautious Use:* history of drug hypersensitivities. *See also Phenytoin.*

ADVERSE/SIDE EFFECTS. Drowsiness, dizziness, skin and mucous membrane manifestations (exfoliative dermatitis, erythema multiforme, toxic epidermal necrolysis, other skin rashes), blood dyscrasias (leukopenia, neutropenia, agranulocytosis, thrombocytopenia, aplastic anemia), hepatic damage, periarteritis nodosa, systemic lupus erythematosus syndrome. *See also Phenytoin.*

ROUTE AND DOSAGE. Oral: Adults and children: initially 50 to 100 mg daily during first week; increased weekly by same amount until maintenance level. Maintenance: **Adults:** 200 to 600 mg daily administered in 3 equally divided doses (some patients require 800 mg daily). **Children:** 100 to 400 mg/daily administered in 3 equally divided doses.

NURSING IMPLICATIONS

Patients should be kept under close supervision at all times, since drug is associated with severe adverse effects. Serious blood dyscrasias have occurred 2 weeks to 30 months after initiation of therapy.

Screening tests of liver function, total white cell count, and differential count should precede initiation of therapy.

Blood studies should be performed every 2 weeks and should be continued until patient is on maintenance dosage for 2 weeks; then they should be repeated monthly for 1 year, and thereafter every 3 months (unless neutrophil count drops to 2500/mm^3 or 1600/mm^3, then performed every 2 weeks).

Medication should be discontinued if neutrophil count falls to 1600/mm^3.

The most frequent side effect of mephenytoin therapy is drowsiness, usually diminished by reduction of dosage. Caution patient to avoid hazardous activities until reactions to the drug has been determined. Supervision of ambulation and bedsides may be indicated for some patients during early therapy.

Advise patients to report immediately the onset of drowsiness, ataxia, skin rash, sore throat, fever, mucous membrane bleeding, or glandular swelling. All are indications of developing toxic reaction.

When mephenytoin replaces another antiepilepsy agent, the dosage of mephenytoin should be gradually increased while the drug being discontinued is gradually decreased over period of 3 to 6 weeks.

Discontinuation of mephenytoin should be accomplished gradually to minimize the risk of precipitating seizures or status epilepticus.

See Phenytoin (prototype anticonvulsant).

MEPHOBARBITAL

(Mebaral, Methylphenobarbital)

(me-foe-bar′bi-tal)
Anticonvulsant
Sedative
Barbiturate
C IV

M

ACTIONS AND USES. Long-acting barbiturate with pharmacologic properties similar to those of phenobarbital (qv); however, larger doses are required to produce comparable anticonvulsant effects. Exerts strong sedative action, but relatively mild hypnotic effect. Clinical uses, contraindications, precautions, and adverse reactions are as for phenobarbital.

Used to control grand mal and petit mal epilepsy, alone or in combination with other anticonvulsant agents, and for sedative effect in management of delirium tremens and other acute agitation and anxiety states.

ABSORPTION AND FATE. Approximately 50% absorbed following oral ingestion. Onset of action in 20 to 60 minutes; duration 6 to 8 hours. Half-life: about 34 hours. About 75% metabolized in liver to phenobarbital in 24 hours. Excreted in urine both unchanged and as metabolites. Alkalinization of urine or increase of urinary flow significantly hastens rate of phenobarbital excretion.

CONTRAINDICATIONS AND PRECAUTIONS. Hypersensitivity to barbiturates. Safe use during pregnancy not established. *Cautious Use:* fever, hyperthyroidism, alcoholism; hepatic, renal, or cardiac dysfunction. *See also Phenobarbital.*

ADVERSE/SIDE EFFECTS. CNS: drowsiness, dizziness, unsteadiness, hangover, paradoxical, excitement. **GI:** nausea, vomiting, constipation. **Other:** hypersensitivity reactions, respiratory depression. *See also Phenobarbital.*

ROUTE AND DOSAGE. Oral: *Anticonvulsant:* **Adults:** 400 to 600 mg daily. **Children (under 5 years):** 16 to 32 mg three or four times daily; **(over 5 years):** 32 to 64 mg three or four times daily. *Sedative:* **Adults:** 32 to 100 mg three or four times daily. *Delirium tremens:* 200 mg three times daily. **Children:** 16 to 32 mg three or four times daily.

NURSING IMPLICATIONS

Change from other antiepilepsy agents to mephobarbital should be accomplished by gradually tapering off the former as mephobarbital doses are increased to maintain seizure control.

When mephobarbital is prescribed concurrently with phenobarbital, the dose should be about one-half the amount of each used alone. When prescribed concurrently with phenytoin, the dose of phenytoin is usually reduced.

Mephobarbital may be prescribed as a single dose at bedtime (if seizures generally occur at night) or during the day (if attacks are diurnal).

When mephobarbital anticonvulsant therapy is to be discontinued, dosage should be reduced gradually over 4 or 5 days to avoid precipitating seizures of status epilepticus.

Abrupt cessation after prolonged mephobarbital therapy may result in withdrawal symptoms (tremulousness, weakness, insomnia, delirium, convulsions).

Since mephobarbital may cause drowsiness and dizziness, caution patients to avoid hazardous activities such as driving a car until response to drug has stabilized.

Classified as Schedule IV drug under Federal Controlled Substances Act.

See Phenobarbital (prototype barbiturate).

PROTOTYPE

MEPROBAMATE

(Equanil, Mepriam, Meprospan, Miltown, Neuramate, Neurate-400, Sedabamate, SK-Bamate, Tranmep)

(me-proe-ba′mate)
Psychotropic
Anxiolytic
Carbamate
C IV

M

ACTIONS AND USES. Propanediol carbamate derivative structurally and pharmacologically related to carisoprodol. CNS depressant actions similar to those of barbiturates. Acts on multiple sites in CNS and appears to block cortical-thalamic impulses. Has no effect on medulla, reticular activating system, or autonomic nervous system. Skeletal muscle relaxant effect is probably related to sedative rather than to direct action. Hypnotic doses suppress REM sleep.

Used to relieve anxiety and tension of psychoneurotic states and as adjunct in disease states associated with anxiety and tension. Also used to promote sleep in anxious, tense patients. Available in fixed combination with benactyzine hydrochloride (Deprol); with aspirin (Micrainin); with conjugated estrogens (Miltrate), and with ethoheptazine citrate and aspirin (Equagesic).

ABSORPTION AND FATE. Onset of sedative action within 1 hour following oral administration. Plasma half-life: 6 to 16 hours. Uniformly distributed throughout body; rapidly metabolized in liver. About 8 to 19% of dose is excreted in urine unchanged, and 10% in feces as inactive metabolites, within 24 hours. Induces hepatic microsomal enzymes. Crosses placenta and enters breast milk.

CONTRAINDICATIONS AND PRECAUTIONS. History of hypersensitivity to meprobamate or related carbamates such as carisoprodol and tybamate; history of acute intermittent porphyria; pregnancy, lactation; children under 6 years of age. *Cautious Use:* impaired renal or hepatic function, convulsive disorders, history of alcoholism or drug abuse, patients with suicidal tendencies.

ADVERSE/SIDE EFFECTS. Allergy or idiosyncrasy: itchy, urticarial, or erythematous maculopapular rash; exfoliative dermatitis, petechiae, purpura, ecchymoses, eosinophilia, peripheral edema, angioneurotic edema, adenopathy, fever, chills, proctitis, bronchospasm, oliguria, anuria, Stevens-Johnson syndrome; anaphylaxis. **CNS:** drowsiness and ataxia (most frequent), dizziness, vertigo, slurred speech, headache, weakness, paresthesias, impaired visual accommodation, paradoxic, euphoria and rage reactions, seizures in epileptics, panic reaction, rapid EEG activity. **CV:** hypotensive crisis, syncope, palpitation, tachycardia, arrhythmias, transient ECG changes. **GI:** anorexia, stomatitis, nausea, vomiting, diarrhea. **Hematologic (rare):** leukopenia, agranulocytosis, thrombocytopenia. **Other:** exacerbation of acute intermittent porphyria, grand mal attack, respiratory depression and circulatory collapse (toxic doses).

ROUTE AND DOSAGE. Adults: Oral: 400 mg three or four times daily, or 600 mg two times daily. Doses greater than 2.4 Gm/day not recommended. **Children (6 to 12 years):** 100 to 200 mg 2 or 3 times daily.

NURSING IMPLICATIONS

May be administered with food to minimize gastric distress.

Dispense least feasible amount of drug at a time because of the possibility of suicide attempts. Supervise ingestion of tablets or capsules. Watch to see that patient does not "cheek" the medication for hoarding, or to avoid treatment.

The elderly, and debilitated patients are prone to oversedation and to the hypotensive effects of meprobamate, especially during early therapy. Generally, lower doses are prescribed and dose increases are made gradually.

Caution patient to make position changes slowly, especially from recumbent to upright, and to dangle legs for a few minutes before standing. Supervise ambulation, if necessary.

Hypnotic doses may cause increased motor activity during sleep. Bed rails are advisable.

Therapeutic blood level range is 0.5 to 2 mg%. Blood levels of 3 to 10 mg% usually correspond with symptoms of mild to moderate overdosage (e.g., slurred speech, ataxia, stupor, light coma); levels of 10 to 20 mg% correspond with deep coma, hypotension, respiratory depression, heart failure and frequently lead to death. Levels above 20 mg% are usually lethal.

Continued effectiveness of response to meprobamate should be reassessed by the physician at the end of 4 months.

Warn patient that tolerance to alcohol will be lowered. When meprobamate and alcohol (or another CNS depressant) are taken concomitantly, the CNS depressant actions of each agent are intensified.

Caution patient not to self-dose with OTC drugs without consulting the physician.

Since meprobamate may impair mental and physical abilities, caution patient to avoid driving a car or engaging in other hazardous activities until drug response has been determined.

If daytime psychomotor function is impaired consult physician. A change in regimen or drug may be indicated.

Patients should be instructed to report immediately: onset of skin rash, sore throat, fever, bruising, unexplained bleeding. All are indicators of possible allergic or idiosyncratic reactions or blood dyscrasias.

Patient should be advised that if she becomes pregnant during therapy or intends to become pregnant she should communicate with her physician about the desirability of discontinuing the drug.

Instruct patient to take drug as prescribed; patient should not change dose or dose intervals. Warn patient not to give any of it to another person, and not to use it for a self-diagnosed problem.

Psychic or physical dependence may occur with long-term use of high doses.

Sudden withdrawal in physically dependent patients may precipitate preexisting symptoms or withdrawal reactions within 12 to 48 hours: vomiting, ataxia, muscle twitching, mental confusion, hallucinations, convulsions, trembling, sleep disturbances, increased dreaming, nightmares, insomnia. Symptoms usually subside within 12 to 48 hours.

Treatment of meprobamate physical dependence consists of gradual drug withdrawal over 1 to 2 weeks to prevent onset of withdrawal symptoms.

Classified as a Schedule IV drug under Federal Controlled Substances Act.

Treatment of overdosage: removal of drug from stomach, administration of charcoal slurry; respiratory assistance, CNS stimulants and pressor agents as indicated; careful monitoring of intake–output ratio. Prevent overhydration.

Relapse and death after initial recovery from overdosage may be due to delayed absorption or incomplete gastric emptying.

Store drug at temperature between 15° and 30°C (59° and 86°F), unless otherwise specified by manufacturer.

Diagnostic Test Interferences. Meprobamate may cause falsely high **urinary steroid** determinations.

Drug Interactions. Possibility of additive CNS depressant effects with concurrent use of meprobamate and **alcohol** and other **CNS depressants, imipramine** and other **tricyclic antidepressants.**

PROTOTYPE

MERCAPTOPURINE

(6-MP, 6-Mercaptopurine, Purinethol)

(mer-kap-toe-pyoor'een)
Antineoplastic
Antimetabolite

M

ACTIONS AND USES. Antimetabolite and purine antagonist. Inhibits purine metabolism by unclear mechanism. Blocks conversion of inosinic acid to adenine and xanthine ribotides within sensitive tumor cells. Also inhibits adenine-containing coenzymes, suggesting an influence over multiple cellular reactions. Has delayed immunosuppressive properties and carcinogenic potential.

Used primarily for treatment of acute lymphocytic and myelogenous leukemia. Response in adults is less than in children, but mercaptopurine is initial drug of choice. In chronic granulocytic leukemia, produces temporary remission.

ABSORPTION AND FATE. Oral preparations are erratically and incompletely absorbed without damage to intestinal mucosa. Half-life: 21 minutes in children, 47 minutes in adults. Rapid distribution to sensitive tumor cells; crosses blood–brain barrier. Partial degradation in liver with rapid excretion in urine as metabolites, including 6-thiouric acid and inorganic sulfates. Small proportion excreted for as long as 17 days. Drug is dialyzable.

CONTRAINDICATIONS AND PRECAUTIONS. Prior resistance to mercaptopurine; first trimester of pregnancy, infections. *Cautious Use:* impaired renal or hepatic function, concomitant use with allopurinol.

ADVERSE/SIDE EFFECTS. GI: stomatitis, esophagitis, anorexia, nausea, vomiting, diarrhea, steatorrhea (rare), intestinal ulcerations. **Hematologic:** leukopenia, anemia, eosinophilia, pancytopenia, thrombocytopenia, abnormal bleeding, bone marrow hypoplasia. **Other:** impaired liver function, hyperuricemia, skin rash, oliguria, renal impairment, drug fever.

ROUTE AND DOSAGE. **Highly individualized. Oral: Adults and children (5 years of age and over):** 2.5 mg/kg/day in single or divided doses. If no clinical improvement in 4 weeks, dose is increased to 5 mg/kg/day, if tolerated. Maintenance: 1.5 to 2.5 mg/kg/day; usually continued during remission.

NURSING IMPLICATIONS

Start flow chart at beginning of therapy to record baseline data related to intake–output ratio and pattern and body weight. Dosage determination and clues to onset of renal dysfunction depend on accurate comparative data.

Monitor daily laboratory reports for suggested adaptations in nursing management. Blood picture may change dramatically in a short period, and counts may continue to decrease several days after drug is withdrawn.

During periods of leukopenia, protect patient from exposure to trauma, infections, or other stresses (restrict visitors and personnel who have colds).

Check vital signs daily.

Oral ulcerations are rare; those that occur resemble lesions of thrush (creamy white exudative patches on inflamed painful mucosa). Inspect buccal membranes if patient complains of discomfort. Amphotericin B or nystatin may be ordered for relief. *See Index: Nursing Interventions: stomatitis.*

Nausea, vomiting, and diarrhea are uncommon during drug administration, but they may signal excessive dosage, especially in adults.

In acute leukemia, mercaptopurine may be continued in spite of thrombocytopenia and bleeding. Often, bleeding stops and platelet count rises during treatment.

If thrombocytopenia develops, watch for signs of abnormal bleeding (ecchymoses, petechiae, melena, bleeding gums); report them immediately.

M

Jaundice signals onset of hepatic toxicity and may necessitate terminating use. Report other signs such as clay-colored stools or frothy dark urine. In some instances, jaundice appears and subsequently disappears during mercaptopurine therapy; it may persist days after drug is discontinued.

Weigh patient under standard conditions once weekly and record weight.

Treatment of hyperuricemia includes:

- allopurinol (reduces or prevents hyperuricemia due to increased nucleoprotein breakdown). (Mercaptopurine dosage will be decreased by one-third or one-fourth of usual dosage.)
- increased hydration (10 to 12 glasses of fluid daily). Consult physician about desirable volume, particularly if patient is receiving IV infusions.
- urine alkinization, e.g., with acetazolamide change in intake–output ratio that could suggest renal insufficiency.

Consult physician about plans for disclosure of diagnosis, prognosis, and particulars about treatment so that discussions with family and patient will be supportive and nonconflicting.

Store tablets in light- and air-resistant container.

Drug Interactions. **Allopurinol** retards metabolism of mercaptopurine and therefore enhances antineoplastic activity and toxicity. Hypoprothrombinemic effect of **oral anticoagulants** may be reduced; monitor patient more closely when mercaptopurine is introduced or stopped. Mercaptopurine may reverse neuromuscular blocking effects of nondepolarizing muscle relaxants e.g., **tubocurarine.**

MESORIDAZINE BESYLATE

(Serentil)

(mez-oh-rid′ a-zeen)
Psychotropic
Antipsychotic
Neuroleptic
Phenothiazine

ACTIONS AND USES. Piperidine derivative of phenothiazine. Major tranquilizer with stronger sedative action than produced by chlorpromazine (qv), but has more antiemetic action and lower incidence of extrapyramidal side effects. Produces psychomotor slowing and reduces emotional stress.

Used in treatment of schizophrenia, behavioral problems in mental deficiency and chronic brain syndrome, acute and chronic alcoholism. Also used to reduce symptoms of anxiety and tension associated with many neurotic disorders.

ABSORPTION AND FATE. Well-absorbed from GI tract and from muscle. After oral administration peak blood level, reached in 2 hours, persists 4 to 6 hours; after intramuscular injection, action peaks in 30 minutes and lasts 6 to 8 hours. Elimination through kidneys and bile.

CONTRAINDICATIONS AND PRECAUTIONS. Known sensitivity to other phenothiazines; severely depressed (drug-induced) patient, comatose state, children under 12 years of age. Safe use during pregnancy, and by nursing mothers not established. *Cautious Use:* previously detected cancer of breast, glaucoma, prostatic hypertrophy, urinary retention, history of cardiovascular disease. *See also Chlorpromazine.*

ADVERSE/SIDE EFFECTS. Dizziness, sedation, fainting, blurred vision, xerostomia, nasal congestion, urinary retention, constipation, decreased sweating, contact dermatitis, tachycardia, orthostatic hypotension. *See also Chlorpromazine.*

ROUTE AND DOSAGE. Oral: Adult and children (over 12 years of age): 10 to 50 mg two or three times daily with dose adjustments as needed and tolerated up to maximum: 400 mg/day. **Intramuscular: Adult and children (over 12 years of age):** initial: 25 mg. Dose may be repeated in 30 to 60 minutes if necessary. Usual optimal dosage range: 25 to 200 mg/day. Oral concentrate: 25 mg/ml. **Elderly, debilitated:** usually lower initial dose required; subsequent increases as needed and tolerated.

M

NURSING IMPLICATIONS

Just before administration, dilute oral concentrate in about ½ glass (120 ml) of fluid. Suggested diluents: fruit juices, water, soup, carbonated beverage. Measure drug with calibrated dispenser included in original package. Explain use of dispenser and dose to patient. No change in the regimen should be made unless prescribed.

Caution patient to avoid spilling drug on skin since it may cause contact dermatitis. Thoroughly rinse off with water if spilling occurs.

Inject IM solution slowly and deeply into upper outer quadrant of buttock. Advise patient to lie still for 20 to 30 minutes after the injection to minimize possible dizziness.

Monitor intake–output and bowel elimination patterns and check bladder for distention. The depressed patient often fails to report urinary discomfort or constipation.

Upon discharge, patient should be told what laxative may be used if necessary.

Alcohol should be avoided during mesoridazine therapy.

Warn patient to consult physician before self-dosing with any OTC drug.

Xerostomia discomfort should be attended to, since deprivation of saliva fosters tissue erosion and demineralization of tooth surfaces. Frequent warm water rinses and, if there is salivary response, sugarfree gum or candy may be helpful. Avoid commercial mouth rinses to prevent disturbance of normal oral flora.

If patient complains of blurred vision, report to physician. Periodic ophthalmic examinations are advisable if patient is on long-term therapy with a phenothiazine.

Because of possible dizziness and drowsiness during early period of therapy, advise patient not to drive a car or engage in any activity that requires mental coordination and physical skill until drug response is known.

Drowsiness usually decreases with continued therapy. If it persists and interferes with ADL, consult physician. A change in time of administration or dose may help to prevent interference with normal physical activities.

Slight yellowing of the solution will not change potency; however, darkened solution should be discarded.

Protect solution from light and freezing. Store below 25°C (77°F); refrigeration is not necessary.

See also Chlorpromazine (prototype antipsychotic).

METAPROTERENOL SULFATE

(Alupent, Metaprel)

(met-a-proe-ter′e-nole)

Adrenergic agonist (beta$_2$)
Smooth muscle relaxant (respiratory)
Bronchodilator
Tocolytic

M

ACTIONS AND USES. Potent synthetic sympathomimetic amine similar to isoproterenol in chemical structure and pharmacologic actions. Acts selectively on β_2-adrenergic receptors to relax smooth muscle of bronchi, uterus, and blood vessels supplying skeletal muscles. Reportedly has less stimulant action on β_1 receptors of heart than does isoproterenol.

Used as bronchodilator in symptomatic relief of asthma and reversible bronchospasm associated with bronchitis and emphysema. *Investigational Use:* treatment and prophylaxis of heart block, and to avert progress of premature labor (tocolytic action).

ABSORPTION AND FATE. Only 40% reaches general circulation after oral administration, due to metabolism in liver. Onset of action within 15 minutes after oral ingestion and within 1 minute following inhalation. Peak effects within 1 hour by either route; effects may persist 4 hours or more after single oral dose and 1 to 5 hours after inhalation. Excreted primarily as glucuronic acid and conjugates.

CONTRAINDICATIONS AND PRECAUTIONS. Sensitivity to other sympathomimetic agents; cardiac arrhythmias associated with tachycardia, hypertension, hyperthroidism. Safe use during pregnancy, nursing mothers, and in women of childbearing potential, and children under 12 years of age (for aerosol use) and under 6 years (for oral use) not established. *Cautious Use:* the elderly. *See Isoproterenol.*

ADVERSE/SIDE EFFECTS. Nervousness, weakness, drowsiness, tremor (particularly after oral administration), tachycardia, hypertension, palpitation, nausea, vomiting, bad taste, occasional difficulty in micturition and muscle cramps, cardiac arrest (excessive use). *See Isoproterenol.*

ROUTE AND DOSAGE. Oral: Adults and children (over 9 years): 20 mg every 6 to 8 hours. **Children (6 to 9 years):** 10 mg every 6 to 8 hours. **Inhalation (metered aerosol): Adults:** 2 or 3 inhalations; usually not repeated more often than every 3 or 4 hours. Total daily dosage should not exceed 12 inhalations (each metered dose from inhaler delivers 0.65 mg of metaproterenol).

NURSING IMPLICATIONS

To administer metered aerosol dose: Instruct patient to shake container, exhale through nose as completely as possible, administer aerosol while inhaling deeply through mouth, and hold breath about 10 seconds before exhaling slowly. At least 2 minutes should elapse between inhalations.

Drug may have shorter duration of action after long-term use. Instruct patients to report failure to respond to usual dose.

Warn patients not to increase dose or frequency unless ordered by physician; there is the possibility of serious adverse effects.

Protect from light and heat. Store preferably between 15 and 30°C (59 and 86°F) unless otherwise directed by manufacturer.

See Isoproterenol for additional nursing implications regarding aerosol therapy.

Drug Interactions. Concurrent use of propranolol and possibly other beta-adrenergic blockers may antagonize the bronchodilating effects of metaproterenol.

METARAMINOL BITARTRATE

(Aramine)

(met-a-ram'i-nole)
Adrenergic agonist
(Sympathomimetic)

ACTIONS AND USES. Potent synthetic sympathomimetic amine. Overall effects similar to those of norepinephrine; but metaraminol is not as potent, has more gradual onset and longer duration of action, and usually lacks CNS stimulant effects. Acts directly on α-adrenergic receptors (vasoconstriction) and also directly stimulates β_1 receptors of heart (positive inotropic effect); indirectly causes release of norepinephrine from storage sites. Tachyphylaxis may occur with prolonged use by depletion of epinephrine stores in nerve endings; in addition, metaraminol may function as weak or false neurotransmitter by replacing norepinephrine in sympathetic nerve endings, with resultant worsening of shock state. Vasoconstrictor action increases pulmonary arterial pressure, produces sustained rise in systolic and diastolic pressures, and reduces blood flow to kidneys and other vital organs and probably skin and skeletal muscles.

Used for prevention and treatment of acute hypotensive states occurring with spinal anesthesia, and as adjunct in treatment of hypotension due to hemorrhage, reaction to medication, surgical complications, brain damage, cardiogenic shock, and septicemia. *Investigational Use:* provocative test for diagnosis of familial Mediterranean fever, and to increase cardiac output in pericardial tamponade.

ABSORPTION AND FATE. Onset of pressor effect occurs within 1 to 2 minutes after start of IV infusion, within 10 minutes after IM injection, and in 5 to 20 minutes after administration. Effects last 20 to 90 minutes, depending on route of administration. Drug effects appear to be terminated primarily by uptake into tissues and urinary excretion.

CONTRAINDICATIONS AND PRECAUTIONS. Use with cyclopropane, halothane, within 14 days of MAO inhibitor therapy; peripheral or mesenteric thrombosis; pulmonary edema, cardiac arrest; untreated hypoxia, hypercapnia, and acidosis; as sole therapy in hypovolemia. Safe use during pregnancy not established. *Cautious Use:* digitalized patients, hypertension, thyroid disease, diabetes mellitus, cirrhosis of liver, history of malaria (may produce relapse).

ADVERSE/SIDE EFFECTS. Apprehension, restlessness, headache, tremor, nausea, vomiting, weakness, flushing, pallor, sweating, precordial pain, palpitation, tachycardia, bradycardia, decreased urinary output, metabolic acidosis (hypovolemic patients), hyperglycemia. **Excessive dosage:** severe hypertension, headache, convulsions, acute pulmonary edema, arrhythmias, cardiac arrest. Injection site reactions (especially following SC): abscess formation, tissue necrosis, sloughing. **Prolonged use:** plasma volume depletion with recurrence of shock state.

ROUTE AND DOSAGE. Adults: Subcutaneous, intramuscular: 2 to 10 mg. At least 10 minutes should elapse before additional dose is given, to prevent cumulative effect. **Intravenous (direct):** *for grave emergency:* 0.5 to 5 mg (followed by IV infusion). **Intravenous infusion:** 15 to 100 mg in 500 ml of 5% dextrose injection or sodium chloride injection. **Children: Subcutaneous, intramuscular:** 0.1 mg/kg. **Intravenous (direct):** 0.01 mg/kg. **Intravenous infusion:** 0.4 mg/kg (each 1 mg diluted in 25 ml of 5% dextrose or sodium chloride injection).

NURSING IMPLICATIONS

Except in emergency situations, blood volume should be corrected as fully as possible before therapy is initiated.

Subcutaneous injection is especially likely to cause tissue necrosis and sloughing; therefore, it is generally not prescribed particularly in shock therapy (poor circulation).

Patients receiving drug IV must be constantly attended, with infusion flow rate being closely monitored. Changes in flow rate must be made cautiously, since the drug has cumulative effect and prolonged action.

Intravenous flow rate will be prescribed by physician (usually, systolic blood pressure is maintained at 80 to 100 mm Hg for previously normotensive patients; for previously hypertensive patients, it is maintained at 30 to 40 mm Hg below the usual pressure).

During IV infusion, check blood pressure every 5 minutes until it is stabilized at prescribed level, then every 15 minutes thereafter throughout therapy. Also note pulse rate and quality. Continue monitoring at regular intervals for several hours after infusion is complete.

When infusion is to be discontinued, flow rate should be reduced gradually, and abrupt withdrawal avoided. Equipment for reinstituting therapy should be immediately available.

Care should be taken to avoid extravasation during IV infusion. Injury to local tissue and necrosis may result. *See Index: Nursing Interventions: extravasation.*

Have on hand phentolamine (may be used to decrease pressor effects), propranolol (to treat cardiac arrhythmias), atropine (for bradycardia).

Observe intake–output ratio and pattern. Keep physician informed of renal response. Urinary output may decrease initially, then increase as blood pressure approaches normal levels. With excessive dosage, output may again decrease.

Metaraminol may cause diuresis in patients with cirrhosis of liver. Patients should be carefully monitored for excessive losses of water, sodium, and potassium.

Patients with diabetes should be closely monitored for loss of diabetes control.

Avoid exposure of drug to excessive heat, and protect it from light.

Drug Interactions. There may be an enhanced pressor response to metaraminol in patients receiving (parenteral) **ergot alkaloids, furazolidone, guanethidine, MAO inhibitors,** or **tricyclic antidepressants.** Concurrent use of these drugs generally avoided. **Digitalis glycosides** may sensitize myocardium to the effects of metaraminol. Response to metaraminol may be altered by **reserpine** (based on limited studies). IV administration of metaraminol during use of

cyclopropane or **halothane** or related general anesthetics may lead to serious ventricular arrhythmias.

METHACYCLINE HYDROCHLORIDE

(Rondomycin)

(meth-a-sye'kleen)
Antiinfective
Antibiotic
Tetracycline

ACTIONS AND USES. Synthetic broad-spectrum antibiotic derived from oxytetracycline. Similar to tetracycline (qv) in actions, uses, contraindications, precautions, and adverse side effects.

ABSORPTION AND FATE. Readily but incompletely absorbed; bound to plasma proteins to variable degree. Half-life: 16 hours. About 50% excreted unchanged in urine and about 5% in feces over 72 hours.

ROUTE AND DOSAGE. Oral: Adults: 150 mg every 6 hours or 300 mg every 12 hours. **Children (8 years or older):** 6 to 12 mg/kg daily divided into two or four equally spaced doses. *Syphilis* (when penicillin is contraindicated): 18 to 24 gm in equally divided doses over period of 10 to 15 days. *Eaton Agent (PPLO) pneumonia:* 900 mg/day for 6 days.

NURSING IMPLICATIONS

Check expiration date before administration. Outdated tetracyclines can cause serious reactions.

Food–Drug Interaction: Food and selected minerals interfere with absorption. Administer methacycline at least 1 hour before or 2 hours following meals. Do not give with milk or with antacids containing aluminum, calcium, or magnesium.

Therapy should be continued for at least 24 to 48 hours after symptoms and fever have subsided.

Preserved in tight, light-resistant containers preferably between 15° and 30°C (59° and 86°F) unless otherwise directed by manufacturer.

See Tetracycline (prototype tetracycline).

METHADONE HYDROCHLORIDE

(Dolophine)

(meth'a-done)
Narcotic analgesic
Opiate agonist
C II

ACTIONS AND USES. Synthetic diphenylheptane derivative with pharmacologic properties qualitatively similar to those of morphine (qv), but is orally effective and has longer duration of action. A single oral dose produces less sedation and euphoria than does morphine, but repeated doses produce marked sedation (cumulative action). Causes less constipation than morphine, but respiratory depressant effect (principal danger of overdosage) and antitussive actions are comparable. Highly addictive, with abuse potential that matches that of morphine; abstinence syndrome develops more slowly; withdrawal symptoms are less intense, but more prolonged.

Used to relieve severe pain; used for detoxification and temporary maintenance treatment in hospital. Also used in federally controlled maintenance programs for ambulatory patients with narcotic abstinence syndrome.

ABSORPTION AND FATE. Well absorbed from GI tract. Following single oral dose, onset of action in 30 to 60 minutes, with duration of 6 to 8 hours; following parenteral administration: onset of action in 10 to 20 minutes, and peak effects in 1 to 2 hours. Duration of action (cumulative effect): 22 to 48 hours. Widely distributed to tissues; about 85% firmly bound to plasma proteins. Half-life: 15 to 25 hours. Metabolized chiefly in liver. Metabolites excreted primarily in urine; less than 10% excreted unchanged in urine. Crosses placenta and enters breast milk.

CONTRAINDICATIONS AND PRECAUTIONS. Obstetric analgesia. Safe use during pregnancy, in nursing mothers, and for treatment of narcotic addiction in patients under 18 years not established. *Cautious Use:* hepatic, renal, or cardiac dysfunction. *See also Morphine.*

ADVERSE/SIDE EFFECTS. Drowsiness, nausea, vomiting, dry mouth, constipation, lightheadedness, dizziness, transient fall in blood pressure, bone and muscle pain, hallucinations, impotence. *See also Morphine.*

ROUTE AND DOSAGE. Oral, subcutaneous, intramuscular: *Analgesic:* **Adults:** 2.5 to 10 mg; repeated, if necessary, every 3 to 4 hours. Parenteral doses larger than 10 mg not recommended. *Detoxification treatment:* 15 to 40 mg; once daily; highly individualized and adjusted to keep withdrawal symptoms at a tolerable level. *Maintenance treatment:* 20 to 120 mg daily; highly individualized. Special state and federal approval required for doses in excess of 120 mg daily, and for use in patients under 18 years of age.

NURSING IMPLICATIONS

M

For analgesic effect, methadone should be administered in the smallest effective dose to minimize the possibility of tolerance and physical and psychic dependence.

IM route is preferred when repeated parenteral administration is required (SC injections may cause local irritation and induration). Aspirate carefully before injecting drug to avoid inadvertent IV administration. Rotate injection sites.

Evaluate the patient's continued need for methadone for pain. With repeated use (and because of cumulative effects), adjustment of dosage and lengthening of between-dose intervals may be possible.

Orthostatic hypotension, sweating, constipation, drowsiness, GI symptoms, and other transient side effects of therapeutic doses appear to be more prominent in ambulatory patients. Most side effects disappear over a period of several weeks.

Instruct patients to make position changes slowly, particularly from recumbent to upright position, and to sit or lie down if they feel dizzy or faint.

Patients should be informed that methadone may impair mental and physical abilities required for performance of potentially hazardous activities, such as driving a car or operating machinery.

Principal danger of overdosage, as with morphine, is extreme respiratory depression.

Due to the cumulative effects of methadone, *abstinence symptoms* may not appear for 36 to 72 hours after last dose and may last 10 to 14 days. Symptoms are usually of mild intensity (anorexia, insomnia, anxiety, abdominal discomfort, weakness, headache, sweating, hot and cold flashes). Purposive behavior is prominent by the sixth day.

In detoxification treatment, methadone is administered in decreasing doses (oral formulation is preferred) over a period not exceeding 21 days, to suppress abstinence symptoms during narcotic withdrawal. If more than 21 days of treatment are required, patient is said to be on maintenance.

Narcotic antagonists such a naloxone, naltrexone, and levallorphan terminate methadone intoxication by competing for narcotic binding sites. Since antagonist action is shorter (1 to 3 hours) than that of methadone (36 to 48 hours or more), repeated doses for 8 to 24 hours may be required. Patient should be watched closely for recurrence of respiratory depression.

Methadone maintenance program consists of substituting stable doses of oral methadone to eliminate compulsive craving and euphoric effects of parenterally administered narcotics.

Treatment frequently begins with daily doses at an ambulatory clinic. Later, take-home doses of methadone may be dispensed as oral liquid (dissolved in juice to discourage parenteral injection).

Since opiate dependence is symptomatic of a wide variety of individual and social problems, methadone maintenance programs usually include coordinated psychiatric, social, and vocational rehabilitation services.

Methadone is classified as a Schedule II drug under Federal Controlled Substances Act. Also subject to strict regulations by Food and Drug Administration and state authorities; use for treatment of narcotic addiction is restricted to approved local programs.

Preserved in tight, light-resistant containers at room temperature (betweem 59° and 86°F) unless otherwise directed by manufacturer.

See Morphine Sulfate.

Drug Interactions. Methadone is used with caution and in reduced dosage in patients concurrently receiving other **CNS depressants** (including **alcohol**), and cimetidine (Tagamet). Patients addicted to heroin or those who are on methadone maintenance may experience withdrawal symptoms when given barbiturates, **pentazocine,** phenytoin (Dilantin) and other hydantoins, **rifampin,** urinary acidifiers e.g., ammonium chloride.

M

METHAMPHETAMINE HYDROCHLORIDE

(Desoxyephedrine Hydrochloride, Desoxyn, Methampex)

(meth-am-fet'a-meen)
Central stimulant
(Sympathomimetic)
Anorexogenic
Amphetamine
C II

ACTIONS AND USES. Sympathomimetic amine chemically related to amphetamine and ephedrine. CNS stimulant actions (mood elevation, depression of appetite, decreased fatigue) approximately equal to those of amphetamine, but accompanied by less peripheral activity. However, larger doses produce increased cardiac output, possibly reflex slowing of heart rate, and sustained increase in blood pressure, chiefly by cardiac stimulation. Excessive doses depress myocardium. *See also Amphetamine Sulfate.*

Used as short-term adjunct in management of exogenous obesity, as adjunctive therapy in attention deficit disorders, narcolepsy, epilepsy, and postencephalitic parkinsonism, and in treatment of certain depressive reactions, especially when characterized by apathy and psychomotor retardation.

ABSORPTION AND FATE. Readily absorbed from GI tract; duration of effects 6 to 12 hours, but may continue up to 24 hours after large oral doses. From 55 to 70% of dose excreted unchanged in urine; 6 to 7% eliminated as amphetamine. Excretion is markedly increased in acid urine.

CONTRAINDICATIONS AND PRECAUTIONS. During pregnancy, especially first trimester; use as anorexiant in children under age 12; patients receiving MAO inhibitors; arteriosclerotic parkinsonism. *Cautious Use:* mild hypertension; psychopathic personalities; hyperexcitability states; history of suicide; elderly or debilitated patients. *See also Amphetamine Sulfate.*

ADVERSE/SIDE EFFECTS. CNS (stimulation): restlessness, tremor, hyperreflexia, insomnia, headache, nervousness, anxiety, dizziness, euphoria or dysphoria. **CV:** palpitation, arrhythmias, hypertension, hypotension, circulatory collapse. **GI:** dry mouth, unpleasant taste, nausea, vomiting, diarrhea, constipation. **Other:** psychotic episodes (rare), depression. *See also Amphetamine Sulfate.*

ROUTE AND DOSAGE. Oral: Adults: 2.5 to 5 mg one to three times daily. Long-acting form: 10 to 15 mg once a day in the morning. Usual dose range: 2.5 to 30 mg daily. **Children:** attention deficit disorders: Initial: 2.5 to 5 mg once or twice daily; may be increased by 5 mg increments weekly until optimum response achieved. Usual effective dose: 20 to 25 mg daily. *Obesity:* **Adults and children over 12 years:** 5 mg thirty minutes before each meal.

NURSING IMPLICATIONS

If possible, medication should be taken early in the day to avoid insomnia.

When used for treatment of obesity, drug is administered 30 minutes before each meal. If insomnia results, advise patient to inform physician.

Duration of methamphetamine use in treatment of obesity should not exceed a few weeks.

Paradoxic increase in depression or agitation sometimes occurs in depressed patients. Report immediately; drug should be withdrawn.

Tolerance develops readily, and prolonged use may lead to drug dependence. High abuse potential. Commonly known as "speed" or "crystal" among drug abusers.

Withdrawal after prolonged use is frequently followed by lethargy that may persist several weeks.

Classified as Schedule II drug under Federal Controlled Substances Act.

Preserved in tight, light-resistant containers.

See Amphetamine sulfate (prototype amphetamine).

METHANDRIOL

(meth-an′dree-ole)
Anabolic

(Anabol, Andriol, Cellubolic, Durabolic, Methabolic, Methydiol, Steribolic)

ACTIONS AND USES. Synthetic steroid closely related to testosterone; has stronger anabolic than androgenic activity; however, androgenic effects cannot be dissociated, especially when used in children. Promotes body tissue building processes; reverses catabolic or tissue depleting processes. Can decrease bone resorption in patient with osteoporosis and improve calcium balance.

Used as a "possibly effective" adjunctive agent in treatment of senile and postmenopausal osteoporosis, and in children for treatment of delayed puberty. *See Ethylestrenol for absorption, fate, limitations, contraindications, and adverse/side effects.*

ROUTE AND DOSAGE. Intramuscular: Adult: 10 to 40 mg daily or 50 to 100 mg once or twice weekly. **Children:** 5 to 10 mg daily or less frequently, until susceptibility to androgenic effects has been ruled out.

NURSING IMPLICATIONS

If used for children, observe for androgenic effects: prepubic hair development, phallic enlargement, increased frequency of erections in boys, and clitoral enlargement in girls. Report these signs; dosage regimen will need to be reviewed.

Anabolic steroids should be used very carefully in children who are small but otherwise healthy and normal. Rate of skeletal maturation may exceed linear growth rate, producing premature epiphyseal closure.

Anabolic steroid therapy for delayed puberty requires careful evaluation by the physician and the complete understanding of parents.

The younger the child the greater the risk for compromising future mature height. Usually anabolic therapy in the young child is undertaken as a last resort.

Urge parent to keep appointments for x-ray analysis of bone growth of the child during methandriol therapy.

Anabolic steroids do not enhance athletic ability. Their use for this purpose is hazardous and has been condemned by medical experts.

See Ethylestrenol.

METHANTHELINE BROMIDE

(Banthine)

(meth-an'tha-leen)
Anticholinergic
(Parasympatholytic)
Antispasmodic

M

ACTIONS AND USES. Synthetic quaternary ammonium compound chemically related to propantheline. Peripheral effects, contraindications, precautions, and adverse reactions similar to those of atropine (qv). Differs from atropine in having a greater ratio of ganglionic blocking activity to antimuscarinic activity.

Used as adjunct in management of peptic ulcer, pylorospasm, spastic colon, pancreatitis, ureteral and bladder spasms, excessive sweating, urinary frequency.

ABSORPTION AND FATE. Onset of effects in 30 to 45 minutes, persisting 4 to 6 hours after oral administration. Excreted through all body fluids, but chiefly through urine and bile.

CONTRAINDICATIONS AND PRECAUTIONS. Hypersensitivity to methantheline or propantheline. Safe use during pregnancy (category c) and lactation not established. *Cautious Use:* prostatic hypertrophy, coronary heart disease, hypertension. *See Atropine.*

ADVERSE/SIDE EFFECTS. Urinary retention, anhidrosis, dry mouth, constipation, mydriasis, blurred vision, dizziness, drowsiness, impotence, flushing, postural hypotension, tachycardia, palpitation, respiratory paralysis (large doses). *See also Atropine.*

ROUTE AND DOSAGE. Oral: **Adults:** 50 to 100 mg four times daily at 6-hour intervals; maintenance generally one-half initial dose. **Children (over 1 year):** 12.5 to 50 mg four times daily; **(under 1 year):** 12.5 mg two to four times daily.

NURSING IMPLICATIONS

Generally administered about 10 minutes before meals or with meals and at bedtime. Advise patient not to chew tablet as it is extremely bitter.

Urinary retention may be avoided by having patient void just prior to each dose.

Patients receiving parenteral therapy should be observed closely for curarelike effect on skeletal muscles, particularly respiratory depression or paralysis. Equipment for artificial respiration should be readily available.

Restlessness, euphoria, fatigue, and occasionally acute psychotic episodes occur in some patients.

Advise patient to report appearance of skin rash to physician.

Increase in fluid intake (if allowed) may help to prevent constipation.

Sugarless hard candy or gum, frequent rinsing mouth with warm water, and mouth care after meals may help to relieve mouth dryness.

See Atropine sulfate (prototype anticholinergic).

METHARBITAL

(Gemonil, Metharbitone)

(meth ar'bi tal)
Anticonvulsant
Barbiturate
C III

ACTIONS AND USES. Long-acting barbiturate derivative with greater sedative effect and less anticonvulsant activity than phenobarbital. Actions, contraindications, precautions, and uses as for phenobarbital (qv).

Used alone or in combination with other anticonvulsants for control of grand mal, petit mal, myoclonic, and mixed-type seizures.

ABSORPTION AND FATE. Onset of action in 2 to 4 hours; duration 6 to 12 hours. Demethylated in liver to barbital, which is then excreted in urine; less than 2% of dose is excreted unchanged.

ADVERSE/SIDE EFFECTS. Usually infrequent and mild: drowsiness, dizziness, increased irritability, skin rash, gastric distress. *See Phenobarbital.*

ROUTE AND DOSAGE. Oral: Adults: Initial: 100 mg one to three times daily; gradually increased to level required to control seizures; dose range 100 to 800 mg daily. **Children:** 5 to 15 mg/kg/day.

NURSING IMPLICATIONS

Not to be confused with mephobarbital.

Abrupt discontinuation of drug in patients taking regular daily doses may precipitate status epilepticus.

Classified as Schedule III drug under Federal Controlled Substances Act of 1970.

See Phenobarbital (prototype barbiturate).

METHAZOLAMIDE

(Neptazane)

(meth-a-zoe'la-mide)
Carbonic anhydrase inhibitor
Sulfonamide derivative

ACTIONS AND USES. Nonbactericidal sulfonamide derivative similar to acetazolamide, but with slower onset and longer duration of action. Appears to cause more drowsiness and fatigue than does acetazolamide, and has less diuretic activity. Actions, contraindications, precautions, and adverse reactions as for acetazolamide (qv).

Used as adjunctive treatment in chronic simple (open-angle) glaucoma and secondary glaucoma and preoperatively in acute-angle-closure glaucoma when delay of surgery is desired in order to lower intraocular pressure. May be used concomitantly with miotic and osmotic agents.

ABSORPTION AND FATE. Intraocular pressure begins to fall within 2 to 4 hours, with peak effect in 6 to 8 hours, duration of action 10 to 18 hours. Distributed in plasma, erythrocytes, aqueous humor, extracellular and cerebrospinal fluids, and bile. Partially metabolized in liver. About 20 to 30% of dose is excreted in urine as active substance; fate of remainder not known. Crosses placenta.

CONTRAINDICATIONS AND PRECAUTIONS. Glaucoma due to severe peripheral anterior synechiae, severe or absolute glaucoma, hemorrhagic glaucoma, hypokalemia, hyponatremia. *See also Acetazolamide.*

ADVERSE/SIDE EFFECTS. Malaise, drowsiness, fatigue, lethargy, mild GI disturbance, anorexia, headache, vertigo, paresthesias, mental confusion, depression. *See also Acetazolamide.*

ROUTE AND DOSAGE. **Oral:** 50 to 100 mg every 8 hours.

NURSING IMPLICATIONS

See Acetazolamide (prototype carbonic anhydrase inhibitor).

M

METHDILAZINE HYDROCHLORIDE

(Dilosyn, Tacaryl)

(meth-dill'a-zeen)
Antipruritic
Antihistamine
H_1-receptor antagonist
Phenothiazine derivative

ACTIONS AND USES. Phenothiazine derivative antihistamine with antipruritic activity and prominent sedative and anticholinergic (drying) side effects similar to promethazine (qv) in pharmacologic properties.

Used for symptomatic relief of pruritic symptoms in urticaria.

CONTRAINDICATIONS AND PRECAUTIONS. Acute asthmatic attack, comatose states, bone marrow depression, jaundice, nursing mothers. Safe use during pregnancy not established. *Cautious Use:* narrow-angle glaucoma, prostatic hypertrophy, GI or GU obstructions, within 14 days of MAOI therapy, children, elderly patients, acute or chronic respiratory impairment, cardiovascular disease, impaired liver function, history of ulcer disease.

ADVERSE/SIDE EFFECTS. Drowsiness, dizziness, lassitude, tinnitus, incoordination, nausea, excitation (in children); hypotension, syncope, confusion, excessive sedation (elderly patients); dry mouth and throat, urinary frequency, urinary retention, dysuria, nasal stuffiness, suppression of cough reflect, thickening of bronchial secretions. Shares toxic potential of other phenothiazines. *See Promethazine Hydrochloride.*

ROUTE AND DOSAGE. **Oral:** **Adults:** 8 mg two to four times daily. **Children (over 3 years):** 4 mg two to four times daily. Available as tablet, chewable tablet, syrup.

NURSING IMPLICATIONS

Chewable tablets should be thoroughly chewed and swallowed promptly. They should not be swallowed whole.

Inform patient that methdilazine will potentiate or prolong the sedative actions of alcohol, barbiturates, and narcotics.

Since methdilazine has an antiemetic effect, bear in mind that it may mask drug or disease-induced nausea and vomiting.

Caution patient to avoid driving and other potentially hazardous activities until reaction to drug is known.

Instruct elderly patients particularly to make position changes slowly from recumbent to upright posture and to dangle and move feet and ankles for a few minutes before ambulating.

Methdilazine should be discontinued about 4 days before skin testing procedures for allergy are performed because of false-negative reactions.

Stored in light-resistant containers.

See Promethazine hydrochloride (prototype antipruritic agent).

METHENAMINE HIPPURATE

(meth en'a-meen hip'yoo-rate)

(Hip-Rex, Urex)

Antiinfective (urinary tract)

ACTIONS AND USES. Chemical combination of methenamine (44%) and hippuric acid (56%). Antibacterial action depends on formaldehyde, which is liberated from methenamine in acidic urine; hippuric acid contributes to urinary acidification and also provides weak antibacterial action. *See Methenamine Mandelate for actions, uses, contraindications, precautions, and adverse effects.*

ABSORPTION AND FATE. Over 90% of single dose is excreted in urine within 24 hours. *See Methenamine mandelate.*

ROUTE AND DOSAGE. **Oral:** **Adults and children (over 12 years):** 1 Gm twice daily (morning and night). **Children (6 to 12 years):** 0.5 to 1 Gm twice daily (morning and night).

NURSING IMPLICATIONS

Elevated serum transaminase levels have been reported; therefore periodic liver function studies are recommended.

See Methenamine mandelate.

METHENAMINE MANDELATE

(meth-en'a-meen man'de-late)

(Mandelamine, Sterine)

Antiinfective (urinary tract)
Acidifier (urinary)

ACTIONS AND USES. Chemical combination of methenamine (48%) and mandelic acid (52%). Antibacterial action depends on liberation of formaldehyde from methenamine in acidic (pH 5.5 or less) urine. Mandelic acid contributes to urine acidification and also provides weak antibacterial action. Active against a variety of gram-negative and gram-positive organisms, including *Escherichia coli, Staphylococcus aureus, S. albus,* and certain streptococci. Drug activity diminishes in infections caused by urea-splitting organisms such as *Pseudomonas* and *Proteus,* since they raise urinary pH.

Used for prophylactic or suppressive treatment of bacteriuria associated with chronic urinary tract infections. Sometimes used prophylactically prior to urinary tract instrumentation and catheterization.

ABSORPTION AND FATE. Readily absorbed from GI tract. Half-life: approximately 4 hours. Rapidly excreted in urine by glomerular filtration and tubular secretion. In acidic urine, methenamine is hydrolyzed to ammonia and formaldehyde.

CONTRAINDICATIONS AND PRECAUTIONS. Impaired renal function, hepatic disease (because ammonia is produced), severe dehydration, combined therapy with sulfonamides. Safe use during pregnancy not established.

ADVERSE/SIDE EFFECTS. Stomatitis, gastric upset, abdominal discomfort, dysuria, hypersensitivity (skin rash, urticaria, pruritus), tinnitus, muscle cramps. Large doses: bladder irritation, frequent and painful urination, albuminuria, hematuria, crystalluria, generalized edema (rare).

ROUTE AND DOSAGE. Oral: **Adults and children over (12 years):** 1 Gm four times daily, after meals and at bedtime. **Children (6 to 12 years):** 0.5 Gm four times daily; **(under 6 years):** 0.25 Gm/14 kg four times daily.

NURSING IMPLICATIONS

Periodic urine culture and susceptibility tests should be performed.

Administration of drug after meals may minimize gastric distress.

Methenamine oral suspension (e.g., Mandelamine) contains a vegetable oil base and therefore should be administered with caution to elderly or debilitated patients because of the possibility of lipid (aspiration) pneumonia.

Monitor intake and output. Methenamine is reportedly most effective when fluid intake is maintained at 1500 or 2000 ml/day and urinary pH is kept at 5.5 or below; consult physician. Increased urine volume (through increased fluid intake or diuretics) and a urinary pH over 5.5 significantly decrease the formaldehyde concentration in urine, an essential for antibacterial action.

Food–Drug Interactions: Urinary pH should be monitored during methenamine therapy. Supplementary urinary acidification, if required, may be achieved by limiting intake of *alkaline-producing foods* such as vegetables, milk, peanuts, and fruits and fruit juices (except cranberry, plum, and prune, which are acid-forming) as well as by concomitant administration of acidifying drugs, e.g., ascorbic acid, ammonium chloride.

Patients should be taught to check urine pH with Nitrazine paper to ensure consistent acidification. Some physicians instruct patients to adjust urine acidity by use of prescribed acidifying drug or special diet when necessary.

Diagnostic Test Interferences. Methenamine may produce falsely elevated values for **urinary catecholamines** and **urinary steroids** (17-hydroxycorticosteroids) (by Reddy method). Possibility of false urine glucose determinations with Benedict's test. Methenamine interferes with **urobilinogen** and possibly **urinary VMA** determinations.

Drug Interactions. Drugs that alkalinize urine decrease methenamine effectiveness, e.g., **acetazolamide, sodium bicarbonate, sodium citrate, thiazide diuretics.** Formaldehyde liberated from methenamine reacts with **sulfonamides** to form insoluble precipitates in urine (crystalluria).

METHICILLIN SODIUM
(Celbenin, Staphcillin)

(meth-i-sill′in)
Antiinfective
Antibiotic (beta lactam)
Penicillin

ACTIONS AND USES. Semisynthetic salt of penicillin with antimicrobial spectrum similar to that of penicillin G (qv); differs from the latter in its high resistance to penicillinase-producing strains of staphylococci. Not as effective as penicillin G against non-penicillinase-producing staphylococci, streptococci, or pneumococci. A growing number of methicillin-resistant strains are reported to be developing.

Used primarily in infections caused by penicillinase-producing staphylococci. May be used to initiate therapy in suspected staphylococcal infections pending results of culture and sensitivity tests.

ABSORPTION AND FATE. Peak plasma concentrations within 30 minutes to 1 hour following IM injection and within 15 minutes after IV injection; serum levels decline within 4 hours after IM and within 2 hours after IV administration. Well distributed in various body tissues and fluids. Little diffusion to cerebrospinal fluid unless meninges are inflamed. About 40% bound to plasma proteins. Approximately two-thirds of 1-Gm dose is eliminated unchanged in urine in 4 hours; 20% or more excreted in feces via bile (rate of elimination is extremely slow in infants). Crosses placenta.

CONTRAINDICATIONS AND PRECAUTIONS. Hypersensitivity to penicillins or cephalosporins. IV dosage in infants and children not established. Safe use during pregnancy (category B) not established. *Cautious Use:* history of allergy, asthma; nursing women, pediatric use, impaired renal function. *See Penicillin G.*

M

ADVERSE/SIDE EFFECTS. Hypersensitivity reactions: skin rash, pruritus, urticaria, eosinophilia, serum sickness, anaphylactic reaction, acute interstitial nephritis. Also reported: bone marrow depression (anemia, neutropenia, granulocytopenia, agranulocytosis), neuropathy, interstitial nephritis, irritation at IM site, thrombophlebitis (following IV administration); oral, rectal, vaginal candidal superinfections. *See Penicillin G.*

ROUTE AND DOSAGE. Intramuscular: Adults: 1 Gm every 4 to 6 hours. **Children:** 25 mg/kg every 6 hours. **Intravenous: Adults:** 1 Gm every 6 hours (in 0.9% sodium chloride) at rate of 10 ml/minute.

NURSING IMPLICATIONS

Culture and susceptibility tests should be performed initially and periodically during therapy.

A careful history must be obtained concerning previous hypersensitivity reactions to penicillins, cephalosporins, or any other allergens.

Reportedly well tolerated by deep intragluteal injection, although it may be painful. Rotate injection sites.

Observe all injection sites for evidence of irritation or inflammation.

Periodic assessment of renal, hematopoietic, and hepatic function are advised during prolonged therapy.

Frequent blood level measurements are advised in infants, since urinary excretion of drug is slower in this age group.

Febrile reactions are reported to occur in some patients 1 to 2 hours following IV administration.

Monitor patients for signs and symptoms of *interstitial nephritis,* a hypersensitivity reaction that occurs 2 to 4 weeks following initiation of therapy: spiking fever, anorexia, skin rash, oliguria, hematuria, cloudy urine (pyuria, albuminuria), eosinophilia. Usually reversible following prompt termination of drug.

Monitor for signs and symptoms of superinfections (sore mouth, foul smelling vaginal discharge, diarrhea, anogenital itching, fever, cough).

Drug therapy is generally continued at least 48 hours, or in the case of serious systemic infections, for at least 1 to 2 weeks after patient has become afebrile and asymptomatic and cultures are negative. Treatment of osteomyelitis may require several weeks of intensive therapy.

Methicillin is reconstituted with sterile water for injection or sodium chloride injection. Shake vial vigorously before withdrawing contents.

Reconstituted methicillin solutions are stable for 24 hours at room temperature (59° to 86°F) and for 4 days under refrigeration (36° to 46°F). Solutions gradually darken to a deep orange color and acquire a distinctive hydrogen sulfide odor upon standing for prolonged periods at room temperature. Discard such solutions.

Methicillin is reported to be incompatible with many drugs including other antibiotics. Use only solutions recommended by manufacturer.

See also Penicillin G (prototype penicillin).

Drug Interactions: Pharmacologic and toxic effects of **digitalis glycosides** may be increased; hypoprothrombinemic effects of **oral anticoagulants** may be reduced.

METHIMAZOLE

(Tapazole)

(meth-im'a-zole)

Antithyroid agent

M

ACTIONS AND USES. Thioamide with actions and uses similar to those of propylthiouracil (qv), but 10 times as potent. Actions are less consistent, but effects appear more promptly than those of propylthiouracil. *For contraindications, and adverse side effects, see Propylthiouracil.*

Used to treat hyperthyroidism in pregnancy, adjunctively with thyroid to prevent hypothyroidism in fetus and mother, and prior to surgery or radiotherapy of the thyroid.

ABSORPTION AND FATE. Onset of action in 30 to 40 minutes; duration 2 to 4 hours. Plasma half-life: 1 to 2 hours. *See also Propylthiouracil.*

ROUTE AND DOSAGE. Oral: Adults: Initial: 15 to 60 mg daily every 8 hours; maintenance 5 to 15 mg daily. **Children:** Initial: 0.4 mg/kg body weight daily divided into 3 doses and given at 8-hour intervals; maintenance approximately half initial dose.

NURSING IMPLICATIONS

Take medication at same time each day relative to meals.

Instruct patient to adhere to established dosage regimen, i.e., not to double, decrease, or omit doses and not to alter the interval between doses.

Dosage may be suspended about 2 weeks before anticipated delivery and restored in postpartum period if required.

Skin rash or swelling of cervical lymph nodes indicates need to discontinue drug and change to another antithyroid agent.

Notify physician promptly if the following symptoms appear: bruising, unexplained bleeding, sore throat, fever, jaundice.

Advise patient who has had drug-induced jaundice that it may persist up to 10 weeks after withdrawal of methimazole.
Methimazole does not induce hypothyroidism.
Store drug in light-resistant container at temperature between 15° and 30°C (59° and 86°F).
See also Propylthiouracil (prototype antithyroid agent).

METHOCARBAMOL

(Delaxin, Marbaxin-750, Metho-500, Robaxin)

(meth-oh-kar'ba-mole)
Skeletal muscle relaxant
(Centrally acting)

ACTIONS AND USES. Propanediol-derivative monocarbamate with actions similar to those of carisoprodol, but it produces higher plasma levels more rapidly and for longer periods. Exerts skeletal muscle relaxant action by depressing multisynaptic pathways in spinal cord and possibly by sedative effect. Has no direct action on skeletal muscles.

Used as adjunct to physical therapy and other measures in management of discomfort associated with acute musculoskeletal disorders. Also used intravenously as adjunct in management of neuromuscular manifestations of tetanus.

ABSORPTION AND FATE. Rapidly absorbed following oral administration. Onset of action: 30 minutes with peak plasma concentrations after about 2 hours. Muscle relaxant effects usually apparent within 10 minutes after IV injection. Metabolized in liver. Half-life: 1 to 2 hours. Excreted in urine.

M

CONTRAINDICATIONS AND PRECAUTIONS. Hypersensitivity to any of the ingredients; comatose states, CNS depression, acidosis, renal dysfunction (injectable methocarbamol contains polyethylene glycol 300 in vehicle, which may cause urea retention and acidotic problems). Safe use during pregnancy and lactation and in women of childbearing potential and children under age 12 (except for tetanus) not established. *Cautious Use:* epilepsy.

ADVERSE/SIDE EFFECTS. Allergic manifestations (parenteral or oral use): urticaria, pruritus, rash, conjunctivitis, nasal congestion, headache, blurred vision, fever, anaphylactic reaction. **Oral use:** drowsiness, dizziness, lightheadedness, syncope (rare), headache, nausea. **Parenteral use:** thrombophlebitis, pain, sloughing (with extravasation), flushing, metallic taste, syncope, hypotension, bradycardia, convulsions. **Other:** slight reduction of white cell count with prolonged therapy.

ROUTE AND DOSAGE. Adults: Oral: Initial: 1.5 Gm four times daily; maintenance 1 Gm four times daily, or 750 mg every 4 hours, or 1.5 Gm three times daily. **Intramuscular:** 0.5 to 1 Gm (5 to 10 ml) repeated at 8-hour intervals, if necessary. **Intravenous:** 1 to 3 Gm daily. Maximum rate (direct): IV is 300 mg (3 ml) per minute. *Intravenous infusion:* 1 Gm diluted to not more than 250 ml with sodium chloride injection or 5% dextrose injection. Parenteral doses not to exceed 3 Gm/day or to be given for more than 3 consecutive days, except in treatment of tetanus. *Tetanus:* **Adults:** Initial: 1 to 2 Gm (10 to 20 ml) administered directly into IV tubing; up to 3 Gm may be given. May be repeated every 6 hours until nasogastric tube insertion is possible. **Via nasogastric tube:** total daily dose up to 24 Gm (tablets should be crushed and suspended in water or saline). **Children:** Initial: 15 mg/kg repeated every 6 hours as indicated.

NURSING IMPLICATIONS

Patient should be recumbent during and for at least 15 minutes following IV injection in order to reduce the possibility of orthostatic hypotension and other adverse reactions. Monitor vital signs and IV flow rate.

Supervise ambulation following parenteral administration. Advise patient to make position changes slowly, particularly from recumbent to upright position, and to dangle legs before standing.

Care should be taken to avoid extravasation of IV solution, which may result in thrombophlebitis and sloughing.

IM dose should not exceed 5 ml (0.5 Gm) into each gluteal region. Insert needle deep, and carefully withdraw plunger to make sure needle is not in blood vessel. Inject drug slowly. Rotate injection sites, and observe daily for evidence of irritation.

Methocarbamol should not be administered subcutaneously.

Oral administration should replace parenteral use as soon as feasible. Keep physician informed of patient's response to therapy.

Adverse reactions following oral administration are usually mild and transient and subside with dosage reduction. Caution patients regarding drowsiness and dizziness. Advise against activities requiring mental alertness and physical coordination until response to drug action is known.

Periodic WBC counts are advised during prolonged therapy.

Urine may darken to brown, black, or green on standing.

Store preferably between 15° and 30°C (59° and 86°F) unless otherwise directed by manufacturer.

Diagnostic Test Interferences. Methocarbamol may cause false increases in **urinary 5-HIAA** (with nitrosonaphthol reagent) and **VMA** (Gitlow method).

Drug Interactions. Inform patient that concurrent administration of methocarbamol with other CNS depressants including **alcohol** produces enhanced CNS depression (drowsiness and impaired judgment and coordination).

M

METHOHEXITAL SODIUM

(Brietal, Brevital Sodium)

(meth-oh-hex′i-tal)
Anesthetic (general)
Barbiturate
C IV

ACTIONS AND USES. Rapid, ultra-short-acting barbiturate anesthetic agent. More potent than thiopental (qv), but has less cumulative effect and shorter duration of action, and recovery is more rapid. Abnormal muscle movements, coughing, sneezing, and laryngospasm reportedly occur more frequently than with thiopental. *See Thiopental for Absorption and Fate, Contraindications and Precautions, Adverse/Side Effects.*

Used for induction of anesthesia, as supplement for other anesthetics, and as general anesthetic for brief operative procedures.

ROUTE AND DOSAGE. Intravenous *(induction):* 5 to 12 ml of 1% solution (50 to 120 mg) at rate of 1 ml every 5 seconds; maintenance: 2 to 4 ml (20 to 40 mg) every 4 to 7 minutes as required. *Continuous drip* (0.2% solution): flow rate 1 drop per second.

NURSING IMPLICATIONS

Patient should be recumbent during drug administration.
Fall in blood pressure may occur in susceptible patients receiving drug in upright position.
Hiccups are not uncommon, particularly with rapid injection; they sometimes persist after anesthesia.
Facilities for assisting respiration and administration of oxygen should be readily available.
Stable in sterile water for injection at room temperature for at least 6 weeks. Solutions prepared with isotonic sodium chloride injection or 5% dextrose injection are stable for about 24 hours. Only clear, colorless solutions should be used.
Classified as Schedule IV drug under the Federal Controlled Substances Act.
Methohexital solution is incompatible with acid solutions, e.g., atropine and with silicone. Do not allow contact with rubber stoppers or parts of syringes treated with silicone.
See Thiopental sodium.

METHOTREXATE
(Amethopterin, Folex, Mexate, MTX)
METHOTREXATE SODIUM

(meth-oh-trex'ate)
Antineoplastic
Antimetabolic
Folic acid antagonist
Antipsoriatic

M

ACTIONS AND USES. Antimetabolite and folic acid antagonist. Blocks folinic acid (active principle of folic acid) participation in nucleic acid synthesis, thereby interfering with mitotic process. Rapidly proliferating tissues (malignant cells, bone marrow) are sensitive to this effect. In psoriasis, reproductive rate of epithelial cells is higher than in normal cells. Methotrexate controls the psoriatic process by its effect on mitosis. Some evidence of toxicity usually accompanies therapeutic response. Induces remission slowly; use often preceded by other antineoplastic therapies.

Used principally in combination regimens to maintain induced remissions in neoplastic diseases. Effective in treatment of gestational choriocarcinoma and hydatidiform mole and as immunosuppressant in kidney transplantation, for acute and subacute leukemias and leukemic meningitis, especially in children. Used in lymphosarcoma, in certain inoperable tumors of head, neck, and pelvis, and in mycosis fungoides. Also used to treat severe psoriasis nonresponsive to other forms of therapy.

ABSORPTION AND FATE. Rapidly absorbed from GI tract; peak serum levels 1 to 2 hours after oral administration and 30 to 60 minutes after parenteral administration. Serum half-life 2 to 4 hours after IM and oral administration; approximately one-half of drug is bound to serum proteins. Wide distribution, with highest concentrations in kidneys, gallbladder, spleen, liver, skin. Unchanged drug is retained several weeks in impaired kidneys, several months in the liver, and about 6 days in cerebrospinal fluid following intrathecal injection. Up to 90% of drug is cleared by kidneys; small amounts also excreted in stools through enterohepatic route. Crosses placenta; minimal passage across blood–brain barrier.

CONTRAINDICATIONS AND PRECAUTIONS. Pregnancy, hepatic and renal insufficiency, men and women in childbearing age, concomitant administration of hepatotoxic drugs and hematopoietic depressants, alcohol, ultraviolet exposure to psoriatic lesions, preexisting blood dyscrasias. *Cautious Use:* infections, peptic ulcer, ulcerative colitis, very young or old patients, cancer patients with preexisting bone marrow impairment, poor nutritional status.

ADVERSE/SIDE EFFECTS. Dose-related and reversible: **Dermatologic:** erythematous rashes, pruritis, uticaria, folliculitis, vasculitis, photosensitivity, depigmentation, hyperpigmentation, alopecia. **GI:** hepatotoxicity, GI ulcerations and hemorrhage, ulcerative stomatitis, glossitis, gingivitis, pharyngitis, nausea, vomiting, diarrhea, hepatic cirrhosis. **Hematologic:** marked myelosuppression, aplastic bone marrow, telangiectasis, thrombophlebitis at intraarterial catheter site, hypogammaglobulinemia, hyperuricemia. **Neurologic:** headache, drowsiness, blurred vision, dizziness, aphasia, hemiparesis, convulsions (after intrathecal administration), mental confusion, tremors, ataxia, coma. **Urogenital:** defective oogenesis or spermatogenesis, nephropathy, hematuria, menstrual dysfunction, infertility, abortion, fetal defects. **Other:** malaise, undue fatigue, systemic toxicity (after intrathecal and intraarterial administration), chills, fever, decreased resistance to infection, septicemia, osteoporosis, metabolic changes precipitating diabetes and sudden death, pneumonitis.

ROUTE AND DOSAGE. **Oral, intramuscular, intravenous, intraarterial, intrathecal:** dosage individualized according to disease being treated, concurrent drug therapy, response, and tolerance of patient. *Severe psoriasis:* **Oral:** 2.5 mg daily for 5 days followed by 2 day rest period. Maximum: 6.25 mg/day. **Intramuscular, intravenous:** 10 to 25 mg/week until adequate response is achieved. Maximum: 50 mg/week.

NURSING IMPLICATIONS

A test dose (5 to 10 mg parentally) one week before therapy, precedes treatment of psoriasis.

Avoid skin exposure and inhalation of drug particles.

Oral preparations should be given 1 to 2 hours before or 2 to 3 hours after meals.

Preserve drug in tight, light-resistant container.

Hepatic and renal function tests, blood tests (including blood type and group, bleeding time, coagulation time) and chest x-rays should be part of the health data base in case of emergency surgery or need for transfusion during therapy. Tests are repeated at weekly intervals during methotrexate therapy.

Hepatic function tests may be abnormal 1 to 3 days after methotrexate administration, and GI symptoms may be absent.

Monitor all laboratory reports daily as indicators for adaptations in nursing and drug regimens.

Patient should be fully informed of dangers of this drug and warned to report promptly any abnormal symptoms.

Alcohol ingestion increases the incidence and severity of methotrexate hepatotoxicity.

Leucovorin calcium (citrovorin factor) given within 12 hours after methotrexate protects normal tissues from lethal effects of the drug (leucovorin "rescue").

If an overdosage of methotrexate is given, leucovorin may be employed as antidote (must be given within the first hour of overdosage).

Prolonged treatment with small frequent doses may lead to hepatotoxicity, which is best diagnosed by liver biopsy.

Ulcerative stomatitis with glossitis and gingivitis, often the first signs of toxicity, necessitate interruption of therapy or dosage adjustment. Inspect mouth daily; report patchy necrotic areas, bleeding and discomfort, or overgrowth (black, furry tongue).

Fastidious mouth care prevents infection, provides comfort, and is essential to maintenance of adequate nutritional status. *See Index: Nursing interventions: stomatitis.*

In presence of hyperuricemia, patient may be kept well hydrated (about 2000 ml/24 hours) to dilute hyperuric fluids and given allopurinol to prevent urate deposition.

Monitor intake–output ratio and pattern. Severe nephrotoxicity (hematuria, dysuria, azotemia, oliguria) fosters drug accumulation and renal damage and requires dosage adjustment or discontinuation.

During leukopenic periods, prevent patient exposure to personnel and visitors with infections or colds. Be alert to onset of agranulocytosis (cough, extreme fatigue, sore throat, chills, fever), and report symptoms promptly. Methotrexate therapy will be interrupted and appropriate antibiotic drugs prescribed.

Be alert for and report symptoms of thrombocytopenia: ecchymoses, petechiae, epistaxis, melena, hematuria, vaginal bleeding, slow and protracted oozing following trauma.

Contraceptive measures should be used both during and for at least 8 weeks following therapy.

Alopecia is reversible; hair regrowth begins after drug discontinuation, but it may require several months. *See Index: Nursing intervention: alopecia.*

Methotrexate may precipitate gouty arthritis. Instruct the patient to report joint pains to physician.

Bloody diarrhea necessitates interruption of therapy to prevent perforation or hemorrhagic enteritis. Report to physician.

Warn patient not to self-medicate with vitamins. Some over-the-counter compounds may include folic acid (or its derivatives), which alters methotrexate response.

Diabetes may be precipitated; therefore, tests for glucosuria should be performed periodically, and significant symptoms such as polydipsia and polyuria should be reported.

Instruct patient to notify physician if psoriasis worsens.

Burning and erythema may occur in psoriatic areas after each dose of methotrexate.

Concomitant exposure to ultraviolet light and to sunlight may aggravate psoriatic lesions in patients on methotrexate therapy.

Advise patient to adhere to dosage schedule; i.e., not to omit, increase, or decrease dose or change dose intervals.

Deaths have been reported with use of this agent in the treatment of psoriasis.

Consult physician about plans for disclosure of diagnosis, prognosis, and treatment so that discussions with patient and family will be supportive and nonconflicting.

M

Diagnostic Test Interferences. Severe reactions may occur when **live vaccines** are administered because of immunosuppressive activity of methotrexate.

Drug Interactions. **Salicylates, sulfonamides, phenylbutazone, phenytoin, tetracycline, chloramphenicol,** and **PABA** displace methotrexate from plasma protein binding, causing increased toxicity. Studies suggest that large doses of **penicillin** and **probenecid** increase methotrexate plasma levels, with resultant increase in its toxicity. **Vitamin preparations** containing **folic acid** and derivatives may alter response to methotrexate. Hepatotoxicity caused by methotrexate is increased by concomitant administration of **alcohol.** Hypoprothrombinemia produced by **anticoagulants** is enhanced by methotrexate. Oral aminoglycoside antibiotics may reduce absorption of oral methotrexate.

METHOTRIMEPRAZINE

(Levoprome, Nozinan)

(meth-oh-trye-mep'ra-zeen)
Nonnarcotic analgesic
Phenothiazine derivative

ACTIONS AND USES. Aliphatic (propylamino) derivative of phenothiazine with CNS actions similar to those of chlorpromazine (qv). In addition to tranquilizing and sedative effects also has prominent analgesic properties. Extrapyramidal symptoms and dry mouth reportedly uncommon, but orthostatic hypotension and sedation effects are more prominent. Also exhibits antiemetic, antipruritic, weak anticholinergic, and local anesthetic properties. Raises pain threshold and may also produce amnesia. Nearly as potent as morphine in analgesic effect (15 mg of methotrimeprazine is reportedly equal to 10 mg of morphine). Unlike morphine-type analgesics, psychic and physical dependence not reported with methotrimeprazine, it has no antitussive activity, and it rarely produces respiratory depression.

Used to relieve moderate to severe pain in nonambulatory patients, and for analgesia and sedation when respiratory depression is to be avoided, as in obstetrics, and pre- and postoperatively.

ABSORPTION AND FATE. Maximum analgesic effects within 20 to 40 minutes, peaks in 1 to 2 hours; duration about 4 hours. Enters cerebrospinal fluid. Probably metabolized in liver. Metabolites exhibit some activity, but less than parent drug. Excreted slowly in urine and feces, primarily as metabolites and about 1% as unchanged drug. Elimination in urine may continue 1 week after a single dose. Crosses placenta; small amounts may enter breast milk.

CONTRAINDICATIONS AND PRECAUTIONS. Hypersensitivity to phenothiazines and to ingredients in the formulation,e.g., bisulfite; severe cardiac, renal, or hepatic disease; history of convulsive disorders; significant hypotension; comatose states; premature labor; children under 12 years of age; concomitant use with antihypertensive agents, including MAO inhibitors. *Cautious Use:* elderly and debilitated patients with heart disease; women of childbearing potential; use during early pregnancy.

ADVERSE/SIDE EFFECTS. CNS: excessive sedation, drowsiness, amnesia, disorientation, euphoria, delirium, extrapyramidal symptoms. **CV:** orthostatic hypotension with faintness, weakness, dizziness; tachycardia, bradycardia, palpitation. **EENT:** blurred vision, nasal congestion. **GI:** nausea, vomiting, abdominal discomfort, dry mouth. **GU:** dysuria, hematuria. **Other:** headache, slurred speech, fever, chills, hypotonic uterine inertia (rare), injection site reactions, elevated serum bilirubin (rare), respiratory depression (infrequent). With prolonged high dosage: increased weight, jaundice, severe blood dyscrasias including agranulocytosis and pancytopenia.

M

ROUTE AND DOSAGE. Intramuscular: *Sedation, analgesia:* 10 to 20 mg every 4 to 6 hours, if necessary. *Preoperative medication:* 2 to 20 mg 45 minutes to 3 hours before surgery. *Postoperative analgesia:* Initial: 2.5 to 7.5 mg is suggested every 4 to 6 hours as necessary since residual effects of anesthetic may be present. **Elderly patients:** 5 to 10 mg.

NURSING IMPLICATIONS

Administer IM injection deep into large muscle mass (subcutaneous injection causes severe local irritation). Carefully withdraw plunger to prevent inadvertent injection into blood vessel.

Pain at injection site and local inflammatory reaction commonly occur. Rotate injection sites and observe daily.

Orthostatic hypotension with faintness, weakness, and dizziness may occur within 10 to 20 minutes after drug administration and may last 4 to 6 hours and occasionally up to 12 hours. Ambulation should be avoided or carefully supervised for at least 6 hours, but preferably 12 hours. Tolerance to these effects usually develops with successive doses.

Excessive sedation and amnesia also occur commonly during early drug therapy.

Blood pressure and pulse should be checked frequently until dosage requirements and response are stabilized. Elderly and debilitated patients require close monitoring.

Severe hypotensive effects have been treated with phenylephrine or methoxamine; levarterenol is reserved for hypotension not reversed by other vasopressors. Epinephrine is specifically contraindicated (may cause paradoxic decrease in blood pressure).

Methotrimeprazine is rarely administered beyond 30 days, except when narcotic drugs are contraindicated or in terminal illness.

When drug is used for prolonged periods, periodic blood studies and liver function tests are recommended.

Although it is not subject to narcotic controls, drug abuse is a possibility.

Injection formulation contains bisulfite, an allergen for some individuals.

The manufacturer states that methotrimeprazine may be mixed in the same syringe with either atropine or scopolamine, but not with any other drugs. (Dosage of atropine or scopolamine should be reduced.)

Protect drug from light.

Drug Interactions: Methotrimeprazine

Plus	Interactions
Anticholinergic agents (e.g., atropine, scopolamine, and others)	Aggravation of extrapyramidal symptoms, CNS stimulation, delirium
Antihypertensive agents (e.g., guanethidine, methydopa, reserpine, and others)	Additive hypotensive effect
CNS depressants (ethyl alcohol, analgesics, general anesthetics, antianxiety agents, antihistamines, barbiturates and other sedatives, hypnotics, narcotics, other phenothiazines)	Enhanced CNS depression
Epinephrine	Methotrimeprazine reverses vasopressor effect of epinephrine
MAO inhibitors	Possibility of severe toxic reaction; additive hypotensive effect
Skeletal muscle relaxants, surgical (e.g., succinylcholine, tubocurarine)	Prolonged muscle relaxation

METHOXAMINE HYDROCHLORIDE

(Vasoxyl)

(meth-ox'a meen)
Alpha-adrenergic agonist
Sympathomimetic
Antiarrhythmic

ACTIONS AND USES. Direct-acting sympathomimetic amine pharmacologically related to phenylephrine. Acts almost exclusively on α-adrenergic receptors. Pressor action is due primarily to direct peripheral vasoconstriction, which in turn causes rise in arterial blood pressure. Has no direct effect on heart, but tends to slow ventricular rate by vagal stimulation in response to elevated blood pressure. Large doses may produce bradycardia. Markedly reduces renal blood flow. Free of CNS stimulating action. True tachyphylaxis not reported.

Used for supporting, restoring, or maintaining blood pressure during anesthesia and to terminate some episodes of paroxysmal supraventricular tachycardia.

ABSORPTION AND FATE. Acts within 15 minutes following IM injection; effects may persist 1.5 hours. Acts almost immediately after IV injection and lasts about 1 hour. Widely distributed in body fluids. Excreted in urine.

CONTRAINDICATIONS AND PRECAUTIONS. Severe coronary or cardiovascular disease; hypovolemia, in combination with local anesthetics for tissue infiltration; within 2 weeks of MAO inhibitors. *Cautious Use:* history of hypertension or hyperthyroidism; following use of ergot alkaloids.

ADVERSE/SIDE EFFECTS. Paresthesias, feeling of coldness (particularly with high dosage), high blood pressure with projectile vomiting, severe headache, pilomotor erection (goose-flesh), urinary urgency, bradycardia.

ROUTE AND DOSAGE. Adults: Intramuscular: 10 to 15 mg, repeated if necessary, but not before about 15 minutes. **Intravenous:** injected slowly: *(emergencies):* 3 to 5 mg; *tachycardia:* 10 mg. **Pediatrics: Intramuscular:** 0.25 mg/kg. **Intravenous:** one-third of IM dose (slowly).

NURSING IMPLICATIONS

Patients should be under close supervision.

Monitor vital signs. Report any increase in blood pressure above level prescribed by physician; report slowing of heart rate.

Have atropine on hand for excessive bradycardia.

Be alert for sudden changes in blood pressure and pulse after drug has been discontinued.

Methoxamine injection contains a bisulfite, an allergen for some patients.

Antidote for extravasation: Area should be infiltrated as soon as possible with 10 to 15 ml of normal saline solution containing 5 to 10 mg phentolamine. *See Index: Nursing Interventions: extravasation.*

Monitor intake and output. Urinary frequency with retention is a possibility. Report oliguria or change in intake–output ratio.

Protect drug from light.

Drug Interactions. Hypertension (increase in alpha adrenergic effects of methoxamine) may occur in patients receiving **furazolidone, guanethidine, methyldopa, oxytocic drugs, rauwolfia alkaloids, tricyclic antidepressants.** Pressor effect (alpha adrenergic actions of methoxamine) may be decreased by **lithium.**

METHOXSALEN
(8-MOP, Oxsoralen)

(meth-ox′ a-len)
Pigmenting agent
Photochemotherapeutic agent
Psoralen

ACTIONS AND USES. A psoralen derivative with strong photosensitizing effects: used with ultraviolet light (UVA) in therapeutic regimens called PUVA therapy ((P)-psoralen). Following photoactivation by long wave-length UVA methoxsalen combines with epidermal cell DNA causing photo-damage (cytotoxic action) and inhibition of the rapid and uncontrolled epidermal cell turnover characteristic of psoriasis, and an inflammatory reaction with erythema. Methoxsalen is also strongly melanogenic. Skin color depends on melanin, product of melanocytes in the basal layer of epidermis. UVA energizes the intracellular oxidation of tyrosine to melanin precursor dihydroxyphenylalamine; methoxsalen enhances the reaction. Repigmentation induced by PUVA appears to be the result of several mechanisms including

M

increased synthesis of melanin, increased number and hypertrophy of functioning melanocytes, stimulation of migration of melanocytes up the follicles to repopulate the epidermis. Long-term effects of PUVA treatment include increased risk of cutaneous cancer. The safe total cumulative dose of UVA in PUVA therapy over a period of time has not been established.

Used with controlled exposure to UVA to repigment vitiliginous skin and for symptomatic treatment of severe disabling psoriasis that is refractory to other forms of therapy. *Investigational Use:* (PUVA therapy) mycosis fungoides.

ABSORPTION AND FATE. Maximum bioavailability: 1½ to 3 hours after administration; action lasts up to 8 hours. Half-life: ½ to 1 hour. Preferentially taken up by epidermal cells but distribution is throughout body including eye lens. Metabolized in liver; excreted in urine within 24 hours.

CONTRAINDICATIONS AND PRECAUTIONS. Sun burn, sensitivity (or its history) to psoralens, diseases associated with photosensitivity (e.g., LE, albinism, melanoma or its history), invasive squamous cell cancer, cataract, aphakia, previous exposure to arsenic or ionizing radiation, pregnancy (category C); safe use (oral) in children not established. *Cautious Use:* hepatic insufficiency, GI disease, chronic infection, treatment with known photosensitizing agents *(see Drug Interactions):* immunosuppressed patient, cardiovascular disease, nursing mothers; safe use (lotion) in children under 12 not established.

ADVERSE/SIDE EFFECTS. CV: hypotension. **Dermatologic:** *phototoxic effects:* severe edema and erythema, pruritus, painful blisters; burning, peeling, thinning, freckling, and accelerated aging of skin; hyper- or hypopigmentation; severe skin pain (lasting 1 to 2 months). *Also:* malignant melanoma (rare), cell carcinoma, cutaneous neuritis, photoallergic contact dermatitis (with topical use), exacerbation of latent photosensitive dermatoses. **GI:** cheilitis, nausea and other GI disturbances, toxic hepatitis. **Neurologic:** nervousness, dizziness, headache, mental depression or excitation, vertigo, insomnia, cataract formation, ocular damage. **Other:** transient loss of muscular coordination, edema, leg cramps, systemic immune effects; acute myeloid leukemia, preleukemia.

ROUTE AND DOSAGE. Oral: *Vitiligo:* 20 mg (2 capsules). *Psoriasis:* 10 to 70 mg (dose determined by body weight). *Mycosis fungoides:* 30 to 50 mg. Dose administered 2 to 4 hours before UVA exposure according to established UVA protocol. **Topical:** Lotion 1% (1 mg/ml): 1 to 2 hours before exposure to UVA light, usually at weekly intervals.

NURSING IMPLICATIONS

Methoxsalen *(PUVA therapy)* should be under the complete control of a physician with special competence and experience in photochemotherapy.

To prevent GI distress, oral doses are best administered with milk or food.

Food–Drug Interactions: Maintain a consistent time relationship between food–drug ingestion. Food digestion and absorption appear to affect drug serum levels.

Methoxsalen is always administered on an alternate day schedule because the full extent of a phototoxic reaction may be delayed for up to 48 hours.

Sunlight is sometimes used as the UV light source with the exposure time factor well controlled by prescription.

Following drug ingestion and UVA exposure, additional exposure to UV light (direct or indirect) should be avoided for at least 8 hours.

After topical methoxsalen application and UVA exposure, the patient should not expose skin to additional UV light for 24 to 48 hours.

If sunlight cannot be avoided after the treatment, sunscreen lotion (with SPF 15 or higher) and protective clothing (hat, gloves) should cover all exposed areas including lips, to prevent burning or blistering.

Sunscreen lotions containing benzophenone (e.g., Solbar) appear to give best protection from drug-induced phototoxicity.

During PUVA therapy, sunscreen lotion is applied to the skin for about one-third of the initial exposure time until there is sufficient tanning. It should not be applied to psoriatric areas before the treatment.

Sunbathing is contraindicated for at least 48 hours after PUVA treatment. Sunburn and photochemotherapy are additive in the production of burning and erythema.

Erythema from PUVA differs from sunburn in severity and depth. UV light from the sun does not penetrate skin cell layers as deeply as the UV light used in PUVA.

During maintenance treatment, the patient's tan and erythematous dose level may be gradually decreased.

Lotion is never dispensed to the patient for self-care. It is applied by the physician.

Only small (less than 10 cm^2), well-defined areas are treated with lotion. Systemic treatment is used for large areas.

The lotion is applied with cotton swabs, allowed to dry 1 to 2 minutes, then reapplied. Borders of the lesion should be protected with petrolatum and sunscreen lotion to prevent hyperpigmentation.

Finger cots or gloves should be used to apply lotion to prevent photosensitization and burned skin.

Following topical application, the initial sunlight exposure is limited to 1 minute, with subsequent gradual and incremental exposures by prescription. The patient should fully understand the intended schedule.

A systemic response to lotion has not been reported.

Repigmentation is more rapid on fleshy areas i.e., face, abdomen, buttocks, than on hands or feet.

Effective repigmentation may require 6 to 9 months of treatment; periodic treatment usually is necessary to retain pigmentation. If, after 3 months of treatment, there is no apparent response, methoxsalen is discontinued.

Wraparound UVA opaque goggles are worn during PUVA treatment. After treatment, wraparound sunglasses with UVA absorbing properties must be worn both indoors and outdoors during daylight hours for 24 hours.

Warn patient not to substitute prescription sunglasses or photosensitive darkening glasses; they may actually increase danger of cataract formation.

A pretreatment ophthalmologic exam is performed to rule out cataract; it should be repeated periodically during treatment and at yearly intervals thereafter. UVA exposure to a drug-loaded lens leads to drug–protein binding and cataract formation.

Complete blood count, renal and hepatic function tests, and antinuclear antibody tests are monitored during oral psoralen therapy.

Instruct patient to alert physician to appearance of new psoriatic areas, to flares, or to regressed cleared skin areas should they occur during treatment and maintenance periods. If any area is more than 5% of the originally involved body areas, the maintenance schedule will be adjusted.

Fair-skinned patients appear to be at greatest risk for photochemotherapeutic toxicity from PUVA therapy.

In acute overdosage, immediate emesis is induced (effective only if accomplished within 2 to 3 hours after ingestion). Patient is placed in darkened room for at least 24 hours or until cutaneous reactions subside; burn therapy is given as required.

Oral methoxsalen contains tartrazine, which can cause allergic-type reactions, including bronchial asthma, in susceptible individuals. Frequently such persons are also hypersensitive to aspirin.

Rarely is it more important for a patient to understand a treatment fully than with PUVA therapy. Discuss the regimen with the physician to facilitate reemphasis and clarification of information given to the patient.

It is not known if PUVA treatment affects fertility.

Store lotion and capsules in light-resistant containers at temperature of 15° to 30°C (59° to 86°F) unless otherwise directed by manufacturer.

Drug Interactions: Methoxsalen

Plus	Interactions
Other systemic or topical photosensitizing agents (e.g., anthralin, coal tar derivatives, griseofulvin, phenothiazines, nalidixic acid, halogenated salicylanilides (bacteriologic soaps), sulfonamides, tetracyclines, thiazides, or certain organic stains, e.g., methylene blue, toluidine blue, rose bengal, methyl orange)	Additive photosensitizing effects

M

METHOXYPHENAMINE HYDROCHLORIDE

(Orthoxine)

(meth ox-ee-fen′a-meen)
Beta-adrenergic agonist
Smooth muscle relaxant (respiratory)
Bronchodilator

ACTIONS AND USES. Direct-acting synthetic amine structurally and pharmacologically related to ephedrine (qv). Main sympathomimetic action is on beta receptors of bronchial smooth muscles. Causes fewer cardiovascular effects than does ephedrine and has less pressor activity, but bronchodilator effect is greater and more prolonged. Has minimal CNS stimulant action and alpha receptor activity, and exhibits weak antihistaminic properties.

Used in treatment of bronchial asthma, acute urticaria, allergic rhinitis, GI allergy, and allergic headaches.

ABSORPTION AND FATE. Readily absorbed from GI tract. Effects appear within 30 minutes and may persist 3 to 4 hours.

CONTRAINDICATIONS AND PRECAUTIONS. History of previous adverse reactions to the drug; use within 2 weeks of MAO inhibitors; pregnancy, lactation. *Cautious Use:* hypertension, hyperthyroidism, thyrotoxicosis, acute coronary disease, cardiac decompensation, diabetes mellitus, elderly patients. *See Ephedrine.*

ADVERSE/SIDE EFFECTS. Nausea, dizziness, drowsiness, faintness, dry mouth. With high doses: palpitation, psychomotor stimulation, anxiety, wakefulness.

ROUTE AND DOSAGE. Oral: Adults: 50 to 100 mg every 3 to 4 hours, if necessary. **Children:** 25 to 50 mg every 4 to 6 hours, if necessary.

NURSING IMPLICATIONS

See Ephedrine sulfate.

METHSCOPOLAMINE BROMIDE

(Pamine)

(meth-skoe-pol'a meen)
Anticholinergic
(Parasympatholytic)
Antispasmodic

ACTIONS AND USES. Quaternary ammonium derivative of scopolamine, but lacks scopolamine's CNS actions. Its spasmolytic and antisecretory actions are quantitatively similar to those of atropine, but they last longer. Has greater selectivity in blocking vagal impulses from GI tract than either scopolamine or atropine (qv).

Used as adjunct in treatment of peptic ulcer, irritable bowel syndrome, and a variety of other GI conditions. Also may be used to control excessive sweating and salivation, migraine headaches, and premenstrual cramps.

ABSORPTION AND FATE. Erratic absorption following oral administration; effects appear in about 1 hour and persist 4 to 6 hours. Excreted primarily in urine and bile; some unchanged drug excreted in feces.

CONTRAINDICATIONS AND PRECAUTIONS. Hypersensitivity to any of the drug's constituents, prostatic hypertrophy, pyloric obstruction, intestinal atony, tachycardia, cardiac disease. Safe use during pregnancy not established. *See also Atropine. Cautious Use:* elderly and debilitated patients.

M

ADVERSE/SIDE EFFECTS. Dry mouth, blurred vision, dizziness, drowsiness, constipation, flushing of skin, urinary hesitancy or retention. *See Atropine.*

ROUTE AND DOSAGE. Adults: Oral: 2.5 to 5 mg before meals and at bedtime.

NURSING IMPLICATIONS

Oral preparation is usually administered 30 minutes before meals and at bedtime.

Incidence and severity of side effects are generally dose-related and therefore may be controlled by dosage reduction. Dosage is usually maintained at a level that produces slight dryness of mouth.

Since methscopolamine may cause dizziness and drowsiness, warn patients not to engage in activities requiring mental alertness, such as driving a car, until response to drug is known. Caution patient to make position changes slowly and in stages.

Dryness of mouth may be relieved by sugarless chewing gum or candy or by frequent rinsing of mouth with water.

Preserved in tight, light-resistant containers.

See Atropine sulfate (prototype anticholinergic).

Drug Interactions. Concurrent use of methscopolamine and the slow-dissolving brand of **digoxin** may cause increased serum digoxin levels (decreased GI motility enhances digoxin absorption). Interaction is not likely to occur with liquid digoxin formulation or with fast-dissolving brand of digoxin. Methscopolamine may increase the pharmacological effects of **atenolol**

(Tenormin), **levodopa** (Dopar, Larodopa), **thiazide diuretics,** and decrease the pharmacological effects of **cimetidine** (Tagamet).

METHSUXIMIDE

(Celontin)

(meth-sux'i-mide)
Anticonvulsant
Succinimide

ACTIONS AND USES. Succinimide derivative with actions, contraindications, precautions, and adverse reactions similar to those of ethosuximide (qv). Associated with high incidence of adverse effects.

Used for control of absence (petit mal) seizures refractory to other anticonvulsants. May be used in combination with other anticonvulsants in mixed types of epilepsy.

ABSORPTION AND FATE. Rapidly absorbed and metabolized. Peak plasma levels in 1 to 3 hours. Plasma half-life: 2 to 4 hours. Not significantly bound to plasma proteins. Metabolized in liver to an active metabolite tentatively believed to be responsible for anticonvulsant action. Excreted in urine as active and inactive metabolites; less than 1% excreted unchanged.

CONTRAINDICATIONS AND PRECAUTIONS. Hypersensitivity to succinimides; drug allergies; hepatic or renal disease; blood dyscrasias. *See also Ethosuximide.*

ADVERSE/SIDE EFFECTS. CNS (most frequent): drowsiness, dizziness, ataxia; also headache, insomnia, diplopia, photophobia, severe mental depression, behavioral changes. **GI** (frequent): nausea, vomiting, anorexia, diarrhea, constipation, epigastric or abdominal pain, weight loss. **Hypersensitivity:** skin eruptions, fever, hiccups, periorbital edema and hyperemia, blood dyscrasias including aplastic anemia, systemic lupus erythematosus. **Other:** renal and hepatic damage. *See also Ethosuximide.*

M

ROUTE AND DOSAGE. Adults and children: Oral: initially 300 mg daily for first week. If required, dosage may be increased by 300 mg at weekly intervals to maximum daily dosage of 1.2 Gm daily administered in divided doses. Highly individualized.

NURSING IMPLICATIONS

Drug tolerance varies among patients. Patient must be closely observed when dosage is increased or decreased, or when adding or eliminating other medication.

Advise patient to report immediately the onset of adverse effects (often controlled by dosage reduction). Development of a rash may herald more serious reactions.

Observe patient closely for behavioral changes. Drug should be withdrawn (slowly) at first appearance of depression, aggression, or other unusual behavioral manifestations in order to prevent progression to acute psychosis.

Abrupt drug withdrawal may precipitate petit mal seizures.

Periodic blood cell counts, tests of liver function, and urinalysis should be performed during therapy.

Since drug may cause drowsiness, dizziness, and visual disturbances, caution patients to avoid potentially hazardous activities such as driving a car until drug response is known.

Celontin contains *tartrazine* which can cause allergic reactions including bronchial asthma in susceptible individuals, who may also be sensitive to aspirin.

Advise patient to carry a wallet identification card or jewelry indicating that patient has epilepsy and is taking medication.

Store capsules away from heat preferably between 15° and 30°C (59° and 86°F) unless otherwise directed by manufacturer.

METHYCLOTHIAZIDE

(Aquatensen, Duretic, Enduron, Ethon)

(meth-i-kloe-thye'a-zide)
Diuretic
Antihypertensive
Thiazide

ACTIONS AND USES. Benzothiadiazine (thiazide) derivative. Similar to chlorothiazide (qv) in actions, uses, contraindications, adverse reactions and interactions.

Used as primary (step 1) agent in stepped care approach to antihypertensive treatment, and adjunctively in the management of edema associated with congestive heart failure, renal pathology and hepatic cirrhosis. Available in fixed combination with reserpine (Diutensen-R); with pargyline (Eutron); and with deserpidine (Enduronyl). *See also Chlorothiazide.*

ABSORPTION AND FATE. Diuretic effect begins within 2 hours, peaks in 6 hours and lasts more than 24 hours. Excreted unchanged by kidneys. Passes placenta; appears in breast milk.

CONTRAINDICATIONS AND PRECAUTIONS. Hypersensitivity to thiazides, sulfonamide derivatives; anuria, hypokalemia, pregnancy, lactation. *Cautious Use:* impaired renal or hepatic function, gout, SLE, hypercalcemia, diabetes mellitus. *See also Chlorothiazide.*

ADVERSE/SIDE EFFECTS. Postural hypotension, sialadenitis, unusual fatigue, dizziness, paresthesias, yellow vision, hypokalemia, agranulocytosis. *See also Chlorothiazide.*

ROUTE AND DOSAGE. Oral: Adults: *Diuretic:* 2.5 to 5 mg once daily or once daily 3 to 5 times a week. *Antihypertensive:* 2.5 to 10 mg once daily. **Pediatric:** 0.05 to 0.2 mg/kg once daily.

NURSING IMPLICATIONS

Administer drug early in AM after eating (to reduce gastric irritation) to prevent sleep interruption because of diuresis. If 2 doses are ordered, administer second dose no later than 3 PM.

Antihypertensive effects may be noted in 3 to 4 days, maximal effects may require 3 to 4 weeks.

Monitor blood pressure and intake–output ratio during first phase of antihypertensive therapy. Report a sudden fall in BP which may initiate severe postural hypotension and potentially dangerous perfusion problems, especially in the extremities.

Monitor patient for hypokalemia: dry mouth, anorexia, thirst, paresthesias, muscle cramps, cardiac arrhythmias. Report promptly. Physician may change dose and institute replacement therapy.

Hypokalemia is rarely severe in most patients even on long-term therapy with thiazides if they eat a balanced diet. To prevent onset, urge patient to eat K-rich foods (potatoes, whole grain cereals, beef, fruit juices, skim milk) and to include a banana (about 370 mg K) and at least 6 ounces orange juice (about 330 mg K) every day. Collaborate with dietitian and arrange for patient–dietitian planning for an individualized diet.

The prediabetic or diabetic patient should be watched carefully for loss of diabetes control or early signs of hyperglycemia: drowsiness, flushed, dry skin; fruitlike breath odor, polyuria, anorexia, polydipsia. The symptoms are slow to develop and to recognize. Check urine for glycosuria. Notify physician.

Counsel patient to avoid use of OTC drugs unless approved by the physician. Many preparations contain both K and Na and if misused or if patient overdoses, electrolyte imbalance side effects may be induced.

The elderly are more responsive to excessive diuresis than young people because of changes in the cardiovascular and renal systems with aging. Orthostatic hypotension may be a problem.

Instruct patient with orthostatic hypotension to change from recumbency to upright positions slowly and in stages; to avoid hot baths or showers, extended exposure to sunlight, and standing still. Provide assistance as necessary to prevent falling. Consult physician about use of support panty hose or knee socks.

Advise patient to avoid driving a vehicle or working with dangerous equipment until adjustment to the hypotensive effects of this drug has been made.

Store drug at temperature between 15° and 30°C (59° and 86°F) unless otherwise instructed by manufacturer.

See Chlorothiazide (prototype thiazide diuretic).

METHYL SALICYLATE

(Betula Oil, Gaultheria Oil, Oil of Wintergreen, Sweet Birch Oil)

Analgesic (topical)
Salicylate

ACTIONS AND USES. Relieves pain in muscles and joints by increasing cutaneous blood flow, thereby producing sensation of warmth and comfort. It is thought that systemic analgesic effects and toxicity can occur from local absorption.

Applied topically to provide temporary symptomatic relief of minor discomforts of osteoarthritis, rheumatoid arthritis, and low back pain.

ADVERSE/SIDE EFFECTS. Redness, rash, burning sensation, blistering. Systemic poisoning: salicylism, *see Aspirin.*

ROUTE AND DOSAGE. **Topical use** *only:* **Adults** *only:* Applied as ointment, or liniment by gentle massage, several times a day. (10 to 25% concentrations commonly used, but available in higher strengths.) Most preparations are intended to be rubbed well into skin. Follow manufacturer's directions.

M

NURSING IMPLICATIONS

Avoid getting medication into eyes or on mucous membranes, open wounds, irritated or broken skin. Do not apply to large areas of the body.

Do not bandage or apply heat to affected part.

Wash hand thoroughly with soap and water after applying medication.

Discontinue medication if excessive redness or irritation develops.

Keep out of the reach of children. Wintergreen odor and taste may invite a child to ingest methyl salicylate. Ingestion of as little as one teaspoonful of pure methyl salicylate can be fatal.

Methyl salicylate is a common ingredient in many external analgesic preparations, e.g., Ben Gay, Heet, Musterole, Sloan's Liniment, and many others.

METHYLCELLULOSE

(Cologel, Isopto-Plain)

(meth-ill-sell′yoo-lose)
Laxative, bulk forming

ACTIONS AND USES. Hydrophilic semisynthetic cellulose derivative. Oral preparation swells on contact with water to form a demulcent nonabsorbable gel that facilitates passage of stool and reflexly stimulates peristalsis.

Used orally as adjunct in treatment of chronic constipation. Also used in ophthalmic preparations for relief of dry eyes and eye irritation associated with deficient tear production, for corneal exposure from half-open eye during coma, and used as ocular lubricant for artificial eyes and contact lenses.

CONTRAINDICATIONS AND PRECAUTIONS. Nausea, vomiting, abdominal pain, intestinal obstruction, ulceration or stenosis, diarrhea.

ADVERSE/SIDE EFFECTS. **Oral form:** diarrhea, nausea, vomiting, fecal impaction, esophageal obstruction.

ROUTE AND DOSAGE. **Oral:** **Adults:** 5 to 20 ml, three times/day. **Children:** 5 to 10 ml once or twice daily. **Ophthalmic** (0.25% to 1%): 1 to 3 drops in eye three or four times daily or as needed.

NURSING IMPLICATIONS

Each oral dose should be taken with 1 or more glasses of water; additional fluids should be taken during the day. Fecal impaction can occur if fluid intake by mouth is insufficient.

Caution the patient not to chew the tablet form because it may start to swell in the esophagus and cause obstruction.

Laxation generally occurs in 12 to 24 hours; however, some patients may require 2 or 3 days of medication.

Review proper bowel hygiene: adequacy of fluid and dietary intake, exercise, habit time.

Ophthalmic preparations *(artificial tears)* are sterile, viscous, water-soluble, nongreasy lubricant combinations of methyl cellulose with buffers and preservatives, e.g., Tears Naturale, Isopto, Methopto, Muracel, and others.

Advise patient to discontinue use of ophthalmic preparation if eye discomfort or irritation occurs and to report to physician.

M

METHYLDOPA

(meth-ill-doe'pa)

(Aldomet, Alpha-Methyldopa, Apo-Methyldopa, Dopamet, Medimet)

(meth-ill-doe'pate)

Antihypertensive (centrally acting)

METHYLDOPATE HYDROCHLORIDE

ACTIONS AND USES. Structurally related to catecholamines and their precursors. Exact mechanism of action unknown; metabolic product of the drug appears to act on both CNS and peripheral vasculature by displacing norepinephrine from its storage sites. Has weak neurotransmitter properties; inhibits decarboxylation of dopa, thereby reducing concentration of dopamine, a precursor of norepinephrine; also inhibits the precursor of serotonin. Lowers standing and supine blood pressures, and unlike adrenergic blockers, it is not so prone to produce orthostatic hypotension, diurnal blood pressure variations, or exercise hypertension. Reduces renal vascular resistance; maintains cardiac output without acceleration, but may slow heart rate; tends to support sodium and water retention. Although it has sedative effect, it also increases REM sleep.

Used as a step 2 agent in stepped care approach in treatment of sustained moderate to severe hypertension, particularly in patients with renal dysfunction. Also used in selected patients with carcinoid disease. Parenteral form has been used for treatment of hypertensive crises but is not preferred because of its slow onset of action. Methyldopa is commercially available in combination with chlorothi azide (Aldoclor) and hydrochlorothiazide (Aldoril).

ABSORPTION AND FATE. About 50% of oral dose is absorbed from GI tract. Maximal antihypertensive effect in 4 to 6 hours; action may persist 24 hours after single oral dose. Following IV injection, major decline in blood pressure occurs within 4 to 6 hours; duration 10 to 16 hours. Weakly bound to plasma proteins. Metabolized in GI tract and liver. About 85% excreted in urine within 24 hours; some unabsorbed oral drug excreted in feces. Crosses placenta: appears in breast milk.

CONTRAINDICATIONS AND PRECAUTIONS. Hypersensitivity to methyldopa, active hepatic disease, pheochromocytoma, blood dyscrasias, mild or labile hypertension amenable to treatment with mild sedation or thiazide diuretics. Safe use in women of childbearing potential and during pregnancy not established. *Cautious Use:* history of impaired liver or renal function or disease; angina pectoris, history of mental depression, young or elderly patients.

ADVERSE/SIDE EFFECTS. Allergic: fever, skin eruptions, ulcerations of soles of feet, flu-like symptoms, lymphadenopathy, eosinophilia. **CV:** orthostatic hypotension, syncope (carotid sinus hypersensitivity), aggravation of angina pectoris, bradycardia, myocarditis, edema, weight gain (sodium and water retention), paradoxic hypertensive reaction (especially with IV administration). **GI:** diarrhea, constipation, abdominal distention, malabsorption syndrome, nausea, vomiting, dry mouth, sore or black tongue, sialadenitis. **Hematologic:** positive direct Coombs' test (common especially in blacks), hemolytic anemia (rare), granulocytopenia, agranulocytosis. **Hepatotoxicity (believed to be allergic reaction):** abnormal liver function tests, jaundice, hepatitis. **Neuropsychiatric:** sedation, drowsiness, sluggishness, headache, weakness, fatigue, dizziness, vertigo, paresthesias, Bell's palsy, decrease in mental acuity, inability to concentrate, amnesia-like syndrome, involuntary choreoathetotic movements, parkinsonism, mild psychoses, depression, nightmares. **Other:** nasal stuffiness (common), gynecomastia, lactation, decreased libido, impotence, hypothermia (large doses), positive tests for lupus and rheumatoid factors, granulomatous skin lesions, pancreatitis.

ROUTE AND DOSAGE. Adults: Oral: 250 mg two or three times a day for first 48 hours; daily dosage may then be increased or decreased, preferably at intervals of not less than 2 days, until adequate response is achieved. Maintenance: 500 mg to 2 Gm in 2 to 4 divided doses daily. Maximum recommended daily dosage 3 Gm. **Intravenous (methyldopate hydrochloride):** 250 to 500 mg at 6-hour intervals, as required. Maximum recommended dose 1 Gm every 6 hours. Desired dose usually added to 100 ml of 5% dextrose injection and given slowly over 30 to 60 minutes. **Children: Oral:** 10 up to 65 mg/kg/24 hours given in 2 to 4 divided doses. **Intravenous:** 20 up to 65 mg/kg/24 hours in 4 equally divided doses at 6-hour intervals.

NURSING IMPLICATIONS

During period of dosage adjustment, physician may request blood pressures to be taken at regular intervals in lying, sitting, and standing positions.

During IV infusion of methyldopate, check blood pressure and pulse at least every 30 minutes until stabilized, and observe for adequacy of urinary output.

Transient sedation and drowsiness, sometimes associated with mental depression, weakness, and headache, commonly occur during first 24 to 72 hours of therapy or whenever dosage is increased. Symptoms tend to disappear with continuation of therapy or with dosage reduction.

To minimize daytime sedation, physician may prescribe dosage increases to be made in the evening. Some patients maintain adequate blood pressure control with a single evening dose.

Orthostatic hypotension with dizziness and lightheadedness may occur during period of dosage adjustment; this indicates need for dosage reduction. Elderly patients and patients with impaired renal function are particularly likely to manifest this drug effect. Supervision of ambulation may be advisable.

Caution patient that hot baths and showers, prolonged standing in one position, and strenuous exercise may enhance orthostatic hypotension. Instruct patient to make position changes slowly, particularly from recumbent to upright posture and to dangle legs a few minutes before standing.

Monitor intake and output. Report oliguria and changes in intake–output ratio.

Weigh patient daily under standard conditions, and check for edema. Concomitant administration of a diuretic is usually prescribed because methyldopa favors sodium and water retention.

Methyldopa hepatoxicity (reversible) resembles viral hepatitis and commonly develops in 2 to 4 weeks, but it may occur from 1 week to 1 year after start of therapy. It is manifested by flu-like symptoms: chills, fever, headache, pruritus, dark urine, fatigue, GI upset and anorexia and is sometimes associated with rash, arthralgia, enlarged liver, and positive Coombs' test. (Occurs commonly in postmenopausal women.) Report to physician; drug should be discontinued.

Baseline and regularly scheduled blood counts and liver function tests are advised during first 6 to 12 weeks of therapy or if patient develops unexplained fever.

Be alert to symptoms of mental depression and report their appearance to physician: anorexia, insomnia, inattention to personal hygiene, withdrawal. Drug-induced depression may persist even after drug is withdrawn.

Positive Coombs' test may or may not indicate hemolytic anemia; it usually develops between 6 to 12 months of therapy and may remain positive for several months after drug is discontinued. If for any reason the need for transfusion arises, both direct and indirect Coombs' tests should be performed. Positive tests may interfere with accurate cross-matching of blood.

Tolerance to drug effect may occur during the second or third week of therapy (manifested by rising blood pressure). Report to physician. Effectiveness may be restored by adding a diuretic or increasing dosage of methyldopa.

Caution patient that methyldopa may affect ability to perform activities requiring concentrated mental effort, especially during first few days of therapy or whenever dosage is increased; patient should avoid potentially hazardous tasks such as driving a car or operating machinery, until reaction to drug is known.

Inform the patient that urine may darken on standing (thought to be due to breakdown product of drug or its metabolite) and that urine contaminated with a hypochlorite toilet bleaching agent may first turn red, then brown and black. Both are possible simple tests for checking patient compliance.

Compliance tends to be poor in patients receiving antihypertensive agents, for a variety of reasons. Urge the patient to keep follow-up visits. Some patients acquire tolerance about the second or third month of therapy, necessitating dosage increases, and rebound hypertension has been reported as a result of acute methyldopa withdrawal.

Advise patient not to take OTC medications for coughs, colds, or allergy unless approved by physician (many contain sympathomimetic agents that may increase blood pressure).

Diagnostic Test Interferences. Methyldopa may interfere with **serum creatinine** measurements using alkaline picrate method, **SGOT** by colorimetric methods, and **uric acid** measurements by phosphotungstate method (in patients with high methyldopa blood levels); it may produce false elevations of **urinary catecholamines,** and increase in **serum amylase** in patients with methyldopa-induced sialadenitis.

Drug Interactions: Methyldopa

Plus	Interactions
Amphetamines Antidepressants, tricyclics	Reduce antihypertensive effect of methyldopa
Ephedrine	Methyldopa may inhibit effectiveness of ephedrine
Haloperidol (Haldol)	Adverse psychiatric symptoms may result
Levodopa (Dopar, Larodopa)	Methyldopa may inhibit therapeutic response to levodopa
Lithium	Increased risk of lithium toxicity
Methotrimeprazine (Levoprome)	Additive hypotensive effect
MAO inhibitors	Hallucinations (based on limited clinical evidence)
Norepinephrine (Levophed)	Slight increase in pressor response to norepinephrine
Phenothiazines Propranolol (Inderal) and possibly other beta-adrenergic blockers	Paradixic hypertensive response may occur
Phenoxybenzamine (Dibenzyline)	Methyldopa augments sympatholytic activity of phenoxybenzamine to cause urinary incontinence
Tolbutamide, and possibly other sulfonylureas	Hypoglycemic effects may be increased by methyldopa

M

METHYLENE BLUE
(Urolene Blue)

(meth'i-leen)
Antiinfective (urinary tract)
Antidote to cyanide poisoning
Diagnostic agent

ACTIONS AND USES. Mildly antiseptic dye with oxidation-reduction action and tissue-staining property. In relatively high concentrations, it oxidizes ferrous iron of reduced hemoglobin to the ferric form, thus producing methemoglobin which complexes with cyanide. In contrast, low concentrations act as catalytic intermediary electron acceptor in conversion of methemoglobin to hemoglobin. Prolonged administration accelerates destruction of erythrocytes.

Used for idiopathic and drug-induced methemoglobinemia and as antidote for cyanide poisoning; used as diagnostic agent, indicator dye, and for medical and surgical marking. Also used in management of oxalate phosphate urinary tract calculi. *Investigational Use:* cutaneous viral infections, for diagnosis of gastroesophageal reflux in pediatrics.

ABSORPTION AND FATE. Poorly absorbed from GI tract. Rapidly reduced in tissues to leuko form, which is excreted slowly in urine together with about 75% unchanged drug. Also excreted in bile and feces.

CONTRAINDICATIONS AND PRECAUTIONS. History of allergy to methylene blue, renal insufficiency. Safe use during pregnancy not established. Methylene blue is ineffective in patients with G6PD deficiency.

ADVERSE/SIDE EFFECTS. Bladder irritation, nausea, vomiting, diarrhea, abdominal pain, hemolysis (patients with G6PD deficiency). Large IV doses: fever, profuse sweating, precordial pain, methemoglobinemia, cardiovascular abnormalities. With continued administration: marked anemia.

ROUTE AND DOSAGE. Oral: 65 to 130 mg two or three times daily after meals.

NURSING IMPLICATIONS

Should be administered after meals with full glass of water.

Inform patients that drug may impart blue-green color to urine and feces.

Since continued administration may cause marked anemia, frequent hemoglobin determinations are advised.

Methylene blue stain may be removed with a hypochlorite solution. Consult pharmacist.

Diagnostic Test Interferences. Methylene blue may interfere with tests for urinary pH.

METHYLERGONOVINE MALEATE

(Methergine)

(meth ill-er-goe-noe′veen)
Oxytocic
Ergot alkaloid

ACTIONS AND USES. Ergot alkaloid and congener of LSD. Induces rapid, sustained titanic uterine contraction that shortens third stage of labor and reduces blood loss. Has minimal vasoconstrictive activity. *For absorption, fate, contraindications, and adverse/side effects, see Ergotamine tartrate.*

Used for routine management after delivery of placenta and for postpartum atony, subinvolution, and hemorrhage. With full obstetric supervision, may be used during second stage of labor.

ROUTE AND DOSAGE. Oral: 0.2 mg three to four times daily in puerperium for maximum of 1 week. **Intramuscular:** 1 ml (0.2 mg) every 2 to 4 hours as necessary after delivery of placenta, after delivery of anterior shoulder, or during puerperium. **Intravenous (emergency use only):** 1 ml (0.2 mg), given slowly over 60-second period.

NURSING IMPLICATIONS

Ampuls containing discolored solution or visible particles should not be used. Store at room temperature between 15° and 30°C (59° and 86°F) unless otherwise directed by manufacturer. Protect from light.

Onset of action after oral administration, 5 to 10 minutes; after IV, immediate; after IM injection, 2 to 5 minutes. Duration of action after oral and IM: 3 hours; after IV: 45 minutes.

Monitor vital signs (particularly blood pressure) and uterine response during and following parenteral administration of methylergonovine until partum period is stabilized (about 1 or 2 hours).

Notify physician if blood pressure suddenly increases or if there are frequent periods of uterine relaxation.

See also Ergotamine tartrate (prototype ergot alkaloid).

M

METHYLPHENIDATE HYDROCHLORIDE

(Ritalin)

(meth-ill-fen'i-date)
Central stimulant
Piperidine
C II

ACTIONS AND USES. Piperidine derivative with pharmacologic actions and abuse potential qualitatively similar to those of amphetamine. Acts mainly on cerebral cortex. Exerts mild CNS and respiratory stimulation, with potency intermediate between those of amphetamine and caffeine. Effects more prominent on mental than on motor activities. Also believed to have an anorexiant effect.

Used as adjunctive therapy in attention deficit disorders or syndrome in hyperkinetic children, narcolepsy, mild depression, and apathetic or withdrawn senile behavior.

ABSORPTION AND FATE. Well absorbed from GI tract. Effects may persist 3 to 6 hours. Widely distributed in body fluids; crosses blood–brain barrier. Excreted in urine as metabolites.

CONTRAINDICATIONS AND PRECAUTIONS. Known hypersensitivity to the drug, marked anxiety, tension, agitation, severe depression, glaucoma, treatment of normal fatigue states, seizure disorders, EEG abnormalities. Safe use during pregnancy and in women of childbearing potential and children under age 6 not established. *Cautious Use:* history of convulsive disorders, hypertension, patients receiving pressor agents or MAO inhibitors, emotionally unstable patients (e.g., history of drug dependence, alcoholism).

ADVERSE/SIDE EFFECTS. Anorexia, dizziness, drowsiness, headache, insomnia, nervousness, blood pressure and pulse changes, palpitation, angina, tachycardia, arrhythmias, hypersensitivity reactions, visual disturbances, dyskinesia, seizures, abdominal pain, weight loss (especially in children). Also reported: leukopenia, anemia, scalp hair loss. *Overdosage:* hypertension, arrhythmias, vomiting, agitation, toxic psychosis, dry mucous membranes, mydriasis, hyperpyrexia, hyperreflexia, convulsions.

M

ROUTE AND DOSAGE. Oral: Adults: 10 mg two or three times a day; usual dose range 20 to 40 mg daily. *Highly individualized.* **Children:** Initial: 5 mg before breakfast and lunch, with gradual increments of 5 to 10 mg weekly. Daily dosage above 60 mg not recommended.

NURSING IMPLICATIONS

Administer 30 to 45 minutes before meals. To avoid insomnia, last dose should be taken before 6 PM.

Nervousness and insomnia (most common side effects) may require reduction of dosage or omission of afternoon or evening dose; however, they may diminish with time. Advise patients to report these and other adverse effects or paradoxic aggravation of symptoms.

Blood pressure and pulse should be monitored at appropriate intervals.

Advise patients to check weight at least two or three times weekly and to report weight loss. Height and weight should be checked in children, and failure to gain in either should be reported.

Periodic CBC and differential and platelet counts are advised during prolonged therapy.

Drug therapy in children should not be indefinite. If improvement is not observed after 1 month, drug should be discontinued. During prolonged therapy, periodic drug-free periods are recommended to assess the child's condition

Chronic abusive use can lead to tolerance, psychic dependence, and psychoses.

Careful supervision is required for drug withdrawal following prolonged use. Abrupt withdrawal may result in severe depression and psychotic behavior.

Classified as Schedule II drug under Federal Controlled Substances Act.

Drug Interactions. Methylphenidate may inhibit metabolism and thus potentiate the actions of **anticonvulsants, coumarin anticoagulants, phenylbutazone, tricyclic antidepressants,** and **vasopressors** (reduced dosage of these drugs may be required when given concomitantly with methylphenidate). Methylphenidate may decrease the hypotensive effect of **guanethidine.** There is possibility of hypertensive crisis with **furazolidone** and **MAO inhibitors.** Methylphenidate may be antagonized by **phenothiazine derivatives** and **propoxyphene.**

METHYLPREDNISOLONE
(Medrol)
METHYLPREDNISOLONE ACETATE
(depMedalone, Depo-Medrol, Depopred-40, Duralone, Medralone-40, Medrone-40; Mepred, Methylone, Pre-Dep, and others)
METHYLPREDNISOLONE SODIUM SUCCINATE
(A-MethaPred, Solu-Medrol)

(meth-ill-pred-niss'oh-lone)
Corticosteroid
Glucocorticoid

ACTIONS AND USES. Intermediate acting synthetic adrenal steroid with similar glucocorticoid activity but considerably less sodium and water retention effects than those of hydrocortisone (qv). On weight basis, 4 mg methylprednisolone is equivalent to 20 mg hydrocortisone. Acetate has longer duration of action and more rapid onset of activity than parent compound. Sodium succinate is characterized by rapid onset of action and is used for emergency therapy of short duration. *See Hydrocortisone.*

Used as an antiinflammatory agent in the management of acute and chronic inflammatory diseases, for palliative management of neoplastic diseases, and for control of severe acute and chronic allergic processes. High dose short-term therapy: management of acute, bronchial asthma, prevention of fat embolism in patient with long bone fracture.

M

ABSORPTION AND FATE. Peak effect: oral, 1 or 2 hours; IM, 4 to 8 days; intraarticular, intralesional, 7 days. Duration of effect: oral, 1.25 to 1.5 days; IM, 1 to 4 weeks, intraarticular, intralesional, 1 to 5 weeks. Plasma half-life: more than 3.5 hours. HPA (hypothalamic–pituitary–adrenal) axis suppression: 18 to 36 hours.

CONTRAINDICATIONS AND PRECAUTIONS. Systemic fungal infections. Safe use by children, during pregnancy (category C), and lactation not established. *Cautious Use:* Cushing's syndrome, GI ulceration, hypertension, varicella, vaccinia, diabetes mellitus, emotional instability or psychotic tendencies. *See also Hydrocortisone.*

ADVERSE/SIDE EFFECTS. Severe hypokalemia, congestive heart failure, euphoria, insomnia, delayed wound healing. *See also Hydrocortisone.*

ROUTE AND DOSAGE. All dosages are individualized according to severity of disease and response of patient. **Pediatric:** less than adult dosage and governed by severity of the condition rather than by a specific dose according to weight and age. **Oral:** 4 to 48 mg/day in single or divided doses. *Acetate:* **Intraarticular:** 4 to 80 mg (depending on size of joint); **Intralesional:** 20 to 60 mg; **Intramuscular:** 40 to 120 mg (every 1 to 4 weeks as necessary). **Rectal (retention enema):** 40 mg three to seven times/week for 2 or more weeks. **Topical Ointment:** 0.25 or 1% applied two or three times daily. *Sodium Succinate:* **Intramuscular, intravenous (direct or infusion):** Initial: 10 to 40 mg; may be repeated every 6 hours if necessary.

NURSING IMPLICATIONS

Tablet may be crushed before administration and taken with fluid of patient's choice.

The oral preparation will be less irritating if given with food.

Do not confuse Solu-Medrol (succinate salt) with Solu-Cortef (hydrocortisone sodium succinate).

Direct intravenous injection should be administered over one to several minutes.

Alternate day therapy *(see Index)* may be employed when methylprednisolone is given over long period of time.

Methylprednisolone sodium succinate solution should be used within 48 hours after preparation.

Avoid contacting eyes with the ointment. *See Hydrocortisone for nursing implications regarding use of topical formulation.*

Instruct patient not to alter established dosage regimen, i.e., not to increase, decrease or omit doses or change dose intervals. Withdrawal symptoms (rebound inflammation, fever) can be induced with sudden discontinuation of therapy.

Monitor urine for glucosuria. The diabetic may require increased doses of insulin or sulfonyl urea agent.

Instruct patient to report immediately onset of signs of hypocorticism adrenal insufficiency: fatigue, nausea, anorexia, joint pain, muscular weakness, dizziness, fever.

Medrol (methylprednisolone) contains tartrazine which can cause allergic reaction, including asthma in susceptible individuals. Frequently these people have a sensitivity to aspirin also.

Store at temperature 15° to 30° C (59° or 86°F). Prevent freezing.

See also Hydrocortisone (prototype glucocorticoid) for additional nursing implications and drug interactions.

METHYLTESTOSTERONE

(Android, Metandren, Oreton Methyl, Testred, Virilon)

(meth-ill-tess-toss'te-rone)
Androgen
Anabolic agent
Hormone

ACTIONS AND USES. Orally effective, short-acting steroid with androgen/anabolic activity ratio (1:1) similar to that of testosterone (qv), but less effective than its esters. Fails to produce full sexual maturation when administered to preadolescent male with complete testicular failure unless preceded by testosterone therapy.

Used as treatment for hypogonadism that starts in adult life after puberty; also used alone or combined with estrogen to treat menopausal symptoms and functional menstrual disorders. *See Testosterone.*

ABSORPTION AND FATE. Absorbed from oral mucosa and GI tract. All metabolites excreted in urine.

CONTRAINDICATIONS AND PRECAUTIONS. Hepatic dysfunction. *See also Testosterone.*

ADVERSE/SIDE EFFECTS. Cholestatic hepatitis with jaundice. *See also Testosterone.*

ROUTE AND DOSAGE. Oral: *Replacement:* 10 to 40 mg/day in divided doses, given after full androgenic effects are established by IM testosterone. *Postpartum breast engorgement:* 80 mg/day for 3 to 5 days. *Breast cancer:* 200 mg/day for duration of therapeutic response or for no longer than 3 months if no remission. **Buccal:** one-half oral dose.

NURSING IMPLICATIONS

Buccal tablet should be placed in upper or lower buccal pouch between cheek and gum. Instruct patient not to chew or swallow tablet and to avoid eating, drinking, or smoking until absorption is complete. Tablet requires at least 60 minutes to dissolve. Change location of absorption site with each dose.

Good oral hygiene should be stressed as a means to decrease infection of cheek membranes irritated by buccal formulation.

Instruct patient to report inflamed or painful oral membranes. In addition to physical discomfort, absorption rate is changed by altered mucosal surface.

Creatinuria is a frequent finding with use of this drug, but its significance is unclear. (Normal *urinary creatinine:* 15 to 25 mg/kg/24 hours.)

Treatment of breast cancer is usually restricted to women who are more than 1 year but less than 5 years postmenopause. If androgen treatment is going to be effective, it will be apparent within 3 months after therapy is instituted. When the disease again becomes progressive, therapy is stopped.

Since dosage sufficient to produce remission in breast cancer is quantitatively similar to that used for androgen replacement in the male, the female patient should be prepared for distressing and undesirable side effects of virilization *(see Index: Clinical signs and symptoms.)*

Advise female patient to report promptly if signs of virilism appear. Voice change and hirsutism may be irreversible, even after drug is withdrawn.

Instruct the male patient to report priapism or other signs of excess sexual stimulation. The physician will terminate methyltestosterone therapy.

Jaundice with or without pruritus appears to be dose-related. Instruct patient to report symptoms to physician. If liver function tests are altered at the same time, this drug will be withdrawn.

See also Testosterone (prototype androgen).

M

METHYPRYLON

(Noludar)

(meth-i-prye'lon)
Hypnotic
Piperidine
C III

ACTIONS AND USES. Piperidine derivative structurally related to glutethimide. Produces CNS depressant effects similar to those of short-acting barbiturates. Hypnotic doses suppress REM sleep.

Used as hypnotic for relief of simple insomnia. Sometimes used as sedative, but value for this purpose not established.

ABSORPTION AND FATE. Hypnotic dose induces sleep within 45 minutes; duration 5 to 8 hours. Plasma half-life 3 to 6 hours. Conjugated in liver; metabolites are secreted in bile and reabsorbed. Most of dose is excreted in urine as metabolites and their glucuronide conjugates; approximately 3% excreted unchanged.

CONTRAINDICATIONS AND PRECAUTIONS. Porphyria, known hypersensitivity to methyprylon, patient who is hallucinating or who is psychotic. Safe use during pregnancy and in women of childbearing potential, nursing mothers, and children under 12 years of age not established. *Cautious Use:* hepatic or renal impairment, addiction-prone individuals, mental depression, history of suicidal tendencies.

ADVERSE/SIDE EFFECTS. Infrequent: morning drowsiness, dizziness, nausea, vomiting, diarrhea, esophagitis, headache, paradoxic excitation, skin rash, exacerbation of intermittent porphyria. Reported, but causal relationship not established: neutropenia, thrombocytopenia. **Acute toxicity:** somnolence, confusion, constricted pupils, hyperpyrexia, hypothermia, shock, pulmonary edema, respiratory depression; occasionally during recovery: excitation, convulsions, delirium, hallucinations.

ROUTE AND DOSAGE. Oral: Adults: 200 to 400 mg before retiring; total daily dose should not exceed 400 mg. **Pediatric (over 12 years):** Initial: 50 mg at bedtime, increased up to 200 mg if required.

NURSING IMPLICATIONS

Hypnotic dose is administered 15 minutes before retiring. Prepare patient for sleep before administering drug.

In some patients, suppression of REM sleep may cause irritability, tension, confusion, and tremors.

Although tolerance develops to suppression of REM sleep, during chronic administration REM rebound may occur when drug is withdrawn: increased dreaming, nightmares, insomnia, hallucinations.

Tolerance may develop to hypnotic and sedative effects, but not to toxic effects.

Psychologic and physical dependence may occur, especially after prolonged use of large doses. Patient's continued need for methyprylon should be evaluated regularly.

Periodic blood counts are advised if drug is used repeatedly or over prolonged periods.

Warn patients about possible additive effects with alcohol and other CNS depressants.

Caution patient to avoid driving a car or engaging in other activities requiring mental alertness, until response to drug is known.

Gradual drug withdrawal is advised after prolonged use. Sudden discontinuation of drug may result in *withdrawal symptoms* similar to those following barbiturate dependence: confusion, marked nervousness, insomnia, sweating, polyuria, hyperreflexia, delirium, miosis, hallucinations, convulsion, death.

Treatment of overdosage: gastric lavage, general supportive measures (airway maintenance, assisted respiration, oxygen, IV fluids), pressor agent (levarternol, metaraminol), short-acting barbiturate for convulsions and excitation, close monitoring of vital signs and urinary output.

Classified as Schedule III drug under Federal Controlled Substances Act.

Preserved in tightly closed, light-resistant containers.

Diagnostic Test Interferences: Methyprylon may interfere with urinary steroid determinations.

METHYSERGIDE
(Sansert)

(meth-i-ser′jide)
Antimigraine
Ergot alkaloid

ACTIONS AND USES. Ergot derivative and congener of LSD. Unlike ergotamine (qv), has weak vasoconstrictor and oxytoxic actions. Action mechanism in migraine prevention unclear. Serotonin (a strong vasoconstrictor) levels are reduced during an attack. Methysergide replaces serotonin on cranial artery receptor sites during an attack, thereby preserving vasoconstriction afforded by serotonin. Ineffective treatment of acute attacks. Prolonged use has been known to promote fibrotic processes.

Used in prophylactic management of severe recurrent migraine, cluster, and other vascular headaches unresponsive to other antimigraine drugs. Also has been used to combat diarrhea and malabsorption associated with GI hypermotility in carcinoid disease, as well as for postgastrectomy dumping syndrome.

ABSORPTION AND FATE. Metabolic fate unknown, but thought to be well absorbed. Widely distributed to all tissues, and metabolized in liver.

CONTRAINDICATIONS AND PRECAUTIONS. Fibrotic processes, pulmonary or collagen diseases, edema, serious infections, debilitated states. *See also Ergotamine Tartrate.*

ADVERSE/SIDE EFFECTS. CNS: insomnia, drowsiness, vertigo, mild euphoria, confusion, excitement, feelings of unreality or depersonalization, distortions of body image, depression, anxiety, hallucinations, nightmares, ataxia, hyperesthesia, paresthesia. **CV:** peripheral edema, thrombophlebitis, claudication, impaired circulation, angina of effort, ECG changes, postural hypotension, tachycardia. **Dermatologic:** facial flushing, telangiectasia, rash, excessive hair loss. **Fibrotic complications:** *retroperitoneal fibrosis* (fatigue, malaise, fever, urinary obstruction with girdle or flank pain, dysuria, oliguria, polyuria, increased BUN and sedimentation rate), *pleuropulmonary fibrosis* (dyspnea, chest pain and tightness, pleural friction rubs and effusion) and *cardiac fibrosis* (fibrotic thickening of cardiac valves with murmurs). **GI:** nausea, vomiting, heartburn, hyperchlorhydria, abdominal pain, diarrhea, constipation. **Other:** neutropenia, eosinophilia, weakness, arthralgia, myalgia, weight gain, scotomata, nasal stuffiness, positive direct Coombs' test.

ROUTE AND DOSAGE. Oral: 4 to 8 mg daily in divided doses.

M

NURSING IMPLICATIONS

GI side effects can frequently be prevented by gradual introduction of medication and by administering drug with meals.

One or 2 days of drug therapy are required before protective drug action is realized; at end of therapy, protection continues 2 days beyond last dose.

Therapeutic trial period of 3 weeks is advised to determine patient's response to methysergide. If no response occurs in this time, it is unlikely that longer administration will be of benefit.

Pretreatment and periodic assessments of cardiac status, renal function, blood count, and sedimentation rate are advised.

Since incidence of side effects is relatively high (usually reversible with discontinuation of drug), patient should be examined regularly for development of fibrotic and vascular complications: auscultate heart and lungs; check peripheral pulses, and auscultate major vessels for bruits; observe for signs of phlebitis or venous obstruction. Also, observe and question patient concerning presence of CNS symptoms and other possible adverse effects *(see Adverse/Side Effects).*

Instruct patient to report the following immediately: onset of abdominal, back, or chest pain; dyspnea; leg pains while walking; cold, numb, or painful extremities; fever; dysuria or other urinary problems; edema; weight gain; other unusual signs and symptoms.

Counsel patient to weigh self daily, and teach patient how to check extremities for edema.

Caloric restriction and reduction of salt intake may be prescribed. Consult physician and instruct patient accordingly.

Since postural hypotension is a possible side effect, advise patient to make position changes slowly, particularly from recumbent to upright posture, and to dangle legs a few minutes before standing. Also instruct patient to lie down if faintness occurs.

Continuous administration of methysergide should not exceed 6 months without a medication-free interval of 3 to 4 weeks. Drug may be readministered after drug-free interval, if necessary.

To avoid "headache rebound," drug should be withdrawn gradually over 2- or 3-week period preceding discontinuation. Caution patient not to stop medication abruptly because of this possibility.

Contains *tartrazine* which may cause allergic-type reaction including bronchial asthma in susceptible individuals, who often are also sensitive to aspirin.

Patients with migraine should be helped to identify underlying emotional and physical stresses that may precipitate attacks and should learn how to deal with them. Adequate relaxation, recreation, and sleep may help to reduce severity and frequency of attacks.

Preserved in tight, light-resistant containers preferably at 15° to 30°C (59° to 86°F) unless otherwise directed by manufacturer.

METOCLOPRAMIDE HYDROCHLORIDE

(Maxeran, Reglan)

(met-oh-kloe-pra′mide)
Cholinergic
(Parasympathomimetic)
Antiemetic

M

ACTIONS AND USES. Potent central dopamine receptor antagonist. Structurally related to procainamide but has little antiarrhythmic or anesthetic activity. Exact mechanism of action not clear, but appears to sensitize GI smooth muscle to effects of acetylcholine by direct action. Increases resting tone of esophageal sphincter (thereby increasing lower esophageal sphincter pressure), and increases tone and amplitude of upper GI contractions. As a result, gastric emptying and intestinal transit are accelerated with little effect if any on gastric, biliary or pancreatic secretions. Antiemetic action results from drug-induced elevation of CTZ threshold and enhanced gastric emptying (which blocks the gastric stasis that precedes vomiting). Has no apparent effect on seizure threshold. Inhibits central and peripheral effects of apomorphine and indirectly stimulates release of prolactin. Directly stimulates secretion of aldosterone, but has no effect on plasma renin activity, plasma K or cortisol concentrations. High doses produce neuroleptic actions similar to those of antipsychotic agents (e.g., phenothiazines). Metoclopramide actions can be reduced or abolished by anticholinergics. Mutagenicity and carcinogenicity potential not known.

Used for management of diabetic gastric stasis (gastroparesis); to prevent nausea and vomiting associated with emetogenic cancer chemotherapy (e.g., cisplatin, dacarbazine); to facilitate intubation of small bowel. *Unlabeled Uses:* symptomatic treatment of gastroesophageal reflux, treatment of acute and postsurgical gastric stasis and peptic ulcer; prevention of nausea and vomiting associated with drugs other than antineoplastics, and with radiation therapy.

ABSORPTION AND FATE. Rapidly absorbed after oral administration (except in presence of gastric paresis). Onset of action in 30 to 60 minutes following oral, 10 to 15 minutes following IM, and 1 to 3 minutes following IV dose. Duration of effects 1 to 2 hours. Subject to first-pass metabolism following oral administration; bioavailability 30 to 100%; protein-binding: 13 to 22%. Half-life: 4 hours. Distributed to most body tissues and fluids including milk. Crosses blood–brain and placenta barriers. Minimally metabolized by liver; excreted in urine and feces (via bile); minimally removed by hemodialysis or peritoneal dialysis.

CONTRAINDICATIONS AND PRECAUTIONS. Sensitivity or intolerance to metoclopramide; history of seizure disorders, concurrent use of drugs that can cause extrapyramidal symptoms; pheochromocytoma, presence of mechanical GI obstruction or perforation, patient with history of breast cancer. Safe use during pregnancy (category B), in fertile women, and in nursing mothers not established. *Cautious Use:* congestive heart failure, hypokalemia, renal dysfunction, GI hemorrhage, history of intermittent porphyria.

ADVERSE/SIDE EFFECTS. CNS: mild sedation (50% patients), fatigue, restlessness, agitation, headache, insomnia, disorientation, extrapyramidal symptoms (acute dystonic type). **CV (rare):** hypotension, supraventricular tachycardia. **GI:** nausea, constipation, diarrhea, dry mouth. **Other:** urticarial or maculopapular rash, glossal or periorbital edema, methemoglobinemia, galactorrhea, gynecomastia, amenorrhea, impotence.

ROUTE AND DOSAGE. *For diabetic gastroparesis:* **Oral:** 10 mg four times daily for 2 to 8 weeks. *Small bowel intubation; radiologic examination:* **Intravenous: Adult:** 10 mg (2 ml) as single dose over 1 to 2 minutes. **Children (6 to 14 years):** 2.5 to 5 mg (0.5 to 1 ml); **(under 6 years):** 0.1 mg/kg. *Prophylaxis for cancer drug-induced emesis:* **Oral:** 2 mg/kg 1 hour before antineoplastic administration; repeated if necessary three times at 2-hour intervals after initial dose. **Intravenous infusion:** 2 mg/kg 30 minutes before; repeated if necessary twice at 2-hour intervals after initial dose.

NURSING IMPLICATIONS

Oral form is usually taken 30 minutes before meals and at bedtime.

Each ml of the injection form contains about 0.14 mEq of sodium (sodium bisulfite and NaCl).

The compatibility of metoclopropamide with other admixtures depends upon multiple factors including temperature, drug concentration, and pH. Consult pharmacist for needed information.

The PVC bags of metoclopramide should be protected from light during infusion (use of aluminum foil or a thick cotton cover).

Discard open ampules; do not store for future use.

The injection form contains sodium metabisulfite as antioxidant. If patient has history of allergy to *sulfiting agents,* this product should be avoided.

Extrapyramidal symptoms *(see Index)* are most likely to occur in children, young adults and with high dose treatment of vomiting associated with cancer chemotherapy. Report immediately the onset of restlessness, involuntary movements, facial grimacing, rigidity, or tremors. Usual treatment: 50 mg diphenhydramine IM.

Therapeutic effectiveness in patient with diabetic gastroparesis is indicated by relief of anorexia, nausea, vomiting, persistent fullness after meals.

During early treatment period, serum aldosterone may be elevated; however, after prolonged administration periods, it returns to pretreatment level.

Monitor for possible Na retention and hypokalemia especially if patient has congestive heart failure or cirrhosis.

Adverse reactions associated with increased serum prolactin concentration (galactorrhea, menstrual disorders, gynecomastia) usually disappear within a few weeks or months after drug treatment is stopped.

Caution patients to avoid driving and other potentially hazardous activities for a few hours after drug administration.

Therapy beyond 12 weeks has not been evaluated sufficiently to recommend prolonged use.

Store in light-resistant bottle at 15° to 30°C (59° to 86°F). Tablets are stable for 3 years; solutions and injections, for 5 years.

Diagnostic Test Interferences. Metoclopramide increases **serum prolactin** levels, and may increase **aldosterone** (during early treatment period) and **thyrotropin** levels.

Drug Interactions: Metoclopramide

Plus	Interactions
Acetominophen, alcohol, levodopa, Tetracyclines	Accelerated intestinal absorption: unpredictable onset of action
Alcohol and other CNS depressants (including antianxiety agents)	Additive sedation
Anticholinergics (e.g., atropine); opiate analgesics	Antagonize metoclopromide's effect on GI motility
Digoxin (slow release) (brand specific)	Decreased pharmacologic effects of digoxin. (Not a problem in USA.) Interaction can be minimized by use of rapidly dissolving preparations, e.g., Lanoxicaps or Lanoxin
Psychotropics (e.g., phenothiazines)	Promotion of extrapyramidal symptoms

METOCURINE IODIDE

(Metubine)

(met-oh-kyoo'reen)

Skeletal muscle relaxant (nondepolarizing)

M

ACTIONS AND USES. Semisynthetic nondepolarizing neuromuscular blocking agent. Pharmacologic effects almost identical to those of tubocurarine but is reportedly two to three times more potent. Has a slightly shorter duration of action, less histamine-releasing effect, and produces less ganglionic blockade.

Used as adjunct to anesthesia to induce skeletal muscle relaxation. Has been used to reduce intensity of skeletal muscle contractions in drug- or electrically-induced convulsions and to facilitate endotracheal intubation.

ABSORPTION AND FATE. Peak effect within 3 to 5 minutes following IV administration. Duration of neuromuscular blockade: 35 to 90 minutes depending on dose and general anesthesia used. Half-life: 3.6 hours; about 35% bound to plasma proteins. Approximately 50% excreted unchanged in urine; small amounts excreted in bile. Crosses placenta.

CONTRAINDICATIONS AND PRECAUTIONS. Hypersensitivity to metocurine or to iodides; allergy, asthma. *Cautious Use:* myasthenia gravis, renal, hepatic, or pulmonary impairment, respiratory depression, electrolyte disturbances. *See also Tubocurarine.*

ADVERSE/SIDE EFFECTS. Same toxic potential as for tubocurarine (qv). Hypotension, dizziness increased salivation, bronchospasm, respiratory depression, decreased GI motility and tone, hypersensitivity reactions.

ROUTE AND DOSAGE. Intravenous: Dose depends on type anesthetic used, e.g., cyclopropane: 2 to 4 mg; ether: 1.5 to 3 mg; nitrous oxide: 4 to 7 mg. Drug is administered over 30 to 60 seconds. Subsequent doses: 0.5 to 1 mg as required. *Electroshock therapy:* 1.75 to 5.5 mg.

NURSING IMPLICATIONS

Complete recovery from IV dose may require several hours.

A peripheral nerve stimulator may be used to monitor response.

Metocurine is incompatible with alkaline solutions. Do not administer in same syringe with barbiturates, meperidine, or morphine because a precipitate will form.
Metocurine solution should be protected from prolonged exposure to heat and direct sunlight.
Store at controlled room temperature preferably between 15° and 30°C (59° and 86°F).
See Tubocurarine chloride (prototype nondepolarizing skeletal muscle relaxant).

METOLAZONE

(Diulo, Zaroxolyn)

(me-tole'a-zone)
Diuretic
Antihypertensive
Sulfonamide derivative

ACTIONS AND USES. Quinazoline derivative diuretic, structurally and pharmacologically similar to chlorothiazide (qv). Appears to be more effective as a diuretic than thiazides in patients with severe renal failure.

Used in management of hypertension as sole agent or to enhance effectiveness of other antihypertensives in severe form of hypertension; also used in treatment of edema associated with congestive heart failure and renal disease.

ABSORPTION AND FATE. Incompletely absorbed (65% in normal subjects, 40% of patients with cardiac disease). Diuresis begins in 1 hour, peaks in 2 hours and lasts for 12 to 24 hours. Half-life (normal kidneys) 5.3 hours. Enterohepatic cycling and high degree of protein binding prolongs duration of action. 79 to 95% drug excreted in urine. Crosses placenta and enters breast milk.

CONTRAINDICATIONS AND PRECAUTIONS. Anuria, hypokalemia, hepatic coma or precoma; hypersensitivity to metolazone and sulfonamides; pregnancy, lactation. *Cautious Use:* history of gout, allergies, concomitant use of digitalis glycosides, renal and hepatic dysfunction. *See also Chlorothiazide.*

ADVERSE/SIDE EFFECTS. Cholestatic jaundice, vertigo, orthostatic hypotension, venous thrombosis, leukopenia, dehydration, hypokalemia, hyperuricemia, hyperglycemia. *See also Chlorothiazide.*

ROUTE AND DOSAGE. Oral: Adult: *Edema of cardiac failure:* Initial: 5 to 10 mg once daily; *edema of renal failure:* 5 to 20 mg once daily. Maintenance: dose lowered to minimum effective level. *Hypertension:* Initial: 2.5 to 5 mg daily in morning. Maintenance: dose determined by patient's blood pressure response. *Highly individualized.*

NURSING IMPLICATIONS

Schedule doses to avoid nocturia and interrupted sleep. Administer oral drug early in AM after eating to prevent gastric irritation; (if given in two doses, schedule second dose no later than 3 PM).
Geriatric patients may be more sensitive to effects of usual adult dose; thus overdosage and adverse reactions should be anticipated.
When adverse reactions are moderate to severe, metolazone therapy should be terminated.
Antihypertensive effects may be observed in 3 or 4 days, but 3 to 4 weeks are required for maximum effect.
Warn patient not to drink alcohol while taking metolazone since it potentiates orthostatic hypotension.

Photosensitivity, paresthesias, agranulocytosis, pancreatitis (adverse reactions of most thiazides) do not appear to be problems with use of this drug.
Collaborate with dietitian with respect to a palatable well-planned diet. Antihypertensive therapy may require as adjunct a high-K, low-Na, and low-calorie diet.
Serum K should be determined at regular intervals while patient is on maintenance therapy. Prolonged treatment with metolazone and inadequate K intake increase potential for hypokalemia (muscle weakness and cramps, thirst, nausea, vomiting, mental confusion polyuria).
Hypokalemia is rarely severe in most patients on prolonged therapy with thiazides, if present at all. To prevent onset, urge patient to eat a normal diet (usually includes K-rich foods such as potatoes, fruit juices, cereals, skim milk) and to include a banana (about 370 mg K) and at least 6 ounces orange juice (about 330 mg K) every day.
If hypokalemia develops, dietary K supplement of 1000 to 2000 mg (25 to 50 mEq) is usually an adequate treatment.
Store tablets in tightly closed container at 15° to 30°C (59° to 86°F) unless otherwise specified by manufacturer.
See Chlorothiazide (prototype thiazide).

METOPROLOL TARTRATE
(Betaloc, Lopressor)

(me-toe'proe-lole)
Antihypertensive
Beta-adrenergic blocking agent

M

ACTIONS AND USES. Relatively selective $beta_1$-adrenergic blocking agent. Like propranolol, comparatively inhibits access of catecholamines to $beta_1$-adrenergic receptors, especially within myocardium (cardioselective action). Suppresses conduction velocity through SA and AV nodes and decreases myocardial automaticity. Mechanism of antihypertensive action not known but may be related to decrease in cardiac output and to reduction in peripheral resistance by blocking norepinephrine release. Reportedly as effective as propranolol in reducing both standing and supine blood pressures. In contrast to propranolol, has little or no membrane-stabilizing quinidinelike effect on heart and also does not block $beta_2$-adrenergic receptors located chiefly in vascular and bronchial smooth muscle except at higher doses. Also unlike propranolol, causes less inhibition of glycogenolysis in skeletal and cardiac muscles, less blocking of insulin release, and does not significantly inhibit isoproterenol-induced bronchodilation. Therefore, generally preferred for use in patients prone to bronchospasm (together with a $beta_2$ agonist such as terbutaline), Raynaud's disease, and diabetes mellitus. Metoprolol decreases plasma renin levels.

Used as step 2 agent in stepped care approach in management of mild to severe hypertension alone or concomitantly with diuretic therapy (usually a thiazide) and/or a vasodilator (e.g., hydralazine or prazosin). *Investigational Use:* prophylactic management of stable angina pectoris.

ABSORPTION AND FATE. Rapidly and almost completely absorbed from GI tract. Undergoes about 50% first-pass metabolism. Peak effects in 1½ to 4 hours. Duration of action (dose related): 13 to 19 hours; with chronic therapy, antihypertensive effect may persist up to 4 weeks. Widely distributed to body tissues. Highest concentrations in heart, liver, lungs, and saliva. Crosses blood–brain barrier. About 11 to 12% protein bound. Half-life: 3 to 4 hours. Extensively metabolized in liver. Eliminated by kidney primarily as minimally active metabolites and about 3 to 10% unchanged drug. Approximately 95% of single dose excreted within 72 hours. Crosses placenta. Enters breast milk.

CONTRAINDICATIONS AND PRECAUTIONS. Cardiogenic shock, sinus bradycardia, heart block greater than first degree, overt cardiac failure, right ventricular failure secondary to pulmonary hypertension. Safe use during pregnancy (category C), in women of childbearing potential, in nursing mothers, and in children not established. *Cautious Use:* impaired hepatic or renal function, cardiomegaly, congestive heart failure controlled by digitalis and diuretics; A-V conduction defects, bronchial asthma and other bronchospastic diseases, history of allergy, thyrotoxicosis, diabetes mellitus, peripheral vascular disease.

ADVERSE/SIDE EFFECTS. **Allergic:** erythematous rash, fever, muscle aches, sore throat, laryngospasms, respiratory distress. **CNS:** dizziness, fatigue, headache, insomnia, nightmares, increased dreaming, hallucinations, mental depression. **CV:** bradycardia, palpitation, cold extremities, Raynaud's phenomenon, intermittent claudication, angina pectoris, congestive heart failure, intensification of AV block, AV dissociation, complete heart block, cardiac arrest. **Dermatologic:** dry skin, pruritus, alopecia (reversible), skin eruptions. **EENT:** visual disturbances, inflamed conjunctiva and eyelids, punctate keratitis, keratoconjunctivitis, corneal ulcerations, dry eyes (decreased tear production), tinnitus. **GI:** nausea, heartburn, gastric pain, diarrhea or constipation, flatulence. **Hematologic:** eosinophilia, agranulocytosis, thrombocytopenic and nonthrombocytopenic purpura. **Other:** dry mouth and mucous membranes, sweating, restless legs; hypoglycemia, bronchospasm (with high doses), Peyronie's disease (rare). *See also Propranolol.*

ROUTE AND DOSAGE. **Oral:** Initial: 50 mg twice daily. May be increased at weekly (or longer) intervals until optimum blood pressure reduction obtained. Maintenance: 100 mg twice daily (range 100 to 450 mg/day in divided doses). Available in 50 and 100 mg tablets.

NURSING IMPLICATIONS

Reportedly, ingestion with food slightly enhances absorption of metoprolol. However, administration with food is not essential, but it is important that drug be given with or without food consistently to minimize possible variations in bioavailability.

Take apical pulse before administering drug. If blood pressure is not stabilized also take this reading before giving drug. Report to physician significant changes in rate, rhythm, or quality of pulse or variations in blood pressure.

Patient receiving metoprolol at home should be informed about usual pulse rate and should be instructed to take radial pulse before each dose. Advise patient to report to physician if it is slower than base rate or becomes irregular. Consult physician for parameters.

Baseline and regularly scheduled evaluations should be made of blood cell counts, blood glucose (diabetic patients), cardiac function, hepatic and renal function.

Insomnia or increased dreaming may be reduced by avoiding late evening doses.

For patients with hypertension, take several readings close to the end of a 12-hour dosing interval to evaluate adequacy of dosage, particularly in patients on twice daily doses. Some patients require doses three times a day to maintain satisfactory control.

Maximal effect on blood pressure reduction is achieved usually after 1 week of therapy.

Hypertensive patients with congestive heart failure controlled by digitalis and diuretics must be closely observed for impending heart failure: dyspnea on exertion, orthopnea, night cough, edema (tight shoes or rings, puffiness), distended neck veins. Monitor intake and output, daily weight; auscultate daily for pulmonary rales.

Patients with diabetes mellitus should be monitored closely. Metoprolol may mask typical symptoms of hypoglycemia such as blood pressure changes and increased pulse rate; may prolong hypoglycemia. Alert patient to other possible signs of hypoglycemia not affected by metoprolol that should be reported: sweating, fatigue, hunger, inability to concentrate.

Since metoprolol masks signs of hyperthyroidism (tachycardia), patients with thyrotoxicosis must be closely monitored. Abrupt withdrawal may precipitate thyroid storm.

Instruct patient to wear warm clothing during cold weather, to avoid prolonged exposure to cold, and not to smoke. Advise patient to report cold, painful, or tender feet or hands or other symptoms of Raynaud's disease (intermittent pallor, cyanosis or redness, paresthesias). Physician may prescribe a vasodilator.

Inform patient that most adverse effects tend to be mild and transient and that they generally disappear with continued therapy.

Instruct patient to report immediately to physician the onset of ocular symptoms.

If mouth dryness is bothersome, advise patient that the following measures may provide relief: rinse mouth frequently with clear warm water; increase noncalorie liquid intake if it has been inadequate; sugarless gum or lemondrops. If these measures fail, consult physician about use of artificial saliva, e.g., Xero-Lube, Moi-stir, Salivart (available OTC).

Eye dryness may be relieved by use of sterile artificial tears, e.g., Tears Naturale, among others (available OTC).

Since metoprolol may cause dizziness, particularly during early therapy, advise patient to avoid driving and other potentially hazardous activities until drug effects are known.

Emphasize importance of compliance and caution patient not to alter established dosage regimen, i.e., not to omit, increase or decrease dosage or change dosage interval without consent of physician.

Whether or not metoprolol should be withdrawn prior to surgery remains controversial. Anesthetist should be informed about metoprolol use prior to general anesthesia.

When metoprolol is to be discontinued, dosage should be reduced gradually over a period of 1 to 2 weeks. Sudden withdrawal can result in increase in anginal attacks and myocardial infarction in patients with angina pectoris and thyroid storm in patients with hyperthyroidism.

M

Because of beta blocking action usual rise in pulse rate may not occur in response to stress situations such as fever or following vigorous exercise. Activity programs must be highly individualized. Consult physician for guidelines.

Drug should be withdrawn if patient presents symptoms of mental depression because it can progress to catatonia. Possible symptoms of depression: disinterest in people, surroundings, food, personal hygiene; withdrawal, apathy, sadness, difficulty in concentrating, insomnia.

Advisable for patients on prolonged metoprolol therapy to wear or carry medical identification such as Medic Alert. Instruct patient to inform dentist or surgeon that he is taking metoprolol.

Stored in tight, light-resistant container.

Diagnostic Test Interferences. In common with other beta-blockers, metoprolol may cause elevated **BUN** and **serum creatinine levels** (patients with severe heart disease), elevated **serum transaminase, alkaline phosphatase, lactate dehydrogenase,** and **serum uric acid.**

Drug Interactions: Metoprolel

Plus	Interactions
Barbiturates Indomethacin Rifampin	Possibility of decreased pharmacologic effects of metoprolol
Cimetidine Methimazole Propylthiouracil Oral contraceptives	Possibility of increased pharmacologic effects of metoprolol

Plus (cont.)	Interactions (cont.)
Lidocaine, Prazosin	Metoprolol may increase pharmacologic effects of these drugs
Digitalis and other cardiac glycosides	Additive bradycardia
Hydralazine	Pharmacologic effects of both drugs may be increased. Can cause pulmonary hypertension in patients with uremia
MAO inhibitors	Concurrent use not recommended (based on theoretical considerations)
Reserpine and other catecholamine-depleting drugs	Additive hypotension and bradycardia
Sympathomimetics	Mutually antagonistic

PROTOTYPE

METRONIDAZOLE

(Flagyl, Metryl, Neo-Tric, Novonidazol, Protostat, Satric)

(me-troe-ni'da-zole)
Antiinfective
Antiprotozoal
Amebicide

ACTIONS AND USES. Synthetic compound with direct trichomonicidal and amebecidal activity against *Trichomonas vaginalis* (causes a venereal disease), *Entamoeba histolytica,* and *Giardia lamblia.* Also exhibits antibacterial activity against obligate anaerobic bacteria, gram-negative anaerobic bacilli and *Clostridia.* Microaerophilic streptococci and most aerobic bacteria are resistant. Metronidazole enters bacterial cells more readily under aerobic conditions; after reduction in the cell, it binds to and degrades DNA. Frequency of postoperative infection and nonspore forming anaerobic infections reported to be decreased with prophylactic use of the drug before and up to 7 days after surgery.

Used in treatment of asymptomatic and symptomatic trichomoniasis in both females and males; acute intestinal amebiasis and amebic liver abscess. *Investigational Uses:* include preoperative prophylaxis in colorectal surgery, elective hysterectomy or vaginal repair, and emergency appendectomy.

ABSORPTION AND FATE. Well absorbed after oral administration. Peak serum concentration usually in 1 to 2 hours. Distributed widely to all tissues including brain; therapeutic levels achieved in abscesses, bile, cerebrospinal fluid, empyema fluid, breast milk, and saliva. Only slightly bound (1 to 8%) to human plasma protein. Elimination half-life range: 6.2 to 11.5 hours. Accumulates in presence of impaired renal function; major route of elimination in urine. Rapidly crosses placenta and is secreted in breast milk. Concentration in saliva and breast milk during treatment approximates that in serum.

CONTRAINDICATIONS AND PRECAUTIONS. History of hypersensitivity to metronidazole, blood dyscrasias, active CNS disease, first trimester of pregnancy, nursing mothers. *Cautious Use:* coexistent candidiasis, second and third trimesters of pregnancy.

ADVERSE/SIDE EFFECTS. Allergic: rash, urticaria, pruritus, flushing. **CNS:** vertigo, headache, ataxia, incoordination (rare), confusion, irritability, depression, restlessness, weakness, fatigue, drowsiness, insomnia, sensory neuropathy, paresthesias. **Genitourinary:** polyuria, dysuria, pyuria, incontinence, cystitis, decreased libido, dyspareunia, dryness of vagina and vulva, sense of pelvic pressure. **GI:** nausea, vomiting, anorexia, epigastric distress, abdominal cramps, diarrhea, constipation, dry mouth, metallic or bitter taste. **Other:** moderate neutropenia, leukopenia; nasal congestion, fever, fleeting joint pains, ECG changes (flattening of T wave); fungal overgrowth of *Candida;* proctitis.

ROUTE AND DOSAGE. Oral: *Trichomoniasis:* One day therapy: 2 Gm in single or two divided doses. Seven day course: 250 mg three times daily for 7 days. *Amebiasis:* **Adults:** 500 to 750 mg three times daily for 5 to 10 days. **Children:** 35 to 50 mg/kg/24 hours in 3 equal doses for 10 days. *Anaerobic infections:* **Intravenous:** Loading dose: 15 mg/kg infused over 1-hour period. Maintenance: 7.5 mg/kg IV or PO every 6 hours. (First maintenance dose should be 6 hours after loading dose.) Maximum recommended dose: 4 Gm/24 hours.

NURSING IMPLICATIONS

Tablets may be crushed before ingestion if patient cannot swallow them whole.

Administer oral preparation immediately before, with, or immediately after meals or with food or milk to reduce Gi distress.

Dosage regimens are individualized sometimes on the basis of anticipated compliance. Some patients cannot be relied upon to take eight tablets in 1 day. Caution the patient to adhere closely to the established regimen without schedule interruption or changing the dose.

Parenteral administration:

- Do not give direct IV bolus injection because of low pH of reconstituted product.
- Sequence for preparing solution *(important):* (a) reconstitution, (b) dilution in IV solution, (c) pH neutralization with sodium bicarbonate injection.
- Avoid use of aluminum-containing equipment when manipulating drug IV product (including syringes equipped with aluminum needles or hubs).
- Avoid admixtures with metronidazole.
- CO_2 will be generated when neutralized with sodium bicarbonate; release of pressure within container may be necessary.
- A precipitate may signify a higher pH than desired (i.e., above 7.0).
- Precipitation occurs if neutralized solution is refrigerated. Use diluted and neutralized solution within 24 hours of preparation.

The 7-day regimen for trichomoniasis reportedly has a higher cure rate than the single day schedule. In addition, with the extended treatment period, reinfection of the female may be minimized long enough to treat sexual contacts.

Presence of trichomonads should be confirmed by wet smear and/or by cultures prior to start of therapy for trichomoniasis and prior to a course of retreatment.

Total and differential leukocyte counts are recommended before, during and after therapy, especially if a second course is necessary.

During therapy for trichomoniasis it is recommended that the patient refrain from intercourse unless the male partner wears a condom to prevent reinfection.

Sexual partners should receive concurrent treatment. Asymptomatic trichomoniasis in the male is a frequent source of reinfection of the female; therefore, it is recommended that treatment be given even if the male partner has a negative culture.

Therapy should be discontinued immediately if symptoms of CNS toxicity develop, e.g., ataxia, tremor, incoordination, paresthesias, numbness, impairment of pain or touch sensation.

Warn patient that ingestion of alcohol during metronidazole therapy may induce a disulfiram reaction (sweating, flushing, vomiting, headache, abdominal cramps).

Inform patient that urine may appear dark or reddish brown (especially with higher than recommended doses). This is thought to be caused by a metabolite and appears to have no clinical significance.

Women with trichomoniasis should be advised not to wear pantyhose or tight underwear and to avoid bubble baths. Also review perineal hygiene technique.

Advise patient to report symptoms of candidal overgrowth: furry tongue, color changes of tongue, glossitis, stomatitis; vaginitis, curdlike, milky vaginal discharge; proctitis. Treatment with a candicidal agent may be indicated.

Therapy instituted during the second or third trimester of pregnancy should be over a 7-day period. The 1-day course of treatment produces a high serum level that may reach fetal circulation.

4 to 6 weeks are allowed to elapse before the decision is made to repeat treatment.

Repeated feces examinations, usually up to 3 months, are necessary to assure that amebae have been eliminated.

Methods of controlling and preventing amebiasis include health education in personal hygiene, particularly hand washing after defecation and before preparing or eating food, sanitary disposal of feces, sanitary water supply, and fly control. *See Index: Nursing Interventions: amebiasis.*

Diagnostic Test Interferences: Metronidazole may interfere with certain chemical analyses for SGOT, resulting in decreased values.

Store drug in tightly closed, light-resistant containers preferably at 15° to 30°C (59° and 86°F) unless otherwise directed by manufacturer. Do not freeze.

Drug Interactions: Metronidazole

Plus	Interactions
Alcohol	Disulfiram reaction
Disulfiram	Acute psychotic reaction due to combined toxicity
Warfarin	Potentiation of hypoprothrombinemic effect of warfarin

M

METYROSINE

(Alpha-methyltyrosine, Alpha-MT, AMPT, Demser)

(me-tye'roe-seen)
Enzyme inhibitor

ACTIONS AND USES. By blocking the enzyme tyrosine hydroxylase, metyrosine inhibits the conversion of tyrosine to DOPA (dihydroxyphenylalanine), which is the initial and rate-setting step in synthesis of catecholamines (dopamine, epinephrine, norepinephrine). In patients with pheochromocytoma (adrenal tumor that causes overproduction of catecholamines, mainly epinephrine and norepinephrine), catecholamine synthesis may be reduced by as much as 80%, resulting in amelioration of hypertensive attacks and associated symptoms *(see Nursing Implications).*

Used for short-term management of phenochromocytoma until surgery is performed, in long-term control when surgery is contraindicated, and in patients with malignant phenochromocytoma. Has been used in selected patients with schizophrenia to potentiate antipsychotic effects of phenothiazines.

ABSORPTION AND FATE. Well-absorbed from GI tract. Maximal lowering of blood pressure during first 2 days after administration, with returns to pretreatment level usually within 2 or 3 days. Peak reduction in urinary catecholamines in 2 or 3 days (with multiple doses) and return to pretreatment values in 3 or 4 days. Half-life: 3.4 to 3.7 hours. Minimally metabolized. About 53 to 85% of dose excreted in urine as unchanged drug.

CONTRAINDICATIONS AND PRECAUTIONS. Hypersensitivity to metyrosine; use for control of essential hypertension. Safe use during pregnancy, in nursing women, and in children under 12 years not established. *Cautious Use:* impaired hepatic or renal function.

ADVERSE/SIDE EFFECTS. CNS: sedation, fatigue; extrapyramidal signs: drooling, difficulty in speaking (dysarthria), tremors, jaw-stiffness (trismus); frank parkinsonism, psychic disturbances (anxiety, depression, hallucinations, disorientation, confusion), headache, muscle spasms. **GI:** diarrhea, nausea, vomiting, abdominal pain, dry mouth. **Hypersensitivity:** rash, urticaria. **Renal:** transient dysuria, oliguria, crystalluria, urolithiasis, hematuria, enuresis. **Reprod:** impotence, failure of ejaculation, breast swelling, galactorrhea. **Other:** peripheral edema, nasal stuffiness, shortness of breath, eosinophilia, increased AST (SGOT).

ROUTE AND DOSAGE. Oral: Adults and children (over 12 years): Initial: 250 mg four times daily; increased by 250 to 500 mg daily, if necessary. Not to exceed 4 Gm/day in divided doses. Maintenance: 2 to 3 Gm/day in four divided doses. When used for preoperative preparation, optimum effective dosage given for at least 5 to 7 days.

NURSING IMPLICATIONS

Advise patient to take each dose with a full glass of water and to be consistent about time medication is to be taken.

Supervise ambulation. Sedative effects occur commonly within the first 24 hours after drug is started. Maximal sedative effects in 2 or 3 days after which time they begin to subside (usually within 1 week). Sedation may persist in patients taking over 2 Gm/day.

Monitor intake–output ratio and pattern. Fluid intake must be enough, e.g., 10 to 12 glasses or more (8 ounces each) to maintain urinary output of 2000 ml or more, to minimize risk of crystalluria.

Routine urinalysis should be performed (includes microscopic examination for evidence of crystalluria). If crystals occur fluid intake should be increased further. If crystalluria persists, metyrosine dosage should be decreased or drug discontinued.

Baseline and regularly scheduled measurements should be made of urinary catecholamines and their metabolites (metanephrines and VMA). Metabolite excretion should decrease in patients with phenochromocytoma in response to drug therapy. Normal values: metanephrines 1.3 mg, VMA (vanillylmandelic acid) up to 9 mg/24 hours. Other baseline and regular determinations should include vital signs, ECG, renal and hepatic function tests (in patients with dysfunction), BMR, and blood and urine sugar tests.

Contact clinical laboratory for information about 24-hour urine collection: container to use, need for preservative, refrigeration, and whether record of timing for each voiding is wanted. Also inform them of all drugs patient is taking.

In addition to reduction of urinary metanephrines and VMA, clinical effectiveness of metyrosine in patients with pheochromocytoma is determined by: decrease in frequency of hypertensive attacks and associated symptoms (elevated blood pressure, headache, nausea, vomiting, sweating, tachycardia), and possibly reduction of hyperglycemia, glycosuria, and BMR.

During anesthesia and surgery, blood pressure and ECG should be monitored continuously. Life-threatening arrhythmias and hypertensive crisis may occur during manipulation of tumor. Have on hand a beta-blocking agent, e.g., propranolol, lidocaine, and an alpha-adrenergic blocker, e.g., phentolamine.

Following tumor removal and into the postoperative period, large volumes of plasma may be required to maintain blood pressure and central venous pressure.

Nursing Interventions in the Postoperative Care Plan:

- ✓ Vital signs must be closely monitored.
- ✓ Check dressing for hemorrhage at least every ½ hour (adrenal gland is highly vascular).
- ✓ Measure and record intake and output. Check urinary output every ½ hour. Notify physician if it is less than 15 ml/30 minutes or less than 30 ml/hour.
- ✓ Control environmental stimuli so that patient can rest.
- ✓ Maintain IV fluid administration as prescribed.
- ✓ Have emergency equipment and supplies readily available to treat shock and hemorrhage.

Patient on prolonged metyrosine therapy should be strongly advised to carry medical identification and to notify all physicians and dentists involved in care about drug regimen.

Advise patient to notify physician if the following metyrosine side effects occur: diarrhea, particularly, if it is severe or persists, painful urination, jaw stiffness, drooling, difficult speech, tremors, disorientation. Dosage reduction or discontinuation of drug may be indicated.

Caution patient to avoid driving and other potentially hazardous activities until reaction to drug is determined.

Abrupt discontinuation of metyrosine may result in psychic stimulation, feeling of increased energy, temporary changes in sleep pattern (usually insomnia). Symptoms may last for 2 or 3 days.

Store preferably between 15° and 30°C (59° and 86°F), unless otherwise directed by manufacturer.

Diagnostic Test Interferences. False increases in **urinary catecholamines** may occur because of catechol metabolites of metyrosine.

Drug Interactions: Metyrosine

Plus	Interactions
Alcohol (Ethanol) and other CNS depressants; Tricyclic antidepressants	Additive sedative and other CNS depressant effects. Concurrent use generally avoided
Butyrophenones, e.g., droperidol (Inapsine), haloperidol (Haldol); Phenothiazines	Potentiation of extrapyramidal effects. Used with caution
Levodopa	Effects of levodopa may be reduced. Dosage adjustments may be necessary

MEXILETINE

(Mexitil)

(mex-il'e-teen)

Antiarrhythmic (Class I)

ACTIONS AND USES. Analogue of lidocaine with potent anesthetic action and Class IB electrophysiologic properties similar to those of tocainide. Shortens action potential duration and refractory period and improves resting potential. Has little or no effect on atrial tissue and produces modest suppression of sinus node automatically and AV nodal conduction. Prolongs the His to ventricular interval (HQ) only if patient has preexisting conduction disturbance (consistent with selective effect of Class IB agents on abnormal tissue). It should be noted that lidocaine response is not a reliable predictor of mexiletine effectiveness. Produces modest negative inotropic and hypotensive effects.

Used to treat acute and chronic ventricular arrhythmias and to prevent recurrent cardiac arrests; to suppress PVCs due to ventricular tachyarrhythmias. Also used in treatment of Wolff–Parkinson–White syndrome, and supraventricular arrhythmias.

ABSORPTION AND FATE. Rapidly absorbed from GI tract with about 88% bioavailability after oral dose. Metabolized in liver; half-life: about 12 hours (lengthened in acute MI). Less than 10% unchanged drug eliminated in urine; renal elimination increases with urine acidification. Excreted in breast milk.

CONTRAINDICATIONS AND PRECAUTIONS. Severe left ventricular failure, cardiogenic shock, severe bradyarrhythmias. *See also Tocainide.*

ADVERSE/SIDE EFFECTS. Dose related, and readily reversible after drug is discontinued: tremor, blurred vision, atoxia. *See also Tocainide.*

ROUTE AND DOSAGE. Oral: 200 to 400 mg every 6 to 8 hours. Dose gradually increased until desired response or side effects occur. **Intravenous:** Loading dose: 150 to 250 mg over 5 to 10 minutes followed by IV infusion of 0.5 to 1.5 mg/minute.

NURSING IMPLICATIONS

Effective serum concentration: 0.5 to 2 mcg/ml.

Administered with food or milk to reduce gastric distress.

During IV administration, connect patient to cardiac monitor, monitor ECG waveforms and be alert for dysrhythmias. Have resuscitative equipment ready.

Check pulse and blood pressure before administration of mexiletine, until both are stabilized. Patient should understand that changes in pulse rate and regularity may signal decreasing clinical effectiveness of drug.

Instruct patient about pulse parameters to be reported: i.e., changes in rhythm, and rate (bradycardia = pulse below 60); symptomatic bradycardia (lightheadedness, syncope, dizziness), and postural hypotension.

Adverse reactions are more common with IV administration than with oral doses, especially if the loading dose was administered too rapidly.

CNS adverse reactions predominate (intention tremors, nystagmus, blurred vision, dizziness, ataxia, confusion, nausea). Supervise ambulation in the weak, debilitated patient or the elderly during drug stabilization period.

Drug compliance with mexiletine is affected particularly by the distressing side effects of tremor, ataxia, and eye symptoms.

Check with patient about adherence to drug regimen frequently. If side effects are increasing, consult physician. Dose adjustment or discontinuation may be needed.

See Tocainide for additional Nursing Implications and Drug Interactions.

M

MEZLOCILLIN SODIUM
(Mezlin)

(mez-loe-sill'in)
Antiinfective
Antibiotic (beta lactam)
Penicillin

ACTIONS AND USES. Semisynthetic acylureidopenicillin with extended spectrum. Structurally resembles ampicillin (qv), and has similar but wider antibacterial spectrum than either ampicillin, carbenicillin, or tricarcillin. In common with other penicillins, mezlocillin is bactericidal and acts by interfering with bacterial cell wall synthesis. Active against a wide variety of gram-negative and gram-positive bacteria including aerobic and anaerobic strains. Broadened spectrum of activity includes strains of pathogenic aerobic gram-negative bacteria, e.g., *Bacteroides, Enterobacter, Escherichia, Haemophilus, Klebsiella, Pseudomonas, Proteus,* and *Serratia,* and gram-positive organisms such as *Streptococcus faecalis* (enterococcus). Inactive against penicillinase-producing strains of *Staphylococcus aureus.* Contains 1.85 mEq (42.6 mg) of sodium per gram.

Used primarily for serious infections caused by *Pseudomonas aeruginosa* alone or in combination with an aminoglycoside or a cephalosporin. Also used to treat other infections caused by susceptible strains.

ABSORPTION AND FATE. Rapidly absorbed following IM or IV administration. Serum levels peak in about 45 minutes after IM and within 5 minutes following IV injection. Well-distributed into most body tissues and fluids; highest concentrations in urine and bile. Adequate CSF penetration if meninges are inflamed. Approximately 16 to 42% bound to plasma proteins. Half-life: 50 to 55 minutes (longer in patients with renal impairment). Only slightly metabolized in liver. Excreted primarily by kidney; 55 to 65% of dose eliminated as unchanged drug within 6 hours, and less than 10% as inactive metabolite. Up to 25% of dose excreted in bile. Crosses placenta. Small amounts excreted in breast milk.

CONTRAINDICATIONS AND PRECAUTIONS. History of hypersensitivity to penicillins or cephalosporins. Safe use during pregnancy (category B) and in nursing mothers not established. *Cautious Use:* patients with known or suspected allergies to drugs or other substances, renal impairment.

ADVERSE/SIDE EFFECTS. **CNS:** convulsive seizures, neuromuscular hyperirritability. **GI:** abnormal taste sensations, nausea, vomiting, diarrhea. **Hematologic:** neuropenia, leukopenia, eosinophilia, thrombocytopenia (infrequent), hypokalemia (rare); increases in AST (SGOT), ALT (SGPT), alkaline phosphatase, serum bilirubin, creatinine, BUN; decreased Hct and Hgb. **Hypersensitivity:** rash, pruritus, urticaria, drug fever, anaphylactic reactions. *Local:* pain (following IM), thrombophlebitis (IV injection), superinfections.

ROUTE AND DOSAGE. **Adults:** *uncomplicated urinary tract infections:* **Intravenous or intramuscular:** 1.5 to 2 Gm every 6 hours (100 to 125 mg/kg/day). *Severe infections:* 3 Gm every 6 hours IV (150 to 200 mg/kg/day). *Life-threatening infections:* 4 Gm every 4 hours IV. *Maximum:* 24 Gm/day. **Infants (beyond 1 month) and children (up to 12 years):** 50 mg/kg every 4 hours IV.

NURSING IMPLICATIONS

Before initiation of therapy a detailed history should be obtained to determine previous hypersensitivity especially to penicillins, cephalosporins, but also to other substances.

Culture and susceptibility tests should be performed before and periodically during therapy to monitor drug effectiveness and possible bacterial resistance. Generally used concurrently with an aminoglycoside antibiotic pending test results. (Aminoglycoside should not be physically mixed with mezlocillin; they must be administered separately.)

Check expiration date on label.

IM injections should be made into a relatively large muscle such as the gluteus maximus (upper outer quadrant). Aspirate carefully before injecting drug to avoid inadvertent entry into blood vessel. Discomfort associated with IM administration may be lessened by making injection slowly (over 12 to 15 seconds). Do not exceed 2 Gm per IM injection.

Intravenous administration may be made by IV push (direct injection of reconstituted solution into vein or IV tubing, over 3 to 5 minutes), or by intermittent infusion over 30 minutes. Primary infusion should be temporarily withheld during infusion of mezlocillin. Observe IV sites for evidence of inflammation.

See manufacturer's directions for reconstitution, compatible solutions, and stability information.

Be prepared to administer emergency therapy for anaphylactic reaction whenever a penicillin antibiotic is administered. Have on hand epinephrine, IV steroids, oxygen, equipment for respiratory assistance and airway maintenance.

Bleeding abnormalities (thrombocytopenia), although rare, are particularly likely to occur in patients with impaired renal function. Observe and report ecchymoses, petechiae, bleeding gums, nosebleeds, or any other evidence of bleeding. Monitor coagulation tests (e.g., bleeding time, platelet aggregation, prothrombin time).

Be alert to signs of superinfections: white patches in mouth or black hairy tongue, foul-smelling stools or vaginal discharge, diarrhea, vaginitis, anogenital itching.

Baseline and regularly scheduled studies of blood, renal, and hepatic function should be performed during long-term therapy.

Therapy generally continues for at least 2 days after signs and symptoms of infection have subsided. Usual duration of therapy for serious infections is 7 to 10 days, but it may be longer in complicated infections.

Antibiotic therapy for group A beta-hemolytic streptococcal infections should continue for at least 10 days, to reduce risk of rheumatic fever or glomerulonephritis.

Store unopened vials and infusion bottles at or below 30°C (86°F), unless otherwise directed by manufacturer. Powder and reconstituted solutions may darken slightly, but this does not indicate loss of potency. Solutions should be clear. If a precipitate should form under refrigeration, warm to 37°C (98.6°F) in a water bath and shake well.

Diagnostic Test Interferences. Possibility of false-positive **urine protein** determinations (when mezlocillin concentration in urine is high) using sulfosalicylic acid and boiling test, acetic acid test, biuret reaction, nitric acid test; bromophenol blue reagent test (Multi-stix) is not affected.

Drug Interaction: Mezlocillin

Plus	Interactions
Anticoagulants (oral and parenteral)	Possibility of additive anticoagulant effects. Monitor closely
Aminoglycoside (parenteral)	Synergistic action possible. However, inactivation of aminoglycoside can occur (1) if physically mixed with penicillin and (2) with excessively high penicillin serum levels in patients with impaired renal function
Chloramphenicol (Chloromycetin) Erythromycin Tetracyclines	Possibility of interference with antimicrobial effectiveness of penicillins. Concurrent administration generally avoided
Probenecid	Increases mezlocillin serum levels and half-life. Used therapeutically

MICONAZOLE NITRATE

(Micatin, Monistat)

(mi-kon′a-zole)
Antiinfective
Antibiotic
Antifungal

ACTIONS AND USES. Broad-spectrum agent with fungicidal activity against *Candida albicans* and other species of this genus. Inhibits growth of common dermatophytes *Trichophyton rubrum, Trichophyton mentagrophytes, Epidermophyton floccosum* and organism responsible for tinea versicolor *(Melassezia furfur).* Mode of action unclear, but appears to inhibit uptake of components essential for cell reproduction and growth and to alter cell wall structure, thus promoting cell death.

Used for treatment of vulvovaginal candidiasis, tinea pedis (athlete's foot), tinea cruris, tinea corporis, and tinea versicolor caused by dermatophytes. Also useful (parenteral) for treatment of severe systemic fungal infections including coccidioidomycosis, candidiasis, cryptococcosis, paracoccidioidomycosis, and for treatment of chronic mucocutaneous candidiasis. IV infusion is inadequate therapy for urinary bladder infections or for fungal meningitis; these conditions require supplements of miconazole by intrathecal administration and bladder irrigation.

ABSORPTION AND FATE. Following absorption, rapid hepatic metabolism. About 90% protein bound; phasic half-lives: 0.4, 2.1, 24.1 hours. Metabolized in liver. Excreted in urine and feces principally as inactive metabolites.

CONTRAINDICATIONS AND PRECAUTIONS. Known sensitivity to miconazole. Safe use in children under 1 year of age, during pregnancy after first trimester, and in nursing women not established. *Cautious Use:* hepatic or renal impairment.

ADVERSE/SIDE EFFECTS. Tachycardia, cardiac arrhythmias (with rapid IV injection); vulvovaginal burning, itching or irritation, pelvic cramps, hives, skin rash, and headache. (With parenteral use): phlebitis, pruritus, rash, nausea, vomiting, diarrhea, febrile reaction, drowsiness, flushing, hyponatremia (transient), decreased hematocrit; thrombocytopenia, hyperlipemia, arrhythmias, anaphylaxis.

ROUTE AND DOSAGE. **Intravaginal:** 1 applicator of cream or suppository into vagina daily at bedtime for 7 days; may be repeated if necessary. **Topical:** cover affected area generously, morning and evening, and once daily in patients with tinea versicolor. **Intravenous: Adult:** 200 to 3600 mg day (usually divided into 3 infusions). **Children:** 20 to 40 mg/kg/day in divided doses. Maximum dose: 15 mg/kg/infusion. **Intrathecal:** 20 mg undiluted injection every 3 to 7 days. **Bladder instillation:** 200 mg diluted solution (10 mg/200 ml).

NURSING IMPLICATIONS

Treatment with miconazole is preferably started in hospital to permit careful monitoring of drug response. Culture and susceptibility studies should be performed.

If nausea is a problem, the patient may be premedicated with an antiemetic or antihistamine.

The castor oil vehicle may cause transient elevation in serum cholesterol and triglycerides.

Ask physician about how to cleanse affected area prior to application of cream or lotion.

Massage affected area gently until cream disappears.

Persistent vulvovaginitis should be reevaluated if 3 to 4 weeks does not bring relief. Advise patient to report to physician for urine and blood glucose studies, since vaginitis may be a symptom of unrecognized diabetes mellitus.

Infections caused by dermatophytes require about 1 week of treatment with miconazole.

Use lotion rather than cream for intertriginous areas, to prevent maceration.

The full course of treatment should be completed in order to assure recovery.

M

Clinical improvement from topical application should be expected in 1 or 2 weeks. If no improvement in 4 weeks, the diagnosis is reevaluated. Tinea pedis infection should be treated for 1 month to assure permanent recovery.

Avoid contact of drug with eyes.

Pathogens causing vaginitis should be identified before treatment since miconazole is effective only against candidal vulvovaginitis.

Instruct patient to insert applicator of drug high into the vagina and to use a sanitary napkin to prevent staining.

Advise patient to avoid sexual intercourse during treatment period to prevent reinfection.

Hypersensitivity test should be performed prior to IV administration. An initial test dose of 200 mg is administered by physician. Monitor patient for hypersensitivity reactions. Have immediately available emergency drugs and resuscitation equipment.

Hgh, Hct, electrolytes, triglycerides and cholesterol values should be determined initially and periodically during therapy.

IV administration should be slow (over a period of 30 to 60 minutes) to prevent nausea and risk of arrhythmias or tachycardia. Physician must prescribe flow rate.

Drug is diluted for IV injection in at least 200 ml Isotonic Saline or 5% Dextrose solution. A 20-ml ampul contains 10 mg/ml drug. Following dilution, solution is stable at room temperature for 48 hours. If solution darkens in color, discard it. This is a sign of deterioration.

Miconazole is stored preferably at 15° to 30°C (59° to 86°F) unless otherwise directed by manufacturer.

Drug Interactions. Miconazole may enhance **oral anticoagulant** effects. When combined with **amphotericin B,** antifungal activity of the combination is less than that of either drug used alone.

MICROFIBRILLAR COLLAGEN HEMOSTAT

(Avitene, MCH)

Hemostatic (topical)

ACTIONS AND USES. Absorbable topical hemostatic agent derived from purified collagen from skin of cattle. On contact with a bleeding surface, platelets adhere to its fibrils and undergo a reaction that triggers their aggregation into thrombi. Reportedly does not interfere with bone regeneration or healing. Hemostatic effect is not inhibited by heparin or aspirin. Not effective in systemic clotting disorders such as hemophilia.

Used as adjunct to hemostasis when control of bleeding by ligature is ineffective or impractical, as in superficial injuries of spleen or liver, large oozing surfaces, and anastomotic sites.

CONTRAINDICATIONS AND PRECAUTIONS. Closure of skin incisions, use in contaminated wounds. Safe use during pregnancy not established.

ADVERSE/SIDE EFFECTS. Potentiation of infection, hematoma, abscess formation, wound dehiscence (separation), adhesion formation, mediastinitis, allergic reactions, foreign body reactions.

ROUTE AND DOSAGE. Topical: Applied directly to source of bleeding (site compressed with dry sponge immediately before application). Followed by pressure with dry sponge for 1 to 5 or more minutes, depending on severity of bleeding. Excess material gently removed by blunt forceps and irrigation.

NURSING IMPLICATIONS

Gloves and forceps used to handle product must be dry since the drug will readily adhere to a moist surface.

Material is inactivated by autoclaving.

This product should not be resterilized.

MINERAL OIL

Laxative

(Agoral; Kondremul: Light and Heavy Mineral Oil; Liquid Petrolatum, Neo-Cultol, Nujol, Petrogalar, Plain)

ACTIONS AND USES. Mixture of hydrocarbons obtained from petroleum. Lubricates and softens feces, retards water absorption from fecal content, eases passage of stool.

Used for temporary relief of constipation, and when straining at stool is contraindicated (e.g., hypertension, certain cardiac disorders, following anorectal surgery), to relieve fecal impaction and to avoid possible adverse effects of oral administration. Also used as pharmaceutical solvent and vehicle. Available in fixed combination with milk of magnesia (Haley's MO), and with phenophthalein (Agoral).

ABSORPTION AND FATE. Limited absorption from intestinal tract with distribution to mesenteric lymph nodes, intestinal mucosa, liver, spleen. Eliminated in stool in 6 to 10 hours, or within 12 hours after bedtime dose.

CONTRAINDICATIONS AND PRECAUTIONS. Nausea, vomiting, abdominal pain, intestinal obstruction, oral administration to dysphagic patients, use with emollients. *Cautious Use:* oral use in elderly or debilitated patients, during pregnancy.

M

ADVERSE/SIDE EFFECTS. Occasionally: pruritus ani; interference with postoperative anorectal wound healing; with aspiration: pulmonary granuloma, lipid pneumonitis. Prolonged use: anorexia, nausea, vomiting, nutritional deficiencies, hypoprothrombinemia.

ROUTE AND DOSAGE. Oral: 15 to 30 ml. **Rectal (retention enema): Adults:** 90 to 120 ml; **Children: (6 years or older):** 5 to 15 ml once a day.

NURSING IMPLICATIONS

Usually administered in the evening. Digestion and passage of food from stomach may be delayed if taken within 2 hours of mealtime.

Potential of lipid pneumonia from aspiration of orally administered mineral oil is especially high in the elderly and debilitated patient. Administer with patient in upright position, and avoid giving just before patient retires.

Mineral oil is tasteless and odorless when cold (store in refrigerator).

Although tasteless, consistency may be objectionable. Many patients prefer to drink orange juice or suck on slice of orange after taking oil; others prefer to mix it in orange juice.

Emulsified preparations are reportedly more palatable; however, this form may enhance absorption of oil through intestinal mucosa.

Prolonged use (more than 2 weeks) can reduce absorption of fat-soluble vitamins A, D, E, and K, carotene, calcium, and phosphates. For these reasons, mineral oil base for low-calorie salad dressings is not advised.

Repeated oral use or rectal administration may result in oil seepage from rectum with

soiling of clothing or bedding. Forewarn patient to be prepared for this possibility to avoid embarrassment.
Administration of retention enema is generally followed by a cleansing enema in 30 minutes to 1 hour. Consult physician.
Application of mineral oil to nasal passages to relieve dryness should be avoided because of danger of migration of droplets from pharynx into lungs, with resulting lipid pneumonia. Aqueous vehicles are safer.
Frequent or prolonged use of mineral oil may result in dependence. *See Bisacodyl for patient teaching points concerning management of chronic constipation.*

Drug Interactions. By reducing absorption of **vitamin K,** mineral oil may potentiate effect of **oral anticoagulants:** on the other hand, ingestion of large amounts of mineral oil may decrease effectiveness of **oral anticoagulants** by impairing absorption (opposing mechanisms). Mineral oil may interfere with action of nonabsorbable **sulfonamides.**

MINOCYCLINE HYDROCHLORIDE

(Minocin)

(mi-noe-sye'kleen)
Antiinfective
Tetracycline

ACTIONS AND USES. Semisynthetic tetracycline derivative with actions, uses, contraindications, precautions, and adverse reactions as for tetracycline (qv). Appears to be active against strains of staphylococci resistant to other tetracyclines, and photosensitivity occurs only rarely. Reported to be more completely absorbed than other tetracyclines because it is more lipid-soluble.

M

ABSORPTION AND FATE. Well absorbed by oral route. About 70 to 75% bound to plasma proteins. Serum half-life following single 200-mg dose approximately 11 to 17 hours. Slow renal clearance. About 12% of dose excreted in urine; remainder persists in body in fatty tissues. Crosses placenta, and appears in breast milk.

CONTRAINDICATIONS AND PRECAUTIONS. Hypersensitivity to tetracyclines, oral administration in meningococcal infections. Safe use during pregnancy not established. *Cautious Use:* renal impairment. *See Tetracycline.*

ADVERSE/SIDE EFFECTS. Most frequent: CNS side effects (weakness, lightheadedness, ataxia, dizziness or vertigo), nausea, cramps, diarrhea, flatulence. *See also Tetracycline.*

ROUTE AND DOSAGE. Adults: Oral: 200 mg followed by 100 mg every 12 hours; alternatively, 100 or 200 mg initially, followed by 50 mg 4 times daily. **Intravenous:** 200 mg followed by 100 mg every 12 hours. Not to exceed 400 mg/24 hours. See manufacturer's directions for preparation of parenteral solution. **Children over 8 years old: Oral:** 4 mg/kg initially, followed by 2 mg/kg every 12 hours.

NURSING IMPLICATIONS

Check expiration date. Outdated tetracyclines can cause severe adverse side effects.
Studies to date indicate that minocycline is not significantly influenced by food and dairy products, in contrast to other tetracyclines.
Since lightheadedness, dizziness, or vertigo occur frequently, caution patient to avoid driving vehicles and other hazardous activities while on minocycline. (Lightheadedness is usually transient and often disappears during therapy.)

Advise patient to report vestibular side effects (CNS symptoms). They usually occur within first week of therapy and are reversible when drug is stopped.
Serum drug level determinations are advised in patients receiving prolonged therapy.
Reconstituted solution is stable for 24 hours at room temperature, but final dilution for administration should be used immediately.
See Tetracycline hydrochloride (prototype tetracycline).

MINOXIDIL
(Loniten)

(mi-nox'i-dill)
Antihypertensive
Vasodilator (peripheral)

ACTIONS AND USES. Direct-acting vasodilator similar to other drugs of this class, e.g., hydralazine, diazoxide, prazosin, but hypotensive effect is more pronounced. Appears to act by blocking calcium uptake into cell membrane. Reduces systolic and diastolic blood pressures in supine and standing positions, and decreases peripheral vascular resistance by direct vasodilating action on arteriolar vessels. Has little or no effect on venous system. Hypotensive action is accompanied by reflex activation of sympathetic, vagal inhibitory, and renal homeostatic mechanisms; increased sympathetic stimulation also activates the renin-angiotensin-aldosterone system. The net result is increased heart rate and cardiac output, sodium retention, and edema formation which usually necessitates concomitant supportive drug therapy. Does not affect vasomotor reflexes and therefore does not produce orthostatic hypotension. Has a greater lowering effect on elevated blood pressures than on blood pressures approaching the normal range.

Used as step 4 agent in stepped care approach to treat severe hypertension that is symptomatic or associated with damage to target organs and is not manageable with maximum therapeutic doses of a diuretic plus two other antihypertensive drugs. Used with a diuretic to prevent fluid retention and a beta-adrenergic blocking agent (e.g., propranolol) or sympathetic nervous system suppressant (e.g., clonidine or methyldopa) to prevent tachycardia.

ABSORPTION AND FATE. Rapidly and well absorbed from GI tract. Onset of antihypertensive effect in 30 minutes; peak action in 2 to 3 hours, with duration of 10 to 12 hours in most patients and up to 75 hours in some (significant interindividual variability reported). Widely distributed throughout body; not bound to plasma proteins. Plasma half-life: approximately 4.2 hours (but drug effects persist significantly longer). About 90% of drug metabolized to minimally active metabolites. Approximately 97% excreted in urine and feces; less than 10% excreted as unchanged drug.

CONTRAINDICATION AND PRECAUTIONS. Pheochromocytoma. Safe use during pregnancy or in women of childbearing potential, or in nursing mothers or children not established. *Cautious Use:* severe renal impairment, recent myocardial infarction (within preceding month), coronary artery disease, chronic congestive heart failure.

ADVERSE/SIDE EFFECTS. **CV:** tachycardia, angina pectoris, ECG changes (especially in direction and magnitude of T-waves), pericardial effusion and tamponade, rebound hypertension (following drug withdrawal), pulmonary hypertension (causal relationship not established), intermittent claudication; edema, including pulmonary edema; congestive heart failure (salt and water retention). **Dermatologic:** hypertrichosis, darkening of skin, transient pruritus, Stevens–Johnson syndrome, hypersensitivity rash. **Other:** nausea, headache, fatigue, breast tenderness, gynecomastia, polymenorrhea, thrombocytopenia.

ROUTE AND DOSAGE. Oral: Adults and children (over 12 years): Initial: 5 mg once daily. If necessary, increased gradually after at least 3-day interval to 10, 20, and then 40 mg/day in single or divided doses. (When rapid management of blood pressure is indicated adjustments may be made every 6 hours if patient is closely monitored.) Maximal recommended dosage 100 mg daily. **Children (under 12 years):** Initial: 0.2 mg/kg of body weight (maximum 5 mcg) once daily. Usual dosage range: 0.25 to 1 mg/kg/day in 1 or 2 divided doses. Maximal recommended dosage: 50 mg day. Available in 2.5 and 10 mg tablets.

NURSING IMPLICATIONS

Minoxidil may be taken without regard to meals or food.

Take blood pressure and apical pulse before administering medication and report significant changes. Consult physician for parameters.

Monitor blood pressure and pulse at regular intervals during therapy. Abrupt reduction in blood pressure can result in cerebrovascular accident and myocardial infarction. Keep physician informed.

Patients with malignant hypertension, particularly those receiving guanethidine, should have initial treatment in a hospital setting.

Since experience with children taking minoxidil is limited, dosage must be very carefully titrated.

Patients on home care should be told usual pulse rate and instructed to count radial pulse for one full minute before taking drug. Advise patient to report an increase of 20 or more beats/minute.

Fluid and electrolyte balance should be closely followed throughout therapy. Sodium and water retention commonly occurs in patients receiving minoxidil. Consult physician regarding sodium restriction. If patient is on diuretic therapy, potassium intake and serum potassium levels will require monitoring.

Monitor intake and output and daily weight. Report unusual changes in intake–output ratio or daily weight gain of 3 or 4 or more pounds.

For patients who develop refractory fluid retention, some clinicians withdraw drug for 1 or 2 days and then resume therapy aimed at more vigorous diuresis.

Observe patient daily for edema and auscultate lungs for rales. Be alert to signs and symptoms of congestive heart failure: night cough, dyspnea on exertion, orthopnea, distended neck veins.

Also observe patient for symptoms of pericardial effusion or tamponade. Symptoms are similar to those of congestive failure but additionally patient may have paradoxical pulse (normal inspiratory reduction in systolic blood pressure may fall as much as 10 to 20 mm Hg). Diagnosis is confirmed by echocardiographic studies.

Note possible adverse reactions of drugs that are given in conjunction with minoxidil.

Patient should be thoroughly informed of possibility of *hypertrichosis* (elongation, thickening, and increased pigmentation of fine body hair, especially of face, arms, and back). It develops 3 to 9 weeks after start of therapy and occurs in approximately 80% of patients. It is reportedly not an endocrine disorder and is reversible within 1 to 6 months following discontinuation of minoxidil. In addition to shaving, depilatory creams containing calcium thioglycolate are effective in removing unwanted hair. Vitamin E therapy has been used to reduce severity of this side effect.

Instruct patient to notify physician promptly if the following signs or symptoms appear: increase of 20 or more beats per minute in resting pulse; breathing difficulty; dizziness; lightheadedness; fainting; edema (tight shoes or rings, puffiness, pitting); weight gain, chest pain, arm or shoulder pain; easy bruising or bleeding.

Review package insert with patient (dispensed with product). Emphasize importance of taking drug as prescribed and caution patient not to skip or alter dosage and not to discontinue medication without consulting physician.

Rebound hypertension has followed minoxidil withdrawal. Conversion to conventional therapy must be accomplished gradually and with close observation of patient.

Treatment of toxicity: have on hand phenylephrine, dopamine, and vasopressin to reverse hypotension.

Stored in tightly covered container preferably at 15° to 30°C (59° to 86°F) unless otherwise directed by manufacturer.

Diagnostic Test Interferences. **Hematocrit, hemoglobin,** and **erythrocyte count** usually decrease (about 7%) during early therapy; **serum alkaline phosphatase, BUN,** and **creatinine** may increase during early therapy.

Drug Interactions: Minoxidil

Plus	Interactions
Epinephrine, Norepinephrine	Excessive cardiac stimulant action
Guanethidine	Profound orthostatic hypotension; if possible guanethidine should be withdrawn gradually 1 to 3 weeks before minoxidil therapy

MITOMYCIN

(Mitomycin-C, MTC, Mutamycin)

(mye-toe-mye'sin)
Antineoplastic
Antibiotic

ACTION AND USES. Potent antibiotic antineoplastic compound produced by *Streptomyces caespitosus* with wide range of antibacterial activity. Described extensively in the literature as Mitomycin-C. Effective in certain tumors nonresponsive to surgery, radiation or other chemotheraputic agents. Action mechanism not clear but reportedly combines with DNA (attachment site unknown), thereby interfering with cellular and enzymatic RNA and protein synthesis. Mitomycin has been shown to be carcinogenic in mice and rats; thus selected patients must be aware of the inherent risk in spite of possible therapeutic benefits.

Used in combination with other chemotherapeutic agents in palliative, adjunctive treatment of disseminated adenocarcinoma of breast, pancreas, or stomach, squamous cell carcinoma of head, neck, lung, and cervix. Not recommended to replace surgery and/or radiotherapy, nor as a single primary therapeutic agent.

ABSORPTION AND FATE. Following IV injection. Mitomycin is cleared rapidly from blood by hepatic metabolism. Half-life: 17 minutes. Approximately 10% dose secreted unchanged in urine.

CONTRAINDICATIONS AND PRECAUTIONS. Hypersensitivity or idiosyncracy reaction; thrombocytopenia; coagulation disorders or bleeding tendencies; pregnancy. *Cautious Use:* renal impairment, myelosuppression.

ADVERSE/SIDE EFFECTS. Bone marrow toxicity (thrombocytopenia, leukopenia occurring 4 to 8 weeks after treatment onset); fever, anorexia, stomatitis, nausea, vomiting, alopecia; desquamation, induration, pruritus, pain, bleeding, paresthesias, necrosis, cellulitis at injection site; hemoptysis, dyspnea, nonproductive cough, pneumonia, elevated BUN. Following symptoms may or may not be drug induced: headache, blurred vision, drowsiness, fatigue, edema, syncope, confusion, thrombophlebitis, anemia, hematemesis, diarrhea, pain.

ROUTE AND DOSAGE. Intravenous: 2 mg/m²/day for 5 days; after drug-free interval of 2 days: 2 mg/m²/day for 5 days; cycle may be repeated every 6 to 8 weeks on basis of hemolytic response; thereafter dosage and schedule highly individualized.

NURSING IMPLICATIONS

Patient receiving mitomycin should be hospitalized so that emergency treatment and laboratory facilities will be available.

Avoid extravasation when drug is administered, to prevent extreme tissue reaction (cellulitis) to the toxic drug. *See Index: Nursing Interventions: extravasation.*

Because of cumulative myelosuppression, laboratory studies of platelet counts, prothrombin and bleeding times, differential and hemoglobin studies, serum creatinine are performed frequently during treatment and for at least 7 weeks after treatment is terminated.

Usually drug is not administered if serum creatinine is greater than 1.7 mg%.

If platelet count falls below 75,000 and WBC down to 3000 or prothrombin or bleeding times are prolonged, treatment is suspended or modified.

Monitor intake–output ratio and pattern. Any sign of impaired kidney function should be reported: change in ratio, dysuria, hematuria, oliguria, frequency, urgency. Keep patient hydrated (at least 2000 to 2500 ml orally daily if tolerated). Drug is nephrotoxic.

Observe closely for signs of infection. Monitor body temperature frequently. Instruct patient to report immediately if signs of common cold present.

See Mechlorethamine for nursing implications related to stomatitis.

M

MITOTANE

(Lysodren)

(mye'toe-tane)
Antineoplastic
Antihormona

ACTIONS AND USES. Cytotoxic agent with suppressant action on the adrenal cortex. Modifies peripheral metabolism of steroids, and reduces production of adrenal steroids. Extraadrenal metabolism of cortisol is altered leading to reduction in 17-hydroxycorticosteroids (17-OHCS); however, plasma levels of corticosteroids do not fall. Apparently increases formation of 6-beta-hydroxycortisol.

Used for treatment of inoperable adrenal cortical carcinoma (functional and nonfunctional).

ABSORPTION AND FATE. Approximately 40% of oral dose is absorbed; 10% is excreted in urine as unchanged drug and metabolite; a small amount is excreted in bile; and remainder deposits in most body tissues, especially in fatty tissue. When administered parenterally about 25% of drug is excreted in urine.

CONTRAINDICATIONS AND PRECAUTIONS. Hypersensitivity to mitotane; pregnancy and lactation only after risk-benefit ratio to mother and fetus has been assessed. *Cautious Use:* hepatic disease.

ADVERSE/SIDE EFFECTS. CNS: vertigo, dizziness, drowsiness, tiredness, depression, sedation, brain damage, impaired neurologic function. **CV:** hypertension, hypotension, flushing. **GI:** anorexia, nausea, vomiting, diarrhea. **GU:** hematuria, hemorrhagic cystitis, albuminuria. **Other:** adrenocortical insufficiency, blurred vision, diplopia, lens opacity, toxic retinopathy, generalized aching, fever, cutaneous eruptions and pigmentation, muscle twitching, hypersensitivity reactions, puritus, hyperpyrexia.

ROUTE AND DOSAGE. Oral: 9 to 10 Gm/day in divided doses, three to four times daily. Dose is reduced or increased on basis of side effects as tolerated. Aim is to give as high a dose as tolerated. Maximum tolerated dose varies from 2 to 16 Gm/day.

NURSING IMPLICATIONS

Mitotane treatment is started and continued in the hospital until stable dosage regimen is established. Drug is continued at least 3 months to determine efficacy.

Nausea and vomiting may be reduced or alleviated by antiemetic therapy before and during drug therapy.

To reduce possibility of infarction and hemorrhage in a tumor due to drug action, all possible tumor tissue is surgically removed from large metastatic masses before mitotane treatment is started.

Mitotane does not cure but reduces tumor mass; reduces pain, weakness, anorexia, and steroid symptoms.

Long-term continuous treatment with high doses may lead to brain damage. Neurologic and behavioral assessments should be made at regular intervals throughout therapy.

Symptoms of *adrenal insufficiency* (weakness, fatigue, orthostatic hypotension, pigmentation, weight loss, dehydration, anorexia, nausea, vomiting and diarrhea) should be reported to physician. Adrenal cortical steroids (both mineralocorticoid and glucocorticoid) will be needed for replacement therapy.

The patient frequently fails to respond to mitotane after the third or fourth course of therapy.

Contraceptive measures are advised during therapy because of teratogenic properties of the drug. If the woman suspects she is pregnant, she should notify the physician.

Medication causes aching muscles, fever, flushing, and muscle twitching. If these symptoms persist and become more severe, the physician should be notified.

Advise patient to use caution when driving or performing hazardous tasks requiring alertness because of drug-induced drowsiness, tiredness, dizziness. These symptoms tend to recede with continuation in therapy.

Monitor the obese patient for symptoms of adrenal hypofunction. Because a large portion of the drug deposits in fatty tissue, this person is particularly susceptible to prolonged side effects. A higher than average dose may be necessary.

Observe for symptoms of hepatoxicity: jaundice, pruritis, and GI disturbances. Report promptly since reduced hepatic capacity can increase toxicity of mitotane, and because dose may have to be decreased.

Monitor pulse and blood pressure for early signs of shock (adrenal insufficiency).

If a medical–surgical emergency occurs, mitotane may be temporarily withdrawn since adrenal suppression is its prime action. Exogenous steroids may be required until the already depressed adrenal starts secreting steroids.

If no clinical benefits are seen in 3 months, the treatment is considered a failure. About 10% of patients have reportedly shown continued response beyond 3 months of treatment (maintenance of clinical status or slowed growth of metastatic lesions).

Stored in tight, light resistant containers, preferably between 15° and 30°C (59° and 86°F) unless otherwise directed by manufacturer.

Diagnostic Test Interferences. Mitotane decreases **protein-bound iodide (PBI)** and **urinary 17-OHCS levels.**

Drug Interactions. Mitotane may alter metabolism of *corticosteroid* requiring higher doses.

M

MOLINDONE HYDROCHLORIDE

(Moban)

(moe-lin'done)
Psychotropic
Antipsychotic
Neuroleptic

ACTIONS AND USES. Dihydroindolone derivative tranquilizer, structurally unrelated but pharmacologically similar to the piperazine phenothiazines. Has less sedative but comparable anticholinergic activity and greater incidence of extrapyramidal side effects than chlorpromazine (qv). EEG studies suggest that ascending reticular system is chief site of action. Reportedly lowers convulsive threshold and produces tranquilization without compromising alertness.

Used in the management of manifestations of psychotic disorders.

ABSORPTION AND FATE. Rapidly absorbed; peak plasma levels achieved in 1½ hours; half-life 1.5 hours. Duration of effects from single dose: 24 to 36 hours. Hepatic metabolism: 90% excreted in urine and feces within 24 hours. May appear in breast milk but it is not known if drug crosses placenta.

CONTRAINDICATIONS AND PRECAUTIONS. Known hypersensitivity to molindone or to phenothiazines; severe CNS depression, comatose states; children under 12. Safe use during pregnancy, by women who might become pregnant, and by nursing mothers has not been established. *Cautious Use:* persons who may be harmed by increase in physical activity, prostatic hypertrophy, cardiovascular disease, previously detected cancer of breast. *See also Chlorpromazine.*

ADVERSE/SIDE EFFECTS. Transient drowsiness, insomnia, extrapyramidal symptoms (dose-related), tinnitus, blurred vision, nasal congestion, xerostomia, constipation, urinary retention, euphoria, mild photosensitivity, tachycardia, change in weight, SLE-like syndrome, heavy menses, amenorrhea, galactorrhea, gynecomastia, increased libido, premature ejaculation, hepatotoxicity. *See also Chlorpromazine.*

M

ROUTE AND DOSAGE. **Oral: Adults and children (over 12 years of age):** initial: 50 to 75 mg/day to be increased to 100 mg/day in 3 to 4 days. (Dose adjustment made on basis of severity of symptoms.) **Elderly, debilitated:** started on lower dosage. Maintenance: 5 to 15 mg three or four times daily; adjusted as needed and tolerated up to 225 mg/day. Oral concentrate: 20 mg/ml.

NURSING IMPLICATIONS

In early treatment be alert to onset of parkinsonian (extrapyramidal) symptoms: rigidity, immobility, reduction of voluntary movements, tremors, fine vermicular tongue movements. Withhold dose and report promptly to physician. Usually a change in dose will interrupt progressive development of extrapyramidal side effects.

Counsel patient to take drug as prescribed: the patient should not alter the dose regimen or stop the medication without consulting his or her physician. In addition, patient should not give any of it to another person.

Dizziness during early therapy usually disappears as treatment continues.

Caution patient not to drive or engage in other activities requiring mental or physical coordination until response to the drug is known.

Instruct patient to withhold dose and consult with physician if the following symptoms occur: tremor, involuntary twitching, exaggerated restlessness, changes in vision, light-colored stools, sore throat, fever, rash.

Warn patient to avoid alcohol and self-medication with other depressants during therapy. Patient should receive the physician's approval before using any OTC drug.

Xerostomia may be relieved by frequent rinses with warm water, and by increasing noncaloric fluid intake. Avoid use of commercial mouth rinses which can change oral flora leading to candida infection and tissue erosion. Use of a saliva substitute also helps to keep oral surfaces moist (e.g., Moi-stir, Xero-lube). Discuss with physician.

Monitor bowel pattern and urinary output. The depressed patient may not report constipation or urinary retention, both side effects of this medicine.

Antiemetic action may mask signs of intestinal obstruction, brain disease, or drug toxicity.

Have available seizure precaution measures if patient has history of convulsive disease.

Resumption of menses in previously amenorrheic patients has been reported.

Lens opacities and retinopathy have not been reported, but it is recommended that the patient on long-term treatment have periodic ophthalmic examinations.

Conditioned avoidance behavior is suppressed by molindone, thus increasing the danger of falling and receiving burns from hot water in tub or bottles, or from heating pads.

Since this drug increases motor activity, supervise ambulation and other activities of daily living in the elderly or debilitated or patient with impaired vision, to prevent injury or falling.

Caution patient with angina to avoid overexertion and to report increase in frequency of precordial pain.

The tablet contains calcium sulfate as an excipient and may interfere with absorption of phenytoin or tetracyclines.

Lidone capsules and concentrate contain tartrazine which can cause allergic-type reactions (including bronchial asthma) in susceptible persons who are frequently also sensitive to aspirin.

Store medication in tightly capped, light-resistant bottles. Protect from heat and moisture.

See also Chlorpromazine (prototype antipsychotic).

M

Drug Interactions: Molindone

Plus	Interactions
Phenytoin Tetracyclines	Molindone may interfere with GI absorption of these drugs

PROTOTYPE

MORPHINE SULFATE

(Roxamol, RMS Uniserts)

(mor'feen)
Narcotic analgesic
Opiate agonist
C II

ACTIONS AND USES. Suggested mechanisms of analgesic action include elevation of pain threshold, interference with pain conduction or CNS response to pain, or altered pain perception. Relieves pain without obtunding other sensory modalites, and may produce euphoria; drowsiness occurs commonly, and higher doses promote deep sleep. Also depresses respiratory center and cough reflex and may induce nausea and vomiting by increasing vestibular sensitivity and by CTZ stimulation (initial doses stimulate and subsequent doses depress vomiting center). Causes constriction of pupils, even in total darkness, and greatly enhances pupillary response to light (tolerance to miotic effect is rare). Generally, has no major effect on blood pressure, heart rate or rhythm when patient is supine; however, orthostatic hypotension may occur in head-up position, possibly by dilatation of peripheral vessels (histamine release) or by depression of medullary vasomotor center. Delays digestion by decreasing stomach motility and hydrochloric acid, biliary and pancreatic secretions. Decreases intensity and frequency of propulsive peristalsis, and enhances amplitude of nonpropulsive contractions, thus causing desiccation of feces and resultant constipation. Increases tone of smooth muscles and sphincters in GI, biliary, and genitourinary systems. Reduction of urinary outflow may be mediated by antidiuretic hormone release or by decreased renal blood flow. Release of ACTH, FSH, LH, and TSH may be suppressed.

Used for symptomatic relief of severe pain after nonnarcotic analgesics have failed and as preanesthetic medication; also used to relieve dyspnea of acute left ventricular failure and pulmonary edema and pain of myocardial infarction. *Unlabeled Use:* Treatment of acute and chronic pain by intrathecal, epidural, and continuous IV routes.

ABSORPTION AND FATE. Absorption from GI tract is complete, but variable in rate. Well absorbed following parenteral injection. Peak analgesia within 50 to 90 minutes following subcutaneous administration and 20 minutes after IV injection. Analgesia may be maintained up to 7 hours. Wide distribution, with concentration mainly in kidney, liver, lung, spleen; lower concentrations in brain and muscle. Plasma half-life: 2.5 to 3 hours. Metabolized chiefly in liver. About 90% of dose is excreted in urine within 24 hours, largely in conjugated form, with small amounts as unchanged drug; 7 to 10% excreted via bile through feces. Crosses placenta; small amounts appear in breast milk.

CONTRAINDICATIONS AND PRECAUTIONS. Hypersensitivity to opiates, increased intracranial pressure, convulsive disorders, acute alcoholism, acute bronchial asthma, chronic pulmonary diseases, severe respiratory depression, chemical-irritant-induced pulmonary edema, prostatic hypertrophy, undiagnosed acute abdominal conditions, pancreatitis, acute ulcerative colitis, severe liver or renal insufficiency, Addison's disease, hypothyroidism. Safe use during pregnancy not established. *Cautious Use:* toxic psychosis, cardiac arrhythmias, cardiovascular disease, emphysema, kyphoscoliosis, cor pulmonale, severe obesity, reduced blood volume; very old, very young, or debilitated patients; use during labor.

M

ADVERSE/SIDE EFFECTS. **Acute intoxication:** deep sleep, coma, marked miosis, severe respiratory depression (as low as 2 to 4/minute) or arrest, pulmonary edema, hypothermia, skeletal muscle flaccidity, oliguria, hypotension, bradycardia, convulsions (infants and children), cardiac arrest. **Allergic:** pruritus, skin rashes, contact dermatitis, urticaria, hemorrhagic urticaria (rare), sneezing; wheal, flare, and pain over injection site; edema, anaphylactoid reaction (rare). **CNS:** respiratory depression, decreased cough reflex, euphoria, dysphoria, paradoxic CNS stimulation (restlessness, tremor, delirium, insomnia), drowsiness, dizziness, weakness, headache, miosis, hypothermia. **CV:** bradycardia, orthostatic hypotension, syncope, flushing of face, neck, and upper thorax. **GI:** nausea, vomiting, anorexia, constipation, dry mouth, biliary colic. **GU:** urinary retention or urgency, dysuria, reduced libido and/or potency (prolonged use). **Other:** sweating, prolonged labor and respiratory depression of newborn, decreased urinary VMA excretion, elevated transaminase levels, precipitation of porphyria.

ROUTE AND DOSAGE. **Oral:** 10 to 20 mg every 4 hours. **Subcutaneous, intramuscular:** **Adults:** 5 to 20 mg every 4 hours, if necessary. **Children:** 0.05 to 0.2 mg/kg per dose (single dose not to exceed 15 mg). **Intravenous** (rarely used): **Adults:** 4 to 10 mg in 4 to 5 ml water for injection, administered slowly over a 4- to 5-minute period. **Rectal:** 10 to 20 mg every 4 hours or as directed.

NURSING IMPLICATIONS

Narcotic analgesics should be given in smallest effective dose and for the shortest time compatible with patient's needs.

Evaluate the patient's need for p.r.n. medication, and check time of last dose and validity of physician's order. Follow health facility policy regarding time limit on narcotic orders. Record time of onset, duration, and quality of pain (preferably in patient's own words).

Fullest analgesic effect is achieved if drug is administered before the patient experiences intense pain (morphine relieves continuous dull pain more effectively than sharp intermittent pain, which generally requires higher doses).

Note that the patient's cultural background may influence response to pain. Some patients tend to be stoic, but others may overtly show that they feel pain.

Elevated pulse or respiratory rate, restlessness, anorexia, or drawn facial expression may indicate need for analgesia.

Differentiate among restlessness as a sign of pain and the need for medication, restlessness associated with hypoxia, and restlessness caused by morphine-induced CNS stimulation (a paradoxic reaction that is particularly common in women and elderly patients).

Provide maximum comfort measures, and reduce environmental stimuli before preparing medication.

Before administering the drug, note respiratory rate, depth, and rhythm and size of pupils. Respirations of 12/minute or below and miosis are signs of toxicity (miosis is replaced by pupillary dilatation in asphyxia). Withhold drug and report these signs to physician.

Pupillary size is best judged in good room light (with patient facing away from window light) rather than by flashlight, which causes immediate miosis.

Caution patients not to smoke or ambulate without assistance after receiving the drug. Bedsides may be advisable.

When given parenterally in repeated doses, the intramuscular route is recommended. Repeated subcutaneous injections can cause local tissue irritation.

Monitor vital signs at regular intervals. Morphine-induced respiratory depression may occur even with small doses, and it increases progressively with higher doses (generally reaching maximum within 90 minutes following SC, 30 minutes after IM, and 7 minutes after IV administration). However, respiratory minute volume may remain below normal 4 to 5 hours following therapeutic doses.

Narcotic analgesics also depress cough and sigh reflexes and thus may induce atelectasis, especially in postoperative patients. Purposefully encourage changes in position, deep breathing, and coughing (unless contraindicated) at regularly scheduled intervals.

Narcotic antagonists (e.g., naloxone, Naltrexone) and facilities for oxygen and support of respiration should be available.

Nausea and orthostatic hypotension (with lightheadedness and dizziness) most often occur in ambulatory patients or when a supine patient assumes the head-up position or in patients not experiencing severe pain. (Morphine decreases the ability of the cardiovascular system to respond to gravitational shifts.)

Transient fall in blood pressure (even in the supine position) is apt to occur in patients with acute myocardial infarction.

Monitor intake–output ratio and pattern. Report oliguria or urinary retention. Morphine may dull perception of bladder stimuli; therefore, encourage the patient to void at least every 4 hours. Palpate lower abdomen to detect bladder distention.

Monitor bowel pattern. Inattention to the defecation reflex and desiccation of feces contribute to the constipating effects of morphine. Check for abdominal distention and intestinal peristaltic sounds during postoperative period.

Record relief of pain and duration of analgesia. Evaluate the patient's continued need for morphine. If indicated, suggest that the physician prescribe a less potent analgesic.

Tolerance as well as physiologic and psychologic dependence may develop with repeated use. There is high abuse liability.

Be alert to purposive behavior (manipulations) to get more drug; this usually begins shortly before next scheduled dose. Such behavior may signal the onset of tolerance and addiction.

Abrupt cessation of drug use in the presence of physiologic dependence initiates the *abstinence syndrome,* usually within 24 to 48 hours after last dose. Without treatment, withdrawal symptoms ("cold turkey") develop, with increasing intensity and a common sequence: drug craving and anxiety (within 6 hours of last dose); irritability, perspiration, yawning, rhinorrhea, itchy nose, sneezing, lacrimation (within 14 hours); pupil dilation, piloerection ("gooseflesh"), tremulousness, muscle jerks, bone and muscle aches, nausea, hot and cold flashes, tossing, restless sleep ("yen"), elevated systolic blood pressure, dilated pupils, elevated temperature, pulse, and respiration rates (within 24 to 36 hours); curled-up position, vomiting, diarrhea, weight loss, hemoconcentration, increased blood sugar, spontaneous ejaculation or orgasm (within 36 to 48 hours).

Severity and character of withdrawal symptoms depend on the interval between doses, duration of drug use, total daily dose, and health and personality of the addicted individual.

Classified as Schedule II drug under Federal Controlled Substances Act.

Morphine is reported to be physically and chemically incompatible with many solutions. Do not mix with other drugs without the advice of a pharmacist.

Preserved in tight, light-resistant containers.

M

Diagnostic Test Interferences. False-positive **urine glucose** determinations may occur using Benedict's solution. **Plasma amylase** and **lipase** determinations may be falsely positive for 24 hours after use of morphine.

Drug Interactions. CNS depressant effects of morphine and other narcotic analgesics may be exaggerated and prolonged by concurrent administration of **alcohol,** general **anesthetics, antianxiety drugs, phenothiazines, tricyclic antidepressants, barbiturates,** other **sedatives, hypnotics,** and **MAO inhibitors.** Narcotic analgesics may enhance the neuromuscular blocking action of **skeletal muscle relaxants.**

MOXALACTAM DISODIUM

(Moxam)

(mox'a-lak-tam)
Antiinfective
Antibiotic (beta-lactam)
Cephalosporin

ACTIONS AND USES. Synthetic, broad spectrum beta-lactam antibiotic with prolonged action; usually classified as third generation cephalosporin. In general, spectrum of activity resembles that of other third generation members, particularly cefotaxime. Like cefotaxime, is less active than first and second generation cephalosporins against gram-positive cocci (e.g., *Staphylococcus aureus,* group A and B streptococci, *Streptococcus pneumonia*). Active against most gram-negative aerobes especially *Escherichia coli, Klebsiella pneumoniae,* and *Serratia marcescens.* Activity against *Pseudomonas aeruginosa* is variable, and it is usually not active against *Acinetobacter.* More highly resistant to inactivation by beta-lactamases (cephalosporinase and penicillinase) than cefotaxime and other cephalosporins. In common with other cephalosporins, acts by inhibiting cell wall synthesis, and lacks activity against fungi and viruses. Moxalactam may affect vitamin K-dependent clotting factors and platelet function possibly by eliminating K-producing gut bacteria from GI tract. Unlike other cephalosporins, crosses blood–brain barrier whether or not meninges are inflamed. Action is not prolonged by probenecid. Contains 3.8 mEq of sodium per gram.

Used for treatment of serious infections of lower respiratory and urinary tracts, skin and skin structure, bone and joint, and for intraabdominal infections, septicemia, and meningitis. Used alone or with an aminoglycoside.

ABSORPTION AND FATE. Well-absorbed following IM or IV administration and widely distributed to most body tissues and fluids. Serum levels peak in ½ to 2 hours following IM injection, and at the end of IV infusion. Half-life: 2 to 2½ hours (longer in patients with renal dysfunction). Crosses blood–brain barrier; drug concentrations in CSF: 10 to 30% of those in serum (higher when meninges are inflamed), and half-life is twice as long. Does not appear to be metabolized. Approximately 80% excreted in urine within 24 hours as unchanged drug; small amounts appear in stool via bile. Crosses placenta. Distribution to breast milk not known.

CONTRAINDICATIONS AND PRECAUTIONS. History of hypersensitivity to moxalactam or other cephalosporins, or to any ingredient in the formulation, e.g., mannitol. Safe use during pregnancy (category C), and in nursing women not established. *Cautious Use:* history of type I hypersensitivity to penicillins (urticaria, angioedema, anaphylaxis), history of other allergies, particularly to drugs, impaired renal or hepatic function, history of bleeding disorders or GI diseases, particularly colitis.

ADVERSE/SIDE EFFECTS. GI: anorexia, diarrhea, nausea, vomiting, pseudomembranous colitis. **Hematologic:** anemia, mild transient neutropenia, leukopenia, granulocytopenia, thrombocytopenia, thrombocytosis, eosinophilia, elevation of hepatic enzymes, hypoprothrombonemia. **Hypersensitivity:** skin rash, purpura, fever, urticaria, pruritus, serum sickness-like reactions, dyspnea, angioedema. **Renal** (causal relationships not established): hematuria, pyuria, proteinuria, increases in BUN and serum creatinine. **Other:** seizures, bleeding problems including pulmonary hemorrhage. *Local (site) reactions:* mild burning pain (IM site); phlebitis, thrombophlebitis (following IV administration).

M

ROUTE AND DOSAGE. Intramuscular, intravenous: Adults: 2 to 6 Gm/day in divided doses every 8 to 12 hours for 5 to 10 days or up to 14 days. Life-threatening infections: 4 Gm every 8 hours. **Children:** 50 mg/kg every 6 to 8 hours. **Neonates:** 50 mg/kg every 8 to 12 hours. Maximum recommended dosage for neonates and children: 200 mg/kg/day up to 12 Gm daily.

NURSING IMPLICATIONS

Culture and susceptibility tests should be performed prior to and periodically during therapy to monitor drug effectiveness and bacterial resistance. Therapy may be instituted pending test results.

Before therapy is initiated, a careful inquiry should be made regarding previous hypersensitivity reactions to cephalosporins, penicillins, and history of previous allergies, particularly to drugs.

IM injections should be made deeply into large muscle mass such as the upper outer quadrant of gluteus maximus. Aspirate carefully to avoid inadvertent entry of drug into blood vessel. Rotate injection sites.

For IM administration, moxalactam should be diluted with either sterile or bacteriostatic water, sterile or bacteriostatic 0.9% sodium chloride for injection, or 0.5 or 1.0% lidocaine hydrochloride injection (by prescription).

For direct intermittent IV administration, injections should be made slowly over 3 to 5 minutes, directly into vein or through tubing of a free-flowing compatible IV infusion solution.

Refer to manufacturer's directions for reconstitution, compatible solutions, storage, stability information, and for specific recommendations for IV administration.

Be prepared to administer emergency therapy for hypersensitivity reactions. Have on hand: epinephrine, IV steroids, oxygen, equipment for respiratory assistance and airway maintenance.

Report promptly the onset of loose stools or diarrhea. Pseudomembranous colitis, a potentially life-threatening complication, should be considered a possible cause of diarrhea. Most patients respond to replacement of fluids, electrolytes, and protein. *See Index: Nursing Interventions: Rehydration.* Discontinuation of drug may be required.

Monitor intake and output ratio and pattern in patients with impaired renal function, or who are receiving high dosages or an aminoglycoside antibiotic concomitantly. Renal status (serum creatinine, BUN, creatinine clearance) and bleeding time should be evaluated at regular intervals in these patients.

Baseline and periodic hematologic, renal, and hepatic function tests should be performed for all patients during prolonged therapy. Patients receiving concomitant therapy with an aminoglycoside antibiotic should also have periodic audiometric tests. Bleeding time (BT), prothrombin, and partial thromboplastin time (PPT) should be monitored in patients receiving over 4 Gm/day for more than 3 days and in patients with significantly impaired renal function.

Prophylactic doses of vitamin K (e.g., 10 mg per week) may be prescribed to reduce possibility of bleeding problems associated with hypoprothrombinemia. Observe patient for signs of bleeding and be alert to complaints that suggest bleeding tendencies: petechiae, ecchymoses, nosebleeds, bleeding gums, hemoptysis, bleeding from IM or IV sites, cloudy urine (possibly hematuria).

Platelet dysfunction and prolonged bleeding time are dose-dependent and usually can be avoided by limiting dosage to 4 Gm/day.

If bleeding occurs, and prothrombin time (PT) is prolonged, vitamin K should be prescribed. Some patients require fresh frozen plasma, packed red blood cells, or platelet concentrates. If bleeding is due to platelet dysfunction, which may be manifested by prolonged PT and PPT times and prolonged BT, drug should be discontinued.

Bleeding abnormalities associated with hypoprothrombinemia are most commonly due to low vitamin K reserves, such as occurs in the debilitated and malnourished, in postoperative patients, patients with renal or hepatic disease, or malabsorption syndromes.

Moxalactam-induced bleeding must be distinguished from disseminated intravascular coagulation (DIC) since both may occur in patients with sepsis, severe trauma or shock, extensive cancer, and renal and hepatic dysfunction. This coagulation disorder is also associated with severe platelet depletion and profuse bleeding, and can be ruled out by appropriate laboratory blood studies.

Observe for and report onset of superinfections: fever, sore mouth or throat, white patches in mouth, black hairy tongue, diarrhea, foul-smelling stools or vaginal discharge, vaginitis, anogenital itching, candidiasis (moniliasis): fungal infection of skin, vagina, bronchi, lungs.

Advise patient to abstain from alcohol or alcohol containing beverages during drug therapy with moxalactam and for several days after last dose. Alcohol and moxalactam may cause a disulfiram reaction (nausea, vomiting, palpitation, tachycardia, flushing, sweating).

Frozen solutions of moxalactam should be allowed to thaw naturally at room temperature, without warming. Do not refreeze.

Store vials below 26°C (78°F), unless otherwise directed by manufacturer. Protect from light.

Diagnostic Test Interferences. Positive **direct Coombs' test** may occur (can interfere with hematologic and crossmatching procedures). Unlike other cephalosporins, moxalactam does not interfere with **urine glucose** tests.

Drug Interactions: Moxalactam

Plus	Interactions
Alcohol (Ethanol) and alcohol-containing solutions	Disulfiram reaction as late as 48 hours after last dose (moxalactam inhibits acetaldehyde dehydrogenase)
Aminoglycosides	Possibility of increased risk of nephrotoxicity and ototoxicity. Used with caution. Aminoglycoside must be administered separately and not mixed with moxalactam
Anticoagulants, oral, and heparin in high doses (over 20,000 units/day) Aspirin	Risk of bleeding may be increased. Used with caution

N

NADOLOL
(Corgard)

(nay-doe'lole)
Beta-adrenergic blocking agent
Antihypertensive
Antianginal

N

ACTIONS AND USES. Nonselective beta-adrenergic blocking agent pharmacologically and chemically similar to propranolol (qv). Inhibits response to adrenergic stimuli by competitively blocking beta-adrenergic receptors within heart. As a result, reduces heart rate and cardiac output at rest and during exercise, and also decreases conduction velocity through AV node and myocardial automaticity. Unlike propranolol, has no membrane-stabilizing activity and little direct myocardial depressant effect. Suppression of $beta_2$-adrenergic receptors in bronchial and vascular smooth muscle can cause bronchospasm and a Raynaud's-like phenomenon. Decreases standing and supine blood pressures by an unknown mechanism. Reduces plasma renin activity.

Used in treatment of hypertension either alone or in combination with a diuretic. Also used for long-term prophylactic management of angina pectoris.

ABSORPTION AND FATE. About 30 to 40% absorbed from GI tract. Peak plasma levels in 2 to 4 hours; duration 17 to 24 hours. Widely distributed in body tissues. Half-life 10 to 24 hours. Approximately 30% protein bound. Not metabolized. About 70% eliminated unchanged via kidneys. Also excreted unchanged in bile and breast milk.

CONTRAINDICATIONS AND PRECAUTIONS. Bronchial asthma, severe chronic obstructive pulmonary disease, inadequate myocardial function, sinus bradycardia, greater than first-degree conduction block, overt cardiac failure, cardiogenic shock. Safe use during pregnancy, in nursing mothers, and in children under 18 years of age not established. *Cautious Use:* congestive heart failure, diabetes mellitus, hyperthyroidism, renal impairment.

ADVERSE/SIDE EFFECTS. Allergic: rash, pruritus, fever, sore throat, laryngospasm, respiratory disturbances. **CNS:** dizziness, fatigue, sedation, headache, paresthesias, behavioral changes; rare: mental depression, hallucinations, disorientation. **CV:** bradycardia, peripheral vascular insufficiency (Raynaud's type), palpitation, postural hypotension, conduction or rhythm disturbances, congestive heart failure. **EENT:** blurred vision, nasal stuffiness, tinnitus, vertigo, dry mouth, dry eyes. **GI:** nausea, vomiting, anorexia, diarrhea, constipation, abdominal cramps, bloating, flatulence, dry mouth. **Hematologic:** agranulocytosis, thrombocytopenia. **Other:** weight gain, sleep disturbances, dry skin, impotence.

ROUTE AND DOSAGE. Oral: *Angina pectoris:* Initial: 40 mg once daily; gradually increased by 40 to 80 mg increments at 3- to 7-day intervals until optimum response or pronounced slowing of heart rate. Maintenance: 80 to 240 mg once daily. *Hypertension:* Initial: 40 mg once daily. If necessary, increased by 40 to 80 mg increments until optimum response. Maintenance: 80 to 320 mg once daily. Rarely, up to 640 mg daily.

NURSING IMPLICATIONS

May be administered without regard to food. Presence of food in GI tract does not affect rate or extent of absorption.

Usually administered no more than once daily because it has a long half-life.

Blood pressure determinations and apical pulse rate should be used as guides to dosage.

Patient should know usual pulse rate and be taught to check it before taking each dose. Instruct patient to withhold medication and to consult physician if pulse rate drops below 60 or becomes irregular.

Excessive bradycardia may be treated with IV atropine. If ineffective isoproterenol IV may be necessary. Hypotension may be treated with a vasopressor such as dobutamine, dopamine, epinephrine, or norepinephrine. Aminophylline may be used to treat bronchospasm.

Monitor intake–output ratio and creatinine clearance in patients with impaired renal function or with cardiac problems. Dosage intervals will be lengthened with decreases in creatinine clearance values.

Monitor weight. Advise patient to report weight gain of 3 to 4 pounds in a day and any other possible signs of congestive heart failure: breathing difficulty, cough, fatigue and dyspnea with exertion, rapid pulse, edema, anxiety.

Therapeutic effectiveness for patients with angina is evaluated by reduction in frequency of anginal attacks and improved exercise tolerance. Improvement should coincide with steady state serum concentration which is generally reached within 6 to 9 days. Keep physician informed of drug effect.

Emphasize importance of compliance and caution patient not to stop medication or alter dosage without consulting physician.

If nadolol is to be discontinued, dosage should be reduced over a 1- to 2-week period. Abrupt withdrawal can precipitate myocardial infarction or thyroid storm in susceptible patients.

Caution patient to avoid driving and other potentially hazardous activities until reaction to drug is known.

Patients with diabetes mellitus should be closely monitored. Beta-adrenergic blockade produced by nadolol may prevent important clinical manifestations of hypoglycemia, e.g., tachycardia, blood pressure changes.

Necessity of withdrawing nadolol before surgery is controversial. Manufacturer recommends withdrawal if possible. If drug is not withheld, anesthetist must be informed.

Protect drug from light. Store at room temperature.

See also Propranolol (prototype beta-adrenergic blocker).

NAFCILLIN, SODIUM

(Nafcil, Unipen)

(naf-sill'in)
Antiinfective
Antibiotic (beta-lactam)
Penicillin

ACTIONS AND USES. Semisynthetic, acid-stable, penicillinase-resistant penicillin. Mechanism of bactericidal action, contraindications, precautions, and adverse reactions as for penicillin G. Effective against both penicillin-sensitive and penicillin-resistant strains of *Staphylococcus aureus.* Also active against pneumococci and group A beta-hemolytic streptococci. Highly active against penicillinase-producing staphylococci, but less potent than penicillin G against penicillin-sensitive microorganisms and generally ineffective against methicillin-resistant staphylococci.

Used primarily in treatment of infections caused by penicillinase-producing staphylococci. May also be used to initiate treatment in suspected staphylococcal infections pending culture and sensitivity test results. As with other penicillins, serum concentrations are considerably enhanced by concurrent use of probenecid.

ABSORPTION AND FATE. Incompletely and irregularly absorbed after oral administration. Peak serum levels within 30 to 60 minutes following oral and IM administration; duration 4 hours following oral and 4 to 6 hours following IM injection. Penetrates pleural, pericardial, and synovial fluids, with predominant concentration in liver. About 90% bound to plasma proteins. Half-life: 1 hour. Enters enterohepatic circulation. Primarily eliminated in bile; 10 to 30% of dose is excreted unchanged in urine.

CONTRAINDICATIONS AND PRECAUTIONS. Hypersensitivity to penicillins, cephalosporins, and other allergens; use of oral drug in severe infections, gastric dilatation, cardiospasm, or intestinal hypermotility; IV use in neonates and infants. Safe use during pregnancy (category B) not established. *Cautious Use:* history of or suspected atopy or allergy (eczema, hives, hay fever, asthma). *See also Penicillin G.*

ADVERSE/SIDE EFFECTS. Nausea, vomiting, diarrhea. **Allergic reactions:** urticaria, pruritus, rash, eosinophilia, drug fever, anaphylaxis (particularly following parenteral therapy), allergic interstitial nephritis. Pain and tissue irritation and increase in serum transaminase activity (following IM); hypokalemia (with high IV doses); thrombophlebitis following IV; neutropenia (long-term therapy). *See also Penicillin G.*

ROUTE AND DOSAGE. **Oral: Adults:** 250 mg to 1 Gm every 4 to 6 hours; **Infants and children:** 25 to 50 mg/kg/day in four divided doses; **Neonates:** 10 mg/kg 3 or 4 times daily. **Intramuscular: Adults:** 500 mg every 4 to 6 hours; **Infants and children:** 25 mg/kg twice daily. **Neonates:** 10 mg/kg twice daily. **Intravenous: Adults:** 500 mg to 1 Gm every 4 hours; **Children:** 50 mg/kg/day in 4 equally-divided doses.

N

NURSING IMPLICATIONS

Culture and sensitivity tests should be performed prior to and periodically during therapy.

A careful history should be obtained before therapy to determine any prior allergic reactions to penicillins, cephalosporins, and other allergens.

Oral dose is best taken on an empty stomach (at least 1 hour before or 2 hours after meals). Although nafcillin is acid-stable, food interferes with absorption. Additionally, GI absorption of nafcillin is erratic.

Oral solution should be dated after reconstitution and refrigerated. Discard unused portions after 1 week.

For IM injection reconstitute with sterile water for injection, 0.9% sodium chloride injection, or bacteriostatic water for injection (with benzyl alcohol or parabens). Follow manufacturer's directions for attaining desired concentration.

Following reconstitution, IM solutions are stable for 7 days under refrigeration and for 3 days at room temperature. Vial should be so labeled and dated.

IM injection in adults: administered by deep intragluteal injection. Make certain solution is clear. Select site carefully. Injection into or near major peripheral nerves or local vessels can result in neurovascular damage. Check for blood backflow before injecting drug to avoid intraarterial administration. Rotate injection sites.

IM injection in children: intragluteal injection is contraindicated in young children because gluteal muscles are underdeveloped. In general, the preferred IM site in children under 3 years of age is the midlateral or anterolateral thigh. Follow agency policy.

For IV injection, required dose should be diluted with 15 to 30 ml sterile water for injection or isotonic sodium chloride for injection and administered over 5- to 10-minute period, either directly or into tubing of running IV infusion.

For continuous IV infusion, concentration of drug should be within range of 2 to 40 mg/ml. Physician will prescribe infusion rate. Rate and volume of infusion should be adjusted so that desired dose is administered before solution loses its stability.

Compatible IV infusion solutions include isotonic sodium chloride; 5% dextrose in water or in 0.4% sodium chloride; Ringer's injection, or M/6 sodium lactate (30 mg/ml concentration). Discard unused portions 24 hours after reconstitution.

IV therapy is usually not given for more than 24 to 48 hours, because of the possibility of thrombophlebitis, particularly in the elderly. Inspect IV site for inflammatory reaction. (The acronym SHARP is a guideline for identifying signs of inflammation: Swelling, Heat, Arrested motion, Redness, Pain.) Also check IV site for leakage, potentially more apt to occur in the elderly patient since loss of tissue elasticity with aging may promote extravasation around the needle.

Allergic reactions, principally rash, occur most commonly. Nausea, vomiting, and diarrhea may occur with oral therapy. Twice weekly differential white blood cell counts are strongly advised in patients receiving IV nafcillin therapy for longer than 2 weeks. Nafcillin-induced neutropenia (agranulocytosis) occurs commonly during third week of therapy. It may be associated with malaise, fever, sore mouth, or throat. Advise patient to report these symptoms promptly.

Periodic assessments of hepatic, renal, and hematopoietic functions are advised during prolonged therapy.

Infections caused by beta-hemolytic streptococci should be treated for at least 10 days to prevent possible development of acute rheumatic fever.

Be alert for signs of bacterial or fungal superinfections in patient on prolonged therapy.

Nafcillin sodium contains approximately 3 mEq of sodium per gram.

See Penicillin G (prototype penicillin).

Diagnostic Test Interferences. Nafcillin in large doses can cause false-positive **urine protein** tests, using sulfosalicylic acid method. *See also Penicillin G.*

NALBUPHINE HYDROCHLORIDE

(Nubain)

(nal'byoo-feen)

Analgesic (nonnarcotic)

Opiate agonist (partial)

ACTIONS AND USES. Synthetic narcotic analgesic with agonist and weak antagonist properties. Structurally similar to naloxone and oxymorphone, but pharmacologic effects are like those of pentazocine and butorphanol. Analgesic potency in about 3 or 4 times greater than that of pentazocine and approximately equal to that produced by equivalent doses of morphine. On a weight basis, produces respiratory depression about equal to that of morphine; however, in contrast to morphine, doses higher than 30 mg produce no further respiratory depression. Antagonistic potency is approximately one-fourth that of naloxone and about 10 times greater than that of pentazocine.

Used for symptomatic relief of moderate to severe pain. Also used to provide preoperative sedation analgesia, and as a supplement to surgical anesthesia.

ABSORPTION AND FATE. Duration of analgesia approximately 3 to 6 hours. Half-life: about 5 hours. Metabolized in liver.

CONTRAINDICATIONS AND PRECAUTIONS. History of hypersensitivity to drug. Safe use during pregnancy and in patients under age 18 years not established. *Cautious Use:* history of emotional instability or drug abuse; head injury, increased intracranial pressure; impaired respirations, impaired renal or hepatic function, myocardial infarction, biliary tract surgery.

ADVERSE/SIDE EFFECTS. Most common: sedation; sweaty, clammy skin; nausea, vomiting, dizziness, vertigo. **CNS:** nervousness, depression, restlessness, crying, euphoria, dysphoria, distortion of body image, unusual dreams, confusion, hallucinations; numbness and tingling sensations. **CV:** hypertension, hypotension, bradycardia, tachycardia, flushing. **GI:** abdominal cramps, bitter taste. **Hypersensitivity:** pruritus, urticaria, burning sensation. **Respiratory:** dyspnea, asthma, respiratory depression. **Other:** speech difficulty, urinary urgency, blurred vision.

ROUTE AND DOSAGE. **Subcutaneous, intramuscular, intravenous:** 10 to 20 mg every 3 to 6 hours, as necessary. Not to exceed 160 mg/day.

NURSING IMPLICATIONS

Caution patient to avoid driving and other potentially hazardous activities until reaction to drug is determined.

Inform patient that concurrent use of alcohol and other CNS depressants may result in additive effects.

Use of drug during labor and delivery may cause respiratory depression of newborn.

Although nalbuphine is not subject to the Federal Controlled Substances Act, it does have some potential for abuse.

Abrupt termination of nalbuphine following prolonged use may result in symptoms similar to narcotic withdrawal: nausea, vomiting, abdominal cramps, lacrimation, nasal congestion, piloerection, fever, restlessness, anxiety.

Management of overdosage: IV administration of naloxone hydrochloride (Narcan); supportive measures: oxygen, IV fluids, vasopressors.

Protect nalbuphine from excessive light and store between 15° and 30°C (59° and 86°F) unless otherwise directed by manufacturer.

NALIDIXIC ACID

(NegGram)

(nal-i-dix'ik)

Antiinfective (urinary tract)

ACTIONS AND USES. Synthetic naphthyridine derivative with marked bactericidal activity against gram-negative organisms, including majority of *Proteus* strains, *Klebsiella,* Enterobacter *(Aerobacter)*, and *Escherichia coli*. Ineffective against *Pseudomonas* species. Gram-positive bacteria are relatively resistant. Appears to act by inhibiting DNA and RNA synthesis. Bacterial resistance has occurred.

Used in treatment of urinary tract infections caused by susceptible gram-negative organisms.

ABSORPTION AND FATE. Rapidly and almost completely absorbed from GI tract. Peak serum levels may occur in 1 to 2 hours, but unpredictably because of high plasma protein binding (93 to 97%). Mostly metabolized in liver. Approximately 80% of single dose is excreted in urine within 24 hours as intact drug and conjugates. Small amounts are excreted in feces. Crosses placenta; negligible excretion in breast milk.

CONTRAINDICATIONS AND PRECAUTIONS. Known hypersensitivity to nalidixic acid, history of convulsive disorders, first trimester of pregnancy, infants younger than 3 months of age. *Cautious Use:* second and third trimesters of pregnancy, renal or hepatic disease, epilepsy, severe cerebral arteriosclerosis.

ADVERSE/SIDE EFFECTS. **Allergic:** photosensitivity, angioedema, pruritus, urticaria, rash, fever, arthralgia (with joint swelling), eosinophilia, anaphylactoid reaction (rare). **CNS:** drowsiness, dizziness, vertigo, muscle weakness, myalgia, visual disturbances; (with overdosage): headache, intracranial hypertension, convulsions, toxic psychosis (rare), 6th cranial nerve palsy (lateral rectus muscle of eye). **GI** (common): nausea, vomiting, abdominal pain, diarrhea; *(occasionally):* bleeding. **Other reported:** cholestasis; metabolic acidosis (with overdosage); paresthesias; thrombocytopenia, leukopenia, hemolytic anemia (especially in glucose-6-phosphate dehydrogenase deficiency); increased BUN and SGOT; glycosuria and hyperglycemia (overdosage).

ROUTE AND DOSAGE. **Oral: Adults:** Initial: 1 Gm four times a day for 1 or 2 weeks; reduced to 500 mg four times a day for prolonged therapy. **Children (over 3 months to age 12):** Initial: 55 mg/kg/day in four equally divided doses; for prolonged therapy, may be reduced to 33 mg/kg/day.

NURSING IMPLICATIONS

Culture and sensitivity tests are advised prior to initiation of treatment and periodically during therapy. Bacterial resistance sometimes develops within 48 hours after start of therapy. Follow-up cultures are also advised to determine if infection is eliminated.

Reportedly, blood levels are higher when drug is administered on empty stomach than when taken with food, but how this affects outcome of urinary level is unknown (because of high plasma protein binding). May be administered with food or milk if patient complains of GI distress.

CNS reactions tend to occur 30 minutes after initiation of treatment or after second or third dose. Infants, children, and geriatric patients are especially susceptible. Observe for and report immediately the onset of marked irritability, vomiting, bulging of anterior fontanelle (infants), headache, excitement or drowsiness, papilledema, vertigo.

Subjective visual disturbances may occur during first few days of therapy. Report to physician. Symptoms usually disappear promptly with reduction of dosage or discontinuation of therapy.

Blood counts and renal and hepatic function tests are recommended if therapy is continued longer than 2 weeks.

Caution patient to avoid exposure to direct sunlight or ultraviolet light while receiving drug. Therapy should be discontinued if photosensitivity occurs (erythema or bullae on exposed skin surfaces). Susceptible patients may continue to be photosensitive up to 3 months after termination of drug.

See Index: Nuring Interventions: urinary tract infection.

Diagnostic Test Interferences. False-positive urine tests for **glucose** with copper reduction methods (e.g., Benedict's, Clinitest, Fehling's), but not with glucose oxidase methods (e.g., Clinistix, Tes-Tape). May cause elevation of **urinary 17-ketosteroids** (Zimmerman method).

Drug Interactions. Absorption of nalidixic acid may be decreased by **antacids;** however, **sodium bicarbonate** may increase absorption (clinical significance not determined). **Nitrofurantoin** may antagonize effect of nalidixic acid. Nalidixic acid may enhance effects of **oral anticoagulants** (by displacing them from protein binding sites).

NALOXONE HYDROCHLORIDE

(Narcan)

(nal-ox'one)
Narcotic antagonist

ACTIONS AND USES. *N*-allyl analog of oxymorphone. A "pure" narcotic antagonist, essentially free of agonistic (morphinelike) properties. Thus, unlike the narcotic antagonist levallorphan, produces no significant analgesia, respiratory depression, psychotomimetic effects, or miosis when administered in the absence of narcotics, and possesses more potent narcotic antagonist action. Not effective against non-opioid-induced respiratory depression. Tolerance and psychic or physical dependence not reported.

Used in treatment of narcotic overdosage and to reverse respiratory depression induced by natural and synthetic narcotics, and by pentazocine, and propoxyphene. Drug of choice when nature of depressant drug is not known, and for diagnosis of suspected acute opioid overdosage.

N

ABSORPTION AND FATE. Onset of action following IV injection occurs within 2 minutes and within 2 to 5 minutes after subcutaneous or IM administration. Duration of action 3 to 5 hours, depending on dosage and route. Plasma half-life 60 to 90 minutes. Rapidly metabolized in liver, primarily by conjugation with glucuronic acid. Based on limited studies, 25 to 40% of IV dose is excreted in urine as metabolites in 6 hours and 60 to 70% in 72 hours. Readily crosses placenta.

CONTRAINDICATIONS AND PRECAUTIONS. Known hypersensitivity to naloxone; respiratory depression due to non-opioid drugs. Safe use during pregnancy (other than labor) not established. *Cautious Use:* in neonates and children; known or suspected narcotic dependence; cardiac irritability.

ADVERSE/SIDE EFFECTS. *Excessive dosage in narcotic depression:* reversal of analgesia, increased blood pressure, tremors, hyperventilation, slight drowsiness, elevated partial thromboplastin time. *Too rapid reversal:* nausea, vomiting, sweating, tachycardia.

ROUTE AND DOSAGE. Subcutaneous, intramuscular, intravenous: Adults: 0.4 mg; may be repeated IV at two- to three-minute intervals, if necessary, for 2 or 3 doses, then a 1- to 2-hour interval, if necessary. **Pediatric:** 0.01 mg/kg; may be repeated as for adult administration.

NURSING IMPLICATIONS

Resuscitative measures such as maintaining airway, artificial ventilation, cardiac massage, and vasopressor agents may be required.

Monitor respirations and other vital signs. In some patients, respirations may "overshoot" to higher level than that prior to respiratory depression.

Duration of action of some narcotics may exceed that of naloxone; therefore, patient must be closely observed. Keep physician informed; repeat naloxone dose may be necessary.

Narcotic abstinence symptoms induced by naloxone generally start to diminish 20 to 40 minutes after administration and usually disappear within 90 minutes.

Do not mix naloxone with preparations containing a metabisulfite or bisulfite, long chain or high molecular weight anions (e.g., dextran) or solutions with alkaline pH. Compatible admixtures should be used within 24 hours.

Surgical and obstetric patients should be closely monitored for bleeding. Naloxone has been associated with abnormal coagulation test results. Also observe for reversal of analgesia, which may be manifested by nausea, vomiting, sweating, tachycardia.

Protect drug from excessive light.

NALTREXONE HYDROCHLORIDE

(Trexan)

(nal-trex'one)
Narcotic antagonist

N

ACTIONS AND USES. A pure opioid antagonist with prolonged pharmacologic effect; structurally and pharmacologically similar to naloxone. Weakens or completely and reversibly blocks the subjective effects (the "high") of IV opioids and analgesics possessing both agonist and antagonist activity (e.g., butorphanol). Mechanism of action not clearly delineated but it appears that competitive binding at opioid receptor sites reduces euphoria and drug craving without supporting the addiction. Since the antagonist action is provided by competition, it is surmountable; but only with dangerously large doses of a narcotic. When administered chronically with morphine, it blocks physcial dependence on morphine. In general, efficacy of this nonaddicting drug depends on its pure antagonist effect and upon a motivated, relatively opiate-free subject ("post-addict").

Used as adjunct to the maintenance of an opioid-free state in detoxified addicts who are and desire to remain narcotic-free. *Investigational Use:* treatment of two other compulsive consumption syndromes: alcoholism and obesity.

ABSORPTION AND FATE. Following oral administration: peak level achieved in 1 hour; pharmacologic effects persist for 24 to 72 hours (depending on dose). Undergoes extensive first-pass hepatic metabolism (chief metabolite: 6-beta-naltrexol is also a pure antagonist). Protein binding: 21%. Half-life of naltrexone: about 4 hours; of 6-beta-naltrexol: about 13 hours. Excreted primarily by kidneys as unchanged drug (1%) and metabolites. Does not accumulate during chronic dosing.

CONTRAINDICATIONS AND PRECAUTIONS. Patient who is receiving opioid analgesics or is in acute opioid withdrawal; the opioid-dependent patient; acute hepatitis, liver failure. Also contraindicated in any individual who: (1) fails naloxone challenge, (2) has a positive urine screen for opioids, or (3) has a history of sensitivity to naltrexone. Safe use during pregnancy (category C), by children under 18 years, or by nursing mothers not established.

ADVERSE/SIDE EFFECTS. CNS: difficulty sleeping, nightmares, bad dreams, anxiety, headache, reduced or increased energy, irritability, dizziness, depression, fatigue, drowsiness, restlessness, confusion, hallucinations, paranoia. **CV:** epistaxis, phlebitis, edema, hypertension, palpitations, tachycardia, nonspecific ECG changes. **Dermatologic:** skin rash, urticaria, pruritus, oily skin, acne, alopecia. **GI:** dry mouth, anorexia, nausea, vomiting, diarrhea, constipation, abdominal cramps/pain, excess gas, hemorrhoids, ulcer, hepatotoxicity. **GU:** delayed ejaculation, decreased potency; increased frequency, painful urination, changed libido. **Musculoskeletal:** muscle and joint pains, tremors. **Respiratory:** nasal congestion, rhinorrhea, sneezing, sore throat, excess mucus, sinus trouble, hoarseness, cough, chest pain. **Special senses:** blurred vision; burning, light sensitivity; swollen, aching, strained eyes; "clogged" or aching ears, tinnitus. **Other:** weight gain or loss, chills, increased thirst, yawning, fever, inguinal pain, cold feet, excessive sweating.

ROUTE AND DOSAGE. Naltrexone administration is preceded by a naloxone challenge test *(see Nursing Implications).* **Oral:** Initial: 25 mg. If no withdrawal signs within 1 hour, followed by an additional 25 mg. Once patient is started on 50 mg/24 hours, maintenance regimen is flexible: e.g., 100 mg on Monday, 100 mg on Wednesday, and 150 mg on Friday; or 50 mg every weekday with 100 mg on Saturday; or 100 mg every other day; or 150 mg every third day. (Doses as high as 800 mg/day have been tolerated without toxicity.)

NURSING IMPLICATIONS

Naltrexone treatment is adjunctive to a prolonged psychotherapeutic or counseling program.

Young addicts with a relatively short history of addiction have proved to be especially good candidates for naltrexone treatment. Patients from lower socioeconomic groups previously on a methadone program seem to have less success than naltrexone-treated healthy professionals and business executives.

If *narcotic abstinence therapy* is to be effective, the patient must be very highly motivated to stay drug free because the drug does not suppress the urge to experience a high from opiates.

Treatment is not started until naloxone challenge is negative, patient has been opioid free 7 to 10 days (as verified by urine analysis for opioids), and patient reports or manifests no withdrawal symptoms.

Compliance may be improved by establishing a maintenance schedule of dosing every 48 to 72 hours.

Liver function tests are checked before the treatment is started, at monthly intervals for 6 months, and then periodically as indicated.

The Naloxone Challenge Test (administered IV or SC) is given before starting the abstinence program with naltrexone:

- A portion of the IV dose is injected and with the needle left in place the patient is observed for 30 seconds for withdrawal symptoms. If none, remainder of dose is injected and patient is observed for the next 20 minutes.
- The SC dose is followed by an observation period of 45 minutes for symptoms of withdrawal.
- Question patient during observation periods to assist in recognition of withdrawal should it occur.
- *Interpretation:* Evidence of withdrawal symptoms indicates that the patient is a potential risk and should not enter a naltrexone program. If no signs or symptoms appear, drug therapy can begin. In case of doubt that the patient is opioid free, confirmatory rechallenge is done.

Withdrawal symptoms include: stuffiness or runny nose, tearing, yawning, sweating, tremors, vomiting, gooseflesh, feeling of temperature change, bone, joint, and muscle pains, abdominal cramps.

Heroin addiction has been successively treated with methadone, although disadvantages are serious: it causes euphoria or sedation, is addictive, and is dangerous in overdosage. Transfer from methadone to naltrexone may be desirable and can be done after gradual withdrawal and final discontinuation of methadone.

Opioid overdose produces a syndrome comprising coma, flaccid paralysis, miosis, and respiratory depression. Discuss with the patient the danger of overdosing with an opiate while on naltrexone therapy. Small doses even at frequent intervals will give no desired effects; however, a dose large enough to surmount naltrexone action (i.e., to produce a high) is very dangerous and may be fatal.

Accidental ingestion of naltrexone by an opioid-dependent individual causes withdrawal symptoms to appear within 5 minutes and to remain for as long as 48 hours. Fluid therapy to replace losses by vomiting and diarrhea, monitoring for respiratory and cardiac symptoms, and protective treatment measures because of changes in mental state are provided during the recovery period.

The patient should be instructed to report promptly onset of signs of hepatotoxicity (naltrexone is a direct hepatotoxin): jaundice, dark urine, pruritus. The drug will be discontinued.

Advise patient not to self-dose with OTC drugs for treatment of cough, colds, diarrhea, or analgesia. Many available preparations contain small doses of an opioid. Consult physician for safe drugs if they are needed.

A doctor or dentist who treats a naltrexone user should be informed of the drug use. In an emergency, when administration of an opioid analgesic seems unavoidable, the opioid dose will be greater than usual and the respiratory depression will be deeper and prolonged.

Advise patient to wear identification jewelry indicating naltrexone use.

N

NANDROLONE DECANOATE

(Anabolin LA, Analone, Androlone-D, Deca-Durabolin, Hybolin)

(nan'droe-lone)
Anabolic

NANDROLONE PHENPROPIONATE

(Anabolin IM, Androlone, Durabolin, Hybolin Improved, Nandrolin)

ACTIONS AND USES. Synthetic steroid with high ratio of anabolic activity to androgenic activity. Both esters have same actions and uses, but differ in action duration: decanoate actions last 3 to 4 weeks; phenpropionate ester continues to exert anabolic effect for 1 to 3 weeks. *See Ethylestrenol for actions, uses, and limitations.*

ROUTE AND DOSAGE. Intramuscular: Adults: 50 to 100 mg *decanoate* every 3 to 4 weeks (100 to 200 mg weekly may be required for severe disease states); 25 to 50 mg *phenpropionate* weekly; 50 to 100 mg weekly may be required for severe disease states. **Children (2 to 13 years):** 25 to 50 mg *decanoate* every 3 to 4 weeks; 12.5 to 25 mg *phenpropionate* every 2 to 4 weeks.

NURSING IMPLICATIONS

Inject drug deep IM, preferably into gluteal muscle in adult; follow agency policy regarding IM site in small child.

Intermittent therapy is usually recommended (4-month course of treatment followed by 6 to 8 weeks rest period).

See also Ethylestrenol (prototype anabolic).

PROTOTYPE

NAPHAZOLINE HYDROCHLORIDE

(Ak-Con, Albalon, Allerest Eye Drops, Clear Eyes, Degest-2, Naphcon, Privine VasoClear, Vasocon)

(naf-az'oh-leen)
Alpha-adrenergic agonist
Sympathomimetic
Decongestant

ACTIONS AND USES. Direct-acting imidazoline derivative with marked alpha-adrenergic activity. Produces rapid and prolonged vasoconstriction of arterioles, thereby decreasing fluid exudation and mucosal engorgement. Differs from other sympathomimetic amines in that systemic absorption may cause CNS depression rather than stimulation.

Used topically as nasal decongestant and as topical ocular vasoconstrictor.

CONTRAINDICATIONS AND PRECAUTIONS. Hypersensitivity to any ingredients of preparation; narrow-angle glaucoma; concomitant use with MAO inhibitors or tricyclic antidepressants. Safe use during pregnancy or in infants or children not established. *Cautious Use:* hypertension, cardiac irregularities, advanced arteriosclerosis, diabetes, hyperthyroidism, elderly patients.

ADVERSE/SIDE EFFECTS. Nasal use: transient stinging or burning, dryness of nasal mucosa, hypersensitivity reactions. **Ophthalmic use:** pupillary dilation, increased intraocular pressure. **Overdosage (systemic absorption):** headache, lightheadedness, hypertension, palpitation, tachycardia, arrhythmias, hyperglycemia, marked sedation (accidental swallowing in children), hypothermia, cardiovascular collapse, respiratory depression.

ROUTE AND DOSAGE. Topical: Nasal solution (0.05%): 2 drops in each nostril, no more frequently than every 3 hours. Nasal spray (0.05%): 2 sprays in each nostril every 4 to 6 hours. Ophthalmic solution (0.012 to 0.1%): 1 or 2 drops into conjunctival sac of affected eye every 3 or 4 hours (frequency depends on response).

NURSING IMPLICATIONS

Note that some commercial nasal solution preparations are designed to instill 2 drops with a single compression of dropper bulb (maximum dose is 2 drops).

Insomnia has not been reported; one dose may be scheduled at bedtime.

Proper technic of nose blowing: blow with both nostrils open.

Instill nasal spray with patient in upright position. If administered in reclining position, a stream rather than a spray may be ejected, with possibility of systemic reaction.

Naphazoline is incompatible with aluminum. Do not use atomizers made of aluminum or that have moving aluminum parts.

When *instilling nose drops,* the amount of drug swallowed can be minimized by taking care not to direct the flow toward nasopharynx and by proper positioning of patient. Position used depends on condition being treated. Consult physician. *Parkinson position:* patient supine, head over edge of bed and turned to affected side (used for treating nasal passages and frontal and maxillary sinuses). *Proetz position:* patient supine, with head hanging straight back over edge of bed (used to treat ethmoid and sphenoid sinuses). Both positions can also be accomplished by placing pillow under patient's shoulders.

Following nasal instillation of spray, rinse dropper or spray top in hot water to prevent contamination of solution.

Rebound congestion and chemical rhinitis can occur with frequent and continued use.

Advise patient not to exceed prescribed regimen. Explain that systemic effects can result from swallowing excessive medication.

If nasal congestion is not relieved after 5 days, advise patient to discontinue medication and to contact physician.

To prevent contamination of eye solution, care should be taken not to touch eyelid or surrounding area with dropper tip.
Warn patient to keep drug out of reach of children.
Preserved in tight container preferably at 15° to 30°C (59° to 86°F) unless otherwise specified by manufacturer. Protect from freezing.

Drug Interactions. Possibility of enhanced pressor effect when administered concomitantly with or within 2 weeks of **MAO inhibitors** or with **tricyclic antidepressants.**

NAPROXEN
(Naprosyn)
NAPROXEN SODIUM
(Anaprox)

(na-prox'en)
Antiinflammatory (nonsteroidal), analagesic, antipyretic

ACTIONS AND USES. Nonsteroidal antiinflammatory drug with analgesic and antipyretic properties similar to other arylacetic acid derivatives, e.g., fenoprofen (qv). Mechanism of action not known but thought to be related to ability to inhibit prostaglandin synthesis. In common with other drugs of this group, inhibits platelet aggregation and prolongs bleeding time, but does not alter whole blood clotting or prothrombin time or platelet count. Cross-sensitivity with other nonsteroidal antiinflammatory drugs (NSAID) has been reported. Naproxen sodium contains about 25 mg (1 mEq) sodium; it is more rapidly absorbed than naproxen.

Used for antiinflammatory and analgesic effects in symptomatic treatment of acute and chronic rheumatoid arthritis, and for treatment of primary dysmenorrhea. Also has been used in management of ankylosing spondylitis, osteoarthritis, and gout.

ABSORPTION AND FATE. Almost completely absorbed when taken on an empty stomach. Plasma levels peak in 2 to 4 hours; analgesic effect may last up to 12 hours; 99% bound to plasma protein. Half-life: 12 to 15 hours; metabolized in liver to inactive metabolites. Excreted in urine within 5 days mostly as inactive metabolites and about 10% unchanged drug. Less than 1% eliminated in feces. Crosses placenta; appears in breast milk.

CONTRAINDICATIONS AND PRECAUTIONS. Hypersensitivity to naproxen; active peptic ulcer, individuals with manifest symptoms of rhinitis, asthma, or nasal polyps (aspirin triad) associated with use of aspirin or other nonsteroidal antiinflammatory drugs. Safe use during pregnancy, in nursing mothers and in children not established. *Cautious Use:* history of upper GI tract disorders, impaired renal, hepatic, or cardiac function, patients on sodium restriction (naproxen sodium).

ADVERSE/SIDE EFFECTS. CNS: headache, drowsiness, dizziness, lightheadedness, depression. **CV:** palpitation, dyspnea, peripheral edema. **EENT:** blurred vision, tinnitus, hearing disturbances. **GI:** anorexia, heartburn, indigestion, nausea, vomiting, GI bleeding. **Hematologic:** agranulocytosis, thrombocytopenia. **Skin:** pruritus, rash, ecchymosis. **Other:** thirst, menstrual disturbances, nephrotoxicity, jaundice. *See also Fenoprofen.*

ROUTE AND DOSAGE. Oral: *musculoskeletal pain:* 250 to 375 mg naproxen (275 mg naproxen sodium) twice daily not to exceed 1000 mg (1100 mg naproxen sodium). *Acute gout:* Initial: 750 mg naproxen followed by 250 mg every 8 hours until attack subsides. *Juvenile arthritis:* 10 mg/kg/day in two divided doses. *Dysmenorrhea:* 500 mg naproxen, followed by 250 mg every 6 to 8 hours (550 mg naproxen sodium followed by 275 mg every 6 to 8 hours).

NURSING IMPLICATIONS

May be administered with food or an antacid (if prescribed) to reduce incidence of GI upset. Food and some antacids, e.g., magnesium oxide and aluminum hydroxide, delay absorption of naproxen but apparently not total amount absorbed. Absorption is reportedly enhanced by sodium bicarbonate.

Patients with arthritis may experience symptomatic relief (reduction in joint pain, swelling, stiffness) within 24 to 48 hours with sodium naproxen therapy and in 2 to 4 weeks with naproxen.

Note that naproxen sodium should not be used concomitantly with the related drug naproxen since they both circulate in plasma as the naproxen anion.

Important to take a detailed drug history prior to initiation of therapy. *See Contraindications and Precautions.*

Since naproxen may cause dizziness and drowsiness, advise patient to exercise caution when driving or performing other potentially hazardous activities.

Baseline and periodic evaluations of hemoglobin, renal and hepatic function, and auditory and ophthalmic examinations are recommended in patients receiving prolonged or high dose therapy.

Inform patient that alcohol and aspirin may increase risk of GI ulceration and bleeding tendencies and, therefore, should be avoided, unless otherwise advised by physician.

Since naproxen may prolong bleeding time, caution patient to inform dentist or surgeon that patient is taking this drug.

See Fenoprofen Drug Interactions; see Aspirin (prototype NSAID).

Diagnostic Test Interferences. Transient elevations in **BUN** and serum **alkaline phosphatase** may occur. Naproxen may interfere with some urinary assays of **5-HIAA** and may cause falsely **high urinary 17-KGS** levels (using n-dinitrobenzene reagent). Suggested that naproxen be withdrawn 72 hours before adrenal function tests.

NATAMYCIN

(Natacyn)

(na-ta-mye′sin)
Antiinfective
Antibiotic (macrolide)
Antifungal

ACTIONS AND USES. Tetraene polyene compound derived from *Streptomyces natalensis.* Effective against may yeasts and filamentous fungi including *Candida, Aspergillus, Cephalosporium, Fusarium,* and *Penicillium.* Action mechanism simulates that of amphotericin B and nystatin: by binding to sterols in the cell membrane, structure and integrity is changed leading to loss of intracellular K and other essential constituents, and destruction of the organism. Has some activity in vivo against *Trichomonas vaginalis;* is not active against gram-positive or gram-negative bacteria or viruses. Has low order of toxicity.

Used topically to treat blepharitis, conjunctivitis, and keratitis caused by susceptible fungi. Initial drug of choice for treatment of *F. solani* keratitis. *Investigational Use:* treatment of oral, cutaneous, and vaginal candidiasis; treatment (intranasal) of pulmonary aspergillosis.

ABSORPTION AND FATE. Following topical application to the eye, drug adheres to ulcerated surfaces of cornea and is retained in conjunctival fornices. Penetration to the deep stromal structures or into the aqueous humor is not usual. Does not appear to be absorbed significantly from intact or debrided mucous membrane or from GI tract.

CONTRAINDICATIONS AND PRECAUTIONS. Hypersensitivity to any component of the formulation; concomitant administration of a corticosteroid. Safe use during pregnancy not established.

ADVERSE/SIDE EFFECTS. Reports scanty. Blurred vision, photophobia, eye pain. Uneven adherence of suspension to epithelial ulcerations or in fornices.

ROUTE AND DOSAGE. **Topical instillation** (5% suspension): *Fungal keratitis.* Initial: 1 drop in conjunctival sac of infected eye every 1 or 2 hours. After first 3 or 4 days, dose can be reduced to 1 drop every 6 to 8 days and eventually to 1 drop every 4 to 7 days. Usual course of treatment: 14 to 21 days or until no evidence of infection remains. *Fungal conjunctivitis and blepharitis:* 1 drop four to six times a day.

NURSING IMPLICATIONS

Initial diagnosis and sustained treatment should be based on clinical laboratory diagnosis by an ophthalmologist.

Lack of improvement in keratitis within 7 to 10 days suggests that causative organisms may not be susceptible to natamycin. Reevaluation is indicated and possibly change in therapy.

Inspect eye for response and tolerance at least twice weekly.

Administration of eye drops *(see Index: Drug administration: eye drops).*

If eye pain occurs, the drug should be discontinued.

Temporary photophobia should be anticipated. Tell patient to be prepared to wear sunglasses outdoors after drug administration and perhaps for a few hours indoors.

Instruct patient to return to ophthalmologist for reevaluation of eye problem if symptoms of conjunctivitis appear: pain, discharge, itching, scratching "foreign body sensation," changes in vision.

Thorough handwashing before and after treatment is imperative. Infection is easily transferred from infected to noninfected eye, and to other individuals.

Facecloths and hand towels should be used only by the patient to prevent transmission of the fungal infection.

Encourage patient to keep hands away from eyes, even if discomfort begs for scratching, rubbing, etc.

Store ophthalmic suspension preferably at 2° to 24°C (36° to 75°F) unless otherwise directed by manufacturer. Shake well before using.

NEOMYCIN SULFATE

(Mycifradin Sulfate, Myciguent, Neobiotic)

(nee-oh-mye′sin)
Antiinfective
Antibiotic
Aminoglycoside

ACTIONS AND USES. Aminoglycoside antibiotic obtained from *Streptomyces fradiae;* reported to be the most potent in neuromuscular blocking action and the most toxic of this group. Broad spectrum of antibacterial activity, and actions similar to those of gentamicin (qv).

Used in treatment of severe diarrhea caused by enteropathogenic *Escherichia coli;* and for preoperative intestinal antisepsis; used to inhibit nitrogen-forming bacteria of GI tract in patients with cirrhosis or hepatic coma and for treatment of urinary tract infections caused by susceptible organisms. Also used topically for short-term treatment of eye, ear, and skin infections. Available in a variety of creams, ointments, and sprays in combination with other antibiotics and corticosteroids.

ABSORPTION AND FATE. About 3% absorbed from GI tract following oral administration (neonates and prematures may absorb up to 10%). Peak plasma levels in 1 to 4 hours; still present in low levels at 8 hours. Half-life: about 3 hours (longer in patients with renal impairment and premature infants). About 90% bound to serum proteins. May be absorbed through ear, eye, denuded or inflamed skin, and body cavities following topical applications. Wide distribution in body tissues and fluids following IM administration; 30 to 50% of dose is excreted unchanged in urine, and about 97% of oral dose is excreted unchanged in feces.

CONTRAINDICATIONS AND PRECAUTIONS. History of sensitivity to topical or systemic neomycin or to any ingredient in formulations; use of oral drug in patients with intestinal obstruction; ulcerative bowel lesions; topical applications over large skin areas; parenteral use in patients with renal disease or impaired hearing; myasthenia gravis. Safe use during pregnancy not established. *Cautious Use:* topical otic applications in patients with perforated eardrum. *See also Gentamicin.*

ADVERSE/SIDE EFFECTS. Oral use: mild laxative effect, diarrhea, nausea, vomiting; prolonged therapy: malabsorptionlike syndrome including cyanocobalamin (vitamin B_{12}) deficiency, low serum cholesterol. **Systemic absorption:** nephrotoxicity, ototoxicity, neuromuscular blockade with muscular and respiratory paralysis, hypersensitivity reactions. *See Kanamycin.* **Topical use:** redness, scaling, pruritus, dermatitis.

ROUTE AND DOSAGE. Adults: Oral: *Intestinal antisepsis:* 1 Gm every hour for 4 doses, then 1 Gm every 4 hours for balance of 24 hours; alternatively 88 to 100 mg/kg daily in six divided doses for not more than 3 days. *Hepatic coma:* four to 12 Gm daily in 4 divided doses for 5 or 6 days. *Diarrhea:* 50 mg/kg in four divided doses for 2 or 3 days (average 3 Gm/day in divided doses). **Intramuscular:** 1.3 to 2.6 mg/kg every 6 hours (infrequently used). **Topical (5 mg/Gm):** ointment, cream. **Children: Oral:** *Intestinal antisepsis:* 10.3 mg/kg every 4 hours for 3 days. *Hepatic coma:* 437.5 mg to 1.225 Gm/m^2 every 6 hours for 5 or 6 days. *Diarrhea:* 8.75 mg/kg every 6 hours for 2 or 3 days.

NURSING IMPLICATIONS

Patients with renal or hepatic dysfunction receiving IM or extended oral neomycin therapy should have audiometric studies twice weekly, daily urinalysis for albumin, casts, and cells, and BUN every other day. Baseline determinations should be done before initiation of therapy. Serum drug levels also advised (toxic levels reportedly range from 8 to 30 mcg/ml, although individual variations exist).

Neomycin can cause irreversible damage to auditory branch of 8th cranial nerve (occurs more frequently than vestibular damage). At first, loss of hearing most often involves high-frequency sounds, then may progress to include normal hearing frequencies. In general, severity and persistence of ototoxic symptoms depend on dosage and duration of drug therapy; these have occurred in patients on prolonged therapy even when serum drug levels have been low. Early reporting is essential.

Advise patient to report any unusual symptom related to ears or hearing: e.g., tinnitus, roaring sounds, loss of hearing acuity, dizziness.

For treatment of diarrhea: Neomycin is used as adjunct to fluid and electrolyte replacement and bed rest.

Patients with hepatic coma: When neomycin therapy is initiated, protein is usually restricted from diet, and carbohydrate intake is increased. Diuretics are generally withheld. As symptoms subside and cerebral functions clear (e.g., handwriting improves), protein intake is gradually increased.

Neomycin retention enema is sometimes prescribed for patients with hepatic coma. Recommended dilution for adults: 200 ml to 1 liter of 1% solution or 100 ml of 2% solution, to be retained for 20 minutes to more than 1 hour, as prescribed.

Monitor intake and output in patients receiving oral or parenteral therapy. Report oliguria or changes in intake–output ratio. Inadequate neomycin excretion results in high serum drug levels and risk of nephrotoxicity and ototoxicity.

Preoperative bowel preparation: Low-residue diet should be prescribed. Saline laxative is generally given immediately before neomycin therapy is initiated. Daily enemas may also be ordered.

Topical use: The possibility of systemic absorption and sensitization should be considered. High incidence of allergic dermatitis is associated with topical neomycin. Sensitivity may be manifested as persistent dermatitis. Caution patient to stop treatment and report to physician if irritation occurs.

Patients who develop sensitivity should be informed that they will probably continue to be sensitive to neomycin and to other aminoglycoside antibiotics (gentamicin, kanamycin, neomycin, streptomycin).

For applications to skin. Consult physician about what to use for cleansing the part to be treated before each neomycin application.

Topical therapy of external ear is most effective if canal is clean and dry prior to instillation of neomycin. Consult physician. Duration of treatment should be limited to 7 to 10 days.

Caution patient not to exceed prescribed dosage or duration of therapy.

Parenteral solutions should be stored in refrigerator (2° to 15°C) to minimize possibility of contamination and discoloration and should be used as soon as possible, preferably within 1 week after reconstitution.

Drug Interactions. Neomycin may reduce **cyanocobalamin** (vitamin B_{12}) absorption. *See also Gentamicin.*

N

PROTOTYPE

NEOSTIGMINE BROMIDE
(Prostigmin Bromide)

NEOSTIGMINE METHYLSULFATE
(Prostigmin Methylsulfate)

(nee-oh-stig′meen)
Cholinergic (indirect acting)
Parasympathomimetic
Cholinesterase inhibitor
Antidote

ACTIONS AND USES. Synthetic quaternary ammonium analog of physostigmine, but less likely to cause disturbing side effects. Produces reversible cholinesterase inhibition or inactivation, and thus allows intensified and prolonged effect of acetylcholine at cholinergic synapses (basis for use in myasthenia gravis). Also produces generalized cholinergic response, including miosis, increased tonus of intestinal and skeletal muscles, constriction of bronchi and ureters, slower pulse rate, and stimulation of salivary and sweat glands. Has direct stimulant action on voluntary muscle fibers and possibly on autonomic ganglia and CNS neurons. Use in amenorrhea or as pregnancy test is based on premise that delayed menstruation may be due to diminished vascular responsiveness to acetylcholine.

Used to prevent and treat postoperative abdominal distention and urinary retention; for symptomatic control of and sometimes for differential diagnosis of myasthenia gravis; and to reverse the effects of nondepolarizing muscle relaxants, e.g., tubocurarine. Also has been used for treatment of delayed menstruation and as screening test for early pregnancy. *Investigational Use:* treatment of supraventricular tachycardia resulting from overdosage of tricyclic antidepressants.

ABSORPTION AND FATE. Poorly and irregularly absorbed from GI tract. Onset of action in 2 to 4 hours following oral administration and in 10 to 30 minutes following parenteral injection; duration of effect is 2.5 to 4 hours. Does not cross blood–brain barrier, except at extremely high doses. Metabolized in liver by microsomal enzymes. Excreted in urine.

CONTRAINDICATIONS AND PRECAUTIONS. Known hypersensitivity to neostigmine or bromide (oral formulation); mechanical, intestinal, or urinary obstruction; megacolon; peritonitis; acute peptic ulcer; urinary tract infection; hyperthyroidism. Safe use during pregnancy not established. *Cautious Use:* bronchial asthma, bradycardia, cardiac arrhythmias, hypotension, recent coronary occlusion, epilepsy, vagotonia, patients receiving other anticholinergic drugs.

ADVERSE/SIDE EFFECTS. **Cholinergic crisis (overdosage):** any or all of the above; with extremely high doses, also CNS stimulation, fear, agitation, restlessness. **Muscarinic effects:** nausea, vomiting, eructation, epigastric discomfort, abdominal cramps, diarrhea, involuntary or difficult defecation or micturition, increased salivation (common) and bronchial secretions, tightness in chest, sneezing, cough, dyspnea, diaphoresis, lacrimation, miosis, blurred vision, bradycardia, hypotension. **Nicotinic effects:** muscle cramps, fasciculations (common), twitching, pallor, elevated blood pressure, fatigability, generalized weakness, respiratory depression and paralysis.

ROUTE AND DOSAGE. Neostigmine bromide: **Oral:** *Myasthenia gravis:* Initial: 15 to 30 mg three or four times daily, increased gradually until maximum benefit obtained. Maintenance dose range: 15 to 375 mg daily, depending on patient's needs and tolerance. Neostigmine methylsulfate: **Subcutaneous, intramuscular:** *Myasthenia gravis:* 0.5 mg; subsequent doses based on individual response. *Myasthenia gravis diagnosis:* 0.022 mg/kg IM. *To prevent postoperative distention and urinary retention:* 0.25 mg SC or IM every 4 to 6 hours for 2 or 3 days. *Abdominal distention:* 0.5 to 1 mg SC or IM. *Urinary retention:* 0.5 to 1 mg SC or IM; dose may be repeated every 3 hours for five doses after bladder has been emptied. *Screening test for pregnancy:* 1 mg IM daily for 3 successive days. *Antidote for non-depolarizing skeletal muscle relaxants:* 0.5 to 2 mg IV administered slowly, repeated as required up to total dose of 5 mg.

NURSING IMPLICATIONS

Note that size of oral dose is considerably larger than that of parenteral dose because drug is poorly absorbed when taken orally (15 mg of oral drug is approximately equivalent to 0.5 mg of parenteral form).

Check pulse before giving drug to bradycardic patients. If below 80/minute, consult physician. Atropine will be ordered to restore heart rate.

For treatment of myasthenia gravis: monitor pulse, respiration, and blood pressure during period of dosage adjustment.

If patient has difficulty chewing, physician may prescribe oral neostigmine 30 to 45 minutes before meals. If patient has difficulty swallowing, the parenteral form may be necessary. Some patients require a nasogastric tube.

GI (muscarinic) side effects occur especially during early therapy and may be reduced by taking drug with milk or food. Physician may prescribe atropine or other anticholinergic agent with each dose or every other dose to suppress side effects (*note:* these drugs may mask toxic symptoms of neostigmine).

Regulation of dosage interval is extremely difficult; dosage must be adjusted for each patient to deal with unpredictable exacerbations and remissions.

Report promptly and record accurately the onset of myasthenic symptoms and drug side effects in relation to last dose in order to assist physician in determining lowest effective dosage schedule.

Encourage patient to keep a diary of "peaks and valleys" of muscle strength.

Frequently, drug therapy is required both day and night, with larger portions of total dose being given at times of greater fatigue, as in the late afternoon and at mealtimes.

All activities should be appropriately spaced to avoid undue fatigue.

Deep breathing, coughing, and range-of-motion exercises should be regularly scheduled. Consult physician.

Respiratory depression may appear abruptly in myasthenic patients. Report unusual apprehension (a frequent manifestation of inadequate ventilation), and be alert for tachypnea, tachycardia, restlessness, rising blood pressure.

Have the following immediately available: atropine, facilities for endotracheal intubation, tracheostomy, suction, oxygen, assisted respiration.

In myasthenic patients, the time that muscular weakness appears may indicate whether patient is in cholinergic or myasthenic crisis. Weakness that appears approximately 1 hour after drug administration suggests *cholinergic crisis (overdosage)* and is treated by prompt withdrawal of neostigmine and immediate administration of atropine. Weakness that occurs 3 hours or more after drug administration is more likely to be due to *myasthenic crisis (underdosage or drug resistance)* and is treated by more intensive anticholinesterase therapy.

Manifestations of neostigmine overdosage often appear first in muscles of neck and those involved in chewing and swallowing, with muscles of shoulder girdle and upper extremities affected next.

Signs and symptoms of myasthenia gravis that may be relieved by neostigmine: lid ptosis; diplopia; drooping facies; difficulty in chewing, swallowing, breathing, or coughing; weakness of neck, limbs, and trunk muscles. Record drug effect and duration of action.

Lid ptosis, especially in the elderly, may continue despite drug therapy. Often, patients are helped by means of an adhesive lid crutch attached to rim of eyeglasses.

Some patients become refractory to neostigmine after prolonged use and require change in dosage or medication.

Drug therapy for myasthenia gravis is lifesaving and must be continued throughout patient's life. Patient may require help to overcome psychologic problems associated with prolonged disability.

Patient and responsible family members should be taught to keep an accurate record for physician of patient's response to drug, as well as how to recognize side effects, how to modify dosage regimen according to patient's changing needs, or how to administer atropine if necessary. They should be aware that certain factors may require an increase in size or frequency of dose (e.g., physical or emotional stress, infection, menstruation, surgery), whereas remission requires a decrease in dosage.

Advise patient to wear identification bracelet (such as Medic Alert) indicating the presence of myasthenia gravis. Also inform patient and family of educational resources provided by Myasthenia Gravis Foundation, Inc., New York Academy of Medicine Building, 2 East 103rd Street, New York, N.Y. 10029.

Neostigmine test for myasthenia gravis: The neostigmine test has been largely replaced by the edrophonium (Tensilon) test. All anticholinesterase medications should be discontinued at least 8 hours before test. Accurate recordings are made of grip strength, vital capacity, range of extraocular movements, ptosis, etc, before test (usually, atropine sulfate 0.6 mg IM is given prior to or concomitantly with neostigmine methylsulfate to prevent muscarinic effects). After neostigmine is given, muscle strength is retested at 15-minute intervals for 1 hour. Objective and subjective improvement in strength and movement indicates positive test. Nonmyasthenic patient may experience weakness, abdominal cramps, diarrhea, diaphoresis, dysuria.

When neostigmine is used as antidote for tubocurarine or other nondepolarizing neuromuscular blocking agents (usually preceded by atropine), monitor respiration, maintain airway or assisted ventilation, and give oxygen as indicated. Respiratory assistance is continued until recovery of respiration and neuromuscular transmission is assured.

For relief of postoperative abdominal distention: Rectal tube (prescribed by physician) is inserted following drug administration to facilitate expulsion of gas. Lubricated tube is inserted just past rectal sphincter and kept in place for about 1 hour. In some cases, a small low enema may be prescribed. Record results: passage of flatus, decrease in abdominal distention, pain, rigidity.

For relief of urinary retention: Report to physician if patient does not urinate within 1 hour after first dose. Generally, catheterization will be prescribed if patient fails to void.

Screening test for early pregnancy and treatment of delayed menstruation: Patient is assumed to be pregnant if bleeding does not occur within 72 hours after third consecutive daily dose, providing other causes are ruled out. Positive diagnosis of pregnancy is not made until results are checked by biologic tests.

Drug Interactions. Parenteral neostigmine antagonizes the effects of **nondepolarizing neuromuscular blocking agents,** e.g., **gallamine, metocurine, pancuronium, tubocurarine** (interaction used therapeutically). Upward adjustment of neostigmine dosage may be required in myasthenic patients receiving drugs that interfere with neuromuscular transmission, e.g., **aminoglycoside antibiotics (gentamicin, kanamycin, neomycin, streptomycin), local anesthetics** and some **general anesthetics,** and **antiarrhythmic agents,** e.g., **procainamide, quinidine** (all used with extreme caution, if at all). Neostigmine may prolong the action of depolarizing muscle relaxants, e.g., **decamethonium, succinylcholine.** Muscarinic effects of neostigmine are antagonized by **atropine** (interaction used therapeutically).

N

NETILMICIN SULFATE

(Netromycin)

(ne-til-mye'sin)
Antiinfective
Antibiotic
Aminoglycoside

ACTIONS AND USES. Rapid acting, broad spectrum, semisynthetic aminoglycoside derivative of sisomicin. In common with other aminoglycosides, appears to act by interfering with protein synthesis of bacterial cell wall. Spectrum of activity comparable to that of gentamicin, but netilmicin is also effective against gentamicin-resistant bacteria. Not inactivated by most strains of bacteria resistant to other aminoglycosides. Bactericidal action primarily against gram-negative organisms including *Citrobacter, Enterobacter, Escherichia coli, Klebsiella, Proteus mirabilis, Pseudomonas aeruginosa, Salmonella, Serratia,* and certain gram-positive bacteria such as *Staphylococcus pyogenes* and *Streptococcus faecalis.* Like other aminoglycosides, not effective against most anaerobic bacteria (*Bacteroides* and *Clostridium* species), viruses, or fungi. Reportedly less ototoxic and nephrotoxic than other aminoglycosides, but has high potential for neuromuscular blocking action.

Used for short-term treatment of serious or life-threatening infections including septicemia, peritonitis, intraabdominal abscess, lower respiratory tract infections, and complicated urinary tract infection, infections of bones and joints, skin and its structures. May be administered in conjunction with a beta lactam antibiotic (e.g., a penicillin or cephalosporin) for synergistic effect pending results of susceptibility testing.

ABSORPTION AND FATE. Rapidly and completely absorbed following IM or IV administration. Serum levels peak within 30 to 60 minutes (still measurable for 12 hours) following IM, and at the end of 1 hour after IV infusion. Promptly distributed into tissues, normal body fluids, (including urine, sputum, bile, pericardial, peritoneal, pleural, synovial), and abscess and blister fluid. Poor distribution to adipose tissue and to CSF, unless meninges are inflamed. Protein binding: 0 to 30%. Half-life: 2 to 3.4 hours (prolonged to about 30 or more hours in impaired renal function); in children: inversely related to weight and age. About 75 to 90% of dose excreted unchanged in urine within 24 hours; minimal amounts eliminated in bile. Crosses placenta. Small quantities distributed into breast milk.

CONTRAINDICATIONS AND PRECAUTIONS. History of hypersensitivity or toxic reaction to netilmicin, or other aminoglycosides, or to bisulfites or any other ingredient in the formulation, pregnancy (category D), nursing infants, use for minor infections. *Cautious Use:* impaired renal function, prematures, neonates, the elderly, patients with ascites, edema, dehydration, severe burns, cystic fibrosis, fever, anemia, myasthenia gravis, parkinsonism, history of ear disease; infant botulism.

ADVERSE/SIDE EFFECTS. Low incidence in patients with normal renal function. **CNS (neurotoxicity):** headache, lethargy, drowsiness, paresthesias, tremors, muscle twitching, peripheral neuritis, disorientation, seizures, neuromuscular blockade; musculoskeletal weakness or paralysis, respiratory depression or paralysis, ototoxicity *(see ENT below).* **CV:** palpitation, hypotension. **Dermatologic (hypersensitivity):** rash, pruritus. **ENT:** ototoxicity (usually irreversible: 8th cranial nerve auditory branch: tinnitus, hearing loss, ringing, buzzing or fullness in ears: vestibular branch: vertigo, nystagmus, ataxia, nausea and vomiting. **GI:** nausea, vomiting, diarrhea, stomatitis, proctitis, enterocolitis (possibly superinfections). **Hematologic:** increases in: SGPT (ALT), SGOT (AST), alkaline phosphatase, bilirubin; anemia, eosinophilia, neutropenia, thrombocytopenia, thrombocytosis, prolonged PT, agranulocytosis, leukopenia, leukemoid reaction, hyperkalemia. **Ophthalmic:** blurred vision. **Renal (nephrotoxicity):** increase in serum creatinine and BUN; decrease in creatinine clearance; hematuria, proteinuria, urinary frequency, oliguria, polyuria. **Other:** fever, edema, arthralgia; pain, induration and hematoma at injection site.

N

ROUTE AND DOSAGE. Intramuscular, intravenous infusion: Adults: *Serious systemic infections:* 1.3 to 2.2 mg/kg every 8 hours or 2 to 3.25 mg/kg every 12 hours. *Complicated urinary tract infections:* 1.5 to 2 mg/kg every 12 hours. **Infants and Children (6 weeks through 12 years):** 1.8 to 2.7 mg/kg every 8 hours or 2.7 to 4 mg/kg every 12 hours. **Neonates (less than 6 weeks):** 2 to 3.5 mg/kg every 12 hours. For patients with compromised renal function, initial or loading dose is generally the same as for patients with normal renal function. Subsequent dosage determined by serum drug levels and/or renal function studies.

NURSING IMPLICATIONS

Netilmicin sulfate (Netromycin) containing 100 mg/ml and preserved with benzyl alcohol should not be used for neonates, infants or children (benzyl alcohol may be toxic to this age group). Netromycin pediatric injection 25 mg/ml and Netromycin neonatal injection 10 mg/ml do not contain benzyl alcohol. All preparations contain a metabisulfite or bisulfite to which some individuals may be allergic.

Culture and sensitivity tests should be done prior to initiation of therapy. Therapy may begin before test results are available.

Obtain patient's pretreatment weight so that physician can calculate dosage. For obese patients, dosage should be based on ideal body weight (IBW) for males = 50 kg + (2.3 kg × inches over 5 feet); for females = 45 kg + (2.3 kg × inches over 5 feet).

Renal function should be evaluated before and periodically during therapy: serum creatinine, creatinine clearance rate, BUN, urinalysis including specific gravity. Close attention to these values is particularly important for high risk patients, i.e., renal function impairment, the elderly, dehydrated patients, burn patients, and patients receiving high doses or prolonged therapy.

Monitor intake–output ratio and pattern and report significant changes. Keep patient well hydrated throughout therapy to minimize possibility of chemical irritation of renal tubules, and to reduce risk of toxicity. Consult physician for guidelines.

Dosage adjustments for patients with impaired renal function are based on creatinine clearance rates, serum creatinine, or on peak and trough serum drug levels. (These patients tend to accumulate toxic concentrations of netilmicin.) Creatinine clearance is either measured or estimated from published nonograms or equations. See manufacturer's package insert.

To determine peak serum drug levels, blood is drawn 1 hour after IM injection or 1 hour after IV infusion begins. To determine trough serum drug levels, blood is drawn just before next scheduled dose. Desirable peak values: 6 to 10 mcg/ml; desirable trough values; 0.5 to 2 mcg/ml. Peak values over 16 mcg/ml and trough above 4 mcg/ml are associated with a high potential for toxicity.

Close monitoring or serum drug concentrations is especially important for patients with fever, edema, severe burns, and anemia. Peak serum drug levels tend to be significantly reduced in these patients, possibly due to alterations in extracellular fluid volume.

Urinalysis may be done daily in high risk patients to determine presence of albumin, casts, white or red blood cells, and lowering of specific gravity. All represent signs of renal irritation and the need for increased hydration.

Patients should be evaluated before and during therapy for hearing acuity and vestibular status. Loss of higher frequency sounds, an early sign of cochlear damage, can be detected only by audiometric testing. Notify physician promptly if patient complains of any hearing loss, tinnitus, vertigo, or ataxia.

Serial audiometric tests may be done for patients at high risk for ototoxicity: patients with impaired renal function, history of hearing, or vestibular problems, concomitant therapy with other potentially ototoxic drugs, patients in high dose or prolonged netilmicin therapy.

If therapeutic effectiveness is not evident within 3 to 5 days, bacterial susceptibility tests should be repeated.

For most patients, therapy may last 7 to 14 days. However, carefully selected patients with complicated infections may require longer therapy.

Have on hand calcium salts and equipment for mechanical respiratory assistance, to reverse neuromuscular blockade.

Watch for signs of superinfection especially of upper respiratory tract. Also suspect overgrowth of opportunistic organisms if patient develops sore rectum, diarrhea, vaginal discharge, sore mouth, fever.

For adults, prescribed dose for IV infusion is diluted with 50 to 200 ml of compatible IV solution *(see manufacturer's package insert);* volume of diluent should be less, according to patient's fluid requirement. Solution may be infused over 30 minutes to 2 hours, as prescribed.

See manufacturer's package insert for list of compatible diluents and stability of prepared solutions. Solutions retain potency for up to 72 hours when stored in glass containers either at room temperature or refrigerated. Do not use solutions that are discolored or that contain particulate matter.

Avoid mixing netilmicin with other drugs without first consulting pharmacist or specialized references for compatibility.
Store between 2° and 30°C (36° to 86°F) unless otherwise directed by manufacturer. Avoid freezing.

Diagnostic Test Interferences. Concomitant netilmicin–cephalosporin therapy may cause false elevations of **creatinine** determinations. Concomitant use of beta-lactam antibiotics (cephalosporins, penicillins) may result in falsely low **aminoglycoside levels** (mutual inactivation may continue in body fluid specimen unless promptly assayed, or frozen, or treated with beta-lactamase).

Drug Interactions: Netilmicin

Plus	Interactions
Aminoglycosides, other	Increased potential for nephrotoxicity, ototoxicity, and neuromuscular blockade. Concurrent or sequential use generally avoided
Amphotericin B (Fungizone)	Synergistic nephrotoxic effects; used concomitantly, e.g., with caution
Antibiotics (polypeptides) e.g., bacitracin (parenteral), capreomycin (Capastat), colistimethate (Coly-Mycin M), polymyxin B (Aerosporin)	Possibility of additive neuromuscular blocking action. Used with extreme caution
Cephalosporins	Additive nephrotoxic effects. Used concomitantly, e.g., only with caution
Cisplatin (Platinol)	Additive nephrotoxicity and ototoxicity. Concurrent or sequential use generally avoided
Citrate-anticoagulated blood	Enhancement of neuromuscular blocking action. Concurrent use generally avoided
Dimenhydrinate	May mask symptoms of ototoxicity. Used with caution
Diuretics (loop) e.g., bumetanide (Bumex), ethacrynic acid (Edecrin), furocemide (Lasix)	Increased risk of ototoxicity, particularly with parenteral diuretics. Concurrent use generally avoided.
Methoxyflurane (Penthrane)	Possibility of additive nephrotoxicity. Aminoglycosides generally avoided 3 days before and following methoxyflurane
Penicillins	Synergistic effects, however, physiochemical inactivation can occur depending on contact time. Scheduling 1 hour apart may help
Succinylcholine (depolarizing muscle relaxant) tubocurarine and other nondepolarizing muscle relaxants	Possibility of additive neuromuscular blocking action. Used with extreme caution
Vancomycin (Vancocin)	Additive neurotoxicity and nephrotoxicity. Concurrent or sequential use requires careful monitoring

NIACIN

(nye'a-sin)
Vitamin

(Niac, Nicobid, Nico-400, Nicolar, Nico-Span, Nicotinex, Nicotinic acid, Novoniacin, Span-Niacin-150, Tega-Span, Vitamin B_3)

ACTIONS AND USES. Water-soluble, heat-stable B-complex vitamin (B_3). Functions with riboflavin as a control agent in coenzyme system that converts protein, carbohydrate, and fat to energy through oxidation-reduction. Produces vasodilation (primarily of cutaneous vessels) by direct action on vascular smooth muscles. Inhibits hepatic synthesis of VLDL, cholesterol and triglyceride, and, indirectly, LDL. Large doses effectively reduce elevated serum cholesterol and total lipid levels in hypercholesterolemia and hyperlipidemic states. Unclear whether drug-induced reduction of cholesterol and lipids has a beneficial effect on morbidity or mortality caused by atherosclerosis or coronary heart disease.

Used in prophylaxis and treatment of pellagra, usually in combination with other B-complex vitamins, and in deficiency states accompanying carcinoid syndrome, isoniazid therapy, Hartnup's disease, and chronic alcoholism. Also used in adjuvant treatment of hyperlipidemia (elevated cholesterol and/or triglycerides) in patient who does not respond adequately to diet or weight loss. Also used as vasodilator in peripheral vascular disorders, Meniere's disease, and labyrinthine syndrome, as well as to counteract LSD toxicity and to distinguish between psychoses of dietary and nondietary origin.

ABSORPTION AND FATE. Rapid absorption from GI tract. Peak serum level: 20 to 70 minutes. Therapeutic plasma concentration of 0.5 to 1.0 mcg/ml required for active antilipidemic action. Plasma half-life: about 45 minutes. Major metabolites from hepatic degradation: nicotinuric acid, *N*-methylnicotinamide and 2-pyridone. About ⅓ oral dose excreted in urine unchanged.

CONTRAINDICATIONS AND PRECAUTIONS. Hypersensitivity to niacin, hepatic impairment, severe hypotension, hemorrhaging or arterial bleeding, active peptic ulcer. Used during pregnancy and lactation only if benefits outweigh risks to fetus or nursing infant. *Cautious Use:* history of gallbladder disease, liver disease, and peptic ulcer; glaucoma, angina, coronary artery disease, diabetes mellitus, predisposition to gout, allergy.

ADVERSE/SIDE EFFECTS. CNS: transient headache, tingling of extremities, syncope; (with chronic use): nervousness, panic, toxic amblyopia, proptosis, blurred vision, loss of central vision. **CV:** generalized flushing with sensation of warmth, postural hypotension, vasovagal attacks, cardiac arrhythmias (rare). **Dermatologic:** increased sebaceous gland activity, dry skin, skin rash, pruritus, keratitis nigricans. **GI:** abnormalities of hepatic function tests; jaundice, bloating, flatulence, hunger pains, nausea, vomiting, GI disorders, activation of peptic ulcer, xerostomia. **Other:** hyperuricemia, allergy, hyperglycemia, glycosuria, hypoprothrombinemia, hypoalbuminemia.

ROUTE AND DOSAGE. Oral: Adults: *Niacin deficiency:* 50 to 100 mg daily. *Pellagra:* up to 500 mg daily. *Hyperlipidemia:* 1 to 2 Gm three times a day, with or following meals. If necessary increased incrementally over period of several weeks to maximum of 6 Gm daily. **Parenteral (subcutaneous, intramuscular, slow intravenous):** *Niacin deficiency:* 100 mg to 3 Gm/daily in divided doses every 2 to 3 hours until desired dose has been given. Oral niacin may be given concomitantly with parenteral administration in a combined dose of 300 mg to 3 Gm daily. *Vasodilation:* 50 mg three times daily.

NURSING IMPLICATIONS

Parenteral therapy is continued until patient can take a complete well-balanced diet and oral niacin.

Take oral drug with meals to decrease GI distress.

Take with cold water (not hot beverage) if necessary to facilitate swallowing.

After oral dose, plasma free fatty acid concentration is lowered within 30 minutes, plasma triglyceride levels within hours; however, cholesterol levels do not decline for several days.

Therapeutic response usually begins within 24 hours. Note and record effect of therapy on clinical manifestations of deficiency (fiery red tongue, sialorrhea and infection of oral membranes, nausea, vomiting, diarrhea, confusion).

For treatment of niacin deficiency, small doses given frequently during the day are more effective than a single large daily dose, since a considerable amount of the latter is excreted in urine.

In treatment of hyperlipidemia, dosage is individualized according to effect on serum lipid levels.

Diabetics, potential diabetics, and patients on high doses will require close monitoring. Hyperglycemia, glycosuria, ketonuria, and increased insulin requirements have been reported.

Baseline and periodic tests of blood glucose and liver function should be performed in patients receiving prolonged high dose therapy.

Inform patient that cutaneous warmth and flushing in face, neck, and ears may occur within first 2 hours after oral ingestion (and immediately after parenteral administration) and may last several hours. Effects are usually transient and subside as therapy continues.

Caution patient to sit or lie down and to avoid sudden posture changes if weakness or dizziness is experienced. These symptoms and persistent flushing should be reported to the physician. Relief may be obtained by reduction of dosage, increasing subsequent doses in small increments, or by changing to sustained-action formulation.

N

Alcohol and large doses of niacin cause increased flushing and sensation of warmth. Alcohol should be limited if patient is being treated for hypertriglyceridemia.

Observe patient closely for evidence of hepatic dysfunction (jaundice, dark urine, light-colored stools, pruritus) and hyperuricemia in patient predisposed to gout (flank, joint, or stomach pain; altered urine excretion pattern).

Caution patient with skin manifestations to avoid exposure to direct sunlight until lesions have entirely cleared.

Subclinical niacin deficiency is often associated with poverty, chronic alcoholism, dietary fads, pregnancy, cachexia or malignancy, isoniazid therapy, and chronic GI disease.

RDA for niacin: infants: 6 to 8 mg; *children 4 to 6:* 11 mg; *adult males:* 18 mg; *adult females:* 13 mg; additional 2 mg during pregnancy and an additional 5 mg during lactation are required.

Collaborate with physician, dietitian, patient, and a responsible family member in development of a teaching plan that includes total nutritional needs. Niacin deficiency is invariably accompanied by deficiencies in other B-complex vitamins.

Rich niacin food sources: liver, kidney, lean meats, poultry, fish, brewer's yeast, wheat germ, peanuts, and other legumes. Milk and eggs contain small amounts, but they are excellent sources of tryptophan, a percursor of niacin (1 mg niacin is derived from each 60 mg dietary tryptophan).

Patient may be restricted in intake of saturated fats, sugars and/or cholesterol.

Store drug at temperature between 15° and 30°C (59° and 86°F) in light- and moisture-proof container.

Diagnostic Test Interferences. Niacin causes elevated serum **bilirubin, uric acid, alkaline phosphatase, SGOT, SGPT, LDH** levels, and may cause **glucose intolerance.** Decreases **serum cholesterol** 15 to 30%, and may cause false elevations with certain fluorometric methods of determining **urinary catecholamines.** Niacin may cause false-positive **urine glucose** tests using copper sulfate reagents, e.g., Benedict's solution.

Drug Interactions. Niacin potentiates hypotensive effects of **antihypertensives** (ganglionic blocking type). **Clonidine** may inhibit niacin-induced skin flushing.

NIACINAMIDE

(Nicotinamide)

(nye-a-sin'a-mide)
Vitamin

ACTIONS AND USES. Amide of niacin used as alternative in prevention and treatment of pellagra. Has same actions as those of niacin (qv). Preferred to niacin in treatment of deficiency because it lacks unpleasant vasodilatory action, and the hypolipemic, hepatic, and GI effects of niacin.

ROUTE AND DOSAGE. **Oral, subcutaneous, intramuscular, intravenous:** 50 mg three to ten times daily. Highly individualized.

NURSING IMPLICATIONS

See Niacin.

N

NICLOSAMIDE

(Niclocide)

(ni-kloe'sa-mide)
Antiinfective
Anthelmintic

ACTIONS AND USES. Salicylanilide derivative reportedly effective against most tapeworms that infect man. Acts by inhibiting oxidative phosphorylation in mitochondria of cestodes. On contact, kills scolex and proximal segments of tapeworm, which may then be partially or fully digested in intestines. Lacks ovicidal action and is not effective in larval or tissue encystment stage of tapeworm infections, e.g., cysticercosis.

Used in treatment of intestinal tapeworm (cestode) infections, e.g., *Taenia saginata* (beef tapeworm), *Diphyllobothrium latum* (fish tapeworm), *Hymenolepis nana* (dwarf tapeworm), *H. diminuta* (rat tapeworm), and *Dipylidium caninum* (dog or cat tapeworm).

ABSORPTION AND FATE. Pharmacokinetic information scanty. Minimally absorbed from GI tract. Excreted in feces.

CONTRAINDICATIONS AND PRECAUTIONS. Hypersensitivity to niclosamide or to any ingredients in the formulation. Safe use during pregnancy (category B), in nursing women, and in children under 2 years not established.

ADVERSE/SIDE EFFECTS. CNS: Drowsiness, dizziness, headache, irritability. **Dermatologic:** Skin rash, pruritus ani, alopecia, sweating, urticaria (rare). **GI:** Nausea, vomiting, abdominal discomfort, anorexia, diarrhea, constipation, oral irritation, bad taste, rectal bleeding. **Other:**

Fever, weakness, edema of an arm, backache, palpitation. Rare: Transient rise in SGOT (AST).

ROUTE AND DOSAGE. Oral: *Beef and fish tapeworms:* **Adults:** 4 tablets (2 Gm) in single dose. **Children [over 34 kg (75 lb)]:** 3 tablets (1.5 Gm); **Children [11 to 34 kg (25 to 75 lb)]:** 2 tablets (1 Gm) in a single dose. *Dwarf tapeworm:* **Adults:** 4 tablets (2 Gm) daily for 7 days. **Children (over 34 kg):** 3 tablets (1.5 Gm) daily for 6 days; **Children (11 to 34 kg):** 2 tablets (1 Gm) daily for 6 days.

NURSING IMPLICATIONS

Administered after a light meal, e.g., after breakfast. Instruct patient to chew tablet thoroughly, then swallow with a little water.

For young children, tablet may be crushed to a fine powder and mixed with sufficient water to form a paste for ease of ingestion. Niclosamide is vanilla-flavored and reportedly not unpleasant to the taste.

Dietary restrictions and purgation before or after drug therapy, and hospitalization during treatment are not usually necessary. Some patients may require a laxative if constipation is a problem, or for recovery of scolex to determine cure.

Fish tapeworm (Diphyllobothrium): diagnosis is based on presence of ova in stools; adult stage in humans, usually only one worm. *Source of infection:* fresh water flea to fish to humans. *Prophylaxis:* proper disposal of excreta and avoiding ingestion of raw or undercooked fish. *Cure:* Presence of ova or segments in stools on 7th day after therapy indicates treatment failure and need for second course of therapy.

Beef tapeworm (Taenia saginata): diagnosis based on presence of eggs and tapeworm segments (moglotids) and ova in stools; require interum host in life cycle, usually only one worm. *Source of infection:* infected beef. *Cure:* presence of ova or segments in stool on 7th day after therapy indicates treatment failure and need for second course of therapy.

Dwarf tapeworm (Hymenolepis nava): Diagnosis based on presence of adult worms and cysts; complete life cycle in numerous worms. *Source of infection:* fecal contamination of food. *Prophylaxis:* proper disposal of excreta. Instruct patient to use meticulous personal and environmental hygiene. Autoinfection occurs commonly. Niclosamide is more effective against adult worm than larval.

Stool examinations for presence of scolex, proglottids (tapeworm segments), and ova may be required at 1 and 3 months following therapy to determine cure. No patient is considered cured unless stools have been negative for ova and proglottids for at least 3 months.

Treatment of niclosamide toxicity: fast-acting laxative, enema. Do *not* induce emesis.

Store preferably at temperature below 30°C (86°F), protected from light, unless otherwise directed by manufacturer.

N

NICOTINE RESIN COMPLEX

(Nicorette)

(nik'to-teen)
Cholinergic
Smoking deterrant

ACTIONS AND USES. A chewing gum containing nicotine, available by prescription only. Nicotine resin complex is a formulation of 2 mg of nicotine bound to the cation exchange resin polacrilin, buffered to pH 8.5. Each piece of gum contains about 0.44 mEq Na. The nicotine is a highly purified extract from dried tobacco leaves and is primarily classified as a ganglionic cholinergic receptor agonist. Its pharmacologic activity is complex and varied resulting in both adrenergic and cholinergic effects. Thus exposure to nicotine produces widespread responses: stimulant and depressant effects on peripheral and central NS, respiratory stimulation, peripheral vasoconstriction; increased heart rate, contractile force, output and stroke volume; increased tone and motor activity of GI tract smooth muscle; and more specifically nausea, vomiting, diarrhea, hypersalivation; increase in bronchial secretion (initially), and antidiuretic activity. The heavy smoker is tolerant to most of these effects; but exposure to nicotine (as in the gum) can cause the nonsmoker to experience tachycardia, symptoms of CNS stimulation, and increased blood pressure. Rational for use of nicotine resin complex is that smoking is partially due to physical dependence on nicotine as evidenced by appearance of withdrawal symptoms during nicotine deprivation. For some smokers, nicotine gum seems to relieve the desire for nicotine and reduces withdrawal symptoms, permitting the patient then to focus attention on overcoming the habit features of smoking. Success rate with nicotine gum use appears to be greatest in smokers with a high "physical" type of nicotine dependence.

Used in conjunction with a medically supervised behavior modification program, as a temporary and alternate source of nicotine by the nicotine-dependent smoker who is withdrawing from cigarette smoking.

ABSORPTION AND FATE. Approximately 90% of the nicotine in a piece of gum is released slowly over a 15- to 30-minute period of chewing; variable rate of release is controlled by vigor and duration of chewing. Absorption from buccal mucosa is facilitated by high oral alkylinization from the buffer component of the resin complex. Blood nicotine levels are variable (depending on nature of chewing). Distribution parameters not fully described, but there is evidence that nicotine is retained in brain cells, crosses placenta and is distributed into milk. May induce its own metabolism to some extent. Metabolism occurs principally in liver (small portion in kidneys and lungs), and is qualitatively the same for bucally absorbed or oral inhalated nicotine. Major metabolites: nicotine-1'-*N*-oxide and cotinine. Wide variability in plasma nicotine accumulation. Biphasic half-life: initial, 2 to 3 minutes; terminal, 30 to 120 minutes. Approximately 10 to 20% of an absorbed dose of nicotine excreted unchanged. Urinary excretion increased in acid urine and by high urine output.

CONTRAINDICATIONS AND PRECAUTIONS. Nonsmokers, immediate post-MI infarction period, life-threatening arrhythmias, active temporomandibular joint disease, severe angina pectoris, women with childbearing potential (unless effective contraception is used). Risk–benefit associated with use during pregnancy must be carefully considered (category X). Safe use by children and adolescents not established. *Cautious Use:* vasospastic disease (e.g., Buerger's disease, Prinzmetal variant angina), cardiac arrhythmias, hyperthyroidism, type I (IDDM) diabetes mellitus, pheochromocytoma, esophagitis, oral and pharyngeal inflammation; use by patient with dentures, denture caps and partial bridges. Use in hypertension and peptic ulcer disease (active or inactive) and use by mother only if benefit of a smoking cessation program outweighs risks.

ADVERSE/SIDE EFFECTS. CV: arrhythmias, tachycardia, palpitations. **GU:** air swallowing, jawache, belching, salivation, anorexia, dry mouth, laxative effects, constipation, indigestion. **Neurologic:** headache, dizziness, light-headedness, insomnia, irritability, dependence on nicotine resin complex. **Other:** sore mouth or throat, coughing, hiccups, hoarseness; injury to mouth, teeth, temporomandibular joint. Acute overdose *("nicotine intoxication"):* nausea, vomiting, sialorrhea, abdominal pain, diarrhea, perspiration, severe headache, dizziness, disturbed hearing and vision, mental confusion, severe weakness, fainting, hypotension, dyspnea, weak, rapid irregular pulse, seizures, death (from respiratory failure secondary to drug-induced respiratory muscle paralysis).

ROUTE AND DOSAGE. Oral: one piece of 2-mg chewing gum when patient has an urge to smoke; may be repeated. *(See Nursing Implications.)* Average daily dose (during first month of treatment): 10 pieces (20 mg nicotine). Maximum dosage should not exceed 30 pieces (60 mg nicotine) per day.

NURSING IMPLICATIONS

Nicotine is known to be one of the most toxic of all poisons. While the gum is being used to help the patient overcome a health hazard, it also must be considered a hazardous drug vehicle.

Smoking is thought to be due in part to physical dependence on nicotine; therefore when a patient stops smoking, he or she experiences withdrawal symptoms which can be minimized by a gradual reduction in nicotine intake.

Nicotine resin complex presumably helps the smoker stop smoking by facilitating a gradual reduction in cigarette use while preventing withdrawal symptoms.

Psychosocial counseling provided by physician or in smoking clinic focuses on breaking an intense habit. Self-help pamphlets are available from local affiliates of the American Cancer Society, the American Lung Association, and the American Heart Association.

Smoking a cigarette causes a rapid rise in serum nicotine which peaks within 2 minutes after the cigarette, then rapidly decreases. Chewing nicotine gum causes a slow increase in serum nicotine over a period of 15 to 30 minutes.

Chewing one piece of 2-mg gum per hour produces a nicotine level less than ½ that produced by smoking one cigarette/hour, but provides relief from abstinence symptoms.

Treatment with nicotine resin gum is at first slightly aversive to most patients and may lead to noncompliance in the patient with low motivation or in one who tries to quit without the support of behavior modification.

Smokers that seem to benefit most from use of nicotine gum and antismoking programs have a high "physical" type of nicotine dependence characterized by: preferring cigarette brands with nicotine levels over 0.9 mg; finding the first cigarette in AM the hardest to give up; smoking the first cigarette within 15 minutes of arising; smoking most in the AM; smoking over 15 cigarettes/day; inhaling smoke; having difficulty giving up smoking where it is forbidden; smoking heavily even when bedridden.

Specific written instructions are packaged with the gum. Review these carefully with the patient to establish understanding of chewing method and of the important fact that chewing the gum is a means of admitting medication into the body system.

The patient must stop smoking immediately before starting therapy with nicotine resin complex in order to prevent overdose.

If patient becomes pregnant during cessation therapy she should be informed of the potential hazard to the fetus. Nicotine resin complex has been associated with depressed fetal respirations.

Chewing many pieces of gum simultaneously or in rapid succession may cause an acute nicotine overdose (nicotine intoxication).

Treatment of overdose (there is no antidote): empty the stomach by an emetic or lavage; activated charcoal; saline cathartic; supportive treatment if hypotension and/or cardiovascular collapse is present; IV diazepam to control seizures, and assisted pulmonary ventilation if necessary.

To prevent transference of nicotine dependence from cigarette to gum, patient should be encouraged to gradually decrease number of pieces chewed in 24 hours. Usually a period of 3 months is allowed before patient is advised to taper use of gum.

Although the manufacturer suggests no more than a 3-month period of gum use, some clinicians have prescribed its use for as long as 6 months.

Usually a medical evaluation is done at least once a month to reinforce progress and/or to determine if patient should continue the cessation therapy.

Most adverse local effects (irritation of tongue, mouth and throat, jaw-muscle aches, dislike of taste) are transient and subside in a few days. Modification of the chewing technique may help.

If nicotine resin is swallowed whole, most of the nicotine remains bound to the complex and is excreted in the feces. However, patient should be advised not to swallow the gum.

Withdrawal or abstinence symptoms (usually appear within 24 hours after the last cigarette) include craving for tobacco, anxiety, difficulty in concentration, headache, GI disturbances, irritability.

Abstinence symptoms may persist for days or weeks after the patient stops smoking. The craving to smoke (most common and clinically important withdrawal symptom) may last for years.

Gum may stick and damage dental work (dentures, bridges, restorations) depending on materials from which they were made. If this occurs patient should stop use of the gum. Have patient demonstrate chewing when program is started to determine if gum is going to stick.

Teach the Following Measures to Prevent Gum from Sticking:

- Take gum out of mouth when ingesting hot food or liquids.
- Avoid chewing a piece of gum more than 45 minutes because it gets stiffer and tougher on the teeth with prolonged chewing.
- If gun sticks to dental work or dentures, chill with ice or cold water or place dentures in the freezer for a few minutes.
- Cold gum is brittle and easy to remove.

Patient-Teaching Summary:

- ✓ The process of chewing controls the amount of nicotine that enters the body.
- ✓ When urge to smoke is experienced, chew one piece of gum very slowly until nicotine is tasted and/or there is a slight tingling in the mouth (usually after 15 chews); stop chewing until taste and/or tingling disappears, then again chew slowly until taste reappears.
- ✓ The full dose of nicotine from a piece of gum is obtained through approximately 30 minutes of the interrupted chewing process.
- ✓ Chew only one piece of gum at a time.
- ✓ Chewing gum too rapidly can cause excessive buccal absorption and lead to adverse effects: nausea, hiccoughs, throat irritation.
- ✓ Patient must learn to self-regulate nicotine gum dose to minimize adverse effects.
- ✓ A supply of gum should be carried by the patient at all times to treat a sudden urge to smoke.
- ✓ One smoke can erase all progress in the cessation program no matter how long abstinence has been maintained.

Protect from light (nicotine is photosensitive and will turn brown when exposed to light). Store at room temperature less than 30°C (86°F).

Drug Interactions. (Smoking cessation with or without smoking substitutes may alter response to medications being taken concurrently by exsmokers.) It may reverse reported effects of smoking–drug interactions thus requiring dose adjustments. Nicotine resin complex:

Plus	Interactions
Caffeine Imipramine (Tofranil) Pentazocine (Talwin) Theophylline	Decreased metabolism and increased blood levels of these drugs
Furosemide (Lasix)	Increased diuretic effects
Glutethimide (Doriden)	Decreased absorption
Propoxyphene (Darvon)	Decreased first-pass metabolism (may lead to higher serum levels)
Propranolol (Inderal)	Hypotension; increased cardiac output

NICOTINYL ALCOHOL
(Roniacol)

(nik-oh-tin'ill)
Vasodilator (peripheral)

ACTIONS AND USES. Almost identical to niacin (nicotinic acid, qv), in pharmacologic properties, but reportedly has more prolonged action. Oxidized to niacin in body. Produces peripheral vasodilation by direct action on vascular smooth muscle. Acts particularly on cutaneous vessels of face, neck, ears, and chest. Also reported to have antilipemic activity in higher doses, but may intensify carbohydrate intolerance. Has been used in high doses to treat hypercholesterolemia.

Used in conditions associated with deficient circulation, as in peripheral vascular disease, vascular spasm, varicose ulcers, decubital ulcers, chilblains, Meniere's syndrome, and vertigo.

ABSORPTION AND FATE. Onset of action following oral tablet administration: within 5 to 30 minutes; duration 10 to 60 minutes. Onset following extended release tablet: within 30 minutes; duration: 6 to 12 hours. Onset following elixir: 5 to 10 minutes; duration: 10 to 60 minutes.

CONTRAINDICATIONS AND PRECAUTIONS. Active peptic ulcer or gastritis, severe cerebrovascular disease, predisposition to glaucoma. Safe use during pregnancy not established.

ADVERSE/SIDE EFFECTS. Flushing of face and neck, nausea, paresthesias, vomiting, heartburn, diarrhea, minor skin rashes, allergic reaction (urticaria, angioedema), dizziness, faintness, orthostatic hypotension, increased hair loss. With large doses for prolonged periods: impaired carbohydrate metabolism (patients with hypercholesterolemia), hepatocellular toxicity with jaundice, edema.

ROUTE AND DOSAGE. Oral: 50 to 100 mg three times daily. Time-release form (nicotinyl tartrate): 150 or 300 mg twice daily, morning and night. Available as tablets, timed release tablet, and elixir.

NURSING IMPLICATIONS

Administered before meals.

Timed-release tablet must be swallowed whole and not crushed or chewed.

Inform patient to expect flushing and sensation of warmth.

Caution patient that alcohol and large doses of niacin (in vitamin preparations) used simultaneously may produce additive vasodilation and dizziness.

Tolerance may develop with prolonged use.

See Index: Nursing Interventions: peripheral vasospastic disorders.
See also Niacin.

N

NIFEDIPINE

(Procardia)

(nye-fed'i-peen)
Vasodilator (coronary)
Antiarrhythmic
Antianginal
Calcium channel blocking agent

ACTIONS AND USES. Calcium channel blocking agent similar to verapamil (qv) in actions, uses, and limitations. Selectively blocks calcium ion influx across cell membranes of cardiac muscle and vascular smooth muscle without changing serum calcium concentrations. Reduces myocardial oxygen utilization and supply and relaxes and prevents coronary artery spasm. In contrast to verapamil and diltiaxem, has little or no effect on SA and AV nodal conduction with therapeutic dosing. Decreases peripheral vascular resistance and increases cardiac output.

Used in management of vasospastic or "variant" angina and effort-associated angina (class IV antiarrhythmic). *Unlabeled Uses:* treatment of mild to moderate hypertension alone or in combination with a diuretic (step 2, 3, 4 of stepped-care approach in antihypertensive therapy); to decrease lower esophageal sphincter pressure; tolytic to prevent preterm labor; treatment of vascular headaches, and vasospasm in Raynaud's phenomenon; treatment of dysmenorrhea.

ABSORPTION AND FATE. Rapidly and fully absorbed (about 9%) after oral administration. Onset of action within 10 minutes; peak levels in 30 minutes. Metabolized in liver. Highly bound (92 to 98%) to plasma protein; half-life: 2 to 5 hours. Effects of renal or hepatic impairment on metabolism and excretion of nifedipine not known. 1 to 2% dose excreted unchanged in urine.

CONTRAINDICATIONS AND PRECAUTIONS. Known hypersensitivity to nifedipine. Safe use during pregnancy (category C) and in children not established. *Cautious Use:* concomitant use with hypotensives; congestive heart failure, lactating women.

ADVERSE/SIDE EFFECTS. CNS: dizziness, nervousness, mood changes, jitteriness, sleep disturbances, blurred vision, retinal ischemia, difficulty in balance, headache. **CV:** hypotension (may be excessive), facial flushing, heat sensation, palpitation. **GI:** nausea, heartburn, diarrhea, constipation, cramps, flatulance, cholestasis (rare). **Musculoskeletal:** inflammation, joint stiffness, muscle cramps. **Other:** hyperglycemia, hypokalemia, sore throat, weakness, dermatitus, pruritus, urticaria, gingival hyperplasia, fever, sweating, chills, febrile reaction, sexual difficulties, peripheral, edema. **Overdosage:** prolonged systemic hypotension.

ROUTE AND DOSAGE. (Dosage established by titration, usually over a 7 to 14 day period.) **Oral: Adult:** Initial: 10 mg three times daily. Usual effective dose range: 10 to 20 mg three times a day; doses above 180 mg/day not recommended. A single dose should rarely exceed 30 mg.

NURSING IMPLICATIONS

May be co-administered with sublingual nitroglycerin and with long-acting nitrates.

Occasionally a patient has developed increased frequency, duration and severity of angina on starting treatment with this drug or when dosage is increased. Counsel patient to keep a record of nitroglycerin use and to report promptly if changes in previous pattern occur.

Careful monitoring of blood pressure during titration period is indicated. Severe hypotension may be produced, especially if patient is also taking other drugs known to lower blood pressure.

N

Warn patient not to change nifedipine dosage regimen without consulting physician; i.e., patient should not omit, increase, decrease dose, or change the dose interval. Withdrawal symptoms may occur with abrupt discontinuation of the drug (chest pain, increase in anginal episodes, myocardial infarction, dysrhythmias).

Monitor the blood sugar in patient who is diabetic. Nifedipine has diabetogenic properties.

Smoking–Drug Interaction. It has been shown that smoking decreases the efficacy of nifedipine and that it has direct and adverse effects on the heart in the patient on nifedipine treatment.

Treatment of overdosage calls for active cardiovascular support, monitoring of cardiac and respiratory function and intake and output ratio and pattern; elevation of extremities; administration of a vasoconstrictor such as norepinephrine.

Discontinuation of drug should be gradual with close medical supervision to prevent severe hypotensive and other side effects.

Protect capsules from light and moisture; store at temperature between 15° and 25°C (59° and 77°F).

See also Verapamil: prototype calcium channel blocking agent.

Diagnostic Test Interferences. Nifedipine may cause mild to moderate increases of **alkaline phosphatase, CK, LDH, SGOT (AST), SGPT (ALT).**

Drug Interactions. Nifedipine and hypotensive may increase likelihood of congestive heart failure, severe hypotension, exacerbation of angina. *See also Verapamil.*

NIKETHAMIDE

(Coramine)

(ni-keth'a-mide)
Central stimulant (respiratory)
Analeptic

N

ACTIONS AND USES. Diethyl derivative of nicotinamide, the pellagra-preventive vitamin. Similar to doxapram in actions and toxic effects (qv), but generally regarded to be less effective and to have less margin of safety.

Used to overcome CNS depression, respiratory depression, and circulatory failure, particularly when due to CNS depressant drugs. May be combined with electroshock therapy to restore respiration more quickly and to reduce number of required treatments.

ABSORPTION AND FATE. Readily absorbed following oral or IM administration; maximum effect in 20 to 30 minutes; duration about 1 hour. Duration of action following IV is 5 to 10 minutes, but may increase with succeeding doses. Converted in part to nicotinamide in body. Metabolic excreted in urine.

ADVERSE/SIDE EFFECTS. Burning or itching, especially at back of nose, is the most common side effect. *See also Doxapram.*

ROUTE AND DOSAGE. Adults: Intravenous, intramuscular: 5 to 10 ml of 25% solution (250 mg/ml). **Oral** (maintenance): 3 to 5 ml of 25% oral solution every 4 to 6 hours; may be repeated with 5 ml every 30 to 60 minutes as necessary.

NURSING IMPLICATIONS

Difference between clinically effective dose and that producing side effects is often small. Therefore, any side effects should be construed to be the result of overdosage.

Widespread CNS stimulation may occur with repeated doses. Observe for and report increases in vital signs, coughing, sneezing, flushing, itching, nausea, vomiting, tremors, muscle rigidity.

See Doxapram hydrochloride (prototype central respiratory stimulant).

NITROFURANTOIN

(nye-troe-fyoor'an-toyn)
Antibacterial (urinary)
Nitrofuran

(Furadantin, Furalan, Furan, Furatoin, Macrodantin, Nephronex, Nitrofan, Nitrofor, Novofuran, Sarodant, Trantoin, Urotoin, and others)

NITROFURANTOIN SODIUM

(Furadantin Sodium, Ivadantin)

ACTIONS AND USES. Synthetic nitrofuran derivative related to nitrofurazone. Active against wide variety of gram-negative and gram-positive microorganisms, including strains of *Escherichia coli, Staphylococcus aureus, Streptococcus faecalis,* enterococci, and *Klebsiella-Aerobacter. Pseudomonas aeruginosa* and many strains of *Proteus* are resistant. Presumed to act by interfering with several bacterial enzyme systems. Highly soluble in urine and reportedly most active in acid urine. Antimicrobial concentrations in urine exceed those in blood.

Used in treatment of pyelonephritis, pyelitis, and cystitis caused by susceptible organisms.

ABSORPTION AND FATE. Rapidly and almost completely absorbed from GI tract (macrocrystalline form appears to be absorbed more slowly than conventional tablets, but urinary concentrations are not significantly reduced). Half-life: 18 minutes to 1 hour. Crosses blood–brain barrier. Degraded by all body tissues (except blood) to inactive metabolites. Excreted rapidly in urine, about 40% of dose as unchanged drug; small amounts may be eliminated in feces. Crosses placenta; enters breast milk.

N

CONTRAINDICATIONS AND PRECAUTIONS. Known hypersensitivity to nitrofuran derivatives, anuria, oliguria, significant impairment of renal function (creatinine clearance under 40 ml/minute), patients with G6PD deficiency, infants under 3 months of age, parenteral use in children under 12 years of age. Safe use in women of childbearing potential, during pregnancy, pregnancy at term, and in nursing mothers not established. *Cautious Use:* history of asthma, anemia, diabetes, vitamin B deficiency, electrolyte imbalance, debilitating disease.

ADVERSE/SIDE EFFECTS. GI (most frequent): anorexia, nausea, vomiting, abdominal pain, diarrhea. **Hematologic (rare):** hemolytic or megaloblastic anemia (especially in patients with G6PD deficiency), granulocytosis. **Hypersensitivity:** allergic pneumonitis, eosinophilia, skin eruptions, pruritus, urticaria, angioedema, anaphylaxis, asthmatic attack (patients with history of asthma), drug fever, arthralgia, cholestatic jaundice. **Neurologic:** peripheral neuropathy, headache, nystagmus, drowsiness, vertigo. **Others:** transient alopecia, genitourinary superinfections (especially with *Pseudomonas*), tooth staining from direct contact with oral suspension and crushed tablets (infants), crystalluria (elderly patients); pulmonary sensitivity reactions (interstitial pneumonitis and/or fibrosis).

ROUTE AND DOSAGE. Oral: Adults: 50 to 100 mg four times daily; for long-term suppressive dosage: 25 to 50 mg four times daily. **Children (over 3 months):** 5 to 7 mg/kg/24 hours divided into four equal doses.

NURSING IMPLICATIONS

Drug must be given at equally spaced intervals around the clock to maintain therapeutic urinary drug levels.

Administer oral drug with meals or milk to minimize gastric irritation.

Nausea occurs fairly frequently and may be relieved by using macrocrystalline preparation (Macrodantin) or by reduction in dosage. Consult physician.

Because of the possibility of tooth staining associated with direct contact of drug with teeth advise patient to avoid crushing tablets to dilute oral suspension in milk, infant formula, water, or fruit juice, and to rinse mouth thoroughly after taking drug.

Forewarn patient that IM injection of nitrofurantoin may be painful (pain may be severe enough to warrant discontinuation of drug by this route).

Inform patient that nitrofurantoin may impart a harmless brown color to urine (due to drug metabolite).

Monitor intake and output. Report oliguria and any change in intake–output ratio. Drug should be discontinued if oliguria or anuria develops or *creatinine clearance* falls below 40 ml/minute. (Normal: 115 ± 20 ml/minute.)

Consult physician regarding fluid intake. Generally, fluids are not forced, since drug is highly soluble; however, intake should be adequate.

Culture and sensitivity tests are performed prior to therapy and are recommended in patients with recurrent infections.

Be alert to signs of urinary tract superinfections: milky urine, foul-smelling urine, perineal irritation, dysuria.

Acute pulmonary sensitivity reaction usually occurs within first week of therapy and appears to be more common in the elderly. May be manifested by mild to severe flulike syndrome: fever, dyspnea, cough, chest pains, chills, decreased breath sounds, rhonchi and crepitant rates on auscultation. Eosinophilia generally develops in a few days. Recovery usually occurs rapidly after drug is discontinued.

Subacute or chronic pulmonary sensitivity reaction is associated with prolonged therapy. Commonly manifested by insidious onset of malaise, cough, dyspnea on exertion, altered pulmonary function (x-ray findings: interstitial pneumonitis and/or fibrosis).

Peripheral neuropathy can be severe and irreversible. Be alert for and advise the patient to report onset of muscle weakness, tingling, numbness, or other sensations. Reportedly, these are most likely to occur in patients with renal impairment, anemia, diabetes, electrolyte imbalance, vitamin B deficiency, or debilitating disease. Drug should be discontinued immediately.

Treatment is continued for at least 3 days after sterile urines are obtained. Course of treatment for acute infections rarely exceeds 14 days.

Dispensed in amber-colored containers; strong light darkens drug. Nitrofurantoin decomposes on contact with metals other than stainless steel or aluminum.

Diagnostic Test Interferences. Nitrofurantoin metabolite may produce false-positive **urine glucose** test results with Benedict's reagent.

Drug Interactions. Drugs that tend to alkalinize urine (e.g., **acetazolamide, thiazides**) may decrease the effect of nitrofurantoin. There is the possibility that **antacids** may delay absorption of nitrofurantoin. Nitrofurantoin may antagonize the effects of **nalidixic acid.** Concomitant administration with **probenecid** (particularly in high doses) and possibly **sulfinpyrazone** may increase nitrofurantoin in serum to toxic levels by decreasing renal clearance (also decreasing effectiveness in urinary tract infections). Antimicrobial effectiveness of nitrofurantoin may be reduced by **magnesium** containing drugs.

NITROFURAZONE

(Furacin, Nitrofural)

(nye-troe-fyoor'a-zone)
Antiinfective (topical)
Nitrofuran

ACTIONS AND USES. Synthetic nitrofuran related to nitrofurantoin. Bactericidal against most microorganisms causing surface infections, including many that have developed antibiotic resistance. Activity against *Pseudomonas aeruginosa* and certain strains of *Proteus* is limited; has no activity against fungi or viruses. Acts by inhibiting aerobic and anaerobic cycles in bacterial carbohydrate metabolism.

Used topically as adjunctive therapy to combat bacterial infection in second- and third-degree burns; used to prevent infection of skin grafts and/or donor sites. Has been used orally in other countries for treatment of late stage of African trypanosomiasis. Available in combination with other drugs for treatment of bacterial urethritis.

CONTRAINDICATIONS AND PRECAUTIONS. History of sensitization to nitrofurazone. Safe use in women of childbearing potential and during pregnancy not established. *Cautious Use:* known or suspected renal impairment, patients with G6PD deficiency.

ADVERSE/SIDE EFFECTS. Allergic contact dermatitis (most frequently reported), irritation, sensitization, superinfections.

ROUTE AND DOSAGE. Topical (available in 0.2% soluble dressing, (ointment) solution, cream): *Soluble dressing:* applied directly to lesions or placed on gauze; reapplied once daily or weekly. *Solution:* sprayed on painful lesions or burns; 1:1 dilution used for saturating dressing for skin grafts. *Cream:* applied directly to lesion or placed on gauze; reapplied once daily or every few days.

NURSING IMPLICATIONS

Dressing removal may be facilitated by flushing the gauze with sterile isotonic saline solution.

Confine applications of nitrofurazone to the part being treated. When wet dressings are used, normal skin surrounding the wound should be protected with an agent such as sterile petrolatum, petrolatum gauze, or zinc oxide. Consult physician.

Consult physician regarding procedure for cleaning wound following each dressing removal.

Drug should be discontinued with onset of symptoms of sensitization or allergy (redness, itching, burning, swelling, rash, failure to heal), and superinfections, e.g., black furry tongue, thrush, malodorous vaginal discharge, anogenital itching, diarrhea.

Preserved in tight, light-resistant containers, away from heat. Drug darkens slowly on exposure to light, but reportedly this does not appreciably affect potency. Autoclaving more than once not recommended.

PROTOTYPE

NITROGLYCERIN

(Ang-O-Span, Glyceryl Trinitrate, Klavichordal, Niong, Nitro-bid, Nitrocap, Nitrodisc, Nitro-Dur, Nitrodyl, Nitroglyn, Nitrol, Nitrolin, Nitrong, Nitrospan, Nitro-T.D., Nitrostat, Nitrotym, NTG, Transderm-Nitro, Trates, Tridil)

(nye-troe-gli'ser-in)
Vasodilator (Coronary)
Antiangina
Nitrate

ACTIONS AND USES. Organic nitrate produced from volatile liquid with explosive potential, rendered nonexplosive by addition of carbohydrates. Relaxes all smooth muscle by direct action, with most prominent effect on vascular smooth muscle. Resulting vasodilation promotes pooling of blood, produces lowered peripheral resistance, fall in blood pressure, and decreased cardiac output due to reduced venous return to heart. Precise mechanism of action in treatment of angina pectoris not established, but appears to be due to reduction in myocardial oxygen consumption. Cross tolerance with other nitrites and nitrates may occur.

Used in prevention and treatment of acute anginal episodes. Sustained release tablets available for longer prophylaxis. Topical application used particularly for patients who fear nocturnal anginal attack. Has been used for temporary pain relief of biliary colic and to relieve paroxysmal nocturnal dyspnea. Intravenous or topical nitroglycerin has been used for treatment of refractory congestive heart failure and to reduce extent of infarction during acute MI.

ABSORPTION AND FATE. Sublingual tablet acts in 1 to 3 minutes; duration up to 30 minutes. Transmucosal form acts in 3 minutes; duration: 10 to 30 minutes. Sustained release tablet acts in about 1 hour; action peaks in 3 to 4 hours and persists 8 to 12 hours. Topical ointment acts in 15 to 30 minutes with duration of 3 or more hours (response is variable). Transdermal system acts in 30 to 60 minutes with duration of about 24 hours. IV nitroglycerin acts immediately; duration of effects: variable. Rapidly metabolized in liver; excreted in urine mostly as inactive metabolites.

CONTRAINDICATIONS AND PRECAUTIONS. Hypersensitivity, idiosyncrasy, or tolerance to nitrites; early myocardial infarction; severe anemia, hypotension, increased intracranial pressure, glaucoma (sustained release forms). Safe use during pregnancy and in children not established. *Cautious Use:* hepatic or renal disease, hyperthyroidism.

ADVERSE/SIDE EFFECTS. Transient headache, dizziness, flushing, postural hypotension, palpitation, increased heart rate, nausea, vomiting. **Hypersensitivity:** skin rash, exfoliative dermatitis, blurred vision, dry mouth, weakness, restlessness, pallor, perspiration, collapse. **Overdosage:** violent headache, syncope, tachycardia, paradoxical angina, circulatory collapse, convulsions, coma, respiratory failure; methemoglobinia (toxic doses).

N

ROUTE AND DOSAGE. **Sublingual:** 0.15 to 0.6 mg.Individualized dosage. Sustained release form: 1 capsule or tablet (1.3 to 9 mg) every 8 to 12 hours (usually before breakfast and at bedtime. **Topical (2% ointment):** 1 to 2 inches (25 to 50 mm) as squeezed from tube, every 8 hours; some patients may require 4 or 5 inches (100 to 125 mm) every 4 hours. **Transdermal system:** dosage increases are made either by using larger sized system or by using a combination of systems. **Intravenous infusion:** Initial: 5 mcg in 5% dextrose or 0.9% sodium chloride injection, with increments of 10 to 20 mcg/minute every 3 to 5 minutes, as necessary.

NURSING IMPLICATIONS

Sublingual Tablet (Discuss the Following Points with Physician):

Instruct patient to sit or lie down upon first indication of oncoming anginal pain, and to place tablet under tongue or in buccal pouch (hypotensive effect of drug is intensified in the upright position). Recumbent position should be avoided since venous blood return to the heart may increase. Advise patient to allow tablet to dissolve naturally and not to swallow until drug is entirely dissolved.

As soon as pain is completely relieved, any remaining tablet may be expelled from mouth, especially if patient is experiencing unpleasant side effects such as headache.

Advise patient to relax for 15 to 20 minutes after taking tablet to prevent dizziness or faintness.

If pain is not relieved after one tablet, additional tablets may be taken at 5 minute intervals, but not more than 3 tablets should be taken in a 15-minute period. Taking more tablets than necessary can further decrease coronary blood flow by producing systemic hypotension.

Pain not relieved by 3 tablets over a 15 minute period may indicate acute myocardial infarction or severe coronary insufficiency. Advise patient to contact physician immediately or have someone take patient directly to emergency room.

For hospitalized patient, tablets should be kept at bedside. Allocate a specific number (usually 10 tablets) in an appropriate container, label, and make sure patient knows location and use. Request patient to report all attacks. Count tablets at 7 AM and 7 PM.

Transient headache a frequent side effect, usually lasts about 5 minutes after sublingual administration and seldom longer than 20 minutes. Report to physician if persistent or severe. (Patients who do not have coronary disease may experience severe disabling headaches.)

Sublingual tablets may be taken prophylactically 5 to 10 minutes prior to exercise or other stimulus known to trigger anginal pain (drug effect will last up to 30 minutes).

Instruct patient to keep record for physician of number of anginal attacks, number of tablets required for relief of each attack, and possible precipitating factors.

Patient Instruction for Care of Sublingual Tablets:

Federal regulations require that tablets be dispensed in original unopened container.

Note expiration date on label.

Once bottle is opened, remove cotton filler. Keep bottle tightly capped.

Store stock supply in cool, dry place or at controlled room temperature not exceeding 30°C (86°F). Inactivation of nitroglycerin is increased by time, heat, air, moisture.

Inform family members of location of stock supply.

Open stock bottle once weekly to remove week's supply of tablets. Do not handle tablets since moisture will hasten deterioration. Carry these on person at all times, away from body heat (e.g., in jacket pocket, handbag).

An empty nitroglycerin bottle is an ideal container for carrying week's supply (amber colored bottle with metal cap). Tablets lose considerable potency in containers made of metal, plastic, or cardboard and when mixed with other capsules or tablets.

References vary with respect to how long stock supply retains potency: it is generally recommended that unused tablets be discarded 6 months after bottle is opened. An indication of potency is suggested if drug produces a burning or stinging sensation under patient's tongue. However, many elderly patients are unable to detect this sensation; additionally, this effect may not be experienced with the newer, more stable sublingual preparations.

Nitrostat is reportedly more stable than other sublingual tablets, but it must be specifically prescribed.

Sustained release oral tablet or capsule:

- Should be taken on an empty stomach (1 hour before or 2 hours after meals), with a full glass of water, and swallowed whole.
- Sustained release form helps to prevent anginal attacks; it is not intended for immediate relief of angina.

Nitroglycerin Ointment (Discuss the Following Points with Physician):

Before initiation of treatment take baseline blood pressure and heart rate, with patient in sitting position. (Have patient rest approximately 10 minutes before taking measurements.)

One hour after medication has been applied, check blood pressure and pulse again with patient in sitting position. Report measurements to physician. (Appropriate dosage is that which produces 10 mm Hg fall in BP, or 10 beat rise in resting heart rate.)

Application of ointment: Squeeze prescribed dose onto special measuring application supplied by manufacturer and use it, *not fingers* to spread ointment. Apply prescribed dose in a thin, uniform layer to premarked 6 by 6 inch square nonhairy skin surface. Areas commonly used: chest, abdomen, anterior thigh, forearm. Do not massage or rub in ointment as this increases absorption and thus interferes with drug's sustained action.

Area may be covered with transparent kitchen wrap and secured with tape to protect clothing.

Rotate application sites to prevent dermal inflammation and sensitization. Remove ointment from previously used sites before reapplication.

To determine optimal dose, physician may initially prescribe ½ or 1 inch of ointment and increase dose ¼ or ½ inch at a time until headache (a definitive sign of overdosage) occurs, then gradually reduce dose to that which does not cause headache.

If treatment is to be terminated, dosage and frequency of application must be reduced gradually over period of 4 to 6 weeks to prevent withdrawal reactions (pain, severe myocardial ischemia).

Keep ointment container tightly closed and store in cool place.

Transdermal system:

- is a nitroglycerin impregnated unit which when applied to skin releases continuous and controlled dosage over 24 hour period.
- System is applied at the same time each day, preferably to skin site free of hair and not subject to excessive movement. Avoid abraded, irritated or scarred skin. Clip hair if necessary.
- Change application site each time to prevent skin irritation and sensitization.
- Contact with water, e.g., bathing, swimming does not affect the unit.
- If faintness, dizziness or flushing occurs, advise patient to remove unit immediately from skin and notify physician. (Consult physician about this teaching point.)

Intravenous nitroglycerin:

- Must be diluted in 5% dextrose or 0.9% sodium chloride injection prior to infusion.
- Stable for at least 48 hours when stored at controlled room temperature between 15° and 30°C (59° and 86°F), and mixed and stored in a glass container.
- Nitroglycerin preparations for IV administration vary in concentration and volume. Check manufacturer's labeling information carefully for dilution and dosage particularly if change is made from one product to another.
- Use only glass containers for making dilutions, for IV administration and for storage of medication. Polyvinyl chloride (PVC) plastic can absorb nitroglycerin and therefore should not be used.
- Non-polyvinyl chloride (non-PVC) sets are recommended or provided by manufacturer.
- Regular IV tubing can absorb 40 to 80% of nitroglycerin. If patient has been receiving nitroglycerin in regular tubing and change is made to non-PVC tubing, dosage should be adjusted.
- Close monitoring of non-PVC infusion sets is essential because of the possibility of inaccuracies reportedly associated with regulation of flow rates.
- IV dosage titration requires careful and continuous monitoring of blood pressure, heart rate, and pulmonary capillary wedge pressure in some patients.

General Points:

- Advise patient to report blurred vision or dry mouth. Both reactions warrant discontinuation of nitroglycerin.
- Pain of angina is usually described as a squeezing, choking, tight or heavy substernal discomfort. Pain may radiate to arms, shoulders, neck and lower jaw and is of short duration, usually less than 10 minutes.

- Dizziness, lightheadedness, and syncope (due to postural hypotension) occur most frequently in the elderly. Recovery may be hastened by head-low position, deep breathing, and movement of extremities. Advise patient to make position changes slowly and to avoid prolonged standing.
- Inform patient that a shock-like syndrome (sharp drop in blood pressure, vertigo, flushing or pallor) may occur if alcohol is ingested too soon after taking nitroglycerin.
- Tolerance to nitroglycerin rarely occurs with usual intermittent use, but is possible with repeated administration. It may be prevented by using smallest effective dose. Temporary withdrawal (few days) usually restores original response to drug.
- Advise patient to report to physician any evidence of refractoriness, i.e., increase in frequency, duration or severity of attacks.
- Each patient must learn to identify stimuli that precipitate anginal pain in him, and pace his activities accordingly. Known factors that may provoke an attack include: emotional distress, heavy meals, smoking, temperature extremes, excessive use of coffee, tea, colas; sudden burst of physical activity; climbing stairs, especially while talking or carrying heavy bundles.
- Regular program of graduated daily exercises is generally recommended as well as control or reduction of body weight, and low cholesterol diet.
- Withdrawal following prolonged use must be accomplished gradually to prevent precipitating anginal attacks.
- Advise patient to carry medical information card or other suitable identification indicating that patient is taking nitroglycerin. (May be purchased in drug store or through Medic Alert; *see Index for address.*)

Diagnostic Test Interferences. Nitroglycerin may cause increases in determinations of **urinary catecholamines,** and **VMA.**

Drug Interactions. Combined use of nitroglycerin and **alcohol** or **antihypertensive agents** may potentiate orthostatic hypotension, from additive vasodilation. Chronic administration of **pentaerythritol tetranitrate** or other long-acting nitrites may impair response to subsequently administered nitroglycerin, by producing tolerance. Nitroglycerin may potentiate hypotensive effects of **tricyclic antidepressants,** and may increase the pharmacologic effects of **ergot alkaloids.**

N

NITROPRUSSIDE, SODIUM

(Nipride, Nitropress)

(nye-troe-pruss-'ide)
Antihypertensive
Vasodilator (peripheral)

ACTIONS AND USES. Potent, rapid-acting hypotensive agent with effects similar to those of nitrates. Acts directly on vascular smooth muscle to produce peripheral vasodilation, with consequent marked lowering of arterial blood pressure, associated with slight increase in heart rate, mild decrease in cardiac output, and moderate lowering of peripheral vascular resistance. Thiocyanate metabolite may inhibit uptake and binding of iodine, with prolonged therapy.

Used for short-term, rapid reduction of blood pressure in hypertensive crises and for producing controlled hypotension during anesthesia to reduce bleeding.

ABSORPTION AND FATE. Onset of hypotensive effect usually occurs within 2 minutes; effect lasts 1 to 10 minutes after infusion is terminated. Rapidly converted to cyanogen (cyanides) in erythrocytes and tissue, which is metabolized to thiocyanate in liver. Excreted in urine, primarily as thiocyanate metabolite.

CONTRAINDICATIONS AND PRECAUTIONS. Use in treatment of compensatory hypertension, as in atriovenous shunt or coarctation of aorta, or for producing controlled hypotension in patients with inadequate cerebral circulation. Safe use during pregnancy and in women of childbearing potential and children not established. *Cautious Use:* hepatic insufficiency, hypothyroidism, severe renal impairment, hyponatremia, elderly patients with low vitamin B_{12} plasma levels or with Leber's optic atrophy.

ADVERSE/SIDE EFFECTS. Usually associated with too rapid reduction in blood pressure: nausea, retching, abdominal pain, nasal stuffiness, diaphoresis, headache, dizziness, apprehension, restlessness, muscle twitching, retrosternal discomfort, palpitation, increase or transient lowering of pulse rate. **Other:** irritation at infusion site, hypothyroidism with prolonged therapy (rare), increase in serum creatinine, fall or rise in total plasma cobalamins. **Overdosage (thiocyanate toxicity):** profound hypotension, tinnitus, blurred vision, fatigue, metabolic acidosis, pink skin color, absence of reflexes, faint heart sounds, loss of consciousness.

ROUTE AND DOSAGE. Intravenous infusion (only): average dose 3 mcg/kg/minute, range 0.5 to 10 mcg/kg/minute; usually infusion rate rarely exceeds 10 mcg/minute. 5% dextrose in water and reportedly, sterile water *without preservative* may be used preparing solutions.

NURSING IMPLICATIONS

Solutions must be freshly prepared and used no later than 4 hours after reconstitution.

Following reconstitution, solutions usually have faint brownish tint; if highly colored do not use. Promptly wrap container with aluminum foil or other opaque material to protect drug from light.

Administered by infusion pump, micro-drip regulator, or similar device that will allow precise measurement of flow rate.

Constant monitoring is required to titrate IV infusion rate to blood pressure response. If concomitant oral hypertensive therapy is given, IV infusion rate will require further adjustment.

Adverse effects *(see Adverse/Side Effects)* are usually relieved by slowing IV rate or by stopping drug; they may be minimized by keeping patient supine.

Monitor intake and output.

Monitoring blood thiocyanate level is recommended in patients receiving prolonged treatment or in patients with severe renal dysfunction (levels usually are not allowed to exceed 10 mg/dl). Determination of plasma cyanogen level following 1 or 2 days of therapy is advised in patients with impaired hepatic function *(see Absorption and Fate)*.

No other drug should be added to sodium nitroprusside infusion.

Treatment of overdosage: amyl nitrite inhalations for 15 to 30 seconds each minute pending preparation of 3% sodium nitrite solution (injection rate not to exceed 2.5 to 5 ml/minute, up to total dose of 10 to 15 ml, followed by IV sodium thiosulfate 12.5 Gm in 50 ml of 5% dextrose in water over 10-minute period; may be repeated at one-half the above doses, if necessary). Have on hand vasopressor agents. Patient must be closely observed for several hours, since signs of overdosage may reappear.

Protect drug from light, heat, and moisture; store preferably at 15° to 30°C (59° to 86°F) unless otherwise directed by manufacturer.

NOREPINEPHRINE BITARTRATE

(Levarterenol, Levophed, Noradrenaline)

(nor-ep-i-nef'rin)
Alpha-adrenergic agonist (direct-acting)
Catecholamine

ACTIONS AND USES. Direct-acting sympathomimetic amine identical to body catecholamine norepinephrine. Acts directly and predominantly on alpha-adrenergic receptors; little action on beta-receptors except in heart ($beta_1$ receptors). Main therapeutic effects are vasoconstriction and cardiac stimulation. Has powerful constrictor action on resistance and capacitance blood vessels. Reduces blood flow to kidney, other vital organs, skin, and skeletal muscle. Peripheral vasoconstriction (alpha-adrenergic action) and moderate inotropic stimulation of heart (beta-adrenergic action) result in increased systolic and diastolic blood pressure, myocardial oxygenation, coronary artery blood flow, and work of heart. Cardiac output varies reflexly with systemic blood pressure. Reflex increase of vagal activity in response to pronounced effect on arterial blood pressure may cause bradycardia. Causes less CNS stimulation and has less effect on metabolism than does epinephrine; however, in large doses it can increase glycogenolysis and inhibit pancreatic insulin release, with resulting hyperglycemia. May cause contraction of pregnant uterus.

Used to restore blood pressure in certain acute hypotensive states such as sympathectomy, pheochromocytomectomy, spinal anesthesia, poliomyelitis, myocardial infarction, septicemia, blood transfusion, and drug reactions. Also used as adjunct in treatment of cardiac arrest.

ABSORPTION AND FATE. Pressor activity occurs rapidly and lasts 1 to 2 minutes following termination of IV infusion. Pronounced localization in sympathetic nerve endings. Inactivated in liver and other tissues, primarily by catechol-*o*-methyl transferase and to smaller extent by monamine oxidase. Excreted in urine mainly as inactive metabolites; 4 to 16% of dose is excreted unchanged. Crosses placenta.

CONTRAINDICATIONS AND PRECAUTIONS. Use as sole therapy in hypovolemic states, except as temporary emergency measure; mesenteric or peripheral vascular thrombosis; profound hypoxia or hypercarbia; pregnancy; use during cyclopropane or halothane anesthesia. *Cautious Use:* hypertension, hyperthyroidism, severe heart disease, elderly patients, within 14 days of MAOI therapy, patients receiving tricyclic antidepressants.

N

ADVERSE/SIDE EFFECTS. Headache, palpitation, hypertension, reflex bradycardia, fatal arrhythmias (large doses), respiratory difficulty, restlessness, anxiety, tremors, dizziness, weakness, insomnia, pallor, tissue necrosis at injection site (with extravasation), swelling of thyroid gland (rare). **With prolonged administration:** plasma volume depletion, edema, hemorrhage, intestinal, hepatic, and renal necrosis. **Overdosage or individual sensitivity:** blurred vision, photophobia, hyperglycemia, retrosternal and pharyngeal pain, profuse sweating, vomiting, severe hypertension, violent headache, cerebral hemorrhage, convulsions.

ROUTE AND DOSAGE. Highly individualized according to response of patient. **Intravenous infusion:** Initial: 8 to 12 mcg of base/minute. Average maintenance dose: 2 to 4 mcg of base/minute.

NURSING IMPLICATIONS

IV infusion of norepinephrine in saline alone is not recommended. Dextrose (in distilled water or saline solution) is used to prevent oxidation and thus loss of potency.

Risk of extravasation is reportedly reduced if infusion is administered through a plastic catheter inserted deep into vein (preferably antecubital). Catheter tie-in technique is not recommended, as it promotes stasis.

A double-bottle setup is advisable (1 bottle without norepinephrine) so that IV can be kept running in the event that norepinephrine must be stopped.

In patients with severe hypotension after myocardial infarction, the physician may prescribe addition of heparin to norepinephrine infusion to prevent thrombosis of infused vein and perivenous reaction.

An infusion pump or apparatus to control norepinephrine flow rate is generally used. Regulation of flow rate is determined by blood pressure response. Consult physician for specific guidelines.

Blood volume depletion must be continuously corrected by appropriate fluid and electrolyte replacement therapy to maintain tissue perfusion and to avoid recurrence of hypotension when norepinephrine is stopped.

Whole blood or plasma is incompatible with norepinephrine and therefore should be administered separately.

Patient should be attended constantly while receiving norepinephrine. Take baseline blood pressure and pulse before start of therapy, then every 2 minutes from initiation of drug until stabilization occurs at desired level, then every 5 minutes during drug administration.

In normotensive patients it is recommended that flow rate be adjusted to maintain blood pressure at low normal (usually 80 to 100 mm Hg systolic). In previously hypertensive patients, systolic is generally maintained no higher than 40 mm Hg *below* preexisting systolic level.

In addition to vital signs, carefully observe and record mentation (index of cerebral circulation), skin temperature of extremities, and color (especially of earlobes, lips, nail beds).

Flow rate must be constantly monitored. Check infusion site frequently for free flow (adhesive tape should not obscure injection site). Report immediately any evidence of extravasation: blanching along course of infused vein (may occur without obvious extravasation), cold, hard swelling around injection site.

Antidote for extravasation ischemia: Phentolamine, 5 to 10 mg in 10 to 15 ml normal saline injection, is infiltrated throughout affected area (using syringe with fine hypodermic needle) as soon as possible. Some physicians prefer to add phentolamine (5 to 10 mg) to each liter of infusion solution as a preventive against sloughing should extravasation occur.

Monitor intake and output. Urinary retention and renal shutdown are possibilities, especially in hypovolemic patients. Urinary output is a sensitive indicator of the degree of renal perfusion. Report decrease in urinary output or change in intake–output ratio.

Be alert to patient's complaints of headache, vomiting, palpitation, arrhythmias, chest pain, photophobia, and blurred vision as possible symptoms of overdosage. Reflex bradycardia may occur as a result of rise in blood pressure.

Emergency drugs should be immediately available in the event of cardiac irregularities. Atropine is an antidote for bradycardia; cardiac arrhythmias may be treated with propranolol.

If therapy is to be prolonged, it is advisable to change infusion sites at intervals to allow effect of local vasoconstriction to subside.

When therapy is to be discontinued, infusion rate is slowed gradually. Abrupt withdrawal should be avoided. Continue to monitor vital signs and observe patient closely after cessation of therapy for clinical sign of circulatory inadequacy.

Do not use solution if discoloration or precipitate is present. Protect from light.

N

Drug Interactions. Norepinephrine should be used cautiously and in small doses in patients receiving drugs that may potentiate its pressor effects: some **antihistamines** (especially **dexchlorpheniramine, diphenhydramine, tripelennamine**), **parenteral ergot alkaloids, guanethidine, methyldopa,** and **tricyclic antidepressants.** Norepinephrine should be administered with extreme caution in patients receiving **MAO inhibitors** (possibility of severe and prolonged hypertension in some patients). Concurrent administration of norepinephrine with **cyclopropane** or **halothane** and related general anesthetics may lead to ventricular arrhythmias. Administration of norepinephrine to patients already receiving **propranolol** may result in high elevations of blood pressure.

NORETHINDRONE
(Aygestin, Micronor, Norlutin, Nor-Q.D.)
NORETHINDRONE ACETATE
(Norlutate)

(nor-eth-in'drone)
Progestin
Contraceptive, progestin-only

ACTIONS AND USES. Synthetic progestational hormone with androgenic, anabolic, and estrogenic properties. (The acetate form is the most potent anabolic agent available with approximately double the progestational potency of norethindrone.) May produce excess estrogenic effect. Mechanism for prevention of contraception unclear. Progestin-only contraceptives alter cervical mucus, exert progestational effect on endometrium, interfere with implantation, and, in some cases, suppress ovulation.

Used to treat amenorrhea, abnormal uterine bleeding due to hormonal imbalance in absence of organic pathology; endometriosis. Also used in combination with an estrogen for birth control (Norinyl, Norlestrin, Ortho-Novum, Brevicon, Ovcon, Loestrin) *See Progesterone for absorption, fate, and limitations.*

ADVERSE/SIDE EFFECTS. Weight gain, acne, hirsutism, deepening of voice; bleeding irregularities. *See also Progesterone.*

ROUTE AND DOSAGE. Oral: Norethindrone (Norlutin): *Amenorrhea:* 5 to 20 mg on day 5 through day 25 of menstrual cycle. *Endometriosis:* Initial: 10 mg daily for 2 weeks; increase with increments of 5 mg daily every 2 weeks up to 30 mg daily. Therapy may remain at this level 6 to 9 months or until breakthrough bleeding demands temporary interruption. *Progestin-only contraception:* 0.35 mg daily on the first day of menstrual flow; one tablet from then on, each day of the year (even during menstruation). **Norethindrone acetate:** doses approximately half those of norethindrone when used to treat amenorrhea and endometriosis.

N

NURSING IMPLICATIONS

It may take 2 or 3 months for effects of hormonal contraception to wear off; pregnancy during this period could result in a child with birth defects, such as heart and limb deformities.

If patient is exposed to norethindrone during first 3 to 4 months of pregnancy she should be apprised of the potential teratogenic risk to the fetus.

Instruct patient to report promptly prolonged vaginal bleeding or amenorrhea.

Notify the pathologist that patient is on hormonal therapy when relevant specimens are submitted for study.

Continuous regimen with progestin-only contraception (mini-pill). e.g., Micronur, Nor-Q-D.:

- When starting the mini-pill regimen, the patient should use a second method of birth control for the first cycle or for 3 weeks, to insure full protection.
- The mini-pill can be started right after delivery in the nonnursing mother; however, she should be aware of an increased risk of thromboembolic disease during the postpartum period.

- Advise patient to wait at least 3 months before becoming pregnant after stopping the mini-pill, to prevent birth defects. A nonhormonal method of contraception should be employed until pregnancy is desired.
- Failure rate of the progestin-only contraceptive is about 3 times higher than that of the norethindrone-estrogen combinations.
- In the event of a missed menstrual period: (a) if patient has not adhered to prescribed dosing regimen, the possibility of pregnancy should be considered after 45 days from the last menstrual period; progestin-only contraceptive should be withheld until pregnancy is ruled out; (b) if patient has adhered to prescribed regimen and misses 2 consecutive periods, pregnancy should be ruled out, and a nonhormonal method of birth control should be used before continuing the regimen.

Teach patient self-breast examination (SBE).

Urge patient to keep appointments for physical checkups (every 6 to 12 months) during period of hormonal birth control.

Review package insert with the patient to assure understanding of use of norethindrone.

Store at temperature between 15° and 30°C (59° and 86°F); protect drug from light and from freezing.

See Progesterone (prototype progestin).

NORGESTREL

(Ovrette)

(nor-jess'trel)
Progestin
Contraceptive, progestin-only

ACTIONS AND USES. Potent antiestrogenic progestational hormone with little or no androgenic or anabolic properties. *See Progesterone for absorption, fate, contraindications, adverse reactions.*

Used as a progestin-only contraceptive (mini-pill).

ROUTE AND DOSAGE. Oral: 0.075 mg (one tablet) daily every day of the year, beginning on first day of menstruation.

NURSING IMPLICATIONS

Mini-pill is to be taken at same time each day, even if user is menstruating.

Amount and duration of flow, cycle length, breakthrough bleeding, spotting, and amenorrhea vary greatly with use of the progestin-only contraceptive.

Continuous regimen with progestin-only contraception:

- When starting the mini-pill regimen, the patient should use a second method of birth control for the first cycle or for 3 weeks, to insure full protection.
- The mini-pill can be started right after delivery in the nonnursing mother; however, she should be aware of an increased risk of thromboembolic disease during the postpartum period.
- Advise patient to wait at least 3 months before becoming pregnant after stopping the mini-pill, to prevent birth defects. A nonhormonal method of contraception should be employed until pregnancy is desired.
- Failure rate of the progestin-only contraceptive is about three times higher than that of the combination contraceptives.

- In the event of a missed menstrual period: (a) if patient has not adhered to prescribed dosing regimen, the possibility of pregnancy should be considered after 45 days from the last menstrual period; progestin-only contraceptive should be withheld until pregnancy is ruled out; (b) if patient has adhered to prescribed regimen and misses 2 consecutive periods, pregnancy should be ruled out and a nonhormonal method of birth control should be used before continuation of the regimen.

The commercial preparation contains *tartrazine* which may cause allergic reaction in susceptible individuals. Frequently these patients also have aspirin hypersensitivity.

Teach patient self-breast examination (SBE).

Store at temperature between 15° and 30°C (59° and 86°F) in a well-closed container.

Review package insert with patient to assure understanding about use of norgestrel.

See Progesterone.

NORTRIPTYLINE HYDROCHLORIDE

(Aventyl, Pamelor)

(nor-trip'ti-leen)
Psychotropic
Antidepressant
Tricyclic

ACTIONS AND USES. Dibenzocycloheptane derivative of amitriptyline. Tricyclic antidepressant (TCA) with less sedative and anticholinergic effects than imipramine (qv). Action mechanism unclear; mood elevation may be due to its inhibition of reuptake of norepinephrine at the presynaptic membrane.

Used to treat endogenous depression. Similar in actions, uses, limitations, and interactions to imipramine.

ABSORPTION AND FATE. Hepatic metabolism; 95% protein binding. Serum half-life: 31 ± 13 hours. Effective plasma levels: 50 to 150 ng/ml. Excreted primarily in urine. Crosses placenta; excreted in breast milk.

CONTRAINDICATIONS AND PRECAUTIONS. Children under 12 years of age; pregnancy, lactation, during or within 14 days of MAO inhibitors therapy; acute recovery period after myocardial infarction. *Cautious Use:* narrow-angle glaucoma, hyperthyroidism, concurrent administration of thyroid medications, concurrent use with electroshock therapy. *See also Imipramine.*

ADVERSE/SIDE EFFECTS. Urinary retention, paralytic ileus, orthostatic hypotension, drowsiness, confusional state (especially in the elderly and with high dosage), agranulocytosis, tremors, hyperhydrosis, dry mouth, blurred vision, photosensitivity reaction. *See also Imipramine.*

ROUTE AND DOSAGE. Oral: Adult: 25 mg three or four times daily; increased gradually according to patient response to regimen; doses above 100 mg daily not recommended. **Elderly; adolescents:** 30 to 50 mg daily in divided doses. Oral solution: 5 ml contains equivalent to 10 mg nortriptyline.

NURSING IMPLICATIONS

Administer drug with food to decrease gastric distress.

Oral solution does not require dilution. Aventyl is a 4% alcohol solution.

Supervise drug ingestion to be sure patient does not "cheek" the drug.

Because of the danger of suicidal intent in a severely depressed patient, limit access to the drug.

N

Nortriptyline has a narrow therapeutic plasma level range, a characteristic called "therapeutic window." Note that drug levels either above or below the therapeutic window of this drug are associated with decreased rate of response.

Therapeutic response may not occur for 2 weeks or more.

Monitor blood pressure and pulse rate during adjustment period of TCA therapy. If systolic BP falls more than 20 mm Hg or if there is a sudden increase in pulse rate, withhold medication and notify the physician.

Monitor bowel elimination pattern and intake–output ratio. Urinary retention and severe constipation are potential problems especially in the elderly. Advise increased fluid intake; consult physician about stool softener (if necessary) and a high-roughage diet.

Inspect oral membranes daily if patient is on high doses of TCA. Urge outpatient to report symptoms of stomatitis, sialoadenitis, xerostomia.

If xerostomia is a problem, institute symptomatic therapy. *See Imipramine.* Sore mouth interferes with speaking, mastication, swallowing, and can be a major cause of poor nutrition and noncompliance. Consult physician about use of a saliva substitute (e.g., VA-Oralube, Moi-stir).

If psychotic signs increase, notify physician. Because of the therapeutic window effect of nortriptyline, a substitute TCA may be prescribed rather than an increase in dosage.

Caution patient that ability to perform tasks requiring alertness and skill may be impaired.

Urge patient not to use OTC drugs unless physician approves.

The actions of both alcohol and nortriptyline are potentiated when used together during therapy and for up to 2 weeks after the TCA is discontinued. Consult physician about safe amount of alcohol, if any, that can be taken.

If a patient uses excessive amounts of alcohol it should be borne in mind that the potentiation may increase the danger of overdosage or suicide attempt.

The effects of barbiturates and other CNS depressants are enhanced by nortriptyline.

Observe patient with history of glaucoma. Symptoms that may signal acute attack (severe headache, eye pain, dilated pupils, halos of light, nausea, vomiting) should be reported promptly.

Fine tremors, a distressing extrapyramidal side effect, may be reduced or alleviated by propranolol. Report symptom to physician.

Store drug in tightly closed container preferably between 15° and 30°C (59° and 86°F) unless otherwise specified by manufacturer.

See Imipramine (prototype antidepressant).

N

NOSCAPINE
(Tusscapine)

(noss'ka-peen)
Antitussive (nonnarcotic)

ACTIONS AND USES. Nonaddictive benzylisoquinoline alkaloid of opium, related to papaverine. Antitussive potency reportedly equivalent to that of codeine, but lacks its side effects. Suppresses cough reflex; has no central action.

Used for temporary relief of nonproductive cough. Included in several proprietary cough mixtures, e.g., Conar.

CONTRAINDICATIONS AND PRECAUTIONS. History of allergy to noscapine, children under 2 years of age.

ADVERSE/SIDE EFFECTS. *Infrequently, with high dosage:* nausea, drowsiness, slight dizziness, headache, allergic reaction (conjunctivitis and vasomotor rhinitis).

ROUTE AND DOSAGE. Oral: Adult: 15 to 30 mg every 4 to 6 hours; not to exceed 120 mg/24 hours. **Children (6 to 12 years):** 15 mg 3 or 4 times daily; **(2 to 6 years):** 7.5 to 15 ml three or four times daily. Available in chewable tablet (adults), and syrup (children).

NURSING IMPLICATIONS

Effect of a single dose usually lasts up to 4 hours.

Noscapine may cause drowsiness. Caution patient to avoid driving and other potentially hazardous activities until reaction to drug is known.

See Benzonatate for nursing implications of cough therapy.

NOVOBIOCIN SODIUM

(Albamycin)

(noe-voe-bye′o-sin)
Antiinfective
Antibiotic

ACTIONS AND USES. Antibiotic obtained from cultures of *Streptomyces niveus* or *S. spheroides.* Bacteriostatic action appears to involve interference with synthesis of bacterial cell wall and inhibition of bacterial protein and nucleic acid synthesis. Cell membrane stability and integrety is also affected due to complexing of drug with magnesium within cell wall. Active in vitro against many gram-positive bacteria including *Staphalococcus aureus, S. pneumoniae,* group A streptococci, and viridans streptococci and against some gram-positive bacilli. Enterococci are usually resistant to novobiocin. Also active against gram-negative bacteria including *H. influenzae* and *N. gonorrhoeae.* Resistant strains of *S. aureus* may develop rapidly during therapy. Cross-resistance between novobiocin and other antiinfectives has not been reported.

Used in treatment of serious infections due to susceptible organisms in patients unresponsive to less toxic or sensitive to other antiinfectives. Drug is usually given with a penicillin.

N

CONTRAINDICATIONS AND PRECAUTIONS. Known sensitivity to novobiocin; neonates, during pregnancy.

ADVERSE/SIDE EFFECTS. GI: nausea, vomiting, diarrhea, anorexia, abdominal distress. **Hematologic:** pancytopenia, agranulocytosis, anemia, thrombocytopenia, hemolytic anemia, positive direct and indirect antiglobin (Coombs') test. **Hepatic:** jaundice, elevated serum bilirubin. **Hypersensitivity reactions:** urticaria, maculopapular dermatitis, swollen joints, Stevens-Johnson syndrome, erythema multiforme, pruritus, fever, eosinophilia. **Other:** dizziness, drowsiness, light-headedness. Causal relationship not established: allergic pneumonitis, myocarditis, alopecia, intestinal hemorrhage, suprainfections.

ROUTE AND DOSAGE. Oral: Adult: 250 mg every 6 hours or 500 mg every 12 hours. In severe infections, 500 mg every 6 hours or 1 Gm every 12 hours. Maximum recommended dosage for adults: 2 Gm/day. **Children:** 15 to 45 mg/kg daily given in two or four divided doses.

NURSING IMPLICATIONS

Novobiocin is an extremely potent sensitizing agent. Side effects should be reported promptly.

Drug resistance may develop rapidly. Advise patient to report if there is a reversal in prior evidence of therapeutic response to drug therapy.

Duration of therapy depends on the infection but inform patient that it will continue about 48 hours after febrile condition is past or when evidence of the infection is eradicated. Patient should not stop treatment just because he or she feels better.

Patient should not alter regimen without consulting physician; sensitivity and adverse effects may occur as well as a loss of therapeutic effects.

Warn patient not to use leftover novobiocin to self-medicate for another infection.

A yellow metabolite of novobiocin can cause jaundice-like skin coloration. Differentiation of drug-induced effect from frank jaundice will have to depend on other signs of hepatic dysfunction (i.e., dark urine, pruritus, elevated serum bilirubin). Advise patient to report symptoms promptly.

Inspect skin for signs of thrombocyte dyscrasia: petechiae, ecchymoses, easy bruising; these signs and/or epistaxis or bleeding for unexplained reason should be reported promptly.

Symptoms of superinfections and/or suprainfections should receive prompt attention. Reportable symptoms include: sore mouth with white mucosal patches, black furry tongue; malodorous vaginal discharge, diarrhea. *See Index: Nursing Intervention: superinfections.*

Drug Test Interferences. A yellow metabolite may appear in serum interferes with **serum bilirubin** determinations (Evelyn–Malloy method).

Drug Interactions. **Tetracyclines** may reduce novobiocin effectiveness.

NYLIDRIN HYDROCHLORIDE

(Arlidin, Rolidrin)

(nye'li-drin)

Beta-adrenergic agonist
Sympathomimetic
Vasodilator (peripheral)

N

ACTIONS AND USES. Sympathomimetic amine (phenylisopropylamine) similar to ephedrine. Acts predominantly on beta-adrenergic receptors. Increases blood flow to skeletal muscle by direct vasodilating action on arteries and arterioles; also causes slight increase in cerebral blood flow. Produces increase in cardiac output and some increase in heart rate; systolic blood pressure usually rises slightly, and diastolic may fall. Effect on cutaneous blood flow is negligible. Clinical value not established.

Used in treatment of vasospastic disorders such as peripheral vascular disease, e.g., acrocyanosis, Raynaud's syndrome, frostbite, night leg cramps, thromboangiitis obliterans, ischemic ulcer, diabetic vascular disease, Meniere's disease, circulatory disturbances of inner ear.

ABSORPTION AND FATE. Readily absorbed from GI tract, but slowly metabolized; therefore, action is prolonged. Excreted slowly in urine.

CONTRAINDICATIONS AND PRECAUTIONS. History of recent myocardial infarction, cardiac disease such as tachyarrhythmias, uncompensated heart failure, angina pectoris, thyrotoxicosis, peptic ulcer. *Cautious Use:* hypertension, peptic ulcer, cardiac disorders.

ADVERSE/SIDE EFFECTS. Trembling, nervousness, weakness, dizziness, palpitation, nausea, vomiting, postural hypotension (not reported, but possible).

ROUTE AND DOSAGE. Oral: 3 to 12 mg three or four times daily.

NURSING IMPLICATIONS

Palpitation is a prominent side effect that usually disappears with continued therapy; if it persists, reduction in dosage may be necessary.

Inform the patient that the benefits of nylidrin may not be apparent until after several weeks of therapy.

Observe for clinical response to therapy. For patients with peripheral vascular disease, note relief of rest pain or intermittent claudication and nail growth. For patients with circulatory disturbances of inner ear, note relief of dizziness, nausea, and nystagmus.

Hygienic care of extremities, properly fitting shoes and stockings, abstinence from smoking, avoidance of exposure to cold, and guidelines regarding acceptable activities are essential aspects of care in patients with peripheral vascular disease.

See Isoxsuprine hydrochloride for additional patient-teaching points.

Drug Interactions. Nylidrin may enhance the activity of **phenothiazines.**

NYSTATIN

(Korostatin, Mycostatin, Nilstat, O-V Statin)

(nye-stat′-in)
Antifungal
Antiinfective

ACTIONS AND USES. Antifungal antibiotic produced by *Streptomyces noursei.* Has fungistatic and fungicidal activity against a variety of yeasts and fungi; not appreciably active against bacteria, viruses, or protozoa. Thought to act by binding to sterols in fungal cell membrane, thereby changing membrane potential and allowing leakage of intracellular components. Reportedly nontoxic, topical preparations are nonstaining even with prolonged administration.

Used to treat infections of skin and mucous membranes caused by *Candida (Monilia) albicans* and other *Candida* species, as in oral thrush, paronychia, and cutaneous, vulvovaginal, and intestinal candidiasis. Available commercially in combination with corticosteroids (e.g., Mycolog) and tetracycline (e.g., Terrastatin).

ABSORPTION AND FATE. Poorly absorbed following oral administration; no detectable blood levels at recommended doses. Excreted in stool as unchanged drug. Not absorbed from intact skin or mucous membrane.

CONTRAINDICATIONS AND PRECAUTIONS. Hypersensitivity to nystatin or to any components in formulation.

ADVERSE/SIDE EFFECTS. Usually mild: nausea, vomiting, epigastric distress, diarrhea (especially with high oral doses), hypersensitivity reactions (rare).

ROUTE AND DOSAGE. Oral tablet: Adults: 500,000 to 1,000,000 units three times daily. **Oral suspension** (100,000 units/ml): **Adults and children:** 400,000 to 600,000 units four times daily. **Infants:** 200,000 units four times daily; **premature and low-weight infants:** 100,000 units four times daily. **Vaginal tablet: Adults:** 1 to 2 tablets (100,000 units each) deposited high in vagina with supplied applicator. **Topical:** cream, ointment, powder containing 100,000 units/Gm.

NURSING IMPLICATIONS

Management of factors predisposing to candidiasis is equally as important as treatment in preventing reinfection and eliminating deep-seated infections.

Avoid contact of drug with hands. Hypersensitivity reactions occur rarely with nystatin alone; reportedly, preservatives used in some formulations are associated with a high incidence of contact dermatitis.

Advise patient to report onset of redness, swelling, or irritation. Drug should be discontinued if these symptoms occur.

Oral candidiasis (thrush): Divide prescribed dose of oral suspension so that one-half is placed in each side of mouth. Mouth should be clear of food debris before drug administration. Instruct patient to keep medication in contact with oral mucosa for at least several minutes, if possible before swallowing. For infants, medication may be applied by means of swab.

Advise patient to brush teeth, or at least to rinse mouth thoroughly after each meal, and to floss teeth daily. (Patients with dentures should remove and clean them also after each meal.) Overuse of commercial mouth washes tends to change oral flora and therefore should be avoided.

In elderly patients, oral candidiasis has been associated with poorly fitting dentures. If this is a problem, advise patient to contact dentist.

Treatment of oral candidiasis should be continued for at least 48 hours after symptoms have subsided and mouth cultures are normal. Pending laboratory confirmation, articles contaminated by mouth contact should be kept isolated for the patient's use or concurrently disinfected.

Candidiasis of feet, skin, and nails: For candidal infection of feet, instruct patient to dust shoes and stockings, as well as feet, with nystatin dusting powder.

Proper hygiene and skin care to prevent spread of infection and reinfection are essential aspects of therapy. Advise patient to change stockings and underclothing daily and to use own linen and towels.

Occlusive dressings (including tight-fitting underclothing) or applications of ointment preparation to moist, dark areas of body favor growth of yeast and therefore should be avoided.

Cream formulation is preferred to the ointment for intertriginous areas. For very moist lesions, powder formulation is usually prescribed. Consult physician.

Infected areas should be cleaned gently before each application. Use of harsh soaps and vigorous scrubbing are contraindicated. Some physicians prescribe moist compresses with cool water for 15 minutes prior to application of medication (for soothing and drying action). Consult physician for specific guidelines.

Treatment of cutaneous candidal infections is usually continued for at least 2 weeks; discontinued only after two negative tests for *Candida*.

Paronychia: Advise patient to keep hands out of water as much as possible. Medication should be applied to nails and paronychial folds. Chronic paronychia may require several months of therapy to achieve clinical and mycologic cure. Relapses may be due to reinfection from *Candida* in intestinal tract.

Intestinal candidiasis: To prevent relapse, therapy is continued for at least 48 hours after symptoms have disappeared (vomiting, diarrhea, abdominal cramps, esophagitis).

Vulvovaginal candidiasis: Inform patient that medication should be continued during menstruation. In most cases 2 weeks of therapy are sufficient; however, some patients may require longer treatment.

In pregnant patients, vaginal tablets may be continued for 3 to 6 weeks before term in order to prevent thrush in newborns.

Cleansing douches may be used by nonpregnant patients if desired for aesthetic purposes (therapeutic douches, i.e., with antiinfective medication, are not necessary and may be inadvisable).

Possible predisposing factors should be considered, e.g., diabetes, pregnancy, infection by sexual partner, use of birth control pills, history of antibiotic therapy (candidal infections have occurred 6 to 8 weeks after therapy), corticosteroid therapy, use of tight-fitting nylon pantyhose.

Nystatin is preserved in tightly covered, light-resistant containers, away from heat. Expiration dates vary with manufacturer.

Mycostatin vaginal tablets should be stored at temperatures below 15°C (59°F) but avoid freezing.

O

OPIUM ALKALOIDS HYDROCHLORIDES

(Pantopon)

(oh'pee-um)
Opium preparation
Narcotic analgesic
Opiate agonist
C II

ACTIONS AND USES. A mixture of opium alkaloids in the same proportions as found in the natural opium powder. Contains about 50% anhydrous morphine or about 5 times the amount found in opium powder. The commercially available injection contains alcohol, glycerin, and parabens as preservatives. Analgesic activity results from the morphine component of the mixture; small doses have antidiarrheal effects. *See Morphine.*

Used to relieve severe pain; Pantopon, however, has been replaced largely by other narcotics.

ABSORPTION AND FATE. Following parenteral administration, activity is similar to that of morphine: peak analgesia occurs in 50 to 90 minutes following SC injection; 30 to 60 minutes following IM injection. Duration of analgesia: up to 7 hours. After rectal administration, opium in suppository form begins action in 15 to 30 minutes; analgesia is maintained for 3 to 5 hours. Hepatic metabolism; excretion in urine.

ROUTE AND DOSAGE. Intramuscular, subcutaneous: Adult: 5 to 20 mg every 4 or 5 hours.

NURSING IMPLICATIONS

A dose of 20 mg hydrochlorides is therapeutically equivalent to 15 mg morphine.

Classified as Schedule II drug under Federal Controlled Substances Act.

See Morphine (prototype narcotic analgesic).

OPIUM, POWDERED
OPIUM TINCTURE, DEODORIZED
(Laudanum)

(oh'pee-um)
Opium preparation
Opiate agonist
Antidiarrheal agent
C II

ACTIONS AND USES. Opium obtained from the unripe capsules of *Papaver somniferum* or *album* contains several natural alkaloids including morphine, codeine, papaverine. Powdered opium contains 10 to 10.5% anhydrous morphine with added inert diluents, and is light brown or yellowish-brown in color. *Opium tincture* is an alcoholic solution containing 50 mg anhydrous morphine/5 ml (19% alcohol). Antidiarrheal effects (primarily due to morphine content) result from decreased digestive secretions, increased GI smooth muscle tone, inhibition of GI motility and propulsion. These actions lead to prolonged transit of intestinal contents, dessication of feces, and constipation. Available fixed combinations: deodorized opium tincture with homatropine and pectin [Dia-Quel] (with alcohol 10%); Parelixir (with alcohol 18%)]; and opium powder with ipecac and lactose (Dover's powder).

Used in symptomatic treatment of acute diarrhea and to treat severe withdrawal symptoms in neonates born to women addicted to opiates.

ABSORPTION AND FATE. Following oral administration, there is variable absorption. Plasma levels of morphine in deodorized opium tincture are lower than those achieved following parenteral administration of morphine (qv). Metabolized in liver with formation of glucuronide metabolites. Eliminated in urine (about 75% of dose of morphine excreted within 48 hours).

CONTRAINDICATION AND PRECAUTIONS. Diarrhea caused by poisoning (until poison is completely eliminated). *Cautious Use:* history of opiate agonist dependence; asthma, severe prostatic hypertrophy, hepatic disease.

ADVERSE/SIDE EFFECTS. Nausea, and other GI disturbances (infrequent). *Acute toxicity:* depression of CNS.

ROUTE AND DOSAGE. (Opium tincture: 0.6 ml is therapeutically equivalent to 6 mg morphine.) **Oral: Adult:** 0.6 ml four times daily. *Range:* 0.3 to 1 ml four times a day. Single doses should not exceed 1 ml. *Maximum dose:* 6 ml/day. **Neonatal withdrawal syndrome:** 1:25 aqueous dilution: 3 to 6 drops every 3 to 6 hours as needed; or *initial:* 0.2 ml every 3 hours. Dosage may be increased by approximately 0.05 ml every 3 hours until withdrawal symptoms are controlled. Dose greater than 0.7 ml rarely needed. After withdrawal symptoms are stabilized for 3 to 5 days, dose is decreased gradually over a 2- to 4-week period.

NURSING IMPLICATIONS

Do not confuse this preparation with camphorated opium tincture (Paregoric) which contains only 2 mg anhydrous morphine/5 ml thus requiring a higher dose volume than that required for therapeutic dose of deodorized opium tincture.

If respirations are 12 per minute or below or have changed in character and rate, report to physician before administering medication.

Give drug diluted with about one-third glass of water to assure passage of entire dose into stomach.

Note character and frequency of stools; drug should be discontinued as soon as diarrhea is controlled.

If diarrhea is not accompanied by emesis and if there has been only minimal (if any) weight loss, uncomplicated measures are indicated to maintain fluid balance during acute phase of diarrhea. Frequently offer small amounts of fluid but attempt to maintain 3000 to

4000-ml fluid total in 24 hours. Appropriate fluids in acute phase: low fat liquids (no milk products), weak tea with honey, popsicle (about 30 to 70 ml liquid), scoop of fruit ice (about 120 ml), Gatorade (good source of potassium), bouillon, cola beverages, jello, water in which rice has been cooked. Soft solids in small frequent amounts progressing to bland low fat diet should be offered as soon as tolerated. Normal diet should gradually be resumed.

Monitor body weight, intake and output ratio and pattern, and temperature. If patient develops fever of 38.8°C (102°F) or above, electrolyte and hydration levels may need to be evaluated. Consult physician. *See Index: Nursing Intervention: rehydration.*

Inform patient that constipation may be a consequence of antidiarrheal therapy, but that normal habit pattern usually is reestablished with resumption of normal dietary intake.

Keep opium tincture out of possible reach of children.

Addiction is possible with prolonged use or with drug abuse.

Classified as schedule II drug under Federal Controlled Substances Act.

Preserved in tight, light-resistant containers. *See Morphine.*

OPIUM TINCTURE

(Deodorized Opium Tincture, Laudanum)

(oh'pee-um)

Antiperistaltic, antidiarrheal

C II

ACTIONS AND USES. Hydroalcoholic solution containing 1% morphine (or 10% opium) and 19% alcohol. Contains 25 times more morphine than does Paregoric. General pharmacologic properties are like those of morphine (qv). Increases tone and spasticity of the large bowel, but decreases propulsive peristalsis, causing constipation. Used in symptomatic relief of diarrhea.

ROUTE AND DOSAGE. Oral: 0.3 to 1 ml (equivalent to 3 to 10 mg of morphine) up to four times daily.

NURSING IMPLICATIONS

Not to be confused with paregoric (camphorated tincture of opium), which is given in much larger dosages than opium tincture.

If respirations are 12 per minute or below or have changed in character and rate, report to physician before administering medication.

Give drug diluted with about one-third glass of water to assure passage into stomach.

Note character and frequency of stools; drug should be discontinued as soon as diarrhea is controlled.

Addiction is possible with prolonged use.

Classified as Schedule II drug under Federal Controlled Substances Act.

Preserved in tight, light-resistant containers.

See Paregoric.

ORAL CONTRACEPTIVES (ESTROGEN–PROGESTIN COMBINATIONS)

Hormones

(Brevicon, Demulen, Enovid, Loestrin, Modicon, Norinyl, Norlestrin, Ortho-Novum, Ovcon, Ovral)

ACTIONS AND USES. Fixed combination of estrogen and progestin produces contraception by preventing ovulation and rendering reproductive tract structures hostile to sperm penetration and zygote implantation. Estrogen suppresses release of gonadotropins: follicle-stimulating hormone (FSH) and luteinizing hormone (LH). Progestin causes structural and secretory changes in endometrium and inhibits ferning of cervical secretions, thus supporting an impenetrable mucoid network. Efficacy and many adverse side effects of oral contraceptives (OCs) are due largely to estrogen component (see Estradiol, prototype for estrogens), while differences between combinations are due to relative potency and dominance of either progestational or estrogenic activity. **All combination products incorporate an estrogen** (ethinyl estradiol or mestranol) **with one of 6 progestins** (norethynodrel, norethindrone, norethindrone acetate, ethynodiol diacetate, levonorgestrel, norgestrel). Claims are made that by supplying a varied progestin dosage in the OC cyclic regimen similar to changes in endogenous progestin levels, the risk of serious cardiovascular complications may be decreased, and breakthrough bleeding, bloating, edema and menstrual tension may be increased. Three types of estrogen/progestin combinations are available monophasic: fixed dosage of estrogen/progestin throughout the cycle; biphasic: amount of estrogen remains the same throughout cycle, less progestin in first half of cycle (supports endometrial proliferation) and increased progestin in second half (allows adequate secretory development); triphasic: estrogen amount is the same or varies throughout cycle, progestin amount varies.

Used to prevent conception and to treat hypermenorrhea and endometriosis.

ABSORPTION AND FATE. All preparations well absorbed from GI tract. Metabolism of individual components apparently not changed by simultaneous administration. Small amounts of estrogen and progestin are detected in breast milk.

CONTRAINDICATIONS AND PRECAUTIONS. Pregnancy (category X), lactation, missed abortion. Familial or personal history of or existence of breast or other estrogen-dependent neoplasm, recurrent chronic cystic mastitis, history of or existence of thrombophlebitis or thromboembolic disorders, cerebral vascular or coronary artery disease, myocardial infarction, serious hepatic dysfunction, hepatic neoplasm, family history of hepatic porphyria, undiagnosed abnormal vaginal bleeding, women age 40 and over, adolescents with incomplete epiphyseal closure. *Cautious Use:* history of depression, preexisting hypertension, or cardiac or renal disease; impaired liver function, history of migraine, convulsive disorders, or asthma; multiparous women with grossly irregular menses, diabetes, or familial history of diabetes; gallbladder disease, lupus erythematosus, rheumatic disease, varicosities. *Also see Estradiol and Progesterone.*

ADVERSE/SIDE EFFECTS. CV: malignant hypertension, thrombotic and thromboembolic disorders, increase in size of varicosities. **GI:** cholelithiasis, gall bladder disease, cholestatic jaundice, benign hepatic adenomas; diarrhea, constipation, abdominal cramps. **GU:** ureteral dilation, increased incidence of urinary tract infection, hemolytic uremia syndrome, renal failure. **Metabolic:** decreased glucose tolerance, pyridoxine deficiency *(see also Diagnostic Test Interferences).* **Ophthalmic:** unexplained loss of vision, optic neuritis, proptosis, diplopia, change in corneal curvature (steepening), intolerance to contact lenses, retinal thrombosis, papilledema. **Reproductive:** increased risk of congenital anomalies, decreased quality and quantity of breast milk, dysmenorrhea, increased size of preexisting uterine fibroids, menstrual disorders. (Dose-related): **Estrogen excess:** nausea (common); bloating, menstrual tension, cervical mucorrhea, polyposis, chloasma (melasma), hypertension, migraine headache, breast fullness or tenderness, edema. **Estrogen deficiency:** hypomenorrhea, early or midcycle breakthrough bleeding, increased spotting. **Progestin excess:** hypomenorrhea, breast regression, vaginal candidiasis, depression, fatigue, weight gain, increased appetite, acne, oily scalp, hair loss. **Progestin deficiency:** late-cycle breakthrough bleeding, amenorrhea. **Other:** Rash (allergic), paresthesias, photosensitivity (photoallergy or phototoxicity), acute intermittent porphyria.

ROUTE AND DOSAGE. **Oral** *(see Patient Package Insert available with product).*

NURSING IMPLICATIONS

Positive evidence associates increased risk of thromboembolic and cardiovascular problems, and increased incidence of gall bladder disease with OC use. Recent studies performed by Centers for Disease Control (CDC) report that OCs (1) provide a protective effect against endometrial and ovarian cancer, (2) are not associated with breast cancer, and (3) do not increase risk of cancer in women with benign breast disease or family history of breast cancer.

Complete medical and family history should be taken prior to initiating oral contraceptive therapy. Baseline and periodic physical examination should include blood pressure, breasts, abdomen, pelvis, Pap smear, and other relevant tests.

Pregnancy should be ruled out before beginning oral contraceptive therapy.

Urge patient not to skip scheduled visits for physical checkups (at least annually) while on contraceptive therapy. Teach breast self-examination and emphasize importance of doing this every month.

Tablets should be taken regularly at same time of day to assure intervals of 24 hours (e.g., with a meal or at bedtime). Stress that strict adherence to dosage schedule is essential for efficacy of medication.

Nausea with or without vomiting occurs in approximately 10% of patients during the first cycle and is reportedly one of the major reasons for voluntary discontinuation of therapy. Most side effects tend to disappear in third or fourth cycle of use. Instruct user to report symptoms that persist after fourth cycle. Dose adjustment or a different product may be indicated.

In the first week of the initial cycle of oral contraceptive (OC) use, patient should also use an additional method of birth control.

If user forgets to take a tablet, she should take it as soon as she remembers or should take two tablets the next day. If two consecutive tablets are omitted, she should take two tablets daily for the next two days, then resume the regular schedule. If three consecutive tablets are missed, she should begin a new compact of tablets, starting 7 days after the last tablet was taken.

Use an additional form of birth control for 7 days after two missed doses or 14 days after three missed doses.

Ovulation is unlikely with omission of one daily dose; however, the possibility of escaping ovulation, spotting, or breakthrough bleeding increases with each missed dose.

If intracycle bleeding resembling menstruation occurs, patient should discontinue medication, then begin taking tablets from a new compact on day 5. If bleeding persists, advise patient to see physician to rule out nonfunctional cause. Amount, duration of flow, and placement in drug regimen are important diagnostic parameters to be reported.

If prescribed regimen has been followed, and two consecutive periods are missed, user should see physician to rule out pregnancy before continuing hormone contraception. If schedule has not been followed, the possibility of pregnancy should be considered after first missed period, and OC should be withheld until pregnancy has been ruled out.

When pregnancy is desired, hormone contraception is discontinued, and patient is advised to use alternate method for at least 3 months to avoid risk of breakthrough pregnancy and congenital defects in fetus.

If possible, hormone contraception should not be used until infant is weaned; alternate method of birth control should be used during this period.

Oral contraception can be started immediately after delivery in the nonnursing mother, if desired.

Oral contraception may mask onset of climacteric. To determine if it has started, physician may advise patient to discontinue pill and to use alternate method of contraception. If menstruation occurs, the pill is indicated.

Anovulation or amenorrhea following termination of oral contraceptive regimen may persist more than 6 months. The user with pretreatment oligomenorrhea or secondary amenorrhea is most apt to have oversuppression syndrome.

Hirsutism and loss of hair are reversible with discontinuation of oral contraceptive or by change of selected combination.

Acne may improve, worsen, or develop for first time. In women on oral contraceptive for at least 1 year, postcontraceptive acne sometimes occurs 3 to 4 months after stopping drug and may continue for 6 to 12 months.

Menstrual tension, bloating, and tender breasts may be relieved by diuretics, sedation, and low salt intake.

If feasible, OC should be discontinued at least one cycle prior to surgery, or anticipated prolonged immobilization, and prior to diagnostic oral glucose tolerance test.

The pathologist should be informed that OC is being taken when relevant tissues are to be examined. Also inform dentist if oral surgery is anticipated.

To avoid later fertility and menstrual problems, hormone contraception is not advised for the adolescent until after at least 2 years of well-established menstrual cycles and completion of physiologic maturation.

An estrogen-dominant agent is the best choice for the adolescent with scanty menses, moderate or severe acne, or candidiasis. A progestin-dominant agent is the best choice for the adolescent with dysmenorrhea, hypermenorrhea, fibrocystic disease of breast, or cyclic premenstrual weight gain.

O

Teach patient how to elicit Homans' sign *(See Index: Clinical signs and symptoms)* and to be alert to other manifestations of thrombotic or thromboembolic disorders: severe headache (especially if persistent and recurrent), dizziness, blurred vision, leg or chest pain, respiratory distress, unexplained cough. Advise patient to withhold drug if any of these symptoms appear and to report promptly to physician.

Sudden abdominal pain should be reported immediately to rule out hepatic adenoma or ectopic pregnancy. Oral contraception is more effective in preventing intrauterine than ectopic pregnancy.

Users with clinical conditions worsened by fluid retention should report exacerbation of symptoms promptly; a preparation with less estrogen may be substituted. Frequent weight checks should be recorded to permit early recognition of fluid retention.

Ophthalmic sequelae can occur as soon as 24 hours after initiation of oral contraception. Advise patient to stop the drug and contact physician if unexplained partial or complete, sudden or gradual loss of vision, protrusion of eyeballs (proptosis), or diplopia occurs.

Astigmatic error and myopic refractive error may be increased twofold to threefold, usually after 6 months of oral contraceptive therapy. Changes in ocular contour and lubricant quality of tears may necessitate change in size and shape of contact lenses.

Chloasma (more marked in dark-skinned women) seems to be aggravated by sunlight and may persist beyond period of pill use. With anticipated exposure (as in summer), taking pill at bedtime will reduce circulating hormone level in daytime.

Leukorrhea is an expected physical reaction to the oral contraceptive; however, if accompanied by vaginal itching and irritation, candidiasis should be ruled out. Caution patient to report discomfort promptly.

Check blood pressure periodically. In some women changes in blood pressure occur within each cycle; in others slow increase of pressure, particularly diastolic, over several months is significant. Drug-induced hypertension is usually reversible with discontinuation of oral contraception.

Instruct the diabetic user to report positive urine or blood glucose test to physician. Adjustment of antidiabetic medication may be necessary. The potential diabetic (family history) should also be closely observed for onset of diabetes and probably should not use mestranol combinations.

Advise user with history of premenstrual and other kinds of depression to report to physician if symptoms recur. A responsible family member should also be alerted to observe carefully.

Caution user against exposure to ultraviolet light or prolonged exposure to sunlight. Use sunscreen lotion (SPF of 12 or above) on exposed skin when outdoors.

Smoking–Drug Interaction: OC users who smoke have about a 5-fold increased risk of fatal MI compared to nonsmoking OC users, and a 10-fold increased risk compared to nonusers who are nonsmokers. This risk increases with age (marked in women over 35) and with heavy smoking (15 or more cigarettes/day). Smoking also increases risk of CVA in OC users. Women on OCs should be made completely aware of this important intervention.

Overdosage: Serious effects have not been reported following acute overdosage of OC in young children. Nausea may result, and withdrawal bleeding may occur in females.

Ortho-Novum contains *tartrazine* which produces allergic reactions (including bronchospasm) in susceptible persons. Such individuals are frequently sensitive to aspirin.

Naegele's rule for estimating date of delivery does not work for the user of OC. Ovulation is delayed 2 weeks after OC is discontinued. The first bleeding after stopping taking the hormonal contraceptive is withdrawal, not menstrual bleeding. Therefore, a delay of spontaneous labor of at least 2 weeks must be anticipated.

Labor should never be induced in a former OC user whose delivery appears to exceed 42 weeks.

Selecting the optimum combination OC should take into account user's response to the estrogen–progestin ratio, e.g., *estrogen-dominant preparations:* Enovid-E, Enovid-5 mg, Norinyl 2 mg, Ortho-Novum 2 mg, Ovulen; *progestin-dominant preparations:* Demulen, Ovral. Other marketed products are intermediate with respect to estrogen–progestin ratio.

O

Diagnostic Test Interferences. Oral contraceptives *increase* **BSP** retention, **prothrombin** and **coagulation factors** VII, VIII, IX, X; **platelet aggregability, thyroid-binding globulin, PBI, T_4;** blood **transcortin;** corticosteroid, triglycerides and phospholipid levels. OCs *decrease* **antithrombin III, T_3** uptake, serum **folate,** and reduce the **metyrapone test response.**

Drug Interactions: Oral contraceptives (OCs)

Plus	**Interactions**
Acetaminophen, lorazepam, oxazepam	Metabolism may be increased by OCs
Aminocaproic acid	May increase clotting factors leading to hypercoagulable state

Plus (cont.)	Interactions (cont.)
Analgesics, antihistamines, antimigraine preparations, barbiturates, chloramphenicol, griseofulvin, isoniazid, neomycin, nitrofurantoin, penicillin V, phenylbutazone, phenytoin, primidone, rifampin sulfonamides, tetracyclines	Reduced efficacy of OC and increased incidence of breakthrough bleeding
Antibiotics (broad-spectrum)	Failure of oral contraception
Anticoagulants, oral	Decreased hypoprothrombinemic effect of anticoagulant
Anticonvulsants	Effectiveness decreased by OC
Antihypertensives	*See anticonvulsants*
Caffeine, diazepam, chlordiazepoxide, metoprolol, propranolol, corticosteroids, imipramine, phenytoin, phenylbutazone	Metabolism may be impaired by OCs
Chenodiol	Effectiveness decreased by OCs
Hypoglycemic agents	*See anticonvulsants*
Tricyclic antidepressants	*See anticonvulsants*
Troleandomycin	May cause jaundice
Vitamins	*See anticonvulsants*

ORPHENADRINE CITRATE

(Banflex, Flexoject, Flexon, Marflex, Myolin, Norflex, X-Otag)

ORPHENADRINE HYDROCHLORIDE

(Disipal)

O

(or-fen′a-dreen)
Anticholinergic
(Parasympathomimetic)
Antiparkinsonian agent
Skeletal muscle relaxant (centrally acting)

ACTIONS AND USES. Tertiary amine anticholinergic agent and centrally acting skeletal muscle relaxant. Structurally similar to diphenhydramine (qv), and also closely related to chlorphenoxamine. Relaxes tense skeletal muscles indirectly, possibly by analgesic action or by atropine-like central action. Has some local anesthetic and antihistaminic activity, but less than that of diphenhydramine. Also produces slight euphoria.

Used as the citrate to relieve muscle spasm discomfort associated with acute musculoskeletal conditions. The hydrochloride is used as an adjunct in the treatment of all forms of parkinsonism (arteriosclerotic, idiopathic, postencephalitic). Orphenadrine citrate is available in combination with aspirin and caffeine (Norgesic).

ABSORPTION AND FATE. Readily absorbed following oral administration. Peak effect in about 2 hours; duration: approximately 4 to 6 hours. Rapidly distributed in tissues. Plasma half-life: 14 hours. Extensively metabolized; 60% excreted in urine within 3 days, 8% as unchanged drug.

CONTRAINDICATIONS AND PRECAUTIONS. Narrow-angle glaucoma, pyloric or duodenal obstruction, stenosing peptic ulcers, prostatic hypertrophy or bladder neck obstruction, myasthenia gravis, cardiospasm (megaloesophagus). Safe use during pregnancy, in women of childbearing potential, and in the pediatric age group not established. *Cautious Use:* history of tachycardia, cardiac decompensation, arrhythmias, coronary insufficiency.

ADVERSE/SIDE EFFECTS. CNS: Drowsiness, weakness, headache, dizziness; mild CNS stimulation (high doses): restlessness, anxiety, tremors, confusion, hallucinations, agitation, tachycardia, palpitation, syncope. **GI:** dry mouth, nausea, vomiting, abdominal cramps, constipation. **GU:** urinary hesitancy or retention. **Hypersensitivity:** pruritus, urticaria, rash, anaphylactic reaction (rare). **Ophthalmic:** increased ocular tension, dilated pupils, blurred vision. **Other:** aplastic anemia (rare): causal relationship not established.

ROUTE AND DOSAGE. *Orphenadrine citrate:* **Oral:** 100 mg two times daily (in the morning and in the evening). **Intramuscular, intravenous:** 60 mg; may be repeated every 12 hours, if necessary. *Orphenadrine hydrochloride:* **Oral:** 50 mg three times daily. Doses up to 250 mg daily if necessary and tolerated.

NURSING IMPLICATIONS

Note that orphenadrine citrate and orphenadrine hydrochloride are not interchangeable. *See Route and Dosage.*

Periodic studies of blood, urine, and liver function are recommended with prolonged therapy.

Complaints of mouth dryness, urinary hesitancy or retention, headache, tremors, GI problems, palpitation, or rapid pulse should be communicated to physician. Dosage reduction or drug withdrawal is indicated.

Mouth dryness may be relieved by frequent rinsing with clear tepid water, increasing noncaloric fluid intake, sugarless gum or lemondrops. If these measures fail, a saliva substitute may help: Xero-lube, Moi-stir, Orex (all available OTC). Consult physician.

Keep physician informed of therapeutic drug effect. In the patient with parkinsonism, orphenadrine reduces muscular rigidity, but has little effect on tremors. Some reduction in excessive salivation and perspiration may occur and patient may appear mildly euphoric.

Caution patient to avoid driving and other potentially hazardous activities until reaction to drug is known.

Warn patient that concomitant use of alcohol and other CNS depressants may result in potentiation of depressant effects.

The elderly patient is particularly sensitive to anticholinergic effects (urinary hesitancy, constipation) and therefore should be closely observed. Have patient void before taking drug.

Protect orphenadrine from light.

Drug Interactions. Based on limited clinical studies, concomitant use with **phenothiazines** may result in reduced phenothiazine levels or hypoglycemia, and patients receiving propoxyphene and orphenadrine concomitantly may manifest confusion, anxiety, tremors.

OXACILLIN SODIUM

(Bactocill, Prostaphlin)

(ox-a-sill'in)
Antiinfective
Antibiotic (Beta-lactose)
Penicillin

ACTIONS AND USES. Semisynthetic, acid-stable, penicillinase-resistant isoxazoyl penicillin. Mechanism of bacteriocidal action, contraindications, precautions, and adverse reactions as for penicillin G (qv). In common with other isoxazolyl penicillins (cloxacillin, dicloxacillin), it is highly active against most penicillinase-producing staphylococci, is less potent than penicillin G against penicillin-sensitive microorganisms, and is generally ineffective against gram-negative bacteria and methicillin-resistant staphylococci.

Used primarily in treatment of infections caused by penicillinase-producing staphylococci and penicillin-resistant staphylococci. May be used to initiate therapy in suspected staphylococcal infections pending culture and sensitivity test results. As with other penicillins, serum concentrations are enhanced by concurrent use of probenecid.

ABSORPTION AND FATE. Rapidly, but incompletely absorbed after oral administration. Serum levels peak in 30 minutes to 1 hour after oral drug and IM injection, and in 5 minutes following IV administration; serum concentrations extremely low after 4 to 6 hours. Oral solutions produce slightly higher serum levels than do capsules. About 90 to 95% protein-bound. Distributed to bile, synovial and pleural fluid, bronchial secretions; also detectable in peritoneal and pericardial fluid. Penetrates cerebrospinal fluid only when meninges are inflamed. Half-life: 30 to 60 minutes. Excreted rapidly by kidneys as intact drug and metabolite; also eliminated in bile. Crosses placenta; appears in breast milk.

CONTRAINDICATIONS AND PRECAUTIONS. Hypersensitivity to penicillins or cephalosporins. Safe use during pregnancy not established. *Cautious Use:* history of or suspected atopy or allergy (hives, eczema, hay fever, asthma); premature infants, neonates. *See Penicillin G.*

ADVERSE/SIDE EFFECTS. Nausea, vomiting, flatulence, diarrhea. **Hypersensitivity reactions:** pruritus, rash, urticaria, wheezing, sneezing, fever, anaphylaxis; hepatocellular dysfunction (elevated SGOT, SGPT, hepatitis), eosinophilia, leukopenia, thrombocytopenia, granulocytopenia, agranulocytosis; neutropenia (reported in children). **Neurotoxicity** (high-dose therapy), interstitial nephritis, transient hematuria, albuminuria, azotemia (newborns and infants on high doses); thrombophlebitis (IV therapy), superinfections. *See also Penicillin G.*

ROUTE AND DOSAGE. Oral, intramuscular, intravenous: Adults and Children (weighing over 40 kg): 250 mg to 1 Gm every 4 to 6 hours for a minimum of 5 days. For severe infections, up to 20 Gm/daily IM or IV. Direct IV administration should be made slowly over a 10-minute period; **(under 40 kg):** 50 to 100 mg/kg every 6 hours.

NURSING IMPLICATIONS

Careful inquiry should be made concerning hypersensitivity reactions to penicillins, cephalosporins, and other allergens.

Oral oxacillin is best administered with a full glass of water on an empty stomach (either 1 hour before meals or 2 hours after meals). Food reduces absorption. Consult physician.

Following reconstitution of oral solution (by pharmacist), it is stable for 3 days at room temperature and for 14 days if refrigerated. Container should be so labeled and dated.

Instruct patient to take the oral medication around the clock, not to miss a dose, and to continue taking it until it is all gone unless otherwise directed by physician.

For IM administration, reconstitute with sterile water for injection (as directed in product monograph), and indicate date and time of reconstitution on vial. Shake vial vigorously until drug is completely dissolved. Discard unused portions after 3 days at room temperature or 7 days under refrigeration. *Do not use undated vials.*

Administer IM to adults by deep intragluteal injection. Follow agency policy for appropriate IM site in young children and infants. Select site carefully. Injection into or near a major peripheral nerve or blood vessel can cause neurovascular damage. Rotate injection sites.

For direct IV administration, reconstitute with sterile water for injection or isotonic sodium chloride (as directed in product monograph). For IV infusion, the reconstituted solution is added to a compatible IV solution, e.g., isotonic sodium chloride, 5% dextrose in water or normal saline, lactated Ringer's injection, or others recommended by manufacturer.

Refer to manufacturer's package insert for instructions on storage of intravenous solutions. Following reconstitution, solutions prepared from "piggyback" IV package are reportedly stable for 24 hours at room temperature. Solutions prepared for IV infusion (as described above) are stable for 6 hours at room temperature.

The total sodium content (including that contributed by buffer) in each gram of oxacillin is approximately 3.1 mEq or 71 mg.

Instruct patient to report to physician the onset of hypersensitivity reactions (hives, pruritus, rash, wheezing), and superinfections (black, hairy tongue; glossitis, stomatitis, anal itching; loose, foul-smelling stools; vaginal itching or discharge).

Hepatic dysfunction (possibly a hypersensitivity reaction) has been associated with IV oxacillin; it is reversible with discontinuation of drug. Symptoms may resemble viral hepatitis or general signs of hypersensitivity and should be reported promptly: hives, rash, fever, nausea, vomiting, abdominal discomfort, anorexia, malaise, jaundice (with dark yellow to brown urine, light-colored or clay-colored stools, pruritus).

Patients on prolonged therapy should be instructed to report symptoms of agranulocytosis: sore throat, elevated temperature, adenopathy, malaise.

Drug therapy is continued for a minimum of 5 days for mild to moderate infections. Infections caused by group A beta-hemolytic streptococci, however, should be treated for a minimum of 10 days to prevent acute rheumatic fever. For severe infections therapy may be continued at least 1 to 2 weeks after patient is afebrile and cultures are negative. Osteomyelitis may require several months of drug therapy.

See Penicillin G (prototype penicillin).

Diagnostic Test Interferences. Oxacillin in large doses can cause false-positive **urine protein tests** using sulfosalicylic acid methods. *See also Penicillin G.*

O

OXAMINIQUINE

(Vansil)

(ox-am'ni-kwin)
Antiinfective
Anthelmintic

ACTIONS AND USES. Tetrahydroquinone derivative prepared in the presence of *Aspergillus sclerotiorum.* Mechanism of action not fully explained, but it appears that drug-induced strong contractions and paralysis of worm musculature leads to immobilization of their suckers and dislodgement from their usual residence in mesenteric veins to the liver. Normal blood flow passively carries dead and dying worms to the liver where they are retained and subsequently elicit host tissue reactions (e.g., phagocytosis). Dislodgment of schistosomes begins about 2 days after single oral dose of oxamniquine; movement is not complete until 6 days after treatment with the drug. After treatment, surviving unpaired females return to mesenteric vessels; however oviposition (egg laying) seems to stop in 24 to 48 hours after drug treatment, reducing egg load and removing principle cause of pathology associated with schistosomal infection. Is not crecaricidal. Drug metabolites do not possess antischistosomal activity.

Used to treat all stages of *Schistosoma mansoni* infection, including acute and chronic phases with hepatosplenic involvement.

ABSORPTION AND FATE. Well absorbed. Plasma concentrations reach a peak at 1 to 1½ hours after therapeutic dose. Half-life: 1 to 2½ hours. Extensively metabolized to inactive acidic metabolites, which are largely excreted in the urine.

CONTRAINDICATIONS AND PRECAUTIONS. Safe use during pregnancy (category C) and lactation or in children not established. *Cautious Use:* History of convulsant disorders.

ADVERSE/SIDE EFFECTS. CNS: transitory dizziness, drowsiness, headache, epileptic convulsions (rare); insomnia, malaise, reversible amnesia (rare); persistent fever (in patients being treated in Egypt); EEG abnormalities. **GI:** anorexia, nausea, vomiting, abdominal pain. **Hematologic:** increased erythrocyte sedimentation rate, reticulocyte count, and increased or decreased leukocyte count. **Other:** urticaria, elevated liver enzyme concentrations, convulsions, serum alkaline phosphatase, AST, ALT (not considered drug-related).

ROUTE AND DOSAGE. Adult: 12 to 15 mg/kg as a single dose in patient with Western hemisphere strains of *S. mansoni.* **Children (less than 30 kg):** 20 mg/kg in two divided doses of 10 mg/kg at 2- to 8-hour intervals.

NURSING IMPLICATIONS

Administer with food to reduce GI distress.

Because drug can cause dizziness or drowsiness, advise patient to use caution while driving or performing other tasks requiring alertness.

Inform patient that drug may change the normal urine color to a harmless orange red.

If patient has a history of seizures, be alert to the possibility that they may recur again because of drug action. (Occur within the first few hours of drug administration.)

See Index: Nursing Intervention: parasitic infection.

Store product in well-closed container at controlled room temperature less than 30°C (86°F).

O

OXANDROLONE

(Anavar)

(ox-an′droe-lone)
Anabolic

ACTIONS AND USES. Synthetic steroid with strong anabolic and low androgenic activity.

Used to promote weight gain in patients who have lost weight after extensive surgery, chronic infections, or severe trauma; used to reduce bone pain associated with osteoporosis and to offset protein catabolism accompanying prolonged corticosteroid administration.

ROUTE AND DOSAGE. Oral: Adult: 2.5 mg two to four times daily for 2 to 4 weeks (dosage may range from 2.5 to 20 mg daily), repeated intermittently if necessary. **Children:** 0.25 mg/kg/day for 2 to 4 weeks.

NURSING IMPLICATIONS

A course of therapy of 2 to 4 weeks is usually adequate. Therapy for adults and children should not exceed 3 months.

Does not enhance athletic ability.

See Ethylestrenol (prototype anabolic steroid).

OXAZEPAM

(Ox-Pam, Serax, Zapex)

(ox-a'ze-pam)
Psychotropic
Anxiolytic
Benzodiazepine
C IV

ACTIONS AND USES. Benzodiazepine derivative related to chlordiazepoxide with which it shares actions, uses, limitations and interactions. Has shorter duration of action, and causes fewer adverse/side effects than chlordiazepoxide (qv).

Used in management of anxiety and tension, associated with a wide range of emotional disturbances. Also used to control acute withdrawal symptoms in chronic alcoholism.

ABSORPTION AND FATE. Following absorption from GI tract, peak plasma concentrations occur in 2 to 4 hours. About 90% protein bound. Metabolized in liver. Plasma half-life: 3 to 21 hours. Excreted slowly in urine, primarily as glucuronide, and in feces as unchanged drug. Most of a given dose is excreted within 2 days.

CONTRAINDICATIONS AND PRECAUTIONS. Hypersensitivity to oxazepam and other benzodiazepines; psychoses, pregnancy, lactation, children under age 12, acute-angle glaucoma, acute alcohol intoxication. *Cautious Use:* elderly and debilitated patients; impaired renal and hepatic function, addiction-prone patients, COPD, mental depression.

ADVERSE/SIDE EFFECTS. Usually infrequent and mild. **CNS:** drowsiness, dizziness, mental confusion, vertigo, ataxia, headache, lethargy, syncope, tremor, slurred speech, paradoxic reaction (euphoria, excitement). **GI:** nausea, xerostomia, jaundice. **Other:** skin rash, edema, hypotension, leukopenia, altered libido, edema.

ROUTE AND DOSAGE. **Oral:** *Anxiety:* 10 to 30 mg, three or four times per day. *Acute alcohol withdrawal:* 15 to 30 mg, three or four times per day. **Elderly, debilitated:** initial dose: 10 mg three times per day, increased cautiously to 15 mg three or four times per day if necessary.

NURSING IMPLICATIONS

Continued effectiveness of response to oxazepam should be reassessed at end of 4 months. Urge patient to keep appointments with physician.

Elderly patients should be observed closely for signs of overdosage. Report to physician if daytime psychomotor function is depressed.

Mild paradoxic stimulation of affect and excitement with sleep disturbances may occur within the first 2 weeks of therapy. Report promptly. Dosage reduction is indicated.

Liver function tests and blood counts should be performed on a regular planned basis.

Instruct patients not to change dose or dose schedule. Furthermore, they should not give any of the drug to another person and should refrain from using it to treat a self-diagnosed condition.

Advise patient to consult physician before self-medicating with OTC drugs.

Caution patient against driving a car or operating dangerous machinery until response to drug has been evaluated.

Warn patient not to drink alcoholic beverages while being treated with oxazepam. The CNS depressant effects of each agent may be intensified.

Patient should be advised that if she becomes pregnant during therapy or intends to become pregnant she should communicate with her physician about the desirability of discontinuing the drug.

Excessive and prolonged use may cause physical dependence.

Following prolonged therapy, drug should be withdrawn slowly to avoid precipitating with-

drawal symptoms (seizures, mental confusion, nausea, vomiting, muscle and abdominal cramps, tremulousness, sleep disturbances, unusual irritability, hyperhydrosis).
Serax contains *tartrazine,* which can cause an allergic reaction including bronchial asthma in susceptible individuals. Frequently such persons are also sensitive to aspirin.
Classified as Schedule IV drug under Federal Controlled Substances Act.
Store in well-closed container at temperature between 15° and 30°C (59° and 86°F) unless otherwise specified by manufacturer.
See also Chlordiazepoxide (prototype anxiolytic agent).

OXIDIZED CELLULOSE

Hemostatic (local)

(Novocell, Oxycel, Surgicel)

ACTIONS AND USES. Sterile, absorbable hemostatic material prepared from cellulose. On contact with blood, it swells into a brownish or black gelatinous mass that acts as artificial clot. Gradually absorbed from tissue bed, usually within 2 to 7 days; complete absorption of large amounts may require up to 6 weeks or more.

Used to control capillary, venous, and small arterial hemorrage when suture or ligation is impractical or ineffective.

CONTRAINDICATIONS AND PRECAUTIONS. Use as wadding or packing; use for implantation in bone defects, including fractures and laminectomy procedures (interferes with callus formation, and may cause cysts and nerve damage); hemorrhage from large arteries or nonhemorrhagic oozing surfaces; impregnation with antiinfective materials or other hemostatic substances.

ADVERSE/SIDE EFFECTS. Foreign-body reactions, burning, stinging sensations, sneezing (when used for rhinologic procedures), necrosis due to tight packing, prolonged drainage.

ROUTE AND DOSAGE. Using aseptic technique, apply to bleeding surface with mild pressure until hemostasis is obtained. Available as pellets, pads, strips.

NURSING IMPLICATIONS

Hemostatic effect is greater when material is applied dry.
Hemostatic effect is not enhanced by thrombin (activity of thrombin is destroyed by low pH of oxidized cellulose). Absorption may be prevented by previous applications of silver nitrate or other escharotic materials.
Only as much as necessary for hemostasis should be used; material is applied to bleeding site or held firmly in place until bleeding stops.
Once hemostasis is achieved, oxidized cellulose is usually removed from site of application. Removal is facilitated by irrigation with sterile water or saline. Observe wound site for bleeding following removal.
Oxidized cellulose is off-white or dusty yellow in color, but it may darken in its sealed container with age. Reportedly this does not affect its hemostatic action.
Material is supplied as a sterile preparation and cannot be resterilized. Autoclaving or other forms of heat sterilization cause physical breakdown. Discard unused portions.

OXTRIPHYLLINE

(Choledyl, Choline Theophyllinate, Chophylline)

(ox-trye'fi-lin)
Bronchodilator
Xanthine

ACTIONS AND USES. Choline salt of theophylline, with similar actions, uses, and limitations as other theophylline derivatives. Contains 64% theophylline. Compared to aminophylline, reportedly more stable, more soluble, and more uniformly and predictably absorbed, and produces less gastric irritation. Development of tolerance reported infrequently; therefore useful in long-term therapy.

CONTRAINDICATIONS AND PRECAUTIONS. Safe use in women of childbearing potential and during pregnancy and lactation not established.

ROUTE AND DOSAGE. Oral: Adults: 200 mg four times a day. **Children (2 to 12 years):** 100 mg/60 lb four times a day. Available as tablets, elixir (100 mg/5 ml), and pediatric syrup (50 mg/5 ml).

NURSING IMPLICATIONS

Preferably administered after meals and at bedtime.

Advise patient to report gastric distress, palpitation, and CNS stimulation (irritability, restlessness, nervousness, insomnia). Reduction in dosage may be indicated.

Preserved in well-closed containers, away from heat. Elixir should be protected from light.

See Theophylline (prototype xanthine bronchodilator).

OXYBUTYNIN CHLORIDE

(Ditropan)

(ox-i-byoo'ti-nin)
Anticholinergic
Antispasmodic (urinary tract)

ACTIONS AND USES. Synthetic tertiary amine with prominent antispasmodic activity. Exerts direct antispasmodic (papaverine-like) action, and inhibits muscarinic effects of acetylcholine on smooth muscle. Animal studies have shown that anticholinergic activity is about ⅕ that of atropine, but antispasmodic action is four to ten times more potent.

Used to relieve symptoms associated with voiding in patients with uninhibited neurogenic bladder and reflex neurogenic bladder. Also has been used to relieve pain of bladder spasm following transurethral surgical procedures.

ABSORPTION AND FATE. Onset of action in 30 minutes to 1 hour. Peak action in 3 to 4 hours; duration: 6 to 10 hours. Probably enters enterohepatic circulation. Metabolized by liver. Excreted primarily in urine.

CONTRAINDICATIONS AND PRECAUTIONS. Glaucoma, myasthenia gravis, partial or complete GI obstruction, paralytic ileus, intestinal atony (especially elderly or debilitated patients), megacolon, severe colitis, GU obstruction, unstable cardiovascular status. Safe use during pregnancy, and in children under 5 years not established. *Cautious Use:* the elderly, autonomic neuropathy, hiatus hernia with reflex esophagitis, hepatic or renal dysfunction, urinary infection, hyperthyroidism, congestive heart failure, coronary artery disease, hypertension, prostatic hypertrophy.

ADVERSE/SIDE EFFECTS. CNS: drowsiness, dizziness, weakness, insomnia, restlessness, psychotic behavior (overdosage). **CV:** palpitation, tachycardia, flushing. **GI:** dry mouth, nausea, vomiting, constipation, bloated feeling. **GU:** urinary hesitancy or retention, impotence. **Hyper-**

sensitivity: severe allergic reactions including urticaria, skin rashes. **Ophthalmic:** mydriasis, blurred vision, cyclopegia, increased ocular tension. **Other:** suppression of lactation, decreased sweating, fever.

ROUTE AND DOSAGE. Oral: Adults: 5 mg two or three times daily; maximum 5 mg four times daily. **Children (over 5 years):** 5 mg two times daily; maximum 5 mg three times daily.

NURSING IMPLICATIONS

The diagnosis of neurogenic bladder is confirmed before initiation of therapy by cystometric and other appropriate diagnostic procedures.

Periodic interruptions of therapy are recommended to determine patient's need for continued treatment. Tolerance has occurred in some patients.

Keep physician informed of expected responses to drug therapy, e.g., effect on urinary frequency, urgency, urge incontinence, nocturia, completeness of bladder emptying.

Patients with colostomy or ileostomy should be closely monitored: abdominal distention and the onset of diarrhea in these patients may be early signs of intestinal obstruction or of toxic megacolon.

Since oxybutynin may cause dizziness, drowsiness, and blurred vision; caution patient to avoid driving and other potentially hazardous activities until reaction to drug is known.

Advise patient to avoid hot environments. By suppressing sweating, oxybutynin can cause fever and heat stroke.

Treatment of overdosage: immediate gastric lavage; IV physostigmine 0.5 to 2 mg not to exceed total dosage of 5 mg; 2% sodium thiopental or chloral hydrate 100 to 200 ml of a 2% solution by rectal infusion; symptomatic treatment of fever, artificial respiration as necessary.

Store in tightly covered containers at room temperature, preferably between 15° and 30°C (59° and 86°F), unless otherwise directed by manufacturer.

OXYCODONE HYDROCHLORIDE
OXYCODONE TEREPHTHALATE

(ox-i-koe'done)
Narcotic analgesic
Opiate agonist
C II

ACTIONS AND USES. Semisynthetic derivative of opium alkaloid thebaine with actions qualitatively similar to those of morphine (qv). Most prominent actions involve CNS and organs composed of smooth muscle. Binds with stereospecific receptors in various sites of CNS to alter both perception of pain and emotional response to pain, but precise mechanism of action not clear. Appears to be more effective in relief of acute than long-standing pain. As potent as morphine and 10 to 12 times more potent than codeine; withdrawal symptoms match those of morphine. Produces mild sedation, but has little or no effect on cough reflex.

Used for relief of moderate to moderately severe pain such as may occur with bursitis, dislocations, simple fractures and other injuries, and neuralgia. Relieves postoperative, postextractional, and postpartum pain. *Available in U.S. only in combination with other drugs.*

ABSORPTION AND FATE. Analgesic effects of oxycodone occur within 10 to 15 minutes, peak in 30 to 60 minutes and persist 4 to 5 hours. Detoxified by liver and kidney. Excreted primarily in urine; crosses placental barrier.

CONTRAINDICATIONS AND PRECAUTIONS. Hypersensitivity to oxycodone and principal drugs with which it is combined; pregnancy, lactation, children under 6 years. *Cautious Use:* alcoholism, renal or hepatic disease, viral infections, Addison's disease, cardiac arrhythmias, chronic ulcerative colitis, history of drug abuse or dependency, gallbladder disease, acute abdominal conditions, head injury, intracranial lesions, hypothyroidism, prostatic hypertrophy, respiratory disease, urethral stricture, elderly or debilitated patients; peptic ulcer or coagulation abnormalities (combination products containing aspirin).

ADVERSE/SIDE EFFECTS. Lightheadedness, dizziness, sedation, anorexia, nausea, vomiting, constipation, euphoria, dysphoria, shortness of breath, pruritus, skin rash, bradycardia, unusual bleeding or bruising, jaundice, dysuria, frequency of urination, urinary retention. *See also morphine sulfate.*

ROUTE AND DOSAGE. Oral: *Percocet-5* (oxycodone hydrochloride 5 mg with acetaminophen 325 mg): one tablet every 6 hours as needed. *Percodan* (oxycodone hydrochloride 4.5 mg, oxycodone terephthalate 0.38 mg with aspirin 325 mg): 1 tablet every 6 hours as needed. *Percodan-Demi* (oxycodone hydrochloride 2.25 mg, oxycodone terephthalate 0.19 mg with aspirin 325 mg): **Adults:** 1 or 2 tablets every 6 hours as needed. **Children (12 years or older):** ½ tablet every 6 hours as needed; **(6 to 12 years):** ¼ tablet every 6 hours as needed. *Tylox* (oxycodone hydrochloride 4.5 mg, oxycodone terephthalate 0.38 mg with acetaminophen 500 mg): **Adults:** 1 capsule every 6 hours as needed. Should not be given to children of any age.

NURSING IMPLICATIONS

In evaluating actions, adverse reactions, and interactions of combination drugs each ingredient must be considered.

Administer after meals or with milk to reduce gastric irritation.

Do not use Percodan if strong vinegar-like odor; this formulation contains aspirin.

Nausea may occur during first few days of therapy; if it continues consult physician.

Lightheadedness, dizziness, sedation, or fainting appear to be more prominent in ambulatory than in nonambulatory patients and may be alleviated if patient lies down.

Warn patient not to alter dosage regimen by increasing, decreasing, or shortening intervals between doses. Habit formation and liver damage may be induced.

Evaluate patient's continued need for oxycodone preparations. Psychic and physical dependence and tolerance may develop with repeated use. The potential for drug abuse is high.

Caution patient to avoid potentially hazardous activities such as driving a car or operating machinery while using oxycodone preparation.

The ingestion of large doses of Percodan and Percodan-Demi can result in acute salicylate intoxication. An overdose of Tylox or Percocet-5 could lead to acetaminophen poisoning.

Serious overdosage of any oxycodone preparation presents problems associated with a narcotic overdose (respiratory depression, circulatory collapse, extreme somnolence progressing to stupor or coma). Skeletal muscle flaccidity also occurs. The narcotic antagonist naloxone, oxygen, IV fluids, vasopressors, and other supportive measures are indicated.

Tell patient to inform surgeon or dentist that oxycodone preparation is being taken before any surgical procedure is undertaken.

Caution patient that taking large amounts of alcoholic beverages while using oxycodone preparation increases risk of liver damage.

Instruct patient to check with physician before taking OTC drugs for colds, stomach distress, allergies, insomnia, or pain while also taking oxycodone.

Laboratory studies of hepatic function and hematologic status should be checked periodically in patients on high dosage.

Classified as Schedule II drug under Federal Controlled Substances Act.
Store this dangerous medication in a place inaccessible to children at temperature between 15° and 30°C (50° and 86°F). Protect from light.
See Morphine sulfate (prototype Narcotic analgesic).

Diagnostic Test Interferences. **Serum amylase** levels may be elevated because oxycodone causes spasm of sphincter of Oddi. **Blood glucose determinations:** false decrease (measured by glucose oxidase/peroxidase method). **5-HIAA determination:** false positive with use of nitrosonaphthol reagent (quantitative test is unaffected).

Drug Interactions: Oxycodone

Plus	Interactions
Anticholinergics	Paralytic ileus a possibility
Other CNS depressants (including alcohol, antianxiety agents, phenothiazines, sedative hypnotics)	Additive CNS depressive effects of oxycodone
See also Morphine sulfate.	

OXYMETAZOLINE HYDROCHLORIDE

(Afrin, Dristan, Duramist, Duration, Sinex)

(ox-i-met-az′oh-leen)
Alpha-adrenergic agonist
Decongestant

ACTIONS AND USES. Imidazoline-derivative sympathomimetic agent structurally and pharmacologically related to naphazoline. Direct action on alpha receptors of sympathetic nervous system produces constriction of smaller arterioles in nasal passages and prolonged decongestant effect. Has no effect on beta receptors.

Used for relief of nasal congestion in a variety of allergic and infectious disorders of the upper respiratory tract; used as nasal tampon to facilitate intranasal examination or before nasal surgery. Also used as adjunct in treatment and prevention of middle ear infection by decreasing congestion of eustachian ostia.

CONTRAINDICATIONS AND PRECAUTIONS. Hypersensitivity to drug components; use in children under 6 years of age. Safe use in women of childbearing potential and during pregnancy not established. *Cautious Use:* within 14 days of MAO inhibitors, coronary artery disease, hypertension, hyperthyroidism, diabetes mellitus.

ADVERSE/SIDE EFFECTS. Burning, stinging, dryness of nasal mucosa, sneezing. With excessive use: headache, lightheadedness, drowsiness, insomnia, palpitation, rebound congestion.

ROUTE AND DOSAGE. Topical: Adults and Children (over 6 years of age): 2 to 4 drops or 2 to 4 sprays of 0.05% solution into each nostril in the morning and at bedtime; **(2 to 5 years):** nose drops (0.025%): 2 to 3 drops in each nostril twice a day for 3 to 5 days.

NURSING IMPLICATIONS

Usually administered in the morning and at bedtime. Effects appear within 30 minutes and last about 6 to 7 hours.

If necessary, patient should blow nose gently with both nostrils open to clear nasal passages before administration of medication.
Nasal spray is delivered with patient in upright position. Place spray nozzle in nostril without occluding it, and have patient bend head slightly forward and sniff briskly during administration.
Lateral, head-low position is recommended for instillation of nose drops.
Rinse dropper or spray tip in hot water after each use to prevent contamination of solution by nasal secretions.
Caution patient not to exceed prescribed or recommended dosage. Rebound congestion (chemical rhinitis) may occur with prolonged or excessive use.
Systemic effects can result from swallowing excessive medication.
Advise patient to keep drug out of reach of children and not to permit use of the medication by anyone.

OXYMETHOLONE

(Anadrol, Anapolon)

(ox-i-meth′oh-lone)
Androgen
Anabolic

ACTIONS AND USES. Potent steroid with androgenic:anabolic activity ratio approximately 1:3. Actions, absorption, fate, contraindications, and adverse reactions are similar to those of ethylestrenol (qv).

Used to treat aplastic anemia, osteoporosis, catabolic conditions.

ROUTE AND DOSAGE. *Osteoporosis:* **Oral: Adults:** 5 to 10 mg daily; doses up to 30 mg/day may be employed. *Aplastic anemia:* **Adults and children:** 1 to 5 mg/kg body weight per day. Highly individualized.

NURSING IMPLICATIONS

Periodic liver function tests are especially important for the geriatric patient. Drug should be stopped with first sign of liver toxicity (jaundice).
Oxymetholone does not replace supportive measures for treatment of anemia (such as transfusions and correction of iron, folic acid, vitamin B_{12}, or pyridoxine deficiency).
A course of therapy for treatment of osteoporosis is 7 to 21 days.
For treatment of anemias, a minimum trial period of 3 to 6 months is recommended, since response tends to be slow.
Optimal effects in treatment of osteoporosis are usually experienced in 4 to 6 weeks.
See Ethylestrenol (prototype anabolic agent).

O

OXYMORPHONE HYDROCHLORIDE

(Numorphan)

(ox-i-mor-fone)
Narcotic analgesic
Opiate agonist
C II

ACTIONS AND USES. Semisynthetic phenanthrene derivative structurally and pharmacologically related to morphine (qv). Analgesic action of 1 mg is reportedly equivalent to that of

10 mg of morphine. Produces mild sedation and, unlike morphine, has little antitussive action. In equianalgesic doses, may cause less constipation and antitussive effect than does morphine, but more nausea, vomiting, and euphoria.

Used for relief of moderate to severe pain, preoperative medication, obstetric analgesia, support of anesthesia, and relief of anxiety in patients with dyspnea associated with acute ventricular failure and pulmonary edema.

ABSORPTION AND FATE. Onset of analgesic action usually occurs in 10 to 15 minutes after subcutaneous or IM, 5 to 10 minutes after IV, and 15 to 30 minutes after rectal administration. Peak action in about 1 to 1.5 hours; duration 3 to 6 hours. Metabolized primarily in liver; excreted in urine. Crosses placenta.

CONTRAINDICATIONS AND PRECAUTIONS. Use for pulmonary edema resulting from chemical respiratory irritants. Safe use during pregnancy (other than labor) and in children under 12 years of age not established. *See also Morphine.*

ADVERSE/SIDE EFFECTS. Nausea, vomiting, euphoria, dizziness. *See also Morphine.*

ROUTE AND DOSAGE. **Subcutaneous, intramuscular:** Initial: 1 to 1.5 mg every 4 to 6 hours, as needed; for obstetric analgesia 0.5 to 1 mg IM every 4 to 6 hours as necessary. **Intravenous:** Initial: 0.5 mg. **Rectal suppository:** 5 mg every 4 to 6 hours, as needed.

NURSING IMPLICATIONS

Evaluate patient's continued need for narcotic analgesic. Prolonged use can lead to dependence of morphine type.

Classified as Schedule II drug under Federal Controlled Substances Act.

Protect drug from light. Store suppositories in refrigerator (2° to 15°C).

See Morphine sulfate (prototype narcotic analgesic).

OXYPHENBUTAZONE

(Oxalid, Oxybutazone, Tandearil)

(ox-i-fen-byoo'ta-zone)
NSAID
Antirheumatic
Pyrazolone

ACTIONS AND USES. Pyrazolone derivative and metabolite of phenylbutazone. Shares actions, uses, absorption, fate, contraindications, precautions, and adverse reactions of phenylbutazone (qv). Has less ulcerogenic activity than phenylbutazone.

ROUTE AND DOSAGE. **Oral:** 100 to 600 mg daily in three or four divided doses (usual range 100 to 400 mg daily).

NURSING IMPLICATIONS

Tablet may be crushed and mixed with food or liquid before swallowing if patient cannot swallow it whole.

Administer immediately before or after meals or with glass of milk. Physician may prescribe concurrent sodium-free antacid to reduce incidence of gastric distress.

A trial period of one week is considered adequate to determine clinical effectiveness.

See also Phenylbutazone (prototype pyrazolone).

Drug Interactions. **Methandrostenolone** may increase oxyphenbutazone plasma levels, possibly by displacing it from plasma protein binding. *See also Phenylbutazone.*

OXYPHENCYCLIMINE HYDROCHLORIDE

(Daricon)

(ox-i-fen-sye'kli-mean)
Anticholinergic
(Parasympatholytic)
Antispasmodic

ACTIONS AND USES. Synthetic tertiary amine with clinical effects qualitatively similar to those of atropine (qv). As with most tertiary amines, exerts direct spasmolytic action on smooth muscle, but has little effect on skeletal, neuromuscular, or ganglionic transmission.

Used as adjunct in management of peptic ulcer, spastic and inflammatory conditions of GI tract, spasms of ureter or bladder, biliary tract disease.

ABSORPTION AND FATE. Onset of effects in 1 to 2 hours; duration 8 to 12 hours.

CONTRAINDICATIONS AND PRECAUTIONS. Narrow-angle glaucoma, obstructive uropathy, obstructive disease of GI tract, severe ulcerative colitis, myasthenia gravis, unstable cardiovascular status. Safe use in children under 12 years not established. *Cautious Use:* debilitated patients with chronic lung disease; elderly patients; renal, hepatic, or biliary disease; autonomic neuropathy. *See also Atropine.*

ADVERSE/SIDE EFFECTS. Atropine-like effects. High doses: CNS stimulation. *See Atropine.*

ROUTE AND DOSAGE. Oral: 5 to 10 mg twice daily. Maximum dosage 50 mg daily in divided doses.

NURSING IMPLICATIONS

Administered preferably in morning and at night before retiring.

Elderly patients are particularly sensitive to even small doses of anticholinergic drugs. Observe closely for excitement, drowsiness, or other untoward effects.

Incidence and severity of side effects are generally dose-related.

Onset of diarrhea in patients who have had ileostomy or colostomy may be an early sign of intestinal obstruction. Report immediately.

Caution patient not to perform activities requiring mental alertness or skill while taking oxyphencyclimine.

In presence of high environmental temperature, heat prostration can occur with use of oxyphencyclimine.

See Atropine sulfate (prototype anticholinergic).

O

OXYPHENONIUM BROMIDE

(Antrenyl)

(ox-i-fen-oh'nee-um)
Anticholinergic
Parasympatholytic
Antimuscarinic
Antispasmodic

ACTIONS AND USES. Potent synthetic quaternary ammonium compound with antimuscarinic properties. Pharmacologic effects qualitatively similar to those of atropine (qv), but has greater incidence of side effects. CNS activity is generally lacking. Toxic doses may block neuromuscular transmission (curarelike action).

Used in adjunctive management of peptic ulcer and other GI disorders associated with hyperacidity, hypermotility, and spasm. Also has been used as preanesthetic antisecretory agent in patients hypersensitive to atropine; used to relieve smooth-muscle spasm in bronchial asthma and to control excessive perspiration.

ABSORPTION AND FATE. Usually acts within 30 minutes, with peak action in about 2 hours; duration of action 4 to 6 hours. Mean half-life: 3.2 hours. Excreted unchanged in urine. Does not penetrate CNS or eyes.

CONTRAINDICATIONS AND PRECAUTIONS. Glaucoma, obstructive uropathy, obstructive diseases of GI tract, biliary tract disease, ulcerative colitis, unstable cardiovascular status, myasthenia gravis. Safe use during pregnancy and lactation and in children not established. *Cautious Use:* debilitated patients with chronic lung disease, elderly patients, renal or hepatic disease, autonomic neuropathy. *See also Atropine.*

ADVERSE/SIDE EFFECTS. Blurred vision, dry mouth, hyperthermia, dizziness, impaired micturition. Toxic dose: respiratory depression, muscle weakness, cardiac disturbances. *See Atropine.*

ROUTE AND DOSAGE. Oral: Adults: Initial: 10 mg four times daily for several days; dosage then reduced according to patient's response.

NURSING IMPLICATIONS

Preferably administered before meals and at bedtime.

Elderly patients are particularly sensitive to even small doses of anticholinergic drugs. Report complaints of nausea, dizziness, constipation, urinary retention, weakness, or other unusual symptoms. Physiologic response versus toxicity may need to be differentiated.

Onset of diarrhea in patients who have had ileostomy or colostomy may be an early sign of intestinal obstruction. Report promptly.

In presence of high environmental temperature, heat prostration can occur with use of this drug.

Caution patient not to engage in activities requiring mental alertness and skill while taking oxyphenonium.

Have on hand the antidote neostigmine in the event of severe toxic reactions.

See Atropine sulfate (prototype anticholinergic).

OXYTETRACYCLINE
(Oxymycin, Terramycin)

OXYTETRACYCLINE CALCIUM
(Terramycin Calcium)

OXYTETRACYCLINE HYDROCHLORIDE
(Terramycin, Uri-Tet)

(ox-i-tet-ra-sye'kleen)
Antiinfective
Antibacterial
Tetracycline

ACTIONS AND USES. Broad-spectrum antibiotic with actions, uses, contraindications, precautions, and adverse reactions similar to those of tetracycline (qv).

ABSORPTION AND FATE. Adequately but incompletely absorbed from GI tract; peak plasma concentrations in 2 to 4 hours. Appears to concentrate in hepatic system. Half-life: 6 to 9 hours. Excreted in bile, feces, and urine in active form. Crosses placenta.

CONTRAINDICATIONS AND PRECAUTIONS. Hypersensitivity to tetracyclines; during tooth development (last half of pregnancy, infancy, childhood to age 8). *Cautious Use:* impaired renal function. *See Tetracycline.*

ADVERSE/SIDE EFFECTS. Nausea, vomiting, diarrhea, stomatitis, skin rash, superinfections, renal toxicity. *See Tetracycline.*

ROUTE AND DOSAGE. Adults: Oral: 250 to 500 mg every 6 to 12 hours. **Intramuscular:** 100 mg every 8 to 12 hours; (For severe infections): 250 mg every 24 hours or 300 mg at 8 to 12 hour intervals. **Intravenous:** 250 to 500 every 12 hours, not to exceed 500 mg every 6 hours. **Children: Oral:** 25 to 50 mg/kg daily in 4 equal doses. **Intramuscular:** 15 to 25 mg/kg daily in 2 or 3 divided doses. No single injection should exceed 250 mg. **Intravenous:** 10 to 20 mg/kg daily in 2 divided doses.

NURSING IMPLICATIONS

Check expiration date. Degradation products of outdated tetracyclines can be highly nephrotoxic. Instruct patient to discard unused drug when course of therapy has ended.

Food may interfere with rate and extent of absorption of oral drug. Administer at least 1 hour before or 2 hours following meals. Do not give with antacids, milk, milk products, or other calcium-containing foods.

Caution patient to avoid excessive exposure to sunlight.

Dosage will require readjustment in the presence of renal dysfunction.

Dry powder for parenteral use is stable at room temperature. Reconstituted solutions are stable for 48 hours at refrigerated temperatures (2° to 8°C).

The commercially available solution for IM use only contains 2% lidocaine.

Syrup formulation (oxytetracycline calcium) should be stored in a cool place protected from light.

See Tetracycline Hydrochloride (prototype tetracycline).

O

OXYTOCIN INJECTION
(Pitocin, Syntocinon)
OXYTOCIN NASAL SOLUTION

(ox-i-toe'sin)
Hormone
Oxytocic

ACTIONS AND USES. Synthetic, water-soluble polypeptide consisting of 8 amino acids, identical pharmacologically to the oxytocic principle of posterior pituitary. Oxytocic activity: 10 USP posterior pituitary units per milliliter. By direct action on myofibrils, produces phasic contractions characteristic of normal delivery. Promotes milk ejection (letdown) reflex in nursing mother, thereby increasing flow (not volume) of milk; also facilitates flow of milk during period of breast engorgement. Uterine sensitivity to oxytocin increases during gestation period and peaks sharply before parturition. Exerts slight intrinsic ADH-like effect in large doses. Not used for elective induction of labor.

Used to initiate or improve uterine contraction at term only in carefully selected patients and only after cervix is dilated and presentation of fetus has occurred; used to stimulate letdown reflex in nursing mother and to relieve pain from breast. Uses include: management of inevitable, incomplete, or missed abortion; stimulation of uterine contractions during third stage of labor; stimulation to overcome uterine inertia; control of postpartum hemorrhage and promotion of postpartum uterine involution. Also used to induce labor in cases of maternal diabetes, preeclampsia, eclampsia, and erythroblastosis fetalis.

ABSORPTION AND FATE. Uterine response following IM injection is evidenced in 3 to 7 minutes, with duration of 30 to 60 minutes; after IV injection, response occurs within 1 minute, with shorter duration; following nasal spray, in 5 to 10 minutes. Plasma half-life is 1 minute to several minutes (shorter during late pregnancy and lactation). Rapidly removed from plasma by mammary gland, kidney, and liver and inactivated, perhaps by oxytocinase, an enzyme produced in placenta and uterine tissue during pregnancy. Small portion of dose is excreted in active form by kidney.

CONTRAINDICATIONS AND PRECAUTIONS. Hypersensitivity to oxytocin, significant cephalopelvic disproportion, unfavorable fetal position or presentations which are undeliverable without conversion before delivery, obstetric emergencies where benefit-to-risk ratio for mother or fetus favors surgical intervention, fetal distress where delivery is not imminent, prematurity, placenta previa, prolonged use in severe toxemia or uterine inertia, hypertonic uterine patterns, previous surgery of uterus or cervix including cesarean section, conditions predisposing to thromboplastin or amniotic fluid embolism (dead fetus, abruptio placentae), grand multiparity, invasive cervical carcinoma, primipara over 35 years of age, past history of uterine sepsis or of traumatic delivery, intranasal route during labor, simultaneous administration of drug by two routes. *Cautious Use:* concomitant use with cyclopropane anesthesia or vasoconstrictive drugs.

ADVERSE/SIDE EFFECTS. **Fetus:** bradycardia and other arrhythmias, hypoxia, intracranial hemorrhage, trauma from too rapid propulsion through pelvis, neonatal jaundice, death. **Mother:** hypersensitivity leading to uterine hypertonicity, tetanic contractions, uterine rupture, anaphylactic reactions, postpartum hemorrhage, cardiac arrhythmias, pelvic hematoma, nausea, vomiting, hypertensive episodes, subarachnoid hemorrhage, increased blood flow, fatal afibrinogenemia, ADH effects leading to severe water intoxication and hyponatremia, hypotension, ECG changes, PVCs anxiety, dyspnea, precordial pain, edema, cyanosis or redness of skin, cardiovascular spasm and collapse. *Citrate:* parabuccal irritation.

ROUTE AND DOSAGE. *Stimulation or induction of labor:* **Intravenous infusion (drip method):** 1 to 2 mU/minute (0.001 to 0.002 U/minute). Gradually increase dose by increments of no more than 1 to 2 mU/minute until a contraction pattern is established which simulates normal labor. *Control of postpartum uterine bleeding:* **Intravenous infusion (drip method):** 10 to 40 U added to 1000 ml nonhydrating diluent at rate needed to control uterine atony. **Intramuscular:** 5 to 10 U after delivery of placenta. *Milk letdown:* **Nasal spray (40 units/ml):** one spray into one or both nostrils 2 to 3 minutes before nursing or pumping of breasts.

NURSING IMPLICATIONS

When diluting oxytocin for IV infusion, rotate bottle gently to distribute medicine throughout solution.

Before instituting treatment, start flow charts to record maternal blood pressure and other vital signs, intake–output ratio, weight, strength, duration, and frequency of contractions, as well as fetal heart tone and rate.

Oxytocin administration should be supervised by persons having thorough knowledge of the drug and the skill to identify complications. A qualified physician should be immediately available to manage complications.

Time of administration of ocytocin in relation to delivery of baby or placenta varies with physician's preference. The nurse should have a clear understanding of when drug is to be administered with respect to progress of labor. Infusion flow rates are established by physician. Accurate control by infusion pump (or other device) is critical.

Use of a Y connection to infusion tubing is advised to allow oxytocin solution to be discontinued if necessary while vein is kept open.

Oxytocin is incompatible with infusions of fibrinolysin, levarterenol bitartrate, prochlorperazine edisylate, protein hydrolysate, and warfarin sodium.

During infusion period, monitor fetal heart rate and maternal blood pressure and pulse at least every 15 minutes; evaluate tonus of myometrium during and between contractions and record on flow chart. Report change in rate and rhythm immediately.

If contractions are prolonged (occurring at less than 2-minute intervals) and if monitor records contractions about 50 mm Hg, or if contractions last 90 seconds or longer, stop infusion to prevent fetal anoxia, turn patient on her side, and notify physician. Stimulation will wane rapidly within 2 to 3 minutes. Oxygen administration may be necessary.

The fundus should be checked frequently during the first few postpartum hours and several times daily thereafter.

Knowledge of time factors related to onset and duration of effects *(see Absorption and Fate)* is essential for prevention of fetal and maternal crises.

Oxytocin should never be administered by more than one route at a time.

Incidence of hypersensitivity or allergic reactions is higher when oxytocin is given by IM or IV injection rather than by IV infusion (diluted solution).

During delivery, IM oxytocin is most easily injected deep into deltoid muscle (using needle length). Massage injection site to assist quick absorption.

If IM oxytocin is used, magnesium sulfate (10 ml of 20%) solution should be available for relaxation of the myometrium.

Nasal spray: Instruct patient to clear nasal passages well before administration. Hold squeeze bottle upright, and spray solution into nostril with patient's head in a vertical position.

When oxytocin is given to stimulate the letdown reflex, provide measures that support a beneficial response: quiet nonstressful environment, maternal confidence through knowledge and freedom from worry and pain.

If local or regional (caudal, spinal) anesthesia is being given to the patient receiving oxytocin, be alert to the possibility of hypertensive crisis: sudden intense occipital headache, palpitation, marked hypertension, stiff neck, nausea, vomiting, sweating, fever, photophobia, dilated pupils, bradycardia or tachycardia, constricting chest pain.

Monitor intake and output during labor. If patient is receiving drug by prolonged IV infusion, watch for symptoms of water intoxication (drowsiness, listlessness, headache, confusion, anuria, weight gain). Report changes in alertness and orientation and changes in intake–output ratio, i.e., marked decrease in output with excessive intake.

Unless otherwise directed by manufacturer, store oxytocin solution in refrigerator but do not freeze.

Drug Interactions. **Ephedrine, methoxamine,** and **other vasopressors** can cause severe hypertension when administered at same time as oxytocin.

P

PANCREATIN
(Viokase)

(pan′kree-a-tin)
Enzyme
Digestant

ACTIONS AND USES. Pancreatic enzyme concentrate of bovine or porcine origin containing principally lipase, protease, and amylase in standardized amounts. Assists in digestion of starch, protein, and fats; decreases nitrogen and fat content of stool.

Used as digestive aid in conditions associated with exocrine pancreatic deficiency such as chronic pancreatitis, pancreatectomy or gastrectomy, and cystic fibrosis. Also has been used as a presumptive test for pancreatic function.

CONTRAINDICATIONS AND PRECAUTIONS. *Cautious Use:* history of hypersensitivity reactions to beef or pork products. Safe use during pregnancy not established.

ADVERSE/SIDE EFFECTS. With large doses: anorexia, nausea, vomiting, diarrhea, buccal and anal soreness (particularly in infants), hyperuricosuria, hypersensitivity reactions (sneezing, lacrimation, skin rashes).

ROUTE AND DOSAGE. Oral: Adults: 325 mg to 1 Gm (as high as 12 Gm daily may be prescribed in divided doses at 1- or 2-hour intervals or before, during, or within 1 hour after meals, with an extra dose taken with any food eaten between meals. **Pediatric:** 300 to 600 mg three times daily. Available in tablets and powder.

NURSING IMPLICATIONS

Since pancreatin is inactivated by gastric pepsin and acid pH, it may be prescribed to be taken with or after an antacid or cimetidine.

Monitor patient for symptoms of diabetes mellitus (polyuria, thirst, hunger, pruritus). Insulin-dependent diabetes frequently occurs in these patients.

Avoid inhalation of powder formulation.

Enteric-coated tablets are to be swallowed whole, not crushed or chewed.

Monitor intake and output and weight. Note appetite, quality of stools, weight loss, abdominal bloating (pancreatic insufficiency may present as diabetes mellitus, steatorrhea, bulky stools).

For pancreatic insufficiency, a special diet high in protein and carbohydrates and low in fat (50 Gm/day) is generally recommended to avoid indigestion. Multivitamin supplements may also be prescribed.

Periodic measurement of fecal fat and nitrogen, serum carotene and calcium, and prothrombin activity may be made to evaluate response to drug therapy.

Stored in tight containers at room temperature not exceeding 30°C (86°F).

Drug Interactions. Pancreatin may inhibit absorption of **oral iron; cimetidine** may enhance enzyme effects.

PANCRELIPASE

(Cotazym, Ilozyme, Ku-Zyme-Hp, Pancrease)

(pan-kre-li'pase)
Enzyme
Digestant

ACTIONS AND USES. Pancreatic enzyme concentrate of porcine origin standardized for lipase content. Similar to pancreatin, but on a weight basis, has 12 times the lipolytic activity and at least 4 times the trypsin and amylase content of pancreatin.

Used as replacement therapy in symptomatic treatment of malabsorption syndrome due to cystic fibrosis and other conditions associated with exocrine pancreatic insufficiency. A component of Accelerase and Ro-Bile.

CONTRAINDICATIONS AND PRECAUTIONS. *Cautious Use:* history of allergy to hog protein or enzymes. Safe use during pregnancy not established.

ADVERSE/SIDE EFFECTS. High doses: anorexia, nausea, vomiting, diarrhea, hyperuricosuria.

ROUTE AND DOSAGE. Oral: Adults: 1 to 3 capsules or tablets or 1 or 2 packets of powder just prior to or with each meal or snack as prescribed. **Pediatric:** 1 or 2 capsules or tablets with each meal. In severe deficiencies, frequency may be increased to hourly intervals.

NURSING IMPLICATIONS

Enteric coated preparations are not to be crushed or chewed.

Avoid inhalation of powder formulation.

For children, powder form may be sprinkled on food.

Cimetidine or an antacid may be prescribed to be given before pancrelipase to prevent its destruction by gastric pepsin and acid pH.

Dosage is usually determined by fat content in diet (suggested ratio: 300 mg pancrelipase for each 17 Gm dietary fat).

Proper balance between fat, protein, and starch intake must be maintained to avoid temporary indigestion.

Monitor intake and output and weight. Note appetite and quality of stools, weight loss, abdominal bloating, polyuria, thirst, hunger, itching. Pancreatic insufficiency is frequently associated with steatorrhea, bulky stools and insulin dependent diabetes.

PANCURONIUM BROMIDE

(Pavulon)

(pan-kyoo-roe'nee-um)
Skeletal muscle relaxant (nondepolarizing)

ACTIONS AND USES. Synthetic curariform nondepolarizing neuromuscular blocking agent. Similar to tubocurarine chloride (qv) in actions, uses, and limitations. Reported to be approximately 5 times as potent as tubocurarine, but produces little or no histamine release or ganglionic blockade, and thus does not cause bronchospasm or hypotension. In high doses, has direct blocking effect on acetylcholine receptors of heart, and may cause increased heart rate, cardiac output, and arterial pressure.

Used as an adjunct to anesthesia to induce skeletal muscle relaxation. Also used to facilitate management of patients undergoing mechanical ventilation.

ABSORPTION AND FATE. Onset of action (dose-dependent) within 30 to 45 seconds, with peak effect in about 3 to 5 minutes, and 90% recovery within 1 hour. Small amount metabolized and eliminated in bile. Excreted primarily unchanged by kidneys.

CONTRAINDICATIONS AND PRECAUTIONS. Hypersensitivity to the drug or bromides; tachycardia. Safe use in women of childbearing potential and during pregnancy not established. *Cautious Use:* debilitated patients, myasthenia gravis, pulmonary, hepatic or renal disease, fluid or electrolyte imbalance.

ADVERSE/SIDE EFFECTS. Increased pulse rate and blood pressure, ventricular extrasystoles, transient acneiform rash, burning sensation along course of vein, salivation, skeletal muscle weakness, respiratory depression.

ROUTE AND DOSAGE. **Intravenous:** 0.04 to 0.1 mg/kg body weight. Additional doses starting at 0.01 mg/kg may be administered at 30- to 60-minute intervals, if necessary.

NURSING IMPLICATIONS

Administered only by or under supervision of experienced clinicians.

Plastic syringe may be used for administration, but drug may adsorb to plastic with prolonged storage.

Facilities for intubation, artificial respiration, controlled ventilation, and oxygen therapy should be immediately available. Also have on hand pyridostigmine bromide, neostigmine, and atropine to reverse action of pancuronium.

Observe patient closely for residual muscle weakness and signs of respiratory distress during recovery period. Monitor blood pressure and vital signs.

Peripheral nerve stimulator may be used to assess the effects of pancuronium and to monitor restoration of neuromuscular function.

See Tubocurarine chloride (prototype nondepolarizing skeletal muscle relaxant).

Diagnostic Test Interferences. Pancuronium may decrease **serum cholinesterase** concentrations.

Drug Interactions. Action of pancuronium is antagonized by **acetylcholine, anticholinesterases,** and **potassium** ion. Drugs known to produce neuromuscular blockade may enhance blockade produced by pancuronium, e.g., **aminoglycoside antibiotics (amikacin, gentamicin, kanamycin, neomycin, paromomycin, streptomycin, tobramycin), bacitracin, magnesium salts, polymyxins (colistin, polymyxin B), quinidine, quinine,** and other **surgical skeletal muscle relaxants.** *See also Tubocurarine Chloride.*

PAPAIN

(pa-pay'in)

(Panafil, Soflens)

Proteolytic enzyme

ACTIONS AND USES. Combination of proteolytic enzymes extracted from *Carica papaya.* At recommended doses, does not affect uninjured cells or tissues.

Used topically for enzymatic debridement, promotion of normal healing, and deodorization of surface lesions. An ingredient in Panafil. Soflens is used as an enzymatic cleaner of contact lenses.

CONTRAINDICATIONS AND PRECAUTIONS. History of allergy to papaya. Tablet formulation: systemic infection or severe blood clotting disorders; concomitant use of anticoagulants. Safe use during pregnancy not established. *Cautious Use:* severe renal or hepatic disease. Topical preparation not to be used in eyes.

ADVERSE/SIDE EFFECTS. Topical use: occasional stinging or itching. Tablet formulation: nausea, vomiting, diarrhea, dizziness, pruritus, rash, urticaria, mild local tingling at site of buccal absorption.

ROUTE AND DOSAGE. **Topical (ointment 10%):** apply locally to lesion once or twice daily.

NURSING IMPLICATIONS

Topical preparations may be covered with gauze.

Before each application of ointment irrigate wound with mild (prescribed) cleansing solution to remove accumulated debris.

Hydrogen peroxide inactivates topical papain and therefore should not be used as an irrigating solution.

Itching or stinging sensation sometimes occurs when papain is first applied. If symptoms persist, report to physician.

Store at controlled room temperature, preferably between 15° and 30°C (59° and 86°F) unless otherwise directed by manufacturer.

PAPAVERINE HYDROCHLORIDE

(pa-pav′er-een)
Vasodilator (peripheral)

(BP-Papaverine, Cerebid, Cerespan, Cirbed, Delapav, Dilart, Kavrin, Lapav, Myobid, Papacon, Pap-Kaps-150, P-A-V, Pavabid, Pavacap, Pavacen Pavaclor, Pavacron, Pavadel, Pavadur, Pavadyl, Pava-Par, Pava-Rx, Pavased, Pavasule, Pava-Wol, Paverolan, Pavex, PT-300, Ro-Papav, Vasal, Vasocap, Vasospan, Vazosan)

ACTIONS AND USES. Benzylisoquinoline alkaloid prepared synthetically or from opium. Lacks pharmacologic properties of narcotics; reportedly does not promote tolerance or habituation, and has little if any analgesic effect. Exerts nonspecific direct spasmolytic effect on smooth muscles unrelated to innervation. Action is especially pronounced on coronary, cerebral, pulmonary, and peripheral arteries when spasm is present. Like quinidine, acts directly on myocardium, depresses conduction and irritability, and prolongs refractory period. Stimulates respiration by action on carotid and aortic body chemoreceptors. Relaxes smooth muscles of bronchi, GI tract, ureters, and biliary system. Objective proof of therapeutic value is reportedly lacking.

Used primarily for relief of cerebral and peripheral ischemia associated with arterial spasm and myocardial ischemia complicated by arrhythmias. Also has been used for visceral spasm as in ureteral, biliary, and GI colic.

P

ABSORPTION AND FATE. Readily absorbed following oral administration. Peak plasma levels in 1 to 2 hours, falling to low levels after 6 hours with regular tablets and 12 hours after extended-release forms. Low and erratic plasma concentrations reported with extended-release preparations. About 90% bound to plasma proteins. Half-life: approximately 90 minutes. Rapidly metabolized in liver; excreted in urine chiefly as metabolites.

CONTRAINDICATIONS AND PRECAUTIONS. Parenteral use in complete AV block. Safe use during pregnancy, in nursing mothers, and in children not established. *Cautious Use:* glaucoma, myocardial depression, angina pectoris, recent stroke.

ADVERSE/SIDE EFFECTS. **Oral:** nausea, anorexia, constipation, diarrhea, abdominal distress, dizziness, drowsiness, headache. **Parenteral:** (low incidence): general discomfort, facial flushing, sweating, dry mouth and throat, pruritus, skin rash, dizziness, headache, excessive drowsiness and sedation (large doses), slight rise in blood pressure, increased depth of respiration, paroxysmal tachycardia, transient ventricular ectopic rhythms, hepatotoxicity (jaundice, eosinophilia, abnormal liver function tests); with rapid IV administration: respiratory depression, AV block, arrhythmias, fatal apnea. **Overdosage:** diplopia, nystagmus, weakness, drowsiness, coma, respiratory depression.

ROUTE AND DOSAGE. Oral: Adult: 100 to 300 mg three to five times daily; timed-release forms: 150 mg every 8 to 12 hours. **Intramuscular, intravenous:** 30 to 120 mg, repeated every 3 hours, as indicated. **Pediatric: Intramuscular, intravenous:** 6 mg/kg/24 hours divided into 4 doses. Available in tablets, timed-release capsules, elixir, and solution for injection.

NURSING IMPLICATIONS

Oral formulations may be taken with or following meals, milk or antacid (prescribed) to reduce possibility of nausea.

Timed-release forms should be swallowed whole and must not be chewed or crushed.

Aspirate carefully before injecting IM, to avoid inadvertent entry into blood vessel, and administer slowly.

When given IV, papaverine must be administered slowly over 1 to 2 minutes.

Monitor pulse, respiration, and blood pressure in patients receiving drug parenterally. If significant changes are noted, withhold medication and report promptly to physician.

Hepatic function and blood tests should be performed periodically. Hepatotoxicity (thought to be a hypersensitivity reaction) is reversible with prompt drug withdrawal.

Instruct patient to notify physician if any side effect persists or if GI symptoms, jaundice, or skin rash appear. Hepatic function tests may be indicated. Because of the possibility of drowsiness and dizziness, advise patient to avoid driving and other potentially hazardous tasks until reaction to drug is known. Alcohol may increase drowsiness and dizziness.

Smoking-Drug Interaction: Since nicotine constricts blood vessels, patients with vascular problems should be advised not to smoke.

Preserved in tightly covered, light-resistant containers.

Parenteral papaverine is incompatible with lactated Ringer's injection (forms precipitate).

Drug Interactions. Concurrent use may decrease **levodopa** effectiveness with worsening of parkinsonism, and may enhance hypotensive effects of **antihypertensives. Morphine** antagonizes smooth muscle relaxant effect of papaverine.

P

PARALDEHYDE

(Paracetaldehyde, Paral)

(par-al'de-hyde)
Sedative, hypnotic
C IV

ACTIONS AND USES. Cyclic ether formed by polymerization of acetaldehyde. Potent CNS depressant with sedative and hypnotic actions similar to those of alcohol, barbiturates, and chloral hydrate.

Used as sedative and hypnotic in acute agitation due to alcohol withdrawal; used to control convulsions arising from tetanus, eclampsia, status epilepticus, and drug poisoning. Has been used rectally to induce basal anesthesia, particularly in children.

ABSORPTION AND FATE. Absorbed well from all routes. Hypnotic action within 10 to 15 minutes; effects last 6 to 8 hours or more. Average half-life: 7.5 hours. Approximately 70 to 80% of dose is metabolized by liver. Significant amounts (11 to 28%) excreted unchanged through lungs; traces eliminated unchanged in urine. Readily crosses placenta.

CONTRAINDICATIONS AND PRECAUTIONS. Severe hepatic insufficiency, respiratory disease, GI inflammation or ulceration, disulfiram therapy.

ADVERSE/SIDE EFFECTS. Irritation of mucous membrane (oral and rectal routes), nausea, vomiting, unpleasant taste and odor, hangover, dizziness, ataxia, erythematous skin rash; occasionally confusion and paradoxical excitement. IM injection: pain, sterile abscess, necrosis, muscle irritation; thrombophlebitis following IV administration. **Prolonged Use:** toxic hepatitis, nephrosis, metabolic acidosis. **Overdosage:** rapid labored breathing, respiratory depression, pulmonary hemorrhage and edema, hypotension, bleeding gastritis, renal and liver damage, acidosis, dilation and failure of right heart, cardiovascular collapse.

ROUTE AND DOSAGE. Each 1 ml contains approximately 1 Gm paraldehyde. **Adults: Oral, rectal:** *Sedative:* 5 to 10 ml. *Hypnotic:* 10 to 30 ml. **Intramuscular, intravenous:** 5 ml IM; 3 to 5 ml IV. For IV injection, 5 ml of drug should be diluted with at least 100 ml of 0.9% sodium chloride injection and administered at rate not exceeding 1 ml/minute. **Children: Oral, rectal, intramuscular:** *Sedative:* 0.15 ml/kg body weight. *Hypnotic:* twice the sedative dose.

NURSING IMPLICATIONS

Paraldehyde is a colorless clear liquid with a strong characteristic odor and a burning, disagreeable taste.

On exposure to light, air, and heat, drug liberates acetaldehyde, which oxidizes to acetic acid. Do not use solution if it is colored in any way or smells of acetic acid (vinegar odor).

Decomposed paraldehyde is extremely corrosive to tissues and can cause fatal poisoning. Discard unused contents of any container that has been opened for more than 24 hours.

Do not use plastics for measuring or administering paraldehyde. Contact with plastic syringes, catheters, measuring or drinking cups, or other plastic materials can result in decomposition of paraldehyde to toxic compounds. Parenteral preparation should be drawn into a glass syringe; use rubber catheter for rectal administration.

Give oral drug well diluted in iced fruit juice or milk to reduce irritation of GI tract and mask odor and taste. Oral capsules are available.

When given rectally, drug should be diluted with at least two volumes of olive oil or cottonseed oil or dissolved in 200 ml of 0.9% sodium chloride solution to prevent rectal irritation.

IM injection should be made deep into upper outer quadrant of buttock well away from nerve trunks. Paraldehyde can cause nerve injury and paralysis. Aspirate carefully before injecting drug, and massage injection site well. Rotate injection sites. Not to exceed 5 ml per injection site.

When given by IV route (infrequently used), CNS depression may be preceded by a brief period of excitement and coughing. The coughing that sometimes occurs when paraldehyde is given IV may be due to untoward effects on pulmonary capillaries. Monitor patient closely for hypotension and respiratory depression.

In some hospitals, physicians administer parenteral paraldehyde because of danger of circulatory collapse or pulmonary edema, sterile abscesses, nerve injury, and paralysis.

Paraldehyde is not analgesic; therefore, it should not be given to relieve pain. The drug may produce excitement or delirium in the presence of pain.

Bronchial secretions may be increased. Keep the patient turned on side to prevent aspiration. Suctioning may be necessary.

Advise bed rest and no smoking. Bedsides are indicated.

Keep patient's room well ventilated to control the strong, pungent odor of exhaled drug.

The odor may attract flies in the summer. Patient's breath will have a characteristic odor for several hours.
Tolerance and physical and/or psychologic dependence can occur with prolonged use. Paraldehyde addiction resembles alcoholism.
Rapid withdrawal after prolonged use may produce delirium tremens and hallucinations.
Treatment of overdosage: gastric lavage for oral ingestion (if endotracheal tube with cuff is in place to prevent aspiration of vomitus) or rectal lavage for rectal overdosage, followed by demulcent such as mineral oil (orally or by nasogastric tube).
Classified as Schedule IV drug under Federal Controlled Substances Act.
Stock drug should be checked periodically for purity as defined by USP.
Preserved in tight, light-resistant containers in amounts not exceeding 30 ml and at temperatures not over 25°C (77°F). Keep away from heat, open flames, and sparks.

Diagnostic Test Interferences. Chronic use of alcohol (ethanol) and paraldehyde may cause false-positive **serum ketones** (nitroprusside tube dilution method) and **urine ketones** (Acetest) and may interfere with **urinary steroid** (17-OHCS) determinations by modification of Reddy, Jenkins, Thorn procedure.

Drug Interactions. Theoretically, **disulfiram** may increase blood levels of paraldehyde by inhibiting its metabolism. Paraldehyde may increase the possibility of **sulfonamide** crystalluria (with the less soluble drugs such as sulfadiazine, sulfapyridine, sulfamerazine). Additive effects may result when administered concomitantly with other **CNS depressant drugs,** such as **alcohol, general anesthetics.**

PARAMETHADIONE

(Paradione)

(par-a-meth-a-dye′one)
Anticonvulsant

P

ACTIONS AND USES. Oxazolidinedione (dione-type) anticonvulsant agent with pharmacologic actions, uses, contraindications, precautions, and adverse reactions similar to those of trimethadione (qv). Unlike trimethadione, chronic administration is not associated with myasthenia-gravis-like syndrome, and although incidence of other toxic reactions is lower, it is reportedly less effective. Causes slightly greater sedative effect than trimethadione.
Used to control absence (petit mal) seizures refractory to other drugs.

ABSORPTION AND FATE. Rapidly absorbed following oral administration. Metabolized by hepatic microsomal enzymes to active metabolites which are excreted slowly in urine.

CONTRAINDICATIONS AND PRECAUTIONS. Hypersensitivity to oxazolidinedione anticonvulsants; severe blood dyscrasias, renal and hepatic dysfunction. Safe use during pregnancy and in nursing mothers not established. *Cautious Use:* retinal or optic nerve disease.

ADVERSE/SIDE EFFECTS. Common: sedation, drowsiness. Infrequent: ataxia, headache, dizziness, paresthesias, vaginal bleeding, changes in blood pressure, visual symptoms, GI distress, rash, alopecia, lympadenopathy, abnormal liver function tests, albuminuria. Same potential for toxicity as trimethadione (qv).

ROUTE AND DOSAGE. Oral: Adult: Initial: 300 mg three times daily; dosage then increased by additional 300 mg/day at weekly intervals until seizures are controlled or toxic symptoms intervene. Not to exceed 2.4 Gm daily. **Children (over 6 years):** 300 mg three or four times a day; **(2 to 6 years):** 200 mg three times a day; **(up to 2 years):** 100 mg three times a day. Available as capsules and oral solution.

NURSING IMPLICATIONS

Capsule form contains an oily liquid and must be swallowed whole and not chewed or crushed.

The 300-mg capsule contains *tartrazine* which may cause an allergic type reaction including bronchial asthma in susceptible individuals. The reaction is seen frequently in patients with aspirin hypersensitivity.

Advise patient to measure oral solution with graduated dropper provided by manufacturer.

Oral solution contains alcohol 65% and should be diluted with water before administration.

Liver function tests, urinalysis, and complete blood count should be done prior to and at monthly intervals during therapy. If blood counts remain normal for 12 months, intervals may be increased. Blood counts are done more frequently if neutrophil count drops to less than 3000, and drug is withdrawn if count drops to 2500 or less.

Since drug may cause drowsiness and visual symptoms, caution patient to avoid driving and other potentially hazardous activities until reaction to drug is known.

Instruct patient to report any unusual symptom to physician. Drug should be discontinued if patient develops scotomata, jaundice, swollen glands, skin rash, hair loss, unexplained fever, fatigue, tendency to bleed or bruise, or sore mouth or throat.

Drug should be withdrawn gradually to avoid precipitating seizure activity.

Stored in tightly covered containers at controlled room temperature preferably between 15° and 30°C (59° and 86°F) unless otherwise directed by manufacturer. Solution should be stored in light-resistant container.

See also Trimethadione (prototype oxazolidinedione anticonvulsant).

PARAMETHASONE ACETATE

(Haldrone)

(par-a-meth'a-sone)
Corticosteroid
Glucocorticoid

ACTIONS AND USES. Long-acting synthetic steroid with antiinflammatory action, but very little sodium-retaining potency. On weight basis, 2 mg paramethasone is equivalent to 20 mg hydrocortisone. Has no particular advantages over other corticosteroids. Similar to hydrocortisone (qv) in actions, uses, absorption, and fate.

P

ABSORPTION AND FATE. Rapidly absorbed; peak effect is 1 to 2 hours after administration. Duration of effect: 2 days. Half-life (plasma) 3 to 45 hours; HPA (hypothalamus–pituitary–adrenal) axis suppression: 36 to 54 hours.

CONTRAINDICATIONS AND PRECAUTIONS. Systemic fungal infections, in presence of ocular herpes simplex, keratitis; safe use during pregnancy (category C), lactation, and by children less than 6 years old not established. *Also see Hydrocortisone.*

ADVERSE/SIDE EFFECTS. Increase in appetite, growth retardation, hypocalcemia, (prolonged treatment). Psychic derangement. Also see Hydrocortisone.

ROUTE AND DOSAGE. Oral: Adults: Initial: 2 to 24 mg daily in divided doses until satisfactory response is achieved; dose is then decreased by small amounts to lowest therapeutic level for maintenance (1 to 8 mg daily; highly individualized). **Children:** 58 to 800 mcg/kg body weight daily, as a single dose or in 3 or 4 divided doses.

NURSING IMPLICATIONS

At high dosage (above 15 mg daily), urinary excretion of calcium and nitrogen increases significantly.

If drug is to be stopped after long-term therapy, it should be withdrawn gradually to prevent onset of hypocortisolism.

Store drug in light-resistant container at temperature between 15° and 30°C (59° and 86°F).

See Hydrocortisone (prototype glucocorticoid).

PARATHYROID

(par-a-thye′roid)
Diagnostic aid
Hormone

ACTIONS AND USES. Protein hormone extracted from bovine parathyroid glands standardized to potency not less than 100 USP units per milliliter; regulates calcium (Ca) metabolism and Ca ion plasma concentration. Increases renal clearance of phosphates, stimulates Ca reabsorption from renal tubules, and (by promoting bone resorption) fosters Ca and phosphate release to serum. Conserves body magnesium, but increases excretion of water, sodium, and bicarbonate. By facilitating renal conversion of vitamin D to its active form, dihydroxycholecalciferol, provides the catalyst required for Ca absorption from small intestine. In deficiency states parenteral administration raises serum Ca levels, thereby restoring normal threshold of excitability in polarized membranes, and decreases serum phosphorus levels.

Used as short-term treatment of acute hypoparathyroidism with tetany, and in Ellsworth-Howard test which establishes diagnosis of idiopathic and postoperative hypoparathyroidism, and differentiates pseudoparathyroidism from hypoparathyroidism.

ABSORPTION AND FATE. Phosphatemic response follows IV injection within 15 minutes. Serum Ca rises in about 4 hours, peaks in 12 to 18 hours, and returns to pretreatment levels after 20 to 24 hours. Binds to plasma proteins; plasma half-life: about 20 minutes. Degradation sites not clear, but possibly in kidney and liver. Only 1% of dose is excreted in urine.

P

CONTRAINDICATIONS AND PRECAUTIONS. Hypercalcemia, hypercalciuria, tetany unrelated to parathyroid failure. *Cautious Use:* sarcoidosis, renal or cardiac disease, digitalized patients. Information about use during pregnancy not available.

ADVERSE/SIDE EFFECTS. **Hypercalcemia (overdosage):** muscular weakness, deep bone and flank pain, lethargy, headache, anorexia, nausea, vomiting, diarrhea, abdominal cramps, vertigo, tinnitus, ataxia, exanthema. **Hypercalcemic crisis:** dehydration, stupor, coma, azotemia. **Other:** subcutaneous site inflammation, vasodilation, decreased blood pressure, bradycardia, cardiac arrhythmias, syncope, cardiac arrest.

ROUTE AND DOSAGE. **Subcutaneous, intramuscular, intravenous:** **Adults:** 20 to 40 U every 12 hours, if necessary, for acute tetany secondary to hypoparathyroidism. *Diagnosis:* 200 U intravenously.

NURSING IMPLICATIONS

Before hormone is given IV, sensitivity should be tested by injecting a small amount subcutaneously or by instilling it into conjunctival sac.

IV flow rate should be slow in case of sensitivity, even though preliminary test may have been negative. Check with physician. Have epinephrine available for emergency treatment when adding parathyroid to another IV fluid; it is recommended that 2.5 to 5% dextrose be used rather than saline in order to prevent precipitation.

Calcium gluconate IV and by mouth is usually ordered with parathyroid injection, particularly during interim before parathyroid effect is established.

If prolonged therapy is indicated, vitamin D_2 and oral Ca are used in preference to parathyroid. Patient soon becomes refractory to the hormone injection.

IM route is preferable to subcutaneous because there is less irritation at injection site.

Frequent determinations of serum Ca and phosphorus levels should be performed during therapy. Most physicians prefer to maintain serum Ca levels at 9 to 11 mg/dl, with 12 mg/dl the outside limit. Normal serum phosphorus level is 3 to 4.5 mg/dl.

Therapy of the deficiency state relieves latent tetany (muscular fatigue) and manifest tetany (paresthesias of extremities, carpopedal spasm, laryngospasm with dyspnea and cyanosis, and spasm of eye muscles, bronchi, stomach, intestines, or urinary bladder, as well as grand mal convulsions).

Until dosage has effectively restored Ca level, prepare for possibility of convulsions: padded bedrails, padded tongue blade, quiet and nonstimulating environment (reduced noise and lights, even temperature levels).

Calcium deficiency is tested by two signs:

Chvostek's sign: Tap seventh cranial nerve (facial) anterior to parotid gland. Muscle contraction of ipsilateral orbicularis oculi, or orbicularis oris, occurs if latent tetany exists.

Trousseau's sign: Grasp patient's wrist so as to constrict circulation for a few minutes, or inflate sphygmomanometer cuff on upper arm to systolic reading. Resulting ischemia of peripheral nerves increases excitability and causes spasm of muscles of lower arm and hand. Carpal spasm occurs in presence of latent tetany.

Be alert for symptoms of drug-induced hypercalcemia. Should they occur (may be due to adrenal insufficiency), discontinue parathyroid injection, Ca salts, and vitamin D. A low-calcium diet, forced fluids, and administration of a phosphate or sulfate laxative may give relief if hypercalcemia is mild.

Monitor intake–output ratio. Increased fluid intake may be ordered to prevent formation of renal stones.

If high-Ca, low-phosphorus diet is prescribed, the patient will be given a drug that blocks absorption of dietary phosphorus (e.g., calcium carbonate or lactate, or aluminum hydroxide suspension) because most foods high in calcium are also high in phosphorus. *See Index for foods high in calcium.*

Store ampules at 2° to 8°C (36°C to 46°F); avoid freezing.

P

Drug Interactions: Parathyroid

Plus	Interactions
Androgens	Decrease of bone resorption activity of parathyroid
Anticonvulsants	Decrease phosphatemic effect of parathyroid
Hydrocortisone	Antagonizes parathyroid effect on Ca absorption from the gut
Dactinomycin	Inhibits bone resorption activity of parathyroid
Thiazide diuretics	Promote hypercalcemia

PROTOTYPE

PAREGORIC

(Opium Tincture, Camphorated)

Opium preparation
Opiate agonist
Antidiarrheal
C III

ACTIONS AND USES. Contains 2 mg anhydrous morphine, alcohol, benzoic acid, camphor, and anise oil. Pharmacologic activity is due to morphine content. Increases smooth muscle tone of GI tract, decreases motility and effective propulsive peristalsis, and diminishes digestive secretions. Delayed transit of intestinal contents results in desiccation of feces and constipation. Available in fixed combination as Brown Mixture: a 12% Paregoric solution with glycyrrhiza fluid extract, antimony potassium tartrate and alcohol.

Used as short-term treatment for symptomatic relief of acute diarrhea and abdominal cramps, and for treatment of neonatal withdrawal syndrome.

ABSORPTION AND FATE. Readily absorbed following oral administration. Duration of action 4 to 5 hours. Metabolized in liver. Half-life: 2 to 3 hours. Excreted in urine.

CONTRAINDICATIONS AND PRECAUTIONS. Hypersensitivity to opium alkaloids, diarrhea caused by poisons (until eliminated). *Cautious Use:* asthma, hepatic disease, history of opiate agonist dependence, severe prostatic hypertrophy.

ADVERSE/SIDE EFFECTS. GI: anorexia, nausea, vomiting, constipation, abdominal pain. **Other (with high doses):** dizziness, faintness, drowsiness, facial flushing, sweating, physical dependence.

ROUTE AND DOSAGE. Oral: *Antidiarrheal:* **Adults:** 5 to 10 ml after bowel movement (may be administered every 2 hours if necessary, up to but not exceeding four times daily until diarrhea is controlled). **Children:** 0.25 to 0.5 ml/kg one to four times daily. *Neonatal withdrawal syndrome:* 3 to 6 drops every 3 to 6 hours as needed, with dose adjustment to control withdrawal symptoms, or *initial:* 0.2 ml every 3 hours with dose increase if needed by about 0.05 ml every 3 hours until symptoms are controlled. Rarely necessary to exceed 0.7 mg/dose. After withdrawal symptoms are stabilized for 3 to 5 days, dose is decreased gradually over a 2- to 4-week period.

NURSING IMPLICATIONS

Not to be confused with opium tincture, deodorized which contains 25 times more anhydrous morphine than the camphorated tincture.

Instruct patient to adhere strictly to prescribed dosage schedule.

Administer Paregoric in sufficient water (2 or 3 swallows) to assure its passage into the stomach (mixture will appear milky).

Possible cause of diarrhea and its duration and accompanying symptoms (e.g., fever, abdominal pain, and passage of mucus or blood) should be investigated. Potential etiologic factors: acute food or chemical poisons; viral, parasitic, or bacterial contamination of food or water; dietary indiscretion; inflammatory disease of GI tract.

Many clinicians feel that Paregoric can worsen the course of diarrhea by delaying the elimination of pathogens.

Bed rest is advisable if diarrhea is severe with a high level of fluid loss.

Replacement of fluids and electrolytes is a vital adjunct to drug therapy for diarrhea. Instruct patient to drink warm clear liquids and to avoid dairy products, concentrated sweets, and cold drinks until diarrhea stops. Physicians generally recommend a bland diet for 2 or 3 days (potato, rice, cooked cereals, eggs, custard, fluid), progressing gradually to normal diet. *(See Index: Nursing Interventions: rehydration.)*

Advise patient to observe character and frequency of stools. Drug should be discontinued as soon as diarrhea is controlled. Urge patient to report promptly to physician: if diarrhea persists more than 3 days, if fever is above 38.8°C (102°F), abdominal pain develops, or if mucus or blood is passed.

Inform patient that constipation is often a consequence of antidiarrheal treatment and that normal habit pattern is usually established as dietary intake increases.

Although the volume of morphine in Paregoric is small (0.4 mg/ml), prolonged use or excessive amounts can lead to physical dependence. Parents should be warned not to use Paregoric to quiet an irritable child or to sooth sore gums during teeth eruption.

Symptoms of *neonatal withdrawal syndrome* (tremulousness, irritability, excessive crying, reduced sleep periods, high pitched cry) may appear immediately after umbilical cord is cut, if a narcotic antagonist is given to the infant for presumed depression due to intrapartum sedative administration.

Addiction to heroin will appear within 4 days after birth (occasionally 7 days after birth). Withdrawal from methodone is usually evident within first few days but may be delayed for 2 to 4 weeks.

Drug treatment of neonatal withdrawal syndrome is augmented by close monitoring of vital signs and intake and output, and by increased fluids and calories as required by the effects of diarrhea, vomiting, sweating, increased motor activity.

Paregoric reportedly restores the sucking reflex to normal, more rapidly than other nonselective sedatives. However, because Paregoric contains camphor and benzoic acid (may cause potential adverse effects), some clinicians recommend use of diluted deodorized opium tincture instead.

Keep Paregoric out of possible reach of children.

Paregoric is classified as a Schedule III drug under the Federal Controlled Substances Act. Commercial preparations containing small amounts of Paregoric are classified under Schedule V (in certain circumstances they may be dispensed without prescription unless additional state regulations apply): e.g., Diabismul.

Preserved in tight, light-resistant container, at controlled room temperature preferably between 15° and 30°C (59° and 86°F), unless otherwise directed by manufacturer.

PARGYLINE HYDROCHLORIDE

(Eutonyl)

(par'gi-leen)
Antihypertensive
MAO inhibitor

ACTIONS AND USES. Nonhydrazine MAO inhibitor with pharmacologic actions similar to those of other MAO inhibitors. Like phenelzine (qv), but reportedly less hepatotoxic. Exerts hypotensive effect and reportedly produces mood elevation. Mechanism of hypotensive activity not known but thought to be related in part to modification of ganglionic transmission. Most prominent effect is orthostatic (hypotensive).

Used in treatment of moderate to severe hypertension. May be used concurrently with other antihypertensive agents such as thiazides and/or rauwolfia alkaloids. Commercially available in fixed-dose combination with methyclothiazide (e.g., Eutron).

ABSORPTION AND FATE. Excreted primarily in urine as unchanged drug.

CONTRAINDICATIONS AND PRECAUTIONS. Mild, labile, or malignant hypertension; hyperactive or excitable individuals; paranoid schizophrenia; hyperthyroidism; pheochromocytoma; advanced renal failure. Safe use during pregnancy, lactation, in women of childbearing potential, and in children under 12 years of age not established. *Cautious Use:* liver disease, arteriosclerosis, coronary artery disease, parkinsonism, diabetes mellitus.

ADVERSE/SIDE EFFECTS. Orthostatic hypotension, sweating, dry mouth, fluid retention, congestive heart failure, increased appetite, weight gain, nausea, vomiting, mild constipation, headache, arthralgia, difficulty in micturition, impotence or delayed ejaculation, rash, purpura, nightmares, hyperexcitability, muscle twitching and other extrapyramidal symptoms, drug fever (rare), hypoglycemia (optic atrophy not reported, although it is associated with use of other MAO inhibitors). *Overdosage:* agitation, confusion, hallucinations, mania, hyperreflexia, convulsions, hyperextension or hypotension.

ROUTE AND DOSAGE. Oral: Initial: 25 mg once daily; may be increased once a week by 10-mg increments until desired response is obtained. Total daily dose not to exceed 200 mg. **Elderly or sympathectomized patients:** Initial 10 to 25 mg daily for first 2 weeks. **Addition to established antihypertensive regimen:** initial dose should not exceed 25 mg (less in elderly or sympathectomized patients). Maintenance: 50 to 75 mg daily.

NURSING IMPLICATIONS

Dosage adjustments are based on blood pressure in standing position.

Instruct patient to report symptoms of orthostatic hypotension (dizziness, weakness, palpitation, fainting); dosage adjustment is indicated.

Warn patient to make position changes slowly, especially when getting out of bed, and to lie or sit down immediately if feeling dizzy or faint.

Pargyline may unmask psychotic symptoms in some patients with preexisting emotional problems.

Febrile illnesses can potentiate the hypotensive effect of pargyline. Temporary drug withdrawal may be necessary.

Dry mouth may be relieved by frequent rinsing with clear water, increasing noncaloric fluid intake if inadequate (and if allowed), or by sugarless gum or lemondrops. If these measures fail, consult physician about use of a saliva substitute, e.g., VA-Ora-Lube, Moi-stir, Xero-Lube.

Advise patient not to take alcohol, sedatives, tranquilizers, or other CNS depressants without prior approval of physician.

Actions of pargyline are cumulative. Maximal therapeutic effect may occur in 4 days, but it may not appear for 3 weeks or more; action may persist for 3 weeks after therapy is discontinued.

Instruct patient to keep daily record of weight and to check ankles and tibias for edema. Pargyline tends to promote weight gain from fluid retention as well as nonfluid retention (increased appetite).

Patients with impaired renal function should be closely observed for signs of cumulative drug effects. Monitor intake and output and BUN in these patients.

Although optic damage has not been reported with pargyline, patients on prolonged therapy should be checked periodically for changes in color perception, visual fields, fundi, and visual acuity.

Patients with diabetes may require adjustment in antidiabetic medication. Severe drug-induced hypoglycemia can occur.

Since drug may suppress anginal pain, patient should be warned not to increase physical activity in response to drug-induced sense of well-being.

Urinalyses, liver function tests, and complete blood counts should be performed periodically during therapy.

Tolerance to pargyline develops rapidly. Urge patient to keep scheduled follow-up appointments.

Drug may augment hypotensive effects of anesthetic agents, and therefore should be discontinued at least 2 weeks prior to elective surgery.

If drug therapy is temporarily interrupted for any reason, it should be reinstituted at a lower dosage level.

Caution patient not to add any medication to drug regimen without consulting physician. OTC preparations containing dextromethorphan or sympathomimetic amines can precipitate hypertensive crisis (e.g., appetite suppressants, nasal decongestants, cold and hay fever remedies).

Acute hypertensive reaction (severe headache, marked hypertension, chest pain, palpitation, tachycardia, bradycardia) can result from ingestion of foods or liquids high in tyramine or tryptophan. Provide family or responsible family member with list of foods to avoid *(see Phenelzine for Food–Drug Interactions).*

See Phenelzine (prototype MAO inhibitor).

PAROMOMYCIN SULFATE

(Humatin)

(par-oh-moe-mye'sin)

Antiinfective

Antibiotic, amebicide

Aminoglycoside

ACTIONS AND USES. Aminoglycoside antibiotic produced by certain strains of *Streptomyces rimosus* with broad spectrum of antibacterial activity closely parallelling that of kanamycin and neomycin (qv). Exerts direct bactericidal and amebicidal action, primarily in lumen of GI tract. Ineffective against extraintestinal amebiasis. Reportedly produces significant reduction in serum cholesterol.

Used for treatment of acute and chronic intestinal amebiasis and to rid bowel of nitrogen-forming bacteria in patients with hepatic coma; used preoperatively to suppress intestinal flora. Also has been used for tapeworm infestation.

ABSORPTION AND FATE. Poorly absorbed from intact GI tract; almost 100% of dose is recoverable in feces.

P

CONTRAINDICATIONS AND PRECAUTIONS. History of hypersensitivity to paromomycin; intestinal obstruction, impaired renal function. *Cautious Use:* GI ulceration.

ADVERSE/SIDE EFFECTS. CNS: headache, vertigo. **GI:** (frequent): diarrhea, abdominal cramps, steatorrhea, nausea, vomiting, heartburn, secondary enterocolitis. **Skin:** exanthema, rash, pruritus. **Other:** ototoxicity, nephrotoxicity (in patients with GI inflammation or ulcerations), eosinophilia, overgrowth of nonsusceptible organisms.

ROUTE AND DOSAGE. Oral: *Intestinal amebiasis:* **Adults and children:** 25 to 35 mg/kg divided in 3 doses, for 5 to 10 days. *Hepatic coma:* **Adults:** 4 Gm daily in divided doses, given at regular intervals for 5 or 6 days.

NURSING IMPLICATIONS

Usually administered after meals to prevent gastric distress.

Be alert for appearance of any new infection (superinfection) during therapy, e.g., foul-smelling stools or vaginal discharge, anal or vaginal itching.

Patients with history of GI ulceration must be closely monitored for nephrotoxicity and ototoxicity. Drug absorption can take place through diseased mucosa.
Patients receiving drug for intestinal amebiasis should be excluded from preparing, processing, and serving food until treatment is complete. Isolation is not required.
Emphasize personal hygiene, particularly handwashing after defecation and before eating food, and sanitary disposal of feces.
Criterion of cure is absence of amebae in stool specimens examined at weekly intervals for 6 weeks after completion of treatment, and thereafter at monthly intervals for 2 years.
Possible sources of contamination (e.g., water, food, infected persons) should be investigated.
Household members and other suspected contacts should have microscopic examination of feces for amebae.
See Metronidazole (prototype amebicide).

Diagnostic Test Interferences. Prolonged use of paromomycin may cause reduction in **serum cholesterol.**

PEMOLINE

(Cylert, Pioxol)

(pem'oh-leen)
Central stimulant
C IV

ACTIONS AND USES. Oxazolidinone derivative with pharmacologic actions qualitatively similar to those of amphetamine and methylphenidate, but with weak sympathomimetic activity. Capable of producing increased motor activity, mental alertness, diminished sense of fatigue, and mild euphoria. Also thought to have anorexigenic effect.

Used as adjunctive therapy to other remedial measures (psychologic, educational, social) in minimal brain dysfunction (hyperkinetic behavior disorders) in carefully selected children. *Investigational Use:* as a mild stimulant for geriatric patients.

ABSORPTION AND FATE. Absorbed from GI tract. Peak serum levels within 2 to 4 hours. CNS stimulation effect peaks within 4 hours and lasts at least 8 hours. Serum half-life about 12 hours. Approximately 50% bound to plasma proteins. Distribution unknown. Probably metabolized in part by liver to active and inactive metabolites; 75% excreted in urine (43% unchanged, 22% as conjugates) within 24 hours.

CONTRAINDICATIONS AND PRECAUTIONS. Known hypersensitivity to pemoline; children younger than 6 years of age. Safe use during pregnancy and lactation not established. *Cautious Use:* impaired hepatic and renal function, history of drug abuse, psychosis, emotional instability.

ADVERSE/SIDE EFFECTS. Insomnia, anorexia, abdominal discomfort, malaise, nausea, diarrhea, skin rash, irritability, fatigue, mild depression, dizziness, headache, drowsiness, dyskinetic movements of eyes or other parts of body; convulsions. *Overdosage:* nervousness, tachycardia, hallucinations, excitement, agitation, restlessness. *Also reported:* elevated SGOT, SGPT, and alkaline phosphatase (after several months of therapy); jaundice, reversible hepatic damage (rare).

ROUTE AND DOSAGE. Oral: Children (6 years of age and older): Initial: 37.5 mg daily; may be increased by 18.75 mg at weekly intervals until desired clinical response is obtained. Effective dose range: 56.25 mg to 75 mg daily. Maximum recommended daily dose 112.5 mg.

NURSING IMPLICATIONS

Administer drug in morning to provide maximal effectiveness during waking hours and to avoid insomnia.

Chewable tablet form may be chewed or swallowed whole.

Insomnia and anorexia (most frequent side effects) appear to be dose-related.

Monitor weight and height (growth rate) throughout therapy. Anorexia is often accompanied by weight loss, particularly during first few weeks of therapy. Although growth suppression has not been reported with pemoline, it has been associated with other CNS stimulants used in children.

Caution patient to avoid potentially hazardous activities until the reaction to drug is known.

Significant benefits of drug therapy may not be evident until third or fourth week of drug administration.

Careful clinical evaluation and supervision of patient are essential. Patients receiving long-term therapy should have periodic liver function studies.

Occasional interruption of drug therapy is advised to determine if behavioral symptoms recur.

Pemoline can produce tolerance and physical and psychologic dependence.

Classified as Schedule IV drug under Federal Controlled Substances Act.

Store at controlled room temperature, preferably between 15° and 30°C (59° and 86°F) unless otherwise directed by manufacturer.

PENICILLAMINE

(pen-i-sill'a-meen)

(Cuprimine, Depen)

Chelating agent

ACTIONS AND USES. Thiol compound prepared by hydrolysis of penicillin but lacking antibacterial activity. Forms stable soluble chelate with copper, zinc, iron, lead, mercury, and possibly other heavy metals and promotes their excretion in urine. Also combines chemically with cystine to form a soluble disulfide complex which prevents stone formation and may even dissolve existing cystitic stones. Mechanism of action in rheumatoid arthritis not known, but appears to be related to inhibition of collagen formation. Cross-sensitivity between penicillin and penicillamine can occur.

Used to promote renal excretion of excess copper in Wilson's disease (hepatolenticular degeneration). Also used in patients with active rheumatoid arthritis who have failed to respond to conventional therapy, and in treatment of moderate asymptomatic lead poisoning. *Investigational Use:* in the management of scleroderma, primary biliary cirrhosis, and porphyria cutanea tarda.

ABSORPTION AND FATE. Well absorbed from GI tract. Peak blood levels in 1 hour. Probably metabolized in liver. Readily excreted in urine and feces primarily as inactive disulfides. Crosses placenta.

CONTRAINDICATIONS AND PRECAUTIONS. Hypersensitivity to penicillamine or to any penicillin; history of penicillamine-related aplastic anemia or agranulocytosis, patients with rheumatoid arthritis who have renal insufficiency or who are pregnant, during pregnancy in patients with cystinuria, concomitant administration with drugs that can cause severe hematologic or renal reactions, e.g., antimalarials, gold salts, immunosuppressants, oxyphenbutazone, phenylbutazone. *Cautious Use:* allergy-prone individuals.

ADVERSE/SIDE EFFECTS. Allergic: generalized pruritus, urticaria, early and late occurring rashes, pemphiguslike rash, fever, arthralgia, lymphadenopathy, thyroiditis, systemic-lupus-erthematosus-like syndrome. **GI:** anorexia, nausea, vomiting, epigastric pain, diarrhea, oral lesions, reduction or loss of taste perception (particularly salt and sweet), metallic taste, activation of peptic ulcer. **Hematologic:** thrombocytopenia, leukopenia, agranulocytosis, thrombotic thrombocytopenic purpura, hemolytic anemia, aplastic anemia. **Hepatotoxicity:** cholestatic jaundice. **Nephrotoxicity:** membranous glomerulopathy, Goodpasture's syndrome, proteinuria, hematuria. **Other:** tinnitus, optic neuritis, thrombophlebitis, hyperpyrexia, alopecia, myasthenia gravis syndrome, mammary hyperplasia, alveolitis, skin friability, excessive skin wrinkling, pancreatitis, pyridoxine deficiency, tingling of feet, ptosis, weakness.

ROUTE AND DOSAGE. Oral: Adults: *Wilson's disease:* 250 mg four times daily. **Children:** 20 mg/kg/day divided into 4 doses. *Cystinuria:* **Adults:** 250 mg four times daily. **Children:** 30 mg/kg/day divided into 4 doses. Dosages individualized to amount that limits cystine excretion to 100 to 200 mg/day in patients with no history of stones, and below 100 mg/day in those who have had stone formation or pain. *Rheumatoid arthritis:* Initial: 125 or 250 mg daily. Dosage increases of 125 or 250 mg/day at 1- to 3-month intervals, if necessary. Maximum daily dosage up to 1 to 1.5 Gm daily.

NURSING IMPLICATIONS

Not to be confused with penicillin.

Administered on an empty stomach (30 to 60 minutes before or 2 hours after meals) to avoid absorption of metals in foods by penicillamine.

If patient cannot swallow capsules or tablets, contents may be administered in 15 to 30 ml of chilled fruit juice.

All patients should be closely monitored throughout therapy. Penicillamine can produce severe toxic reactions involving skin, blood, kidneys, and liver. Most reactions respond favorably if drug is discontinued.

Allergic reactions occur in about one-third of patients receiving penicillamine. Temporary interruptions of therapy increase possibility of sensitivity reactions.

Temperature should be taken nightly during first few months of therapy. Fever is a possible early sign of allergy.

White and differential blood cell counts, direct platelet counts, hemoglobin, and urinalyses should be done prior to initiation of therapy and every 3 days during the first month of therapy then every 2 weeks thereafter. Liver function tests and eye examinations should be performed before start of therapy and at least twice yearly thereafter.

Instruct patient to observe skin over pressure sites: knees, elbows, shoulder blades, toes, buttocks. Penicillamine increases skin friability. Report unusual bruising or bleeding, sore mouth or throat, fever, skin rash, or any other unusual symptoms.

For patients undergoing elective surgery, physician may reduce dosage because penicillamine tends to retard tissue healing by inhibiting collagen and elastin formation.

Physician may prescribe prophylactic doses of pyridoxine (vitamin B_6) because penicillamine interferes with the metabolism of this vitamin.

Clinical evidence of therapeutic effectiveness may not be apparent until 1 to 3 months of drug therapy.

Wilson's disease: Physician may prescribe sulfurated potash before each meal to minimize absorption of copper.

Patients with Wilson's disease will require a low copper diet (less than 2 mg copper daily). Foods high in copper that should be avoided include: alcoholic beverages, chocolate, tea, all organs meats, all shellfish, duck, goose, meat gelatin, molasses, mushrooms, nuts, dried beans, dried lentils, bran products.

Drinking water should be analyzed for copper content. Demineralized water should be used if copper content is more than 0.1 mg/L.

Therapeutic effectiveness in Wilson's disease is indicated by improvement in psychiatric and neurologic symptoms, visual symptoms, and hepatic function. In some patients, neurologic symptoms become more prominent during initial therapy and then subside.

Optimal dose for patients with Wilson's disease is determined by quantitative analysis of urinary copper. Urine must be collected in copper-free container.

Cystinuria: Penicillamine may be used alone or in addition to conventional therapy, maintenance of urinary pH at 7.5 to 8 by administration of alkalis, sufficient fluids (3000 to 4000 ml/24 hours) to keep urine specific gravity below 1.010, and a low methionine diet. (Cystine is the end product of methionine metabolism.) Low methionine diet is not recommended in children or during pregnancy because it is low in protein.

If 4 equally divided doses are not possible, the larger dose should be given at bedtime. When adjustments in dosage must be made, the bedtime dose should be retained.

Patients with cystinuria should be instructed to drink a pint (500 ml) of water at bedtime and again during the night because urine tends to be more acidic and concentrated at night.

Rheumatoid arthritis: Record evidence of drug effectiveness such as improvement in grip strength, decrease in stiffness following immobility, reduction of pain, decrease in sedimentation rate and rheumatoid factor.

Dosage should be reduced or drug discontinued if the patient with rheumatoid arthritis develops proteinuria greater than 1 Gm (some clinicians accept up to 2 Gm), or if platelet count drops to less than 100,000/m^3 or platelet count falls below 3500 to 4000/mm^3, or neutropenia occurs.

Drug Interactions. Potentiation of hematologic and renal adverse effects may occur with **antimalarials, cytotoxics, gold therapy, oxyphenbutazone,** and **phenylbutazone.** Oral iron may inhibit absorption of penicillamine. (Space as far apart as possible.)

PENICILLIN G BENZATHINE

(Bicillin, Bicillin L-A, Megacillin Suspension, Permapen)

(pen-i-sill'in)
Antiinfective
Antibiotic (Beta-lactam)
Penicillin

P

ACTIONS AND USES. Acid-stable, penicillinase-sensitive, repository (long-acting) form of penicillin G. Because it has extremely low water solubility, it is absorbed slowly in body. Produces lower blood concentrations than other penicillin G compounds, but has the longest duration of antimicrobial activity of all other available parenteral or repository penicillins. Has local anesthetic effect comparable to that of penicillin G procaine. Like penicillin G (qv) in actions, uses, contraindications, precautions, and adverse reactions.

Used in the treatment of infections highly susceptible to penicillin G, such as streptococcal, pneumococcal, and staphylococcal infections, veneral disease such as syphilis (including early late and congenital forms), and nonvenereal diseases, e.g., yaws, bejel, and pinta. Also used in prophylaxis of rheumatic fever.

ABSORPTION AND FATE. Absorption rate is not reliable following oral administration; however, effective blood levels may last up to 6 hours. When given IM, forms tissue depot from which penicillin is slowly released; serum levels peak in about 12 to 24 hours. Average duration of therapeutic blood levels is 26 days, but may persist for 4 weeks. Converted by hydrolysis to penicillin (qv) in body. Distributed throughout body tissue and fluids. Highest levels in kidneys; lesser amounts in liver, skin, intestines, and spinal fluid. Approximately 60% bound to serum proteins. Excreted slowly by kidneys. Urinary excretion is considerably delayed in patients with impaired renal function and in young infants.

CONTRAINDICATIONS AND PRECAUTIONS. Hypersensitivity to penicillins or cephalosporins. *Cautious Use:* history of or suspected atopy or allergy (eczema, hives, hay fever, asthma).

ADVERSE/SIDE EFFECTS. Local pain, tenderness, and fever associated with IM injection, Jarisch-Herxheimer reaction in patients with syphilis *(see Penicillin G)*. **Hypersensitivity reactions:** (pruritus, urticaria and other skin eruptions, chills, fever, wheezing, anaphylaxis, eosinophilia, hemolytic anemia and other blood abnormalities, neuropathy, nephrotoxicity); myocarditis (rare), superinfections. *See Penicillin G.*

ROUTE AND DOSAGE. Adults and Children (12 years and over): Oral: 400,000 to 600,000 units every 4 to 6 hours; *rheumatic fever prophylaxis;* 200,000 units every 12 hours, on a continuing basis. **Intramuscular:** 1.2 to 2.4 million units as single dose: *rheumatic fever prophylaxis:* 1.2 million units once a month or 600,000 units every 2 weeks. **Children (under 12 years): Oral:** 25,000 to 90,000 units/kg/day in 3 to 6 equally divided doses. **Intramuscular:** 600,000 to 1.2 million units as a single dose to 1.2 million units monthly.

NURSING IMPLICATIONS

Careful inquiry should be made concerning previous hypersensitivity reactions to penicillins, cephalosporins, or other allergens.

Not to be confused with preparations containing penicillin G benzathine in combination with procaine penicillin G (e.g., Bicillin C-R).

As with other penicillins, therapy should be guided by bacteriologic studies, susceptibility test, and clinical response.

Absorption of oral tablet is not significantly affected by food.

Instruct patient to take medication around the clock, not to miss a dose, and to continue taking medication until it is all gone.

Shake multiple-dose vial vigorously before withdrawing desired IM dose. Shake prepared cartridge unit vigorously before injecting drug.

IM injection should be made deep into upper outer quadrant of buttock. In infants and small children, the preferred site is the midlateral aspect of the thigh.

Select IM site with care. Injection into or near a major peripheral nerve can result in nerve damage.

Check for blood backflow before injecting drug; if blood appears, remove needle and select another site. Inadvertent intravascular administration has resulted in arterial occlusion and cardiac arrest.

Injections should be made at a slow steady rate to prevent needle blockage.

Instruct patient to report immediately to physician the onset of an allergic reaction. There is great risk of severe and prolonged reactions, because drug is absorbed so slowly.

See Penicillin G.

PROTOTYPE

PENICILLIN G POTASSIUM
(M-Cillin B, Pentids, Pfizerpen, SK-Penicillin G)
PENICILLIN G SODIUM

Antiinfective
Antibiotic
Penicillin

ACTIONS AND USES. Acid-labile, penicillinase-sensitive, natural penicillin derived from cultures of *Penicillium notatum* or related molds. Antimicrobial spectrum is relatively narrow compared to that of the semisynthetic penicillins. Bactericidal at therapeutic serum levels; bacteriostatic at lower concentrations. Acts by interfering with synthesis of mucopeptides essential to formation and integrity of bacterial cell wall. Effective primarily on immature cell walls of rapidly growing and dividing cells; minimally or ineffective on dormant or mature organisms. Action is inhibited by penicillinase; therefore penicillin G is ineffective against many strains of *Staphylococcus aureus.* Highly active against **gram-positive cocci** (e.g., nonpenicillinase-producing *Staphylococcus,* Streptococcus groups A,C,G,H,L,M, and *S. pneumoniae*); and **gram-negative cocci** *(Neisseria gonorrhoeae, N. meningitidis).* Also effective against **gram-positive bacilli** *(Bacillus anthracis, Clostridium* species including gas gangrene and tetanus, and certain species of *Corynebacterium, Erysipelothrix,* and *Listeria*); **gram-negative bacilli** (Fusobacterium, Pasteurella, Streptobacillus, and *Bacteroides* species. Parenteral penicillin G is effective against most strains of *Escherichia coli,* all strains of *Proteus mirabilis, Salmonella,* and *Shigella,* and some strains of *Enterobacter aerogenes,* and *Alcaligenes faecalis*); **Spirochetes** *(Treponema pallidum, T. pertenue, Leptospira);* **Actinomycetes** *(A. bovis, A. israelii).* The penicillins are not active against fungi, plasmodia, amebae, rickettsiae, and viruses. In large doses, penicillin G is capable of inhibiting platelet aggregation and may also act as a CNS irritant.

Used in treatment of infections caused by penicillin-sensitive microorganisms: actinomycosis, anthrax, diphtheria (carrier state), empyema, erysipelas, gas gangrene, gonorrheal infections, leptospirosis, mastoiditis, meningitis, acute osteomyelitis, otitis media, pinta, pneumonia, rat-bite fever, sinus infections; certain staphylococcal infections; streptococcal infections, including scarlet fever; syphilis (all stages), tetanus, urinary tract infections, Vincent's gingivostomatitis, yaws. Also used as prophylaxis in patients with rheumatic or congenital heart disease. Since oral preparations are absorbed erratically and thus must be given in comparatively high doses, this route is generally used only for mild or stabilized infections or long-term prophylaxis.

ABSORPTION AND FATE. Absorption following oral administration is irregular and incomplete and occurs chiefly in the duodenum. Only about 30% of oral dose absorbed (susceptible to destruction by gastric acid and penicillinase-producing intestinal bacteria). Absorption may be more complete in patients with low gastric acidity, e.g., infants, the elderly. Readily absorbed following IM administration; serum levels peak in 15 to 30 minutes and persist 3 to 5 hours. Diffuses rapidly into most body fluids and tissues including kidneys, liver, skin, bile, lymph; peritoneal, pleural, pericardial, and joint spaces; small amounts of saliva, and prostatic secretion. Adequate absorption into cerebrospinal fluid and eye occurs when inflammation is present. About 45 to 65% bound to plasma proteins. Half-life: 30 to 60 minutes. Excreted in urine mostly as unchanged drug (approximately 60 to 90% of IM dose eliminated within 5 hours). Excretion delayed in neonates, young infants, the elderly, and patients with impaired renal function. Small amounts excreted in feces. Crosses placenta. Appears in breast milk.

CONTRAINDICATIONS AND PRECAUTIONS. Hypersensitivity to any of the penicillins or cephalosporins; administration of oral drug to patients with severe infections, nausea, vomiting, hypermotility, gastric dilatation, cardiospasm. Pentids (Squibb) contains tartrazine to which some patients may be allergic (notably, patients with aspirin hypersensitivity); use of penicillin G sodium in patients on sodium restriction. *Cautious Use:* history of or suspected atopy or allergy, (asthma, eczema, hay fever, hives); renal or hepatic dysfunction, myasthenia gravis, epilepsy, neonates, young infants. Use in nursing mothers may lead to sensitization of infants.

ADVERSE/SIDE EFFECTS. **Electrolyte imbalance:** hyperkalemia (penicillin G potassium); hypokalemia, alkalosis, hypernatremia, congestive heart failure (penicillin G sodium). **Hypersensitivity reactions.** **(1) immediate** (usually occurs within 2 to 30 minutes after drug administration); *localized anaphylaxis:* itchy palms or axilla or generalized pruritus or urticaria, flushed skin, coughing, sneezing, feeling of uneasiness; *systemic anaphylaxis:* fever, vomiting, diarrhea, severe abdominal cramps, widespread increase in capillary permeability and vasodilation with resulting edema (mouth, tongue, pharynx, larynx), laryngospasm, bronchospasm, hypotension, circulatory collapse (anaphylactic shock), cardiac arrhythmias, cardiac arrest. **(2) Accelerated** (occurs in 1 to 72 hours): malaise, fever, urticaria, erythema or other skin reactions and (less commonly) angioneurotic and laryngeal edema, asthma. **(3) Delayed or late** (develops after 72 hours): *serum sickness* (fever, malaise, pruritus, urticaria, lymphadenopathy, arthralgia, angioedema of face and extremities, neuritis prostration, eosinophilia). Skin rashes ranging from urticaria to exfoliative dermatitis, Stevens-Johnson syndrome, fixed-drug eruptions, contact dermatitis; hemolytic anemia, granulocytopenia, neutropenia, leukopenia, thrombocytopenia, SLE-like syndrome, interstitial nephritis, Loeffler's syndrome, vasculitis. **Injection site reactions:** pain, inflammation, abscess, phlebitis, thrombophlebitis. **Superinfections:** especially with Candida and gram-negative bacteria (e.g., *Proteus, Pseudomonas*). **Toxicity:** bone marrow depression, granulocytopenia, hepatitis (infrequent), neuromuscular irritability: twitching, lethargy, confusion, stupor, hyperreflexia, multifocal myoclonus, localized or generalized seizures, coma. **With oral therapy:** nausea, vomiting, epigastric distress, diarrhea, flatulence, dark discoloration of tongue, sore mouth or tongue. **Other:** increased bleeding time, Jarisch-Herxheimer reaction (syphilis).

ROUTE AND DOSAGE. **Oral:** **Adults and Children (over 12 years):** 200,000 to 500,000 units every 6 to 8 hours. *For prophylaxis:* 200,000 to 400,000 units twice daily. **Children (under 12 years):** 25,000 to 90,000 units/kg daily in 3 to 6 divided doses. **Intramuscular, intravenous (slowly by continuous infusion):** **Adults:** 1 to 20 million units daily. Doses of 80 million units daily have been used for serious infections. **Children:** 50,000 to 250,000 units/kg daily in 4 to 6 divided doses (up to 10 million units daily have been infused IV).

P

NURSING IMPLICATIONS

Before treatment with penicillin is initiated, an exact history should be obtained of patient's previous exposure and sensitivity to penicillins and cephalosporins, and other allergic reactions of any kind.

Patients who have a history of mild sensitivity to penicillin may be given a scratch test and/or intradermal test to assess the risk of penicillin therapy. Special antigens are used for the test, e.g., Benzylpenicilloyl-polylysine, abbreviated BPO-PL (Pre-Pen).

Check expiration date on penicillin container or package label. Also note whether physician has prescribed penicillin G potassium or sodium.

Penicillin G potassium contains approximately 1.7 mEq of potassium/and 0.3 mEq of sodium/million units. Penicillin G sodium contains 2 mEq of sodium/million units.

The patient should be informed that he or she is going to receive penicillin therapy.

Oral penicillin G should be taken on an empty stomach, at least 1 hour before or 2 hours after meals, to reduce possibility of destruction by gastric acid and delay in absorption by food.

Administer with a full glass of water. Instruct patient to avoid acidic beverages 1 hour before and after taking oral penicillin G.

Measure liquid dosage form with specially marked measuring device. Household teaspoons vary in measure and therefore are not advised.

When used for infection, penicillin is to be taken around the clock (i.e., 3 times/day means every 8 hours, four times/day every 6 hours, etc.) Instruct patient not to miss any doses and to continue taking the medication until it is all gone, unless otherwise directed by the physician.

Culture and sensitivity tests should be done to determine course of therapy; however, treatment may be started before results are known.

Parenteral administration: See manufacturer's labeling for directions on preparation of initial dilution. Loosen powder by tapping vial against palm of hand. Holding vial horizontally, rotate it while directing stream of diluent against wall of vial. Shake vial vigorously until powder is completely dissolved. (For IV administration, the initial dilution should be further diluted with 0.9% sodium chloride or 5% dextrose for IV use.)

Carefully select IM site. Accidental injection into or near a nerve can cause irritation with severe pain and dysfunction. IM injection is made deep into a large muscle mass. Before injecting drug, check for blood back-flow to avoid entering a blood vessel. Inject slowly. Rotate injection sites.

Lidocaine hydrochloride 1% or 2% (without epinephrine) may be prescribed by the physician to minimize pain associated with IM injection.

In high doses, IV penicillin G should be administered slowly to avoid electrolyte imbalance from potassium or sodium content. Physician will prescribe specific flow rate.

Penicillin is a highly sensitizing substance. Contact dermatitis can occur in certain susceptible individuals who are frequently in contact with the drug. Babies whose mothers are receiving penicillin therapy can be sensitized through breast milk.

The incidence of hypersensitivity to penicillin among adults in the U.S. is estimated to be between 1% and 5% (reports vary).

Allergy to penicillin is unpredictable. It has occurred in patients with a negative history of penicillin allergy and also in patients with no known prior contact with penicillin (sensitization may have occurred from penicillin used commercially in foods and beverages, e.g., Roquefort or bleu cheese, fowl, beer). Paradoxically, some patients with mild sensitivity have tolerated penicillin at a later date.

Hypersensitivity reactions are more likely to occur with parenteral penicillin but may also occur with the oral drug. Skin rash is the most common type allergic reaction and should be reported promptly to physician.

Reactions to penicillin may be rapid in onset or may not appear for days or weeks *(see Adverse/Side Effects).* Symptoms usually disappear fairly quickly once drug is stopped, but in some patients may persist for 5 days or more and require hospitalization for treatment.

Observe all patients closely for at least one-half hour following administration of parenteral penicillin. The rapid appearance of a red flare or wheal at the IM or IV injection site is a possible sign of sensitivity. Report to physician. Also suspect an allergic reaction if patient becomes irritable, has nausea and vomiting, breathing difficulty, or sudden fever.

Have on hand tourniquet, epinephrine, an antihistamine, e.g., diphenhydramine (Benadryl), and aminophylline, hydrocortisone (e.g., Solu-Cortef), suction, and equipment for endotracheal intubation and tracheostomy.

If patient is found to be allergic to penicillin, note this in prominent place on chart, Kardex, and at the bedside. Advise patient to carry a Medic Alert or similar type bracelet and wallet card with this information and to be sure to communicate it to the attending physician at any future time.

Neuromuscular irritability occurs most commonly in patients receiving parenteral penicillin in excess of 20 million units/day who have renal insufficiency, hyponatremia, or underlying CNS disease, notably myasthenia gravis or epilepsy. Seizure precautions are indicated. Symptoms usually begin with twitching, especially of face and extremities *(see also Adverse /Side Effects).*

Some patients receiving penicillin for treatment of syphilis develop Jarisch-Herxheimer reaction. This reaction resembles penicillin allergy, but is thought to be due to the toxic products released from spirochetes killed by penicillin. It occurs 8 to 24 hours following treatment with penicillin and is characterized by headache, chills, fever, myalgia, arthralgia, malaise, and worsening of syphilitic skin lesions. Advise patient to notify physician if these symptoms appear. The reaction is usually self-limiting.

Monitor intake and output particularly in patients receiving high parenteral doses. Report oliguria, hematuria, and changes in intake–output ratio. Consult physician regarding optimum fluid intake. Dehydration increases the concentration of drug in kidneys and can cause renal irritation and damage.

Neonates, young infants, the elderly, and patients with impaired renal function receiving high-dose penicillin therapy should be closely observed for signs of toxicity *(see Adverse /Side Effects).* Urinary excretion of penicillin is significantly delayed in these patients.

Patients with diabetes who are receiving massive doses of penicillin should be advised of the possibility of obtaining false-positive urine glucose test results *(see Diagnostic Test Interferences).*

It is reported that therapeutic failure has occurred in some adult diabetic patients receiving IM penicillin G. Close monitoring is indicated.

Patients on high-dose therapy should be closely observed for evidence of bleeding, and bleeding time should be monitored. (In high doses, penicillin interferes with platelet aggregation.)

Patients receiving prolonged treatment should have evaluations of renal, hepatic, and hematologic systems at regular intervals. Additionally, electrolyte balance and cardiovascular status should be checked periodically in patients receiving high parenteral doses.

Instruct patient to take medication around the clock, not to miss a dose, and to continue taking medication until it is all gone, unless otherwise directed by physician.

Instruct patient to report signs and symptoms of superinfection: black, furry overgrowth on tongue, rectal or vaginal itching, vaginal discharge, loose, foul-smelling stools, unusual odor to urine.

Advise patient to check with physician if symptoms do not improve within a few days or if they get worse.

At least 10 days of continuous treatment is recommended for streptococcal infections to prevent possible sequelae such as rheumatic fever. Cultures should be taken following completion of treatment to determine need for further medication. Impress on patient the importance of medical follow-up; present evidence suggests that glomerulonephritis, a possible complication of streptococcal infection, may not be prevented by penicillin.

The stability of penicillin G is affected by changes in pH (most stable at pH 6.0 to 7.0) and, therefore, it is physically incompatible with many drugs. Be guided by product information brochures and by pharmacist concerning incompatibilities.

Store penicillin G tablets at room temperature in tightly-closed containers. Avoid excessive heat. Store oral suspensions and syrups in refrigerator and discard unused portions after 14 days. The dry powder (for parenteral use) may be stored at room temperature. After reconstitution (initial dilution), solutions may be stored for 1 week under refrigeration. Intravenous infusion solutions containing penicillin G are stable at room temperature for at least 24 hours.

Diagnostic Test Interferences. **Blood grouping and compatibility tests:** Possible interference associated with penicillin doses greater than 20 million units daily. **Urine glucose:** Massive doses of penicillin may cause false-positive test results with Benedict's solution and possibly Clinitest, but not with glucose oxidase methods, e.g., Clinistix, Diastix, Tes-Tape. **Urine protein:** Massive doses of penicillin can produce false-positive results when turbidity measures are used (e.g., acetic acid and heat, sulfosalicylic acid); Ames reagent reportedly not affected. **Urinary PSP excretion tests:** False decrease in urinary excretion of PSP. **Urinary steroids:** Large IV doses of penicillin may interfere with accurate measurement of urinary 17-OHCS (Glenn-Nelson technique not affected).

Drug Interactions: Penicillin G

Plus	Interactions
Alcohol, ethyl	Reportedly enhances degradation of the penicillins
Antacids	Tend to delay absorption of oral penicillins; however, they also may protect penicillins from destruction by gastric acids
Antibiotics: Chloramphenicol (Chloromycetin), Erythromycins, Tetracyclines	Bacteriostatic antibiotics antagonize bactericidal actions of the penicillins by slowing rate of bacterial growth *(see Actions and Uses)*
Anticoagulants	Penicillins may enhance bleeding tendency by inhibiting platelet aggregation
Aspirin (salicylates), Indomethacin (Indocin)	Increase serum levels of penicillins by displacing them from plasma protein binding sites
Neomycin	Oral neomycin may decrease absorption of oral penicillins presumably by producing a malabsorption syndrome
Phenylbutazone	Increases serum levels of penicillins by displacing them from plasma protein binding sites
Probenecid (Benemid), Sulfinpyrazone (Anturane)	Decrease renal excretion of penicillins with resulting higher and more prolonged penicillin blood levels

PENICILLIN G PROCAINE SUSPENSION, STERILE

(Crysticillin A.S., Duracillin A.S., Procaine Benzylpenicillin, Pfizerpen-AS)

Antiinfective
Antibiotic
Penicillin

ACTIONS AND USES. Repository (long-acting) form of penicillin G. The procaine salt has low solubility and thus creates a tissue depot from which penicillin is slowly absorbed. Accordingly, the number of injections required to maintain effective blood levels is reduced. Also, procaine exerts a local anesthetic effect. Same actions and antibacterial activity as for Penicillin G and is similarly inactivated by penicillinase and gastric acids. Onset of action is slower and produces lower serum concentrations than equivalent doses of penicillin G, but has longer duration of action. Prepared in aqueous or oil suspension. The oil suspension (Procaine Penicillin G in oil with 2% aluminum monostearate) is no longer available in the U.S.

Used in moderately severe infections due to penicillin G-sensitive microorganisms *(see Penicillin G)* that are susceptible to low but prolonged serum penicillin concentrations. Commonly used for uncomplicated pneumococcal pneumonia, one-day treatment of uncomplicated gonorrheal infections, and for all stages of syphilis. May be used concomitantly with penicillin G or probenecid when more rapid action and higher blood levels are indicated.

ABSORPTION AND FATE. Slowly released from IM injection site. Hydrolyzed to penicillin G in body. Blood levels peak in 1 to 3 hours, plateau in almost 4 hours and decrease slowly over the next 15 to 20 hours. Widely distributed in body with highest concentrations in kidneys and lesser amounts in liver, skin, intestines, and cerebrospinal fluid. Approximately 60% bound to plasma proteins. Excreted rapidly via kidneys; 60 to 90% of dose (aqueous suspension) eliminated within 24 to 36 hours. Excretion may be delayed in neonates, young infants, the elderly, and in other patients with impaired renal function.

CONTRAINDICATIONS AND PRECAUTIONS. History of hypersensitivity to any of the penicillins, cephalosporins, or to procaine or any other "caine-type" local anesthetics; neonates. *Cautious Use:* history of or suspected atopy or allergy. *See Penicillin G.*

ADVERSE/SIDE EFFECTS. Hypersensitivity reactions. *Procaine toxicity:* mental disturbances (anxiety, confusion, depression, combativeness, hallucinations), expressed fear of impending death, weakness, dizziness, headache, tinnitus, unusual tastes, palpitation, changes in pulse rate and blood pressure, seizures. *See also Penicillin G.*

ROUTE AND DOSAGE. **Intramuscular (only): Adults:** 600,000 to 1.2 million units daily. *Uncomplicated gonorrheal infections:* 4.8 million units divided between 2 different injection sites, at one visit; preceded by probenecid 1 Gm orally, just before to 30 minutes before the injections. *Syphilis (primary, secondary, latent):* 600,000 units daily for 8 days; *(late latent, tertiary, and neurosyphilis):* same dose for 15 days. **Children:** 500,000 to 1 million units/m^2/once daily.

NURSING IMPLICATIONS

Before treatment is initiated, an exact history should be obtained of patient's previous exposure and sensitivity to penicillins, cephalosporins, and to procaine, and other allergic reactions of any kind.

If sensitivity to procaine is suspected, physician may test patient by injecting 0.1 ml of 1 to 2% procaine hydrochloride, intradermally. The appearance of a wheal, flare, or eruption indicates procaine sensitivity.

Note expiration date. Multiple-dose vial should be shaken thoroughly before withdrawing medication, to ensure uniform suspension of drug.

Administer IM deeply into upper outer quadrant of gluteus muscle; in infants and small children midlateral aspect of thigh is generally preferred. Injections are almost painless because of local anesthetic action of procaine. Select IM site carefully. Accidental injection into or near major peripheral nerves and blood vessels can cause neurovascular damage. Subcutaneous or intraarterial injection is contraindicated.

Aspirate carefully before injecting drug, to avoid entry into a blood vessel. Inadvertent IV administration reportedly has resulted in pulmonary infarcts and death. Inject drug at a slow, but steady rate to prevent needle blockage. Rotate injection sites.

If nondisposable syringe is used, remove needle and plunger immediately after injection to prevent "freezing" of any remaining medication; rinse thoroughly with water.

Be alert to the possibility of a transient toxic reaction to procaine particularly when large single doses are administered. The reaction manifested by mental disturbance and other symptoms *(see Adverse/Side Effects)* occurs almost immediately and usually subsides after 15 to 30 minutes.

Therapy is guided by culture and sensitivity tests and clinical response.

Report the following to the physician: onset of rash, pruritus, fever, chills or other symptoms of an allergic reaction *(see Penicillin G)*. Reactions may be difficult to treat because drug action is relatively prolonged.

Note manufacturer's directions for storage. Generally, penicillin G procaine aqueous suspension (A.S.) is stored in refrigerator. Avoid freezing.

See Penicillin G Potassium (prototype penicillin).

PENICILLIN V
PENICILLIN V POTASSIUM

Antiinfective
Antibiotic (Beta-lactam)
Penicillin

(Beepen VK, Betapen-VK, Deltapen-VK, Ledercillin VK, Nadopen-V, Novopen-VK, Penapar VK, Penicillin VK, Pen-Vee K, Pfizerpen VK, Repen-VK, Robicillin VK, SK-Penicillin VK, Uticillin VK, V-Cillin K, Veetids)

ACTIONS AND USES. Acid-stable phenoxymethyl analog of penicillin G (qv) with which it shares actions; is bactericidal, and is inactivated by penicillinase. Less active than penicillin G against gonococci and other gram-negative microorganisms.

Used for mild to moderate infections caused by susceptible streptococci, pneumococci, and staphylococci. Also used in treatment of Vincent's infection and as prophylaxis in rheumatic fever.

ABSORPTION AND FATE. Rapidly absorbed from GI tract. Serum concentrations peak in 30 to 60 minutes and are maintained for 6 or more hours. Highest levels in kidneys. Approximately 50 to 80% bound to plasma proteins. Half-life: 30 minutes. Excreted in urine as rapidly as absorbed; excretion is delayed in neonates, young infants, and patients with impaired renal function. Appears in breast milk.

CONTRAINDICATIONS AND PRECAUTIONS. Hypersensitivity to any penicillin or cephalosporin. History of or suspected atopy or allergy (hay fever, asthma, hives, eczema). *See also Penicillin G.*

P

ADVERSE/SIDE EFFECTS. Nausea, vomiting, diarrhea, epigastric distress; hypersensitivity reactions: flushing, pruritus, urticaria or other skin eruptions, eosinophilia, anaphylaxis; hemolytic anemia, leukopenia, thrombocytopenia, neuropathy, superinfections.

ROUTE AND DOSAGE. Oral: Adults and Children (over 12 years): 125 to 500 mg every 6 to 8 hours. **Children (under 12 years):** 15 to 50 mg/kg/day in three to six equally divided doses. (Each 125 mg = 200,000 units.)

NURSING IMPLICATIONS

It is reported that drug may be better absorbed and result in higher blood levels when taken after a meal than on an empty stomach.

Culture and sensitivity tests should be obtained prior to initiation of therapy and at regular intervals throughout therapy.

Before therapy begins, careful inquiry should be made concerning hypersensitivity reactions to penicillins, cephalosporins, and other allergens.

Following reconstitution (by pharmacist), oral solution is stable for 14 days under refrigeration. Date and time of reconstitution and discard date should appear on container. Shake well before pouring.

If oral liquid preparation is not dispensed with a specially marked measuring device, question pharmacist. The average household measure is not accurate enough for this formulation.

Inform patient that in order to maintain a constant blood level, penicillin V should be given around the clock at specific intervals. If it is not prescribed in this way the physician should be asked to clarify the order.

Instruct patient not to miss any doses and to continue taking medication until it is all gone, unless otherwise directed by the physician.

Patients receiving prolonged therapy should have evaluations of renal, hepatic, and hematologic systems at regular intervals.

As with other penicillin preparations, advise patient to withhold medication and to report promptly to physician the onset of hypersensitivity reactions and superinfections.

See Penicillin G.

PENTAERYTHRITOL TETRANITRATE

(Duotrate, P.E.T.N., Pentol, Pentraspan, Pentritol, Pentylan, Peritrate, Vaso-80, and others)

(pen-ta-er-ith′ri-tole)
Vasodilator (coronary)
Antianginal
Nitrate

ACTIONS AND USES. Nitric acid ester of a tetrahydric alcohol. Actions, contraindications, precautions, and adverse/side effects as for nitroglycerin (qv). Slower acting than nitroglycerin but duration of action is longer. Not effective for control of acute attacks. Tolerance can occur, and cross tolerance with other nitrites and nitrates is possible.

Used prophylactically for long-term management of angina pectoris.

ABSORPTION AND FATE. Onset of hemodynamic effects in 20 to 60 minutes; duration 4 to 5 hours. Action of sustained release forms may persist up to 12 hours. Largely metabolized in liver prior to entering general circulation. Half-life: about 10 minutes. Excreted in urine; small amounts in feces.

P

ROUTE AND DOSAGE. (Dose titrated to individual's response.) **Oral: Adult:** initial: 10 or 20 mg four times daily and titrated upward to 40 mg four times daily. Sustained-release forms: 30 to 80 mg every 12 hours. **Pediatric:** dosage not established.

NURSING IMPLICATIONS

Not to be used to relieve an acute episode of anginal pain.

Administered at least 30 minutes before or 1 hour after meals and at bedtime. Sustained release forms also administered on an empty stomach (one dose on arising and second dose 12 hours later).

Advise patient to report onset of skin rash or persistent headaches to physician. Discontinuation of therapy may be required.

Inform patient that alcohol may enhance drug hypotensive effect.

Orthostatic hypotension can be particularly dangerous for the elderly. Evaluate incidence; if troublesome, notify physician.

Chronic administration may produce tolerance and may impair response to nitroglycerin or other concomitantly administered nitrites or nitrates. Advise patient to report signs of decreasing therapeutic effect.

Avoid sudden discontinuation of pentaerythritol therapy; coronary vasospasm may be induced.
Protect drug from exposure to heat and moisture to prevent loss of potency.
Store at temperature between 15° and 30°C (59° and 86°F).
See Nitroglycerin.
In presence of high environmental temperature, heat prostration can occur with use of this drug, especially in the elderly.
Caution patient not to engage in activities requiring mental alertness and skill until drug response has stabilized.
Have on hand the antidote neostigmine in the event of severe toxic reactions.
See Atropine [prototype anticholinergic (antimiscarinic)].

PENTAMIDINE ISOETHIONATE

(Pentam 300)

(pen-tam'i-deen)
Antiinfective

ACTIONS AND USES. Aromatic diamide antiprotozoal drug effective against the sporozoan parasite *Pneumocystis carinii.* Action mechanism is unclear, but drug appears to block parasite reproduction by interfering with nucleotide (DNA, RNA), phospholipid, and protein synthesis. This parasite rarely causes infection in the general population, but if the patient is immunocompromised [e.g., acquired immune deficiency syndrome (AIDS)] carinii pneumocystosis can be fatal. Pentamidine also has trypanosomicidal and leishmonicidal activity but required doses for these conditions are quite toxic. Has an assigned orphan drug status (FDA) with specifically identified use as treatment for *P. carinii* pneumonia (PCP), an often fatal opportunistic disease in an immunocompromised individual.

Used to treat PCP. *Unlabeled Use:* treatment of African trypanosomiasis and visceral leishmoniasis. (Drug supply for the latter uses is through the Centers for Disease Control, Atlanta, GA.)

ABSORPTION AND FATE. Well absorbed after IM administration. Leaves bloodstream rapidly to bind extensively to tissue. About one-half to two-thirds of a dose excreted unchanged in urine in first 6 hours; small amounts found in urine for as long as 6 to 8 weeks following administration of a single dose. Accumulates in renal failure.

CONTRAINDICATIONS AND PRECAUTIONS. Safe use in pregnancy (category C) not established. *Cautious Use:* hypertension, hypotension, hyperglycemia, hypoglycemia, hypocalcemia, blood dyscrasias, hepatic or renal dysfunction, diabetes mellitus.

ADVERSE/SIDE EFFECTS. CV: sudden, severe hypotension, cardiac arrhythmias, ventricular tachycardia, phlebitis. **GI:** anorexia, nausea, vomiting, unpleasant taste. **Hematologic:** leukopenia, thrombocytopenia, anemia. **Metabolic:** hypoglycemia, hypocalcemia, hyperkalemia. **Neurologic:** confusion, hallucinations, neuralgia, dizziness, sweating. **Other:** Stevens–Johnson syndrome, acute renal failure, facial flush (with IV injection), local reactions at injection site.

ROUTE AND DOSAGE. Intramuscular, intravenous: Adults and children: 4 mg/kg once a day for 14 days. Infuse diluted IV solution over a 60-minute period.

NURSING IMPLICATIONS

Preparation of pentamidine solution for administration: IM: dissolve contents of 1 vial (300 mg) in 3 ml sterile water for injection. IV: dissolve contents of 1 vial in 3 to 5 ml sterile water for injection or 5% dextrose solution.

P

The intramuscular injection is painful and frequently causes local reactions (pain, induration, swelling). Select alternate sites for daily doses and institute local treatment if indicated.

Severe sudden hypotension may develop after a single dose. The patient should be in a supine position while receiving the drug. Monitor blood pressure continuously during the infusion, every half hour for 2 hours thereafter, and then every 4 hours until BP stabilizes.

Renal, cardiac, and hepatic function may be changed by pentamidine.

Measure and record intake–output ratio and pattern and check patient's pulse (to detect arrhythmia) at least twice daily.

Dosage adjustment is indicated in renal failure; therefore signs of impending dysfunction should be promptly reported (e.g., changed input–output ratio, oliguria, edema).

Characteristics of pneumonia in the immunocompromised patient include constant fever, scanty (if any) sputum, dyspnea, tachypnea, and cyanosis. (Patient has few inflammatory cells and cannot "mount" a local response.)

Fever is a constant symptom in *P. carinii* pneumonia but it may be rapidly elevated [as high as 40°C (104°F)] shortly after drug infusion. Monitor temperature changes and institute measures to lower the temperature as indicated.

Give physical support to the patient's chest if coughing, but do not urge to cough. Institute measures to reduce nonproductive coughing in order to decrease energy expenditure and chest pain. *(See Benzonatate for Nursing Implications and for Patient Teaching.)*

The immunocompromised patient must be protected from additional infections and other stress. Design nursing care to:

- reduce patient's expenditure of energy to a minimum
- prevent invasive procedures if possible (i.e., IMs, IVs, intubation)
- protect patient from additional infection
- support normal physiologic functions

One of the most important methods for interruption and prevention of spread of disease is thorough hand washing before and after contact with the patient (liquid soap is advised; *see Nursing Intervention: handwashing).* Another important rule for the care-giver to follow is to maintain optimum personal health.

Consult physician and hospital infection control nurse about appropriate techniques and policies designed to protect the patient and care-giver: e.g., visitors, environment control, protective clothing.

Keep in mind that recovery from a severe infection requires adequate nutrient intake. Collaborate with dietician to meet the patient's dietary needs and preferences. Invite a member of the family to share in the important effort to restore normal nutrition.

Since advice regarding availability and use of this drug is usually immediately desirable, a 24-hour hot-line for emergency assistance has been established by the manufacturer: (312)-34-LYPHO.

IV solutions of 1.0 to 2.5 mg/ml prepared in 5% dextrose injection are stable at room temperature for up to 24 hours. Dry product should be stored at 2° and 8°C (35° to 46°F). Protect solution and drug product from light. Discard unused portions.

PENTAZOCINE HYDROCHLORIDE

(Talwin)

(pen-taz'oh-seen)
Narcotic analgesic
C IV

ACTIONS AND USES. Synthetic benzomorphan analgesic structurally related to phenazocine. On a weight basis, analgesic potency approximately one-third that of morphine, and somewhat greater than that of codeine. In general, adverse reactions are qualitatively similar to those of morphine (qv). Unlike morphine, large doses may cause increase in blood pressure and heart rate. Also, acts as weak narcotic antagonist of meperidine and morphine, and has sedative properties. Available in combination with aspirin (Talwin Compound).

Used for relief of moderate to severe pain; also used in obstetrics and for preoperative analgesia or sedation.

ABSORPTION AND FATE. Onset of action 15 to 30 minutes following oral, IM, or subcutaneous administration, and 2 to 3 minutes after IV administration. Duration of action for parenteral preparations: 2 to 3 hours (about 4 to 5 hours or longer for oral form). Extensively metabolized in liver. About 60% of dose is eliminated in urine within 24 hours; small amounts excreted unchanged in urine and feces. (Individual variability in rate of drug metabolism.) Crosses placenta.

CONTRAINDICATIONS AND PRECAUTIONS. Head injury, increased intracranial pressure, emotionally unstable patients, or history of drug abuse. Safe use during pregnancy (other than labor) and in children under 12 years of age not established. *Cautious Use:* impaired renal or hepatic function, respiratory depression, biliary surgery, patients with myocardial infarction who have nausea and vomiting.

ADVERSE/SIDE EFFECTS. Drowsiness, sweating, flushing, dizziness, lightheadedness, nausea, vomiting, constipation (infrequent), dry mouth, alterations of taste, urinary retention, visual disturbances, allergic reactions, injection-site reactions (induration, nodule formation, sloughing, sclerosis, cutaneous depression). High doses: respiratory depression, hypertension, palpitation, tachycardia, psychotomimetic effects, confusion, anxiety, hallucinations, disturbed dreams, bizarre thoughts, euphoria and other mood alterations.

ROUTE AND DOSAGE. Oral: initially 50 mg every 3 to 4 hours. Total daily oral dosage not to exceed 600 mg. **Intramuscular, subcutaneous, intravenous:** (excluding patients in labor); 30 mg every 3 to 4 hours as needed. Doses exceeding 60 mg IM or subcutaneously or 30 mg IV not recommended. Total daily parenteral dosage not to exceed 360 mg. *Patients in labor:* 20 to 30 mg IM; 20 mg may be repeated one or two times at 2- to 3-hour intervals as needed.

NURSING IMPLICATIONS

IM administration is preferable to subcutaneous route when frequent injections over an extended period are required. Rotation of injection sites (upper outer quadrant, midlateral thighs, deltoid) are recommended. Observe injection sites daily for signs of irritation or inflammation.

Pentazocine may produce acute withdrawal symptoms in some patients who have been receiving opioids on a regular basis.

Caution ambulatory patients to avoid potentially hazardous activities such as driving a car or operating machinery until response to drug is known.

Tolerance to analgesic effect sometimes occurs. Psychologic and physical dependence have been reported in patients with history of drug abuse, but rarely in patients without such history. Addiction liability matches that of codeine.

Abrupt discontinuation of drug following extended use may result in chills, abdominal and muscle cramps, yawning, rhinorrhea, lacrimation, itching, restlessness, anxiety, drug-seeking behavior.

Overdosage is treated by supportive measures such as oxygen, IV fluids, vasopressors, assisted or controlled ventilation as necessary, and narcotic antagonist naloxone (levallorphan is not effective for respiratory depression).

Do not mix pentazocine in same syringe with soluble barbiturates, because precipitation will occur.

Classified as Schedule IV drug under Federal Controlled Substances Act.

Preserved in tight, light-resistant containers.

PENTOBARBITAL

(Nembutal)

PENTOBARBITAL SODIUM

(Novopentabsorb, Nembutal Sodium, Pentagen)

(pen-toe-bar'bi-tal)
Sedative, hypnotic
Barbiturate
C II

ACTIONS AND USES. Short-acting barbiturate with actions, contraindications, precautions, and adverse reactions as for other barbiturates *(see Phenobarbital).* Potent respiratory depressant.

Used as sedative or hypnotic for preanesthetic medication, induction of general anesthesia, adjunct in manipulative or diagnostic procedures, and emergency control of acute convulsions.

ABSORPTION AND FATE. Following oral administration, onset of action in 15 to 30 minutes; peak plasma levels in 30 to 60 minutes; duration of action 3 to 6 hours. Onset of action within 10 to 15 minutes after IM injection, and within 1 minute after IV administration. Approximately 35 to 45% bound to plasma proteins. Metabolized primarily in liver to inactive metabolites. Excreted in urine. Crosses placenta.

ADVERSE/SIDE EFFECTS. With rapid IV: respiratory depression, laryngospasm, bronchospasm, apnea, hypotension. *See also Phenobarbital.*

P

ROUTE AND DOSAGE. Oral: *Sedation:* **Adults:** 20 to 30 mg three or four times daily. **Children:** 8 to 30 mg/day in divided doses. *Insomnia:* **Adults:** 100 mg. **Rectal (suppository): Adults:** 120 to 200 mg. **Children:** 30 to 120 mg depending on weight and age. **Intramuscular: Adults:** 150 to 200 mg. **Children:** 25 to 80 mg. **Intravenous: Adults:** initial: 100 mg, increased if necessary to 500 mg. **Children:** reduced proportionately.

NURSING IMPLICATIONS

Do not use parenteral solutions that appear cloudy or in which a precipitate has formed.

Parenteral solution is highly alkaline. Extreme care should be taken to avoid extravasation and intraarterial injection. Necrosis may result.

IV administration should be slow; subsequent injections should be at least 1 minute *(see Adverse/Side Effects).*

During IV administration monitor blood pressure, pulse, and respiration every 3 to 5 minutes. Observe patient closely; maintain airway. Equipment for artificial respiration should be immediately available.

Caution ambulatory patients against operating a motor vehicle or machinery for the remainder of day, after taking drug.

IM injections should be made deep into large muscle mass, preferably upper outer quadrant of buttock. Aspirate carefully before injecting to prevent inadvertent entry into blood vessel. No more than 5 ml (250 mg) should be injected in any one site because of possible tissue irritation.
After IM administration of hypnotic dose, observe patient closely for adverse effects for at least 30 minutes.
Classified as Schedule II drug under Federal Controlled Substances Act.
See Phenobarbital.

PENTOXIFYLLINE
(Trental)

(pen-tox-i′fi-leen)
Hemorheologic agent

ACTIONS AND USES. Dimethyl xanthine derivative with hemorheologic properties. Useful in restoration of blood flow through nutritive capillary microcirculation which has been compromised by structural and flow dynamic changes in cerebral and peripheral vascular disorders. Action mechanism is not clear but pentoxifylline administration is followed by decreased blood viscosity and improved blood flow, with consequent reduction of tissue hypoxia. *Specific effects:* (1) increased deformability (flexibility) of RBC, thereby easing their passage through microcirculatory capillaries; (2) decreased RBC hyperaggregation; (3) decreased synthesis of thromboxane A_2, leading to reduced platelet aggregation; (4) increased cell membrane permeability, which promotes nutrient exchange at tissue level; and (5) increased blood fibrinolytic activity (watchdog property that prevents intravascular coagulation). Drug action (appears to be unrelated to vasodilation) interrupts the vicious cycle of tissue hypoxia, sludging and stasis of capillary blood flow, microthrombotic activity, reduced O_2 delivery to ischemic cells. With increased blood flow to the extremities, the limiting pain and paresthesia of intermittent claudication is reduced; further, psychopathologic conditions associated with cerebral hypoxia are improved.

Used to treat intermittent claudication associated with occlusive peripheral vascular disease, and to treat diabetic angiopathies. *Unlabeled Use:* to improve psychopathologic symptoms in patient with cerebral vascular insufficiency and to reduce incidence of stroke in the patient with recurrent TIAs.

ABSORPTION AND FATE. Rapidly absorbed from GI tract with peak plasma levels, achieved in 2 to 4 hours, remaining high for an extended period of time. Undergoes first-pass effect. Hepatic degradation produces several metabolites. Half-life: (pentoxifylline): 0.4 to 0.8 hours; (metabolites): 1 to 1.6 hours. Hepatic enzyme induction or accumulation during multiple dosing have not been reported. Eliminated mainly in urine.

CONTRAINDICATIONS AND PRECAUTIONS. Intolerance to pentoxifylline or to xanthines (caffeine and theophylline). Safe use in pregnancy (category C), lactation, or in children under 18 not established. *Cautious Use:* angina, hypotension, arrhythmias, cerebrovascular disease.

ADVERSE/SIDE EFFECTS. CNS: agitation, nervousness, dizziness, drowsiness, headache, insomnia, tremor, confusion. **CV:** angina, chest pain, dyspnea, arrhythmias, palpitations, hypotension, edema, flushing. **Dermatologic:** brittle fingernails, pruritus, rash, urticaria. **GI:** abdominal discomfort, belching, flatus, bloating, diarrhea, dyspepsia, nausea, vomiting. **Ophthalmic:** blurred vision, conjunctivitis, scotomata. **Other:** earache, unpleasant taste, excessive salivation, leukopenia, malaise, sore throat, swollen neck glands, weight change. (Rare, causal relationship unknown): arrhythmia, tachycardia, hepatitis, jaundice, decreased serum fibrinogen, pancytopenia, purpura, thrombocytopenia. **Overdosage:** fever, flushing, hypotension, convulsions, somnolence, loss of consciousness.

NURSING IMPLICATIONS

When given with food, absorption is delayed but total amount absorbed is not affected; serum levels are lowered, however. Administer on an empty stomach or if taken with food, be consistent with time of day and relationship to food in establishing the daily regimen.

Therapeutic effects may be evident within 2 to 4 weeks, but treatment is continued at least 8 weeks before therapeutic failure is admitted.

Successful treatment provides relief from pain and cramping in calf muscles, buttocks, thighs, and feet during exercise, and improves walking performance (time and duration).

Since tolerance to pentoxifylline does not develop, it is expected that drug-induced relief will continue during long-term therapy.

If patient is also on antihypertensive treatment, monitor blood pressure. Pentoxifylline may slightly decrease an already stabilized blood pressure, necessitating a reduced dose of the hypotensive drug.

Emphasize the use of self-help measures to augment drug therapy in occlusive peripheral vasospastic disorders: e.g., establish plan for regular exercise, give up smoking, control weight and diet (low fat, low cholesterol). *(See also Index: Nursing intervention: peripheral vasospastic disorders.)*

Before patient reestablishes walking as exercise, the patient should be checked by the physician to determine CV status and capacity.

Overdosage symptoms are dose related and may occur 4 to 5 hours after ingestion and last about 12 hours *(see Adverse/Side Effects). Treatment of overdose* (symptomatic): gastric lavage, activated charcoal, supported respiratory and CV function and preparation for seizure control.

Because of potential side effects (i.e., somnolence, blurred vision, dizziness) advise patient to avoid driving or working with dangerous machinery until drug response has stabilized.

No drug interactions have been reported.

Store tablets at controlled room temperature 15° to 30°C (59° to 86°F).

PERPHENAZINE

(Phenazine, Trilafon)

(per-fen'a-zeen)
Psychotropic
Antipsychotic
Antiemetic
Phenothiazine

ACTIONS AND USES. Piperazine phenothiazine similar to chlorpromazine in actions, absorption and fate, contraindications, precautions, adverse reactions and interactions. Effects all parts of CNS, particularly the hypothalamus. Produces less sedation and hypotension, greater antiemetic effects, higher incidence of extrapyramidal effects and lower levels of anticholinergic side effects than chlorpromazine (qv).

Used in management of the manifestations of psychotic disorders and for control of nausea and vomiting, intractable hiccoughs, or acute conditions such as violent retching during surgery.

CONTRAINDICATIONS AND PRECAUTIONS. Hypersensitivity to perphenazine and other phenothiazines; preexisting liver damage, suspected or established subcortical brain damage, comatose states, blood dyscrasias, bone marrow depression, pregnancy, nursing mothers, women who may become pregnant, children under 12 years of age. *Cautious Use:* previously diagnosed breast cancer; renal dysfunction, alcohol withdrawal, epilepsy, psychic depression, patients with suicidal tendency, and those who will be exposed to extreme heat in work, or exposed to phosphorous insecticides. *See also Chlorpromazine.*

ADVERSE/SIDE EFFECTS. Extrapyramidal effects, convulsions, constipation, xerostomia, nasal congestion, decreased sweating, tachycardia, bradycardia, adynamic ileus, hypotension, photosensitivity. *See also Chlorpromazine.*

ROUTE AND DOSAGE. Oral: Adult and Children (over 12 years of age): *Nonhospitalized:* 4 to 8 mg three times daily; reduce as soon as possible. *Hospitalized:* 8 to 16 mg two to four times daily up to maximum dosage of 64 mg/day. Oral concentrate: 16 mg/5 ml. **Intramuscular:** Initial: 5 to 10 mg repeated every 6 hours if necessary. Recommended total daily dose: 15 mg for ambulatory patient or 30 mg for hospitalized patient. **Intravenous (fractional injection or slow drug infusion):** Initial: 5 mg doses, or in divided doses: dilute to 0.5 mg/ml and give 1 mg/minute until symptoms subside. **Elderly, debilitated and emaciated patients:** lower initial dose which is then gradually increased as needed and tolerated.

NURSING IMPLICATIONS

If the patient is also receiving antacid or antidiarrheal medication, schedule the phenothiazine to be taken at least 1 hour before or 1 hour after the other medication.

Extended release tablet (not recommended for children) should be swallowed whole.

Each 5 ml (16 mg) of oral concentrate should be diluted with 60 ml water, orange juice, milk, or carbonated beverage. Color changes and precipitate may occur with cola drinks, black coffee, tea, grape juice, or apple juice.

Administer intramuscular injection deep into upper outer quadrant of the buttock with patient in recumbent position. Advise patient to continue lying down for at least 1 hour after injection. Monitor blood pressure and pulse. Usually patient can be transferred to the oral formulation (equal or higher doses) within 24 to 48 hours.

IV perphenazine is seldom required and is used with caution; given only to recumbent hospitalized adults.

The elderly and pediatric patients should be observed very carefully during parenteral therapy for hypotensive and extrapyramidal reactions.

Blood pressure and pulse should be monitored continuously during IV administration. Keep patient supine until assured that vital signs are stable. Have on hand levarterenol. (Epinephrine is contraindicated.)

A high incidence of extrapyramidal effects accompanies use of perphenazine particularly with high doses and IV administration. Report restlessness, weakness of extremities, dystonia of neck and shoulder muscles, abnormal positioning, excessive salivation, and other unusual symptoms.

The patient on long-term therapy (especially the elderly female patient) is at high risk for tardive dyskinesia. Watch for early signs: fine vermicular movement or rapid protrusions of the tongue. Report immediately when noticed. Discontinue medication.

Warn patient not to spill oral concentrate on skin or clothing. Wash well with soap and water if it occurs. Contact dermatitis has been reported.

If jaundice appears in the 2nd to 4th week, suspect hypersensitivity; withhold drug and report to physician.

Monitor intake–output ratio and bowel elimination pattern. The depressed patient is apt to drink too little fluid and may not seek help for constipation.

Alcohol potentiates drug effect and consequently may increase danger of overdose. Consult physician about permissible amount.
A significant unexplained rise in body temperature suggests individual intolerance to perphenazine and should be reported.
Be alert to the patient's altered tolerance to environmental temperature changes. Provide extra clothing if necessary but be cautious with external heat devices. Conditioned avoidance behavior may be depressed, and a severe burn could result.
Pigmentation of skin, especially on exposed areas (and in women on large doses) may result in blue-gray discoloration (photosensitivity reaction). Caution patient to avoid long exposure in sunlight, even on cloudy days. Use of sun screen lotion (SPF above 12) is advisable.
Caution patient to avoid potentially hazardous activities such as driving a car or operating machinery, since drug may produce drowsiness or dizziness.
Antiemetic effect of this drug may obscure signs of toxicity due to overdosage of other drugs, or make it more difficult to diagnose conditions with nausea as a primary symptom.
Blood, hepatic, and renal laboratory studies should be checked periodically. Urge patient to keep appointments for evaluation of clinical status.
Caution patient to avoid OTC drugs unless physician specifically prescribes them.
Review dosage regimen with patient: urge him or her to adhere to it precisely and to consult physician before changing it for any reason.
Perphenazine may discolor urine reddish brown.
Protect solutions from light. Do not use precipitated or darkened parenteral solution; however, slight discoloration does not alter potency or therapeutic effects.
Store drug at temperature between 15° and 30°C (59° and 86°F) unless otherwise specified by manufacturer. Protect from freezing.
See Chlorpromazine.

PHENACEMIDE

(Phenurone)

(fe-nass'e-mide)
Anticonvulsant
Hydantoin

P

ACTIONS AND USES. Potent structural analog of the hydantoins. Prevents or modifies seizure by elevating threshold for minimal convulsive activity. Found to be equal to or more effective than other antiseizure agents, but high toxicity potential removes it from first choice category.

Used alone or with other anticonvulsants to treat severe epileptic states, especially mixed forms of psychomotor seizures refractory to other drugs.

ABSORPTION AND FATE. Well absorbed from GI tract. Duration of action about 5 hours. Metabolized by liver. Excreted by kidneys as inactive metabolites.

CONTRAINDICATIONS AND PRECAUTIONS. Safe use in women of childbearing potential, during pregnancy or lactation not established; severe personality disorders. *Cautious Use:* liver impairment, allergies, concomitant use with another anticonvulsant.

ADVERSE/SIDE EFFECTS. CNS: headache, drowsiness, insomnia, dizziness, paresthesias, personality changes, suicidal tendencies, toxic psychoses. **GI:** nausea, anorexia, weight loss, hepatitis. **Hematologic:** leukopenia, aplastic anemia, agranulocytosis. **Other:** skin rash; nephritis with marked albuminuria, drowsiness, ataxia, hepatitis, and coma.

ROUTE AND DOSAGE. Oral: Adults: Initial: 250 to 500 mg 3 times daily; after first week, additional 500 mg on arising may be added if necessary to control seizures; in third week, additional 500 mg at bedtime may be added. Effective total daily dose range: from 1.5 to 5 Gm. **Children (5 to 10 years):** approximately one-half adult dosage and given at same intervals.

NURSING IMPLICATIONS

Administration of drug with food may minimize GI side effects.

Complete blood counts, liver function tests, and urine tests should be performed before and at monthly intervals during therapy. If no abnormalities appear after 12 months, intervals may be widened.

Patient and responsible family members should be advised of need for close medical supervision, because drug has high potential for serious toxicity.

Personality changes, including attempts at suicide, are possible drug effects. Instruct patient and family to report changes in behavior, e.g., depression, apathy, aggressiveness, paranoia, and severe headaches. All are indications for drug withdrawal which should be gradual.

Advise patient and family to report immediately the onset of fever, sore mouth or throat, and malaise, skin rash or other allergic manifestations, easy bruising or unexplained bleeding (symptoms of developing blood dyscrasia).

Counsel patient to be cautious about driving or engaging in any activity requiring alertness until response to phenacemide is known.

Teach patient and family to observe for and report evidence of jaundice: yellow skin and sclerae, petechiae, pruritus, dark amber urine with yellow froth.

Treatment of overdosage: emesis, gastric lavage as alternative or adjunct, general supportive measures. Follow-up evaluation of liver and kidney function, mental state, and blood-forming organs should be made.

Physician may prescribe vitamin K for infants born to mothers treated with anticonvulsants. These agents appear to reduce levels of vitamin-K-dependent clotting factors in the newborn.

PHENAZOPYRIDINE HYDROCHLORIDE

(fen-az-oh-peer′-i-deen)

(Azodine, Azo-Standard, Baridium, Di-Azo, Phenazodine, Pyridium)

Analgesic (urinary tract)

P

ACTIONS AND USES. Azo dye with local anesthetic action on urinary tract mucosa. Precise mechanism of action not known. Imparts little or no antibacterial activity.

Used for symptomatic relief of pain, burning, frequency, and urgency arising from irritation of urinary tract mucosa, as from infection, trauma, surgery, or instrumentation. Available in fixed combination with methenamine mandelate (Azolate, Azo Mandelamine, Uritral), sulfamethizole (Microsul-A, Thiosulfil-A), sulfamethoxazole (Azo Gantanol), sulfisoxazole (Azo Gantrisin).

ABSORPTION AND FATE. Partly metabolized, probably in liver and other tissues. Excreted by kidney within 20 hours; about 65% excreted unchanged. Small amounts eliminated in feces. Trace amounts believed to cross placenta.

CONTRAINDICATIONS AND PRECAUTIONS. Renal insufficiency, glomerulonephritis, pyelonephritis during pregnancy, severe hepatitis. *Cautious Use:* GI disturbances, glucose-6-phosphate dehydrogenase deficiency.

ADVERSE/SIDE EFFECTS. Infrequent: headache, vertigo, mild GI disturbances; (in patients with impaired renal function or with high dosage or prolonged therapy): methemoglobinemia, hemolytic anemia, skin pigmentation, renal stones, transient acute renal failure.

ROUTE AND DOSAGE. Oral: Adults: 200 mg three times daily. **Children:** 12 mg/kg/24 hours in 3 divided doses.

NURSING IMPLICATIONS

Administer phenazopyridine after meals.

Inform patient that drug will impart an orange to red color to urine and may stain fabric. Fabric stains may be removed by soaking in 0.25% solution of sodium dithionate or sodium hydrosulfite. Consult pharmacist.

Appearance of yellowish tinge to skin or sclerae may indicate drug accumulation due to renal impairment. Advise patient to report immediately. Drug should be discontinued.

Phenazopyridine should be discontinued when pain and discomfort are relieved (usually 3 to 15 days). Instruct patient to keep physician informed.

Diagnostic Test Interferences. Phenazopyridine may interfere with any urinary test that is based on color reactions or spectrometry: **Bromsulphalein** and **phenolsulfonphthalein** excretion tests; urinary **glucose** test using Clinistix or Tes-Tape (copper-reduction methods such as Clinitest and Benedict's test reportedly not affected); **bilirubin** using "foam test" or Ictotest; **ketones** using nitroprusside (e.g., Acetest, Ketostix, or Gerhardt ferric chloride); urinary **protein** using Albustix, Albutest, or nitric acid ring test; urinary **steroids; urobilinogen;** assays for **porphyrins.**

PHENDIMETRAZINE TARTRATE

(fen-dye-me'tra-zeen)
Anorexiant
C III

(Adphen, Bacarate, Bontril PDM, Di-Ap-Trol, Limit, Melfiat, Metra, Obalan, Obeval, Obezine, PDM, Phenzine, Plegine, Sprx 1, Statobex, Trimstat, Weightrol)

P

ACTIONS AND USES. Sympathomimetic amine with actions similar to those of other amphetamine-like compounds.

Used as adjunct to control endogenous obesity.

ABSORPTION AND FATE. Peak blood levels within 1 hour after regular tablet; effects persist about 4 hours, approximately 12 hours after sustained-release form.

CONTRAINDICATIONS AND PRECAUTIONS. Hypersensitivity to sympathomimetic amines, pregnancy, children under 12 years of age, severe coronary artery disease, moderate to severe hypertension, cardiac decompensation, hyperthyroidism, glaucoma, agitated persons, history of drug abuse, concomitant use with MAO inhibitors, CNS stimulants.

ADVERSE/SIDE EFFECTS. Occasional: nervousness, insomnia, dizziness, mouth dryness, glossitis, stomatitis, nausea, mydriasis, blurring of vision, difficulty in starting urination, cystitis, constipation, abdominal cramps, palpitation, tachycardia, elevation of blood pressure. *See also Amphetamine.*

ROUTE AND DOSAGE. Oral: 35 mg two or three times daily, or one sustained-release capsule (105 mg) once daily.

NURSING IMPLICATIONS

Administer 1 hour before meals. Sustained-release form is administered in the morning. Give last dose at least 6 hours before patient retires in order to avoid insomnia.

Psychogenic dependence is a possibility, as with all amphetaminelike compounds.

Classified as Schedule III drug under Federal Controlled Substances Act.

See Amphetamine Sulfate.

PROTOTYPE

PHENELZINE SULFATE

(Nardil)

(fen'el-zeen)
Antidepressant
MAO inhibitor
Hydrazine

ACTIONS AND USES. Potent hydrazine MAO inhibitor with amphetaminelike pharmacologic properties. Precise mode of action not known. Antidepressant and diverse effects believed to be due to irreversible inhibition of MAO (mitochondrial enzyme involved in degradation and excretion of sympathomimetic amines), thereby permitting increased concentrations of endogenous epinephrine, norepinephrine, serotonin, and dopamine within presynaptic neurons and at receptor sites. Also thought to inhibit hepatic microsomal drug-metabolizing enzymes; thus may intensify and prolong the effects of many drugs. Termination of drug action depends on regeneration of MAO, which occurs 2 to 3 weeks after discontinuation of therapy. Exerts paradoxic hypotensive effect (apparently by ganglionic blocking action), suppresses REM sleep, and reportedly may decrease serum cholinesterase. MAO inhibitor has unpredictable effect on convulsive threshold in epilepsy.

Used in management of endogenous depression, depressive phase of manic-depressive psychosis, and severe exogenous (reactive) depression not responsive to more commonly used therapy.

ABSORPTION AND FATE. Readily absorbed from GI tract and rapidly metabolized. Excreted in urine as metabolites and unchanged drug.

CONTRAINDICATIONS AND PRECAUTIONS. Hypersensitivity to MAO inhibitors, pheochromocytoma, hyperthyroidism, congestive heart failure, cardiovascular or cerebrovascular disease, impaired renal function, hypernatremia, atonic colitis, glaucoma, history of frequent or severe headaches, history of liver disease, abnormal liver function tests, elderly or debilitated patients, paranoid schizophrenia. Safe use during pregnancy and lactation and in women of childbearing potential and children under 16 years of age not established. *Cautious Use:* epilepsy, pyloric stenosis, diabetes, depression accompanying alcoholism or drug addiction, manic-depressive states, agitated patients, suicidal tendencies, chronic brain syndromes, history of angina pectoris.

ADVERSE/SIDE EFFECTS. Constipation, dry mouth, dizziness or vertigo, headache, orthostatic hypotension, drowsiness or insomnia, weakness, fatigue, nausea, vomiting, anorexia, weight gain, edema, tremors, twitching, hyperreflexia, mania, hypomania, confusion, memory impairment, blurred vision, hyperhidrosis, skin rash. **Hypertensive crisis:** intense occipital headache, palpitation, marked hypertension, stiff neck, nausea, vomiting, sweating, fever, photophobia, dilated pupils, bradycardia or tachycardia, constricting chest pain, intracranial bleeding. **Less common:** glaucoma, nystagmus, incontinence, dysuria, urinary frequency or retention, transient impotence, galactorrhea, gynecomastia, black tongue, hypernatremia, transient respiratory and cardiovascular depression, jaundice, delirium, hallucinations, euphoria, acute anxiety reaction, akathisia, ataxia, toxic precipitation of schizophrenia, convulsions, possibility of optic damage, peripheral neuropathy, spider telangiectasis, photosensitivity, hypoglycemia, decreased 5-HIAA and VMA, normocytic and normochromic anemia, leukopenia. **Severe overdosage:** faintness, hypotension or hypertension, hyperactivity, marked agitation, anxiety, seizures, trismus, opisthotonos, respiratory depression, coma, circulatory collapse.

ROUTE AND DOSAGE. Oral: Initial: 15 mg three times a day. Increased gradually until maximum benefit is achieved, dosage reduced slowly over several weeks to maintenance level: 15 mg daily or every other day, as long as required. Maximum recommended daily dose: 75 mg.

NURSING IMPLICATIONS

Before initiation of phenelzine treatment, it is advisable to evaluate patient's blood pressure in standing and recumbent positions. Baseline blood cell counts and liver function tests should also be performed.

Many adverse reactions associated with MAO inhibitors are dose-related. Physician will rely on accurate observations and prompt reporting of patient's response to therapy to determine spacing and lowest effective dosage.

In titrating initial dosages, blood pressure and pulse should be monitored between doses, and patient should be closely observed for evidence of adverse drug effects. Thereafter, monitor at regular intervals throughout therapy.

Elastic stockings and elevation of legs when sitting may minimize hypotensive effects of drug (discuss with physician).

Instruct patient to make position changes slowly, especially from recumbent to upright posture, and to dangle legs over bed a few minutes before ambulating. Also caution against standing still for prolonged periods. Patient should avoid hot showers and baths (resulting vasodilatation may potentiate hypotension) and should lie down immediately if feeling lightheaded or faint. Supervise ambulation.

Headache and palpitation, prodromal symptoms of hypertensive crisis, indicate need to discontinue drug therapy. Instruct patient to report immediately the onset of these symptoms or any other unusual effects.

Ingestion of foods and beverages containing tyramine or tryptophan (form pressor amines in body) or drugs containing pressor agents can result in severe hypertensive reactions. Provide patient and responsible family members with a list of foods and beverages that may cause reactions (see below). These substances should be avoided during drug therapy and for at least 2 to 3 weeks after therapy has been discontinued.

Food and beverages to avoid: avocado, bananas, canned figs, raisins, licorice, chocolate, cheeses (particularly cheddar and other strong and aged varieties), yogurt, cream, sour cream, broad bean pods, liver (especially chicken liver), aged meats, pickled or kippered herring, yeast and meat extracts, soy sauce, meat tenderizers, game. Alcoholic beverages in general should be avoided (since tyramine content is difficult to determine), especially Chianti, other wines, and beer. Also advise against excessive amounts of caffeine beverages (e.g., coffee, tea, cocoa, or cola) and cyclamates (believed to be converted in body in part to a pressor amine).

Treatment of hypertensive crisis: Have on hand short-acting α-adrenergic blocking agent (e.g., phentolamine) to lower blood pressure; external cooling for hyperpyrexia.

Treatment of overdosage: Gastric lavage if performed early; maintain airway, hydration, and electrolyte balance. Have on hand phenothiazine tranquilizer (for agitation). Toxic effects may be delayed and prolonged; therefore, patient must be closely observed for at least 1 week after overdosage.

Advise patient to avoid self-medication. OTC preparations containing dextromethorphan, sympathomimetic agents, or antihistamines (e.g., cough, cold, and hay fever remedies, appetite suppressants) can precipitate severe hypertensive reactions if taken during therapy or within 2 or 3 weeks after discontinuation of an MAO inhibitor.

Monitor intake–output ratio and pattern until dosage is stabilized to identify indirect indices of edema and urinary dysfunction. Report changes and abnormalities; impaired renal function increases the possibility of toxicity from cumulative effects.

Instruct patient to check weight two or three times weekly and report unusual gain.

Dry mouth may be relieved by sugarless candy or gum or by rinsing mouth with clear water.

Attempt at suicide by the depressed person is particularly possible when the response to drug therapy begins (i.e., near end of depressive cycle). Careful observation of patient should be maintained until depression is controlled. Watch to see that drug is swallowed, not "cheeked" or hoarded.

In manic-depressive states, observe closely for rapid swing to manic phase. Patients with schizophrenia may present with excessive stimulation.

Hypomania (exaggeration of motility, feelings, and ideas) may occur as depression improves, particularly in patients with hyperkinetic symptoms obscured by a depressive affect. This reaction may also appear at higher than recommended doses or with long-term therapy. Report immediately.

Observe for and report therapeutic effectiveness of drug: improvement in sleep pattern, appetite, physical activity, interest in self and surroundings, as well as lessening of anxiety and bodily complaints.

If no therapeutic response occurs after 3 or 4 weeks, drug is usually discontinued. Maximum antidepressant effects generally appear in 2 to 6 weeks and persist several weeks after drug withdrawal.

Patient with diabetes should be closely observed for signs of hypoglycemia. Reduced dosage of insulin or oral antidiabetic drug may be necessary *(see Drug Interactions).*

MAO inhibitors should be discontinued at least 10 days before elective surgery to allow time for recovery of MAO before anesthetics are given.

Patients on prolonged therapy should be checked periodically for altered color perception, visual fields, and fundi. Changes in red-green vision may be the first indication of eye damage.

Instruct patient to report jaundice. Hepatotoxicity is believed to be a hypersensitivity reaction unrelated to dosage or duration of therapy.

Periodic hematologic studies and liver function tests are recommended during prolonged therapy and high dosage.

MAO inhibitors may suppress anginal pain that would otherwise serve as a warning sign of myocardial ischemia. Caution patient to avoid overexertion while receiving drug therapy.

Rapid withdrawal of MAO inhibitors should be avoided, particularly after high dosage, since a rebound effect may occur (headache, excitability, hallucinations, and possibly depression).

Preserved in tightly covered containers away from heat and light.

Diagnostic Test Interferences. Phenelzine may cause a slight false increase in **serum bilirubin.**

Drug Interactions. Hypertensive reaction and related symptoms may result from use (concurrently or within 2 weeks) of MAO inhibitors with amines having indirect sympathomimetic action: **amphetamines, cyclopentamine, ephedrine, metaraminol, methylphenidate, phenylephrine, phenylpropanolamine, pseudoephedrine.** Similar interactions are reportedly possible with **cyclamates, dextromethorphan, levodopa, methyldopa, methotrimeprazine, reserpine, tricyclic antidepressants, tryptamine,** and **tyramine**-rich foods and beverages.

With the exception of **dopamine** (contraindicated), direct-acting sympathomimetic amines (**epinephrine, isoproterenol, levarterenol, methoxamine**) are not significantly affected by MAO inhibitors; however, cautious administration is advised.

MAO inhibitors may potentiate the effects of **barbiturates;** potentiate adverse cardiovascular effects of **doxapram** (theoretical possibility); antagonize antihypertensive effects of **guanethidine** (concurrent use avoided); enhance or prolong hypoglycemic action of **insulin** and **oral antidiabetic agents;** cause severe CNS excitation and depression leading to coma and death with **meperidine,**—thus concurrent use is to be avoided (other **narcotic analgesics** used only with extreme caution and in small doses); increase extrapyramidal reactions of **phenothiazines;** enhance the effect of **succinylcholine** by reducing its breakdown by plasma pseudocholinesterase; produce hypotension when used with **thiazide diuretics.**

PHENMETRAZINE HYDROCHLORIDE

(Preludin)

(fen-met′ra-zeen)
Adrenergic, anorexiant
C II

ACTIONS AND USES. Sympathomimetic agent chemically and pharmacologically related to amphetamine (qv), but reportedly produces less CNS stimulation.

Used solely for short-term management of endogenous obesity.

ABSORPTION AND FATE. Peak serum concentration occurs about 2 hours after administration of conventional tablet; duration of action about 4 hours. Duration of action for sustained-release form approximately 12 hours.

CONTRAINDICATIONS AND PRECAUTIONS. History of hypersensitivity to sympathomimetic amines, hypertension, advanced arteriosclerosis, symptomatic cardiovascular disease, hyperthyroidism, glaucoma (narrow angle), hyperexcitable or psychotic states, concomitant use of CNS stimulants, during or within 2 weeks of MAO inhibitors. Safe use in women in childbearing potential, during pregnancy, and in children under 12 years of age not established.

P

ADVERSE/SIDE EFFECTS. CNS: nervousness, dizziness, insomnia, headache. **CV:** palpitation, tachycardia, elevated blood pressure. **EENT:** blurred vision, dry mouth. **GI:** nausea, abdominal cramps, constipation. **Other:** sweating, frequent urination, urticaria, changes in libido, impotence. Large doses for prolonged periods: marked insomnia, irritability, severe dermatoses, hyperactivity, severe mental depression, personality changes, psychosis.

ROUTE AND DOSAGE. Oral: 25 mg two or three times daily; maximum dosage 75 mg/day. Sustained-release form: 50 to 75 mg tablet once daily.

NURSING IMPLICATIONS

Conventional tablet is administered at least 1 hour before meals. Schedule last dose of day at an appropriate time so that insomnia is avoided *(see Absorption and Fate).*

Sustained-release form may be taken in the morning; administration time should be determined by period of day anorexiant effect is needed (generally taken at least 12 hours before bedtime). Advise patient to swallow tablet whole.

Blood pressure checks before and periodically during treatment are advised.

For maximal results, drug therapy should be used as part of a plan that includes reeducation of patient with respect to eating habits and attention to possible underlying psychologic factors.

Since drug may cause blurred vision and dizziness, caution patient to avoid potentially hazardous activities such as driving a car or operating machinery until reaction to drug is known.

Instruct patient to notify physician if nervousness, dizziness, or palpitation occur.

Mouth dryness may be relieved by rinsing with warm water or by increasing noncaloric fluid intake (if allowed) and particularly if inadequate. Sugarless gum or lemondrops may also help. Notify physician if symptom is pronounced.

Advise patient against excessive use of CNS stimulants such as coffee, tea, and cola drinks.

Instruct patient not to exceed recommended dosage. Tolerance to drug effects usually develops in a few weeks; drug should be discontinued when this occurs.

As with other amphetamines, physical and psychic dependence and tolerance may develop with prolonged use.

Sustained release tablets contain tartrazine which may cause allergic type reactions including bronchial asthma in susceptible individuals. This reaction is frequently seen in patients with aspirin hypersensitivity.

Classified as Schedule II drug under Federal Controlled Substances Act.

See Amphetamine Sulfate.

PROTOTYPE

PHENOBARBITAL

(Barbita, Gardenal, Luminal, PBR/12, Sedadrops, SK-Phenobarbital, Solfoton)

PHENOBARBITAL SODIUM

(Luminal Sodium)

(fee-noe-bar'bi-tal)
CNS depressant
Sedative, hypnotic
Anticonvulsant
Barbiturate
C IV

P

ACTIONS AND USES. Long-acting barbiturate. Sedative and hypnotic effects of barbiturates appear to be due primarily to interference with impulse transmission of cerebral cortex by inhibition of reticular activating system (concerned with both sleep and arousal mechanisms). Initially, barbiturates suppress REM sleep, but with chronic therapy REM sleep returns to normal. Has no analgesic properties, and small doses may increase reaction to painful stimuli. CNS depression may range from mild sedation to coma, depending on dosage, route of administration, degree of nervous system excitability, and drug tolerance. Phenobarbital limits spread of seizure activity by increasing threshold for motor cortex stimuli. Anticonvulsant action of phenobarbital is shared by mephobarbital, but not other barbiturates, and is reportedly unrelated to sedative effect. Phenobarbital has a bilirubin lowering effect, by inducing production of glucuronyl transferase; also increases excretion and flow of bile salts. Barbiturates are habit forming. Tolerance, physical, and psychologic dependence may occur especially with long-term use. Use in the elderly is generally being replaced by shorter-acting agents.

Used in long term management of tonic-clonic (grand mal) seizures and partial seizures; status epilepticus, eclampsia, febrile convulsions in young children. Also used as a sedative in anxiety/tension states, e.g., essential hypertension, cardiac failure, hypothyroidism, motion sickness, acute labyrinthitis, nausea and vomiting of functional origin; in pediatrics as preoperative and postoperative sedation and to treat pylorospasm in infants. Also used in treatment and prevention of hyperbilirubinemia in neonates and in the management of chronic cholestasis.

ABSORPTION AND FATE. Absorbed slowly following all routes of administration. Peak serum concentrations reached in 8 to 12 hours; peak brain concentration in 10 to 15 hours. Widely distributed in tissues and body fluids. Hypnotic doses produce sleep within 20 to 60 minutes; duration varies from 6 to 10 hours. About 40 to 60% bound to plasma proteins and also to tissues, including brain. Half-life 53 to 118 hours (somewhat shorter and more variable in children). Small amount metabolized in liver; excreted in urine largely as unchanged drug. Alkalinization of urine and hydration enhance renal excretion. Readily crosses placenta; enters breast milk.

CONTRAINDICATIONS AND PRECAUTIONS. Sensitivity to barbiturates, manifest hepatic, or familial history of porphyria, severe respiratory or renal disease, history of previous addiction to sedative hypnotics, uncontrolled pain, women of childbearing potential, pregnancy (particularly early pregnancy), nursing mothers, timed release formulation for children under 12 years of age. *Cautious Use:* impaired hepatic, renal, cardiac, or respiratory function, history of allergies, elderly or debilitated patients, patients with fever, hyperthyroidism, diabetes mellitus, or severe anemia, during labor and delivery, lactation, patient with borderline hypoadrenal function.

ADVERSE/SIDE EFFECTS. CNS: somnolence, nightmares, insomnia, "hangover", headache, anxiety, thinking abnormalities, dizziness, nystagmus, irritability, paradoxic excitement and exacerbation of hyperkinetic behavior (in children); confusion or depression or marked excitement (elderly or debilitated patients); ataxia, **CV:** bradycardia, syncope, hypotension. **Dermatologic:** mild maculopapular, morbilliform rash; (rare) exfoliative dermatitis, erythema multiforme, Stevens–Johnson syndrome. **GI:** nausea, vomiting, constipation, diarrhea, epigastic pain. **Hypersensitivity:** rash, angioneurotic edema, fever, serum sickness, urticaria; hypoventilation, apnea, laryngospasm, bronchospasm, circulatory collapse. **Injection site (extravasation):** thrombosis, gangrene transient pain, tenderness, redness. **Intravenous:** coughing, hiccuping, laryngospasm. **Other:** liver damage, megaloblastic anemia, hypocalcemia, osteomalacia, rickets, myalgic, neuralgic, arthritic pain (rare); agranulocytosis, thrombocytopenia, folic acid deficiency, vitamin D deficiency. **Overdosage (acute intoxication):** *see Nursing Implications.*

ROUTE AND DOSAGE. Adults: *Sedative:* **Oral:** 15 to 32 mg two to four times/day. *Hypnotic:* **Oral:** 50 to 100 mg. **Parenteral (subcutaneous, IM, IV):** 100 to 320 mg/day; not to exceed 600 mg/24 hours; IV rate not greater than 60 mg/minute. *Anticonvulsant:* **Oral:** 50 to 100 mg. **Parenteral:** 100 to 320 mg/day. **Children:** *Sedative:* **Oral, rectal suppository:** 2 mg/kg/24 hours in 3 equally divided doses. *Hypnotic:* 3 to 6 mg/kg. *Anticonvulsant:* 16 to 50 mg two or three times daily. Timed release: one in AM; one in PM.

NURSING IMPLICATIONS

Phenobarbital and other long acting barbiturates may be cumulative in action. Doses in excess of 400 mg/day for more than 90 days are likely to cause some degree of physical dependence.

Therapeutic serum concentrations of 10 to 20 mcg/ml produce anticonvulsant activity in most patients. These values are usually attained after 2 or 3 weeks of therapy with a dose of 100 to 200 mg/day.

Serum concentrations greater than 50 mcg/ml may cause coma; concentrations in excess of 80 mcg/ml are potentially lethal.

Because of the long half-life, steady-state plasma level may not be reached until after 3 or 4 weeks of therapy with phenobarbital.

Preparation of IV solution: slowly introduce sterile water for injection into ampul with sterile syringe. Rotate ampul to hasten dissolving drug (may take several minutes). If solution not clear in 5 minutes or if a precipitate remains, discard.

Commercially prepared solutions for injection (sodium phenobarbital) may be diluted with most IV infusion solutions. If not absolutely clear, discard.

Administer reconstituted solution no later than 30 minutes after preparation.

Administer IM deep into large muscle mass; volume should not exceed 5 ml at any one site. Patients receiving large doses should be closely observed for at least 30 minutes to assure that narcosis is not excessive.

Keep patient under constant observation when drug is administered IV, and record vital signs at least every hour or more often if indicated. Administration rate: no greater than 60 mg/minute. Resuscitation equipment and drugs should be immediately available.

Extravasation of IV phenobarbital may cause necrotic tissue changes that may necessitate skin grafting. (Addicts who use IV phenobarbital for a "high" have been known to lose a finger from the damage of intraarterial injections.) Frequently check the injection site. *(See Nursing Interventions: extravasation.)*

When administering oral barbiturates, observe that patient actually swallows the pill and does not "cheek" it.

If patient cannot swallow pill, it may be crushed before administration, then mixed with a fluid or with food. (Do not permit patient to swallow dry crushed drug.)

Barbiturates do not have analgesic action, and they may be expected to produce restlessness when given to patients in pain.

Patients receiving anticonvulsant therapy may experience drowsiness during first few weeks of treatment, but this usually diminishes with continued use of the barbiturate.

The elderly or debilitated patient and children sometimes have parodoxical response to barbiturate therapy: i.e., irritability, marked excitement (inappropriate tearfulness and aggression in children), depression and confusion. Be alert to unexpected responses and report promptly. Protect the elderly patient from falling, irrational behavior and effects of depression (anorexia, social withdrawal).

The elderly patient receiving a barbiturate is predisposed to bedsore development (decreased body movement in sleep). Total multidrug therapy, if necessary, is difficult to control because of altered hepatic microsomal enzyme function with aging.

Caution patient to avoid potentially hazardous activities requiring mental alertness such as driving a car or operating machinery, until response to drug is known.

Alcohol in any amount given with a barbiturate may severely impair judgment and abilities; it should not be consumed by a patient on barbiturate therapy.

Food-Drug Interaction:

- Phenobarbital increases vitamin D metabolism leading to subtherapeutic levels and possible onset of osteomalacia, or rickets (long-term therapy). Advise patient to increase vitamin D fortified foods (e.g., milk products). A vitamin D supplement may be prescribed.
- Long-term therapy may result in nutritional folate deficiency (barbiturates inhibit intestinal tract deconjugase enzymes that prepare dietary folic acid for absorption). Laboratory confirmation is the basis for urging patient to maintain adequate dietary folate intake: fresh vegetables (especially green leafy), fresh fruits, whole grains, liver. A supplement of folic acid may be prescribed.

Caution patient to adhere to drug regimen: i.e., intervals between doses should not be changed and doses should not be increased or decreased without advice.

Warn patient not to stop taking drug abruptly because of danger of withdrawal symptoms which can be fatal: (8 to 12 hours after last dose): apprehension, hand and finger tremors, weakness, dizziness, disturbed vision, nausea, vomiting, sweating, orthostatic hypotension, insomnia. More severe symptoms may develop 2 to 8 days after withdrawal: delirium, convulsion, status epilepticus (patient with epilepsy). Withdrawal symptoms may occur after a course of therapy with 600 to 800 mg daily for 35 days and may last up to 15 days after abrupt cessation of drug therapy.

Be alert to adverse reactions in the patient who apparently has tolerated phenobarbital in the past:

Chronic toxicity (dependence; drug abuse):

- Behavior simulates that of the chronic alcoholic): desire or need to continue taking the drug without physician's knowledge; self-limited abstinence periods; patient begins to see a number of physicians never admitting to multiple prescriptions.
- Symptoms: ataxia, slurred speech, irritability, poor judgment, slight dysarthria, nystagmus on vertical gaze, confusion, insomnia, somatic complaints.
- *Treatment* (detoxification): cautious, gradual withdrawal of the drug in a drug-free, inpatient setting (because of the severity of withdrawal symptoms). Several regimens are used (e.g., substitution of 30 mg phenobarbital for each 100 to 200 mg dose of barbiturate patient has been using and its administration in 3 or 4 equally divided doses/day. Prescription, adapting treatment to patient by protocol, and administration of phenobarbital are medically supervised.
- During withdrawal period, long range plans for support of abstinence (professional counseling, rehabilitation) should be made. Patient and family need to be involved in the planning.

Acute toxicity (intoxication): (serum concentration in excess of 80 mcg/ml):

- Profound CNS depression, respiratory depression which may progress to Cheyne–Stokes respirations, hypoventilation, cyanosis; cold, clammy skin; hypothermia, pupils constricted (but may be dilated in severe intoxication), shock, oliguria, tachycardia, hypotension, respiration arrest, circulatory collapse, death. Frequently, pressure sores are on skin surfaces pressured by the unconscious patient's body weight; these may develop within 4 hours after drug ingestion.
- *Treatment:* If patient is conscious and still has gag reflex: emesis induction with ipecac; when vomiting is completed, activated charcoal (30 Gm in a glass of water) is given. If emesis is contraindicated: gastric lavage with cuffed endotracheal tube in place with patient in face-down position. Multiple-dose nasogastric administration of charcoal has been effective, or charcoal may be left in the emptied stomach and a saline cathartic administered. Supportive measured for respiratory function and blood pressure, warming blanket, urinary alkalization, hemodialysis or hemoperfusion.
- Monitor vital signs, intake–output ratio and pattern; roll patient from side to side every 30 minutes.
- Frequent complications of acute toxicity: pulmonary edema, aspiration pneumonia. Prevent aspiration of vomitus by proper positioning and by having someone in constant attendance during vomiting period.

It is important that pregnancy be avoided in patients receiving barbiturates (reportedly teratogenic). Patients on prolonged therapy should consider alternative methods of contraception in addition to or instead of oral contraceptives to prevent unplanned pergnancy. *(see Drug Interactions).* The neonate born of mother who received barbiturate therapy throughout the last trimester may show withdrawal symptoms for 1 to 14 days after birth. Symptoms resemble congenital opiate withdrawal symptoms: hyperactivity, restlessness, tremor, hyperreflexia, disturbed sleep.

Hepatic function and hematology tests and determinations of serum folate and vitamin D levels are advised during prolonged therapy.

Instruct patients on prolonged therapy to report to physician the onset of fever, sore throat or mouth, malaise, easy bruising or bleeding, petechiae, jaundice, rash.

Advise patients taking barbiturates at home not to keep drug on bedside table or in a readily accessible place. Patients have been known to forget having taken the drug, and in half-wakened conditions have accidentally overdosed themselves.

Classified as Schedule IV drug under Federal Controlled Substances Act.

Slang names for barbiturates include "barbs," "sleepers," "downs," "phennies," "peanuts," among many others. Addicts frequently use barbiturates to boost the effects of weak heroin.

Barbiturates increase the metabolism of many drugs leading to decreased pharmacologic effects of those drugs. Whenever a barbiturate is added to an established regimen of another drug close observation for changes in effectiveness of the first drug is essential, at least during early phase of barbiturate use.

Barbiturates decrease or reduce pharmacologic effects of the following drugs (groups); anticoagulants (coumarins), carbamazepine, corticosteroids, digitoxin, doxycycline, estradiol, griseofulvin, oral contraceptives, quinidine, phenothiazines, tricyclic antidepressants. Clinical significance is not always delineated (e.g., griseofulvin). *See specific drug interactant for more information.*

Store at 15° to 30°C (59° to 86°F) unless otherwise directed by manufacturer.

Diagnostic Test Interferences. Barbiturates may affect **bromsulphalein** retention tests (by enhancing hepatic uptake and excretion of dye) and increase **serum phosphatase.**

Drug Interactions: Phenobarbitol

Plus	Interactions
Alcohol and other CNS depressants	Additive depressant effects
Anesthetics	
Chloramphenicol, Valproic acid, Disulfiram	Prolonged barbiturate action
Nondepolarizing skeletal muscle relaxants (e.g., tubocurarine)	Additive respiratory depression
Furosamide	May aggravate or produce orthostatic hypotension
Phenytoin	Increased/decreased effects of either drug
Sulfonamides	May increase effects of barbiturates

PHENOLPHTHALEIN

(fee-nol-thay'leen)

(Alophen, Correctol, Evac-U-Gen, Evac-U-Lax, Ex-Lax, Feen-a-Mint, Fructines-Vichy, Phenolax, Prulet)

Laxative, stimulant

ACTIONS AND USES. Diphenylmethane laxative similar to bisacodyl in pharmacologic properties. Common ingredient in several OTC fixed combination laxative drugs. Used for temporary relief of simple constipation.

P

ABSORPTION AND FATE. Acts in 6 to 8 hours. Excreted in feces. Up to 15% of dose absorbed and eliminated primarily by kidney in conjugated form; some enters the enterohepatic cycle before excretion in the feces.

CONTRAINDICATIONS AND PRECAUTIONS. Hypersensitivity to phenolphthalein; abdominal pain, nausea, vomiting, fecal impaction, intestinal obstruction or perforation.

ADVERSE/SIDE EFFECTS. Allergic reactions: skin eruptions, urticaria, Stevens-Johnson syndrome, lupus erythematosus-like syndrome. Large doses or chronic use: electrolyte imbalance, impaired glucose tolerance from potassium loss.

ROUTE AND DOSAGE. Oral: 30 to 200 mg.

NURSING IMPLICATIONS

All preparations are OTC drugs.

Usually administered at bedtime to produce effect the next morning (approximately 6 to 8 hours later).

Since drug enters enterohepatic circulation, inform patient that laxative effect may persist for several days.

Advise patient to avoid prolonged or frequent use. Dependence on drug action, as well as electrolyte imbalance, can occur.

Drug may impart reddish or purplish pink discoloration to alkaline urine or feces (made alkaline by soapsuds enema). Inform patient of this possibility.

Instruct patient to discontinue drug immediately if skin rash appears.

Skin lesions resulting from allergic reaction may persist for months or years and may leave residual pigmentation.

Phenolax contains tartrazine which may cause allergic-like reactions including bronchial asthma in susceptible persons. Such individuals are frequently sensitive to aspirin.

Caution patient to store drug out of reach of children; fatalities have occurred when drug was eaten as candy.

See Bisacodyl.

Diagnostic Test Interferences. Phenolphthalein may interfere with **BSP excretion** test.

PHENOXYBENZAMINE HYDROCHLORIDE

(Dibenzyline)

(fen-ox-ee-ben'za-meen)

Antihypertensive

Alpha-adrenergic blocking agent

ACTIONS AND USES. Long-acting alpha-adrenergic blocking agent. Apparently produces noncompetitive blockade ("chemical sympathectomy") of alpha-adrenergic receptor sites at postganglionic synapse. Alpha receptor sites are thus unable to react to endogenous or exogenous sympathomimetic agents. Blocks excitatory (alpha) effects of epinephrine, including vasoconstriction, but does not affect adrenergic cardiac inhibitory (beta) actions. Produces dilatation of muscular, cutaneous, and pulmonary vascular systems, but does not significantly alter cardiac output or renal, hepatic, and cerebral blood flow. Causes orthostatic hypotension in both normotensive and hypertensive patients, and also blocks pupillary dilation and retraction of eyelids.

Used in management of pheochromocytoma and to improve circulation in peripheral vasospastic conditions such as Raynaud's acrocyanosis and frostbite sequelae. *Investigational Use:* for adjunctive treatment of shock.

ABSORPTION AND FATE. About 30% of oral dose is absorbed. Onset of action in 2 hours; peak effects within 4 to 6 hours. Alpha-adrenergic blockade persists for 3 or 4 days. Half-life approximately 24 hours. About 80% excreted in urine and bile in 24 hours.

CONTRAINDICATIONS AND PRECAUTIONS. When fall in blood pressure would be dangerous; compensated congestive failure. *Cautious Use:* marked cerebral or coronary arteriosclerosis, renal insufficiency, respiratory infections. Safe use during pregnancy not established.

ADVERSE/SIDE EFFECTS. Nasal congestion, dry mouth, miosis, drooping of eyelids, postural hypotension, tachycardia, palpitation, dizziness, fainting, inhibition of ejaculation, drowsiness, sedation, tiredness, weakness, lethargy, confusion, headache, GI irritation, vomiting, shock, CNS stimulation (large doses), allergic contact dermatitis.

ROUTE AND DOSAGE. **Oral: Adults:** Initial: 10 mg daily in a single dose; dosage may be increased by increments of 10 mg daily at 4-day intervals to desired dose. Maintenance: 20 to 60 mg daily in single or divided doses. **Children:** Initial: 0.2 mg/kg daily in a single dose. Maintenance: 0.4 mg/kg daily.

NURSING IMPLICATIONS

Giving the drug with milk or in divided doses may reduce gastric irritation.

During period of dosage adjustment, monitor blood pressure and note pulse quality, rate, and rhythm in recumbent and standing positions. (Hypotension and tachycardia are most likely to occur in standing position.) Patient should be closely observed for at least 4 days from one dosage increment to the next.

Instruct patient to make position changes slowly, particularly from recumbent to upright posture, and to dangle legs and exercise ankles and feet for a few minutes before standing.

Advise patient to lie down or sit down in head-low position immediately at the onset of faintness or weakness. Physician may prescribe support stockings and abdominal support to help prevent orthostatic hypotension. Miosis, nasal stuffiness, and inhibition of ejaculation generally decrease with continued therapy.

Inform patient that postural hypotension and palpitation usually disappear with continued therapy, but they may reappear under conditions that promote vasodilation, such as strenuous exercise or ingestion of a large meal or alcohol.

Since phenoxybenzamine has cumulative action, onset of therapeutic effects may not occur until after 2 weeks of therapy, and full therapeutic effects may not be apparent for several more weeks. (Drug action lasts several days after discontinuation of therapy.)

Therapeutic effectiveness in patients with pheochromocytoma is indicated by decreases in blood pressure, pulse, and sweating. In patients with peripheral vasospastic problems, observe for improvement in skin color, temperature, and quality of peripheral pulses, as well as less sensitivity to cold.

Treatment of overdosage: recumbent position with legs elevated (keep patient flat for 24 hours or more if necessary); application of leg bandages and abdominal binder. For severe hypotensive reaction, IV infusion of norepinephrine may be given. Epinephrine is *contraindicated* because it may cause further drop in blood pressure.

Advise patient not to take OTC medications for coughs, colds, or allergy without approval of physician. (Many contain sympathomimetic agents that cause blood pressure elevation.)

Preserved in airtight containers, protected from light.

PHENPROCOUMON
(Liquamar)

(fen-proe-koo'mon)
Anticoagulant, oral
Coumarin

ACTIONS AND USES. Long-acting coumarin derivative. Qualitatively similar to other drugs of this class in actions, uses, contraindications, precautions, and adverse reactions. *See Warfarin.*

Used generally to maintain anticoagulant effect initiated by other anticoagulants.

ABSORPTION AND FATE. Peak prothrombin time effect in 48 to 72 hours. Half-life: 6.5 days. Normal values may not return for 7 to 14 days after cessation of drug.

ADVERSE/SIDE EFFECTS. Relatively frequent: nausea, diarrhea, dermatitis. Less frequent: bleeding, agranulocytosis, hepatitis, renal damage, alopecia, hypersensitivity reaction. *See also Warfarin.*

ROUTE AND DOSAGE. Oral: first day: 21 mg; second day: 9 mg; maintenance: 0.5 to 6 mg daily according to prothrombin time determinations.

NURSING IMPLICATIONS

Prothrombin time should be determined prior to and 24 hours after administration of initial dose.

During period of dosage adjustment, prothrombin time results should be measured every 24 to 48 hours; results should be checked by physician and dosage order obtained. Follow agency policies for administration of anticoagulants.

Thereafter, prothrombin time is usually measured once or twice weekly for the next 3 or 4 weeks, and at 2- to 4-week intervals for patients on long-term therapy.

Advise patient to report diarrhea. Dosage adjustment or drug withdrawal may be indicated.

Prolonged duration of drug action may add to the dangers of anticoagulant therapy, since hemorrhage will be more difficult to control if it occurs.

Instruct patient to withhold drug and to report immediately the onset of bleeding, fever, chills, sore throat or mouth, malaise, marked fatigue, or any other unusual sign or symptom.

Caution patient not to start or stop taking any other medication without approval of physician.

Counsel patient not to engage in contact sports or other activities with high risk of injuries.

Advise patient to tell all doctors and dentists who may administer care that patient is taking an anticoagulant.

Stress importance of avoiding unusual changes in diet or life-style without consulting physician.

Store drug in tightly-closed container at temperature between 15° and 30°C (59° and 86°F).

See also Warfarin.

PHENSUXIMIDE
(Milontin)

(fen-sux'i-mide)
Anticonvulsant
Succinimide

ACTIONS AND USES. Succinimide derivative reportedly less potent and less effective than other drugs of this class. *See Ethosuximide for actions, contraindications, precautions, and adverse reactions.*

Used in management of petit mal epilepsy (absence seizures) and with other anticonvulsants when other forms of epilepsy coexist with petit mal.

ABSORPTION AND FATE. Absorbed promptly; peak plasma levels in 1 to 4 hours. Not bound to plasma proteins. Half-life about 5 to 12 hours. Metabolized in liver; excreted in urine as active and inactive metabolites.

CONTRAINDICATIONS AND PRECAUTIONS. Intermittent porphyria.

ADVERSE/SIDE EFFECTS. Drowsiness, dizziness, ataxia, alopecia, muscle weakness, anorexia, nausea, flushing, periorbital edema, pruritus, skin rash, reversible nephropathy, granulocytosis. *See also Ethosuximide.*

ROUTE AND DOSAGE. Oral: Adult: 0.5 to 1 Gm two or three times daily. Highly individualized. **Pediatric:** 0.6 to 1.2 Gm two or three times daily. Total dosage, regardless of age, may vary between 1 and 3 Gm/day.

NURSING IMPLICATIONS

Shake oral suspension well before pouring to assure uniform dosage.

Caution against potentially hazardous tasks such as driving a car or operating machinery until response to drug is known.

Advise patient to report onset of skin rash or other unusual symptoms to physician.

Stress importance of keeping scheduled appointments for blood, urine, and liver function studies.

Caution patient not to change drug regimen, i.e., reduce, increase or omit doses. Patient should not change dose intervals, and should not share the drug with another person.

Concomitant use of OTC drugs must be discouraged unless the physician approves; loss of seizure control can be induced by ingredients in some popular OTC drugs.

Inform patient that phensuximide may color urine pink, red, or red brown.

Store at temperature between 15° and 30°C (59° and 86°F) unless otherwise advised by manufacturer.

Protect from light and heat.

See Ethosuximide.

P

PHENTERMINE HYDROCHLORIDE

(fen′ter-meen)

(Adipex, Fastin, Ionamin, Obe-Nix, Obephen, Obermine, Paramine, Phentrol, Rolaphent, Unifast, Wilpowr)

Anorexiant
Sympathomimetic
C IV

ACTIONS AND USES. Sympathomimetic amine related chemically and pharmacologically to amphetamine (qv). Cardiovascular actions and CNS stimulant effects are less prominent than those of amphetamine. Available as the hydrochloride salt and as a complex with a cationic-exchange resin of sulfonated polystyrene. Resin complex reacts with cations in GI tract and is designed to give controlled release of drug over 10- to 14-hour period. Effects of conventional oral tablet (hydrochloride) persist about 4 hours.

Used as short-term (a few weeks) adjunct in management of exogenous obesity.

CONTRAINDICATIONS AND PRECAUTIONS. History of hypersensitivity to sympathomimetic amines; during or within 14 days of MAO inhibitor use; glaucoma, angina, children 12 years or less. Safe use during pregnancy not established. *Cautious Use:* advanced arteriosclerosis, symptomatic cardiovascular disease, moderate to severe hypertension, hyperthyroidism, glaucoma, agitated states, history of drug abuse.

ADVERSE/SIDE EFFECTS. Nervousness, dizziness, insomnia, dry mouth, nausea, constipation, hypertension, palpitation, tachycardia, decreased sexual desire, impotence; severe dermatoses, marked insomnia, irritability, hyperactivity, psychoses. Abrupt cessation following prolonged high dosage: extreme fatigue, depression, changes in sleep EEG patterns.

ROUTE AND DOSAGE. Oral: Adult: Extended release capsule (resin complex): 15 to 30 mg once a day before breakfast. Hydrochloride: 8 mg three times daily ½ hour before meals.

NURSING IMPLICATIONS

Not to be confused with chlorphentermine, also an anorexiant, but given at much higher dosages. Caution patient not to change established dose regimen, i.e., not to increase, decrease or omit doses. Warn against use of the drug for any purposes other than the one for which it is prescribed.

To prevent insomnia, late evening medication should be avoided.

Avoid caffeine drinks which increase amphetaminelike and related amine effects.

Tolerance to anorexigenic effect usually occurs within a few weeks. Drug should be discontinued when this occurs.

Caution patient to avoid potentially hazardous activities such as driving a car or operating machinery until his response to the drug is known.

Instruct patient to notify physician if palpitation, nervousness or dizziness occur.

Renal excretion is enhanced by urinary acidification; reabsorption and recycling are enhanced by alkaline urine. A high alkaline-ash diet could potentially increase side effects. *See Index.*

Severe psychologic dependence has occurred in patients who have exceeded recommended dosage.

Classified as Schedule IV drug under Federal Controlled Substances Act.

See also Amphetamine.

P

Drug Interactions: Phentermine Hydrochloride

Plus	Interactions
Acetozolamide, sodium bicarbonate	Increased renal reabsorption of phentermine
Ammonium chloride, ascorbic acid	Decreased phentermine effects
MAO inhibitors	Severe hypertension
Phenothiazines, haloperidol	Decreased effect of psychotropics

PHENTOLAMINE HYDROCHLORIDE

(Regitine Hydrochloride)

(fen-tole'a-meen)

Antihypertensive diagnostic aid
Alpha-adrenergic blocking agent

ACTIONS AND USES. Imidazoline alpha-adrenergic blocking agent structurally related to tolazoline, but has more potent blocking effects. Competetively blocks alpha-adrenergic receptors, but action is transient and incomplete. Prevents hypertension resulting from elevated levels of circulating epinephrine and/or norepinephrine. Causes vasodilation, and decreases general vascular resistance and pulmonary arterial pressure, primarily by direct action on vascular smooth muscle. Through stimulation of beta-adrenergic receptors, produces positive inotropic and chronotropic cardiac effects, and increases cardiac output. Also has histamine-like action that stimulates gastric secretions.

Used in diagnosis of pheochromocytoma and to prevent or control hypertensive episodes prior to or during pheochromocytomectomy. Also used to prevent dermal necrosis and sloughing following IV administration or extravasation of norepinephrine. *Investigational Use:* to treat hypertensive crises caused by certain foods or drugs.

ABSORPTION AND FATE. Maximum effect on blood pressure following IV administration in 2 minutes (persists 10 to 15 minutes), and in 15 to 20 minutes after IM (blood pressure returns to preinjection level in 3 to 4 hours).

CONTRAINDICATIONS AND PRECAUTIONS. Hypersensitivity to phentolamine or related drugs; myocardial infarction (previous or present). Safe use during pregnancy and lactation not established. *Cautious Use:* gastritis, peptic ulcer, coronary artery disease.

ADVERSE/SIDE EFFECTS. Weakness, dizziness, flushing, orthostatic hypotension, nasal stuffiness, conjunctival infection. GI side effects (common): abdominal pain, nausea, vomiting, diarrhea, exacerbation of peptic ulcer. With parenteral administration especially: acute and prolonged hypotension, tachycardia, anginal pain, cardiac arrhythmias, myocardial infarction, cerebrovascular spasm, shocklike state.

ROUTE AND DOSAGE. **Oral:** **Adults:** *Prevention of hypertensive episodes:* 50 mg four to six times daily. **Children:** 25 mg four to six times daily; alternatively, 5 mg/kg body weight, divided into 4 to 6 doses. **Intravenous, intramuscular:** **Adults:** 5 mg. **Children:** 1 mg; alternatively, 0.1 mg/kg. *To prevent necrosis:* 10 mg to each L of IV fluid containing levarterenol. *To treat extravasation:* 5 to 10 mg in 10 ml of 0.9% sodium chloride injection injected into affected area, within 12 hours after extravasation. *Test for pheochromocytoma:* 5 mg.

NURSING IMPLICATIONS

Reconstitute 5 mg vial with 1 ml of sterile water for injection. Manufacturer recommends that reconstituted solutions be used immediately.

Patient should be in supine position when receiving drug parenterally. Monitor blood pressure and pulse every 2 minutes until stabilized.

Test for pheochromocytoma: (1) Medications not deemed absolutely essential should be withheld at least 24 hours, preferably 48 to 72 hours; antihypertensive agents withheld until blood pressure returns to pretreatment level (rauwolfia drugs withdrawn at least 4 weeks prior to testing). (2) Keep patient at rest in supine position throughout test, preferably in quiet darkened room. (3) Take blood pressure every 10 minutes for at least 30 minutes; when blood pressure stabilizes, injection should be administered by physician. (4) IV administration: record blood pressure immediately after injection and at 30-second intervals for first 3 minutes, then at 1-minute intervals for next 7 minutes. IM administration: blood pressure determinations at 5-minute intervals for 30 to 45 minutes.

Test results: Positive response (indicated by drop in systolic pressure of at least 35 mm Hg and 25 mm Hg diastolic) suggests pheochromocytoma. Presumptive negative response: blood pressure is unchanged, elevated, or reduced less than 35 mm Hg systolic and 25 mm Hg diastolic. Advise patient to avoid sudden changes in position, particularly from recumbent to upright posture and to dangle legs and exercise ankles and toes for a few minutes before ambulating.

Instruct patient to lie down or sit down in head-low position immediately if feels lightheaded or dizzy.

Treatment of overdosage (evidenced by precipitous drop in blood pressure): Keep patient recumbent with head lowered; supportive measures; IV fluids; IV infusion of levarterenol, carefully titrated. *Epinephrine is contraindicated,* since paradoxic fall in blood pressure may result.

Phentolamine hydrochloride is preserved in well-closed, light-resistant containers.

PHENYLBUTAZONE

(fen-ill-byoo'ta-zone)

(Algoverine, Azolid, Buffazone, Butazolidin, Intrabutazone, Nadozone, Novobutazone, Phenbuff)

NSAID
Antirheumatic
Pyrazolone

ACTIONS AND USES. Pyrazolone derivative with antiinflammatory, antipyretic, analgesic, and mild uricosuric properties. Specific antiinflammatory action mechanism unknown but appears to be associated with prostaglandin synthesis, leukocyte migration, and release or activity of lysosomal enzymes. Inhibits platelet aggregation. Does not cure inflammatory condition but produces effective short-term symptomatic relief of pain and disability. Should not be used as a general analgesic or antipyretic.

Used in short-term treatment of acute gouty arthritis, active rheumatoid arthritis and ankylosing spondylitis, and short-term treatment of painful acute osteoarthritis of joints not responsive to other treatments.

ABSORPTION AND FATE. Readily absorbed from GI tract with onset of action in 30 to 60 minutes. Peak plasma levels in 2 hours; duration of action 3 to 5 days. Repeated daily doses produce plateau in plasma levels in 3 to 5 days. Metabolized in liver to several active metabolites including oxyphenbutazone and hydroxyphenylbutazone. 98% protein-bound; half-life: 50 to 100 hours (increased to 149 hours with hepatic dysfunction). Distributed to most body tissues. Excreted slowly in urine as unchanged drug (1%) and metabolites. Crosses placenta; enters breast milk, and synovial spaces (with concentration equal to about 50% that in plasma). Has potential cumulative toxicity.

CONTRAINDICATIONS AND PRECAUTIONS. Phenylbutazone or oxyphenbutazone sensitivity and idiosyncracy, history of peptic ulcer, GI inflammatory disease, pancreatitis, stomatitis, aspirin hypersensitivity, drug allergy, blood dyscrasias, renal disease, hepatic dysfunction, left ventricular failure, borderline cardiac failure, severe hypertension, edema, polymyalgia rheumatica, temporal arteritis, concomitant use with other drugs such as chemotherapeutic agents, use with long-term anticoagulants (oral) therapy, children under age 14, senile patient. Safe use during pregnancy especially during third trimester not established. *Cautious Use:* glaucoma, patients over age 40, asthma.

ADVERSE/SIDE EFFECTS. CV: hypertension, palpitation, pericarditis, cardiac decompensation. **Dermatologic:** fixed drug eruptions, erythema nodosum and multiforme, nonthrombocytopenic purpura. **Ear/Eye:** Optic neuritis, retinal hemorrhage and detachment, oculomotor palsy, toxic amblyopia, blurred vision, conjunctivitis, scotomata; hearing loss, tinnitus. **Endocrine/metabolic:** hyperglycemia, thyroid hyperplasia, toxic goiter, myxedema; sodium, chloride and fluid retention; rapid plasma volume expansion with plasma dilution, metabolic acidosis, respiratory alkalosis. **GI:** recurring dyspepsia (including heartburn and indigestion), nausea, vomiting, constipation, diarrhea, xerostomia, ulcerative stomatitis and esophagitis, salivary gland enlargement, epigastric pain, constipation, abdominal distention with flatulence, ulceration of bowel, reactivation of peptic ulcer, hepatitis (fatal and nonfatal), pancreatitis. **Hematologic:** bone marrow depression, pancytopenia, thrombocytopenia, agranulocytosis, aplastic anemia (sometimes fatal), leukopenia, leukemia. **Hypersensitivity:** asthma, urticaria, anaphylaxis, drug fever, serum sickness, Stevens-Johnson syndrome, activation of SLE, Lyell's syndrome. **Renal:** hematuria, proteinuria, glomerulonephritis, renal failure, nephrotic syndrome, renal calculi, azotemia. **Other:** trembling, nervousness, taste disturbances.

ROUTE AND DOSAGE. Oral: *Rheumatoid arthritis, acute attacks of degenerative joint disease:* Initial: 300 to 600 mg three to four times daily. Maximum therapeutic response usually obtained with daily dose of 400 mg. *Acute gout and gouty arthritis:* Initial: 400 mg followed by 100 mg every 4 hours until relief of symptoms (usually 4 to 7 days).

NURSING IMPLICATIONS

Steady state therapeutic serum levels: 95 mcg/ml reached in 3 to 4 days.

Possible GI irritation can be minimized by administering drug with meals or with full glass of milk.

Tablet may be crushed and capsule may be emptied if patient cannot swallow them whole. Mix crushed powder or capsule contents with fluid of patient's choice or mix with food. Should not be swallowed dry.

Careful, detailed history and complete physical and laboratory examinations (including GI diagnostic tests in patient with persistent or severe dyspepsia) are advised prior to initiating therapy.

Frequent regular blood studies are advisable when drug is given beyond 1 week, the usual treatment period.

Urge patient to report for all scheduled blood studies. Hematologic toxicity may occur suddenly or many days or weeks after drug use has been terminated.

Any significant change in hematology: i.e., total white count depression, relative decrease in granulocytes, appearance of blast forms, fall in hematocrit, signals the necessity to stop treatment pending complete hematology studies.

If a drug with lower percentage protein-binding is given with phenylbutazone, the actions and toxicity of that drug may be increased because it will be displaced from its binding to protein thereby increasing its serum concentration (free drug).

Although phenylbutazone increases action of oral anticoagulants when given concomitantly, it does not affect prothrombin activity when administered alone; however, the combination of antiplatelet and ulcerogenic action of phenylbutazone contributes to the hazard of serious hemorrhage during drug therapy.

Patients should be closely followed during therapy and made fully aware of potential adverse reactions. Symptoms of phenylbutazone toxicity are insidious in onset, and should be reported promptly.

Keep physician informed of patient's response to medication. If favorable response is not noted in 1 week drug is discontinued. When improvement occurs (usually begins in 3 to 4 days), dosage is reduced and discontinued as soon as symptomatic relief dictates.

Adverse reactions are both age- and dose-related. If the patient is over age 60, longer than a 1-week treatment period is not recommended because of high risk of severe, fatal, toxic reactions in this age group.

Check with physician about alcohol ingestion. Alcohol impairs motor coordination in the patient receiving phenylbutazone (probably an additive effect). This action should be pointed out to the patient especially with respect to driving.

Warn patient to discontinue drug therapy immediately and report to physician: fever, stomatitis, oral ulcerations, salivary gland enlargement, severe sore throat, epigastric pain, dyspepsia, unusual unexplained bleeding and bruising, tarry stools, skin rashes, edema, pruritus, jaundice.

Any eye symptom should be investigated. Be sure patient understands this, because (especially with the elderly person) adaptation to blurring may be subconscious at first. Drug should be discontinued and a complete ophthalmic examination scheduled.

Keep in mind that the presenting symptom of leukemia (an adverse effect of phenylbutazone) can be arthritic-like pain; therefore reappearance of acute joint pain after satisfactory response to treatment, should be differentially evaluated.

Monitor patient with asthma especially if patient is also sensitive to aspirin. This drug like others with prostaglandin synthetase inhibition activity may precipitate an acute asthma attack.

Urge patient not to self-dose with OTC drugs unless advised to do so by physician. Many pain relief OTC preparations contain aspirin.

Symptoms of overdosage: prompt onset of respiratory or metabolic acidosis with hyperventilation which can progress to trismus, tonic-clonic seizures, shock, coma, hypotension, oliguria. Other symptoms include: nausea, vomiting, epigastric pain, excessive perspiration, euphoria, psychoses, headache, vertigo, insomnia, tinnitus, edema, cyanosis, agitation, hallucinations, convulsions, hematuria. Buccal or GI mucosal ulcerations are late manifestations of massive overdosage.

Treatment of overdosage: if patient is alert: induce emesis, followed by lavage of stomach and administration of activated charcoal. In obtunded patient: maintain vital functions, treat shock with appropriate supportive measures. Respiratory stimulants not advised. Control seizures with IV benzodiazipines (e.g., diazepam) or short-acting barbiturates; hemodialysis may be effective if renal function is impaired.

Phenylbutazone may cause drowsiness; therefore, advise patient to observe caution while driving or performing tasks requiring alertness until response to drug is known.

Warn patient to adhere to dosage regimen, i.e., not to double, reduce, or omit doses nor to change dose intervals without the physician's approval.

Food (Nutrient)-Drug Interaction: Phenylbutazone interferes with absorption of folates, tryptophane and other amino acids.

Smoking-Drug Interaction: Smoking shortens half-life and increases clearance rate of phenylbutazone. It is possible that the heavy smoker may require an adjusted dosage regimen.

Instruct patient to keep a record of daily weights and to check for lower leg, ankle, or facial edema. Advise patient to report sudden weight gain (i.e., gain of 2 to 3 pounds within 2 to 3 days). Edema may signify hepatic or renal dysfunction or electrolyte imbalance and may indicate necessity of stopping therapy. In the elderly, a reduction of dose may suffice to reduce edema of ankles and face.

Store drug at temperature between 15° and 30°C (59° and 86°F) in light and moisture-resistant container.

P

Diagnostic Test Interferences. Phenylbutazone reduces **iodine uptake** by thyroid gland.

Drug Interactions: Phenylbutazone

Plus	Interactions
Alcohol	Increased phenylbutazone-induced ulcerogenic effects
Antiinflammatory agents (other NSAIDs)	Displaced from protein-binding sites with resulting increase in pharmacologic and toxic effects of displaced drug; the reverse is also true: i.e., phenylbutazone may be displaced, increasing its serum concentration and potential toxicity

Plus (cont.)	Interactions (cont.)
Anticoagulants, coumarins	Increased anticoagulant effect; increased risk of serious hemorrhage. Concomitant use should be avoided
Aspirin	Increases ulcerogenic effects of phenylbutazone
Beta-blocking agents	May reduce antihypertensive effects of the beta-blocker
Desipramine	Decreases phenylbutazone serum level, thereby reducing clinical effects
Digitalis glycosides	Enhances metabolism of digitalis leading to underdigitalization
Hydantoins (e.g., phenytoin)	Increased risk of phenytoin toxicity
Hypoglycemics, sulfonylureas (e.g., Folbutamide, glipizide)	Increased hypoglycemic effects
Insulin	Potentiation of hypoglycemic action of insulin
Methofrexate	Increased response to methotrexate possibly leading to toxicity. Concomitant use should be avoided
Salicylates	Antagonizes uricosuric activity
Sulfonamides	*See antiinflammatory agents*
Thyroid hormone	*See antiinflammatory agents*

PHENYLEPHRINE HYDROCHLORIDE

(AK-Dilate, Alconefrin, Allerest, Coricidin, Efricel, Isopto Frin, Mydrin, Neo-synephrine, Nostril, Prefrin, Rhinall, Sinarest, Sinex, Vacon, and others)

(fen-ill-ef′rin)
Adrenergic (vasoconstrictor)
Alpha-adrenergic

ACTIONS AND USES. Potent, noncatecholamine, direct-acting sympathomimetic with strong alpha-adrenergic and weak beta-adrenergic cardiac stimulant actions. Produces little or no CNS stimulation. Elevates systolic and diastolic pressures through arteriolar constriction; also constricts capacitance vessels and increases venous return to heart. Rise in blood pressure causes reflex bradycardia. Topical applications to eye produce vasoconstriction and prompt mydriasis of short duration, usually without causing cycloplegia. Reduces intraocular pressure by increasing outflow and decreasing rate of aqueous humor secretion. Nasal decongestant action qualitatively similar to that of epinephrine, but more potent and has longer duration of action.

Used parenterally to maintain blood pressure during anesthesia, to treat vascular failure in shock, and to overcome paroxysmal supraventricular tachycardia. Used topically for rhinitis of common cold, allergic rhinitis, and sinusitis; in selected patients with wide-angle glaucoma; as mydriatic for ophthalmoscopic examination or surgery, and for relief of uveitis.

ABSORPTION AND FATE. IV: immediate effects lasting 20 to 30 minutes. SC: IM: effects last 45 to 60 minutes. Maximum mydriasis achieved within 60 minutes; recovery usually occurs approximately 6 hours later. Decongestant effect (direct vasoconstriction) with use of nasal preparations: prompt and lasts for several hours.

CONTRAINDICATIONS AND PRECAUTIONS. Severe coronary disease, severe hypertension, ventricular tachycardia; narrow-angle glaucoma (ophthalmic preparations). *Cautious Use:* hyperthyroidism, diabetes mellitus, myocardial disease, cerebral arteriosclerosis, bradycardia, elderly patients; 21 days before or following termination of MAO inhibitor therapy. *10%*

ophthalmic solution: elderly patients with preexisting cardiovascular disease, or patients with diabetes mellitus, hypertension or hyperthyroidism; patients with aneurysms, infants.

ADVERSE/SIDE EFFECTS. Intranasal: rebound congestion (hyperemia and edema of mucosa), burning, stinging, dryness, sneezing. **Ophthalmic:** transient stinging, lacrimation, browache, headache, blurred vision, conjunctival allergy (pigmentary deposits on lids, conjunctiva, and cornea with prolonged use), increased sensitivity to light. **Systemic effects:** palpitation, tachycardia, bradycardia (overdosage), extrasystoles, hypertension, trembling, sweating, pallor, sense of fullness in head, tingling of extremities, sleeplessness, dizziness, lightheadedness, weakness.

ROUTE AND DOSAGE. Parenteral: *Hypotension:* **Intramuscular, subcutaneous:** 2 to 5 mg (range 1 to 10 mg) initial dose not to exceed 5 mg every 10 to 15 minutes as needed. **Intravenous infusion (10 mg/500 ml Dextrose Injection or NaCl Injection):** 100 to 180 drops/minute until blood pressure stabilizes, then 40 to 60 drops/minute for maintenance. **Intravenous injection:** 0.2 to 0.5 mg; subsequent doses no more often than 10 to 15 minutes at increments of up to 0.2 mg. **Ophthalmic preparations:** *Ophthalmoscopy:* **Adult (2.5 or 10% solution); children (2.5% solution):** 1 drop to conjunctiva; repeated once in 5 minutes if necessary. *Chronic mydriasis:* 1 drop, two or three times daily. *Vasoconstrictor* (0.02 to 0.15%): 1 drop every 3 to 4 hours as necessary. **Intranasal:** Nasal jelly: **Adult:** small amount placed into each nostril every 3 or 4 hours as needed. Nasal solution or spray: **Adult:** (0.25 to 0.5%): 2 or 3 drops or 1 or 2 sprays into each nostril every 3 to 4 hours as needed. **Children (up to 6 years):** (0.125%): 2 or 3 drops every 3 to 4 hours as needed. **(6 to 12 years):** (0.25%): 2 or 3 drops every 3 to 4 hours as needed. Spray: (0.25%) 1 or 2 sprays every 3 to 4 hours as needed.

NURSING IMPLICATIONS

During IV administration, monitor pulse, blood pressure and central venous pressure (every 2 to 5 minutes). Control flow rate and dosage to prevent excessive increases.

IV overdoses can induce ventricular dysrhythmias.

Have on hand phentolamine to treat hypertensive emergency with IV administration; levodopa to reduce excess mydriatic effect of ophthalmic preparation.

Caution patient not to exceed recommended dosage regardless of formulation; i.e., patient should not double, decrease or omit doses nor should patient change dose intervals unless told to do so by the physician.

If no relief is experienced from preparation in 5 days, patient should inform the physician.

Systemic absorption from nasal and conjunctival membranes can occur, though infrequently *(See Adverse/Side Effects).* Stop the drug and report to the physician.

Nasal preparations: Instruct patient to blow nose gently (with both nostrils open) to clear nasal passages well, before administration of medication.

- *Instillation (Drops):* tilt head back while sitting or standing up, or lie on bed and hang head over side. Stay in position a few minutes to permit medication to spread through nose.
- *(Spray):* with head upright, squeeze bottle quickly and firmly to produce 1 or 2 sprays into each nostril; wait 3 to 5 minutes, blow nose and repeat dose.
- *(Jelly):* place in each nostril and sniff it well back into nose.

Ophthalmic preparations *(See Index for administration instructions):*

- To avoid excessive systemic absorption, tell patient to apply pressure to lacrimal sac during and for 1 to 2 minutes after instillation of drops.
- Inform patient that after instillation of ophthalmic preparation, pupils of eyes will be very large and eyes may be more sensitive to light than usual. Advise patient to use

sunglasses in bright light and to stop medication and notify physician if this sensitivity persists beyond 12 hours after drug has been discontinued.
- Instillation of 2.5 to 10% strength solution frequently can cause burning and stinging.
- Observe for congestion or rebound miosis after topical administration to eye.
- A local anesthetic may be instilled before the phenylephrine to reduce discomfort of stinging and burning.
- Caution patient that some ophthalmic solutions may stain contact lenses.

Avoid swallowing solutions or jelly; systemic effects may be induced.

Cleanse tips and droppers of nasal solution dispensers with hot water after use to prevent contamination of solution. Droppers of ophthalmic solution bottles should not touch any surface including the eye.

Do not allow anyone other than the patient to use the prescribed supply of phenylephrine.

Phenylephrine is incompatable with butacaine, oxidizing agents, ferric salts, metals, and alkalies.

Solutions and jelly change color to brown, form a precipitate and lose potency with exposure to air, strong light or heat. Do not transfer solutions from original container to another.

Store in original container at temperature between 15° and 30°C (59° and 86°F) protected from freezing, strong light and exposure to air.

Drug Interactions: Phenylephrine Hydrochloride

Plus	Interactions
Ergot alkaloids, guanethidine, reserpine, tricyclic antidepressants	Increase pressor effects of phenylephrine
Halothane, digitalis, mercurial diuretics	Cardiac arrhythmias
MAO inhibitors	Hypertensive crisis
Oxytoxics	Persistence hypertension

P

PHENYLPROPANOLAMINE HYDROCHLORIDE

(Acutrim, Control, Diadax, Dietac, Propagest, Propadrine, Rhidecon)

(fen-ill-proe-pa-nole'a-meen)
Adrenergic (vasoconstrictor)
Alpha-adrenergic

ACTIONS AND USES. Indirect-acting sympathomimetic amine with prominent peripheral adrenergic effects similar to those of ephedrine (qv), but its action is more prolonged and it causes less CNS stimulation. Acts by stimulating alpha-adrenergic (excitatory) receptors of vascular smooth muscles, causing vasoconstriction and blanching of nasal mucosa. Also depresses appetite center in CNS.

Used in symptomatic relief of nasal congestion associated with allergies, hay fever, common cold, sinusitis, nasopharyngitis. Used parenterally as vasopressor during surgery, particularly during spinal anesthesia. Available in fixed combination with dextromethorphan (Ornacol) and many other OTC drugs used as decongestants and expectorants.

CONTRAINDICATIONS AND PRECAUTIONS. Concomitant use with MAO inhibitors. *Cautious Use:* hypertension, cardiovascular disease, hyperthyroidism, diabetes, prostatic enlargement, tricyclic antidepressants.

ADVERSE/SIDE EFFECTS. Larger doses: hypertension, tachycardia, palpitation, nervousness, restlessness, insomnia. **Overdosage:** tachycardia, rapid respirations, disorientation, kidney failure, dilated pupils, headache, CNS stimulation, nausea, vomiting, anorexia. *See also Ephedrine.*

ROUTE AND DOSAGE. Oral: Adults: 25 mg at 4-hour intervals or 50 mg at 8-hour intervals, as indicated. **Children (6 to 12 years):** 25 mg at 8-hour intervals; **(2 to 6 years):** 12.5 mg every 8 hours. Also available as elixir: 20 mg/ml.

NURSING IMPLICATIONS

Caution patient not to exceed recommended dosage.

Several OTC anorexiants, cold preparations and decongestants contain sizable amounts of phenylpropanolamine (e.g., Phen-Lets, 100 mg; Rhindecon, 75 mg). Since 75 mg of this drug can produce a significant rise in blood pressure in healthy normotensive adults, no more than one capsule containing 50 mg or less of phenylpropanolamine (e.g., Contac, Allerest Timed Release Caps, Supres, Dexatrim) should be taken at one time.

The use of OTC combination drugs without physician's approval while patient is receiving phenylpropanolamine should be discouraged.

Preserved in tight, light-resistant containers.

See Ephedrine.

Drug Interactions: Phenylpropanolamine Hydrochloride

Plus	Interactions
Bethanidine, Guanethidine	Antagonizes hypotensive effects of bethanidine and guanethidine
MAO inhibitors	May cause hypertensive crisis
Reserpine	Antagonizes therapeutic effects of phenylpropanolamine
Tricyclic antidepressants	Enhances pressor effects of phenylpropanolamine

See also Ephedrine.

P

PROTOTYPE

PHENYTOIN
(Dilantin, Novophenytoin)

PHENYTOIN SODIUM
(Dilantin Kapseals, Diphenylan)

(fen'i-toy-in)
Anticonvulsant
Antiarrhythmic
(Class IB)
Hydantoin

ACTIONS AND USES. Hydantoin derivative chemically related to phenobarbital. Precise mechanism of anticonvulsant action not known but drug use is accompanied by reduced voltage, frequency, and spread of electrical discharges within the motor cortex, resulting in prevention or reduction in severity and frequency of epileptiform attacks. Unlike phenobarbital, has little hypnotic action, is ineffective for control of drug-induced seizures, and has limited ability to modify threshold in electroconvulsive seizures. Has Class IB antiarrhythmic properties similar to those of lidocaine and tocainamide (also Class IB agents): in abnormal tissue causes slight increase in A-V conduction velocity depressed by digitalis glycosides, prolongs effective refractory period, suppresses ventricular pacemaker, automaticity and may slow conduction or cause complete block in abnormal ventricular fibers. Shortens action potential duration and improves resting potential. Membrane stabilizing effect on pancreas may inhibit effective insulin release. Induces hepatic microsomal enzymes and therefore affects the metabolism of many other drugs. Like other hydantoin derivatives, increases metabolic inactivation of vitamin D and has antifolate properties.

Used to control grand mal, psychomotor and nonepileptic seizures (e.g., Reye's syndrome, post-head trauma). Is not effective for absence seizures. *Unlabeled Use:* treatment of paradoxical atrial tachycardia, ventricular arrhythmias, particularly those associated with digitalis toxicity, and symptomatic treatment of rheumatoid arthritis.

ABSORPTION AND FATE. Slowly absorbed following oral administration (rate of absorption may vary widely among products by different manufacturers). Peak plasma concentrations (oral): 3 to 12 hours; phenytoin sodium: 2 to 3 hours. Onset of action: 3 to 5 minutes following IV injection. Drug precipitates at IM injection site and is slowly and erratically absorbed. Wide distribution to all tissues with highest concentrations in liver and fat; 70 to 95% bound to plasma proteins (mainly albumin). Half-life: 8 to 60 (average: 20 to 30) hours after initiation of therapy with oral daily dose of 300 mg (may be longer in black patients). Biotransformation in liver primarily, with excretion in bile as inactive metabolites which are reabsorbed from GI tract (enterohepatic circulation). Renal excretion (enhanced by alkaline urine) as glucuronides. Less than 5% excreted unchanged. Crosses placenta; enters breast milk.

CONTRAINDICATIONS AND PRECAUTIONS. Hypersensitivity to hydantoin products, skin rash, seizures due to hypoglycemia, during lactation, sinus bradycardia, complete or incomplete heart block, Adams-Stokes syndrome. *Cautious Use:* impaired hepatic or renal function, alcoholism, blood dyscrasias, hypotension, heart block, bradycardia, myocardial insufficiency, impending or frank heart failure, elderly, debilitated, gravely ill patients; pancreatic adenoma, pregnancy, diabetes mellitus, hyperglycemia, respiratory depression.

ADVERSE/SIDE EFFECTS. CNS (most common, usually dose-related): nystagmus, diplopia, blurred or dimmed vision, lethargy, drowsiness, ataxia, dizziness, slurred speech, mental confusion, tremors, insomnia, headache; peripheral neuropathy, encephalopathy; **CV:** With rapid IV injection: ventricular fibrillation, bradycardia, hypotension, cardiovascular collapse, cardiac (and respiratory) arrest. Also: phlebitis, injection site pain. **GI:** nausea, vomiting, constipation, epigastric pain, dysphagia, loss of taste, weight loss, hepatitis, liver necrosis. **Hematologic:** thrombocytopenia, leukopenia, leukocytosis, agranulocytosis, pancytopenia, eosinophilia, macrocytosis, megaloblastic anemia. **Hypersensitivity:** pruritus, fever, arthralgia, measles-like rash; exfoliative, purpuric or bullous dermatitis; Stevens-Johnson syndrome, lymphadenopathy, acute renal failure. **Metabolic:** hyperglycemia, glycosuria, transient increase in serum thyrotropic (TSH) level. **Ophthalmic:** photophobia, conjunctivitis, visual disturbances. **Other:** gingival hyperplasia, hirsutism (especially young females), keratosis, edema, osteomalacia or rickets associated with hypocalcemia and elevated alkaline phosphatase activity; pulmonary fibrosis, periarteritis nodosum; acute systemic lupus erythematosus; tissue necrosis; lymphadenopathy, craniofacial abnormalities (especially in young people) after long-term use, neonatal hemorrhage.

ROUTE AND DOSAGE. Oral: Adults: usual range: 100 mg three times daily. Dose limit up to 600 mg/day. Doses may be given once a day or in 3 divided doses after maintenance dose is established. **Pediatrics:** usual range: 4 to 8 mg/kg/day divided into 2 or 3 doses, or as single dose. **Intravenous:** (given by direct injection; rate not to exceed 40 mg/minute): **Adults:** *Antiarrhythmic:* 50 to 100 mg every 10 to 15 minutes as necessary, not to exceed total dose of 1 Gm/24 hours. *Anticonvulsant:* 150 to 250 mg then 100 to 150 mg after 30 minutes if necessary, at rate not to exceed 50 mg/minute. **Pediatric:** *Anticonvulsant:* 5 mg/kg as single dose or divided into 2 doses.

NURSING IMPLICATIONS

Therapeutic serum concentration: 10 to 20 mcg/ml; *toxic levels:* 30 to 50 mcg/ml; *lethal level:* 100 mcg/ml. Steady state therapeutic levels are not achieved for at least 7 to 10 days.

The sodium content of phenytoin sodium is 0.35 mEq (8 mg) per 100-mg capsule and 0.2 mEq (4.5 mg)/ml for injectable form.

If patient cannot take a whole tablet or capsule, the tablet may be crushed or the capsule may be emptied prior to administration. Drug should be mixed with food or fluid; have patient swallow a fluid first, then follow with the diluted or mixed drug along with a full glass of water, milk, or with food. This drug is strongly alkaline, and should not be swallowed without prior preparation prevent esophageal and gastric direct contact.

Shake suspension vigorously before pouring to ensure uniform distribution of drug.

Inform patient that drug may impart a harmless pink or red to red-brown coloration to urine.

All brands of phenytoin now are classified as prompt release or extended release (one product Dilantin Kapseals).

Prompt release capsules and chewable tablets are not intended for once-a-day dosage since drug is too quickly bioavailable and can therefore lead to toxic serum levels.

Extended-release capsules are used for once-a-day dosage regimens.

Two chewable tablets are not dose-exchangeable for one 100-mg capsule of phenytoin sodium: capsules contain 92 mg but tablet contains 50 mg drug.

Intramuscular injection is not recommended because of high alkalinity of solution (pH 12). If used however, when patient is returned to oral regimen, dosage is reduced by 50% of original oral dosage for 1 week to compensate for sustained release of medication.

Solubility of phenytoin is pH dependent; therefore, avoid mixing with other drugs or adding to any infusion solution, to prevent precipitation.

A slightly yellowed injectable solution may be used safely. Precipitation may be caused by refrigeration, but slow warming to room temperature restores clarity. Do not administer unclear solution.

During IV phenytoin administration, observe injection site frequently to prevent increase in rate of infusion and infiltration. Local soft tissue irritation may be serious leading to erosion of tissues and possible decrease in ROM for affected hand lasting as long as 3 weeks. The elderly woman, especially if peripheral vascular disease is present, seems to be at high risk.

To minimize local venous irritation, 0.9% saline solution is introduced after the drug injection through the same in-place catheter or needle.

To reduce side effects, lower doses than the usual adult range are given to geriatric, severely ill, debilitated patients or those with liver damage and the flow rate is reduced to 50 mg over a 2- to 3-minute period.

Margin between toxic and therapeutic IV dose is relatively small. Closely monitor vital signs and symptoms during IV infusion and for an hour afterward. If patient is elderly or has cardiac disease constant observation and a cardiac monitor are necessary.

Observe patient closely for CNS side effects. Have on hand oxygen, atropine, vasopressor, assisted ventilation, seizure precaution equipment (padded side rails, mouth gag, nonmetal airway, suction apparatus).

Phenytoin can unmask a low thyroid reserve. Advise patient on long-term therapy to report symptoms of fatigue, dry skin, deepening voice.

Caution patient to report promptly onset of liver dysfunction as evidenced by jaundice. Since the drug is largely metabolized in the liver, impairment of function leads to increased serum levels of phenytoin, and toxicity. Early recognition of a toxic reaction may save the patient's life.

Liver and thyroid function tests, blood counts, and urinalyses are recommended prior to therapy, at monthly intervals during early therapy, and at regular periods during prolonged therapy.

Caution patient not to alter prescribed drug regimen. Abrupt drug discontinuation may precipitate seizures and status epilepticus.

Withdrawal and discontinuation of phenytoin must be done gradually, over a period of 1 to 3 or more months and in relation to serum drug levels and EEGs.

Advise patient not to ask for another drug brand when refilling prescription. Differences in dissolution and absorption rates of different products can alter serum levels of phenytoin.

Gingival hyperplasia appears most commonly in children and adolescents; never occurs in edentulous patients. Condition can be minimized by daily brushing with soft toothbrush, careful flossing to remove dental plaque, and gum massage. Parents must brush and floss teeth (waxed floss) for children once daily up to at least 6 to 8 years of age when child should be able to do it alone. Advise patient/parent to inform dentist that patient is taking phenytoin, gingivectomy is sometimes necessary.

Use of electric toothbrush may assure better compliance in young children. For babies with erupting teeth, mechanical stimulation and relief of discomfort may be provided by nonimported, approved teething ring with frozen liquid.

Caution patient to avoid hazardous activities particularly during early therapy, and not to drive a car until approval is given by physician. Many states now permit a patient with epilepsy to obtain a driver's license provided he or she has physician's certificate stating patient has been seizure-free for a period of time (usually 1 to 2 years).

Warn patient about the effects of alcohol: alcohol intake may increase phenytoin serum levels leading to phenytoin toxicity. The chronic alcoholic may decrease serum levels of the drug with alcohol ingestion leading to loss of or erratic seizure control. Doses will need to be higher than for the nonalcoholic patient.

Phenytoin should be discontinued immediately if a measles-like skin rash appears. Therapy may be resumed when rash disappears. If exfoliative, purpuric, or bullous, drug treatment is not usually resumed.

Anticonvulsant therapy during pregnancy, lactation or in the woman of childbearing age must be weighed carefully as to benefit–risk to both mother and unborn child. Multiple congenital anomalies in the newborn of a mother on phenytoin during pregnancy have been reported.

Notify physician if pregnancy is suspected or planned. Seizure frequency during pregnancy increases in a large number of women because of changes in absorption or metabolism of phenytoin.

If patient is receiving phenytoin to prevent major seizures it probably will not be stopped during pregnancy because of the risk of precipitated status epilepticus with attendant hypoxia, a danger to both mother and fetus.

Be certain patient realizes she needs the drug and counsel her about risk to fetus if she interrupts drug therapy without physician's advice. Urge her to keep appointments for frequent serum concentration evaluations during pregnancy.

An attempt may be made to discontinue anticonvulsant treatment before and during pregnancy if the nature, frequency, and severity of seizures do not pose a threat to the woman. Whether or not slight seizures affect the fetus is not clearly established.

Anticonvulsants taken during pregnancy appear to pose a threat of coagulation defect that may cause neonatal bleeding (usually within 24 hours). Vitamin K_1 may be given to the mother one month before and during delivery and to the infant (IV) immediately after birth.

Marked hypoglycemic states may cause severe convulsive seizures. If hypoglycemia is present or suspected as with pancreatic adenoma, blood sugar studies should be followed.

Patients with diabetes should be monitored regularly for symptoms of hyperglycemia (polydipsia, polyuria, lethargy, drowsiness, psychotic manifestations, glycosuria). Adjustment of phenytoin dosage (for patients on insulin) or adjustment of oral hypoglycemic dosage may be necessary.

Hydration may be a sufficient factor in seizure control. Mild dehydration has been associated with decline in number of seizures. Discuss with physician.

A well balanced diet is an important adjunct to effective anticonvulsant therapy. Collaborate with dietitian, patient/family in diet planning. Urge patient to eat regularly and to avoid overeating.

Food/Nutrient–Drug Interactions:

- Patients on prolonged therapy should have adequate intake of vitamin D containing foods (e.g., fortified milk, margarine, butter, liver, egg yolk, fish such as salmon, sardines, herring), and sufficient exposure to sunlight.
- Periodic checks are indicated for decrease in serum Ca levels (sign of bone demineralization and potential rickets or osteomalacia). Particularly susceptible: black children, patients receiving other anticonvulsants concurrently, patients who are inactive, have limited exposure to sunlight, or whose dietary intake is inadequate.
- Hydantoin derivatives interfere with metabolism of folic acid, a nutrient with doubled requirements during pregnancy (could lead to megaloblastic anemia). Observe patient for symptoms of folic acid deficiency: neuropathy, mental dysfunction, psychiatric disorders. Serum folate levels should be determined at onset of symptoms.
- Daily supplements (if required) with phenytoin therapy: vitamin K, vitamin D, folic acid may be prescribed.

Influenza vaccine during phenytoin treatment may cause an increase in seizure activity. The patient should be alerted in case a change in dose is necessary.

P

After patient has been well stabilized on maintenance regimen of divided doses, physician may prescribe single daily phenytoin dose of same amount.

Duration of phenytoin treatment is extremely variable. In some patients, a lifetime of drug therapy is necessary; in others, physician may attempt to withdraw drug after a seizure-free period (including auras) of 2 to 5 years.

Instruct responsible family member how to take care of patient during a seizure, what to observe and record. Advise to call for emergency help if patient has one seizure after another, has trouble breathing, or has sustained an injury. *General instructions:* Do not attempt to restrain patient, but protect from injury, e.g., pillow, blanket, or clothing under head, loosen constricting clothing. Place padded tongue depressor, or anything firm and soft between teeth. If teeth are clenched, do not force them open because they could be broken and aspirated. After convulsion is over, turn patient on side to facilitate drainage of oropharyngeal secretions. Record sequence of various phenomena during seizure (describe location and type movements; position of head, eyes, extremities; pupil size; duration of seizure, behavior following seizure to help physician to localize area of brain involved) Notify physician that patient had a seizure.

Patient/family may require help with emotional reaction to epilepsy, problems of stigmatized discrimination that may occur, and required life style adjustments.

Most states have local chapters or state associations concerned with special problems of the epileptic; e.g., Epilepsy Foundation of America (EFA), one among other nonprofit organizations, provides information and services related to life insurance, legal problems, training and placement, school children, low-cost prescriptions, educational literature. Contact local chapter if available, or national headquarters: 1828 L Street, N.S., Washington, D.C., 20036.

Patient–Family Teaching Plan. Construct plan in collaboration with physician, dietitian, and other relevant health team members emphasizing the following points:

- ✓ Reason for taking medication.
- ✓ Take drug precisely as prescribed.
- ✓ Adverse reactions.
- ✓ What to do in the event of a seizure.
- ✓ Avoid colds, infections: if they occur, notify physician.
- ✓ Importance of regularity and moderation in life style.
- ✓ Well-balanced diet; avoid overeating and overhydration.
- ✓ Avoid OTC drugs.
- ✓ Alcohol restriction (consult physician regarding allowable amount).
- ✓ Moderation in physical activity; avoid high risk sports.
- ✓ Avoid emotional stress; talk problems out with physician, nurse, or significant other.
- ✓ Keep follow-up appointments.
- ✓ Carry identification card or jewelry with pertinent medical data (may be procured from local pharmacy, Medic Alert Foundation, or AMA).

Diagnostic Test Interferences. Phenytoin (hydantoins) may produce lower than normal values for dexamethasone or metyrapone tests; may increase serum levels of glucose, BSP and alkaline phosphatase; and may decrease PBI levels and urinary steroid levels.

Drug Interactions: Phenytoin

Plus	Interactions
Alcohol, chronic abuse Antacids (aluminum, calcium magnesium compounds) Antihistamines (H_1-receptor antagonists) Antioneoplastics (cisplatin, vinblastine, bleomycin) Barbiturates Calcium gluconate Carbamazepine (Tegretol) CNS depressants Folic acid (Folvite) Oxacillin Reserpine Rifampin	Decreased serum levels: decreased phenytoin effects

P

Plus (cont.)	Interactions (cont.)
Alcohol (acute intake) Aminosalicylic acid (PAS) Aminodarone Anticoagulants, coumarins Anticonvulsants, other e.g., trimethoidione, ethotoin Benzodiazepines (e.g., diazepain, flurazepam) Chloramphenicol (Chloromycetin) Cimetidine (Tagamet) Dexamethozone Disulfiram (Antabuse) Estrogens (including oral contraceptives) Ethosuximide Halothane Isoniazid Methylphenidate (Ritalin) Phenothiazines (e.g., chlorpromazine, thioridazine) Pyrazolones (e.g., phenylbutazone) Salicylates Sulfonamides Tolbutamide	Increased serum levels: increased risk of toxicity; loss of seizure control; increased phenytoin effects
Lidocaine Propranolol	Additive cardiac depressant effects
Sympathomimetics	Sudden hypotension and bradycardia
Valproic acid	May cause increased or decreased phenytoin serum concentration

P

PHYSOSTIGMINE SALICYLATE
(Antilirium, Isopto Eserine)
PHYSOSTIGMINE SULFATE
(Eserine Sulfate)

(fi-zoe-stig′meen)
Cholinergic, ophthalmic
Miotic

ACTIONS AND USES. Reversible anticholinesterase and tertiary amine. Alkaloid of West African calabar or ordeal bean, *Physostigma venenosum.* Chief effect: increases concentration of acetylcholine at cholinergic transmission sites; prolongs and exaggerates its action. Similar to neostigmine (qv) in actions and adverse effects, but produces greater secretion of glands, constriction of pupil and effect on blood pressure, and less action on skeletal muscle. Also has direct blocking action on autonomic ganglia. Parenteral physostigmine can produce transient decrease in manic symptoms as well as precipitate mental depression. Topical application to conjunctiva produces constriction of ciliary muscle (spasm of accommodation) and iris sphincter (miosis) as result of which the iris is pulled away from anterior chamber angle, thus facilitating drainage of aqueous humor, with lowering of intraocular pressure.

Used to reverse CNS and cardiac effects of tricyclic antidepressant overdose, to reverse CNS toxic effects of atropine, scopolamine, and similar anticholinergic drugs and to antagonize CNS depressant effects of diazepam. Applied topically to eye to reduce intraocular tension in glaucoma.

ABSORPTION AND FATE. Readily absorbed from mucous membranes, muscle, and subcutaneous tissue. Onset of action following oral and parenteral administration occurs in 5 minutes; duration is 30 minutes to 5 hours. Readily passes blood–brain barrier; widely distributed throughout body. Largely hydrolyzed and inactivated by cholinesterases. Excretion not fully understood; only small amounts found in urine. Following instillation into conjunctival sac, action begins within 2 minutes, peaks in 1 to 2 hours, and persists 12 to 36 hours. Renal impairment does not require dose adjustment.

CONTRAINDICATIONS AND PRECAUTIONS. Asthma, diabetes mellitus, gangrene, cardiovascular disease, mechanical obstruction of intestinal or urogenital tract, any vagotonic state, secondary glaucoma, inflammatory disease of iris or ciliary body, concomitant use with choline esters (e.g., methacholine, bethanechol) or depolarizing neuromuscular blocking agents (e.g., decamethonium, succinylcholine). Safe use during pregnancy not established. *Cautious Use:* epilepsy, parkinsonism, bradycardia, hyperthyroidism, peptic ulcer, hypotension.

ADVERSE/SIDE EFFECTS. Acute toxicity: cholinergic crisis. *(See Neostigmine.)* **CNS:** restlessness, hallucinations, twitching, tremors, sweating, weakness, ataxia, convulsions, collapse, respiratory paralysis, pulmonary edema. With rapid IV: bradycardia, hyperactivity, respiratory distress, convulsions. **Ophthalmic:** headache, eye and brow pain, marked miosis, twitching of eyelids, lacrimation, dimness and blurring of vision; prolonged use: changes in pigmented epithelium of iris, chronic conjunctivitis, follicular cysts, contact allergic dermatitis. **Systemic absorption:** nausea, vomiting, epigastric pain, diarrhea, involuntary urination or defecation, miosis, salivation, sweating, lacrimation, rhinorrhea, dyspnea, bronchospasm, irregular pulse, palpitation, bradycardia, rise in blood pressure.

ROUTE AND DOSAGE. Oral: Adults: 1 to 2 mg three times/day. **Intramuscular, intravenous (salicylate):** 0.5 to 4 mg. **Pediatric (emergency use only):** initial: 0.5 mg by very slow IV injection of at least one minute. If necessary, dose may be repeated at 5 to 10 minute intervals until therapeutic effects attained or maximum dose of 2 mg is reached. **Topical** (instilled in conjunctival sac): ophthalmic ointment (0.25%): 1 cm strip one to three times daily. Ophthalmic solution (0.25% or 0.5%): 1 or 2 drops, three times daily.

NURSING IMPLICATIONS

The patient with brown or hazel irides may require a stronger ophthalmic solution, or more frequent instillation for desired effects than the patient with blue irides.

Physostigmine ophthalmic ointment may be prescribed at bedtime for patients with glaucoma to prevent nocturnal rise in ocular tension.

When used as topical agent, be alert to symptoms of systemic absorption *(see Adverse/Side Effects)*. Dosage should be reduced or drug discontinued.

To reduce the possibility of systemic effects, apply gentle pressure over lacrimal sac during and for 1 or 2 minutes following instillation. Instruct patient to avoid squeezing lids together. Blot excess medication with clean tissue.

Inform patient that physostigmine ophthalmic preparations may produce annoying lid twitching, temporary blurring of vision, and difficulty in seeing in dimmed light; therefore, necessary safety precautions should be taken. Hospitalized patients will require supervised ambulation.

Emphasize the need for following prescribed drug regimen for glaucoma, and urge patient to remain under medical supervision. Untreated glaucoma can cause blindness.

Tolerance may develop with long-term use. Effectiveness can be regained by substituting another miotic for a short time and then resuming treatment with physostigmine.

Teaching plan for patients with glaucoma should include the following: proper administration of eyedrops; adverse symptoms to be reported; caution about not wearing constricting clothing, such as tight collar, belt, or girdle; activities to avoid that could provoke increase in intraocular pressure, such as heavy exertion, forceful nose blowing or coughing, straining at stool, crying, and emotionally upsetting situations.

Patient should be advised to wear identification tag indicating the presence of glaucoma and the medication being taken.

Closely monitor vital signs and state of consciousness in patients receiving drug for atropine poisoning. Since physostigmine is usually rapidly destroyed, patient can lapse into delirium and coma within 1 to 2 hours; repeat doses may be required.

Monitor closely for side effects related to CNS and for signs of sensitivity to physostigmine. Have atropine sulfate readily available for clinical emergency.

When used parenterally or orally the following symptoms indicate need to discontinue drug: excessive salivation, emesis, frequent urination, or diarrhea. Excessive sweating or nausea may be eliminated by dose reduction.

IV administration should be at a slow rate, no more than 1 mg/minute. Rapid administration and overdosage can cause a cholinergic crisis (muscle cramps, hypertension, respiratory depression and paralysis, diaphoresis, nausea, vomiting, diarrhea, involuntary micturation, CNS stimulation, fear, agitation, restlessness).

Preserved in tightly covered, light-resistant containers. Use only clear, colorless solutions. Red-tinted solution indicates oxidation, and such solutions should be discarded.

Store at temperature between 15° and 30°C (59° and 86°F).

See also Neostigmine.

Drug Interactions: Physostigmine

Plus	Interactions
Echothiophate, isoflurophate	Actions inhibited by prior instillation

P

PHYTONADIONE

(fye-toe-na-dye'one)

(AquaMEPHYTON, Konakion, Mephyton, Phylloquinone, Vitamin K_1)

Vitamin prothrombogenic

ACTIONS AND USES. Fat-soluble naphthoquinone derivative chemically identical to, and with similar degree of activity as naturally occurring vitamin K. Vitamin K is essential for hepatic biosynthesis of blood clotting factors II (prothrombin), VII (proconvertin), IX (plasma thromboplastin component), and X (Stuart factor). Promotes liver synthesis of clotting factors by unknown mechanism. Antagonizes inhibitory effects of coumarin and indandione anticoagulants on the hepatic synthesis of these clotting factors. Does not reverse anticoagulant action of heparin. Pharmacologically more active than menadione and derivatives, and action is more prompt and prolonged. Reportedly demonstrates wide margin of safety when used in newborns.

Drug of choice as antidote for overdosage of coumarin and indandione oral anticoagulants. Also used to reverse hypoprothrombinemia secondary to administration of oral antibiotics, quinidine, quinine, salicylates, sulfonamides, excessive vitamin A, and secondary to inadequate absorption and synthesis of vitamin K (as in obstructive jaundice, biliary fistula, ulcerative colitis, intestinal resection, prolonged hyperalimentation). Also used in prophylaxis and therapy of neonatal hemorrhagic disease.

ABSORPTION AND FATE. Adequate absorption from intestinal lymph after oral administration, only if bile is present. Drug response following oral intake: 6 to 12 hours; after IM injection: 1 to 2 hours; and after IV administration: 15 minutes. Hemorrhage usually controlled within 3 to 8 hours. Normal prothrombin level may be obtained in 12 to 14 hours after parenteral administration. Concentrates in liver briefly after absorption; only small amounts accumulate in body tissues. Rapidly metabolized; metabolites excreted in urine and bile. Crosses placenta.

CONTRAINDICATIONS AND PRECAUTIONS. Hypersensitivity to phytonadione or its components; severe liver disease. Effect on fertility and teratogenic potential not known.

ADVERSE/SIDE EFFECTS. Gastric upset, headache (after oral dose). *Following IV:* hypersensitivity or anaphylaxis-like reaction: facial flushing, cramplike pains, convulsive movements, chills, fever, diaphoresis, weakness, dizziness, peculiar taste sensation, bronchospasm, dyspnea, sensation of chest constriction, shock, cardiac arrest, respiratory arrest. *Injection site reactions:* pain, hematoma, and nodule formation, erythematous skin eruptions (with repeated injections). Paradoxic hypoprothrombinemia (patients with severe liver disease). *Newborns* (following large doses): hyperbilirubinemia, severe hemolytic anemia, kernicterus, brain damage, death.

ROUTE AND DOSAGE. **Adults:** *Anticoagulant overdose:* **Oral:** Initial: 2.5 to 10 mg; rarely, up to 50 mg daily. Oral dose may be repeated after 12 to 24 hours. **Subcutaneous, intramuscular:** 0.5 to 10 mg up to maximum 25 mg; repeat after 6 to 8 hours if prothrombin time has not shortened satisfactorily. **Intravenous (emergency only):** 0.5 to 10 mg; may be repeated in 4 hours for treatment of bleeding (injection rate not to exceed 1 mg/minute). *Hemorrhagic disease of newborn: prophylaxis:* 0.5 to 1 mg IM immediately after delivery. Although less desirable, 1 to 5 mg SC or IM may be given to mother 12 to 24 hours before delivery. *Treatment:* 1 to 2 mg IM or SC. *Other prothrombin deficiencies:* **Infants:** 2 mg IM or SC; **Older Infants and Children:** 5 to 10 mg IM or SC.

NURSING IMPLICATIONS

Frequency, dose, and therapy duration are guided by prothrombin times and clinical response. One-stage prothrombin time is commonly used to monitor vitamin K therapy; prothrombin and proconvertin (P and P) test of Owren is also used, but results may not be reliable in newborns.

Patients with bile deficiency receiving oral phytonadione will require concomitant administration of bile salts to assure adequate absorption.

If possible, drugs that inhibit or interfere with vitamin K activity (e.g., oral antibiotics, salicylates) may be discontinued or given at reduced dosages as an alternative or addition to phytonadione therapy.

In adults and older children, IM injection should be given in upper outer quadrant of buttocks. For infants and young children, anterolateral aspect of thigh or deltoid region is preferred. Carefully aspirate to avoid intravascular injection *(see Adverse/Side Effects)*. Apply gentle pressure to site following injection. Swelling (internal bleeding) and pain sometimes occur with SC or IM administration.

Note that *Konakion* (which contains a phenol preservative) is intended for IM use only. AquaMEPHYTON may be given subcutaneously, IM, or IV as prescribed.

For IV infusion, dilution may be made with 0.9% sodium chloride, 5% dextrose, or 5% dextrose in 0.9% sodium chloride injection. *Other diluents should not be used.* Administer solution immediately after dilution. Discard unused solution and contents in open ampul.

Phytonadione is photosensitive. Protect infusion solution from light by wrapping container with aluminum foil or other opaque material.

Severe reactions, including fatalities, have occurred during and immediately after IV injection *(see Adverse/Side Effects).* Patient should be under constant surveillance. Monitor vital signs.

Severe blood loss or delayed response to phytonadione may necessitate supplementary therapy with fresh whole blood, frozen plasma, or plasma concentrate of vitamin K-dependent clotting factors.

Some patients with liver disease, especially women, develop an itchy erythematous rash at injection sites following repeated IM doses. The rash is at first localized and later may spread, and corresponds to inadequate control of prothrombin time. It appears within a few days to several weeks after initiation of therapy, and subsides with scaling in 2 to 12 weeks. A change to another form of vitamin K such as menadiol sodium diphosphate (Synkayvite) has resolved the problem.

Therapeutic responses to phytonadione: shortened prothrombin, bleeding, and clotting times, as well as decreased hemorrhagic tendencies.

Normal prothrombin time: 12 to 14 seconds; bleeding time (Ivy): 1 to 6 minutes; clotting time: 5 to 15 minutes.

Use of phytonadione to correct anticoagulant-induced prothrombin deficiency may promote the same clotting hazards that existed prior to anticoagulant therapy.

Patients on large doses may develop temporary resistance to coumarin- or indandione-type anticoagulants. If oral anticoagulant is reinstituted, larger than former doses of anticoagulant may be needed. Some patients may require change to heparin, which acts on a different principle.

Estimated minimum daily requirement of vitamin K for adults is 0.03 mcg/kg body weight and up to 10 mcg/kg for infants. Since vitamin K is synthesized by intestinal bacteria and is present in a wide variety of foods, deficiency in normal individuals is improbable.

Advise patient stabilized on phytonadione to maintain consistency in diet, and to avoid significant increases in daily intake of vitamin K-rich foods. High sources of vitamin K: asparagus, broccoli, cabbage, lettuce, turnip greens, pork or beef liver, green tea, spinach, watercress, tomatoes.

The American Academy of Pediatrics recommends routine administration of phytonadione to infants at birth to prevent the decline in clotting factors that occurs a few days following birth.

Overdosage of phytonadione is treated with heparin.

Stored in tight, light-resistant containers in a dark place, at 15° to 30°C (59° to 86°F). Protect from light at all times.

Diagnostic Test Interferences. Falsely elevated **urine steroids** (by modifications of Reddy, Jenkins, Thorn procedure).

Drug Interactions: Phytonadione

Plus	Interactions
Antibiotics, oral (broad spectrum) long-term therapy	Potentiate hypoprothrombinemia by suppressing vitamin K-producing intestinal bacteria
Anticoagulants, oral	Vitamin K significantly antagonizes effects of anticoagulants
Cholestyramine (Questran) Mineral Oil	Inhibit GI absorption of vitamin K

PILOCARPINE HYDROCHLORIDE

(Adsorbocarpine, Akarpine, Almocarpine, Isopto Carpine, Miocarpine, Ocusert, Pilo, Pilocar, Pilocel, Pilokair, Piloptic)

(pye-loe-kar'peen)
Cholinergic (parasympathomimetic)
Miotic

ACTIONS AND USES. Tertiary amine derived from chief alkaloid of *Pilocarpus jaborandi.* Acts directly on cholinergic receptor sites, thus mimicking acetylcholine. Induces miosis, spasm of accommodation, and fall in intraocular pressure (IOP) that may be preceded by a transitory rise. Decrease in IOP results from stimulation of ciliary and pupillary sphincter muscles which pull iris away from filtration angle thus facilitating outflow of aqueous humor. Also decreases production of aqueous humor.

Used for medical management of open-angle and angle-closure glaucomas; to reduce IOP and to protect the lens during surgery and laser iridotomy; to counteract effects of mydriatics and cycloplegics following surgery or ophthalmoscopic examination. Available in fixed combination with epinephrine (E-Pilo-1) and with physostigmine salicylate (Miocel, Isopto P-ES).

ABSORPTION AND FATE. Penetrates cornea rapidly. Miosis begins in 10 to 30 minutes, peaks in about 30 minutes and lasts 4 to 8 hours. IOP reduction begins in 60 minutes, peaks in 75 minutes and persists 4 to 14 hours. Spasms of accommodation begin in 15 minutes and last 2 to 3 hours. Ocular therapeutic system: ocular hypotensive effect is fully developed with 1½ to 2 hours after placement in cul-de-sac and is continuously maintained for 7 days. Tolerance may develop with prolonged use.

CONTRAINDICATIONS AND PRECAUTIONS. Hypersensitivity to drug components, secondary glaucoma, acute iritis, acute inflammatory disease of anterior segment of eye. Safe use during pregnancy and lactation has not been established. *Cautious Use:* bronchial asthma, hypertension. Ocular therapeutic system: not used in acute infectious conjunctivitis, keratitis, retinal detachment, or when intense miosis is required.

ADVERSE/SIDE EFFECTS. Generally well tolerated. Ciliary spasm with brow ache, twitching of eyelids, eye pain with change in eye focus, miosis, diminished vision in poorly illuminated areas, blurred vision, reduced visual acuity, sensitivity. *Infrequent:* contact allergy, lacrimation, follicular conjunctivitis, conjunctival irritation, cataract, retinal detachment. *Systemic:* nausea, vomiting, abdominal cramps, diarrhea, epigastric distress, salivation, bronchospasm, tachycardia, tremors, increased sweating.

ROUTE AND DOSAGE. Ocular therapeutic system (Ocusert): Adult, Pediatric: 1 ocular system (20 to 40 mcg) every 7 days. **Ophthalmic solution:** (many strengths ranging from 0.25 to 10%): **Adult, Pediatric:** *Acute glaucoma:* (1 to 2% solution): 1 drop every 5 to 10 minutes for three to six doses, then 1 drop every 1 to 3 hours until intraocular pressure is reduced. *Chronic glaucoma:* (0.5 to 4%): 1 drop four times daily. *Miotic* (1%): 1 drop.

NURSING IMPLICATIONS

During acute phase, physician/ophthalmologist may prescribe instillation of drug into unaffected eye also, to prevent bilateral attack of acute glaucoma.

Wash hands thoroughly with soap and water before and after instilling eyedrops or placing the ocular therapeutic system in the cul-de-sac.

When instilling eye drops, care should be taken to prevent contamination of dropper tip and solution, and to avoid touching eyelids or surrounding area with the dropper tip.

Immediately after instillation of drops, apply gentle digital pressure to periphery of nasolacrimal drainage system for 1 to 2 minutes to prevent delivery of drug to nasal mucosa and general circulation. Excess solution around eye or on hands should be removed immediately with a tissue. *(See Index: Drug administration for additional notes about ophthalmic instillation.)*

P

Hourly tonometric tests may be done during early treatment with pilocarpine because drug may cause an initial transitory increase in IOP.

The patient should understand that therapy for glaucoma is prolonged and that adherence to established regimen is crucial to prevent blindness.

Since drug causes blurred vision and difficulty in focusing, caution patient to avoid hazardous activities such as driving a car or operating machinery until vision clears.

Brow pain and myopia tend to be more prominent in younger patients and generally disappear with continued use of drug.

Inform patient to withhold medication if symptoms of irritation or sensitization persist and to report to physician/ophthalmologist.

Ocular Therapeutic System (Ocusert):

- Releases 20 mcg pilocarpine/hour for 7 days. The elliptical-shaped unit is placed in the eye cul-de-sac where it remains for a week. Slow release of drug provides a nonfluctuating concentration of pilocarpine in the ciliary body and iris.
- The 20-mcg unit is 5.7 mm × 13.4 mm on its axes and 0.3 mm thick: the 40 mcg unit is 5.5 mm × 13 mm and 0.5 m thick.
- The 20 mcg/hour system produces reduction in IOP about equal to that produced by topical application of 28 mg pilocarpine as a 2% solution every 6 hours.
- Induced myopia, miosis, and spasm of accommodation is less than that produced by eyedrops. However, since transient blurring and dimness of vision may occur following Ocusert insertion, have patient do so at bedtime; myopia will be at a stable level in the AM.
- After the first several hours following Ocusert insertion, induced myopia decreases to a low base level (about 0.5 diopters) that persists for the life of the therapeutic system.
- Conjunctival irritation with mild erythema and increase in mucus secretion may accompany early use of Ocusert. Usually these symptoms subside, but if they do not, notify physician/ophthalmologist.
- If the system contacts an unclean surface, wash it with cool tap water before replacing it into cul-de-sac.
- If retention of the system is a problem, the superior conjunctival cul-de-sac may be a preferred site for insertion. This location is also preferred during sleep.
- Ocusert may be transferred from the lower conjunctival sac to the superior sac by closing eyelids, rolling the eye toward the nose and, with gentle digital pressure through the closed eyelid, directly moving the system. Avoid moving it over the colored part of the eye.
- If an unexpected increase in drug action occurs (sudden miosis, ciliary spasm, decreased visual acuity), the system should be removed and replaced with a new one.
- If system ruptures, is deformed or grossly contaminated, discard and replace with another.
- Instruct patient to check for presence of Ocusert before retiring at night and upon rising. If the ocular system slips out during sleep, its ocular hypotensive effect following loss safely continues for a short time. Epinephrine ophthalmic solution or carbonic anhydrase inhibitor may be used concurrently if necessary.
- While IOP increases immediately with removal of Ocusert, it does not reach uncontrolled levels for 2 to 3 days.

Information about inserting the ocular system is included in the drug package. Review these directions carefully with patient, and ask for demonstration to test patient's ability to adjust, insert, and remove the system.

Advise patient to keep follow-up appointments.

Store ocular system form at 2° to 8°C (35° to 46°F); avoid freezing. Store solutions in tight, light-resistant containers.

Drug Interactions. The actions of pilocarpine and carbarchol are additive when used concomitantly.

PIMOZIDE
(Orap)

(pi'moe-zide)
Psychotropic
Antipsychotic agent (neuroleptic)
Butyrophenone

ACTIONS AND USES. Orphan neuroleptic agent; analogue of the butyrophenones and derivative of meperidine-like analgesics. A potent central dopamine antagonist that causes altered release and turnover of central dopamine stores; has no effect on turnover of norepinephrine. Blockade of CNS dopaminergic receptors results in suppression of the motor and phonic tics that characterize Tourette's disorder. Produces less sedation and extrapyramidal reactions than haloperidol (qv); lowers seizure thershold. Animal studies suggest that pimozide may be tumorigenic in humans.

Used to suppress severe motor and phonic tics in patient with Tourette's disorder who has failed to respond satisfactorily to standard treatment (e.g., haloperidol).

ABSORPTION AND FATE. More than 50% of dose absorbed after ingestion; significant first-pass metabolism. Peak serum levels attained in 6 to 8 hours after dose is administered. Metabolized chiefly in liver with production of two major metabolites. Half-life: about 55 hours. Excreted in urine.

CONTRAINDICATIONS AND PRECAUTIONS. Hypersensitivity to pimozide, treatment of simple tics other than those associated with Tourette's disorder; drug-induced tics; history of cardiac dysrrhythmias and conditions marked by prolonged QT syndrome, patient taking drugs that may prolong QT interval (e.g., quinidine), severe toxic CNS depression. Safe use in children under 12 years of age, during pregnancy (category C), and by nursing mothers not established. *Cautious Use:* renal and hepatic dysfunction; patients receiving anticonvulsant therapy.

ADVERSE/SIDE EFFECTS. CNS: headache, sedation, drowsiness, insomnia, akathisia, speech disorder, handwriting changes, akinesia, grand mal seizures, fainting, hyperpyrexia, persistent tardive dyskinesia, oculogyric crisis, hyperreflexia; neuroleptic malignant syndrome: extrapyramidal dysfunction, hyperthermia, autonomic dysfunction; tachycardia, labile blood pressure, diaphoresis, dyspnea, urinary incontinence; elevated CPK, WBC, liver function enzymes; respiratory failure, acute renal failure, stupor. **CV:** prolongation of QT interval, inverted or flattened T wave, appearance of U wave. **Dermatologic:** sweating, skin irritation. **Special senses:** visual disturbances, photosensitivity, decreased accommodation, blurred vision, cataracts. **Urogenital:** loss of libido, impotence, nocturia, urinary frequency. **Other:** weight changes, asthenia, chest pain, periorbital edema.

ROUTE AND DOSAGE. (Slow, gradual introduction.) **Oral:** Initial: 1 to 2 mg/day in divided doses: then dose increased every other day. Maintenance (usual): less than 0.2 mg/kg/day or 10 mg/day, whichever is less. Maximum dose: 0.3 mg/kg/day or 20 mg/day.

NURSING IMPLICATIONS

Advise patient to adhere to established drug regimen, i.e., dose or intervals should not be changed and dose should be discontinued only with physician's guidance.

P

Risk of tardive dyskinesia appears to be greatest in women, in the elderly, and those on high dosage. Both patient and family should be alerted to the earliest symptom ("flycatching"—an involuntary movement of the tongue) which should be reported promptly to the physician.

When drug is to be discontinued, the regimen should be adjusted by prescription: slow, gradual changes over a period of days or weeks (drug has a long half-life). Sudden withdrawal may cause reemergence of original symptoms (motor and phonic tics) and of neuromuscular side effects of the drug.

If neuromuscular reactions are too distressing, an antiparkinsonian agent (e.g., benztropine, trihexphenidyl), may be prescribed.

Warn patient that drug-caused hand tremors, drowsiness, and blurred vision may impair alertness and ability to safely drive a car or to engage in dangerous activities.

The syndrome of tardive dyskinesia can be unmasked by reinstitution of drug therapy after a drug holiday, by increasing dosage, or by switching to another antipsychotic drug. Be alert to symptoms at these particular times.

Extrapyramidal reactions often appear within the first few days of therapy, are dose-related, and usually occur when dose is high. Dose reduction may alleviate symptoms, but if not, drug should be discontinued.

Pseudoparkinsonian symptoms (drooling, mask facies, rigidity and tremors especially of hands) are usually mild and reversible with dose adjustment.

ECG baseline data should be obtained at beginning of therapy and checked periodically, especially during period of dosage adjustment.

Urge patient to return for periodic assessments of therapy benefit and cardiac status.

One of the adverse effects is widening of the QT interval (QRS complex and T wave), representing both ventricular depolarization and repolarization. Widening or prolongation of the interval suggests developing cardiotoxicity.

Anticholinergic effects (dry mouth, constipation) may increase as dose is increased. Check with patient about their occurrence. Discuss measures to help patient tolerate dry mouth (frequent rinsing with water, saliva substitute, increased fluid intake) and constipation (increased dietary fiber, drink 6 to 8 glasses of water daily). Other anticholinergic symptoms (urinary retention, ataxia, dizziness) are indicators for dose adjustment or drug therapy. Discuss with physician.

The physician will periodically attempt to reduce pimozide dosage to see if tics persist. An increase in frequency and intensity may be due to a withdrawal-like phenomenon rather than reemergence of disease symptoms. Usually 1 to 2 weeks are allowed to elapse before clinical differentiation between drug withdrawal or disease etiology can be made.

Moderation or abstinence from alcohol is advised, to prevent augmenting CNS depressant effects of pimozide.

See also Haloperidol for nursing implications of drug therapy with an antipsychotic agent.

Drug Interactions: Pimozide

Plus	Interactions
Alcohol, sedatives, hypnotics	Increased CNS depressant action of pimozide
Anticholinergics	Increased anticholinergic effects of pimozide
Phenothiazines, tricyclic antidepressants, antiarrhythmics	Increased risk of QT prolongation
Anticonvulsants	Loss of seizure control; increased CNS depressant effects

PINDOLOL

(Visken)

(pin′-oe-lole)
Antihypertensive
Beta-adrenergic blocking agent (nonselective)

ACTIONS AND USES. Nonselective beta-adrenergic blocking agent. Possesses slight intrinsic sympathomimetic activity (ISA) or partial beta-agonist effect in therapeutic dose ranges. Thus pindolol exerts vasodilator as well as hypotensive effects. Hypotensive action mechanism similar to that of propranolol (qv): competitively blocks beta-adrenergic receptors primarily in myocardium, and beta receptors within bronchial and smooth muscle. Membrane-stabilizing or anesthetic-like action has been demonstrated but only at plasma levels above therapeutic safety. Has negative chronotropic and inotropic properties and slows conduction in AV node (but to lesser extent than other beta-blockers). Does not consistently affect cardiac output, resting heart rate, or renin release; it does, however, decrease peripheral vascular resistance, perhaps the major factor in pindolol's hypotensive effect. The ISA effect can be completely reversed by other beta-antagonists.

Used in the management of hypertension (in stepped-care approach: step 1) concurrently with a thiazide diuretic or as single agent. Used in patient who has failed to respond to diet, exercise, and/or weight reduction. *Investigational Use:* stress/exercise-induced chronic stable angina pectoris.

ABSORPTION AND FATE. Rapid absorption from GI tract. Bioavailability 50 to 95% (less in uremic patient). Peak plasma concentrations achieved 1 to 2 hours after administration of a single 20 mg dose. Action duration: begins within 3 hours after administration and lasts for 24 hours. 40 to 60% protein bound. Half-life: 3 to 4 hours; increased to 3 to 11 hours in renal failure, 7 to 15 hours in geriatric patient, and varies from 2½ to 30 hours in hepatic cirrhosis. 60 to 65% of dose metabolized in liver to glucuronide and sulfate metabolites. 35 to 50% excreted unchanged. Secreted into breast milk.

CONTRAINDICATIONS AND PRECAUTIONS. Bronchospastic diseases, severe bradycardia, cardiogenic shock, cardiac failure. Safe use in pregnancy (category B), nursing mothers, and children not established. *Cautious Use:* nonallergic bronchospasm, CHF, diabetes mellitus, hyperthyroidism, impaired hepatic and renal function. *See also Propranolol.*

ADVERSE/SIDE EFFECTS. *See Propranolol.*

ROUTE AND DOSAGE. Oral: Adult: *Hypertension:* 5 mg two or three times a day. If blood pressure reduction is inadequate in 3 to 4 weeks, dosage is gradually increased by 10 mg in daily increments at 3- to 4-week intervals as necessary up to maximum dosage of 60 mg/day. Usual adult dosage: 10 to 30 mg/day in 3 divided doses. Chronic stable angina pectoris: 15 to 40 mg/day in 3 to 4 divided doses.

NURSING IMPLICATIONS

Food does not decrease bioavailability but may increase rate of absorption. Advise patient to take drug at same time of day each day with respect to time of food intake.

Pindolol masks the dizziness and sweating premonitory symptoms of hypoglycemia less than other beta-blockers; however, this drug action should be understood by the patient/primary care provider as a potential problem during regulation period of antidiabetic therapy.

Hypotensive effect may begin within 7 days but is not therapeutically maximum until about 2 weeks after beginning of treatment with pindolol.

Abrupt withdrawal of drug might precipitate a thyroid crisis in a patient with hyperthyroidism, and angina in the patient with ischemic heart disease and lead to an MI. Warn any patient on pindolol to adhere to the prescribed drug regimen. If a change is desired, consult physician first.

Withdrawal or discontinuation of treatment is gradual over a period of 1 to 2 weeks.

Because of the vasodilating action of this drug, the cold extremities side effect observed with other beta-blockers is rarely a problem.

See Propranolol: prototype beta-adrenergic blocking agent for additional nursing implications, drug test interferences and drug interactions.

PIPERACILLIN SODIUM

(Pipracil)

(pi-per'a-sill-in)
Antiinfective
Antibiotic (beta-lactam)
Penicillin

ACTIONS AND USES. Extended-spectrum parenteral penicillin with antibiotic activity against most gram-negative and many gram-positive anaerobic and aerobic organisms including members of *Clostridium, Bacteroides, Klebsiella, Enterobacter, Pseudomonas, Proteus, Serratia* species, and the anaerobic and aerobic cocci. Action mechanism is similar to that of other penicillins: by interference with bacterial cell wall synthesis, promotes loss of membrane integrity leading to osmotic instability and death of the organism. Penicillins do not affect human cells in this way because of the differences in cell wall structure. Less active than penicillin G (qv) against pneumococci and group A streptococcus but comparable to ampicillin against enterococci. Penicillinase-producing staphalococci are resistant to piperacillin. Contains less Na and is therefore less likely to cause fluid retention than carbenicillin or ticarcillin.

Used to treat susceptible organisms that cause gynecologic, skin and skin structure, gonococcal and streptococcal infections; lower respiratory tract, intraabdominal and bone and joint infections; septicemia, UTI (urinary tract infections). Also used prophylactically prior and during surgery, and as empiric antiinfective therapy in granulocytopenic patients.

ABSORPTION AND FATE. Approximately 70 to 80% IM dose absorbed from injection site. Peak serum concentrations attained within 30 to 50 minutes (30 to 36 mcg/ml after a 2-Gm dose). Distribution (after both IV and IM dose) into pleural, peritoneal, wound and synovial fluids, sputum, and bone (low concentrations). Minimal distribution to CSF unless meninges are inflamed. (Concurrent administration with oral probenecid increases CSF concentration.) Protein binding: 16 to 22%; hepatic metabolism is slight. Half-life is biphasic: initial, 0.7 to 0.33 hours; terminal, 0.6 to 1.35 hours; prolonged in severe renal and hepatic impairment. Rapidly excreted in urine and partly in feces via bile. Readily crosses placenta; distributed into milk. Removed by hemodialysis, but not appreciably by peritoneal dialysis.

CONTRAINDICATIONS AND PRECAUTIONS. Hypersensitivity to penicillins, cephalosporins, or other drugs. Safe use in children younger than 12 years, lactating mother, and during pregnancy not established. *Cautious Use:* hepatic and renal dysfunction. *See also Penicillin G.*

ADVERSE/SIDE EFFECTS. *Rare:* abnormal platelet aggregation and prolonged prothrombin time (with high doses). *See also Penicillin G.*

ROUTE AND DOSAGE. Intramuscular; intravenous: Adult: *Serious infections:* 12 to 18 Gm/day IV in divided doses every 4 to 6 hours. *Complicated UTIs:* 8 to 16 Gm IV in divided doses every 6 to 8 hours. *Gonorrheal infection (uncomplicated):* **Intramuscular:** 2 Gm single dose.

NURSING IMPLICATIONS

Although safe doses for children less than 12 years old have not been firmly established, pipericillin has been given by IV infusion in dosages of 76 to 100 mg/kg daily.

Duration of therapy depends on type and severity of infection but usually continues for at least 48 to 72 hours after patient is asymptomatic and evidence that infection is eradicated has been obtained.

Doses and frequency are usually modified if creatinine clearance is less than 40 ml/minute.

Patients undergoing hemodialysis usually receive a maximum dosage of 2 Gm piperacillin every 8 hours and an additional 1-Gm dose after each dialysis period.

IM injections should be limited to 2 Gm/site. Use the gluteal muscle, preferably. The deltoid muscle should be used only if well developed; lower or midthird of arm should not be used. Diluents for reconstitution of drug include sterile or bacteriostatic water for injection, bacteriostatic NaCl injection, lactated Ringer's injection for IVs and sterile lidocaine HCl injection 0.5 to 1.0% without epinephrine for IM. When reconstituted, solution contains 1 Gm/2.5 ml.

Do not mix piperacillin with an aminoglycoside in a syringe or infusion bottle; aminoglycoside will be inactivated.

Store reconstituted solution at room temperature for 24 hours; up to 1 week refrigerated, and up to 1 month frozen.

See Penicillin G (prototype penicillin) for additional nursing implications, drug test interferences, and drug interactions.

PIPERAZINE CITRATE

(pi′per-a-zeen)
Anthelmintic

(Antepar, Bryrel, Entacyl, Vermazine)

PIPERAZINE PHOSPHATE

PIPERAZINE TARTRATE

(Razine Tartrate)

P

ACTIONS AND USES. Appears to act by producing muscle paralysis in parasite, thus promoting elimination through intestinal peristalsis.

Used in treatment of pinworm disease *(Enterobius vermicularis)* and roundworm or ascariasis *(Ascaris lumbricoides)* infestations.

ABSORPTION AND FATE. Variable GI absorption. Excreted essentially unchanged in urine within 24 hours.

CONTRAINDICATIONS AND PRECAUTIONS. Hypersensitivity to piperazine or its salts, impaired renal or hepatic function, convulsive disorders. Safe use during pregnancy not established. *Cautious Use:* malnutrition, anemia.

ADVERSE/SIDE EFFECTS. Low toxicity. Usually with excessive dosage: **CNS:** headache, vertigo, ataxia, tremors, choreiform movements, muscular weakness, hyporeflexia, paresthesia, sense of detachment, memory defect, EEG abnormalities, convulsions. **EENT:** blurred vision, paralytic strabismus, nystagmus, cataracts, lacrimation, rhinorrhea, accomodative defects. **GI:** nausea, vomiting, abdominal cramps, diarrhea. **Hypersensitivity:** urticaria, erythema multiforme, photosensitivity, purpura, fever, productive cough, bronchospasm, arthralgia.

ROUTE AND DOSAGE. *Roundworms:* Once daily for 2 consecutive days: **Adults:** 3.5 Gm. **Children:** 75 mg/kg; maximum daily dose 3.5 gm. When repeated therapy is not practical, single dose of 70 mg/lb body weight up to maximum of 3 Gm may be given. *Pinworms:* **Adults and Children:** single daily dose of 65 mg/kg with maximum daily dose of 2.5 Gm for 7 or 8 consecutive days.

NURSING IMPLICATIONS

Drug may be given with food to reduce gastric distress.

Use of laxatives or enema and dietary restrictions are usually not necessary.

Caution patient or parent not to exceed recommended schedule because of danger of neurotoxicity with high dosages.

Instruct patient to withhold medication if CNS, GI, or hypersensitivity reactions occur and report to physician.

In severe infections, course of therapy may be repeated after 1-week rest period.

It is not unusual for an entire family to be infested with pinworms. Positive diagnosis in one family member warrants stool examination of other members to prevent reinfestation.

Specimens for pinworms are best obtained immediately on arising in the morning (female worm lays eggs at night around anal region). Obtain specimen by applying cellulose tape swab to perianal region; eggs can then be transferred to glass slide and examined microscopically.

Roundworm ova are examined in routine stool specimens.

Pinworms and roundworms are transmitted by direct and indirect transfer of ova, e.g., by hands, food, and contaminated articles. *Instruct patient and family in personal hygiene:* washing hands after defecation and before touching food; sanitary disposal of feces; daily change of underwear and bedding (for pinworms). Ova are destroyed by household washing machine.

Store at controlled room temperature protected from heat and light.

Drug Interactions. There is a possibility that piperazine may exaggerate extrapyramidal effects of **phenothiazines.**

PIPOBROMAN

(Vercyte)

(pi-poe-broe′man)

Antineoplastic (alkylating agent)

ACTIONS AND USES. Dicarboxylic acid neutral amide of piperazine with toxic hematopoietic depressant properties. Exact mechanism of action unknown, but classified as a polyfunctional alkylating agent. Blocks DNA, RNA, and protein synthesis in rapidly proliferating cells.

Used primarily to treat polycythemia. Also used to produce remissions in chronic myelocytic leukemia.

ABSORPTION AND FATE. Readily absorbed from GI tract. Metabolic fate and excretion unknown.

CONTRAINDICATIONS AND PRECAUTIONS. Children under 15 years of age, myelosuppression from radiation or previous cytotoxic chemotherapy, pregnancy, women in childbearing years.

ADVERSE/SIDE EFFECTS. Nausea, vomiting, abdominal cramps, diarrhea, anorexia (transient), skin rash, leukemia, thrombocytopenia, anemia.

ROUTE AND DOSAGE. Oral: *Polycythemia:* Initial: 1 mg/kg daily for at least 30 days; may be increased to 1.5 to 3 mg/kg if no previous response; maintenance dose 0.1 to 0.2 mg/kg/day. *Chronic myelocytic leukemia:* Initial: 1.5 to 2.5 mg/kg daily until optimal therapeutic response occurs; maintenance dose 7 to 175 mg daily (highly individualized).

NURSING IMPLICATIONS

Since patient requires close observation, therapy is initiated in the hospital.

Bone marrow studies should be performed prior to therapy and repeated at time of maximum hematologic response. Liver and kidney function tests should also be performed before and during therapy.

Leukocyte and thrombocyte counts are advised every other day and complete blood counts weekly until desired response is obtained or toxic effects intervene.

Therapy is interrupted when platelet or WBC count falls to 150,000/mm^3 or to 3,000/mm^3, respectively.

Anemia (dose-related) is treated with blood replacement without interrupting therapy, but therapy is discontinued if rapid drop in hemoglobin, increased bilirubin levels, and reticulocytosis occur.

Monitor laboratory values for indicators of specific nursing actions.

Observe carefully for ecchymoses, petechiae, purpura, melena, and hemoptysis and report to physician promptly.

If nausea, vomiting, diarrhea, and skin rash persist, therapy will be interrupted.

Myelosuppression may not appear for 4 weeks or more after treatment begins.

Maintenance therapy is usually started when hematocrit is reduced 50 to 55% in polycythemia vera, or when leukocyte count approaches 10,000/mm^3 in chronic myelocytic leukemia.

Therapy is continued for as long as needed to maintain a satisfactory clinical response.

PIROXICAM
(Feldene)

(peer-ox'i-kam)
NSAID
Analgesic, antipyretic, antirheumatic

P

ACTIONS AND USES. Oxicam nonsteroidal antiinflammatory drug (NSAID) with analgesic, antipyretic, as well as antiinflammatory properties. Exact mechanism of action not clear. Produces strong inhibition of enzyme cyclooxygenase, biogenic catalyst of prostaglandin synthesis. (Prostaglandins are naturally occurring mediators of the inflammatory process, are found throughout the body, and formed in every tissue; therefore the potential loci for NSAID action is vast.) Drug-induced reduction in prostaglandin levels is associated with decreased inflammatory processes in bone–joint disease (including crystal disorders), and with possible interference with platelet aggregation. Reportedly has lower incidence of gastric erosion and fecal blood loss than aspirin. Habituation, tolerance, and addiction data not reported.

Used for acute and long-term relief of mild to moderate pain and for symptomatic treatment of osteoarthritis and rheumatoid arthritis.

ABSORPTION AND FATE. Well-absorbed after oral administration. Analgesic action begins in about 1 hour, peaks in 3 to 5 hours, and lasts 48 to 72 hours. Antirheumatic action: onset, up to 7 days; peak action, 2 to 4 weeks. Hepatic metabolism; highly protein bound. Half-life: 30 to 86 hours (average 50 hours); is unaffected by age but effects of impaired renal or hepatic disease have not been established. Piroxicam and its metabolites are excreted primarily in urine; small amounts in feces. Less than 5% of dose excreted unchanged.

CONTRAINDICATIONS AND PRECAUTIONS. Hypersensitivity to piroxicam, hemophilia; syndrome (bronchospasm, nasal polyps, angioedema) precipitated by aspirin or other NSAID; active peptic ulcer, GI bleeding. Safe use in children, during pregnancy, and during lactation not established. *Cautious Use:* history of upper GI disease including ulcerative colitis, renal dysfunction, compromised cardiac function, hypertension or other conditions predisposing to fluid retention; coagulation disorders.

ADVERSE/SIDE EFFECTS. CNS: somnolence, dizziness, vertigo, depression, insomnia, nervousness. Causal relationships not established: akathisia, depression, hallucinations, dream abnormalities, mental confusion paresthesias. **CV/Respiratory:** peripheral edema, hypertension, worsening of congestive heart failure, exacerbation of angina. **Dermatologic:** urticaria, erythema multiforme, maculopapular, vesiculobullous rash; photosensitivity, sweating, Stevens-Johnson syndrome, brusing, dermatitis. **ENT:** tinnitus, hearing loss. **GI:** nausea, vomiting, dyspepsia, GI bleeding, diarrhea, constipation, flatulence, dry mouth, peptic ulceration, anorexia, jaundice, hepatitis. **Hematologic:** anemia, decreases in Hgb, Hct; leukopenia, eosinophilia, aplastic anemia; thrombocytopenia. **Ophthalmic:** blurred vision, reduced visual acuity, changes in color vision, scotomata, corneal deposits, retinal disturbances. **Other:** bronchospasm, allergic rhinitis, angioedema, fever, hypoglycemia, hyperglycemia, hyperkalemia, weight gain; causal relationships not established: dysuria, dyspnea, palpitations, syncope, muscle cramps, fever, hypersensitivity reactions.

ROUTE AND DOSAGE. Oral: (capsule): **Adult:** 20 mg/day. If desired, may be given in divided doses.

NURSING IMPLICATIONS

Patient should take drug at the same time every day.

Administration of capsule with food or fluid may help to reduce GI irritation.

Concomitant administration of an antacid to reduce gastric distress; does not interfere with piroxicam absorption or action.

Piroxicam plasma levels after repeated daily dosing (for 7 to 12 days) usually stabilize at 3 to 8 mcg/ml.

Implications of the long half-life (30 to 86 hours) of piroxicam:

- Permits maintenance of a stable plasma concentration through the day on a once daily dose.
- Dose adjustments, usually made on basis of clinical response, are made at intervals of weeks rather than days in order to prevent overdosage.
- Appearance of adverse/side effects may be delayed for 7 to 10 days after start of therapy (except for an allergic reaction).
- Evaluation of antirheumatic effect cannot be made for at least 7 days.
- If an adverse/side effect occurs, it may continue after drug withdrawal requiring treatment for several days.

Clinical evidence of benefits from drug therapy: pain relief in motion and in rest, reduction in night pain, stiffness, and swelling; increased ROM (range of motion) in all joints.

Check to be sure patient is not self-dosing with aspirin or any other OTC drug without physician's advice. For example: there is no evidence that aspirin in combination with piroxicam increases relief from pain; but the possibility of intensified side effects has not been completely ruled out.

If patient misses a dose, advise taking the drug when omission is discovered if it is 6 to 8 hours before the next scheduled dose. Otherwise, omit the dose and reestablish regimen at next scheduled hour.

Warn patient not to increase dosage beyond prescribed regimen. Patient should understand the reasons for delayed therapeutic effect and need to adhere to the established regimen. Higher than recommended doses are associated with increased incidence of GI irritation and peptic ulcer. If dose appears to be ineffective, physician should be consulted.

Incidence of GI bleeding with this drug is relatively high. Instruct patient to promptly report symptoms of melena, hematemesis, or severe gastric pain.

Because peptic ulceration side effect has a high incidence, some clinicians advise endoscopy before and some weeks after a course of therapy.

Be alert to symptoms of drug-induced anemia: profound fatigue, skin and mucous membrane pallor, lethargy. Drug will be discontinued if diagnosis is confirmed (Hgb, Hct studies).

Because most of the drug is excreted by the kidneys, impaired renal function could increase danger of toxicity and overdose. Encourage patient to maintain adequate fluid intake, i.e., at least 6 to 8 full glasses of water daily (if allowed) and to report signs of compromised renal function: peripheral edema, changed intake and output ratio and pattern, dysuria, unusual weight gain.

Advise patient to report immediately to the physician the onset of eye problems; ophthalmologic studies may be indicated.

If piroxicam is used concomitantly with an anticoagulant be alert to signs of hypoprothrombinemia during and for several days after therapy has been discontinued: ecchymoses, petechiae, unexplained bleeding, epistaxis, hematuria.

Since side effects, i.e., blurred vision, vertigo, dizziness, may impair ability to perform activities requiring mental alertness, caution patient to avoid driving a car or engaging in hazardous activities until response to drug is known.

Since alcohol may intensify the risk of gastric mucosal erosion (GI bleeding), it is advisable to avoid or at least to moderate its use.

Severe hepatic reactions have occurred with other NSAIDs. The most sensitive laboratory indicator is the ALT serum level. Advise patient/family observer to report onset of clinical symptoms (jaundice, pruritus) of hepatitis (sometimes insidious in development). Drug will be discontinued.

Periodic laboratory test levels (BUN, ALT, AST) as well as cell counts, Hgb, and Hct, should be evaluated in patient (especially the elderly) receiving piroxicam for an extended period of time.

Overdosage reports are few. If it occurs, treatment would follow standard procedures: evacuate stomach promptly by emesis or gastric lavage and administer symptomatic and supportive treatment as indicated. If absorption has already occurred, patient should be observed for 4 to 6 days after overdosage because of the long plasma half-life.

Store in tightly closed container at 15° to 30°C (59° to 86°F), unless otherwise directed by manufacturer.

P

Drug Interactions: Piroxicam

Plus	**Interactions**
Alcohol	May augment risk of GI bleeding
Anticoagulants (coumarins)	Slight increase in hypoprothrombinemic response
Aspirin	Slight reduction in piroxicam plasma level

Plus (cont.)	Interactions (cont.)
Diazepam (Valium) Propranolol (Inderal) Phenylbutazone (Butazolidin) Other highly protein-bound drugs	May be displaced by piroxicam leading to their increased therapeutic and toxic serum levels
Lithium (Eskalith)	Possible increase in therapeutic and toxic levels of lithium

---

PLASMA PROTEIN FRACTION

(Plasmanate, Plasma-Plex; Plasmatein, PPF, Protenate)

Plasma volume expander

ACTIONS AND USES. 5% solution of stabilized human plasma proteins in NaCl containing approximately 88% albumin, 7% alpha-globulin, and 5% beta-globulin. Each liter contains about 145 mEq sodium, 85 mEq chloride, and 2 mEq potassium. Oncotic action approximately equivalent to that of human plasma; does not provide coagulation factors or γ-globulins. Heat-treated to minimize hazard of transmitting serum hepatitis; risk of sensitization is reduced since it lacks cellular elements. Does not require cross-matching.

Used in emergency treatment of hypovolemic shock due to burns, trauma, surgery, and infections; used as temporary measure in treatment of blood loss when whole blood is not available; used to replenish plasma protein in patients with hypoproteinemia (if sodium restriction is not a problem).

CONTRAINDICATIONS AND PRECAUTIONS. Severe anemia, cardiac failure; patients undergoing cardiopulmonary bypass surgery. *Cautious Use:* patients with low cardiac reserve; absence of albumin deficiency; hepatic or renal failure.

ADVERSE/SIDE EFFECTS. *Low incidence:* nausea, vomiting, hypersalivation, headache. *Hypersensitivity:* tingling, chills, fever, cyanosis, chest tightness, backache, urticaria, erythema, shock (systemic anaphylaxis). *With rapid IV infusion:* circulatory overload, pulmonary edema.

P

ROUTE AND DOSAGE. Intravenous: *Hypovolemic shock:* **Adults:** 250 to 500 ml, administered at rate up to 10 ml/minute; **Infants and children:** 4.5 to 6.8 ml/kg at rate of 5 up to 10 ml/minute. *Hypoproteinemia:* **Adults:** 1 to 1.5 L (50 to 75 Gm protein) daily; rate not to exceed 5 to 8 ml/minute.

NURSING IMPLICATIONS

Check expiration date on label. Solutions that show a sediment or appear turbid should not be used.

Once container is opened, solution should be used within 4 hours because it contains no preservatives. Discard unused portions.

Rate of infusion and volume of total dose will depend on patient's age, diagnosis, degree of venous and pulmonary congestion, Hct and Hgb determinations. Specific flow rate should be prescribed by physician.

As with any oncotically active solution, infusion rate should be relatively slow. Range may vary from 1 to 10 ml/minute *(see Route and Dosage).*

Monitor blood pressure and pulse. Frequency of readings will depend on patient's condition. Flow rate adjustments are made according to clinical response and blood pressure. Slow or stop infusion if patient suddenly becomes hypotensive.

Observe patient closely during and after infusion for signs of hypervolemia or circulatory overload (distended neck veins, shortness of breath, cyanosis, persistent cough with or without frothy sputum, abnormal rises in blood pressure, pulse, and central venous pressure; sense of chest pressure, edema). Report these symptoms immediately to physician.

A widening pulse pressure (difference between systolic and diastolic) correlates with increase in cardiac output and should be reported.

Make careful observations of patient who has had either injury or surgery in order to detect bleeding points that failed to bleed at lower blood pressure.

Report changes in input–output ratio and pattern.

Serum hepatitis and interference with blood typing or cross-matching procedures have not been reported.

Plasma protein fraction is reportedly incompatible with solutions containing alcohol or norepinephrine (levarterenol bitartrate).

PLICAMYCIN

(Mithracin)

(plik-a-mi′-cin)

Antineoplastic hypocalcemic agent

Antibiotic

ACTIONS AND USES. Cytotoxic antibiotic produced by *Streptomyces plicatus,* with minimal immunosuppressive activity. Complexes with DNA, thus inhibiting DNA-directed RNA synthesis. May lower serum calcium levels by unclear mechanism. Appears to block hypercalcemic action of vitamin D, and may inhibit parathyroid hormone effect on osteoclasts. Interferes with synthesis of various clotting factors. High toxicity with low therapeutic index limits clinical use.

Used to treat hospitalized patients with hypercalcemia or hypercalciuria associated with advanced neoplasms and to treat testicular malignancy.

ABSORPTION AND FATE. Information on absorption, fate, and excretion is limited. Crosses blood–brain barrier, and appears to localize in areas of active bone resorption; excreted in urine. Has cumulative and irreversible toxicity.

P

CONTRAINDICATIONS AND PRECAUTIONS. Bleeding and coagulation disorders, myelosuppression, electrolyte imbalance (especially hypocalcemia, hypokalemia, hypophosphatemia), pregnancy, women of childbearing age. *Cautious Use:* patients with prior abdominal or mediastinal radiology; liver or renal impairment.

ADVERSE/SIDE EFFECTS. GI: stomatitis, anorexia, nausea, vomiting, diarrhea, widespread intestinal hemorrhage. **Hematologic:** thrombocytopenia, bleeding and coagulation disorders (dose-related) leukopenia (mild). **Other:** fever, drowsiness, irritability, dizziness, weakness, headache, mental depression, marked facial flushing, hemoptysis, nonspecific or acneiform skin rash, phlebitis, hypophosphatemia, hypokalemia, hypocalciuria, abnormal liver and renal function (reflected in laboratory values).

ROUTE AND DOSAGE. Intravenous: dosage and duration of therapy highly individualized on basis of hematologic and clinical responses. *Typical dosage:* 25 to 30 mcg/kg/day. Daily doses should not exceed 30 mcg/kg; a course of therapy beyond 10 daily doses not recommended.

NURSING IMPLICATIONS

When edema, ascites, or hydrothorax is present, drug dose is based on ideal body weight.

Watch IV flow rate (established by physician); GI side effects increase when rate is too fast.

Terminate infusion if extravasation occurs. Apply moderate heat to disperse the drug and to minimize tissue irritation. Infusion should be restarted in another vein.

Tumor response to therapy is usually observed within 3 to 4 weeks.

Electrolyte imbalance will be corrected prior to instituting or restarting mithramycin therapy; thereafter, weigh patient daily under standard conditions.

Establish flow chart at beginning of therapy, permitting continuous record of weight, intake–output ratio and pattern, and bowel pattern for comparative data on which to base patient care plan.

Frequent assessments of liver, hematologic (platelet count, bleeding and prothrombin times), and renal function are performed throughout therapy and for several days after last dose.

An antiemetic drug given before and concomitantly with drug administration may prevent nausea and vomiting.

Therapy is interrupted if leukocyte count is below 4000/mm^3, if platelet count is below 150,000/mm^3, or if prothrombin time is more than 4 seconds higher than control. (Normal: 12 to 14 seconds.)

Thrombocytopenia, frequently evidenced by a single or persistent episode of epistaxis or hematemesis, may be rapid in onset during or after a course of treatment. Report marked facial flushing, which is often an early symptom.

Inspect skin daily for signs of purpura. Hemoptysis may occur because of bleeding into metastasis; report this immediately.

Rebound hypercalcemia (normal: 9 to 10.6 mg/dl) following mithramycin-induced hypocalcemia may persist 2 to 4 days. *Hypercalcemia symptoms:* nausea, vomiting, GI atony, polyuria, nocturia, thirst, skeletal muscle weakness, confusion, drowsiness, shortened Q-T interval, bradycardia.

The hypercalcemia patient may be dehydrated. Monitor intake–output ratio to assure adequate fluid intake. Encourage increased oral intake.

A single intravenous dose may be sufficient to reduce elevated serum calcium to normal level within 24 to 48 hours for 3 to 15 days.

Signs of antiblastic action on GI mucosal cells (hematemesis, melena) necessitate stopping drug use.

Check patient's bowel function daily to prevent high fecal impaction due to diminished action of intestinal musculature.

Consult physician about dietary calcium intake, and coordinate dietary planning with dietitian, patient, and family.

P

Drug Interactions. Concomitant administration of **vitamin D** may enhance hypercalcemia.

POLOXAMER 188

(Alaxin)

(pol-ox'a-mer)
Laxative
Emollient (fecal softener)

ACTIONS AND USES. Nonionic surfactant with emulsifying and wetting properties similar to those of dioctyl sodium sulfosuccinate. Lowers surface tension of intestinal fluids, thereby softening feces and allowing passage of feces without straining.

Used for short-term treatment of constipation associated with dry, hard stools, or when straining is to be avoided, e.g., hypertension, heart disease, history of stroke, hernia, hemorrhoids.

ABSORPTION AND FATE. Probably absorbed in small amounts in small intestines and subsequently eliminated in bile.

CONTRAINDICATIONS AND PRECAUTIONS. Symptoms of appendicitis, rectal bleeding, congestive heart failure, fecal impaction, intestinal obstruction.

ADVERSE/SIDE EFFECTS. Gastric or intestinal cramping, skin rash.

ROUTE AND DOSAGE. Oral: Adults: 2 or 3 capsules (240 mg each) daily for not more than 5 to 7 days.

NURSING IMPLICATIONS

Usually administered after meals with a full glass (240 ml) of water or other liquid.

It is important for patient to drink at least 6 to 8 glasses of liquid per day for optimum drug effect.

Several days (3 to 5) of drug therapy may be required for full stool-softening effect. Drug should be discontinued after desired effects are obtained.

Advise patient not to take poloxamer within 2 hours of any other medication.

Poloxamer 188 may increase absorption of mineral oil and other fat-soluble substances.

See Bisacodyl for patient-teaching points.

POLYCARBOPHIL

(Mitrolan)

(pol-i-kar'boe-fil)
Laxative: bulk forming
Antidiarrheal agent

ACTIONS AND USES. Calcium polycarbophil is hydrophilic. Absorbs free water in intestinal tract and opposes dehydrating forces of bowel by forming a gelatinous mass, thereby restoring more normal moisture level and motility in the lower GI tract. Produces well-formed stool and reduces diarrhea. Contains negligible amount of sodium (0.02 mEq, or 0.46 Na/tablet) and is dextrose free.

Used to treat constipation or diarrhea associated with acute bowel syndrome, diverticulosis, irritable bowel, and in patients who should not strain during defecation. Also used to treat choleretic diarrhea, diarrhea caused by small bowel surgery or vagotomy, and disease of terminal ileum.

ABSORPTION AND FATE. Not absorbed from GI tract. Onset of action within 12 to 24 hours after administration; full effect may not be apparent for 1 to 3 days.

CONTRAINDICATIONS AND PRECAUTIONS. Partial or complete GI obstruction, fecal impaction, dysphagia, acute abdominal pain, rectal bleeding, undiagnosed abdominal pain, or other symptoms pathognomonic of appendicitis, poisonings, before radiologic bowel examinaton, bowel surgery. Use in children under 3 years of age not established.

ADVERSE/SIDE EFFECTS. GI: esophageal blockage, intestinal impaction, abdominal fullness. **Other:** low serum K, elevated blood glucose levels (with extended use), asthma, skin rash.

ROUTE AND DOSAGE. (Individualized) **Oral: Adults:** 1 Gm four times/day or as needed; not to exceed 6 Gm/24 hours. **Children (6 to 12 years):** 500 mg three times/day or as needed; not to exceed 3 Gm/24 hours. **Children (3 to 6 years):** 500 mg twice daily or as needed; not to exceed 1.5 Gm/24 hours.

NURSING IMPLICATIONS

Crush tablets before administration or have patient chew tablets well before swallowing.

Each dose should be administered with a full glass (8 ounces) of water or other liquid.

In severe diarrhea, dose may be repeated every 1/2 hour up to the maximum dose in 24 hours.

Abdominal fullness may be prevented by taking smaller doses more frequently during the day.

If sudden changes in bowel habit persist more than 1 week, or action is minimal or ineffective for 1 week, or if there is no antidiarrheal action within 2 days, consult physician.

Extended use may cause dependence on the drug for normal bowel function.

Polycarbophil is not an appropriate agent when prompt or thorough evacuation of the bowel is necessary.

Diet and exercise as well as medication are important in a plan designed to restore a more normal bowel habit.

Dietary fiber may increase intraluminal colonic pressure, enhance motility and increase stool size; its addition to patient's daily diet could help to restore normal function. Abuse of dietary fiber intake, however, can lead to loss of significant quantities of trace elements (e.g., zinc). Consult physician and dietitian regarding supplementation of diet with high-fiber intake.

Examples of high-fiber foods include peas, beans, broccoli, prunes, apricots, bran, wheat, all bran, shredded wheat, almonds, peanuts, jams.

If patient is being treated for diarrhea, determine duration and severity of diarrhea before medical treatment in order to anticipate signs of fluid–electrolyte losses.

Monitor and record number and consistency of stools per day, presence and location of abdominal discomfort (i.e., tenderness, distention) and bowel sounds.

If diarrhea is profuse and watery and if patient is not nauseated, replace fluid losses orally (tepid nondairy fluids) and withhold solids.

Monitor and record intake–output ratio and pattern. Dehydration is indicated if urine specific gravity is above 1.030 and if output is less than 30 ml/hour.

Daily weights provide a rough estimate of fluid loss. Record for reference.

Dehydration from an episode of diarrhea appears rapidly in young children and the elderly. Inspect oral cavity for dryness, and be alert to systemic signs, e.g., thirst and fever.

If rehydration with oral intake is not tolerated, IV fluids may be prescribed.

As patient responds to medication (with decreased diarrhea) dietary intake should be augmented by bland, low-fat, low-carbohydrate foods (if allowed) for 2 or 3 days. Consult physician and dietitian.

If patient is also taking an oral anticoagulant, digitalis, salicylates, or nitrofurantoin, warn against discontinuing polycarbophil unless physician advises patient to do so. Established serum concentrations (and drug effects) may be altered by physical binding of any of these drugs to polycarbophil. Be alert to potential changes in expected pharmacological action if dose titration is altered: e.g., change in weight and pulse (digitalis), onset of pain and tenderness in leg (oral anticoagulant).

This OTC medication is packaged with manufacturer's directions for use. Inform patient, and review with patient if necessary.

Store in tightly closed container at temperature of 15° to 30°C (59° to 86°F), unless otherwise directed by manufacturer.

See Bisacodyl for patient-teaching points related to drug therapy of constipation.

Drug Interactions: Polycarbophil

Plus	Interactions
Antibiotics Anticoagulants, oral Digitalis preparations Nitrofurantoin Salicylates	May decrease absorption, and alter clinical effects of these drugs
Tetracyclines	Impaired absorption (by calcium released from polycarbophil)

POLYESTRADIOL PHOSPHATE

(Estradurin)

(pol-ee-ess-tra-dye′ole)
Antineoplastic
Hormone
Estrogen

ACTIONS AND USES. Estrogen derivative. Provides a continuous active level of exogenous estradiol that functions to alter the hormonal milieu of a tumor originating from hormone-responsive tissue. Polyestradiol suppresses pituitary secretion of luteinizing or interstitial cell stimulating hormone (LH), an action that in turn depresses ("turns off") androgen secretion by the testes (antitumor effect). Tumor growth is interrupted, but existing neoplastic cells are not killed.

Used as palliative treatment of an inoperable, progressing prostatic carcinoma.

ABSORPTION AND FATE. Injected solution leaves bloodstream within 24 hours; passively stored in reticuloendothelial system. As circulating estradiol level drops, more enters bloodstream from storage sites to provide continuous therapeutic effects. *See Estradiol for contraindications, adverse/side effects.*

ROUTE AND DOSAGE. Intramuscular: 40 mg every 2 to 4 weeks or less frequently depending on patient response. Dose may be increased to as much as 80 mg if necessary.

NURSING IMPLICATIONS

Reconstitute solution with sterile diluent; swirl gently to produce clear solution; do not shake vigorously. Discard cloudy solution.

Administer drug deeply into large muscle mass (gluteus). A transitory burning sensation may occur, but this usually does not continue with subsequent doses. If it continues, thereafter the dose may be given with local anesthetic.

Increasing the dosage prolongs action but does not increase blood level.

Clinical response should be apparent within 3 months. Hormone should be continued until disease is again progressive, then stopped. 30% of patients may have another period of improvement (rebound regression).

Store reconstituted solution at room temperature, away from direct light. Stability remains about 10 days, as long as solution is clear.

See Estradiol (prototype estrogen).

PROTOTYPE

POLYMYXIN B SULFATE

(Aerosporin)

(pol-i-mix'in)
Antiinfective
Antibiotic (polypeptide)
Polymyxin

ACTIONS AND USES. Basic polypeptide antibiotic of the polymyxin group derived from strains of *Bacillus polymyxa.* Bactericidal against susceptible gram-negative organisms, particularly most strains of *Pseudomonas aeruginosa, Escherichia coli, Haemophilus influenzae, Enterobacter aerogenes,* and *Klebsiella pneumoniae.* Most species of *Proteus* and *Neisseria* are resistant, as are all gram-positive organisms and fungi. Spectrum of antibacterial activity is similar to that of colistin derivatives, complete cross-resistance but reportedly more nephrotoxic; and cross-sensitivity reported. Binds to lipid phosphates in bacterial membranes, and through cationic detergent action changes permeability to permit leakage of cytoplasm. Neuromuscular blocking action usually associated with high serum levels, intracellular potassium deficit, or low serum calcium concentration.

Used topically and in combination with other antiinfectives and/or corticosteroids for various superficial infections of eye, ear, mucous membrane, and skin. Concurrent systemic antiinfective therapy may be required for treatment of intraocular infection and severe progressive corneal ulcer. Commercially available in fixed-dose combination with neomycin and hydrocortisone (Cortisporin); available with neomycin alone (Statrol Ophthalmic) and with neomycin and gramicidin (Neosporin). Also available in combination with oxytetracycline (Terramycin with Polymyxin B); and with bacitracin zinc (Polysporin).

Used parenterally only in hospitalized patients for treatment of severe acute infections of urinary tract, bloodstream, and meninges. Also used parenterally in combination with neosporin for continuous bladder irrigation to prevent bacteremia associated with use of indwelling catheter.

P

ABSORPTION AND FATE. Does not appear to be significantly absorbed from normal GI tract, mucous membranes or skin. Plasma concentrations of 1 to 8 mcg/ml reached in about 2 hours following IM injection of 20,000 to 40,000 units/kg body weight. Serum half-life: 4.3 to 6 hours. Serum levels higher in patients with renal impairment and in infants and children. (In renal impairment, half-life may be 2 to 3 days.) Widely distributed in body following IM or IV administration, but not evident in cerebrospinal fluid, synovial fluid, or aqueous humor. Not highly bound to plasma proteins, but possibly bound to phospholipids of cell membranes in various tissues. About 60% of dose is excreted unchanged in urine; excretion continues 1 to 3 days after single dose. Not removed appreciably by peritoneal dialysis or by hemodialysis.

CONTRAINDICATIONS AND PRECAUTIONS. Hypersensitivity to polymyxin antibiotics: concurrent and sequential use of other nephrotoxic and neurotoxic drugs; concurrent use of skeletal muscle relaxants, ether, or sodium citrate *(see Drug Interactions).* Safe use during pregnancy not established. *Cautious Use:* impaired renal function, myasthenia gravis.

ADVERSE/SIDE EFFECTS. **Hypersensitivity:** drug fever, dermatoses, pruritus, urticaria, local irritation and burning (topical use), eosinophilia, anaphylactoid reaction (rarely). **Nephrotoxicity:** rising blood drug levels without increase in dosage; albuminuria, cylinduria, azotemia, hematuria. **Neurotoxicity:** irritability, facial flushing, drowsiness, dizziness, vertigo, ataxia, circumoral, lingual, and peripheral paresthesias (stocking-glove distribution); blurred vision, nystagmus, slurred speech, dysphagia, ototoxicity (vestibular and auditory) with high doses; convulsions, coma; neuromuscular blockade (generalized muscle weakness, respiratory depression or arrest); meningeal irritation, increased protein and cell count in cerebrospinal fluid, fever, headache, stiff neck (intrathecal use). **Other:** GI disturbances, severe pain (IM site), thrombophlebitis (IV site), superinfections, electrolyte disturbances (prolonged use; also reported in patients with acute leukemia).

ROUTE AND DOSAGE. Dosages reduced for patients with renal impairment. **Intramuscular:** **Adults and children:** 25,000 to 30,000 units/kg/day; may be divided and given at 4- to 6-hour intervals. **Infants:** up to 40,000 units/kg/day. **Intravenous (infusion):** **Adults and children:** 15,000 to 25,000 units/kg/day, divided and given every 12 hours. **Infants:** up to 40,000 units/kg/day. **Intrathecal:** **Adults and children (over 2 years of age):** 50,000 units once daily for 3 or 4 days, then every other day for at least 2 weeks after negative cerebrospinal fluid sugar and cultures; **Children (under 2 years of age):** 20,000 units once daily for 3 or 4 days followed by 25,000 units every other day for at least 2 weeks after negative cerebrospinal fluid sugar and cultures. **Topical:** *Ophthalmic drops:* 1 to 2 drops of 0.1 to 0.25% (10,000 to 25,000 units)/ml every hour; intervals increased as response indicates. *Otic drops:* 3 or 4 drops in affected ear 3 or 4 times daily. Total topical and systemic dose should not exceed 2 million units/day.

NURSING IMPLICATIONS

Aerosporin Sterile Powder is used to prepare solutions for parenteral (IM, IV, intrathecal) and/or ophthalmic administration. Follow manufacturer's directions for dilution and storage.

Baseline serum electrolytes and renal function tests should be performed prior to parenteral therapy. Frequent monitoring of renal function and serum drug levels is advised during therapy.

Electrolytes should be monitored at regular intervals during prolonged therapy. Patients with low serum calcium and low intracellular potassium are particularly prone to develop neuromuscular blockade.

Baseline and periodic culture and susceptibility tests are essential to determine continuing sensitivity of causative organisms.

Dosage is reduced (as indicated by creatinine clearance) in the patient with renal impairment. For example, when creatinine clearance is 5 to 20 ml/minute, the dose is reduced by 50% to be given every 12 hours.

Routine administration by IM route not recommended because it causes intense discomfort, particularly in infants and children. Pain, described as "aching" or "drawing," radiates along peripheral nerve distribution, 40 to 60 minutes after IM injection. Reportedly, addition of procaine may not prevent its occurrence. (Procaine must not be used for IV or intrathecal administration.)

In adults, IM injection should be made deep into upper outer quadrant of buttock. Select IM site carefully to avoid injection into nerves or blood vessels. Rotate injection sites. Follow agency policy for IM site used in children.

Advise patient to inspect tongue every day. Polymixin therapy supports the growth of opportunistic organisms (superinfection). Symptoms: black, furry tongue or white patches on tongue and oral membranes; malodorous vaginal discharge with pruritus, anorectal itching. Report symptoms promptly. An appropriate antiinfective will be prescribed.

Some degree of renal toxicity usually occurs within first 3 or 4 days of therapy even with therapeutic doses. Monitor intake and output. Fluid intake should be sufficient to maintain daily urinary output of at least 1500 ml. Consult physician.

Decreases in urine output (change in intake–output ratio), proteinuria, cellular casts, rising BUN, serum creatinine, or serum drug levels (not associated with dosage increase) can be interpreted as signs of nephrotoxicity. If any of these signs occurs, withhold drug and report findings to physician.

Nephrotoxicity is generally reversible, but it may progress even after drug is discontinued. Therefore, close monitoring of kidney function is essential, even following termination of therapy.

Warn patient to report promptly onset of stiff neck and headache, (possible symptoms of neurotoxic reactions, including neuromuscular blockade). This response is usually associated with high serum drug levels and/or nephrotoxicity. Drug-induced neuromuscular blockade is difficult to reverse. Calcium chloride has been used as an antagonist.

Respiratory arrest has occurred with first dose and also as long as 45 days after initiation of therapy. It occurs most commonly in patients with renal failure and high plasma drug levels, and is often preceded by dyspnea and restlessness.

Encourage patient to report immediately signs of muscle weakness, shortness of breath, dyspnea, depressed respiration. These symptoms are rapidly reversible if drug is withdrawn immediately. Resuscitative equipment, oxygen, and intravenous calcium chloride should be available at all times.

Transient neurologic disturbances (paresthesias, numbness, formication, dizziness) occur commonly and usually respond to dosage reduction. Report promptly. Supervise ambulation.

Protect unreconstituted product and reconstituted solution from light and freezing. Store in refrigerator at 2° to 8°C (36° to 46°F). Parenteral solutions are stable for 1 week when refrigerated. Discard unused portion after 72 hours.

Drug Interactions: Polymyxin B Sulfate

Plus	Interactions
Nephrotoxic drugs:	
Aminoglycosides (e.g., kanamycin, streptomycin, cephaloridine); Polypeptide antibiotics (e.g., bacitracin, capreomycin); Quinidine (parenteral)	Intensified nephrotoxicity and neurotoxicity associated with polymixins
Quinine (parenteral); Sodium citrate	Intensified nephrotoxicity and neurotoxicity associated with polymixins
Skeletal muscular relaxants (e.g., succinylcholine, tubocurarine); Anesthetics	Prolonged neuromuscular blockade effect; may precipitate respiratory paralysis

POLYTHIAZIDE

(Renese)

(pol-i-thye'a-zide)
Diuretic, antihypertensive
Thiazide

ACTIONS AND USES. Benzothiadiazine (thiazide) derivative. Similar to chlorothiazide (qv) in actions, uses, contraindications, adverse reactions, and interactions.

Used as primary agent in stepped care approach to antihypertensive treatment, and adjunctively in the management of edema associated with congestive heart failure, renal pathology, and hepatic cirrhosis. Available in fixed combination with prazosin (Minizide) and with reserpine (Renese-R). *See also Chlorothiazide.*

ABSORPTION AND FATE. Diuretic effect begins in 2 hours, peaks in 6 hours, and lasts 24 to 48 hours. Highly bound to plasma proteins. Excreted unchanged in urine. *See Chlorothiazide.*

CONTRAINDICATIONS AND PRECAUTIONS. Hypersensitivity to other thiazides or sulfonamides; anuria, pregnancy, lactation. *Cautious Use:* renal and hepatic dysfunction, SLE, gout, diabetes mellitus. *See Chlorothiazide.*

ADVERSE/SIDE EFFECTS. Agranulocytosis, vascular thrombosis, hyperuricemia, hypokalemia, hyperglycemia, orthostatic hypotension, hepatic encephalopathy, photosensitivity. *See also Chlorothiazide.*

ROUTE AND DOSAGE. Oral: Adult: *diuretic:* 1 to 4 mg daily, once every other day, or once a day 3 to 5 times weekly. *Antihypertensive:* 2 to 4 mg daily. **Pediatric:** 0.02 to 0.08 mg/kg/day.

NURSING IMPLICATIONS

Administer drug early in AM after eating (to reduce gastric irritation) and to prevent interrupted sleep because of diuresis.

Antihypertensive effects may be noted in 3 to 4 days, maximal effects may require 3 to 4 weeks. Effects persist for at least 1 week after use of drug is discontinued.

Elderly patients may be more sensitive to the average adult therapeutic dose. Excessive diuresis may induce sudden hypotension and serious electrolyte imbalance.

If orthostatic hypotension is a clinical problem, instruct patient to change from recumbency to upright positions slowly and in stages; to avoid hot baths or showers, extended exposure to sunlight, and standing still. Provide assistance if necessary to prevent falling. Consult physician about use of elastic panty hose or support knee socks.

Warn patient about the possibility of photosensitivity reaction and to notify physician if it occurs. Thiazide-related photosensitivity is considered a photoallergy (ultraviolet radiation changes drug structure and makes it allergenic for some individuals) and occurs 1½ to 2 weeks after initial sun exposure. Advise use of a sunscreen lotion with a high sun protection factor (SPF 12 to 15).

Urge patient to include specific sources of K in daily diet such as a banana (about 370 mg K) and at least 6 ounces orange juice (about 330 mg K). Other K-rich foods include whole grain cereals, fruits, vegetables such as broccoli, potatoes, carrots, nuts.

Counsel patient to avoid OTC drugs unless approved by the physician. Many preparations contain both potassium and sodium and if misused, or if patient overdoses, electrolyte side effects could be induced.

If K deficiency develops, the physician may change dosage or add a K-sparing diuretic (spironolactone, triamterene) to the regimen. Symptoms of hypokalemia include dry mouth, nausea, vomiting, anorexia, paresthesias, muscle cramps.

Advise patient to maintain prescribed dosage regimen. Patient should not skip, reduce or double doses or change dose intervals.

Store drug in tightly closed container at temperature between 15° to 30°C (59° and 86°F) unless otherwise instructed by manufacturer.
See Chlorothiazide.

POTASSIUM CHLORIDE

(Cena-K, Kaochlor, Kaon-Cl, Kato, Kay Ciel, KK-10, KK-20, K-Lor, Klor-10%, KLOR-Con, Kloride, Klorvess, Klotrix, K-Lyte/Cl, K-tab, Pan-Kloride, Rum-K, SK-Potassium Chloride, Slow-K)

(poe-tass'ee-um)
Electrolyte replenisher

POTASSIUM GLUCONATE

(Kalinate, Kaon, Kao-Nor, Kaylixir, K-G Elixir)

ACTIONS AND USES. Potassium (K), the principle intracellular cation, is essential for maintenance of intracellular isotonicity, transmission of nerve impulses, contraction of cardiac, skeletal and smooth muscles, maintenance of normal renal function, and for enzyme activity. In the steady state, K movement is physiologically coupled with that of sodium (Na): entry of K into cells is associated with energy-driven extrusion of Na from cell; K secretion-excretion in distal convoluted tubule is accompanied by Na resorption. Normally, intracellular concentration is about 150 mEq/L; plasma concentration (adult) is 3.5 to 5 mEq/L (neonate, 7.7 mEq/L). Plays a prominent role in both genesis and correction of imbalances in acid-base metabolism; thus, K salts assume special importance as therapeutic agents, but are also very dangerous if improperly prescribed and administered.

Used to prevent and treat K deficit secondary to diuretic or corticosteroid therapy. Also indicated when K is depleted by severe vomiting, diarrhea; intestinal drainage, fistulas, or malabsorption; prolonged diuresis, diabetic acidosis. Effective in the treatment of hypokalemic alkalosis (chloride, not the gluconate).

ABSORPTION AND FATE. Nearly all dietary K absorbed from upper GI tract; enters cells from extracellular fluid by active transport. Excreted by kidneys (90%) and in feces (10%). Amount of K excreted in urine (normal: 25 to 100 mEq/24 hours) essentially equals dietary K intake. During excessive K intake, amount secreted into colon and excreted in feces increases.

CONTRAINDICATIONS AND PRECAUTIONS. Severe renal impairment, severe hemolytic reactions, untreated Addison's disease, crush syndrome, early postoperative oliguria (except during GI drainage); adynamic ileus, acute dehydration, heat cramps, hyperkalemia, patients receiving K-sparing diuretics, digitalis intoxication with AV conduction disturbance. *Cautious Use:* cardiac or renal disease, systemic acidosis, slow-release K preparations in presence of delayed GI transit or Meckel's diverticulum; extensive tissue breakdown (such as severe burns).

ADVERSE/SIDE EFFECTS. Nausea, vomiting, diarrhea, abdominal distention and pain, skin rash (rare), oliguria. *Hyperkalemia* (serum K above 5.5 mEq/L): mental confusion, irritability, listlessness, paresthesias of extremities, muscle weakness and heaviness of limbs, difficulty in swallowing, flaccid paralysis, anuria, respiratory distress, hypotension, bradycardia; cardiac depression, arrhythmias, or arrest; altered sensitivity to digitalis glycosides. *ECG changes* (in hyperkalemia): tenting (peaking) of T wave (especially in right precordial leads), lowering of R with deepening of S waves and depression of RST; prolonged P-R interval, widened QRS complex, decreased amplitude and disappearance of P-waves, prolonged Q-T interval, signs of right and left bundle block, deterioration of QRS contour and finally ventricular fibrillation and death.

ROUTE AND DOSAGE. *Highly individualized.* (1 Gm KCl furnishes 13.41 mEq K; 1 Gm potassium gluconate furnishes 4.27 mEq K). **Oral: Adult:** (solution) 20 mEq (1.5 Gm) two to four times daily up to 100 mEq (7.5 Gm) daily. **Pediatric:** 1 to 3 mEq (75 to 225 mg)/kg daily in divided doses. **Adults:** enteric coated tablet (although not recommended are used occasionally): 8 to 13.4 mEq (600 mg to 1 Gm) three times daily. Extended-release tablets: 10 to 20 mEq (750 mg to 1.5 Gm) three times daily. Not recommended for children. **Intravenous infusion (usually administered in dextrose solution):** (manufacturer's recommendations) **Adults:**

If serum K is:	Maximum concentration:	Maximum infusion rate:	Maximum 24-hr dose:
2.5 mEq/L	30 mEq/L	10 mEq/hr (750 mg)	200 mEq
2.0 mEq/L	80 mEq/L	40 mEq/hr (3 Gm)	400 mEq

Pediatric: maximum 24-hour dose: 3 mEq/kg or 40 mEq/m^2 body surface. (Volume of administered fluid adjusted to body size.) *Maximum infusion rate:* no more than 0.02 mEq/kg/minute. *Potassium gluconate:* elixir (20 mEq/15 ml) **Adults:** 20 mEq, 2 to 4 times daily. **Pediatric:** 20 to 40 mEq/m^2 daily in divided doses.

NURSING IMPLICATIONS

Some patients find it difficult to swallow the large sized KCl tablet. Be sure it is taken while patient is sitting up or standing (never in recumbent position) to prevent drug-induced esophagitis.

No potassium salt tablets should be crushed and then taken dry, or chewed. Be certain patient does not suck tablet (oral ulcerations have been reported if tablet is allowed to dissolve in mouth). Whole tablet should be swallowed with large glass of water or fruit juice (if allowed, since it is another source of K) to wash drug down and to start esophageal peristalsis.

Counsel patient to follow instructions regarding dilution. In general, each 20 mEq K (chloride, gluconate) should be diluted in at least 90 ml water or juice. Liquids, powders, and effervescent tablets must be completely dissolved in a large glass of water or fruit juice before administration. Allow "fizzing" to stop, then sip slowly with meal or immediately after eating, over a 5 to 10 minute period. Dilution minimizes saline cathartic effect, gastric distress and unpleasant taste.

Dilute elixir as directed before giving it through nasogastric tube.

Effervescent tablets (e.g., Klorvess) and K elixir (e.g., Pan-Kloride) are sugar free. Most other formulations, except enteric-coated tablets, are sugar coated.

Effervescent formulations deliver K and Cl ions that are derived from a fixed combination of several K salts.

Enteric-coated KCl (rarely prescribed) carries high risk of stenosis by release of highly concentrated KCl on small tissue segment. If used, be alert to symptoms of obstruction or ulceration (abdominal pain, distention, tarry stools). Stop drug and report to physician; alternate formulation may be prescribed.

The extended-release tablet (e.g., Slow-K) utilizes a wax matrix as carrier for KCl crystals. After absorption of drug, the tablet carcass appears in the stool. Inform the patient that this is no cause for alarm.

Use of extended-release tablets reduces the danger of bowel ulcerations and potential compliance problems. However, esophageal and gastric ulceration in cardiac patients with esophageal compression from left atrial enlargement have been reported with use of this formulation. Report signs (esophageal or epigastric pain or hematemesis). A liquid preparation in such a patient could be more tolerable.

An antacid may improve the tolerance of KCl by decreasing its irritating effect on GI mucosa. 10 ml KCl flavored syrup mixed with 15 ml antacid has given relief. Consult physician.

KCl is never administered by IV "push" or IM or in concentrated amounts by any route. Add the drug to infusion fluid with plastic bag in upright (noninfusion) position to prevent delivery of excessive amount of KCl in first few minutes of the treatment.

Added parenteral drug to infusion solution should be noted on label. When IV concentration is 40 mEq/L or more, there is danger of irritation to veins.

Extreme care should be taken to prevent extravasation and infiltration. Palpate entry site occasionally to confirm needle position. *Signs of infiltration:* swelling (may or may not be painful), coolness, absence of blood back flow, sluggish flow rate. At first sign, discontinue infusion and immediately remove needle or catheter. If infiltration is small, apply ice; if otherwise, the physician may order area infiltration with 1% procaine HCl, to which hyaluronidase may be added to reduce venospasm and dilute the K remaining in local tissue. Apply heat to stimulate and increase microcirculation in area.

K infusion should be administered slowly to prevent fatal hyperkalemia. Flow rate will be prescribed according to serial ECG and serum electrolyte determinations.

Irregular heartbeat is usually the earliest clinical indication of hyperkalemia. Care of patient receiving parenteral potassium demands close surveillance of the cardiac monitor.

Monitor intake–output ratio and pattern in patients receiving the parenteral drug. If oliguria occurs, stop infusion promptly and notify physician.

When K supplement is prescribed for a patient with anorexia or reduced dietary intake of K, or for an elderly patient whose dietary intake is substandard, compliance may be a problem. Factors that reenforce "slippage" in maintaining drug regimen include: unpalatability and delivery form of drug, gastric distress following ingestion of drug, or mental confusion (associated with hypokalemia). Teach patient/family importance of this drug and adherence to established dose regimen.

The established regimen should be followed without manipulation by the patient: patient should not skip, reduce, or double doses.

Before discharge from medical supervision, help patient to design an acceptible, feasible dosing schedule for KCl and other drugs being taken concomitantly (e.g., digitalis, diuretics).

Patient should be well informed about sources of K with special reference to foods and OTC drugs, because their selection and intake are controlled by the patient.

The physician may want to augment therapeutic K intake by diet. Arrange an opportunity for patient/family to discuss diet with dietitian before patient is discharged.

Suggested daily requirement for K is 0.8 to 1.3 Gm. The normal diet provides 2 to 4 Gm daily. K-rich foods include avocado, lima beans, broccoli, carrots, potato, peanut butter, nuts, fruits (especially banana, orange, grapefruit, apricot, melons, prunes); whole grain cereals; instant coffee, cocoa, molasses.

Advise patient to include a banana (about 370 mg K) and at least 6 ounces orange juice (about 330 mg K) in diet each day. Patient should avoid licorice, since large amounts can cause both hypokalemia and sodium retention.

Salt substitutes contain a substantial amount of K and electrolytes other than Na. Excessive use can be dangerous for the patient who borders on the hyperkalemic state. Instruct patient not to use any substitute unless it is specifically ordered by the physician. Examples: Co-Salt and Neocurtasal: both deliver 50 to 60 mEq K and 0.5 mg Na per teaspoon; Morton's Lite Salt furnishes approximately 35 mEq K and 1100 mg Na per teaspoon.

Discuss self-medication habits with patient. Point out that many OTC drugs contain K: multiple vitamin preparations (Gevral), antacids (Alka-Seltzer), analgesics (Neocylate). Advise consulting physician before continuing or starting to use any OTC preparation.

Caution patient not to self-prescribe laxatives. Chronic laxative use has been associated with diarrhea-induced K loss.

Large losses of K can also occur because of persistent vomiting. If this occurs, notify physician.

Urge patient on long-term replacement therapy to report continuing signs of K deficit: weakness, fatigue, disturbances in cardiac rhythm, polyuria, polydipsia.

If K supplement is given in conjunction with a diuretic it may be preferable to give the K on days other than when diuretic is given.

The risk of hyperkalemia with K supplement increases: (1) in the elderly because of decremental changes in kidney function associated with aging, (2) when dietary intake of K suddenly increases, and (3) when renal function is significantly compromised.

Potassium intoxication (hyperkalemia) may result from any therapeutic dosage and the patient may be asymptomatic. Monitoring of K level is of extreme importance. Urge patient to keep appointments for periodic evaluation of electrolyte status.

When detected, hyperkalemia demands immediate attention since lethal levels can be reached in a few hours.

Treatment of K intoxication: Eliminate all K-containing foods and medications. Have available parenteral calcium to overcome cardiotoxicity (not used in patient receiving digitalis); parenteral sodium bicarbonate, glucose infusion with regular insulin (facilitates shift of K into cell), cation exchange resins (hasten K elimination). Hemodialysis and peritoneal dialysis may be required.

Counsel patient to assume responsibility for informing dentist or new physician that a potassium drug has been prescribed as maintenance therapy.

Kaon-Cl and Klor-Con contain tartrazene which may cause allergic reactions (including bronchial asthma) in susceptible individuals (frequently those who are also sensitive to aspirin).

Foil-wrapped powders and tablets should not be opened before use.

Unless manufacturer advises otherwise, store all preparations of KCl at temperatures between 15° and 30°C (59° and 86°F). Protect from light, and do not freeze.

Color in some commercial oral solutions fades with exposure to light, but drug effectiveness is reportedly not altered.

Drug Interactions: Potassium Chloride

Plus	Interactions
K-sparing diuretics (triamterene, spironolactone); Penicillin G potassium	Severe hyperkalemia

P

PROTOTYPE

POTASSIUM IODIDE

(KI, Pima, SSKI, Thyro-Block)

Expectorant
Supplement (iodine)
Protectant (radiation)

ACTIONS AND USES. Pharmacologic use primarily related to iodide portion of molecule. Exact mechanism not clear but it is believed that by direct action on bronchial tissue, potassium iodide (KI) increases secretion of respiratory fluids, thereby decreasing mucus viscosity. If patient is euthyroid, excess iodide (i.e., beyond dietary intake) causes minimal change in thyroid gland mass. Conversely, when thyroid is hyperplastic, excess iodide temporarily inhibits secretion of thyroid hormone, fosters colloid accumulation in thyroid follicles, and decreases vascularity of gland. "Escape" from temporary effects (i.e., return of thyrotoxic symptoms) may occur after 10 to 14 days continuous treatment; consequently iodide administration for hyperthyroidism is limited to short-term therapy. Contains 6 mEq (234 mg) of potassium per gram.

Used to facilitate bronchial drainage and cough in emphysema, asthma, chronic bronchitis, bronchiectasis, and respiratory tract allergies characterized by difficult-to-raise sputum. Also used alone for treatment of hyperthyroidism or in conjunction with antithyroid drugs and propranolol in treatment of thyrotoxic crisis; in immediate preoperative period for thyroidectomy to decrease vascularity, fragility, and size of thyroid gland and for treatment of persistent or recurring hyperthyroidism that occurs in Graves disease patients. Used as a radiation protectant in patients receiving radioactive iodine, and to shield the thyroid from radiation in the wake of a serious nuclear plant accident. (Use as an expectorant has been largely replaced by other agents.)

ABSORPTION AND FATE. Following adequate absorption from GI tract, iodide enters circulation and is cleared from plasma by renal excretion or by thyroid uptake. If patient is euthyroid, renal clearance rate is two times that of the thyroid. Crosses placenta.

CONTRAINDICATIONS AND PRECAUTIONS. Hypersensitivity or idiosyncrasy to iodine, hyperthyroidism, hyperkalemia, acute bronchitis. Safe use during pregnancy (category D) and in nursing mothers and children not established. *Cautious Use:* renal impairment, cardiac disease, pulmonary tuberculosis, Addison's disease.

ADVERSE/SIDE EFFECTS. GI: Diarrhea, nausea, vomiting, stomach pain, nonspecific small bowel lesions (associated with enteric coated tablets). **Hypersensitivity:** angioneurotic edema, cutaneous and mucosal hemorrhage, fever, arthralgias, lymph node enlargement, eosinophilia. **Iodine poisoning (iodism):** metallic taste, stomatitis, salivation, coryza, sneezing; swollen and tender salivary glands (sialadenitis), frontal headache, vomiting (blue vomitus if stomach contained starches, otherwise yellow vomitus), bloody diarrhea. **Metabolic:** hyperthyroid adenoma, goiter, hypothyroidism, collagen-disease-like syndromes. **Other:** irregular heart beat, mental confusion, acneiform skin lesions (prolonged use), weakness, paresthesias, productive cough, pulmonary edema, periorbital edema, flare-up of adolescent acne.

ROUTE AND DOSAGE. Oral (solution, syrup, tablets, enteric-coated tablets). Available oral solution strength: 1 Gm/ml. **Adults:** *Expectorant:* 300 to 600 mg three or four times daily as needed. *Iodine replacement:* 300 mg 3 times daily. *Protectant, radiation:* **Oral:** 0.13 ml SSKI immediately before or after initial exposure; same dose 3 hours after exposure and for up to 10 days (under continuous medical surveillance. 100 to 150 mg every 24 hours before and for 3 to 10 days after administration of radionuclides. *Prior to thyroidectomy:* 5 drops of SSKI (approximately 250 mg) three times daily for 10 days before surgery, administered concurrently with antithyroid agent. Usual maximum dose for adults: up to 12 Gm/day. **Pediatric:** *Expectorant:* 2.5 to 5 ml four to six times a day.

P

NURSING IMPLICATIONS

To disguise salty taste and to minimize gastric distress, administer drug after meals in a full glass (240 ml) of water, milk, or fruit juice, and at bedtime with food or milk.

Enteric-coated tablets are not commonly used because they reportedly cause small bowel lesions and possibly obstruction, perforation, and hemorrhage. If patient is using this form, instruct patient to swallow tablet whole and not to crush or chew it. Precede swallowing with a swallow of fluid, then take tablet with a full glass of water (or other fluid).

Advise patient to report promptly the occurrence of GI bleeding, abdominal pain, distention, nausea, or vomiting.

People who are likely to receive more than 25 rem to the thyroid from radioiodine released into the environment should receive potassium iodide under direction of a public health officer. Warn patient not to self-dose with KI (an OTC drug). Recommend daily dose for adults and children over 1 year: 130 mg; children under 1 year: 65 mg.

Instruct patient to report clinical signs of iodism *(see Adverse/Side Effects).* Usually symptoms will subside with dose reduction and lengthened intervals between doses.

Serum potassium levels should be determined before and periodically during therapy. (Normal serum K: 3.6 to 5.5 mEq/L.)

When iodide is administered to prepare thyroid gland for surgery, strict adherence to schedule and accurate dose measurements are essential, particularly at end of treatment period when possibility of "escape" (from iodide) effect on thyroid gland increases.

Sudden withdrawal following prolonged use may precipitate thyroid storm.

Warn patient to avoid use of OTC drugs without consulting physician. Many preparations contain iodides and could augment prescribed dose, e.g., cough syrups, gargles, asthma medication, salt substitutes, cod liver oil, multiple vitamins (often suspended in iodide solutions).

Foods rich in iodine to be avoided if patient develops iodism: vegetables growing near seacoast, seafoods, fish liver oils, iodized salt.

Impress on the patient taking KI as an expectorant that optimum hydration is the best expectorant. Encourage increased daily fluid intake.

Keep physician informed about characteristics of spectum: quantity, consistency, color.

If crystals form in the solution, they may be dissolved by placing container in warm water and gently agitating it.

Solutions may turn brownish yellow on standing, especially if exposed to light, because of liberated trace of free iodine. Discard such solutions.

Store in airtight, light-resistant container at controlled room temperature preferably between 15° and 30°C (59° and 86°F) unless otherwise directed by manufacturer.

Diagnostic Test Interferences. Potassium iodide may alter thyroid function test results, and may interfere with **urinary 17-OHCS** determinations.

Drug Interactions: Potassium Iodide

Plus	Interactions
Antithyroid drugs (others), Lithium	Potentiated hypothyroid and goitrogenic action of KI
Diuretics, K-sparing, Potassium preparations	Increased risk of hyperkalemia, cardiac arrhythmias, cardiac arrest

P

POVIDONE-IODINE

(poe′vi-done eye′oh-din)

(Betadine, Bridine, Isodine, Proviodine)

Antiinfective, topical

ACTIONS AND USES. Water-soluble iodine complex (iodophor) with nonselective broad microbiocidal spectrum that includes gram-positive, gram-negative, and antibiotic-resistant organisms, fungi, viruses, protozoa, and yeast. On contact with skin, liberates free iodine, maintains germicidal action in presence of blood, serum, and pus. Unlike iodine, it is virtually nonstinging and nonirritating to skin and mucous membrane and nonstaining to skin and clothing. Reportedly not as effective as aqueous solutions or tincture of iodine.

Used for prevention and treatment of surface infections, as antiseptic for burns, lacerations, abrasions, and other minor wounds, and in management of vaginitis (monilial, trichomonas vaginalis, and nonspecific forms).

CONTRAINDICATIONS AND PRECAUTIONS. Sensitivity to iodine; use as vaginal antiseptic during pregnancy. *Cautious Use:* extensive burns, particularly in patients with metabolic acidosis or renal dysfunction.

ADVERSE/SIDE EFFECTS. Systemic absorption can occur with extensive burns: ioderma, metabolic acidosis, renal impairment.

ROUTE AND DOSAGE. Topical: aerosol, antiseptic gauze pads, gargle, ointment, perineal wash, shampoo, skin cleanser, solution, surgical scrub, treated applicators, gauze pads, swabsticks, vaginal douche, vaginal gel, whirlpool concentrate.

NURSING IMPLICATIONS

Avoid contact with eyes.
Treated areas can be bandaged.
Use should be discontinued if irritation, redness, or swelling develops.
Available OTC.

Diagnostic Test Interferences. Urine contaminated with povidone-iodine (as might occur following surgical skin prep or vaginal use) can cause false-positive test for **occult blood.** There is possibility of interference with **PBI** levels (study results are conflicting).

PRALIDOXIME CHLORIDE

(PAM, Protopam Chloride)

(pra-li-dox'eem)
Cholinesterase reactivator

P

ACTIONS AND USES. Quaternary ammonium oxime. Reactivates cholinesterase inhibited by phosphate esters (e.g., organophosphorous insecticides and related compounds) by displacing the enzyme from its receptor sites; the free enzyme then can resume its function of degrading accumulated acetylcholine thereby restoring normal neuromuscular transmission. Less effective against carbamate anticholinesterases (ambenonium, neostigmine, pyridostigmine). More active against effects of anticholinesterases at skeletal neuromuscular junction than at autonomic effector sites or in CNS respiratory center; therefore, atropine must be given concomitantly to block effects of acetylcholine and accumulation in these sites. Effective against nicotinic effects of anticholinesterase poisoning (muscle twitching, fasciculations, cramps, weakness), but action against muscarinic effects (bronchoconstriction, increased secretions, diarrhea) is less striking than that of atropine.

Used as antidote in treatment of poisoning by organophosphate insecticides and pesticides with anticholinesterase activity (e.g., parathion, TEPP, sarin) and to control overdosage by anticholinesterase drugs used in treatment of myasthenia gravis (cholinergic crisis). *Investigational Use:* to reverse toxicity of echothiophate ophthalmic solution.

ABSORPTION AND FATE. Variable and incomplete absorption after oral administration. Peak plasma levels in 2 to 3 hours after oral administration, 5 to 15 minutes after IV, and 10 to 20 minutes after IM injection. Distributed throughout extracellular fluids; crosses blood–brain barrier only very slowly, if at all. Not bound to plasma proteins. Plasma half-life approximately 1.7 hours. Probably metabolized in liver. Rapidly excreted in urine, partly as unchanged drug (80 to 90% of IV or IM dose excreted within 12 hours).

CONTRAINDICATIONS AND PRECAUTIONS. Use in poisoning by carbamate insecticide Sevin, inorganic phosphates, or organophosphates having no anticholinesterase activity; asthma, peptic ulcer, severe cardiac disease, patients receiving aminophylline, theophylline, morphine, succinylcholine, reserpine, or phenothiazines. Safe use during pregnancy not established. *Cautious Use:* myasthenia gravis, renal insufficiency, concomitant use of barbiturates in organophosphorous poisoning.

ADVERSE/SIDE EFFECTS. *Most commonly following IV use* (usually mild and transient): dizziness, nausea, blurred vision, diplopia, impaired accommodation, tachycardia, hypertension (dose-related), hyperventilation, headache, drowsiness, muscular weakness. *With rapid IV:* tachycardia, laryngospasm, muscle rigidity.

ROUTE AND DOSAGE. Adults: *Organophosphorus poisoning:* **Intravenous infusion (preferred):** 1 or 2 Gm in 100 ml isotonic NaCl injection, infused over 15 to 30 minutes. **Direct IV injection:** administered as 5% solution in sterile water for injection *(without preservative)* over not less than 5 minutes; second dose of 1 to 2 Gm repeated after 1 hour if muscle weakness not relieved; additional doses given cautiously, if indicated. **Subcutaneous, intramuscular:** when IV administration is not feasible. **Oral:** 1 to 3 Gm every 5 hours. **Children:** 20 to 40 mg/kg repeated every 10 to 12 hours if needed. *Anticholinesterase overdosage in myasthenia gravis:* **Intravenous:** 1 or 2 Gm followed by increments of 250 mg every 5 minutes, as indicated.

NURSING IMPLICATIONS

Generally used only in hospitalized patients. Have on hand respirator, suction apparatus, tracheostomy set, oxygen, IV sodium thiopental (2.5% solution) for control of convulsions, atropine, gastric lavage equipment for ingested poison. ECG monitoring may be required in severe poisoning.

Treatment is most effective if started within a few hours after organophosphate poisoning has occurred. If exposure to poison was through skin, initial measures should include removal of contaminated clothing and washing skin thoroughly with sodium bicarbonate solution or alcohol.

Pralidoxime is started at the same time as atropine. Atropine sulfate 2 to 4 mg (adult) or 0.5 to 1 mg (pediatric) is given IV (given IM if cyanosis is present) at 5 to 10 minute intervals until signs of atropinism appear: flushing, dry mouth and throat, dilated pupils, rapid pulse, restlessness, disorientation. Some degree of atropinism is usually maintained for at least 48 hours.

Monitor blood pressure, vital signs, and intake and output. Report oliguria or changes in intake–output ratio.

It is difficult to differentiate toxic effects of organophosphates or atropine from toxic effects of pralidoxime. Be alert for these signs and report them immediately: reduction in muscle strength, onset of muscle twitching, changes in respiratory pattern, altered level of consciousness, increases or changes in heart rate and rhythm.

Infusion should be stopped or IV rate reduced if hypertension occurs. Have on hand phentolamine mesylate (Regitine).

Excitement and manic behavior reportedly may occur following recovery of consciousness. Observe necessary safety precautions.

Patient should be kept under close observation for 48 to 72 hours, particularly when poison was ingested, because of likelihood of continued absorption of organophosphate from lower bowel.

Pralidoxime is relatively short-acting. In patients with myasthenia gravis, overdosage with pralidoxime may convert cholinergic crisis into myasthenic crisis *(see Index)*. Have on hand edrophonium chloride (Tensilon).

PRAZEPAM

(Centrax)

(pra'ze-pam)
Antianxiety agent (minor tranquilizer)
Benzodiazepine
C IV

ACTIONS AND USES. Benzodiazepine derivative structurally and pharmacologically related to chlordiazepoxide (qv). Has hypnotic and sedative effects.

Used for management of anxiety disorders or for short-term relief of symptoms of anxiety.

ABSORPTION AND FATE. Absorbed readily from GI tract. Peak level of action in 6 hours; duration of effect up to 48 hours. Serum half-life: 30 to 100 hours; protein binding: 85%. First pass hepatic biotransformation produces active metabolite desmethyldiazepoxide. Excreted by kidneys. Crosses placenta and appears in breast milk.

CONTRAINDICATIONS AND PRECAUTIONS. Hypersensitivity to prazepam and other benzodiazepines; psychoses, concomitant use during or within 14 days of MAO inhibitors, patient under age 18, acute narrow-angle glaucoma, acute alcohol intoxication, pregnancy, lactation. *Cautious Use:* elderly and debilitated patients; impaired renal and hepatic function, addiction-prone patients, mental depression.

ADVERSE/SIDE EFFECTS. Usually mild. **CNS:** blurred vision, drowsiness, fatigue, dizziness, mental confusion, vertigo, ataxia, headache, lethargy, syncope, slurred speech, tremor, paradoxic reaction (excitement, euphoria). **GI:** nausea, vomiting, xerostomia, gastric pain, diarrhea, constipation, jaundice. **Other:** skin rash, edema, hypotension, leukopenia, weight gain, altered libido.

ROUTE AND DOSAGE. Oral: *Hypnotic:* 20 to 40 mg at bedtime. *Sedation:* 10 mg three times daily. Individualized according to patient's response. **Elderly, debilitated:** initial dose: 10 to 15 mg daily in divided doses.

NURSING IMPLICATIONS

Continued effectiveness of response to prazepam should be reassessed at end of 4 months. Urge patient to keep appointments with physician.

Elderly patients should be observed closely for signs of overdosage. Report to physician if daytime psychomotor function is depressed.

Instruct patient not to change dose or dose schedule. Furthermore, patient should not give any of the drug to another person and should refrain from using it to treat a self-diagnosed condition.

Patient should be advised that if she becomes pregnant during therapy or intends to become pregnant she should communicate with her physician about the desirability of discontinuing the drug.

Advise patient to consult physician before self-medicating with OTC drugs.

Caution patient against driving a car or operating dangerous machinery until response to drug has been evaluated.

Warn patient not to drink alcoholic beverages while being treated with prazepam. The CNS depressant effects of each agent may be intensified.

Following prolonged therapy drug should be withdrawn slowly to avoid precipitating withdrawal symptoms (seizures, mental confusion, nausea, vomiting, muscle and abdominal cramps, tremulousness, unusual irritability, hyperhydrosis).

Liver function tests and blood counts should be performed on a regularly planned basis.

Classified as Schedule IV drug under Federal Controlled Substances Act.
Store in tightly closed container at temperature between 15° and 30°C (59° and 86°F) unless otherwise specified by manufacturer.
See also Chlordiazepoxide.

PRAZIQUANTEL

(Biltricide)

(pray-zi-kwon'tel)
Antiinfective
Anthelmintic

ACTIONS AND USES. Synthetic agent with broad spectrum of anthelmintic activity against all developmental stages of schistosomes and other trematodes (flukes) and against cestodes (tapeworm). Increases permeability of parasite cell membrane to calcium. Drug-induced influx of Ca ions induces strong contractions and paralysis of worm musculature, leading to immobilization of their suckers and dislodgement from their residence in blood vessel walls. Normal blood flow passively carries dead and dying worms to the liver, where they are retained and subsequently elicit host tissue reactions (e.g., phagocytosis). Praziquantel is active against all developmental stages of schistosomes, including cercaria (free-swimming larvae that emerge from the intermediate snail host). Activity against other trematodes (flukes) not fully understood; activity against cestodes (tapeworms) not clear but may be similar to that against schistosomes.

Used for treatment of all stages of schistosomiasis (bilharziasis) caused by all schistosoma species pathogenic to humans. *Unlabeled Uses:* treatment of other trematode infections caused by Chinese liver fluke, lung, intestinal, sheep liver, and intestinal flukes, and treatment of tapeworm infections.

ABSORPTION AND FATE. Approximately 80% absorbed from GI tract following oral administration but extensive first-pass metabolism limits amount of unchanged praziquantel that reaches systemic circulation. Peak serum concentration: 1 to 3 hours after oral administration. Rapid and extensive hepatic metabolism. Serum half-life: 0.8 to 1.5 hours; half-life of metabolites: 4 to 5 hours (if renal and hepatic function are normal). 70 to 80% of dose excreted in urine within 24 hours as metabolites; less than 0.1% of dose excreted unchanged. Enters CSF and breast milk (concentration in breast milk: about 1/4 that of maternal serum).

CONTRAINDICATIONS AND PRECAUTIONS. Hypersensitivity to drug; ocular cysticercosis. Safe use in children less than 4 years of age not established; use during pregnancy (category B) only when clearly needed. Women should not nurse on day of praziquantel therapy or for 72 hours after last dose of drug.

ADVERSE/SIDE EFFECTS. GI: abdominal pain or discomfort with or without nausea; vomiting, anorexia, diarrhea. **Hepatic:** increased AST, ALT (slight). **Neurologic:** dizziness, headache, malaise, drowsiness, lassitude, giddiness, CSF reaction syndrome (exaccerbation of neurologic signs and symptoms such as seizures, increased CSF protein concentration, increased anticysticercal IgG levels, hyperthermia, intracranial hypertension) in patient treated for cerebral cysticercosis. **Other:** pruritus, urticaria, fever, sweating, symptoms of host-mediated immunologic response to antigen release from worms (fever, eosinophilia).

ROUTE AND DOSAGE. Oral: individualized dosage according to patient's weight and type of infection. *Schistosomiasis:* 60 mg/kg in 3 equally divided doses at 4- to 6-hour intervals

P

on same day (treatment may be repeated in 2 or 3 months after exposure). *Other trematodes:* 75 mg/kg in 3 doses on same day. Cestodiasis (adult or intestinal stage): 10 to 20 mg/kg as single dose. (Larval or tissue stage): 50 mg/kg in 3 divided doses daily for 14 days.

NURSING IMPLICATIONS

Tablets are easily divided because of three scores (four segments). If ¼ tablet is required, break the segment from the outer end.

Administer oral dose preferably with food and fluids. Tablets can be broken into quarters but should not be chewed. Advise patient to take sufficient fluid to wash down the medication. tablets are very soluble in water; gagging or vomiting because of bitter taste may result if tablets are retained in the mouth. Check to see that they are swallowed, if necessary.

Note: Doses of praziquantel are the same for adults and for children more than 4 years of age.

Generally the patient with cerebral cysticerosis is hospitalized for the duration of praziquantel treatment.

Prior to treatment, discuss drug history with patient *(see Diagnostic Test Interferences).* Inform patient that any drug other than prescribed drugs should be avoided for the duration of therapy to prevent interference with assessment of treatment success.

If experience with treatment of parasitic infections is lacking, there should be consultation with a specialist and/or with a local state disease control center or with the Centers for Disease Control, Atlanta, Georgia 30333.

Schistosomiasis can be acquired by swimming in cercaria-infested freshwater in many parts of the world, especially Africa and the Middle East (larvae enter the body through the skin). Diarrhea, urinary disturbances, hematuria, hepatic cirrhosis, chronic dysentery are the most common symptoms. Ova in urine, stool, and rectal and liver biopsy confirm the diagnosis.

Drug-induced dislodgement of schistosomes to the liver is rapid, occurring within 1 hour after drug administration.

Usually all schistosomal worms are dead 7 days following treatment with praziquantel.

Cure rates are generally lower in children and in patients with the heavy worm burden characteristic of massive infection.

Treatment for cestodiasis (tapeworm) may be followed by gentle purgation 2 hours after drug administration to facilitate rapid removal of tapeworms and ova. The patient should be reexamined in 2 or 3 months to ensure complete eradication of the infections.

Instruct patient being treated for cestodes infection to contact physician if patient develops a sustained headache or high fever. Conjunctive treatment with corticosteroids may be employed for treatment of cerebral cysticercosis (caused by pork tapeworm) to hasten recovery and reduce symptoms of CSF reaction syndrome *(see Adverse/Side Effects).*

Adverse/side effects are frequent, mild to moderate, and transient and usually do not require treatment. Many effects are similar to disease-produced effects.

In spite of the slight increases in serum AST and ALT, serious drug-induced adverse hepatic effects have not been reported, even in the patient with severe hepatosplenic involvement from a schistosomal infection.

Because of potential drug-induced dizziness and drowsiness, the patient should be warned not to drive a car or operate hazardous machinery on day of praziquantel treatment or the following day.

Only limited information is available about acute toxicity and the lethal dose is unknown. However, the manufacturer states that a fast-acting laxative should be given following ingestion of an overdose.

Travelers to developing countries with questionable sanitation are especially susceptible to "geographic illnesses" such as parasitic infections. Preventive advice includes: avoid eating raw crayfish, snails, fish; raw vegetables or fruits (unless they can be peeled); and avoid drinking water unless proven potable. Laboratory clearance of parasitic infection (stool and blood studies) should assume priority upon return to the U.S.

See Index: Nursing Interventions: parasitic infections (for additional nursing implications and patient teaching points).

Store tablets in tight containers at room temperature less than 30°C (86°F).

Diagnostic Test Interferences. Be mindful that selected drugs may interfere with stool studies for ova and parasites: iron, bismuth, oil (mineral or castor), **metamucil** (if ingested within 1 week of test), **barium, antibiotics, antiamebic** and **antimalarial drugs,** and gallbladder dye (if administered within 3 weeks of test).

PRAZOSIN HYDROCHLORIDE

(Minipress)

(pra'zoe-sin)
Antihypertensive
Alpha-adrenergic blocking agent

ACTIONS AND USES. Quinazoline derivative and alpha-adrenergic blocking agent structurally unrelated to other antihypertensive drugs. Mode of action not fully understood. Appears to cause peripheral vasodilation mainly on resistance vessels (arterioles) by blockade of postsynaptic alpha-adrenergic receptors with resulting reduction in total peripheral vascular resistance. Reduces orthostatic and supine blood pressures, with most pronounced effect on diastolic. Does not significantly change cardiac output, heart rate, renal blood flow, or glomerular filtration, and does not increase plasma renin activity.

Used in treatment of hypertension as initial agent or in conjunction with a diuretic and/or another antihypertensive drug, and conjunctively in treatment of congestive heart failure. Available in fixed-dose combination with polythiazide (Minizide).

ABSORPTION AND FATE. Peak plasma levels in 2 to 3 hours in fasting patients (plasma levels usually do not correlate with therapeutic effect). Plasma half-life: 2 to 3 hours. Approximately 97% bound to plasma proteins. Blood pressure begins to decrease within 2 hours, with maximum reduction in 2 to 4 hours; antihypertensive effect lasts less than 24 hours. Widely distributed to body tissues. Probably metabolized in liver and excreted mainly in bile and feces; about 6 to 10% excreted in urine.

P

CONTRAINDICATIONS AND PRECAUTIONS. Hypersensitivity to prazosin. *Cautious Use:* chronic renal failure. Safe use in women of childbearing potential, during pregnancy and lactation, and in children not established.

ADVERSE/SIDE EFFECTS. CV: edema, dyspnea, syncope, orthostatic hypotension, tachycardia, angina. **CNS (rare):** nervousness, vertigo, depression, paresthesia, insomnia. **Dermatologic:** rash, pruritis, alopecia, lichen planus. **EENT:** blurred vision, epistaxis, tinnitus, reddened sclerae, dry mouth, nasal congestion. **GI:** vomiting, diarrhea, constipation, abdominal discomfort, and/or pain. **GU:** urinary frequency, incontinence, priapism (especially patients with sickle cell trait), impotence. **Most common:** dizziness, lightheadedness, headache, drowsiness, fatigue, weakness, palpitation, nausea. **Other:** diaphoresis, arthralgia, transient leukopenia, increased serum uric acid and BUN.

ROUTE AND DOSAGE. Oral: Initial: 1 mg two or three times daily. Maintenance: dosage may be increased slowly to total of 20 mg daily in divided doses. Up to 40 mg daily in divided doses may be required. Highly individualized according to blood pressure response and tolerance. When diuretic or other antihypertensive drug is added, dosage should be reduced to 1 or 2 mg three times per day, and then retitration should be carried out.

NURSING IMPLICATIONS

Reportedly, food may delay absorption, but does not affect degree of absorption. It has been suggested that the frequency of faintness and dizziness may be reduced by taking drug with food.

"First-dose phenomenon" is a transient, dose-related syndrome manifested by dizziness, weakness, lightheadedness, and syncope. It may be especially severe in patients with low serum sodium. It commonly occurs within 30 minutes to 2 hours after initial dose is given, and may usually be prevented by administering initial dose at bedtime.

Caution patient to avoid situations that would result in injury should syncope occur. In most cases, effect does not recur after initial period of therapy; however, it has occurred during acute febrile episodes.

Syncope is also associated with rapid dosage increases or addition of another antihypertensive drug to regimen.

Instruct patient to make position changes slowly, particularly from recumbent to upright posture, and to dangle legs and move ankles a few minutes before standing.

Caution patient to lie down immediately if feeling weak or faint and to avoid potentially hazardous activities such as driving a car or operating machinery until reaction to drug is known. Side effects usually disappear with continuation of therapy, but they may require dosage reduction.

Patient-Teaching Points:

- ✓ Take drug at same times each day.
- ✓ Maintain optimum weight.
- ✓ Control sodium intake.
- ✓ Comply with established medical regimen.
- ✓ Keep follow-up appointments.

Advise patient not to take OTC medications, especially those that may contain a sympathomimetic agent (e.g., remedies for coughs, colds, allergy) without first consulting physician.

Full therapeutic effect of prazosin may not be achieved until after 4 to 6 weeks of therapy.

P

Drug Interactions. Hypotensive effect of prazosin is increased when given concomitantly with other **antihypertensive agents,** particularly **propranolol** (may be used therapeutically; permits reduction in dosage of each drug).

PREDNISOLONE

(Cordrol, Cortalone, Delta-Cortef, Inflamase, Novoprednisolone, Predoxine, Sterane, and others)

(pred-niss'oh-lone)
Corticosteroid
Glucocorticoid

PREDNISOLONE ACETATE

(Meticortelone, Predcor-25, Savacort, and others)

PREDNISOLONE SODIUM PHOSPHATE

(Hydeltrasol, PSP-IV)

PREDNISOLONE TEBUTATE

(Hydeltra-T.B.A., Metalone TBA, Nor-Pred TBA, Predcor-TBA)

ACTIONS AND USES. Intermediate-acting synthetic dehydrogenated analog of hydrocortisone (qv) with three to five times greater potency. Mineralocorticoid properties are minimal and potential for sodium and water retention and potassium loss is reduced. HPA suppression: 24 to 36 hours; half-life: about 130 minutes. Side effects minimal, but insomnia sometimes occurs during first few days of treatment. Compared with hydrocortisone, prednisolone and its esters have greater tendency to produce gastric irritation, gastroduodenal ulceration, ecchymotic skin lesions, vasomotor symptoms. Safe use during pregnancy (category C), by lactating women, or children not established.

Used principally as an antiinflammatory and immunosuppressant agent.

ADVERSE/SIDE EFFECTS. Hirsutism (occasional), perforation of cornea (with topical drug), sensitivity to heat, fat embolism, adverse effects on growth and development of the individual and on spermatozoa; hypotension and shocklike reactions. *See also Hydrocortisone.*

ROUTE AND DOSAGE. Oral: Adult: 5 to 60 mg/day as single or divided doses. **Pediatric:** 140 mcg to 2 mg/kg/day. **Intramuscular: Adult:** 4 to 60 mg/day. **Pediatric:** 40 to 250 mcg/kg one or two times daily. **Intralesional, intraarticular, intrasynovial:** 2 to 60 mg repeated at weekly intervals as needed. **Intravenous (phosphate): Adult:** 4 to 60 mg/day. **Pediatric:** 40 to 250 mcg/kg once or twice daily. Drug also available in aerosol, creams, ointment, ophthalmic-otic dosage forms and are usually applied three to four times daily (adult), once or twice daily (pediatric).

NURSING IMPLICATIONS

Administer with meals to reduce gastric irritation. If distress continues, consult physician about possible adjunctive antacid therapy.

Advise patient to adhere to established dosage regimen, i.e., should not increase, decrease, or omit doses; or change dose intervals.

Since topical corticosteroid treatment may increase intraocular pressure in susceptible individuals, it is usual to have frequent tonometric exams during prolonged therapy.

In diseases caused by microorganisms, infection may be masked, activated, or enhanced by corticosteroids. Be alert to subclinical signs of lack of improvement such as continued drainage, low-grade fever, and interrupted healing. Observe and report exacerbation of symptoms after short period of therapeutic response.

Alternate Day Therapy (ADT) (for Patient on Long-Term Therapy):

- ADT minimizes suppression of HPA axis and adverse/side effects associated with long-term treatment, while maintaining the desired therapeutic effect.
- ADT dosing mimics the normal diurnal variation of plasma cortisol and provides a period of rest and recovery from the effects of elevated plasma glucocorticoid levels.
- The patient's 48-hour requirement for steroids is administered as a single dose every

other morning: after the condition being treated has been controlled for divided daily or single daily dose.
- If patient becomes symptomatic (during period of switching to dose consolidation) on the off or drugless day, a single small dose of glucocorticoid should be given on the off day and gradually reduced.
- If an acute flare is precipitated (high fever, reactivation of inflammatory condition being treated), ADT may have to be abandoned.
- ADT is not used for replacement glucocorticoid treatment.

Temporary local discomfort may follow injection of prednisolone into bursa or joint.
Reconstituted solution should not be autoclaved.
Preserve in airtight containers; protect from light. Store at temperature 15° to 30°C (59° to 86°F); do not freeze.
See Hydrocortisone (prototype corticosteroid) for contraindications, additional nursing implications, and drug interactions.

PREDNISONE

(pred'ni-sone)

(Colisone, Cortan, Deltasone, Meticorten, Novoprednisone, Orasone, Panasol, Prednicen, Sterapred Winpred)

Corticosteroid
Glucocorticoid

ACTIONS AND USES. Immediate acting synthetic analog of hydrocortisone (qv). Effect depends on biotransformation to prednisolone, a conversion that may be impaired in patient with liver dysfunction. Has less mineralocoid activity than hydrocortisone but Na (therefore fluid) retention and K depletion can occur. Shares actions, uses, absorption and fate, contraindications, adverse/side effects with hydrocortisone. On weight basis 5 mg prednisone is equivalent to 5 mg prednisolone, 20 mg hydrocortisone, and 25 mg cortisone. Safe use by pregnant women (category C), children, or during lactation, not established.

Used as single agent or conjunctively with antineoplastics in cancer therapy; also used in treatment of myasthenia gravis. *See Hydrocortisone.*

ABSORPTION AND FATE. Peak effect: 1 to 2 hours; duration, 1 to 1½ days. Plasma half-life: 3.4 to 3.8 hours; HPA (hypothalamic–pituitary–adrenal) axis suppression: 24 to 36 hours.

P

ROUTE AND DOSAGE. Oral: Adult: Initial: 5 to 60 mg/24 hours in single or divided doses until desired clinical response; then gradual decremental dose (5 to 10 mg) adjustment every 4 to 5 days to lowest effective maintenance level: usually 5 to 20 mg//24 hours. **Pediatric (about 1/5 cortisone dose):** 0.1 to 0.15 mg/kg/24 hours or 4 to 5 mg/m²/24 hours divided every 12 hours. Doses highly individualized.

NURSING IMPLICATIONS

Tablet may be crushed before administration and taken with fluid of patient's choice.
Administer prednisone after meals and at bedtime.
Alternate day drug administration may be advised to keep daily dose at minimal levels and to reduce degree of "steroid rebound" with withdrawal.
Periodic blood K levels are recommended. Urge patient to keep scheduled appointments for medical supervision.
Monitor weight to detect onset of fluid accumulation, especially if patient is on unrestricted salt intake and does not receive K supplement. Report if weight gain is more than 5 pounds/week.

When patient is on an extended therapy regimen, incidence of oral candida infection is high. Inspect mouth daily for symptoms: white patches, black furry tongue, painful membranes and tongue.

Advise patient to report symptoms of K deficit (anorexia, paresthesias, drowsiness, muscle weakness, nausea, polyuria, postural hypotension, mental depression).

Protect drug from light and air in tightly closed dark container.

Store at temperature between 15° and 30°C (59° and 86°F).

See Hydrocortisone (prototype glucocorticoid) for contraindications, additional nursing implications and drug interactions.

PRIMAQUINE PHOSPHATE

(prim'a-kween)
Antimalarial

ACTIONS AND USES. Synthetic 8-aminoquinoline that acts on primary exoerythrocytic forms of *Plasmodium vivax* and *P. falciparum* by an incompletely known mechanism. Destroys late tissue forms of *P. vivax* and thus effects radical cure (prevents relapse). Also has gametocidal activity against all species of plasmodia that infect man, and thus can interrupt transmission of malaria. For treatment of acute attacks, always used in conjunction with a 4-aminoquinolone schizontocide such as chloroquin, which destroys erythrocytic parasites.

Used to prevent relapse ("radical" or "clinical" cure) of *P. vivax* and *P. ovale* malarias and to prevent attacks after departure from areas where *P. vivax* and *P. ovale* malarias are endemic.

ABSORPTION AND FATE. Absorbed well from intestine. Peak plasma levels in about 6 hours; only trace amounts detectable after 24 hours. Biodegradation products of primaquine are the active antimalarial and hemolytic agents. Concentrates in liver, lungs, heart, brain, and skeletal muscle. About 1% excreted unchanged in urine.

CONTRAINDICATIONS AND PRECAUTIONS. Rheumatoid arthritis, lupus erythematosus, hemolytic drugs, concomitant or recent use of agents capable of bone marrow depression, e.g., quinacrine; patients with G-6-PD deficiency. NADH methemoglobin reductase deficiency, pregnancy.

P

ADVERSE/SIDE EFFECTS. Hematologic reactions including granulocytopenia and acute hemolytic anemia in patients with G6PD deficiency. *Overdosage:* nausea, vomiting, epigastric distress, abdominal cramps, pruritus, methemoglobinemia (cyanosis): headache, confusion, mental depression, hypertension, arrhythmias (rare), moderate leukocytosis or leukopenia, anemia, granulocytopenia, agranulocytosis, disturbances of visual accommodation.

ROUTE AND DOSAGE. Oral: *Relapse prevention:* **Adults:** 15 mg (base). **Pediatric:** 0.3 mg (base)/kg. Doses given daily for 14 days concomitantly or consecutively with chloroquine, hydroxychloroquine, or amodiaquine which are given on first 3 days of an acute attack. *Prophylaxis:* **Adults:** 15 to 30 mg (base). **Pediatric:** 0.3 mg (base)/kg. Doses given daily for 14 days beginning immediately after person has left malarious area. Each 26.3 mg tablet = 15 mg base.

NURSING IMPLICATIONS

Administration of drug at mealtime or with an antacid (prescribed) may prevent or relieve gastric irritation. Notify physician if GI symptoms persist.

Primaquine may precipitate acute hemolytic anemia in persons with G6PD deficiency, an inherited error of metabolism carried on the X chromosome, present in about 10% American black males and certain Caucasian ethnic groups: Sardinians, Sephardic Jews, Greeks, and Iranians and those with personal or family history of favism. Caucasians manifest more intense expression of hemolytic reaction than do blacks.

Patients whose ethnic origin indicate the possibility of G6PD deficiency should be screened prior to initiation of therapy.

Advise all patients to examine urine after each voiding and to report darkening of urine, red-tinged urine and decrease in urine volume. Also report chills, fever, precordial pain, cyanosis (all are suggestive signs of hemolytic reaction). Sudden reductions in hemoglobin or erythrocyte count suggest impending hemolytic reaction.

Repeated hematologic studies (particularly blood cell counts and hemoglobin) and urinalyses should be performed during therapy.

Preserve in well-closed, light-resistant containers.

Drug Interactions. **Quinacrine** potentiates toxicity of primaquine and other 8-aminoquinolone antimalarial agents.

PRIMIDONE

(pri′mi-done)

(Myidone, Mysoline, Primoline, Sertau)

Anticonvulsant

ACTIONS AND USES. Not a true barbiturate, but closely related chemically and with similar mechanism of action. Converted in body to phenobarbital (qv) metabolite. Appears to increase metabolism of vitamin D so that more is needed to fulfill normal requirements. May also impair calcium, folic acid and vitamin B_{12} metabolism and utilization.

Used alone or concomitantly with other anticonvulsant agents in the prophylactic management of complex partial (psychomotor) and generalized tonic–clonic (grand mal) seizures. *Investigational Use:* essential tremor.

ABSORPTION AND FATE. Approximately 60 to 80% of dose absorbed from GI tract. Peak serum levels reached in 4 hours. Slowly metabolized in liver to two active metabolites: phenobarbital and phenylethylmalonamide (PEMA). Protein binding varies from 0 to 19%, but phenobarbital metabolite is 50% bound. Primidone plasma half-life varies from 3 to 24 hours, that of PEMA 24 to 48 hours and that of phenobarbital 72 to 144 hours. Excreted in urine, approximately 15 to 25% as unchanged drug (40% in children). Appears in breast milk.

P

CONTRAINDICATIONS AND PRECAUTIONS. Safe use in women of childbearing potential, during pregnancy, and in nursing mothers not established. Hypersensitivity to barbiturates, porphyria. *Cautious Use:* chronic lung disease, hepatic or renal disease, hyperactive children.

ADVERSE/SIDE EFFECTS. CNS: drowsiness, sedation, vertigo, ataxia, headache, excitement (children), confusion, unusual fatigue, hyperirritability, emotional disturbances, acute psychoses (usually patients with psychomotor epilepsy). **GI:** nausea, vomiting, anorexia. **Hematologic:** leukopenia, thrombocytopenia, eosinophilia, decreased serum folate levels, megaloblastic anemia (rare). **Ophthalmic:** diplopia, nystagmus, swelling of eyelids. **Other:** alopecia, impotence, maculopapular or morbilliform rash, edema, lupus erythematosus-like syndrome, lymphadenopathy, osteomalacia.

ROUTE AND DOSAGE. Oral: Adults and Children (over 8 years): Initial: 250 mg daily; increased by 250 mg weekly to tolerance or therapeutic effect, or to maximum of 2 Gm daily divided into 2 to 4 doses. **Children (under 8 years):** 125 mg daily increased by 125 mg weekly up to maximum of 1 Gm daily divided into 2 to 4 doses.

NURSING IMPLICATIONS

Tablet may be crushed before administration and taken with fluid of patient's choice.

If drug causes GI distress, take it with meals.

Because drowsiness, dizziness, and ataxia may be severe at beginning of treatment, advise patient to avoid driving and other potentially hazardous activities. Symptoms tend to disappear with continued therapy; if they persist, dosage reduction or drug withdrawal may be necessary.

Transition from another anticonvulsant to primidone should not be completed in less than 2 months.

Baseline and periodic studies should be made of CBC, SMA-12 (every 6 months), and primidone and phenobarbital blood levels. (Therapeutic blood level for primidone: 5 to 10 mcg/ml; for phenobarbital: 15 to 40 mcg/ml.)

Dosage may be adjusted with reference to primidone or phenobarbital metabolite plasma levels (concentrations of primidone greater than 10 mg/ml are usually associated with significant ataxia and lethargy).

Therapeutic response may not be evident for several weeks.

Neonatal hemorrhage has been reported in newborns whose mothers were taking primidone. Monitor closely for bleeding.

Presence of unusual drowsiness in nursing newborns of primidone-treated mothers is an indication to discontinue nursing.

Pregnant women should receive prophylactic vitamin K therapy for 1 month prior to and during delivery to prevent neonatal hemorrhage.

Observe for signs and symptoms of folic acid deficiency: mental dysfunction, psychiatric disorders, neuropathy, megaloblastic anemia. When indicated, serum folate levels should be determined.

Megaloblastic anemia responds to folic acid 15 mg daily, without necessity of interrupting primidone therapy.

Caution patient not to take OTC medications unless approved by physician.

Primidone withdrawal should be done gradually to avoid precipitating status epilepticus.

Advise patient to avoid alcohol and other CNS depressants unless otherwise directed by physician.

Advise patient to carry medical information card or jewelry with name of drug, physician's name, and telephone number.

Drug Interactions. Concomitant use of **barbiturates** may result in excessive phenobarbital blood levels *(see Absorption and Fate).* **Isoniazid** may inhibit primidone metabolism with resulting high blood levels. **Phenytoin** may cause increase in phenobarbital blood levels probably by stimulating conversion of primidone to phenobarbital. *See also Phenobarbital: prototype anticonvulsant.*

PROBENECID

(Benemid, Benuryl, Probalan, SK-Probenecid)

(proe-ben'e-sid)
Antigout agent
Uricosuric
Sulfonamide derivative

ACTIONS AND USES. Sulfonamide-derivative renal tubular blocking agent. In sufficiently high doses, competitively inhibits renal tubular reabsorption of uric acid, thereby promoting its excretion and reducing serum urate levels (subtherapeutic doses may depress uric acid excretion). Prevents formation of new tophaceous deposits, and causes gradual shrinking of old tophi. Since it has no analgesic or antiinflammatory activity, it is of no value in acute gout, and may exacerbate and prolong acute phase. Increases plasma levels of weak organic acids, including beta-lactam antibiotics, by competitively inhibiting their renal tubular secretion.

Used for treatment of hyperuricemia in chronic gouty arthritis and tophaceous gout, and as adjuvant to therapy with penicillin G and penicillin analogs to elevate and prolong plasma concentrations of these antibiotics. *Unlabeled Use:* to promote uric acid excretion in hyperuricemia secondary to administration of thiazides and related diuretics, furosemide, ethycrinic acid, pyrasinamide; in the diagnosis of Parkinson's syndrome; mental depression.

ABSORPTION AND FATE. Rapidly and completely absorbed from GI tract. Maximal renal clearance of uric acid in 30 minutes; effect on penicillin levels after about 2 hours. Plasma levels peak in 2 to 4 hours and persist for 8 hours. Plasma half-life 8 to 10 hours. About 75 to 95% bound to plasma proteins. Metabolized by liver. Excreted in urine after 2 days as metabolites and unchanged drug. Urine alkalinization decreases reabsorption of probenecid and increases uric acid solubility. Crosses placenta.

CONTRAINDICATIONS AND PRECAUTIONS. Hypersensitivity to probenecid, blood dyscrasias, uric acid kidney stones, during or within 2 to 3 weeks of acute gouty attack, overexcretion of uric acid (over 1000 mg/day), patients with creatinine clearance less than 50 mg/minute, use with penicillin in presence of known renal impairment, use for hyperuricemia secondary to cancer chemotherapy. Safe use during pregnancy, in nursing mothers, and in children under 2 years of age not established. *Cautious Use:* history of peptic ulcer.

ADVERSE/SIDE EFFECTS. Headache, nausea, vomiting, anorexia, sore gums, urinary frequency, flushing, dizziness, anemia, hemolytic anemia (possibly related to G6PD deficiency). Nephrotic syndrome, hepatic necrosis, and aplastic anemia (rare). Exacerbations of gout, uric acid kidney stones. **Hypersensitivity:** dermatitis, pruritus, fever, anaphylaxis. **Overdosage:** CNS stimulation, convulsions, respiratory depression.

ROUTE AND DOSAGE. Oral: *Gout therapy:* first week 0.25 Gm twice daily for 1 week, followed by 0.5 Gm twice daily. For patients with renal impairment: 1 Gm; daily dosage may be increased by 0.5 Gm increments every 4 weeks (usually not above 2 gm/day) if symptoms are not controlled or 24-hour urate excretion is not above 700 mg. *Penicillin or cephalosporin therapy:* **Adults:** 0.5 Gm four times daily. **Children (2 to 14 years):** Initial: 25 mg/kg; maintenance 40 mg/kg/day divided into 4 doses; children weighing over 50 kg may receive adult dosage. *Gonorrhea* (uncomplicated): 1 Gm concurrently with single dose of oral ampicillin 3.5 Gm or IM aqueous procaine penicillin G 4.8 million units divided into at least 2 doses injected at different sites.

P

NURSING IMPLICATIONS

GI side effects minimized by taking drug after meals, with food, milk, or with antacid (prescribed). If symptoms persist, dosage reduction may be required.

Increased uric acid excretion promoted by probenecid predisposes to renal calculi. Therefore, during early therapy, high fluid intake (approximately 3000 ml/day) is recommended to maintain daily urinary output of at least 2000 ml or more.

Oral sodium bicarbonate (3 to 7.5 Gm/day) or potassium citrate (7.5 Gm/day) may be prescribed to alkalinize urine until serum uric acid levels return to normal range (3 to 7 mg/dl).

When urinary alkalinizers are used, periodic determinations of acid–base balance are advised. Some physicians prescribe acetazolamide at bedtime to keep urine alkaline and dilute throughout night.

Physician may advise restriction of high-purine foods during early therapy until uric acid level stabilizes. Foods high in purine: organ meats (sweetbreads, liver, kidney), meat extracts, meat soups, gravy, anchovies, sardines. Moderate amounts in other meats, fish, seafood, asparagus, spinach, peas, dried legumes, wild game.

Alcohol may increase serum urate levels and therefore should be avoided.

Caution patient not to stop taking drug without consulting physician. Irregular dosage schedule may cause sharp elevation of serum urate level and precipitation of acute gout.

Urate tophaceous deposits should decrease in size with probenecid therapy. Classic locations are in cartilage of ear pinna and big toe, but they can occur in bursae, tendons, skin, kidneys, and other tissues.

Because frequency of acute gouty attacks may increase during first 6 to 12 months of therapy, physician may prescribe concurrent prophylactic doses of colchicine for first 3 to 6 months of probenecid therapy (probenecid alone aggravates acute gout). Probenecid is available in combination with colchicine, e.g., ColBenemid.

When gouty attacks have been absent for 6 months or more and serum urate levels are controlled, daily dosage may be cautiously decreased by 0.5 Gm every 6 months to lowest effective dosage that maintains stable serum urate levels.

Lifelong therapy is usually required in patients with symptomatic hyperuricemia. Advise patient to keep scheduled appointments with physician and appointments for studies of renal function and hematology.

Instruct patient to report symptoms of hypersensitivity to physician. Discontinuation of drug is indicated.

Patients taking oral hypoglycemics may require dosage adjustment. Probenecid enhances hypoglycemic actions of these drugs. *See also Diagnostic Test Interferences.*

Advise patient not to take aspirin or other OTC medications without consulting physician. If a mild analgesic is required, acetaminophen is usually allowed.

Tablets should be stored in well-closed containers at 15° to 30°C (59° to 86°F). Expiration date is 3 to 5 years after date of manufacture.

P

Diagnostic Test Interferences. Probenecid may decrease excretion of **urinary 17-ketosteroids** and may increase **BSP** retention and inhibit **urinary PSP** excretion. False-positive results **urine glucose** tests are possible with Benedict's solution or Clinitest (glucose oxidase methods not affected, e.g., Clinistix, Tes-Tape).

Drug Interactions: Probenecid

Plus	Interactions
Aminosalicylic acid (PAS), dapsone, clofibrate, pantothenic acid, indomethacin, rifampin, methotrexate, naproxen Sulfonylureas Sulfonamides	Probenicid inhibits renal excretion and raises the plasma concentration of these drugs thus increasing their potential for toxicity

Plus (cont.)	Interactions (cont.)
Nitrofurantoin Alcohol Diazoxides Diuretics Salicylates Pyraxinamide	Decreased antiinfective activity of nitrofurantoin Increased serum urate levels, therefore increased dosage of probenecid may be necessary

---

PROBUCOL

(Lorelco)

(proe′byoo-kole)
Antilipemic

ACTIONS AND USES. Lowers serum cholesterol levels by reducing low density lipoprotein (LDL) concentrations. Therapeutic action thought to be due to inhibition of early stages of cholesterol synthesis, and to increased bile acid excretion in feces, and (minimal) inhibition of dietary cholesterol absorption. Serum triglyceride (VLDL) levels are not appreciably lowered by this agent. It is not known whether a cholesterol lowering drug has an effect, no effect, or a detrimental effect on morbidity or mortality related to atherosclerosis or coronary heart disease.

Used to lower elevated cholesterol concentrations in patients with type II hyperlipoproteinemia, especially type IIa and type III. Use is adjunctive to diet and is indicated for patients who fail to respond adequately to diet, weight reduction, and control of diabetes mellitus.

ABSORPTION AND FATE. Less than 10% oral dose is absorbed; plasma levels are higher and less variable when drug is administered with meals. Continuous oral administration leads to gradual accumulation in adipose tissue; maximum blood levels reached in 1 to 3 months. Half-life: 24 hours to 20 days. Drug may remain in fat and blood for 6 months or longer after last dose. Elimination via bile and feces; renal clearance is negligible.

CONTRAINDICATIONS AND PRECAUTIONS. Hypersensitivity to probucol; pregnancy, nursing mothers, women in childbearing years, children; patient with unresponsive congestive heart failure, frequent multifocal or paired ventricular extrasystoles, primary biliary cirrhosis. *Cautious Use:* patients behaviorally incapable of strict adherence to diet therapy; impaired hepatic function, cholelithiasis.

P

ADVERSE/SIDE EFFECTS. CNS: headache, dizziness, paresthesias, peripheral neuritis, decreased sense of taste and smell. **EENT:** blurred vision, tinnitus, conjunctivitis, tearing. **GI:** nausea, vomiting, anorexia, heartburn, GI bleeding, diarrhea, flatulance, adominal pain. **Hematologic:** eosinophilia, low HGE, Hct, thrombocytopenia. **Idiosyncracy:** dizziness, palpitation, syncope, chest pains, nausea, vomiting. **Other:** rash, pruritus, impotence, enlargement of multinodal goiter, nocturia, hyperhidrosis, fetid sweat, angioneurotic edema.

ROUTE AND DOSAGE. Oral: Adult: 500 mg twice daily.

NURSING IMPLICATIONS

Administer drug with morning and evening meals to enhance its action.

The patient should fully understand that this drug does not reduce necessity to adhere to special diet.

Baseline data to be established before treatment begins include existing serum cholesterol and triglyceride levels.
Serum cholesterol levels (normal 150 to 280 mg/dl) should be checked frequently during first month of therapy. Usually a favorable decline in levels is observed within 2 months of probucol therapy. If not observed within 4 months, drug is discontinued.
If there is a sustained rise in serum triglycerides (normal 40 to 150 mg/dl), investigate degree of compliance with special diet, carbohydrate and caloric intake, and alcohol intake. Reinforce and emphasize importance of strict adherance to dietary regimen. Probucol will be withdrawn if hypertriglyceridemia persists.
The dosage of oral anticoagulant or oral hypoglycemic agents is not altered when used concomitantly with probucol.
Strict birth control measures should be used by women in childbearing years during probucol therapy. If pregnancy is desired, it is recommended that birth control be practiced at least 6 months after the drug is withdrawn to insure its complete elimination before conception.
Monitor pulse during early therapy. Irregularity in rhythm and strength should be evaluated by ECG. (If patient has history of or existing myocardial damage or dysrhythmia periodic ECG evaluations should accompany therapy with probucol.) Drug is discontinued if pronounced QT interval prolongation or arrhythmias are observed.
Alcohol intake is usually not allowed during probucol therapy.
GI side effects are generally transient and seldom require treatment or discontinuation of drug therapy. If persistent, however, patient should report to the physician because of danger of fluid and electrolyte imbalance and dehydration.
Any unexplained bleeding (ecchymoses, petechiae, epistaxis, black stools) must be reported to physician as soon as observed.
Swelling of face, oral membranes, hands or feet and symptoms of angioneurotic edema should be reported; drug will be discontinued.
Counsel patient not to change dose intervals of probucol. Patient should not increase or decrease doses, nor discontinue taking the drug without the physician's approval.
Xanthelasama and xanthomata may disappear or reduce in size during probucol therapy. Keep physician informed.
Instruct patient to check with the physician before self-dosing with OTC medications.
Store in light- and moisture-proof container at temperature between 15° and 30°C (59° and 86°F) unless otherwise specified by the manufacturer.

P

Diagnostic Test Interferences. Probucol therapy is accompanied by transient elevations in serum transaminases (**AST, ALT**), **bilirubin, alkaline phosphatase, creatine, phosphokinase, uric acid, BUN** and **blood glucose. Hematocrit, hemoglobin** and **eosinophil values** may be decreased.

PROCAINAMIDE HYDROCHLORIDE

(Procan, Promine, Pronestyl, Sub-Quin)

(proe-kane-a'mide)
Antiarrhythmic (class I)
Vasodilator

ACTIONS AND USES. Amide analogue of procaine hydrochloride with cardiac actions very similar to those of quinine. Depresses excitability of myocardium to electrical stimulation, reduces conduction velocity in atria, ventricles and His-Purkinje system. Increases duration of refractory period especially in the atria. Unless myocardial damage is present, contractility of cardiac muscle and cardiac output are changed only slightly by procainamide; however, automaticity of His-Purkinje-ventricular muscle is suppressed. In the absence of dysrhythmia, therapeutic doses may accelerate heart rate, suggesting that procainamide may have anticholinergic properties. Produces peripheral vasodilation and hypotension, especially with IV use. Larger doses can induce AV block and ventricular extrasystoles that may proceed to ventricular fibrillation. ECG changes reflecting these effects include: prolonged PR and QT intervals. Also has local anesthetic properties equal to but more sustained than those of procain and produces less CNS stimulation than does procain. Prolonged administration often leads to development of positive antinuclear antibodies (ANA) in about 50% of patients.

Used prophylactically to maintain normal sinus rhythm following conversion of atrial flutter or fibrillation by other methods. Also used to prevent recurrence of paroxysmal atrial fibrillation and tachycardia, paroxysmal AV junctional rhythm, ventricular tachycardia, and ventricular and atrial premature contractions. Also used to treat cardiac arrhythmias associated with surgery and anesthesia. *Unlabeled Use:* malignant hyperthermia.

ABSORPTION AND FATE. Rapidly absorbed, except for extended-release form. Plasma levels peak within 15 to 60 minutes after IM; within 30 to 60 minutes after PO administration; duration of effects about 3 hours (about 8 hours for extended release form). Protein binding 20%; plasma half-life: about 3 hours (5 to 8 hours in patients with cardiac disease, 11 to 20 hours in presence of renal dysfunction). Approximately 25% of dose acetylated in liver to produce active metabolite N-acetylprocainamide (NAPA) with half-life of 6 hours. About 60% of drug excreted in urine unchanged. NAPA is entirely cleared by kidneys.

CONTRAINDICATIONS AND PRECAUTIONS. Myasthenia gravis, hypersensitivity to procainamide or procaine; blood dyscrasias, complete AV block, second and third degree AV block unassisted by pacemaker. *Cautious Use:* patient who has undergone electrical reversion to sinus rhythm, hypotension, cardiac enlargement, congestive heart failure, myocardial infarction, coronary occlusion, ventricular dysrhythmia from digitalis intoxication, hepatic or renal insufficiency, electrolyte imbalance, bronchial asthma, history of systemic lupus erythematosis (SLE). Safe use in pregnancy or lactation not established.

ADVERSE/SIDE EFFECTS. CNS: dizziness, mental depression, psychosis with hallucinations. **CV:** severe hypotension, pericarditis, ventricular fibrillation (parenteral use); tachycardia, flushing. **GI:** (mostly oral); bitter taste, nausea, vomiting, diarrhea, anorexia. **Hematologic:** agranulocytosis with repeated use; thrombocytopenia. **Hypersensitivity:** fever, muscle and joint pain, angioneurotic edema, maculopapular rash, pruritus, eosinophilia, rarely: generalized or digital vasculitis, proximal myopathy, and Sjögren's syndrome. **Other:** *SLE-like syndrome* (40% of patients on large doses for one year): polyarthralgias, pleuritic pain, pleural effusion, erythema, skin rash, myalgia, fever.

P

ROUTE AND DOSAGE. (Oral route preferred; IV use limited to extreme emergencies). **Oral: Adults:** *Ventricular tachycardia:* initial: 1 Gm followed by 6 mg/kg every 3 hours. *Premature ventricular contractions:* initial: 50 mg to 1.25 Gm; maintenance: 50 mg/day in divided doses every 3 hours. *Atrial fibrillation* and *paroxysmal atrial tachycardia:* initial: 1.25 Gm followed in 1 hour by 0.75 Gm if no ECG changes. Additional doses of 0.5 to 1 Gm every 2 hours until normal rhythm is restored or toxicity manifests. Maintenance: 0.5 to 1 Gm every 4 to 6 hours. **Pediatric:** dose not established by manufacturer. **Intramuscular: Adult:** *Arrhythmias:* 0.5 to 1 Gm every 4 to 6 hours until oral dose is feasible. *Cardiac arrhythmias associated with anesthesia or surgery:* 100 to 500 mg. **Intravenous (direct): Adult:** 100 mg doses every 5 minutes given slowly at rate of 25 to 50 mg/minute until arrhythmia is controlled or toxic symptoms appear or maximum dose of 1 Gm has been given; maintenance: intravenous infusion of 2 to 6 mg/minute adjusted to body weight, circulatory and renal function criteria. Sustained-release tablet (500 mg) is used for maintenance dosing. Usual dose: 500 mg to 1 Gm every 6 hours.

NURSING IMPLICATIONS

Patients at particular risk to adverse effects are those with severe heart, hepatic or renal disease, and hypotension. Dosage adjustment is based on individual requirements, response, general condition and cardiovascular status.

Administer oral preparation on empty stomach 1 hour before or 2 hours after meals with a full glass of water to enhance absorption. If drug causes gastric distress, administer with food.

Tablet may be crushed if patient is unable to swallow it whole. Capsule may be emptied and contents swallowed with water or mixed with food.

Instruct patient to swallow sustained-release tablet whole. It uses a wax matrix which is not absorbed but appears in the stool.

Fever sometimes occurs during the first few days of therapy and may necessitate discontinuation of drug. Monitor temperature and report elevation.

Procainamide administration by IV infusion pump requires constant monitoring by qualified personnel to maintain desired flow rate and to detect special problems. Keep patient in supine position. Be alert to signs of *"speed shock"* (because of too rapid administration of drug): irregular pulse, tight feeling in chest, flushed face, headache, loss of consciousness, shock, cardiac arrest. Usual procedure: stop medication; start in-line infusion of 5% dextrose in water at KVO (keep vein open) rate, to permit later emergency treatment. Obtain rhythm strip and notify physician immediately.

A complication of procainamide infusion given to treat atrial dysrhythmia is the onset of ventricular tachycardia (a lethal arrhythmia) evidenced by increased rate to as high as 200 beats per minute.

If symptoms of ventricular dysrhythmia develop during IV therapy, talk with patient to gauge responsiveness. Be prepared to defibrillate immediately if beginning to lose consciousness.

Ventricular dysrhythmias are usually abolished within a few minutes after IV dose and within an hour after oral or IM administration.

IV dosage over a period of several hours is controlled by assessment of procainamide plasma levels: effective nontoxic therapeutic level: 3 to 10 mcg/ml. (Eight to 16 mcg/ml is potentially toxic and toxicity is common at plasma levels above 16 mcg/ml).

Drug is temporarily discontinued when the following occur: (1) arrhythmia is interrupted, (2) severe toxic effects present, (3) QRS complex is excessively widened, (greater than 50%) (4) PR interval is prolonged, or (5) blood pressure drops 15 mm Hg or more. Obtain rhythm strip and notify physician.

Hypotensive effects of IV infusion are treated with dopamine phenylephredine or norepinephrine overdosage is managed by fluid volume replacement, vasopressors, hemodialysis or resin hemoperfusion.

When patient with acute myocardial infarction is changed from parenteral to oral dosage form, the first oral dose may coincide with one elimination half-life. Consult physician about precise time.

Apical-radial pulses should be checked before each dose of procainamide during period of adjustment to the oral route.

Digitalization may precede procainamide in patients with atrial arrhythmias. Cardiotonic glycosides may induce sufficient increase in atrial contraction to cause dislodgement of atrial mural emboli with subsequent pulmonary embolism. Report promptly patient complaints of chest pain, dyspnea and anxiety.

Procainamide blood levels and that of its active metabolite (NAPA) are reached in approximately 24 hours if kidney function is normal, but are delayed several days in presence of renal impairment.

In renal pathology or congestive heart failure dosage may be reduced to prevent procainamide build-up (and potential toxicity). Theoretically antidysrhythmic action is maintained even with a lower dose because hepatic acetylation continues to release NAPA (also antiarrhythmic) with its longer half-life.

Advise patient to monitor and report immediately evidence of kidney dysfunction: changes in intake–output ratio and body weight, local edema (tight shoes or rings). Encourage keeping a record of weekly weight for comparison purposes. If weight gain of 2 pounds or more is accompanied by local edema, patient should notify the physician.

LE (lupus erythematosus) test and ANA titers are evaluated regularly when patient is on long-term maintenance dosage or if SLE-like symptoms appear. Approximately 60 to 70% of all patients will have elevated ANA titers, and 20 to 30% will develop clinical symptoms in 1 month to 1 year.

Urge the patient on long-term therapy to keep appointments for periodic evaluations of blood counts, hepatic and renal function, and ECG studies.

SLE-like syndrome, unlike the spontaneous form of SLE, has no symptoms of nervous system or renal dysfunction; hematopoietic disorders occur rarely, and are reversible. Syndrome symptoms that should be reported by the patient: polyarthralgia, pleuritic pain, cough, and fever. If ANA titer is also high, drug will be discontinued and substituted by quinidine; steroid therapy may be used if symptoms are severe. Clinical manifestations of the syndrome may remain for years after cessation of therapy.

The physician may want patient who has had drug-induced SLE to wear a medical bracelet with information about the SLE incidence. Such a patient needs to understand that procainamide therapy should be avoided in the future.

Instruct patient on maintenance doses to record and report date, time and duration of fibrillation episodes (lightheadedness, giddiness, weakness, or syncope): such symptoms suggest changed ventricular rhythm. Evaluation of ECG rhythm strips and procainamide plasma levels will be necessary.

Consult with physician regarding patient monitoring own pulse and how often it should be done.

Patient-Teaching Points for Pulse-Taking:

- ✓ Establish a base-line pulse range for comparison purposes.
- ✓ Show patient how to "feel" and count radial pulse rate.
- ✓ Take a resting pulse rate, i.e., just before getting out of bed each AM.
- ✓ Count pulse for 1 full minute.
- ✓ Avoid taking carotid pulse: may cause arrhythmias or asytole.
- ✓ Keep a record of pulse rates.
- ✓ Report changes in rate or quality (i.e., if pulse is too rapid or too slow, faint or irregular).

Instruct patient or family to report to the physician if signs of reduced procainamide control occur: weakness, irregular pulse, unexplained fatiguability, anxiety.

Adequacy of oral dosage may be evaluated by 24-hour Holter ECG recordings.

If Holter monitoring is ordered, discuss with the patient importance of noting relationships, feelings, and subjective symptoms to assure that diary recordings will be as accurate as possible.

The characteristic symptoms of agranulocytosis (soreness of mouth, gums and throat; upper respiratory tract infection, fatigue, and unexplained fever) should be reported promptly to permit appropriate differential diagnosis (leukocyte counts) and treatment. Discontinuation of procainamide therapy may be required because of the danger of severe or even fatal infection.

Although bleeding disorders are uncommon, the patient should be aware of the possibility. Any unexplainable bleeding (melena, petechiae, purpura, ecchymosis, bruising, epistaxis) should be investigated.

Consult physician about whether patient should discontinue drinking caffeine beverages (tea, coffee, cola, hot chocolate).

Caution the patient to adhere to dosage schedule as planned by the physician. At no time should a dose be doubled nor should an interval be changed because a previous dose was missed. Procainamide should be taken at evenly spaced intervals around the clock unless otherwise prescribed.

Before discharge, work with patient to design a 24-hour dosing schedule for procainamide and all other prescribed drugs that will best fit into activities of daily living at home.

Check patient's self-medication habits. If patient has been in the habit of taking OTC medications for nasal congestion, allergy, pain, or obesity, instruct patient to discuss with physician about continued need and safe substitutes, if necessary.

If surgery is anticipated, and in an emergency situation, the patient should inform doctor or dentist that procainamide is being taken.

Caution patient to avoid driving car until risk of lightheadedness and fainting has been eliminated.

Advise patient to carry medical identification card or bracelet stating that procainamide is being taken.

Pronestyl tablets contain tartrazine which may cause allergic reactions (including bronchial asthma) in susceptible individuals (frequently people who also have a hypersensitivity to aspirin).

Procainamide solution is stable for 24 hours at room temperature and for 7 days under refrigeration at 2° to 8°C (36° to 46°F). Avoid freezing the solution. Refrigeration will retard color changes in solution. Slight yellowing does not alter drug potency, but discard if markedly discolored or precipitated.

Store tablets in dark airtight containers. Procainamide is hygroscopic: therefore do not store in bathroom medicine cabinet or in refrigerator where moisture levels are high.

Diagnostic Test Interferences. Procainamide increases the plasma levels of **alkaline phosphatase, bilirubin, lactic dehydrogenase** and **SGOT** (serum glutamic oxaloacetic transaminase). It may also alter results of the **edrophonium test.**

Drug Interactions: Procainamide Hydrochloride

Plus	Interactions
Acetazolamide	Increases effect of procainamide
Antiarrhythmics	Additive effect of both procainamide and the other antiarrhythmics
Anticholinergic agents	Additive anticholinergic effects
Antihypertensives	Additive hypotensive effect
Cholinergics	Antagonizes effects of cholinergic drugs
Kanamycin, magnesium salts, Noemycin Neuromuscular blockers (nondepolarizing and depolarizing) Sodium bicarbonate	Enhances muscle relaxation produced by these agents

PROCAINE HYDROCHLORIDE *(proe'kane)*

(Anduracaine, Anuject, Durathesia, Novocain) *Anesthetic (local)*

ACTIONS AND USES. Ester of benzoic acid with anesthetic properties. Blocks sodium ion transport across members thereby preventing the initial depolarization that generates a nerve action potential. Inhibits subsequent transmission of nerve impulses thus leading to local anesthesia. Relatively nontoxic but fairly high incidence of allergic reactions. Lacks surface anesthetic action.

Used for spinal anesthesia (10% solution) in general surgery, obstetric anesthetic at term, or in dental surgery. 1 to 2% solution used to produce local anesthesia by infiltration injection, nerve block or other peripheral blocks.

ABSORPTION AND FATE. Readily absorbed following parenteral administration; hydrolyzed by plasma cholinesterase to para-amino-benzoic acid (PABA) and diethylaminoethanol. Onset of action: 2 to 5 minutes; duration of action: 30 to 90 minutes, depending on type of block, drug concentration, anesthetic technique and the patient. Excreted as metabolites in urine.

CONTRAINDICATIONS AND PRECAUTIONS. Known hypersensitivity to procaine or to other drugs of similar chemical structure or PABA or its derivatives. Generalized septicemia, inflammation, or sepsis at proposed injection site; cerebrospinal diseases (meningitis, syphilis); heart block, concomitant use with a sulfonamide drug. Safe use in women of childbearing potential and early pregnancy (category B) have not been established. *Cautious Use:* debilitated, elderly, acutely ill patients; obstetric delivery, increased intraabdominal pressure, known drug allergies and sensitivities, disturbances of cardiac rhythm, shock.

ADVERSE/SIDE EFFECTS. Allergic reactions: cutaneous lesions of delayed onset, or urticaria, edema and other manifestations of allergy. **CNS:** (excitatory) nervousness, dizziness, blurred vision, tremors, drowsiness, convulsions, unconsciousness, postspinal headache, meningismus, arachnoiditis, palsies, spinal nerve paralysis. **CV:** depressed myocardium, hypo- or hypertension, bradycardia, cardiac arrest. **GI:** nausea, vomiting. **Respiratory:** respiratory impairment or paralysis.

ROUTE AND DOSAGE. (The lowest dose required to provide effective anesthesia should be administered.) **Infiltration anesthesia (0.25 or 0.5%):** 350 to 600 mg as single dose. *Peripheral nerve block* (0.5% solution): up to 200 ml; (1% solution): up to 100 ml; (2% solution) up to 50 ml. Usual initial dose: should not exceed 1000 mg. **Spinal anesthesia:** *Surgical, dental and obstetric anesthesia* (10% solution): initial dose: should not exceed 1000 mg. Rate of injection: 1 ml/5 seconds. **Rectal anesthesia:** 1.25 to 1.5% solution.

P

NURSING IMPLICATIONS

Avoid use of disinfecting agents containing heavy metals which cause release of specific ions, e.g., mercury, copper, on skin or mucous membranes; such solutions have been related to swelling and edema.

To prepare 60 ml of a 0.5% solution (5 mg/ml) dilute 30 ml of 1% solution with 30 ml sterile distilled water. 0.5 to 1 ml epinephrine 1:1000/100 ml anesthetic solution may be added for vasoconstrictive effect (1:200,000 to 1:100,000).

Do not use solutions that are cloudy or that contain precipitated drug.

Discard unused portion of the drug.

Injection should be slow, with frequent aspirations to avoid inadvertent intravascular (and therefore systemic) administration which can lead to toxicity.

Rectal administration of procaine is for local effect only, for proctology.

When used during obstetric delivery, fetal heart rate should be monitored prior to and during paracervical block. Fetal distress, prematurity, and toxemia of pregnancy add to the risk of using this drug.

Fetal bradycardia following paracervical block may indicate high fetal blood concentrations of procaine which could lead to fetal acidosis.

Hypersensitivities and anaphylactic reaction are not usually dose-related. Resuscitation equipment and drugs should be immediately available when procaine is used.

Keep in mind that addition of epinephrine to procaine solution increases the risk of precipitating arrhythmias. Monitor patient closely during the anaesthesia period.

When chemical disinfection of multiple dose vials is needed, use undiluted isopropyl alcohol (91%) or 70% ethyl alcohol. However, heat sterilization (autoclaving) of intact ampuls and vials before opening is recommended. Autoclave once at 15 pounds pressure at 121°C (250°F) for 15 minutes.

Do not autoclave procaine solutions containing epinephrine.

Reautoclaving increases the potential for crystal formation in vial or ampul.

Store at 10° to 30°C (59° to 86°F). Avoid freezing.

Drug Interactions. Procaine may delay action of **sulfonamide antibiotics.**

PROCARBAZINE HYDROCHLORIDE

(Matulane, MIH, Natulan)

(proe-kar'ba-zeen)
Antineoplastic
Hydrazine

ACTIONS AND USES. Hydrazine derivative with antimetabolite properties; cell cycle-specific for the S phase of cell division. Precise mechanism of action unknown. Suppresses mitosis at interphase, and causes chromatin derangement. Highly toxic to rapidly proliferating tissue. Has immunosuppressive properties, and exhibits MAO inhibitory activity. May cause delayed myelosuppression. No cross-resistance with radiotherapy, steroids, or other antineoplastics has been demonstrated. Reportedly does not affect survival time, but may produce remissions of at least 1 month's duration.

Used as adjunct in palliative treatment of Hodgkin's disease. *Investigational Use:* treatment of solid tumors.

P

ABSORPTION AND FATE. Readily absorbed from GI tract. Wide distribution through body fluids, with concentrations in liver, kidneys, intestinal wall, and skin. Half-life in plasma and cerebrospinal fluid about 1 hour. Metabolized in liver; excreted in urine (25 to 42% appearing during first 24 hours after administration) as unchanged drug and metabolites, and from respiratory tract as methane and CO_2.

CONTRAINDICATIONS AND PRECAUTIONS. Hypersensitivity to procarbazine; myelosuppression; alcohol ingestion; foods high in tyramine content; sympathomimetic drugs. MAO inhibitors should be discontinued 14 days prior to therapy; tricyclic antidepressants, 7 days before therapy. Safe use during pregnancy and lactation and in women of childbearing potential not established. *Cautious Use:* concomitant administration with CNS depressants; hepatic or kidney impairment; following radiation or chemotherapy before at least 1 month has elapsed, hepatic and renal inpairment, infection, diabetes mellitus.

ADVERSE/SIDE EFFECTS. CNS: myalgia, arthralgia, paresthesias, weakness, fatigue, lethargy, drowsiness. **Dermatologic:** dermatitis, pruritus, herpes, hyperpigmentation, flushing, alopecia. **GI:** severe nausea and vomiting (common), anorexia, stomatitis, dry mouth, dysphagia, diarrhea, constipation, jaundice. **Hematologic:** bone marrow suppression (leukopenia, anemia, thrombocytopenia), hemolysis, bleeding tendencies. **Infrequent:** confusion, neuropathies, headache, dizziness, depression, apprehension, insomnia, nightmares, hallucinations, psychosis, slurred speech, ataxia, footdrop, decreased reflexes, tremors, coma, convulsions. **Other:** ascites, pleural effusion, cough, hoarseness, hypotension, tachycardia, chills, fever, sweating, gynecomastia, depressed spermatogenesis, atrophy of testes; (rare): edema, nystagmus, photophobia, retinal hemorrhage, diplopia, papilledema; altered hearing; photosensitivity; intercurrent infections.

ROUTE AND DOSAGE. Oral: Adults: during first week; 2 to 4 mg/kg daily in single or divided doses then 4 to 6 mg/kg daily until WBC count falls below 4000/mm³ or platelets below 100,000/mm³ or maximum response obtained. Drug is then discontinued until recovery is satisfactory. Treatment is again started at 1 to 2 mg/kg daily. **Children:** highly individualized dosage; during first week, 50 mg daily; then maintained at 100 mg/m² body surface (to nearest 50 mg) until leukopenia, thrombocytopenia or maximum response occurs. Drug is then withdrawn until hemotologic recovery, then maintenance dosage is started: 50 mg daily.

NURSING IMPLICATIONS

Toxicity is a serious problem and demands that patient be hospitalized and under close medical and nursing supervision during treatment induction period.

Hematologic status (hemoglobin, hematocrit, WBC, differential, reticulocyte, and platelet counts) should be determined initially and at least every 3 to 4 days. Hepatic and renal studies (transaminase, alkaline phosphatase, BUN, urinalysis) are also indicated initially and at least weekly during therapy.

Start flow sheet, and record baseline blood pressure, weight, temperature, pulse, and intake–output ratio and pattern.

Since procarbazine has MAO inhibitory activity, OTC nose drops, cough medicines, and antiobesity preparations containing sympathomimetic drugs (e.g., ephedrine, amphetamine, epinephine) and tricyclic antidepressants should be avoided because they may cause hypertensive crises. Warn patient not to use OTC preparations without physician's approval.

Intake of foods high in tyramine content should also be avoided *(see Index: Food sources).* Warn patient that ingestion of any form of alcohol may precipitate a disulfiram-like reaction.

Be alert to signs of hepatic dysfunction: jaundice (yellow skin, sclerae, and soft palate), frothy or dark urine, clay-colored stools.

Patient's hematologic status should be monitored carefully for indicators that suggest special nursing interventions and need for dosage adjustment or drug withdrawal.

As patient approaches nadir of leukopenia (below 4000/mm³), protect patient from exposure to infection and trauma. Visitors and personnel with common colds should not visit. Alert patient to report any sign of impending infection. Note and report changes in voiding pattern, hematuria, and dysuria (possible signs of urinary tract infection). Intake–output ratio and temperature should be closely monitored.

Tolerance to nausea and vomiting (most common side effects) usually develops by end of first week of treatment. Doses are kept at a minimum during this time. If vomiting persists, therapy will be interrupted.

Symptoms of pleural effusion, an allergic reaction to procarbazine (chills, fever, weakness, shortness of breath, productive cough) should be reported promptly. Drug will be discontinued.

Instruct patient to report immediately signs of hemorrhagic tendencies: bleeding into skin and mucosa, epistaxis, hemoptysis, hematemesis, hematuria, melena, ecchymoses, petechiae. Bone marrow depression often occurs 2 to 8 weeks after start of therapy.

Prompt cessation of therapy is usual with appearance of CNS signs and symptoms (paresthesias, neuropathies, confusion), leukopenia (WBC count under 4000/mm^3), thrombocytopenia (platelet count under 100,000/mm^3), hypersensitivity reaction, the first small ulceration or persistent spot soreness of oral cavity, diarrhea, and bleeding. Patient should be warned to report promptly any signs and symptoms of toxicity.

See Mechlorethamine for nursing implications of stomatitis and xerostomia.

Advise patient to avoid excessive exposure to the sun because of potential photosensitivity reaction: cover as much skin area as possible with clothing, and use sunscreen lotion (SPF above 12) on all exposed skin surfaces.

Since drowsiness, dizziness, and blurred vision are possible side effects, warn patient to use caution while driving or performing hazardous tasks until response to drug is known.

Advise use of contraceptive measures during procarbazine therapy.

Diagnostic Test Interference. Procarbazine may enhance the effects of **CNS depressants.** A disulfiram-like reaction may occur following ingestion of **alcohol.**

Drug Interactions: Procarbazine Hydrochloride

Plus	Interactions
Alcohol	Additive CNS depressant effects; disulfiramlike reaction
Antidepressants, tricyclics, MAO inhibitors, tyramine foods	Hypertensive crisis, hyperpyrexia, convulsions and death
Antihistamines, belladonna alkaloids, antiparkinsonism agents	Potentiate atropinelike effects of procarbazine
Antihypertensives	Enhance hypotensive effects of procarbazine
Guanethidine, levodopa, methyldopa, reserpine	Excitement and hypertension
Insulin, oral hypoglycemics	Augmented hypoglycemic effects
Phenothiazines	Increased CNS depression
Sympathomimetics (indirect-acting) e.g., amphetamines, ephedrine, phenylpropanoline	Severe hypertension and hyperpyrexia
Thiazide diuretics	Enhance hypotensive effects of procortrozine

P

PROCHLORPERAZINE
(Compazine)
PROCHLORPERAZINE EDISYLATE
(Compazine)
PROCHLORPERAZINE MALEATE
(Chlorazine, Compazine)

(proe-klor-per'a-zeen)
Psychotropic
Antipsychotic (neuroleptic)
Antiemetic
Phenothiazine

ACTIONS AND USES. Piperazine phenothiazine derivative with similar actions, contraindications, and interactions as chlorpromazine (qv). Has greater extrapyramidal effects and antiemetic potency but less sedative, hypotensive and anticholinergic effects than chlorpromazine. Not as effective in treatment for vertigo or motion sickness.

Used in management of manifestations of psychotic disorders, of excessive anxiety, tension and agitation, and to control severe nausea and vomiting. Available in fixed combination with dextroamphetamine (Eskatrol) and isopropamide iodide (Combid).

ABSORPTION AND FATE. Onset of action: oral tablet: 30 to 40 minutes (duration 3 to 4 hours); extended-release form: 30 to 40 minutes (duration 10 to 12 hours); rectal suppository: 60 minutes (duration 3 to 4 hours); IM: 10 to 20 minutes (duration up to 12 hours). Crosses placenta; appears in breast milk.

CONTRAINDICATIONS AND PRECAUTIONS. Hypersensitivity to phenothiazines, bone marrow depression, comatose or severely depressed states, children under 20 pounds or 2 years of age, pediatric surgery, short-term vomiting in children or vomiting of unknown etiology, Reye's syndrome or other encephalopathies, history of dyskinetic reactions or epilepsy. *Cautious Use:* patient with previously diagnosed breast cancer, children with acute illness or dehydration. *See also Chlorpromazine.*

ADVERSE/SIDE EFFECTS. Drowsiness, dizziness, hypotension, contact dermatitis, galactorrhea, amenorrhea, blurred vision, cholestatic jaundice, leukopenia, agranulocytosis, extrapyramidal reactions (akathesia, dystonia or parkinsonism), persistent tardive dyskinesia, acute catatonia. *See also Chlorpromazine.*

ROUTE AND DOSAGE. Adults: *Severe nausea, vomiting, anxiety:* **Oral:** 5 to 10 mg three or four times daily. Sustained-release: 10 to 15 mg every 12 hours. **Rectal (suppository):** 25 mg twice daily. **Intramuscular:** 5 to 10 mg repeated every 3 to 4 hours not to exceed 40 mg/day. *Surgery:* **Intramuscular:** 5 to 10 mg 1 to 2 hours before anesthesia induction, or to control acute symptoms during and after surgery. **Intravenous infusion:** 20 mg/L isotonic solution; add to IV infusion 15 to 30 minutes before induction. *Psychiatry:* **Oral:** 5 to 10 mg three or four times daily. Dosage increased in small increments every 2 to 3 days to maximum of 100 to 150 mg/day. **Intramuscular:** 10 to 20 mg repeated if necessary every 2 to 4 hours (usually 2 to 4 doses are sufficient). Patient then is switched to oral formulation. **Pediatric:** individualized according to weight and condition being treated. *Nausea, vomiting:* **Oral and rectal:** (usually 1 day's treatment is sufficient): 2.5 mg one to three times daily or 5 mg twice daily (not to exceed 15 mg/day). *Psychiatry:* 2.5 mg two or three times daily; dose up to 25 mg daily. *Nausea, vomiting, psychiatry:* **Intramuscular:** 0.06 mg/lb.

NURSING IMPLICATIONS

P

Strength of liquid formulations: syrup: 5 mg/5 ml; oral concentrate: 10 mg/1 ml. Do not confuse the preparations.

Note dosage of pediatric suppository. Do not confuse 2.5 mg for 25 mg (adult dose size).

Oral concentrate is intended for institutional use only and is not to be administered to children.

To ensure stability and palatability of oral concentrate add prescribed dose to 60 ml or more of diluent just prior to administration. Suggested diluents: tomato or fruit juice, carbonated drinks, water, semisolid foods, e.g., puddings, soups, etc.

Avoid skin contact with oral concentrate or injection solution because of possibility of contact dermatitis.

Minimum effective dosage is advised. Keep physician informed of patient's response to drug therapy.

Most elderly and emaciated patients and children, especially those with dehydration or acute illness, appear to be particularly susceptible to extrapyramidal effects. Be alert to onset of symptoms: in early therapy watch for pseudoparkinson's and acute dyskinesia. After 1 to 2 months, be alert to akathisia. *See Chlorpromazine.*

Dosage for elderly, emaciated patients, and for children should be advanced very slowly.

Counsel patient to take drug as prescribed and not to alter dose or schedule. Consult physician before stopping the medication.

Keep in mind that the antiemetic effect may mask toxicity of other drugs or make it difficult to diagnose conditions with a primary symptom of nausea, such as intestinal obstruction, brain disease.

IM injection in adults should be made deep into the upper outer quadrant of the buttock. Do not mix IM solution in the same syringe with other agents. Follow agency policy regarding IM injection site for children.

Postoperative patients who have received prochlorperazine should be carefully positioned to prevent aspiration of vomitus. Keep in mind that the cough reflex is depressed.

Since drug may impair mental and physical abilities, especially during first few days of therapy, caution patient to avoid hazardous activities such as driving a car until response to drug is known.

It has been reported that although patient is not responsive during acute catatonia (side effect) everything that happens during the episode can be recalled.

Exposure to high environmental temperature, to sun's rays, or to a high fever associated with serious illness places this patient at risk for heat stroke. Be alert to signs: red, dry, hot skin, full bounding pulse, dilated pupils, dyspnea confusion, temperature over 105°F (40.6°C), elevated blood pressure. Inform physician and institute measures to reduce body temperature rapidly.

Monitor intake–output ratio and elimination pattern. Depressed patients frequently cut back on fluid intake and do not seek help for constipation.

This drug may color urine reddish brown. It also may cause the sun-exposed skin to turn a gray-blue color.

Advise patient to protect skin from direct sun's rays and to use a sunscreen lotion (SPF above 12) to prevent photosensitivity reaction.

Patient on long-term antipsychotic therapy should be evaluated periodically for possibility of decreasing dose or discontinuating therapy.

Treatment of overdosage: early gastric lavage, airway maintenance, general supportive measures. Have available antiparkinson drugs, barbiturates, and diphenhydramine. Emesis should not be induced because it may precipitate dystonic reactions of head and neck with possible aspiration of vomitus.

Instruct patient to withhold dose and report to the physician if the following symptoms persist more than a few hours: tremor, involuntary twitching, exaggerated restlessness. Other reportable symptoms include: light-colored stools, changes in vision, sore throat, fever, rash.

Prochlorperazine tablets contain tartrazine which can cause allergic reaction (including bronchial asthma) in susceptible individuals. Frequently such persons are also sensitive to aspirin.

Slight yellowing does not appear to alter potency; however, markedly discolored solutions should be discarded. Protect drug from light; do not freeze. Store at temperature between 15° and 30°C (59° and 86°F) unless otherwise instructed by manufacturer.

See Chlorpromazine (prototype phenothiazine psychotropic).

PROCYCLIDINE HYDROCHLORIDE

(Kemadrin, Procyclid)

(proe-sye'kli-deen)
Anticholinergic (parasympatholytic)
Antimuscarinic
Antiparkinsonian agent

ACTIONS AND USES. Centrally acting synthetic anticholinergic agent with actions similar to those of atropine (qv); closely related to trihexyphenidyl.

Used to relieve parkinsonism, including postencephalitic, arteriosclerotic, and idiopathic types, and drug-induced extrapyramidal symptoms.

ABSORPTION AND FATE. Onset of action in 30 to 45 minutes; duration 4 to 6 hours.

CONTRAINDICATIONS AND PRECAUTIONS. Angle-closure glaucoma. Safe use during pregnancy (category C) and use in women of childbearing potential, in nursing mothers, and in children not established. *Cautious Use:* hypotension, mental disorders, tachycardia, prostatic hypertrophy.

ADVERSE/SIDE EFFECTS. Dry mouth, blurred vision, mydriasis, palpitation, tachycardia, flushing of skin, headache, lightheadedness, nausea, vomiting, epigastric distress, dizziness, urinary retention, feeling of muscle weakness, constipation, acute suppurative parotitis, skin eruptions; (occasionally): mental confusion, psychotic-like symptoms.

ROUTE AND DOSAGE. Oral: initial: 2 to 2.5 mg three times daily after meals; if tolerated, dosage gradually increased to 4 to 5 mg 3 times daily; additional 4 to 5 mg at bedtime may be prescribed for some patients.

NURSING IMPLICATIONS

Side effects may be minimized by administration of drug during or after meals.

Drug-induced dryness of mouth may be relieved by sugarless gum or hard candy, and by frequent rinses with warm water or by increasing noncaloric fluid intake. If these measures fail a saliva substitute may help, e.g.; Moi-Stir, Orex, Xero-Lube. All are available OTC.

If urinary hesitancy or retention is a problem, advise the patient to void before taking drug.

Drug occasionally causes mental confusion, disorientation, agitation, and psychoticlike symptoms, particularly in elderly patients who have low blood pressure. Report these symptoms to physician.

Since procyclidine may cause blurred vision and dizziness, caution the patient to avoid potentially hazardous activities until reaction to drug is known.

Report palpitation, tachycardia, or decreasing blood pressure. Dosage adjustment or discontinuation of drug may be indicated.

Since dosage is guided by clinical response, observe and record improvement (or lack of it) that accompanies therapy.

Advise patient to avoid alcohol and not to take other CNS depressants unless otherwise advised by physician.

Procyclidine is usually more effective in controlling rigidity than tremors. Tremors may temporarily appear to be exaggerated as rigidity is relieved, especially in patients with severe spasticity.

Store in tightly closed containers at controlled room temperature, preferably between 15° and 30°C (59° and 86°F) unless otherwise directed by manufacturer.

Drug Interactions. Procyclidine may partially inhibit the therapeutic effects of **haloperiodol** (possibly by delaying gastric emptying time and increasing its metabolism in GI tract) and

phenothiazines (possibly by interfering with their absorption). *See also Atropine sulfate (prototype anticholinergic).*

PROTOTYPE

PROGESTERONE

(proe-jess'ter-one)
Progestin
Hormone

(Bay Progest, Femotrone, Gesterol, Progestasert, Progestoject, Progestronaq)

ACTIONS AND USES. Steroid hormone synthesized and released by testes, ovary, adrenal cortex, and placenta. Has antiestrogenic, anabolic, and androgenic activity. Physiologic precursor to estrogens, androgens, and adrenocortical steroids. Transforms endometrium from proliferative to secretory state; suppresses pituitary gonadotropin secretion thereby blocking follicular maturation and ovulation. Acting with estrogen, promotes mammary gland development without causing lactation and increases body temperature 1°F at time of ovulation (thermogenic action). Stimulates endocervical secretion of glycogen and thick mucus. Relaxes estrogen-primed myometrium and prohibits spontaneous contraction of uterus. Sudden drop in blood levels of progestin (and estradiol) causes "withdrawal bleeding" from endometrium. Intrauterine placement of progesterone (intrauterine progesterone contraceptive system) hypothetically inhibits sperm capacity or survival, alters uterine milieu so as to prevent nidation and suppresses endometrial proliferation (antiestrogenic effect).

Used to treat secondary amenorrhea, functional uterine bleeding, endometriosis, and investigationally to treat premenstrual syndrome. As an intrauterine agent (Progestasert) and in combination with estrogens provides fertility control. Largely supplanted by new progestins which have longer action and oral effectiveness.

ABSORPTION AND FATE. Rapid absorption follows injection. Plasma half-life approximately 5 minutes; duration of action about 24 hours. Biotransformation takes place during one pass through liver; after enterohepatic circulation, portion of metabolites excreted in feces. Urinary excretion of remainder as pregnanediol provides indirect index of natural progesterone secretion. Small amounts excreted in breast milk. Intrauterine progesterone contraceptive system (Progestasert): continuous delivery of progesterone into uterine cavity.

CONTRAINDICATIONS AND PRECAUTIONS. Hypersensitivity to progestins, known or suspected breast or genital malignancy; thrombophlebitis, thromboembolic disorders; cerebral apoplexy (or its history), impaired liver function or disease, undiagnosed vaginal bleeding, missed abortion, first 4 months of pregnancy, nursing mother. Progestasert: pregnancy or suspicion of pregnancy. *Cautious Use:* anemia, diagnostic test for pregnancy; diabetes mellitus, cardiac and renal dysfunction, epilepsy, asthma, migraine, history of psychic depression; persons susceptible to acute intermittent porphyria, previous ectopic pregnancy, presence or history of salpingitis, venereal disease, unresolved abnormal Pap smear, genital bleeding of unknown etiology, previous pelvic surgery.

ADVERSE/SIDE EFFECTS. CNS: partial or complete loss of vision, proptosis, diplopia, migraine, mental depression. **CV:** thromboembolic disorders, pulmonary embolus. **Intrauterine progesterone contraceptive system (in addition to the foregoing):** endometritis, spontaneous abortion, septic abortion, septicemia, perforation of uterus and cervix, pelvic infection, cervical erosion, vaginitis, leukorrhea, ectopic pregnancy, pregnancy, uterine embedment, difficult removal, anemia, amenorrhea or delayed menses, dysmenorrhea, backaches, dyspareunia. **Reproductive:** mammary nodules, benign and malignant; gynecomastia, galactorrhea, masculinization of female fetus, changes in cervical erosion and secretions, and in menstrual pattern; amenorrhea, breakthrough bleeding, spotting, pruritus vulvae, changes in libido. **Other:** fatigue, headache, acne, alopecia, hirsutism, urticaria, photosensitivity, allergic rash, pruritus cholestatic jaundice, edema, changes in weight, candidiasis, pain at injection site, melasma or chloasma.

ROUTE AND DOSAGE. **Intramuscular (sesame oil vehicle):** *Amenorrhea:* 5 to 10 mg for 6 to 8 consecutive days. If proliferative endometrium has been produced, withdrawal bleeding is expected in 48 to 72 hours after last injection. This may be followed by spontaneous normal cycles. *Functional uterine bleeding:* 5 to 10 mg daily for 6 days. Bleeding is expected to stop within 6 days. When estrogen is also given, progesterone is started after 2 weeks of estrogen therapy. If menses begin during course of injections stop the drugs. **Intrauterine:** *Contraception* (Progestasert): delivers progesterone 65 mcg/day into uterine cavity for one year.

NURSING IMPLICATIONS

Protect medication vial from light.

Immerse vial in warm water momentarily to redissolve crystals and to facilitate aspiration of drug into syringe.

Inject deeply IM. Injection site may be irritated by drug in oil. Inspect used sites carefully and rotate areas systematically.

A physical examination with special reference to pelvic organs, breasts, as well as Pap smear should precede therapy with a progestin. Urge patient to keep appointments for physical check-ups at established intervals.

Baseline data for comparative value about patient's weight, intake–output ratio, blood pressure, and pulse should be recorded at onset of progestin therapy. Deviations should be reported promptly.

Progestins may cause some degree of fluid retention. Monitor conditions that may be worsened by edema: epilepsy, migraine, asthma, cardiac or renal dysfunction.

Treatment with a progestin may mask onset of the climacteric.

Progestins reportedly may precipitate attack of acute intermittent porphyria in susceptible patients. (Common manifestations include acute colicky, severe abdominal pain; vomiting, distention, diarrhea, constipation.)

Instruct patient to notify physician if she suspects pregnancy while receiving progestational therapy. She should be apprised of the potential risk to the fetus from progestin exposure.

Serious mental depression may signal a recurrence of previous psychiatric disorder. Alert family or significant other to this potential side effect and give instructions for prompt reporting. The drug will be discontinued if mental changes are severe.

Instruct a diabetic user of progestin or progestin combination drug to monitor clinical signs of loss of diabetes control. If urine tests become positive, or hypoglycemic symptoms occur, the physician should be consulted.

Caution patient to avoid exposure to ultraviolet light and prolonged periods of time in the sun. Photosensitivity severity is related to both time of exposure and dose. A phototoxic drug reaction usually looks like an exaggerated sunburn but may also produce acute eczematous or urticarial reactions. The reaction can occur within 5 to 18 hours after exposure to sun and is maximal by 36 to 72 hours.

Advise use of a sunscreen lotion (SPF above 12) which contains para-amino-benzoic acid (PABA) on exposed skin surfaces whenever patient goes outdoors, even on dark days.

Side effects that warrant medical attention should be clearly identified for the patient. Inform physician promptly if any of the following occur: sudden severe headache or vomiting, dizziness or fainting, numbness in an arm or leg, pain in calves accompanied by swelling, warmth and redness; visual disturbance, acute chest pain or dyspnea.

Progestins can affect endocrine and hepatic function tests. An interval of up to 60 days following cessation of therapy with the drug may be necessary before laboratory results can be considered definitive.

Progestins are no longer recommended for use in pregnancy tests because of potential teratogenic effects.

Inform pathologist of progestin therapy when relevant specimens are submitted. Instruct patient to tell the dentist if extraction is anticipated and the surgeon in an emergency situation.

Intrauterine Progesterone Contraceptive System (Progestasert):

- This is a medication-releasing type of intrauterine device (IUD).
- A physical examination should precede insertion of the system with especial attention to the breasts and pelvic regions, Pap smear, gonorrhea culture (and if indicated, tests for other forms of veneral disease), hematocrit.
- Progestasert is a T-shaped unit containing a reservoir of 38 mg progesterone with barium sulfate dispersed in medical-grade silicone oil.
- Observe patient carefully during insertion of the system; a neurovascular episode may occur (syncope, bradycardia).
- During the first 2 months of Progestasert use, another method of birth control (foam or condom) should be used.
- Advise patient to return to the physician 3 months after insertion of the system for evaluation of its placement and efficacy.
- Spotting, cramping, and discomfort during first 3 months can be relieved by nonnarcotic analgesics.
- Regular cyclic pattern of ovulation continues while Progestasert is in place.
- The menstrual period during Progestasert use is frequently heavier and longer than usual. If increased menstrual bleeding continues, however, patient should consult her physician. Loss of excess blood can be dangerous for the anemic patient.
- The Progestasert threads should be checked frequently during first few months and after menstruation (times when expulsion is most likely to occur). If patient can't feel threads, she should go to physician for an examination and prescription for another method of birth control.
- Warn against pulling on threads for any reason. If the IUD is partially expelled, it should be removed; however, the user should not try to remove it herself nor allow her partner to attempt to do so.
- Instruct patient to consult with physician if a period is missed and pregnancy is suspected. The device should be removed during pregnancy.
- Fever, acute pelvic pain and tenderness, unusual bleeding, severe cramping are symptoms that indicate infection. The Progestasert user should report to the physician for immediate treatment.
- To prevent pregnancy, the system must be replaced 1 year after insertion. Pelvic examination must be done. Pap smear, breast examination, hematocrit evaluation.
- Teach patient self-breast examination (SBE).
- Review package insert with patient using progesterone to assure complete understanding.
- Store drug at temperature between 15° and 30°C (59° and 86°F) unless otherwise specified by manufacturer. Protect from freezing and light.

Diagnostic Test Interferences. Progestins may increase levels of **urinary pregnanediol, serum alkaline phosphatase, plasma amino acids, urinary nitrogen.** They also decrease **glucose toler-**

ance (may cause false-positive **urine** glucose tests) and lower **HDL** (high density lipoprotein) levels.

PROMAZINE HYDROCHLORIDE

(Promanyl, Prozine, Sparine)

(proe'ma-zeen)
Psychotropic
Antipsychotic
(Neuroleptic)
Phenothiazine

ACTIONS AND USES. Aliphatic (ethylamino) derivative of phenothiazine. Compared with chlorpromazine (qv) has weak antipsychotic activity and extrapyramidal effects occur less frequently. Although drug-induced agranulocytosis is rare, it occurs more often than with other phenothiazines.

Used in management of manifestations of psychotic disorders and for reducing agitation and paranoia associated with alcohol withdrawal. Also used to control postoperative nausea and vomiting and that caused by therapy with cytotoxic drugs.

CONTRAINDICATIONS AND PRECAUTIONS. Hypersensitivity to phenothiazines, myelosuppression, CNS depression, children under 12 years of age, Reye's syndrome. Safe use during pregnancy and by nursing mothers not established. *Cautious Use:* prostatic hypertrophy, cardiovascular or hepatic disease, paralytic ileus, xerostomia, angle closure glaucoma, persons exposed to extremes in temperature or to organophosphorous insecticides, convulsive disorders. *See also Chlorpromazine.*

ADVERSE/SIDE EFFECTS. *Common:* Drowsiness, orthostatic hypotension. Also, blurred vision, constipation, epileptic seizures in susceptible individuals, leukopenia, agranulocytosis (rare). *See also Chlorpromazine.*

ROUTE AND DOSAGE. *Psychotic disorders:* **Oral, intramuscular: Adults:** (individualized according to severity of condition being treated): 10 to 200 mg at 4 to 6 hour intervals. Usual dose limit: 1000 mg/day. Dose adjusted gradually as needed and tolerated. **Children (over 12 years):** 10 to 25 mg every 4 to 6 hours. **Elderly, debilitated, emaciated patients:** Lower initial dose; then increase as needed by gradual increments. *Antiemetic:* **Oral: Adults:** 25 to 50 mg every 4 to 6 hours. **Intramuscular:** 50 mg. **Intravenous:** (infrequently used): administered slowly in concentrations no greater than 25 mg/ml.

P

NURSING IMPLICATIONS

Oral route should be used whenever possible. Parenteral administration is reserved for acutely disturbed or uncooperative patients or those who cannot tolerate an oral preparation.

Absorption is inhibited by antacids; therefore administer promazine 1 hour before or 1 hour after antacid.

Syrup (10 mg/5ml) or oral concentrate (30 mg/ml) may be prescribed when tablet is unsuitable or refused. Dilute the concentrate immediately before administration with fruit juice, chocolate-flavored drinks, carbonated drinks or soup. (For best taste, 10 ml of diluent for each 25 mg of drug.) Avoid coffee or tea ingestion near time of taking oral preparation. Explain dosage and dilution to patient if drug is to be self-administered.

Parenteral administration is seldom given to the ambulatory patient except to treat an acute psychotic condition.

IM injection is made deep into upper outer quadrant of buttock. Tissue irritation can occur if given SC. Carefully aspirate before injecting drug slowly. Intraarterial injection can cause arterial or arteriolar spasm and consequent impairment of local circulation. Rotate injection sites.

IV route is reserved only for hospitalized patients; routine use not recommended. Localized cellulitis, thrombophlebitis, and gangrene have occurred because of improper drug dilution, extravasation, or injections made into previously damaged blood vessels. Palpate entry site occasionally to confirm needle position.

Incidence of postural hypotension and drowsiness is particularly high after parenteral administration. Monitor blood pressure and pulse before administration and between doses. Keep patient recumbent for about 1 hour after dose is given.

Warn patient that dizziness or faintness may occur on arising. Advise making all position changes slowly, particularly from recumbent to upright position.

Monitor intake–output ratio and bowel elimination pattern. Check for abdominal distention and pain. Encourage adequate fluid intake as prophylaxis for constipation and xerostomia. The depressed patient may not seek help for either symptom, or for urinary retention.

Warn patient to avoid alcohol during therapy.

OTC drugs should be approved by physician during antipsychotic therapy.

Promazine may cause contact dermatitis. Caution patient to avoid spilling oral solutions on hands or clothing. Wash exposed skin well with soap and water.

Symptoms suggesting agranulocytosis should be reported promptly: sore throat, fever, malaise, other signs of infection.

Promazine may color urine pink to red to reddish brown.

Store medication in light-resistant container at temperature between 15° and 30°C (59° and 86°F) unless otherwise directed by manufacturer.

See Chlorpromazine (prototype phenothiazine).

PROTOTYPE

PROMETHAZINE HYDROCHLORIDE

(proe-meth'a-zeen)

(Histantil, Ganphen, K-Phen, Pentazine, Phenazine, Phencen, Phenergan, Phenoject-50, Promine, Prorex, Prothazine, Remsed, V-Gan)

Antihistamine
H1-receptor antagonist
Antiemetic
Phenothiazine

P

ACTIONS AND USES. Long-acting ethylamino derivative of phenothiazine with marked antihistaminic activity and prominent sedative, amnesic, antiemetic, and anti-motion-sickness actions. Unlike other phenothiazine derivatives, it is relatively free of extrapyramidal side effects; however, in high doses it carries same potential for toxicity. In common with other antihistamines, exerts antiserotonin, anticholinergic, and local anesthetic action. Prevents most actions of histamine by competing with it for H_1-receptor sites on effector cells. Antiemetic action thought to be due to depression of CTZ in medulla. Reported to have slight antitussive activity, but this may be due to anticholinergic and CNS depressant effects.

Used for symptomatic relief of various allergic conditions, to ameliorate and prevent reactions to blood and plasma, and in prophylaxis and treatment of motion sickness, nausea, and vomiting. Used for preoperative, postoperative, and obstetric sedation, and as adjunct to analgesics for control of pain.

ABSORPTION AND FATE. Well absorbed from GI tract and parenteral routes. Antihistaminic effects occur within 20 minutes following oral, rectal, and IM and within 3 to 5 minutes after IV administration. Duration of action generally 4 to 6 hours; antihistaminic activity sometimes persists for 12 hours. Widely distributed in body tissues. Metabolized by liver; excreted slowly in urine and feces, primarily as inactive metabolites.

CONTRAINDICATIONS AND PRECAUTIONS. Hypersensitivity to phenothiazines, narrow-angle glaucoma, stenosing peptic ulcer, pyloroduodenal obstruction, prostatic hypertrophy, bladder neck obstruction, epilepsy, bone marrow depression, comatose or severely depressed states, pregnancy (except labor), nursing mothers, newborn or premature infants, acutely ill or dehydrated children. *Cautious Use:* impaired hepatic function, cardiovascular disease, asthma, acute or chronic respiratory impairment (particularly in children), hypertension, elderly or debilitated patients.

ADVERSE/SIDE EFFECTS. **Acute toxicity:** deep sleep, coma, convulsions, cardiorespiratory symptoms, extrapyramidal reactions, nightmares (in children), CNS stimulation, abnormal movements, respiratory depression. Toxic potential as for other phenothiazines. *See Chlorpromazine for complete description of symptoms.* **CNS:** sedation drowsiness, confusion, dizziness, disturbed coordination, restlessness, tremors. **CV:** transient mild hypotension or hypertension. **GI:** anorexia, nausea, vomiting, constipation. **Hematologic:** leukopenia, agranulocytosis. **Other:** photosensitivity, irregular respiration, blurred vision, urinary retention; dry mouth, nose, or throat.

ROUTE AND DOSAGE. **Adults:** **Oral, rectal suppository, intramuscular, intravenous:** *nausea and vomiting:* 12.5 to 25 mg in a single dose, or repeated at 4- to 6-hour intervals if necessary. Highly individualized. *Sedation:* 12.5 to 50 mg. *For motion sickness,* 25 mg repeated at 8- to 12-hour intervals if necessary. **Children:** **Oral, rectal, parenteral:** 0.25 to 0.5 mg/kg 12.5 to 25 mg one or two times daily; alternatively 0.25 to 0.5 mg/kg every 4 to 6 hours, if necessary. *Intravenous concentration* should be no greater than 25 mg/ml, at rate not exceeding 25 mg/minute.

NURSING IMPLICATIONS

Administration of oral medication with food, milk or a full glass of water may minimize GI distress.

Tablet may be crushed and mixed with water or food before swallowing.

Oral doses for allergy are generally prescribed before meals and on retiring or as single dose at bedtime.

When administered as prophylaxis against motion sickness, initial dose should be taken 30 minutes to 1 hour before anticipated travel and repeated at 8 to 12 hour intervals if necessary. For duration of journey, repeat dose on arising and again at evening meal.

Inspect parenteral drug before preparation. Discard if it is darkened or contains precipitate.

IM injection is made deep into large muscle mass. Aspirate carefully before injecting drug. Intraarterial injection can cause arterial or arteriolar spasm, with resultant gangrene. Subcutaneous injection (also contraindicated) can cause chemical irritation and necrosis. Rotate injection sites and observe daily.

When administered by IV infusion, wrap IV bottle with aluminum foil to protect drug from light.

Promethazine injection is reportedly incompatible with several drugs, especially those with alkaline pH. Consult pharmacist for specific information.

Promethazine sometimes produces marked sedation and dizziness. Bedsides and supervision of ambulation may be advisable.

Advise ambulatory patient to avoid driving a car or engaging in other activities requiring mental alertness and normal reaction time until response to drug is known.

Bear in mind that antiemetic action may mask symptoms of unrecognized disease and signs of drug overdosage as well as dizziness, vertigo, or tinnitus associated with toxic doses of aspirin or other ototoxic drugs.

Patients in pain may develop involuntary (athetoid) movements of upper extremities following parenteral administration. These symptoms usually disappear after pain is controlled.

Respiratory function should be monitored in patients with respiratory problems, particularly children. Promethazine may suppress cough reflex and cause thickening of bronchial secretions.

Dry mouth may be relieved by frequent rinses with warm water or by increasing noncaloric fluid intake (if allowed), or by sugarless gum or lemon drops. If these measures fail a saliva substitute may help, e.g., Moi-Stir, Orex, Xero-Lube.

Promethazine may cause photosensitivity. Advise patient to avoid sunlamps or prolonged exposure to sunlight. A sunscreen lotion may be advisable during initial drug therapy.

Advise patient not to take OTC medications without physician's approval, and caution against alcohol and other CNS depressants.

Treatment of overdosage: early gastric lavage (endotracheal tube with cuff in place to prevent aspiration of vomitus). Emesis should not be induced because dystonic reactions of head and neck may result in aspiration. Have on hand: antiparkinson drugs, barbiturates, diazepam, diphenhydramine, phenylephrine, norepinephrine.

Store in tight, light-resistant container at controlled room temperature, preferably between 15° and 30°C (59° and 86°F) unless otherwise directed by manufacturer.

Diagnostic Test Interferences. Promethazine may interfere with **blood grouping** in ABO system and may produce false results with **urinary pregnancy tests** (Gravindex, false-positive; Prepurex and Dap tests, false-negative). Promethazine can cause significant alterations of flare response in **intradermal allergen tests** if performed within 4 days of receiving promethazine, and can cause elevations in **blood glucose.**

Drug Interactions. Additive sedative action may result when promethazine is given concurrently with drugs that have CNS depressant effect, e.g., **alcohol,** other **antihistamines, barbiturates, narcotic analgesics,** and antipsychotics. Promethazine reverses vasopressor effect of **epinephrine** and may cause further lowering of blood pressure in patients with hypotension. **MAO inhibitors** intensify and prolong the anticholinergic effects of promethazine.

PROPANTHELINE BROMIDE

(Banlin, Norpanth, Noropropanthil, Pro-Banthine, Propanthel)

(proe-pan'the-leen)
Anticholinergic
Parasympatholytic
Antimuscarinic

ACTIONS AND USES. Synthetic quaternary ammonium compound. Similar to atropine (qv) in peripheral effects, contraindications, precautions, and adverse reactions. Potent in antimuscarinic activity and in nondepolarizing ganglionic blocking action. Very high doses block neurotransmission at myoneural junction.

Used as adjunct in treatment of peptic ulcer, irritable bowel syndrome, pancreatitis, ureteral and urinary bladder spasm. Also used prior to radiological diagnostic procedures to reduce duodenal motility.

ABSORPTION AND FATE. Incompletely absorbed from GI tract. Onset of effects following oral administration in 30 to 45 minutes, persisting 4 to 6 hours. Metabolism: 50% in GI tract before absorption; 50% hepatic. Excreted through all body fluids, but chiefly in urine and bile.

ADVERSE/SIDE EFFECTS. Constipation, difficult urination, dry mouth, blurred vision, mydriasis, increased intraocular pressure, drowsiness, decreased sexual activity. *See Atropine.*

ROUTE AND DOSAGE. Adults: Oral: 15 mg with meals and 30 mg at bedtime. For geriatric patients or patients of small stature: 7.5 mg three times daily. Usual adult prescribing limit: 120 mg daily. **Intramuscular, intravenous:** 30 mg or more every 6 hours. **Pediatric: Oral:** 0.375 mg/kg four times daily. Maintenance: one-half initial dose, same administration intervals.

NURSING IMPLICATIONS

Oral preparation is generally administered 30 to 60 minutes before meals and at bedtime. Advise the patient not to chew tablet; drug is very bitter.

Sustained release tablets should not be crushed or chewed. Regular tablets may be crushed and mixed with fluid or food before swallowing.

If patient is also receiving an antacid (or antidiarrheic agent), propantheline should be taken at least 1 hour before or 1 hour after the other drug.

Parenteral drug is reconstituted with 1 ml Sterile Water for Injection for IM administration and with 10 ml NaCl Injection for IV administration. It is advisable to administer reconstituted solution immediately after preparation; however, if protected from contamination, prepared solution may be kept under refrigeration up to 2 weeks with safety.

When drug is administered parenterally, observe the patient closely for curarelike distress or paralysis. Equipment for respiratory support should be readily available.

Alcoholic beverages should be avoided while patient is receiving propantheline.

Urinary hesitancy or retention (especially likely to occur in elderly patients) may be avoided by advising patient to void just prior to each dose. Instruct the patient to note daily urinary volume and to report voiding problems to physician.

The elderly or debilitated patient may respond to a usual dose with agitation, excitement, confusion, drowsiness. If these symptoms are observed, stop the drug and report to physician.

Dry mouth may be relieved by frequent rinsing with warm tap water, by sugar-free gum or hard candy. If symptoms persist, report to physician.

Caution patient to maintain adequate fluid and high fiber food intake to prevent constipation.

Patients with cardiac disease should have periodic checks of blood pressure, heart sounds and rhythm.

Postural hypotension and tachycardia may occur during early therapy. Instruct the patient to make all position changes slowly and to lie down immediately if faintness, weakness, or palpitation occurs. Advise the patient to report these symptoms to the physician.

Caution the patient to avoid potentially hazardous activities such as driving a car or operating machinery until response to drug is known.

Store dry powder and tablets at temperature between 15° and 30°C (59° and 86°F), protected from freezing and moisture.

See Atropine (prototype antimuscarinic/antispasmodic agent).

PROPIOMAZINE HYDROCHLORIDE

(Largon)

(proe-pee-oh'ma-zeen)
Sedative
Phenothiazine

ACTIONS AND USES. Ethylamino derivative of phenothiazines with prominent sedative effects. General properties similar to those of other phenothiazines. *See Chlorpromazine.* Action relieves apprehension and promotes sleep, from which patient can be easily aroused.

Used for sedative and antiemetic effects preoperatively, postoperatively and during labor. Also used as adjunct to local, nerve block, or spinal anesthesia.

ABSORPTION AND FATE. Peak sedative effect within 15 to 30 minutes following IV infusion and in 40 to 60 minutes after IM injection. Duration of effect 3 to 6 hours.

CONTRAINDICATIONS AND PRECAUTIONS. Safe use during 1st trimester of pregnancy not established comatose patient, hypertensive crisis. *See Chlorpromazine.*

ADVERSE/SIDE EFFECTS. Hypersensitivity to phenothiazines. Dry mouth, tachycardia, GI upsets, skin rash, dizziness, confusion, amnesia; restlessness, akathisia, respiratory depression (high doses); elevated blood pressure, hypotension. Also irritation and thrombophlebitis at injection site with extravasation.

ROUTE AND DOSAGE. Intramuscular, intravenous: Adults: 20 to 40 mg repeated in 3 hours if necessary. **Children (up to 27 kg):** 0.55 to 1.1 mg/kg; **(2 to 4 years):** 10 mg; **(4 to 6 years):** 15 mg; **(6 to 12 years):** 25 mg.

NURSING IMPLICATIONS

Avoid combining propiomazine solution with barbiturate salts or other alkaline substances.

Do not use solution if it is cloudy or if it has a precipitate.

Administer IM deep into large muscle mass, preferably upper outer quadrant of buttock. Avoid SC injection. Aspirate carefully before injecting drug; intraarterial injection is specifically contraindicated because it may cause vascular spasm and tissue damage.

Rotate injection sites. Administer the IV solution slowly into undamaged vein. Palpate injection site periodically to detect extravasation. Chemical irritation can be severe enough to cause necrosis.

Check blood pressure and pulse before drug administration, and monitor between doses.

Elderly patients may experience dizziness, confusion, and amnesia. Bedsides and supervision of ambulation may be indicated.

Restlessness or akathisia is usually dose-related. Report promptly to physician. Symptoms may last 30 minutes to 4 hours.

Caution patient to avoid driving or hazardous activity requiring physical and mental alertness until response to drug is known.

If patient requires a vasopressor agent, norepinephrine may be used. Epinephrine is contraindicated, because it may augment the hypotensive effect of propiomazine.

Store drug at temperature between 15° and 30°C (59° and 86°F) protected from light.

See Chlorpromazine (prototype phenothiazine).

PROPOXYPHENE HYDROCHLORIDE

(Darvon, Doxaphene, Novopropoxyn, Profene, Propoxyphene Napsylate)

PROPOXYPHENE NAPSYLATE

(Darvon-N)

(proe-pox'i-feen)
Narcotic analgesic
(Opiate agonist)
C IV

ACTIONS AND USES. Centrally acting opioid (narcoticlike substance) structurally related to methadone. Analgesic potency about ½ to ⅔ that of codeine. Unlike codeine, propoxyphene has little or no antitussive effect and abuse liability is somewhat lower. Has no significant antiinflammatory or antipyretic actions. The hydrochloride is freely soluble in water and is more rapidly and completely absorbed than the napsylate, which is only slightly water-soluble. Lower incidence of GI side effects reported with the napsylate salt.

Used for relief of mild to moderate pain. *Investigational Use:* to suppress narcotic withdrawal symptoms.

ABSORPTION AND FATE. Absorbed chiefly in upper part of small intestines. Peak serum levels within 2 hours (hydrochloride) and within 3 hours (napsylate). Onset of analgesic effects in 15 to 30 minutes; duration 4 to 6 hours. Half-life of metabolite 30 to 36 hours; of propoxyphene: 6 to 12 hours. Degraded primarily in liver. Excreted in urine within 6 to 48 hours as metabolites and traces of unchanged drug. Crosses placenta; low levels detected in breast milk.

CONTRAINDICATIONS AND PRECAUTIONS. Hypersensitivity to drug, suicidal individuals, alcoholism, dependence on opiates. Safe use during pregnancy and in children not established. *Cautious Use:* renal or hepatic disease.

ADVERSE/SIDE EFFECTS. CNS: dizziness, lightheadedness, drowsiness, sedation, unusual fatigue or weakness, restlessness, tremor, euphoria, dysphoria, headache, paradoxic excitement. **GI:** nausea, vomiting, abdominal pain, constipation. **Other:** minor visual disturbances, headache, skin eruptions (hypersensitivity), hypoglycemia (patients with impaired renal function); liver dysfunction. **Overdosage:** mental confusion, toxic psychosis, coma, convulsions, respiratory depression, pulmonary edema, acidosis, pinpoint pupils (dilate with advancing hypoxia), circulatory collapse, ECG abnormalities, nephrogenic diabetes insipidus.

ROUTE AND DOSAGE. Oral (hydrochloride): 65 mg every 4 hours, as needed. Available in capsule form. (Napsylate): 100 mg every 4 hours, as needed. Available in tablet and suspension forms. (100 mg of the napsylate is equivalent to 65 mg of the hydrochloride.)

NURSING IMPLICATIONS

Capsules may be emptied and contents mixed with water or food before swallowing.

Absorption may be somewhat delayed by presence of food in stomach.

Evaluate patient's need for continued use of this drug. Propoxyphene is commonly abused.

Tremulousness, restlessness ("speeding"), and mild euphoria (effects desired by many addicts) occur frequently.

Dizziness, lightheadedness, drowsiness, nausea, and vomiting appear to be more prominent in the ambulatory patient. Symptoms may be relieved if patient lies down.

Caution ambulatory patients not to drive a car and to avoid other potentially hazardous activities.

Treatment of overdosage: Fatalities occur commonly within first hour following overdosage, therefore prompt action is required: immediate emesis or gastric lavage; activated charcoal slurry. Maintain airway (apnea occurs quickly). Have on hand: narcotic antagonist naloxone (preferred), levallorphan, or nalorphine to combat respiratory depression; assisted ventilation equipment, oxygen, anticonvulsants, IV therapy, as indicated. Analeptic drugs (e.g., amphetamines, caffeine) are not used because they tend to precipitate fatal convulsions. Cardiac function, blood gases, pH, and electrolytes should be monitored.

Propoxyphene in excessive doses, alone or in combination products, ranks second only to barbiturates as a major cause of drug-related deaths.

Caution patient not to exceed recommended dose and to avoid alcohol and other CNS depressants.

Tolerance and physical and psychic dependence of the morphine type can occur with excessive use.

Classified as Schedule IV drug under the Federal Controlled Substances Act. (Many professionals are urging additional controls.)

Effectiveness of propoxyphene may be reduced in smokers. Smoking induces liver enzymes responsible for metabolizing propoxyphene.

Propoxyphene hydrochloride is available in fixed combination with acetaminophen: Dolacet, Dolene, SK-65, Wygesic, and with aspirin: Darvon with A.S.A., Darvon Compound (also contains phenacetin and caffeine). The napsylate is marketed in fixed combination with acetaminophen: Darvocet-N, and with aspirin: Darvon-N with A.S.A.

When propoxyphene is included in combination products, precautions relative to each drug ingredient must be considered.

Store at 15° to 30°C (59° to 86°F) unless otherwise directed by manufacturer.

Drug Interactions: Propoxyphene Napsylate

Plus	Interactions
Alcohol and CNS depressants	Additive CNS depression: drowsiness, stupor; respiratory depression
Anticoagulants, oral	Potentiates warfarin by reducing its metabolism
Carbamazepine (Tegretol)	Potentiates carbamazepine toxicity by reducing its metabolism
Orphenadrine (Norflex)	Increased CNS stimulation: anxiety, tremors, confusion (symptoms similar to hypoglycemic reaction)

P

PROTOTYPE

PROPRANOLOL HYDROCHLORIDE

(Inderal, Novopranol)

(proe-pran'oh-lole)

Antihypertensive

Beta-adrenergic blocking agent (non-selective)

Antiarrhythmic

Antianginal

Antiplatelet

ACTIONS AND USES. Nonselective beta blocker of both cardiac ($beta_1$) and bronchial ($beta_2$) adrenoreceptors which competes with epinephrine and norepinephrine for available beta-receptor sites. Blocks cardiac effects of beta-adrenergic stimulation; as a result, reduces heart rate, myocardial irritability (class II antiarrhythmic) and force of contraction, depresses automaticity of sinus node and ectopic pacemaker, and decreases AV and intraventricular conduction velocity. In higher doses, exerts direct quinidinelike effects which depress cardiac function. Propranolol also blocks bronchodilator effect of catecholamines and reduces plasma levels of free fatty acids, and tends to promote retention of sodium; therefore, a diuretic is frequently given concurrently. Inhibition of epinephrine, the result of beta-adrenergic blockade, prevents premonitory signs of hypoglycemia in the diabetic and may also augment hypoglycemia by interfering with catecholamine-induced glycogenolysis. Propranolol may also block insulin release from pancreas with resulting hyperglycemia. Lowers both supine and standing blood pressures in hypertensive patients. Hypotensive effect (i.e., lowered systolic and diastolic blood pressure) is associated with decreased cardiac output, suppressed renin activity, as well as beta-blockade. Increases exercise tolerance by blocking sympathetic effects of exertion and decreases myocardial oxygen requirements in patients with frequent anginal attacks. Also decreases platelet aggregability. Mechanism of antimigraine action unknown but thought to be related to inhibition of cerebral vasodilation and arteriolar spasms.

Used in management of cardiac arrhythmias, myocardial infarction, tachyarrhythmias associated with digitalis intoxication, anesthesia, and thyrotoxicosis, hypertrophic subaortic stenosis, angina pectoris due to coronary atherosclerosis, pheochromocytoma; also treatment of hypertension alone, but generally with a thiazide or other antihypertensive as Step 1 agent. Available in fixed-dose combination with hydrochlorothiazide (Inderide). *Unlabeled Use:* anxiety states, migraine prophylaxis, essential tremors, schizophrenia, tardive dyskinesia, acute panic symptoms (e.g., stage fright), recurrent GI bleeding in cirrhotic patients, treatment of aggression and rage, vaginal contraceptive.

ABSORPTION AND FATE. Almost completely absorbed from GI tract following oral administration. Much of drug is metabolized during first pass through liver; about 30 to 60% may reach systemic circulation. With chronic administration less drug is removed during first pass; accordingly half-life gradually increases. Onset of action within 30 minutes, peak plasma levels in 1 to 1½ hours (marked interindividual variations in plasma levels); duration about 6 hours. Following IV administration, action begins within 2 minutes, peaks in about 15 minutes, with duration of 3 to 6 hours; plasma levels more consistent. Half-life: 3 to 5 hours. Widely distributed in body tissues; more than 90% bound to plasma proteins. Excreted in urine as free and conjugated propranolol, and active metabolites; 1 to 4% excreted in feces. Crosses placenta and blood–brain barrier; small amounts may appear in breast milk.

CONTRAINDICATIONS AND PRECAUTIONS. Greater than 1st degree heart block, congestive heart failure, right ventricular failure secondary to pulmonary hypertension; sinus bradycardia, cardiogenic shock, significant aortic or mitral valvular disease, bronchial asthma or bronchospasm, severe COPD, allergic rhinitis during pollen season; concurrent use with adrenergic-augmenting psychotropic drugs or within 2 weeks of MAO inhibition therapy. Safe use in women of childbearing potential, during pregnancy (category C), in nursing mothers and in children not established. *Cautious Use:* peripheral arterial insufficiency, history of allergy, history of systemic insect sting reaction, patients prone to nonallergenic bronchospasm (e.g., chronic bronchitis, emphysema); major surgery; renal or hepatic impairment, diabetes mellitus, patients prone to hypoglycemia, myasthenia gravis, Wolff-Parkinson-White syndrome.

ADVERSE/SIDE EFFECTS. Allergic: erythematous, psoriasislike eruptions, pruritus, fever, pharyngitis, respiratory distress. **CNS:** drug-induced psychosis, sleep disturbances, depression, confusion, agitation, giddiness, light-headedness, fatigue, vertigo, syncope, weakness, drowsiness, insomnia, vivid dreams, visual hallucinations, delusions, reversible organic brain syndrome. **CV:** palpitation, profound bradycardia, AV heart block, cardiac standstill, hypotension, angina pectoris, tachyarrhythmia, acute congestive heart failure, peripheral arterial insufficiency resembling Raynaud's disease, myotonia, paresthesia of hands. **Dermatologic:** reversible alopecia; hyperkeratoses of scalp, palms, feet; nail changes, dry skin. **EENT:** dry eyes (gritty sensation), visual disturbances, conjunctivitis, tinnitus, hearing loss, nasal stuffiness. **GI:** dry mouth, cheilostomatitis, nausea, vomiting, heartburn, diarrhea, constipation, flatulence, abdominal cramps, mesenteric arterial thrombosis, ischemic colitis. **Hematologic:** transient eosinophilia, thrombocytopenic or nonthrombocytopenic purpura, agranulocytosis, hypoglycemia, hyperglycemia (rare); hypocalcemia (patients with hyperthyroidism). **Respiratory:** dyspnea, laryngospasm, bronchospasm. **Other:** brown discoloration of tongue (rare), pancreatitis, weight gain, impotence or decreased libido, Peyronie's disease (rare), LE-like reaction, cold extremities, leg fatigue.

ROUTE AND DOSAGE. Oral: *Hypertension:* 40 mg twice daily (at 6- to 8-hour intervals); increased until optimum response obtained. Maintenance: 120 to 240 mg/day in divided doses; up to 640 mg/day may be required. *Angina pectoris:* initial: 10 to 20 mg three or four times daily; dosage gradually increased at 3 to 7 day intervals until optimum response obtained (average optimum dosage: 160 mg/day). *Arrhythmias:* 10 to 30 mg three to four times daily. *Hypertrophic subaortic stenosis:* 20 to 40 mg three to four times daily. *Migraine prevention:* initial: 80 mg daily in divided doses. Maintenance: 160 to 240 mg daily in divided doses. *Pheochromocytoma:* 20 mg three times daily, 3 days prior to surgery (concomitantly with alpha adrenergic blocking agent); *inoperable pheochromocytoma:* 10 mg three times daily. **Intravenous** (for life-threatening arrhythmias): 1 to 3 mg at rate not exceeding 1 mg/minute; may be repeated after 2 minutes, if necessary. Thereafter, additional drug not given in less than 4 hours. Available as 10, 20, 40, and 80 mg tablets and sterile solution for injection.

NURSING IMPLICATIONS

Manufacturer recommends giving oral propranolol before meals and at bedtime. Reports to date are conflicting relative to whether food enhances or delays bioavailability of propranolol. Advise patient to be consistent with regard to taking propranolol with food or on an empty stomach, to minimize variations in absorption.

Tablet may be crushed before administration and taken with fluid of patient's choice.

Careful medical history and physical examination are essential to rule out allergies, asthma, and other obstructive pulmonary disease. Propranolol can cause bronchiolar constriction even in normal subjects.

Take apical pulse before administering drug; if blood pressure is not stabilized, also take this reading before giving drug.

Apical pulse, respiration, blood pressure, and circulation of extremities should be closely monitored throughout period of dosage adjustment. Consult physician regarding acceptable parameters.

Patient receiving propranolol at home should be informed about usual pulse rate and should be instructed to take radial pulse before each dose. Advise patient to report to physician if it is slower than base level or becomes irregular. (Consult physician for parameters.)

Response to propranolol is reported to be associated with a high degree of individual variability. Therefore, sensitive observations are critically essential for establishing the patient's optimal dosage level.

For patients being treated for hypertension, checking blood pressure near end of dosage interval or before administration of next dose is a way of evaluating if control is adequate or whether more frequent dosage intervals are indicated.

Bradycardia is the most common adverse cardiac effect especially in patients with digitalis intoxication and Wolff-Parkinson-White syndrome.

When administered by IV route careful monitoring must be made of ECG, blood pressure, and pulmonary wedge pressure. Reduction in sympathetic stimulation caused by beta blocking action can result in cardiac standstill.

Adverse reactions generally occur most frequently following IV administration; however, incidence is also high following oral use in the elderly and in patients with impaired renal function. Reactions may or may not be dose-related and commonly occur soon after therapy is initiated.

Treatment of toxicity or exaggerated response may include use of the following drugs: atropine, epinephrine, isoproterenol, aminophylline, dobutamine, and glucagon. Cardiac failure is treated by digitalization and diuresis.

Intake and output ratio and daily weight are significant indices for detecting fluid retention and developing heart failure: dyspnea on exertion, orthopnea, night cough, pulmonary rales, distended neck veins, edema (tight shoes or rings, puffiness).

Plasma volume may increase with consequent risk of congestive failure if dietary sodium is not restricted in patients receiving propranolol without concomitant diuretic therapy. Consult physician regarding allowable salt intake.

Patients with diabetes should be closely monitored. Propranolol suppresses clinical signs of hypoglycemia (e.g., blood pressure changes, increased pulse rate) and may prolong hypoglycemia. Patient should be alert to other possible signs of hypoglycemia not affected by propranolol such as excessive sweating, hunger, fatigue, inability to concentrate. Instruct patient to report these easily overlooked and tolerated symptoms. Adjustment in dosage of insulin or other hypoglycemic agents may be necessary.

Fasting for more than 12 hours may induce hypoglycemic effects fostered by propranolol.

Because of beta blocking action, usual rise in pulse rate may not occur in response to stress situations, such as fever or following vigorous exercise. Activity programs must be highly individualized. Consult physician for guidelines.

In patients taking propranolol for angina pectoris, exercise performance studies and ECGs are recommended before therapy to establish baseline data, and during therapy to determine dosage requirements and need to continue treatment. Therapy is not continued unless there is reduced pain and increased work capacity.

When propranolol is to be discontinued, dosage is reduced gradually over a period of 1 to 2 weeks and patient closely monitored.

Abrupt discontinuation of propranolol can precipitate withdrawal syndrome: tremulousness, sweating, severe headache, malaise, palpitation, rebound hypertension, myocardial infarction, and life-threatening arrhythmias (in patients with angina pectoris), and hyperthyroidism in patients with thyrotoxicosis.

Because propranolol impairs reflex responses of the heart, manufacturer recommends that it be withdrawn gradually 48 hours prior to major surgery, with exception of patients with pheochromocytoma. (However, many clinicians prefer to continue the beta blocker at lower doses.)

Anesthetist should be informed about propranolol use prior to general anesthesia.

Caution patient to avoid prolonged exposure of extremities to cold. If patient complains of cold, painful, or tender feet or hands examine them carefully for evidence of impaired circulation. Peripheral pulses may still be present even though circulation is impaired.

Stress importance of compliance and warn patient not to alter established regimen, i.e., not to omit, increase or decrease dosage, or change dosage interval.

Normotensive patients on prolonged therapy should be cautioned that propranolol may cause mild hypotension (experienced as dizziness or light-headedness). Advise patient to make position changes slowly and to avoid prolonged standing and to notify physician if these symptoms persist.

Since propranolol may cause dizziness and light-headedness, caution patient to avoid driving and other potentially hazardous activities until reaction to drug is known.

When given for prolonged periods, periodic determinations should be made of hematologic, renal, hepatic, and cardiac function.

Counsel patient to avoid excesses of alcohol. Heavy alcohol consumption (i.e., more than 2 ounces/day) may elevate arterial pressure; therefore to maintain treatment effectiveness, patient should either avoid alcohol or drink moderately (less than 2 ounces/day). Consult physician.

Moderation in sodium (salt) intake is advisable for the hypertensive patient. Give information about food sources to be avoided *(see Index: Food sources).* A consultation with the dietician regarding a diet for weight control (if necessary) should be arranged before patient is discharged.

Smoking–Drug Interaction. Smoking has a direct and adverse effect on the myocardium: (increased heart rate and myocardial oxygen requirements). Additionally it increases hepatic metabolism of propranolol leading to unpredictable or lack of drug effects. Advise patient to stop smoking; but if it continues, more frequent monitoring for clinical effects of the drug is indicated.

Advise patient to consult physician before self-medicating with OTC drugs.

It is advisable for patient on prolonged propranolol therapy to wear or carry medical identification such as Medic Alert. Instruct patient to inform dentist, surgeon, or ophthalmologist (propranolol lowers normal and elevated intraocular pressure) that he or she is taking propranolol.

Patient-Teaching Points. (**Pharmacologic therapy of hypertension,** *see Index: Nursing Intervention: hypertension.*) **Nonpharmacologic therapy of hypertension:** Discuss the following with the patient:

- ✓ weight reduction
- ✓ modification of dietary sodium intake
- ✓ moderation in alcohol consumption
- ✓ avoidance of tobacco
- ✓ controlled exercise program
- ✓ behavior modification (biofeedback, relaxation therapy).

Preserve in tightly closed, light-resistant containers at temperature 15° to 30°C (59° to 86°F).

Diagnostic Test Interferences. Beta-adrenergic blockers may produce false-negative test results in exercise tolerance ECG tests, and elevations in: **serum potassium, peripheral platelet** count, **serum uric acid, serum transaminase, alkaline phosphatase, lactate dehydrogenase, serum creatinine, BUN,** and an increase or decrease in **blood glucose** levels in diabetic patients.

P

Drug Interactions: Propranolol Hydrochloride

Plus	**Interactions**
Antacids	Delay absorption if administered concomitantly; space several hours apart
Antiarrhythmics, other: e.g., lidocaine, phenytoin, procainamide, quinidine	Additive cardiac depressant effects; additive toxic effects
Antidiabetic drugs (insulins and oral hypoglycemics)	Prolonged hypoglycemic effects of insulin and coumarins
Barbiturates Rifampin	Enhance metabolism of propranolol (by inducing hepatic microsomal enzymes), thereby reducing pharmacologic effects of propranolol
Clonidine	Severity of rebound hypertension caused by abrupt discontinuation of clonidine may be increased

Plus (cont.)	Interactions (cont.)
Digitalis glycosides	Potentiation of bradycardic effect (additive depression of AV conduction)
Epinephrine (adrenalin) (intravenous)	Possibility of hypertension and excessive bradycardia
Cimetidine Chlorpromazine Contraceptives, oral Furosemide Hydralazine	Increased hypotensive effects (inhibition of hepatic metabolism therefore increased bioavailability of propranolol)
Ergot alkaloids	Possible additive peripheral vasoconstrictors
Glucagon	Propranolol may partially inhibit glucagon-induced hyperglycemia
Indomethacin Salicylates	May inhibit antihypertensive response (inhibition of prostaglandin synthesis)
Isoproterenol Dobutamine Epinephrine Dopamine	May reverse beta blockade; severe hypotension is possible
Phenothiazines	Additive hypotensive effects
Reserpine (and other catecholamine-depleting drugs)	Additive hypotensive and bradycardic effects
Skeletal muscle relaxants, e.g., gallamine, pancuronium, tubocurarine	Intensified neuromuscular blockade
Tricyclic antidepressants Antimuscarinics (e.g., atropine)	May antagonize cardiac depressive activity of propranolol

PROTOTYPE

P

PROPYLTHIOURACIL

(Propacil, Propyl-Thyracil, PTU)

(proe-pill-thye-oh-yoor'a-sill)

Antithyroid agent

ACTIONS AND USES. Relatively nontoxic thioamide. Interferes with organification of iodine and blocks synthesis of thyroxine (T_4) and triiodothyronine (T_3). Does not interfere with release and utilization of stored thyroid; thus antithyroid action is delayed days and weeks until preformed T_3 and T_4 are degraded. Drug-induced hormone reduction results in compensatory release of thyrotropin (TSH), which causes marked hyperplasia and vascularization of thyroid gland. With good adherence to drug regimen, chemical euthyroidism can be achieved 6 to 12 weeks after start of thioamide therapy.

Used in medical treatment of hyperthyroidism, to establish euthyroidism prior to surgery or radioactive iodine treatment, and for palliative control of toxic nodular goiter. Also used to treat iodine-induced thyrotoxicosis and hyperthyroidism associated with thyroiditis.

ABSORPTION AND FATE. Absorption of effective amounts within 30 minutes after oral dose. Duration of action 2 or 3 hours; plasma half-life: 3 to 5 hours; protein binding: 80%. 30 to 35% of drug is excreted in urine within 24 hours; some excretion through bile. Crosses placenta, inhibits fetal thyroid function, and is excreted in breast milk.

CONTRAINDICATIONS AND PRECAUTIONS. Hypersensitivity or idiosyncrasy to propylthiouracil, last trimester of pregnancy, lactation, concurrent administration of sulfonamides or coal tar derivatives such as aminopyrine or antipyrine. *Cautious Use:* infection, concomitant administration of anticoagulants or other drugs known to cause agranulocytosis; bone marrow depression, impaired hepatic function.

ADVERSE/SIDE EFFECTS. CNS: ototoxicity (rare), paresthesias, headache, vertigo, drowsiness, neuritis. **Dermatologic:** skin rash, urticaria, pruritus, hyperpigmentation, lightening of hair color, abnormal hair loss. **GI:** nausea, vomiting, diarrhea, dyspepsia, loss of taste, sialoadenitis, hepatitis. **Hematologic:** myelosuppression, lymphadenopathy, periarteritis, hypoprothrombinemia, thrombocytopenia, leukopenia, agranulocytosis. **Hypothyroidism (goitrogenic):** enlarged thyroid, reduced GI motility, periorbital edema, puffy hands and feet, bradycardia, cool and pale skin, worsening of ophthalmopathy, sleepiness, fatigue, mental depression, dizziness, vertigo, sensitivity to cold, paresthesias, nocturnal muscle cramps, changes in menstrual periods, unusual weight gain. **Other:** drug fever, lupuslike syndrome, arthralgia, myalgia.

ROUTE AND DOSAGE. All doses usually administered in 3 equal doses at 8-hour intervals. **Oral: Adults:** initial: 300 to 900 mg/day. Maintenance: 100 to 150 mg. **Pediatric (6 to 10 years):** 50 to 150 mg/day. **Children (10 years or older):** 150 to 300 mg/day. Maintenance dose individualized.

NURSING IMPLICATIONS

Administer PTU at the same time each day with relation to meals. Food may alter drug response by changing absorption rate.

About 10% of patients with hyperthyroidism have leukopenia of less than 4000 cells/mm^3 and relative granulopenia.

If drug is being used to improve thyroid state before radioactive iodine (RAI) treatment, PTU should be discontinued 3 or 4 days before treatment to prevent interference with RAI uptake. PTU therapy may be resumed if necessary 3 to 5 days after the RAI administration.

Iodine (Lugol's solution or SSKI) is usually added to PTU treatment for 7 to 10 days before surgery to reduce drug-induced thyroid vascularity and friability.

Objective signs of clinical response to PTU (usually within 2 or 3 weeks): significant weight gain, reduced pulse rate, reduced serum T_4.

When thyroid gland is greatly enlarged, satisfactory euthyroid state may be delayed for several months.

Generally duration of therapy covers a period of 6 months to several years, followed by remission in 25% of patients. Medication is then stopped in the hope that natural remission will occur.

Long-term PTU therapy is usually monitored by follow-up examinations and hematologic studies every 2 to 3 months. As soon as patient is euthyroid, thyroid hormone (especially T_3) may be added to regimen to prevent goitrogenic-induced hypothyroidism and to suppress TSH production.

If surgery fails to render patient euthyroid, PTU treatment may be reinstituted.

PTU given during pregnancy may be withdrawn 2 or 3 weeks before delivery to prevent excess drug passage across the placenta and the accompanying danger of cretinism and goiter in fetus.

To prevent hypothyroidism in mother, thyroid may be given concomitantly with PTU throughout pregnancy and after delivery with little effect on fetus.

Postpartum patients receiving PTU should not nurse their babies. Exacerbation of hyperthyroidism 3 to 4 months postpartum in the mother is common; PTU therapy can be reinstituted.

The goitrogenic hypothyroid state (excess dosage) develops insidiously, and in some cases it may be noted only after an infrequent observer calls attention to changes such as periorbital edema.

Important diagnostic signs of excess dosage: contraction of a muscle bundle when pricked, mental depression, hard and nonpitting edema, and need for high thermostat setting and extra blankets in winter (cold intolerance).

Urticaria may occur (3 to 7% of patients) during period from second to eighth week of treatment. If mild, symptomatic treatment with an antihistamine may be started; switching to another thioamide is usual if rash is severe.

Advise patient to report severe skin rash or swelling of cervical lymph nodes. Therapy may be discontinued.

Warn patient to report sore throat, fever, and rash immediately (most apt to occur in first few months of treatment). Drug will be discontinued and hematologic studies initiated. If agranulocytosis is diagnosed, patient may be given broad-spectrum antibiotics and placed on reverse isolation.

Be alert to signs of hypoprothrombinemia: ecchymoses, purpura, petechiae, unexplained bleeding. Warn ambulatory patients to report these signs promptly.

Advise patients to avoid use of OTC drugs for asthma, coryza, or cough treatment without checking with the physician. Iodides sometimes included in such preparations are contraindicated.

Teach patient how to take pulse accurately. Advise daily check.

Clinical response is monitored through changes in weight and pulse. Advise patient to chart weight two or three times weekly. Continued tachycardia, diarrhea, fever, irritability, listlessness, vomiting, weakness, should be reported as signs of inadequate therapy or thyrotoxicosis.

Instruct patient in remission to continue monitoring and recording weight and pulse rate. Patient should report onset of tremor, anxiety state, gradual ascending pulse rate, and loss of weight to the physician (signs of hormone deficiency).

Some young females may have been "outeating" their hyperthyroidism and gaining weight prior to seeking treatment. Restoration of euthyroid state may be accompanied by further obesity; reduced caloric intake may be prescribed for these patients. Consult physician.

Urge patient not to alter drug regimen: not increase, decrease or omit doses nor change administration intervals.

If compliance is a problem, the physician may prescribe a once-a-day regimen.

Check with physician about use of iodized salt and inclusion of seafood in the diet.

Store drug in light-resistant container at temperature between 15° and 30°C (59° and 86°F).

P

Diagnostic Test Interferences. Propylthiouracil may elevate **prothrombin time** and serum **alkaline phosphatase, SGOT (AST), SGPT (ALT)** levels.

Drug Interactions: Propylthiouracil

Plus	**Interactions**
Anticoagulants, oral Heparin	May enhance anticoagulant effect

PROTAMINE SULFATE

(proe'ta-meen)
Antidote

ACTIONS AND USES. Purified mixture of simple, low molecular weight proteins obtained from sperm or testes of suitable fish species. When used alone, has anticoagulant effect. Since it is strongly basic, protamine combines with strongly acidic heparin to produce a stable complex, and thus anticoagulant effect of both drugs is neutralized.

Used as antidote for heparin calcium or heparin sodium overdosage (after heparin has been discontinued). *Unlabeled Use:* antidote for heparin administration during extracorporeal circulation.

ABSORPTION AND FATE. Onset of heparin neutralization (IV) occurs within 5 minutes. Duration of action is about 2 hours (dose-dependent).

CONTRAINDICATIONS AND PRECAUTIONS. Hemorrhage not induced by heparin overdosage. Human reproductive studies have not been performed. *Cautious Use:* cardiovascular disease, history of allergy to fish.

ADVERSE/SIDE EFFECTS. Abrupt drop in blood pressure, bradycardia, dyspnea, nausea, vomiting, lassitude; transient flushing and feeling of warmth; bleeding: protamine overdose or "heparin rebound" (hyperheparinemia); hypersensitivity reactions.

ROUTE AND DOSAGE. Intravenous: Dosage guided by blood coagulation studies. Administered slowly; not to exceed 50 mg in any 10-minute period. Each 1 mg of protamine sulfate neutralizes the activity of approximately 90 USP units of heparin derived from lung tissue or the activity of about 115 USP units of heparin from intestinal mucosa. If heparin was administered by deep SC injection, 1 to 1.5 mg of protamine is given for each 100 U heparin. *Loading dose:* 25 to 50 mg by slow IV injection; then rest of dose by continuous IV infusion over 8 to 16 hours or expected duration of absorption of heparin. To neutralize heparin administration during extracorporeal circulation, 1.5 mg protamine is usually given for each 100 U of heparin administered.

NURSING IMPLICATIONS

Monitor blood pressure and pulse every 15 to 30 minutes, or more often if indicated. Continue for at least 2 to 3 hours after each dose, or longer as dictated by patient's condition. Be prepared to treat patient for shock as well as hemorrhage.

Since protamine has a longer half-life than heparin and also has some anticoagulant effect of its own, dose must be carefully titrated to prevent excess anticoagulation.

Protamine is not used if only minor bleeding occurs during heparin therapy because withdrawal of heparin will usually correct minor bleeding within a few hours.

The effect of protamine in neutralizing heparin is monitored by APTT (activated partial thromboplastin time) or ACT (activated coagulation time) values. Coagulation tests are usually performed 5 to 15 minutes after administration of protamine and again in 2 to 8 hours, if desirable.

Patients undergoing extracorporeal dialysis or patients who have had cardiac surgery must be observed carefully for bleeding (heparin rebound). Even with apparent adequate neutralization of heparin by protamine, bleeding may occur 30 minutes to 18 hours after surgery. Monitor vital signs closely. Additional protamine may be required in these patients.

Protamine sulfate injection should be stored at 2° to 8°C (36° to 46°F); protamine powder for injection and reconstituted solution at 15° to 30°C (59° to 86°F). Avoid freezing. Solutions are stable for 72 hours at this temperature.

PROTEIN HYDROLYSATE

(A/G-Pro, Protinex, Pro-Mix, Propac)

Parenteral nutrient
Protein

ACTIONS AND USES. Contains amino acids and short-chain peptides derived from hydrolysis of protein (casein or fibrin). Commercial preparations differ in composition of essential and nonessential amino acids and electrolytes. Composition of most products: 60% free amino acids, 40% peptides. Sufficient nonprotein caloric source (in the form of dextrose) must be maintained during therapy to prevent utilization of protein hydrolysate for energy rather than for protein synthesis (nitrogen-sparing effect). Oral formulations, e.g., A/G-Pro, PDP, Liquid Protein, Pro-Mix, Protinex are nonprescription (OTC) products. *See Amino Acid Injection for uses, contraindications, adverse reactions and interactions.*

ADVERSE/SIDE EFFECTS. (When used for weight reduction): thrombophlebitis of lower extremities, orthostatic hypotension, arrhythmias. *See also Amino Acid Injection.*

ROUTE AND DOSAGE. Dosage depends on patient's metabolic needs and clinical response. Administered by **intravenous infusion.**

NURSING IMPLICATIONS

Protein hydrolysates are rarely used as prescription drugs because of increasing popularity of Amino Acid Injection.

Administration by IV infusion for hyperalimentation or total parenteral nutrition introduces hypertonic solution of dextrose and protein hydrolysate into superior vena cava via subclavian or internal jugular vein. Solution provides nutrients without exceeding daily fluid requirement.

Hyperalimentation requires specialized knowledge of fluid and electrolyte balance and nutritional and clinical expertise to recognize potential complications.

OTC protein hydrolysates (designation includes at least 50 brand names), have low biologic value, i.e., they lack some of the essential amino acids, vitamins, and minerals needed during rapid weight loss.

Use of OTC formulations to lose weight is dangerous. FDA regulated labels (as of 1980) indicate that liquid protein low caloric diets (below 800 calories/day) may cause serious illness or death, are not to be used by infants, children and pregnant and nursing mothers, nor should they be used without medical supervision or with monitoring of serum K, Na, Ca, phosphate and ECG.

Inform patients that stools will be reduced in size and frequency while receiving hyperalimentation therapy.

See Amino Acid Injection.

P

PROTRIPTYLINE HYDROCHLORIDE

(Triptil, Vivactil)

(proe-trip′te-leen)
Psychotropic, antidepressant
Tricyclic

ACTIONS AND USES. Dibenzocycloheptene derivative tricyclic antidepressant (TCA) with more rapid onset of action than imipramine (qv). Has little if any sedative properties characteristic of most other TCAs, but causes tachycardia, CNS stimulation, and strong anticholinergic activity; orthostatic hypotension occurs frequently. Actions, limitations, and interactions are similar to those of imipramine.

Used for symptomatic treatment of endogenous depression in patient under close medical supervision. Particularly effective for depression manifested by psychomotor retardation, apathy, and fatigue.

ABSORPTION AND FATE. Completely absorbed from GI tract. Peak levels reached in 24 to 30 hours. Effective therapeutic plasma level 115 to 210 ng/ml; 92% protein binding. Serum half-life: 54 to 98 hours. Hepatic metabolism. Steady state reached in 10 days. Cumulative effects are due to slow excretory rate: after 16 days, 50% of drug still persists in urine. Crosses placenta.

CONTRAINDICATIONS AND PRECAUTIONS. Use in children; concurrent use of MAO inhibitors; during acute recovery phase following myocardial infarction. *Cautious Use:* hepatic, cardiovascular, or renal dysfunction; diabetes mellitus, hyperthyroidism, patients with insomnia. *See also Imipramine.*

ADVERSE/SIDE EFFECTS. Allergic: photosensitivity, edema (general or of face and tongue). *See Imipramine.* **Anticholinergic:** xerostomia, blurred vision, constipation, paralytic ileus, urinary retention, confusional states. **CNS:** insomnia, headache, confusion. **CV:** change in heat or cold tolerance; orthostatic hypotension, tachycardia.

ROUTE AND DOSAGE. Oral: 15 to 40 mg daily in 3 or 4 divided doses; maximum 60 mg/day. **Adolescent and elderly patients:** 5 mg three times/day with gradual increase, if necessary.

NURSING IMPLICATIONS

Tablet may be crushed before administration and taken with fluid or mixed with food.

Has fairly rapid onset of initial effect characterized by increased activity and energy, usually within 1 week after therapy is initiated.

Increase in dosage should be made in the morning dose to prevent sleep interference, and because this TCA has psychic energizing action.

Last dose of day should be taken no later than midafternoon; insomnia rather than drowsiness is a frequent side effect.

If the elderly patient has a dose higher than 20 mg/day, monitor CV system responses closely.

Maximum antidepressant effect may not occur for 2 weeks or more after therapy begins.

To reduce possibility of relapse, maintenance therapy is generally continued at least 3 months after satisfactory improvement is noted.

Monitor vital signs closely during early therapy, particularly in patients with cardiovascular disorders and in elderly patients receiving daily doses in excess of 20 mg. If BP falls more than 20 mm Hg and if there is a sudden increase in pulse rate, withhold drug and inform physician.

Suicide is an inherent risk with any depressed patient and may remain until there is significant improvement. Supervise patient closely during early treatment period.

Anticholinergic effects are prominent (xerostomia, blurred vision, constipation, paralytic ileus, urinary retention, delayed micturition).

During early therapy and when patient is on large doses, monitor intake and output ratio and question patient about bowel regularity.

Xerostomia can interfere with patient's appetite, fluid intake and integrity of tooth surfaces. Assess condition of oral membranes frequently; institute symptomatic treatment if necessary. *See Imipramine.*

Photosensitivity reactions may occur. Until this possibility is ruled out, advise patient to avoid exposure to the sun without protecting skin with sunscreen lotion (SPF 12 or above), if allowed, and to avoid sun between the hours of 10 and 3 when sun's rays are nearest.

The actions of both alcohol and protriptyline are potentiated when used together during therapy and for up to 2 weeks after the TCA is discontinued. Consult physician about safe amount of alcohol, if any, that can be taken.

If a patient uses excessive amounts of alcohol it should be borne in mind that the potentiation of TCA effects may increase the danger of overdosage or suicide attempt.

Smoking–Drug Interaction: Smoking increases the metabolism of TCAs and therefore reduces its effectiveness. Urge patient to stop or to reduce smoking. Monitor the heavy smoker's response; apparent treatment failure may be due to the nicotine effect.

Advise patient to consult physician before taking any OTC medications.

The effects of barbiturates and other CNS depressants are enhanced by TCAs.

Caution patient to avoid hazardous activities requiring alertness and skill until response to drug is known.

Patients receiving large doses for prolonged periods or in combination with other drugs should have periodic determinations of liver function and blood cell counts.

Store drug in tightly closed container at temperature between 15° and 30°C (59° and 86°F) unless otherwise directed by manufacturer.

See Imipramine (prototype tricyclic antidepressant).

PSEUDOEPHEDRINE HYDROCHLORIDE

(soo-doe-e-fed'rin)

(Cenafed, Dorcol Pediatric Formula, Halofed, Neofed, Novafed, Profedrine, Robidrine, Sudafed, Sudrin, and others)

Adrenergic agonist (sympathomimetic)
Decongestant

ACTIONS AND USES. Sympathomimetic amine that, like ephedrine, produces decongestion of respiratory tract mucosa by action on sympathetic nerve endings. Unlike ephedrine, also acts directly on smooth muscle and constricts renal and vertebral arteries. Has fewer side effects, less pressor action and longer duration of effects than ephedrine. Produces little, if any, congestive rebound or irritation that occur with nasal sprays and solutions.

Used for symptomatic relief of nasal congestion associated with rhinitis, coryza, and sinusitis and for eustachian tube congestion.

P

ABSORPTION AND FATE. Onset of action within 15 to 30 minutes, and persists for 4 to 6 hours; 8 to 12 hours after extended-release form. Partially metabolized in liver. Enters breast milk.

CONTRAINDICATIONS AND PRECAUTIONS. Hypersensitivity to sympathomimetic amines, severe hypertension, coronary artery disease, use within 14 days of MAO inhibitors, nursing mother, glaucoma, hyperthyroidism, prostatic hypertrophy. Safe use during pregnancy, lactation, and in children under 6 not established. *Cautious Use:* hypertension, heart disease.

ADVERSE/SIDE EFFECTS. Transient stimulation, tremulousness, difficulty in voiding, arrhythmias, palpitation, tachycardia, nervousness, dizziness, headache, sleeplessness, numbness of extremities, anorexia, dry mouth, nausea, vomiting.

ROUTE AND DOSAGE. Oral: Adults and children (12 years and older): 60 mg every 4 to 6 hours; timed-release form: 120 mg every 12 hours. **Children (6 to 11 years):** 30 mg every 4 to 6 hours; **(2 to 6 years):** 15 mg every 4 to 6 hours up to 60 mg/day.

NURSING IMPLICATIONS

Tablet may be crushed before administration and taken with fluid of patient's choice.

Since drug may act as a stimulant, advise patient to avoid taking it within 2 hours of bedtime.

Warn patient against concomitant use of OTC medications, many contain ephedrine or other sympathomimetic amines and might intensify action of pseudoephedrine. Consult physician.

Advise patient to withhold medication if extreme restlessness or signs of sensitivity occur and to consult physician.

See Ephedrine sulfate.

PSYLLIUM HYDROPHILIC MUCILOID

(sill'i-um)

(Hydrocil, Konsyl, Metamucil, Modane Bulk, Mucilose, Plova, Pro-Lax, Regacilium, Reguloid, Serutan, Siblin, Syllact, V-Lax)

Laxative (bulk forming)

ACTIONS AND USES. Highly refined colloid of blond psyllium seed *(Plantago ovata)* with equal amount of dextrose added as dispersing agent. On contact with water, produces bland, lubricating, gelatinous bulk, which promotes peristalsis and natural elimination. Contains negligible amounts of sodium and about 14 calories/dose (instant-mix effervescent form is flavored and contains 0.25 Gm sodium and 43 calories/dose). Reportedly, chronic use may reduce plasma cholesterol, possibly by interfering with reabsorption of bile acids.

Used in treatment of chronic atonic or spastic constipation and in constipation associated with rectal disorders or anorectal surgery.

CONTRAINDICATIONS AND PRECAUTIONS. Esophageal and intestinal obstruction, fecal impaction, undiagnosed abdominal pain.

ADVERSE/SIDE EFFECTS. Eosinophilia, nausea and vomiting, diarrhea, with excessive use; GI tract strictures when drug used in dry form, abdominal cramps.

ROUTE AND DOSAGE. Oral: Adults: 1 to 2 rounded teaspoonfuls or 1 packet (instant mix) one or three times a day. **Children (6 years and over):** 1 rounded teaspoonful in ½ glass liquid once or twice a day.

NURSING IMPLICATIONS

Instruct patient to fill an ordinary 8-oz. (240 ml) water glass with cool water, milk, fruit juice, or other liquid, sprinkle powder into liquid, stir briskly, and drink immediately (if effervescent form is used, add liquid to powder). Granules should not be chewed.

If patient complains of retrosternal pain after taking the drug, report promptly to physician. The drug may be lodged as a gelatinous mass (because of poor mixing) in the esophagus.

Best results are obtained if each dose is followed by an additional glass of liquid.

Note sugar and Na content of preparation if patient is on low sodium or low caloric diet.

Na content of metamucil instant mix: 0.25 Gm/packet; effersyllium instant mix: 7 Gm/teaspoon; Hydrocil Instant Powder: 10 mg/packet.

Be cautious with elderly patient who may aspirate the drug.

Laxative effect usually occurs within 12 to 24 hours. Administration for 2 or 3 days may be needed to establish regularity.
Inform patient that drug may reduce appetite if taken before meals.
See Bisacodyl for patient-teaching points about drug therapy and constipation.

PYRANTEL PAMOATE

(Antiminth, Combantriln)

(pi-ran′tel)
Antiinfective
Anthelmintic

ACTIONS AND USES. Exerts selective depolarizing neuromuscular blocking action, which results in spastic paralysis of worm; also inhibits cholinesterases.

Used in *Enterobius vermicularis* (pinworm) and *Ascaris lumbricoides* (roundworm) infestations. *Unlabeled Use:* hookworm infestations; treatment of trichostrongyliasis.

ABSORPTION AND FATE. Partially absorbed from GI tract. Plasma levels of unchanged drug, which are low, peak in 1 to 3 hours. Metabolized in liver. Over 50% excreted in feces unchanged within 24 hours; about 7% eliminated in urine as free drug and metabolites.

CONTRAINDICATIONS AND PRECAUTIONS. Safe use during pregnancy and in children under 2 years of age not established. *Cautious Use:* liver dysfunction, malnutrition, dehydration, anemia.

ADVERSE/SIDE EFFECTS. CNS: dizziness, headache, drowsiness, insomnia. **GI:** anorexia, nausea, vomiting, abdominal distention, diarrhea, tenesmus, transient elevation of SGOT (AST). **Other:** skin rashes.

ROUTE AND DOSAGE. Oral: Adults and Children: 11 mg/kg (5 mg/lb) body weight administered in a single dose. Maximum total dose 1 Gm.

NURSING IMPLICATIONS

Shake suspension well before pouring to assure accurate dosage.
May be taken with milk or fruit juices and without regard to prior ingestion of food or time of day.
Purging is not necessary before, during, or after therapy.
Store at temperature below 30°C (86°F). Protect from light.
See Mebendazole for patient-teaching points.

Drug Interactions. There is a possibility that pyrantel and **piperazine** are mutually antagonistic.

PYRAZINAMIDE

(peer-a-zin′a-mide)
Antiinfective
Antituberculosis agent

ACTIONS AND USES. Pyrazinoic acid amide, analog of nicotinamide and bacteriostatic against *Mycobaterium tuberculosis.* When employed alone, resistance may develop in 6 to 7 weeks;

therefore, administration with other effective agents is recommended. Appears to interfere with renal capacity to concentrate and excrete uric acid; thus may cause hyperuricemia.

Used for short-term therapy of advanced tuberculosis before surgery and to treat patients unresponsive to primary agents (e.g., isoniazid, streptomycin).

ABSORPTION AND FATE. Readily absorbed from GI tract. Peak serum concentrations in about 2 hours, declining thereafter; half-life: 9 to 10 hours, prolonged in patient with impaired hepatic and renal function. Metabolized in liver. Slowly excreted in urine; 30% eliminated as metabolites and 4% as unchanged drug within 24 hours.

CONTRAINDICATIONS AND PRECAUTIONS. Severe hepatic damage. Safe use in children not established. *Cautious Use:* presence or family history of gout or diabetes mellitus, impaired renal function, history of peptic ulcer, acute intermittent porphyria.

ADVERSE/SIDE EFFECTS. Arthralgia, active gout, difficulty in urination, headache, photosensitivity, urticaria, skin rash (rare), sideroblastic or hemolytic anemia, splenomegaly, lymphadenopathy, fatal hemoptysis, aggravation of peptic ulcer, rise in serum uric acid, hepatotoxicity, abnormal liver function tests, acute yellow atrophy of liver, decreased plasma prothrombin.

ROUTE AND DOSAGE. Oral: 20 to 35 mg/kg/day in 3 or 4 divided doses; maximal dose 3 Gm/day.

NURSING IMPLICATIONS

The patient receiving pyrazinamide requires close observation and medical supervision. He or she should receive at least one other effective antituberculosis agent concurrently.

Drug should be discontinued if hepatic reactions (jaundice, pruritis, icteric sclerae, yellow skin), or hyperuricemia with acute gout (severe pain in great toe and other joints) occur. (Normal serum uric acid: 3 to 7 mg/dl).

Patients should be examined at regular intervals and questioned about possible signs of toxicity: liver enlargement or tenderness, jaundice, fever, anorexia, malaise, impaired vascular integrity (ecchymoses, petechiae, abnormal bleeding).

Hepatic reactions appear to occur more frequently in patients receiving high doses.

Liver function tests (especially AST, ALT, serum bilirubin) should be done prior to and at 2- to 4-week intervals during therapy. Blood uric acid determinations are advised before, during, and following therapy.

Report to physician the onset of difficulty in voiding. Patient should be urged to keep fluid intake at a 2000-ml/day level, if possible.

Aspirin in large doses (e.g., 3 to 5 Gm/day) or other uricosuric agents may be prescribed to control hyperuricemia.

Patients with diabetes should be closely monitored for possible loss of control.

Store tablets in well-closed container at temperature 15° to 39°C (59° to 56°F).

Diagnostic Test Interferences. Pyrazinamide may produce a temporary decrease in **17-ketosteroids** and an increase in **protein-bound iodine.**

PYRETHRINS

(peer′e-thrins)
Pediculocide

(A-200 Pyrinate, Barc, Blue, Pyrin-Aid, Pyrinyl, R & C, Rid, TISIT, Triple X)

ACTIONS AND USES. Pediculocide solution composed of pyrethrins and piperonyl butoxide in deodorized kerosene. Acts as a contact poison affecting the parasite's nervous system causing paralysis and death. Controls head lice, pubic (crab) lice, and body lice and their eggs (nits). Used for external treatment of *Pediculus humanus* infestations.

CONTRAINDICATIONS AND PRECAUTIONS. Sensitivity to solution components; skin infections and abrasions. *Cautious Use:* ragweed sensitized patient, infants, children.

ADVERSE/SIDE EFFECTS. Irritation with repeated use.

ROUTE AND DOSAGE. Solution supplied in 2- and 4-ounce bottles with special fine-toothed comb and patient instructions; gel in 1-ounce tube. *See Nursing Implications for dosage.*

NURSING IMPLICATIONS

Pyrethrins should not be swallowed, inhaled, or allowed to contact mucosal surfaces or the eyes.

Do not apply to eyebrows or eyelashes without consulting physician.

In accidental contact of eyes, flush with copious amounts of warm water.

If treated area becomes irritated, discontinue use and consult physician.

Application of Drug:

- Apply enough solution to completely wet infested area, including hair.
- Allow to remain on area for 10 minutes.
- Wash and rinse with large amounts of warm water.
- Use fine-toothed comb to remove lice and eggs from hair.
- Shampoo hair to restore body and luster.
- Treatment may be repeated if necessary once in a 24-hour period.
- Repeat treatment in 7 to 10 days to kill newly hatched lice.

Patient-Teaching Points:

✓ Each family member should be examined carefully; if infested, he or she should also be treated immediately to prevent spread or reinfestation of previously treated patient.
✓ Dry clean, boil, or otherwise treat contaminated clothing.
✓ Sterilize (soak in pyrithrins) comb and brushes used by patient.
✓ Teach patient not to share comb, brush, or headgear with another person.
✓ Inform patient/family that patient information booklet should have been included with packaged drug. Review with patient and family.

PYRIDOSTIGMINE BROMIDE

(peer-id-oh-stig′meen)
Cholinergic (parasympathomimetic)
Cholinesterone inhibitor

(Mestinon, Regonal)

ACTIONS AND USES. Indirect-acting cholinergic with anticholinesterase activity. Synthetic quaternary ammonium compound similar to neostigmine (qv) in actions, contraindications, precautions, and adverse reactions. Has longer duration of action than does neostigmine, and reportedly produces less GI and other muscarinic side effects.

Used to improve muscle strength in symptomatic treatment of myasthenia gravis. Used parenterally to reverse the effects of neuromuscular blocking agents.

ABSORPTION AND FATE. Poorly absorbed from GI tract; onset of action (improved muscle strength) in 20 to 30 minutes, with duration of 3 to 6 hours. Action begins within 15 minutes following IM and 2 to 5 minutes after IV injection. Metabolized in liver. Excreted in urine as metabolites and free drug up to 72 hours after a single IV dose. Reportedly metabolized and excreted more rapidly in patients with severe myasthenia. Crosses placenta.

CONTRAINDICATIONS AND PRECAUTIONS. Hypersensitivity to anticholinesterase agents or to bromides. Safe use in women of childbearing potential and use during pregnancy (category C) or lactation not established. *Cautious Use:* bronchial asthma, cardiac dysrhythmias. *See Neostigmine.*

ADVERSE/SIDE EFFECTS. Acneiform (bromide) rash, thrombophlebitis (following IV administration). With large doses: *Muscarinic effects:* nausea, vomiting, diarrhea, miosis, excessive salivation and sweating, increased bronchial secretion, bronchoconstriction, bradycardia, weakness, fasciculation and hypotention. *See also Neostigmine.*

ROUTE AND DOSAGE. **Oral (myasthenia gravis): Adults:** dosage range 60 mg to 1.5 Gm daily, spaced according to requirements and response of patient. Sustained-release tablets: 1 to 3 180 to 540 mg tablets once or twice daily, at intervals of at least 6 hours. **Children:** 7 mg/kg/24 hours divided into 5 or 6 doses. **Intramuscular, intravenous: Adults:** approximately 1/30 of usual (myasthenic) oral dose; (for reversal of muscle relaxants): IV 10 to 20 mg, immediately preceded by IV atropine. **Neonates:** IM 0.05 to 0.15 mg/kg.

NURSING IMPLICATIONS

Failure of patient to show improvement may reflect either underdosage or overdosage. Report increasing muscular weakness, cramps, or fasciculations. *See Neostigmine for differentiation between myasthenic and cholinergic crises.*

Have the following immediately available: IV atropine, facilities for endotracheal intubation and respiratory assistance, tracheostomy, suction, oxygen.

Observe for cholinergic reactions, particularly when drug is administered IV.

Duration of drug action reportedly may vary with physical and emotional stress, as well as with severity of disease.

Sustained-release tablets are generally prescribed only at bedtime for patients who complain of weakness on awakening.

Neonates of myasthenic mothers who have received pyridostigmine should be closely observed for difficulty in breathing, swallowing, or sucking.

When used as muscle relaxant antagonist, patient should be continuously observed. Airway and respiratory assistance must be maintained until full recovery of voluntary respiration and neuromuscular transmission is assured. Complete recovery usually occurs within 30 minutes.

Report onset of rash. Drug discontinuation may be indicated.

Sustained-release tablets may become mottled in appearance; this does not affect their potency.

Pyridostigmine syrup should be protected from light.

See Neostigmine (prototype cholinesterase inhibitor).

Drug Interactions. Pyridostigmine antagonizes the effect of nondepolarizing muscle relaxants (e.g., tubocurarine, gallamine, pancuronium). Atropine antagonizes the muscarinic effects of pyridostigmine. *See also Neostigmine.*

PYRIDOXINE HYDROCHLORIDE

(peer-i-dox'een)

(Beesix, Hexa-Betalin, NesFrex, Vitabee-6)

Vitamin B_6

ACTIONS AND USES. Water-soluble complex of three closely related compounds (pyridoxine and its active derivatives pyridoxamine and pyridoxal) with B_6 activity. Considered essential to human nutrition, although a deficiency syndrome is not well defined. Converted in body to pyridoxal, a coenzyme that functions in protein, fat, and carbohydrate metabolism and in facilitating release of glycogen from liver and muscle. In protein metabolism, participates in many enzymatic transformations of amino acids and conversion of tryptophan to niacin and serotonin. Aids in energy transformation in brain and nerve cells, and is thought to stimulate heme production.

Used in prophylaxis and treatment of pyridoxine deficiency, as seen with inadequate dietary intake, drug-induced deficiency (e.g., isoniazid, oral contraceptives), and inborn errors of metabolism (vitamin B_6-dependent convulsions or anemia). Also has been used to prevent chloramphenicol-induced optic neuritis, to treat acute toxicity caused by overdosage of cycloserine, hydralzine, isoniazid (INH); to treat alcoholic polyneuritis, sideroblastic anemia associated with high serum iron concentration. Has been used for management of many other conditions ranging from nausea and vomiting in radiation sickness and pregnancy, to suppression of postpartum lactation.

ABSORPTION AND FATE. Readily absorbed following oral and parenteral administration. Half-life: 15 to 20 days. Degraded in liver and excreted in urine primarily as 4-pyridoxic acid.

CONTRAINDICATIONS AND PRECAUTIONS. History of hypersensitivity to pyridoxine. Safe use of large doses in pregnancy (category A), during lactation, and in children not established.

ADVERSE/SIDE EFFECTS. Rarely: paresthesias, somnolence (particularly following large parenteral doses), slight flushing or feeling of warmth, low folic acid levels, temporary burning or stinging pain in injection site.

P

ROUTE AND DOSAGE. Oral, intramuscular, intravenous: *dietary deficiency:* 2.5 to 10 mg daily for 3 weeks; followed with oral therapeutic multivitamin containing 2 to 5 mg pyridoxine daily for several weeks. *Vitamin B_6 deficiency syndrome:* 600 mg/day may be required; maintenance: 50 mg for life. *Isoniazid-induced deficiency:* 100 to 200 mg daily for 3 weeks; maintenance: 25 to 100 mg daily. Drug-induced pyridoxine deficiency and acute drug toxicity: 10 to 50 mg daily.

NURSING IMPLICATIONS

Normal serum concentrations of vitamin B_6 are 30 to 80 ng/ml. Total body store is estimated to be 16 to 27 ng.

Therapeutic effectiveness of vitamin B_6 therapy is evaluated by improvement of deficiency manifestations: nausea, vomiting, skin lesions resembling those of riboflavin and niacin deficiency (seborrhealike lesions about eyes, nose, and mouth, glossitis, stomatitis), edema, CNS symptoms (depression, irritability, peripheral neuritis, convulsions), hypochromic microcytic anemia.

Collaborate with physician, dietitian, patient, and a responsible family member in planning for diet teaching. A complete dietary history should be recorded so that poor eating habits can be identified and corrected (a single vitamin deficiency is rare; patient can be expected to have multiple vitamin deficiencies).

Recommended dietary allowance (RDA) of pyridoxine: 2.2 mg for adults; 2.6 mg during pregnancy and lactation. Need for pyridoxine increases with amount of protein in diet.

Rich dietary sources of vitamin B_6 include yeast, wheat germ, whole grain cereals, muscle and glandular meats (especially liver), legumes, green vegetables, bananas.

Advise patient not to self-medicate with vitamin combinations (OTC) without first consulting physician.

Preserved in tight, light-resistant containers at temperature 15° to 30°C (59° to 86°F). Avoid freezing.

Drug Interactions. Pyridoxine (in doses of 5 mg or more daily) appears to enhance the peripheral metabolism of **levodopa** and thus may greatly reduce or abolish its therapeutic effects; may decrease serum concentrations of phenobarbital and phenytoin. Pyridoxine requirements may be increased by INH, cycloserine, penicillamine, hydralazine, and oral contraceptives.

PYRIMETHAMINE

(Daraprim)

(peer-i-meth'a-meen)

Antiinfective

Antimalarial

Folic acid antagonist

ACTIONS AND USES. Long-acting folic acid antagonist chemically related to metabolite of chloroguanide. Selectively inhibits action of dehydrofolic reductate in parasite with resulting blockade of folic acid metabolism. Has no gametocidal activity, but prevents development of fertilized gametes in mosquito and thus helps to prevent transmission of malaria. Because action against blood-borne schizonts is slow in onset, has little value as single agent in treatment of acute primary malarial attack. Cross-resistance with chloroguanide may occur. Available in fixed combination with sulfadoxine (Fansidar).

Used for prophylaxis of malaria due to susceptible strains of plasmodia. May be used conjointly with fast-acting schizonticide (e.g., chloroquine, quinacrine, quinine) to initiate transmission control and suppressive cure. Used with a sulfonamide *(see above)* to provide synergistic action in treatment of toxoplasmosis.

P

ABSORPTION AND FATE. Well-absorbed from GI tract; peak plasma concentrations in about 2 hours. Concentrates mainly in kidneys, lungs, liver, spleen. Slowly excreted in urine; excretion may extend over 30 days or longer. Appears in breast milk.

CONTRAINDICATIONS AND PRECAUTIONS. Chloroguanide-resistant malaria. Safe use during pregnancy not established. *Cautious Use:* patients with convulsive disorders receiving high doses of an anticonvulsant (e.g., phenytoin).

ADVERSE/SIDE EFFECTS. With large doses or prolonged therapy: anorexia, vomiting, atrophic glossitis, skin rashes, folic acid deficiency (megaloblastic anemia, leukopenia, thrombocytopenia, pancytopenia, diarrhea). Acute toxicity: CNS stimulation including convulsions, respiratory failure.

ROUTE AND DOSAGE. Oral: *Malaria chemoprophylaxis:* **Adults and children (over 10 years):** 25 mg once weekly; **Children (4 through 10 years):** 12.5 mg once weekly; **Infants and children (under 4 years):** 6.25 mg once weekly. *Toxoplasmosis:* **Adults:** initial: 50 to 75 mg daily (together with 1 to 4 Gm of a sulfonamide) (or as combination product) for 1 to 3 weeks, depending on patient's tolerance and response; dosage may then be reduced by one-half for each drug and continued an additional 4 or 5 weeks. **Children:** 1 mg/kg/day divided into 2 equal daily doses (used together with sulfonamide); similar regimen as for adults.

NURSING IMPLICATIONS

GI distress may be minimized by taking drug with meals. If symptoms persist, dosage reduction may be necessary.

For malaria prophylaxis, drug should be taken on same day each week. Administration should begin when individual enters malarious area and should continue for 10 weeks after leaving the area.

Dosages required for treatment of toxoplasmosis approach toxic levels. Blood counts, including platelets, should be performed twice weekly during therapy. If hematologic abnormalities appear, dosage should be reduced or drug discontinued; parenteral leucovorin (folinic acid) (leucovorin rescue) will be administered until blood counts return to normal.

Some physicians prescribe leucovorin concurrently for patients on high-dosage therapy to prevent the hematologic complications of folic acid deficiency.

Food–Drug Interaction: Folic acid deficiency may occur with long-term use of pyrimethamine. Instruct patient to report symptoms: weakness, and pallor (from anemia), ulcerations of oral mucosa, superinfections, glossitis; GI disturbances such as diarrhea and poor fat absorption, fever. Folate (folinic acid) replacement may be prescribed. Encourage patient to increase food sources of folates (if allowed) in diet. *(See Index: Food sources.)*

Caution patient to keep drug out of reach of children. Fatalities from accidental poisoning have been reported.

Treatment of overdosage: gastric lavage: Have on hand parenteral short-acting barbiturate, leucovorin (folinic acid), and facilities for artificial respiration.

Drug Interactions. Antitoxoplasmic effects of pyrimethamine may be decreased by **folic acid** and **para-aminobenzoic acid.** Pyrimethamine may increase **quinine** blood levels (displaces quinine from plasma binding sites).

P

PYRVINIUM PAMOATE

(Pamovin, Povan, Vanquin)

(peer-vin′ee-um)
Antiinfective
Anthelmintic

ACTIONS AND USES. Cyanine dye. Appears to kill parasite by depleting carbohydrate stores; prevents parasite from using exogenous carbohydrate.

Used to control pinworm *(Enterobius vermicularis)* infestations. *Investigational Use:* treatment of strongyloidiasis.

ABSORPTION AND FATE. Not appreciably absorbed from GI tract. Approximately 60% of dose is excreted in feces; small amounts appear in urine, blood, bile.

CONTRAINDICATIONS AND PRECAUTIONS. Inflammatory conditions of GI tract, intestinal obstruction. Safe use during pregnancy not established. *Cautious Use:* children weighing less than 15 kg, renal or hepatic disease.

ADVERSE/SIDE EFFECTS. Nausea, vomiting, cramps, diarrhea, hypersensitivity reactions including photosensitivity, erythema multiforme, dizziness.

ROUTE AND DOSAGE. Oral: Adults, Children: 5 mg/kg body weight, as a single dose (maximum adult dosage 350 mg). If necessary, dose may be repeated in 2 to 3 weeks.

NURSING IMPLICATIONS

Administer drug before or after a meal.

Caution patient to swallow tablets whole or take emulsion form through straw to avoid staining teeth (bright red).

GI side effects appear to occur more frequently with emulsion than with tablets, as well as in older children and in adults receiving high dosages.

Inform the patient that drug will cause a harmless bright red staining of stools and vomitus and that suspension form will stain clothing if spilled.

Pyrvinium (Povan) tablets should not be used in individuals sensitive to aspirin because of possible cross-sensitivity between tartrazine in tablet coating, and aspirin. Suspension may be used.

When pinworm infection is found in a single member of a family or institutional group, treatment of all members should be considered.

Pinworms are transmitted by direct transfer of infective eggs on hands (from anus) to mouth, or indirectly by clothing, bedding, food, or other contaminated articles. Dust-borne infection by inhalation is also possible in heavily contaminated households.

Instruct patient and family in personal hygiene: wash hands (avoid sharing bar soap) after defecation and before eating or preparing foods; keep nails short and avoid biting nails; daily bathing (showers preferable to tub baths); change bed linen and underwear daily (eggs are destroyed by household washing solutions).

Follow-up examination for pinworm ova should be done at least 5 weeks after end of treatment. Specimens are best procured on arising in the morning, before bathing, breakfast, or defecation. Female worms lay eggs at night in perianal region. Specimen is obtained by applying cellulose tape swab to contaminated areas; they are then transferred to glass slide for microscopic examination.

Protect suspension form from light.

See also Index: Nursing Interventions: parasite infestations.

QUINACRINE HYDROCHLORIDE

(Atabrine)

(kwin′a-kreen)
Antiinfective
Anthelmintic

ACTIONS AND USES. Acridine dye derivative. Eradicates beef, pork, dwarf, and fish tapeworm and *Giardia lamblia* by causing worm scolex to detach from intestinal tract. Acts as suppressive agent and controls clinical attacks of malaria, but is not a true causal prophylactic agent, nor does it produce radical cure.

Used in treatment of tapeworm infestations and giardiasis. Use as antimalarial has been largely superseded by more effective and less toxic drugs.

ABSORPTION AND FATE. Readily absorbed from GI tract. Peak concentrations in plasma within 8 hours. Widely distributed in tissues, and accumulates when administered chronically. Concentrates in liver, lungs, pancreas, erythrocytes. Excreted slowly, primarily in urine; small amounts eliminated in sweat, saliva, bile, milk. Significant amounts still detectable in urine for at least 2 months after discontinuation of oral drug. Crosses placenta.

CONTRAINDICATIONS AND PRECAUTIONS. Psoriasis, porphyria, pregnancy, concomitant use of primaquine, intracavitary use in patients with pneumothorax, psoriasis, porphyria. *Cautious Use:* patients over age 60, children under 1 year, history of psychosis, hepatic disease, alcoholism, concomitant use with hepatotoxic drugs, patients with G6PD deficiency.

ADVERSE/SIDE EFFECTS. CNS stimulation: restlessness, confusion, irritability, emotional changes, insomnia, nightmares, psychotic reactions, convulsions (large doses). **Dermatologic:** yellow pigmentation, urticaria, exfoliative dermatitis, contact dermatitis, lichen-planus-like eruptions. **GI:** nausea, vomiting, anorexia, diarrhea, abdominal cramps. **Neuropsychiatric:** headache, dizziness, vertigo. **Other (usually with prolonged therapy):** aplastic anemia, agranulocytosis, hepatitis, corneal edema or deposits (reversible), retinopathy (rare), fever.

ROUTE AND DOSAGE. Oral: *Beef, pork or fish tapeworm:* **Adults and children (over 14 years):** 200 mg given 10 minutes apart for four doses; sodium bicarbonate 600 mg with each dose. **Children (5 to 10 years):** total dose 400 mg; **(11 to 14 years):** total dose 600 mg, divided into three or four doses administered 10 minutes apart; sodium bicarbonate 300 mg may be given with each dose. *Dwarf tapeworm:* **Adults:** 900 mg in three portions 20 minutes apart, then 100 mg three times daily for 3 days. **Children (4 to 8 years):** initial: 200 mg, then 100 mg after breakfast for 3 days; **(8 to 10 years):** initial: 300 mg, then 100 mg twice daily for 3 days; **(11 to 14 years):** initial: 400 mg, then 100 mg three times daily for 3 days. *Giardiasis:* **Adults:** 100 mg three times daily for 5 days. **Children:** 7 mg/kg/day in 3 divided doses (maximum 300 mg/day). *Malaria suppression:* **Adults:** 100 mg once daily. **Children:** 50 mg daily.

NURSING IMPLICATIONS

General Information:

Inform patients that drug imparts a reversible yellow coloration to skin (not jaundice) and urine (if acid) and sometimes may cause a grayish blue tinge to ears, nasal cartilage, and fingernail beds resembling cyanosis. Skin discoloration usually disappears in about 2 weeks after drug is discontinued.

Complete blood counts and ophthalmoscopic examinations should be done periodically in patients on prolonged drug therapy.

Advise patients to report immediately the onset of skin eruptions or visual disturbances; e.g., halos of light, focusing difficulties, blurred vision.

Be alert for symptoms of drug-induced behavioral changes and psychosis. Psychotic reactions may last 2 to 4 weeks after drug is stopped.

Caution patients to keep drug out of reach of children.

Tapeworm infestations:

Patient is given a bland liquid or no-residue semisolid, nonfat diet for 24 to 48 hours before start of drug therapy, with fasting after evening meal before and on morning of treatment.

Generally, a saline purge and cleansing enema are given before treatment to reduce amount of stool that must be examined for scolex. Saline purge is repeated 1 to 2 hours after quinacrine is administered. Sodium bicarbonate is prescribed with each dose of quinacrine to reduce tendency to nausea and vomiting.

Entire stool specimen is collected for 48 hours and passed through sieve or cheesecloth to find the scolex (worm head). Provide receptacle for toilet paper, which should not be put in bedpan. Search for scolex is facilitated by using ultraviolet light (worm becomes fluorescent when it absorbs quinacrine). Worm is usually passed within 4 to 10 hours, alive, stained yellow, in one piece or segmented. Cure is presumed if scolex of beef, pork, or fish tapeworm is found; dwarf tapeworm infestations are usually multiple and require more persistent treatment.

If scolex is not found, stools should be examined periodically; stools must be free of worm eggs or segments for 3 to 6 months to be certain of cure.

For pork tapeworm *(Taenia solium),* drug is administered by duodenal tube to prevent vomiting. Vomiting may cause passage of worm segments (proglottids) into stomach, with subsequent release of ova and invasion of tissue (cysticercosis).

Giardiasis:

Administer quinacrine after meals; stools are examined 2 weeks after last dose. Repeat course may be given, if indicated.

Antimalarial use:

Quinacrine should be taken after meals with a full glass of water, tea, or fruit juice.

For suppression of malaria, medication should be taken for 1 to 3 months.

Diagnostic Test Interferences. Possibility of false-positive **adrenal function tests** using Mattingly method (quinacrine is fluorescent in aqueous media).

Drug Interactions. Concurrent use of **alcohol** with quinacrine may result in disulfiram-like reaction (due to accumulation of acetaldehyde). Quinacrine enhances toxicity of **primaquine.**

QUINESTROL

(Estrovis)

(kwin-ess'trole)
Estrogen
Hormone

ACTIONS AND USES. Long-lasting orally effective estrogen derived from ethinyl estradiol. Actions, uses, contraindications, and adverse reactions similar to those of estradiol (qv).

CONTRAINDICATIONS AND PRECAUTIONS. Thrombophlebitis, cancer of breast. *Cautious Use:* hypertension, diabetes mellitus. *See also Estradiol.*

ADVERSE/SIDE EFFECTS. CNS: headache, dizziness, depression. **CV:** thromboembolism, increased risk of stroke, pulmonary edema, myocardial infaction. **EENT:** intolerance to contact lenses. **GI:** nausea, vomiting, abdominal cramps, anorexia. **Hepatic:** cholestatic jaundice. **Other:** hyperglycemia, hypercalcemia, folic acid deficiency, leg cramps, purpura. *See also Estradiol.*

ROUTE AND DOSAGE. Oral: initial: 100 mcg once daily for 7 days. Maintenance: 100 mcg weekly (1 tablet) beginning 2 weeks after inception of treatment. Dose may be increased to 200 mcg/week if necessary.

NURSING IMPLICATIONS

Advise the diabetic patient to report altered blood and urine glucose tests. Estrogen activity may increase requirement for hypoglycemic medication.

Explain to patient receiving quinestrol for postmenopausal symptoms that menstrual-like bleeding may occur, but does not indicate return of fertility.
Teach or reinforce previous teaching of self-examination of the breast.
Attempts to discontinue or taper medication should be made at 3- to 6-month intervals.
Urge patient to read package insert to assure understanding of estrogen therapy.
Store at temperature between 15° and 30°C (59° and 86°F) in a tightly capped container.
See Estradiol (prototype estrogen).

QUINETHAZONE

(Aquamox, Hydromox)

(kwin-eth'a-zone)
Diuretic, antihypertensive
Sulfonamide

ACTIONS AND USES. Sulfonamide derivative diuretic, with structural and pharmacologic properties similar to those of the thiazides. Inhibits renal tubular reabsorption of Na, chloride, and to a lesser degree, K thus promoting excretion of the electrolytes with an accompanying volume of water. Antihypertensive effect may result from the diuresis and Na loss, and/or possibly from decreased peripheral resistance. Available in fixed combination with reserpine (Hydromox R).

Used with other antihypertensives to enhance effect, to treat edema associated with congestive heart failure, and renal pathology. *See Chlorothiazide.*

ABSORPTION AND FATE. Rapidly absorbed from GI tract. Diuretic effect begins in 2 hours, peaks in 6 hours and continues for 18 to 24 hours. Excreted unchanged in urine. Crosses placenta and appears in breast milk.

CONTRAINDICATIONS AND PRECAUTIONS. Anuria, hypersensitivity to sulfonamide-derived drugs, pregnancy, lactation. *Cautious Use:* history of allergy, renal and hepatic disease, gout, diabetes mellitus, sympathectomy. *See also Chlorothiazide.*

ADVERSE/SIDE EFFECTS. Hypokalemia, hyperuricemia, hyperglycemia, orthostatic hypotension, exacerbation of SLE, photosensitivity, yellow vision, agranulocytosis. *See also Chlorothiazide.*

ROUTE AND DOSAGE. Oral: Adult: 50 to 100 mg once daily. *Dose limit:* up to 200 mg/day in divided doses.

NURSING IMPLICATIONS

Administer drug early in AM after eating (to reduce gastric irritation) and to prevent interrupted sleep because of diuresis. If 2 doses are ordered, schedule second dose no later than 3 PM.
Antihypertensive effects may be noted in 3 to 4 days; maximal effects may require 3 to 4 weeks.
Sensitivity reactions are more apt to occur in patients with a history of allergy or bronchial asthma.
Potassium depletion is a possibility. As a preventive measure, urge patient to include specific sources of K in daily diet such as a banana (about 370 mg K) and at least 6 ounces orange juice (about 330 mg K). Other K-rich foods include whole grain cereals, fruits, vegetables such as potatoes, carrots, broccoli, nuts, meat.

Counsel patient to avoid OTC drugs unless approved by the physician. Many preparations contain both K and Na and if misused, or if patient overdoses, electrolyte imbalance side effects may be intensified.

Asymptomatic hyperuricemia can be produced because of interference with uric acid excretion, although acute gout is rarely precipitated. Report joint pain (especially at night) and limitation of motion. A patient with history of gout may be continued on quinethazone with adjusted doses of a uricosuric agent.

Monitor blood pressure and intake–output ratio and pattern during first phase of antihypertensive therapy. Report a sudden fall in BP which may initiate severe postural hypotension and potentially dangerous perfusion problems, especially in the extremities.

Instruct patient to weigh self daily. Consult physician about acceptable range of weight change. Report sudden gain of 2 or more pounds within 2 to 3 days.

Store tablets in tightly closed container at temperature between 15° and 30°C (59° and 86°F) unless otherwise specified by the manufacturer.

See Chlorothiazide (prototype thiazide diuretic).

QUINIDINE GLUCONATE

(Duraquin, Quinaglute Dura-Tabs, Quinatime, Quin-Release, Quinate)

(kwin'i-deen)
Cardiac depressant
Antiarrhythmic

ACTIONS AND USES. Dextro isomer of quinine; Group I-A antiarrhythmic agent. Similar to quinidine sulfate (qv) in actions, uses, contraindications, and adverse reactions. Parenteral form used when oral therapy not feasible or when rapid effects are required. Contains 62.3% anhydrous quinidine alkaloid base.

ABSORPTION AND FATE. Onset of action in 15 minutes following IM injection; peak effect in 30 to 90 minutes; duration of action 6 to 8 hours. Protein binding: 60 to 80%; half-life: 6 to 7 hours (prolonged by hepatic dysfunction and in the elderly). Excreted in urine. Crosses placenta; enters breast milk.

CONTRAINDICATIONS AND PRECAUTIONS. Safe use during pregnancy (category C), during lactation, and by children not established. *See Quinidine sulfate.*

ADVERSE/SIDE EFFECTS. Particularly with IV use: nausea, vomiting, abdominal cramps, urge to defecate or urinate, cold sweat, apprehension, severe hypotension. *See Quinidine sulfate.*

ROUTE AND DOSAGE. *Highly individualized.* **Oral (maintenance and prophylaxis):** extended-release form, 1 or 2 tablets every 12 hours, or every 8 hours. Each tablet contains 324 mg quinidine gluconate. **Intramuscular (acute tachycardia):** initial: 600 mg; subsequently 400 mg may be repeated as often as every 2 hours, depending on need and response of patient. **Intravenous:** 200 to 750 mg. Suggested rate of administration: 1 ml/minute.

NURSING IMPLICATIONS

Instruct patient not to crush or chew tablet before swallowing.

Examine parenteral solution before preparation; use only if clear and colorless.

Some physicians give an initial test dose (50 to 200 mg IM) or 1 tablet po to determine sensitivity. If positive, patient will display symptoms of cinchonism: tinnitus, headache, nausea, visual disturbances, particularly if patient has not received quinidine before and if time permits.

Continuous monitoring of ECG and blood pressure and frequent determinations of plasma quinidine levels are advised when drug is administered intravenously.
Observe monitor before administration of each parenteral dose.
The following are indications to stop quinidine; report their onset immediately to physician: (1) worsening of minor side effects; (2) restoration of sinus rhythm; (3) prolongation of QRS complex (beyond 25%); (4) changes in QT or refractory period; (5) disappearance of P waves; (6) sudden onset of or increase in PVCs; (7) decrease in heart rate to 120 beats/minute.
When administering drug IM, aspirate carefully before injection to avoid inadvertent entry into blood vessel.
Severe hypotension is most likely to occur in patients receiving drug IV. Supine position during drug administration is advisable.
Observe patient closely following each parenteral dose. Amount of subsequent dose is gauged by response to preceding dose.
Extended-action tablet is used only for maintenance and prophylactic therapy. Advise patient to swallow tablet whole.
Quinidine plasma levels are generally higher when oral dose is given on an empty stomach (i.e., 1 hour before or 2 hours after meals). GI distress may be minimized by administration of oral drug with food, however.
Oral quinidine gluconate is considerably more expensive than quinidine sulfate.
Protect solutions from light and heat to prevent brownish discoloration and possibly precipitation.
See also Quinidine sulfate.

QUINIDINE POLYGALACTURONATE
(Cardioquin)

(kwin'i-deen)
Antiarrhythmic

ACTIONS AND USES. Reported to have lower incidence of GI irritation than quinidine sulfate (qv). Peak plasma level achieved within 6 hours after dose; duration of action: 6 to 8 hours.

ROUTE AND DOSAGE. Oral: initial: 1 to 3 tablets every 3 or 4 hours for four or more doses. (Each 275-mg tablet equivalent to 200 mg of quinidine sulfate); maintenance: 1 tablet two or three times a day.

Q

NURSING IMPLICATIONS

See Quinidine sulfate.

QUINIDINE SULFATE
(Cin-Quin, Quinidex Exstentabs, Quinora, SK-Quinidine Sulfate)

(kwin'i-deen sul-fate)
Antiarrhythmic

ACTIONS AND USES. Dextro isomer of quinine and alkaloid of *Cinchona.* Group I-A antiarrhythmic. Like quinine, exhibits some antimalarial, antipyretic, and oxytocic properties. Contains 83% anhydrous quinidine alkaloid. Cardiac actions similar to those of procainamide. At the cellular level, decreases sodium influx during depolarization and potassium efflux in repolarization; also reduces calcium transport across cell membrane. Depresses myocardial excitability, contractility, automaticity, and conduction velocity, and prolongs effective refractory period. Anticholinergic action blocks vagal stimulation of AV node, thus tending to increase ventricular rate, particularly in larger doses. Also exerts muscle relaxant action by decreasing effective transmission across neuromuscular junction. Hypotensive effect is produced primarily by peripheral vasodilation and in part by alpha-adrenergic blockade.

Used in treatment of premature atrial, AV junctional, and ventricular contraction; paroxysmal atrial tachycardia, chronic ventricular tachycardia (when not associated with complete heart block); maintenance therapy after electrical conversion of atrial fibrillation or flutter.

ABSORPTION AND FATE. Almost completely absorbed following oral administration. Peak plasma level within ½ to 1 hour; persisting 6 to 8 hours or more; (about 12 hours for extended-release form). Widely distributed in body tissues, except brain. At therapeutic serum levels (3 to 6 mcg/ml) about 60 to 80% strongly bound to plasma albumin. Unbound fraction is increased in hepatic insufficiency. Accumulation occurs in most tissues except brain. Plasma half-life: 4 to 10 hours (prolonged in congestive heart failure and in the elderly). Metabolized in liver. Approximately 10 to 30% excreted in urine within 24 hours as unchanged drug, and remainder as metabolites. Urinary pH influences excretion rate (alkalinization decreases and acidification increases excretion).

CONTRAINDICATIONS AND PRECAUTIONS. Hypersensitivity or idiosyncrasy to quinidine or *Cinchona* derivatives; safe use during pregnancy (category C), during lactation, or in children not established. Thrombocytopenic purpura resulting from prior use of quinidine, intraventricular conduction defects, complete AV block, ectopic impulses and rhythms due to escape mechanisms, thyrotoxicosis, acute rheumatic fever, subacute bacterial endocarditis, extensive myocardial damage, frank congestive heart failure, hypotensive states, myasthenia gravis, digitalis intoxication. *Cautious Use:* incomplete heart block, impaired renal or hepatic function, bronchial asthma or other respiratory disorders, myasthenia gravis, potassium imbalance.

ADVERSE/SIDE EFFECTS. CNS: headache, fever, tremors, apprehension, dilirium, syncope with sudden loss of consciousness, and ventricular arrhythmias, disturbed hearing (tinnitus, auditory acuity). **CV:** hypotension, congestive heart failure, widened QPS complex, bradycardia, heart block, atrial flutter, ventricular flutter, fibrillation or tachycardia; quinidine syncope. **Dermatologic:** rash, urticaria, cutaneous flushing with intense pruritus, photosensitivity. **GI:** nausea, vomiting, diarrhea, abdominal pain, hepatic dysfunction. **Hematologic:** acute hemolytic anemia, hypoprothrombinemia, thrombocytopenic purpura (rare), leukopenia, agranulocytosis (rare). **Hypersensitivity or idiosyncrasy:** may include symptoms of cinchonism plus angioedema, acute asthma, respiratory depression, vascular collapse. **Ophthalmic:** mydriasis, blurred vision, disturbed color perception, reduced visual field, photophobia, diplopia, night blindness, scotomata, optic neuritis. **Other:** SLE; *Cinchonism:* nausea, vomiting, headache, dizziness, fever, tremors, vertigo, tinnitus, visual disturbances. **Overdosage:** hypokalemia, cinchonism, tachyarrhythmias, seizures.

ROUTE AND DOSAGE. Dosages individualized according to patient's requirements and responses. **Oral: Adults:** *Test dose:* **Intramuscular:** 200 mg. **Oral:** *Ectopic beats:* 200 to 300 mg three or four times daily. *Ventricular tachycardia:* 400 to 600 mg every 2 or 3 hours until paroxysms terminate. *Atrial flutter:* patient digitalized before receiving quinidine; highly individualized dosage. *Atrial fibrillation* (various schedules): 200 mg every 2 or 3 hours for 5 to 8 doses; subsequent daily increase of individual dose until sinus rhythm restored or toxic effects intervene (ventricular rate and/or congestive failure controlled by digitalis prior to quinidine therapy). Total daily dose not to exceed 3 to 4 Gm. Maintenance: 200 to 300 mg three or four times daily at 6-hour intervals. Sustained-release forms: 300 to 600 mg every 8 to 12 hours. **Children:** *Test dose:* 2 mg/kg. *Therapeutic dose:* 6 mg/kg five times daily.

NURSING IMPLICATIONS

Test dose is used by some physicians to determine idiosyncrasy before establishing full dosage schedule.

For optimum absorption, quinidine is taken preferably with a full glass of water on an empty stomach (i.e., 1 hour before or 2 hours after meals). If GI symptoms occur (nausea, vomiting, diarrhea are most common), administer drug with food.

Sustained-release tablet is usually reserved for maintenance and prophylactic therapy.

Continuous monitoring of ECG and blood pressure is required. Close observation of patient (check sensorium and be alert for any sign of toxicity) and frequent determinations of plasma quinidine concentrations are indicated when large doses (more than 2 Gm/day) are used or when quinidine is given parenterally (e.g., quinidine gluconate).

Observe cardiac monitor and report immediately the following conversion to cardiotoxic effects: (1) sinus rhythm; (2) widening QRS complex in excess of 25% (i.e., greater than 0.12 seconds); (3) changes in QT interval or refractory period; (4) disappearance of P waves; (5) sudden onset of or increase in ectopic ventricular beats (extrasystoles, PVCs); (6) decrease in heart rate to 120 beats/minute. Also report immediately any worsening of minor side effects. All are indications for stopping quinidine, at least temporarily.

Dosage is adjusted to maintain plasma concentration between 3 and 6 mcg/ml. Levels of 8 mcg/L or more are associated with myocardial toxicity.

During acute treatment, monitor vital signs every 1 to 2 hours (frequency depends on individual patient requirements and dosage used). Count apical pulse for a full minute. Report any change in pulse rate, rhythm, or quality or any fall in blood pressure.

Severe hypotension is most likely to occur in patients receiving high oral doses or parenteral quinidine.

Reversion to sinus rhythm in long-standing fibrillation, or when complicated by congestive failure, involves some risk of embolization from dislodgement of atrial mural emboli.

Quinidine can cause unpredictable rhythm abnormalities in the digitalized heart. Patients with atrial flutter or fibrillation may be pretreated with digitalis (until ventricular rate is 100 bpm) to increase AV nodal block and thus reduce possibility of paradoxic tachycardia.

Monitor intake and output. Diarrhea occurs commonly during early therapy; most patients become tolerant to this side effect. If symptoms become severe, serum electrolytes and acid–base, and fluid balance should be evaluated. Dosage adjustment may be required.

During long-term therapy, periodic blood counts, serum electrolyte determinations, and kidney and liver function tests are advised.

Food–Drug Interaction: A diet high in alkaline ash foods (vegetables, citrus fruit, milk) renders urine alkaline may prolong half-life of quinidine by decreasing its excretion and increasing danger of toxicity. Advise patient to eat a balanced diet: i.e., no excesses in fruit or fruit juices, milk, or a vegetarian diet.

Hypersensitivity reactions usually appear 3 to 20 days after drug is started. Fever occurs commonly and may or may not be accompanied by other symptoms.

Instruct patient to report feeling of faintness ("quinidine syncope") caused by quinidine-induced changes in ventricular rhythm resulting in decreased cardiac output and syncope.

Advise patient not to self-medicate with OTC drugs without advice from physician.

Discuss medication schedule with patient. Advise patient not to increase, decrease, skip, or discontinue doses without consulting physician.

Also advise patient to notify physician immediately of disturbances in vision, ringing in ears, sense of breathlessness, onset of palpitation, and unpleasant sensation in chest and to note time of occurrence and duration of chest symptoms.

Overdosage Treatment: Induce vomiting or give lavage; charcoal (even many hours after ingestion because of quinidine long half-life). Monitor CV status. Prepare for seizures (IV diazepam); sodium bicarbonate IV, adrenergic stimulants; hemodialysis or resin hemoperfusion.

Patient-Teaching Points Should Be Included in the Discharge Plan (Consult Physician):

- ✓ Reason for taking drug.
- ✓ Specific dosage schedule.
- ✓ Use of calendar check-off sheet when dose is taken.
- ✓ Symptoms to report.
- ✓ Allowable planned physical activities.
- ✓ Importance of spaced rest periods.
- ✓ Diet and weight control.
- ✓ Things to avoid, e.g., fatigue, excessive caffeine (coffee, tea, cola), alcohol, smoking, heavy meals, (avoid excessive citrus juices) stressful situations, OTC medications (unless approved by physician).
- ✓ Advisability of wearing medical identification such as Medic-Alert.

Preserve in tight, light-resistant containers away from excessive heat.

Diagnostic Test Interferences. Possibility of false increases in **urinary catecholamines** (using Sobel and Henry modification of trihydroxyindole method); quinidine may also interfere with **urinary steroid (17-OHCS)** determinations made with the Reddy, Jenkins, Thorn procedure.

Drug Interactions: Quinidine sulfate

Plus	Interactions
Antiarrhythmics (other)	Additive cardiac depressant effects
Phenothiazines, reserpine	
Anticholinergic blocking agents	Additive vagolytic effect
Anticoagulants: coumarins	Decreased prothrombin levels and clotting factor concentrations possibly resulting in hemorrhage
Anticonvulsant (hydantoins): Phenobarbital, Rifampin	Quinidine half-life shortened by up to 50%; dose adjustment of quinidine may be necessary when adding any one of these agents to quinidine regimen
Carbonic anhydrase inhibitors: Sodium bicarbonate, Thiazide diuretics, Antacids	Prolonged half-life of quinidine leading to decreased excretion and increased potential for toxicity
Cholinergics	Antagonized by quinidine
Digoxin	Increased digoxin levels leading to necessity to decrease dose of digoxin or use another antiarrhythmic
Nifedipine	Decreased quinidine serum concentrations with breakthrough ventricular tachycardia
Skeletal muscle relaxants (e.g., tubocurarine, decamethonium, succinylcholine)	Potentiates neuromuscular blocking effects in ventilatory depression of patient receiving relaxants
Verapamil	Significant hypotensive effects

Q

QUININE SULFATE

(kwye'nine)

(Novoquinine, Quinamm, Quine, Quinite, Quiphile, Strema)

Antiinfective, antimalarial

ACTIONS AND USES. Chief alkaloid from bark of cinchoma tree. Exact mechanism of antimalarial action uncertain. Inhibits protein synthesis, and depresses many enzyme systems in malaria parasite. Has schizonticidal action and is gametocidal with *Plasmodium vivax* and *P. malariae,* but not *P. falciparum.* Resembles salicylates in analgesic and antipyretic properties, and exerts curarelike skeletal-muscle relaxant effect. Also has oxytocic action and hypoprothrombinemic effect. Qualitatively similar to quinidine in cardiovascular effects. Generally replaced by less toxic and more effective agents in treatment of malaria.

Used for treatment of chloroquine-resistant falciparum malaria and in combination with other antimalarials for radical cure of relapsing vivax malaria; also used for relief of nocturnal recumbancy leg cramps.

ABSORPTION AND FATE. Rapidly and completely absorbed from GI tract. Peak plasma concentrations in 1 to 3 hours. Oral dose of 1 Gm/day produces therapeutic plasma concentration of 7 mcg/ml. Approximately 70% bound to plasma proteins. Plasma half-life: 4 to 5 hours. Metabolized primarily in liver. Excreted in urine in about 24 hours, mostly as inactive metabolites; small amount eliminated in saliva, gastric juice, bile, and feces. Renal excretion is decreased when urine is alkaline. Crosses placenta. Dialyzable by hemodialysis and by hemoperfusion.

CONTRAINDICATIONS AND PRECAUTIONS. Hypersensitivity or idiosyncrasy to quinine, patients with tinnitus, optic neuritis, myasthenia gravis, G6PD deficiency, pregnancy (category X). *Cautious Use:* cardiac arrhythmias. Same precautions as for quinidine when used in patients with cardiovascular conditions.

ADVERSE/SIDE EFFECTS. **Cinchonism:** tinnitus, decreased auditory acuity, dizziness, vertigo, headache, visual impairment, nausea, vomiting, diarrhea, fever. **CNS:** confusion, excitement, apprehension, syncope, delirium. **CV:** angina. **Hematologic:** leukopenia, thrombocytopenia, agranulocytosis, hypoprothrombinemia, hemolytic anemia. **Hypersensitivity:** cutaneous flushing, visual impairment, pruritus, skin rash, fever, gastric distress, dyspnea, tinnitus. **Toxicity:** decrease in blood pressure and respiration, tachycardia, hypothermia, convulsions, cardiovascular collapse, coma, blackwater fever (extensive intravascular hemolysis with renal failure), death. **Other:** urticaria, acute asthma.

ROUTE AND DOSAGE. **Oral:** **Adults:** 650 mg every 8 hours for 10 to 14 days. **Children:** 25 mg/kg/day in divided doses every 8 hours for 10 to 14 days. *Nocturnal leg cramps:* 260 to 300 mg at bedtime or after evening meal.

NURSING IMPLICATIONS

Administer drug with or after meals or a snack to minimize gastric irritation. Quinine has potent local irritant effect on gastric mucosa. Advise patients not to crush capsule; drug is not only irritating but also extremely bitter.

Patients should be informed about possible adverse reactions and advised to report promptly the onset of any unusual symptom.

Be alert to rising plasma concentration of quinine: tinnitus and hearing impairment usually do not occur until concentration is 10 mcg/ml or more.

Treatment of overdosage: Prompt emesis or gastric lavage is imperative because drug is rapidly absorbed; oxygen, support of respiration, and blood pressure.

Preserved in tight, light-resistant containers.

Diagnostic Test Interferences. Quinine may interfere with determinations of **urinary catecholamines** (Sobel and Henry modification procedure) and **urinary steroids** (17-hydroxycorticosteroids) (modification of Reddy, Jenkins, Thorn method).

Drug Interactions. Quinine absorption from GI tract may be delayed by **aluminum containing antacids.** Quinine enhances hypoprothrombinemic action of **oral anticoagulants** and may decrease anticoagulant action of **heparin.** Excessive quinine blood levels may result from concomitant use of **pyrimethamine,** or **quinidine** or urinary alkalizers (e.g., acetozolamide) (decrease urinary excretion of quinine). Use of quinine with **skeletal muscle relaxants** may prolong respiratory depression and apnea.

R

RANITIDINE HYDROCHLORIDE

(Zantac)

(ra-nye'te-deen)
Antihistamine
H_2-receptor antagonist
Enzyme inhibitor

ACTIONS AND USES. A potent antiulcer drug that competitively and reversibly inhibits histamine action at H_2-receptor sites on parietal cells. Blocks daytime and nocturnal basal gastric acid secretion stimulated by histamine and reduces gastric acid release in response to food, pentogastrin, and insulin. Indirectly reduces pepsin secretion but appears to have minimal effect on fasting and postprandial serum gastrin concentrations, or secretion of gastric intrinsic factor or mucus. Increases gastric bacterial flora (nitrate-reducing organisms), reduces hepatic blood flow and delays gastric emptying, but clinical significance of these actions is unclear. Lacks antiandrogenic activity and does not appear to alter mean daily insulin requirement in patients with type I (IDDM) diabetes mellitus. Does not interact with hepatic cytochrome P450 (microsomal) enzyme system; therefore drug interaction potential is minimal; can be given with drugs metabolized by oxidation in the liver without concern for interference with their clearance, e.g., phenytoin, warfarin, theophylline, diazepam, propranolol. It is not known whether ranitidine alters ulcer recurrence rates; however, it appears that the clinical response it produces outlasts that of cimetidine (H_2-receptor inhibitor), permitting a twice daily regimen.

Used for short-term treatment of active duodenal ulcer; to treat pathologic GI hypersecretory conditions (e.g., Zollinger-Ellison syndrome, systemic mastocytosis, and postoperative hypersecretion), and "short-gut" syndrome.

ABSORPTION AND FATE. Absorption rate following 150 mg oral does is slow but constant, promoting maintenance of blood levels for up to 8 hours. Bioavailability is low (50%); peak levels of 440 to 545 ng/ml reached in 2 to 3 hours; duration of action: 8 to 12 hours. Half-life: 2 to 3 hours. Minimal penetration of CSF. Excreted in the urine with 30% dose collected in the urine as unchanged drug in 24 hours. Metabolites make up 6% of dose; remainder is found in the stool. Secreted in human milk; removed by hemodialysis.

CONTRAINDICATIONS AND PRECAUTIONS. Known hypersensitivity to ranitidine. Safe use during pregnancy (category B), lactation, and in children under age 12 not established. *Cautious Use:* hepatic and renal dysfunction.

ADVERSE/SIDE EFFECTS. (Generally infrequent) **CV:** (rare): tachycardia, bradycardia, PVCs. **GI:** constipation, nausea, abdominal pain, diarrhea; hepatotoxicity (rare). **CNS:** headache, malaise, dizziness, somnolence, insomnia, vertigo. Rare: mental confusion, agitation, depression, hallucinations in elderly patients; increased intraocular pressure (ocluar pain, blurred vision). **Reproductive:** (rare): gynecomastia, impotence. **Other:** rash, reversible decreases in WBC and platelet counts (clinically unimportant); hypersensitivity reactions, anaphylaxis (rare).

ROUTE AND DOSAGE. Oral: Adult: *Duodenal ulcer:* 150 mg twice daily (smaller doses may be as effective). Pathologic hypersecretory conditions: 150 mg twice daily. Doses up to 6.3 Gm/day have been employed in patients with severe disease. Adjust doses in patient with impaired renal function.

NURSING IMPLICATIONS

Simultaneous administration of food or low dose antacids (neutralizing capacity of 10 to 15 mEq HCl/10 ml) does not appear to reduce ranitidine absorption or serum concentrations.

It has been shown that to inhibit 50% of the stimulated gastric acid secretion, serum concentrations of ranitidine need to be 36 to 94 ng/ml. Concentrations in this range are maintained after a 150 mg dose for up to 12 hours.

If patient is having hemodialysis treatments, the scheduled ranitidine dose should coincide with the end of hemodialysis.

Long duration of action provides ulcer pain relief that is maintained through the night as well as the day.

Adjunctive antacid treatment of pain may be necessary and can be given without affecting action of ranitidine. Administer the antacid 2 hours before or after ranitidine.

Endoscopic examination is usually performed at end of 2 weeks of therapy because about 37% of patients have been completely healed in that time.

Most patients have healed ulcers by 4 weeks; however, if healing cannot be confirmed endoscopically, treatment may be continued for up to 8 weeks.

Even if symptomatic relief is provided by ranitidine, this should not be interpreted as absence of gastric malignancy. Follow-up examinations will be scheduled after therapy is discontinued.

The potential for toxicity resulting from decreased clearance (elimination) and therefore prolonged action, is greatest in the elderly patient or the patient with hepatic or renal dysfunction.

The incidence of hepatotoxicity is low (and thought to be a hypersensitivity reaction), but be alert to early signs: jaundice (dark urine, pruritus, yellow sclera and skin), elevated transaminases (especially ALT) and LDH.

Onset of jaundice may lack subjective symptoms and since a family member ordinarily recognizes it quicker than the patient, discuss these possible symptoms with patient and family. Urge adherence to scheduled periodic laboratory checkups during ranitidine treatment.

Creatinine clearance is monitored if renal dysfunction is present or suspected. When clearance is less than 50 ml/min, manufacturer recommends reduction of the dose to 150 mg once every 24 hours with cautious and gradual reduction of the interval to every 12 hours or less, if necessary.

Instruct patient not to supplement therapy with OTC remedies for gastric distress or pain without physician's advice (e.g., Mylanta II reduces ranitidine absorption).

Smoking–Drug Interaction: Smoking has been shown to decrease ranitidine efficacy and adversely affect ulcer healing, i.e., it has been associated with increased frequency of duodenal ulcers and decreased rate of ulcer healing. Smoking itself, rather than the number of cigarettes smoked per day, is the key factor. Urge patient to stop smoking, informing him or her that giving it up may be more important in preventing ulcer recurrence than the medication.

Food–Drug Interaction: Long-term ranitidine therapy may lead to vitamin B_{12} deficiency.

Overdosage is treated by removing unabsorbed drug from GI tract (emesis, lavage), clinical monitoring, supportive treatment and hemodialysis if necessary.

Store tablets in light-resistant, tightly capped container at controlled room temperature in a dry place.

Drug Test Interferences. Ranitidine may produce slight elevations in **serum creatinine** (without concurrent increase in BUN); (rare) increases in **AST (SGOT), ALT (SGPT), alkaline phosphatase, LDH** and total **bilirubin.** Produces false-positive tests for **urine protein** with Multistix (use sulphosalicylic acid instead).

Drug Interactions. Propantheline delays absorption and increases peak concentration of ranitidine, thus increasing its bioavailability.

RAUWOLFIA SERPENTINA

(Hiwolfia, Raudixin, Raufola, Rauserpin, Rauval, Rauverid, Serfolia, Wolfina, and others)

(rah-wool'fee-a ser-pen-tee'na)
Antihypertensive
Antipsychotic
Rauwolfia alkaloid

ACTIONS AND USES. Powdered whole root of *Rauwolfia serpentina.* Contains reserpine (among other rauwolfia alkaloids) which is responsible for about half of its total activity. Actions, uses, contraindications, precautions, and adverse reactions are essentially the same as those of reserpine (qv).

Used in treatment of mild to moderate hypertension and adjunctive therapy with other antihypertensive agents for the more severe forms. Also has been used to relieve symptoms in selected patients in agitated psychotic states. Commercially available in fixed-dose combination with bendroflumethiazide (Rauzide).

ABSORPTION AND FATE. Crosses placenta; appears in breast milk. *See Reserpine.*

R

CONTRAINDICATIONS AND PRECAUTIONS. Hypersensitivity to rauwolfia alkaloids; mental depression, acute peptic ulcer, acute ulcerative colitis, patients receiving electroconvulsive therapy, bronchial asthma or other allergies, other respiratory problems, pheochromocytoma. Safe use in women of childbearing potential, during pregnancy, and in nursing women and children not established. *Cautious Use:* Impaired renal function, epilepsy, gallstones, severe cardiac or cardiovascular disease.

ADVERSE/SIDE EFFECTS. CNS: mental depression, drowsiness, dizziness, nervousness, lethargy, vivid dreams, nightmares. **CV:** bradycardia, edema, excessive hypotension, cutaneous flushing (overdosage). **EENT:** nasal stuffiness, epistaxis, dry mouth. **GI:** nausea, vomiting, reactivation of peptic ulcer (hypersecretion), increased appetite. **Hypersensitivity:** pruritus, rash. **Other:** impotence, decreased sexual interest; weight gain. *See also Reserpine.*

ROUTE AND DOSAGE. Oral: initial: 200 to 400 mg daily as single dose or in 2 divided doses; maintenance: 50 to 300 mg/day in single or two divided doses.

NURSING IMPLICATIONS

Administer with meals or with milk or other food to minimize possibility of gastric irritation.

Withdrawal of rauwolfia derivatives prior to surgery is not considered necessary. However, anesthesiologist should be informed that patient is receiving such therapy.

Record blood pressure and pulse at intervals prescribed by physician. Compare readings with baseline determinations and keep physician informed. Antihypertensive effect is commonly associated with bradycardia.

Because rauwolfia preparations are cumulative in action, dosage adjustments, when necessary, are usually made at 7- to 14-day intervals.

Mental depression can be sufficiently severe to lead to suicide. It may not appear until after 2 to 8 months of therapy and may last for several months after drug is withdrawn. Instruct patient and responsible family members to report beginning symptoms of depression; early morning insomnia, nightmares or vivid dreams, impotence or decreased sexual interest, self deprecation, mood swings, despondency, loss of appetite. Hospitalization may be necessary.

Advise patient to record weight and to check for edema daily. A gain of 3 to 5 pounds in 1 week should be reported to physician.

Orthostatic hypotension occurs infrequently with usual oral doses. Instruct patient to report symptoms of dizziness, lightheadedness to physician. Dosage reduction may be indicated. Advise patient to make position changes slowly, particularly from recumbent to upright posture and to lie down or sit down (head-low position) if patient feels faint. Also advise patient not to take hot showers or tub bath, to avoid hot environments, and not to stand still for prolonged periods.

Mouth dryness may be relieved by frequent rinsing with warm water, increase in noncaloric fluid intake, if allowed, particularly if fluid intake has been inadequate, sugarless gum, or lemon drops. If these measures fail, a saliva substitute may help (e.g., Moi-stir). Consult physician.

Advise patient not to take OTC drug without prior approval of physician. Many medications for nasal congestion, colds, hay fever, or other allergies contain sympathomimetic agents that may interfere with the effects of rauwolfia derivatives.

Warn patient that drug may enhance depressant effects of alcohol, barbiturates, and other CNS depressants, and to consult physician before taking these drugs.

Advise patient to avoid driving and other potentially hazardous activities until reaction to drug is determined.

Certain formulations, e.g., Raudixin, Rauserpin, contain tartrazine which may cause an allergic-type reaction in certain individuals. Such persons have aspirin hypersensitivity.

Store in tightly covered light-resistant container preferably between 15° and 30°C (59° and 86°F) unless otherwise directed by manufacturer.

See Reserpine: prototype rauwolfia alkaloid.

RESCINNAMINE

(Moderil)

(re-sin'a-meen)
Antihypertensive
Antipsychotic
Rauwolfia alkaloid

ACTIONS AND USES. Extracted from *Rauwolfia serpentina* and other *Rauwolfia* alkaloids. Actions, contraindications, precautions, and adverse reactions as for reserpine (qv). Sedation and bradycardia may occur less frequently and in milder form than with reserpine.

Used for treatment of mild essential hypertension; used as adjunct with other antihypertensive agents for the more severe forms.

ABSORPTION AND FATE. *See Reserpine.*

CONTRAINDICATIONS AND PRECAUTIONS. Hypersensitivity to rauwolfia alkaloids, history of mental depression, acute peptic ulcer, acute ulcerative colitis, patients receiving electroconvulsive therapy. *See also Reserpine.*

ADVERSE/SIDE EFFECTS. CNS: drowsiness, sedation, nervousness, anxiety, nightmares, mental depression, dizziness, headache, extrapyramidal tract symptoms. **CV:** excessive hypotension, bradycardia, anginalike symptoms. **EENT:** nasal congestion, conjunctival injection, dry mouth or increased salivation. **GI:** nausea, vomiting, diarrhea, reactivation of peptic ulcer, hypersecretion. **Hypersensitivity:** pruritus, rash. **Other:** muscle aches, impotence, dysuria, purpura. *See also Reserpine.*

ROUTE AND DOSAGE. Oral: initial: 0.5 mg twice daily up to 2 weeks, increased gradually if necessary; maintenance: 0.25 to 0.5 mg daily.

NURSING IMPLICATIONS

Administered with meals or with milk or other foods to minimize gastric irritation.

Since rescinnamine has a slow onset of action and a sustained duration of effects, dosage adjustments when necessary are usually made at 7- to 14-day intervals.

Take blood pressure and pulse at intervals prescribed by physician. Blood pressure lowering may be accompanied by bradycardia. Keep physician informed.

Rescinnamine may cause drowsiness and dizziness during early therapy. Caution patient to avoid driving or other potentially hazardous activities until reaction to drug is determined.

Drug should be discontinued promptly if patient shows signs of mental depression: early morning insomnia, inability to concentrate, anorexia, despondency, self-deprecation, detached attitude, mood swings, impotence.

Advise patient to check for edema and to record weight daily. Distinction must be made between weight gain from edema and weight gain from increased appetite.

Dry mouth may be relieved by rinsing with warm water or by increasing noncaloric fluid intake, if allowed (particularly if intake has been inadequate) or by sugarless gum or lemon drops. If these measures do not provide relief, a saliva substitute may help (e.g., Xero-Lube, Moi-stir).

Advise patient not to take OTC medications without first consulting physician or pharmacist.

Preserved in tight, light-resistant containers preferably between 15° and 30°C (59° and 86°F) unless otherwise directed by manufacturer.

See Reserpine: prototype rauwolfia alkaloid.

PROTOTYPE

RESERPINE

(Novoreserpine, Releserp, Reserfia, Sandril, Serpalan, Serpasil, Serpate, Sk-Reserpine, Zepine, and others)

(re-ser′peen)
Antihypertensive
Antipsychotic
Rauwolfia alkaloid

ACTIONS AND USES. Principal alkaloid of *Rauwolfia serpentina* (Indian snakeroot). Interferes with binding of 5-hydroxytryptamine (serotonin) at receptor sites, decreases synthesis of norepinephrine by depleting dopamine (their precursor), and competitively inhibits their reuptake in storage granules. Causes depletion of these biogenic amines (norepinephrine, serotonin) in brain, peripheral nervous system, heart, and other organs and tissues. Sympathetic inhibitory action is reflected in small but persistent decrease in blood pressure, frequently associated with bradycardia, and reduced cardiac output. Usually does not cause orthostatic hypotension, and has no marked effect on renal blood flow. Central effect results in tranquilization and sedation similar to that produced by chlorpromazine.

Used orally in treatment of mild essential hypertension and as adjunctive therapy with other antihypertensive agents in the more severe forms of hypertension. Used parenterally for treatment of hypertensive emergencies, such as acute hypertensive encephalopathy, and occasionally to initiate treatment in psychiatric emergencies. Also used in agitated psychotic states, primarily in patients intolerant to phenothiazines or patients who also require antihypertensive medication. *Investigational Use:* to reduce vasospastic attacks in Raynaud's phenomenon and other peripheral vascular disorders, and for symptomatic treatment of thyrotoxicosis. Available in fixed-dose combination with a diuretic, e.g., chlorothiazide (Diupres), quinethazone (Hydromox R), hydrochlorothiazide (Hydropres), trichlormethiazide (Metatensin, Naquival), chlorthalidone (Regroton), and others.

ABSORPTION AND FATE. Slow onset of action after oral administration; antihypertensive effect begins in 3 to 6 days; duration 2 to 6 weeks. Following IM, action begins in 2 to 3 hours, peaks in 3 to 6 hours and persists 10 to 12 hours. Well distributed in body. Tightly bound to catecholamine storage sites. Extensively metabolized in liver. Slowly excreted in urine (about 10%) and feces (30 to 60%) mainly as inactive metabolites and some unchanged alkaloids. Crosses blood–brain barrier and placenta. Appears in breast milk.

CONTRAINDICATIONS AND PRECAUTIONS. Hypersensitivity to rauwolfia alkaloids; history of mental depression; acute peptic ulcer, ulcerative colitis, patients receiving electroconvulsive therapy; within 7 to 14 days of MAO inhibitor therapy. Safe use during pregnancy and in women of childbearing potential and nursing mothers not established. *Cautious Use:* renal insufficiency, cardiac arrhythmias, cardiac damage, cerebrovascular accident, epilepsy, bronchitis, asthma, elderly patients, debilitated patients, gallstones, obesity, chronic sinusitis, parkinsonism, pheochromocytoma.

ADVERSE/SIDE EFFECTS. CNS: drowsiness, sedation, lethargy, mental depression, nervousness, anxiety, nightmares, increased dreaming, headache, dizziness, increased appetite, dull sensorium; prolonged use of large doses: CNS stimulation (parkinsonian syndrome): tremors, muscle rigidity; respiratory depression, convulsions, hypothermia. **CV:** bradycardia, flushing (parenteral), edema, congestive heart failure (rare), orthostatic hypotension, increased AV conduction time (prolonged therapy); anginalike symptoms, arrhythmias. **EENT:** nasal congestion, epistaxis, lacrimation, blurred vision; miosis, ptosis, conjunctival congestion (acute toxicity); causal relationship not established: glaucoma, uveitis, optic atrophy, deafness. **GI:** dry mouth or excessive salivation, nausea, vomiting, abdominal cramps, diarrhea, reactivation of peptic ulcer (hypersecretion), heartburn, biliary colic. **Hematologic:** thrombocytopenic purpura, anemia, prolonged BT. **Hypersensitivity:** pruritus, rash, asthma. **Reproductive:** menstrual irregularities, breast engorgement, galactorrhea, gynecomastia, feminization (males), impaired sexual function, impotence. **Other:** muscle aches, dysuria, fixed-drug eruptions.

ROUTE AND DOSAGE. Adults: Oral: *Hypertension:* initial: 0.25 to 0.5 mg daily for 1 to 2 weeks; maintenance: 0.1 to 0.25 mg daily. *Psychiatric disorders:* initial: 0.5 mg; dosage adjusted upward or downward according to patient's response (range 0.1 to 1 mg daily). **Pediatric:** *Hypertension: psychiatric use:* **Oral:** 0.02 mg/kg/24 hours or 0.6 mg/m²/24 hours. May be divided into 2 doses. Available in capsule, tablet, and elixir.

NURSING IMPLICATIONS

Reserpine (oral) is administered with meals or with milk or other food to minimize possibility of gastric irritation (drug increases gastric secretions).

Take blood pressure and pulse at intervals prescribed by physician. Both should be taken before each parenteral dose. Compare readings with baseline determinations and keep physician informed. (Note: drop in blood pressure may be accompanied by bradycardia.)

Advise patient to take drug at the same time each day, not to skip or double doses, and not to stop therapy without advice of physician.

Since drowsiness, sedation, and dizziness are possible side effects, caution patient to avoid driving and other potentially hazardous activities until reaction to drug has been determined.

Counsel patient regarding possible side effects and importance of prompt reporting. Untoward effects are usually minimal with proper dosage and adequate supervision.

Because rauwolfia alkaloids are cumulative and have a long duration of action, dosage adjustments when necessary are usually made at 7- to 14-day intervals.

Full therapeutic effect of oral drug for hypertension may not occur until 2 to 3 weeks of therapy, and effects may persist for as long as 4 to 6 weeks after drug is discontinued. Special precautions should be observed when reserpine is prescribed for the elderly and the obese patient (half-life is reportedly prolonged in obese patients).

Mental depression is a serious side effect and may be sufficiently severe to lead to suicide. It occurs most commonly in high dosage regimens, e.g., 0.5 to 1 mg or more daily; may not appear until 2 to 8 months of therapy, and may last for several months after drug is withdrawn. Instruct patient and responsible family members to report the following possible beginning symptoms of depression: early morning insomnia, anorexia, inability to concentrate, despondency, self-deprecation, attitude of detachment, mood swings, or impotence. Hospitalization may be necessary.

Monitor intake and output especially in patients with impaired renal function. Report changes in intake–output ratio and pattern.

Postural hypotension occurs rarely with usual oral doses, but is not uncommon in patients receiving large parenteral doses. Supervise ambulation as indicated. Instruct patient to report symptoms of dizziness, light-headedness to physician. Dosage reduction may be indicated. Advise patient to make position changes slowly, particularly from recumbent to upright posture, and to lie down or sit down (head-low position) if patient feels faint. Also advise patient not to take hot showers or hot tub baths, to avoid hot environments, and not to stand still for prolonged periods.

Advise patient to check for edema and to record weight daily. Distinction must be made between weight gain from edema and that from increased appetite. Consult physician about gain of 3 to 5 lb in 1 week.

Dry mouth may be relieved by rinsing with warm water, by increasing noncaloric fluid intake if allowed (particularly if intake has been inadequate), or by sugarless gum or lemon drops. If these measures do not provide relief, a saliva substitute may help, (e.g., Xero-Lube, Moi-stir). Consult physician.

Consult physician regarding diet regimen, allowable salt intake, and physical activity program.

If a vasopressor is needed for treatment of hypotension, levarterenol (or other direct-acting sympathomimetic amine) is preferred to ephedrine, which is indirect-acting (i.e., it relies on release of catecholamines for action).

Rauwolfia alkaloids tend to lower the threshold for convulsions. Patients with epilepsy should be monitored for possible need of adjustment in anticonvulsant dosage.

It is not necessary to discontinue rauwolfia alkaloids prior to surgery because cardiovascular stability does not appear to be adversely affected. However, the anesthesiologist should be informed of such therapy.

Rauwolfia alkaloids should be discontinued 1 week before electroconvulsive therapy.

Advise patient not to take OTC medications without prior approval of physician or pharmacist. Many preparations for coughs and colds contain adrenergic agents that affect the actions of rauwolfia alkaloids.

Preserved in tight, light-resistant containers, preferably between 15° and 30°C (59° and 86°F), unless otherwise directed by manufacturer.

Patient-Teaching Points:

✓ *Medication:* Explain how medication works; help plan convenient schedule (the same time[s] each day); review drugs that may aggravate blood pressure, e.g., sympathomimetics (found in nasal decongestants and medications for coughs, cold, asthma); contraceptives. Do not take OTC drugs without first consulting physician or pharmacist. Adverse drug effects; what to report; possible need for lifelong therapy and medical follow-up, importance of compliance; what to do about a missed dose (discuss with physician beforehand); anticipate when supply of medication will need refilling; request physician to write an extra prescription for emergency use.

✓ No smoking.

✓ *Exercise:* Planned, graduated aerobic exercise program, e.g., bicycling, swimming, brisk walking. (Discuss with physician.)

✓ *Diet:* Keep record of weights; reduce excess weight; gradual reduction of salt intake (drastic reduction may cause paradoxical water retention), omit salty "finger foods" (potato chips, pretzels, peanuts), do not add salt at the table; collaborate with physician and dietitian; recommended daily salt intake commonly prescribed is 3 to 5 Gm.

✓ Avoid undue stress; relaxation procedures: deep breathing several times daily; some patients benefit by referral for biofeedback methods, yoga, transcendental meditation, or psychotherapy.

✓ *Medical follow-up:* Advise patient to carry all medications for review; show physician record of weights, blood pressure and pulse at each visit.

✓ *Medical identification:* Carry Medic Alert or other appropriate identification at all times.

Diagnostic Test Interferences. Possibility of elevated **blood glucose** values; however, it is also reported that reserpine may decrease thiazide-induced hyperglycemia. Increase in **serum prolactin** with chronic administration of rauwolfia alkaloids; overdoses may cause initial increase in **urinary catecholamines** excretion; decreases with chronic administration. Large doses may cause initial rise in **urinary 5 HIAA** excretion. Initial IM doses may increase **urinary VMA** excretion followed by decrease by end of third day of therapy (with oral or parenteral administration). Possible interference with **urinary steroid** colorimetric determinations: **17-OHCS** and **17-KS.**

Drug Interactions: Reserpine

Plus	Interactions
Alcohol, barbiturates and other CNS depressants	Additive CNS depressant effects
Digitalis glycosides	Risk of cardiac arrhythmias
Diuretics	Additive hypotensive effect
Ephedrine, amphetamines and other indirect-acting sympathomimetic agents	Rauwolfia alkaloids inhibit their action
Epinephrine, isoproterenol norepinephrine (levarterenol) and other direct-acting sympathomimetics	Rauwolfia alkaloids may prolong their action (theoretical); preferred for use in hypotensive episodes
Levodopa	Diminished response to levodopa (concurrent use usually avoided)
MAO inhibitors	Excessive sympathetic response, excitation and hypertension (concurrent use avoided)
Methotrimeprazine (Levoprome)	Additive hypotension (concurrent use usually avoided)
Propranolol (Inderal) and other beta-adrenergic blockers as well as other antihypertensives	Additive hypotensive effects
Procainamide, Quinidine	Risk of additive cardiac depression, arrhythmias

RIBOFLAVIN

(Riobin-50, Vitamin B_2)

(rye'boo-flay-vin)

Vitamin B_2

ACTIONS AND USES. Water-soluble vitamin and component of the flavoprotein enzymes that work together with a wide variety of proteins to catalyze many cellular respiratory reactions by which the body derives its energy.

Used to prevent riboflavin deficiency and to treat ariboflavinosis also used to heat microcytic anemia, as supplement to other B vitamins in treatment of pellagra and beriberi.

ABSORPTION AND FATE. Readily absorbed from upper GI tract and from parenteral sites. Distributed to all tissues, with highest concentrations in liver, kidney, and heart. Half-life: 66 to 84 minutes. Little is stored. 60% protein-bound. Amounts in excess of body needs excreted unchanged in urine. In amounts approaching minimal daily requirements, approximately 9% excreted in urine; metabolic fate of remainder unknown.

CONTRAINDICATIONS AND PRECAUTIONS. Children under 12.

ADVERSE/SIDE EFFECTS. Apparently nontoxic.

ROUTE AND DOSAGE. Oral: 5 to 10 mg daily. **Intramuscular:** deficiency: 50 mg daily.

NURSING IMPLICATIONS

Administer oral preparation with food to enhance absorption.

Inform patient receiving large doses that an intense yellow discoloration of urine may occur.

Therapeutic effectiveness of vitamin B_2 therapy is evaluated by improvement of clinical manifestations of deficiency: digestive disturbances, headache, burning sensation of skin (especially "burning" feet), cracking at corners of mouth (cheilosis), glossitis, seborrheic dermatitis (often at angle of nose and anogenital region) and other skin lesions, mental depression, corneal vascularization (with photophobia, burning and itchy eyes, lacrimation, roughness of eyelids), anemia, neuropathy.

Recommended daily allowances of riboflavin: infants, 0.4 to 0.6 mg; children, 0.8 to 1.4 mg; adult males, 1.6 mg; adult females, 1.2 mg; pregnancy and lactation, 1.5 and 1.7 mg, respectively.

Rich dietary sources of riboflavin: liver, kidney, heart, eggs, milk and milk products, yeast, whole-grain cereals, and green vegetables.

Collaborate with physician, dietitian, patient, and responsible family member in planning for diet teaching. A complete dietary history is an essential part of vitamin replacement so that poor eating habits can be identified and corrected. Additionally, deficiency in one vitamin is usually associated with other vitamin deficiencies.

Preserved in airtight containers protected from light.

Diagnostic Test Interferences. In large doses, riboflavin may produce yellow green fluorescence in **urine** and thus cause false elevations in certain fluorometric determinations of **urinary catecholamines.**

Drug Interactions. Riboflavin decreases activity of **tetracyclines.**

RIFAMPIN

(Rifadin, Rifamycin, Rimactane, Rofact)

(rif′am-pin)
Antiinfective
Antibiotic
Antituberculosis agent

ACTIONS AND USES. Semisynthetic derivative of rifamycin B, an antibiotic derived from *Streptococcus mediterranei,* with bacteriostatic and bactericidal actions. Inhibits DNA-dependent RNA polymerase activity in susceptible bacterial cells, thereby suppressing RNA synthesis. Active against *Mycobacterium tuberculosis, Neisseria meningitidis,* and a wide range of gram-negative and gram-positive organisms. Since resistant strains emerge rapidly when it is employed alone, it is used in conjunction with other antitubercular agents in treatment of tuberculosis.

Used primarily as adjuvant with other antituberculosis agents in initial treatment and retreatment of clinical tuberculosis, and as short-term therapy to eliminate meningococci from nasopharynx of asymptomatic carriers when risk of meningococcal meningitis is high. *Investigational Use:* chemoprophylaxis in contacts of patients with *Haemophilus influenzae* type B infection; alone or in combination with dapsone in treatment of epilepsy; treatment of infections caused by susceptible gram-negative and gram-positive bacteria that fail to respond to other antiinfectives; in combination with erythromycin or tetracycline for treatment of Legionnaire's disease.

ABSORPTION AND FATE. Well absorbed from GI tract. Peak plasma concentrations in 2 to 4 hours following 600-mg dose; still detectable for 24 hours. Widely distributed in body tissues and fluids, including CSF and saliva, with highest concentrations in liver, gallbladder wall, and kidneys. About 80 to 90% protein bound. Half-life: about 3 hours (higher and more prolonged in hepatic dysfunction, and may be decreased in patients receiving isoniazid concomitantly). Rapidly deacetylated in liver to active and inactive metabolites; enters bile via enterohepatic circulation; 60 to 65% excreted in feces. Up to 30% of dose is excreted in urine, about half as free drug. Rifampin induces microsomal enzymes and thus may inactivate certain drugs. Crosses placenta; appears in breast milk.

CONTRAINDICATIONS AND PRECAUTIONS. Hypersensitivity to rifamycin derivatives; obstructive biliary disease, intermittent rifampin therapy. Safe use during pregnancy and in children under 5 years of age not established. *Cautious Use:* hepatic disease, history of alcoholism, concomitant use of other hepatotoxic agents.

ADVERSE/SIDE EFFECTS. CNS: fatigue, drowsiness, headache, ataxia, confusion, dizziness, inability to concentrate, generalized numbness, pain in extremities, muscular weakness, visual disturbances, transient low-frequency hearing loss (infrequent), conjunctivitis. **GI:** heartburn, epigastric distress, nausea, vomiting, anorexia, flatulence, cramps, diarrhea, pseudomembranous colitis. **Hematologic:** thrombocytopenia, transient leukopenia, anemia, including hemolytic anemia. **Hypersensitivity:** fever, pruritus, urticaria, skin eruptions, soreness of mouth and tongue, eosinophilia, hemolysis. **Renal:** hemoglobinuria, hematuria, acute renal failure. **Other:** hemoptysis, light-chain proteinuria, flu-like syndrome, menstrual disorders, hepatorenal syndrome (with intermittent therapy), transient elevations in liver function tests (bilirubin, BSP, alkaline phosphatase, SGOT (AST), SGPT (ALT)), pancreatitis (infrequent). **Overdosage:** GI symptoms, increasing lethargy, liver enlargement and tenderness, jaundice, brownish-red or orange discoloration of skin, sweat, saliva, tears, and feces; unconsciousness.

ROUTE AND DOSAGE. Oral: *Pulmonary tuberculosis* (used in conjunction with at least one other antituberculosis agent): **Adults:** 600 mg once daily; used in conjunction with other antitubercular agent(s). **Children:** 10 to 20 mg/kg/day, not to exceed 600 mg/day. *Meningococcal carriers:* **Adults:** 600 mg once daily for 4 consecutive days. **Children:** 10 to 20 mg/kg once daily for 4 consecutive days, not to exceed 600 mg/day.

NURSING IMPLICATIONS

Capsule may be emptied and contents swallowed with fluid or mixed with food, if desired.

Administered 1 hour before or 2 hours after a meal. Peak serum levels are delayed and may be slightly lower when given with food.

A desiccant should be kept in bottle containing capsules; they become unstable with moisture.

Caution patient not to interrupt prescribed dosage regimen. Hepatorenal reaction with flu-like syndrome has occurred when therapy has been resumed following interruption.

Serology and susceptibility testing should be performed prior to and in the event of positive cultures.

Inform patients that drug may impart a harmless red-orange color to urine, feces, sputum, sweat, and tears. Soft contact lens may be permanently stained.

Periodic hepatic function tests are advised. Patients with hepatic disease must be closely monitored.

Instruct patients to report onset of jaundice (yellow skin, sclerae, and posterior portion of hard palate; pruritus), hypersensitivity reactions, and persistence of GI adverse effects.

Patients taking oral contraceptives (OC) should consider alternative methods of contraception *(see Drug Interactions).* Concommitant use of rifampin and OC leads to decreased effectiveness of the contraceptive and to menstrual disturbances (spotting, breakthrough bleeding).

If patient is also receiving an anticoagulant, prothrombin times should be performed daily or as necessary to establish and maintain required anticoagulant activity.

Caution patient to keep drug out of reach of children.

Treatment of overdosage: Gastric lavage in absence of vomiting, followed by activated charcoal slurry; antiemetic to control severe nausea and vomiting. Forced diuresis, with measurement of intake and output ratio, to promote drug excretion. Hemodialysis may be required.

Diagnostic Test Interferences. Rifampin interferes with contrast media used for **gallbladder study,** therefore test should precede daily dose of rifampin. May also cause retention of **BSP.** Inhibits standard assays for **serum folate** and **vitamin B_{12}.** Possible interference with **contrast media** used for gallbladder study; may also cause retention of **BSP.**

Drug Interactions: Rifampin

Plus	Interactions
Alcohol	Increased risk of hepatotoxicity
Aminosalicylic acid (PAS)	Decreased serum concentration of rifampin
Barbiturates, benzodiazepines, clofibrate, corticosteroids, dapsone, digitoxin, methadone, metoprolol; oral anticoagulants, antidiabetic agents, and contraceptives; progestins, propranolol, quinidine	Decreased plasma concentrations of these drugs leading to potential of treatment failure and necessity to adjust dosage
Isoniazid (INH)	May result in hepatotoxicity

PROTOTYPE

RITODRINE HYDROCHLORIDE

(Yutopar)

(ri'toe-dreen)
Adrenergic agonist (sympathominetic)
Tocolytic agent
Uterine relaxant

ACTIONS AND USES. Beta$_2$-adrenergic agonist clinically effective in preventing or delaying of preterm labor. Preferentially stimulates beta$_2$-receptors in uterine smooth muscle resulting in reduced intensity and frequency of uterine contractions and lengthening gestation period. (Actions may be eliminated by beta-adrenergic blocking agents.) Beta$_2$-receptor stimulation also results in bronchial relaxation and slight effect on vascular smooth muscles. Transitory cardiovascular effects including increased cardiac output, increased maternal and fetal heart rates, and widening of maternal pulse pressure (beta$_1$-stimulation) are common. Administered parenterally in individualized doses with beginning of contractions, and continued until they are inhibited. Oral medication then given until delivery of a mature infant is assured. Safety and effectiveness during advanced labor has not been established. Animal studies have shown no teratogenic or carcinogenic effects, but drug is used only when clearly warranted by clinical condition.

Used to manage premature labor in selected patients.

ABSORPTION AND FATE. Following oral administration, 30% of drug absorbed; maximum serum levels of 5 to 15 ng/ml reached within 30 to 60 minutes. Serum levels of 32 to 52 ng/ml reached after IV infusion at rate of 0.15 mg/minute for 1 hour. 32% protein-bound. Half-life (triphasic): initial: 6.9 minutes, second phase: 1.7 to 2.6 hours, third phase: more than 10 hours. Metabolized in liver. 90% excretion completed in 24 hours. Crosses placenta.

CONTRAINDICATIONS AND PRECAUTIONS. Mild to moderate preeclampsia or eclampsia, intrauterine infection, cervix dilated 4 or more centimeters (in a singleton pregnancy); hypertension, diabetes mellitus; use prior to 20th week or after 36 weeks of pregnancy or if continuation of pregnancy would be hazardous to mother and fetus (e.g., antepartum hemorrhage, eclampsia, intrauterine fetal death, maternal cardiac disease, pulmonary hypertension, maternal hyperthyroidism, severe diabetes mellitus). Also hypovolemia, cardiac arrhythmias associated with tachycardia or digitalis intoxication, uncontrolled hypertension, thyrotoxicosis, bronchial asthma being treated with betamimetics and/or steroids. *Cautious Use:* concomitant use of potassium depleting diuretics, cardiac disease.

ADVERSE/SIDE EFFECTS. More pronounced and frequent following IV infusion: altered maternal and fetal heart rates and maternal blood pressure (dose-related); temporary hyperglycemia, palpitations, arrhythmias, tremor, nausea, vomiting, headache, erythema; nervousness, restlessness, anxiety, malaise, chest pain, pulmonary edema. Infrequent: anaphylactic shock, rash, epigastric distress, ileus, bloating, constipation, diarrhea, dyspnea, hyperventilation, glycosuria, hemolytic icterus, sweating, chills, drowsiness, weakness, myotomic muscular dystrophy.

ROUTE AND DOSAGE. **Intravenous:** 50 to 100 mcg/minute administered by means of a calibrated constant-rate infusion pump. Dose gradually increased by 50 mcg/minute every 10 minutes until adequate uterine relaxation is achieved. Effective dose range: 150 to 350 mcg/minute. May be continued for 12 hours after uterine contractions cease. **Oral (started 30 minutes prior to termination of infusion):** 10 mg every 2 hours for first 24 hours; thereafter, 10 to 20 mg every 4 to 6 hours up to but not exceeding 120 mg daily.

NURSING IMPLICATIONS

Hospitalization is advised during treatment with ritodrine.

Preparation of IV solution: 150 mg ritodrine is added to 500 ml 5% dextrose or normal saline solution giving a final concentration of 0.3 mg/ml.

IV solution should be clear and should not be administered if cloudy or if a precipitate is present.

Place patient in left lateral recumbent position throughout the infusion period to reduce risk of hypotension.

Monitor IV infusion flow rate to prevent circulation overload.

Pronounced dose-related side effects in cardiovascular system require continuous monitoring of maternal and fetal heart rates and maternal blood pressure while infusion is running.

Occult cardiac disease has been unmasked by use of ritodrine.

Uterine contractions will decrease in frequency and intensity during treatment.

If patient is also on steroid therapy, hospitalization for treatment with ritodrine is advised. Be alert to signs and symptoms of pulmonary edema *(see Index)*.

Store drug at controlled room temperature preferably below 30°C (80°F). Do not freeze.

R

Diagnostic Test Interferences. Ritodrine (intravenous route) may produce an increase in **serum** levels of **glucose, insulin** and **free fatty acids,** and a decrease in **serum potassium.** It temporarily elevates results of **glucose tolerance test.**

Drug Interactions: Ritodrine Hydrochloride

Plus	Interactions
Anesthetics, general	Potentiated hypotensive effects of general anaesthetic
Corticosteroids	Pulmonary edema in mother; action is antagonized by beta-adrenergic blocking agents, e.g., propranolol, and is potentiated by other sympathomimetics

S

SALICYLIC ACID

(Calicylic, Hydrisalic, Keralyt, Saligel, Salonil)

Keratolytic
Salicylate

ACTIONS AND USES. Causes swelling and softening of keratin, cornified epithelium and scales, thereby facilitating their removal. Has weak bacteriostatic and fungistatic actions. May be destructive to tissues in concentrations above 6%.

Used as topical aid in hyperkeratotic skin disorders such as psoriasis and various ichthyoses, calluses, warts, and to produce exfoliation in superficial fungal infections, acne, and seborrheic dermatitis. Available in plaster form or as ether-alcohol solution (with 20% salicylic acid and collodion) for removal of warts, corns, and calluses.

CONTRAINDICATIONS AND PRECAUTIONS. Sensitivity to salicylates or to any ingredient in preparation; applications over large areas or for prolonged periods. Use of high concentrations or collodion preparations on moles, birthmarks, warts with hairs, inflamed or infected skin, patients with diabetes mellitus, peripheral vascular disease. Concurrent use of other keratolytic agents (acne preparations) or peeling agents. *Cautious Use:* children under 12 years of age.

ADVERSE/SIDE EFFECTS. Irritation, burning of skin. Systemic absorption (salicylism): dizziness, tinnitus, impaired hearing, mental confusion, headache, hyperventilation. *See also Aspirin.*

ROUTE AND DOSAGE. Topical: cream, gel, liquid, ointment, plaster. Compounded in concentrations of 1 to 60% depending upon formulation.

NURSING IMPLICATIONS

Physician should prescribe specific dosage form, strength, and details of application.

Avoid contact of medication with eyes and mucous membranes.

Advise patients to wash hands thoroughly following use of cream, gel, lotion, or ointment forms unless hands are also being treated.

Caution patient to use drug as directed. Systemic absorption has been reported. Also application to normal skin can cause irritation and burning.

Physician may prescribe hydration of part (wet packs, soaks, or baths) before or after application and an occlusive dressing at night to enhance drug effect. Use medication only as directed.

Advise patient to keep medication out of the reach of children.

Whitfield's ointment contains benzoic acid 12%, and salicylic acid 16%.

Salicylic acid is incorporated into several OTC acne preparations: Fostex, Komed, Microsyn, Stridex; and in corn and callus remedies: Dr. Scholl's, Freezone; wart removers: Compound W, and other preparations.

For implications of possible systemic effects, see Aspirin.

SALSALATE

(Artha-G, Disalcid, Mono-Gesic)

NSAID
Salicylate
Antirheumatic

ACTIONS AND USES. Action similar to those of other salicylates. *See Aspirin.* Clinical studies suggest that salsalate does not produce significant gastric irritation, and it has not been associated with reactions causing asthmatic attacks in susceptible individuals. The incidence of side effects in general appears to be lower than that of other salicylates. Unlike aspirin it does not appear to inhibit platelet aggregation.

Used for symptomatic treatment rheumatoid arthritis, osteoarthritis, and related rheumatic disorders.

ABSORPTION AND FATE. Insoluble in gastric acid. Completely absorbed from small intestine and partially hydrolyzed in liver; almost totally excreted in urine. Half-life: about 1 hour.

CONTRAINDICATIONS AND PRECAUTIONS. Hypersensitivity to salicylates, chronic renal insufficiency, peptic ulcer, pregnancy (category C), children under 12 years. *See also Aspirin.*

ADVERSE/SIDE EFFECTS. Occasionally, nausea, dyspepsia, heartburn. **Overdosage:** (salicylism) tinnitus, hearing loss (reversible), vertigo, flushing, headache, confusion, drowsiness, hyperventilation, sweating, vomiting, diarrhea. *See also Aspirin.*

ROUTE AND DOSAGE. Oral: 325 to 3000 mg daily in divided doses adjusted to the individual.

NURSING IMPLICATIONS

Administer with a full glass of water or with food or milk to reduce GI side effects.

Symptom relief is gradual (may require 3 to 4 days to establish steady-state salicylate level).

Warn patient not to take another salicylate (e.g., aspirin) while on salsalate therapy.

See Aspirin, prototype NSAID.

SCOPOLAMINE

(Transderm-scōp)

SCOPOLAMINE HYDROBROMIDE

(Hyoscine, Isopto-Hyoscine, Murocoll)

(skoe-pol′a-meen)
Anticholinergic (parasympathalytic)
Antimuscarinic
Belladonna alkaloid, mydriatic

ACTIONS AND USES. Alkaloid of belladonna with peripheral actions resembling those of atropine (qv). In contrast to atropine, produces CNS depression, with marked sedative and tranquilizing effects, and is less effective in preventing reflex bradycardia during anesthesia (tends to slow heart even in large doses). More potent in mydriatic and cycloplegic actions and in inhibiting secretions of salivary, bronchial, and sweat glands, but has less prominent effect on heart, intestines, and bronchial muscles.

Used in obstetrics with morphine to produce amnesia and sedation ("twilight sleep"), and as preanesthetic medication. Used to control spasticity (and drooling) in postencephalitic parkinsonism, paralysis agitans, and other spastic states, as prophylactic agent for motion sickness and as mydriatic and cycloplegic in ophthalmology. Therapeutic system (Transderm-Scōp) is used to prevent nausea and vomiting associated with motion sickness.

ABSORPTION AND FATE. Well-absorbed from GI tract. Bound to plasma proteins. Peak mydriatic effect in 20 to 30 minutes, lasting 3 to 7 days; peak cycloplegic effect in 30 minutes to 1 hour, lasting 5 to 7 days.

CONTRAINDICATIONS AND PRECAUTIONS. Asthma, hepatitis, toxemia of pregnancy. *Cautious Use:* cardiac disease, patients over 40 years of age. *See also Atropine.*

ADVERSE/SIDE EFFECTS. Sense of fatigue, dizziness, drowsiness, dry mouth and throat, constipation, urinary retention, disorientation, decreased heart rate, dilated pupils, photophobia, depressed respiration. **Ophthalmic:** local irritation, follicular conjunctivitis. *See also Atropine.*

ROUTE AND DOSAGE. Oral: Adults: 0.5 to 1 mg. *Motion sickness:* 0.25 to 0.6 mg 1 hour before anticipated travel. **Subcutaneous, intramuscular, intravenous (with suitable dilution):** 0.3 to 0.6 mg. **Topical (ophthalmic): Adult:** 1 or 2 drops of 0.5 to 1% solution. **Children:** 0.006 mg/kg orally or subcutaneously; 0.2 to 0.25% solution (ophthalmic) or ointment twice daily for 2 days before refraction. Transdermal therapeutic system delivers 0.5 mg scopolamine over 3 days applied 3 to 12 hours before anticipated travel.

NURSING IMPLICATIONS

Some patients manifest excitement, delirium, disorientation, and garrulousness shortly after drug is administered, until sedative effect takes hold. Observe patient closely for these effects.

Bedsides are advisable, particularly for the elderly, because of amnesic effect of scopolamine.

In the presence of pain, scopolamine may cause delirium, restlessness, and excitement unless given with an analgesic.

Tolerance may develop with prolonged use.

To minimize possibility of systemic absorption, apply pressure against lacrimal sac during and for 1 or 2 minutes following installation of eye drops.

When used as mydriatic or cycloplegic, caution the patient that vision will be blurred; the patient should avoid potentially hazardous activities such as driving a car or operating machinery until vision clears.

Ophthalmic use should be terminated if local irritation, edema, and conjunctivitis occur.

Therapeutic system (Transderm-Scōp) (a controlled release system):

- Wash and dry hands thoroughly before and after application of the disc.
- Place on dry surface behind the ear.
- If system becomes dislodged, it can be replaced by another on another site behind the ear.
- Effective if applied as soon as 2 to 3 hours before anticipated motion; however, therapeutic effect with 12 hours of application is best.

Advise patient to place it on skin site the night before an expected trip.

Many OTC "sleep aids" contain scopolamine in small doses, e.g., Compoz, Nytol, Sominex.

Preserved in tight, light-resistant containers.

See Atropine sulfate (prototype belladonna alkaloid).

S

SECOBARBITAL
(Seconal)
SECOBARBITAL SODIUM
(Seconal Sodium)

(see-koe-bar′bi-tal)
Hypnotic, sedative
Barbiturate
C II

ACTIONS AND USES. Short-acting barbiturate with CNS depressant effects and anticonvulsant action similar to that of phenobarbital (qv). Available in fixed combination with amobarbital (Tuinal).

Used as hypnotic for simple insomnia, and preoperatively to provide basal hypnosis for general, spinal, or regional anesthesia. Effective in the emergency control of acute convulsive conditions (e.g., tetanus, toxic reactions to poisons) and in the management of acute agitated behavior.

ABSORPTION AND FATE. Approximately 90% absorbed from GI tract following oral ingestion. Full hypnotic effect in 15 to 30 minutes after oral or rectal administration, 7 to 10 minutes after IM, and 1 to 3 minutes after IV injection. Duration: 3 to 5 hours following oral or rectal; 15 minutes following IV. 30 to 45% protein bound. Half-life: 30 hours. Metabolized by liver; excreted in urine as inactive metabolites and small amounts of unchanged drug. Crosses placenta. Enters breast milk.

CONTRAINDICATIONS AND PRECAUTIONS. History of sensitivity to barbiturates, use during parturition, fetal immaturity, uncontrolled pain. Use of sterile injection containing polyethylene glycol vehicle in patients with renal insufficiency. *Cautious Use:* pregnant women with toxemia or history of bleeding. *See also Phenobarbital.*

ADVERSE/SIDE EFFECTS. Drowsiness, lethargy, hangover, paradoxical excitement in the elderly patient; respiratory depression, laryngospasm, fall in blood pressure (with rapid IV). *See also Phenobarbital.*

ROUTE AND DOSAGE. Adults: Oral (sedative): 30 to 50 mg 3 times per day; (preoperative sedative): 100 to 300 mg 1 or 2 hours before surgery; (hypnotic): 100 to 200 mg orally or IM. **Intramuscular, intravenous** (acute convulsive episodes): 5.5 mg/kg repeated every 3 to 4 hours, if needed. **Children: Oral, rectal suppository** (sedative): 4 to 6 mg/kg/24 hours, divided into 3 doses; (hypnotic): 3 to 5 mg/kg. **Intramuscular** (acute convulsive episodes): 3 to 5 mg/kg.

NURSING IMPLICATIONS

Discard parenteral solutions that are not clear or that contain a precipitate.

Aqueous solutions of secobarbital sodium for injection are not stable; they must be freshly prepared and used within 30 minutes after container is opened. Reconstitute secobarbital sodium powder with sterile water for injection (incompatible with bacteriostatic water for injection or lactated Ringer's injection). Following addition of water, rotate ampul; do not shake it. Several minutes are required to dissolve drug completely. If solution is not completely clear within 5 minutes, do not use. Consult package literature for details.

Secobarbital sodium injection in aqueous polyethylene glycol vehicle is more stable than aqueous solution. It should be refrigerated (2° to 8°C). May be diluted with sterile water for injection, 0.9% sodium chloride, or Ringer's injection (*not* lactated). Consult package literature for details.

Administer IM injection deep into large muscle mass. Carefully aspirate before injecting drug to avoid inadvertent entry into blood vessel.

Following IM injection of large hypnotic dose, observe patient closely for 20 to 30 minutes to assure that hypnosis is not excessive.

Elderly and debilitated patients may manifest excitement, depression, or confusion with usual adult dose.

An occasional patient may become irritable, uncooperative, and restive after a subhypnotic dose of a short-acting barbiturate.

Patients receiving drug IV must be kept under constant observation. Monitor blood pressure, pulse, and respiration every 3 to 5 minutes. Maintain patient airway. Equipment for respiratory support should be immediately available.

When administered to pregnant patient, fetal heart beat should be closely monitored. Report slowing or irregularities.

Following administration to a patient in ambulatory service or physician's office, the patient should not attempt to go home unescorted. Caution the patient to avoid driving a car or other potentially hazardous activities for the remainder of day.

Classified as Schedule II drug under Federal Controlled Substances Act except for suppository which is classified under Schedule III.

See Phenobarbital (prototype barbiturate) for additional nursing implications and drug interactions.

SENNA

Laxative (stimulant)
Anthraquinone

(Black Draught, Nitolox, Senexon, Senokot, Senolox, X-Prep)

ACTIONS AND USES. Anthraquinone derivative prepared from dried leaflet of *Cassia acutifolia* or *Cassia angustifolia.* Similar to cascara sagrada, but with more potent action. Senna glycosides are converted in colon to active aglycones, which stimulate Auerbach's plexus to induce peristalsis. Available as crude drug (e.g., Black Draught) crystalline senna glycosides (sennosides A and B, e.g., nitotox), and as standardized senna concentrate (e.g., Senokot, X-Prep). Standardized concentrate is purified and standardized for uniform action and is claimed to produce less colic than crude form.

Used for relief of acute constipation and for preoperative and preradiographic bowel evacuation.

ABSORPTION AND FATE. Cathartic action usually occurs in 6 to 10 hours; may not act before 24 hours in some patients metabolized in liver; excreted in feces (some may be eliminated in urine).

CONTRAINDICATIONS AND PRECAUTIONS. Irritable colon, nausea, vomiting, abdominal pain, intestinal obstruction, nursing mothers.

ADVERSE/SIDE EFFECTS. Abdominal cramps, flatulence, nausea. *Prolonged use:* watery diarrhea, excessive loss of water and electrolytes, weight loss, melanotic segmentation of colonic mucosa (reversible).

ROUTE AND DOSAGE. Oral: *Crude Senna leaf or fruit:* **Adults:** 0.5 to 2 Gm; **Children:** 4 mg/kg. *Senna fluid extract:* **Adults:** 2 ml; **Children:** 0.04 ml/kg. *Senna syrup:* **Adults:** 8 ml; **Children:** 0.15 mg/kg. *Sennocides A and B:* **Adults and children (over 10 years):** 12 to 36 mg; **Children (6 to 10 years):** 12 mg. *Standardized senna concentrate:* **Adults:** 2 tablets (187 mg each); granules, 1 teaspoon (326 mg/tsp). **Rectal suppository:** 625 mg. **Children (over 60 lb):** approximately one-half the usual adult dose.

S

NURSING IMPLICATIONS

Generally administered at bedtime for relief of constipation.

When given for preoperative or prediagnostic bowel preparation, usually prescribed to be taken between 2 and 4 PM on day prior to procedure. Diet is then confined to clear liquids.

Some patients may experience considerable griping; if medication is to be repeated, dose reduction may be indicated.

Inform patient that drug may impart yellowish brown color (in acid urine) or reddish brown color (in alkaline urine). Feces may be similarly colored.

Caution patient that continued use may lead to dependence. If constipation persists, consult physician.
Avoid exposure of drug to excessive heat; fluidextracts should be protected from light.
See Bisacodyl for patient-teaching points.

PROTOTYPE

SILVER NITRATE
($AgNO_3$)
SILVER NITRATE, TOUGHENED
(Lunar Caustic, Silver Nitrate Pencil)

Antiinfective
Caustic

ACTIONS AND USES. Has bactericidal, astringent, and caustic properties. Contact of silver ion with chloride in tissue results in precipitation to silver chloride, which limits its effectiveness and penetrating ability. Bactericidal action thought to be due to ability to interfere with essential metabolic actions of microbial cells. Degree of action depends on concentration used and period of time drug is allowed to remain in contact with tissue. Silver nitrate ophthalmic solution is used to prevent and treat ophthalmia neonatorum. Weak solutions are also used to irrigate bladder and urethra. Strong concentrations and toughened silver nitrate are used to cauterize mucous membranes, wounds, granulomatous tissue, and warts. *Unlabeled Use:* (0.1 to 0.5%, solution) wet dressings in burns and on lesions.

ADVERSE/SIDE EFFECTS. Transient chemical irritation of eyes (redness, edema, discharge) expected reaction following eye instillations. Argyria (silver discoloration of tissue with prolonged use).

ROUTE AND DOSAGE. Topical (silver nitrate ophthalmic solution 1%): *Ophthalmia neonatorum:* 2 drops instilled into eye. Eyelids are first cleaned with sterile cotton and sterile water to remove blood, mucus, or meconium. Drug should remain in contact with whole conjunctival sac for 30 seconds or longer. (Irrigation of eyes following instillation of silver nitrate is not recommended by National Society for Prevention of Blindness.) *For cauterization:* silver nitrate solution 10, 25, 50%.

NURSING IMPLICATIONS

Use only silver nitrate ophthalmic solution for the eyes.
Many states by law require instillation of silver nitrate solution to prevent ophthalmia neonatorum (Credé prophylaxis). However, the American Academy of Pediatrics currently supports the use of a topical tetracycline or topical erythromycin as an alternative treatment.
Follow agency policy or physician's directions for ophthalmic instillation in newborns.
For wound cauterization, area to be treated should first be cleaned to remove organic matter (may interfere with drug action). If toughened silver nitrate (silver nitrate pencil) is used, it should be dipped in water and applied to area for period of time according to degree of action desired. Treated area will appear grayish black (silver stain).
Medication should be confined to specific area to be treated. If healthy skin is accidentally touched, it may be washed with physiologic salt solution (the chloride in salt solution forms insoluble precipitate with silver nitrate and thus cancels its action).

Handle silver nitrate with care. Solutions leave gray or black stain on skin, clothing, and utensils. Skin stains (argyria) usually persist indefinitely or disappear only very slowly. Argyria may be exaggerated by exposure to sunlight. Concentrations of silver nitrate 5% and higher are caustic.

Preserved in tight, light-resistant containers.

SILVER PROTEIN, MILD

(Argyrol S.S., Solargentum)

Antiinfective

ACTIONS AND USES. Colloidal compound of silver and a protein derivative. Contains less concentration of ionized silver than silver nitrate, and consequently is less irritating to tissues. Has antimicrobial activity against both gram-nagative and gram-positive organism. *See Silver Nitrate for actions and adverse reactions.*

Used preoperatively in eye surgery to stain and coagulate mucus, which can then be removed by irrigation, and for mild inflammatory conditions of eye, nose, and throat.

ROUTE AND DOSAGE. **Topical (ophthalmic solution 10 to 20%):** *Preoperatively in eye surgery:* 2 or 3 drops, then rinsed out with sterile irrigating solution. *Mild inflammatory conditions:* (10% solution): 1 to 3 drops into eye at 3- to 4-day intervals for several days.

NURSING IMPLICATIONS

Stored in tightly-covered light resistant containers.

See Silver Nitrate.

SILVER SULFADIAZINE

(Silvadene)

(sul-fa-dye'a-zeen)
Antiinfective
Sulfonamide

ACTIONS AND USES. Produced by reaction of silver nitrate with sulfadiazine. Mechanism of action differs from that of either component. Silver salt is released slowly and exerts bactericidal effect only on bacterial cell membrane and wall, rather than by inhibiting folic acid synthesis; antibacterial activity is not inhibited by *p*-amino-benzoic acid (PABA). Contact with sodium chloride in body tissues and fluids results in slow release of sulfadiazine, which may be systemically absorbed from application site. Has broad antimicrobial activity including many gram-negative and gram-positive bacteria and yeast. Does not affect electrolyte balance, and reportedly does not alter acid-base balance.

S

Used for prevention and treatment of sepsis in second- and third-degree burns.

CONTRAINDICATIONS AND PRECAUTIONS. Hypersensitivity to silver sulfadiazine and components (and possibly other sulfonamides), patients with glucose-6-phosphate dehydrogenase deficiency, women of childbearing potential, use during pregnancy, pregnant women at term, prematures and newborn infants under 2 months of age. *Cautious Use:* impaired renal or hepatic function.

ADVERSE/SIDE EFFECTS. Pain (occasionally), burning, itching, rash, reversible leukopenia. Potential for toxicity as for other sulfonamides. *See Sulfisoxazole.*

ROUTE AND DOSAGE. Topical: (micronized) cream (1%) applied once or twice daily to thickness of approximately 1/16 inch.

NURSING IMPLICATIONS

Silver sulfadiazine cream is water-soluble and white in color; if darkening occurs, do not use.

Applied with sterile, gloved hands to cleansed, debrided burned areas. Cream should be reapplied to areas where it has been removed by patient activity; burn wounds should be covered with medication at all times.

Dressings are not required, but may be used if necessary. Silver sulfadiazine does not stain clothing.

Occasionally, pain is experienced on application; intensity and duration depend on depth of burn. Analgesic may be required.

If burned area is fairly extensive, protective isolation is indicated.

When drug is applied to extensive areas, serum sulfa concentrations, urinalysis, and kidney function tests should be monitored, since significant quantities of drug may be absorbed. Observe patient for reactions attributed to sulfonamides.

Observe for and report hypersensitivity reaction manifested by rash, itching, or burning sensation in unburned areas.

If possible, patient should be bathed daily (in whirlpool or shower or in bed) as aid to debridement.

Unless adverse reactions occur, treatment should continue until satisfactory healing or until burn site is ready for grafting.

Preserved at room temperature away from heat.

See nursing implications, diagnostic test interferences, and drug interactions for Sulfisoxazole (prototype Sulfonamide).

Drug Interactions. Silver sulfadiazine reacts with most **heavy metals,** with possible release of silver and darkening of cream. Topically applied **proteolytic enzymes** may be inactivated by the silver in silver sulfadiazine.

SIMETHICONE

(si-meth'i-kone)

(Gas-x, Mylicon, Silain)

Antiflatulent

ACTIONS AND USES. A surfactant (surface-active agent) claimed to defoam gastric juice by causing small gas bubbles to break up and coalesce so they can be more easily removed by belching or passing flatus.

Used to relieve flatulence and functional gastric bloating.

ROUTE AND DOSAGE. Oral: 40 to 100 mg after meals and at bedtime, as needed.

S

NURSING IMPLICATIONS

Shake suspension well before pouring.

Instruct patient to chew tablet form thoroughly before swallowing.

Simethicone is available alone or in combination with antacids such as aluminum hydroxide gel and magnesium hydroxide mixtures, e.g., Di-Gel Liquid, Gelusil, Maalox Plus, Mylanta, Silain Gel, Simeco.

SODIUM BICARBONATE

("Baking Soda", Bell/ans, $NaHCO_3$, Soda Mint)

Antacid
Alkalizer (systemic)
Electrolyte

ACTIONS AND USES. Short-acting, potent systemic antacid. Rapidly neutralizes gastric acid to form sodium chloride, carbon dioxide, and water. After absorption, plasma alkali reserve is increased and excess sodium and bicarbonate ions excreted in urine, thus rendering it less acid. Not suitable for treatment of peptic ulcer because it is short-acting, high in sodium and may cause gastric distention (from CO_2 release), systemic alkalosis and possibly acid-rebound. In the presence of acidosis, replaces bicarbonate ions and thus restores buffering capacity of body. Each gram of sodium bicarbonate contains approximately 12 mEq of sodium.

Used as systemic alkalizer to correct metabolic acidosis (as occurs in diabetes mellitus, shock, cardiac arrest, or vascular collapse), to minimize uric acid crystallization associated with uricosuric agents, to increase antimicrobial effectiveness of aminoglycosides, and the solubility of sulfonamides, and to enhance renal excretion of barbiturate and salicylate overdosage. Commonly used as home remedy for relief of occasional heartburn, indigestion, or sour stomach. Used topically as paste, bath or soak to relieve itching and minor skin irritations such as sunburn, insect bites, prickly heat, poison ivy, sumac, or oak. Sterile solutions are used to buffer acidic parenteral solutions to prevent acidosis. Also as a buffering agent in many commercial products (e.g., mouthwashes, douches, enemas, ophthalmic solutions).

ABSORPTION AND FATE. Completely absorbed following oral administration: rapid onset of action; short duration of action (8 to 10 minutes). Following IV administration, acts within 15 minutes; duration of action 1 to 2 hours. Excreted in urine within 3 to 4 hours.

CONTRAINDICATIONS AND PRECAUTIONS. Prolonged therapy with sodium bicarbonate, patients losing chlorides (as from vomiting, GI suction, diuresis), heart disease, hypertension, renal insufficiency, peptic ulcer. *Cautious Use:* presence of edema, sodium-retaining disorders, elderly patients.

ADVERSE/SIDE EFFECTS. GI: belching, gastric distention, flatulence. **Metabolic:** *systemic alkalosis* (anorexia, abdominal cramps, nausea, vomiting, dizziness, headache, irritability, muscle cramps, pain, twitching, weakness, depressed respirations, convulsions); electrolyte imbalance: sodium overload (pulmonary edema), hypocalcemia (tetany), hypokalemia. **Rapid IV in neonates:** hypernatremia, reduction in CSF pressure, intracranial hemorrhage. **Other:** milk–alkali syndrome *(see Nursing Implications),* severe tissue damage following extravasation of IV solution, dehydration, renal calculi or crystals, impaired renal function, renal calculi.

ROUTE AND DOSAGE. Adults: *Antacid:* **Oral:** 300 mg to 2 Gm (tablets) one to four times daily, or ½ teaspoon (powder) in glass of water. Each ½ teaspoon dose contains 20.9 mEq (0.476 Gm) sodium. *Urinary alkalizer:* 325 mg to 2 Gm, one to four times daily usually before meals and at bedtime. Not to exceed 16 Gm daily. *Cardiac arrest:* **Intravenous (bolus):** 200 to 300 mEq as the 7.5 or 8.4% solution, administered rapidly. Further doses based on arterial blood gas determinations. *Metabolic acidosis:* 2 to 5 mEq/kg by IV infusion over a 4- to 8-hour period. **Topical use for skin problems:** *See Nursing Implications.* **Infants (up to 2 years):** By IV infusion up to 8 mEq/kg/day as a 4.2% solution. *Note:* daily dosage should not exceed 200 mEq or (8) ½ teaspoons of powder for individuals under 60 years, and up to 100 mEq or (4) ½ teaspoons for individuals over 60.

NURSING IMPLICATIONS

Antacid use: Antacid tablets should be chewed thoroughly and taken with a full glass of water. The powder form should be dissolved in a full glass of water.

Instruct patient to wait until effervescent product has dissolved and stopped bubbling before drinking it.

Chronic administration of oral preparation with milk or calcium can cause milk–alkali syndrome: anorexia, nausea, vomiting, headache, mental confusion, hypercalcemia, hypophosphatemia, soft tissue calcification, renal and ureteral calculi, renal insufficiency, metabolic alkalosis.

Caution patient who self-medicates that even routine doses of sodium bicarbonate or soda mints may be sufficient to cause sodium retention and alkalosis especially when renal function is impaired. Antacids should not be taken longer than 2 weeks except under advise and supervision of a physician.

For urinary alkalinization: Urinary pH should be monitored as a guide to dosage (pH testing with nitrazine paper may be done at intervals throughout the day and dosage adjustments made accordingly).

Metabolic acidosis: patient should be closely monitored by observations of clinical condition and by measurements of acid-base status (blood pH, Po_2, Pco_2, HCO_3^-, and other electrolytes are usually made several times daily during acute period). Observe for signs of alkalosis (overtreatment). *See Adverse/Side Effects.*

If symptoms of alkalosis develop they sometimes can be reversed by having patient rebreathe expired air in a paper bag or rebreathing mask. Have on hand parenteral calcium gluconate and 2.14% ammonium chloride solution for treatment of severe alkalosis and tetany.

Observe for and report improvement or reversal in signs and symptoms of metabolic acidosis: dry skin and mucous membranes, polyuria, polydipsia, nausea, vomiting, abdominal pain, air hunger, (Kussmaul's) respiration, hyperpnea.

Infusion should be stopped immediately if extravasation occurs. Severe tissue damage has followed tissue infiltration.

Topical use (manufacturer's directions): *Bath or soak:* ½ cup or more into tub of warm water. *Footsoak:* 4 tablespoons/quart warm water; soak 5 to 10 minutes. *Paste:* 3 parts sodium bicarbonate to 1 part water. Solutions in water slowly decompose: decomposition is accelerated by agitating or warming the solution.

Commonly used OTC antacid products containing sodium bicarbonate: *Alka-Seltzer* (also contains aspirin 325 mg and citric acid); *Alka-Seltzer without aspirin; Bi-So-Dol* (also contains calcium and magnesium carbonates, magnesium oxide, or hydroxide); *Bromo-Seltzer* (also contains acetaminophen and citric acid); *Fizrin* also contains aspirin 324 mg, citric acid and sodium carbonate. *Gaviscon* (also contains aluminum hydroxide, magnesium trisilicate and alginic acid).

Avoid adding sodium bicarbonate to infusion solutions containing other drugs without consulting pharmacist.

Store in airtight containers. Note expiration date.

S

Diagnostic Test Interferences. Small increase in **blood lactate** levels (following IV infusion of sodium bicarbonate); false-positive **urinary protein** determinations (using Ames reagent, sulfoacetic acid, heat and acetic acid or nitric acid ring method); elevated **urinary urobilinogen** levels (urobilinogen excretion increases in alkaline urine).

Drug Interactions: Sodium Bicarbonate

Plus	Interactions
Amphetamines Mecamylamine (inversine) Pseudoephedrine, quinidine Quinine	By rendering urine alkaline, sodium bicarbonate decreases renal excretion and enhances effects of these drugs
Lithium Phenobarbital Salicylates	Urinary alkalinization increases renal excretion and thus reduces drug effect
Methenamine compounds	Urinary alkalinization inhibits antibacterial activity of methenamine
Tetracyclines	Increase in gastric pH may reduce absorption of oral tetracyclines

SODIUM FLUORIDE

Prophylactic: dental caries

(Fluor-A-Day, Fluoral, Fluorineed, Fluorinse, Fluoritab, Fluotic, Flura, Flura-Drops, Karidium, Karigel, Kari-Rinse, Luride, Pediaflor, Point-Two, Thera-Flur, Thera-Flur-N)

ACTION AND USES. Source of the fluoride ion (F), a trace element. Its incorporation into developing tooth enamel hardens surfaces and increases resistance against cariogenic microbial processes. Topical application reduces acid production by bacteria in dental plaque and promotes remineralization of acid-damaged enamel. Application to exposed root surfaces supports formation of insoluble materials within dentinal tubules, thereby blocking transport of offending stimuli. Arrests rapid dental decay associated with drug-, radiation-, or age-related xerostomia. One of the few agents known that stimulates osteoblastic activity, leading to increased bone mass.

Used to prevent periodontal disease and dental caries, to treat dental cervical hypersensitivity, and to control dental caries associated with xerostomia. *Investigational Use:* with calcium and vitamin D, or calcium and an estrogen in treatment of osteoporosis, and in the management of bone lesions in multiple myeloma.

ABSORPTION AND FATE. Following absorption, F is stored in bones and teeth (particularly in outer surface layer). Small amounts distributed into sweat, saliva, tears, and hair. Crosses placenta and is distributed into milk (0.05 to 0.13 ppm) in amounts unrelated to F content of mother's serum or drinking water. Rapidly excreted principally in urine; small amount in feces.

S

CONTRAINDICATIONS AND PRECAUTIONS. When daily intake of fluoride from drinking water exceeds 0.7 ppm, low-sodium or sodium-free diets, hypersensitivity to fluoride, use of gels or dental rinses by child under 6 years, use of 1-mg tablet or rinse in child under 3 years of age, or 1-mg rinse in child under 6 years of age, pregnancy.

ADVERSE/SIDE EFFECTS. (Rare): rash, atopic dermatitis, urticaria, stomatitis, GI and respiratory allergic reactions. *Acute toxicity:* GI symptoms: salty or soapy taste, dehydration, thirst, excessive salivation, muscle weakness, rash, tremors, transient epileptiform seizures (rare), shock, death from cardiac and respiratory failure. *Chronic overdose:* dental fluorosis (brown or white mottling of tooth enamel), osseous fluorosis (patchy mineralization and possible decrease in bone strength). *Fatal dose:* 500 mg in children; 5 to 10 Gm in untreated adults.

ROUTE AND DOSAGE. **Oral (Water supply less than 0.3 ppm):** **Children (2 years or under):** 0.25 mg; **(2 to 3 years):** 0.5 mg; **(3 to 12 years):** 1.0 mg. (Water supply 0.3 to 0.7 ppm): one half above dose. **Topical (0.05%):** **Children (6 to 12 years):** 5 to 10 ml. **Adults and children (over 12):** (Hypersensitivity, Xerostomia) rinse or gel: 10 ml, once daily. (One ppm fluoride is equal to 1 mg F/L.)

NURSING IMPLICATIONS

All F preparations should be applied or taken after thorough brushing and flossing and preferably at bedtime.

To be effective, F supplementation must be consistent and continuous, i.e., from infancy until 12 to 14 years of age.

A high F content in drinking water and water used in food processing in addition to prescribed fluoride therapy may be a cause of dental fluorosis.

If the family moves or if there is a change in water supply, consult dentist about continuation of fluoride therapy. (Mottling may occur if drinking water has F in excess of 1.5 ppm.)

Fluoride intake is related to concentration in drinking water and foods processed in water. In cold climates, recommended fluoride level in the public water supply is higher than in hot climates because of lower consumption of drinking water.

Recommended daily F intake: Adults: 1.5 to 4 mg; children: 4 years to adolescent: 2.5 mg; Children 1 to 4 years: 0.5 to 1.5 mg; first year of life: 0.1 mg.

Diets high in certain foods (e.g., fish, mineral waters, tea) can provide more than 5 mg F daily.

Acidulated fluoride (Thera-Flur) may dull porcelain or ceramics; neutral fluoride (Thera-Flur-N) is recommended if patient has restorations made of such materials.

Dental fluorosis occurs only during tooth development but remains throughout life. If mild, it appears as opaque paper-white areas on tooth surfaces; if moderate, as brown stains with pitting.

Patient-Teaching Points (Drug Use):

Systemic:

- ✓ Drops or tablets are given preferably after meals. Drops may be taken undiluted or mixed with fluids.
- ✓ Tablets may be allowed to dissolve in the mouth or chewed, before swallowing. Administer with water or fruit juice, or add to water used in preparation of infant formula.

Food–Drug Interaction: Avoid giving sodium fluoride with milk or dairy products. Calcium from these products combines with F, decreasing its absorption.

- ✓ Children under 6 years may not have full control of swallowing reflex. Supervise use of toothpaste, gel, or rinse to prevent swallowing the preparation.

Topical:

- ✓ Topical F treatment for sensitive teeth can be used for all age groups regardless of whether the water supply is fluoridated or not.
- ✓ Topically applied, or rinse preparations are not to be swallowed.
- ✓ If patient's mouth is sore, the neutral preparation is better tolerated.
- ✓ Treatment for hypersensitivity: swish oral solution around and between teeth for 1 minute, then expectorate. If gel is used, apply a few drops to toothbrush and brush gently onto affected surfaces.
- ✓ Gel-drops may also be applied using applicators supplied by the dentist. Spread gel on inner surfaces of applicators which are then placed over lower and upper teeth at

the same time. Instruct user to bite down lightly for 6 minutes. Remove applicators; rinse mouth thoroughly. Applicators are cleansed with cold water.

✓ Do not eat, drink, or rinse mouth for at least 30 minutes after treatment.

Advise patient not to exceed recommended dosage. If mottling of teeth occurs, notify dentist.

Large-dose emetic effect offers some protection in case of oral overdose of sodium fluoride.

Acute toxicity usually is the result of accidental ingestion of rodenticides or insecticides containing fluoride salts.

Treatment: oral or IV calcium, aluminum hydroxide gel, cardiac monitoring, hemodialysis.

Patient-Teaching Points:

Prophylactic F Regimen:

✓ Parent should clean child's teeth as soon as they erupt, with moist gauze-covered fingers.

✓ Supervision of child under 6 in oral hygiene (i.e., techniques and schedule for proper brushing and flossing).

✓ Appropriate eating habits (i.e., well-balanced diet, avoidance of high-carbohydrate snacks).

✓ Regular visits to dentist starting shortly after eruption of primary dentition for treatment and prevention guidance.

Sodium fluoride gel or solution used in orthodontic treatment regimen is applied immediately before attachment or reattachment of the tooth-encircling bands.

Exploratory use with calcium therapy to treat osteoporosis (unlabeled use) is accompanied by increased retention of Ca, and reduction in bone demineralization.

Pregnant or lactating women should consult physician about continuing F therapy.

Some products contain tartrazine, which can cause allergic-type reaction in susceptible persons, especially if aspirin sensitivity is present.

Keep sodium fluoride preparations out of the reach of children.

Store in plastic or paraffin-lined glass containers (sodium fluoride reacts with ordinary glass at a slow but appreciable rate) at room temperature.

SODIUM IODIDE I-131

(Iodotope I-131, Oriodide, Theriodide)

Antineoplastic, antithyroid
Radiopharmaceutical

ACTIONS AND USES. Radiopharmaceutical with relatively long half-life (8.06 days). Processed in form of sodium iodide (NaI) from products of uranium fission or neutron bombardment of tellurium. Chemically and physiologically identical to stable, naturally occurring iodide. Affords relatively simple, effective, economic means of treating hyperthyroidism (Graves' disease) by ablation without surgery. Therapeutic doses of radioactive iodine (RAI) deliver ionizing radiation to follicular cells, thereby damaging and destroying thyroid and neoplastic tissues. About 10% of oral radiation is caused by gamma radiation and 90% by beta radiation.

Used to treat hyperthyroidism and thyrotoxicosis, and to suppress neoplastic disease of thyroid. As a diagnostic aid, tracer doses are used in thyroid function studies and imaging to evaluate suspected hyperthyroidism and to visualize thyroid malignancy and metastasis.

S

ABSORPTION AND FATE. Following oral administration, absorbed from GI tract; evident in blood within 3 to 6 minutes. Physical half-life: 8.06 days. Concentrates in thyroid gland and small amounts in salivary glands and stomach. Iodide secretion from these organs permits radioactivity detection in nasal secretion, oral cavity, trachea, female breast, gallbladder, liver, and intestines. Excreted primarily by kidneys, with small amounts in sweat and feces. Crosses placenta and appears in breast milk. Disintegrates by beta and gamma emission. Radiation of therapeutic dose is expended within 56 days.

CONTRAINDICATIONS AND PRECAUTIONS. Acute hyperthyroidism, large nodular goiter, preexisting vomiting or diarrhea, use of antithyroid, thyroid hormone or iodine-containing preparations within 15 days, recent myocardial infarction, pregnancy, lactation, sensitivity to iodine, patients younger than 30 years of age unless indications are exceptional. *Cautious Use:* patients in childbearing age, impaired renal and cardiac function.

ADVERSE/SIDE EFFECTS. Primary hypothyroidism, thyroid nodules, thyroid cancer (in children), angioedema, petechiae, transient thyroiditis (marked thyroid tenderness with swelling, feeling of fullness, fever, malaise, aching of teeth, headache, transient decrease in erythrocyte sedimentation rate, pain referred to ear, chest, or throat), alopecia (reversible), genetically transmissible chromosomal abnormalities, myelosuppression, blood dyscrasias.

ROUTE AND DOSAGE. Oral (solution and capsules): *Hyperthyroidism:* 4 to 10 mCi single dose; second dose, if necessary, 6 weeks later. *Carcinoma of thyroid:* 50 mCi; subsequent dose: 100 to 150 mCi if necessary.

NURSING IMPLICATIONS

All antithyroid, thyroid, or iodine-containing medications are stopped 5 to 7 days before I-131 dose. After treatment, antithyroid drugs are not resumed but other drugs taken to treat hyperthyroidism symptoms (e.g., propranolol) can be resumed until onset of full therapeutic effect of I-131 (normally 5 to 6 weeks).

Presence of food may delay absorption; therefore patient should fast overnight prior to RAI administration.

When administering oral liquid I-131, rinse container two or three times to ensure delivery of total dose. Glass or plastic cups are preferable to wax cups or paper cups.

Urge patient to empty bladder frequently after therapeutic dosages of ^{131}I to reduce gonadal radiation.

Given only during or 10 days after menstruation.

Expected pattern of response to therapy: first 2 weeks, minimal chemical or clinical change in thyrotoxicosis; next 4 to 8 weeks, decrease in thyroid function reaching nadir (acute effects of radiation) between 8 to 12 weeks post-treatment.

If patient is hyperthyroid following treatment, RAI is repeated in 16 weeks and every 3 to 4 months thereafter until euthyroid state is achieved.

Emphasize need for rest following RAI therapy. Consult physician for activity guides.

Frequently, thyroxine replacement is instituted after patient achieves euthyroid state, as prophylaxis against myxedema. Patient should understand that this will be lifelong medication and that patient will need to return to physician at least once a year for medical surveillance. Consult physician about when to discuss this with the patient and family.

Teach the patient the symptoms of hypothyroidism (enlarged thyroid gland, reduced GI motility, periorbital edema, puffy hands and feet, cool and pale skin, fatigue, vertigo, nocturnal muscle cramps) and advise to be sensitive to verbalized observations of friends who may see a change in appearance. Myxedema develops insidiously over a period of years; objective and subjective symptoms are difficult to detect in oneself.

Urge patient to force fluids for first 48 hours after treatment to aid in flushing out the radiopharmaceutical.

Transient thyroiditis *(see Adverse/Side Effects)* may occur within a week after RAI treatment. Patient should report symptoms promptly to permit treatment.

Temporary thinning of hair may begin 2 or 3 months after treatment.

The patient receiving thyroid cancer treatment is usually confined to a single room. A radiation survey is made of bedding, furnishings, and equipment when patient is discharged. No special precautions are indicated when dose less than 30 mCi is given.

Urine is slightly radioactive for 24 hours, but may be flushed down toilet. Saliva and vomiting is highly radioactive for 6 to 8 hours. Urge patient to refrain from expectorating and avoid coughing for 24 hours, if possible. Urine, saliva, and perspiration remain radioactive for 3 days.

Be fully knowledgeable about agency policies designed to protect patient and health personnel. Work in patient area and body contact with patient should be guided by the principle that radioactivity can be neither neutralized nor destroyed.

If patient is receiving treatment for thyroid cancer, plan patient side activities so as to keep time spent at the bedside at a minimum.

Limit contact to 30 minutes per shift per person the first day; increase time to 1 hour second day. The nurse should not be pregnant. The nurse should wear gloves when handling urine or contaminated linen. Contaminated bed linens and clothing of patient should be monitored and handled separately. Disposable items, such as Kleenex, are also considered radioactive waste.

Decay time for ^{131}I is about 3 months. Radioactive contaminated articles may be stored for controlled decay for the 3-month RAI decay time. Liquid wastes may be disposed of in the sewer if certain AEC or state regulations are met.

Instruct visitors to remain several feet away from the patient who is on therapeutic RAI. Usually visiting is restricted the first day after treatment with more than 30 mCi.

If patient is discharged before 7 days after treatment he or she should be instructed about the following:

- Avoid extended contact with small children (do not cuddle or hold on lap) until 7 days after treatment with ^{131}I.
- Avoid sleeping in same room with spouse until after 7 days from the treatment date.
- Use of the same bathroom facilities as the rest of the family is safe.

Solution is clear and colorless; however, on standing, bottle and solution may darken (without interfering with efficacy).

SODIUM POLYSTYRENE SULFONATE

(Kayexalate, SPS)

(pol-ee-stye'reen)

Resin exchange agent (cation exchange)

ACTIONS AND USES. Sulfonic cation-exchange resin. Removes potassium from body by exchanging sodium ion for potassium, particularly in large intestine; potassium-containing resin is then excreted. Small amounts of other cations such as calcium and magnesium may be lost during treatment.

Used in treatment of hyperkalemia.

S

CONTRAINDICATIONS AND PRECAUTIONS. *Cautious Use:* acute or chronic renal failure; patients receiving digitalis preparations; patients who cannot tolerate even a small increase in sodium load, e.g., actual or impending heart failure, hypertension, edema.

ADVERSE/SIDE EFFECTS. Hypokalemia, hypocalcemia, sodium retention, anorexia, nausea, vomiting, constipation, fecal impaction, diarrhea (occasionally).

ROUTE AND DOSAGE. **Oral: Adults:** 15 Gm (4 *level* teaspoons) one to four times daily; **Infants and small children:** calculated on exchange rate of 1 mEq of potassium per gram of resin.

Rectal enema: **Adults:** 30 to 50 Gm (suspended in 100 sorbitol 20% dextrose in water) every 6 hours.

NURSING IMPLICATIONS

Oral dose should be given as a suspension in a small quantity of water or in syrup. Usual amount of fluid ranges from 20 to 100 ml or approximately 3 to 4 ml/Gm of drug.

Serum potassium levels should be determined daily throughout therapy. Acid–base balance, electrolytes, and minerals should also be monitored in patients receiving repeated doses.

Serum potassium levels do not always reflect intracellular potassium deficiency. Therefore, observe patient closely for early clinical signs of severe *hypokalemia:* irritability, confusion, delayed thought process, muscular pain and weakness. ECGs are also recommended.

Usually a mild laxative is prescribed to prevent constipation (common side effect) and fecal impaction. Check bowel function daily. Elderly patients are particularly prone to fecal impaction.

Since drug contains approximately 100 mg (4.1 mEq) of sodium per gram (1 teaspoon, 15 mEq sodium) sodium content from dietary and other sources may be restricted. Consult physician.

Retention Enema:

- Use warm fluid (as prescribed) to prepare the emulsion. Do not heat sodium polystyrene sulfonate, since this may alter its exchange properties.
- Administer at body temperature and introduce by gravity, keeping suspension particles in solution by stirring. Flush suspension with 50 to 100 ml of fluid; then clamp tube and leave it in place.
- If back leakage occurs, elevate hips with pillows or place patient temporarily in a knee–chest position.
- Do not introduce a thicker solution, because this reduces exchange surface area.
- Urge patient to retain enema at least 30 to 60 minutes but as long as several hours, if possible.
- Irrigate colon (after enema solution has been expelled) with 1 or 2 quarts flushing solution (should be non-sodium containing). Drain returns constantly through a Y-tube connection.

Store remainder of prepared solution for 24 hours, then discard.

Drug Interactions. Potassium-exchange capability of sodium polystyrene sulfonate may be reduced by concomitant use of **antacids** or **laxatives** containing magnesium or calcium.

SODIUM SALICYLATE

(Uracel-5)

NSAID
Salicylate
Antirheumatic

S

ACTIONS AND USES. Properties similar to those of aspirin (qv), but less effective. Liberates free salicylic acid in the stomach and therefore tends to cause gastric irritation. Unlike aspirin, does not inhibit platelet aggregation. Increases prothrombin time, like aspirin, but reportedly associated with less occult blood loss.

Used primarily in treatment of acute rheumatic fever. May be used as an alternative in individuals hypersensitive to aspirin.

CONTRAINDICATIONS AND PRECAUTIONS. Hypersensitivity to other salicylates, severe renal disease, heart failure, patients on low-sodium diets. *See also Aspirin.*

ADVERSE/SIDE EFFECTS. Tinnitus, diminished hearing, nausea, vomiting, hypersensitivity reactions, thrombophlebitis (with rapid infusion), sloughing of soft tissues (with extravasation), pulmonary edema in patients with rheumatic fever. *See also Aspirin.*

ROUTE AND DOSAGE. Oral: Adults: 325 to 650 mg every 4 to 6 hours, as needed. *For arthritis:* 3.6 to 5.4 Gm daily in divided doses. **Pediatric:** 1.5 Gm/m^2/daily, in 4 to 6 divided doses. **Intravenous: Adults:** 500 mg as slow infusion (over 4 to 8 hours); not to exceed 1 Gm daily. Entire coated tablets are available.

NURSING IMPLICATIONS

Administer with food, milk, or a full glass (240 ml) of water to minimize risk of gastric irritation. Caution patient not to chew or crush tablet.

Some physicians prescribe concurrent administration of sodium bicarbonate or other antacid to prevent gastric irritation, although it may increase urinary excretion of salicylate and thus lower blood salicylate levels.

Dosage in children younger than 2 years is individualized.

In the symphomotic treatment of rheumatic fever. The dosage of sodium solicylate is the same as that employed with aspirin.

Serum salicylate levels may be required as a guide for adequate dosing of patients on long-term therapy.

For patients receiving sodium salicylate IV, frequent checks of infusion site for extravasation and prescribed infusion rate (should be slow) are advised.

Sodium salicylate is incompatible with mineral acids and ferric salts.

There are 2 mEq (46 mg) of sodium in each 325 mg tablet of sodium salicylate; therefore, large doses are not appropriate for patients on low-salt diets.

Warn patient not to self-dose with aspirin or any other OTC drug during sodium salicylate therapy.

Keep medication out of the reach of children.

Store in light-resistant containers. Turns pink on exposure to light.

See Aspirin (prototype NSAID and salicylate).

SODIUM THIOSALICYLATE

(-thye-oh-sul'fate)

(Arthrolate, Asproject, Jecto-Sal, Nalate, Rexolate, Thiocyl, Thiosul, Tusal)

NSAID, salicylate

S

ACTIONS AND USES. Sodium salt of thiosalicylic acid with analgesic activity that may be due to interference with transmission of peripheral pain impulse reaching cerebral level.

Used to ameliorate moderate pain in arthritis; also used in rheumatic fever. Has been used for acute gout, but other agents are more effective.

ABSORPTION AND FATE; CONTRAINDICATIONS AND PRECAUTIONS; ADVERSE/SIDE EFFECTS: *See Aspirin: prototype salicylate.*

ROUTE AND DOSAGE. Intramuscular: Adult: *Acute gout:* 100 mg over 3 to 4 hours, then 100 mg/day. *Analgesia:* (Musculoskeletal pain): 50 to 100 mg/day or on alternate days. *Rheumatic fever:* 100 to 150 mg every 4 to 6 hours for 3 days then reduce to 100 mg twice daily. Continue until patient is asymptomatic.

NURSING IMPLICATIONS

See Aspirin (prototype salicylate).

SOMATROPIN

(Asellacrin, Crescormon, Somatotropin)

(soe-ma-troe'pin)
Anabolic hormone

ACTIONS AND USES. Anterior pituitary growth hormone (GH) extracted from human anterior pituitary at necropsy. Elicits all pharmacologic responses produced by endogenous human growth hormone (GH). Anabolic effect is equated with accelerated linear growth rate in children with GH deficiency and with increased body weight and muscle mass. Increases intracellular transport and utilization of amino acids and retention of potassium, nitrogen, phosphorus, sodium, magnesium, chloride, and calcium. With respect to calcium, increased urinary loss appears to be augmented by increased absorption from intestinal mucosa. Stimulates synthesis of chondroitin sulfate and collagen; increases serum concentration of alkaline phosphatase and urinary excretion of hydroxyproline. In large doses, may exert diabetogenic effect by causing hepatic gluconeogenesis, increased blood glucose levels, decreased glucose tolerance, and decreased sensitivity to exogenous insulin, particularly in diabetes. In some patients serum insulin concentration is increased. Promotes utilization of depot fat (increases circulating fatty acids), and appears to reduce serum cholesterol levels while increasing triglyceride concentrations. May induce bone marrow activity, increase hemoglobin synthesis, and elevate serum levels of immunoglobulin G and transferrin.

Used to treat growth failure due to GH deficiency; as replacement therapy prior to epiphyseal closure in patients with idiopathic GH deficiency. Also to treat GH deficiency secondary to intracranial tumors or panhypopituitarism.

ABSORPTION AND FATE. Plasma half-life: 15 to 50 minutes, but pharmacotherapeutic effects persist several days. More than 90% of drug metabolized in liver; approximately 0.1% of dose is excreted unchanged in urine. Does not cross placenta.

CONTRAINDICATIONS AND PRECAUTIONS. Patient with closed epiphyses; underlying progressive intracranial tumor. *Cautious Use:* diabetes mellitus or family history of the disease, concomitant or prior use of thyroid and/or androgens in prepubertal male; hypothyroidism.

ADVERSE/SIDE EFFECTS. Pain, swelling at injection site; myalgia, early morning headache (rare), hypercalciuria (frequent); oversaturation of bile with cholesterol, induction of hypothyroidism (rare), high circulating GH antibodies with resulting treatment failure, allergic reactions (rare), hyperglycemia, ketosis, accelerated growth of intracranial tumor.

ROUTE AND DOSAGE. Intramuscular: 2 IU or 0.05 to 0.1 IU/kg body weight three times weekly with a minimum of 48 hours between injections. If at any time during continuous administration growth rate does not exceed 2.5 cm (1 inch) in a 6-month period, dose may be doubled for next 6 months (with or without presence of antibodies).

NURSING IMPLICATIONS

Reconstitute each vial (containing 10 IU of drug) with 5 ml bacteriostatic water for injection only. Record date of reconstitution on vial.

Subcutaneous injection should be avoided because it may enhance development of neutralizing antibodies, with resulting treatment failure. Also it may cause local lipoatrophy (localized fat atrophy) or lipodystrophy (defective nutrition of subcutaneous tissue).

Rotate IM sites to prevent tissue damage.

Before initiating treatment, careful documentation is made of growth rate for at least 6 to 12 months. In addition, GH deficiency may be confirmed by demonstrating failure of plasma GH levels to exceed 5 to 7 ng/ml in response to two standard stimuli (e.g., insulin, hypoglycemia, IV arginine, oral levodopa, or IM glucagon). Thyroid, adrenal, and gonadal functions are also evaluated to rule out multiple pituitary hormone deficiency.

Danger of premature epiphyseal closure with somatropin therapy is usually minimal because acceleration of bone age progression is not as marked as that of linear growth rate. However, annual bone age assessments are advised in all patients and especially those also receiving concurrent thyroid and/or androgen treatment, since these drugs may precipitate early epiphyseal closure. Urge parent to take child for bone age assessment on appointed annual dates.

During first 6 months of successful treatment, linear growth rates may be increased 8 to 16 cm or more per year (average about 7 cm/year). Additionally, subcutaneous fat diminishes, but returns to pretreatment value later.

Instruct parent of child under treatment to record accurate height measurements at regular intervals and to report to physician if rate is less than expected.

In general, growth response to somatropin is inversely proportional to duration of treatment. Somatropin should be discontinued when patient has reached satisfactory adult height, when epiphyses have fused, or when patient fails to exhibit growth response.

Hypercalciuria, a frequent side effect in the first 2 to 3 months of therapy, may be symptomless; however, it may be accompanied by renal calculi, with these reportable symptoms: flank pain and colic, GI symptoms, urinary frequency, chills, fever, hematuria.

In patients who respond initially but who later fail to respond to somatropin therapy, test for circulating GH antibodies (antisomatropin antibodies) should be performed.

Diabetic patients or those with family history of diabetes should be observed closely. Regular testing of urine for glycosuria or fasting blood glucose levels is recommended.

Patient with GH deficiency secondary to intracranial lesion should be examined frequently for progression or recurrence of underlying disease process.

Store drug in refrigerator (2° to 8°C). Discard after 1 month.

Drug Interactions. Concomitant treatment with **thyroid hormone** and/or **androgens** may precipitate epiphyseal closure. **Corticosteroids** may diminish growth response to somatropin and act synergistically with it in increasing blood glucose levels and decreasing sensitivity to exogenous insulin.

SPECTINOMYCIN HYDROCHLORIDE

(Trobicin)

(spek-ti-noe-mye'sin)
Antiinfective
Antibiotic
Aminoglycoside

S

ACTIONS AND USES. Aminocyclitol antibiotic produced by *Streptomyces spectabilis.* Antibacterial action results from selective binding of 30S subunits of bacterial ribosomes, thereby inhibiting protein synthesis. Variable activity against a wide variety of gram-negative and gram-positive organisms. Inhibits majority of *Neisseria gonorrhoeae* strains. Not effective against syphilis.

Used only for treatment of uncomplicated gonorrhea, particularly in patients sensitized or resistant to penicillin or other effective drugs.

ABSORPTION AND FATE. Rapidly absorbed after IM injection. Plasma concentration peaks in 1 to 2 hours; appreciable levels persist 8 hours or more. Half-life: 1 to 3 hours; minimal binding to plasma proteins. Active form excreted in urine within 48 hours after injection.

CONTRAINDICATIONS AND PRECAUTIONS. Hypersensitivity to spectinomycin. Safe use during pregnancy and in infants and children not established. *Cautious Use:* history of allergies.

ADVERSE/SIDE EFFECTS. Soreness at injection site, uticaria, dizziness, nausea, chills, fever, insomnia. Following multiple doses: decrease in hemoglobin, hematocrit, or creatinine clearance; elevated alkaline phosphatase, SGPT (ALT), BUN; decrease in urine output.

ROUTE AND DOSAGE. **Intramuscular:** 2 to 4 Gm (4 Gm dose should be divided and administered at 2 different gluteal sites). Reconstitute with accompanying diluent.

NURSING IMPLICATIONS

Shake vial vigorously immediately after adding diluent and before withdrawing drug. Following reconstitution, solution should be used within 24 hours.

Administer IM injection deep into upper outer quadrant of buttock. No more than 5 ml should be injected into single site (20-gauge needle is recommended). Injection may be painful.

Observe patient for 45 to 60 minutes after injection. Systemic anaphylaxis has been reported (apprehension, pruritus, hypertension, abdominal pain, collapse).

All patients with gonorrhea should have serologic tests for syphilis at time of diagnosis and again after 3 months.

Clinical effectiveness of drug should be monitored to detect antibiotic resistance.

SPIRONOLACTONE

(Aldactone)

(speer-on-oh-lak'tone)
Diuretic (potassium-sparing)
Aldosterone antagonist

ACTIONS AND USES. Steroidal compound and specific pharmacologic antagonist of aldosterone. Presumably acts by competing with aldosterone for cellular receptor sites in distal renal tubule. Promotes sodium and chloride (and water) excretion without concomitant loss of potassium. Diuretic effect reportedly not associated with hyperuricemia or hyperglycemia. Activity depends on presence of endogenous or exogenous aldosterone. Lowers systolic and diastolic pressures in hypertensive patients by unknown mechanism. Potentially mutagenic and tumorigenic.

Used in clinical conditions associated with augmented aldosterone production, as in essential hypertension, refractory edema due to congestive heart failure, hepatic cirrhosis, nephrotic syndrome, and idiopathic edema. May be used to potentiate actions of other diuretics and antihypertensive agents or for its potassium-sparing effect. Also used for treatment of (and as presumptive test for) primary aldosteronism. *Investigational Use:* treatment of hirsutism in women with polycystic ovary syndrome or idiopathic hirsutism; adjunct in treatment of myasthenia gravis and familial periodic paralysis. Commercially available in combination with hydrochlorothiazide (Aldactazide).

ABSORPTION AND FATE. Rapidly and extensively metabolized. Peak plasma levels of active metabolite (canrenone) within 2 to 4 hours. Half-life following multiple doses: between 13 and 24 hours. (90% protein bound.) Maximal diuretic effect attained in about 3 days; activity persists 2 or 3 days after discontinuation of drug. Metabolites excreted slowly, primarily in urine, and also in bile. Crosses placental barrier.

CONTRAINDICATIONS AND PRECAUTIONS. Anuria, acute renal insufficiency, progressing impairment of renal function, hyperkalemia. Safe use in women of childbearing potential, during pregnancy and lactation not established. *Cautious Use:* BUN of 40 mg/dl or greater, hepatic disease.

ADVERSE/SIDE EFFECTS. CNS: lethargy, mental confusion, fatigue (with rapid weight loss), headache, drowsiness, ataxia. **Dermatologic:** maculopapular or erythematous rash, urticaria. **Endocrine:** gynecomastia (both sexes), inability to achieve or maintain erection, androgenic effects (hirsutism, irregular menses, deepening of voice); parathyroid changes, decreased glucose tolerance. **GI:** abdominal cramps, nausea, vomiting, anorexia, diarrhea. **Other:** fluid and electrolyte imbalance (particularly hyperkalemia and hyponatremia); evelated BUN, mild acidosis, drug fever, agranulocytosis, SLE, hypertension (postsympathectomy patient), hyperuricemia, gout.

ROUTE AND DOSAGE. Oral: *Essential hypertension:* **Adults:** initial: 50 to 100 mg daily in divided doses, continued for at least 2 weeks; subsequent dosage adjusted according to patient's response. *Edema:* **Adults:** initial: 25 to 200 mg daily in divided doses, continued for at least 5 days; dosage then adjusted to optimal therapeutic or maintenance level; if there is no response, a diuretic that acts on proximal renal tubule may be added; **Children:** 1.5 to 3.3 mg/kg body weight daily in 4 divided doses. *Primary aldosteronism (therapy):* 100 to 400 mg daily in divided doses; *(long test):* 400 mg daily for 3 to 4 weeks; *(short test):* 400 mg daily for 4 days.

NURSING IMPLICATIONS

Administer with food to enhance absorption.

Tablet may be crushed before administration and taken with fluid of patient's choice.

Serum electrolytes should be monitored, especially during early therapy.

Food–Drug Interaction: Potassium supplementation is not indicated in spironolactone therapy (unless patient is also receiving another diuretic and a corticosteroid). Patient is generally instructed to avoid excessive intake of high-potassium foods and salt substitutes *(see Index: Food sources).* If hyperkalemia develops, patient is usually placed on restricted dietary intake of potassium. Consult physician regarding allowable potassium and sodium intake.

Inform patient that maximal diuretic effect may not occur until third day of therapy and that diuresis may continue for 2 or 3 days after drug is withdrawn.

Monitor daily intake and output and check for edema. Report lack of diuretic response or development of edema; both may indicate tolerance to drug action.

Weigh patient under standard conditions before therapy begins and daily throughout therapy. Weight is a useful index of need for dosage adjustment. For patients with ascites, physician may want measurements of abdominal girth.

Check blood pressure before initiation of therapy and at regular intervals throughout therapy.

Be alert for signs of fluid and electrolyte imbalance, and instruct patient to report dry mouth, thirst, abdominal cramps, lethargy, and drowsiness (symptoms of hyponatremia, most likely to occur in patients with severe cirrhosis), as well as paresthesias, confusion, weakness, or heaviness of legs (symptoms of hyperkalemia).

Observe for and report immediately the onset of mental changes, lethargy, or stupor in patients with hepatic disease.

Adverse reactions are generally reversible with discontinuation of drug. Gynecomastia appears to be related to dosage level and duration of therapy; it may persist in some patients even after drug is stopped.
Presumptive diagnosis of primary aldosteronism is made if short test produces serum potassium increase during spironolactone administration followed by decrease when it is discontinued or if long test results in correction of hypertension and hypokalemia with spironolactone.
Preserved in tight, light-resistant containers. Suspension formulation is stable for 1 month under refrigeration.

Diagnostic Test Interferences. Spironolactone may produce marked increases in **plasma cortisol determinations** by Mattingly fluorometric method; these may persist for several days after termination of drug (spironolactone metabolite produces fluorescence). There is the possibility of false elevations in measurements of **digoxin serum levels** by radioimmunoassay procedures.

Drug Interactions. Combinations of spironolactone and acidifying doses of **ammonium chloride** may produce systemic acidosis; use these combinations with caution. Diuretic effect of spironolactone may be antagonized by **aspirin** and other **salicylates** (possibly by competing for same receptor sites). Spironolactone potentiates the actions of other **antihypertensives,** particularly **ganglionic blocking agents** (dosage of these drugs should be reduced by at least 50% when spironolactone is added), and other **diuretics.** Patients receiving spironolactone and **digitoxin** or similar **cardiac glycosides** concurrently should be monitored for decreased effect of cardiac glycoside (spironolactone shortens its half-life, possibly by acting as enzyme inducing agent). Hyperkalemia may result with **potassium supplements** (spironolactone conserves potassium).

STANOZOLOL

(Winstrol)

(stan-oh'zoe-lole)
Anabolic

ACTIONS AND USES. Synthetic steroid with relatively strong anabolic and weak androgenic activity.

Used primarily to increase hemoglobin in selected cases of aplastic anemia. *See Ethylestrenol for actions, indications, and limitations.*

ROUTE AND DOSAGE. Oral: Adults: 2 mg 3 times daily; for young women, 2 mg once or twice daily. **Children: (under 6 years):** 1 mg 2 times daily; **Children (6 to 12 years):** 2 mg 3 times daily.

NURSING IMPLICATIONS

Administer just before or with meals to reduce incidence of gastric distress.
Smaller dose for young women is given to prevent virilizing effects of the drug. If such effects appear (early sign: change of voice), physician should be notified.
Patient may need to be on a restricted salt intake. Check with the physician.
Used with high caloric, high protein diet unless contraindicated.
Be alert to symptoms of hypercalcemia. *(See Index: Clinical sign, symptoms.)*
Stanozolol does not enhance athletic ability.
See Ethylestrenol (prototype anabolic).

STREPTOKINASE

(Kabikinase, Streptase)

(strep-toe-kye'-nase)
Thrombolytic
Enzyme

ACTIONS AND USES. Derivative of the purified filtrates of beta-hemolytic streptococci. Promotes thrombolysis by activating the conversion of plasminogen to plasmin, the enzyme that degrades fibrin, fibrinogen, and other procoagulant proteins into soluble fragments. This fibrinolytic activity is effective both outside and within the formed thrombus/embolus. Decreases blood and plasma viscosity and erythrocyte aggregation tendency thus increasing perfusion of collateral blood vessels. Bacterial source bestows strong antigenic properties: support of antibody formation and high potential for allergic reactions. Use has been associated with altered platelet function. Streptokinase (SK) activity is expressed in international units (IU): one IU equals amount of drug required to activate enough blood plasminogen to lyse a standard fibrin clot within 10 minutes under standard conditions.

Used for treatment of acute extensive deep venous thrombosis, acute arterial thrombosis or embolism, acute pulmonary embolus, coronary artery thrombosis, and arteriovenous cannula occlusion.

ABSORPTION AND FATE. Plasminogen activation begins promptly with infusion or instillation; SK itself is rapidly removed from circulation by antibodies and reticuloendothelial system. Biphasic half-life: initial, 18 minutes (due to antibody action); then 83 minutes. Does not cross placenta but its antibodies do. Anticoagulation effect may persist 12 to 24 hours after infusion is discontinued.

CONTRAINDICATIONS AND PRECAUTIONS. Active internal bleeding, very recent cardiopulmonary resuscitation; recent (within 2 months) intraspinal, intracranial, intraarterial procedures; intracranial neoplasm; CVA, severe uncontrolled hypertension; history of allergic response to SK, recent streptococcal infection, obstetrical delivery; diabetic hemorrhagic retinopathy, ulcerative colitis, diverticulitis; any condition in which bleeding presents a hazard or would be difficult to manage because of location; pregnancy (category A); safe use during lactation or in children, not established. *Cautious Use:* patient with preexisting hemostatic deficits, conditions accompanied by risk of cerebral embolism, septic thrombophlebitis, uremia, hepatic failure.

ROUTE AND DOSAGE. (Volumetric-controlled infusion device and 0.22 or 0.45 micron filter used.) **Intravenous:** loading dose: 250,000 IU over 30 minutes. Maintenance (continuous infusion): 100,000 IU/hour: pulmonary embolus: 24 hours; deep venous thrombosis: 24 to 72 hours. **Intracoronary:** initial: 10,000 to 20,000 IU followed by 2000 to 4000 IU/minute until lysis occurs, then 2000 IU/minute for 1 hour. *Arteriovenous cannulae occlusion:* 250,000 IU.

ADVERSE/SIDE EFFECTS. Allergic: major (12%) (bronchospasm, periorbital swelling, angioneurotic edema, anaphylaxis); mild (urticaria, itching, headache, musculoskeletal pain, flushing, nausea, pyrexia). **Hematologic:** phlebitis, bleeding or oozing at sites of percutaneous trauma; prolonged systemic hypocoagulability; spontaneous bleeding (GU, GI, retroperitoneal); unstable blood pressure; reperfusion atrial or ventricular dysrhythmias, acute CVA or MI (causal relationship not established).

S

NURSING IMPLICATIONS

Prolonged infusion time may seriously deplete plasminogen pool leading to reduced fibrinolytic capacity of the blood (reduced drug response).

Thrombi more than 7 days old respond poorly to SK therapy; therefore IV infusion is started as soon as possible after the thrombotic event.

Effectiveness of intracoronary instillation to prevent extension of myocardial infarct decreases rapidly after 5 to 6 hours.

Since exposure to streptococci is common, SK antibodies (resistance) are normally present in the blood. A loading dose is required to override antibody neutralization of the drug-induced thrombolysis.

Before SK treatment is started, heparin is discontinued and baseline control levels are established for thrombin time (TT), activated partial thromboplastin time (APTT), prothrombin time (PT), Hct, and platelet count. Treatment is delayed until TT and APTT are less than two times the normal control level.

The patient is frequently premedicated with a corticosteroid that can be repeated during the treatment to minimize pyrogenic or allergic reaction.

Heparin is contraindicated during IV infusion of streptokinase, but may be continued during intracoronary administration. After SK infusion and when TT has decreased to less than twice normal control value (usually 4 hours after discontinuation of therapy), anticoagulation therapy is restarted. After intracoronary use, heparin therapy is continued (or instituted). Eventually an oral anticoagulant is substituted for heparin.

Streptokinase is reconstituted with 5 ml 0.9% NaCl Injection (preferred) or 5 ml 5% Dextrose Injection. Roll or tilt vial; avoid shaking to prevent foaming or increase in flocculation. Reconstituted solution may be carefully diluted again, avoiding shaking or agitation of the solution. Slight flocculation does not interfere with drug action; discard solution with large amount of flocculant.

An occluded arteriovenous cannula should be carefully cleared with heparinized saline solution. If adequate flow is not reestablished, instill SK solution into each occluded limb at a constant rate over a 25- to 35-minute period; clamp off cannula for 2 hours, then aspirate contents of limb, flush with saline, and reconnect.

Spontaneous bleeding occurs about twice as often with SK as with heparin. Protect patient from invasive procedures: IM injections are contraindicated. Also prevent undue manipulation during thrombolytic therapy to prevent bruising.

If a blood gas determination is needed, select the radial rather than femoral artery because of greater ease in applying a pressure dressing to control oozing. Pressure to puncture sites, if necessary, should be maintained 15 to 30 minutes.

Support thrombosed extremity for proper alignment and reduce unnecessary movement to prevent infusion site bleeding.

During treatment with SK, TT is generally kept at about two times or more baseline value and checked every 3 to 4 hours.

Report signs of potential serious bleeding; gum bleeding, epistaxis, hematoma, spontaneous ecchymoses, oozing at catheter site, increased pulse, pain from internal bleeding. SK infusion should be interrupted, then resumed when bleeding stops.

Observe infusion site frequently. If phlebitis occurs, it can usually be controlled by diluting the infusion solution.

Monitor for excessive bleeding every 15 minutes for the first hour of therapy, every 30 minutes for second to eighth hour, then every 8 hours.

Complete bed rest is usual during entire treatment.

Check patient's temperature during treatment. A slight elevation, 0.8°C (1.5°F), perhaps with chills, occurs in about one-third of the patients. An elevation to 40°C (104°F) or more requires symptomatic treatment.

If an analgesic/antipyretic is indicated, avoid giving aspirin because of its antiplatelet action; instead acetaminophen or corticosteroids may be prescribed.

Monitor blood pressure. Mild changes can be expected, but report substantial changes (greater than ±25 mm Hg). Therapy may be discontinued.

Report promptly symptoms of a major allergic reaction; therapy will be discontinued and emergency treatment instituted. Minor symptoms (e.g., itching, nausea) respond to concurrent antihistamine and/or corticosteroid treatment without interruption of SK administration.

Check pulse frequently. Be alert to changes in cardiac rhythm, especially during intracoronary instillation. Dysrhythmias signal need to stop therapy at once.

Have readily available for treatment of serious bleeding: typed and cross-matched fresh whole blood, packed RBCs, cryoprecipitate or fresh frozen plasma (dextran should not be used); aminocaproic acid (SK antidote).

Patient is at risk for postthrombolytic bleeding for 2 to 4 days after intracoronary SK treatment. Continue monitoring vital signs until laboratory tests confirm anticoagulant control.

Reconstituted solution should be stored at 2° to 4°C (36° to 39°F). Discard after 24 hours. Store unopened vials at 15° to 30°C (59° to 86°F).

Diagnostic Test Interferences: Streptokinase promotes increases in **TT, APTT,** and **PT.**

Drug Interactions: Streptokinase

Plus	Interactions
Aminocaproic acid	Inhibition of streptokinase-induced activation of plasminogen
Anticoagulants (including oral anticoagulants); Antiplatelet agents (e.g., indomethacin, phenylbutazone, salicylates)	Increased risk of hemorrhage

PROTOTYPE

STREPTOMYCIN SULFATE

(strep-toe-mye'sin)
Antiinfective
Antituberculostatic
Aminoglycoside

ACTIONS AND USES. Aminoglycoside antibiotic derived from *Streptomyces griseus,* with bactericidal and bacteriostatic actions. Appears to act by interfering with normal protein synthesis in susceptible bacteria by binding to 30S subunits of ribosomes. Active against a variety of gram-positive, gram-negative, and acid-fast organisms. Because of rapid emergence of resistant strains when used alone, most commonly used concurrently with other antimicrobial agents. Reportedly, the least nephrotoxic of aminoglycosides. In common with other aminoglycosides, has weak neuromuscular blocking effect.

Used only in combination with other antitubercular drugs in treatment of all forms of active tuberculosis caused by susceptible organisms. Used alone or in conjunction with tetracycline for tularemia, plaque, and brucellosis. Also used with other antibiotics in treatment of subacute bacterial endocarditis due to enterococci and streptococci (viridans group) and *Haemophilus influenzae* and in treatment of peritonitis, respiratory tract infections, granuloma inguinale, and chancroid when other drugs have failed. *Investigational Use:* treatment of bilateral Meniere's disease.

ABSORPTION AND FATE. Following IM administration, peak serum levels in 1 to 2 hours; levels slowly diminish by about 50% after 5 to 6 hours, but are still measurable up to 8 to 12 hours. About one-third of dose is bound to plasma proteins. Half-life: about 2 to 3 hours for young adults; longer in newborns, and up to 27 hours in impaired renal function. Diffuses rapidly into most body tissues and extracellular fluids and penetrates tuberculous cavities and caseous tissue. Does not diffuse into CSF unless meninges are inflamed. Excreted rapidly, primarily by glomerular filtration; 30 to 90% of dose is excreted within 24 hours. Small amounts excreted in saliva, sweat, tears, bile, and milk. Crosses placenta.

CONTRAINDICATIONS AND PRECAUTIONS. History of toxic reaction or hypersensitivity to aminoglycosides, labyrinthine disease, during pregnancy or lactation, myasthenia gravis, concurrent or sequential use of other neurotoxic and/or nephrotoxic agents. *Cautious Use:* impaired renal function (given in reduced dosages), use in the elderly and in prematures, neonates, and children.

ADVERSE/SIDE EFFECTS. Hypersensitivity: skin rashes, pruritus, angioedema, drug fever, eosinophilia, exfoliative dermatitis, stomatitis, enlarged lymph nodes, anaphylactic shock, blood dyscrasias: leukopenia, thrombocytopenia (rare), neutropenia, pancytopenia, hemolytic or aplastic anemia, agranulocytosis (rare). **Ototoxicity:** labyrinthine damage (most frequent), auditory damage. **Other neurotoxic effects:** paresthesias (peripheral, facial. **Other:** myocarditis (rare), nephrotoxicity (uncommon), hepatotoxicity, transient bleeding (due to inhibition of factor and especially circumoral), headache, inability to concentrate, lassitude, muscular weakness, optic nerve toxicity (scotomata, V), systemic lupus erythematosus, pain and irritation at IM site, superinfections, neuromuscular blockade (respiratory dimmed or blurred vision), arachnoiditis, encephalopathy, CNS depression syndrome (infants): stupor, flaccidity, coma, paralysis, cardiac arrest). respiratory depression.

ROUTE AND DOSAGE. Intramuscular: Adults: Tuberculosis therapy (various regimens used): up to 1 Gm daily in conjunction with other antitubercular drugs; when sputum becomes negative, either streptomycin is discontinued or dosage is reduced to 1 Gm 2 to 3 times weekly for duration of therapy. For other disease conditions (highly individualized): 1 to 4 Gm daily in divided doses every 6 to 12 hours. **Pediatric:** 20 to 40 mg/kg/day in divided doses. (Doses are modified in renal impairment on basis of creatinine clearance.)

NURSING IMPLICATIONS

Administer IM deep into large muscle mass to minimize possibility of irritation. Injections are painful.

Avoid direct contact with drug; sensitization can occur. Rubber or plastic gloves are advised when preparing drug.

Culture and sensitivity tests are done prior to and periodically during course of therapy.

Patient should be instructed to report any unusual symptom. Adverse reactions should be reviewed periodically, especially in patients on prolonged therapy.

Caloric stimulation and audiometric tests should be performed before, during, and 6 months after discontinuation of streptomycin. Periodic renal and hepatic function tests are also recommended.

Although drug fever is uncommon, it is life-threatening. Monitor temperature and blood pressure. If either are altered, report to physician.

Monitor intake and output. Report oliguria or changes in intake–output ratio (possible signs of diminishing renal function). Sufficient fluids to maintain urinary output of 1500 ml/24 hours are generally advised. Consult physician.

In patients with impaired renal function, drug accumulation reportedly occurs if administered more frequently than every 8 to 12 hours (intervals of 1 to 2 days are recommended if creatinine clearance is 10 ml/minute or greater, and 3 to 4 days if less than 10 ml/

minute). Physician may prescribe an alkalinizing agent to reduce possibility of renal irritation. Frequent determinations of serum drug concentrations and periodic renal and hepatic function tests are advised (serum concentrations should not exceed 25 mcg/ml in these patients).

Be alert for and report immediately symptoms suggestive of ototoxicity. Symptoms are most likely to occur in patients with impaired renal function, patients receiving high doses (1.8 to 2 Gm daily) or other ototoxic or neurotoxic drugs, and the elderly. If drug is not discontinued promptly, irreversible damage may occur.

Damage of vestibular portion of eighth cranial nerve (higher incidence than auditory toxicity) appears to occur in three stages: *Acute stage:* may be preceded for 1 or 2 days by moderately severe headache, then followed by nausea, vomiting, vertigo in upright position, difficulty in reading, unsteadiness, and positive Romberg; lasts 1 to 2 weeks and ends abruptly. *Chronic stage:* characterized by difficulty in walking or in making sudden movements and ataxia; lasts approximately 2 months. *Compensatory stage:* symptoms are latent and appear only when eyes are closed. Full recovery may take 12 to 18 months; residual damage is permanent in some patients.

Auditory nerve damage is usually preceded by vestibular symptoms and high-pitched tinnitus, roaring noises, impaired hearing (especially to high-pitched sounds), sense of fullness in ears. Audiometric test should be done if these symptoms appear, and drug should be discontinued if indicated. Hearing loss can be permanent if damage is extensive. Tinnitus may persist several days to weeks after drug is stopped.

Refer patients receiving drug for tuberculosis to visiting nurse for home supervision and continued teaching, and encourage examination of contacts.

Except for tuberculosis and subacute bacterial endocarditis, streptomycin is rarely administered for more than 7 to 10 days.

Commercially prepared IM solution is intended *only* for intramuscular injection (contains a preservative, and therefore is not suitable for other routes). Stable at room temperature; expiration date 1 to 2 years depending on manufacturer.

Solutions made from streptomycin sulfate powder are preferably used immediately after reconstitution. If necessary, Lilly product may be stored up to 48 hours at room temperature or in refrigerator (2° to 8°C) for 14 days; Pfizer states that reconstituted solutions may be stored up to 4 weeks without significant loss of potency. Check package insert.

Exposure to light may cause slight darkening of solution, with no apparent loss of potency.

Diagnostic Test Interferences. Streptomycin reportedly produces false-positive **urinary glucose** tests using copper sulfate methods (Benedict's solution, Clinitest), but not with glucose oxidase methods (e.g., Clinistix, Tes-Tape). False increases in protein content in urine and **CSF** using Folin-Ciocalteau reaction and decreased **BUN** readings with Berthelot reaction may occur from test interferences. **Culture and sensitivity** tests may be affected if patient is taking salts such as sodium and potassium chloride, sodium sulfate and tartrate, ammonium acetate, calcium and magnesium ions.

Drug Interactions. Streptomycin may produce additive anticoagulant effect in patients receiving **oral anticoagulants** (it is thought that streptomycin interferes with synthesis of intestinal vitamin K and stimulates production of factor V inhibitor). *See Gentamicin: prototype aminoglycoside.*

STREPTOZOCIN
(Zanosar)

(strep-toe-zoe'sin)
Antineoplastic: antibiotic
Alkylating agent
Nitrosurea

ACTIONS AND USES. Antineoplastic antibiotic (produced naturally by *Streptomyces achromogenes*). Therapeutic product is synthetic and is similar to other nitrosurea antineoplastics (e.g., carmustine) but with weaker alkylating effects. Not used therapeutically as an antibiotic because of its potent cytotoxic properties. In general this drug is highly toxic and has a low therapeutic index; thus a clinically effective response is likely to be accompanied by some evidence of toxicity. Inhibits DNA synthesis in both bacterial and mammalian cells and prevents progression of cells into mitosis, affecting all phases of the cell cycle (cell-cycle nonspecific). Appears to have minimal effects on RNA or protein synthesis. Delays repair of DNA damaged by nitrosurea-induced alkylation. Unlike other nitrosureas has markedly significant specificity for pancreas beta and exocrine cells; however, it does not appear to have clinically important diabetogenic properties. Has mild to moderate myelosuppressive activity, is mutagenic, and potentially carcinogenic. Use is limited by high incidence of nephrotoxicity (more than 50%) and strong emetogenic potential.

Used to treat metastatic functional and nonfunctional islet cell carcinoma of pancreas, as single agent or in combination with fluorouracil. *Unlabeled Use:* treatment of a variety of other malignant neoplasms including metastatic carcinoid tumor or carcinoid syndrome, refractory advanced Hodgkin's disease, metastatic colorectal cancer and others. *Investigational Use:* being evaluated in other combination chemotherapeutic regimens.

ABSORPTION AND FATE. Administered by IV infusion; disappears rapidly from plasma and is undetected after 3 hours. Distribution into body tissues and fluid has not been described. Does not cross blood–brain barrier although metabolites are distributed into CSF within 2 hours. Extensive hepatic and renal metabolism. Biphasic half-life: initial, 5 minutes; terminal, 35 to 40 minutes. 60 to 70% IV dose excreted in urine within 24 hours as metabolites, approximately 10% of dose excreted unchanged; 1% excreted in feces, 5% in expired air.

CONTRAINDICATIONS AND PRECAUTIONS. Safe use in pregnancy (category C), during lactation, and in children has not been established; hepatic and renal dysfunction.

ADVERSE/SIDE EFFECTS. GI: nausea, vomiting, diarrhea, duodenal ulcer (rare). **Hematologic:** (rare): mild to moderate myelosuppression (leukopenia, thrombocytopenia, anemia); asymptomatic eosinophilia. **Hepatic:** transient increase in AST, ALT, and/or alkaline phosphatase; hypoalbuminemia, severe liver dysfunction. **Metabolic:** glucose tolerance abnormalities (moderate and reversible); insulin shock with hypoglycemia, glycosuria without hyperglycemia; fever. **NS:** confusion, lethargy, depression. **Renal:** nephrotoxicity: azotemia, anuria, proteinuria, hypophosphatemia, hyperchloremia; Fanconi-like syndrome (proximal renal tubular reabsorption defects, alkaline pH of urine, glucosuria, acetonuria, aminoaciduria); hypokalemia, hypocalcemia. **Other:** local necrosis following extravasation.

ROUTE AND DOSAGE. Intravenous injection, infusion, or intermittent intravenous infusion (over 15 minutes to 6 hours): dosage is given according to published protocols. Continuous-day regimen: 500 mg/m^2 daily for 5 consecutive days every 6 weeks until optimal benefit or toxicity occur. Weekly regimen: single IV dose: 1 Gm/m^2 week for 2 weeks, then dose increased, if necessary, to 1.5 Gm/m^2/week provided toxicity does not occur. Maximum single dose should not exceed 1.5 Gm/m^2. Duration of maintenance therapy for either schedule has not been established.

NURSING IMPLICATIONS

Used only under constant supervision by physician experienced in therapy with cytotoxic agents and only when the benefit: risk ratio is fully and thoroughly understood by patient and family. Hospitalization may not be necessary but (because of drug toxicity) there should be easy access for the compromised patient to a facility with clinical laboratory and other supportive resources.

Intraarterial administration has been used investigationally, but is not recommended because adverse effects can be evoked too rapidly.

When patient is receiving medication on a weekly dosing regimen, onset of therapeutic response usually occurs about 17 days after start of therapy, reaching maximum response in about 35 days.

Response to therapy is evidenced by reduction in organomegaly, lymph nodes, or masses.

Functional islet cell tumors produce and secrete a variety of hormones including glucagon, insulin, calcitonin, serotonin, and others. Successful therapy with streptozocin (alone or in combination) produces a biochemical response evidenced by decreased secretion of hormones as well as measurable tumor regression. Thus, serial fasting insulin levels during treatment indicate response to the antineoplastic.

Although this drug has minimal, if any, diabetogenic action, advise patient to report hypoglycemia symptoms (diaphoresis, light-headedness, tremulousness).

Renal function must be adequate to prevent drug toxicity. Serial urinalyses and determinations of BUN, creatinine clearance, and serum electrolytes are obtained prior to and weekly during therapy, then for 4 weeks after termination of therapy.

Dosage adjustment may be made on basis of creatinine clearance. If it is 10 to 50 ml/minute, 75% of usual dose is given; if clearance is less than 10 ml/minute, usual dose is reduced to 50%.

Evidence of drug-induced declining renal function should be reported promptly; changes are dose-related and cumulative.

Early laboratory evidence of renal dysfunction: hypophosphatemia and mild proteinurea. Other evidence includes: changes in intake and output ratio and pattern, urinary retention, hematuria, oliguria, and signs of edema. Instruct patient to report any change promptly.

Mild adverse renal effects may be reversible following discontinuation of streptozocin, but nephrotoxicity may be irreversible, severe, or fatal.

Encourage adeqate fluid intake (2000 to 3000 ml/day). Hydration has been used to give protection against drug toxicity effects; however, the role of hydration in decreasing streptozocin-induced nephrotoxicity has not been established.

Complete blood counts should be performed at least weekly, and liver function tests at least prior to each course of therapy. Dosage adjustment or discontinuation may be required if there is evidence of decreased hepatic or bone marrow function.

Myelosuppression is severe in 10 to 20% of patients and may be cumulative and more severe if patient has had prior exposure to radiation or to other antineoplastics. Be alert to symptoms of sepsis and superinfections (leukopenia) and/or increased tendency to bleed (thrombocytopenia).

Platelet and leukocyte nadirs generally occur 1 or 2 weeks after beginning therapy with streptozocin.

Patient-Teaching Points About Bleeding Precautions:

✓ No aspirin.
✓ Use electric shaver (avoid razor).
✓ Prevent injury, abrasions.

✓ Gentle brushing and flossing of teeth *(See Index: Nursing Interventions: Xerostomia).*
✓ Report hematuria, epistaxis, ecchymoses, petechiae promptly.

Instruct patient to report symptoms that suggest anemia: short of breath; pale mucous membranes and nail beds; exhaustion, rapid pulse.

Superinfection in the oral cavity is evidenced by black furry tongue (fungal overgrowth), or by white, round to irregularly shaped patches that adhere to underlying epithelium (Candidiasis). Inspect mouth daily during therapy.

Monitor and record temperature pattern to promptly recognize impending sepsis.

90% of patients receiving this antineoplastic drug experience severe nausea and vomiting within 1 to 4 hours after drug therapy begins. It may last up to 24 hours and occasionally necessitates discontinuation of treatment.

The anticipation of vomiting, which has previously been experienced with antineoplastic therapy, is sufficient in some patients to influence acceptance of therapy. An antiemetic given routinely every 4 or 6 hours and prophylactively 30 minutes before a treatment may provide sufficient control to maintain the treatment regimen (even if it is reduction but not complete elimination of nausea and vomiting). *(See Index: Nursing Intervention: nausea and vomiting.)*

Antiemetics that have been effective adjuncts to chemotherapy include prochlorperazine (Compazine), metoclopramide (Reglan), trimethobenzamide (Tigan), droperidol (Inapsine), hydroxyzine (Vistaril).

Persons handling streptozocin should wear gloves to protect against topical exposure which may pose a carcinogen hazard. If solution or powder comes in contact with skin or mucosa, promptly flush the area thoroughly with soap and water.

Reconstitute streptozocin powder for injection with 9.5% ml Dextrose Injection or 0.9% Sodium Chloride Injection; resulting solution will contain 100 mg/ml streptozocin and will be pale gold color. Dilute solution further if desired with the same diluents.

Inspect injection site frequently and recognize signs of extravasation: patient complaints of stinging or burning at site, swelling around site, no blood return or questionable blood return.

If extravasation occurs, area requires immediate attention to prevent necrosis. Remove needle, apply ice, and contact physician regarding further treatment to infiltrated tissue. Teach patient to inspect site at weekly intervals and to report changes in tissue appearance.

Protect reconstituted solution and vials of drug from light.

Repeat courses of streptozocin treatment are not given until patient's hepatic, renal, and hematologic functions are within acceptable limits.

Storage: stability is assured for at least 3 years if unopened vials are stored at 2° to 8°C (35° to 46°F). Reconstituted solutions should be discarded after 12 hours (contains no preservative and not intended for multidose use).

Drug Interactions: Streptozocin

Plus	Interactions
Doxorubicin	Doxorubicin half-life prolonged. If used concomitantly, doxorubicin dose is reduced
Myelosuppressive nitrosurea agents (e.g., carmustine)	Synergistic hematologic toxicity of both agents
Nephrotoxic drugs	Increased toxicity of both agents
Phenytoin (Dilantin)	May reduce cytotoxic effect of streptozocin on pancreatic beta cells; concurrent administration is avoided

STRONG IODINE SOLUTION

Suppressant (iodine)

(Lugol's Solution, Strong Iodine Tincture)

ACTIONS AND USES. Inorganic iodide solution; usually contains 5 to 7% elemental iodine dissolved in aqueous KI 5 to 10%. In the toxic thyroid gland, interferes with proteolysis of thyroglobin; thus blocks release of thyroid hormones (T_3 and T_4). Decreases size and vascularity of thyroid gland caused by previous thioamide medication. Suppresses mild hyperthyroidism completely, and partially suppresses more severe hyperthyroidism.

Used to prepare thyroid gland for surgery; may be used with an antithyroid drug in the treatment of thyrotoxic crisis.

ABSORPTION AND FATE. After absorption from GI tract, inorganic iodide enters circulation, from which it is cleared by renal excretion or thyroid uptake to be utilized in hormone synthesis. Small amounts excreted in urine; more than 70% reabsorbed by renal tubules and distributed to tissues. Degradation principally in liver; glucuronide metabolites excreted in bile to feces. Fecal loss regulated by degree of absorption of oral iodide, liver function, intestinal motility, and fecal volume. Readily crosses placenta.

CONTRAINDICATIONS AND PRECAUTIONS. Marked sensitivity to iodine, tuberculosis, hypothyroidism.

ADVERSE/SIDE EFFECTS. Iodism *(see Index: Clinical Signs and Symptoms),* goiter with hypothyroidism (rare).

ROUTE AND DOSAGE. Oral: 0.1 to 0.3 ml (2 to 5 drops) three to four times daily for 10 to 14 days prior to thyroid surgery.

NURSING IMPLICATIONS

Administer solution well diluted in fruit juice, milk, or water after meals.

Teach patients the symptoms of iodism and advise prompt reporting if they appear. Symptoms usually subside rapidly with discontinuation of iodine solution.

Store in airtight container.

See Potassium iodide.

PROTOTYPE

SUCCINYLCHOLINE CHLORIDE

(suk-sin-ill-koe'leen)

(Anectine, Quelicin, Sucostrin, Sux-Cert)

Skeletal muscle relaxant (depolarizing)
Neuromuscular blocking agent

S

ACTIONS AND USES. Synthetic, ultrashort-acting depolarizing neuromuscular blocking agent with high affinity for acetylcholine (ACh) receptor sites. Initial transient contractions and fasciculations are followed by sustained flaccid skeletal muscle paralysis produced by state of accomodation that develops in adjacent excitable muscle membranes. Rapidly hydrolyzed by plasma pseudocholinesterase. May increase vagal tone initially, particularly in children and with high doses, and subsequently produce mild sympathetic stimulation. Intraocular pressure may increase slightly and may persist after onset of complete paralysis. Reported to have histamine-releasing properties. Has no known effect on consciousness or pain threshold.

Used to produce skeletal muscle relaxation as adjunct to anesthesia, to facilitate intubation and endoscopy, to increase pulmonary compliance in assisted or controlled respiration, and to reduce intensity of muscle contractions in pharmacologically-induced or electroshock convulsions.

ABSORPTION AND FATE. Following IV administration, complete muscle relaxation occurs within 1 minute, persists 2 or 3 minutes, returns to normal in 6 to 10 minutes. Following IM injection, action begins in 2 to 3 minutes and lasts 10 to 30 minutes. Plasma level falls rapidly by redistribution. Rapidly hydrolyzed by plasma pseudocholinesterases to succinylmonocholine (a mildly active nondepolarizing muscle relaxant), and then more slowly to succinic acid and choline. Excreted in urine primarily as active and inactive metabolites; 10% excreted as unchanged drug. Does not readily cross placenta.

CONTRAINDICATIONS AND PRECAUTIONS. Hypersensitivity to succinylcholine; family history of malignant hyperthermia. Safe use in pregnancy and in women of childbearing potential not established. *Cautious Use:* during delivery by cesarean section; renal, hepatic, pulmonary, metabolic, or cardiovascular disorders; dehydration, electrolyte imbalance, digitalized patients, severe burns or trauma, fractures, spinal cord injuries, degenerative or dystrophic neuromuscular diseases, low plasma pseudocholinestarase levels (recessive genetic trait, but often associated with severe liver disease, severe anemia, dehydration, marked changes in body temperature, exposure to neurotoxic insecticides, certain drugs); collagen diseases, porphyria, intraocular surgery, glaucoma.

ADVERSE/SIDE EFFECTS. CV: bradycardia, tachycardia, hypotension, hypertension, arrhythmias, sinus arrest. **Neuromuscular:** muscle fasciculations, profound and prolonged muscle relaxation, muscle pain. **Respiratory:** respiratory depression, bronchospasm, hypoxia, apnea. **Other:** malignant hyperthermia, increased intraocular pressure, excessive salivation, enlarged salivary glands, myoglobinemia, hyperkalemia; hypersensitivity reactions (rare); decreased tone and motility of GI tract (large doses).

ROUTE AND DOSAGE. Intravenous: (surgical and anesthetic procedures): 25 to 75 mg administered over 10 to 30 seconds: (prolonged muscle relaxation): continuous infusion (0.1 to 0.2% solution): 2.5 to 4.3 mg/minute. **Intramuscular:** 2.5 mg/kg body weight; total dose not to exceed 150 mg. Highly individualized.

NURSING IMPLICATIONS

Only freshly prepared solutions should be used; succinylcholine hydrolyzes rapidly with consequent loss of potency.

Primarily administered by anesthesiologist or under direct observation.

Some physicians order plasma pseudocholinesterase activity determinations before administering succinylcholine.

Initial small test dose may be given to determine individual drug sensitivity and recovery time.

IM injections are made deeply, preferably high into deltoid muscle. Baseline serum electrolyte determinations advised. Electrolyte imbalance (particularly potassium, calcium, magnesium) can potentiate effects of neuromuscular blocking agents.

Transient apnea usually occurs at time of maximal drug effect (1 to 2 minutes); spontaneous respiration should return in a few seconds, or at most, 3 or 4 minutes.

Facilities for emergency endotracheal intubation, artificial respiration, and assisted or controlled respiration with oxygen should be immediately available. A nerve stimulator may be used to assess nature and degree of neuromuscular blockage.

Selective muscle paralysis following drug administration develops in the following sequence:

levator eyelid muscles, mastication, limbs, abdomen, glottis, intercostals, diaphragm. Recovery generally occurs in reverse order.
Adverse effects are primarily extensions of pharmacologic actions.
Patient may experience postprocedural muscle stiffness and pain (caused by initial fasciculations following injection) for as long as 24 to 30 hours. Inform patient that hoarseness and sore throat are common even when pharyngeal airway has not been used.
Monitor vital signs and keep airway clear of secretions. Observe for and report residual muscle weakness.
Tachyphylaxis (reduced response) may occur after repeated doses. Expiration date and storage before and after reconstitution varies with the manufacturer.

Drug Interactions. Agents that may potentiate or prolong neuromuscular blockage of skeletal muscle relaxants: **acetylcholine, certain antibiotics** (gentamicin, kanamycin, neomycin, streptomycins); **benzodiazepines, cholinesterase inhibitors, colistin, cyclophosphamide, cyclopropane, echothiophate iodide, halothane, lidocaine, magnesium salts, methotrimeprazine, narcotic analgesics, organophosphamide insecticides, pantothenyl alcohol, phenelzine, phenothiazines, polymixins, procainamide** (possibly); **procaine, propranolol quinidine, quinine, thio-tepa** (possibly). Succinylcholine may increase risk of cardiac arrhythmias in patients receiving **digitalis glycosides. Diazepam** may decrease neuromuscular blockade of succinylcholine.

SUCRALFATE

(soo-kral'fate)

(Carafate)

Enzyme inhibitor

ACTIONS AND USES. A complex of aluminum hydroxide and sulfated sucrose structurally related to heparin but lacks its anticoagulant activity. Its action is chemically unlike any other drug used for antiulcer therapy. Following oral administration, sucralfate and gastric acid react to form a viscous, adhesive, pastelike substance that is resistant to further reaction with acid. This "paste" adheres to the GI mucosa with a major portion binding electrostatically to the positively charged protein molecules in the damaged mucosa of an ulcer crater or an acute gastric erosion caused by alcohol or other drugs. Sucralfate absorbs bile, inhibits (inactivates) the enzyme pepsin, and blocks back diffusion of H^+ ions (acid). These actions plus adherence of the pastelike complex protect damaged mucosa against further destruction from ulcerogenic secretions and drugs. The aluminum ions released as sucralfate reacts with HCl are partly responsible for sucralfate-poor absorption from GI tract. May decrease rate of gastric emptying; has no effect on activity of trypsin or pancreatic amylase.

Used for short-term (up to 8 weeks) treatment of duodenal ulcer. *Unlabeled Uses:* short-term treatment of gastric ulcer, treatment of aspirin-induced erosions.

S

ABSORPTION AND FATE. Minimally absorbed from GI tract (less than 5% of dose). Duration of action (depends on contact time with damaged tissue) up to 6 hours. 30% of dose retained in GI tract for at least 3 hours; the small amount that is systemically absorbed is excreted unchanged within 48 hours. It is not known if sucrose sulfate crosses placenta or is distributed into milk.

CONTRAINDICATIONS AND PRECAUTIONS. Safe use during pregnancy (category B), by nursing mothers, or by children has not been established.

ADVERSE/SIDE EFFECTS. GI: nausea, gastric discomfort, constipation, diarrhea, dry mouth. **NS:** dizziness, sleepiness, vertigo. **Other:** rash, pruritus, back pain, hypophosphatemia (rare).

ROUTE AND DOSAGE. Oral: Adult: 1 Gm four times daily on empty stomach (1 hour before meals and at bedtime).

NURSING IMPLICATIONS

If drug is to be administered through nasogastric tube, it should be solubilized in an appropriate diluent by a pharmacist. A poorly crushed and dissolved tablet can cause a bezoar.

Antacids may be prescribed for pain relief if needed. Administer ½ hour before or after sucralfate.

Successful short-term course of sucralfate therapy does not seem to alter the tendency of the duodenal ulcer to heal and then to recur.

Sucralfate apparently binds to certain compounds *(see Drug Interactions)* in the intestinal tract, thereby reducing their bioavailability. To prevent this action separate administration of these agents from that of sucralfate by 2 hours.

Although healing has occurred within the first 2 weeks of therapy, treatment is usually continued 4 to 8 weeks (in absence of healing as demonstrated by x-ray or endoscopic examination).

If constipation is a drug-related problem, investigate patient's food–fluid–exercise habits. Relief and prevention of constipation may result from the following measures (unless contraindicated): increase water intake to 8 to 10 glasses/day; increase physical exercise, increase dietary bulk, avoid laxative abuse. Consult physician: a suppository or bulk-producing laxative (e.g., Metamucil) may be prescribed.

Emphasize need to adhere to sucralfate regimen: patient should not omit, increase, or decrease dosage or change administration times.

Advise patient to stop smoking. Research findings indicate that smoking is a major factor in recurrence of duodenal ulcer. Further, it is suggested that giving up smoking may be more important in prevention of recurrence of the ulcer than medication.

Store in tight container at room temperature. Stable for 2 years after manufacture.

Drug Interactions: Sucralfate

Plus	Interactions
Cimetidine (Tagamet) Phenytoin (Dilantin) Tetracyclines	Decreased bioavailability of these drugs

---

SUFENTANIL CITRATE

(Sufenta)

(soo-fen'ta-nil)
Analgesic
Opiate agonist
Anesthetic
C II

S

ACTIONS AND USES. Potent synthetic opioid related to fentanyl (Sublimaze) and with similar pharmacologic actions, but about seven times more potent. Onset of action and recovery from anesthesia occur more rapidly with sufentanil than with fentanyl. Like fentanyl, does not appear to have significant effect on histamine release (believed to be responsible in part for peripheral vasodilation and hypotension induced by opiate agonists). Reported to be especially useful as a primary anesthetic for patients with coronary insufficiency because it inhibits sympathetic responses to surgical stress, such as excessive rise in blood pressure, by producing dose-related decrease in catecholamine release particularly norepinephrine. In common with other opiate agonists, sufentanil can cause respiratory depression and suppression of cough reflex.

Used as analgesic adjunct to general anesthesia and also as a primary anesthetic.

ABSORPTION AND FATE. Immediate onset of action following IV administration. Approximately 93% protein bound. Half-life: almost 2 minutes. Metabolized in liver and small intestines. About 80% of dose eliminated in urine and feces within 24 hours; 2% excreted unchanged.

CONTRAINDICATIONS AND PRECAUTIONS. Hypersensitivity to sufentanil. Safe use during pregnancy (category C) and in nursing women not established. *Cautious Use:* pulmonary disease, reduced respiratory reserve, impaired hepatic or renal function.

ADVERSE/SIDE EFFECTS. CV: bradycardia, tachycardia, hypotension, hypertension. **GI:** nausea, vomiting, constipation. **Respiratory:** bronchospasm, respiratory depression, apnea. **Other:** skeletal muscle rigidity (especially of trunk), chills, itching, spasms of sphincter of Oddi, urinary retention.

ROUTE AND DOSAGE. Intravenous: *Adjunct to general anesthesia:* **Adults:** 1 to 8 mcg/kg, depending on duration of surgery. *As primary anesthetic:* **Adults:** 8 to 30 mcg/kg. **Children (under 12 years):** 10 to 25 mcg/kg administered with 100% oxygen; supplemental doses up to 25 to 50 mcg each for maintenance.

Dosages determined on basis of lean body weight. Reduced dosages for elderly and debilitated patients. Used in conjunction with neuromuscular blocking agent (muscle relevant), administered prior to or concomitantly with sufentanil.

NURSING IMPLICATIONS

Sufentanil is administered only by qualified personnel, specifically prepared in the use of IV anesthesia and in the management of respiratory depression.

Equipment of resuscitation and intubation should be immediately available.

Have on hand naloxone to reverse respiratory depression.

Monitor vital signs. Observe for skeletal muscle rigidity, especially of chest wall, and respiratory depression, particularly in the elderly, and in patients who are obese, debilitated, or who have received high doses.

Because sufentanil is an opioid, the need for preoperative analgesia is generally reduced.

If naloxone is given to reverse respiratory depression bear in mind that the duration of sufentanil-induced respiratory depression may exceed the duration of naloxone.

Tolerance, physical, and psychologic dependence can occur with prolonged use. Classified as Schedule II drug under the Federal Controlled Substances Act.

Store preferably at 15° to 30°C (59° to 86°F), unless otherwise directed by manufacturer. Protect from light during storage. Examine solution for particulate matter and discoloration (solution should be clear) before administration.

S

Drug Interactions: Sufentanil

Plus	Interactions
CNS depressants, e.g., barbiturates, general anesthetics, other opioid tranquilizers	Possibility of additive CNS depression. Dose of one or the other should be reduced

SULFACETAMIDE SODIUM

(Bleph-10, Cetamide, Isopto Cetamide, Sebizon, Sulf-10)

(sul-fa-see'ta-mide)
Antiinfective
Sulfonamide

ACTIONS AND USES. Highly soluble sulfonamide effective against a wide range of gram-positive and gram-negative microorganisms. Exerts bacteriostatic effect by interfering with bacterial utilization of para-aminobenzoic acid (PABA) thereby inhibiting folic acid biosynthesis required for bacterial growth.

Ophthalmic preparations are used for treatment of conjunctivitis, corneal ulcers, and other superficial ocular infections, and as adjunct to systemic sulfonamide therapy for trachoma. The topical lotion is used to treat scaly dermatoses, seborrheic dermatitis, seborrhea sicca, and other bacterial skin infections.

CONTRAINDICATIONS AND PRECAUTIONS. Hypersensitivity to sulfonamides or to any ingredients in the formulation. *Cautious Use:* application of lotion to denuded or debrided skin.

ADVERSE/SIDE EFFECTS. Temporary stinging or burning sensation (common with eye preparation), retardation of corneal healing associated with long-term use of ophthalmic ointment; hypersensitivity reactions: Stevens-Johnson syndrome, lupuslike syndrome; superinfections with nonsusceptible organisms.

ROUTE AND DOSAGE. **Ophthalmic solution (10, 15, 30%):** Initial: 1 or 2 drops into lower conjunctival sac every 1 to 4 hours during the day and less frequently during the night. Interval increased as condition responds. **Ophthalmic ointment 10%:** ½ to 1 inch into lower conjunctival sac every 6 hours and at bedtime. (Also commonly used at night, with drops being used during day.) **Topical scalp and skin lotion 10%:** Apply to scalp at bedtime and allow to remain overnight. If hair and scalp are oily, application should be preceded by a nonirritating shampoo so that drug will be in intimate contact with affected areas. In severe cases, lotion may be applied to scalp twice daily. Skin: apply to affected skin 2 to 4 times daily until infection has cleared.

NURSING IMPLICATIONS

Note strength of medication prescribed and also note that ophthalmic preparations and skin lotion are not interchangeable.

Instruct Patient or Responsible Family Member How to Instill Eye Drops:

- Wash hands thoroughly with soap and running water (before and after instillation).
- Patient should be sitting or lying down if another person is to administer medication. If patient is to instill own medication, have patient stand in front of mirror.
- Examine eye medication; discard if cloudy or dark in color. Avoid contaminating any part of eye dropper that is inserted in bottle.
- With head tilted back, pull down lower lid. At the same time, have patient look up while drop is being instilled into conjunctival sac.
- Immediately apply gentle pressure to punctum (inner canthus next to nose) for 1 minute.
- As soon as pressure is applied to punctum, patient should close eyes gently, so as not to squeeze out medication.
- Blot excess medication with clean facial tissue.

Drug should be discontinued if symptoms of hypersensitivity appear (erythema, skin rash, pruritus, urticaria).

Report purulent eye discharge. Sulfacetamide sodium is inactivated by purulent exudates.
Solutions of sulfacetamide sodium are incompatible with silver preparations (e.g., silver nitrate, mild silver protein).
Store in tightly closed containers in a cool place, preferably between 8° and 15°C (46° to 59°F), unless otherwise directed by manufacturer. On long standing, solutions may darken in color. If this occurs, medication should be discarded.

Drug Interactions. Local anesthetics, which are derivatives of paraaminobenzoic acid (PABA), e.g., **tetracaine,** may antagonize antibacterial activity of sulfonamides.

SULFACYTINE

(Renoquid)

(sul-fa-sye'teen)
Antiinfective: sulfonamide

ACTIONS AND USES. Short-acting sulfonamide bacteriostatic agent. Blocks bacterial synthesis of folic acid from para-aminobenzoic acid (PABA), thereby preventing synthesis of nucleic acids, essential building blocks of the bacterial cell. Effective against infections caused by *Escherichia coli, Klebsiella-Enterobacter, staphylococcus, Proteus mirabilis, Proteus vulgaris.* The increased frequency of resistant microorganisms is limiting usefulness of this agent.

Used to treat acute urinary tract infections (in absence of foreign bodies or obstructive uropathy) when due to susceptible strains of the mentioned microorganisms.

ABSORPTION AND FATE. Rapid absorption following single doses; peak blood level in 2 to 3 hours. Half-life: 4 hours. Protein binding: 86%. Rapidly excreted by kidneys. Following single dose of 500 mg, 88% of dose recovered in urine at end of 24 hours, 95% by end of 5 days; after a dose of 250 mg four times a day for 7 days, excretion distribution: 79% free drug, 21% metabolites. (Free form is therapeutically active.)

CONTRAINDICATIONS AND PRECAUTIONS. Hypersensitivity to sulfonamides, children less than 14 years of age, pregnancy at term, nursing mothers. *Cautious Use:* impaired renal or hepatic function, severe allergies, bronchial asthma, pregnancy.

ADVERSE/SIDE EFFECTS. *See Sulfisoxazole.*

ROUTE AND DOSAGE. Oral: Adult: Initial: 500 mg (loading dose), then 250 mg four times daily, for 10 days.

NURSING IMPLICATIONS AND DRUG INTERACTIONS

See Sulfisoxizole (prototype sulfonamide).

S

PROTOTYPE

SULFADIAZINE

(Microsulfon)

(sul-fa-dye'a-zeen)
Antiinfective
Sulfonamide

ACTIONS AND USES. Short-acting sulfonamide, slightly less soluble than sulfisoxazole (qv). Shares actions, uses, contraindications, precautions, and adverse reactions of other sulfonamides.

ABSORPTION AND FATE. Readily absorbed from GI tract. Detected in urine within 30 minutes following oral administration. Peak serum levels in 3 to 6 hours after oral ingestion. Distributed to most body tissues; readily diffuses into CSF. About 32 to 56% bound to plasma proteins; 10 to 40% in plasma is acetylated. Approximately 50% of single dose is excreted in urine within 72 hours, 43 to 60% as intact drug and 15 to 40% as N_4 acetyl metabolite. *See also Sulfisoxazole.*

ROUTE AND DOSAGE. Oral: Adults: initial: 2 to 4 Gm, followed by 2 to 4 Gm daily in 3 to 6 equally divided doses. **Children (over 2 months):** initial: 75 mg/kg, followed by 150 mg/kg in 4 to 6 equally divided doses; total daily dose not to exceed 6 Gm. Rheumatic fever prophylaxis: 0.5 to 1 Gm daily.

NURSING IMPLICATIONS

Fluid intake must be sufficient to support urinary output of at least 1500 ml/day. If this cannot be accomplished, urinary alkalinizer such as sodium bicarbonate may be prescribed to reduce risk of crystalluria and stone formation.

Preserved in tight, light-resistant containers.

See Sulfisoxazole.

SULFAMETHIZOLE

(Proklar, Thiosulfil)

(sul-fa-meth'i-zole)
Antiinfective
Sulfonamide

ACTIONS AND USES. Short-acting sulfonamide with actions, contraindications, precautions, and adverse reactions as for other sulfonamides. Like sulfisoxazole (qv), excreted in high antibacterial concentrations, mostly in active rather than acetylated form. Most effective against *Escherichia coli, Klebsiella-Aerobacter, Staphylococcus aureus,* and *Proteus mirabilis.*

Used primarily in treatment of acute and chronic urinary tract infections.

ABSORPTION AND FATE. Readily absorbed from GI tract. Peak blood levels within 2 hours. Approximately 2 to 11% in blood is in acetylated form. Distributed to most body tissues; does not appear to diffuse into CSF. Approximately 90% protein bound. Excreted rapidly. About 60% of dose eliminated in 5 hours, only 5 to 7% as N_4 acetylated derivative. *See also Sulfisoxazole.*

ROUTE AND DOSAGE. Oral: Adults: 0.5 to 1 Gm 3 to 4 times daily. **Children (over 2 months):** 30 to 45 mg/kg/24 hours divided into 4 doses.

NURSING IMPLICATIONS

Fluid intake sufficient to support urinary output of at least 1500 mg/day is usually prescribed. Urinary alkalinization generally is unnecessary.

Preserved in tight, light-resistant containers at 15° to 30°C (59° to 80°F). Do not freeze.

See Sulfisoxazole (prototype sulfonamide).

SULFAMETHOXAZOLE

(Gamazole, Gantanol, SMZ, Urobak)

(sul-fa-meth-ox'a-zole)
Antiinfective
Sulfonamide

ACTIONS AND USES. Intermediate-acting sulfonamide closely related chemically to sulfisoxazole and similar to it in actions, uses, contraindications, precautions, and adverse reactions. Intestinal absorption and urinary excretion are somewhat slower than those of sulfisoxazole, and thus it is given less frequently to avoid excessive blood levels. Marketed in fixed-dose combinations with trimethoprim to enhance antibacterial effect (Co-trimoxazole) *(See Nursing Implications)* and with phenazopyridine (Azo Gantanol) for relief of associated dysuria in urinary tract infections.

ABSORPTION AND FATE. Readily absorbed from GI tract. Peak serum concentrations in 3 to 4 hours (12 to 20% in blood is in N_4 acetylated form. About 50 to 70% protein bound. Half-life: 7 to 12 hours, increased to 22 to 50 hours in renal dysfunction. Metabolized primarily in liver. 25 to 75% of dose excreted in 24 hours as unchanged drug (20%) and metabolites.

ROUTE AND DOSAGE. Oral: Adults: initial: 2 Gm, followed by 1 Gm 2 or 3 times daily (8- to 12-hour intervals), depending on severity of infection. **Children (over 2 months):** initial: 50 to 60 mg/kg, then 25 to 30 mg/kg morning and evening (12-hour intervals); not to exceed 75 mg/kg/24 hours.

NURSING IMPLICATIONS

Tablet may be crushed prior to administration and taken with fluid of patient's choice.

Fluid intake must be sufficient to support urinary output of at least 1500 mg/24 hours. Concomitant administration of urinary alkalinizer may be prescribed to reduce possibility of crystalluria and stone formation.

Trimethoprim–sulfisoxizole (TMP–SMZ) is a fixed combination of synergistic antiinfection effective against urinary and middle ear pathogens, and *Pneumocystis carinii pneumonitis* (PCP) in the immuncompromised patient. Its use is associated with increased incidence of fungal infection. Available as: Septra, Co-trimoxazole, Bactrim, Cotrim.

Preserved in tight, light-resistant containers at 15° to 30°C (59° to 86°F). Do not freeze.

See Sulfisoxazole (prototype sulfonamide).

SULFAPYRIDINE

(Dagenan)

(sul-fa-peer'i-deen)
Sulfonamide

S

ACTIONS AND USES. Intermediate-acting sulfonamide with actions, contraindications, precautions, and adverse reactions as for other sulfonamides *(see Sulfisoxazole)*. Mechanisms of action in ability to suppress dermatitis herpetiformis unknown. Not used as an antiinfective because of its toxicity.

Use largely restricted to treatment of dermatitis herpetiformis when sulfones are not tolerated or contraindicated.

ABSORPTION AND FATE. Irregularly and slowly absorbed from GI tract. Peak blood levels within 5 to 7 hours. Distributed to most body tissues; readily enters CSF. Approximately 10 to 45% bound to plasma proteins; up to 75% in blood present as N_4 acetylated form. Urinary excretion rate irregular, but usually complete within 72 to 96 hours; up to 60% excreted as metabolites, 18 to 59% as unchanged drug.

ROUTE AND DOSAGE. Oral: 500 mg four times per day until improvement is noted; daily dose then reduced by 500 mg at 3-day intervals until symptom-free maintenance is achieved. Minimum effective dose used for maintenance.

NURSING IMPLICATIONS

Fluid intake must be sufficient to support urinary output of at least 1500 mg/day. Urinary alkalinizer is usually prescribed to reduce risk of crystalluria and stone formation.

Toxic effects occur commonly, e.g., hepatotoxicity, renal dysfunction, erythema multiforme, epidermal necrolysis, agranulocytosis, aplastic anemia. Close observation of patient and early recognition and reporting of adverse reactions are critically essential.

Preserved in tight, light-resistant containers. Store at 15° to 30°C (59° to 86°F). Do not freeze.

See Sulfisoxazole (prototype Sulfonamide).

SULFASALAZINE

(sul-fa-sal'a-zeen)

(Azaline, Azulfidine, S.A.S.-500)

Antiinfective

Sulfonamide

ACTIONS AND USES. Locally acting sulfonamide. Believed to be converted by intestinal microflora to sulfapyridine (which has antibacterial action) and 5-aminosalicylic acid (which may exert antiinflammatory effect). Other proposed mechanisms of action include: inhibition of prostaglandins known to cause diarrhea and affect mucosal transport, interference with absorption of fluids and electrolytes from colon, and reduction in *Clostridium* and *Escherichia coli* in the stools. Contraindications, precautions, and adverse/side effects are as for other sulfonamides *(see Sulfisoxazole).*

Used in treatment of ulcerative colitis and relatively mild regional enteritis. *Investigational Use:* treatment of granulomatous colitis, Crohn's disease, scleroderma.

ABSORPTION AND FATE. About one-third of dose absorbed from small intestine as unchanged drug; remaining two-thirds absorbed from colon, where it is converted to sulfapyridine (SP), most of which is absorbed, and 5-aminosalicylic acid (5-ASA), 30% of which is absorbed, with remainder being excreted in urine. Peak serum levels in 1.5 to 6 hours for parent drug and 6 to 24 hours for SP (serum levels tend to be higher in slow acetylator phenotypes). Half-life: 5 to 10 hours. Excreted in urine as unchanged drug, SP, 5-ASA, and acetyl derivatives.

CONTRAINDICATION AND PRECAUTIONS. Sensitivity to sulfasalazine and other sulfonamides; agranulocytosis, children under 2 years of age, intestinal and urinary tract obstruction. *See also Sulfisoxazole.*

ADVERSE/SIDE EFFECTS. Frequent: nausea, vomiting, bloody diarrhea; anorexia, arthralgia, rash, anemia, infertility (reversible), blood dyscrasias, hepatic injury, infectious mononucleosis-like reaction, SLE (rare), allergic reactions (common). *See also Sulfisoxazole.*

ROUTE AND DOSAGE. Oral: Adults: initial: 1 to 2 Gm daily, then 3 to 4 Gm daily (up to 8 Gm daily) in equally divided doses; maintenance: 2 Gm daily in 4 divided doses. **Children:** 40 to 60 mg/kg/24 hours in 3 to 6 divided doses; maintenance: 30 mg/kg/24 hours in 4 divided doses.

NURSING IMPLICATIONS

If possible, drug should be administered after eating food to provide longer intestine transit time for the drug.

Sulfasalazine should be given in evenly divided doses over each 24-hour period. Intervals between nighttime doses should not exceed 8 hours.

If GI intolerance occurs after first few doses, symptoms are probably due to irritation of stomach mucosa. Symptoms may be relieved by spacing total daily dose more evenly over the day or by administration of enteric-coated tablets. Consult physician.

Some patients pass enteric-coated tablets intact in feces, possibly because they lack enzymes capable of dissolving them. Advise patient to examine stools and report to physician if tablet is intact. Conventional tablet will be ordered.

GI symptoms that develop after a few days of therapy may indicate need for dosage adjustment. If symptoms persist, physician may withhold drug for 5 to 7 days and restart it at a lower dosage level.

High doses (more than 2 Gm/day) reduce tissue folate stores as shown by measurement of RBC folate. In addition the disease condition itself compromises an adequate dietary intake of folates. Therefore, food sources cannot be depended upon to restore normal levels. A daily supplement may be prescribed.

Desensitization of patient who has an allergic reaction to sulfasalazine can be accomplished safely to permit continued use of the drug. Usually the process is started with one-eighth tablet daily; dose is doubled every 3 to 7 days.

Adverse reactions generally occur within a few days to 12 weeks after start of therapy and are most likely to occur in patients receiving high doses (4 Gm or more).

Forewarn patient that drug may impart an orange-yellow color to alkaline urine and to skin.

Advise patient to remain under close medical supervision. Relapses occur in about 40% of patients after initial satisfactory response. Response to therapy and duration of treatment are governed by endoscopic examinations.

Preserved in tight, light-resistant containers; store at 15° to 30°C (59° to 86°F).

See Sulfisoxazole (prototype Sulfonamide).

Drug Interactions. **Antibiotics** may alter metabolism of sulfasalazine by altering intestinal flora. By chelating **iron,** sulfasalazine absorption may be inhibited, with resulting lower blood levels. Sulfasalazine inhibits **folic acid** absorption. **Phenobarbital** administered concomitantly may decrease urinary excretion of sulfasalazine. *See also drug interactions for Sulfisoxazole.*

S

SULFINPYRAZONE

(Antazone, Anturan, Anturane, Novopyrazone, Zynol)

(sul-fin-peer'a-zone)
Uricosuric
Pyrazolone

ACTIONS AND USES. Potent pyrazolone-derivative renal tubular blocking agent structurally related to phenylbutazone. At therapeutic doses, promotes urinary excretion of uric acid and reduces serum urate levels by competitively inhibiting tubular reabsorption of uric acid. Like all uricosurics, low doses may inhibit tubular secretion of uric acid and cause urate retention. Inhibits release of adenosine diphosphate and 5-hydroxytryptophan, and thus decreases platelet adhesiveness and increases platelet survival time; has no effect on prothrombin or blood clotting time. May cause slight but significant decrease in serum cholesterol. Since it has no apparent analgesic or antiinflammatory activity, it is not used for relief of acute gout. Reportedly not associated with cumulative effects, development of tolerance, or electrolyte imbalance.

Used for maintenance therapy in chronic gouty arthritis and tophaceous gout. *Investigational Use:* to treat drug-induced hyperuricemia, to decrease platelet aggregation and increase their survival in prevention of TIAs and stroke.

ABSORPTION AND FATE. Readily and completely absorbed from GI tract. Peak plasma levels in 1 to 2 hours. Duration of action 4 to 6 hours, but may persist to 10 hours. About 98% bound to plasma proteins. Half-life: 3 hours (range 1 to 9 hours). Rapidly metabolized by liver to active and inactive metabolites. After 2 days, 45% of single dose is excreted as unchanged drug and metabolites.

CONTRAINDICATIONS AND PRECAUTIONS. Known hypersensitivity to pyrazoline derivatives, active peptic ulcer, concurrent administration of salicylates, patients with creatinine clearance less than 50 mg/minute, treatment of hyperuricemia secondary to neoplastic disease or cancer chemotherapy. *Cautious Use:* impaired renal function, pregnancy, history of healed peptic ulcer, use in conjunction with sulfonamides and sulfonylurea, hypoglycemic agents.

ADVERSE/SIDE EFFECTS. GI disturbances (common): nausea, vomiting, diarrhea, epigastric pain, blood loss, reactivation or aggravation of peptic ulcer, ataxia, dizziness, vertigo, tinnitus; edema, labored respirations, convulsions, coma, hypersensitivity, reactions (skin rashes, fever), blood dyscrasias (rare: anemia, leukopenia, agranulocytosis, thrombocytopenia), jaundice, precipitation of acute gout, urolithiasis, renal colic.

ROUTE AND DOSAGE. Oral (first week of therapy): 100 to 200 mg initially twice daily, gradually increased as needed to full maintenance range of 200 to 400 mg twice daily; after serum urate levels are controlled, dosage may be reduced to 200 mg daily in divided doses. Patients previously controlled with other uricosuric agents may begin sulfinpyrazone at full maintenance dosage.

NURSING IMPLICATIONS

Administered with meals, milk, or antacid (prescribed) to prevent local drug irritant effect. Severity and frequency of symptoms increase with dosage. Persistence of GI symptoms may require discontinuation of drug.

During early therapy, fluid intake should be sufficient to support urinary output of at least 2000 to 3000 ml/day (consult physician), and urine should be alkalinized (e.g., with large doses vitamin C) to increase solubility of uric acid and minimize risk of uric acid stones.

Serum urate levels are used to monitor therapy. Aim of therapy is to lower serum urate levels to about 6 mg/dl and thus to reduce joint changes, tophi formation, and frequency of acute attacks and to improve renal function.

Patient must remain under close medical supervision while taking sulfinpyrazone. Therapy is continued indefinitely.

Caution patient to avoid experimentation with dosage, since subtherapeutic doses may enhance urate retention, and large doses may increase risk of toxicity.

Periodic blood cell counts are advised during prolonged therapy. Patients with impaired renal function should have periodic assessments of renal function.

Anturane capsules contain tartrazine which may cause allergic-type reactions including bronchial asthma in susceptible individuals who also may be sensitive to aspirin.

Sulfinpyrazone may increase the frequency of acute gouty attacks during first 6 to 12 months of therapy, even when serum urate levels appear to be controlled. Physician may prescribe prophylactic doses of colchicine concurrently during first 3 to 6 months of treatment to prevent or at least lessen severity of attacks.

Sulfinpyrazone therapy should be continued without interruption even when patient has an acute gouty attack, which may be treated with full therapeutic doses of colchicine or other antiinflammatory agent.

Caution patient to avoid aspirin-containing medications *(see Drug Interactions)*. If an analgesic is required (in patients with normal renal function), generally acetaminophen is recommended.

Patients receiving oral hypoglycemic agents should be supervised closely *(see Drug Interactions)*.

Diagnostic Test Interferences. Sulfinpyrazone decreases urinary excretion of **aminohippuric acid** and **phenolsulfonphthalein.**

Drug Interactions. Possibility of additive uricosuric effects with **allopurinol** (may be used therapeutically). The uricosuric action of sulfinpyrazone is antagonized by **aspirin** and other **salicylates.** Sulfinpyrazone may affect urinary excretion of weak organic acids with resulting higher serum levels, e.g., **aminosalicylic acid, cephalosporins, dapsone, indomethacin, nitrofurantoin, penicillins. Probenecid** may increase toxicity of sulfinpyrazone by inhibiting its renal excretion. Sulfinpyrazone may potentiate hypoglycemia by interfering with renal excretion of **sulfonylurea** hypoglycemic agents. There is the possibility that sulfinpyrazone may enhance hypoprothrombinemic effect of **warfarin** and **other coumarin-type anticoagulants.** Concomitant administration of drugs that tend to increase serum urate levels may necessitate higher sulfinpyrazone dosage, e.g., **alcohol, aluminum nicotinate, diazoxide,** most **diuretics, mecamylamine, pyrazinamide.** Cholestyramine may delay absorption of sulfinpyrazone (administer sulfinpyrazone at least 1 hour before or 4 to 6 hours after cholestyramine). There is the possibility of increased risk of blood dyscrasias with concomitant use of sulfinpyrazone and **colchicine.**

PROTOTYPE

SULFISOXAZOLE

(sul-fi-sox'a-zole)

(Gantrisin, Lipo Gantrisin, Novosoxazole, SK-Soxazole)

Antiinfective
Sulfonamide

S

ACTIONS AND USES. Short-acting derivative of sulfanilamide. In common with other sulfonamides, has broad antimicrobial spectrum against both gram-positive and gram-negative organisms. Bacteriostatic action believed to be by competitive inhibition of *p*-aminobenzoic acid (PABA), thereby interfering with folic acid biosynthesis required for bacterial growth. Increase in resistant organisms is a limitation to usefulness of sulfonamides; cross-resistance to other sulfonamides is possible. Since sulfisoxazole and its derivatives are highly soluble in alkaline urine and slightly acidic urine and are excreted rapidly, the risk of crystalluria is small.

Used in treatment of acute, recurrent, and chronic urinary tract infections, chancroid, used as adjunctive therapy in trachoma, chloroquine-resistant strains of malaria, acute otitis media due to *Haemophilus influenzae,* and meningococcal and *H. influenzae* meningitis. Ophthalmic preparations used in treatment of conjunctivitis, corneal ulcer, and other superficial eye infections and as adjunct to systemic sulfonamide therapy for trachoma. Topical vaginal preparation used for *H. vaginalis* vaginitis.

ABSORPTION AND FATE. Sulfisoxazole and diolamine forms readily absorbed. Peak blood levels within 2 to 4 hours after oral and IM administration and within 30 minutes after IV injection;

wide variations in blood levels. About 85% protein-bound (65 to 72% in nonacetylated form). Distributed only into extracellular fluids. Half-life: 4 to 7 hours. Deacetylation of acetyl sulfisoxazole by enzymes in GI tract results in slower absorption and lower peak levels than equal oral doses of sulfisoxazole. Metabolized chiefly in liver. Major metabolite (N_4 acetyl) is less soluble in acid urine, has no antibacterial activity, and has same toxic potential as parent drug (concentrations in blood and urine approximately 30%). Up to 95% of single dose is excreted in urine within 24 hours (70% as free drug). Small amounts eliminated in feces, sweat, saliva, tears, breast milk, and intestinal and other secretions. Crosses placenta.

CONTRAINDICATIONS AND PRECAUTIONS. History of hypersensitivity to sulfonamides, salicylates, or chemically related drugs; use in treatment of group A beta-hemolytic streptococcal infections; infants less than 2 months of age (except in treatment of congenital toxoplasmosis), pregnant women at term, nursing mothers; porphyria; advanced renal or hepatic disease; intestinal and urinary obstruction. *Cautious Use:* impaired renal or liver function, severe allergy, bronchial asthma, blood dyscrasias, patients with G6PD deficiency.

ADVERSE/SIDE EFFECTS. Low toxicity level, but may include the following: **Blood dyscrasias:** acute hemolytic anemia (especially in patients with G6PD deficiency), aplastic anemia, methemoglobinemia, agranulocytosis, thrombocytopenia, leukopenia, eosinophilia, hypoprothrombinemia. **CNS:** headache, peripheral neuritis, peripheral neuropathy, tinnitus, hearing loss, vertigo, insomnia, drowsiness, mental depression, acute psychosis, ataxia, convulsions, kernicterus (newborns). **GI:** nausea, vomiting, diarrhea, abdominal pains, hepatitis, jaundice, pancreatitis, stomatitis, impaired folic acid absorption. **Hypersensitivity:** headache, fever, chills, arthralgia, malaise, pruritus, urticaria, conjunctival or scleral infection, erythema multiforme including Stevens-Johnson syndrome, exfoliative dermatitis, allergic myocarditis, serum sickness, anaphylactoid reactions, photosensitivity, vascular lesions. **Renal:** crystalluria, hematuria, proteinuria, anuria, toxic nephrosis. **Other:** conjunctivitis, goiter, hypoglycemia, diuresis, overgrowth of nonsusceptible organisms, lupus erythematosus phenomenon, retardation of corneal healing (ophthalmic ointment), alopecia, reduction in sperm count, lymphadenopathy, local reaction following IM injection, fixed drug eruptions.

ROUTE AND DOSAGE. Oral: Adults: initial: 2 to 4 Gm, followed by 4 to 8 Gm divided into 4 to 6 doses per 24 hours. **Children (over 2 months):** initial: 75 mg/kg/24 hours; maintenance: 150 mg/kg divided into 4 to 6 doses per 24 hours; not to exceed 6 Gm/24 hours. Extended-release preparation: total daily dosage given in 2 equally divided doses. **Intravenous, intramuscular, subcutaneous: Adults and children (over 2 months):** initial: 50 mg/kg/24 hours; maintenance: 100 mg/kg/24 hours, divided into 4 doses per 24 hours for IV and given by slow injection or IV drip, divided into 2 or 3 doses per 24 hours for IM. No dilution required for IM, but subcutaneous and IV must be diluted (follow manufacturer's directions.) **Topical:** *Vaginal cream:* 250 to 500 mg (½ to 1 applicator) into vagina twice daily (morning and on retiring) up to 2 weeks; course may be repeated. *Ophthalmic* (4% solution): 1 to 3 drops 3 or more times daily; (4% ointment): small amount into lower conjunctival sac 1 to 3 times a day and at bedtime.

NURSING IMPLICATIONS

Tablet may be crushed before administration and taken with full glass of water (or other fluid) of patient's choice.

Administration with food appears to delay, but reportedly does not reduce amount of drug absorbed.

Monitor intake and output. Report oliguria and changes in intake and output ratio. Fluid intake should be adequate to support urinary output of at least 1500 ml/day to prevent crystalluria and stone formation.

Since a fall in urinary pH (more acidic) increases risk of crystalluria, daily check of urine pH with Nitrazine paper or Labstix is advisable.

Report increasing acidity. If urine is highly acidic, physician may prescribe a urinary alkalinizer, e.g., acetazolamide (routine alkalinization of urine not necessary with sulfisoxazole).

Monitor temperature. Sudden appearance of fever may signify sensitization (serum sickness) or hemolytic anemia (frequent in patients with G6PD deficiency, which is most common among black males and Mediterranean ethnic groups). These reactions generally develop within 10 days after start of drug. Agranulocytosis may develop after 10 days to 6 weeks of therapy.

Fever with sore throat, malaise, unusual fatigue, joint pains, pallor, bleeding tendencies, rash, and jaundice are early manifestations of blood dyscrasias or hypersensitivity reactions.

Skin lesions, papular or vesiculobullous lesions, especially on sun-exposed areas, Stevens-Johnson syndrome (severe erythema multiforme) may be preceded by high fever, severe headache, stomatitis, conjunctivitis, rhinitis, urticaria, balanitis (inflammation of penis or clitoris). Treatment: systemic steroids, local wet dressings every 4 hours on ruptured blisters, and zinc oxide ointment between local treatment periods. Termination of drug therapy is indicated.

Frequent kidney function tests and urinalyses (including microscopic examination) are recommended; complete blood tests and hepatic function tests are advised, especially in patients receiving sulfonamides for longer than 2 weeks.

Determinations of drug blood levels are advised, particularly in patients receiving high doses. Therapeutically effective blood level ranges from 5 to 15 mg/dl; levels above 20 mg/dl are usually associated with adverse reactions.

Bacterial sensitivity tests are not always reliable and therefore must be closely correlated with bacteriologic studies and accurate assessments of clinical response.

Diabetic patients receiving oral hypoglycemic agents should be closely observed for hypoglycemic reactions *(see Drug Interactions).* Monitor urine and blood sugar frequently, as necessary, during and after concurrent treatment. Determinations of blood glucose levels are advised before and shortly after initiation of sulfonamide therapy.

Advise patients to avoid exposure to ultraviolet light and excessive sunlight to prevent photosensitivity reaction, during therapy and for several months after treatment is discontinued.

The patient should understand clearly that the established dosage regimen must be followed: patient should not omit, increase, interrupt, or decrease dose. The full course of treatment should be completed.

Caution patients not to take OTC medications without consulting physician. Many proprietary analgesic mixtures contain aspirin in combination with *p*-aminobenzoic acid *(see Drug Interactions).* Inform patients that excessive doses of vitamin C acidify urine and therefore should be avoided (to prevent crystalluria).

Advise patients using topical applications to stop treatment if local irritation or sensitivity reaction develops and to report to physician. Patient should be informed that sensitization to topical application precludes future systemic use of sulfonamides.

Recent studies suggest that recurrent dysuria may be due to overuse of soap when washing female genitalia, rather than to bacteriuria. Cleansing with water only may prevent this "urethral syndrome."

Oral contraceptives may be unreliable while patient is receiving a sulfonamide. Advise abstinence from intercourse or use of an alternate method of contraception. Breakthrough bleeding should be considered evidence of an interaction.

Advise patient to inform dentist or new physician of taking a sulfonamide.
Topical applications are inactivated by pus, cellular debris, and blood.
Sulfonamides are incompatible with silver preparations.
Preserved in tight, light-resistant containers. Store at 15° to 30°C (59° to 86°F).

Diagnostic Test Interferences. Sulfonamides may interfere with **BSP** retention and **PSP** excretion tests and may affect results of **thyroid function** tests (**I-131** may be decreased for about 7 days). Large doses of sulfonamides reportedly may produce false-positive **urine glucose** determinations with copper reduction methods (e.g., Benedict's and Clinitest). Sulfonamides may produce false-positive results for **urinary protein** (with sulfosalicylic acid test) and may interfere with **urine urobilinogen** determinations using Ehrlich's reagent or Urobilistix. Follow-up cultures are unreliable unless *p*-aminobenzoic acid is added to culture medium.

Drug Interactionss: Sulfisoxazole

Plus	Interactions
Alkalinizing agents, urinary	Increased excretion of sulfonamide
Anesthetics, local (derived from *p*-aminobenzoic acid)	Antagonize antibacterial activity of sulfonamide
Antacids	May decrease absorption of sulfonamide
Anticoagulants, oral	Increased or prolonged anticoagulant effects
Anitconvulsants (hydantoins)	Increased anticonvulsant effects and potential increase in toxicity of anticonvulsant
Digoxin, folic acid	Decreased absorption when used concurrently with a sulfonamide; dose adjustment may be necessary
Hypoglycemics, oral; methotrexate, phenotoin, thiopental	Increased or prolonged clinical effects leading to increase in potential for toxicity
Methenamine and other acidifying agents	Increased danger of sulfonamide crystallization in urine
Oral contraceptives, Estrogens	May increase risk of pregnancy because of increased hepatic metabolism and reduced absorption of estrogen
Oxyphenbutazone, phenylbutazone	Potentiated effects of the agents
PABA and local anesthetics	May antagonize sulfonamide action
Phenothiazines	May increase toxic effects of sulfonamide
Probenecid, sulfinpyrazone	Decreased excretion of sulfonamide resulting in prolonged antibacterial level and increased potential for toxicity

S

SULINDAC

(Clinoril)

(sul-in'dak)
Analgesic
Antipyretic
NSAID

ACTIONS AND USES. Indene acetic acid derivative structurally and pharmacologically related to indomethacin. Pharmacologic properties are similar to those of aspirin (qv) but chemically unrelated. In common with these drugs, exhibits antiinflammatory, analgesic, and antipyretic properties. Exact mechanism of antiinflammatory action not known but thought to result from inhibition of prostaglandin synthesis. Sulindac is an inactive prodrug converted to an active sulfide metabolite in the liver. Comparable to aspirin in antiinflammatory activity, but has longer half-life, lower incidence of GI intolerance and tinnitus, and less effect on bleeding time and platelet function. May prolong bleeding time, but prothrombin time, whole blood clotting time, and platelet count are not affected. Serum uric acid lowering effect is less than that of aspirin. Cross-sensitivity to other nonsteroidal antiinflammatory drugs (NSAID) has been reported.

Used for acute and long-term symptomatic treatment of osteoarthritis, rheumatoid arthritis, ankylosing spondylitis; for acute painful shoulder (acute subacromial bursitis or supraspinatus tendinitis), and acute gouty arthritis.

ABSORPTION AND FATE. Approximately 90% absorbed following oral administration. Plasma concentration peaks within 2 hours in fasting state and within 3 to 4 hours if drug is taken with food. About 99% protein bound. Metabolized in liver to active (sulfide) (responsible for most of its pharmacologic activity) and to inactive (sulfone) metabolites. Half-life of unchanged drug and active sulfide metabolite: 7.8 and 16.4 hours, respectively. Sulindac and its metabolites undergo extensive enteroheptic recirculation. Approximately 50% excreted in urine as unchanged drug and inactive metabolites, and about 25% excreted in feces primarily as active and inactive metabolites. Minimal if any passage of drug across placenta; enters breast milk.

CONTRAINDICATIONS AND PRECAUTIONS. Hypersensitivity to sulindac; hypersensitivity to aspirin (patients with "aspirin triad": acute asthma, rhinitis, nasal polyps) or to other NSAIDs; significant renal or hepatic dysfunction. Safe use during pregnancy, in nursing mothers, and in children not established. *Cautious Use:* history of upper GI tract disorders, compromised cardiac function, hypertension, hemophilia or other bleeding tendencies.

ADVERSE/SIDE EFFECTS. CNS: drowsiness, dizziness, headache, anxiety, nervousness. **CV:** palpitation, peripheral edema, congestive heart failure (patients with marginal cardiac function). **EENT:** blurred vision, amblyopia, vertigo, tinnitus, decreased hearing. **GI:** abdominal pain, dyspepsia, nausea, vomiting, constipation, diarrhea, ulceration, flatulence, anorexia; stomatitis, sore or dry mucous membranes, dry mouth; rarely: gastritis, gastroenteritis, peptic ulcer, GI bleeding. **Hematologic:** prolonged bleeding time, aplastic anemia, thrombocytopenia. **Hypersensitivity** (rare): angioneurotic edema, rash, pruritus, fever, chills, leukopenia, eosinophilia, anaphylaxis. **Other:** Stevens-Johnson toxic epidermal necrolysis syndrome. Causal relationship unknown: hypertension, epistaxis, paresthesias, vaginal bleeding, hematuria.

ROUTE AND DOSAGE. Oral: *osteoarthritis, rheumatoid arthritis, ankylosing spondylitis:* initial: 150 mg twice daily. Subsequent dosage adjusted accordingly to patient's response. Not to exceed 400 mg/daily. *Acute painful shoulder, acute gouty arthritis:* 200 mg twice daily for 7 to 14 days then reduced according to patient's response.

NURSING IMPLICATIONS

If patient cannot swallow tablet, it may be crushed prior to administration.

May be administered with food, milk, or antacid (if prescribed) to reduce possibility of GI upset. However, food retards absorption and results in delayed and lower peak concentrations.

A detailed drug history should be elicited before initiation of therapy. *See Contraindications and Precautions.*

Because sulindac may cause dizziness, drowsiness, and blurred vision, advise patient to exercise caution when driving or performing other potentially hazardous activities.

Baseline and periodic evaluations of hemoglobin, renal and hepatic function, and auditory and ophthalmic examinations are recommended in patients receiving prolonged or high-dose therapy.

Advise patient to report the onset of skin rash, itching, hives, jaundice, black stools, swelling of feet or hands, sore throat or mouth, unusual bleeding or bruising, shortness of breath or night cough.

Since eye changes have been observed with other NSAIDs, their occurrence is possible with sulindac. An ophthalmoscopic examination is recommended if patient has eye complaints.

Therapeutic effectiveness of sulindac may not be evidenced for up to 7 days; peak effect is usually experienced in 2 to 3 weeks: (relief of joint pain and stiffness, reduction in joint swelling, increase in grip strength, and improved mobility).

Inform patient that alcohol and aspirin may increase risk of GI ulceration and bleeding tendencies and, therefore, should be avoided while taking sulindac.

Because sulindac may prolong bleeding time, advise patient to inform dentist or surgeon that patient is taking this drug.

See Aspirin: prototype NSAID.

Diagnostic Test Interferences. Abnormalities in **liver function tests** may occur.

Drug Interactions: Sulindac

Plus	Interactions
Anticoagulants (coumarins)	Prolongation of prothrombin time
Dimethylsulfoxide (DMSO)	Decreased serum levels of sulfide metabolite which could decrease effect of sulindac
Phenobarbital	Decreased effect of sulindac by hepatic enzyme induction
Probenecid	Increased plasma levels of sulindac
Salicylates, e.g., aspirin	Increased GI side effects

SUTILAINS

(Travase)

(soo'ti-lains)

Enzyme

ACTIONS AND USES. Concentrate of proteolytic enzymes produced by *Bacillus subtilis;* available as ointment (white petrolatum and polyethylene base). As a result of enzymatic activity sutilains selectively digests necrotic soft tissue, hemoglobin, and purulent exudate. Moisture and a pH of 6 to 6.8 must be present to support proteolytic activity. Action is unaffected by presence in site of topical bacitracin, gentamicin, mafenide, neomycin, penicillin, silver sulfadiazine, or streptomycin, nor is it affected by appropriate systemic antiinfectives. Action, however, is adversely affected by detergents, compounds with metallic ions, and certain antiseptics *(see Drug Interactions).* There is no consensus about efficacy of sutilains ointment in burn therapy (to remove eschar), although it is used in some medical centers to shorten preparation time for skin grafting.

Used for biochemical debridement of decubitus ulcers, second and third degree burns, pyogenic, incisional or traumatic wounds, ulcers secondary to peripheral vascular disease;

also used adjunctively with other measures to debride necrotic tissue (e.g., mechanical debridement).

ABSORPTION AND FATE. Onset of action after topical application within 1 hour; optimal effects during first 6 hours. Duration of action about 8 to 12 hours.

CONTRAINDICATIONS AND PRECAUTIONS. Wounds communicating with major body cavities, wound containing exposed major nerves or nervous tissue, fungating neoplastic ulcers, bleeding, dermatitis, compromised cardiac or pulmonary reserves. Safe use in wounds during pregnancy or in woman who may become pregnant not established.

ADVERSE/SIDE EFFECTS. Antibody response (to absorbed enzyme material); pain, paresthesia, bleeding, transient dermatitis.

ROUTE AND DOSAGE. **Topical:** Apply ointment three or four times daily. *See Nursing Implications for treatment protocol.*

NURSING IMPLICATIONS

Resuscitation measures to control shock, pain, and electrolyte imbalance should be instituted before starting treatment with sutilains ointment.

Allergic reactions to sutilains has not been reported. Such symptoms should suggest reaction to another agent being used concomitantly.

Maximum effect is usually achieved in 5 to 7 days for burns and wounds, and in 8 to 12 days for ulcers.

When adjunctive therapy has been used and slough is not removed after sutilains treatment for 24 to 48 hours, further application is not likely to be effective. Recheck for break in procedure or for inadvertent use of interacting agents.

If used in treatment of burns, it is most effective before eschar becomes hard and dry.

Drug-induced eschar digestion leads to increased fluid and blood loss in treated area; therefore no more than 10 to 15% of a burned area is treated with sutilanis at one time.

Proteolytic action produces a warm, moist, and nutritious environment for bacteria. Topical antiinfectives are used concomitantly to prevent sepsis if there is extant or threatening systemic invasion.

If ointment gets into the patient's eyes, irrigate promptly and copiously with normal saline or with sterile water.

Inspect wound for bleeding. If it occurs or if pain persists during interval between treatments, sutilains therapy will be discontinued.

Pain induced by the treatment may be reduced by administration of an analgesic beforehand.

If hydrogen peroxide is used to cleanse the wound, it should be used before application of sutilains (not concomitantly).

S

Treatment protocol:

- ✓ Wear gloves.
- ✓ Thoroughly cleanse and irrigate wound area with sterile water or 0.9% saline solution.
- ✓ Gently wipe away dissolved material. Be sure all medication has been removed.
- ✓ Thoroughly moisten wound area (bathing, showering, or saline or sterile water soaks).
- ✓ Change gloves and apply ointment in very thin layer (a small dab will cover an area as large as back of hand).
- ✓ Cover every crevice and crack in wound and extend ointment ¼ to ½ inch beyond areas being debrided.

✓ Apply an appropriate topical antiinfective agent if indicated.
✓ Cover area with loose, wet dressings (not occlusive) to maintain constant moisture.
✓ Repeat entire protocol three or four times a day.
✓ Store in refrigerator at 2° to 8°C (35° to 40°F).

Drug Interactions: Sutilains

Plus	Interactions
Antiinfectives (i.e., benzalkonium chloride, hexachlorophene, nitrofurazone) Detergents Hydrogen peroxide Iodine compounds Silver nitrate Thimerosol	Interfere with enzymatic actions of sutilains

T

TALBUTAL
(Lotusate)

(tal′byoo-tal)
Hypnotic
Barbiturate
C III

ACTIONS AND USES. Short- to intermediate-acting barbiturate with actions, contraindications, precautions, and adverse/side effects as for phenobarbital (qv).

Used as hypnotic in patients with simple insomnia.

ABSORPTION AND FATE. Peak plasma levels within 2 hours following oral dose. Half-life: about 15 hours. Metabolized in liver. Excreted in urine as metabolites and traces of unchanged drug.

ROUTE AND DOSAGE. Oral: *Hypnotic:* 120 mg administered 15 to 20 minutes before retiring. *Sedation:* 30 to 60 mg two or three times daily.

NURSING IMPLICATIONS

Sleep usually occurs in 15 to 30 minutes and lasts 6 to 8 hours.

Prevent hoarding ("cheeking") dose by severely depressed patient.

Avoid alcohol ingestion during therapy with talbutal.

Hypnotic dose should not be given to a patient for treatment of insomnia for period of time exceeding 2 weeks. Action to improve sleep induction and maintenance decreases after this period.

Withdraw drug gradually over a period of weeks after long-term use.

Classified as Schedule III drug under Federal Controlled Substances Act.

See Phenobarbital (prototype barbiturate).

TAMOXIFEN CITRATE

(Nolvadex)

(ta-mox'i-fen)
Antineoplastic
Antiestrogen

ACTIONS AND USES. Nonsteroid gonad-stimulating principle with potent antiestrogenic activity. Competes with estradiol at estrogen receptor sites in target tissues such as breast, uterus, vagina, anterior pituitary, tumor with high concentration of estrogen receptors. Tamoxifen-receptor complexes move into nucleus resulting in decreased DNA synthesis and estrogen responses. Ovulation may be induced by stimulation of the release of hypothalamic gonadotropic-releasing factor. May have oncogenic activity.

Used in palliative treatment of advanced breast cancer in postmenopausal women, and investigationally to stimulate ovulation in selected anovulatory women desiring pregnancy. Patients with recent negative estrogen receptor (ER) assay are unlikely to respond to tamoxifen treatment.

ABSORPTION AND FATE. Blood level following single oral dose reaches peak values approximately 4 to 7 hours after dose administration with only 20 to 30% of drug remaining as tamoxifen. Biphasic half-life: initial: 7 to 14 hours; terminal: 7 days. Hepatic metabolism; enters enterohepatic circulation and is excreted primarily in feces.

CONTRAINDICATIONS AND PRECAUTIONS. Pregnancy especially during first trimester. *Cautious Use:* lactation, vision disturbances, cataracts, leukopenia, thrombocytopenia.

ADVERSE/SIDE EFFECTS. CNS: depression, lightheadedness, dizziness, headache, mental confusion, sleepiness. **CV:** thrombosis. **GI:** nausea and vomiting (about 25% of patients), distaste for food, anorexia. **Hematopoietic:** leukopenia, thrombocytopenia. **Ophthalmic:** retinopathy, corneal changes (infrequent), decreased visual acuity, blurred vision. **Reproductive:** changes in menstrual period, milk production and leaking from breasts, vaginal discharge and bleeding, pruritus vulvae. **Other:** swelling and pain in legs, hands or feet; skin rash or dryness, excessive growth of hair, increased bone pain, and transient local disease flair; loss of hair, weight gain, shortness of breath, photosensitivity, hot flashes, hypercalcemia.

ROUTE AND DOSAGE. Oral: *Advanced breast carcinoma:* 10 to 20 mg twice daily (morning and evening). *Stimulation of ovulation:* 5 to 40 mg twice daily for 4 days.

NURSING IMPLICATIONS

An objective response may require 4 to 10 weeks of therapy, longer if there is bone metastasis.

Bone and tumor pain and local disease flair often necessitate administration of analgesics for pain relief. Reassure patient that this discomfort frequently signals a good tumor response.

Soft tissue disease response to tamoxifen may be local swelling and marked erythema over preexisting lesions and/or the development of new lesions. These symptoms rapidly subside after tamoxifen treatment is initiated.

Complete blood counts including platelet counts are periodically assessed. Transient leukopenia and thrombocytopenia (50,000 to 100,000/mm^3) without hemorrhagic tendency have been reported, but it is uncertain if these effects are caused by tamoxifen.

If side effects are severe, sometimes a simple reduction in dosage gives sufficient relief without losing control of disease.

Report to physician if marked weakness, sleepiness, mental confusion, edema, dyspnea, and blurred vision occur.

Discuss the possibility of drug-induced menstrual irregularities with patient before starting

treatment. She should be advised not to conceive while taking tamoxifen and to notify physician if she suspects pregnancy.
Avoid prolonged sun exposure especially if skin is unprotected. Sun-screen lotions (SFP 12 and above) are available and should be applied to all exposed skin surfaces before going outdoors.
Caution patient not to change established dose schedule, i.e., not to omit, double, interrupt, or divide doses, or change length of dose intervals.
OTC drugs should be avoided unless specifically prescribed by the physician. Discuss with patient, particularly with respect to OTC analgesics.
Report onset of tenderness or redness in an extremity.
Urge patient to adhere to scheduled appointments for clinical evaluation. Medical supervision is necessary during tamoxifen therapy.
Store drug at temperature between 15° and 30°C (59° and 86°F) in container that protects drug from light.

Diagnostic Test Interferences. Tamoxifen may produce transient increase in **serum calcium.**

TEMAZEPAM
(Restoril)

(te-maz'e-pam)
Sedative/Hypnotic
Benzodiazepine
C IV

ACTIONS AND USES. Benzodiazepine derivative with hypnotic, anxiolytic, sedative effects. Principal effect is significant improvement in sleep parameters as evidenced by: reduced night awakenings and early morning awakening, increased total sleep times and absence of rebound effects. Sleep latency is not reduced, and there is minimal change in REM sleep.

Used to relieve insomnia associated with frequent nocturnal awakenings and/or early AM awakenings.

ABSORPTION AND FATE. Absorption nearly complete with detectable blood levels in 20 to 40 minutes and peak concentration reached in 2 to 3 hours; minimal first-pass metabolism. Hepatic metabolism nearly complete with formation of metabolites. Half-life: 10 hours; protein binding: 96%. 80 to 90% dose excreted in urine as inactive metabolites.

CONTRAINDICATIONS AND PRECAUTIONS. Pregnancy (category X); safe use in children below age of 18 not established; narrow angle glaucoma; psychoses. *Cautious Use:* nursing mother, severely depressed patient or one with suicidal ideation, history of drug abuse or dependence, acute intoxication, hepatic or renal dysfunction, elderly patients.

ADVERSE/SIDE EFFECTS. (Usually mild and transient.) **GI:** anorexia, diarrhea. **NS:** drowsiness, dizziness, lethargy, confusion, euphoria, relaxed feeling, weakness; (rare): tremor, ataxia, lack of concentration, loss of equilibrium, hallucination, horizontal nystagmus, paradoxical reaction. **Other:** palpitations.

ROUTE AND DOSAGE. Oral: Adult: 15 to 30 mg at bedtime. **Elderly:** Initial dose: 15 mg.

NURSING IMPLICATIONS

Steady state plasma concentration under research conditions: 26 ng/ml after 24 hours.

Steady state is reached on about the third day of once-a-day regimen. Patient should be advised that improvement in sleep will not occur until after 2 or 3 doses of drug.

If dreams or nightmares (usually occur during REM sleep) interfere with rest, notify physician. An alternate drug or reduced dose may be prescribed.

Since temazepam affects little change in sleep latency, patient may still have difficulty getting to sleep. Drug effect is evidenced by the increased amount of rest once asleep.

If insomnia continues in spite of medication, physician should be consulted. It is possible the complaint is related to a condition for which a more specific treatment is indicated.

Discuss patient's presleep routine and mental activity during attempts to fall asleep. Propose some measures that might help shorten sleep latency:

- Allow time to "unwind" from physical–mental activity of day
- Avoid engaging in mentally stimulating activity just before bedtime
- Go to bed only when sleepy and arise at regular time in the AM
- Gradually increase physical exercise during day (if allowed) but avoid it just before bedtime
- Avoid use of alcohol as a sedative
- Take a warm beverage (e.g., milk) or light snack before bedtime
- Sit upright in bed for 20 to 30 minutes after taking drug; (this may help patient to experience the onset of natural sleepiness)

If patient is elderly, suggest to avoid daytime "catnaps"; but if patient does nap, the time should be added to nighttime sleep (i.e., patient should not believe that 7 to 8 hours of sleep at night are needed in addition to an afternoon nap).

Psychoactive drugs are the most frequent cause of acute confusion in the elderly. Be alert to signs of paradoxical reaction (excitement, hyperactivity, and disorientation) in this age group.

Reduce possibility of confusion during night by providing enough light in the environment, by speaking to patient clearing and simply when it becomes necessary to communicate during period of drug action, by raising bed rails, and by testing patient's understanding about how to call for assistance.

As with any hypnotic drug (and even without medication), onset of sleep culminates a non-conscious progressive, temporally unpredictable process of relaxation. The danger of a lighted cigarette is obvious; therefore no smoking should be allowed after patient begins to prepare for sleep nor after medication is taken.

CNS side effects are more apt to occur in the patient with hypoalbuminemia, liver disease, and the elderly patient. Report promptly incidence of bradycardia, drowsiness, dizziness, clumsiness, lack of coordination. Supervise ambulation, especially at night.

If patient becomes pregnant, she should be advised to stop taking temazepam. If she intends to become pregnant while taking the drug she should discuss the potential risks to the fetus with the physician.

Use by nursing mothers may cause sedation and possibly feeding problems and weight loss in the infant. Neonates metabolize benzodiazepines more slowly than adults, leading to accumulation of both unchanged drug and metabolites.

With long-term use of this drug, hepatic and renal function tests are advised.

Warn patient not to use OTC drugs (especially for insomnia) during temazepam therapy without advise of physician.

Advise patient to consult physician before discontinuing drug especially after long-term use. Gradual reduction of dose may be necessary to avoid withdrawal symptoms.

Use of alcohol and other CNS depressants should be avoided.

Advise patient about using extreme caution when operating machinery or driving a car, because this drug may depress psychomotor skills and causes sedation.

Signs of overdose include weakness, bradycardia, somnolence, confusion, slurred speech, ataxia, coma with reduced or absent reflexes, hypertension, respiratory depression. Treatment includes use of an emetic (if patient is conscious), gastric lavage, and measures to support adequate respiratory function, fluids to encourage diuresis.

Classified as Schedule IV drug under Federal Controlled Substances Act.

Store between 15° and 30°C (59° and 86°F) in tight container, unless otherwise specified by manufacturer.

Drug Interactions: Temazepam

Plus	Interactions
Alcohol and other CNS depressants	Increased sedation; increased effects of both drugs
Hydantoin anticonvulsants (ethotoin, mephenytoin, phenytoin)	Increased serum concentration of hydantoin, leading to toxicity
Levodopa	Decreased antiparkinsonian effect of levodopa
Contraceptives, oral	Pharmacologic effect of temazepam may be increased

---

TERBUTALINE SULFATE
(Brethaire, Brethine, Bricanyl)

(ter-byoo'te-leen)
Adrenergic agonist (sympathomimetic)
Bronchodilator
Tocolytic

ACTIONS AND USES. Synthetic adrenergic stimulant with selective beta$_2$- and negligible beta$_1$-agonist (cardiac) activity. Exerts preferential effect on beta$_2$-receptors in bronchial smooth muscles, inhibits histamine release from mast cells, and increases ciliary motility. These effects lead to relief of bronchospasm in chronic obstructive pulmonary disease (COPD) and significant increase in vital capacity. Other adrenergic effects include relaxation of vaccular smooth muscle, contraction of GI, and urinary sphincters, increase in renin, pancreatic beta-cell secretion, and increase in serum HDL–cholesterol concentration. Increases uterine relaxation (thereby preventing or abolishing high intrauterine pressure).

Used orally or subcutaneously as a bronchodilator in bronchial asthma and for reversible airway obstruction associated with bronchitis and emphysema. *Unlabeled Use:* (oral and IV infusion) to delay delivery in preterm labor.

ABSORPTION AND FATE. Bioavailability is less with oral than SC dose. Onset of action: 30 minutes after oral administration, 6 to 15 minutes after SC, and 5 to 30 minutes after inhalation. Duration of action (bronchodilation): 4 to 8 hours after oral, 1½ to 4 hours after SC, 3 to 6 hours after inhalation. Elimination half-life: 3 to 4 hours; protein binding: 25%. Metabolized in liver and excreted in urine (small amount in feces). Distributed into breast milk.

CONTRAINDICATIONS AND PRECAUTIONS. Known hypersensitivity to sympathomimetic amines, severe hypertension and coronary artery disease, tachycardia with digitalis intoxication, use within 14 days of MAO inhibitor therapy, children under 12 years of age, angle closure glaucoma. Used only after evaluation of risk–benefit ratio in pregnancy, lactation, and in women of childbearing years. *Cautious Use:* angina, stroke, hypertension, diabetes mellitus, thyrotoxicosis, history of seizure disorders, cardiac arrhythmias, the elderly patient, renal and hepatic dysfunction.

ADVERSE/SIDE EFFECTS. (Dose-related.) **CV:** tachycardia, hypotension or hypertension, palpitation, maternal and fetal tachycardia. **GI:** nausea, vomiting. **CNS:** nervousness, tremor, headache, light-headedness, drowsiness, fatigue, seizures. **Other:** sweating, muscle cramps, tinnitus (rare).

ROUTE AND DOSAGE. **Oral:** **Adult:** 2.5 to 5 mg three times daily at 6 hour intervals; not to exceed 15 mg daily. **Children (12 to 15 years):** 2.5 mg three times daily at 6 hour intervals not to exceed 7.5 mg in 24 hours. **Subcutaneous:** **Adults:** 0.25 mg; repeated after 15 to 30 minutes, if necessary. Total dose of 0.5 mg should not be exceeded within 4-hour period. Failure to respond to second 0.25 mg dose within 15 to 30 minutes indicates need to consider other therapeutic measures. **Intravenous infusion:** 10 mcg/minute with titration upward to maximum dose of 80 mcg/minute. IV dosage maintained at minimum effective dose for 4 hours. Oral doses of 2.5 mg every 4 to 6 hours until term. **Inhalation:** **Adults and children (over 12 years):** 2 inhalations separated by 60 seconds at interval of no more than every 4 to 6 hours. (Each actuation delivers about 0.20 mg of terbutaline from the mouthpiece.)

NURSING IMPLICATIONS

Tablet may be crushed before administration and taken with fluid of patient's choice.

Be certain about recommended doses: oral preparation: 2.5 mg; SC: 0.25 mg. A decimal point error can be fatal.

If GI symptoms occur, advise patient to take the tablets with food.

Onset and degree of effect, incidence and severity of side effects of the SC formulation resemble those of epinephrine. Oral terbutaline appears to be equally as effective as ephedrine; however, onset of action is more rapid and it has longer duration of effects.

Teach the ambulatory patient on oral terbutaline how to take own pulse and the limits of change that indicate need to notify the physician.

SC injection is usually administered into lateral deltoid area.

Most side effects are transient and disappear without treatment. However, rapid heart rate may persist for a relatively long time.

Cardiovascular side effects are more apt to occur when drug is given by SC route and when it is used by a patient with cardiac arrhythmia. Check pulse and BP before each dose. If perceptively altered from baseline level, consult physician.

Inhalator Therapy:

- Review and discuss with the patient the instructions for use of inhalator (included in the package).
- Aerosolized terbutaline produces little cardiac stimulation or tremors.
- *See Index: Nursing intervention: inhalation therapy.*
- Contents of the aerosol are under pressure. Warn patient not to puncture container, not to use or store it near heat or open flame, and not to expose it to temperature above 49°C (120°F) may cause bursting. Can should not be discarded into a fire or incinerator. Keep it out of reach of children.
- No other aerosol bronchodilator should be used while the patient is being controlled by aerosol terbutaline. Warn patient not to self-medicate with an OTC aerosol.

Terbutaline appears to have a short clinical period for sustained effectiveness. Advise patient to keep appointments with physician for evaluation of continued drug effectiveness and clinical condition.

If patient has exacerbations of bronchial symptoms, exposure to unknown or unsuspected environmental allergens should be ruled out. Recent studies indicate that the car air-conditioner may harbor respiratory allergens. Make inquiries about exposure to this challenge. The air conditioning system may need to be decontaminated. (Home air conditioning systems have not been implicated.)

Tolerance can develop with chronic use of terbutaline. Consult physician if symptomatic relief wanes. Usually a substitute agent will be prescribed.

Instruct patient to consult the physician if breathing difficulty is not relieved or if it becomes worse within 15 minutes after an oral dose of terbutaline.

The use of an adrenergic aerosol bronchodilator of the stimulant type (e.g., isoetharine) may relieve acute bronchospasm in the patient on chronic oral terbutaline therapy. The physician should outline the schedule for use of both terbutaline and the aerosol bronchodilator.

Tocolytic Therapy:

- Monitor patient for CV signs and symptoms for 12 hours after drug is discontinued.
- Report tachycardia promptly.
- Monitor intake and output ratio. Fluid restriction may be necessary. Consult physician.

Muscle tremor is a fairly common side effect that appears to subside with continued use.

The neonate born of a mother who used terbutaline during pregnancy may have hypoglycemia. Monitor for symptoms if there is reason to suspect this condition.

Instruct patient to adhere to established dosage regimen, i.e., not to change dose intervals or omit, increase, or decrease the dose.

Be alert to the pattern of self-dosing established by the patient on long-term therapy. Caution patient that in the face of waning response increasing the dose may cause overdosage and will not improve the clinical condition. The patient should understand that decreasing relief with continued treatment indicates need for another bronchodilator, not an increase in dose.

Warn the patient not to use OTC drugs unless the physician approves. Many cold and allergy remedies, for example, contain a sympathomimetic agent that when combined with terbutaline may be deleterious to the patient.

Overdosage resulting in enhanced adverse reactions *(see Adverse/Side Effects)* in the alert patient is treated by emptying the stomach (induced emesis and gastric lavage). In the unconscious patient, a cuffed endotracheal tube secures the airway before beginning the lavage. Activated charcoal slurry may be instilled to reduce terbutaline absorption; respiratory and cardiac supportive measures should be readily available.

Store medication at temperature between 15° and 30°C (59° and 86°F). Protect from light and freezing.

Diagnostic Test Interferences. Terbutaline may increase **blood glucose** and free **fatty acids.**

Drug Interactions: Terbutaline Sulfate

Plus	**Interactions**
MAO inhibitors	Concurrent use may cause severe hypertensive crisis
Propranolol	Antagonizes bronchodilating effect of terbutaline
Sympathomimetics, other	May increase effects and potential side effects of sympathomimetics and/or terbutaline; does not preclude, however, use of a stimulant adrenergic bronchodilator for acute bronchospasm *(see Nursing Implications)*

TERPIN HYDRATE ELIXIR
TERPIN HYDRATE AND CODEINE ELIXIR

(ter'pin)
Antitussive
Expectorant
C v

ACTIONS AND USES. Terpin hydrate is a volatile oil derivative claimed to exert direct action on bronchial secretory cells, thereby increasing respiratory tract fluid production and facilitating expectoration.

Commonly used as a vehicle for other cough medications, e.g., terpin hydrate and codeine elixir contains 10 mg codeine in each 5 ml (added for antitussive effect).

CONTRAINDICATIONS AND PRECAUTIONS. Severe diabetes mellitus, peptic ulcer (for self-medication); child younger than 12 years.

ROUTE AND DOSAGE. Oral (terpin hydrate elixir): 5 ml, repeated in 3 to 4 hours, if necessary; (terpin hydrate and codeine elixir): 5 ml three or four times a day.

NURSING IMPLICATIONS

Some patients experience epigastric pain following administration on an empty stomach.

Soothing, local effect of the syrup is enhanced if it is administered undiluted and not immediately followed by water.

Adequate fluid intake and humidification of air will help to liquefy sputum and relieve bronchial irritation.

Because of the high alcoholic content (42.5%) of terpin hydrate elixir, it is undesirable to administer larger doses than recommended.

Terpin hydrate and codeine elixir is classified as a Schedule V drug under the Federal Controlled Substances Act. Warn patient not to exceed recommended dose.

See Benzonatate (prototype antitussive).

TESTOLACTONE
(Teslac)

(tess-toe-lak'tone)
Antineoplastic
Hormone

ACTIONS AND USES. Chemotherapeutic agent with chemical configuration similar to that of certain androgens but devoid of androgenic activity in therapeutic doses. Exact mechanism of antineoplastic action unknown. Action simulates that of androgens without producing virilization in recommended dosage. In breast cancer, effect may result from depression of ovarian function by inhibition of synthesis of pituitary gonadotropin.

Used as adjunctive treatment in palliation of breast carcinoma in postmenopausal women when hormone therapy is indicated. Also effective in women diagnosed before menopause in whom ovarian function has been subsequently terminated.

CONTRAINDICATIONS AND PRECAUTIONS. Pregnancy, premenopausal women, breast cancer in males. *Cautious Use:* hypercalcemia, cardiorenal disease.

ADVERSE/SIDE EFFECTS. CNS: paresthesias. **Dermatologic:** maculopapular erythema, nail growth disturbances. **Endocrine:** deepening of the voice, acne, facial hair growth, clitoral enlargement. **GI:** glossitis, anorexia, nausea, vomiting. **Other:** hypertension, edema in extremities, alopecia (rare and reversible).

ROUTE AND DOSAGE. Oral: 250 mg four times a day.

NURSING IMPLICATIONS

Testalactone treatment is usually continued for a minimum of three months (unless there is active progression of the disease) in order to evaluate response.

Clinical response usually occurs in 6 to 12 weeks and is measured according to the following criteria; decrease in size of tumor, more than 50% of nonosseous lesions decrease in size even though all bone lesions remain static.

Plasma calcium levels are checked routinely and periodically. (Normal serum calcium: 8.5 to 10.6 mg/dl.)

Report signs that may suggest impending *hypercalcemia:* hypotonicity of muscles, bone and flank pain, polyuria, thirst, anorexia, nausea, vomiting, constipation.

Hypercalcemia represents active remission of bone metastasis; if it occurs, appropriate therapy is instituted.

Note intake–output ratio and pattern.

Encourage patient mobility if feasible; if not, assist with passive exercises.

Store at controlled room temperature preferably between 15° and 30°C (59° and 86°F), unless otherwise directed by manufacturer. Protect from freezing.

Diagnostic Test Interferences. **Urinary 17-OHCS** determinations may be elevated.

Drug Interactions. Testolactone may increase effects of **oral anticoagulants.**

PROTOTYPE

TESTOSTERONE

(Andro 100, Android-T, Bay Testone, Histerone, Malogen, Testaqua)

(tess-toss'ter-one)
Androgen
Anabolic steroid
Antineoplastic
Hormone

ACTIONS AND USES. Synthetic steroid compound with both androgenic and anabolic activity (1:1). Controls development and maintenance of secondary sexual characteristics. Androgenic activity: responsible for the growth spurt of the adolescent and for growth termination by epiphyseal closure. In males and some females reduces excretion of phosphorus, nitrogen, potassium, sodium, and chloride. Increases erythropoiesis, possibly by stimulating production of renal or extrarenal erythropoietin, and promotes vascularization and darkening of skin. Antagonizes effects of estrogen excess on female breast and endometrium. Anabolic activity: increases protein metabolism and decreases its catabolism. Large doses suppress spermatogenesis. thereby causing testicular atrophy. Unlike other androgens, testosterone and its esters do not produce cholestatic hepatitis or creatinuria.

Used primarily as androgen replacement in male sex hormone deficiency states, e.g., male climacteric, postpubertal cryptorchidism, oligospermia, impotence. In women, given to treat postpartum breast pain and engorgement (nonnursing mother) (does not suppress lactation), and treatment palliation of androgen-responsive inoperable breast cancer more than one, but less than 5 years postmenopausal. Also used as adjunct in treatment of osteoporosis, and to stimulate growth in prepubertal males. Available in fixed combination with estrogens in many preparations.

TU

ABSORPTION AND FATE. Rapid absorption following oral administration; more prolonged absorption from IM site. In plasma, 98% bound to sex hormone-binding globulin (transcortin) and albumin. Remainder is free and represents magnitude of androgen effects. Serum half-life: 10 to 100 minutes. Metabolites (including andosterone and etiocholanolone) conjugated and excreted through enterohepatic route (about 10%) and urinary route (90%). Crosses placenta; appears in breast milk.

CONTRAINDICATIONS AND PRECAUTIONS. Hypersensitivity or toxic reactions to androgens; pregnancy, lactation, women of childbearing potential (possibility of virilization of female infant); hypercalcemia; known or suspected prostatic or breast cancer in male; benign prostatic hypertrophy with obstruction; patients easily stimulated sexually; elderly, asthenic males who may react adversely to androgenic overstimulation; conditions aggravated by fluid retention; hypertension. *Cautious Use:* cardiac, hepatic and renal disease; prepubertal males, geriatric patients, acute intermittent porphyria.

ADVERSE/SIDE EFFECTS. **Both sexes:** hypersensitivity, anaphylactoid reaction (rare), increased libido, skin flushing and vascularization, acne, excitation and sleeplessness, chills, leukopenia, sodium and water retention (especially in the elderly) with edema; nausea, vomiting, anorexia, diarrhea, gastric pain, jaundice, bladder irritability, hypercalcemia, renal calculi in bedfast or partially immobilized patient, hypercholesterolemia, precipitation of acute intermittent porphyria, aggravation of disease being treated, site irritation and sloughing (pellet implantation), hepatocellular carcinoma (rare). **Female:** suppression of ovulation, lactation, or menstruation; virilism: hoarseness or deepening of voice (often irreversible); hirsutism; oily skin; acne; clitoral enlargement; regression of breasts; male-pattern baldness (in disseminated breast cancer). **Male (post-pubertal):** testicular atrophy, decreased ejaculatory volume, azoospermia, oligospermia (after prolonged administration or excessive dosage), impotence, epididymitis, priapism, gynecomastia; (prepubertal): phallic enlargement, priapism, premature epiphyseal closure.

ROUTE AND DOSAGE. **Intramuscular:** Androgen deficiency: 10 to 25 mg two or three times weekly. *Postpartum breast engorgement:* 25 to 50 mg daily for 3 or 4 days starting at time of delivery. *Metastatic cancer of breast:* 100 mg three times weekly, as long as improvement is maintained.

NURSING IMPLICATIONS

IM injections should be made deep into gluteal musculature. A wet syringe or needle may cloud the solution, but potency of material reportedly is unaffected.

Store IM formulations prepared in oil at room temperature. Warming and shaking vial will redisperse precipitated crystals.

Check intake and output and weigh patient daily during dose adjustment period. Weight gain (due to Na and water retention) suggests need for decreased dosage. When dosage is stabilized, urge patient to check weight at least twice weekly and to report increases, particularly if accompanied by edema in dependent areas. Dose adjustment and diuretic therapy may be started.

Sodium and water retention respond to diuretic therapy; therefore, use of a diuretic differentiates skeletal growth from edema weight gain.

Restoration of positive nitrogen balance, as in patients with metastatic carcinoma, is supported by a diet high in protein and calories. Sodium restriction may be prescribed to control edema. Collaborate with physician and dietitian in developing a dietary teaching plan that includes patient and responsible family members.

Periodic serum cholesterol and calcium determinations as well as cardiac and liver function tests should be performed throughout testosterone therapy.

Improvement from testosterone therapy is slow. Therapeutic response in patients with breast cancer is usually apparent within 3 months after regimen begins. If signs of disease progression appear, therapy should be terminated.

In patients with metastatic breast cancer, hypercalcemia usually indicates progression of bone metastasis. (*Normal serum calcium:* 8.5 to 10.6 mg/dl.)

If serum calcium rises above 14 mg/dl, androgenic therapy is terminated.

Promptly report signs and symptoms of hypercalcemia: nausea, vomiting, constipation, lethargy, asthenia, loss of muscle tone, polydipsia, polyuria, dehydration, increased urine and serum calcium levels. Treatment consists of withdrawing testosterone, providing fluids to assure daily urinary output of 3 to 4 liters or more (to prevent urinary calculi), and appropriate drug therapy. Calcium, phosphate, and BUN levels should be checked daily.

Bedridden patients should be given range-of-motion exercises at least twice daily to prevent mobilization of calcium from bone. The immobilized patient is particularly prone to develop hypercalcemia. Consult physician about daily activity and dietary calcium intake.

Testosterone-induced anabolic action enhances hypoglycemia (hyperinsulinism). Instruct diabetic patient to report sweating, tremor, anxiety, diplopia, vertigo. Dosage adjustment of antidiabetic agent may be required.

Be sensitive to the fact that the patient may find it embarrassing to initiate questions or report symptoms related to sexual organs and functions. Attention to such symptoms should not be delayed by hesitant reporting, since many signify overdosage.

Instruct male patient to report priapism (sustained and often painful erections occurring especially in early replacement therapy), reduced ejaculatory volume, and gynecomastia. The symptoms indicate necessity for temporary withdrawal or discontinuation of testosterone therapy.

Instruct patient to notify physician promptly if pregnancy is suspected or planned. Masculinization of the fetus is most likely to occur if testosterone (androgen) therapy is provided during first semester of pregnancy.

Observe the patient who is on concomitant anticoagulant treatment for signs of overdosage (e.g., ecchymoses, petechiae). Report promptly to physician; anticoagulant dose may need to be reduced.

At dosage required to treat carcinoma, androgens may cause virilism in the female. Advise her to report increase in libido (early sign of toxicity), growth of facial hair, deepening of voice, male-pattern baldness. The onset of hoarseness can easily be overlooked unless its significance as an early and possibly irreversible sign of virilism is appreciated. Reevaluation of treatment plan is indicated.

Prepubertal or adolescent males should be monitored by radiology throughout therapy to avoid precocious sexual development and premature epiphyseal closure. Skeletal stimulation may continue 6 months beyond termination of therapy.

Alterations in clinical laboratory test values persist 2 to 3 weeks after drug discontinuation. Notify laboratory and pathologist that patient is on testosterone.

Diagnostic Test Interferences. Testosterone alters **glucose** tolerance tests; decreases **PBI, thyroxine-binding globulin concentration, creatinine** and **creatinine** excretion (lasting up to 2 weeks after therapy is discontinued), and alters response to **metyrapone test.** It suppresses **clotting factors II, V, VII, X; hematocrit,** increases uptake of **triiodothyronine** by RBC and excretion of **17-ketosteroids.** May increase or decrease **serum cholesterol.**

Drug Interactions: Testosterone

Plus	Interactions
Adrenal steroids, ACTH	Increased testosterone-induced edema
Anticoagulants	Enhanced effect may necessitate reduced dose of anticoagulant
Antidiabetic agents (sulfonylureas and insulin)	Additive hypoglycemic effect; decreased doses of hypoglycemic may be necessary
Oxyphenbutazone	Antiflammatory effects may be enhanced by testosterone (conflicting evidence)

TESTOSTERONE CYPIONATE

(Andro-Cyp, Andronate, depAndro, Depo-Testosterone, Duratest, Testa-C, Testoject-L.A., T-Ionate P.A.)

TESTOSTERONE ENANTHATE

(Anthatest, Andro L.A., Andryl, Android-T, Delatestryl, Everone, Malojex, Testone L.A., Testrin PA, Testostroval P.A., Testoject E.P.)

TESTOSTERONE PROPIONATE

(Textex)

Androgen
Anabolic steroid
Antineoplastic
Hormone

ACTIONS AND USES. Esters of testosterone with similar actions, androgenic/anabolic activity (1:1) and contraindications as parent compound *(see Testosterone).* Duration of action of cypionate and enanthate is longer than that of testosterone. The propionate is more intense in action, but has somewhat shorter duration than testosterone; parenteral route is not suited to long-term treatment.

Uses are indicated under Route and Dosage.

ADVERSE/SIDE EFFECTS. Urticaria at injection site, postinjection induration, furunculosis, virilism. *See also Testosterone.*

ROUTE AND DOSAGE. Intramuscular: Replacement therapy: (propionate): 10 to 25 mg two to three times a week; (cypionate, enanthate): 50 to 400 mg every 2 to 4 weeks. *Delayed puberty* (cypionate, enanthate): 50 to 200 mg for 2 to 4 weeks. *Postpartum breast pain and engorgement* (propionate): 25 to 50 mg/day for 3 or 4 days. *Metastatic breast cancer* (propionate): 100 mg three times/week; (cypionate, enanthate): 200 to 400 mg every 2 to 4 weeks.

NURSING IMPLICATIONS

Inject intramuscular preparation deep into gluteal muscle. Advise patient to report soreness at injection site, since post injection furunculosis may be an associated adverse reaction.

Priapism (persistent erection) and virilization are signs of overdosage and indicate necessity for temporary drug withdrawal. Advise patient to report to physician.

See Testosterone.

PROTOTYPE

TETRACYCLINE
TETRACYCLINE HYDROCHLORIDE

(Achromycin, Cefracycline, Novatetra, Sumycin, Tetracyn, Tetralean, and others)

(tet-ra-sye'kleen)
Antiinfective
Antibiotic
Tetracycline

ACTIONS AND USES. Broad-spectrum antimicrobial effective against a variety of gram-positive and gram-negative bacteria, certain mycoplasma, rickettsiae, protozoa. Believed to act by inhibiting phosphorylation and protein synthesis by susceptible microorganisms. Oral administration results in suppression of intestinal flora, therefore has been used in treatment of vitamin B malabsorption and steatorrhea; also for this purpose in preoperative preparation of bowel for surgery. *Investigational Use:* adjunctively in treatment of acne.

ABSORPTION AND FATE. Irregularly absorbed from GI tract. Peak levels reached in 2 to 4 hours; effective blood levels maintained for at least 6 hours. IM administration produces lower blood levels than oral administration, 20 to 66% protein bound. Half-life: 6 to 10 hours. Well distributed in tissues and body fluids; lower levels in spinal and joint fluids, and higher than plasma concentrations in bile. Excreted mainly in feces and urine. Crosses placenta; enters breast milk.

CONTRAINDICATIONS AND PRECAUTIONS. Liver and renal impairment, hypersensitivity to tetracyclines, use during pregnancy, lactation, infancy and during period of tooth development (4th month of fetal life through 8th year); concomitant administration of potentially hepatotoxic drugs, and penicillins. *Cautious Use:* undernourished patients.

ADVERSE/SIDE EFFECTS. Nausea, anorexia, vomiting, diarrhea, dizziness, thrombophlebitis at site of injection, fever, hypersensitivity reactions, photosensitivity, superimposed candidal growth (skin eruptions, gingivitis, stomatitis, pharyngitis, dysphagia, lingua nigra, anal pruritus, proctitis, vaginal discharge); hepatotoxicity, nephrotoxicity, blood dyscrasias; intracranial hypertension (pseudotumor cerebri): bulging fontanels, impaired vision, papilledema, severe headache; permanent discoloration and inadequate calcification of deciduous teeth, enamel hypoplasia, onycholysis and discoloration of nails; fixed drug eruptions.

ROUTE AND DOSAGE. **Oral: Adults:** 1 to 2 Gm/day in divided doses. **Children (over 8 years):** 25 to 50 mg/kg divided into 2 to 4 equal doses. **Intramuscular: Adults:** 250 mg once every 24 hours or 300 mg daily in divided doses at 8- to 12-hour intervals; **Children (over 8 years):** 15 to 25 mg/kg divided and given at 8- to 12-hour intervals. **Intravenous: Adults:** 250 to 500 mg every 12 hours, not to exceed 500 mg every 6 hours; **Children (over 8 years):** 12 mg/kg/day divided into two doses.

NURSING IMPLICATIONS

Therapy should be designed on basis of culture studies.

Check expiration date before administering drug. Renal injury (Fanconi-like syndrome) has been attributed to administration of outdated tetracyclines.

Children weighing more than 40 kg should receive the adult dose.

Tablet may be crushed before administration and taken with water. Capsule may be emptied and contents swallowed with water or mixed with food.

Tetracycline absorption is inhibited by iron, aluminum, calcium and magnesium. Therefore administer oral doses on an empty stomach (at least 1 hour before or 2 hours after eating).

Avoid concurrent use of antacids; if necessary, however, administer 2 hours before or after tetracycline.

If nausea, anorexia, and diarrhea occur, they are controlled by administering drug with some food (*exception:* foods high in calcium, such as milk, interfere with absorption of tetracycline preparations) or by reducing drug dosage. Consult physician. If symptoms persist, drug should be discontinued.

Deep IM injection into body of a large muscle is recommended. Inadvertent injection into subcutaneous or fat layer may result in painful local irritation; may be relieved by an ice pack.

IV tetracycline is an irritant. Inspect IV site frequently to prevent extravasation. At particular risk are the very young (cannot communicate pain at site), the debilitated and the elderly (aging causes loss of skin elasticity), thereby promoting leakage around the needle.

Be alert for evidence of overgrowth of *nonsensitive organisms (superinfection).* Inspect tongue regularly to note development of black, furry appearance. The incidence of infection by candida may be reduced by meticulous hygienic care of skin and mouth, and by allowing patient to wash perineal area several times a day, particularly after each bowel movement. If superinfection develops, drug is discontinued.

It is important to distinguish between frequent stools resulting from local irritant effect of drug (usually occur early during therapy) and those due to superinfection, which require immediate discontinuation of therapy.

Monitor intake and output. Report oliguria or changes in intake–output ratio (patient can be taught to make rough estimates).

Advise patient to avoid exposure to direct or artificial sunlight during use of tetracyclines. Certain hypersensitive persons develop a phototoxic reaction (exaggerated sunburn) precipitated by exposure to sun or ultraviolet light. Advise use of sun screen lotion (SPF above 12). At the first sign of skin discomfort, drug should be discontinued.

Tetracycline may combine with calcium of developing teeth to cause yellow-gray-brownish discoloration. Its use during bone formation and tooth development periods (prenatally, neonatally, and in childhood) is generally avoided.

The drug is generally administered for 24 to 72 hours after fever and other symptoms have subsided. Warn patient to discard unused tetracycline after therapy is completed.

Solutions prepared for IM injection should be used within 24 hours. Initial reconstituted IV solutions are stable at room temperature for 12 hours, but when final dilution is made, they should be administered immediately.

Tetracyclines decompose with age, with exposure to light, and when improperly stored under conditions of extreme humidity and heat. The resulting product may be toxic.

Diagnostic Test Interferences. Possibility of false increases in **urinary catecholamines** (Hungert method) and false decreases in **urinary urobilinogen.** Parenteral tetracycline containing ascorbic acid may produce false-positive **urinary glucose** determinations by copper reduction methods (e.g., Benedict's and Clinitest) and false-negative values with glucose oxidase methods (e.g., Clinistix, Tes-Tape).

Drug Interactions: Tetracycline

TU

Plus	Interactions
Antacids (aluminum, magnesium, calcium); Iron preparatins	Chelation and interference with tetracycline absorption
Anticoagulants (oral, and heparin)	Augmented anticoagulant effects
Penicillins	Possible decrease in bacterial action of penicillin
Sodium bicarbonate	Interference with tetracycline absorption

TETRAHYDROZOLINE HYDROCHLORIDE

(Murine, Soothe Eye, Tetrasine, Tyzine, Visine)

(tet-ra-hye-drozz'a-leen)
Alpha-adrenergic (sympathomimetic)
Vasoconstrictor

ACTIONS AND USES. Imidazole derivative structurally and chemically related to naphazoline (qv). In common with naphazoline, has more marked alpha-adrenergic than beta-adrenergic activity; large doses cause CNS depression, rather than the stimulation produced by other sympathomimetic amines.

Used for symptomatic relief of minor eye irritation and allergies, and for nasopharyngeal congestion of allergic or inflammatory origin.

CONTRAINDICATIONS AND PRECAUTIONS. Hypersensitivity to any component, use of ophthalmic preparation in glaucoma or other serious eye diseases, use of drug in children under age 2, use of 0.1% or higher strengths in children under age 6, use within 14 days of MAO inhibitor therapy. Safe use during pregnancy not established. *Cautious Use:* hypertension, cardiovascular disease, hyperthyroidism, diabetes mellitus, young children.

ADVERSE/SIDE EFFECTS. Transient stinging, irritation, sneezing, dryness, headache, tremors, drowsiness, lightheadedness, insomnia, palpitation. Overdosage: CNS depression (marked drowsiness, sweating, coma, hypotension, shock, bradycardia).

ROUTE AND DOSAGE. Topical: Ophthalmic: **Adults:** 1 or 2 drops of 0.05% solution in each eye two or three times a day. Nasal: **Adults and children (6 years and over):** 2 to 4 drops of 0.1% solution in each nostril as needed, never more often than every 3 hours; **Children (2 to 6 years):** 2 or 3 drops of 0.05% solution in each nostril as needed, never more often than every 3 hours. (Use of either topical preparation is usually restricted to 3 or 4 days only.)

NURSING IMPLICATIONS

Since drug action lasts 4 to 8 hours, interval between doses is at least 4 to 6 hours.

Instruct patient to discontinue medication and to consult physician if relief is not obtained within 48 hours or if symptoms for which drug was given persist or increase.

Caution patient not to exceed recommended dosage. Rebound congestion and rhinitis may occur with frequent or prolonged use of nasal preparation.

When using squeeze bottle, patient should be in upright position. When reclined, a stream rather than a spray may be ejected, with consequent overdosage.

Nasal drops are usually administered in lateral, head-low position.

See Index: Drug administration.
See also Naphazoline.

PROTOTYPE

THEOPHYLLINE

(Asmalix, Bronkodyl, Duraphyl, Elixicon, Elixophyllin, Gyrocaps, Lanophyllin, Lodrane, Pulmopylline, Quibron-T, Respbid, Slo-Bid, Slo-Phyllin, Somophyllin, Sustaire, Theo-24, Theoclear, Theo-Dur, Theolair, Theolixir, Theon, Theophyl, Theospan, Theostat, Uniphyl, and others)

(thee-off'i-lin)
Smooth muscle relaxant
Bronchodilator
Xanthine

THEOPHYLLINE SODIUM GLYCINATE

(Acet-Am, Sonophylate)

ACTIONS AND USES. Methyl xanthine derivative with pharmacologic actions qualitatively similar to those of other xanthines e.g., caffeine, theobromine; occurs naturally in tea. Relaxes smooth muscle by direct action, particularly of bronchi and pulmonary vessels, and stimulates medullary respiratory center with resulting increase in vital capacity. Also relaxes smooth muscles of biliary and GI tracts. Stimulates myocardium, thereby increasing force of contractions and cardiac output, and stimulates all levels of CNS, but to a lesser degree than caffeine. Produces mild diuresis by increasing renal blood flow and by inhibiting sodium and chloride reabsorption at proximal tubule. At cellular level, xanthines block phosphodiesterase, thereby promoting cyclic AMP accumulation. Cyclic AMP excess promotes catecholamine stimulation of lipolysis, glycogenolysis, and gluconeogenesis and induces release of epinephrine from adrenal medulla cells. Unlike sympathomimetic agents, tolerance to bronchodilator effects of theophylline derivatives rarely develops. Available in combination with ephedrine and phenobarbital (e.g., Tedral, Thalfed). *Investigative Use:* treatment of apnea and bradycardia of prematures and to reduce severe bronchospasm associated with cystic fibrosis and acute descending respiratory infection. Theophylline Sodium Glycinate is a mixture of sodium theophylline and aminoacetic (glycine). Contains 45 to 47% theophylline. Similar actions, uses, adverse reactions, and precautions as other theophylline derivatives, but claimed to produce less gastric irritation.

Used for prophylaxis and symptomatic relief of bronchial asthma, as well as bronchospasm associated with chronic bronchitis and emphysema. Also used for emergency treatment of paroxysmal cardiac dyspnea and edema of congestive heart failure.

ABSORPTION AND FATE. Rate of absorption depends on drug solubility. Oral solution and uncoated tablet are well absorbed from GI tract; peak blood levels in 1 to 2 hours. Absorption following sustained-release forms is variable and incomplete. Peak plasma levels occur in about 5 hours for sustained-release form but this varies with manufacturer. Rapidly distributed throughout extracellular fluid and tissues. About 60% bound to plasma proteins. Plasma elimination half-life: approximately 7 to 9 hours in nonsmokers, 4 to 5 hours in smokers, and 2 to 9 hours in children and 15 to 58 in premature infants. Partially demethylated and oxidized in liver (individual variability in rate of metabolism). About 10% excreted unchanged in urine. Small amount excreted in feces. Readily crosses placenta; appears in breast milk in high concentrations.

CONTRAINDICATIONS AND PRECAUTIONS. Hypersensitivity to xanthines; coronary artery disease or angina pectoris when myocardial stimulation might be harmful; severe renal or liver impairment. Safe use during pregnancy (category C) and lactation and in women of childbearing potential not established. *Cautious Use:* children, compromised cardiac or circulatory function, hypertension, hyperthyroidism, peptic ulcer, prostatic hypertrophy, glaucoma, diabetes mellitus, in the elderly (particularly males) and neonates.

ADVERSE/SIDE EFFECTS. **CNS (stimulation):** irritability, restlessness, insomnia, dizziness, headache, hyperexcitability, muscle twitching, drug-induced seizures. **CV:** palpitation, tachycardia, extrasystoles, flushing, marked hypotension, circulatory failure. **GI:** nausea, vomiting, anorexia, epigastric or abdominal pain, diarrhea, activation of peptic ulcer. **Renal:** transient urinary frequency, albuminuria, kidney irritation. **Respiratory:** tachypnea, respiratory arrest. **Other:** fever, dehydration, possibility of increased urinary catecholamine excretion.

ROUTE AND DOSAGE. Theophylline: **Adults: Oral:** 100 to 200 mg every 6 hours. Sustained-release forms: 200 to 300 mg every 12 hours. **Children: Oral:** 4 to 6 mg/kg every 6 hours. Available as capsules, sustained release capsules, elixir, liquid, syrup, tablet, chewable tablet. Extended-release preparations suitable for dosing every 8 to 12, 12, 24 hours are available. Regimen is individualized. Theophylline Sodium Glycinate: **Oral: Adults:** 330 to 660 mg every 6 to 8 hours. **Children (over 12 years):** 220 to 330 mg; **(3 to 6 years):** 110 to 165 mg; **(1 to 3 years):** 55 to 110 mg.

NURSING IMPLICATIONS

Therapeutic theophylline plasma level ranges from 10 to 20 mcg/ml (a narrow therapeutic range). Levels exceeding 20 mcg/ml are associated with toxicity. Theophylline saliva levels (sometimes used when plasma levels cannot be obtained) are equal to approximately 60% of simultaneous plasma levels.

Sustained-release forms and enteric coated tablets must be swallowed whole. Chewable tablets must be chewed thoroughly before swallowing. Slow-release theophylline sprinkle (Theo-Dur Sprinkle) is dispensed in easy to open capsules for children and adults who cannot swallow tablet or capsule. The microencapsulated granules of theophylline can be taken on an empty stomach or mixed with applesauce or water.

Oral preparations should preferably be administered with a full glass of water and may be given after meals to minimize gastric irritation. Food, and antacids delay but do not reduce extent of absorption. Physician may prescribe an antacid if GI symptoms continue. Dosage reduction may also be indicated.

Timing of dose is critically important. Be certain patient understands the food and drug relationships and the necessity to adhere to the proper intervals between doses.

Patient on a once-daily theophylline dose 900 mg or more is advised to take the drug after fasting overnight and about 2 hours before eating. If patient is not likely to adhere to this regimen, patient will be given alternate therapy (such as twice-a-day dosing).

Once-a-day administration provides patient convenience and increased compliance. However, such a schedule may not adequately control asthmatic patients, smokers, or children. These patients need to have regular frequent serum concentration tests in the beginning of therapy to prevent toxicity.

Variability in rate and extent of absorption and rate of metabolism of xanthines produce peak-to-trough fluctuations in serum concentrations. These variabilities are the primary reasons for subtherapeutic or toxic response to theophylline. Regular monitoring of serum concentrations is required until dose-response has been stabilized.

Although this drug is in category C, recent reports claim its use by pregnant women who are asthmatic is considered safe.

If theophylline is given to a patient with severe cardiac disease, monitor for tachycardia. Conversely, keep in mind that theophylline toxicity may be masked in patients with tachycardia.

Plasma clearance of xanthines may be reduced in patients with heart failure, renal or hepatic dysfunction, alcoholism, high fever. Dosage regulation must be closely monitored particularly in these patients.

Monitor vital signs and intake and output. Improvement in quality of pulse and respiration and diuresis are expected clinical effects.

Observe and report early signs of possible toxicity: anorexia, nausea, vomiting, dizziness, shakiness, restlessness, abdominal discomfort, irritability, palpitation, tachycardia, marked hypotension, cardiac arrhythmias, seizures.

During early therapy, dizziness is a relatively common side effect in the elderly. Take necessary safety precautions and forewarn patient of this possibility.

Urge patient to drink adequate fluids (at least 2000 ml/day) to decrease viscosity of airway secretions.

Warn patient to avoid self-dosing with OTC medications, especially cough suppressants. The physician may prescribe one for short periods, but unsupervised use may cause retention of secretions and CNS depression.

Theophylline does not seem to prolong labor in the pregnant asthmatic user.

In the neonate of a mother using this drug, slight tachycardia, jitteriness, and apnea have been observed.

Since theophylline is distributed into breast milk it may be advisable for the infant to be nursed just before mother takes the drug.

Theophylline metabolism in the infant under 6 months and in prematures is prolonged as is the half-life; therefore close monitoring for side effects is especially crucial in this age group.

Food–Drug Interactions:

- Charcoal broiled foods (high in polycyclic carbon content) may increase theophylline elimination and reduce the half-life as much as 50%.
- Methylxanthines derivatives (coffee, tea, chocolate) can change theophylline metabolism.
- A low carbohydrate, high protein diet is said to increase theophylline elimination (shortens half-life) therefore interfering with dosing. Conversely, a high carbohydrate, low protein diet increases the half-life.

Smoking–Drug Interactions:

- Cigarettes and marijuana smoking induce hepatic microsomal enzyme activity, decreasing serum half-life and increasing body clearance of theophylline. This effect plus the narrow therapeutic range requires close monitoring of drug level in the heavy smoker who will need a larger dose for therapeutic effects. An increase of dosage from 50 to 100% is usual in heavy smokers.
- The heavy smoker may suffer less from drug side effects than nonsmokers because of increased theophylline metabolism.

Chest physiotherapy (postural drainage with rapid percussion of thorax, instruction in coughing, training to prevent airway collapse during expiration, and improved diaphragmatic movement) is a necessary concomitant to adequate response to this drug. Consult physiotherapist or respiratory therapist.

If patient has exacerbations of bronchial symptoms, exposure to unknown or unsuspected environmental allergens should be ruled out. Recent studies indicate that the car air-conditioner may harbor respiratory allergens. Make inquiries about exposure to this challenge. The conditioning system may need to be decontaminated. (Home air-conditioning systems have not been implicated.)

Overdose with prolonged release preparation necessitates observing patient for a longer period of time than if conventional formulation had been ingested. Continued slow absorption leads to sustained high plasma concentrations for a prolonged period. Avoid discharge of the patient from medical supervision too soon.

Treatment of overdosage: induce vomiting with ipecac syrup (gastric lavage if patient has had seizures); activated charcoal; cathartic. IV diazepam for convulsions. Maintain airway, oxygenation, and hydration, tepid water sponges or hypothermic blanket for hyperpyrexia. Monitor vital signs.

Patient-Teaching Points: Clarify or emphasize:

- drug action and expected responses to drug
- dosage schedule: stress adherence to established regimen
- food–drug and smoking–drug interactions
- adequate fluid intake
- humidified environment especially in winter months
- postural drainage (4 to 6 times daily)
- planned physical conditioning program
- avoidance of exposure to infection, chilling, environmental pollutants including smoke and sprays
- avoidance of smoking
- possible need to decontaminate car air conditioner
- maintenance of follow-up appointments

Diagnostic Test Interferences. False-positive elevations of **serum uric acid** (Bittner or colorimetric methods). **Probenecid** may cause false high serum theophylline readings, and spectrophometric methods of determining **serum theophylline** are affected by a furosemide, sulfathiazole, phenylbutazone, probenecid, theobromine.

Drug Interactions: Theophylline

Plus	Interactions
Adrenergics (e.g., epinephrine) Allopurinol Cimetidine Furosamide Influenza virus vaccine	Excessive CNS stimulation especially in children
Macrolide antibiotics (e.g., erythromycin) Thiabendazole Troleandomycin	Increased serum concentrations of theophylline (increased pharmacologic effects and risk of toxicity)
Antacids (aluminum and magnesium products) Anticoagulants, oral	Slowed absorption rate of theophylline (with high doses of theophylline): increased anticoagulant effect
Barbiturates (e.g., phenobarbital)	Decreased therapeutic effects of theophylline
Beta-adrenergic blocking agents (e.g., propranolol)	Antagonistic effects: theophylline produces beta-adrenergic stimulation
Halothane	Cardiac arrhythmias, reduced therapeutic effects of lithium
Phenytoin	Increased theophylline clearance requiring larger than usual doses
Reserpine	Produces tachycardia
Skeletal muscle relaxants, nondepolarizing (e.g., pancuronium)	Reversal of neuromuscular blockade of skeletal muscle relaxants

THIABENDAZOLE
(Mintezol)

(thye-a-ben′da-zole)
Antiinfective
Anthelmintic
Enzyme inhibitor

ACTIONS AND USES. Benzimadazole with vermicidal properties, structurally related to mebendazole. Precise action mechanism not clear, but has wide spectrum of antihelmintic activity. Has been shown to inhibit helminth-specific enzyme fumarate reductase. Demonstrates antiinflammatory, antipyretic, and analgesic effects in animals. Suppresses production of eggs and/or larvae by some parasites and may inhibit subsequent development of eggs or larvae passed in feces.

Used in treatment of enterobiasis (pinworm infestation), ascariasis (roundworm), strongyloidiasis (threadworm), cutaneous larva migrans (creeping eruption), and hookworm infestations caused by *Ancyclostoma duodenale* or *Necator americanus.* Used during invasive stage of trichinosis to relieve symptoms and for mixed helminthic infestations.

ABSORPTION AND FATE. Oral dose rapidly absorbed from GI tract (can also be absorbed from skin). Peak plasma concentration reached in 1 to 2 hours after dose. Metabolized almost completely with most of drug out of plasma within 8 hours; major excretion in first 24 hours. 48 hours after dose about 5% administered dose is recovered from feces and about 90% from urine as glucuronide or sulfate conjugates.

CONTRAINDICATIONS AND PRECAUTIONS. Safe use during pregnancy and lactation not established. *Cautious Use:* hepatic or renal dysfunction, when vomiting can be dangerous, severe dehydration or malnutrition, anemia, children weighing less than 15 kg.

ADVERSE/SIDE EFFECTS. CV: hypotension, bradycardia. **GI:** anorexia, nausea, vomiting, epigastric distress, jaundice, cholestasis, parenchymal liver damage, diarrhea, perianal rash. **NS:** weariness, drowsiness, headache; rarely: tinnitus, abnormal sensation in eyes, blurred vision, zanthopsia. **Renal:** malodor of urine, crystalluria, hematuria, nephrotoxicity, enuresis. **Other:** transient rise in cephalin flocculation and AST, transient leukopenia, hypersensitivity, hyperglycemia, pruritus.

ROUTE AND DOSAGE. Oral: 2 doses/day (dose determined by patient's weight). Patient weighing less than 150 lb: 10 mg (0.1 ml)/lb or 25 mg (0.25 ml)/kg. Weight more than 150 lb: 1.5 Gm (15 ml).

NURSING IMPLICATIONS

If patient is anemic, dehydrated, or malnourished, supportive treatment is indicated prior to start of thiabendazole therapy.

Administer drug after meals. Tablets should be chewed before swallowing. Shake suspension well before pouring.

A special diet or purgation prior to drug administration is not necessary.

Adverse/side effects generally occur 3 to 4 hours after administration, are mild and last for 2 to 8 hours. Incidence tends to be related to dose and duration of treatment.

If hypersensitivity occurs, drug should be discontinued immediately. Symptoms: fever, facial flush, chills, conjunctival injection, skin rashes, erythema multiforme (including Stevens-Johnson syndrome), which can be fatal.

CNS side effects occur frequently and may prevent the patient from driving a car or engaging in activities requiring mental alertness. Warn patient of the possibility.

See Mebendazole for additional Nursing Implications related to drug therapy of helminthic infestation.

THIAMINE HYDROCHLORIDE

(Bay Bee 1, Biamine, Vitamin B_1)

(thye'-a-min)
Vitamin
Antineuritic

ACTIONS AND USES. Water-soluble vitamin and member of B-complex group. Functions as an essential coenzyme in carbohydrate metabolism. Also has role in conversion of tryptophan to nicotinamide.

Used in treatment and prophylaxis of beriberi, to correct anorexia due to thiamine deficiency states, and in treatment of neuritis associated with pregnancy, pellagra, and alcholism, including Wernicke-Korsakoff syndrome. Therapy generally includes other members of vitamin B complex, since thiamine deficiency rarely occurs alone.

ABSORPTION AND FATE. Limited absorption following oral administration, as compared with IM injection, which is rapid and complete. Wide distribution to most body tissues, with highest concentrations in liver, brain, kidney, and heart. Minimal body storage. Excreted in urine as pyrimidine and, with excessive intake, as unchanged drug.

ADVERSE/SIDE EFFECTS. Feeling of warmth, weakness, urticaria, pruritus, sweating, nausea, restlessness, tightness of throat, angioneurotic edema, cyanosis, pulmonary edema, GI hemorrhage, cardiovascular collapse, anaphylaxis. Following rapid IV administration: slight fall in blood pressure.

ROUTE AND DOSAGE. Oral: Replacement: 5 to 30 mg daily. Wet beriberi with myocardial failure: **Intravenous:** 30 mg three times a day. Beriberi: **Intramuscular:** 10 to 20 mg three times a day for 2 weeks. **Intramuscular, intravenous** *(rarely used)*: 30 to 60 mg divided into 3 equal doses.

NURSING IMPLICATIONS

Intradermal test dose is recommended prior to administration in suspected thiamine sensitivity. Deaths have occurred following IV use.

IM injections may be painful. Rotate sites and apply cold compresses to area if necessary for relief of discomfort.

Careful recording of patient's dietary history is an essential part of vitamin replacement therapy. Collaborate with physician, dietitian, patient, and responsible family member in developing a diet teaching plan that can be sustained by patient.

Therapeutic effectiveness is evaluated by improvement of clinical manifestations of thiamine deficiency: anorexia, gastric distress, depression, irritability, insomnia, palpitation, tachycardia, loss of memory, paresthesias, muscle weakness and pain, elevated blood pyruvic acid level (diagnostic test for thiamine deficiency), elevated lactic acid level. Severe deficiency: ophthalmoplegia, polyneuropathy, muscle wasting ("dry" beriberi), edema, serous effusions, congestive heart failure ("wet" beriberi).

Body requirement of thiamine is directly proportional to carboyhydrate intake and metabolic rate; thus, requirement increases when diet consists predominantly of carbohydrates. Total absence of dietary thiamine can produce a deficiency state in about 3 weeks.

Classic beriberi is uncommon in the United States, but it is endemic in Asia. Like deficiencies of other B vitamins, subclinical states often accompany poverty, chronic alcoholism, dietary fads, and pregnancy.

Recommended daily allowance (RDA): children 4 to 6 years of age, 0.9 mg; adult males, 1.4 mg; adult females, 1 mg; pregnancy and lactation, 1.4 mg.

Rich thiamine food sources: yeast, pork, beef, liver, wheat and other whole grains, fresh vegetables, especially peas and dried beans.

Preserved in tight, light-resistant, nonmetallic containers. Thiamine is unstable in alkaline solutions (e.g., solutions of acetates, barbiturates, bicarbonates, carbonates, citrates) and neutral solutions.

THIETHYLPERAZINE MALEATE
(Torecan)

(thye-eth-il-per′a-zeen)
Antiemetic
Phenothiazine

ACTIONS AND USES. Piperazine phenothiazine derivative with contraindications, precautions, and toxic effects similar to those of chlorpromazine (qv). Reported to have higher ratio of antiemetic action to tranquilizing action than other phenothiazines. Acts directly on chemoreceptor trigger zone as well as the vomiting center.

Used to control nausea and vomiting. *Investigational Use:* treatment of vertigo.

ABSORPTION AND FATE. Onset of effects in less than 1 hour following oral or rectal administration and within 30 minutes following IM injection. *See Chlorpromazine.*

CONTRAINDICATIONS AND PRECAUTIONS. Hypersensitivity to phenothiazines, CNS depression or comatose states, pregnancy, IV administration. Safe use in children under age 12, in nursing mothers, or following intracardiac or intracranial surgery not established. *Cautious Use:* renal or hepatic disease. *See also Chlorpromazine.*

ADVERSE/SIDE EFFECTS. Drowsiness, dizziness, headache, dry mouth and nose, blurred vision, tinnitus, restlessness, fever, orthostatic hypotension. Occasionally: extrapyramidal symptoms including convulsions; sialorrhea with altered taste sensations, cholestatic jaundice. *See Chlorpromazine.*

ROUTE AND DOSAGE. **Oral, rectal suppository, intramuscular:** 10 mg one to three times a day.

NURSING IMPLICATIONS

Examine parenteral solution and administer only if it is clear and colorless.

Patient should be recumbent when administering drug IM. Postural hypotension (manifested by weakness, lightheadedness, faintness) and drowsiness may occur, particularly after initial injection. Advise patient to remain in bed for about 1 hour or longer, if indicated, and supervise ambulation. If vasopressor agent is required, levarterenol or phenylephrine is used. Epinephrine is contraindicated.

Administer IM deep into large muscle mass, and aspirate carefully before injecting drug in order to avoid inadvertent entry into a blood vessel. IV administration is specifically contraindicated because it can cause severe hypotension.

Patients who have received drug preoperatively may manifest restlessness or depression during anesthesia recovery.

Tablet formulation contains tartrazine which may cause allergic reactions including bronchospasm. Susceptible individuals are frequently also sensitive to aspirin.

Report immediately the onset of extrapyramidal effects: gait disturbances, difficulty in speaking, muscle spasms, torticollis, deviations in eye movements. Reduction in dosage or discontinuation of medication is indicated.

Caution patient to avoid potentially hazardous activities such as driving a car or operating machinery because of possibility of drowsiness and dizziness.

Stored at room temperature, away from heat, in light-resistant containers. Suppositories should be stored below 77°F.

See Chlorpromazine (prototype phenothiazine).

THIMEROSAL

(Mersol, Merthiolate)

(thye-mer′oh-sal)
Antiinfective
Mercurial

ACTIONS AND USES. Topical organic mercurial with sustained bacteriostatic and fungistatic activity. Ineffective against spore-forming organisms.

Used in first-aid treatment of contaminated wounds, in antisepsis of intact skin, before surgery, and in pustular dermatose; as antifungal agent in athlete's foot for wound irrigations. Ophthalmic preparation is used to treat conjunctivitis and corneal ulcer and for prevention of infection following removal of foreign bodies. Also used as preservative for biologic and pharmaceutical products.

CONTRAINDICATIONS AND PRECAUTIONS. History of sensitivity to thio or mercurial compounds, prolonged use.

ADVERSE/SIDE EFFECTS. **Hypersensitivity reaction:** erythema, papular or vesicular eruptions. Prolonged use: **mercury poisoning** (metallic taste, salivation, stomatitis, lethargy, peripheral neuropathy).

ROUTE AND DOSAGE. **Topical:** 1:1000 cream, glycerite, solution, tincture; aerosol pump 0.33%; ophthalmic solution 1:5000. Application of medication: one to three times a day. Alcohol content: tincture, 50%; aerosol, up to 72%.

NURSING IMPLICATIONS

For first-aid treatment: appropriate cleansing should precede application of antiseptic.

To prevent skin irritation, do not apply bandage or other occlusive dressing until tincture application has completely dried.

Thimerosal is antagonized by whole blood and is incompatible when used concurrently or following applications of boric acid, iodine, strong acids, aluminum, silver, or other salts of heavy metals. It is compatible with sulfonamides.

Reportedly not inactivated by soaps or cotton materials, and action is not significantly diminished by nonsanguinous drainage (plasma, serum) or discharge.

Aqueous Merthiolate contains thimerosal and borate (0.14%). Both are toxic if absorbed systemically. Long-term use, especially as treatment of otitis media, may lead to fatal toxicity due to swallowing of solution.

Preserved in tightly covered, light-resistant containers. Avoid exposure to excessive heat.

THIOGUANINE

(TG, 6-Thioguanine)

(thye-oh-gwah'neen)
Antineoplastic
Antimetabolite

ACTIONS AND USES. Antimetabolite and purine antagonist with immunosuppressive activity. Qualitatively and quantitatively similar to mercaptopurine (qv). A highly toxic drug with a low therapeutic index; therapeutic response is normally accompanied by evidence of toxicity. Delays myelosuppression; has potential mutagenic and carcinogenic properties. Cross-resistance exists between mercaptopurine and thioguanine. *For Contraindications and Adverse/Side Effects, see Mercaptopurine.*

Used in combination with other antineoplastics for remission induction in acute myelogenous leukemia and as treatment of chronic myelogenous leukemia. Has little advantage over mercaptopurine.

ABSORPTION AND FATE. Partially (30%) absorbed from GI tract, with maximum blood levels achieved in 10 to 12 hours. Rapidly detoxified in liver. Biphasic half-life: initial, 15 minutes; terminal, 11 hours; excreted in feces and urine as metabolites. Toxicity is not reduced by hemodialysis.

ROUTE AND DOSAGE. **Oral (dosage depends on clinical and hematologic responses and is highly individualized):** usual initial dose: 2 mg/kg body weight daily; if no clinical improvement occurs after 4 weeks of treatment, dosage is cautiously increased to 3 mg/kg body weight daily administered at one time; usual maintenance dose: 2 mg/kg daily.

NURSING IMPLICATIONS

Unlike mercaptopurine, thioguanine dose schedule may be maintained during concomitant administration of allopurinol.

Blood counts are determined weekly; monitor reports as indicators for adaptations in nursing and drug regimens.

Patient receiving this drug experiences an increased incidence of infections, and possibly hemorrhage complications. Therapy should be discontinued at first sign of altered blood cell counts.

Maintenance doses are continued throughout remissions.

Monitor intake and output ratio and report oliguria.

Observe patient's skin and sclera for *jaundice.* It is thought to be a reversible clinical sign, but it should be reported promptly as a symptom of toxicity; drug will be discontinued promptly.

Expect that the leukocyte count descent may be slow over a period of 2 to 4 weeks. Treatment is interrupted if there is a rapid fall within a few days.

Contraceptive measures should be used during therapy with this drug.

Because there is no known antagonist to thioguanine, prompt discontinuation of the drug is essential in avoiding irreversible myelosuppression when toxicity develops.

Store drug in airtight containers at temperature 15° to 30°C (59° to 86°F).

See Mercaptopurine.

THIOPENTAL SODIUM

(Pentothal)

(thye-oh-pen′tal)
Anesthetic
Sedative/hypnotic
Barbiturate
C III

ACTIONS AND USES. Ultra-short-acting barbiturate. CNS depressant action produces anesthesia, without analgesia, and with insignificant effects at myoneural junctions.

Used to induce hypnosis and anesthesia prior to or as supplement to other anesthetic agents, or as sole agent for brief (15-minute) operative procedures. Also used to control convulsive states following anesthesia and for narcoanalysis and narcosynthesis in psychiatric disorders.

ABSORPTION AND FATE. Hypnotic action within 30 to 40 seconds following IV administration. Absorption from rectum is unpredictable, with onset of action in 8 to 10 minutes and duration of about 1 hour. With repeated doses, fatty tissue acts as reservoir (concentrations 6 to 12 times that of plasma), from which slow release of drug prolongs anesthesia. Metabolized in liver. Half-life: 11.5 hours (increases with age, and during pregnancy). Crosses placenta.

TU

CONTRAINDICATIONS AND PRECAUTIONS. Absolute contraindications: hypersensitivity to barbiturates, absence of suitable veins for IV administration, status asthmaticus, acute intermittent or other hepatic porphyrias. *Cautious Use:* severe cardiovascular disease, hypotension or shock, conditions that may potentiate or prolong hypnotic effect (excessive premedication,

Addison's disease, hepatic or renal dysfunction, myxedema, increased BUN, severe anemia, increased intracranial pressure, asthma, myasthenia gravis).

ADVERSE/SIDE EFFECTS. Respiratory and myocardial depression, cardiac arrhythmias, retrograde amnesia, prolonged somnolence and recovery, sneezing, coughing, bronchospasm, laryngospasm, shivering, muscle irritability, hypersensitivity reactions, pain, neurosis, neuritis, thrombosis, and sloughing at site of IV extravasation, anaphylaxis (rare). *See also Phenobarbital.*

ROUTE AND DOSAGE. Intravenous rectal suspension: Highly individualized by titration against patient's requirements as governed by age, sex, and body weight, preexisting disease, premedication, concurrent nitrous oxide administration.

NURSING IMPLICATIONS

Solution should be freshly prepared and used promptly. If a precipitate is present, discard solution. Unused portions should be discarded within 24 hours.

Prepare solution with one of the following diluents: sterile water, 0.9%, or 5% dextrose for injection. Sterile water for injection is not used if concentration is less than 2.5%. A water solution causes hemolysis.

Resuscitation equipment, endotracheal tube, suction, and oxygen should be readily available for treatment of respiratory depression.

Test dose with 2 ml thiopental is advisable to determine tolerance or unusual sensitivity. Observe patient reaction at least 1 minute.

Physician may prescribe normal saline enema several hours before administration of rectal suspension (soap solution may interfere with drug effect).

If extravasation occurs, the site will require particular attention to prevent tissue and vessel damage. A vasodilator (nitroprusside) or local anesthetic (e.g., chloroprocaine) and local injection of heparin will relieve pain and vascular spasm and promote opening of collateral circulation. Monitor site at regular intervals for signs of progressing tissue or vessel damage; signs of phlebitis or thrombosis may not appear for 24 hours. Consult physician about use of heat or cold applications. Chemical irritant effects and pain can be reduced by local injections of 1% procaine and applications of heat to increase circulation and removal of drug.

Vital signs should be assessed every 3 to 5 minutes before, during, and after drug administration until recovery from anesthesia. Continue to monitor vital signs as scheduled routinely for postoperative period.

Shivering or twitching muscles sometimes progressing to localized or generalized tremors may result from increased sensitivity to cold or from pain. Control environment and provide additional external heat, if necessary.

Monitor for signs of pain (e.g., increased pulse, restlessness). Administer prescribed analgesic before pain is intense.

Classified as Schedule III drug under Federal Controlled Substances Act.

See Phenobarbital (prototype barbiturate).

THIORIDAZINE HYDROCHLORIDE

(Mellaril, Millazine, Novoridazine, Thioril)

(thye-or-rid'a-zeen)
Psychotropic
Antipsychotic
Neuroleptic
Phenothiazine

ACTIONS AND USES. Piperidine phenothiazine with actions, uses, limitations and interactions similar to those of chlorpromazine (qv). Rarely produces extrapyramidal effects. Has weak antiemetic but strong anticholinergic and alpha adrenergic activity and potent sedative action.

Used in management of nonpsychotic behavioral disturbances of senility, manifestations of psychotic disorders, alcohol withdrawal, and in symptomatic treatment of organic brain disease. Used in short-term treatment of moderate to marked depression and for management of hyperkinetic behavior syndrome (attention deficit disorder).

ABSORPTION AND FATE. Absorbed well from GI tract. Half-life: 26 to 36 hours. Hepatic metabolism; excreted by kidneys. Crosses placenta and appears in breast milk.

CONTRAINDICATIONS AND PRECAUTIONS. Hypersensitivity to phenothiazines. Severe CNS depression, CV disease, children under 2 years of age. Safe use by pregnant women and nursing mothers not established. *Cautious Use:* patients with premature ventricular contractions, or previously diagnosed breast cancer; patients exposed to extremes in heat or to organophosphorous insecticides, respiratory disorders. *See also Chlorpromazine.*

ADVERSE/SIDE EFFECTS. Sedation, dizziness, drowsiness, lethargy, nasal congestion, blurred vision, pigmentary retinopathy; xerostomia, constipation, paralytic ileus; amenorrhea, breast engorgement, gynecomastia, galactorrhea, ventricular dysrhythmias. Infrequent: extrapyramidal syndrome, nocturnal confusion, hyperactivity. *See also Chlorpromazine.*

ROUTE AND DOSAGE. Oral: Adults: *Psychotic manifestations:* initial: 25 to 100 mg three times daily with gradual dose adjustment of up to 800 mg/day as needed and tolerated. Once symptoms are controlled, dose is reduced gradually to lowest effective maintenance level (200 to 800 mg/day in 2 to 4 divided doses). *Moderate to marked depression:* initial: 25 mg three times daily; total daily dose range 20 to 200 mg. **Elderly:** initial: 10 mg three times daily; increments up to 200 mg/day if needed and tolerated. Recommended maximum single dose: 100 mg. **Children (over 2 years):** *Psychotic manifestations:* 0.5 to 3 mg/kg/day. If hospitalized: initial: 25 mg two or three times daily; increased gradually until optimum therapeutic effect or maximum dosage is reached.

NURSING IMPLICATIONS

Tablet may be crushed before administration and taken with fluid of patient's choice.

If the patient is also receiving antacid or antidiarrheal medication, schedule the phenothiazine to be taken at least 1 hour before or 1 hour after the other medication.

Liquid concentrate should be diluted just prior to administration with ½ glass of fruit juice, milk, water, carbonated beverage, or soup. Preparation and storage of bulk dilutions are not recommended.

Increases in dose should be added to the first dose of the day to prevent sleep disturbance.

Explain dosage and dilution to patient if responsible for administration.

Warn the patient against spilling drug on skin or clothing because of danger of contact dermatitis. Wash skin well in soap and water if liquid drug is spilled.

Suicide is an inherent risk with any depressed patient, and may remain a problem until there is significant clinical improvement. Supervise patient closely during early course of therapy. Do not permit access to more than one dose of medication and watch to see that the dose is not "cheeked" or hoarded.

Counsel patient to take drug as prescribed and not to alter dosing regimen or stop medication without consulting physician. Additionally, patient should never give the drug to another person.

Alcohol should be avoided during phenothiazine therapy. Concomitant use enhances CNS depression effects.

Warn patient to avoid use of all OTC drugs unless they are approved by the physician.

Orthostatic hypotension may occur in early therapy. Female patients appear to be more susceptible than male patients.

Advise patient to make position changes slowly, particularly from recumbent to upright posture, and to dangle legs a few minutes before standing. Also inform patient that vasodilation produced by hot showers or baths or by long exposure to environmental heat may accentuate hypotensive effect.

The patient may be unable to adjust to extremes of temperature because of drug effect on the heat regulatory center in the hypothalamus. If patient complains of being cold even at average room temperature, heed complaints and furnish additional clothing or blankets if necessary. The elderly patient is particularly susceptible to this modified regulatory function.

Do not apply heating pad or hot water bottles to the body for external heat. Because of depressed conditioned avoidance behaviors, a severe burn may result.

If patient has been exposed to extremes in heat, or has had an elevated temperature for several hours, be alert to the risk of *heat stroke. Signs:* red, dry, hot skin, full bounding pulse, dilated pupils, temperature above 40.6°C (105°F), dyspnea. Report to physician and be prepared to institute measures to reduce temperature rapidly.

Monitor intake and output ratio and bowel elimination pattern. Check for abdominal distention and pain. Encourage adequate fluid intake as prophylaxis for constipation and xerostomia. The depressed patient may not seek help for either symptom, or for urinary retention.

Caution patient to avoid potentially hazardous activities such as driving a car or operating machinery until reaction to drug is known.

Marked drowsiness generally subsides with continued therapy or reduction in dosage.

Instruct patient to report to physician the onset of any change in visual acuity, brownish coloring of vision, or impairment of night vision. These symptoms suggest pigmentary retinopathy (observed primarily in patients receiving extremely high doses). An ophthalmic consultation may be indicated.

Periodic blood and hepatic function tests are advised during therapy.

May turn urine pink-red to reddish brown color.

Preserved in tightly covered, light-resistant containers at temperature between 15° and 30°C (59° and 86°F), unless otherwise indicated by the manufacturer.

See Chlorpromazine (prototype phenothiazine).

THIOTEPA

(TSPA)

(thye-oh-tep'a)
Antineoplastic
Alkylating agent

ACTIONS AND USES. Ethylenimine cell cycle nonspecific alkylating agent that selectively reacts with DNA phosphate groups to produce chromosome cross-linkage and consequent blocking of nucleoprotein synthesis. Nonvesicant, highly toxic hematopoietic agent with a low therapeutic index. Myelosuppression is cumulative and unpredictable, and may be delayed. Has some immunosuppressive activity. Like all alkylating agents thiotepa is carcinogenic, and potentially mutagenic.

Used to produce remissions in malignant lymphomas, including Hodgkin's disease and adenocarcinoma of breast and ovary. Also used in treatment of chronic granulocytic and lymphocytic leukemia, superficial papillary carcinoma of urinary bladder, bronchogenic carcinoma, and for management of malignant effusions secondary to neoplastic disease of serosal cavities. *Investigational Use:* prevention of pterygium recurrences following postoperative beta-irridiation; leukemia.

ABSORPTION AND FATE. Rapidly cleared from plasma following intravenous administration. Slow onset of action, with therapeutic response becoming increasingly evident over period of several weeks. Slowly bound to tissues; significant amounts remain in blood 72 hours after IV administration. Extensively metabolized. About 60% of IV dose eliminated in urine within 24 to 72 hours.

CONTRAINDICATIONS AND PRECAUTIONS. Hypersensitivity to drug; acute leukemia, pregnancy. *Cautious Use* (if at all): chronic lymphocytic leukemia, myelosuppression produced by radiation, with other antineoplastics; bone marrow invasion by tumor cells, impaired renal or hepatic function.

ADVERSE/SIDE EFFECTS. **GI:** anorexia, nausea, vomiting, stomatitis, ulceration of intestinal mucosa. **Hematologic:** leukopenia, thrombocytopenia, anemia, pancytopenia. **Hypersensitivity:** hives, rash, pruritus. **Reproductive:** amenorrhea, interference with spermatogenesis. **Other:** headache, febrile reactions, pain and weeping of injection site, hyperuricemia, alopecia (rare), slowed or lessened response in heavily irradiated area, sensation of throat tightness. Reported with intravesical administration: lower abdominal pain, hematuria, hemorrhagic chemical cystitis, vesical irritability.

ROUTE AND DOSAGE. **Intravenous:** 0.3 to 0.4 mg/kg at 1- to 4-week intervals. **Intratumor:** Initial: 0.6 to 0.8 mg/kg injected directly into tumor (preceded by injection of local anesthetic (same needle, different syringe). Maintenance: 0.07 to 0.8 mg/kg at 1- to 4-week intervals. **Intracavitary:** 0.6 to 0.8 mg/kg (usually through same tubing used for parencentesis) given at intervals of at least 1 week. **Intravesicular:** 60 mg in 30 to 60 ml distilled water instilled into bladder by catheter; to be retained 2 hours. Maintenance: once a week for 4 weeks, then once monthly.

NURSING IMPLICATIONS

Used only under constant supervision by physicians experienced in therapy with cytotoxic agents.

Reconstitute with sterile water for injection. Usual dilution: 1.5 ml of diluent to vial containing 15 mg of drug (resultant solution: 10 mg/ml). Other diluents may result in hypertonic solutions which can cause irritation on injection.

Avoid exposure of skin and respiratory tract to particles of thiotepa during solution preparation.

Following reconstitution, solution may be clear to slightly opaque. If markedly opaque or contains a precipitate do not use.

Reconstituted solutions may be further diluted with sodium chloride, dextrose, dextrose and sodium chloride, Ringer's or lactated Ringer's injection for IV infusion, or for intracavitary or perfusion therapy.

Powder for injection and reconstituted solutions should be stored in refrigerator at 2° to 8°C (35° to 46°F) and protected from light. Reconstituted solutions are stable for 5 days under refrigeration.

Thiotepa may be mixed with procaine 2% and epinephrine 1:1000 for local administration.
Discuss possibility of amenorrhea with patient (usually reversible in 6 to 8 months).
Most patients will manifest some evidence of toxicity; therefore close monitoring is essential.
Because of cumulative effects, maximum myelosuppression may be delayed 3 or 4 weeks after termination of therapy. Warn patient to report onset of fever, bleeding, a cold or illness, no matter how mild; medical supervision may be necessary.
Hemoglobin level and leukocyte and thrombocyte counts should be determined at least weekly during therapy, and for at least 3 weeks after therapy is discontinued.
Manufacturer recommends discontinuing therapy if leukocyte count falls to 3000/mm^3 or below or if platelet count falls below 150,000/mm^3.
Monitor leukocyte and thrombocyte counts as indicators for adaptations in nursing and drug regimens.
Treatment of bladder tumor: patient is dehydrated 8 to 12 hours prior to treatment; 60 mg in 30 to 60 ml distilled water are instilled into bladder by catheter to be retained for 2 hours (if patient cannot retain 60 ml solution, 30 ml dilution is used); if desired, patient is repositioned every 15 minutes for maximal area contact. Usual course of treatment is once a week for 4 weeks; repeated beyond this with caution, because bone marrow depression may increase.
See Mechlorethamine (prototype antineoplastic).

Drug Interactions. Thiotepa increases pharmacologic and toxic effects of **succinylcholine** by decreasing pseudocholinesterase levels.

THIOTHIXENE HYDROCHLORIDE
(Navane)

(thye-oh-thix'een)
Psychotropic, antipsychotic (neuroleptic)
Thioxanthene

ACTIONS AND USES. Thioxanthene derivative chemically and pharmacologically similar to chlorprothixene and the piperazine phenothiazines. Possesses sedative, adrenolytic, antiemetic, and weak anticholinergic activity. *See Chlorpromazine.*

Used to manage manifestations of psychotic disorders. *Investigational Use:* as an antidepressant.

ABSORPTION AND FATE. Oral form slowly absorbed from GI tract. Therapeutic effects following IM injection: 1 to 6 hours, with duration of effect up to 12 hours. Metabolized in liver. Half-life: 34 hours; drug may remain in body several weeks after administration. Excreted in bile and feces. Crosses placenta.

CONTRAINDICATIONS AND PRECAUTIONS. Hypersensitivity to thioxanthenes and phenothiazines, children under 12 years, comatose states, CNS depression, circulatory collapse, blood dyscrasias. Safe use in women of childbearing potential or during pregnancy not established. *Cautious Use:* history of convulsive disorders, patient in state of alcohol withdrawal, glaucoma, prostatic hypertrophy, cardiovascular disease; patients who might be exposed to organophosphorous insecticides or to extreme heat; concomitant use of atropine or related drugs or ototoxic medications (especially ototoxic antibiotics); previously diagnosed breast cancer. *See also Chlorpromazine.*

ADVERSE/SIDE EFFECTS. Drowsiness, insomnia, dizziness, cerebral edema, convulsions, extrapyramidal symptoms (dose related), paradoxical exaggeration of psychotic symptoms; depressed cough reflex; xerostomia, constipation, tachycardia, orthostatic hypotension, impotence, gynecomastia, galactorrhea, amenorrhea, rash, contact dermatitis, photosensitivity, blurred vision, pigmentary retinopathy, decreased serum uric acid levels; sudden death. *See also Chlorpromazine.*

ROUTE AND DOSAGE. Oral: Initial: 2 mg three times daily; increase to 15 mg/day as needed or tolerated. Optimal dose: 20 to 30 mg/day; maximum recommended oral dose: 60 mg/day. **Intramuscular:** 4 mg, two to four times daily. Maximum recommended IM dose: 30 mg/day.

NURSING IMPLICATIONS

Oral concentrate, contains 7% alcohol, must be diluted just before administration in a cupful of water, fruit juice, carbonated beverage, milk, or soup.

Capsule may be emptied and contents swallowed with water or mixed with food, if patient prefers or if unable or unwilling to swallow the capsule.

Administer IM injection deep into upper outer quadrant of buttock. Aspirate carefully before injection to avoid inadvertent entry into blood vessel. Rotate injection sites.

Although therapeutic response can be observed 1 to 6 hours following IM injection, it may be days or several weeks before response with the oral preparations.

When thiothixene is added to the drug regimen of a patient on hypertensive treatment, monitor BP for excessive hypotensive response until drug therapy has been stabilized.

Because of the possibility of orthostatic hypotension, patient receiving IM drug should be recumbent for at least 1 hour following injection. Periodically check blood pressure during this time.

Dosage adjustment may be necessary when patient is changed from IM to oral forms (capsules, concentrate).

Counsel patient to take drug as prescribed and not to alter dosing regimen or stop medication without consulting physician. Abrupt discontinuation can cause delirium.

If patient has suicidal tendency, do not permit access to more than one dose of medication; supervise its ingestion to prevent "cheeking" for hoarding purposes.

Because of danger of light-headedness, advise patient to make position changes slowly, particularly from recumbent to upright, and to sit a few minutes before ambulation. Supervise patient if necessary.

Mild drowsiness, common during first few days of drug therapy, usually subsides with continued treatment. Caution patient to avoid potentially hazardous activities such as driving a car or operating machinery until response to drug is known.

Avoid contact of oral concentrate with skin and clothing to prevent contact dermatitis. If concentrate spills, wash skin promptly with water.

Hyperreflexia has been reported in infants delivered from mothers having received thiothixene.

Periodic ophthalmic examinations, blood and hepatic function tests are advisable in patients on prolonged therapy.

Keep in mind that antiemetic effect may mask toxicity of other drugs or make it difficult to diagnose conditions whose primary symptom is nausea, such as brain tumor, intestinal obstruction, or Reye's syndrome.

Warn patient to avoid alcohol and other depressants during therapy.

The use of all OTC drugs should be approved by the physician during antipsychotic therapy.

Inform patient that although hyperhydrosis is an uncomfortable side effect, it does not indicate need to terminate therapy. Another antipsychotic agent may be substituted, if necessary.

Extrapyramidal effects (pseudoparkinsonism, akathisia, dystonia) may occur during early therapy. Report to physician; dose adjustment or short-term therapy with an antiparkinson agent may provide relief.

Be alert to first symptoms of tardive dyskinesia (tongue protrusion, lateral jaw movements, cheek puffing, lip smacking, etc). *(See Chlorpromazine.)* Discontinue drug immediately and inform physician.

Advise patient to avoid excessive exposure to sunlight to prevent a photosensitivity reaction. If sun exposure is expected, protect skin with sunscreen lotion (SPF 12 or above).

Store medication in light-resistant containers at temperature of 15° to 30°C (56° to 89°F), unless otherwise indicated by the manufacturer.

See Chlorpromazine (prototype phenothiazine).

THROMBIN

Hemostatic (topical)

(Fibrindex, Thrombinar, Thrombostat)

ACTIONS AND USES. Sterile plasma protein prepared from prothrombin of bovine origin. Induces clotting of whole blood or a fibrinogen solution without addition of other substances. Action mechanism: conversion of fibrinogen to thrombin. Potency standardized and expressed in terms of NIH units (1 NIH unit is amount required to clot 1 ml of standardized fibrinogen solution in 15 seconds).

Used when oozing of blood from capillaries and small venules is accessible, as in dental extraction, plastic surgery, grafting procedures, and epistaxis; also used to shorten bleeding time at puncture sites in heparinized patient (i.e., following hemodialysis).

CONTRAINDICATIONS AND PRECAUTIONS. Known hypersensitivity to any of drug components or to material of bovine origin, parenteral use, entry or infiltration into large blood vessels.

ADVERSE/SIDE EFFECTS. Sensitivity, allergic and febrile reactions, intravascular clotting and death when thrombin is allowed to enter large blood vessels.

ROUTE AND DOSAGE. Topical: 100 to 2000 NIH units/ml, depending on extent of bleeding. May be used as solution, in dry form, or by mixing thrombin with blood plasma to form a fibrin "glue." Also used in conjunction with absorbable gelatin sponge: sponge strips of desired size are immersed in thrombin solution; sponge is kneaded vigorously to remove trapped air, then applied and held in place 10 to 15 seconds with dry sterile cotton pledget or gauze sponge. **Oral:** *Upper GI tract hemorrhage: (method 1):* patient is given 60 ml milk to neutralize gastric acid; after 5 minutes, 10,000 to 20,000 NIH units thrombin are administered in 60 ml milk; repeated 3 times daily for 4 or 5 days or until bleeding is controlled; *(method 2):* 60 ml phosphate buffer solution are introduced via Levin tube; stomach contents are aspirated; 60 ml phosphate buffer are repeated; after 5 minutes additional 60 ml of buffer containing 10,000 NIH units thrombin are given; Levin tube is clamped off for 30 minutes, at the end of which time it is aspirated gently; if there is no fresh bleeding, patient is given buffer for 48 hours (15 ml every hour); entire procedure is repeated, if necessary.

NURSING IMPLICATIONS

Be prepared for possible hemorrhage by having patient's blood typed and cross-matched.

Sponge recipient area free of blood before applying thrombin.

Solutions may be prepared in sterile distilled water or isotonic saline.

Thrombin activity is affected by dilute acids, alkalis, heat, and salts of heavy metals.
Solutions should be used within a few hours of preparation. If several hours are to elapse between time of preparation and use, solution should be refrigerated, or preferably frozen, and used within 48 hours.
Store hyophilized preparation at 2° to 8°C (36° to 46°F).

THYROGLOBULIN

(Proloid)

(thye-roe-glob'yoo-lin)
Hormone

ACTIONS AND USES. Obtained from purified extract of hog thyroid; contains levothyroxine (T_4) and liothyronine (T_3) in approximate ratio of 2.5:1. Clinical effects similar to those of thyroid (qv). *For absorption and fate, see Thyroid.*

Used in thyroid replacement therapy of all forms of hypothyroidism. Has no clinical advantage over thyroid.

CONTRAINDICATIONS AND PRECAUTIONS. Myocardial infarction. *Cautious Use:* myxedema (such patients are extremely sensitive to thyroid), uncorrected adrenal insufficiency. *See also Thyroid.*

ADVERSE/SIDE EFFECTS. Signs and symptoms of hyperthyroidism such as menstrual irregularities, nervousness, angina pectoris, cardiac arrhythmias, hypertension. *See also Thyroid.*

ROUTE AND DOSAGE. Oral: start dosage in small amounts; increments at intervals of 1 or 2 weeks; usual maintenance: 32 to 200 mg daily.

NURSING IMPLICATIONS

Tablet may be crushed before administration and taken with fluid or mixed with food.
Dosage highly individualized according to thyroid status.
Thyroid status may be assessed by thyroid function test: free thyroxine index (FTI) and total serum thyroxine concentrations (RT_3U).
Dosage is adjusted to maintain protein-bound iodine at 4 to 8 mcg/dl.
Transfer from thyroglobulin to liothyronine: thyroglobulin is discontinued and therapy initiated with low daily dose of liothyronine; in the reverse situation, thyroglobulin replacement precedes complete withdrawal of liothyronine by several days in order to prevent relapse.
Drug is stable when stored at room temperature.
See also Thyroid.

THYROID

(Armour Thyroid, Thyro-Teric)

(thye'roid)
Hormone

ACTIONS AND USES. Preparation of desiccated animal thyroid gland containing active thyroid hormones, *l*-thyroxine (T_4) and *l*-triiodothyronine (T_3); total iodine content between 0.17 and 0.23%. Action mechanism unknown; T_4 is largely converted to T_3, which exerts principal effects. Influences growth and maturation of various tissues (including skeletal and CNS) at critical periods. Promotes a generalized increase in metabolic rate of body tissues, producing increases in the following: rate of carbohydrate, protein, and fat metabolism, enzyme system activity, oxygen consumption, respiratory rate, body temperature, cardiac output, heart rate, blood volume. Thyroid affects water and ion transport and directly promotes synthesis and transcription of nuclear RNA. Potentiates actions of catecholamines; e.g., many prominent features of hyperthyroidism (tachycardia, lid lag and tremor) represent increased catecholamine effects. Therapeutic actions are slow to develop and prolonged.

Used as replacement or substitution therapy in primary hypothyroidism (cretinism, myxedema, simple goiter, deficiency states in pregnancy and in the elderly) and secondary hypothyroidism caused by surgery, excess radiation, or antithyroid drug therapy. May be given as adjunct to thyroid inhibiting agents when it is desirable to limit release of thyrotropic hormones and to prevent goitrogenesis and hypothyroidism.

ABSORPTION AND FATE. Adequate absorption from GI tract. 99% circulating drug binds competitively and reversibly to plasma transport proteins: thyroxine-binding globulin (TBG), thyroxine-binding prealbumin (TBPA), and albumin. Maximum effect of T_4 (half-life 6.9 days) not reached for several days; that of T_3 (half-life 12 hours) reached in 12 to 24 hours; full effect usually achieved in 10 to 14 days. Excreted in urine and stool in both free and conjugated forms. Fecal excretion (10 to 15%) is variable, depending on hepatic function, luminal contents, and physical state of intestines. Minimal transport across placenta.

CONTRAINDICATIONS AND PRECAUTIONS. Thyrotoxicosis, acute myocardial infarction uncomplicated by hypothyroidism, cardiovascular disease, morphologic hypogonadism, nephrosis, uncorrected hypoadrenalism. *Cautious Use:* angina pectoris, hypertension, elderly patients who may have occult cardiac disease, renal insufficiency, pregnancy, concomitant administration of catecholamines, diabetes mellitus, hyperthyroidism (history of), malabsorption states.

ADVERSE/SIDE EFFECTS. Chronic overdosage: hyperthyroidism. **Massive overdosage:** thyroid storm: high temperature (as high as 106°F), tachycardia, vomiting, shock, coma. **Overdosage (thyrotoxicosis):** staring expression in eyes, congestive heart failure, angina, cardiac arrhythmias, palpitation, tachycardia; weight loss, tremors, headache, nervousness, fever, diarrhea or abdominal cramps, insomnia, warm and moist skin, heat intolerance, leg cramps, menstrual irregularities, shock, changes in appetite, hyperglycemia (usually offset by increased tissue oxidation of sugar).

ROUTE AND DOSAGE. Oral (highly individualized): Adults: *Myxedema:* 16 mg/day for 2 weeks, followed by 32 mg/day for 2 weeks or more, then 65 mg/day; thereafter, dosage increased as clinically indicated; maintenance: 65 to 130 mg/day. *Mild hypothyroidism without myxedema:* initial: 65 mg/day; then increased by 65 mg every 30 days to maintenance dose. *Severe hypothryoidism:* 15 mg/day; dosage increased to 30 mg/day after 2 weeks, then 2 weeks later increased to 60 mg/day. (Usual maintenance: 60 to 180 mg/day.) **Children:** *Cretinism or severe hypothyroidism:* same dosage regimen as for adults with severe hypothyroidism but in children increases in dosage should be at 2-week intervals. Eventual maintenance may be higher in growing children than in adults.

NURSING IMPLICATIONS

Administer as a single dose, preferably before breakfast.

Transfer from thyroid treatment to liothyronine: discontinue thyroid and initiate treatment with low daily dose of liothyronine; transfer in reverse direction: therapy initiated with replacement several days before complete withdrawal of liothyronine in order to avoid collapse.

During institution of treatment, observe patient carefully for untoward reactions such as angina, palpitation, cardiac pain.

Physical examination at monthly intervals and thyroid function tests: free thyroxine index (FTI) and total serum thyroxine concentration (RT_3U) every 3 months are usual during dose adjustment period.

Normal values of laboratory tests used to determine clinical response to thyroid: *Free thyroxine:* 1.4 to 3.5 ng/dl; *thyroid stimulating hormone (TSH) level:* up to 10 μU/ml; and *resin uptake of T_3 in vitro:* 27 to 37% uptake of T_3.

Generally dosage is initiated at low level and systematically increased in small increments to desired maintenance dose.

Be alert for symptoms of overdosage *(see Adverse/Side Effects)* that may occur 1 to 3 weeks after therapy is started. If they develop, treatment should be interrupted for several days and restarted with reduced dosage.

Hypothyroidism is common in the elderly. Women generally require less thyroxine replacement than men; however, if replacement dosage is required the regimen is: initial: 25 mcg/daily with gradual increments, as indicated. Monitor response until regimen is stabilized (e.g., thyroid function tests, weight changes) to prevent iatrogenic hyperthyroidism. In drug-induced hyperthyroidism, there may also be increased bone loss. Such a patient is vulnerable to pathologic fractures. If back or chest (rib) pain is experienced, the physician should be consulted.

Toxic effects of thyroid develop slowly and disappear gradually. T_4 effects require up to 3 to 6 weeks to dissipate; T_3 effects last 6 to 14 days after drug withdrawal.

If patient has taken hormone during pregnancy, dose is frequently discontinued in the postpartum period, with evaluation of thyroid function 6 weeks later.

Serial height measurement of the juvenile being treated with thyroid is an important means of monitoring influence of thyroid on growth. Too rapid growth rate results in premature epiphyseal closure. Urge parent to keep accurate record of height measurements for reporting to physician.

Useful guides of thyroid therapy in children include sleeping pulse and basal morning temperature.

Prepare parent and juvenile hypothyroid for a dramatic response to therapy: excessive shedding of hair, increased assertiveness of previously passive child, initial rapid weight loss and rapid catch-up growth. Symptoms usually disappear with continued therapy.

Earliest clinical response to thyroid (adult) is diuresis, accompanied by loss of weight and puffiness, followed by sense of well-being, increased pulse rate, increased pulse pressure, increased appetite, increased psychomotor activity, loss of constipation, normalization of skin texture and hair, and increased T_3 and T_4 serum levels.

Instruct patient to adhere to established dosage regimen: patient should not double, decrease or omit doses and the dose intervals should not be changed without approval of the physician.

In patient teaching, emphasize that replacement therapy for hypothyroidism is life-long; therefore, continued follow-up surveillance is important. Regular yearly appointments for evaluation are recommended.

Keep in mind that these patients tend to discontinue their medication when they begin to feel well.

Thyroid hormone is no longer used as a therapeutic agent for treatment of obesity, reproductive disorders (e.g., habitual abortion), breast cancer, and depression. The patient should not be taking thyroid at home without medical supervision.

Thyroid drug abuse leading to self-induced hyperthyroidism occurs in persons seeking a short-cut to weight reduction, often among paramedical personnel who have easy access to the drug. Patients have died from overuse of the drug for a period of 6 months or more.

Inadequate dosage in infant hypothyroidism is manifested by bradycardia, circulatory mottling, inactivity, hoarse cry, constipation, delay in relaxation phase of deep tendon reflexes.

Pulse rate is an important clue to drug effectiveness. Count pulse before each dose during period of dosage adjustment. Consult physician if rate is 100 or more, or if there has been a marked change in rate or rhythm.

When patient is euthyroid, teach to take own pulse and to record it periodically. If rate begins to increase or if rhythm changes, patient should notify physician.

Adrenocortical insufficiency may occur with prolonged therapy (dehydration, hypotension, asthenia, hypoglycemia, increased pigmentation of skin and mucous membranes). The diabetic patient receiving thyroid hormone may require increased dosage of insulin or oral hypoglycemic agent. Conversely, decreasing the thyroid dose may cause a hypoglycemic reaction unless insulin dosage is also reduced. Reinforce the necessity of continuing regular testing of urine for sugar and blood glucose level.

The patient should not change brands of thyroid unless physician approves. Hormone content varies among brands.

Thyroid hormones will alter the results of thyroid function tests.

If patient is receiving anticoagulant therapy, a decrease in the requirement usually develops within 1 to 4 weeks after starting treatment with thyroid. Close monitoring of prothrombin time (normal 9 to 11 seconds) is necessary. Warn patient to report evidence of excess anticoagulant, evidenced by ecchymoses, petechiae, purpura, unexplained bleeding.

Onset of chest pain or other signs of aggravated CV disease (dyspnea, tachycardia) should be reported promptly. The physician will decrease dosage.

Steatorrhea and other disease states that interfere with enterohepatic circulation may lead to excessive fecal loss of drug. Patient should be cautioned to report persistent diarrhea.

Teach the patient to avoid exposure to even a small amount of iodine. Instruct patient to avoid application of topical iodine, ingestion of OTC medications with iodides or dentifrices.

Food–Drug Interactions: Advise patient to avoid ingestion of foods high in iodine (e.g., turnip, cabbage, soy beans, some breads, kelp). Iodized salt and iodine-containing multivitamin preparations usually do not interfere with thyroid uptake test.

The physician will want to know if patient has had any procedure requiring radiopaque dyes (e.g., bronchography, myelography, cisternography) during the past 4 to 6 weeks.

Store in dark bottle to minimize spontaneous deiodination. Keep desiccated thyroid dry. Potency in this form reportedly persists for as long as 17 years.

Diagnostic Test Interferences. Thyroid increases basal metabolic rate; may increase **blood glucose levels, creatine phosphokinase, AST, LDH, PBI.** It may decrease **serum uric acid, cholesterol, thyroid stimulating hormone (TSH), I-131** uptake. Many medications may produce false results in thyroid function tests.

Drug Interactions: Thyroid

Plus	Interactions
Antidiabetics (coumarins, warfarin)	Anticoagulant effect may be potentiated (reduction of anticoagulant may be necessary)
Cholestyramine	May decrease thyroid action by interfering with absorption
Digitalis glycosides	Thyroid may increase toxic effects of the glycosides
Epinephrine and other catecholamines	Increased risk of coronary insufficiency
Estrogens	Increases serum thyroxin binding globulin (TBg). Increased dose of thyroid may be necessary

TU

Plus (cont.)	Interactions (cont.)
Insulin and oral hypoglycemics	Increases need for antidiabetic agent
Sympathomimetic agents Tricyclic antidepressants	May increase effects of these medications and of thyroid

THYROTROPIN

(Thytropar)

(thye-roe-troe'pin)
Hormone
Diagnostic agent

ACTIONS AND USES. Highly purified thyrotropic hormone (TSH) isolated from bovine anterior pituitary. Increases iodine uptake by the thyroid, and stimulates formation and secretion of thyroid hormone. May cause hyperplasia of thyroid cells, a rapidly reversible effect.

Used as diagnostic tool to determine subclinical hypothyroidism or low thyroid reserve, to assess need for continued thyroid medication, to differentiate primary and secondary hypothyroidism, and to detect remnants and metastases of thyroid carcinoma. Also used therapeutically in management of selected types of thyroid carcinoma and adjunctively with I-131 to promote uptake of the radioactive substance by the thyroid.

ABSORPTION AND FATE. Following parenteral injection, rapidly cleared by kidney. Half-life: 35 minutes in euthyroid; increased in hypothyroidism, and decreased in hyperthyroidism.

CONTRAINDICATIONS AND PRECAUTIONS. Hypersensitivity to thyrotropin, coronary thrombosis. *Cautious Use:* in presence of angina pectoris, cardiac failure, hypopituitarism, adrenocortical suppression.

ADVERSE/SIDE EFFECTS. Menstrual irregularities, fever, headache, nausea, vomiting, urticaria, transient hypotension, tachycardia, atrial fibrillation, thyroid swelling (especially with large doses), postinjection flare, anaphylactic reactions, induced or exaggerated angina pectoris or congestive heart failure. **Overdosage:** fever, tachycardia, vomiting, shock, coma.

ROUTE AND DOSAGE. **Subcutaneous, intramuscular:** diagnosis: 10 IU for 1 to 3 days; therapy (with I-131) of thyroid carcinoma: 10 U daily for 3 to 8 days. Diagnosis of thyroid cancer remnant: 10 U daily for 3 to 7 days.

NURSING IMPLICATIONS

Ten units lyophilized powder are dissolved in 2 ml sterile physiologic saline solution for injection.

Diagnostic tests may be made even though patient is receiving thyroid hormone therapy.

Thyrotropin is stable at room temperature when kept dry. Retains potency in solution at least 2 weeks if refrigerated.

Diagnostic use: in presence of normal thyroid tissue, stimulation provided by daily doses of 10 IU thyrotropin for 1 to 3 days causes an elevated serum thyroxine level and increased radioactive iodine uptake (RAI) by thyroid gland. If hypothyroidism is primary, there will be no change in RAI uptake following several days of thyrotropin stimulation. Conversely, there will be a significant increase in RAI uptake if hypothyroidism is secondary to hypopituitarism.

Treatment of overdosage: discontinue thyrotropin and supply supportive measures required by shock and potential adrenal insufficiency.

Drug Interactions. **Levodopa** lowers thyrotropin levels.

TICARCILLIN DISODIUM
(Ticar)

(tye-kar-sill'in)
Antiinfective
Antibiotic (beta-lactam)
Penicillin

ACTIONS AND USES. Extended spectrum penicillinase-sensitive, semisynthetic derivative of penicillin. Antibacterial activity closely resembles that of carbenicillin, but reportedly more active against *Pseudomonas aeruginosa* strains. Like carbenicillin, it is primarily effective against gram-negative microorganisms (including *Pseudomonas,* indole-positive and negative; *Proteus* species, *Escherichia coli, Haemophilus influenzae,* some *Enterobacter,* and *Bacteroides fragilis*). Gram-positive spectrum is similar to that of penicillin, but is more active than penicillin against gram-negative infections *(see Penicillin G).* May be appropriately used for mixed infections. In common with penicillin G and carbenicillin, capable of inhibiting platelet aggregation. Cross-resistance between ticarcillin and carbenicillin reported.

Used in treatment of bacterial septicemia, acute and chronic respiratory tract infections, skin and soft tissue infections, and infections of genitourinary tract. May be used to treat infections in patients with impaired immunologic defenses. Sometimes used concomitantly with gentamicin or tobramycin (with which it has synergistic action) in treatment of certain strains of *Pseudomonas.* Probenecid may be used to attain greater and more prolonged ticarcillin serum levels.

ABSORPTION AND FATE. Serum concentrations peak within 1 hour following IM administration, decrease considerably by fourth hour, and are low or absent by sixth hour. Following IV administration, serum concentrations are initially higher than IM levels, but decline more quickly. Widely distributed in body tissues and fluids; some penetration into pleural fluid, CSF (particularly if meninges are inflamed), and bile. Highly concentrated in urine. Approximately 50 to 65% protein bound: serum half-life: about 70 minutes [prolonged in renal (7 to 17 hours) and hepatic (28 hours) dysfunction]. Small amount presumed to be metabolized in liver, then excreted in urine. About 80 to 95% of a 1 Gm IM or IV dose excreted unchanged in urine within 6 to 12 hours. Appears in breast milk. Removed by hemodialysis; minimal amounts removed by peritoneal dialysis.

CONTRAINDICATIONS AND PRECAUTIONS. Hypersensitivity to penicillins or cephalosporins. *Cautious Use:* history of or suspected atopy or allergies (hives, eczema, asthma, hay fever); renal or hepatic disease, coagulation disorders, patients on sodium restriction (cardiac patients; hypertensives). Safe use during pregnancy not established.

ADVERSE/SIDE EFFECTS. CNS (patients with impaired renal function on high-dose therapy): neuromuscular irritability, convulsions. **GI:** nausea, vomiting, diarrhea. **Hematologic:** hemolytic anemia, thrombocytopenia, leukopenia, neutropenia, hemorrhagic manifestations. **Hypersensitivity:** pruritus, urticaria, rash, drug fever, anaphylaxis, eosinophilia. **Other:** hypernatremia, hypokalemia; elevations of: alkaline phosphatase, SGOT (AST), SGPT (ALT); pain, induration (following IM), phlebitis (IV), superinfections, hemorrhagic cystitis. *See also Penicillin G.*

ROUTE AND DOSAGE. Intravenous infusion: *Systemic infections:* **Adults and children (weighing more than 40 kg):** 150 to 300 mg/kg/day in divided doses, every 3, 4, or 6 hours, (or 3 Gm daily in divided doses every 4 to 6 hours). **Children (under 40 kg):** 150 to 200 mg/kg/day in divided doses, every 4 to 6 hours (not to exceed adult dosage). **Neonates:** initial: 100 mg/kg IM or as 10- to 20-minute IV infusion, followed by 75 mg/kg every 4 hours. **Intramuscular, intravenous (direct): Adults and Children (over 40 kg):** 1 Gm every 6 hours. **Children (under 40 kg):** 50 to 100 mg/kg/day in divided doses every 6 to 8 hours. Direct IV injections should be administered as slowly as possible. Intermittent infusions are generally administered over a 30-minute to 2-hour period.

NURSING IMPLICATIONS

Careful inquiry should be made concerning hypersensitivity reactions to penicillins, cephalosporins, and other allergens.

Culture and sensitivity tests should be performed initially and at regular intervals throughout therapy in order to monitor drug effectiveness.

Administer IM deeply into body of a relatively large muscle. IM injections should not exceed 2 Gm per individual injection site. Rotate injection sites.

Pain and other local reactions associated with IM injections may be minimized by reconstituting drug with 1% lidocaine hydrochloride (without epinephrine) or bacteriostatic water for injection containing 0.9% benzyl alcohol. Consult physician.

After reconstitution for IM use, solutions should be discarded after 24 hours when stored at room temperature or 72 hours if refrigerated. Indicate time and date of reconstitution, and discard time on containers.

For IV use, follow manufacturer's directions regarding diluent and amount to use for initial reconstitution and for further dilution, to avoid tissue irritation and phlebitis.

After reconstitution for IV use, storage time depends on drug concentration and nature of diluent. See manufacturer's package insert for details.

Monitor intake and output. Report any change in intake–output ratio and unusual appearance of urine. Consult physician regarding advisable fluid intake.

Patients with impaired renal function are particularly susceptible to nephrotoxicity, neurotoxicity, and hemorrhagic manifestations, and therefore must be observed closely. Doses are generally based on creatinine clearance rates.

Bleeding tendency is most likely to occur in patients with impaired renal function or who are receiving high dose therapy. Observe patient for frank bleeding, hematuria, purpura, petechiae, easy bruising, or ecchymoses. Drug should be stopped if patient shows signs of bleeding. Report promptly to physician.

In patients on prolonged therapy or who are receiving high doses or who have impaired renal or hepatic function, assessments should be made of serum electrolytes (particularly sodium and potassium); cardiac, renal, hepatic, and blood status (including coagulation tests; bleeding time, prothrombin time or platelet aggregation) prior to and at regular intervals during therapy.

Each gram of ticarcillin disodium contains approximately 5.2 to 6.5 mEq of sodium.

Observe patient for symptoms of *hypernatremia:* confusion, neuromuscular excitability, seizures, congestive heart failure (paroxysmal nocturnal dyspnea, cough, edema, dyspnea on exertion, tachycardia), thirst, urine with high specific gravity; and *hypokalemia:* paresthesias, muscle weakness, depressed reflexes, polyuria, polydypsia, disturbances in cardiac rhythm; gastric distention, ileus; postural hypotension, dizziness.

Report immediately signs and symptoms of hypersensitivity reaction *(see Penicillin G for Adverse/Side Effects).* Have on hand epinephrine, IV corticosteroids, oxygen, suction, endotracheal tube, tracheostomy equipment.

Bear in mind that superinfections are particularly likely to occur in patients receiving extended spectrum antibiotics. Report black, furry overgrowth on tongue, stomatitis, glossitis, rectal or vaginal itching, vaginal discharge; loose, foul-smelling stools, unusual odor to urine.

See Penicillin G (prototype penicillin).

Drug Interactions. **Gentamicin** and **tobramycin,** and possibly other aminoglycosides, have synergistic action with ticarcillin when administered concomitantly. (However, these drugs are incompatible with ticarcillin in same infusion fluid.) *See also Penicillin G.*

TIMOLOL MALEATE
(Blocadren, Timoptic)

(tye'moe-lole)
Antihypertensive
Beta-adrenergic blocking agent (nonselective), antiglaucoma agent

ACTIONS AND USES. Nonselective beta-adrenergic blocking agent similar to propranolol (qv) in actions, but approximately 5 to 10 times as potent. Like propranolol, demonstrates antihypertensive, antiarrhythmic, and antianginal properties, and suppresses plasma renin activity. Unlike propranolol, appears to lack quinidinelike (local anesthetic or membrane-stabilizing) effects. When applied topically lowers elevated and normal intraocular pressure by unknown mechanism, but presumed to act by decreasing formation of aqueous humor and possibly by increasing outflow. In contrast to pilocarpine and other miotics, timolol does not constrict pupil and therefore does not cause night blindness, nor does it affect accommodation or visual acuity. Reportedly as effective as pilocarpine or epinephrine in reducing intraocular pressure and produces fewer and less severe adverse effects.

Used topically (ophthalmic solution) to reduce elevated intraocular pressure in chronic, open-angle glaucoma, aphakic glaucoma, secondary glaucoma, and ocular hypertension. May be used alone or in conjunction with epinephrine, pilocarpine or a carbonic anhydrase inhibitor such as acetazolamide. Oral preparation is used as step 1 agent alone or in combination with a thiazide diuretic to prevent reinfarction after MI, and to treat mild hypertension. *Investigational Use:* prophylactic management of stable, uncomplicated angina pectoris and migraine headaches.

ABSORPTION AND FATE. Reduction in intraocular pressure usually occurs in 15 to 30 minutes following instillation into eye. Effects peak in 1 to 2 hours; duration of effects about 24 hours. Over 98% absorbed following oral administration. Hepatic metabolism. Peak action in ½ to 3 hours; duration: approximately 4 hours. Half-life: 4 hours (prolonged with renal failure); 10% protein bound. About 15% excreted in urine as unchanged drug. Not dialyzable.

CONTRAINDICATIONS AND PRECAUTIONS. Hypersensitivity to timolol or to any components in product; bronchospasm, severe COPD, bronchial asthma, heart failure. Safe use during pregnancy (category C), lactation and in children not established. *Cautious Use:* bronchitis, patients subject to bronchospasm; sinus bradycardia, greater than first degree heart block, cardiogenic shock, right ventricular failure secondary to pulmonary hypertension, myasthenia gravis; concomitant use with adrenergic augmenting psychotropic drugs, e.g., MAO inhibitors.

ADVERSE/SIDE EFFECTS. Topical: CNS: fatigue, lethargy, weakness, somnolence, anxiety, headache, dizziness, confusion, psychic dissociation, depression. **GI:** anorexia, dyspepsia, nausea. **Hypersensitivity:** rash, urticaria. **Ophthalmic:** eye irritation including conjunctivitis, blepharitis, keratitis, blurred vision (rare), superficial punctate keratopathy. **Systemic: CV:** palpitation, bradycardia, hypotension, syncope, AV conduction disturbances, congestive heart failure. **Other:** difficulty in breathing, bronchospasm, hypoglycemia, hypokalemia, aggravation of peripheral vascular insufficiency, brown discoloration of finger and toe nails.

ROUTE AND DOSAGE. Topical (ophthalmic solution): *Glaucoma:* 1 drop of 0.25% solution in eye(s) twice a day (usually at 12-hour intervals). If necessary, dose increased to 1 drop of 0.5% solution twice a day. Once intraocular pressure is controlled, dosage reduced to once a day. **Oral:** *Angina prophylaxis:* (investigational use): 10 to 45 mg daily in 2 or 3 divided doses. If necessary, up to 60 mg/day in divided doses. *Hypertension:* initial: 10 mg twice daily. Maintenance: 20 to 40 mg/day. If necessary, dosage increased to maximum of 60 mg/day divided into 2 doses. Interval of at least 7 days between dose increases recommended. *Myocardial infarction:* 10 mg twice daily.

NURSING IMPLICATIONS

Tablet may be crushed before administration and taken with fluid of patient's choice.

Check pulse before administering timolol, topical or oral.

Inform patient that drug may cause slight reduction in resting heart rate. Patient should be informed about usual pulse rate and should be instructed to report significant changes in pulse rate and rhythm. Consult physician for parameters.

Monitor pulse rate and blood pressure at regular intervals in patients with severe heart disease.

Apply gentle pressure to lacrimal sac during and immediately following drug instillation, for about 1 minute, to lessen possibility of systemic absorption. *See Index: Drug administration: eye drops.*

Intraocular pressure (IOP) must be monitored throughout ophthalmic therapy. Normal IOP is in the range of 12 to 20 mm Hg. Readings may vary during the day; pressure tends to be higher at time of waking and lowest in the evening.

Because of diurnal variations in intraocular pressure, patients on once a day drug dosage should have measurements taken at various times during the day.

When drug is instilled in one eye only, intraocular pressure in opposite eye may be reduced slightly also.

Emphasize importance of adhering to prescribed regimen and of keeping follow-up appointments.

Advise patient to report difficulty in breathing promptly. Drug withdrawal may be indicated.

Some patients develop tolerance during long-term therapy.

Systemic use: see Propranolol, Nursing Implications.

Store between 15° and 30°C (59° and 86°F) in tight, light-resistant container unless otherwise directed by manufacturer.

See Propranolol (prototype beta-adrenergic blocking agent antihypertensive) for drug interactions.

TOBRAMYCIN SULFATE

(Nebcin, Tobrex)

(toe-bra-mye'sin)

Antiinfective, antibiotic

Aminoglycoside

ACTIONS AND USES. Aminoglycoside antibiotic derived from *Streptomyces tenebrarius.* Closely related to gentamicin (qv) in spectrum of antibacterial activity and pharmacologic properties. Reportedly causes less nephrotoxicity than gentamicin but incidence of ototoxicity is similar. Cross-allergenicity and some cross-resistance among aminoglycosides have been demonstrated. Has greater antibiotic activity against *Pseudomonas aerugenosa* than other aminoglycosides.

Used in treatment of severe infections caused by susceptible organisms.

ABSORPTION AND FATE. Following IM injection, peak serum concentrations in 30 to 90 minutes in adults and 1 to 2 hours in children. Measurable levels persist up to 8 hours. Serum concentrations higher and more prolonged in patients with reduced kidney function and infants. Widely distributed to body tissues and fluids; significant levels in CSF usually not achieved. Minimal protein binding. Half-life: 2 hours. Not appreciably metabolized in body. Eliminated by glomerular filtration; up to 93% of dose is excreted in urine in 24 hours. Crosses placenta.

CONTRAINDICATIONS AND PRECAUTIONS. History of hypersensitivity to tobramycin and other aminoglycoside antibiotics, concurrent use with other neurotoxic and/or nephrotoxic agents or potent diuretics. Safe use during pregnancy (category D) and in nursing mothers not established. *Cautious Use:* impaired renal function, premature and neonatal infants. *See also Gentamicin.*

ADVERSE/SIDE EFFECTS. Neurotoxicity (including ototoxicity), nephrotoxicity, increased SGOT (AST), and SGPT (ALT), LDH, increased serum bilirubin; anemia, granulocytopenia, thrombocytopenia, fever, rash, pruritis, urticaria, nausea, vomiting, headache, lethargy, superinfections. **Ophthalmic:** burning, stinging of eye after drug instillation; lid itching and edema. Hypersensitivity. *See also Gentamicin.*

ROUTE AND DOSAGE. Intramuscular, intravenous: Adults, children, and older infants with normal renal function: 3 mg/kg/day in 3 equal doses every 8 hours. *Life-threatening infections:* up to 5 mg/kg/day in 3 or 4 equal doses. Total daily dose more than 3 to 5 mg/kg should be reduced as soon as possible. **Neonates (1 week of age or younger):** not to exceed 4 mg/kg/day in equally divided doses every 12 hours. *Patients with impaired renal function:* initial: 1 mg/kg/day; subsequent dosage adjusted either with reduced doses at 8-hour intervals or usual doses at longer intervals. For IV injection, usual volume of diluent (0.9% sodium chloride injection or 5% dextrose injection) is 50 to 100 ml for adults and proportionately less for children, infused in not less than 20 minutes (range 20 to 60 minutes), to avoid neuromuscular blockade. **Topical** (ophthalmic): 1 or 2 drops in affected eye every 4 hours. If infection is severe: 2 drops in the infected eye every hour.

NURSING IMPLICATIONS

Weigh patient before treatment for calculation of dosage (by physician).

Bacterial culture and susceptibility tests are advised prior to and during tobramycin therapy.

As with other aminoglycosides, patient receiving tobramycin must remain under close clinical observation because of the high potential for toxicity, even in conventional doses.

Monitoring of serum drug concentrations is advised to minimize rise of toxicity. Prolonged serum concentrations above 12 mcg/ml are not recommended.

Renal, auditory, and vestibular functions should also be closely monitored, particularly in patients with known or suspected renal impairment and patients receiving high doses.

Drug induced auditory changes are irreversible (may be partial or total); usually bilateral. In cochlear damage, the patient may be asymptomatic and partial or bilateral deafness may continue to develop even after therapy has been discontinued.

Ophthalmic:

- Prolonged use may encourage development of superinfection with nonsusceptible organisms including fungi.
- Wash hands before and after instillation of medication. *(See Index: Drug administration: eye drops.)*
- Apply gentle finger pressure to lacrimal sac for 1 minute after drug has been instilled.
- Overdosage: increased lacrimation, keratitis, edema and itching of eye lids. Report symptoms to physician.

Advise patient to report symptoms of superinfections (black furry tongue or white patches on oral membranes, stomatitis, malodorous vaginal discharge, anorectal itching and irritation). Prompt treatment with an antibiotic or antifungal medication may be necessary.

Monitor patient with neuromuscular disorder (e.g., myasthenia gravis) for muscular weakness. Observe ambulation and assist, if necessary.

Evidence of impaired renal function (increasing BUN or NPN, increasing creatinine, cylinduria, proteinuria, cells, oliguria), auditory toxicity (hearing impairment, tinnitus), or vestibular damage (dizziness, vertigo, nystagmus, ataxia) indicates need for discontinuation of drug or dosage adjustment.

Monitor intake and output. Report oliguria, changes in intake–output ratio, and cloudy or frothy urine (may indicate proteinuria). The elderly patient is especially susceptible to renal toxicity. Patient is usually kept well hydrated to prevent chemical irritation in renal tubules. Consult physician.

Therapy is generally continued for 7 to 10 days. Complicated infection may require longer course of therapy, in which case close monitoring of renal, auditory, and vestibular function and serum drug concentrations is essential.

Prior to reconstitution, vial should be stored at controlled room temperature, preferably between 15° and 30°C (59° and 86°F). After reconstitution, solution may be kept refrigerated and used within 96 hours. If kept at room temperature, use within 24 hours.

Tobramycin should not be mixed with other drugs.

See Gentamicin (prototype aminoglycocide) for drug interactions.

PROTOTYPE

TOCAINIDE HYDROCHLORIDE

(Tonocard)

(toe-kay'nide)
Antiarrhythmic
Anesthetic (local)

ACTIONS AND USES. Antiarrhythmic agent (Class IB) and analog of lidocaine (qv), with similar electrophysiologic characteristics and hemodynamic properties. Effective orally. Suppresses PVCs and may have particular use in arrhythmias associated with a prolonged QT interval that do not respond to quinidine-like antiarrhythmics (Class IA). Decreases active potential duration in Purkinje fibers and slightly decreases resting membrane potential. Shortens effective refractory periods of atria, AV node, and ventricles without affecting AV conduction. QRS and QT intervals do not change. Exerts slight negative inotropic effect and slightly increases pulmonary and peripheral vascular resistance. Chronic oral therapy rarely precipitates cardiac decompensation; however, it has not been shown to prevent sudden death in patients with serious ventricular ectopic activity.

Used in treatment of refractory ventricular arrhythmia. May be combined to increase effectiveness with a Class IA antiarrhythmic (e.g., quinidine, disopyramide), or with propranolol. Also used to prevent ventricular tachyarrhythmia after acute MI.

ABSORPTION AND FATE. Absorption nearly complete from GI tract followed by 95 to 100% bioavailability. Peak plasma levels in approximately 1 hour (range ½ to 3 hours) oral, in 10 to 15 minutes IV. Metabolized in liver; about 10 to 20% protein bound. Elimination half-life: 10 to 17 hours (increases in renal failure to 22 hours and in hepatic dysfunction to 27 hours). About 35 to 40% excreted unchanged by kidneys; remainder excreted as metabolites. Renal elimination of unchanged drug increased by alkalynization of urine.

CONTRAINDICATIONS AND PRECAUTIONS. Hypersensitivity to tocainide and to local anesthetics of the amide type, second- or third-degree AV block (in absence of artificial ventricular pacemaker), hypokalemia, myasthemia gravis, pregnancy (category C), nursing mothers. Safe use in children not established. *Cautious Use:* during multiple drug therapy, known heart failure patient with minimum cardiac reserve, renal or hepatic disease.

ROUTE AND DOSAGE. **Oral:** 400 mg every 8 hours; then dose titrated on basis of clinical response and tolerance. **Usual adult dose:** 1200 to 1800 mg/day. **Intravenous:** 750 mg over 15-minute period; directly followed by 800-mg oral dose.

ADVERSE/SIDE EFFECTS. **CV:** cardiac toxicity (rare): exacerbation of arrhythmias, complete heart block, sinus node slowing (in patient with preexisting conduction system disease); hypotension, palpitations, bradycardia, chest pain, left ventricular failure, PVCs, hot flashes. **Dermatologic** (rare): rash, LE syndrome. **GI:** nausea, vomiting, anorexia, abdominal pain, diarrhea, hepatitis (rare). **Neurologic:** tremors, dizziness, lightheadedness, visual disturbances, vertigo, tinnitus, hearing loss, ataxia, paresthesia; (rare): agitation, memory loss, confusion, convulsions. **Respiratory:** pulmonary fibrosis, edema, embolism and alveolitis; pneumonia, dyspnea. **Other:** alopecia, sweating, night sweats, tiredness/drowsiness, sleepiness, hot/cold feelings, hematologic disorders (leukopenia, agranulocytosis, thrombocytopenia, hypoplastic anemia), lupus, claudication, cold extremities, leg cramps, urinary retention, polyuria, metallic or menthol taste, hiccups.

NURSING IMPLICATIONS

Effective serum concentration: 3.5 to 10 mcg/ml.

Response to lidocaine seems to be a good predictor of tocainide effectiveness.

Prior to beginning treatment, patient should be evaluated by ECG and clinically. Periodic reevaluations during treatment produces essential data to support decision to continue therapy.

Administer with food to decrease GI distress. This also protects against high peak concentration and toxicity because absorption rate is slowed. Bioavailability is not affected by food.

When steady-state drug level is attained (usually in about 70 hours), plasma level monitoring is recommended, especially if patient has renal or hepatic dysfunction.

Onset of tremors is a good clinical indicator that maximum dose is being approached.

When switching a patient from IV lidocaine to oral tocainide, give 600 mg oral dose of tocainide 6 hours before stopping lidocaine and repeat 6 hours later; then proceed to maintenance therapy with tocainide.

Blood pressure should be checked before administration of drug. It may be slightly increased within 5 minutes of IV tocainide but usually returns to normal in about 15 minutes. If patient is hypotensive, question continuing drug administration.

The patient and/or primary care-giver should fully understand what an irregular pulse signifies and how often it should be checked.

Since drug may cause dizziness and drowsiness, warn patient to use caution while driving a car until drug response is known.

Symptomatic bradycardia (pulse below 60, lightheadedness, syncope) should be reported. Dose adjustment or discontinuation will follow.

In patient with kidney or hepatic dysfunction, drug elimination is significantly decreased.

Monitor intake–output ratio and pattern. Instruct patient on self-care to report to physician if symptoms of renal dysfunction occur.

Advise patient to report promptly: chest pain, exertional dyspnea, wheezing, and cough even if no fever is present. Pulmonary fibrosis is a serious side effect and should be ruled out by chest x-ray or pulmonary function tests. Drug is discontinued if pulmonary symptoms persist or if pulmonary disorder is diagnosed.

Drug-induced lupus-like syndrome (rare) may first be evidenced as an inflammatory facial photosensitivity dermatitis with butterfly configuration on malar surfaces. If confirmed by a positive antinuclear antibody (ANA) test, drug will be discontinued.

Anticipate and report evidence of blood dyscrasia: unexplained bruising or bleeding, flu-like symptoms (fever, sore throat, chills).
Blood counts may be monitored during first 6 months of treatment; abnormal counts usually stabilize within 1 month after discontinuing treatment.

Drug Interactions: Tocainide Hydrochloride

Plus	Interactions
Allopurinol	Extends half-life (increases blood level of tocainide)
Metoprolol	Additive effects on wedge pressure and cardiac index
Propranolol	May lead to paranoia

TOLAZAMIDE
(Tolinase)

(tole-az'a-mide)
Antidiabetic
Sulfonylurea (first generation)
Sulfonamide derivative

ACTIONS AND USES. Orally effective sulfonylurea hypoglycemic structurally and pharmacologically related to tolbutamide (qv), but about 5 times more potent in action (potency is about equal to that of chlorpropamide). Lowers blood glucose primarily by stimulating pancreatic beta cells to secrete insulin. As with other sulfonylureas, is ineffective in the absence of functioning beta cells. Contraindications, precautions, pharmacokinetics, and adverse effects as for tolbutamide.

Used in management of mild to moderately severe type II noninsulin-dependent diabetes mellitus (NIDDM) which cannot be controlled by diet and weight reduction, and which is uncomplicated by acidosis, ketosis, coma. Effective in primary or secondary failures to other sulfonylurea.

ABSORPTION AND FATE. More slowly absorbed than tolbutamide, but absorption is complete. Onset of action in 4 to 6 hours; peak blood levels in 4 to 8 hours; duration of maximum hypoglycemic effect 10 to 15 hours. Half-life: 6 to 8 hours; drug accumulates in blood for first 4 to 6 doses, then steady state is reached, after which peak and trough values do not vary appreciably from day to day. Metabolized in liver. Approximately 85% of drug is excreted in urine. Excreted in breast milk.

CONTRAINDICATIONS AND PRECAUTIONS. Known sensitivity to sulfonylureas and to sulfonamides, type I (IDDM) insulin-dependent diabetes, diabetes complicated by ketoacidosis, infection, trauma; pregnancy (category C); safe use in nursing mothers and in children not established. *See also Tolbutamide.*

ADVERSE/SIDE EFFECTS. Nausea, vomiting, hypoglycemia, vertigo, photosensitivity, agranulocytosis, cholestatic jaundice. *See also Tolbutamide.*

ROUTE AND DOSAGE. Oral (individualized): 100 mg to 1 Gm once daily with breakfast; doses exceeding 500 mg should be divided and given twice daily.

NURSING IMPLICATIONS

Tablet may be crushed if patient is unable to swallow it whole. Be sure it is swallowed with an allowable fluid, not dry.
When patient is newly diagnosed, dosage is guided by fasting blood sugar values: if less

than 200 mg%, therapy is started with 100 mg daily with breakfast. If greater than 200 mg%, therapy is started with 250 mg daily with breakfast. Subsequent adjustments are made according to urine and blood tests and physician's evaluations.

Dose increments made at home for geriatric, debilitated, or underweight patients are in the order of 50 to 125 mg daily at weekly intervals.

Patient must be under close medical supervision for first 6 weeks of treatment; should see physician at least once weekly and should check urine daily for sugar and acetone.

Transferral from another sulfonylurea drug usually does not require a priming dose or transitional period.

For conversion from insulin: Patients receiving less than 20 units of insulin can be placed directly on tolazamide 100 mg daily. Patients receiving less than 40 units but more than 20 units can be placed directly on 250 mg daily. For patients receiving more than 40 units of insulin, dosage is reduced 50%, and patient is started on 250 mg of tolazamide. Dosage is then adjusted weekly, or more often in patients who had received 40 units of insulin. Instruct patient to check urine three times daily for glucose and acetone and to report results to physician.

Doses larger than 1000 mg/day rarely provide improvement in diabetic control: patient then usually is maintained on insulin therapy only.

Reduction of dose frequently alleviates most of the mild to moderately severe hypoglycemic symptoms.

Unlike tolbutamide, tolazamide is effective in some patients with a history of ketoacidosis or coma; close observation of these patients is especially important during the early adjustment period.

Caution patient not to self-dose with OTC unless approved or prescribed by physician.

Be certain that patient understands that alcohol can precipitate a disulfiram-like reaction.

No false-positive tests for urinary protein have been reported (these occasionally are noted with other sulfonylureas).

Store below 40°C (104°F) preferably between 15° and 30°C (59° and 86°F) in a well-closed container, unless otherwise directed by manufacturer. Keep drug out of the reach of children.

See Tolbutamide (prototype sulfonylurea antidiabetic agent).

TOLAZOLINE HYDROCHLORIDE
(Priscoline)

(toe-laz'a-leen)
Alpha-adrenergic blocking agent (sympatholytic), vasodilation, peripheral

ACTIONS AND USES. Imidazoline derivative structurally related to phentolamine. In addition to weak alpha-adrenergic blocking activity, beta-adrenergic action, increases cardiac output and rate, cholinergic effect increases GI motility, and histaminelike activity stimulates gastric secretions and peripheral vasodilation. Vasodilation is primarily due to direct relaxant effect on vascular smooth muscle. Inhibits aldehyde dehydrogenase, and may increase or decrease pulmonary artery pressure and total pulmonary resistance.

Used to improve blood flow in thromboangiitis obliterans (Buerger's disease), diabetic arteriosclerosis gangrene, Raynaud's disease, causalgia, scleroderma, postthrombotic conditions, frostbite sequelae, and other peripheral vasospastic disorders. *Investigational Use:* improve visualization of vasculature during arteriography, for treatment of neonatal hypoxemia, as diagnostic agent to differentiate vasospastic and obstruction components in occlusive peripheral vascular disease, and as a provocative test for glaucoma.

ABSORPTION AND FATE. Absorbed well by all routes. Maximal effects in 30 to 60 minutes after IM or SC injection. Effects may persist 3 or 4 hours. Half-life: about 2 hours. Excreted rapidly in urine, largely as unchanged drug.

CONTRAINDICATIONS AND PRECAUTIONS. Hypersensitivity to tolazoline; following cerebrovascular accident; coronary artery disease; alcohol ingestion. Safe use during pregnancy and in nursing mothers not established. *Cautious Use:* gastritis, peptic ulcer (previous or current), mitral stenosis.

ADVERSE/SIDE EFFECTS. CV: tachycardia, arrhythmias, anginal pain, postural hypotension, blood pressure changes, marked hypertension (particularly following parenteral use.) **GI:** nausea, vomiting, diarrhea, epigastric discomfort, abdominal pain (common), exacerbation of peptic ulcer. **Hematologic** (rare): agranulocytosis, leukopenia, thrombocytopenia, pancytopenia. **Intraarterial administration:** feeling of warmth or burning at injection site, transient weakness, postural vertigo, palpitation, formication, apprehension, transient paradoxic impairment of blood supply, peripheral vasodilation. **Severe overdosage:** hypotension progressing to shock. **Skin:** profuse sweating, flushing, increased pilomotor activity with tingling and chilliness, rash. **Other:** mydriasis, edema, headache; rarely: psychiatric reactions, oliguria, hematuria, hepatitis.

ROUTE AND DOSAGE. Subcutaneous, intramuscular, intravenous: 10 to 50 mg four times daily. **Intraarterial:** initial: 25-mg test dose; depending on response, 50 to 75 mg one or two times daily; maintenance: 50 to 75 mg, two or three times weekly.

NURSING IMPLICATIONS

Side effects are generally mild and usually decrease with continued therapy.

During period of dosage adjustment in patients receiving drug orally, check blood pressure and pulse 3 or 4 times during the day, and more frequently if indicated.

Patients should be closely observed for blood pressure changes and excessive cardiac effects. Monitor blood pressure and pulse at 2- to 4-hour intervals as indicated and report changes to physician. Advise patient to remain recumbent for at least 30 minutes after IV administration.

Since postural hypotension is a possibility, instruct patient to make position changes slowly, particularly from recumbent to upright posture, and to dangle legs for a few minutes before standing.

Observe affected limbs for changes in color and skin temperature, and keep physician informed.

Feelings of warmth, flushing, piloerection, (gooseflesh), crawling or chilly sensations in affected limb (or generalized) indicate that effective dosage has been reached. Report to physician immediately.

Intraarterial administration should be done only by those experienced in the procedure. (It is used for local effect, only after maximum benefit has been derived from other routes.)

Patient should be in supine position while receiving tolazoline intraarterially. Histamine may be given prior to injection to prevent paradoxic impairment of blood supply to affected limb. Patient must be closely monitored.

Caution patient to avoid alcohol ingestion since it may cause a severe disulfiram reaction: flushing, tachycardia, hypotension, chest pains, sweating, nausea, vomiting.

Drug effectiveness is enhanced by keeping patient comfortably warm. Avoid exposure and cold environment.

Treatment of overdosage: Hypotension is treated by head-low position and IV fluids. Ephedrine should be administered as needed. *Epinephrine and norepinephrine (levarterenol) are contraindicated. See Drug Interactions.*

Patient-Teaching Points: Discuss the following teaching points concerning peripheral vasospastic disorders with physician for specific patient instruction:
- ✓ Hygienic care of affected parts (frequency and details of care).
- ✓ Avoidance of hot-water bottles, heating pads, garters, as well as smoking and alcohol.
- ✓ Importance of properly fitting shoes and hosiery.
- ✓ Positioning (some physicians prescribe elevation of head of bed on 6-inch blocks to enhance circulation to legs).

Drug Interactions: Tolazoline Hydrochloride

Plus	Interactions
Alcohol, ethyl	May cause disulfiram reaction (acetaldehyde accumulation)
Epinephrine Norepinephrine (levarterenol)	Tolazoline administered concurrently may cause paradoxic fall in blood pressure followed by rebound increase
Antihypertensives	Hypotensive action may be decreased by tolazoline

PROTOTYPE

TOLBUTAMIDE
(Mobenol, Novobutamide, Orinase, Rastinon, SK-Tolbutamide)

TOLBUTAMIDE SODIUM
(Orinase Diagnostic)

(tole-byoo′ta-mide)
Antidiabetic
Sulfonylurea (first generation)
Sulfonamide derivative
Diagnostic agent

ACTIONS AND USES. Short-acting sulfonylurea compound chemically related to sulfonamides, but without antiinfective activity. Lowers blood glucose concentration by stimulating pancreatic beta cells to synthesize and release insulin. No action demonstrated if functional beta cells are absent. During long-term use it is proposed that extrapancreatic effects (increased number of insulin receptors on cell membranes, decreased hepatic uptake of insulin, and increased peripheral utilization of insulin) also contribute to hypoglycemic effect of the sulfonylurea drugs. Responsiveness to blood glucose lowering effects with long-term therapy may decline in some patients. Alternatively, patient who has become poorly responsive to other sulfonylureas may be responsive to tolbutamine. May be mildly goitrogenic without producing clinical hypothyroidism or thyroid enlargement. It has not been established that long-term cardiovascular or neural complications of diabetes can be prevented by the sulfonylureas.

Used in management of mild to moderately severe, stable noninsulin-dependent diabetes (type II, NIDDM) that is not controlled by diet and/or weight reduction alone. Also used in treatment of patients who are unresponsive to other sulfonylureas and adjunctively with insulin to stabilize certain cases of labile diabetes. Used as diagnostic agent to rule out pancreatic islet cell adenoma or diabetes.

ABSORPTION AND FATE. Rapidly absorbed from GI tract; detected in blood in 20 to 60 minutes with peak concentrations in 3 to 5 hours; only small amount detectable in 24 hours. Onset of hypoglycemic action is gradual with peak antidiabetic activity occurring within 5 to 8 hours and lasting 6 to 12 hours. Blood glucose level then gradually returns to pretreatment level within 24 hours. About 95% protein bound. Half-life (considerable interindividual difference): 4 to 25 hours (average: 7 hours). Oxidized in liver to inactive metabolites. Eliminated in urine (85%); about 9% excreted in feces via bile.

CONTRAINDICATIONS AND PRECAUTIONS. Hypersensitivity to sulfonylureas or to sulfonamides, history of repeated episodes of diabetic ketoacidosis (with or without coma), type I (IDDM) diabetes; as sole therapy; diabetic coma; severe stress, infection, trauma, or major surgery; severe renal insufficiency, hepatic or endocrine disease. Safe use during pregnancy (category C) or use in children not established. *Cautious Use:* cardiac, thyroid, pituitary, or adrenal dysfunction, history of peptic ulcer, women of childbearing age who may become pregnant, alcoholism; the elderly, debilitated, malnourished or uncooperative patient.

ADVERSE/SIDE EFFECTS. Dermatologic: allergic skin reactions: pruritus, erythema, urticaria, morbilliform or maculopapular eruptions; porphyria cutanea tarda, photosensitivity. **GI:** cholestatic jaundice (rare); (dose related): nausea, epigastric fullness, heartburn, anorexia, constipation, diarrhea. **Hematologic:** agranulocytosis, thrombocytopenia, leukopenia, hemolytic anemia, aplastic anemia, pancytopenia. **Metabolic:** hepatic porphyria, disulfiram-like reactions. **Other:** taste alterations, headache, vertigo (rare). **Overdosage:** *Hypoglycemia (mild)* without loss of consciousness or neurologic symptoms: unusual fatigue, tremulousness, hunger, drowsiness, GI distress, sweating, anxiety, headache; *(severe):* visual disturbances, ataxia, paresthesias, confusion, tachycardia, seizures, coma.

ROUTE AND DOSAGE. Oral (highly individualized): initial: 1 to 2 Gm daily, subsequently adjusted to minimal dosage for adequate control. Maintenance dose: of more than 2 Gm daily seldom required. **Intravenous (tolbutamide sodium):** 1 Gm given over period of 2 to 3 minutes.

NURSING IMPLICATIONS

Treatment with an oral antidiabetic agent is generally preceded by an appropriate trial of dietary management, including weight control.

Tolbutamide is neither oral insulin nor a substitute for insulin; however, the same diagnostic and therapeutic measures required to insure optimum insulin control of diabetes are required for control by tolbutamide.

Impress on the patient and family that oral antidiabetic drug therapy controls diabetes, but will never cure it.

Total dose may be taken before breakfast but preferably in divided doses after meals.

Tablet may be crushed and taken with full glass of water if patient desires.

Because of danger of nocturnal hypoglycemia, tolbutamide should not be taken at bedtime unless specifically prescribed.

Elderly patients may be hyperresponsive to oral antidiabetic therapy; thus the initial dose should be low and given before breakfast. If blood and urine glucose tests are negative during first 24 hours of therapy, initial dose may be continued on a daily basis; if hypoglycemia occurs, dose is reduced to minimum level or discontinued.

During initial period of therapy, patient should be under close medical supervision until dosage is established (using negative tests for glucosuria, ketonuria, and blood glucose level as criteria). One or 2 weeks of therapy may be required before full therapeutic effect is achieved.

Failure to respond (i.e., blood glucose remains elevated) after 1 to 2 weeks therapy is called primary failure.

Effectiveness of any hypoglycemic agent (including the sulfonylureas) in lowering blood glucose, declines over time (perhaps due to diminished responsiveness to the drug or to progression of severity of diabetes); this phenomenon is called secondary (drug) failure.

Patients most prone to secondary failure may be underweight, erratic in their meal schedules, careless about dosage, or they may have developed drug resistance.

If a patient stabilized on tolbutamide is exposed to stress (e.g., infection, surgery), loss of blood glucose control may occur. Tolbutamide may be discontinued and replaced by insulin.

Transfer from one sulfonylurea compound to another can be effected without transitional period or priming dose.

Transfer from insulin to tolbutamide (sulfonylurea) is best controlled in the hospital. For patients receiving 20 units or less of insulin daily, insulin may be stopped abruptly; oral drug is usually started at maintenance dose.

For patients receiving 20 to 40 units of insulin daily, tolbutamide is started at maintenance level, with concurrent 30 to 50% reduction in insulin dose; further daily decrease of insulin is done gradually until response to tolbutamide observed.

For patients taking more than 40 units of insulin daily, tolbutamide is initiated at maintenance level in conjunction with a 20% reduction in insulin on first day followed by cautious decremental adjustments of insulin to omission.

During the conversion period, hypoglycemia occurs rarely. Urine should be tested for glucose and ketone bodies at least three times daily and reported to the physician. The presence of persistent acetonuria with glycosuria indicates primary failure: patient is type I diabetic and requires insulin therapy.

The patient/family member should fully understand that symptoms of hyperglycemia and ketoacidosis (representing loss of diabetes control) must be reported to the physician promptly. Symptoms include flushed, dry skin, weight loss, fatigue, Kussmaul respiration, double or blurred vision, soft eyeballs, irritability, fruity smelling breath, abdominal cramps, nausea, vomiting, diarrhea, dyspnea, polydipsia, polyphagia, polyuria, headache, hypotension, weak and rapid pulse, positive ketonuria and glycosuria). Report symptoms promptly so that emergency antidiabetic therapy can be instituted.

Hypoglycemia is frequently caused by overdosage of hypoglycemic drug, inadequate or irregular food intake, nausea, vomiting, diarrhea, and added exercise without caloric supplement or dose adjustment. *See Adverse/Side Effects.* Its occurrence indicates need for immediate reevaluation of patient's diet, medication regimen, and compliance. It is most likely to appear in patients over 50 years of age. Report to physician.

A beta-adrenergic agent (e.g., propranolol) blocks hypoglycemia-induced tachycardia, but does not inhibit hypoglycemic sweating. Detection of a hypoglycemic reaction in a diabetic patient also receiving a beta-blocker, especially if elderly, is difficult. Monitor closely during adjustment period watching for other symptoms (e.g., unexplained fatigue, hunger, nausea) of impending hypoglycemia.

Early hypoglycemic reactions can be stemmed quickly by ingestion of soluble glucose (such as orange juice, or other fruit juices, sugar cubes, or table sugar dissolved in water, soft drinks). If symptoms do not subside in 10 to 15 minutes, repeat glucose; if after another 10 to 15 minutes patient still has symptoms and urine test for sugar is negative, notify physician. If feeling faint, advise patient to go to the doctor or hospital.

When hypoglycemic reaction has progressed to grogginess, the patient can be given a teaspoon of honey or corn syrup; the sugar will be rapidly absorbed by oral membranes, and patient should revive enough to drink a glass of fruit juice. Unconsciousness should be treated in the hospital, where IV dextrose in water and clinical supervision will be given until maintenance dose is reestablished. Patient should be observed closely for at least 3 to 5 days.

Hypoglycemic symptoms may be especially vague in the elderly; therefore, check out nondefinitive expressions such as "I don't feel good today" to discover real meaning. Observe patient carefully, especially 2 to 3 hours after eating, check urine for sugar and ketone bodies and capillary blood glucose.

Repetitive complaints of headache and weakness a few hours after eating may signal incipient hypoglycemia. Dosage adjustment may be indicated.

Teach patient that undereating is as hazardous as overeating. Warn that a self-directed, weight-loss regimen, redistribution of dietary carbohydrate, or skipped meals interfere with drug control of diabetes.

Patients using oral contraceptives should be advised to use another form of birth control *(see Drug Interactions).*

Advise patient on tolbutamide who wishes to become pregnant that a transfer to insulin for blood glucose control is recommended by many clinicians.

If tolbutamide is used during pregnancy, it is discontinued at least 2 weeks before the expected delivery date to prevent prolonged severe hypoglycemia (4 to 10 days) in the neonate.

The potential for hypoglycemia in nursing infants presents the necessity to decide whether to discontinue nursing or to temporarily transfer to insulin (if diet alone is inadequate for blood sugar control).

Urge patient to report promptly an injury, severe nausea, vomiting, or diarrhea or if patient feels sick or has a fever or sore throat (common cold symptoms). The physician may want to evaluate quality of imposed stress to determine need for insulin or rule out agranulocytosis by blood studies.

Pruritus and rash, frequently reported side effects, may clear spontaneously; however, if they persist, drug will be discontinued.

Instruct patient to avoid self-medication with OTC drugs unless approved or prescribed by physician.

Alcohol, even in moderate amounts, can precipitate a disulfiram reaction (flushing, sweating, slurred speech, palpitations, headache, abdominal cramps, nausea, vomiting). The patient should be aware of becoming hypoglycemic after ingesting alcohol; an observer may mistakingly think he or she is inebriated and therefore patient may be deprived of necessary emergency treatment.

Because of potential photosensitivity (especially in the alcoholic), it may be wise for the patient to protect exposed skin areas from the sun with a sunscreen lotion (SPF 12 to 15) when outdoors for several hours.

Transient alterations in certain liver function tests during initial period of sulfonylurea therapy reportedly have little clinical significance; fluctuating abnormalities of liver function frequently occur in patients with diabetes.

Advise patient to report promptly signs of hepatic dysfunction (pruritus, jaundice, dark urine, abdominal discomfort), renal insufficiency (dysuria, anuria, hematuria), or blood dyscrasia (easy bruising, unexplained bleeding). All indicate probable reasons for terminating treatment with tolbutamide (perhaps only temporarily).

Advise patient to weigh self at least weekly and to report a progressive gain, especially if edema is present. These signs indicate the necessity to discontinue tolbutamide.

Urine testing: In stabilized patients urine is tested for glucose usually once a day about 2 hours after largest meal. Instruct patient to keep record and to show physician at next visit.

When a drug that affects the hypoglycemic action of sulfonyureas *(see Drug Interaction)* is withdrawn or added to the tolbutamide regimen the patient should be alerted to the added danger of loss of control (hyperglycemia). Urine tests and blood glucose tests and test for ketone bodies should be carefully monitored and possibly increased in frequency for several days to determine if antidiabetic drug dose adjustment is indicated.

Tolbutamide sodium test (IV): differentiates the nondiabetic (rapid, intense hyperinsulin response within 15 to 20 minutes) from the diabetic (gradual hypoglycemic response). If a pancreatic islet cell adenoma is present, a hypoglycemic response is rapid and may persist for as long as 3 hours requiring treatment. Patient must be closely monitored to prevent fatal hypoglycemia. Inspect injection site for local irritation or phlebitis and institute local treatment if present. Consult physician.

A careless, casual attitude toward oral antidiabetic regimen leads to noncompliance and lack of diabetic control. Encourage and support the patient in accepting responsibility for keeping his or her condition under control and for maintaining scheduled visits to the physician for periodic clinical evaluation (CBC, measurement of glycosylated Hgb, etc.)

Instruct the patient to carry medical identification card or jewelry with self at all times (available from most drug stores). Card information should include patient and physician's names and addresses, diagnosis, medication, and dose being taken.

Store below 40°C (104°F), preferably between 15° and 30°C (59° and 86°F) in well-closed container; avoid freezing.

For summary of patient/family teaching plan, see Insulin.

Diagnostic Test Interferences. The sulfonylureas may produce abnormal **thyroid function test** results, and reduced **RAI uptake** (after long-term administration). A tolbutamide metabolite may cause false-positive **urinary protein** values when turbidity procedures are used (such as heat and acetic acid or sulfosalicylic and); Ames reagent strips reportedly not affected.

Drug Interactions: Tolbutamide

Plus	Interactions
Alcohol	Disulfiram-like reactions with concomitant use
Anticoagulants, oral Chloramphenicol MAO inhibitors Probenecid Salicylates and other NSAIDs Sulfonamides	May displace tolbutamide from binding site potentiating its hypoglycemic effects
Beta adrenergic blockers: (e.g., propranolol)	Suppresses rebound increase in blood sugar following tolbutamide-induced hypoglycemia. Concomitant use with caution
Digitalis glycosides (e.g., digoxin)	May decrease metabolism of digitalis agents
Calcium channel blockers (e.g., verapamil) Corticosteroids Contraceptives, oral Estrogens Hydantoins (e.g., phenytoin) Isoniazid Nicotinic acid Phenothiazines Thiazide diuretics Thyroid products	May cause hyperglycemia leading to loss of control (secondary failure)
Pyrazolones (e.g., phenylbutazone)	Inhibit tolbutamide metabolism leading to enhanced hypoglycemic effects

TOLMETIN SODIUM

(Tolectin, Tolectin DS)

(tole'met-in)

Analgesic, nonnarcotic
NSAID
Antirheumatic

ACTIONS AND USES. Pyrrole acetic acid derivative, nonsteroidal antiinflammatory drug (NSAID) structurally and pharmacologically related to indomethacin. Possesses analgesic, antiinflammatory, and antipyretic activity. Exact mode of antiinflammatory action not known. Inhibits prostaglandin synthetase resulting in decreased plasma levels of prostaglandin E, the possible basis for antiinflammatory action. Inhibition of platelet aggregation is less than that produced by equal therapeutic doses of aspirin. Changes in prothrombin and whole blood clotting times not reported. Fecal blood loss studies suggest that tolmetin does not produce blood loss (contrary to findings with aspirin and indomethacin). Comparable to aspirin and indomethacin in antirheumatic activity, but incidence of GI symptoms and tinnitus is less than in aspirin-treated patients, and CNS effects are less than in patients receiving indomethacin. Each tablet contains 18 mg (0.784 mEq) of sodium. Relieves symptomatology but does not seem to alter the course of the disease.

Used in treatment of acute flares and in management of chronic rheumatoid arthritis. May be used alone or in combination with gold or corticosteroids.

ABSORPTION AND FATE. Rapidly and almost completely absorbed. Peak serum levels in 30 to 60 minutes. Approximately 99% bound to plasma protein. Half-life: 1 to 1½ hours. Metabolized in liver; almost entirely excreted in urine within 24 hours, primarily as inactive metabolite, glucuronide, and unchanged drug (about 20%). Animal studies suggest that excretion is enhanced by alkalinization of urine.

CONTRAINDICATIONS AND PRECAUTIONS. History of intolerance or hypersensitivity to tolmetin, aspirin, and other NSAIDs; active peptic ulcer, patients with asthma, nasal polyps, rhinitis ("aspirin triad"), in patients with Functional Class IV rheumatoid arthritis (severely incapacitated, bedridden, or confined to a wheelchair). Safe use not established during pregnancy, in nursing mothers, and in children under 2 years. *Cautious Use:* history of upper GI tract disease, impaired renal function, compromised cardiac function.

ADVERSE/SIDE EFFECTS. CNS: headache, dizziness, vertigo, light-headedness, mood elevation or depression, tension, nervousness, weakness, drowsiness, insomnia, tinnitus, hearing impairment (rare). **CV:** mild edema (about 7% patients), sodium and water retention, mild to moderate hypertension. **Dermatologic:** toxic epidermal necrolysis, morbilliforin eruptions, urticaria, pruritus. **GI:** epigastric or abdominal pain, dyspepsia, nausea, vomiting, heartburn, constipation, peptic ulcer, GI bleeding. **Hematologic:** transient and small decreases in hemoglobin and hematocrit, purpura, petechiae, granulocytopenia, leukopenia, agranulocytosis. **Other:** hypothermia, asthenia, chest pain, fever, anaphylaxis (especially after drug is discontinued and then reinstituted).

ROUTE AND DOSAGE. Oral: Adults: Initial: 400 mg 3 times daily. Maintenance: *Rheumatoid arthritis:* control usually maintained with 600 mg to 1.8 Gm/day in divided doses. Maximum recommended dose: no more than 2 Gm/day. *Osteoarthritis:* control usually maintained with 600 mg to 1.6 Gm/day in 3 or 4 divided doses. Maximum recommended dose: no more than 1.6 Gm/day. **Children (2 years and older):** *Juvenile arthritis:* Initial: 20 mg/kg/day in 3 or 4 divided doses. Maintenance: 15 to 30 mg/kg/day (maximum).

NURSING IMPLICATIONS

Treatment is preferably scheduled to include a morning dose (on arising) and a bedtime dose.

Tablet may be crushed before administration and taken with fluid of patient's choice; capsule may be emptied and contents swallowed with water or mixed with food.

Food delays absorption but does not affect total amount absorbed. If GI disturbances occur, instruct patient to take drug with meals, milk, or antacid (prescribed). Sodium bicarbonate is not recommended since it may enhance drug excretion. Advise patient to notify physician if symptoms persist; dosage reduction may be necessary.

Since other NSAIDs have produced eye changes, it is recommended that ophthalmic examinations be carried out at periodic intervals during chronic treatment.

The patient with renal damage should be closely monitored and perhaps given lower doses. Intake–output ratio should be evaluated and the patient encouraged to increase fluid intake to at least 8 full glasses of fluid/day.

Instruct patient with impaired renal or cardiac function to monitor weight (an increase of more than 4 pounds/week should be reported) and to check for swelling in ankles, tibiae, hands, and feet.

Periodic renal function tests (routine urinalysis, creatinine clearance, and serum creatinine) are recommended for patient on long-term therapy.

Sodium bicarbonate, sometimes taken without prescription by the elderly to "settle the stomach" alkalizes the urine which increases urinary excretion of tolmetin. Thus, degree and duration of effectiveness may be reduced. Check self-medicating habits of the patient.

Therapeutic response in patient during treatment for rheumatoid arthritis or osteoarthritis generally occurs within 1 week with progressive improvement in succeeding week: reduced joint pain and swelling, reduction in duration of morning stiffness, improved functional capacity (increase in grip strength, delayed onset of fatigue, decreased time to walk 50 feet).

If patient is also receiving a corticosteroid, any reduction in steroid dosage should be gradual to avoid withdrawal symptoms.

Because of possible enhanced bleeding, warn patient to inform surgeon or dentist before treatment that patient is taking tolmetin.

Warn patient to report promptly signs of abnormal bleeding (ecchymosis, epistaxis, melena, petechiae), itching, skin rash, persistent headache, edema.

Dizziness and drowsiness are common side effects; therefore, caution the patient to avoid potentially hazardous activities such as driving a car or operating machinery until response to the drug is known.

Overdosage: Stomach should be emptied by induced vomiting or gastric lavage, followed by administration of activated charcoal slurry. Forced alkaline diuresis may be attempted to hasten drug excretion.

Store drug in tightly capped light-resistant container at temperature between 15° and 30°C (59° and 86°F), unless otherwise instructed by manufacturer.

Diagnostic Test Interferences. Tolmetin prolongs **bleeding time,** inhibits **platelet aggregation,** elevates **BUN, alkaline phosphatase,** and **SGOT** (AST) levels; may decrease **hemoglobin** and **hematocrit** values. Metabolites may produce false-positive results for **proteinuria** (with tests that rely on acid precipitation, e.g., sulfosalicylic acid).

Drug Interactions: Tolmetin Sodium

Plus	Interactions
Anticoagulants, oral (e.g., Warfarin)	Enhanced anticoagulant activity (postulated)
NSAIDs, other (e.g., Indomethacin) Phenylbutazone Salicylates	May potentiate ulcerogenic effects of all these drugs and of tolmetin
Sulfonamides, sulfonylureas, hydantoins	May displace tolmetin or be displaced by tolmetin from binding sites leading to increased potential for toxicity

---

TOLNAFTATE

(Aftate, Pitrex, Tinactin)

(tole-naf'tate)
Antiinfective
Antibiotic
Antifungal

ACTIONS AND USES. Synthetic topical antifungal agent. Agent mechanism not clear, but it has been shown that tolnaftate distorts hyphae and stunts mycelial growth on susceptible fungi. Toxicity and susceptibility rates are low. Fungistatic or fungicidal to *Microsporum gypseum, M. canis, M. audouinii, M. japonicum, Trichophyton rubrum, T. Schoenleinii, T. tonsurans,* and *Epidermophyton floccosum,* but ineffective against *Candida albicans, Cryptococcus neoformans, Aspergillus fumigatus,* bacteria, protozoa, and viruses.

Used to treat tinea pedis (athlete's foot), t. cruris (jock itch), t. corporis (body ringworm); also used to treat tinea capitis or tinea unguium if infection is superficial, plantar or palmar lesions adjunctively with kerotolytic agents, and t. versicolor (caused by *Malassezia furfur*).

CONTRAINDICATIONS AND PRECAUTIONS. Hypersensitivity to tolnaftate, skin irritations prior to therapy, nail and scalp infections; safe use during pregnancy and breast feeding or by children under 2 years old not established. *Cautious Use:* excoriated skin.

ADVERSE/SIDE EFFECTS. Local irritation, stinging of skin from aerosol formulation.

ROUTE AND DOSAGE. Topical (to skin): twice daily in morning and evening. Powder, powder aerosols: used alone or adjunctively with cream, solution, or ointment (for mild infection) or as prophylactic agent in normally moist areas. Only small amounts of drug should be applied at one time.

NURSING IMPLICATIONS

Preparations are for topical use only.

Tolnaftate is greaseless, odorless, and does not stain skin or clothing.

Thoroughly cleanse site with water and dry completely before applying tolnaftate. Massage a thin layer of drug gently into skin. Area should not be wet from excess drug after application.

Emphasize importance of personal cleanliness. Daily bathing, thorough rinsing, and complete drying of skin destroys the kind of environment conducive to growth of fungi.

If used by child under 12 years of age, supervise application procedure and personal hygiene measures to prevent recurrence.

Shake aerosol powder container well before use.

The cream and powder are not recommended for nail or scalp infection.

If hair follicles or nail beds are involved, a systemic antifungal (e.g., griseofulvin) will be necessary concomitant treatment.
Liquids (solutions) are recommended for scalp infection or to treat hairy areas.
Powder and powder aerosol are effective in treatment of athlete's foot and in daily hygiene to reduce natural moisture in groin and intertriginous areas.
If patient has athlete's foot, patient should put socks on before putting on underclothes to avoid spread of infection to groin area (jock itch).
Supplementary antiinfective treatment is indicated if infections are complicated by concurrent bacterial or nonsusceptible fungal infections.
Surgical debridement of dead skin and treatment of calluses on feet usually accompanies kerotolytic and tolnaftate treatment of plantar and palmar lesions.
Wet compresses may be prescribed for adjunctive therapy of exudative lesions.
Treatment is frequently continued for 2 to 3 weeks.
In the absence of improvement within 4 weeks, patient should return to physician for reevaluation of etiologic factors and prescribed treatment.
Explain to patient that treatment should be continued for 2 to 3 weeks after disappearance of all symptoms in order to prevent recurrence.
If skin has thickened as a result of the infection, desired clinical response may be delayed for 4 to 6 weeks.
Pruritus, soreness, burning should be relieved within 24 to 72 hours after start of treatment.
Avoid contact of all drug forms with eyes.
If solution solidifies, place container in warm water to liquify contents. Potency is unaffected by these changes.
Do not puncture, use, or store aerosol near heat or an open flame, or expose to temperature above 49°C. Do not place aerosol container in fire or incinerator for disposal.
Store cream, gel, powder, and topical solution in light-resistant containers at 15° to 30°C (59° to 86°F); store aerosol container at 2° to 30°C (38° to 86°F). Avoid freezing and exposure to light.

TRANYLCYPROMINE SULFATE

(Parnate)

(tran-ill-sip′roe-meen)
Psychotropic
Antidepressant
MAO inhibitor

ACTIONS AND USES. Potent nonhydrazine MAO inhibitor structurally similar to amphetamine. Actions and toxicity similar to those of hydrazine MAO inhibitors, but also has rapid and direct amphetamine-like CNS stimulatory action, is less likely to cause hepatotoxicity, and does not produce prolonged MAO inhibition.

Owing to its toxic potential, use is reserved for treatment of severe mental depression in hospitalized patients who have not responded to other antidepressant therapy. *See Phenelzine.*

TU

ADVERSE/SIDE EFFECTS. CNS: vertigo, dizziness, termors, muscle twitching, headache, blurred vision. **CV:** orthostatic hypotension, arrhythmias. **GI:** dry mouth, anorexia, constipation, diarrhea, abdominal discomfort. **Other:** rash, impotence, peripheral edema, sweating. *See also Phenelzine.*

ROUTE AND DOSAGE. Oral: initial: 10 mg in morning and 10 mg in afternoon. This dosage may be continued for 2 weeks. If no response, dosage may be adjusted to 20 mg in morning and 10 mg in afternoon for another week. Following improvement, dosage then is reduced to lowest effective maintenance level. Dosage not to exceed 30 mg daily.

NURSING IMPLICATIONS

Tablet may be crushed before administration and taken with fluid or mixed with food, if patient has difficulty swallowing a pill.

Because of possibility of insomnia, usually not given in the evening.

Incidence of severe hypertensive reactions appears to be greater with tranylcypromine than with other MAO inhibitors.

Food–Drug Interactions: Emphasize importance of avoiding tyramine-containing foods (e.g., aged cheeses, Chianti wine, raisins). *(See Index: Food sources.)*

Inform patient that excessive use of caffeine-containing beverages (chocolate, coffee, tea, cola) can contribute to development of rapid heart beat, arrhythmias, and hypertension.

Instruct patient to make position changes slowly, particularly from recumbent to upright posture.

Usually produces therapeutic response within 3 days, but full antidepressant effects may not be obtained until 2 or 3 weeks of drug therapy.

See Phenelzine sulfate (prototype MAO inhibitor).

TRAZODONE HYDROCHLORIDE

(Desyrel)

(tray'zoe-done)
Psychotropic (antidepressant)
Alpha-adrenergic blocking agent

ACTIONS AND USES. Centrally acting triazolepyridine derivative, chemically and structurally unrelated to tricyclic, tetracyclic, or other antidepressants but has its own profile of actions. Potentiates seratonin (5-HT) effects by selectively blocking its reuptake at presynaptic membranes in CNS. Has little effect on dopamine or norepinpehrine, which may explain low incidence of cardiovascular toxicity and minimal effect on blood pressure with its use. Does not stimulate CNS; causes fewer anticholinergic genitourinary and neurologic effects when compared with incidence with other antidepressants. Produces varying degrees of sedation in normal and mentally depressed patient, increases total sleep time, decreases number and duration of awakenings in depressed patient, and decreases REM sleep. Has anxiolytic effect in severely depressed patient and exhibits mild analgesic, antihistaminic and skeletal muscular relaxant action. Has no anticonvulsant action.

Used to treat both inpatient and outpatient with major depression with or without prominent anxiety. *Unlabeled Uses:* schizophrenic disorders, adjunctive treatment of alcohol dependence, anxiety neuroses, drug-induced dyskinesias.

ABSORPTION AND FATE. Well-absorbed from GI tract. Peak blood concentrations reached in 1 hour if taken on empty stomach, 2 hours if taken with food. Multidose regimen steady state plasma level reached in about 4 days. Extensive hepatic metabolism (oxidation and hydroxylation); 89 to 95% protein-bound. Biphasic half-life: 4.4 hours for first 3 to 10 hours after drug ingestion; 7.5 hours for next 10 to 34 hours. Approximately 75% drug and metabolites are excreted in urine within 72 hours; remainder in feces via bile.

CONTRAINDICATIONS AND PRECAUTIONS. Hypersensitivity to trazodone, initial recovery phase of MI, ventricular ectopy, electroshock therapy. Safe use in children below 18 years of age not established; pregnancy (category C). *Cautious Use:* patient with suicidal ideation, cardiac arrhythmias or disease; nursing mother.

ADVERSE/SIDE EFFECTS. (Appear to be dose-related.) **CV:** hypotension (including orthostatic hypotension), hypertension, syncope, shortness of breath, chest pain, tachycardia, palpitations, bradycardia, PVCs, ventricular tachycardia (short episodes of 3 to 4 beats). **Dermatologic:** skin eruptions, rash, pruritus, acne, photosensitivity. **EENT:** nasal and sinus congestion, blurred vision, eye irritation, sweating or clamminess, tinnitus. **GI:** dry mouth, anorexia, constipation, abdominal distress, nausea, vomiting, dysgeusia, flatulence, diarrhea, hypersalivation (rare). **GU:** hematuria, increased frequency, delayed urine flow, early or absent menses, male priapism, ejaculation inhibition. **Hematologic:** anemia, decreased and neutrophil counts (infrequent). **Musculoskeletal:** skeletal aches and pains, muscle twitches. **NS:** drowsiness, lightheadedness, tiredness, dizziness, insomnia, headache, agitation, impaired memory and speech, disorientation; rarely: hypomania, nightmares, seizures, hallucinations, paresthesias, akathisia. **Other:** increased alkaline phosphatase, AST and ALT; weight gain or loss.

ROUTE AND DOSAGE. (Individualized.) **Oral: Adult:** Initial: 150 mg/day in divided doses. Drug may be increased by 50 mg every 3 to 4 days (depending on clinical response and tolerance). Maximum dosage: not to exceed 600 mg/day (400 mg/day for outpatient). Maintenance: lowest dose to preserve attained antidepressive effect.

NURSING IMPLICATIONS

Food–Drug Interactions. Drug taken with food rather than on an empty stomach increases amount of absorption by 20% and appears to decrease incidence of dizziness or lightheadedness. Urge patient to maintain the same schedule for food–drug intake throughout treatment period to prevent variations in serum concentration (i.e., always with food or snack, or always before or after food intake).

Therapeutic effects usually begin in 1 week but may require 2 to 4 weeks to reach maximum levels. This period, i.e., waiting for desired symptom relief, is the most vulnerable for noncompliant drug-taking behavior. Teach patient importance of adhering to regimen and have family member reenforce this teaching with patient in the home.

Therapy is usually continued on minimum dosage several months beyond optimum clinical response to prevent recurrence of depression.

Urge patient not to alter dose or intervals between doses.

Adherence to follow-up appointment is important to permit dose adjustment or discontinuation, as indicated.

If patient has preexisting cardiac disease, monitor pulse rate and regularity before administration of drug.

When trazodone is given at the same time as an MAO inhibitor, therapy is initiated cautiously and dose is adjusted according to clinical response. No interaction has been documented but the potential for hypertensive crisis is recognized until ruled out.

Adverse/side effects generally are mild and tend to decrease and disappear after the first few weeks of treatment.

Observe patient's level of activity and compare with base or admission level. If it appears to be increasing toward sleeplessness and agitation, with changes in reality orientation report to physician. Manic episodes have been reported.

Ask male patient if he is having inappropriate or prolonged penile erections. If he is, the drug should be discontinued and physician consulted.

Check patient for symptoms of hypotension. If orthostatic, hypotension is troublesome (and it may be, especially in the elderly), suggest measures to reduce danger of falling and to help patient to tolerate the effects. *See Index: Nursing Interventions: hypotension.* Discuss with physician; a reduction of dose or discontinuation of the drug may be prescribed.

If drowsiness becomes a distressing side effect, e.g., interfering with ADL, patient should consult physician. Dose regimen may be adjusted so that largest dose is at bedtime.
Advise patient to limit or abstain from alcohol use. The depressant effects of CNS depressants and alcohol may be potentiated by this drug.
Warn patient not to self-medicate with OTC drugs for colds, allergy, or insomnia treatment without advice of physician. Many of these drugs contain CNS depressants.
Overdosage causes extension of common adverse/side effects: vomiting, lethargy, drowsiness and exaggerated anticholinergic effects. Seizures or arrhythmias are unusual. Death rarely occurs except when other drugs are being given concomitantly (such as alcohol, meprobamate).
Treatment of overdosage (no antidote) is symptomatic and supportive. It is not known whether drug is dialyzable but high protein binding suggests that hemodialysis would not be effective.
Alert dentist, surgeon, or emergency personnel that drug is being used. Trazodone is discontinued as long as possible prior to elective surgery.
Store drug in tightly closed, light-resistant container at temperature of 15° to 30°C (59° to 86°F).

Drug Interactions: Trazodone Hydrochloride

Plus	Interactions
Antihypertensives	May inhibit hypotensive effects requiring reduction of antihypertensive dose
CNS depressants (e.g., alcohol, opiates, barbiturates, anesthetics)	Potentiated or additive depressant effects
Digoxin (Lanoxin)	Increased digoxin level
MAO inhibitors (e.g., isocarboxazid, pargyline, phenelzine)	Intensified hypertensive effect of trazodone
Phenytoin (Dilantin)	Increased serum phenytoin level

TRETINOIN
(Retin-A)

(tret′i-noyn)
Cell stimulant
Cell proliferant
Vitamin A isomer
Retinoid

ACTIONS AND USES. A contact irritant containing retinoic acid and vitamin A acid. Reverses retention hyperkeratosis and comedone formation, primary events in acne pathology. Exact action mechanism unknown but it is suggested that keratinocytes in the sebaceous follicle become less adherent, and turnover of follicular epithelial cells is increased (by stimulated mitosis). These two processes promote easy extrusion of the comedone and prevent it from reformation (comedolytic action). Tretinoin also increases permeability of skin and supports conversion of follicular epithelium into less sturdy and almost fragile condition. Unlike benzoyl peroxide and topical antibiotics, does not reduce surface free fatty acids or bacterial colonization (principally *Propionibacterium acnes*) of skin. Although studies in albino mice suggest that the carcinogenic potential of ultraviolet radiation may be accelerated by tretinoin, the significance to humans is not clear. Long-term animal studies have not been performed.

Used for topical treatment of acne vulgaris grades I–III, especially during early stages when number of comedones is greatest; also used adjunctively in management of associated comedones and in treatment of flat warts. *Investigational Uses:* psoriasis, senile keratosis, ichthyosis vulgaris, keratosis palmaris and plantaris, basal cell carcinoma and other skin conditions.

ABSORPTION AND FATE. Minimal absorption follows topical application: 9 to 18% of preparation penetrates horny layer within 10 minutes to 16 hours, respectively, with lesser penetration of epidermis and dermis. About 0.1% of dose excreted in urine with 24 hours.

CONTRAINDICATIONS AND PRECAUTIONS. Hypersensitivity to any of the formulation ingredients (alcohol, polyethylene glycol, butylated hydroxytoluene); eczema, exposure to sunlight or ultraviolet rays (as with sunlamp); sunburn, pregnancy (category B). *Cautious Use:* patient in an occupation necessitating considerable sun exposure or weather extremes; nursing mothers.

ADVERSE/SIDE EFFECTS. (All reversible with discontinuation of medication): local inflammatory reactions, transient stinging or warmth on site, redness, scaling, severe erythema, blistering, crusting and peeling, temporary hypo- or hyperpigmentation, contact allergy (rare).

ROUTE AND DOSAGE. Topical (cream—0.05%, 0.1%; gel—0.01%, 0.025%; solution—0.05%): Apply once a day before retiring. Individualized regimen.

NURSING IMPLICATIONS

If patient has been using a kerotolytic agent, a waiting period long enough for recovery from its action should intervene before starting treatment with tretinoin.

Cleanse, using a mild bland soap, and thoroughly dry areas being treated before applying drug. Avoid use of medicated, drying or abrasive soaps and cleansers.

Wash hands before and after treatment. Apply drug preparation with fingertip, cotton swab, or gauze pad, being careful not to apply on nonaffected skin area. Excess gel results in pilling; therefore excess application is not usual.

Avoid contact of drug with eyes, mouth, angles of nose, open wounds, mucous membranes.

Time of day and frequency may be changed by prescription on the basis of individual response and preference as treatment progresses.

Inform patient that erythema and desquamation during the first 1 to 3 weeks of treatment do not represent exaccerbation of the skin problem but a probable response to the drug from deep previously unseen lesions.

Urge compliance with therapy even during the first discouraging weeks.

As treatment is continued, lesions gradually disappear leaving an inflammatory background; scaling and redness decrease after 8 to 10 weeks of therapy.

Instruct the patient to wash face no more often than 2 to 3 times daily.

Topical preparations with high concentrations of alcohol, astringents, spices or lime, perfumes and shaving lotions, should not be used during treatment period.

Tretinoin treatment to black individuals may cause unsightly postinflammatory hyperpigmentation; dark-complexioned Caucasians may have a mild hypopigmentary effect. Both are reversible with termination of drug treatment.

Clinical response to tretinoin should be evident in 2 or 3 weeks but a complete and satisfactory response (in 75% of the patients) may require a period of 3 or 4 months. Once achieved, control is maintained by less frequent applications or a change in formulation/dosage.

Inform patient that the drug is not curative; relapses commonly occur within 3 to 6 weeks after treatment has been discontinued. However, most acne spontaneously remits in the second decade.

Nonmedicated cosmetics may be used during therapy, but they should be removed thoroughly before drug is applied.

If exposure to sun cannot be avoided, it is advisable to use a sunscreen product with SPF 15 or higher and protective clothing over treated areas. If sunscreen lotion contains PABA, it should be applied 1 to 2 hours before exposure to the sun and reapplied every 2 hours, particularly if there is profuse sweating.

Exposure to high winds and extremely cold weather increases the drug-induced irritative action on lesions.

Warn patient against self-medication with additional acne treatment. Kerotolytic agents such as salicylic acid, sulfur, resorcinol, or benzoyl peroxide should not be used (unless prescribed) during tretinoin therapy because of danger of drug–drug interactions.

Diet as an etiologic factor in acne vulgaris continues to be debated. However, if patient notices a relationship between a flare-up and certain foods, they should be avoided.

Discuss skin care, emphasizing the following:

- Avoid picking, squeezing, or touching lesions to prevent infection and scarring.
- If hair is oily, shampoo frequently; avoid greasy hair dressing and keep hair away from face.
- Avoid getting sunburned.
- Inform physician if even the mildest side effects occur rather than terminating the treatment prematurely. Keep appointments for assessment of progress to permit regimen adjustment when needed.

Store gel and liquid formulations at temperature below 30°C (86°F) and solution below 27°C (80°F).

TRIAMCINOLONE

(Aristocort, Kenacort)

(trye-am-sin′oh-lone)

Corticosteroid, glucocorticoid

TRIAMCINOLONE ACETONIDE

(Acetospan, Cenocort A-40, Kenalog, Tramacort-40 Tri-kort, Triamonide-40, Trilog)

TRIAMCINOLONE DIACETATE

(Amcort, Cenocort Forte, Cino-40, Tracilon, Triam Forte, and others)

TRIAMCINOLONE HEXACETONIDE

(Aristospan)

ACTIONS AND USES. Immediate acting synthetic fluorinated adrenal corticosteroid with glucocorticoid and antirheumatic activity 7 to 13 times more potent than that of hydrocortisone (qv). Possesses minimal sodium and water retention properties in therapeutic doses. Administered orally, 4 mg triamcinolone is equivalent to 20 mg hydrocortisone on a weight basis. Acetonide formulation has longer duration of action than parent compound; when administered into joint or bursa, pharmacologic activity begins within few hours and may persist a number of weeks. Differs from other corticosteriods in that it does not increase appetite.

Used as an inflammatory or immunosuppressant agent. *Investigational Use:* (orally inhaled): treatment of bronchial asthma in patient who has not responded to conventional treatment. Therapeutic doses do not appear to cause HPA (hypothalamic–pituitary–adrenal) axis suppression.

ABSORPTION AND FATE. Oral preparation rapidly absorbed. IM slowly sbsorbed. Onset of action (oral, IM), 24 to 48 hours; peak effect: 1 to 2 hours. Duration of action: oral; 2.25 days; IM, 1 to 6 weeks; intralesional, intraarticular (hexacetonide) 3 to 4 weeks. Plasma half-life: 2 to 5 hours; HPA axis suppression: 18 to 36 hours.

CONTRAINDICATIONS AND PRECAUTIONS. Safe use during pregnancy (category C), by lactating women, and by children under 6 not established. Renal dysfunction. *See also Hydrocortisone.*

ADVERSE/SIDE EFFECTS. Muscle weakness and loss of tissue mass. Local: burning, itching, folliculitis, hypertrichosis, hypopigmentation. *See also Hydrocortisone.*

ROUTE AND DOSAGE. Oral (triamcinolone and diacetate), subcutaneous, intraarticular, intramuscular, intralesional, intradermal (hexacetonide, diacetate), topical (acetonide): creams, lotions, foam, ophththalmic ointment; Inhalation: 4 inhalatations 4 times/day. Wide dose range dependent on condition being treated and response of patient. Usual initial dose for adults is 4 to 48 mg daily in single or divided doses. **Pediatric:** 3.3 to 50 mg/m²/day in divided doses. Subsequent reduction of dose is gradual and consistent with patient response.

NURSING IMPLICATIONS

Tablet may be crushed before administration and taken with fluid of patient's choice.

This preparation may cause natriuresis, negative nitrogen balance, with weight loss in most patients (along with headache, fatigue, and dizziness) and sodium retention with weight gain and moon facies in others. Adequate diet to counter these effects should be designed. Plan with dietician, patient, and physician. High protein, high K diet is often needed.

If a local infection develops use of occlusive dressing should be discontinued and appropriate antimicrobial treatment started.

Caution patient to adhere to drug regimen: i.e., not to increase or decrease established regimen and not to abruptly discontinue taking or using the drug.

Systemic absorption may occur after topical application, especially in children and if used over extensive areas for prolonged periods of time, or if occlusive dressings are used. Reportable symptoms include hypercortisolism (hypertension, moon facies, hypokalemia), hyperglycemia, glucosuria. If HPA axis suppression occurs, drug will be withdrawn.

Postural hypotension may accompany sodium and weight loss. It may be necessary to keep patient in supine position for 30 minutes after triamcinolone is given. Warn patient to keep this possibility in mind as ambulating.

Kenacort contains tartrazine, which may cause an allergic reaction including bronchial asthma in susceptible persons who may also be sensitive to aspirin.

Protect drug from light. Store at temperature 15° to 30°C (59° to 86°F).

See Hydrocortisone (prototype glucocorticoid) for nursing implications and nursing interactions.

TRIAMTERENE

(Dyrenium)

(trye-am'ter-een)

Diuretic (potassium-sparing)

TU

ACTIONS AND USES. Pteridine derivative structurally related to folic acid. Like spironolactone, has weak diuretic action and a potassium-sparing effect. Promotes excretion of sodium, chloride (to lesser extent), and carbonate, with no excretion or slight excretion of potassium ion. Unlike spironolactone, blocks potassium secretion by direct action on distal renal tubule rather than by inhibiting aldosterone; activity is independent of aldosterone levels. May cause decrease in alkali reserve and slight increase in urinary pH. Does not appear to inhibit excretion of uric acid, but serum uric acid levels may increase in predisposed individuals. Decreased glomerular filtration rate and elevated BUN are associated with daily administration, but seldom with intermittent (every other day) therapy. Has mild hypotensive effect and is a weak competitive inhibitor of dihydrofolate reductase.

Used as adjunct in the management of edema associated with congestive heart failure, hepatic cirrhosis, nephrotic syndrome, idiopathic edema, steroid-induced edema, and edema due to secondary hyperaldosteronism. Also used alone or in conjunction with a thiazide or loop diuretic in patients with hypertension because of its potassium-sparing activity. Commercially available in combination with hydrochlorothiazide (e.g., Dyazide, Maxzide).

ABSORPTION AND FATE. Rapidly and irregularly absorbed from GI tract (individual variability). Onset of diuretic action in 2 to 4 hours; usually tapers off 7 to 9 hours later. Approximately 40 to 70% bound to plasma proteins. Plasma half-life: 90 to 100 minutes. Metabolized by liver to active and inactive metabolites. Excreted by renal filtration and tubular secretion; 10 to 80% of dose is eliminated within 24 hours.

CONTRAINDICATIONS AND PRECAUTIONS. Hypersensitivity to drug; anuria, severe or progressive kidney disease or dysfunction, severe hepatic disease, elevated serum potassium. Safe use during pregnancy (category B), in women of childbearing potential, and in nursing mothers not established. *Cautious Use:* impaired renal or hepatic function, history of gouty arthritis, diabetes mellitus.

ADVERSE/SIDE EFFECTS. Diarrhea, nausea, vomiting, and other GI disturbances; dizziness, headache, dry mouth, pruritus, rash, anaphylaxis, photosensitivity, weakness and hypotension (large doses), muscle cramps, hyperkalemia and other electrolyte imbalances, elevated BUN, elevated uric acid (patients predisposed to gouty arthritis), hyperchloremic acidosis, blood dyscrasias: granulocytopenia, eosinophilia, megaloblastic anemia, patients with reduced folic acid stores (e.g., hepatic cirrhosis).

ROUTE AND DOSAGE. **Oral: Adult:** initial: 100 mg twice daily; titrated to needs of patient. Total daily dosage (adult and pediatric) not to exceed 300 mg. Maintenance: 100 mg/day or every other day. When used with other diuretics, initial dose of each drug is reduced, then adjusted according to patient's response and tolerance. **Children:** 2 to 4 mg/kg in divided doses daily or on alternate days.

NURSING IMPLICATIONS

If patient cannot swallow capsule, it may be emptied and contents swallowed with fluid or mixed with food.

Give drug with or after meals to prevent or minimize nausea. Note that nausea and vomiting are also symptoms of electrolyte imbalance and renal failure and therefore, require careful evaluation. Dosage reduction or discontinuation of drug may be indicated.

Schedule doses to prevent interruption of sleep from diuresis, e.g., with or after breakfast if a single dose is taken, or no later than 6 PM if more than one dose is prescribed. Consult physician.

Monitor blood pressure during period of dosage adjustment. Hypotensive reactions, although rare, have been reported. Implications for ambulation should be noted, particularly for elderly patients.

Weigh patient under standard conditions (preferably before breakfast, after voiding, same scale, same clothing), prior to drug initiation and daily during therapy.

Diuretic response usually occurs on first day of therapy, but maximum effect may not occur for several days.

Monitor and report oliguria and unusual changes in intake–output ratio. Hyperkalemia is reportedly not as likely to occur in patients with adequate urinary output. Consult physician regarding allowable fluid intake.

Renal stone formation has been reported in patients taking high doses, or who have low urine volume and increased urine acidity.

Unlike most diuretics, triamterene promotes potassium retention. Therefore, potassium supplements, potassium-rich diet, and salt substitutes are usually not prescribed.

Generally salt restriction is not stressed because of the possibility of low-salt syndrome (hyponatremia). Consult physician.

Observe for signs and symptoms of hyperkalemia *(see Index),* particularly in patients with renal insufficiency, in patients on high-dose or prolonged therapy, in the elderly, and in patients with diabetes. Baseline and periodic determinations of serum potassium and other electrolytes should be done.

Periodic evaluations of renal function (BUN, serum creatinine) are advised in patients with known or suspected renal insufficiency. Fatigue, insomnia, decreased mental acuity, nausea, vomiting, stomatitis, and unpleasant taste are suggestive symptoms of advancing renal insufficiency.

Patients with cirrhosis are usually hospitalized during triamterene therapy because rapid alterations in fluid and electrolyte balance can precipitate hepatic coma or precoma: irritability, restlessness, confusion, stupor, liver flap (asterixis), coma.

Periodic blood studies are advised in patients on prolonged therapy and in patients with cirrhosis since they are prone to develop megaloblastic anemia, symptoms of which may include: burning, inflamed mouth with bright red tongue, cracked corners of lips, weakness.

Instruct patient to report overpowering fatigue or weakness, malaise, fever, sore throat, or mouth (possible symptoms of granulocytopenia) and unusual bleeding or bruising (thrombocytopenia).

Drug should be withdrawn gradually in patients on prolonged therapy, or patients who have received high doses, in order to prevent rebound kaliuresis (increased urinary excretion of potassium).

Triamterene may increase blood glucose, therefore, it should not be given to a diabetic patient unless blood glucose is controlled, primarily in patients with diabetes. Patients should be closely monitored.

Warn patient that triamterene may cause photosensitivity and therefore to avoid exposure to sun and sunlamps.

Inform patient that triamterene may impart a harmless pale blue fluorescence to urine.

Preserved in tight, light-resistant containers, preferably between 15° and 30°C (59° and 86°F), unless otherwise directed by manufacturer.

Diagnostic Test Interferences. Pale blue fluorescence in urine interferes with fluorometric assay of **quinidine** and **lactic dehydrogenase activity.** Triamterene may cause increases in **blood glucose** levels (diabetic patients), **BUN, serum potassium, magnesium,** and **uric acid** and **urinary calcium excretion.**

Drug Interactions: Triamterene

Plus	Interactions
Antihypertensives	Additive hypotensive effect
Digitalis glycosides	Effects may be decreased by triamterene
Lithium (Eskalith)	Possibility of lithium toxicity due to decreased renal clearance
Indomethacin and other NSAIDs	Combined therapy can cause marked decrease in creatinine clearance
Whole blood and plasma	May contain a significant amount of potassium when stored for more than 10 days. Possibility of hyperkalemia

TRIAZOLAM
(Halcion)

(trye-ay'zoe-lam)
Hypnotic
Benzodiazepine
C IV

ACTIONS AND USES. Benzodiazepine derivative with hypnotic effects similar to those of flurazepam but with fewer residual daytime effects. Enhances inhibitory effects of the neurotransmitter gamma aminobutyric acid (GABA) on pre- and postsynaptic receptors in all CNS regions, but particularly in the brainstem reticular formation. Blockade of cortical and limbic arousal results in hypnotic activity. Drug-induced effects on sleep include decreased sleep latency and number of nocturnal awakenings, decreased total nocturnal wake time, and increased duration of sleep. Reduction of daytime anxiety and carry-over CNS depression is minimal.

Used for short-term management of insomnia characterized by difficulty in falling asleep, frequent wakeful periods and/or early morning wakefulness. Following long-term use, tolerance or adaptation may develop.

ABSORPTION AND FATE. Readily absorbed from GI tract. Onset of action in 15 to 30 minutes with peak effect, 1.3 hours after single dose. Duration of action: 6 to 8 hours. Half-life: 1.7 to 3 hours; protein-binding (high): 89%. Metabolized in liver; excreted with its metabolites in urine.

CONTRAINDICATIONS AND PRECAUTIONS. Hypersensitivity to triazolam and benzodiazepines; pregnancy (category X). *Cautious Use:* depression, elderly and debilitated patients, patient with suicidal tendency, impaired renal or hepatic function, chronic pulmonary insufficiency. *See also Chlordiazepoxide.*

ADVERSE/SIDE EFFECTS. CNS: drowsiness, lightheadedness, headache, dizziness, ataxia, visual disturbances, confusional states, memory impairment, "rebound insomnia," euphoria, anterograde amnesia. **GI:** nausea, vomiting, constipation, and taste alterations (rare). **Other:** paradoxical reactions, minor changes in EEG patterns, tinnitus (rare). *See also Chlordiazepoxide.*

ROUTE AND DOSAGE. Carefully individualized. **Oral: Adults:** Initial dose: 0.125 mg until response is determined. Recommended dose range: 0.25 to 0.5 mg. **Elderly, debilitated patient:** 0.125 to 0.25 mg.

NURSING IMPLICATIONS

Because of short half-life, under normal circumstances dose is usually cleared before next bedtime dose; therefore "morning after" grogginess rarely occurs.

Use prior to or during labor may cause neonatal flaccidity.

Engaging in hazardous activities (driving a car, use of machinery) until drug response has been defined should be avoided.

Periodic blood counts, urinalysis, and blood chemistries are advised during long-term use of triazolam.

Advise patient that use of alcohol or other CNS depressants while on this drug increases sedative effects.

Warn patient not to stop taking drug suddenly, especially if patient is subject to seizures. Withdrawal symptoms may occur. These range from mild dysphoria to more serious symptoms such as tremors, abdominal and muscle cramps, convulsions. Consult physician about schedule for discontinuing therapy.

Signs of developing tolerance or adaptation (with long-term use) include increased daytime anxiety, increased wakefulness during last one third of the night.

Although the drug has minimum abuse potential it should not be used by addiction-prone patients (drug addicts, alcoholics) unless careful surveillance by health personnel is available. Habituation and dependence can occur.

It is recommended that no more than a 1-month supply of triazolam be dispensed to the patient and that a repeat prescription be given only if patient is under medical supervision.

Symptoms of overdosage: slurred speech, somnolence, confusion, impaired coordination, coma. Treatment: immediate gastric lavage; support of respiratory and cardiovascular systems by maintenance of patent airway, and IV fluids if necessary.

Smoking–Drug Interaction. As with other benzodiazepines, smoking may decrease hypnotic effects of triazolam. When preparing patient for sleep, remove cigarettes, not only to assure maximum drug effect but to prevent accidental fire by smoking while drowsy.

Caution patient not to increase dose without physician's advice.

Overdosage (accidental or by intent): four times the maximum recommended therapeutic dose (0.5 mg), or 2 mg.

Subject to control under Federal Controlled Substances Act; classified as Schedule IV drug.

Store at controlled room temperature 15° to 30°C (59° to 86°F).

See also Chlordiazepoxide (prototype benzodiazepine).

Drug Interactions. Triazolam CNS depressant effects are augmented if coadministered with any of the following: **anticonvulsants, antihistamines, ethanol, other psychotropics, other CNS depressants.**

TRICHLORMETHIAZIDE

(trye-klor-meth-eye'a-zide)

(Aquazide, Diurese, Metahydrin, Mono-Press, Naqua, Niazide, Trichlorex)

Diuretic
Antihypertensive
Thiazide

ACTIONS AND USES. Benzothiadiazine (thiazide) derivative. Similar to chlorothiazide (qv) in pharmacologic actions, uses, contraindications, precautions, adverse effects, and interactions.

Used to treat hypertension as sole agent or to enhance the effects of another antihypertensive when given in combination. Also used to treat edema associated with congestive heart failure, renal decompensation, and hepatic cirrhosis. Available in fixed combination with reserpine (Metatensin). *See also Chlorothiazide.*

ABSORPTION AND FATE. Onset of diuretic effect in 2 hours; peak effect in 6 hours; duration 24 hours or longer. Excreted unchanged in urine; crosses placenta; appears in breast milk.

CONTRAINDICATIONS AND PRECAUTIONS. Anuria, hypersensitivity to thiazides, sulfonamides; pregnancy (category B), lactation. *Cautious Use:* history of allergy, renal and hepatic disease; gout, diabetes mellitus. *See also Chlorothiazide.*

ADVERSE/SIDE EFFECTS. Xerostomia, sialadenitis, anorexia, paresthesias, photosensitivity, vasculitis; exacerbation of gout, SLE. *See also Chlorothiazide.*

ROUTE AND DOSAGE. Oral: Adult: *Edema:* Initial: 1 to 4 mg once or twice daily; maintenance: 1 to 4 mg daily. *Antihypertensive:* 2 to 4 mg daily as single dose or divided into 2 doses. **Pediatric:** 0.07 mg/kg daily in single or divided doses. Highly individualized.

NURSING IMPLICATIONS

Administer drug early in AM after eating (to reduce gastric irritation) and to prevent interrupting sleep because of diuresis. If 2 doses are ordered, schedule second dose no later than 3 PM.

Antihypertensive effects may be noted in 3 to 4 days, maximal effects may require 3 to 4 weeks.

Older patients may be more sensitive to the average adult dose.

Monitor blood pressure and intake and output ratio during first phase of antihypertensive therapy. Report a sudden fall in BP which may initiate severe postural hypotension and potentially dangerous perfusion problems, especially in the extremities.

Monitor patient for hypokalemia: dry mouth, anorexia, thirst, unusual fatigue, paresthesias, muscle cramps, cardiac arrhythmias. Report promptly.

Hypokalemia is rarely severe in most patients even on long-term therapy, but the elderly are especially susceptible.

To prevent onset of hypokalemia, urge patient to eat a balanced diet (usually includes K-rich foods such as potatoes, vegetables, whole grain cereals, skim milk, fruits and fruit juices).

The prediabetic or diabetic patient should be watched carefully for loss of control of diabetes or early signs of hyperglycemia: drowsiness, flushed, dry skin; fruitlike breath odor, polyuria, anorexia, polydipsia. These symptoms are slow to develop and to recognize. Check urine for glycosuria.

Counsel patient to avoid use of OTC drugs unless approved by the physician. Many preparations contain both potassium and sodium and if misused, or if patient overdoses, electrolyte imbalance side effects may be induced.

Advise patient to maintain prescribed dosage regimen, not to skip, reduce, or double doses, or change dose intervals.

Antihypertensive effects persist for at least 1 week after termination of therapy with trichlormethiazide.

Store drug in tightly closed container at temperature between 15° and 30°C (59° and 86°F), unless otherwise instructed by the manufacturer.

See Chlorothiazide (prototype thiazide diuretic).

TRIDIHEXETHYL CHLORIDE

(Pathilon)

(trye-dye-hex-eth′ill)
Anticholinergic
Antimuscarinic

TU

ACTIONS AND USES. Synthetic (amine) quaternary ammonium compound pharmacologically related to the belladonna alkaloids. Exhibits selected anticholinergic actions similar to those of atropine (qv). Exerts antimuscarinic activity by binding competitively with acetylcholine at postganglionic cholinergic effector sites. Decreases spasm of smooth muscle of GI tract, an action said to be responsible for relief of pain associated with peptic ulcer disease. However, there are no conclusive data that recommended doses aid in healing, prevent complications, or reduce recurrence rate of peptic ulcers. Also available in fixed combination with meprobamate (e.g., Milpath) or with phenobarbital.

Used as adjunct in the treatment of peptic ulcer disease and irritable bowel syndrome.

ABSORPTION AND FATE. Incompletely absorbed from GI tract. Information about distribution or metabolism not available. Poor lipid solubility and complete ionization prevent penetration of the drug into eye or CNS. Excreted in urine and feces as unchanged drug.

CONTRAINDICATIONS AND PRECAUTIONS. Glaucoma, obstructive uropathy, obstructive disease of GI tract, ulcerative colitis, biliary tract disease, intestinal atony in the elderly or debilitated patient, unstable CV status, myasthenia gravis. Safe use in children not established. *Cautious Use:* potential benefit-to-risk ratio should be weighed before use during pregnancy or lactation; hiatal hernia, diarrhea; patient with nonobstructive prostatic hypertrophy, ileostomy, or colostomy; hyperthyroidism. *See also Atropine.*

ADVERSE/SIDE EFFECTS. GI: xerostomia, nausea, vomiting, antral stasis, constipation. **GU:** urinary hesitancy and retention; impotence. **CNS:** confusion and/or excitement (especially in elderly), loss of taste, blurred vision, cycloplegia, increased ocular tension, headache, decreased sweating. **Other:** severe allergic reaction, urticaria, tachycardia, palpitations, suppression of lactation.

ROUTE AND DOSAGE. Dose is individualized by titration. (Average dose): **Oral: Adults:** Initial: 25 mg three times/day and 50 mg at bedtime; then titrated against patient need and response. Extended-release capsules are available.

NURSING IMPLICATIONS

Decreased GI motility, an expected change in aging may increase the hazard of drug-induced antral stasis in the elderly patient.

A "full" sensation, anorexia, regurgitation, or nausea may be symptomatic of stasis and should be reported. Drug use may be discontinued.

Since delayed emptying (drug-induced) affects the transit of medications and food, space administration intervals in multidrug therapy to avoid drug interaction (e.g., slowed absorption rate, increased metabolism in the GI tract). Take tridihexethyl chloride 1 hour before or 2 hours after meals and other medications, unless otherwise advised.

Check pulse before drug administration. If tachycardia is present, withhold dose and consult physician.

Because of the possibility of drug-induced drowsiness and blurred vision, patient should be warned not to drive a car or engage in dangerous activity until drug response has stabilized without such symptoms.

Decreased sweating may lead to heat prostration (fever, tachycardia, heat stroke) in an extremely warm environment, especially if patient is elderly or debilitated. Check the debilitated or otherwise threatened patient's temperature and pulse daily.

Side effects of quaternary ammonium compounds may be tolerated by young adults but not by the elderly because of reduced efficiency of adaptive mechanisms. Anticipate exaggerted anticholinergic effects: vision and accommodation changes, confusion, excitement, or agitation, as well as constipation and urination problems, especially in the elderly age group. Drug dose adjustment or discontinuation may be prescribed.

Overdosage leads to toxic and exaggerated pharmacologic effects which may differ among individuals. Treatment should include Universal Antidote *(see Index),* lavage, supportive and symptomatic therapy as indicated.

See also Atropine (prototype anticholinergic agent).

Drug Interactions: Tridihexethyl Chloride

Plus	Interactions
Atenolol	May increase pharmacologic effects of atenolol
Cimetidine (Tagamet)	Pharmacologic effects of cimetidine may be decreased
Digoxin (oral) (Lanoxin)	May increase pharmacologic effects of digoxin (product specific)

See also Atropine

TRIFLUOPERAZINE HYDROCHLORIDE

(trye-floo-oh-per'a-zeen)

(Novoflurazine, Solazine, Stelazine, Suprazine, Terfluzine, Triflurin)

Psychotropic
Antipsychotic (neuroleptic)
Phenothiazine

ACTIONS AND USES. Piperazine phenothiazine similar to chlorpromazine (qv) in most actions, uses, limitations, and interactions. Produces less sedative, cardiovascular and anticholinergic effects and more prominent antiemetic and extrapyramidal effects than other phenothiazines. Total pharmacologic effects are more prolonged than those of chlorpromazine. Lowers convulsive threshold.

Used in management of manifestations of psychotic disorders; "possibly effective" control of excessive anxiety and tension associated with neuroses or somatic conditions.

ABSORPTION AND FATE. Rapid onset of action; effects persist for more than 12 hours. Optimum therapeutic dose level reached in 2 to 3 hours. *See also Chlorpromazine.*

CONTRAINDICATIONS AND PRECAUTIONS. Hypersensitivity to phenothiazines, comatose states, CNS depression, blood dyscrasias, children under 6, bone marrow depression, preexisting hepatic disease, pregnancy. *Cautious Use:* previously detected breast cancer; patient with compromised respiratory function; seizure disorders. *See also Chlorpromazine.*

ADVERSE/SIDE EFFECTS. Nasal congestion, dry mouth, sweating, blurred vision, drowsiness, insomnia, dizziness, agitation, extrapyramidal effects, agranulocytosis, photosensitivity, skin rash, constipation, tachycardia, hypotension, pigmentary retinopathy, depressed cough reflex, gynecomastia, galactorrhea. *See also Chlorpromazine.*

ROUTE AND DOSAGE. Oral: Adult: (ambulatory patient): 2 to 5 mg twice daily; more than 4 mg/24 hours rarely necessary; (hospitalized patient): 2 to 5 mg twice daily up to 15 to 20 mg/day (optimal dose). **Children (6 to 12 years of age) (under close medical supervision):** 1 mg one or two times daily to maximum of 15 mg/day. **Intramuscular: Adult:** 1 or 2 mg every 4 to 6 hours; more than 10 mg/24 hours rarely necessary. **Children (6 to 12 years):** 1 mg one or two times daily. **Elderly:** lower dose range: adjusted to need and tolerance.

NURSING IMPLICATIONS

Not to be confused with triflupromazine hydrochloride.

Separate antacid and phenothiazine doses by at least 2 days.

Dilute oral concentrate just before administration with about 60 to 120 ml suitable diluent (e.g., water, fruit juices, carbonated beverage, milk, soups, puddings). Avoid coffee or tea near time of taking oral preparation. Explain dosage and dilution to patient if drug is to be self-administered.

Warn patient to wash hands if undiluted concentrate is spilled on skin to prevent contact dermatosis.

Monitor ingestion of tablet to see that patient does not "cheek" or hoard medication.

Tablet may be crushed before administration and taken with fluid or mixed with food if patient will not or "cannot" swallow a pill.

Administer IM injection deep into upper outer quadrant of buttock. Unlike other phenothiazines this drug apparently causes little if any pain and irritation at injection site. Rotate sites.

Intervals between injections should be no less than 4 hours because of possible cumulative effects. Oral therapy is substituted for IM treatment as soon as feasible.

Hypotension and extrapyramidal effects (especially akathisia and dystonia) are most likely to occur in patients receiving high doses or parenteral administration and in the elderly patient. Stop drug if patient has dysphagia, neck muscle spasm, or if tongue protrusion occurs.

Reduction in dosage or temporary discontinuation of drug usually reverses extrapyramidal symptoms.

Counsel patient to take drug as prescribed and not to alter dosing regimen or stop medication without consulting physician. Additionally, patient should not give any of the drug to another person.

Advise patient to consult physician about use of any OTC drugs during therapy.

Alcohol and other depressants should not be taken during phenothiazine therapy.

Drug-induced antiemetic effect may mask toxicity of other drugs, or block diagnosis of conditions with nausea as the primary symptom (e.g., brain tumor, intestinal obstruction, or Reye's syndrome).

Monitor intake–output ratio and bowel elimination pattern. Check for abdominal distention and pain. Encourage adequate fluid intake as prophylaxis for constipation and xerostomia. The depressed patient may not seek help for either symptom or for urinary retention.

Patient may be unable to adjust to temperature extremes because of drug effect on thermoregulatory center. If patient complains of being cold even at average room temperature, heed complaints, and furnish additional clothing or blankets, if necessary. Do not apply heating pad or hot water bottles; because of depressed conditioned avoidance behaviors, a severe burn may result.

Caution patient to avoid potentially hazardous activities such as driving a car or operating machinery, especially during first days of therapy. (Drowsiness and dizziness may be prominent during this time.)

Since stelazine potentiates analgesics, its use may reduce amount of narcotic required in painful long-term illness such as cancer.

Agitation, jitteriness, and sometimes insomnia may simulate original neurotic or psychotic symptoms. (They may disappear spontaneously.) Dosage should not be increased until side effects have subsided.

Increase in mental and physical activity is an expected result of therapy. Caution patients with angina to avoid overexertion and to report increase in frequency of original pain.

Advise patient to cover as much skin surface as possible with clothing when he or she must be in direct sunlight. A sun screen lotion (SPF above 12) should be applied to exposed skin.

Inform patient that urine may be discolored or reddish brown, and that this is harmless.

Maximum therapeutic response generally occurs within 2 or 3 weeks after initiation of therapy.

Slight yellow discoloration of injectable drug reportedly does not alter potency. If color markedly changed, discard solution.

Store drug in light-resistant container at temperature between 15° and 30°C (59° and 86°F), unless otherwise directed by manufacturer.

See Chlorpromazine (prototype phenothiazine antipsychotic) for drug interactions.

TRIFLUPROMAZINE HYDROCHLORIDE

(Vesprin)

(trye-floo-proe'ma-zeen)
Psychotropic
Antipsychotic (neuroleptic)
Antiemetic
Phenothiazine

ACTIONS AND USES. Aliphatic derivative of phenothiazine similar to chlorpromazine (qv) in actions, limitations, and interactions. Produces moderate to strong extrapyramidal effects and has strong anticholinergic activity.

Used in management of manifestations of psychotic disorders (excluding psychotic depressive reactions) and for prophylaxis and in treatment of severe nausea and vomiting.

ABSORPTION AND FATE. Absorbed well from GI tract; hepatic metabolism. Excreted in urine and feces. Crosses placenta.

CONTRAINDICATIONS AND PRECAUTIONS. Hypersensitivity to phenothiazines, brain damage, comatose states, bone marrow depression, use in children under 2.5 years of age, IV use in children of any age; in children or adolescents with suspected Reye's syndrome. Safe use during pregnancy and in nursing mothers not established. *Cautious Use:* urinary retention, prostatic hypertrophy, peptic ulcer, respiratory disease, especially in children, glaucoma, previously diagnosed breast cancer. *See also Chlorpromazine.*

ADVERSE/SIDE EFFECTS. Xerostomia, constipation, drowsiness, dizziness, nasal congestion, decreased sweating, inhibition of ejaculation, urinary retention, extrapyramidal reactions, tachycardia, hypotension, bizarre dreams, excitement, SLE-like syndrome, pigmentary retinopathy, blurred vision. *See also Chlorpromazine.*

ROUTE AND DOSAGE. *Psychotic disorders:* **Adults: Oral:** 100 to 150 mg/day; maintenance: 30 to 150 mg/day. **Intramuscular:** 60 to 150 mg/day in 2 or 3 divided doses. **Children (over 2.5 years): Oral:** 2 mg/kg up to 150 mg/day in divided doses. **Intramuscular:** 0.2 mg/kg up to 10 mg/day. *Nausea, vomiting:* **Adult: Oral:** 10 to 30 mg/day. **Intramuscular:** 5 to 60 mg/day. **Intravenous:** 1 to 3 mg/day. **Children (over 2.5 years of age): Oral, intramuscular:** 0.2 mg/kg to 10 mg/day. **Elderly, debilitated: Intramuscular:** 2.5 mg to 15 mg/day.

NURSING IMPLICATIONS

Not to be confused with trifluoperazine hydrochloride.

Antacids delay absorption. Give triflupromazine at least 1 hour before or 2 hours after the antacid.

Tablet may be crushed before administration and taken with fluid or mixed with food if patient is unable or unwilling to swallow a tablet.

Counsel patient to take drug as prescribed and not to alter dosing regimen or stop medication

without consulting physician. Additionally, patient should not give any of it to another person.
Permissible amounts of alcohol, if any, should be prescribed by the physician during therapy with phenothiazine.
The use of any OTC drug should be approved by the physician.
Transient hypotension may occur when drug is administered parenterally. Check blood pressure and pulse before administration and between doses. Advise patient to remain recumbent until assured that vital signs are stable.
Extrapyramidal effects are prominent in patients receiving large doses, particularly the elderly and debilitated patient.
Withhold medication and report to the physician if the following extrapyramidal effects are observed: involuntary twitching, exaggerated restlessness (or other involuntary motion), tremor, grimacing.
Tardive dyskinesia may be halted or reversed only if observed promptly and if drug is discontinued. Be alert to the following: fine vermicular movements or rapid protrusions of the tongue, puffing of cheeks, or chewing movements. *See also Chlorpromazine.*
Monitor intake–output ratio and bowel elimination pattern. Check for abdominal distention and pain. Encourage adequate fluid as prophylaxis for constipation and xerostomia. The depressed patient may not seek help for either symptom or for urinary retention.
Caution patient to avoid driving and other potentially hazardous activities until reaction to drug is known.
Vesprin (25- and 50-mg tablets) contain tartrazine which can cause allergic reactions including bronchial asthma in susceptible individuals. Frequently such persons are also sensitive to aspirin.
Instruct patient to withhold dose and report the following symptoms to the physician: light-colored stools, changes in vision, sore throat, fever.
Xerostomia may be relieved by frequent rinses with warm water. The depressed patient may not complain of this side effect; therefore, frequently inspect oral membranes of the hospitalized patient on high doses of the drug. Consult physician regarding the use of a saliva substitute to keep membranes moist (e.g., Xero-Lube). Supervise oral hygiene.
Parenteral solution should be no darker than light amber in color. Discard darkened solution.
Protect liquid preparations from light. Store drug at temperature between 15° and 30°C (59° and 86°F). Avoid freezing.
See Chlorpromazine (prototype phenothiazine antipsychotic).

TRIFLURIDINE

(trye-flure′i-deen)

(Viroptic)

Antiinfective, antiviral

ACTIONS AND USES. Pyrimidine nucleoside structurally related to idoxuridine (qv) and an analog of thymidine. Active against Herpes simplex virus (HSV) types 1 and 2, vaccinia virus, and certain strains of *Adenovirus.* Mechanism of antiviral action not completely known, but appears to involve inhibition of viral DNA synthesis and viral replication. Not effective against bacteria, fungi, or *Chlamydia.*

Used topically to eyes for treatment of primary keratoconjunctivitis and recurring epithelial keratitis caused by Herpes simplex virus types 1 and 2. Also has been used for other herpetic ophthalmic infections including stromal keratitis, uveitis, and for infections caused by vaccinia and *Adenovirus,* but clinical effectiveness has not been established.

TU

ABSORPTION AND FATE. Following topical application to eye, penetrates cornea and aqueous humor (inflammation enhances penetration). Systemic absorption does not appear to be significant.

CONTRAINDICATIONS AND PRECAUTIONS. Hypersensitivity to trifluridine or to any ingredient in the formulation. Safe use during pregnancy and in nursing women not established. *Cautious Use:* dry eye syndrome.

ADVERSE/SIDE EFFECTS. Mild transient burning or stinging, mild irritation of conjunctiva or cornea, photophobia, edema of eyelids and cornea, punctal occlusion, superficial punctate keratopathy, epithelial keratopathy, stromal edema, heratitis sicca, hyperemia, increased intraocular pressure, hypersensitivity reactions (rare).

ROUTE AND DOSAGE. Topical: Ophthalmic solution 1%: 1 drop into affected eye every 2 hours while awake, until healing (reepithelialization) has occurred. Not to exceed 9 drops daily. When healing appears to be complete, dosage reduced to 1 drop every 4 hours while awake for additional 7 days; not to exceed 5 drops daily. Continuous administration beyond 21 days not recommended.

NURSING IMPLICATIONS

See Index: Drug administration: eye drops.

Epithelial eye infections usually respond to therapy within 2 to 7 days with complete healing occurring in 1 to 2 weeks.

If improvement has not occurred after 7 days of treatment, or healing has not taken place after 14 days, other therapy should be considered.

Urge patient to keep physician informed and to keep follow-up appointments. Herpetic eye infection have a tendency to recur and can lead to corneal damage if not adequately treated.

Trifluridine is reportedly compatible with many drugs. Consult pharmacist regarding concurrent use with other typical ophthalmic preparations.

Store under refrigeration preferably at 2° to 8°C (36° to 46°F), unless otherwise directed by manufacturer.

TRIHEXYPHENIDYL HYDROCHLORIDE

(trye-hex-ee-fen′i-dill)

(Aparkane, Aphen, Artane, Tremin, Trihexane, Trihexidyl, Trihexy-2)

Anticholinergic
Antiparkinsonian agent

ACTIONS AND USES. Synthetic tertiary amine anticholinergic agent with actions, contraindications, precautions, and adverse reactions similar to those of atropine (qv). Thought to act by blocking excess of acetylcholine at certain cerebral synaptic sites. Relaxes smooth muscle by direct effect and by atropinelike blocking action on parasympathetic nervous system. Antispasmodic action appears to be one-half that of atropine, and side effects are usually less frequent and less severe.

Used in symptomatic treatment of all forms of parkinsonism (arteriosclerotic, idiopathic, postencephalitic). Also used to prevent or control drug-induced extrapyramidal disorders.

ABSORPTION AND FATE. Rapidly absorbed from GI tract, with onset of action within 1 hour. Peak effects last 2 to 3 hours; duration of action 6 to 12 hours. Metabolic fate not determined. Excreted in urine.

CONTRAINDICATIONS AND PRECAUTIONS. Hypersensitivity to trihexyphenidyl, narrow-angle glaucoma. Safe use during pregnancy, in nursing mothers, and children not established. *Cautious Use:* history of drug hypersensitivities, arteriosclerosis, hypertension; cardiac disease, renal or hepatic disorders, obstructive diseases of GI or genitourinary tracts, elderly patients with prostatic hypertrophy. *See also Atropine.*

ADVERSE/SIDE EFFECTS. Common: dry mouth, dizziness, blurred vision, mydriasis, photophobia, nausea, nervousness. Insomnia, constipation, drowsiness, urinary hesitancy or retention. **CNS (usually with high doses):** confusion, agitation, delirium, psychotic manifestations, euphoria. **CV:** tachycardia, palpitations, hypotension, orthostatic hypotension. Hypersensitivity reactions, angle-closure glaucoma, suppurative parotitis secondary to mouth dryness (infrequent). *See also Atropine.*

ROUTE AND DOSAGE. Highly individualized. **Oral:** *Parkinsonism:* initial: 1 mg; increased by 2 mg increments at 3- to 5-day intervals up to 6 to 10 mg daily in 3 or more divided doses; some patients may require 12 to 15 mg daily. Sustained-release capsule (5 mg each): (dose: same mg for mg as for daily dose with conventional tablets): in single or divided doses.

NURSING IMPLICATIONS

Patient may be switched to sustained release capsules once stabilized on conventional dosage forms to permit once-a-day or twice-a-day dosing.

May be taken before or after meals, depending on how patient reacts. Elderly patients and patients prone to excessive salivation (e.g., postencephalitic parkinsonism) may prefer to take drug after meals. If drug causes excessive mouth dryness, it may be better taken before meals, unless it causes nausea.

Drug-induced mouth dryness may be relieved by ice chips, sugarless gum or hard candy, by frequent sips of water, and by maintaining adequate total daily fluid intake.

Incidence and severity of side effects are usually dose-related and may be minimized by dosage reduction.

CNS stimulation *(see Adverse/Side Effects)* may occur with high doses and in patients with arteriosclerosis or history of hypersensitivity to other drugs. If severe, drug may be discontinued for a few days and then resumed at lower dosage.

If patient develops urinary hesitancy or retention, voiding before taking drug may relieve problem.

In patients with severe rigidity, tremors may appear to be accentuated during therapy as rigidity diminishes.

Gonioscopic evaluations and close monitoring of intraocular pressure at regular intervals are advised.

Caution patient not to engage in activities requiring alertness and skill, as drug causes dizziness, drowsiness, and blurred vision. Supervision of ambulation may be indicated.

Close follow-up care is advisable. Tolerance may develop, necessitating dosage adjustment or use of combination therapy. Patients over age 60 frequently develop sensitivity to trihexyphenidyl action.

See also Atropine sulfate.

Diagnostic Test Interferences. Trihexyphenidyl may partially inhibit the therapeutic effects of **haloperidol** and **phenothiazines** (possibly by delaying gastric emptying time and increasing metabolism in GI tract). Trihexyphenidyl may be potentiated by **MAO inhibitors.** *See also Atropine.*

Drug Interactions: Trihexyphenidyl Hydrochloride

Plus	Interactions
Chlorpromazine, Haloperidol, Phenothiazines	Reduced therapeutic effects of these drugs
Digoxin	Increased bioavailability of digoxin
MAO inhibitors	Potentiated action of trihexyphenidyl

TRIMEPRAZINE TARTRATE

(Panectyl, Temaril)

(trye-mep′ra-zeen)
Antihistaminic
H_1-receptor antagonist
Antipruritic
Phenothiazine

ACTIONS AND USES. Structural analog of the phenothiazines. Similar to chlorpromazine (qv), with prominent antipruritic activity. Also shares sedative and antihistaminic effects of chlorpromazine. In common with antihistamines, exerts both anticholinergic and antiserotonin action. Suppresses the cough reflex; may exert ulcerogenic effect.

Used primarily for symptomatic relief of pruritic symptoms in a variety of dermatologic and nondermatologic conditions. *Investigational Use:* preoperative sedation in children.

CONTRAINDICATIONS AND PRECAUTIONS. Hypersensitivity to phenothiazines; acute asthma attack; pregnancy; infants and under 6 months of age; use of extended-release form in children 6 years of age and younger. *Cautious Use:* hepatic disease; history of GI ulceration; history of convulsive disorders in the elderly or debilitated patient; upper respiratory tract infection. *See Chlorpromazine.*

ADVERSE/SIDE EFFECTS. Drowsiness, dizziness, dry mucous membranes, GI upset, allergic skin reactions, cholestatic jaundice, extrapyramidal reactions, leukopenia, agranulocytosis. In some children: paradoxic hyperactivity, irritability, insomnia, hallucinations. Acute poisoning: CNS depression with hypotension, hypothermia. Toxic potential as for other phenothiazines. *See Chlorpromazine.*

ROUTE AND DOSAGE. Oral: Adults: 2.5 mg 4 times daily; **Children (over 3 years):** 2.5 mg at bedtime or three times daily, if needed; **Children (6 months to 3 years):** 1.25 mg at bedtime or three times daily, if needed. Sustained-release formulation: **Adults:** 5 mg every 12 hours; **Children (over 6 years):** 5 mg daily. Dosages highly individualized according to severity of symptoms and patient response.

NURSING IMPLICATIONS

Usually administered after each meal and at bedtime.

Incidence and severity of adverse effects are generally dose-related; however, in some patients individual sensitivity is involved.

If child (or elderly patient) has a severe upper respiratory tract infection, this drug should be used only with caution because it suppresses the cough reflex.

Caution parents not to administer more than the prescribed dose to children.

Drowsiness occurs frequently, but it generally disappears after a few days of medication.

If it persists, dosage adjustment is indicated. Bedsides and supervision of ambulation may be necessary for some patients.
Warn patient to avoid activities requiring mental alertness and normal reaction time, such as operating a car or other hazardous activities, until drug response is known.
Patient should know that sedative action of trimeprazine is additive to that of alcohol, barbiturates, narcotics, analgesics, and other CNS depressants.
Toxic manifestations of phenothiazine derivatives are most likely to occur between 4 and 10 weeks of therapy.
Preserved in tight, light-resistant containers.
See Chlorpromazine (prototype phenothiazine) for drug interactions.

PROTOTYPE

TRIMETHADIONE

(Tridione)

(trye-meth-a-dye'one)
Anticonvulsant
Oxazolidinedione

ACTIONS AND USES. Oxazolidinedione derivative similar to paramethadione in pharmacologic properties. Elevates seizure threshold in cortex and basal ganglia and reduces synaptic response to repetitive low-frequency impulses. Has high potential for toxicity. Increases solubility of calcium carbonate, the principle constituent of pancreatic stones.

Used for control of absence (petit mal) seizures refractory to other anticonvulsant drugs. May be administered concomitantly with other anticonvulsants when other forms of epilepsy coexist with petit mal. *Investigational Use:* dissolution of pancreatic stones.

ABSORPTION AND FATE. Rapidly and completely absorbed. Peak plasma concentrations in 30 minutes to 2 hours. Uniformly distributed in tissues, including brain. Not significantly bound to plasma proteins. Largely demethylated to active metabolite (dimethadione) by hepatic microsomal enzymes. Metabolite half-life: 6 to 13 days; slowly excreted in urine (excretion rate increases with alkalinization of urine or increased urine volume).

CONTRAINDICATIONS AND PRECAUTIONS. Hypersensitivity to oxazolidinediones, as single agent in treatment of patient with history of grand mal seizures, severe hepatic or renal impairment, blood dyscrasias. Safe use in women of childbearing potential and during pregnancy not established. *Cautious Use:* diseases of retina and optic nerve; renal dysfunction.

ADVERSE/SIDE EFFECTS. CNS: hemeralopia, photophobia, diplopia, vertigo, ataxia, drowsiness, insomnia, headache, fatigue, malaise, paresthesias, irritability, personality changes. **Dermatologic:** exfoliative dermatitis, erythema multiforme, acneiform dermatitis. **GI:** hiccups, nausea, vomiting, abdominal pain, gastric distress, anorexia, weight loss. **Hematopoietic:** severe blood dyscrasias: leukopenia, neutropenia, thrombocytopenia, pancytopenia, agranulocytosis, aplastic anemia. **Hypersensitivity:** lymphadenopathy with splenomegaly, hepatomegaly, pruritus, morbilliform rash. **Renal:** albuminuria, nephrosis, hepatotoxicity, precipitation of grand mal seizures, hair loss (rare). **Other:** bleeding gums, epistaxis, retinal and petechial hemorrhages, vaginal bleeding, systemic lupus erythematosus syndrome, myasthenia-gravis-like syndrome, changes in blood pressure.

ROUTE AND DOSAGE. Oral: Adults: 300 to 600 mg 3 or 4 times daily (therapy generally started at 900 mg daily; dosage then increased by 300 mg/day at weekly intervals until seizures are controlled or toxic symptoms intervene). Maintenance: 0.9 to 2.4 Gm/day in 3 or 4 divided doses. **Children:** 300 to 900 mg in 3 or 4 equally divided doses (depending on age and weight). Maintenance: 1 Gm/m^2/day in 3 or 4 equally divided doses.

NURSING IMPLICATIONS

Because of potential for toxicity, close medical supervision, especially during first year of therapy, is essential.

A transitory increase in number of obscure seizures may occur at beginning of therapy. Instruct patient and responsible family member to keep a record of number, duration, and time of attacks. Clinical improvement usually occurs 1 to 4 weeks after start of therapy.

Visual disturbances are usually controlled by reduction in dosage. Hemeralopia (glare effect or blurring of vision in bright light) is relieved by wearing dark glasses.

Drowsiness tends to diminish with continued therapy, or it can be controlled by dosage reduction or concurrent administration of an amphetamine. Caution patient to avoid potentially hazardous activities such as driving a car or operating machinery until this side effect is controlled.

Instruct patient to report immediately to physician symptoms of agranulocytosis: fever, sore throat or mouth, muscle weakness, joint pains, skin rash, swollen lymph nodes; of hypertoxicity: jaundice; of thrombocytopenia: petechiae, ecchymoses, unexplained bleeding; scotomata, hair loss or other unusual symptoms.

Complete blood and differential counts and urinalyses are recommended at monthly intervals or more frequently if indicated. Therapy should be discontinued if neutrophil count drops to $2500/mm^3$ or below or if albuminuria persists or increases.

Plasma concentrations of dimethadione, active metabolite of trimethadione, may be used as guide to dosage adjustment (usually maintained at about 700 mcg/ml for effective seizure control).

Advise patient to follow prescribed regimen precisely, without interruption, changes in dosage or abrupt discontinuation.

Stress the importance of keeping follow-up appointments.

Advise patient to wear medical identification jewelry or card at all times.

Following prolonged use, withdrawal should be accomplished gradually to avoid precipitating petit mal status or seizures.

Preserved in tightly closed containers in a dry place at temperatures not exceeding 25°C (77°F).

TRIMETHAPHAN CAMSYLATE
(Arfonad)

(trye-meth'a-fan)
Antihypertensive
Ganglionic blocking agent

ACTIONS AND USES. Potent, short-acting nondepolarizing ganglionic blocking agent. Blocks transmission in both adrenergic and cholinergic ganglia by competing with acetylcholine for receptor sites on postganglionic membranes. Adrenergic blockade results in vasodilation, improved peripheral blood flow, and thus decrease in blood pressure. Also has direct peripheral vasodilation action and thus can produce marked hypotension. Blood pressure is significantly lower in head-up position because venous dilation and peripheral pooling causes reduction in cardiac output. Capable of causing histamine release.

Used to produce controlled hypotension for certain surgical procedures (e.g., neurologic, ophthalmic, and plastic surgery) and for short-term treatment of hypertensive crises associated with pulmonary edema. *Unlabeled Use:* management of acute dissecting aneurysm of aorta and ischemic heart disease.

ABSORPTION AND FATE. Effects appear almost immediately following IV administration and may persist 10 to 30 minutes. Thought to be metabolized by pseudocholinesterases. About 20 to 40% excreted in urine. Crosses placenta.

CONTRAINDICATIONS AND PRECAUTIONS. Anemia, hypovolemia, shock, asphyxia, respiratory insufficiency, glaucoma; during pregnancy. *Cautious Use:* history of allergy; elderly and debilitated patients, children, cardiac disease, arteriosclerosis, hepatic or renal disease, degenerative CNS disease, Addison's disease, diabetes mellitus, patients receiving steroids, antihypertensives, anesthetics (especially spinal), and diuretics.

ADVERSE/SIDE EFFECTS. CV: tachycardia or decrease in heart rate, orthostatic hypotension, angina. **GI:** nausea, vomiting, anorexia. **Hypersensitivity:** urticaria, pruritus, histamine-like reaction along course of vein. Symptoms resulting from cholinergic blockade: atony of urinary bladder or GI tract, cycloplegia, mydriasis, dry mouth, suppression of perspiration. **Other:** restlessness, extreme weakness; respiratory depression, respiratory arrest (following large doses).

ROUTE AND DOSAGE. Intravenous infusion: 500 mg (10 ml) of drug in 500 ml of 5% dextrose in water to yield concentration of 1 mg/ml. **Pediatric:** 50 to 150 mcg/kg/minute. Rate of administration 0.3 to 6 mg/minute.

NURSING IMPLICATIONS

IV flow rate is prescribed by physician to maintain desired blood pressure level. Rate of infusion should be monitored constantly. Individuals vary considerably in response to drug.

Use of an infusion pump, microdrip regulator or similar device is recommended for precise measurement of flow rate.

Intensity of hypotensive effect is largely dependent on positioning. Decrease in blood pressure is most marked in sitting or standing position. If blood pressure fails to drop with patient in supine position, physician may prescribe elevation of head of bed. Conversely, excessive hypotension can be reversed by having patient assume head-low position or by elevating legs.

Take vital signs prior to initiation of therapy as a baseline for comparison during drug administration.

Patient must be observed continuously while receiving infusion. Blood pressure should be checked every 2 minutes until stabilized at desired level, then every 5 minutes for duration of treatment. Pulse and respiration should also be monitored closely.

Infusion should be terminated gradually while blood pressure is closely monitored. It is stopped before wound closure in surgery to allow BP to return to normal.

Continue to monitor vital signs at regular intervals after completion of treatment. Since blood pressure returns to pretreatment level within 10 minutes after the infusion is terminated an oral antihypertensive is usually initiated in patients with hypertension as soon as desired blood pressure level is achieved with trimethaphan.

Note: Pupillary dilatation may not necessarily indicate anoxia or depth of anesthesia, but may represent a specific effect of the drug.

Facilities for resuscitation and maintenance of oxygenation and ventilation should be immediately available. Have on hand vasopressor drugs to counteract undesirably low blood pressure, e.g., phenylephrine, mephentermine. Norepinephrine is used only if other vasopressors are not effective.

Some patients become refractory to trimethaphan (tachyphylaxis) within 48 hours after initiation of therapy. Notify physician promptly if blood pressure fails to respond.

Monitor intake and output. Ganglionic blockade may reduce renal blood flow initially as well as voiding contractions and urge to void. Check lower abdomen for bladder distention.

Do not use trimethaphan infusion as a vehicle for administration of other drugs.

Trimethaphan is stable under refrigeration, but freezing should be avoided. Infusion solution should be freshly prepared and any unused portion discarded. Storage: controlled room temperature: 15° to 30°C (59° to 81°F).

Diagnostic Test Interferences. Trimethaphan may decrease **serum potassium** and may prevent elevation of **blood glucose** that usually occur during postoperative period.

Drug Interactions: Trimethaphan

Plus	Interactions
Antihypertensives, other diuretics; Anesthetics	Additive hypotensive effects

TRIMETHOBENZAMIDE HYDROCHLORIDE

(Tegamide, Ticon, Tigan, Tiject-20)

(trye-meth-oh-ben'za-mide)
Antiemetic

ACTIONS AND USES. Structurally related to ethanolamine antihistamines, but in therapeutic doses antihistamine activity is weak. Has sedative and antiemetic actions. Less effective than phenothiazine antiemetics, but produces fewer side effects. Must be used with other agents when vomiting is severe. Primary locus of action is thought to be the chemoreceptor trigger zone (CTZ) in medulla.

Used for control of nausea and vomiting.

ABSORPTION AND FATE. Antiemetic action: following oral administration, within 20 to 40 minutes with duration of 3 to 4 hours; following IM: within 15 minutes with duration of 2 to 3 hours. Approximately 30 to 50% of dose is excreted unchanged in urine within 48 to 72 hours.

CONTRAINDICATIONS AND PRECAUTIONS. Hypersensitivity to drug, for treatment of uncomplicated vomiting in viral illness, parenteral use in children, rectal administration in prematures and newborns, known sensitivity to benzocaine (in suppository) or to similar local anesthetics. Safe use during pregnancy and lactation not established. *Cautious Use:* patients who have recently received other centrally acting drugs; in presence of high fever, dehydration, electrolyte imbalance.

ADVERSE/SIDE EFFECTS. Hypersensitivity reactions (including allergic skin eruptions), extrapyramidal symptoms (including parkinsonism), hypotension, blurred vision, dizziness, drowsiness, headache, depressed mood, disorientation, diarrhea, exaggeration of nausea, acute hepatitis, jaundice, muscle cramps. Rarely: Reye's syndrome; convulsions, opisthotonos, coma; causal relationship not established. **Other:** pain, stinging, burning, redness, irritation at IM site; local irritation following rectal administration.

ROUTE AND DOSAGE. Adults: Oral: 250 mg three or four times daily. **Rectal:** 200 mg three or four times daily. **Intramuscular: Adults only:** 200 mg three or four times daily. **Children (15 to 45 kg): Oral, rectal:** 100 to 200 mg three or four times daily; **Children: (under 15 kg):** 100 mg rectally three or four times daily. Rectal use not recommended in prematures and newborns.

NURSING IMPLICATIONS

Capsule may be emptied and contents swallowed with water or mixed with food (if patient has difficulty swallowing capsule).

Restoration of body fluids and electrolytes is important adjunct to therapy.

Administer IM deep into upper outer quadrant of buttock. To minimize possibility of irritation and pain, avoid escape of solution along needle track. If permitted by agency policy, this can be accomplished by drawing a small bubble of air into syringe after drug is measured; when medication is injected, air bubble will clear needle of drug.

Hypotension is reported, particularly in surgical patients receiving drug parenterally. Monitor blood pressure.

There is some suspicion that use of centrally-acting antiemetics for viral illnesses may contribute to development of Reyes' syndrome.

Possible early signs are similar to reported side effects of this drug: persistent vomiting, hyperpnea, lethargy, confused or irrational behavior. Other early signs of Reye's syndrome: convulsions, coma, and opishotonos may occur, especially in children and the elderly with use of this drug. If an acute febrile illness accompanies or begins during therapy with trimethobenzamide, report promptly and stop drug therapy.

The antiemetic effect of drug may obscure diagnoses of GI or other pathologic conditions or signs of toxicity from other drugs.

Advise patient to report promptly to physician the onset of rash or other signs of hypersensitivity. Drug should be discontinued immediately.

Since drug may cause drowsiness and dizziness, caution patient to avoid driving a car or other potentially hazardous activities.

Advise patient not to drink alcohol or alcoholic beverages during therapy with this drug.

Drug Interactions: Trimethobenzamide

Plus	Interactions
Alcohol, barbiturates and other centrally-acting depressants	Additive depressant activity
Belladonna alkaloids	May intensify anticholinergic side effects
Phenothiazines	May cause expression of extrapyramidal syndrome

PROTOTYPE

TRIMETHOPRIM

(Proloprim, Trimpex)

(trye-meth'oh-prim)
Antiinfective, urinary
Folate antagonist

ACTIONS AND USES. Antiinfective and folate antagonist with slow bactericidal action. Binds to and reversibly blocks enzyme reduction of folic acid to its active metabolite tetrahydrofolic acid, thus preventing bacterial synthesis of thymidine, an essential nucleoside in DNA. This binding and interference with cell growth is 1000 times stronger in bacterial than in mammalian cells. Most pathogens causing urinary tract infection (UTI) are in normal vaginal and fecal flora. Trimethoprim concentration in vaginal secretions is higher than in serum, and sufficient amounts of the drug are excreted in feces to reduce or eliminate susceptible fecal organisms. Thus, drug is effective against most common UTI pathogens, including *Escherichia coli, Enterobacter* species, *Klebsiella pneumoniae, Proteus mirabilis,* most strains of *Haemophilus influenzae, Streptococcus pneumoniae, S. pyrogens, Staphalococcus* organisms (including *S. saprophyticus*). Not effective against *Bacteroides, Lactobacillus* species, *Chlamydia* or *Pneumocystis carinii, Pseudomonus aeroginosa.* Demonstrated resistance is usually chromosomally mediated. Resistant strains of *Enterobacteriaceae (E. coli* and *Klebsiella* and *Proteus* species) may develop during therapy although incidence of resistance in this group of organisms is low. Emergence of trimethoprim-resistant organisms occurs more frequently when it is used alone than when used in combination therapy. Efficacy as treatment of UTI appears to match that of amoxicillin, ampicillin, nitrofurantoin, or sulfisoxazole. Available in fixed combination with sulfamethoxazole (1 part trimethoprim to 2 parts sulfamethoxazole) as Co-Trimoxazalin (Bactrim, Cotrim, Septra, TMP-SMZ).

Used to treat initial episodes of acute uncomplicated UTIs and in the treatment and prophylaxis of chronic and recurrent UTI in both men and women. *Unlabeled Use:* treatment of traveler's diarrhea.

ABSORPTION AND FATE. Readily and almost completely absorbed from GI tract. Peak serum concentration of approximately 1 mcg/ml reached in 1 to 4 hours after single 100-mg dose. Widely distributed into most body tissues and fluids including CSF. (If meninges are inflamed, concentration in CSF increases.) Elimination half-life: 8 to 11 hours in adult with normal renal function; 15 to 26 hours when creatinine clearances are 10 to 30 or 0 to 10 ml/minute respectively. 42 to 46% protein bound. Metabolized in liver; 50 to 60% oral dose rapidly excreted in urine unchanged within 24 hours. Drug concentration in urine decreased in patient with impaired renal function. Crosses placenta and enters amniotic fluid and breast milk. Partial removal by hemodialysis.

CONTRAINDICATIONS AND PRECAUTIONS. Hypersensitivity to trimethoprim, megaloblastic anemia secondary to folate deficiency, creatinine clearance less than 15 ml/min, impaired renal or hepatic function, possible folate deficiency, pregnancy (category C), nursing mothers, children with fragile X chromosome associated with mental retardation. Safe use in infants less than 2 months old and efficacy in children under 12 years old has not been established.

ADVERSE/SIDE EFFECTS. Most serious: hypersensitivity and hematologic reaction (0.5%). **Dermatologic:** rash, pruritus, exfoliative dermatitis. **GI:** epigastric discomfort, nausea, vomiting, glossitis, abnormal taste sensation. **Hematologic (rare):** thrombocytopenia, neutropenia, megaloblastic anemia, methemoglobinemia. **Other:** fever, increased serum transaminases (ALT, AST), bilirubin, creatinine, BUN.

ROUTE AND DOSAGE. Oral: Acute UTI: 100 mg every 12 hours or 200 mg once daily. Dose and frequency modified to individual needs. *Unlabeled Use:* Prophylaxis of chronic/recurrent UTI: 100 mg daily at bedtime for 6 weeks to 6 months.

NURSING IMPLICATIONS

Culture of the causative organism and susceptibility tests are conducted before trimethoprim therapy is initiated; however, therapy may be started before test results have been received.

Antiinfective treatment of acute uncomplicated UTIs is usually continued 10 to 14 days.

Uncomplicated UTIs usually respond to treatment if patient takes all of prescribed medication.

Recurrent UTI may reflect noncompliance with drug therapy. Reinforce initial teaching about importance of adhering to drug regimen at time of checkup visits.

Trimethoprim may worsen the psychomotor regression associated with mental retardation because of potential drug-induced folate deficiency.

Monitor *creatinine clearance tests.* Usually dose reduction is prescribed when clearance values are 15 to 30 ml/minute. (*Normal:* 90 to 120 ml/minute.)

Periodic urine cultures are recommended during therapy for recurrent or chronic UTIs.

Follow-up urine cultures may be ordered after treatment is discontinued to determine whether bacteria have been eliminated.

Symptoms pathognomonic of an emerging hematologic disorder (fever, sore throat, pallor, purpura, ecchymosis) should be reported promptly. Complete blood count should be obtained. If formed elements of blood are reduced, drug will be discontinued.

Leucovorin (folinic acid) will be administered if bone marrow suppression occurs ("leucovorin rescue"). Usually 3 to 6 mg only for 3 days restores normal hematopoiesis.

Discuss fluid intake pattern with the patient. Ordinarily, the elderly tend to restrict fluids; therefore teaching needs to emphasize that amount and frequency of drinking water and other fluids is an important adjunct to drug therapy.

Usually the adult patient should attempt to maintain fluid intake of 2000 to 3000 ml/day (if not contraindicated) to help flush out urinary bacteria.

Assess urinary pattern during treatment. Altered pattern (frequency, urgency, nocturia, retention, polyuria) may reflect emerging drug resistance, necessitating change of drug regimen. Periodically inspect bladder area for distension.

Pain and hematuria should be reported immediately.

Before full drug effects are experienced, patient may have pain and discomfort with voiding which can be relieved by a urinary analgesic.

Tell the male patient not to postpone voiding even though increases in fluid intake may cause more frequent urination.

If patient (especially the elderly) has edema, urge elevation of legs when sitting and physical exercise as tolerated. When patient goes to bed at night, fluid accumulated in the legs during the day reenters the circulatory system and is excreted during the night, resulting in nocturia.

Elderly, malnourished, alcoholic, pregnant, or debilitated patients are especially susceptible to the hematologic toxic effects. Changes in temperature pattern and intake–output ratio and pattern should be recognized and reported.

Drug-induced rash, a common side effect, is usually maculopapular, pruritic, or morbilliform and appears 7 to 14 days after start of therapy with daily doses of 200 mg or less.

To prevent nosocomial infections, aseptic technique during catheter insertion and care is essential. Thoroughly wash hands before and after any procedural interventions.

Inspect perineal areas for evidence of inflammation (sore, red excoriated mucosa). Warm Sitz baths may give relief. Warn patient not to use douching, sprays, or bubble baths during treatment period, and stress careful perineal hygiene to prevent reinfection. Cleansing areas with water (no soap) is advised. Vaginal discharge, dysuria, and pruritus should be reported.

The female patient with recurrent UTIs should be advised to cleanse genital area before sex and to urinate afterwards. If this is not possible, advise her to drink a glass of water before sex.

Overdosage of 1 Gm or more produces symptoms of nausea, vomiting, diarrhea, mental depression, confusion, facial swelling, bone marrow depression, elevated serum transaminases. *Treatment:* induce emesis, lavage stomach, administer supportive and symptomatic treatment, and acidify urine. Hemodialysis is moderately effective.

Drug Interactions. When **trimethoprim** and **phenytoin** are given concomitantly, incidence of folate deficiency increases.

TRIMIPRAMINE MALEATE

(Surmontil)

(tri-mip'ra-meen)
Psychotropic, antidepressant
Tricyclic, antienuretic

ACTIONS AND USES. Tricyclic antidepressant (TCA) pharmacologically similar to imipramine (qv) in actions, uses, absorption and fate, limitations, and interactions. Has moderate anticholinergic and strong sedative effects, therefore useful in depression associated with anxiety and sleep disturbances. More effective in alleviation of endogenous depression than other depressive states. Recent studies suggest strong, active H_2-receptor antagonism is a characteristic of TCAs.

Uses similar to those for imipramine. *Investigational Use:* management of enuresis; treatment of peptic ulcer disease.

CONTRAINDICATIONS AND PRECAUTIONS. Prostatic hypertrophy; during recovery period after myocardial infarction. Safe use during pregnancy and lactation not established. *Cautious Use:* patients with schizophrenia and on electroshock therapy; patients with suicidal tendency; cardiovascular, hepatic, thyroid, renal disease. *See also Imipramine.*

ADVERSE/SIDE EFFECTS. CV: tachycardia, orthostatic hypotension, hypertension. **GI:** xerostomia, constipation, paralytic ileus. **CNS:** seizures, tremor, confusion, sedation, blurred vision. **Other:** urinary retention, photosensitivity, sweating. *See also Imipramine.*

ROUTE AND DOSAGE. Highly individualized. **Oral: Adults** (hospitalized): initial: 100 mg/day in divided doses; gradual increases depending on response and tolerance to maximum recommended dose of 250 to 300 mg/day if necessary. *(Outpatient):* initial: 75 mg/day in divided doses; may be increased gradually to maximum of 200 mg/day. Maintenance: 50 to 150 mg daily at bedtime. **Elderly, adolescents:** 50 mg daily increased to 100 mg/day if necessary. Maintenance: lowest dose that will maintain remission, given preferably at bedtime. Therapy may be continued for 3 months. *Antienuretic action:* **Oral:** initial: 25 mg 1 hour before bedtime; if no response in child under 12: increase dose to 50 mg; if no response in child over 12: increase dose to 75 mg.

NURSING IMPLICATIONS

Administer drug with food to decrease gastric distress.

Supervise drug ingestion to be sure patient does not "cheek" the drug.

Monitor blood pressure and pulse rate during adjustment period of tricyclic antidepressant (TCA) therapy. If blood pressure falls more than 20 mm Hg or if there is a sudden increase in pulse rate, withhold medication, and notify physician.

Drug may cause intolerance to heat or cold. Regulate environmental temperature and patient's clothing accordingly.

The severely depressed patient may need assistance with personal hygiene, particularly because of excessive sweating caused by the drug.

Monitor bowel elimination pattern and intake–output ratio. Severe constipation and urinary retention are potential problems especially in the elderly. Advise increased fluid intake to at least 1500 ml daily (if allowed). Consult physician about stool softener (if necessary) and a high-fiber diet.

Inspect oral membranes daily if patient is on high doses. Urge outpatient to report symptoms of stomatitis, sialoadenitis, xerostomia.

If xerostomia is a problem, institute symptomatic therapy *(see Imipramine).* Sore or dry mouth interferes with speaking, mastication, swallowing, and can be a major cause of poor food intake and noncompliance. Consult physician about use of a saliva substitute (e.g., Moi-stir).

Caution patient that ability to perform tasks requiring alertness and skill may be impaired.

Urge patient not to use OTC drugs unless physician approves.

The actions of both alcohol and trimipramine are potentiated when used together during therapy and for up to 2 weeks after the TCA is discontinued. Consult physician about safe amount of alcohol, if any, that can be taken.

If a patient uses excessive amounts of alcohol it should be borne in mind that the potentiation of TCA effects may increase the danger of overdosage or suicide attempt.

Note that the effects of barbiturates and other CNS depressants may also be enhanced by trimipramine.

Fine tremors, a distressing extrapyramidal side effect, may be reduced or alleviated by propranolol. Report symptom to physician.

Report signs of hepatic dysfunction: yellow skin and sclerae, light-colored stools, pruritus, abdominal discomfort.

Orthostatic hypotension may be sufficiently severe to require protective assistance when patient is ambulating. Instruct patient to change position from recumbency to standing slowly and in stages. Elastic panty hose or support hose may be helpful. Consult physician.

Because of the danger of suicidal intent in a severely depressed patient, limit access to the drug.

Alert patient to the fact that because TCAs have a "lag period" of 2 to 4 weeks, therapeutic response will be delayed. (Increased dosage does not shorten period but rather increases incidence of adverse reactions.) This period is one that fosters noncompliance. Monitor drug intake to see that therapy is not interrupted.

Store drug in tightly closed container at temperature between 15° and 30°C (59° and 86°F), unless otherwise specified by the manufacturer.

See Imipramine (prototype tricyclic antidepressant) for additional Nursing Implications and Drug Interactions.

TRIOXSALEN

(Trisoralen)

(trye-ox'sa-len)
Pigmenting agent
Photochemotherapeutic agent
Psoralen

ACTIONS AND USES. Systemic psoralen derivative structurally and pharmacologically related to methoxsalen (qv) but produces less intense melanogenic and erythemic responses. Produces resistance to solar damage in persons particularly susceptible to painful reactions with exposure to sunlight (e.g., blond persons or persons with fair complexions). This response appears to be related to drug-induced thickening of the horny layer of skin, with retention of melanin, resulting in formation of a stratum lucidum. Accelerates pigmentation only when followed by exposure of skin to sunlight or ultraviolet irradiation, and may reach equivalence of a full summer of sun exposure. Use to produce a cosmetic tan, however, is not advised by some clinicians, because of its high potential for toxicity.

Used in conjunction with controlled exposure to ultraviolet light or sunlight to repigment vitiliginous skin, to improve tolerance to sunlight in patients with albinism, and to enhance pigmentation (debatable use).

ABSORPTION AND FATE. Well absorbed from GI tract. Following single dose, skin sensitivity to long-wavelength ultraviolet light (UVA) occurs in 1 to 2 hours, peaks within 2 to 4 hours, and persists for 7 to 8 hours. Extent of distribution unknown; high concentrations are found in liver, skin, and blood. Rapidly degraded in liver to inactive metabolites; 80% of dose excreted in urine within 8 hours.

CONTRAINDICATIONS AND PRECAUTIONS; ADVERSE/SIDE EFFECTS. *See Methoxsalen.*

ROUTE AND DOSAGE. Oral: (accompanied by some form of UVA light or sunlight). **Adults and Children (over 12 years):** 10 mg daily as single dose, 2 to 4 hours before controlled exposure to UVA or sunlight.

NURSING IMPLICATIONS

Administer with milk or after a meal to reduce gastric distress.

Repigmentation may begin a few weeks after start of treatment but significant effects require 6 to 9 months of therapy.

If repigmentation is not apparent after 3 months of treatment, drug is discontinued.

Following successful repigmentation with (P-psoralen; UVA) (PUVA) therapy, pigmentation can be maintained by periodic exposure to sunlight and trioxsalen.

If trioxsalen is used to increase tolerance of skin to sunlight, treatment is continued no longer than 14 days with dosage not exceeding 140 mg.

Trioxsalen formulation contains tartrazine, which may cause an allergic-type reaction, including bronchial asthma in susceptible persons. Frequently these individuals are also allergic to aspirin.

Federal law prohibits distribution of trioxsalen without a prescription.

Food–Drug Interactions: Concomitant ingestion of furocoumarin-containing foods may intensify adverse reactions. Warn patient to avoid the following foods: figs, limes, parsley, parsnips, mustard, carrots, celery.

Urge patient to adhere to dosage and exposure time prescribed by physician. Severe burning may occur with overdosage.

The lethal dose is six times greater than that of methoxsalen.

Store in tightly closed light resistant container at temperature of 15° to 30°C (59° to 86°F).

See Methoxsalen for additional Nursing Implications and Drug Interactions.

TRIPELENNAMINE HYDROCHLORIDE

(PBZ-SR, Pelamine, Pyribenzamine, Ro-Hist)

(tri-pel-enn'a-meen)
Antihistamine
H_1-receptor antagonist
Enzyme inhibitor

ACTIONS AND USES. Ethylenediamine antihistamine with mild CNS depressant effects and relatively high incidence of GI side effects. Antagonizes histamine action (i.e., increased capillary permeability, edema formation, itching, and constriction of respiratory, GI, and vascular smooth muscle). Does not inhibit gastric secretion. Has antiemetic, antitussive, anticholinergic, and local anesthetic action.

TU

Used to relieve symptoms of various allergic conditions, to ameliorate reactions to blood or plasma, and in anaphylaxis as adjunct to epinephrine and other standard measures after acute symptoms have been controlled. Also has been used to provide oral mucous membrane analgesia in young children with herpetic gingivostomatitis.

ABSORPTION AND FATE. Onset of effects within 15 to 30 minutes; duration of action about 4 to 6 hours (generally, up to 8 hours with sustained-release formulation). Detoxified by liver; excreted in urine.

CONTRAINDICATIONS AND PRECAUTIONS. Hypersensitivity to antihistamines of similar structure; narrow-angle glaucoma; symptomatic prostatic hypertrophy; bladder neck obstruction; GI obstruction or stenosis; lower respiratory tract symptoms, including asthma; within 14 days of MAO inhibitors therapy. Safe use during pregnancy, lactation, and in neonates and prematures not established. *Cautious Use:* history of asthma; convulsive disorders; increased intraocular pressure; hyperthyroidism; cardiovascular disease; hypertension; diabetes mellitus.

ADVERSE/SIDE EFFECTS. **Atropine-like effects:** dry mouth, nose, and throat; thickened bronchial secretions, wheezing, sensation of chest tightness, blurred vision, diplopia, headache; urinary frequency, hesitancy, or retention; dysuria; palpitation, tachycardia, mild hypotension or hypertension. **CNS:** drowsiness, dizziness, tinnitus, vertigo, fatigue, disturbed coordination, tingling, heaviness, weakness of hands, tremors, euphoria, nervousness, restlessness, insomnia. **GI (common):** epigastric distress, anorexia, nausea, vomiting, constipation or diarrhea. Low incidence of other side effects: **Hematologic:** leukopenia, agranulocytosis, hemolytic anemia. **Other:** skin rash, urticaria, photosensitivity, anaphylactic shock. **Overdosage (especially in children):** hallucinations, excitement, fever, ataxia, athetosis, convulsions, coma, cardiovascular collapse.

ROUTE AND DOSAGE. **Oral:** **Adults:** 25 to 50 mg every 4 to 6 hours (as much as 600 mg daily in divided doses, if necessary). Long-acting tablet and sustained-release form: 100 mg morning and evening or every 8 to 12 hours. **Children:** 5 mg/kg/24 hours divided into 4 to 6 doses. Not to exceed 300 mg/24 hours. All dosages highly individualized. Each 5 ml of tripelennamine citrate (elixir) is equal to 25 mg of the hydrochloride.

NURSING IMPLICATIONS

GI side effects may be lessened by administration of drug with or immediately after meals or food or with a glass of milk or water.

Note that the sustained-release formulation (100 mg) is not intended for use in children of any age.

Patients taking the sustained-release tablet should be instructed to swallow tablet whole and not to crush, break, or chew it.

Urinary hesitancy can be reduced if patient voids just before taking drug.

In patients receiving antihistamines for allergic manifestations, a careful history should be taken that includes change from usual pattern of recently ingested foods and drugs, as well as social or emotional stress.

Mild to moderate drowsiness, blurred vision, and dizziness occur in some patients. Caution against operating motor vehicle or engaging in hazardous activities until drug response has been determined.

Dizziness, sedation, and hypotension are more likely to occur in the elderly. Assistance during ambulation may be necessary. Advise patient to touch stable objects while walking, to provide balance.

Patient should know that the effects of antihistamines may be augmented by alcohol ingestion and by use of other CNS depressants.

Caution patient not to take OTC preparations without consulting physician.

Patients receiving long-term therapy with antihistamines should have periodic blood cell counts.

Antihistamines should be discontinued within 4 days prior to skin testing procedure for allergy because they may obscure otherwise positive reactions.

Caution patient to store antihistamines out of reach of children. Fatalities have been reported.
Preserved in tight, light-resistant containers.

Drug Interactions: Tripelennamine

Plus	Interactions
Alcohol, antipsychotics, anxiolytics, barbiturates, hypnotic sedatives, and other drugs with central activity	Potentiated CNS depression
MAO inhibitors	Intensified anticholinergic effects
Propranolol	Beta-adrenergic blocking action of propranolol may be inhibited; quinidine-like effect (myocardial depression) may be increased

TRIPROLIDINE HYDROCHLORIDE

(Actidil, Bayidyl)

(trye-proe'li-deen)
Antihistamine
H_1-receptor antagonist
Enzyme inhibitor

ACTIONS AND USES. Long-acting, potent propylamine (alkylamine) antihistamine, similar to chlorpheniramine (qv) in actions, uses, contraindications, precautions, and adverse effects. Has rapid onset of action, with maximum effect in about 3.5 hours and duration up to 12 hours. Low incidence of drowsiness and other side effects.

ROUTE AND DOSAGE. Oral: Adults: 2.5 mg two or three times daily. **Children (6 to 12 years):** ½ adult dose; **Children (2 to 5 years):** 0.6 mg (syrup only) three or four times daily; **Children (4 months to 2 years):** 0.3 mg (syrup only) three or four times daily.

NURSING IMPLICATIONS

The product Actifed combines the antihistaminic action of triprolidine and the decongestant effect of pseudoephedrine.
Preserved in tight, light-resistant containers.
See Chlorpheniramine (prototype propylamine antihistamine).

TROLEANDOMYCIN

(Tao)

(troe-lee-an-doe-mye'sin)
Antiinfective
Antibiotic (macrolide)

ACTIONS AND USES. Derivative of oleandomycin, a macrolide antibiotic prepared from cultures of *Streptomyces antibioticus.* Chemically related to streptomycin and has similar range of antibacterial activity, but reportedly less effective; has high potential for toxicity. Cross-sensitivity with erythromycin reported.

Used in treatment of acute, severe infections of upper respiratory tract caused by susceptible strains of pneumococci and group A beta-hemolytic streptococci.

ABSORPTION AND FATE. Readily absorbed from GI tract. Peak serum concentration (2 mcg/ml) 2 hours after 500 mg dose; still detectable in serum after 12 hours. Well distributed throughout body fluids; diffusion into CSF is poor, unless meninges are inflammed. Metabolized in liver. Excreted in bile and urine.

CONTRAINDICATIONS AND PRECAUTIONS. Hypersensitivity to drug; use for prophylaxis or for minor infections. Safe use during pregnancy not established. *Cautious Use:* impaired hepatic function.

ADVERSE/SIDE EFFECTS. Abdominal cramps (frequent) and discomfort, nausea, vomiting, diarrhea; allergic reactions (urticaria, skin rash, anaphylaxis); cholestatic jaundice, superinfections.

ROUTE AND DOSAGE. Oral: Adults: 250 to 500 mg every 6 hours. **Children:** 6.6. to 11 mg/kg (125 to 250 mg) every 6 hours. Available as capsules and suspension.

NURSING IMPLICATIONS

Advise patient to take drug on an empty stomach (1 hour before or 2 hours after meals).

To maintain effective blood levels, drug should be taken at evenly spaced intervals throughout the day preferably around the clock.

Periodic liver function tests are advised in patients receiving drug longer than 10 days or in repeated courses.

Some patients develop an allergic type of hepatitis with right upper quadrant pain, fever, nausea, vomiting, jaundice, eosinophilia, and leukocytosis. Liver changes are reversible if drug is discontinued immediately. Instruct patient to report signs of jaundice: acholic stools, pruritus, icteric sclerae.

Generally, drug therapy does not exceed 10 days. For streptococcal infections, therapy should continue for 10 days to prevent development of rheumatic fever or glomerulonephritis.

Instruct patient not to stop drug before full course of therapy is completed. Patient should not interrupt then restart therapy, or increase or decrease dose or interval.

Superinfections are most likely to occur in patients on prolonged or repeated therapy. Drug should be discontinued if symptoms present (sore mouth with white patches or black furry tongue; malodorous creamy, vaginal discharge; anorectal irritation and itching); appropriate therapy should be started.

Diagnostic Test Interferences. Troleandomycin may cause false elevations of **urinary 17-ketosteroids** (Drekter), and **17-hydroxycorticosteroids** (Porter-Silver method).

Drug Interactions: Troleandomycin

Plus	Interactions
Contraceptives, oral	Cholestatic jaundice
Ergotamine-containing drugs	May induce ischemic reactions
Theophyllines (except dyphylline), Carbamazepine, Corticosteroids	Hepatic metabolism may be inhibited by troleandomycin leading to increased risk of toxicity

TROPICAMIDE

(Mydriacyl)

(troe-pik'a-mide)
Anticholinergic (parasympatholytic)
Mydriatic
Cycloplegic

ACTIONS AND USES. Derivative of tropic acid, with pharmacologic properties similar to those of atropine (qv), but mydriatic and cycloplegic effects occur more rapidly and are less prolonged.

Used to induce mydriasis and cycloplegia for ophthalmologic diagnostic procedures.

ABSORPTION AND FATE. Maximal mydriatic effects occur in 20 to 40 minutes maximum cycloplegia in 20 to 35 minutes. Mydriasis may persist for 6 to 7 hours; full recovery of cycloplegia in 50 minutes to 6 hours.

CONTRAINDICATIONS AND PRECAUTIONS. Hypersensitivity to drug and to ingredients of drug; known or suspected glaucoma, angle closure. Safe use in pregnancy not established. *Cautious Use:* infants, children with brain damage or spastic paralysis, Down's syndrome.

ADVERSE/SIDE EFFECTS. CV: tachycardia. **CNS:** psychotic reactions, behavioral disturbances in children, unusual drowsiness or weakness, headache. **Ophthalmic:** transient stinging, photophobia, blurred vision, slight increase in intraocular pressure. **Other:** Sweating, flushing, allergic reactions.

ROUTE AND DOSAGE. Ophthalmic: *For refraction:* 1 or 2 drops of 1% solution in eye; repeated in 5 minutes. If patient is not seen within 20 to 30 minutes an additional drop may be instilled to prolong mydriatic effect. *Examination of fundus:* 1 or 2 drops of 0.5% solution 15 to 20 minutes prior to examination.

NURSING IMPLICATIONS

Forewarn patient that transient stinging may occur on instillation.

Possibility of systemic absorption may be minimized by applying pressure against lacrimal sac during and for 1 or 2 minutes following instillation.

Photophobia may disappear as early as 2 hours after application; if troublesome, advise patient to wear dark glasses.

Caution patient to avoid potentially hazardous activities such as driving a car if vision is blurred.

See also Atropine (prototype mydriatic/cycloplegic agent).

PROTOTYPE

TUBOCURARINE CHLORIDE

(Tubarine)

(too-boe-kyoo-ar'een)
Skeletal muscle relaxant (nondepolarizing)
Neuromuscular blocking agent

ACTIONS AND USES. Curare alkaloid, nondepolarizing neuromuscular blocking agent extracted from the plant *Chondodendron tomentosum.* Produces skeletal muscle relaxation or paralysis by competing with acetylcholine at cholinergic receptor sites on skeletal muscle endplate, and thus blocks nerve impulse transmission. Also has histamine-releasing and ganglionic blocking properties. Has no known effect on intellectual functions, consciousness, or pain threshold.

Used to induce skeletal muscle relaxation as adjunct to general anesthesia, to facilitate management of mechanical ventilation, to reduce intensity of muscle contractions in tetanus and in pharmacologically or electrically induced convulsions, to treat spastic states in children, and for diagnosis of myasthenia gravis when conventional tests have been inconclusive.

ABSORPTION AND FATE. Following IV injection, muscle relaxation begins within seconds. Maximal effects in 2 to 3 minutes; effects usually last 25 to 90 minutes. IM injection is slowly and irregularly absorbed; action time unpredictable. Approximately 40% protein-bound. Half-life: 1 to 3 hours. Minimally degraded in liver and kidney. Approximately 35 to 75% excreted unchanged in urine within 24 hours; about 10% excreted in bile. Crosses placenta.

CONTRAINDICATIONS AND PRECAUTIONS. Hypersensitivity to curare preparations; when histamine release is a hazard; hyperthermia; electrolyte imbalance; acidosis; neuromuscular disease; renal disease. Safe use in women of childbearing potential or during pregnancy not established. *Cautious Use:* impaired cardiovascular, renal, hepatic, pulmonary, or endocrine function; hypotension; carcinomatosis; thyroid disorders; collagen diseases; porphyria; familial periodic paralysis; history of allergies; myasthenia gravis; elderly or debilitated patients.

ADVERSE/SIDE EFFECTS. Slight dizziness, feeling of warmth, profound and prolonged muscle weakness and flaccidity, respiratory depression, hypoxia, apnea, increased bronchial and salivary secretions, bronchospasm, decreased GI motility, hypotension, circulatory collapse, malignant hyperthermia, hypersensitivity reactions.

ROUTE AND DOSAGE. Intravenous: *Adjunct to general anesthesia:* 40 to 60 U at beginning of surgical procedure; then 20 to 30 U in 3 to 5 minutes, if required. *Electroshock therapy:* 0.5 U/lb slowly over a period of 1 to 1.5 minutes. *Diagnosis of myasthenia gravis:* $\frac{1}{15}$ to $\frac{1}{5}$ of average electroshock therapy dose (may vary with manufacturer).

NURSING IMPLICATIONS

Primarily administered by anesthesiologist or under direct observation.

Baseline tests of renal function and determinations of serum electrolytes are generally done before drug administration. Electrolyte imbalance (particularly potassium and magnesium) can potentiate the effects of nondepolarizing neuromuscular blocking agents.

Preparations should be made in advance for endotracheal intubation, suction, or assisted or controlled respiration with oxygen administration. Have on hand atropine and antagonists neostigmine or edrophonium (cholinesterase inhibitors). A nerve stimulator may be used to assess nature and degree of neuromuscular blockade.

Selective muscle paralysis following drug administration occurs in the following sequence: jaw muscles, levator eyelid muscles and other muscles of head and neck, limbs, intercostals and diaphragm, abdomen, trunk. Facial and diaphragm muscles are first to recover, followed in order by legs, arms, shoulder girdle, trunk, larynx, hands, feet, pharynx. Muscle function is usually restored within 90 minutes.

Monitor blood pressure, vital signs, and airway until assured of patient's recovery from drug effects. Ganglionic blockade (hypotension) and histamine liberation (increased salivation, bronchospasm) and neuromuscular blockade (respiratory depression) are known effects of tubocurarine.

Tubocurarine is retained in the body long after effects of neuromuscular blockade appear to have dissipated. Observe for and report residual muscle weakness.

Patient may find oral communication difficult until muscles of head and neck recover.

Measure and record intake–output ratio during day of drug administration. Renal dysfunction will prolong drug action. Peristaltic action may be suppressed. Check for bowel sounds.

Test for myasthenia gravis is considered positive if muscle weakness is exaggerated.
Solutions of drug should not be used if more than faintly discolored.
Tubocurarine is incompatible with solutions that have a high pH such as barbiturates; therefore, do not mix in same syringe.

Drug Interactions. Drugs that may potentiate or prolong neuromuscular blocking action of (katariform) skeletal muscle relaxants: **certain inhalation anesthetics** (cyclopropane, ether, halothane, methoxyflurane); **certain antibiotics,** e.g., amikacin, aminoglycosides, amphotericin B, bacitracin, clindamycin, lincomycin, tetracyclines; also **diazepam; potassium-depleting diuretics, magnesium salts, narcotic analgesics, phenothiazines, procainamide, propranolol, quinidine.**

U

URACIL MUSTARD

(yoor'a-sill)
Antineoplastic
Alkylating agent
Nitrogen mustard

ACTIONS AND USES. Nitrogen mustard agent thought to react selectively with phosphate groups of DNA causing chromosomal cross-linkage and interference with normal mitosis. Lacks vesicant properties; ineffective in treatment of acute leukemia or acute blastic crisis. Has cumulative hematopoietic depressive properties at therapeutic dosage levels. Maximum bone marrow depression may not occur until 2 to 4 weeks after uracil has been discontinued. Like other alkylating agents uracil may be carcinogenic. *See also Mechlorethamine.*

Used for treatment of chronic lymphocytic and myelocytic leukemia, reticulum cell cancer, carcinoma of lung, cervix, or ovary, non-Hodgkin's lymphomas. Beneficial in treatment of early stages of polycythemia vera and in therapy of mycosis fungoides.

ABSORPTION AND FATE. Well absorbed from GI tract. Plasma concentrations decrease rapidly, with no evidence after 2 hours; less than 1% recovered unchanged in urine.

CONTRAINDICATIONS AND PRECAUTIONS. Severe leukopenia, thrombocytopenia, aplastic anemia, pregnancy. *Cautious Use:* patient with history of gout, or urate renal stones, leukopenia thrombocytopenia. *See also Mechlorethamine.*

ADVERSE/SIDE EFFECTS. Dermatologic: Pruritus, dermatitis, partial alopecia (rare), pigmentation. **GI:** anorexia, epigastric distress, nausea, vomiting, diarrhea, oral ulcerations. **Hematologic:** bone marrow depression (sometimes irreversible). **Neurologic:** irritability, nervousness, mental confusion, depression (rare). **Other:** hepatotoxicity, hyperuricemia, amenorrhea, azoospermia. *See also Mechlorethamine.*

ROUTE AND DOSAGE. Oral: Adult: single weekly dose: 0.15 mg/kg/4 weeks. **Children:** single weekly dose: 0.30 mg/kg/4 weeks. Continue dosage until relapse or until clinical improvement. Highly individualized dosage regimens.

NURSING IMPLICATIONS

Administered at least 2 or 3 weeks after maximum effect of previous antineoplastic or radiation has been achieved.

Usually administered at bedtime to alleviate GI side effects.

Uracil capsules contain tartrazine which may produce an allergic-type reaction, including bronchial asthma, to susceptible individuals. These persons are also frequently sensitive to aspirin.

Severe nausea and vomiting may necessitate discontinuation of drug.

In some patients, drug appears to act slowly, and response may not be apparent for 2 to 3 months after drug therapy is initiated.

As total cumulative dose of uracil approaches 1 mg/kg body weight, irreversible bone marrow damage may occur.

Depression of platelets is apt to be more serious than that of leukocytes; watch carefully for beginning signs of bleeding into skin and mucosa and gingival bleeding with tooth brushing. Report immediately.

If possible avoid invasive procedures that could lead to bleeding during thrombocytopenic period (IM, SC, rectal temperatures).

Complete blood counts, including platelets, are advised 1 or 2 times weekly during and at least 1 month after end of therapy. (Maximum bone marrow depression may not occur until 2 to 4 weeks after discontinuation of therapy.)

If the uric acid level is elevated, the dosage regimen for anti-gout medication will need to be reviewed.

Urge patient to increase fluid intake so that renal flushing occurs. Changes in intake and output ratio and pattern, and flank, stomach, or joint pain should be reported promptly.

Notify physician of the following symptoms: fever, chills, oral ulcerations, sore throat, bleeding and bruising, swelling of lower legs and feet.

Frank alopecia is not a usual side effect as with other nitrogen mustards.

Because of the immunosuppression produced by uracil, generalized vaccinia may occur if patient is immunized with small pox.

See Mechlorethamine.

UREA

(yoor-ee'a)

(Carbamide, Dermaflex, Nutraplus, Ureacin-20, Ureaphil, Urisec, Velvelan)

Diuretic
Keratolytic
Aborifacient

ACTIONS AND USES. Diamide salt of carbonic acid. When present in high concentrations in blood, induces diuresis by elevating osmotic pressure of glomerular filtrate, with subsequent decrease in sodium and water reabsorption and promotion of chloride and (to a lesser extent) potassium excretion. Volume and rate of urine flow is increased. Increased blood toxicity results in transudation of fluid from tissue including brain, cerebrospinal, and intraocular fluid, into the blood. When used as an aborifacient, urea (in dextrose) is injected into amniotic sac, followed by IV oxytocin about 400 milliunits/minute or by prostaglandin F_2. Mechanism of action: not clear, but it is suggested that decidual damage due to the hyperosmotic drug may induce the formation of prostaglandins which cause uterine contractions and cervical dilatation. The fetus is usually killed. Topical applications increase water binding capacity of stratum corneum and thus may soften dry scaly skin conditions.

Used to reduce or prevent intracranial pressure (cerebral edema) and intraocular pressure and to prevent acute renal failure during prolonged surgery or trauma. Also used transabdominally for aborting second trimester of pregnancy. Topical preparation used to promote hydration and removal of excess keratin in dry skin and hyperkeratotic conditions. *Investigational Use:* severe migraine attacks; acute sickle cell crisis.

ABSORPTION AND FATE. Following IV administration, maximum reduction of intraocular and intracranial pressures and diuretic effect occur in 1 or 2 hours. Diuresis and intracranial pressure reduction may persist 3 to 10 hours; intraocular pressure lasts 5 to 6 hours then returns to pretreatment levels. After intraamniotic instillation about 10% of drug diffuses rapidly into maternal blood. Distributed widely; good ocular penetration. Half-life: about 1 hour. Excreted in urine essentially unchanged; 50% may be reabsorbed. Crosses placenta; excreted in breast milk.

CONTRAINDICATIONS AND PRECAUTIONS. Severely impaired renal or hepatic function; congestive heart failure; active intracranial bleeding; marked dehydration; IV injection into lower extremeties, especially in elderly patients, topical use for viral skin diseases, or impaired circulation. Safe use in pregnancy (category C) lactation or in children not established. (Contraindications for intraamniotic urea: impaired renal function, frank liver failure, active intracranial bleeding; marked dehydration, diabetes mellitus, sickle cell anemia.) *Cautious Use:* women of childbearing potential; use on face or broken skin.

ADVERSE/SIDE EFFECTS. CNS: somnolence (prolonged use in patients with renal dysfunction), headache, acute psychosis, confusion, disorientation, nervousness. **CV:** tachycardia, hypotension, syncope. **GI:** nausea, vomiting, increased thirst. **Metabolic:** fluid and electrolyte imbalance, dehydration. **Other:** intraocular hemorrhage (rapid IV), pain, irritation, sloughing, venous thrombosis, chemical phlebitis at injection site (infrequent); hyperthermia, skin rash.

ROUTE AND DOSAGE. Intravenous infusion: Adults (30% solution): 1 to 1.5 Gm/kg body weight by slow infusion (over 1 to 2.5 hours); maximum dose: 120 Gm in 24 hours; rate not to exceed 4 ml per minute. **Children:** 0.5 to 1.5 Gm/kg; **Children (up to 2 years):** 0.1 to 0.5 Gm/kg. **Topical cream, lotion (2 to 25%):** apply to affected area 1 or 3 times daily. **Intraabdominal, intraamniotic instillation:** 40 to 50% urea solution in 5% dextrose injection.

NURSING IMPLICATIONS

The parenteral solution may also be used orally. To improve palatability, pour medication over iced fruit juice (unsweetened) or mix with lemon juice or cola flavoring and have patient sip through a straw.

Solution should be freshly prepared for each patient; discard unused portion. May be reconstituted with 5 or 10% dextrose injection or 10% invert sugar in water.

Reconstituted solution should be used within a few hours if stored at room temperature. If refrigerated at 2° to 8°C, solution should be used within 48 hours; prolonged storage leads to ammonia formation. Discard unused portions.

Infusion flow rate will be prescribed by physician. Rapid administration may be associated with increased capillary bleeding and hemolysis.

Urea should not be administered by same IV set through which blood is being infused.

Urea has the potential for causing tissue damage because of its osmotic properties. Extreme care must be taken to avoid extravasation; thrombosis and tissue necrosis can occur. Inspect injection site frequently. If extravasation is suspected, discontinue the IV line stat. Consult physician about removal of needle or cannula. Institute local treatment (according to institution protocol or physician's instructions); elevate part even if extravasation is minor. Use of heat or cold is debatable. Heat induces vasodilation and increases drug distribution and absorption. Cold may decrease circulation and reentry of drug into circulation.

Dosage is individualized on basis of water and electrolyte balance, urinary volume, clinical signs.

Determinations of serum and urinary sodium should be performed every 12 hours. Frequent BUN and kidney function studies are advised, particularly in patients suspected of having renal dysfunction.

Be alert for signs of hyponatremia, hypokalemia, dehydration, or transient overhydration (due to hyperosmotic activity).

Monitor vital signs and mental status; promptly report any changes.

Observe postoperative patients closely for signs of hemorrhage. Urea reportedly may increase prothrombin time and promote internal oozing at suture sites.

Patient should be encouraged to drink fluids so as to hasten excretion or urea. However, if patient complains of a headache do not allow him or her to drink as this will counteract the osmotic effects of the drug. Consult physician about fluid volume parameters.

Monitor intake and output. If diuresis does not occur within 6 to 12 hours following administration, or if BUN exceeds 75 mg/dl, drug should be withheld until renal function is evaluated.

Comatose patients receiving urea should have an indwelling catheter to insure satisfactory bladder emptying.

The mean induction-to-abortion time following administration of urea, with IV oxytocin is 18 to 30 hours; abortion occurs within 76 hours in about 80% of the patients.

There is minimal systemic absorption of intraamniotic-instilled drug when given in the intraamniotic sac and minimal systemic effects. If patient complains of lower abdominal pain, it may be that drug is going into abdomen rather than into the amniotic sac.

Action of topical preparation is enhanced by applying it to skin while still moist following washing or bathing.

See also Mannitol.

Drug Interactions. Urea may increase excretion rate of lithium, thereby decreasing its effectiveness.

UROKINASE

(Abbokinase)

(yoor-oh-kin'ase)
Enzyme
Plasminogen activator

ACTIONS AND USES. Enzyme produced by kidneys and isolated from human kidney tissue cultures. Promotes thrombolysis by direct action on the endogenous fibrinolytic system which results in conversion of plasminogen to the enzyme plasmin, an action that occurs within as well as on the surface of thrombus/embolus. (Plasmin degrades fibrin, fibrinogen, and other procoagulant plasma proteins.) Urokinase also has an anticoagulant effect because its action leads to high plasma levels of fibrin and fibrinogen degradation products. Activity expressed in international units (IU): i.e., ability to cause lysis of a fibrin clot via the in vivo plasmin system. Most effective action is on fresh recently formed thrombi.

Used for lysis of acute massive pulmonary emboli, for lysis of peripheral emboli, and to restore patency in occluded IV catheters (including central venous catheter). *Investigational Use:* treatment of acute myocardial infarction, retinal vessel occlusion, lysis of clot-occluded arteriovenous cannulae, and various other conditions associated with thromboembolization phenomenon.

ABSORPTION AND FATE. Following IV infusion, rapidly cleared from circulation. Adequate activation of fibrinolytic system usually established within 3 to 4 hours after start of therapy. Half-life: 10 to 20 minutes (longer in presence of hepatic dysfunction). Small amount excreted in urine and bile. It is not known if drug crosses placenta. Fibrinolytic effects usually disappear in a few hours after treatment is discontinued, but increased thrombin time (TT), decreased fibrinogen and plasminogen levels, and increased degradation products may persist for 12 to 24 hours.

CONTRAINDICATIONS AND PRECAUTIONS. Pregnancy (category B), during lactation, children. *See also Streptokinase.*

ADVERSE/SIDE EFFECTS. *See Streptokinase.*

ROUTE AND DOSAGE. (Administered through in line 0.22 or 0.45 micron filter, using an infusion pump with 195 ml capacity.) **Intravenous infusion:** 4400 IU/kg as admixture of urokinase with 0.9% NaCl for Injection or 5% Dextrose Injection. Administer over period of 10 minutes (90 ml/hour) followed by continuous infusion of 4400 IU/kg/hour (15 ml/hour) for 12 hours. At end of treatment period, flush remaining admixture from pump with 0.9% NaCl Injection or 5% Dextrose Injection at continuous infusion rate of 15 ml/hour. *Occluded coronary artery:* precede urokinase with bolus of heparin (2500 to 10,000 U IV). Urokinase instillation: 6000 IU/minute for periods up to 2 hours. Continue until artery is maximally opened (usually 15 to 30 minutes using about 500,000 IU). *Central venous catheter clearance:* 5000 IU/ml solution. Instruct patient to exhale and hold breath any time catheter is disconnected from syringe or IV tubing. Avoid excessive pressure of instillation to prevent rupture of catheter or forcing clot into circulation. Follow manufacturer's instructions for procedural details.

NURSING IMPLICATIONS

Urokinase is more expensive than streptokinase (SK) but may be useful in patient with high levels of SK antibodies.

Measurable signs of clinical response may not occur for 6 to 8 hours after therapy is started.

Reconstituted by adding 5.2 ml sterile water for injection to vial containing 250,000 IU (resulting solution contains 50,000 IU/ml). Roll or tilt vial to mix; avoid agitating or shaking to prevent foaming and filament formation. Prepare further dilutions according to manufacturer's literature.

Urokinase should be reconstituted immediately before use. Since the product contains no preservatives discard unused portion. Total volume of administered fluid should not exceed 200 ml.

Avoid adding other medication to urokinase solution.

Anticoagulant therapy with heparin is reinstituted at end of urokinase therapy and when TT has decreased to less than twice normal control value (usually within 3 to 4 hours).

Severe spontaneous bleeding, including fatality from cerebral hemorrhage, has occurred during urokinase treatment. Risk is estimated to be twice that associated with heparin therapy.

Abbokinase formulation also includes mannitol 25 mg and NaCl 45 mg.

Store vials at 2° to 8°C (35° to 47°F).

See also Streptokinase for additional Nursing Implications, Diagnostic Test Interferences, and Drug Interactions.

V

VALPROIC ACID

(Depakene)

(val-proe'ic)
Anticonvulsant

ACTIONS AND USES. Antiepileptic agent unrelated chemically to other drugs used to treat seizure disorders. Mechanism of action unknown; may be related to increased bioavailability of the inhibitory neurotransmitter gamma-aminobutyric acid (GABA) to brain neurones. Inhibits secondary phase of platelet aggregation.

Used alone or with other anticonvulsants in management of absence (petit mal) and mixed epilepsy seizures. Used in the management of status epilepticus refractory to IV diazepam, petit mal variant seizures, febrile seizures in children. *Unlabeled Use:* treatment of other types of seizures including psychomotor (temporal lobe), myoclonic and akinetic epilepsy, photosensitivity epilepsy, and those refractory to other antiepilepsy agents.

ABSORPTION AND FATE. Absorbed rapidly and almost completely from GI tract. Peak plasma levels (wide interindividual variation) are usually reached in 1 to 4 hours following single oral dose. Half-life: 8 to 16 hours; may be increased in patient with cirrhosis or acute hepatitis. Protein binding: 85 to 95%. Widely distributed; may enter enterohepatic circulation. Metabolized in liver; excreted primarily as glucuronic conjugates in urine. Small amount excreted in feces and expired air. Crosses placenta, enters breast milk.

CONTRAINDICATIONS AND PRECAUTIONS. Hypersensitivity to valproic acid; patient with bleeding disorders, hepatic dysfunction or disease. *Cautious Use:* women who are or may become pregnant, nursing mothers, history of renal disease, adjunctive treatment with other anticonvulsants, angina pectoris, active recovery period following myocardial infarction.

ADVERSE/SIDE EFFECTS. CNS: breakthrough seizures, sedation, drowsiness, dizziness, decreased alertness, ataxia, headache, nystagmus, diplopia, "spots before eyes," tremors, asterixis, dysarthria, muscle weakness, incoordination, paresthesias. **GI:** nausea, vomiting, indigestion (transient), hypersalivation, anorexia with weight loss, increased appetite with weight gain, abdominal cramps, diarrhea, constipation, acute pancreatitis, hepatic failure. **Hematologic:** prolonged bleeding time, leukopenia, lymphocytosis, thrombocytopenia, hypofibrinogenemia, bone marrow depression, anemia. **Psychiatric:** depression, hallucinations, hyperactivity, behavioral deterioration in children, aggression, emotional upset. **Other:** enuresis, skin rash, transient hair loss, curliness or waviness of hair, irregular menses, secondary amenorrhea; hyperammonemia (usually asymptomatic); tremor. **Overdosage:** deep coma, pulmonary edema, death.

ROUTE AND DOSAGE. Oral: Adults and children: initial: 15 mg/kg/day. Increase at one week intervals by 5 to 10 mg/kg/day until seizures are controlled or side effects preclude more increases. Maximum recommended dose: 60 mg/kg/day. Divide doses (2 or more times daily) when total daily dose exceeds 250 mg. Syrup: 250 mg valproic acid per 5 ml. Sodium valproate (Depakote) is also available as an enteric-coated tablet.

NURSING IMPLICATIONS

Instruct patient not to chew tablets or capsule. Medication should be swallowed whole. Patient should avoid using a carbonated drink as diluent for the syrup because it will release drug from delivery vehicle. Free drug painfully irritates oral and pharyngeal membranes.

Serious GI side effects can lead to discontinuation of therapy with valproic acid. To reduce gastric irritation administer drug with food. Enteric-coated tablet or syrup formulation are usually well tolerated.

Effective therapeutic serum levels of valproic acid: 50 to 100 mcg/ml.

Inform the diabetic patient that this drug may cause a false-positive test for urine ketones. Should that occur notify the physician; a differential diagnostic blood test may be indicated.

Warn patient to avoid alcohol and self-medicating with other depressants during therapy. The use of all OTC drugs should be approved by the physician during anticonvulsant therapy. Particularly unsafe are combination drugs containing aspirin, sedatives, medications for hay fever or other allergies.

If spontaneous bleeding and/or bruising (petechiae, ecchymotic areas, otorrhagia, epistaxis, melena), occur, notify physician promptly.

Monitor alertness in patient on multiple drug therapy for seizure control. Plasma levels of the adjunctive anticonvulsants should be evaluated periodically as indicators for possible neurologic toxicity.

Platelet counts and bleeding time determinations are recommended prior to initiating treatment and at periodic intervals. Liver function tests, including serum ammonia, should be performed initially and at least every 2 months, especially during the first 6 months of therapy.

Patients on multiple drug therapy are at risk from hyperammonemia (lethargy, anorexia, asterixis, increased seizure frequency, vomiting. These symptoms should be reported promptly. If they persist with decreased dosage, the drug will be discontinued.

Food–Drug Interactions: In presence of hyperammonemia, dietary proteins may be restricted to reduce the exogenous source of nitrogen (ammonia).

Advise patient not to drive a car or engage in other activities requiring mental alertness and physical coordination until reaction to drug is known.

The syrup is red and flavorful. Keep out of the reach of children.

Advise patient to carry medical identification card or jewelry bearing information about medication in use and the epilepsy diagnosis.

Instruct patient to withhold dose and report to the physician if the following symptoms appear: visual disturbances, rash, jaundice, light-colored stools, protracted vomiting, diarrhea. Fatal hepatic failure has occurred in patients receiving this drug.

Increased dosage increases frequency of adverse effects. Monitor patient carefully when dose adjustments are being made and report promptly if side effects persist.

Before any kind of surgery (including dental surgery), the patient should inform the doctor or dentist of taking valproic acid.

Inform patient that abrupt discontinuation of therapy can lead to loss of seizure control. Warn patient not to stop or alter dosage regimen without consulting physician. He or she should also refrain from giving any of the drug to another person.

Diagnostic Test Interferences. Valproic acid produce false-positive results for **urine ketones,** elevated **SGOT (AST), SGPT (ALT), LDH,** and **serum alkaline phosphatase,** prolonged **bleeding time,** altered **thyroid function** tests.

Drug Interactions: Valproic acid

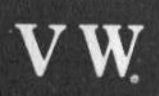

Plus	**Interactions**
Alcohol	Potentiated depressant effects of alcohol
Anticonvulsants	Increased anticonvulsant action
Antidepressants, tricyclic	Potentiated CNS depressant effects

Plus (cont.)	Interactions (cont.)
Aspirin	Potentiated platelet aggregation effect of valproic acid (increases possibility of spontaneous bleeding)
Barbiturates	Increased serum levels of barbiturates; severe CNS depression
Clonazepam	Absence seizures may occur
CNS depressants	Increased depressant action
Dipyridamole	*See Aspirin*
MAO inhibitors	Potentiated CNS depressant effects
Phenytoin	May increase or decrease phenytoin plasma levels; breakthrough seizures may occur. Adjust phenytoin dosage accordingly
Primidone	*See Barbiturates*
Salicylates	Increased valproic acid serum level; increased toxicity
Sulfinpyrazone	*See Aspirin*
Warfarin	*See Aspirin*

VANCOMYCIN HYDROCHLORIDE

(Vancocin)

(van-koe-mye'sin)
Antiinfective
Anitbiotic

ACTIONS AND USES. Glucopeptide antibiotic prepared from *Streptomyces orientalis*, with bactericidal and bacteriostatic actions. Action interferes with cell membrane synthesis in multiplying organisms. Active against many gram-positive organisms, including group A beta-hemolytic streptococci, staphylococci, pneumococci, enterococci, clostridia, and corynebacteria. Gram-negative organisms, mycobacteria, and fungi are highly resistant. Cross-resistance with other antibiotics, or resistance to vancomycin has not been reported.

Used parenterally for potentially life-threatening infections in patients allergic, nonsensitive, or resistant to other less toxic antimicrobial drugs. Used orally only in treatment of staphylococcal enterocolitis (not effective by oral route for treatment of systemic infections).

ABSORPTION AND FATE. Poorly absorbed from GI tract. Peak serum levels of 49 mcg/ml achieved in 5 minutes following IV injection of 1 Gm; trough level of 2 mcg/ml after 12 hours. Oral doses of 2 Gm/day produce serum concentrations less than 1 mcg/ml. Diffuses into pleural, ascitic, pericardial and synovial fluids; penetrates noninflamed meninges, but does not enter CSF if meninges are inflamed. About 10% protein bound. Half-life: 4 to 8 hours in adults; 2 to 3 hours in children; increased to 7 to 8 days in the anuric patient. Accumulation occurs with renal dysfunction. About 80 to 90% of dose excreted in active form in urine within 24 hours. Readily crosses placenta. Not significantly removed by hemodialysis or continuous ambulatory peritoneal dialysis.

CONTRAINDICATIONS AND PRECAUTIONS. Known hypersensitivity to vancomycin, previous hearing loss, concurrent or sequential use of other ototoxic or nephrotoxic agents, IM administration. Safe use during pregnancy not established. *Cautious Use:* neonates, impaired renal function.

ADVERSE/SIDE EFFECTS. Ototoxicity (auditory portion of eighth cranial nerve), nephrotoxicity leading to uremia, hypersensitivity reactions (chills, fever, skin rash, urticaria, shocklike state); transient leukopenia, eosinophilia, anaphylactoid reaction with vascular collapse;

superinfections, severe pain, thrombophlebitis at injection site; nausea, warmth, and generalized tingling following rapid IV infusion.

ROUTE AND DOSAGE. Oral, intravenous: (intermittent infusion (preferred): administer over period of 30 minutes; continuous infusion: over 24 hour period): **Adults:** 500 mg every 6 hours or 1 Gm every 12 hours; **Older children:** 44 mg/kg body weight in divided doses every 6 hours. **Neonates:** 10 mg/kg daily in divided doses every 6 to 12 hours.

NURSING IMPLICATIONS

For oral administration, contents of vial (500 mg) may be diluted in 30 ml of water. It may also be administered at this dilution via nasogastric tube.

Preparation of parenteral drug: reconstitute with 10 ml sterile water for injection for concentration of 500 mg/100 ml. Further dilution required for IV methods of administrations: see manufacturer's directions.

Rapid infusion may cause sudden hypotension. Monitor BP and heart rate continuously through period of drug administration.

Extravasation of IV infusion must be avoided; severe irritation and necrosis can result.

Periodic urinalyses, renal and hepatic function tests, and hematologic studies are advised in all patients.

Serial tests of vancomycin blood levels are recommended in patients with borderline renal function and in patients over age 60 (generally maintained at 10 to 20 mg/ml).

Vancomycin may cause damage to auditory branch (not vestibular branch) of eighth cranial nerve, with consequent deafness, which may be permanent.

Serum levels of 60 to 80 mcg/ml are associated with ototoxicity. Tinnitus and high tone hearing loss may precede deafness which may progress even after drug is withdrawn. The elderly and those on high doses are especially susceptible. Warn patient to report ringing in ears promptly.

Instruct patient to adhere to drug regimen: i.e., not to increase, decrease, or interrupt dosage. The full course of prescribed drug therapy should be completed.

Monitor intake and output; report changes in intake and output ratio and pattern. Oliguria or cloudy or pink urine may be a sign of nephrotoxicity (also manifested by transient elevations in BUN, albumin, and hyaline and granular casts in urine).

Storage: *Oral and parenteral solution:* stable for 14 days in refrigerator; after further dilution, parenteral solution is stable 24 hours at controlled room temperature.

Drug Interactions. Possibility of additive toxicity with other ototoxic and/or nephrotoxic drugs (e.g., **aminoglycoside antibiotics, cephaloridine, colistin, polymyxin B, viomycin**).

PROTOTYPE

VASOPRESSIN INJECTION

(Pitressin)

VASOPRESSIN TANNATE

(Pitressin Tannate)

(vay-soe-press'in)
Hormone
Antidiuretic

VW

ACTIONS AND USES. Polypeptide hormone extracted from animal posterior pituitaries. Possesses pressor and antidiuretic (ADH) principles, but is relatively free of oxytocic properties. Produces concentrated urine by increasing tubular reabsorption of water (ADH activity), thus preserving up to 90% water. May increase Na and decrease K reabsorption, but plays no causative role in edema formation. In doses greater than those required for ADH effects, directly stimulates smooth-muscle contraction (especially in small arterioles and capillaries), thereby decreasing blood flow to splanchnic, coronary, GI, pancreatic, skin, and muscular systems. Small doses may produce anginal pain; large doses may precipitate myocardial infarction, decrease heart rate and cardiac output, and increase pulmonary arterial pressure and blood pressure. Pressor effects on GI system promote increased peristalsis (especially in large bowel), increased GI sphincter pressure, and decreased gastric secretion without effect on gastric acid concentration. Also contracts smooth muscle of gallbladder and urinary bladder; in large doses may stimulate uterine contraction. Promotes release of growth hormone, FSH, and corticotropin. The tannate (in peanut oil) is preferred for chronic therapy; intranasal aqueous vasopressin is effective for daily maintenance of mild diabetes insipidus.

Used as an antidiuretic to treat diabetes insipidus, to dispel gas shadows in abdominal roentgenography, and as prevention and treatment of postoperative abdominal distention. Also given to treat transient polyuria due to ADH deficiency, (related to head injuries or to neurosurgery). *Unlabeled Use:* test for differential diagnosis of nephrogenic, psychogenic, and neurohypophyseal diabetes insipidus; test to elevate ability of kidney to concentrate urine, and provocative test for pituitary release of corticotropin and growth hormone; emergency and adjunct pressor agent in the control of massive GI hemorrhage (e.g., esophageal varices).

ABSORPTION AND FATE. Following IM or SC injection of aqueous preparation, antidiuretic activity maintained 2 to 8 hours. Absorption of IM tannate is cumulative and cannot be determined for days; average duration of action 48 to 72 hours. IV infusion: pressor response for 30 to 60 minutes. Distributed throughout extracellular fluid, with little evidence of plasma protein binding; Half-life: 10 to 20 minutes. Most of drug is destroyed in liver and kidneys. Approximately 5% of subcutaneous dose of aqueous vasopressin is excreted unchanged after 4 hours; following IV administration, 5 to 15% of dose appears in urine.

CONTRAINDICATIONS AND PRECAUTIONS. Intravenous injection, chronic nephritis accompanied by nitrogen retention, ischemic heart disease, PVCs, advanced arteriosclerosis, during first stage of labor. *Cautious Use:* epilepsy, migraine, asthma, heart failure, angina pectoris; any state in which rapid addition to extracellular fluid may be hazardous; vascular disease, preoperative and postoperative polyuric patients, renal disease, goiter with cardiac complications, elderly patients, children, pregnancy.

ADVERSE/SIDE EFFECTS. Infrequent with low doses. **Hypersensitivity reactions:** rash, urticaria, anaphylaxis, tremor, sweating, bronchoconstriction, circumoral and facial pallor, angioneurotic edema, eructations, passage of gas, nausea, vomiting, pounding in head, anginal (in patient with coronary vascular disease), cardiac arrest, uterine cramps, water intoxication (especially with tannate). **Intraarterial infusion:** cardiac arrhythmia, pulmonary edema, bradycardia, gangrene at injection site. **Intranasal:** congestion, rhinorrhea, irritation, mucosal ulceration and pruritus, headache, conjunctivitis, heartburn, postnasal drip, abdominal cramps, increased bowel movements secondary to excessive use. **Large doses:** blanching of skin, abdominal cramps, nausea (almost spontaneously reversible), hypertension, bradycardia, minor arrhythmias, premature atrial contraction, heart block, peripheral vascular collapse, coronary insufficiency, myocardial infarction.

ROUTE AND DOSAGE. Adults: Vasopressin Injection: **Intramuscular, subcutaneous, intranasal (spray or cotton pledgets).** *Abdominal distention:* initial: 5 units IM increased to 10 units every 3 to 4 hours, as required. *Diabetes insipidus:* 5 to 10 units IM, SC, or intranasally, two or three times daily, as necessary. *Abdominal roentgenography:* 10 units IM 2 hours, then ½ hour before films are exposed. *GI hemorrhage* **(intraarterial):** 0.2 to 0.4 units/minute. Vasopressin tannate in oil: **Intramuscular, subcutaneous:** *Diabetes insipidus:* 1.5

to 5 units every 36 to 72 hours. **Pediatric:** (individualized): 2.5 to 10 units IM, SC, or intranasally.

NURSING IMPLICATIONS

Vasopressin tannate should never be administered IV. Before withdrawing drug for IM administration, warm ampul to body temperature and shake vigorously to disperse active principle.

The tannate injection is often painful, and allergic reactions may develop. It is preferred for use in chronic therapy because of its longer duration of action.

Administration of 1 or 2 glasses of water with vasopressin tannate may reduce side effects and improve therapeutic response.

Infants and children are more susceptible to volume disturbances (such as sudden reversal of polyuria) than are adults.

The use of vasopressin to stimulate peristalsis is being replaced largely by cholinergic drugs.

Following vasopressin injection given to relieve abdominal distention, a lubricated rectal tube (prescribed by physician) is inserted just past rectal sphincter and kept in place for about 1 hour. Auscultate abdomen at frequent intervals for peristaltic sounds. Record decrease in distention. Question patient about passage of flatus and return of normal pattern of bowel movements.

Some roentgenologists advise giving an enema before the first dose of vasopressin being used to clear abdomen of gas for x-rays.

Polyuria and thirst of diabetes insipidus are usually controlled for 36 to 48 hours with a single dose of the tannate.

At beginning of therapy, establish baseline data of blood pressure, weight, intake and output pattern and ratio. Monitor both blood pressure and weight throughout therapy. Report sudden changes in pattern to physician.

Patient with vascular disease and diabetes insipidus may receive small doses of vasopressin. Patient should be prepared for possibility of anginal attack and should have available a coronary vasodilator (e.g., nitroglycerin). Such pain should be reported to the physician.

Be alert to the fact that even small doses of vasopressin may precipitate myocardial infarction or coronary insufficiency, especially in elderly patients. Emergency equipment and drugs (antiarrhythmics) should be readily available.

Use of intraarterial vasopressin for emergency treatment of GI hemorrhage should not preclude other measures usually employed: e.g., blood transfusion, esophageal tamponade, ice water gavage, emergency surgery.

Intraarterial infusion constricts the splanchnic and peripheral vasculature and may cause gangrene in the peripheral entry vessel. Inspect infusion site and catheter at hourly intervals for blanching of skin. If noted, stop infusion stat and question physician about immediate local treatment (immediate flushing of catheter with a vasodilator has been prescribed). If vasopressin is to be continued, it should be administered via central venous catheter.

Dose used to stimulate diuresis has little effect on blood pressure.

Check patient's alertness and orientation frequently during therapy. Lethargy and confusion associated with headache may signal onset of water intoxication. Although insidious in rate of development, symptoms can lead to convulsions and terminal coma.

If water intoxication occurs (drowsiness, listlessness, headache, confusion, anuria, weight gain), vasopressin is withdrawn and fluid intake is restricted until specific gravity is at least 1.015 and polyuria occurs. With severe overhydration, osmotic diuresis is effected by drug therapy (e.g., mannitol, alone or in conjunction with furosemide).

Urine output, specific gravity and serum osmolality are monitored while patient is hospitalized. At home, patient must measure and record data related to polydipsia and polyuria. Teach patient to determine specific gravity and how to keep an accurate record of output. Patient should understand that intense thirst should diminish with treatment and undisturbed normal sleep should be restored.

Patient should avoid intake of hypertonic fluids (such as undiluted syrups), since these increase urine volume (increased sodium load).

Vasopressin test (rarely used) to determine functional ability of kidney to concentrate urine: give vasopressin 5 to 10 U IM; measure specific gravity 1 and 2 hours later (results are equivalent to that resulting from 18 hours of water deprivation). Normal response: urine osmolality 600 mOsm/kg or greater; specific gravity greater than 1.020. In diabetes-insipidus-like syndromes, urine remains hyposmotic relative to plasma.

Diagnostic Test Interferences. Vasopressin increases **plasma cortisol** levels.

Drug Interactions: Vasopressin

Plus	Interactions
Alcohol, cyclophosphamide, demeclocycline, epinephrine, heparin, lithium	Decrease antidiuretic activity of vasopressin
Antidiabetic agents, acetominophin, fludrocortisone, ganglionic blocking agents (e.g., guanethidine), neostigmine	Increase action of vasopressin
Chlorpropamide, clofibrate, carbamazepine	Increase antidiuretic activity of vasopressin

---

VECURONIUM

(Norcuon, ORG NC 45)

(vek-yoo-roe′-nee-um)
Skeletal muscle relaxant (nondepolarizing)
Neuromuscular blocking agent

ACTIONS AND USES. Intermediate-acting nondepolarizing skeletal muscle relaxant structurally similar to pancuronium, but about 1 to 1½ times more potent and has shorter duration of action. Unlike older neuromuscular blocking agents, demonstrates negligible histamine release and therefore has minimal direct effect on cardiovascular system. Similar to atracurium in having unique metabolic and excretion pathways (independent of renal function). However, since it relies heavily on biliary excretion, patients with hepatic disease may require dosage adjustment. Although it is four times more potent, it is like atracurium in having negligible cumulative tendencies with subsequent doses, provided recovery begins before dose is repeated. In common with other drugs of this class, inhibits neuromuscular transmission by competitive binding with acetylcholine to motor endplate receptors. Lacks analgesic action and has no apparent effect on pain threshold, consciousness or cerebration; given only after induction of general anesthesia.

Used as adjunct for general anesthesia to produce skeletal muscle relaxation during surgery. Especially useful for patients with severe renal disease, limited cardiac reserve, and history of asthma or allergy. Also used to facilitate endotracheal intubation.

ABSORPTION AND FATE. Prompt onset of action after IV administration (may be delayed in patients with reduced circulation time). Maximal neuromuscular blockade occurs within 3 to 5 minutes after IV injection. Under balanced anesthesia neuromuscular blockade lasts about 25 to 30 minutes. Recovery usually 95% complete in 45 to 65 minutes. Half-life: 65 to 75 minutes. About 60 to 80% bound to plasma proteins. From 30 to 35% excreted in urine in 24 hours. Not metabolized in liver, but undergoes biliary excretion; approximately 30 to 50% eliminated in feces via bile. Crosses placenta. Distribution into breast milk not known.

CONTRAINDICATIONS AND PRECAUTIONS. Hypersensitivity to any ingredient in the formulation; safe use during pregnancy (category C), or in nursing mother or neonate not established. *Cautious Use:* severe hepatic disease, impaired acid–base, fluid, and electrolyte balance, severe obesity, adrenal or neuromuscular disease (myasthenia gravis, Eaton–Lambert syndrome), patients with slow circulation time (cardiovascular disease, old age, edematous states), malignant hyperthermia.

ADVERSE/SIDE EFFECTS. (Generally well tolerated.) *Rarely:* skeletal muscle weakness, respiratory depression, hyperthermia.

ROUTE AND DOSAGE. **Adults and Children (10 to 17 years):** initial: 0.04 to 0.1 mg/kg. Maintenance dose (generally given in 25 to 40 minutes after initial dose if necessary): 0.010 to 0.015 mg/kg may be repeated at 12- to 15-minute intervals, under balanced anesthesia (slightly longer for potent inhalation anesthetics).

NURSING IMPLICATIONS

Administered only by qualified clinicians.

Baseline determinations of serum electrolytes, acid–base balance, renal and hepatic function are generally done as part of preanesthetic assessment.

Peripheral nerve stimulator may be used during and following drug administration to avoid risk of overdosage and to identify residual paralysis during recovery period. It is especially indicated when cautious use of vecuronium is specified *(see Contraindications and Precautions).*

Personnel and equipment for endotracheal intubation, administration of oxygen, artificial respiration, assisted or controlled ventilation should be immediately available.

For treatment of overdosage, have on hand: anticholinesterases such as edrophonium (Tensilon), neostigmine (Prostigmine), or pyridostigmine (Mestinon) to reverse neuromuscular blockade. Also have available atropine or glycopyrolate (Robinul) to counteract muscarinic side effects of anticholinesterase drugs.

Monitor vital signs at least every 15 minutes until stable, then every ½ hour for the next 2 hours. Also monitor airway patency until assured that patient has fully recovered from drug effects. Note rate, depth, and pattern of respirations. Obese patients and patients with myasthenia gravis or other neuromuscular disease may pose ventilation problems.

Evaluate patients for recovery from neuromuscular blocking (curare-like) effects as evidenced by ability to breathe naturally or to take deep breaths and cough, keep eyes open, lift head keeping mouth closed, adequacy of hand grip strength. Notify physician if recovery is delayed. *(See Absorption and Fate.)*

Note that recovery time may be delayed in patients with cardiovascular disease, edematous states, and in the elderly.

Following reconstitution, refrigerate or store solution at room temperature, not to exceed 30° C (86°F), unless otherwise directed by manufacturer. Discard solution after 24 hours.

See Tubocurarine (prototype nondepolarizing skeletal muscle relaxant).

Drug Interactions: Vecuronium

Plus	Interactions
Aminoglycoside antibiotics Bacitracin Colistimethate sodium Colistin B sulfate Enflurane Isoflurane Magnesium salts Polymyxin B (Aerosporin) Quinidine Tetracyclines Tubocurarine (Tubarine) and other nondepolarizing skeletal muscle relaxants	Possibility of enhanced neuromuscular blockade

PROTOTYPE

VERAPAMIL HYDROCHLORIDE

(Calan, Isoptin)

(ver-ap'a-mill)
Vasodilator
Antiarrhythmic
Antianginal
Calcium channel blocking agent

ACTIONS AND USES. Calcium channel blocking agent with short duration of action. Inhibits calcium ion (Ca) influx through slow channels into contractile and conductile myocardial cells and vascular smooth muscle cells. This action blocks release of internal stores of Ca, essential to the sequence that terminates in muscle contraction. Slow channel Ca influx into AV nodal cells results in slowed AV conduction and prolonged refractory period. Inhibits exercise-induced bronchoconstriction and may slow and convert multifocal atrial tachycardia to normal sinus rhythm. Vasodilation effect is reflected by transient, usually asymptomatic reduction in normal systemic arterial pressure, vascular resistance, and contractility and slight increase in left ventricular filling pressure. Coronary vasodilation improves blood flow and oxygen supply to myocardium leading to reduced anginal pain. Does not alter total serum Ca levels. Has local anaesthetic action 1.6 times that of procaine but significance to man is unclear.

Used for treatment of supraventricular tachyarrhythmias and temporary control of rapid ventricular rate in atrial flutter or atrial fibrillation and to relieve variant, rest (Prinzmetal's), and effort angina. *Unlabeled Use:* tocolytic to prevent preterm labor; treatment of vascular headaches; treatment of systemic and pulmonary hypertension, chronic heart failure, peripheral vasospastic disorders, and for myocardial preservation during cardiopulmonary bypass.

ABSORPTION AND FATE. Bolus IV dose produces therapeutic effects in 3 to 5 minutes with duration of action, 10 to 20 minutes. Use in atrial arrhythmias: onset of action on AV node, 1 to 5 minutes; peak action in 10 to 15 minutes with duration of 6 hours. Oral dose almost completely absorbed from GI tract; only 10 to 20% is bioavailable after first-pass hepatic metabolism. Elimination half-life is biphasic: initial: 4 minutes; terminal: 2 to 5 hours. Therapeutic plasma level ranges from 80 to 300 ng/ml. 90% protein binding. Approximately 70% excreted in urine and 16% or more in feces within 5 days. About 3 to 4% excreted as unchanged drug.

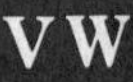

CONTRAINDICATIONS AND PRECAUTIONS. Severe hypotension, cardiogenic shock, cardiomegaly, digitalis toxicity, second- or third-degree AV block, severe congestive heart failure, concomitant IV beta-blockers (unless hours apart) sick sinus syndrome (except in patient with functioning artificial ventricular pacemaker). Safe use during pregnancy (category C for oral, category B for parenteral) or lactation not established. *Cautious Use:* concomitant digitalis, procainamide and quinidine therapy; disopyramide unless administered at least 48 hours before or 24 hours after verapamil, hepatic and renal impairment.

ADVERSE/SIDE EFFECTS. CNS: dizziness, headache; (rarely): vertigo, sleepiness, rotary nystagmus, depression. **CV:** hypotension (symptomatic), congestive heart failure, bradycardia, severe tachycardia. **GI:** nausea, abdominal discomfort, constipation. **Other:** ankle edema, pruritus, flushing, pulmonary edema, muscle fatigue, diaphoresis.

ROUTE AND DOSAGE. Oral: (investigational): *Hypertension:* 480 to 640 mg/day. *Angina:* 80 mg three or four times daily; increase by 80-mg increments weekly until optimal control is achieved. **Intravenous: Adults:** initial: 5 to 10 mg given as IV bolus over 2-minute period. Repeat dose (if necessary): 10 mg, 30 minutes after first dose. **Elderly:** administer dose over at least 3-minute period. **Pediatric:** 0.1 to 0.3 mg/kg over period of 2 minutes. Repeat dose (if necessary): same as initial dose, 30 minutes afterward. Maximum recommended single dose: 10 mg.

NURSING IMPLICATIONS

The initial use of verapamil should be in a treatment setting with facilities for monitoring and resuscitation, including D.C.-cardioversion capabilities.

Establish baseline data before treatment is started: blood pressure, pulse, and laboratory evaluations of hepatic and renal function.

Transient asymptomatic hypotension may accompany IV bolus. Instruct patient to remain in recumbent position for at least 1 hour after the dose is given to diminish subjective effects of hypotension.

During conversion to normal sinus rhythm or marked reduction of ventricular rate, a few benign complexes sometimes resembling PVCs may occur. They apparently have no clinical significance.

If IV verapamil is given concurrently with digitalis preparations monitor for AV block or for excessive bradycardia.

Monitor intake–output ratio during IV and early oral maintenance therapy. Renal function impairment prolongs duration of action increasing potential for toxicity and incidence of side effects.

Adverse reactions occur most frequently after IV administration, in the elderly or in patients with impaired renal function.

During early treatment for hypertension, check blood pressure near end of dosage interval or before administration of next dose to evaluate degree of control or whether dose intervals need to be changed.

Patient receiving verapamil at home should be informed about his or her usual pulse rate and instructed to take radial pulse before each dose. An irregular pulse or one slower than base level should be reported.

Warn patient to adhere to established guidelines for exercise program. Reduced anginal pain because of verapamil action can give a false interpretation of tolerance.

Caution against driving or operating dangerous equipment until patient's response to verapamil is established. Dizziness (experienced as lightheadedness) during early treatment period is common.

Advise patient to decrease caffeine-containing beverage intake (i.e., coffee, tea, chocolate). *(See Drug Interactions.)*

Until tolerance to reduced blood pressure is established, advise patient to change positions slowly from recumbent to standing to prevent falls because of vertigo.

Verapamil should decrease angina frequency, nitroglycerin consumption, hospitalizations, and episodes of ST segment deviation.

Instruct patient to record need for and use of nitroglycerin (activity at time recorded, dose interval, number of tablets needed to give pain relief) as data important to physician for setting the dosage regimen for verapamil with or without continued use of nitroglycerin.

If anginal pain (rest or effort) is not reduced by this drug therapy, the patient should notify the physician.

Stress importance of compliance. Caution patient not to alter established drug regimen, i.e., not to increase, omit or decrease dosage, or change dose intervals without consulting the physician.

Advise patient not to use OTC drugs unless they are specifically prescribed.

Emphasize importance of keeping appointments made for periodic evaluation of efficacy of verapamil and cardiovascular status.

Treatment of overdosage is supportive and may include: beta-adrenergic stimulation or IV Ca solutions to increase transmembrane influx of Ca ion through slow channels; vasopressor agents, cardiac pacing or cardiopulmonary rescusitation.

Inspect parenteral drug preparation before administration. Solution should be clear and colorless.

Store at 15° to 30°C (59° to 86°F) and protect from light.

Diagnostic Test Interferences. Verapamil may cause elevations of serum **AST, AST, alkaline phosphase.**

Drug Interactions: Verapamil

Plus	Interactions
Beta-adrenergic agonists (epinephrine, isoproterenol)	May oppose calcium blocking action of verapamil
Beta-adrenergic blocking agents (e.g., propranolol, metoprolol)	May augment cardiodepressant activity of verapamil
Highly protein-bound drugs: e.g., oral anticoagulants, hydantoins, salicylates, sulfonamides, sulfonylureas	Verapamil could be displaced by or could displace these agents from protein binding sites thus increasing risk of toxicity. Concurrent use with caution
Methylxanthines (caffeine, theophylline)	May oppose Ca blocking effects of verapamil
Digoxin, possibly digitoxin	May elevate digoxin and digitoxin blood levels and increase risk of digitalis toxicity
Quinidine	Increased incidence of symptomatic hypotension

VIDARABINE

(Adenine Arabinoside, ARA-A, Vira-A)

(vye-dare'a-been)
Antiinfective
Antiviral

ACTIONS AND USES. Pyrimidine nucleoside obtained from fermentation cultures of *Streptomyces antibioticus.* Mechanism of action not known, but appears to block early stages of DNA synthesis by inhibiting DNA polymerase. Has antiviral activity against herpes simplex virus types 1 and 2, varicella zoster, vaccinia, cytomegalovirus, hepatitis B virus, and Epstein-Barr virus. Not active against smallpox, adenovirus, DNA or RNA viruses (except Rhabdovirus and Oncornavirus), bacteria, and fungi. A degree of immunocompetence must be present if drug is to be effective. Potentially mutagenic and oncogenic.

Used systemically for treatment of herpes simplex encephalitis and herpes zoster infections in patients with suppressed immunologic responses. Used topically (ophthalmic) for treatment of acute keratoconjunctivitis and recurrent epithelial keratitis caused by herpes simplex virus types 1 and 2. Topical antibiotics and topical corticosteroids may be used concurrently.

ABSORPTION AND FATE. Following topical application to eye, a trace amount of the major metabolite Ara-Hx (ara-hypoxanthine) is found in aqueous humor; no appreciable systemic absorption. Following IV administration, rapidly deaminated to Ara-Hx, which is less active than parent drug; it has mean half-life of 3.3 hours and is 0 to 3% protein-bound. Accumulates in plasma in patient with impaired renal function. Vidarabine half-life: 1.5 hours; 20 to 30% protein bound. Parent drug and metabolite widely distributed in body tissues and fluid and both cross blood–brain barrier. Excreted primarily by kidneys, mostly as the metabolite. Probably crosses placenta. Secretion into breast milk not determined.

CONTRAINDICATIONS AND PRECAUTIONS. Hypersensitivity to vidarabine. Safe use during pregnancy (category C) and breast feeding not established. *Cautious Use:* impaired renal or hepatic function, patients susceptible to fluid overload or cerebral edema.

ADVERSE/SIDE EFFECTS. **Intravenous: CNS** (with high doses): hallucinations, confusion, psychosis, dizziness, ataxia, weakness, tremor, fatal metabolic encephalopathy. **GI** (usually transient): nausea, vomiting, anorexia, diarrhea, weight loss. **Hematologic:** anemia, thrombocytopenia, neutropenia, decrease in WBC, Hgb, Hct. **Hepatic:** elevated bilirubin and SGOT (AST). **Other:** SIADH and hyponatremia (association with vidarabine not determined), malaise, pruritus, painful injection site. *Ophthalmic use:* burning, itching, mild irritation, lacrimation, foreign body sensation, pain, photophobia, punctal occlusion, superficial punctate keratitis. Association with ophthalmic vidarabine not determined: uveitis, stromal edema, secondary glaucoma, trophic defects, corneal vascularization, and hyphema.

ROUTE AND DOSAGE. **Ophthalmic:** approximately ½ inch ribbon into lower conjunctival sac five times daily at 3-hour intervals. After reepithelialization, treatment usually given for an additional 5 to 7 days twice daily. **Intravenous:** 15 mg/kg daily for 10 days.

NURSING IMPLICATIONS

Intravenous administration:

- Dilute the vidarabine just before administration and use within 48 hours.
- Shake vial well before withdrawing dose, and transfer it to appropriate IV fluid. Most IV infusion fluids are suitable. Blood products, protein, or other colloidal fluids should not be used. Follow manufacturer's directions.
- A large volume of fluid is required to dissolve vidarabine since it is only slightly soluble (1 L of IV infusion fluid will solubilize a maximum of 450 mg of vidarabine, or 1 mg of drug to 2.22 ml of IV fluid). Agitate thoroughly until drug is completely dissolved. Prewarming the IV infusion fluid to 35° to 40°C (95° to 100°F) will facilitate dissolution. Once dissolved, subsequent shaking is unnecessary. *Do not refrigerate the dilution.*
- Final dilution is administered through an in-line membrane filter (pore size of 0.45 μ or smaller).
- Infusion should be administered at a constant rate over 12 to 24 hours.
- Diagnosis of meningitis should be established before initiation of therapy by studies

of CSF, brain scan, EEG, or CAT. Vidarabine therapy is reportedly most effective when started before patient becomes semicomatose or comatose.
- Periodic hematologic tests are recommended during therapy: Hgb, Hct, WBC, platelets.

Ophthalmic use:
- Instruct patient to wash hands before and after treatment.
- Caution patient that vision may be temporarily hazy following instillation, and to avoid potentially hazardous activities until vision clears.
- Advise patient that drug may cause sensitivity to bright lights, and to use sunglasses, if necessary.
- Generally, epithelial healing begins in 2 to 4 days with complete healing in 1 to 3 weeks. If patient deviates from this expected course, other forms of therapy may be prescribed. Keep physician informed.
- Caution patient not to exceed recommended dose, frequency and duration of treatment.
- *See Index: Drug administration: eye ointment.*

Drug Interaction. Concurrent therapy with **allopurinol** increases potential for CNS side effects.

VINBLASTINE SULFATE

(Velban, Velbe, VLB)

(vin-blast′een)
Antineoplastic
Mitotic inhibitor

ACTIONS AND USES. Cell cycle specific alkaloid, extracted from periwinkle plant *Vinca rosea.* Arrests mitosis in metaphase by combination with microtubule proteins; may also interfere with other microtubular functions such as phagocytosis and cell mobility. In contrast to vincristine, has potent myelosuppressive and immunosuppressive properties, but produces less neurotoxicity. Spectrum of activity not completely established.

Used for palliative treatment of Hodgkin's disease and non-Hodgkin's lymphomas, choriocarcinoma, lymphosarcoma, neuroblastoma, mycosis fungoides, advanced testicular germinol cell cancer, histiocytosis and other malignancies resistant to other chemotherapy. Used singly or in combination with other chemotherapeutic drugs.

ABSORPTION AND FATE. Following IV administration, rapidly clears bloodstream and concentrates primarily in liver where it is partially metabolized. About 75% protein-bound with additional localization on platelets and leukocytes. Half-life: initial phase: 53 to 98 minutes; terminal phase: 24 hours. Toxicity increases if liver disease is present. Poor penetration of blood–brain barrier. Excreted in bile to feces; less than 5% of dose excreted in urine.

CONTRAINDICATIONS AND PRECAUTIONS. Leukopenia, bacterial infection, pregnancy, men and women of childbearing potential, elderly patients with cachexia or skin ulcers. *Cautious Use:* malignant cell infiltration of bone marrow, obstructive jaundice, hepatic impairment, history of gout; use of small amount of drug for long periods; use in eyes.

ADVERSE/SIDE EFFECTS. Generally dose-related and short-lived. **CNS (uncommon):** mental depression, peripheral neuritis, numbness and paresthesias of tongue and extremities, loss of deep tendon reflexes, headache, convulsions, psychoses (rare). **Dermatologic:** alopecia (reversible), vesiculation. **GI:** vesiculation of mouth, stomatitis, pharyngitis, anorexia, nausea, vomiting, diarrhea, ileus, abdominal pain, constipation, rectal bleeding, hemorrhagic enterocolitis, bleeding of old peptic ulcer. **Hematologic:** leukopenia (most common), agranulocytosis, thrombocytopenia and anemia (infrequent). **Other:** phlebitis, cellulitis, and sloughing following extravasation (at injection site); fever, weight loss, muscular pains, weakness, urinary retention, hyperuricemia, parotid gland pain and tenderness, tumor site pain, aspermia, Raynaud's phenomenon, photosensitivity.

ROUTE AND DOSAGE. After initial dose, subsequent doses (individualized incremental approach) given at 7-day intervals based upon WBC counts or until maximum recommended dose is reached. **Intravenous: Adult:** initial: 3.7 mg/m^2; maximum recommended dose not to exceed 18.5 mg/m^2. **Pediatric:** initial: 2.5 mg/m^2; maximum recommended dose not to exceed 12.5 mg/m^2. Dose is not increased after that dose which reduces white cell count to about 3000 cells/mm^3. The maintenance dose is one increment smaller than the dose that established the above degree of leukopenia.

NURSING IMPLICATIONS

To prepare solution: add 10 ml sodium chloride injection (preserved with phenol or benzyl alcohol) to 10 mg of drug (yields 1 mg/ml). Other diluents not advised.

Drug is usually injected into tubing of running IV infusion over period of 1 minute. If given directly into vein, fresh, dry needle is used (discard needle used to withdraw drug). To ensure no spillage into extravascular tissue, needle and syringe should be rinsed with venous blood before withdrawal from vein.

If extravasation occurs, stop infusion promptly; applications of moderate heat and local injection of hyaluronidase are advised to help disperse extravasated drug. Infusion should be restarted in another vein. Observe injection site; sloughing may occur.

Avoid contact with eyes. Severe irritation and persisting corneal changes may occur. Copious amounts of water should be applied immediately and thoroughly. Wash both eyes; don't assume one eye escaped contamination.

Recovery from leukopenic nadir follows rapidly, usually within 7 to 14 days. With high doses, total leukocyte count may not return to normal for 3 weeks.

Even if 7 days have passed, drug is not administered unless WBC count has not returned to at least 4000/mm^3.

Thrombocyte reduction seldom occurs unless patient has had prior treatment with other antineoplastics. However, be alert to unexplained bruising or bleeding which should be promptly reported.

Classical ABVD regimen used to treat advanced Hodgkin's disease combines rapid simultaneous IV administration of doxorubicin, bleomycin, vinblastine, dacarbazine on days 1 and 14 of each cycle. Reportedly, ABVD regimen can induce complete remission in more than half of the patients with MOPP-resistant disease (mechlorethamine, vincristine, procarbazine, prednisone).

A new treatment protocol in which drug combinations are alternated with significant success in the maintenance of remission in Stage IV Hodgkin's disease involves the systematic switching of MOPP *(see Vincristine)* and ABVD regimens for a minimum of 12 months of treatment (in the absence of disease progression).

In patients receiving alternating combination drug therapy (MOPP with ABVD) vomiting (pronounced because of doxorubicin and dacarbazine), and transient but frank, alopecia secondary to ABVD chemotherapy may occur in about 10% of patients.

An antiemetic agent given before the injection may help to control nausea and vomiting.

Course of therapy may be continued 12 weeks or more for adequate clinical trial. Encourage community-based patient to keep all appointments so that course of treatment is not interrupted.

With exception of epilation, leukopenia and neurologic side effects, adverse reactions seldom persist beyond 24 hours.

Temporary mental depression sometimes occurs on second or third day after treatment begins.

Monitor bowel elimination pattern and bowel sounds to recognize severe constipation or paralytic ileus. A stool softener may be necessary.

Instruct patient to avoid exposure to infection, injury to skin or mucous membranes, and excessive physical stress, especially during leukocyte nadir period.

Alopecia is frequently not total; in some patients, regrowth begins during maintenance therapy period.

Instruct patient to report promptly onset of symptoms of agranulocytosis: profound weakness, high fever, chills, rapid and weak pulse, sore throat, dysphagia, pharyngeal and buccal ulcerations. Appropriate treatment should not be delayed.

Skin surfaces over pressure areas should be inspected daily if patient is not ambulating. Note condition of skin of the elderly especially, since normal aging changes of integument (thinning, decrease in subcutaneous fatty tissue and microcirculation, diminished hydration) promote breakdown under stressed conditions.

Avoid exposure to sunlight unless protected with sunscreen lotion (SPF above 12), and clothing.

See Mechlorethamine for nursing care of stomatitis. Drug should be stopped if oral tissues breakdown.

Preserved in tight, light-resistant containers in refrigerator. Reconstituted solution may be refrigerated up to 30 days without loss of potency.

VINCRISTINE SULFATE

(Oncovin, VCR, LCR)

(vin-kris'teen)
Antineoplastic
Mitotic Inhibitor

ACTIONS AND USES. Cell cycle specific vinca alkaloid (obtained from periwinkle plant *Vinca rosea*); analogue of vinblastine. Antineoplastic mechanism unclear; arrests mitosis at metaphase, thereby inhibiting cell division. In contrast to vinblastine, has relatively low toxic effect on normal cells and thus produces minimal myelosuppression; however, neurologic and neuromuscular effects are more severe.

Used in treatment of acute lymphoblastic and other leukemias, Hodgkin's disease, lymphosarcoma, neuroblastoma, Wilm's tumor, lung and breast cancer, and reticular cell carcinoma, osteogenic and other sarcomas. *Unlabeled Use:* Treatment of idiopathic thrombocytopenic purpura. Used alone or adjunctively with other antineoplastics.

ABSORPTION AND FATE. Following IV administration, rapidly distributed with extensive tissue binding; about 75% plasma protein bound with additional binding to formed blood elements. Half-life: initial: 50 to 155 minutes; terminal: 23 to 85 hours. Hepatic dysfunction increases toxicity. Hepatic metabolism; poor penetration into CSF. Excreted primarily in feces via bile.

CONTRAINDICATIONS AND PRECAUTIONS. Obstructive jaundice, pregnancy, men and women of childbearing age; patient with demyelinating form of Charcot-Marie-Tooth syndrome. *Cautious Use:* leukopenia, preexisting neuromuscular disease, hypertension, infection, patients receiving drugs with neurotoxic potential.

ADVERSE/SIDE EFFECTS. Usually dose-related and reversible. **CNS:** peripheral neuropathy, neuritic pain, paresthesias, especially of hands and feet; foot and hand drop, sensory loss, athetosis, ataxia, loss of deep tendon reflexes, muscle atrophy, dysphagia, weakness in larynx and extrinsic eye muscles, ptosis, diplopia, mental depression. **Dermatologic:** urticaria, rash, alopecia, cellulitis and phlebitis following extravasation (at injection site). **GI:** stomatitis, pharyngitis, anorexia, nausea, vomiting, diarrhea, abdominal cramps, severe constipation (upper-colon impaction), paralytic ileus, (especially in children), rectal bleeding; hepatotoxicity. **GU:** uri nary retention, polyuria, dysuria, SIADH (high urinary Na excretion, hyponatremia, dehydration, hypotension); uric acid nephropathy. **Hematologic** (rare): thrombocytopenia, anemia, leukopenia. **Ophthalmic:** optic atrophy with blindness; transient cortical blindness, ptosis, diplopia, photophobia. **Other:** convulsions with hypertension, malaise, fever, headache, pain in parotid gland area, hyperuricemia, hyperkalemia, weight loss.

ROUTE AND DOSAGE. Various schedules have been used; all are highly individualized. **Intravenous: Adult:** initial: 0.01 mg/kg at weekly intervals. **Children:** initial: 0.05 mg/kg at weekly intervals. When remission is achieved, dose is reduced to maintenance level: **Adult:** 0.02 to 0.05 mg/kg/week. **Children:** 0.05 to 0.75 mg/kg/week.

NURSING IMPLICATIONS

Administration directly into vein or into running infusion should be over a 1 minute period. Syringe and needle should be rinsed with venous blood before needle is withdrawn.

If extravasation occurs, drug administration is discontinued immediately and restarted in another vein. Hyaluronidase should be injected locally into surrounding tissue. Apply moderate heat to the area to disperse drug and to minimize danger of sloughing. Be cautious because of possible sensory loss. Check agency policy or consult physician.

Reconstitute with provided solution (Bacteriostatic Sodium Chloride) or with sterile water or physiological saline to concentrations of 0.01 to 1.0 mg/ml.

Classical MOPP treatment of advanced Hodgkin's disease combines administration of mechlorethamine and vincristine by rapid IV injection on days 1 and 8 of each cycle, and oral procarbazine and oral prednisone each day for 14 days only during each cycle. After blood studies, providing the disease process is not progressing, the next cycle starts on day 29.

Chemotherapy failure with MOPP has been attributed to development of drug resistance. Alternating drug combinations (e.g., MOPP and ABVD) in a cyclical manner has been effective in prolonging remissions *(see Vinblastine).*

Monitor intake–output ratio and pattern, blood pressure, and temperature daily. Record on flow chart as indicators for adaptations in nursing and drug regimen.

Regularly scheduled serum uric acid determinations, adequate hydration, and administration of a uricosuric agent may be prescribed to prevent uric acid nephropathy. Advise patient to report promptly stomach, bone or joint pain, and swelling of lower legs and ankles.

Weigh patient under standard conditions weekly or more often if ordered. In the presence of edema or ascites, patient's ideal weight is used to determine dosage. Report a steady gain or sudden weight change to physician.

A prophylactic regimen against constipation and paralytic ileus (adequate fluids, high fiber diet, laxatives) is usually started at beginning of treatment with vincristine. Encourage patient to report changes in bowel habit as soon as manifested. Paralytic ileus is most likely to occur in young children.

Note that while fluid intake should be encouraged to prevent constipation, if hyponatremia is a problem, fluid deprivation may be necessary. Consult physician for guidelines.

An empty rectum with colicky pain may be misdiagnosed. Physician may order an abdominal flat plate to rule out high fecal impaction. If present, high enemas and laxatives may be effective.

Complete bone marrow remission in leukemia varies widely and may not occur for as long as 100 days after therapy is started.

Care should be taken to distinguish between the depression associated with realization of neoplastic disease and that which is drug-induced.

Toxicity with vincristine occasionally follows an irreversible sequence: sensory impairment and paresthesias, neuritic pain, motor difficulties.

Neuromuscular side effects, most apt to appear in the patient with preexisting neuromuscular disease, usually disappear after 6 weeks of treatment. Occasionally, however, side effects persist for prolonged periods of time after therapy is terminated.

Children are especially susceptible to neuromuscular side effects.

Grasp hands of patient each day to detect onset of hand muscular weakness, and check deep tendon reflexes (depression of Achilles reflex is the earliest sign of neuropathy). Also observe for and report promptly: mental depression, ptosis, double vision, hoarseness, paresthesias, neuritic pain, and motor difficulties.

If patient is bedridden, provide prophylactic measures to prevent footdrop; inspect skin over pressure areas frequently to prevent tissue breakdown.

Walking may be impaired; check patient's ability to ambulate, and supply support if necessary.

Dental caries or periodontal disease should be treated since patient is highly susceptible to superinfections.

See Mechlorethamine for nursing care of stomatitis.

Alopecia (reversible) (up to 70% of patients) is reportedly the most common adverse reaction any may persist for the duration of therapy. However, regrowth of hair may start before end of treatment. Before therapy begins, discuss this side effect with patient so that plans for providing a wig or hair piece can be made if desired. Inform patient that scalp hair will drop out in large clumps on pillow at night. This is a very distressing side effect. Many patients avoid all social contacts because of the loss of hair (self-image problems).

To prevent injury to rectal mucosa, use of rectal thermometer or intrusive tubing should be avoided if possible.

Leukopenia occurs in a significant number of patients; leukocyte count in children usually reaches nadir on 4th day and begins to rise on 5th day after drug administration. Provide special protection against infection or injury during leukopenic days.

Reconstituted solution may be refrigerated for 14 days without loss of potency. Both dry form and solutions should be protected from light. Refrigerate dry powder.

VITAMIN A

vye'ta-min

(Acon, Afaxin, Alphalin, Aquasol A)

Vitamin

ACTIONS AND USES. Synthetic fat-soluble vitamin available for clinical use as retinol (vitamin A alcohol) or retinol esters. Obtained from seawater fish liver oils or prepared synthetically. Formulation includes vitamin A as well as its precursors, alpha, beta, and gamma carotene, and crystoxanthin. Expressed in terms of international units (IU). One IU (equivalent to 1 USP unit) is equal to 0.3 mcg of retinol, 0.34 mcg of vitamin A acetate, or 0.6 mcg of beta carotene (provitamin A). Vitamin A is essential for normal growth and development of bones and teeth, for integrity of epithelial and mucosal surfaces and for synthesis of rhodopsin (visual purple) necessary for visual dark adaptation.

Also, thought to act as cofactor in biosynthesis of adrenal steroids, mucopolysaccharides, cholesterol, and RNA. Stimulates healing of cortisone-retarded wounds when applied topically.

Used in treatment of vitamin A deficiency and as dietary supplement during periods of increased requirements, such as pregnancy, lactation, infancy and infections. Also used as replacement therapy in conditions that affect absorption, mobilization, or storage of vitamin A, e.g., steatorrhea, severe biliary obstruction, hepatic cirrhosis, total gastrectomy. Used in skin disorders [e.g., folliculosis keratosis (Darier's disease), psoriasis], however, other retinoids are being preferentially selected. Also used as a screening test for fat malabsorption.

ABSORPTION AND FATE. Readily absorbed from GI tract (in presence of bile salts, pancreatic lipase, and dietary fat). Aqueous formulations produce more rapid and higher blood concentrations than oil form; absorption of emulsion is moderate. Stored mainly in liver; small amounts also found in kidney and body fat. Metabolites excreted in feces and urine. Does not readily cross placenta, but passes into breast milk.

CONTRAINDICATIONS AND PRECAUTIONS. History of sensitivity to vitamin A or to any ingredient in formulation, hypervitaminosis A, oral administration to patients with malabsorption syndrome. Safe use in amounts exceeding 6000 IU during pregnancy not established. *Cautious Use:* women on oral contraceptives, high doses in nursing mothers.

ADVERSE/SIDE EFFECTS. CNS: irritability, headache, intracranial hypertension (pseudotumor cerebri), increased intracranial pressure, bulging fontanelles, papilledema, exophthalmos, miosis, nystagmus. **Dermatologic:** gingivitis, lip fissures, excessive sweating, drying or cracking of skin, pruritus, increase in skin pigmentation, massive desquamation, brittle nails, alopecia. **Hypervitaminosis A syndrome** (general manifestations): malaise, lethargy, abdominal discomfort, anorexia, vomiting. **Skeletal:** slow growth; deep tender hard lumps (subperiosteal thickening) over radius, tibia, occiput; migratory arthralgia; retarded growth; premature closure of epiphyses. **Other:** hypomenorrhea, hepatosplenomegaly, hypercalcemia, polydipsia, polyurea, jaundice, leukopenia, hypoplastic anemias, vitamin A plasma levels over 1200 IU/dl, elevations of sedimentation rate and prothrombin time; anaphylaxis, death after IV use.

ROUTE AND DOSAGE. Oral: *Severe deficiency:* **Adults and children (over 8 years):** 500,000 IU daily for 3 days, followed by 50,000 IU daily for 2 weeks; follow-up therapy 10,000 to 20,000 IU daily for 2 months. *Dietary supplement:* **Children (4 to 8 years):** 15,000 IU daily; **Children (under 4 years):** 10,000 IU daily. **Intramuscular: Adults:** 100,000 IU daily for 3 days, followed by 50,000 IU daily for 2 weeks. **Children (1 to 8 years):** 17,500 to 35,000 IU daily for 10 days; **infants:** 7500 to 15,000 IU daily for 10 days.

NURSING IMPLICATIONS

Evaluation of dosage is made with consideration of patient's average daily intake of vitamin A. Dietary and drug history is advisable, e.g., intake of fortified foods, dietary supplements, self-administration or prescription drug sources. Women taking oral contraceptives tend to have significantly high plasma vitamin A levels.

Vitamin A deficiency is often associated with protein malnutrition as well as other vitamin deficiencies. May be manifested by night blindness, retardation of growth and development, epithelial alterations, susceptibility to infection, abnormal dryness of skin, mouth, and eyes (xerophthalmia) progressing to keratomalacia (ulceration and necrosis of cornea and conjunctiva), urinary tract calculi.

Recommended daily allowance (RDA): adult females 4000 IU, adult males 5000 IU, lactating women 6000 IU, children 4 to 6 years 2500 IU, infants 2100 IU.

Cause of deficiency should be clearly identified for patient, and he or she and responsible family members should be included in dietary planning.

About half of vitamin A activity in the average American diet comes from carotene (provitamin A), found in yellow and green (leafy) vegetables and yellow fruits. Sources of preformed vitamin A are supplied primarily from livers of cod, halibut, tuna, and shad, fat of dairy products, fortified margarine and milk, and egg yolk.

Avoid use of mineral oil while on vitamin A therapy.

Instruct patient to report to physician symptoms of overdosage: nausea, vomiting, anorexia, drying and cracking of skin or lips, headache, loss of hair.

Patients receiving therapeutic doses should be closely supervised. Inform patient and family that self-medication with vitamin A is potentially harmful.

For treatment of overdosage (hypervitaminosis A), drug should be discontinued immediately. Most signs and symptoms *(see Adverse/Side Effects)* subside within a week, but tender, hard swellings in extremities and occiput may remain for several months.

Caution patient to keep drug out of reach of children. Toxicity (hypervitaminosis A) from a large dose of vitamin A is more common in a child than an adult.

Preserved in tight, light-resistant containers.

Diagnostic Test Interferences. Vitamin A may falsely increase **serum cholesterol** determinations (Zlatkis-Zak reaction); may falsely elevate **bilirubin** determination (with Ehrlich's reagent).

Drug Interactions. Concomitant administration of **mineral oil** may decrease absorption of vitamin A. **Corticosteroids** may increase plasma vitamin A levels.

VITAMIN E

Vitamin

(Aquasol E, CEN-E, Daltose, E-Ferol, Epsilan-M, E-Vital, Pheryl-E, Tocopherol, Vita-Plus E, Viterra-E)

ACTIONS AND USES. Vitamin E refers to a group of naturally occurring fat-soluble substances known as tocopherols (alpha, beta, gamma, and delta). Alpha tocopherol, comprising 90% of the tocopherols, is the most biologically potent and has been synthesized. Prevents peroxidation, a process that adds oxygen to molecules in a way that gives rise to free radicals, highly reactive chemical structures that damage cell membranes and alter nuclear proteins. Some researchers hypothesize that this protective function may be a deterrent to the constant free radical damage thought to be a factor in the initiation and promotion of many cancers. Vitamin E is essential to the digestion and metabolism of polyunsaturated fats; it maintains the integrity of cell membranes, protects against blood clot formation by decreasing platelet aggregation, enhances vitamin A utilization, and promotes normal growth, development, and tone of muscles. Vitamin E deficiency causes no specific disease in humans but has been associated with increased susceptibility of RBC to hemolysis by biologic oxidizing agents and with edema, irritability, and hemolytic anemia in premature neonates. Low serum tocopherol in adults and children appears to be associated with creatinuria, muscle weakness, and decreased RBC survival—conditions that are completely reversed by the administration of vitamin E. Although vitamin E has not been shown to have any therapeutic value, it is prescribed for a number of clinical problems: anemia associated with protein-calorie malnutrition (kwastiorkor), infertility, impotence, habitual abortion, menopausal syndrome, chronic cystic mastitis, peptic ulcer, burns, cancer prevention, skin disorders, heart diseases.

Used to treat and prevent hemolytic anemia due to vitamin E deficiency in premature neonates; to prevent retrolental fibroplasia secondary to oxygen treatment in neonates, and in treatment of diseases with secondary erythrocyte membrane abnormalities, e.g., sickle cell anemia, G6PD deficiency and as supplement in malabsorption syndromes. Used in patients on diets containing large amounts of polyunsaturated fats for long periods and in the patient who abruptly discontinues such a diet. Also used topically for dry or chapped skin and minor skin disorders. *Investigational Use:* muscular dystrophy and a number of other conditions, with no conclusive evidence of value. A component of many multivitamin formulations, and in topical deodorant preparations as an antioxidant.

ABSORPTION AND FATE. Readily and almost completely absorbed from GI tract, if fat absorption is normal, and enters blood via lymph. Distributed to all body tissues and stored in adipose tissue in amounts adequate to meet body requirements for 4 or more years on a deficient diet. Metabolized in liver and excreted primarily in bile. Placental transfer is incomplete.

ADVERSE/SIDE EFFECTS. Appears to be nontoxic at therapeutic dosage range. With excessive doses for prolonged periods: skeletal muscle weakness, headache, blurred vision, fatigue, nausea, diarrhea, intestinal cramps, gonadal dysfunction; increased serum creatine kinase, cholesterol, triglycerides; decreased serum thyroxine and triiodothyromine; increased urinary estrogens, androgens; creatinuria; sterile abscess, thrombophlebitis, contact dermatitis.

ROUTE AND DOSAGE. *Vitamin E deficiency:* **Adults: Oral; intramuscular:** 60 to 75 IU daily. **Children: Oral:** 1 IU/kg daily. *Prophylactic:* **Adults:** 12 to 15 IU daily. **Children:** 7 to 10 IU daily. **Topical:** cream, lotion, ointment.

NURSING IMPLICATIONS

Daily vitamin E requirements are estimated, but are related to the dietary intake of polyunsaturated fatty acids (PUVA) (especially linoleic acid).

Recommended daily dietary allowance (RDA) of vitamin E for infants is 4 IU; for children 4 to 6 years, 9 IU; adult males, 15 IU; adult females, 12 IU; pregnant and lactating women, 15 IU.

Absorption of vitamin E from GI tract requires presence of bile.

The estimated daily requirement is usually provided by the normal adult diet, but requirements are higher with increased intake of unsaturated fats.

Food–Drug Interaction: RDA of vitamin E may be increased if patient is also taking a large dose of iron.

Wheat germ is the richest source of vitamin E; also found in vegetable oils (sunflower, corn, soybean, cottonseed); green leafy vegetables, nuts, dairy products, eggs, cereals, meat, liver.

Preserved in tight containers, protected from light.

Drug Interactions. Concomitant administration of vitamin E may enhance oral anticoagulant activity. Excessive use of **mineral oil** may decrease absorption of vitamin E. Vitamin A absorption, utilization, and storage may be increased by vitamin E (controversial).

W

PROTOTYPE

WARFARIN, POTASSIUM
(Athrombin-K)

WARFARIN SODIUM
(Confarin, Coumadin Sodium, Panwarfin)

(war'far-in)
Anticoagulant, oral
Coumarin

ACTIONS AND USES. Indirectly interferes with blood clotting by depressing hepatic synthesis of vitamin K–dependent coagulation factors: II (prothrombin), VII (proconvertin), IX (Christmas factor or plasma thromboplastin component), and X (Stuart–Prower factor). Deters further extension of existing thrombi and prevents new clots from forming. Has no effect on already synthesized circulating coagulation factors, or on circulating thrombi but may prevent extension of existing thrombi. Does not reverse ischemic tissue damage and has no effect on platelets. Unlike heparin, action is cumulative and more prolonged. Warfarin is not cross allergenic with other coumarin derivatives. Some patients have an inherited resistance to warfarin and other oral anticoagulants (an autosomal dominant derivative) and thus require larger than usual doses to achieve therapeutic effects.

Used for prophylaxis and treatment of deep venous thrombosis, and its extension, pulmonary embolism, treatment of atrial fibrillation with embolization. Also used as adjunct in treatment of coronary occlusion, transient cerebral ischemic attacks, and as a prophylactic in patients with prosthetic cardiac valves. Used extensively as rodenticide.

ABSORPTION AND FATE. Onset of action in 2 to 12 hours; peak prothrombin activity (i.e., after circulating functional coagulation factors are depleted) in 0.5 to 3 days. Duration of action: 2 to 5 days following single dose. Half-life: ½ to 3 days, is independent of dose. (Warfarin contains equal parts of an R and S isomer that differ in potency and rate of metabolism. The S isomer is the more potent and most likely to interact with other drugs.) Approximately 99% weakly bound to plasma albumin. Accumulates mainly in liver where it is metabolized; also distributed to lungs, spleen, kidney. Excreted in urine and feces via bile as inactive metabolites and traces of unchanged drug. Marked individual differences in metabolism and excretion rates. Crosses placenta. Amount in breast milk is negligible.

CONTRAINDICATIONS AND PRECAUTIONS. Hemorrhagic tendencies: vitamin C or K deficiency, hemophilia, coagulation factor deficiencies, dyscrasias; active bleeding, open wounds, active peptic ulcer, visceral carcinoma, esophageal varices, malabsorption syndromes, hypertension (diastolic BP >110 mm Hg), cerebral vascular disease, pregnancy, pericarditis with acute MI, severe hepatic or renal disease, continuous tube drainage of any orifice, subacute bacterial endocarditis, recent surgery of brain, spinal cord, eye, regional or lumbar block anesthesia, threatened abortion, unreliable patients; *Cautious Use:* alcoholism, allergic disorders, during menstruation, nursing mother, elderly, debilitated patients; in *endogenous factors that may increase prothrombin time response* (enhance anticoagulant effect): carcinoma, congestive heart failure, collagen diseases, hepatic and renal insufficiency, diarrhea, fever, pancreatic disorders, malnutrition, vitamin K deficiency, alcoholism, *endogenous factors that may decrease prothrombin time response* (decrease anticoagulant response): edema, hypothyroidism, hyperlipidemia, hypercholesterolemia, chronic alcoholism, hereditary resistance to coumarin therapy.

ADVERSE/SIDE EFFECTS. Major or minor hemorrhage from any tissue or organ. **GI:** anorexia, nausea, vomiting, abdominal cramps, diarrhea, steatorrhea, stomatitis. **Hypersensitivity:** dermatitis, urticaria, pruritus, fever, anaphylaxis (rare). **Other:** increased serum transaminase levels, hepatitis, jaundice, priapism (rare), burning sensation of feet, transient hair loss. With prolonged use of high doses: myalgia, bone pain, osteoporosis. **Overdosage:** internal or external bleeding, paralytic ileus; skin necrosis of toes (purple toes syndrome), tip of nose, buttocks, thighs, calves, female breast, abdomen, and other fat-rich areas.

ROUTE AND DOSAGE. Oral, intramuscular, intravenous: 10 to 15 mg daily for 2 or 5 days, then maintenance dose: 2 to 10 mg daily. Alternatively, initial loading dose: 40 to 60 mg (half this for elderly or debilitated patients); then maintenance: 2 to 10 mg daily. Dosages individualized according to prothrombin time response.

NURSING IMPLICATIONS

Tablet may be crushed before administration and taken with fluid of patient's choice.

Prothrombin time (PT) should be determined before initiation of therapy and then daily until maintenance dosage is established. Daily checks should be made by physician to verify or change dose order.

Start flow chart indicating prothrombin activity data, control values, administered anticoagulant doses.

The one-stage prothrombin time test (PT or Quick) is widely used as a guide for anticoagulant dosage. Usual aim of therapy is to adjust dose so as to maintain prothrombin time at 1½ to 2½ times the control (12 to 15 seconds), or 15 to 35% of normal prothrombin activity.

When patient is receiving maintenance dosage, PT determinations may be prescribed at 1- to 4-week intervals depending upon patient's response. Periodic urinalyses, stool guaiac, and liver function tests are also usually performed. Optimum time to draw blood sample: 12 to 18 hours after last dose.

In an emergency, sodium heparin may be administered initially along with warfarin (both may be given in same syringe). Since heparin may affect PT, blood sample should be drawn just prior to next heparin dose, at least 5 hours after last IV injection, or 24 hours after last SC dose.

Since so many drugs interfere with the activity of anticoagulant drugs, a careful medication history should be obtained before start of therapy and whenever interpreting altered responses to therapy.

Continued anticoagulant therapy is not advised in the absence of laboratory facilities or patient compliance.

Elderly, psychotic, or alcoholic patients require close monitoring because they present serious noncompliance problems.

Patients with greatest risk of hemorrhage include those whose PT is difficult to regulate, who have an aortic valve prostheses, who are receiving long-term anticoagulant therapy and the elderly and debilitated.

Inform patient, without frightening, that bleeding can occur even though PT is within therapeutic range. Advise patient to withhold dose and to notify physician immediately if bleeding or signs of bleeding appear: hematuria, a bright red or black tarry stools, hematemesis, gingival bleeding with toothbrushing, ecchymoses, petechiae (often occurs in ankle areas), epistaxis, bloody sputum, chest pain (hemopericardium), abdominal or lumbar pain or swelling (retroperitoneal bleeding), menorrhagia, pelvic pain, severe or continuous headache, faintness or dizziness (intracranial bleeding); prolonged oozing from any minor injury (e.g., nicks from shaving).

Instruct patient to use a soft toothbrush and to floss teeth gently with waxed floss. Also advise use of electric razor for shaving.

Menstrual flow is generally normal, but may be slightly increased or prolonged. Advise patient to notify physician if there is an unusual increase in bleeding. PT should be checked at least monthly in menstruating women.

If patient becomes pregnant while on anticoagulant therapy, she should be informed of the potential risk of congenital malformations.

Antidote: In the event of bleeding, anticoagulant effect usually is reversed by omitting one or more doses of warfarin and by administration of specific antidote phytonadione (vitamin K_1) 2.5 to 10 mg orally. Physician may advise patient to carry vitamin K_1 with him at all times, but not to take it until after consultation. If bleeding persists or progresses to a severe level, vitamin K_1 5 to 25 mg IV is given or a fresh whole blood transfusion may be necessary.

Resumption of anticoagulatant therapy reverses the effect of vitamin K_1 and a therapeutic hypothrombinemic level can be obtained.

Instruct patient/family to withhold dose and to report immediately: symptoms of hepatitis (dark urine, itchy skin, jaundice, abdominal pain, light stools), or hypersensitivity reaction.

Suspect skin necrosis (local gangrene) and report to physician immediately if area is painful and skin appears purple–black surrounded by redness. Lesions usually occur within 3 days after initiation of therapy. Incidence is high in elderly, obese patients.

Smoking–Drug Interaction: Smoking increases metabolism and therefore may increase dose requirement. Patient should stop smoking or at least greatly modify amount of smoking during anticoagulant therapy.

Influenza vaccine decreases hepatic metabolism of warfarin, leading to augmented anticoagulant effect as evidenced by hemorrhage. Monitor patient. It is believed that the patient is at risk of bleeding for up to 1 month after receiving the vaccine.

Patient-Teaching Points: Alert patient to factors that may affect anticoagulant response:

- ✓ Prothrombin time may be *lengthened* (enhanced anticoagulant effect) by fever, prolonged hot weather, malnutrition, diarrhea, exposure to x-ray.
- ✓ Prothrombin time may be *shortened* (decreased anticoagulant effect) by: edema (reduces drug absorption and distribution), exposure to DDT or chlordane. *(See also Contraindications and Precautions.)*

Food–Drug Interactions: PT may be shortened by a high-fat diet, sudden increase in vitamin K–rich foods (cabbage, cauliflower, broccoli, asparagus, lettuce, turnip greens, onions, spinach, kale, fish, liver, and coffee or green tea, (caffeine), or by tube feedings with high vitamin K content.

Resistance to effects of warfarin may result from a vegetable-rich reducing diet because of high vitamin K content (see above). Some commercial dietary supplements have sufficient vitamin K content to produce resistance.

If a coumarin is administered before, during, or immediately following minor dental or surgical procedures, the dose is adjusted to maintain PT at about 1½ to 2½ times control level. Operative site should be limited enough to permit use of local procedures for hemostasis (absorbable hemostatic agents, sutures, pressure dressing).

When emergency surgery is necessary for a patient receiving a coumarin, blood coagulation can be brought to normal by administration of fresh, whole blood or plasma.

Advise patient to inform dentist or any new physician about anticoagulant therapy and duration of treatment.

Warn patient against taking any other drug unless specifically approved by physician or pharmacist. Anticoagulant action is affected by many prescription drugs as well as commonly used OTC preparations: e.g., antacids, antihistamines, aspirin, mineral oil, oral contraceptives or vitamin C (in large doses).

Urge patient to maintain a well-balanced diet and to avoid excess intake of alcohol. Consult physician regarding allowable amount. Generally an occasional drink is allowed.

Misuse of sodium bicarbonate (self-dosed to decrease dyspepsia) causes the urine to be alkaline, which may result in red-orange coloration of urine.

Patient should carry on his or her person medical identification card or jewelry, such as Medic Alert, that notes medications and physician's name, address, and telephone number. (May be purchased in a pharmacy.)

Recent studies suggest that anticoagulant therapy can be stopped abruptly rather than tapered over a few weeks.

The risk of recurrence of venous thrombosis or thrombophlebitis can be lessened by measures that prevent venous stasis. Discuss the following points with physician before developing a teaching plan for the patient:

- ✓ Avoid standing still.
- ✓ Elevate legs when sitting (avoid jackknife position); interrupt sitting periods with walk breaks about every ½ hour.
- ✓ Do not cross legs; avoid garters, tight girdles, tight pants, and narrow band knee-highs.
- ✓ Wear support hose or antiembolic stockings (must be prescribed by physician and patient must be measured for them). To be put on before getting out of bed in the morning and removed just before going to bed at night. (Review proper foot hygiene.)
- ✓ Planned exercise: have physician specify type (walking, bicycling, etc.), frequency, length of time, and rate of increase of exercise.
- ✓ Maintain optimum weight.
- ✓ Avoid injuring legs.

The patient and a significant family member or friend should be provided with explicit information and guidelines, verbally and in writing, concerning oral anticoagulant therapy:

- ✓ Why drug was prescribed and its expected action. Proper drug storage.
- ✓ Dosage and time of administration. Emphasize importance of taking drug at same time each day (usually late afternoon) and not skipping or changing a dose.
- ✓ Use of OTC drugs only with physician's approval.
- ✓ Avoid brand interchange.
- ✓ Assist patient in setting up a system for keeping track of drug administration and drug-related events, such as a check-off drug calendar or diary.
- ✓ Importance of adhering to schedule of PT determinations, other laboratory procedures, and doctor's appointments: give patient next laboratory date and date patient is to call doctor following laboratory visit, for directions concerning dosage.
- ✓ Adverse drug effects and reportable symptoms.
- ✓ Drug interactions.
- ✓ Factors that may affect anticoagulant response. Importance of maintaining consistency in diet and life-style. Allowable intake of fat, vitamin K–rich foods, alcohol.
- ✓ Necessity of carrying medical information card or jewelry.
- ✓ Keep drug out of the reach of children.

Follow manufacturer's directions for reconstitution and storage of parenteral preparation. Protect all preparations from light and moisture (tablets). Discard discolored or precipitated solutions.

Diagnostic Test Interferences. Warfarin (coumarins) may cause alkyline urine to be red–orange in color, may enhance **uric acid** excretion, cause elevation of **serum transaminases** and may increase **lactic dehydrogenase** activity.

VW

Drug Interactions. In addition to the listed drugs, many other drugs have been reported to alter the expected response to warfarin (prototype coumarin); however, clinical importance of these reports has not been substantiated. The addition or withdrawal of any drug to an established drug regimen should be made cautiously, with more frequent PT determinations than usual, with careful observation of the patient and dose adjustment as indicated.

Drugs that may increase response (i.e., enhance anticoagulant effect):

Acetohexamide
Acetaminophen
Alcohol–acute intoxication*
Alkylating agents
Allopurinol
Aminoglycosides
Aminosalicylic acid
Amiodarone
Anabolic steroids†
Antibiotics (oral)
Antimetabolites
Antiplatelet drugs
Aspirin
Aspiraginase
Bromelains
Chloral hydrate*,†
Chloramphenicol†
Chlorpropamide
Chymotrypsin
Cimetidine
Cincophen
Clofibrate
Co-trimoxazole
Danazol
Dextran
Dextrothyroxine†
Diazoxide
Dietary deficiencies
Disulfiram†
Diuretics*
Drugs affecting blood elements
Erythromycin
Ethacrynic acid
Glucagon
Guanethidine
Hepatotoxic drugs
Influenza vaccine
Isoniazid
MAO inhibitors
Meclofenamate
Mefenamic acid
Methyldopa
Methylphenidate
Metronidazole†
Mineral oil
Miconazole
Nalidixic acid
Neomycin (oral)
NSAIDs (except ibuprofen, naproxen, tolmetin)
Plicamycin
Potassium products
Prolonged narcotics
Propoxyphene
Propylthiouracil
Pyrazolones†
Quinidine
Quinine
Salicylates†
Streptokinase†
Sulindac
Sulfonamides
Sulfonylureas
Tetracyclines
Thiazides
Tolbutamide
Tricyclic antidepressants
Thyroid drugs
Urokinase
Vitamin E

Drugs that may decrease response (i.e., reduce anticoagulant effect):

Alcohol (chronic alcoholism)*,†
Barbiturates†
Carbamazepine
Chloral hydrate*,†
Cholestyramine†
Corticosteroids
Corticotropin
Diuretics
Ethchlorynol
Glutethimide†
Griseofulvin
Laxatives
Mercaptopurine
Oral contraceptives (containing estrogens)†
Rifampin
Spironolactone
Vitamin C
Vitamin K (dietary)

† Avoid concurrent use if possible.
* Increased or decreased response.

X

XYLOMETAZOLINE HYDROCHLORIDE

(Chlorohist, Neosynephrine II, Otrivin, Sinutab L.A.)

(zye-loe-met-az'oh-leen)
Alpha-adrenergic agonist (sympathomimetic)
Decongestant, local

ACTIONS AND USES. Imidazoline derivative with marked alpha-adrenergic activity (vasoconstriction) on dilated arterioles of nasal membrane. Has little or no beta-adrenergic activity. Structurally related to naphazoline (qv). Decreases fluid exudate and mucosial engorgement associated with rhinitis and may open up obstructed eustachian ostia in patient with ear inflammation.

Used for temporary relief of nasal congestion associated with common cold, sinusitis, acute and chronic rhinitis, hay fever and other allergies.

ABSORPTION AND FATE. Local vasoconstriction within 5 to 10 minutes; effects persists for 5 to 6 hours.

CONTRAINDICATIONS AND PRECAUTIONS. Sensitivity to adrenergic substances, angle-closure glaucoma, concurrent therapy with MAO inhibitors or tricyclic antidepressants. Safe use during pregnancy not established. *Cautious Use:* hypertension; hyperthyroidism; heart disease, including angina; advanced arteriosclerosis; use in the elderly, or in children.

ADVERSE/SIDE EFFECTS. Usually mild and infrequent: local stinging, burning, dryness and ulceration, sneezing, headache, insomnia, drowsiness. *With excessive use:* rebound nasal congestion, and vasodilation, tremulousness, hypertension, palpitation, tachycardia, arrhythmia, somnolence, sedation, coma.

ROUTE AND DOSAGE. Topical: Adults: 1 or 2 sprays or 2 or 3 drops of nasal solution (0.1%) in each nostril every 8 to 10 hours. **Children:** 2 or 3 drops of pediatric solution (0.05%) in each nostril every 8 to 10 hours. **Infants less than 6 months of age:** one drop (0.057% solution) in each nostril every 6 hours if necessary.

NURSING IMPLICATIONS

Instruct patient to clear each nostril gently before administering spray or drops.

Patient-Teaching Points: Application of drug:

✓ *Spray:* Do not shake container. Hold tube vertically (spray end up) so that solution is delivered in a fine spray. Head should be erect; spray into each nostril; 3 to 5 minutes later, clear (blow) nose thoroughly.

✓ *Drops:* Patient should be in a lateral, head-low position to permit application of drops to lower nostril surface. Have patient remain in this position for 5 minutes, then apply drops to opposite nostril surface in same manner; or drops may be instilled with patient in reclining position with head tilted back as far as possible.

Systemic effects are possible, particularly when excessive amounts of spray introduced intranasally are swallowed.

To prevent contamination of nasal solution, and to prevent spread of infection; rinse dropper and tip of nasal spray in hot water after each use and restrict use to the individual patient.

Prolonged use may cause rebound congestion and chemical rhinitis. Caution patient not to exceed prescribed dosage and to report to physician if drug fails to provide relief within 3 or 4 days.

Warn patient not to self-medicate with OTC drugs, sprays, or drops without physician's approval.
Excessive use by child may lead to CNS depression. The spray is difficult to apply to child; parent should supervise use and prevent drug abuse (overuse).
Xylometazoline solution should not be stored in aluminum container.
Preserved in tight, light-resistant containers, at 15° to 30°C (59° to 86°F).

Z

ZINC OXIDE

(Zincofax)

Astringent, protectant (topical)

ACTIONS AND USES. Water-insoluble, opaque substance with mildly astringent, protective, antipruritic, and weakly antiseptic properties.

Used topically for minor skin wounds, chafing, eczema, and sunburn and to protect skin from wound drainage, and from sunlight (sunscreen agent). Incorporated in many topical preparations.

CONTRAINDICATIONS AND PRECAUTIONS. Patients being x-rayed or receiving x-ray therapy (zinc, like other metals, may alter dosage of x-ray).

ROUTE AND DOSAGE. **Topical:** cream 15%, ointment 20%, paste 25%.

NURSING IMPLICATIONS

Repeated applications of an ointment can cause skin maceration by interfering with evaporation of perspiration. Folliculitis may result if applied to hairy areas.
Apply zinc oxide sparingly. Before reapplying, gently cleanse skin. Consult physician about appropriate solvent.
Avoid prolonged storage at temperatures greater than 30°C (86°F).

ZOMEPIRAC SODIUM

(Zomax)

(zoe-me-peer'ak)
Analgesic
Antipyretic
NSAID

ACTIONS AND USES. Analgesic and nonsteroidal antiinflammatory agent with pharmacologic properties similar to those of aspirin. In common with other antiinflammatory agents, has antipyretic properties and inhibits prostaglandin synthesis, but complete mode of action is not known. Provides greater analgesic potency than aspirin (50 mg of zomepirac is comparable to 650 mg of aspirin), is nonaddicting, and its use does not lead to tolerance. Has no effect on platelet count or humoral coagulation mechanism but prolongs bleeding time by decreasing platelet adhesiveness and aggregation; however, normal function returns 24 to

48 hours after drug is withdrawn. Does not alter prothrombin time of patients stabilized on warfarin therapy because it does not displace warfarin from its plasma binding sites.

Used for relief of mild to moderately severe pain.

ABSORPTION AND FATE. Rapidly and completely absorbed following oral administration with peak level (4.5 mcg/ml) reached in one hour after a single 100-mg dose. Onset of analgesia within one-half hour, peaks within 1 to 2 hours, and lasts about 4 to 6 hours (or longer in some patients). Half-life: about 4 hours, but following multiple doses may increase to 9.6 hours. Highly protein bound. Excreted primarily in urine as unchanged drug and metabolites.

CONTRAINDICATIONS AND PRECAUTIONS. Hypersensitivity to aspirin and other NSAIDs; during pregnancy, in nursing mothers, children. *Cautious Use:* history of upper GI tract disease, impaired renal function, coagulation disorders, hypertension, heart failure, fluid retention.

ADVERSE/SIDE EFFECTS. CNS: drowsiness, dizziness, insomnia, disorientation, euphoria, anxiety, depression, paresthesias. **CV:** purpura, petechiae, edema, hypertension, arrhythmias, palpitation. **Dermatologic:** toxic epidermal necrolysis, erythema multiforme, pruritus with rash, urticaria, increased sweating, skin pain, angiodema, anaphylaxis. **GI:** nausea, dyspepsia, vomiting, constipation, diarrhea, flatulence, abdominal pain, anorexia, peptic ulcer, GI bleeding with fecal blood loss. **Renal:** (associated with prolonged use): urinary tract infection (UTI) with urinary frequency, dysuria, hematuria, pyuria, increased BUN and serum creatinine, nephrotoxicity, vaginitis. **Other:** prolonged bleeding time, asthenia, tinnitus, taste changes, sodium retention with increased plasma volume (with prolonged use), periorbital edema, mild peripheral edema, abnormal liver function tests, chills (causal relationship not established), suspected tumorigenic potential with chronic use.

ROUTE AND DOSAGE. Oral: 50 to 100 mg every 4 to 6 hours, as necessary. Not to exceed 600 mg/day. For treatment in excess of 3 months duration, doses greater than 400 mg/day not recommended.

NURSING IMPLICATIONS

Zomepirac was temporarily recalled by the manufacturer in 1983 because of reports of severe hypersensitivity reactions and 4 deaths. Now available with new labeling regarding use and adverse/side effects. Available by prescription only.

For maximum effect, zomepirac should be taken on an empty stomach. Food decreases rate and extent of drug absorption.

If patient complains of GI distress, physician may prescribe giving the drug with an antacid (other than sodium bicarbonate). Bioavailability of zomepirac is not affected by antacids.

Baseline and periodic renal function studies are recommended for patients on long-term therapy.

Because ocular changes have occurred with other NSAISs, ophthalmoscopic examinations are advised if patient complains of visual disturbances.

Since zomepirac can cause dizziness and drowsiness, caution patient to avoid driving and other potentially hazardous activities until reaction to drug is known.

Advise patient to report promptly the onset of dark or tarry stools, blood in the urine, or frequent or painful urination.

Keep in mind that the antipyretic and antiinflammatory actions of zomepirac mask warning signs of emergent infection.

Warn patient not to take aspirin or aspirin-containing OTC drugs while on zomepirac therapy. *See Drug Interactions.*

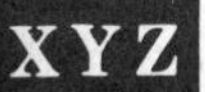

Drug Interactions. **Aspirin** and other **salicylates** decrease binding of zomepirac to plasma proteins and thus increase potential for zomepirac toxicity.

APPENDIX

Abbreviations

ABG	arterial blood gases
a.c.	before meals (ante)
ACh	acetylcholine
ACT	activated clotting time
ACTH	adrenocorticotropic hormone
ADH	antidiuretic hormone
ADL	activities of daily living
ad lib	freely as desired (ad libitum)
ADR	adverse drug reaction
ADT	alternate day therapy
$AgNO_3$	silver nitrate
ALT	alanine aminotransferase (formerly SGPT)
ANA	antinuclear antibodies
APTT	activated partial thromoboplastin time
ASHD	arteriosclerotic heart disease
AST	aspartate aminotransferase (formerly SGOT)
AV	atrioventricular
b.i.d.	two times a day (bis in die)
BBT	basal body temperature
BP	blood pressure
BMR	basal metabolic rate
BSP	bromsulphalein
BT	bleeding time
BUN	blood urea nitrogen
C	centigrade, Celsius
Ca	calcium
CBC	complete blood count
CCr	creatinine clearance
CDC	Centers for Disease Control

CHF	congestive heart failure
Cl	chloride
cm	centimeter
CNS	central nervous system
COMT	catechol-o-methyltransferase
COPD	chronic obstructive pulmonary disease
CPK	creatinine phosphokinase
CPR	cardiopulmonary resuscitation
CSF	cerebrospinal fluid
CT	clotting time
CTZ	chemoreceptor trigger zone
Cu	copper
CV	cardiovascular
CVA	cerebrovascular accident
CVP	central venous pressure
Derm	dermatologic
D&C	dilatation and curettage
DIC	disseminated intravascular clotting
dl	deciliter (100 ml or 0.1 liter)
DM	diabetes mellitus
DNA	deoxyribonucleic acid
DSD	dry sterile dressing
DTRs	deep tendon reflexes
ECG	electrocardiogram
ECT	electroconvulsive therapy
End	endocrine
EEG	electroencephalogram
EENT	eye, ear, nose, throat
ENT	ear, nose, throat
EPS	extrapyramidal symptoms (or syndrome)
ER	estrogen receptor
ESR	erythrocyte sedimentation rate
F	Fahrenheit
FBS	fasting blood sugar
FDA	(U.S.) Food and Drug Administration
Fe	iron
Fl	fluoride

FSH	follicle stimulating hormone
FUO	fever of unknown origin
GABA	gamma-aminobutyric acid
GFR	glomerular filtration rate
GH	growth hormone
GI	gastrointestinal
Gm	gram
gr	grain
GU	genitourinary
Gyn	gynecologic
G6PD	glucose-6-phosphate dehydrogenase (deficiency)
HCG	human chorionic gonadotropin
HCl	hydrochloride
HCO_3	bicarbonate
Hct	hematocrit
HDL	high density lipoprotein
Hem	hematologic
Hg	mercury
Hgb	hemoglobin
5-HIAA	5-hydroxyindoleacetic acid
HMG	human menopausal gonadotropin
HPA	hypothalamic–pituitary–adrenocortical (axis)
h.s.	hour of sleep (hora somni)
HSV	herpes simplex virus
Hx	history
I	iodine
I&O	intake and output
IBW	ideal body weight
Ig	immunoglobulin
IM	intramuscular
IOP	intraocular pressure
IPPB	intermittent positive pressure breathing
IU	international unit
IUD	intrauterine device
IV	intravenous
IVH	intravenous hyperalimentation
K	potassium

kg	kilogram
17-KGS	17-ketogenic steriods
17-KS	17-ketosteriods
KVO	keep vein open
L	liter
lb	pound
LDH	lactic dehydrogenase
LDL	low density lipoprotein
LE	lupus erythematosus
LH	leuteinizing hormone
Li	lithium
LVEDP	left ventricular end-diastolic pressure
m^2	square meter (of body surface area)
MAO	monamine oxidase
MAOI	monamine oxidase inhibitor
MBD	minimal brain dysfunction
MDR	minimum daily requirements
μCi or μC	microcurie
mCi or mC	millicurie
μg or mcg	microgram (1/1000 of a milligram)
mEq	milliequivalent
mg	milligram
Mg	magnesium
MI	myocardial infarction
MIC	minimum inhibitory concentration
ml	milliliter (1/1000 of a liter)
N	nitrogen
N&V	nausea and vomiting
Na	sodium
NaCl	sodium chloride
NAPA	N-acetyl procainamide
ng	nanogram (1/1000 of a microgram)
NPN	nonprotein nitrogen
NPO	nothing by mouth
NS	nervous system
NSAID	nonsteroidal antiinflammatory drug
NSR	normal sinus rhythm

17-OHCS	17-hydroxycorticosteriods
Oph	ophthalmic
OTC	over-the-counter
P	phosphorus
PABA	para-aminobenzoic acid
PAS	para-aminosalicylic acid
PAWP	pulmonary artery wedge pressure
Pb	lead
PBI	protein bound iodine
p.c.	after meals (post cibum)
PERLA	pupils equal, react to light and accommodation
PG	prostaglandin
Ph	hydrogen ion concentration
PKU	phenylketonuria
PND	paroxysmal nocturnal dyspnea
PO	by mouth (per os)
POR	problem oriented record
PPI	patient packet insert
PRN	when required (pro re nata)
PSP	phenolsulfonphthalein
PSVT	paroxysmal supraventricular tachycardia
PT	prothrombin time
PTT	partial thromboplastin time
PVC	premature ventricular contraction
qv	which see (quode vide)
RAI	radioactive iodine
RDA	recommended (daily) dietary allowance
REM	rapid eye movement
Reprod	reproductive
RIA	radioimmunoassay
RNA	ribonucleic acid
ROM	range of motion
RTA	renal tubular acidosis
SA	sinoatrial
SBE	self-breast examination
SC	subcutaneous
SGOT	serum glutamic-oxaloacetic transaminase (*see* AST)

SGPT	serum glutamic-pyruvic transaminase (*see* ALT)
SIADH	syndrome of inappropriate antidiuretic hormone
SL	sublingual
SLE	systemic lupus erythematosus
SMA	sequential multiple analysis
SOAP	subjective, objective, assessment, planning (*see* POR)
SPF	sun protection factor
SR	sedimentation rate
SRS-A	slow-reacting substance of anaphylaxis
t1/2	half-life
TCA	tricyclic antidepressant
TIA	transient ischemic attack
t.i.d.	three times a day (ter in die)
TPN	total parenteral nutrition
TPR	temperature, pulse, respirations
TSH	thyroid-stimulating hormone
URI	urinary tract infection
USP	United States Pharmacopeia
VDRL	veneral disease research laboratory
vital signs	temperature, pulse, respirations, blood pressure
VLDL	very low density lipoprotein
VMA	vanillylmandelic acid
VS	vital signs (qv)
WBC	white blood (cell) count
WBCT	whole blood clotting time
Zn	zinc

Glossary

Acid rebound Hypersecretion of gastric acid induced by excessive buffering of stomach acid (e.g., by calcium carbonate).

Adverse effect An unintended, unpredictable, and potentially injurious response to drug action. Adverse effects generally result from direct toxic drug effects, idiosyncrasies, hypersensitivity reactions, and noncompliance.

Agonist A drug with high affinity for the receptor and high intrinsic activity; causes a pharmacologic effect by its interaction with a specific receptor.

Antagonist A drug with high affinity for the receptor, but minimal or no intrinsic activity. Capable of preventing or reducing activity at the receptor sight.

Antiarrhythmic drug classification Based on the major electrophysiologic action of the drug:

	Examples
Class III:	quinidine, procainamade, lidocain, phenytoin
Class I:	quinidine, procainamide, lidocain, phenytoin
Class II:	propranolol
Class III:	bretylium
Class IV:	verapamil, digoxin

Atopy An inherited predisposition to allergies (e.g., asthma, acute urticaria, allergic dermatitis, hay fever).

Bioavailability The fraction of unchanged drug that reaches the systemic circulation.

Biotransformation Metabolic changes that occur following drug absorption and distribution convert the drug into products that are usually less active and that can be more readily excreted.

Drug abuse Self-administered drug use that deviates from sanctioned medical, social, or cultural patterns. Implicit in the definition is the notion of social disapproval.

Drug addiction *See* Drug dependence.

Drug dependence A state of physical or psychic dependence or both on a drug that occurs following repeated use of that drug. *Physical dependence* is a altered physiologic state that results following repeated drug use such that withdrawal symptoms appear when drug dose is reduced or drug discontinued. *Psychic dependence* is an emotional reliance on a drug. Drug dependence is characterized by compulsive drug seeking and drug taking behavior and a high risk of recurrence following drug withdrawal.

Enterohepatic circulation (A route of elimination) Drugs or drug metabolites released in the bile enter the small intestine where they may be totally or partially reabsorbed, returned to the liver, and again secreted to the bile. The metabolite may be enzymatically broken down by intestinal bacteria to release unchanged drug which is then reabsorbed.

First-pass effect The extensive metabolism of a drug that occurs during its passage through the gut wall and/or through the liver before reaching the systemic circulation. As a result of first-pass metabolism, the amount of drug reaching the active sight is reduced and the effectiveness of the oral drug is decreased.

Fixed drug eruption A drug-induced circumscribed skin lesion that persists or recurs in the same site. Residual pigmentation may remain following drug withdrawal.

Half-life The time required for drug concentration in plasma or total body to decline by one-half. The concept of half-life is important in time determinations of steady state and clearance of drug from the body.

Lipoatrophy Atrophy of subcutaneous fat caused by repeated injections of insulin in the same site, over prolonged periods.

Microsomal enzyme system A catalytic system that generally inactivates drugs and makes them more water soluble so they can be readily eliminated by the kidneys.

Minimum inhibitory concentration (MIC) Minimum drug concentration that inhibits microbial growth.

Nadir Pharmacological expression of the lowest point reached in the blood count; for example, thrombocytes and leukocytes in response to cytotoxic drug effects on hematopoietic tissues.

Pharmacodynamics Study of the time required for drug actions to occur in the body through processes of absorption, distribution, metabolism, and elimination.

Pharmacokinetics The study of how a drug reaches its use of action and is removed from the body through processes of absorption, distribution, metabolism, and elimination.

Photosensitivity Drug-induced skin changes resulting in unusual susceptibility to effects of sun or ultraviolet light.

Physical dependence An altered physiological state resulting from repeated drug use such that withdrawal symptoms appear with dose redirection or when the drug is discontinued.

Pressure effect Hemodynamic effect reflected in changes in blood pressure.

Protein binding A reversable drug-protein complex in equilibrium with free (active) drug in the plasma. Only the free drug can diffuse to the action sight, thus factors that decrease protein binding (for example, displacement of bound drug by another drug, or hypoalbumenism). May raise the potential for increased pharmacological effect.

Psychic dependence An emotional reliance on a drug.

Recall phenomenon Skin reaction due to prior radiotherapy.

Sequential Multiple Analysis (SMA) An automated electronic system that performs comprehensive blood studies rapidly and economically. For example, SMA 12/60 can make 12 determinations on 60 serum specimens in 1 hour.

Side effects An expected or predictable drug response caused by the pharmacological action of a drug.

Smogi effect A rebound phenomenon caused by accelerated release of hormone normally covered with plasma glucose regulation. Smogi effect develops when patient chronically receives unnecessarily large insulin doses. As a result, the body attempts to compensate by producing unrecognized hypoglycemia.

Smoking–drug interaction Interaction which occurs when smoking interferes with the pharmacokinetics of the drug.

Steady-state (plateau) During continued drug administration amount of drug in the body rises until average rate of drug elimination (drug clearance) equals average rate of drug intake. Plateau remains as long as drug intake is maintained.

Tachyphylaxis A sudden resistance to pharmacologic effectiveness of a drug. Initial drug response cannot be restored by increasing the dose.

Therapeutic window Effective serum drug level is close to toxic level.

Tolerance Reduced responsiveness during repeated administration of a drug requiring increasingly larger doses.

Schedules of Controlled Substances

Schedule I High potential for abuse and of no currently accepted medical use. Examples: heroin, LSD, marijuana, mescaline, peyote. Not obtainable by prescription, but may be legally procured for research, study, or instructional use.

Schedule II High abuse potential and high liability for severe psychic or physical dependence. Prescription required and cannot be renewed. Includes opium derivatives, other opioids, and short-acting barbiturates. Examples: amphetamine, cocaine, meperidine, morphine, secobarbital.

Schedule III Potential for abuse is less than for drugs in Schedules I and II. Moderate to low physical dependence and high psychological dependence. Includes certain stimulants and depressants not included in the above schedules, and preparations containing limited quantities of certain opioids. Examples: chlorphentermine, glutethimide, mazindol, paregoric, phendimetrazine. Prescription required.[a]

Schedule IV Lower potential for abuse than Schedule III drugs. Examples: certain psychotropics (tranquilizers), chloral hydrate, chlordiazepoxide, diazepam, meprobamate, phenobarbital. Prescription required.[a]

Schedule V Abuse potential is less than for Schedule IV drugs. Preparations contain limited quantitities of certain narcotic drugs; generally intended for antitussive and antidiarrheal purposes and may be distributed without a prescription provided that:

1. Such distribution is made only by a pharmacist
2. Not more than 240 ml or not more than 48 solid dosage units of any substance containing opium, nor more than 120 ml or not more than 24 solid dosage units of any other controlled substance may be distributed at retail to the same purchaser in any given 48-hour period without a valid prescription order
3. The purchaser is at least 18 years old
4. The pharmacist knows the purchaser or requests suitable identification
5. The pharmacist keeps an official written record of: name and address of purchaser, name and quantity of controlled substance purchased, date of sale, initials of dispensing pharmacist. This record is to be made available for inspection and copying by U.S. officers authorized by the Attorney General
6. Other federal, state, or local law does not require a prescription order

Under jurisdiction of the Federal Controlled Substances Act.
[a]Refillable up to 5 times within 6 months, but only if so indicated by physician.

FDA Pregnancy Categories

The FDA requires that all prescription drugs absorbed systemically or known to be potentially harmful to the fetus be classified according to one of five pregnancy categories (A, B, C, D, X). The identifying letter signifies the level of risk to the fetus and is to appear in the precautions section of the package insert. The categories described by the FDA are as follows:

Category A Controlled studies in women fail to demonstrate a risk to the fetus in the first trimester (and there is no evidence of risk in later trimesters), and the possibility of fetal harm appears remote.

Category B Either animal-reproduction studies have not demonstrated a fetal risk but there are no controlled studies in pregnant women, or animal-reproduction studies have shown an adverse effect (other than a decrease in fertility) that was not confirmed in controlled studies in women in the first trimester (and there is no evidence of a risk in later trimesters).

Category C Either studies in animals have revealed adverse effects on the fetus (teratogenic or embryocidal effects or other) and there are no controlled studies in women, or studies in women and animals are not available. Drugs should be given only if the potential benefit justifies the potential risk to the fetus.

Category D There is positive evidence of human fetal risk, but the benefits from use in pregnant women may be acceptable despite the risk (e.g., if the drug is needed in a life-threatening situation or for a serious disease for which safer drugs cannot be used or are ineffective). There will be an appropriate statement in the "warnings" section of the labeling.

Category X Studies in animals or human beings have demonstrated fetal abnormalities or there is evidence of fetal risk based on human experience, or both, and the risk of the use of the drug in pregnant women clearly outweighs any possible benefit. The drug is contraindicated in women who are or may become pregnant. There will be an appropriate statement in the "contraindications" section of the labeling.

DHHS Drug Experience Report Form

Health care professionals are encouraged to use the following Drug Experience Report form to document significant adverse reactions, either suspected or confirmed. The types of reactions of particular interest to the FDA are those that: 1) are not included in the labeling; 2) are serious, life-threatening, or fatal; and 3) appear to be increasing in number and severity.

DEPARTMENT OF HEALTH AND HUMAN SERVICES
PUBLIC HEALTH SERVICE
FOOD AND DRUG ADMINISTRATION
ROCKVILLE' MD 20857

FORM APPROVED; OMB 0910-0004.

Use of this form is prohibited after 12/31/85.

DRUG EXPERIENCE REPORT

FDA CONTROL NO.

ACCESSION NO.

I. REACTION INFORMATION

1. PATIENT ID/INITIALS (In Confidence)	2. AGE	3. SEX	4. WGT.	5. HT.	6. REPORTING DATE			7. REACTION ONSET DATE		
					MO	DA	YR	MO	DA	YR

8. DESCRIBE SUSPECTED REACTION(S)

9. OUTCOME OF REACTION TO DATE

- ☐ Alive with sequelae
- ☐ Recovered
- ☐ Still under treatment for reaction
- ☐ Died (Give cause/date)

10. TESTS/LABORATORY DATA CONFIRMING REACTION (Include biopsy and/or autopsy results)

11. WAS OUTPATIENT TREATMENT FOR REACTION REQUIRED?

☐ Yes ☐ No

12. WAS HOSPITAL TREATMENT FOR REACTION REQUIRED?

☐ Yes ☐ No

II. SUSPECT DRUG(S) INFORMATION

13. SUSPECT DRUG(S) - TRADE/GENERIC NAME(S), MANUFACTURER, IND/NDA NO.

14. TOTAL DAILY DOSE

15. ROUTE OF ADMINISTRATION

16. INDICATION(S) FOR USE		17. THERAPY DATES *(From/To)*	18. THERAPY DURATION
19a. WAS TREATMENT WITH SUSPECTED DRUG REDUCED IN DOSAGE? ☐ Yes ☐ No OR: ☐ Discontinued	19b. DID REACTION ABATE? ☐ Yes ☐ No	20a. WAS DRUG REINTRODUCED OR DOSE INCREASED? ☐ Yes ☐ No	20b. DID REACTION REAPPEAR? ☐ Yes ☐ No

III. **RECENT/CONCOMITANT DRUGS AND MEDICAL PROBLEMS**

21. OTHER DRUGS	TOTAL DAILY DOSE	ROUTE	DATES/DURATION OF ADMINISTRATION	INDICATIONS

22. DESCRIBE OTHER RELEVANT MEDICAL HISTORY (i.e., allergies, environmental or occupational exposure, previous drug reactions, pregnancy with gravidity/parity, ethnic origin.)

Your cooperation is needed to insure comprehensive, accurate, and timely use and interpretation of these data.

23. MFR NAME/ADDRESS		24. Check one ☐ Initial Report ☐ Follow-up Report	25. REPORTER'S NAME AND ADDRESS (In confidence)
MFR CONTROL NO.	DATE SENT TO FDA		

NOTE: *Required of manufacturers by 21 CFR 310.300, 310.301 and 431.60. Manufacturers may attach additional clinical material and product analyses at their discretion.*

26. MAY THE SOURCE OF THIS REPORT BE RELEASED TO THE ARMED FORCES INSTITUTE OF PATHOLOGY? ☐ Yes ☐ No

☆U.S. GOVERNMENT PRINTING OFFICE 1982 361-176/103

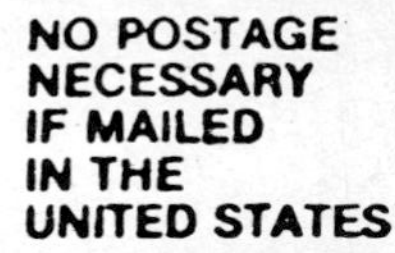

DEPARTMENT OF
HEALTH AND HUMAN SERVICES

Public Health Service
Food and Drug Administration
Rockville, Maryland 20857

Official Business
Penalty For Private Use $300

BUSINESS REPLY MAIL

First Class Permit No. 946 Rockville, MD

Postage Will Be Paid by the Food and Drug Administration

Division of Drug Experience (HFN-730)
Food and Drug Administration
5600 Fishers Lane
Rockville, Maryland 20857

NO POSTAGE
NECESSARY
IF MAILED
IN THE
UNITED STATES

ADDITIONAL INSTRUCTIONS FOR COMPLETING FORM FDA 1639

Use a separate report form for each case. Additional pages may be attached.

I. PATIENT/REACTION INFORMATION (ITEMS 1-12)

Items 2, 3, 4, 5. In case of a congenital malformation, record age, weight and height of the *mother*, and sex of the *baby*.

Item 8. Describe signs, symptoms and course of the drug related event.

Item 9. Indicate the status of the patient as of the reporting date and include discharge summary and/or autopsy findings, if available.

Item 10. Describe all diagnostic tests and exams results done as result of events in Item 8. Pertinent base line values and laboratory normals should be included.

Item 11. If "yes", describe treatment in Item 8.

Item 12. Hospitalization Required: If "yes", describe treatment in Item 8.

II. SUSPECT DRUG INFORMATION (ITEMS 13-20)

Item 13. Trade name and lot number, when available.

Item 14. As of date in Item 7. If drug(s) was given in a different dose or form previously, include dates and total daily dose for each drug exposure.

Item 15. As of the date in Item 7.

III. RECENT/CONCOMITANT DRUGS AND MEDICAL PROBLEMS (ITEMS 21-22)

Item 22. When reporting a congenital malformation, include date of mother's last menstrual period, gravidity, parity and previous abortions.

IV. OTHER INFORMATION (ITEMS 23-26)

Item 24. If this is a follow-up to a previous report, attach copy of initial report.

Item 25. (Record the name, title and address of the provider originating the report. THIS INFORMATION IS KEPT IN CONFIDENCE BY THE FDA AND IS NOT RELEASED UNDER THE FREEDOM OF INFORMATION ACT.)

After completing the form on the other side of this sheet, please tear off the page, triple fold, and staple or seal with tape. No postage is necessary.

Bibliography

Books

AMA Division of Drugs: AMA Drug Evaluations, 5th ed. New York, Wiley, 1983.

American Hospital Formulary Service, Drug Information 85, edited by McEvoy GK, et al. Bethesda, American Society of Hospital Pharmacists, 1985. Updated quarterly.

APhA Staff: Handbook of Nonprescription Drugs, 7th ed. Washington, D.C., American Pharmaceutical Association, 1982.

Avery GS (ed): Drug Treatment: The Principles and Practice of Clinical Pharmacology and Therapeuticals, 2nd ed. New York, Adis, 1980.

Biller JA, Yeager AM (eds): The Harriet Lane Handbook, 9th ed. Chicago, Year Book Medical, 1981.

Billups NF, Billups SM: American Drug Index 1984, 28th ed. Philadelphia, Lippincott, 1984.

Brunner LS, Suddarth DS, et al: The Lippincott Manual of Nursing Practice, 3rd ed. Philadelphia, Lippincott, 1984.

Brunner LS, Suddarth DS: Textbook of Medical Surgical Nursing, 5th ed. Philadelphia, Lippincott, 1984.

Cassileth BR, Cassileth PA: Clinical Care of the Terminal Cancer Patient. Philadelphia, Lea & Febiger, 1982.

Chernecky CC, Ramsey PW: Critical Nursing Care of the Client with Cancer. Norwalk, Connecticut, Appleton-Century-Crofts, 1984.

Covington TR, Walker JI: Current Geriatric Therapy. Philadelphia, Saunders, 1984.

Cox TC, et al: Drugs and Drug Abuse. Toronto, Addiction Research Foundation, 1983.

Donovan MI, Girton SE: Cancer Care Nursing, 2nd ed. Norwalk, Connecticut, Appleton-Century-Crofts, 1984

Drug Information for the Health Care Provider, 1984 USP DI, Vol I. United States Pharmacopeial Convention, Inc. New Jersey, Medical Economics, 1984.

Dukes MNG: Meyler's Side Effects of Drugs, An Encyclopedia of Reactions and Interactions, 10th ed. New York, Eserier, 1984.

Fischbach FT: A Manual of Laboratory Diagnostic Tests, 2nd ed. Philadelphia, Lippincott, 1984.

Frazer G: Crushing Tablets, Opening Capsules: When Is It Safe? In Kohut, Kohut, Fleishman (eds): Reality Orientation for the Elderly. Oradell, New Jersey, Medical Economics, in press.

Gangarosa LP, Ciarlone AE, Jeske AH: Pharmcotherapeutics in Dentistry. Norwalk, Connecticut, Appleton-Century-Crofts, 1983.

Gilman AG, Goodman LS, Gilman A (eds): Goodman and Gilman's The Pharmacological Basis of Therapeutics, 6th ed. New York, Macmillan, 1980

Greenblatt DJ, Shader RI: Pharmacokinetics in Clinical Practice. Philadelphia, Saunders, 1985.

Griffiths MC (ed): USAN and the USP Dictionary of Drug Names. Maryland, United States Pharmacopeial Convention, Inc., 1982.

Guyton AC: Textbook of Medical Physiology, 6th ed. Philadelphia, Saunders, 1981.

Hansten D: Drug Interactions, 5th ed. Philadelphia, Lea & Febiger, 1985.

Harkness R: Drug Interactions Handbook. Englewood Cliffs, New Jersey, Prentice-Hall, 1984.

Harvey AM, et al: The Principles and Practice of Medicine, 21st ed. Norwalk, Connecticut, Appleton-Century-Crofts, 1984.

Hawkins JW, Higgins LP: Maternity and Gynecologic Nursing: Women's Health Care. Philadelphia, Lippincott, 1981.

Kastrup ED (ed): Facts and Comparison. St. Louis, Lippincott (updated monthly).

Katzung BG (ed): Basic and Clinical Pharmacology, 2nd ed. Los Altos, California, Lange Medical, 1984.

Lerman F, Weibert RT: Drug Interactions Index. Oradell, New Jersey, Medical Economics, 1982.

Levine RR: Pharmacology: Drug Actions and Reactions, 3rd ed. Boston, Little, Brown, 1983.

Luckman J, Sorensen KC: Medical-Surgical Nursing. A Psychophysiologic Approach, 2nd ed. Philadelphia, Saunders, 1980.

Martin EW: Hazards of Medication, 2nd ed. Philadelphia, Lippincott, 1978.

Martindale W (edited by Wade A): The Extra Pharmacopoeia, 28th ed. London, The Pharmaceutical Press, 1982.

Melmon KL, Morelli HF (eds): Clinical Pharmacology, 2nd ed. New York, Macmillan, 1978.

Paige DM: Manual of Clinical Nutrition. Pleasantville, New Jersey, Nutrition Publication, 1983.

Physicians Desk Reference, 39th ed. Oradell, New Jersey, Medical Economics, 1985.

Pritchard JA, MacDonald PC, Gant NF: Williams Obstetrics, 17th ed. Norwalk, Connecticut, Appleton-Century-Crofts, 1985.

Rakel RE (ed): Conn's Current Therapy, 1984. Philadelphia, Saunders, 1984.

Ravel R: Clinical Laboratory Medicine, 4th ed. Chicago, Year Book Medical Publishers, 1984.

Reese RE, Douglas RG Jr (eds): A Practical Approach to Infectious Disease. Boston, Little, Brown, 1983.

Rudolph AM (ed): Pediatrics, 17th ed. Norwalk, Connecticut, Appleton-Century-Crofts, 1982.

Shelov SP, et al: Primary Care Pediatrics. Norwalk, Connecticut, Appleton-Century-Crofts, 1984.

Shirkey HC (ed): Pediatric Therapy, 6th ed. St. Louis, Mosby, 1980.

Smith LH, Thier SO: Pathophysiology: The Biological Principles of Disease. Philadelphia, Saunders, 1981.

Waldman RH, Kluge RM (eds): Textbook of Infectious Diseases. New York, Medical Examination, 1984.

Walser M, et al: Nutritional Management, The Johns Hopkins Handbook. Philadelphia, Saunders, 1984.

Schneider HA, Anderson CE, Coursin DB (eds): Nutritional Support of Medical Practice, 2nd ed. Philadelphia, Harper and Row, 1983.

Schrier RW: Clinical Internal Medicine in the Aged. Philadelphia, Saunders, 1982.

Journals and Newsletters

American Journal of Nursing
American Journal of Obstetrics and Gynecology
Canadian Nurse
Consultant
Consumer
Drug Intelligence and Clinical Pharmacology
Drug Therapy
Gastroenterology
Geriatrics
Journal of the American Medical Association
Journal of Clinical Pharmacology
Medical Clinics of North America
Medical Letter on Drug and Therapeutics
Medical Science Bulletin
Modern Medicine
New England Journal of Medicine
Nursing '85
Nursing Clinics of North America
Primary Care & Cancer (formerly, Your Patient & Cancer)
Patient Care
Pediatric Nurse Practitioner
Practical Cardiology
Primary Care
Rational Drug Therapy
RN

PROPRIETARY NAME INDEX

The generic name of the drug appears in parentheses after each trade name. Page numbers in *italic* indicate that the product is available over the counter; in **boldface**, by prescription only.

Anspor (cephradine), **247**
Antabuse (disulfiram), **464**
Antacid (magnesium carbonate), *754*
Antepar (piperazine citrate), **1017**
Anthatest (testosterone enanthate), **1178**
Anthra-Derm (anthralin), **90**
Anthraforte (anthralin), **90**
Anthranol (anthralin), **90**
Antibiopto (chloramphenicol), **257**
Antihemophilic Factor Human (antihemophilic factor), **92**
Antihemophilic Globulin (AHG) (antihemophilic factor), **92**
Antilirium (physostigmine salicylate), **1006**
Antiminth (pyrantel pamoate), **1088**
Antispas (dicyclomine hydrochloride), **422**
Anti-Tuss (guaifenesin), *608*
Antivert (meclizine hydrochloride), **773**
Antrenyl (oxyphenonium bromide), **937**
Antuitrin-S (chorionic gonadotropin), **294**
Anturane (sulfinpyrazone), **1158**
Anuject (procaine hydrochloride), **1058**
Anxanil (hydroxyzine hydrochloride), **660**
APAP (acetaminophen), *2*
Aparkane (trihexyphenidyl hydrochloride), **1238**
Aphen (trihexyphenidyl hydrochloride), **1238**
A.P.L. (chorionic gonadotropin), **294**
Apo-Acetazolamide (acetazolamide), **4**
Apo-Allopurinol (allopurinol), **26**
Apo-Amitriptyline (amitriptyline hydrochloride), 66
Apo-Benzothopine (benztrophine mesylate), 148
Apo-Bisacodyl (bisacodyl), 157
Apo-C (ascorbic acid), 97
Apo-Chlorpropamide (chlorpropamide), **282**
Apo-Cimetidine (cimetidine), 298
Apo-Diazepam (diazepam), **411**
Apo-Flurazepam (flurazepam hydrochloride), 580
Apo-Folic (folic acid), *582*
Apo-Furosemide (furosemide), **585**
Apogen (gentamicin sulfate), **591**
Apo-Hydro (hydrochlorothiazide), 642
Apo-ISDN (isosorbide dinitrate), 712
Apo-Methyldopa (methyldopa), 825
A-poxide (chlordiazepoxide hydrochloride), 260
Apresoline (hydralazine hydrochloride), **639**
Aquachloral Supprettes (chloral hydrate), **253**
AquaMEPHYTON (phytonadione), **1008**
Aquamox (quinethazone), **1098**
Aquasol A (vitamin A), *1277*
Aquasol E (vitamin E), *1279*
Aquatag (benzthiazide), **147**
Aquatensen (methyclothiazide), **823**
Aquazide (trichlormethiazide), **1231**
Aqueous Penicillin G (penicillin G potassium), **961**
ARA-A (vidarabine), **1271**
ARA-C (cytarabine), **366**
Aralen Hydrochloride (chloroquine hydrochloride), **265**
Aralen Phosphate (chloroquine phosphate), **265**
Aramine (metaraminol bitartrate), **797**
Arco-Cee (ascorbic acid), *97*
Arfonad (trimethaphan camsylate), **1242**
Argyrol S.S. (silver protein, mild), **1124**
Aristocort (triamcinolone), **1226**
Aristospan (triamcinolone hexacetonide), **1226**
Arlidin (nylidrin hydrochloride), **914**
Arm-aMed (isoetharine hydrochloride), 703
Armour Thyroid (thyroid), **1198**
Artane (trihexyphenidyl hydrochloride), **1238**
Artha-G (salsalate), **1119**
Arthrolate (sodium thiosalicylate), **1134**
Arthropan (choline salicylate), 293
A.S.A. (aspirin), *103*
Ascorbicap (ascorbic acid), *97*
Asellacrin (somatropin), **1135**
Asendin (amoxapine), **73**
Asmalix (theophylline), **1181**
Asminyl (dyphylline), **483**
A-spas (dicyclomine hydrochloride), **422**
Aspergum (aspirin), *103*
Asproject (sodium thiosalicylate), **1134**
AsthmaHaler (epinephrine bitartrate), *499*
AsthmaNefrin (epinephrine, racemic), *499*
Astrin (aspirin), 103
Atabrine (quinacrine hydrochloride), **1095**
Atarax (hydroxyzine hydrochloride), **660**
Atasol (acetaminophen), 2
Athrombin-K (warfarin, potassium), **1281**
Ativan (lorazepam), 748
Atozine (hydroxyzine hydrochloride), **660**
Atromid-S (clofibrate), **312**
Atropisol (atropine sulfate), **112**
A/T/S (erythromycin), **512**
Aureomycin (chlortetracycline hydrochloride), *286*
Aureomycin Ophthalmic (chlortetracyline hydrochloride), **286**
Aventyl hydrochloride (nortriptyline hydro-

Italic page numbers, OTC; **boldface**, prescription only.

BioCal (calcium carbonate, precipitated), *188*
Biosone (hydrocortisone acetate), **645**
Biotic-T (penicillin G potassium), **961**
Biozyme-C (collagenase), **336**
Biscao-Lax (bisacodyl), 157
Bishydroxycoumarin (dicumarol), **421**
Black Draught (senna), *1122*
Blenoxane (bleomycin sulfate), **160**
Bleph-10 (sulfacetamide sodium), **1153**
Blocadren (timolol maleate), **1205**
Bluboro (aluminum acetate solution), *36*
Blue (pyrethrins), *1090*
Blupav (papaverine hydrochloride), **945**
Bonamine (meclizine hydrochloride), 773
Bonine (meclizine hydrochloride), *773*
Bontril PDM (phendimetrazine tartrate), 978
Boracic Acid (boric acid), *163*
Borofax (boric acid), *163*
BP-Papaverine (papaverine hydrochloride), **945**
Brethaire (terbutaline sulfate), **1171**
Brethine (terbutaline sulfate), **1171**
Bretylate (bretylium tosylate), **164**
Bretylol (bretylium tosylate), **164**
Brevicon [oral contraceptives (estrogenprogestin combinations)], **920**
Brevital Sodium (methohexital sodium), **811**
Bricanyl (terbutaline sulfate), **1171**
Brietal (methohexital sodium), 811
Bristagen (gentamicin sulfate), **591**
British Anti-Lewisite (dimercaprol), **445**
Bromamine (brompheniramine maleate), **169**
Brombay (brompheniramine maleate), **169**
Bromphen (brompheniramine maleate), **169**
Broncaid Mist Suspension (epinephrine), **499**
Bronitin Mist Suspension (epinephrine bitartrate), *499*
Bronkephrine (ethylnorepinephrine hydrochloride), **546**
Bronkodyl (theophylline), **1181**
Bronkometer (isoetharine mesylate), **703**
Bronkosol (isoetharine hydrochloride), **703**
Bryrel (piperazine citrate), **1017**
Bucladin-S Softabs (buclizine hydrochloride), **172**
Buffazone (phenylbutazone), **994**
Buf-Opto Atropine (atropine sulfate), **112**
Bu-Lax (docusate sodium), *468*
Bumex (bumetanide), **173**
Buminate (albumin human), **20**
Burcillin-G (penicillin G potassium), **961**
Burow's Solution (aluminum acetate solution), *36*
Butalan (butabarbital sodium), **177**
Butatran (butabarbital sodium), **177**
Butazolidin (phenylbutazone), **994**
Buticaps (butabarbital sodium), **177**
Butisol Sodium (butabarbital sodium), **177**
Byclomine (dicyclomine hydrochloride), 422

Cabadon M (cyanocobalamin), **345**
Caffedrine (caffeine), *180*
Calan (verapamil hydrochloride), **1269**
Calcibind (cellulose sodium phosphate), **239**
Calciferol (ergocalciferol), **504**
Calcilac (calcium carbonate, precipitated), *188*
Calcimar [calcitonin (salmon)], **184**
Calcium Disodium Versenate (edetate calcium disodium), **488**
Calcium EDTA (edetate disodium calcium), **488**
Calcium Folinate (leucovorin calcium), **727**
CaldeCort (hydrocortisone acetate), **645**
Calderol (calcifediol), **182**
Calglycine (calcium carbonate, precipitated), *188*
Calicylic (salicylic acid), *1118*
Cal-Sup (calcium carbonate, precipitated), *188*
Caltrate (calcium carbonate, precipitated), *188*
Campain (acetaminophen), 2
Camphorated opium tincture (paregoric), 952
Cankaid (carbamide peroxide), *205*
Canthacur (cantharidin), 195
Cantharone (cantharidin), **195**
Cantil (mepenzolate bromide), **785**
Capastat Sulfate (capreomycin sulfate), **197**
Capoten (captopril), **199**
Carafate (sucralfate), **1150**
Carbacel (carbachol), **201**
Carbadon M (cyanocobalamin), **345**
Carbamide (urea), 1257
Carbolith (lithium carbonate), 742
Cardilate (erythrityl tetranitrate), **511**
Cardioquin (quinidine polygalacturonate), **1100**

Italic page numbers, OTC; **boldface**, prescription only.

Cardizem (diltiazem), **443**
Carfusin (carbol-fuchsin topical solution), 214
Carmol HC (hydrocortisone acetate), **645**
Cascara Sagrada Aromatic Fluidextract (cascara sagrada), *220*
Cascara Sagrada Fluidextract (cascara sagrada), *220*
Castaderm (carbol-fuchsin topical solution), **214**
Castellani's Paint (carbol-fuchsin topical solution), **214**
Catapres (clonidine hydrochloride), **319**
CCNU (lomustine), **745**
CDCA (chenodiol), **251**
Ceclor (cefaclor), **222**
Cecon (ascorbic acid), *97*
Cedilanid (lanatoside C), **713**
Cedilanid Injection (deslanoside), **391**
Ceebate (ascorbic acid), 97
CeeNU (lomustine), **745**
Cefadyl (cephapirin sodium), **246**
Cefobid (cefoperazone sodium), **230**
Cefracycline (tetracycline hydrochloride), **1179**
Celbenin (methicillin sodium), **808**
Celestone (betamethasone), **153**
Celestone Phosphate (betamethasone sodium phosphate), **153**
Celestone Soluspan (betamethasone acetate and betamethasone sodium phosphate), **153**
Cellubolic (methandriol), **802**
Celontin (methsuximide), **822**
Cel-U-Jec (betamethasone sodium phosphate), **153**
Cemill (ascorbic acid), *97*
Cenafed (pseudoephedrine hydrochloride), *1086*
Cena-K (potassium chloride), *1032*
Cenalax (bisacodyl), *157*
CEN-E (vitamin E), *1279*
Cenocort A-40 (triamcinolone acetonide), **1226**
Cenocort Forte (triamcinolone diacetate), **1226**
Cenolate (ascorbate, sodium), **97**
Centrax (prazepam), **1040**
Cephulac (lactulose), **725**
Ceporacin (cephalothin sodium), **243**
Cerebid (papaverine hydrochloride), **945**
Cerespan (papaverine hydrochloride), **945**
Cerubidine (daunorubicin hydrochloride), **380**
Cetamide (sulfacetamide sodium), **1153**
Cetane (ascorbic acid), *97*
Cetazol (acetazolamide), **4**
Cevalin (ascorbic acid), *97*
Cevi-Bid (ascorbic acid), *97*
Ce-Vi-Sol (ascorbic acid), **97**
Cevita (ascorbate, sodium), **97**
Cevita (ascorbic acid), **97**
Cevitamic Acid (ascorbic acid), 97
Charcocaps (charcoal, activated), 249
CharcolantiDote (charcoal, activated), *249*
Chealamide (edetate disocium), **490**
Chenic Acid (chenodiol), **251**
Chenix (chenodiol), **251**
Chenodeoxycholic Acid (chenodiol), **251**
Chigger-Tox (benzocaine), *139*
Chlo-Amine (chlorpheniramine maleate), *274*
Chlorate (chlorpheniramine maleate), **274**
Chlorazine (prochlorperazine maleate), **1061**
Chlor-Niramine (chlorpheniramine maleate), *274*
Chlorohist (xylometazoline hydrochloride), *1286*
Chloromycetin (chloramphenicol), **257**
Chloromycetin Palmitate (chloramphenicol palmitate), **257**
Chloromycetin Sodium Succinate (chloromycetin sodium succinate), **257**
Chloronase (chlorpropamide), **282**
Chloroptic (chloramphenicol), **257**
Chloroptic S.O.P. (chloramphenicol), **257**
Chlor-Pro (chlorpheniramine maleate), **274**
Chlorspan (chlorpheniramine maleate), **274**
Chlortab (chlorpheniramine maleate), **274**
Chlor-Trimeton (chlorpheniramine maleate), **274**
Chlorzide (hydrochlorothiazide), **642**
Cholan-DH (dehydrocholic acid), *383*
Choledyl (oxtriphylline), **931**
Choline Theophyllinate (oxtriphylline), 931
Choloxin (dextrothyroxine sodium), **409**
Chooz (calcium carbonate, precipitated), *188*
Chophylline (oxtriphylline), 931
Chorex (chorionic gonadotropin), **294**
Chronulac (lactulose), **725**
Chymex (bentiromide), **135**
Chymodiactin (chymopapain), **295**
Cibalith (lithium carbonate), **742**
Ciclopirox Ethanolamine (ciclopiroxolamine), **297**
Cidomycin (gentamicin sulfate), **591**
Cinobac (cinoxacin), **302**
Cino-40 (triamcinolone diacetate), **1226**
Cin-quin (quinidine sulfate), **1100**
Cirbed (papaverine hydrochloride), **945**

Italic page numbers, OTC; **boldface**, prescription only.

Dermolate and others [hydrocortisone (cortisol)], *645*
Dermophyl (fluocinolone acetonide), 569
Dermoplast (benzocaine), *139*
Dermo-Sterol (benzalkonium chloride), 137
Dermoxyl (benzoyl peroxide), 142
Deronil (dexamethasone), 397
DES (diethylstilbestrol), **425**
Desacetyl-anatoside C (deslanoside), 391
Desferal Mesylate (deferoxamine mesylate), **382**
Desoxyephedrine Hydrochloride (methamphetamine hydrochloride), 801
Desoxyn (methamphetamine hydrochloride), **801**
Desquam-X (benzoyl peroxide), **142**
D-Est 5 (estradiol cypionate), **524**
Desyrel (trazodone hydrochloride), **1222**
Dexacen-4 (dexamethasone sodium phosphate), **397**
Dexameth (dexamethasone), **397**
Dexampex (dextroamphetamine sulfate), 406
Dexasone (dexamethasone), **397**
Dexasone (dexamethasone sodium phosphate), **397**
Dexasone-LA (dexamethasone acetate), **397**
Dexchlor (dexchlorpheniramine maleate), **300**
Dexedrine (dextroamphetamine sulfate), *406*
Dexitac (caffeine), *180*
Dexon (dexamethasone sodium phosphate), **397**
Dexone (dexamethasone), **397**
Dexone (dexamethasone sodium phosphate), **397**
Dexon LA Dexone LA (dexamethasone acetate), **397**
Dextro Calcium Pantothenate (calcium pantothenate), **195**
Dey-Dose (isoproterenol hydrochloride), 708
Dey-Dose Epinephrine (epinephrine, racomic), 499
Dey-Lute (isoetharine hydrochloride), 703
Dezone (dexamethasone), **397**
D.H.E. 45 (dihydroergotamine mesylate), **439**
DHT (dihydrotachysterol), **440**
DiaBeta (glyburide), **600**
Diabinese (chlorpropamide), **282**
Diachlor (chlorothiazide), **267**
Diahist (diphenhydramine hydrochloride), **453**
Dialose (docusate potassium), *468*
Dialume (aluminum hydroxide), *39*
Diamine T.D. (brompheniramine maleate), **169**
Diamox (acetazolamide), **4**
Diamox Parenteral (acetazolamide sodium), 4
Diamox Sequels (acetazolamide), **4**
Diapid (lypressin), **751**
Di-Ap-Trol (phendimetrazine tartrate), 978
Diaqua (hydrochlorothiazide), **642**
Di-Azo (phenazopyridine hydrochloride), *977*
Dibent (dicyclomine hydrochloride), **422**
Dibenzyline (phenoxybenzamine hydrochloride), **988**
Dicarbosil (calcium carbonate, precipitated), *188*
Dicen (dicyclomine hydrochloride), **422**
Didrex (benzphetamine hydrochloride), **144**
Didronel (etidronate disodium), **547**
Dietic (diethylpropion hydrochloride), 424
Digifortis (digitalis leaf), **430**
Dihydrex (diphenhydramine hydrochloride), **453**
Dihydrocodeinone Bitartrate (hydrocodone bitartrate), 644
Dihydroergotoxine (ergoloid mesylates), 506
Diiodhydroxyquinoline (iodoquinol), 698
Diiodohydroxyquin (iodoquinol), 698
Dilantin (phenytoin), **1000**
Dilantin Kapseals (phenytoin sodium), **1000**
Dilart (papaverine hydrochloride), **945**
Dilaudid (hydromorphone hydrochloride), **654**
Dilax (docusate sodium), *468*
Dilin (dyphylline), **483**
Dilocaine (lidocaine hydrochloride), 734
Dilomine (dicyclomine hydrochloride), **422**
Dilor (dyphylline), 483
Dilosyn (methdilazine hydrochloride), 805
Dilyn (guaifenesin), 608
Dimelor (acetohexamide), 7
Dimentabs (dimenhydrinate), *444*
Dimetane (brompheniramine maleate), **169**
Dimetane Extentabs (brompheniramine maleate), **169**
Dinate (dimenhydrinate), **444**
Diocto (docusate sodium), *468*
Diocto-k (docusate potassium), *468*
Dioctyl calcium sulfosuccinate (docusate calcium), 468
Dioval (estradiol valerate), **524**

Italic page numbers, OTC; **boldface**, prescription only.

Dycill (dicloxacillin sodium), **420**
Dyclone (dyclonine hydrochloride), **482**
Dyflex (dyphylline), **483**
Dylline (dyphylline), **483**
Dymelor (acetohexamide), **7**
Dymenate (dimenhydrinate), **444**
Dynapen (dicloxacillin sodium), **420**
Dyrenium (triamterene), 1227
Dysne-Inhal (epinephrine hydrochloride), 499

Easprin (aspirin), **103**
Econochlor (chloramphenicol), **257**
Ecostatin (econazole nitrate), 487
Ecotrin (aspirin), *103*
Edecrin (ethacrynic acid), 530
E.E.S. (erythromycin ethylsuccinate), **515**
E-Ferol (vitamin E), 1279
Efficin (magnesium salicylate), **759**
Efo-Dine (povidone-iodine), 1037
Efricel (phenylephrine hydrochloride), 997
Efudex (fluorouracil), **572**
E-lonate PA (estradiol cypionate), **524**
Elase (fibrinolysin and desoxyribonuclease), **563**
Elavil (amitriptyline hydrochloride), **66**
Eldopaque (hydroquinone), *654*
Eldoquin (hydroquinone), *654*
Elixicon (theophylline), 1181
Elixophyllin (theophylline), 1181
Elspar (asparaginase), **100**
Eltroxin (levothyroxine sodium), 733
Elzyme 303 (pancreatin), 926
Emcyt (estramustine phosphate sodium), **525**
Emete-Con (benzquinamide hydrochloride), **145**
Emitrip (amitriptyline hydrochloride), **66**
Empirin (aspirin), *103*
Emulsoil (castor oil), *221*
E-Mycin (erythromycin), **515**
E-Mycin E (erythromycin ethylsuccinate), **515**
Endep (amitriptyline hydrochloride), **66**
Endrate (edetate disodium), **490**
Enduron (methyclothiazide), **823**
Enovid [oral contraceptives (estrogen–progestin combinations)], **920**
Enovil (amitriptyline hydrochloride), **66**
Enoxa (diphenoxylate hydrochloride with atropine sulfate), 456
Entaegl (piperazine citrate), 1017
Entamide (diloxanide furoate), 442
Entrophen (aspirin), 103
Epifoam (hydrocortisone acetate), **645**
Epifrin (epinephrine hydrochloride), **499**
Epinal (epinephryl borate), **499**
Epipen Auto-Injector (epinephrine), 499
Epitrate (epinephrine bitartrate), 499
Eppy/N (epinephryl borate), **499**
Epsilan-M (vitamin E), 1279
Epsilon-Aminocaproic Acid (EACA) (aminocaproic acid), **55**
Epsom Salts (magnesium sulfate), *759*
Equanil (meprobamate), 791
Equilet (calcium carbonate, precipitated), *188*
Eramycin (erythromycin stearate), **518**
Ergomar (ergotamine tartrate), **508**
Ergostat (ergotamine tartrate), **508**
Ergotrate Maleate (ergonovine maleate), **507**
Eryc (erythromycin), **512**
EryDerm (erythromycin), **512**
Erypar (erythromycin stearate), **518**
Erythrocin (erythromycin), 512
Erythrocin Ethyl Succinate (erythromycin ethylsuccinate), **517**
Erythrocin Lactobionate-I.V. (erythromycin lactobionate), **517**
Erythrocin Piggyback (erythromycin lactobionate), **517**
Erythromid (erythromycin), 512
Eserine Sulfate (physostigmine sulfate), 1006
Esidrix (hydrochlorothiazide), **642**
Eskalith (lithium carbonate), **742**
Estabs (estrogens, esterified), **528**
Estaqua (estrogenic substance aqueous suspension), **528**
Estinyl (ethinyl estradiol), **537**
Estra-D (estradiol cypionate), **524**
Estrace (estradiol), **520**
Estradurin (polyestradiol phosphate), 1027
Estraguard (dienestrol), **423**
Estratab (estrogens, esterified), **528**
Estraval-PA (estradiol valerate), **524**
Estrocon (estrogens conjugoted), 526
Estro-Cyp (estradiol cypionate), **524**
Estrofol (estrogenic substance aqueous suspension), **528**
Estroject-LA (estradiol cypionate), **524**
Estroject-2 (estrogenic substance aqueous suspension), **528**

Italic page numbers, OTC; **boldface**, prescription only.

Fulvicin-U/F (griseofulvin microsize), **606**
Fumasorb (ferrous fumarate), *559*
Fumerin (ferrous fumarate), *559*
Funduscein (fluorescein sodium), **570**
Fungizone (amphotericin B), **79**
Furacin (nitrofurazone), 901
Furadantin (nitrofurantoin), 899
Furadantin Sodium (nitrofurantoin sodium), 899
Furalan (nitrofurantoin), 899
Furamide (diloxanide furoate), **442**
Furan (nitrofurantoin), 899
Furatoin (nitrofurantoin), 899
Furoside (furosemide), 585
Furoxone (furazolidone), **583**
Fynex (diphenhydramine hydrochloride), **453**

Gamastan [immune globulin (intramuscular)], 672
Gamazole (sulfamethoxazole), 1156
Gamimune [immune globulin (intravenous)], 672
Gamma Benzene Hexachloride (lindane), 738
Gamma Globulin [immune globulin (intramuscular)], 672
Gammar [immune globulin (intramuscular)], 672
Gamulin Rh (Rho(D) immune globulin), 674
Ganphen (promethazine hydrochloride), 1069
Gantanol (sulfamethoxazole), 1156
Gantrisin (sulfisoxazole), 1155
Garamycin (gentamicin sulfate), 591
Garamycin Ophthalmic (gentamicin sulfate), 591
Gardenal (phenobarbital), 983
Gas-x (simethicone), 1125
Gaultheria Oil (methyl salicylate), 824
gBh (lindane), 738
Gee-Gee (guaifenesin), *608*
Gelfoam (absorbable gelatin sponge), *1*
Gemonil (metharbital), 804
Genoptic (gentamicin sulfate), 804
Gentran 40 (dextran 40), 402
Gentran 75 (dextran 75), 404
Geocillin (carbenicillin indanyl sodium), 210
Geopen (carbenicillin disodium), 208
Germa-Medica (hexachlorophene), 633
Germicin (benzalkonium chloride), 138
Gesterol (progesterone), 1065
Gesterol L.A. (hydroxyprogesterone caproate), **658**
Glaucon (epinephrine hydrochloride), 499
Globin Insulin (insulin, globin zinc, injection), 572
Globin Zinc Insulin (insulin, globin zinc, injection), 572
Gluco-Fedrin (ephedrine), 496
Glucotrol (glipizide), 593
Glukor (chorionic gonedotropin), 294
Glycerol (glycerin), 601
Glyceryl Guaiacolate (guaifenesin), 608
Glyceryl Trinitrate (nitroglycerin), 901
Glycotuss (guaifenesin), *599*
Gly-Oxide (carbamide peroxide), *204*
Glyrol (glycerin), **601**
Glytuss (guaifenesin), *608*
Gold thioglucose (aurothioglucose), 116
Gonic (chorionic gonadotropin), **294**
Gravigen (estrogenic substance aqueous suspension), **528**
Gravigen in Oil (estrogenic substance in oil), **528**
Grifulvin V (griseofulvin microsize), **606**
Grisactin Ultra (griseofulvin microsize), **606**
Grisovin-FP (griseofulvin microsize), 606
Gris-PEG (griseofulvin ultramicrosize), **606**
Gyne-Lotrimin (clotrimazole), **323**
Gynergen (ergotamine tartrate), **508**
Gynogen (estrogenic substance aqueous suspension), **528**
Gyrocaps (theophylline), 1181

Hal Chlor (chlorpheniramine maleate), **274**
Halciderm (halcinonide), 618
Halcion (triazolam), 1230
Haldol (haloperidol), **618**
Haldrone (paramethasone acetate), 949
Halofed (pseudoephedrine hydrochloride), 1086
Halog (halcinonide), **618**
Halotestin (fluoxymesterone), **575**
Halotex (haloprogin), **621**
Harmonyl (deserpidine), **388**
HBIG (hepatitis B immune globulin), **628**
H-BIG (hepatitis B immune globulin), 628
HCTZ (hydrochlorthiazide), 642
Hematinic (ferrous sulfate), *560*
Hematran (iron dextran), **700**
Hemocyte (ferrous fumanate), 559
Hemofil (antihemophilic factor), **92**
Hemofil T (antihemophilic factor), **92**

Italic page numbers, OTC; **boldface**, prescription only.

Ilopan (dexpanthenol), **397**
Ilosone (erythromycin estolate), **506**
Ilotycin (erythromycin), **504**
Ilotycin Gluceptate (erythromycin gluceptate), **508**
Ilozyme (pancrelipase), 943
Imferon (iron dextran), **700**
Imidazole carboxamide (dacarbazine), 368
Immuglobin [immune globulin (intramuscular], **661**
Immune Serum Globulin [immune globulin (intramuscular)], 672
Imodium (loperamide), 746
Impril (imipramine hydrochloride), 666
Imuran (azathioprine), **121**
Inapsine (droperidol), **477**
Inderal (propranolol hydrochloride), 1075
Indocin (indomethacin), **667**
Inflamase (prednisolone sodium phosphate), 1045
INH (isoniazid), 705
Inocor (amrinone), 85
Insomnal (diphenhydramine hydrochloride), 453
Insulatard NPH (insulin, isophane suspension), *679*
Intal (cromolyn sodium), **342**
Intrabutazone (phenylbutazone), 978
Intralipid (fat emulsion, intravenous), **545**
Intropin (dopamine hydrochloride), **466**
Inversine (mecamylamine hydrochloride), **752**
Iodotope I-131 (sodium iodide I-131), 1114
Ionamin (phentermine hydrochloride), 976
Iron (ferrous fumarate), *559*
Irodex (iron dextran), **700**
ISG [immune globulin (intramuscular)], 672
Ismelin (guanethidine sulfate), **603**
Ismotic (isosorbide), **698**
Isobec (amobarbital), 71
Iso-Bid (isosorbide dinitrate, dilute), **699**
Isodine (povidone-iodine), 1037
Isonicotinic Acid Hydrazide (isoniazid), *705*
Isoptin (verapamil hydrochloride), 1269
Isopto Atropine (atropine sulfate), **112**
Isopto Carbachol (carbachol), **200**
Isopto Carpine (pilocarpine hydrochloride), 1011
Isopto Cetamide (sulfacetamide sodium), 1153
Isopto Eserine (physostigmine salicylate), 1006
Isopto Fenicol (chloramphenicol), 257
Isopto Frin (phenylephrine hydrochloride), 997
Isopto Homatropine (homatropine hydrobromide), 637
Isopto-Hyoscine (scopolamine hydrobromide), 1119
Isopto-Plain (methylcellulose), *808*
Isordil (isosorbide dinitrate, dilute), **699**
Isotamine (isoniazed), 705
Isotrate (isosorbide dinitrate, dilute), **699**
Isovex-100 (ethaverine hydrochloride), **526**
Isuprel (isoproterenol hydrochloride), **708**
Ivadantin (nitrofurantoin sodium), **882**

Janimine (imipramine hydrochloride), **655**
Jecto-Sal (sodium thiosalicylate), 1134
Jenamicin (gentamicin sulfate), 582

Kabikinase (streptokinase), 1140
Kalcinate (calcium gluconate), **190**
Kalinate (potassium gluconate), 1032
Kantrex (kanamycin), **704**
Kaochlor (potassium chloride), 1032
Kaon (potassium gluconate), 1032
Kaon-Cl (potassium chloride), 1032
Kao-Nor (potassium gluconate), 1032
Kaopectate tablets (attapulgite, activated), *115*
Karidium (sodium fluoride), 1128
Karigel (sodium fluoride), 1128
Kari-Rinse (sodium fluoride), 1128
Kasof (docusate potassium), *468*
Kato (potassium chloride), 1032
Kavrin (papaverine hydrochloride), 945
Kay Ciel (potassium chloride), 1032
Kaybovite (cyanocobalamin), *342*
Kayexalate (sodium polystyrene sulfonate), 1132
Kaylixir (potassium gluconate), 1032
Keflex (cephalexin), **240**
Keflin (cephalothin sodium), **242**
Kefzol (cefazolin sodium), **226**
Kellogg's Castor Oil (castor oil), *221*
Kemadrin (procyclidine hydrochloride), 1064
Kemsol (dimethyl sulfoxide), 447
Kenacort (triamcinolone), 1226
Kenalog (triamcinolone acetonide), 1226
Keralyt (salicylic acid), 1118
Kestrin (estrogenic substance aqueous

Italic page numbers, OTC; **boldface**, prescription only.

progestin combinations)], **920**
Lofene (diphenoxylate hydrochloride with atropine sulfate), 456
Lomine (dicyclomine hydrochloride), 422
Lomotil (diphenoxylate hydrochloride with atropine sulfate), 456
Loniten (minoxidil), **855**
Lonox (diphenoxylate hydrochloride with atropine sulfate), 456
Lopid (gemfibrozil), **589**
Lopressor (metoprolol tartrate), **840**
Loprox (ciclopiroxolamine), **298**
Lopurin (allopurinol), **26**
Lorelco (probucol), 1052
Lorfan (levallorphan tartrate), **728**
Lotrimin (clotrimazole), **323**
Lo-Trol (diphenoxylate hydrochloride with atropine sulfate), 456
Lotusate (talbutal), 1167
Low-Quel (diphenoxylate hydrochloride with atropine sulfate), 456
Lowsium (magaldrate), 754
Lotapac (loxapine succinate), **750**
Loxitane (loxapine succinate), **750**
Loxitane C (loxapine hydrochloride), **750**
Lozol (indapamide), **676**
L-Pam (melphalan), 780
L-Sarcolysin (melphalan), 780
l-Sedrin Plain (ephedrine), 496
L-Thyroxine (levothyroxine sodium), 733
Ludiomil (maprotiline hydrochloride), **764**
Lufyllin (dyphylline), **483**
Lugol's Solution (strong iodine solution), 1148
Luminal (phenobarbital), 983
Luminal Sodium (phenobarbital sodium), 983
Lunar Caustic (silver nitrate, toughened), 1123
Luride (sodium fluoride), 1128
LV (penicillin V potassium), 967
Lyderm (fluocinonide), 561
Lyovac (dactinomycin), 370
Lysodren (mitotane), **858**

Macrodantin (nitrofurantoin), **899**
Macrodex (dextran 70), **402**
Magan (magnesium salicylate), **759**
Magnesia Magma (magnesium hydroxide), 756
Magnesia (magnesium hydroxide), 742
Magnesium Carbonate (magadrate), 754
Mag-Ox (magnesium oxide), *758*
Mallamint (calcium carbonate, precipitated), *188*
Mallisol (povidone-iodine), 1037
Malogen (testosterone), 1175
Malojex (testosterone enanthate), 1178
Malotuss (guaifenesin), *608*
Mandelamine (methenamine mandelate), **806**
Mandol (cefamandole nafate), **225**
Maolate (chlorphenesin carbamate), **273**
Maox (magnesium oxide), *758*
Marazide (benzthiazide), **147**
Marbaxin-750 (methocarbamol), 810
Marezine Hydrochloride (cyclizine hydrochloride), **347**
Marezine Lactate (cyclizine lactate), **350**
Marflex (orphenadrine citrate), **924**
Marmine (dimenhydrinate), **444**
Marplan (isocarboxazid), **690**
Marzine (cyclizine lactate), 350
Masoxin (digoxin), 435
Matulane (procarbazine hydrochloride), 1059
Maxeran (metoclopramide hydrochloride), 836
Maxibolin (ethylestrenol), **543**
Maxidex (dexamethasone), 397
Maxiflor (diflorasone diacetate), **427**
Mazaner (mazinidol), 765
MCH (microfibrillar collagen hemostat), 852
M-Cillin B (penicillin G potassium), 961
Measurin (aspirin), *103*
Mebaral (mephobarbital), 790
Meclan (meclocycline sulfosalicylate), **774**
Meclomen (meclofenamate sodium), **775**
Medicinal Charcoal (charcoal, activated), 249
Medihaler Ergotamine (ergotamine tartrate), **508**
Medihaler-Epi (epinephrine bitartrate), **499**
Medihaler-Iso (isoproterenol sulfate), **708**
Medilium (chlordiazepoxide hydrochloride), 260
Medimet (methyldopa), 825
Medralone-40 (methylprednisolone acetate), **831**
Medrol (methylprednisolone), **831**
Medrone-40 (methylprednisolone acetate), **831**
Mefoxin (cefoxitin sodium), **235**
Megace (megestrol acetate), **779**

Italic page numbers, OTC; **boldface**, prescription only.

Italic page numbers, OTC; **boldface**, prescription only.

Italic page numbers, OTC; **boldface**, prescription only.

Persantine (dipyridamole), **460**
Pertofrane (desipramine hydrochloride), **390**
Pethadol (meperidine hydrochloride), 785
Pethidine Hydrochloride (meperidine hydrochloride), 785
P.E.T.N. (pentaerythritol tetranitrate), 968
Petrogalar (mineral oil), **853**
Pferoglylutamic acid (folic acid), 582
Pfizerpen (penicillin G potassium), 961
Pfizerpen VK (penicillin V potassium), 967
Pfizerpen-A (ampicillin), **83**
Pfizerpen-AS (penicillin G procaine suspension, sterile), 965
PGE1 (alprostadil), **33**
PGE2 (dinoprostone), 450
PGF2a (dinoprost tromethamine), 448
Phenazine (perphenazine), 959
Phenazodine (phenazopyridine hydrochloride), 977
Phenbuff (phenylbutazone), 977
Phencen (promethazine hydrochloride), 1069
Phenergan (promethazine hydrochloride), 1069
Phenetron (chlorpheniramine maleate), 274
Phenoject-50 (promethazine hydrochloride), 1069
Phenolax (phenolphthalein), 987
Phentrol (phentermine hydrochloride), 991
Phenurone (phenacemide), 976
Phenylalinine Mustard (melphalen), 780
Phenzine (phendimetrazine tartrate), 978
Pheryl-E (vitamin E), 1279
pHiso Scrub (hexachlorophene), **633**
pHisoHex (hexachlorophene), **633**
Phosphaljel (aluminum phosphate), *42*
Phospholine Iodide (echothiophate iodide), **485**
Phyllocontin (aminophylline), **59**
Phylloquinone (phytonadione), 1008
Pil-Digis (digitalis leaf), 430
Pilocar (pilocarpine hydrochloride), 1011
Pilocel (pilocarpine hydrochloride), 1011
Pilokair (pilocarpine hydrochloride), 1011
Piloptic (pilocarpine hydrochloride), 1011
Pima (potassium iodide), 1035
Piperazine Estrone Sulfate (estropipate), 529
Pipracil (piperacillin sodium), 1016
Pipril (piperazine citrate), 1017
Pitocin (oxytocin injection), **939**
Pitressin (vasopressin injection), 1264
Pitressin Tannate (vasopressin tannate), 1264
Pitrex (tolnaftate), 1220
Placidyl (ethchlorvynol), 535
plain (mineral oil), 853
Plain (mineral oil), 853
Plaquenil Sulfate (hydroxychloroquine sulfate), **657**
Plasbumin (albumin human), **20**
Plasmanate (plasma protein fraction), 1022
Plasma-Plex (plasma protein fraction), 1022
Plasmatein (plasma protein fraction), 1022
Platinol (cisplatin), **303**
Plegine (phendimetrazine tartrate), 978
Plova (psyllium hydrophilic muciloid), 1087
Point-Two (sodium fluoride), 1128
Poladex T.D. (dexchlorpheniramine maleate), **400**
Polaramine (dexchlorpheniramine maleate), **400**
Polycillin (ampicillin), **83**
Polycillin-N (ampicillin sodium), **83**
Polymox (amoxicillin), **75**
Polymyxin E (colistin sulfate), 335
Ponderal (fenfluramine hydrochloride), 555
Pondimin (fenfluramine hydrochloride), 555
Ponstan (mefenamic acid), 778
Ponstel (mefenamic acid), 778
Porcelana (hydroquinone), 654
Pork Protamine (insulin, protamine zinc), *692*
Povan (pyrvinium pamoate), 1094
Poyamin (cyanocobalamin), 345
Precipitated chalk (calcium carbonate, precipitated), 188
Predcor-TBA (prednisolone tebutate), 1045
Predcor-25 (prednisolone acetate), 1045
Pre-Dep (methylprednisolone acetate), **831**
Prednicen (prednisone), 1046
Predoxine (prednisolone), 1045
Prefrin (phenylephrine hydrochloride), 997
Pregnyl (chorionic gonadotropin), **294**
Preludin (phenmetrazine hydrochloride), 982
Premarin (estrogens, conjugated), **526**
Pre-Sate (chlorphentermine hydrochloride), 276
Primatene Mist Solution (epinephrine), *499*
Primatene Mist Suspension (epinephrine bitartrate), *499*
Primoline (primidone), 1048
Principen (ampicillin), **83**
Prioderm (malathion), **761**
Priscoline (tolazoline hydrochloride), 1211
Privine VasoClear (naphazoline hydrochloride), 877

Italic page numbers, OTC; **boldface**, prescription only.

Quarzan (clidinium bromide), **307**
Quelicin (succinylcholine chloride), 1148
Questran (cholestyramine resin), **289**
Quibron-T (theophylline), 1181
Quick Pep (caffeine), *180*
Quiess (hydroxyzine hydrochloride), **660**
Quin III (iodochlorhydroxyquin), *684*
Quinaglute Dura-Tabs (quinidine gluconate), 1099
Quinamm (quinine sulfate), 1100
Quinate (quinidine gluconate), 1099
Quinatime (quinidine gluconate), 1099
Quine (quinine sulfate), 1100
Quinidex Exstentabs (quinidine sulfate), 1100
Quinite (quinine sulfate), 1100
Quinnone (hydroquinone), *654*
Quinora (quinidine sulfate), 1100
Quin-Release (quinidine gluconate), 1099
Quiphile (quinine sulfate), 1100

R & C (pyrethrins), 1090
Racemic Amphetamine Sulfate (amphetamine sulfate), 77
Raudixin (rauwolfia serpentina), 1107
Raufola (rauwolfia serpentina), 1107
Rauserpin (rauwolfia serpentina), 1107
Rauval (rauwolfia serpentina), 1107
Rauverid (rauwolfia serpentina), 1107
Rauwiloid (alseroxylon), **35**
Razine Tartrate (piperazine tartrate), 1017
Rectalad-Aminophylline (aminophylline), 59
Redisol (cyanocobalamin), *345*
Redoxon (ascorbic acid), 97
Regacilium (psyllium hydrophilic muciloid), 1087
Regibon (diethylpropion hydrochloride), 424
Regitine Hydrochloride (phentolamine hydrochloride), 992
Reglan (metoclopramide hydrochloride), **836**
Regonal (pyridostigmine bromide), 1090
Regular Iletin (insulin injection), *682*
Regular Iletin II (insulin injection), **682**
Regular Insulin (insulin injection), 682
Regulex (docusate sodium), 468
Reguloid (psyllium hydrophilic muciloid), 1087
Regutol (docusate sodium), *468*
Reidamine (dimenhydrinate), **444**
Rela (carisoprodol), **216**
Releserp (reserpine), 1110
Remsed (promethazine hydrochloride), 1069
Ren Amin (essential amino acid injection), 519
Renese (polythiazide), 1031
Renoquid (sulfacytine), 1154
Repen-VK (penicillin V potassium), 967
Reponans-10 (chlordiazepoxide hydrochloride), 260
Resectisol (mannitol), 762
Reserfia (reserpine), 1110
Respbid (theophylline), 1181
Restoril (temazepam), 1169
Resyl (guaifenesin), 608
Revimine (dopamine hydrochloride), 469
Rexolate (sodium thiosalicylate), 1134
Rheaban (attapulgite, activated), *115*
Rheomacrodex (dextran 40), **402**
Rhesonativ (Rho(D) immune globulin), 674
Rhidecon (phenylpropanolamine hydrochloride), 999
Rhinalar (flunisolide), 568
Rhinall (phenylephrine hydrochloride), 997
RhoGAM (Rho(D) immune globulin), **674**
Rhulicream (benzocaine), *139*
Rid (pyrethrins), 1090
Rifadin (rifampin), 1114
Rifamycin (rifampin), 1114
Rimactane (rifampin), 1114
Rimifon (isoniazid), 705
Rimso-50 (dimethyl sulfoxide), **447**
Riobin-50 (riboflavin), 1113
Riopan (magaldrate), *754*
Ritalin (methylphenidate hydrochloride), 830
Rival (diazepam), 411
RMS Uniserts (morphine sulfate), 861
Robaxin (methocarbamol), **810**
Robicillin VK (penicillin V potassium), 967
Robidex (dextromethorphan hydrobromide), 408
Robidone (hydrocodone bitartrate), 644
Robidrine (pseudoephedrine hydrochloride), 1086
Robigesic (acetaminophen), 2
Robimycin (erythromycin), **512**
Robinul (glycopyrrolate), **603**
Robinul Forte (glycopyrrolate), 603
Robitussin (guaifenesin), *608*

Italic page numbers, OTC; **boldface**, prescription only.

Italic page numbers, OTC; **boldface**, prescription only.

Italic page numbers, OTC; **boldface**, prescription only.

Italic page numbers, OTC; **boldface**, prescription only.

Italic page numbers, OTC; **boldface**, prescription only.

GENERIC NAME INDEX

Generic names of prototype drugs are *italicized*; major drug categories and areas applicable to patient teaching are set in **boldface.** The reader is referred to the most complete description of all medical-surgical conditions.

Prototype drugs are in *italic*; major drug categories and areas applicable to patient teaching are in **boldface**.

Prototype drugs are in *italic*; major drug categories and areas applicable to patient teaching are in **boldface**.

Prototype drugs are in *italic*; major drug categories and areas applicable to patient teaching are in **boldface**.

Prototype drugs are in *italic*; major drug categories and areas applicable to patient teaching are in **boldface**.

Prototype drugs are in *italic*; major drug categories and areas applicable to patient teaching are in **boldface**.

Prototype drugs are in *italic*; major drug categories and areas applicable to patient teaching are in **boldface**.

Prototype drugs are in *italic*; major drug categories and areas applicable to patient teaching are in **boldface**.

Prototype drugs are in *italic*; major drug categories and areas applicable to patient teaching are in **boldface**.

Prototype drugs are in *italic*; major drug categories and areas applicable to patient teaching are in **boldface**.

Prototype drugs are in *italic*; major drug categories and areas applicable to patient teaching are in **boldface**.